617.601 B69-13
Boyd, Linda D.
Wilkins' clinical practice of the
dental hygienist

EMORY W. MORRIS LIBRARY

W9-CLV-138

617.601
B69-13

13TH EDITION

Wilkins'
Clinical Practice of the
Dental Hygienist

LINDA D. BOYD, RDH, RD, EdD
Professor and Associate Dean
Forsyth School of Dental Hygiene
MCPHS University
Boston, Massachusetts

LISA F. MALLONEE, RDH, RD, LD, MPH
Professor and Graduate Program Director
Caruth School of Dental Hygiene
Texas A&M College of Dentistry
Dallas, Texas

CHARLOTTE J. WYCHE, BSDH, MS
Retired
Department of Periodontics and Oral Medicine
University of Michigan School of Dentistry
Ann Arbor, Michigan

KELLOGG COMMUNITY COLLEGE LRC

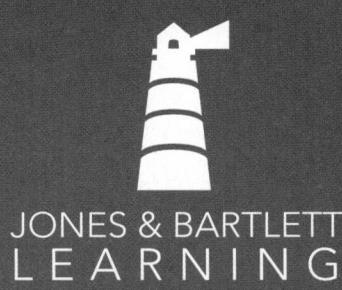

JONES & BARTLETT
LEARNING

6/22

EP

123.95

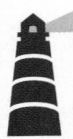

World Headquarters
Jones & Bartlett Learning
5 Wall Street
Burlington, MA 01803
978-443-5000
info@jblearning.com
www.jblearning.com

Jones & Bartlett Learning books and products are available through most bookstores and online booksellers. To contact Jones & Bartlett Learning directly, call 800-832-0034, fax 978-443-8000, or visit our website, www.jblearning.com.

Substantial discounts on bulk quantities of Jones & Bartlett Learning publications are available to corporations, professional associations, and other qualified organizations. For details and specific discount information, contact the special sales department at Jones & Bartlett Learning via the above contact information or send an email to specialsales@jblearning.com.

Copyright © 2021 by Jones & Bartlett Learning, LLC, an Ascend Learning Company

All rights reserved. No part of the material protected by this copyright may be reproduced or utilized in any form, electronic or mechanical, including photocopying, recording, or by any information storage and retrieval system, without written permission from the copyright owner.

The content, statements, views, and opinions herein are the sole expression of the respective authors and not that of Jones & Bartlett Learning, LLC. Reference herein to any specific commercial product, process, or service by trade name, trademark, manufacturer, or otherwise does not constitute or imply its endorsement or recommendation by Jones & Bartlett Learning, LLC and such reference shall not be used for advertising or product endorsement purposes. All trademarks displayed are the trademarks of the parties noted herein. *Wilkins' Clinical Practice of the Dental Hygienist, Thirteenth Edition* is an independent publication and has not been authorized, sponsored, or otherwise approved by the owners of the trademarks or service marks referenced in this product.

There may be images in this book that feature models; these models do not necessarily endorse, represent, or participate in the activities represented in the images. Any screenshots in this product are for educational and instructive purposes only. Any individuals and scenarios featured in the case studies throughout this product may be real or fictitious, but are used for instructional purposes only.

The authors, editor, and publisher have made every effort to provide accurate information. However, they are not responsible for errors, omissions, or for any outcomes related to the use of the contents of this book and take no responsibility for the use of the products and procedures described. Treatments and side effects described in this book may not be applicable to all people; likewise, some people may require a dose or experience a side effect that is not described herein. Drugs and medical devices are discussed that may have limited availability controlled by the Food and Drug Administration (FDA) for use only in a research study or clinical trial. Research, clinical practice, and government regulations often change the accepted standard in this field. When consideration is being given to use of any drug in the clinical setting, the health care provider or reader is responsible for determining FDA status of the drug, reading the package insert, and reviewing prescribing information for the most up-to-date recommendations on dose, precautions, and contraindications, and determining the appropriate usage for the product. This is especially important in the case of drugs that are new or seldom used.

20691-3

Production Credits

VP, Product Management: Amanda Martin
Director of Product Management: Cathy L. Esperti
Product Manager: Sean Fabery
Product Coordinator: Elena Sorrentino
Senior Project Specialist: Vanessa Richards
Digital Project Specialist: Angela Dooley
Director of Marketing: Andrea DeFronzo
VP, Manufacturing and Inventory Control: Therese Connell

Composition & Project Management: S4Carlisle Publishing Services
Cover Design: Kristin E. Parker
Senior Media Development Editor: Troy Liston
Rights Specialist: Rebecca Damon
Cover Image (Title Page, Part Opener, Chapter Opener):
© phyZick/Shutterstock
Printing and Binding: LSC Communications
Cover Printing: LSC Communications

Library of Congress Cataloging-in-Publication Data
Library of Congress Cataloging-in-Publication Data unavailable at time of printing.

LCCN: 2019917179

6048

Printed in the United States of America
24 23 22 21 20   10 9 8 7 6 5 4 3 2

TRIBUTE TO DR. ESTHER M. WILKINS

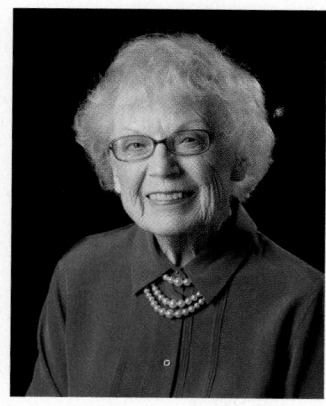

The first edition of Dr. Esther Wilkins' *Clinical Practice of the Dental Hygienist* was published in 1959. Before that, the "book" was provided for Esther's students at the University of Washington as a series of individually copied, topic-related handouts, organized as the book is today, using an easy-to-read outline format. Over the next 60 or so years, Esther wrote and supervised the revision through 12 editions (an average of one new edition every 5 years!).

Anyone who worked with Esther on any of those editions understands the effort and energy she put into making the book as up–to-date and evidence-based as possible. Even in that very first edition, every chapter contained a list of references to support the information in that chapter. A look through any of those previous editions reveals how current Esther's thinking was as she updated each edition. Anyone fortunate enough to be invited to visit Esther in her condo overlooking Boston Common will tell you that her home office was bursting with textbooks and copies of thousands of journal articles, stacked on every available surface and poking out of overfilled file cabinets. Such was her commitment to understanding the current science related to dental hygiene practice. Those of us who worked with her over the years can tell you about her attention to detail and insistence that everything be perfect as we submitted chapter manuscripts for publication.

The editorial and contributor teams who have revised this first new edition since Esther is no longer here to guide us are proud to say that we have done our best to carry forward the integrity, attention to detail, and dedication to the science and art of dental hygiene practice that was Esther's vision for this book.

DEDICATION

The 13th edition of *Clinical Practice of the Dental Hygienist* is dedicated to all past and present students who have studied from the preceding editions. Gratitude is expressed to their teachers in the many different dental hygiene programs around the world, for their leadership in, and devotion to, dental hygiene education.

A very special recognition goes to the students of the first 10 classes in dental hygiene at the University of Washington in Seattle for whom the original "mimeographed" syllabus was created by Dr. Esther Wilkins. They are remembered with much appreciation because their need for text study material made this book possible in the first place.

—Esther M. Wilkins

Gratitude to my husband, who has supported me tirelessly on my academic journey, and to my grandmother, Fay Nelson, who instilled a love of learning. Special thanks to my professional mentors who recognized my potential even when I did not: Dr. John Chirgwin, Dr. Carole Palmer, and last, but never least, Dr. Esther Wilkins. Dr. Wilkins is the wind beneath our wings as educators and dental hygienists! Never forget all she has done for our profession!

—Linda D. Boyd

To my husband Scott and our children, Harper and Layney, who provide me with daily inspiration, love, and support in all that I do. To Dr. Esther Wilkins—it is an honor to play an integral role in moving your legacy for the profession of dental hygiene forward. A special thanks goes to all who have mentored me throughout my career, to my Caruth School of Dental Hygiene family that provide a constant source of encouragement, and to my students—past, present, and future—who motivate me to keep evolving as an educator.

—Lisa F. Mallonee

To Esther, of course.

—Charlotte J. Wyche

Contents

Preface   *xiv*
Contributors   *xvii*
Reviewers   *xx*

SECTION I
ORIENTATION TO CLINICAL DENTAL HYGIENE PRACTICE   1

CHAPTER 1
The Professional Dental Hygienist   **3**
History of the Dental Hygiene Profession   4
Scope of Dental Hygiene Practice   4
Objectives for Professional Practice   11
Standards for Clinical Dental Hygiene Practice   11
Dental Hygiene Process of Care   11
Dental Hygiene Ethics   13
The Code of Ethics   13
Core Values   13
Ethical Applications   14
Legal Factors in Practice   15
Professionalism   15
References   16

CHAPTER 2
Evidence-Based Dental Hygiene Practice   **19**
Evidence-Based Practice   20
A Systematic Approach   21
Approaches to Research   27
Ethics in Research   29
Documentation   30
References   31

CHAPTER 3
Effective Health Communication   **33**
Types of Communication   34
Health Communication   34
Health Literacy   36
Communication Across the Life Span   37
Social and Economic Aspects of Health Communication   39
Cultural Considerations   39
Interprofessional Communication   42
Communication with Caregivers   42
Documentation   43
References   44

CHAPTER 4
Dental Hygiene Care in Alternative Settings   **47**
Alternative Practice Settings   48
Residence-Bound Patients   48
Dental Hygiene Care   49
The Critically Ill or Unconscious Patient   54
The Terminally Ill Patient   56
Documentation   56
References   57

SECTION II
PREPARATION FOR DENTAL HYGIENE PRACTICE   59

CHAPTER 5
Infection Control: Transmissible Diseases   **61**
Standard Precautions   62
Microorganisms of the Oral Cavity   62
The Infectious Process   63
Pathogens Transmissible from the Oral Cavity   65
Tuberculosis   67
Viral Hepatitis   68
Human Herpesvirus Diseases   70
Human Papillomavirus   75
HIV/AIDS Infection   75
Methicillin-Resistant *Staphylococcus aureus*   79
Documentation   79
References   80

CHAPTER 6
Exposure Control: Barriers for Patient and Clinician   **83**
Infection Control   84
Personal Protection for the Dental Team   84
Clinical Attire   84
Use of Face Mask: Respiratory Protection   85
Use of Protective Eyewear   86
Hand Care   87
Hand-Hygiene Principles   89
Methods of Hand Hygiene   89
Gloves and Gloving   91
Latex Hypersensitivity   93
Documentation   94
References   95

CHAPTER 7
Infection Control: Clinical Procedures   97
Infection Control   98
Treatment Room Features   98
Instrument Processing Center   100
Precleaning Procedures   100
Instrument Packing and Management System   102
Sterilization   102
Moist Heat: Steam under Pressure   104
Dry Heat   104
Chemical Vapor Sterilizer   105
Intermediate-Use Steam Sterilization   105
Chemical Liquid Sterilization   105
Care of Sterile Instruments   105
Chemical Disinfectants   106
Barriers and Surface Covers   107
Preparation of the Treatment Room   107
Patient Preparation   110
Summary of Standard Procedures   110
Disposal of Waste   111
Supplemental Recommendations   111
Occupational Postexposure Management   112
Documentation   112
References   113

CHAPTER 8
Patient Reception and Ergonomic Practice   115
Preparation for the Patient   116
Patient Reception   116
Position of the Patient   116
Position of the Clinician   118
Neutral Working Position   118
The Treatment Area   120
Ergonomic Practice   121
Self-Care for the Dental Hygienist   123
Documentation   124
References   125

CHAPTER 9
Emergency Care   127
Emergency Preparedness   128
Prevention of Emergencies   128
Patient Assessment   128
Stress Minimization   130
Emergency Materials and Preparation   130
BLS Certification   136
Oxygen Administration   136
Specific Emergencies   137
Documentation   137
References   145

SECTION III
DOCUMENTATION   147

CHAPTER 10
Documentation for Dental Hygiene Care   149
The Patient Record   150
The Health Insurance Portability and Accountability Act   151

Documenting the Extra- and Intraoral Examination   152
Tooth Numbering Systems   152
Charting of Hard and Soft Tissues   154
Periodontal Records   155
Dental Records   157
Care Plan Records   157
Informed Consent   157
Documentation of Patient Visits   157
References   159

SECTION IV
ASSESSMENT   161

CHAPTER 11
Medical, Dental, and Psychosocial Histories   163
Introduction   164
History Preparation   164
The Questionnaire   165
The Interview   167
Items Included in the History   168
Application of Patient Histories   176
Pretreatment Antibiotic Prophylaxis   178
American Society of Anesthesiologists Determination   179
Review and Update of History   180
Documentation   180
References   182

CHAPTER 12
Vital Signs   183
Introduction   183
Body Temperature   184
Pulse   185
Respiration   186
Blood Pressure   187
Documentation   191
References   192

CHAPTER 13
Extraoral and Intraoral Examination   195
Rationale for the Extraoral and Intraoral Examination   196
Components of Examination   196
Anatomic Landmarks of the Oral Cavity   198
Sequence of Examination   198
Morphologic Categories   204
Oral Cancer   206
Clinical Recommendations for Evaluation of Oral Lesions   207
Documentation   207
References   209

CHAPTER 14
Family Violence   211
Family Violence   212
Child Abuse and Neglect   212
Munchausen Syndrome by Proxy   216
Human Trafficking   217
Elder Abuse and Neglect   217
Intimate Partner Violence   218

Reporting Abuse and/or Neglect   219
Forensic Dentistry   220
Documentation   221
References   223

CHAPTER 15

Dental Radiographic Imaging   **225**
Introduction   226
How X-Rays are Produced   226
Digital Radiography   229
Characteristics of an Acceptable Radiographic Image   231
Factors That Influence the Finished Radiograph   231
Exposure to Radiation   235
Risk of Injury from Radiation   237
Procedures for Image Receptor Placement and
    Angulation of Central Ray   241
Image Receptor Selection for Intraoral Surveys   242
Periapical Survey: Paralleling Technique   243
Bitewing Survey   244
Periapical Survey: Bisecting-Angle Technique   245
Occlusal Survey   245
Panoramic Radiographic Images   246
Infection Control   247
Traditional Film Processing   248
Handheld X-Ray Devices   249
Analysis of Completed Radiographs   249
Ownership   250
Documentation   252
References   253

CHAPTER 16

Hard Tissue Examination of the Dentition   **255**
The Dentitions   256
Hard Tissue Examination Procedure   257
Developmental Enamel Lesions   260
Developmental Defects of Dentin   261
Noncarious Dental Lesions   261
Noncarious Cervical Lesions   261
Fractures of the Teeth   263
Dental Caries   263
Enamel Caries   266
Early Childhood Caries   267
Root Caries   267
Testing for Pulp Vitality   268
Occlusion   269
Occlusion of the Primary Teeth   273
Dynamic or Functional Occlusion   274
Trauma from Occlusion   274
Study Models   275
The Interocclusal Record   275
Documentation   275
References   277

CHAPTER 17

**Dental Soft Deposits, Biofilm, Calculus,
and Stains**   **279**
Dental Biofilm and Other Soft Deposits   280
Acquired Pellicle   281

Dental Biofilm   281
Supragingival and Subgingival Dental Biofilm   284
Composition of Dental Biofilm   284
Clinical Aspects of Dental Biofilm   285
Significance of Dental Biofilm   286
Materia Alba   286
Food Debris   287
Calculus   287
Calculus Composition   289
Calculus Formation   290
Attachment of Calculus   291
Significance of Dental Calculus   291
Clinical Characteristics   291
Prevention of Calculus   293
Dental Stains and Discolorations   293
Significance of Dental Stains   293
Extrinsic Stains   294
Endogenous Intrinsic Stains   297
Exogenous Intrinsic Stains   299
Documentation   300
References   301

CHAPTER 18

The Periodontium   **303**
The Normal Periodontium   303
The Gingival Description   309
The Gingiva of Young Children   314
The Gingiva after Periodontal Surgery   314
Documentation   315
References   316

CHAPTER 19

Periodontal Disease Development   **317**
Periodontal-Systemic Disease Connection   318
Risk Assessment   318
Etiology of Periodontal Disease   318
Risk Factors for Periodontal Diseases   319
Pathogenesis of Periodontal Diseases   323
Gingival and Periodontal Pockets   324
Complications Resulting from Periodontal Disease Progression   325
The Recognition of Gingival and Periodontal Infections   327
Classification of Periodontal Health   328
Classification of Gingivitis   328
Classification of Periodontitis   329
Acute Periodontal Lesions   332
Documentation   333
References   334

CHAPTER 20

Periodontal Examination   **337**
Basic Instruments for Examination   338
The Mouth Mirror   338
Air–Water Syringe   338
Explorers   339
Basic Procedures for Use of Explorers   339
Explorers: Supragingival Procedures   340
Explorers: Subgingival Procedures   340
Periodontal Probe   340

Guide to Periodontal Probing   343
Preliminary Assessment Prior to Periodontal Examination   344
Parameters of Care for the Periodontal Examination   345
Radiographic Changes in Periodontal Disease   353
Other Radiographic Findings   355
Documentation   355
References   356

CHAPTER 21
Indices and Scoring Methods   357
Types of Scoring Methods   357
Indices   358
Oral Hygiene Status (Biofilm, Debris, and Calculus)   359
Gingival and Periodontal Health   365
Dental Caries Experience   371
Dental Fluorosis   375
Community-Based Oral Health Surveillance   376
Documentation   377
References   379

SECTION V
DENTAL HYGIENE DIAGNOSIS
AND CARE PLANNING   381

CHAPTER 22
Dental Hygiene Diagnosis   383
Introduction   384
Assessment Findings   384
The Periodontal Diagnosis and Risk Level   386
Dental Caries Risk Level   388
The Dental Hygiene Diagnosis   388
The Dental Hygiene Prognosis   388
Putting It All Together   389
Documentation   391
References   391

CHAPTER 23
The Dental Hygiene Care Plan   393
Preparation of a Dental Hygiene Care Plan   394
Components of a Written Care Plan   395
Additional Considerations   398
Sequencing and Prioritizing Patient Care   398
Presenting the Dental Hygiene Care Plan   399
Informed Consent   400
Documentation   401
References   402

SECTION VI
IMPLEMENTATION: PREVENTION   403

CHAPTER 24
Preventive Counseling and Behavior Change   405
Steps in a Preventive Program   406
Patient Counseling   406
Patient Motivation and Behavior Change   407
Motivational Interviewing   408

MI Implementation   410
Exploring Ambivalence   413
Eliciting and Recognizing Change Talk   414
Strengthening Commitment (The Plan)   416
MI with Pediatric Patients and Caregivers   417
Motivational Training and Coaching   418
Documentation   418
References   419

CHAPTER 25
Protocols for Prevention and Control
of Dental Caries   421
History of Dental Caries Management   422
The Dental Caries Process   422
Dental Caries Classifications   423
Caries Risk Assessment Systems   424
Implementation of CRA in the Process of Care   427
Caries Risk Management Systems   427
Planning Care for the Patient's Caries Risk Level   427
Continuing Care   429
Documentation   429
References   430

CHAPTER 26
Oral Infection Control: Toothbrushes
and Toothbrushing   433
Development of Toothbrushes   434
Manual Toothbrushes   434
Power Toothbrushes   436
Toothbrush Selection for the Patient   439
Methods for Manual Toothbrushing   439
The Bass and Modified Bass Methods   440
The Stillman and Modified Stillman Methods   441
The Roll or Rolling Stroke Method   442
Charters Method   442
The Horizontal (or Scrub) Method   443
The Fones (or Circular) Method   443
Leonard's (or Vertical) Method   443
Method for Power Toothbrushing   444
Supplemental Brushing Methods   444
Guidelines for Toothbrushing Instructions   446
Toothbrushing for Special Conditions   448
Adverse Effects of Toothbrushing   449
Care of Toothbrushes   450
Documentation   451
References   452

CHAPTER 27
Oral Infection Control: Interdental Care   455
The Interdental Area   456
Planning Interdental Care   456
Selective Interdental Biofilm Removal   457
Interdental Brushes   457
Dental Floss and Tape   459
Aids for Flossing   461
Power Flossers   463
Single-Tuft Brush (End-Tuft Brush)   464

Interdental Tip   464
Toothpick in Holder   465
Wooden Interdental Cleaner   465
Oral Irrigation   466
Documentation   467
References   468

CHAPTER 28
Dentifrices and Mouthrinses   **471**
Chemotherapeutics   472
Dentifrices   472
Preventive and Therapeutic Benefits of Dentifrices   472
Cosmetic Effects of Dentifrices   472
Basic Components of Dentifrices: Inactives   473
Active Components of Dentifrices   474
Selection of Dentifrices   474
Mouthrinses   475
Purposes and Uses of Mouthrinses   475
Preventive and Therapeutic Agents of Mouthrinses   475
Commercial Mouthrinse Ingredients   477
Procedure for Rinsing   478
Emerging Alternative Practices   479
United States Food and Drug Administration   479
American Dental Association Seal of Acceptance Program   479
Documentation   480
References   482

CHAPTER 29
The Patient with Orthodontic Appliances   **485**
Cemented Bands and Bonded Brackets   486
Clinical Procedures for Bonding   487
Dental Hygiene Care   488
Clinical Procedures for Band Removal and Debonding   490
Postdebonding Evaluation   492
Orthodontic Retention   493
Postdebonding Preventive Care   493
Documentation   493
References   495

CHAPTER 30
Care of Dental Prosthesis   **497**
Missing Teeth   498
The Edentulous Mouth   498
Purposes for Wearing a Fixed or Removable Prosthesis   499
Fixed Partial Denture Prostheses   499
Removable Partial Denture Prostheses   500
Complete Denture Prosthesis   501
Complete Overdenture Prostheses   502
Obturator   503
Denture Marking for Identification   503
Professional Care Procedures for Fixed Prostheses   505
Patient Self-Care Procedures for Fixed Prostheses   505
Professional Care Procedures for Removable Partial Prosthesis 506
Patient Self-Care Procedures for Removable Partial Prostheses 507
Professional Care Procedures for Complete Dentures   509
Patient Self-Care Procedures for the Complete Denture   510
Denture-Induced Oral Mucosal Lesions (OMLs)   511
Documentation   513
References   514

CHAPTER 31
The Patient with Dental Implants   **517**
Bone Physiology   518
Osseointegration   518
Implant Interfaces   518
Types of Dental Implants   519
Patient Selection   521
Evaluation for Implant Placement   521
Post-restorative Evaluation   521
Peri-Implant Preventive Care   522
Continuing Care   523
Classification of Peri-Implant Disease   524
Documentation   525
References   526

CHAPTER 32
The Patient with Nicotine Use Disorders   **529**
Health Hazards and Current Trends   530
Components of Tobacco Products and Tobacco Smoke   530
Metabolism of Nicotine   530
Alternative Tobacco Products   531
Systemic Effects   534
Environmental Tobacco Smoke   534
Prenatal and Children   535
Oral Manifestations of Tobacco and Nicotine Use   535
Tobacco and Periodontal Infections   536
Nicotine Addiction   536
Treatment   538
Pharmacotherapies Used for Treatment of Nicotine Addiction   539
Nicotine-Free Therapy   541
Dental Hygiene Care for the Patient Who Uses Tobacco   541
Assessment   542
Clinical Treatment Procedures   542
Tobacco Cessation Program   543
Motivational Interviewing   543
The "5 A's"   543
The Team Approach   546
Advocacy   546
Documentation   547
References   548

CHAPTER 33
Diet and Dietary Analysis   **553**
Nutrient Standards for Diet Adequacy in Health Promotion   554
Oral Health Relationships   555
Counseling for Dental Caries Control   562
The Dietary Assessment   562
Preparation for Additional Counseling   566
Counseling Procedures   567
Evaluation of Progress   569
Documentation   569
References   571

CHAPTER 34
Fluorides   **573**
Fluoride Metabolism   574
Fluoride and Tooth Development   574
Tooth Surface Fluoride   576

Demineralization–Remineralization   576
Fluoridation   577
Effects and Benefits of Fluoridation   578
Partial Defluoridation   579
School Fluoridation   579
Discontinued Fluoridation   579
Fluorides in Foods   579
Dietary Fluoride Supplements   580
Professional Topical Fluoride Applications   581
Clinical Procedures: Professional Topical Fluoride   583
Self-Applied Fluorides   587
Tray Technique: Home Application   587
Fluoride Mouthrinses   588
Brush-On Gel   589
Fluoride Dentifrices   590
Combined Fluoride Program   591
Fluoride Safety   591
Documentation   593
References   595

CHAPTER 35
Sealants   **599**
Introduction   600
Sealant Materials   600
Indications for Sealant Placement   601
Penetration of Sealant   601
Clinical Procedures   603
Maintenance   607
School-Based Dental Sealant Programs   608
Documentation   608
References   609

SECTION VII
IMPLEMENTATION: TREATMENT   611

CHAPTER 36
Anxiety and Pain Control   **613**
Components of Pain   614
Pain Control Mechanisms   614
Nonopioid Analgesics   615
Nitrous Oxide–Oxygen Sedation   615
Characteristics of Nitrous Oxide   615
Equipment for Nitrous Oxide–Oxygen   616
Patient Selection   617
Clinical Procedures for Nitrous Oxide–Oxygen Administration   618
Potential Hazards of Occupational Exposure   620
Advantages and Disadvantages of Nitrous
    Oxide/Oxygen Sedation Anesthesia   620
Local Anesthesia   620
Pharmacology of Local Anesthetics   621
Indications for Local Anesthesia   624
Patient Assessment   625
Armamentarium for Local Anesthesia   627
Clinical Procedures for Local Anesthetic Administration 630
Potential Adverse Reactions to Local Anesthesia   633
Advantages and Disadvantages of Local Anesthesia   635

Noninjectable Anesthesia   635
Topical Anesthesia   636
Application of Topical Anesthetic   637
New Developments in Pain Control   638
Documentation   639
References   640

CHAPTER 37
**Instruments and Principles for
Instrumentation**   **643**
Overview of Periodontal Instruments   644
Instrument Design   645
Grasps and Fulcrum   646
Instrumentation Basics   649
Scalers   651
Curets   652
Periodontal Files   654
Powered Instruments   655
Sonic Scalers   657
Magnetostrictive Ultrasonic Scalers   657
Piezoelectric Ultrasonic Scalers   658
Powered Instrumentation Technique   659
Dexterity Development   660
Cumulative Trauma   662
Documentation   663
References   664

CHAPTER 38
Instrument Care and Sharpening   **667**
Instrument Sharpening   667
Basic Sharpening Principles   669
Sharpening Curets and Scalers   671
Moving Flat Stone: Stationary Instrument   671
Stationary Flat Stone: Moving Instrument   674
Sharpening the File Scaler   675
Care of Sharpening Equipment   675
Documentation   676
References   677

CHAPTER 39
**Nonsurgical Periodontal Therapy and
Adjunctive Therapy**   **679**
Nonsurgical Periodontal Therapy   680
Aims and Expected Outcomes   680
Nonsurgical Periodontal Therapy Treatment Goals   681
Components of Nonsurgical Periodontal Therapy   682
Dental Hygiene Treatment Care Plan for Periodontal
    Debridement   682
Appointment Planning   682
Preparation for Periodontal Therapy   684
Advanced Instrumentation   686
Specialized Debridement Instruments   689
Post-Op Instruction for Periodontal Debridement Appointments   692
Re-Evaluation of Nonsurgical Periodontal Therapy   693
Adjunctive Therapy   694
Antimicrobial Treatment   694
Indications for Use of Local Delivery Agents   695

Types of Local Delivery Agents   696
Documentation   699
References   700

CHAPTER 40
Sutures and Dressings   **703**
Sutures   704
Needles   705
Knots   706
Suturing Procedures   706
Procedure for Suture Removal   706
Periodontal Dressings   709
Types of Dressings   709
Clinical Application   710
Dressing Removal and Replacement   710
Documentation   713
References   714

CHAPTER 41
Dentinal Hypersensitivity   **715**
Hypersensitivity Defined   716
Etiology of Dentinal Hypersensitivity   716
Natural Desensitization   718
The Pain of Dentin Hypersensitivity   719
Differential Diagnosis   720
Hypersensitivity Management   721
Oral Hygiene Care and Treatment Interventions   722
Documentation   726
References   727

CHAPTER 42
Extrinsic Stain Removal   **729**
Introduction   730
Purposes for Stain Removal   730
Science of Polishing   730
Effects of Cleaning and Polishing   730
Indications for Stain Removal   731
Clinical Application of Stain Removal   732
Cleaning and Polishing Agents   733
Procedures For Stain Removal (Coronal Polishing)   735
The Power-Driven Instruments   736
Use of the Prophylaxis Angle   738
Air-Powder Polishing   739
Polishing Proximal Surfaces   741
Historical Perspective: The Porte Polisher   743
Documentation   743
References   744

CHAPTER 43
Tooth Bleaching   **747**
Overview of Tooth Bleaching   747
Vital Tooth Bleaching   748
Nonvital Tooth Bleaching   756
Dental Hygiene Process of Care   757
Documentation   759
References   760

SECTION VIII
EVALUATION   **763**

CHAPTER 44
Principles of Evaluation   **765**
Principles of Evaluation   765
Evaluation Based on Goals and Outcomes   766
Evaluation of Clinical (Treatment) Outcomes   767
Evaluation of Health Behavior Outcomes   767
Comparison of Assessment Findings   767
Standard of Care   767
Self-Assessment and Reflective Practice   768
Documentation   769
References   771

CHAPTER 45
Continuing Care   **773**
Goals of the Continuing Care Program   773
Continuing Care Appointment Procedures   774
Appointment Intervals (Frequency)   776
Methods for Continuing Care Systems   776
Documentation   777
References   778

SECTION IX
PATIENTS WITH SPECIAL NEEDS   **779**

CHAPTER 46
The Pregnant Patient and Infant   **781**
Introduction   782
Fetal Development   782
Oral Findings during Pregnancy   784
Aspects of Patient Care   785
Patient Instruction   788
Special Problems Requiring Referral   789
Transitioning from Pregnancy to Infancy   790
Infant Oral Health   790
Documentation   794
References   795

CHAPTER 47
The Pediatric Patient   **799**
Pediatric Dentistry   800
The Child as a Patient   800
Patient Management Considerations   801
Components of the Dental Hygiene Visit   805
Periodontal Risk Assessment   809
Caries Risk Assessment   809
Anticipatory Guidance   814
Treatment Planning and Consent   819
Documentation   819
References   820

CHAPTER 48
The Older Adult Patient   **823**
Aging   824
Normal Physiologic Aging   824
Pathology and Disease   826

Chronic Conditions Associated with Aging 826
Oral Changes Associated with Aging 831
Dental Hygiene Care for the Older Adult Patient 834
Documentation 838
References 839

CHAPTER 49
The Patient with a Cleft Lip and/or Palate 841
Classification of Clefts 842
Etiology 842
General Physical Characteristics 843
Oral Characteristics 844
Treatment 844
Dental Hygiene Care 846
Documentation 847
References 848

CHAPTER 50
The Patient with a Neurodevelopmental Disorder 849
Neurodevelopmental Disorders Overview 850
Intellectual Disorders 850
Down Syndrome 852
Fragile X Syndrome 854
Autism Spectrum Disorder 855
Dental Hygiene Care 858
Documentation 860
References 862

CHAPTER 51
The Patient with a Disability 865
Disabilities Overview 866
Barrier-Free Environment 870
Risk Assessment 871
Oral Disease Prevention and Control 872
Patient Management 876
Wheelchair Transfer 882
Instruction for Caregivers 885
Group In-Service Education 885
The Dental Hygienist with a Disability 887
Documentation 887
References 889

CHAPTER 52
Neurologic Disorders and Stroke 891
Introduction 892
Neurologic Disorders Associated with Physical Disability 892
Other Conditions that Limit Physical Ability 892
Spinal Cord Injury 892
Cerebrovascular Accident (Stroke) 895
Bell's Palsy (Idiopathic Temporary Facial Paralysis) 897
Amyotrophic Lateral Sclerosis 898
Parkinson's Disease 898
Postpolio Syndrome 899
Cerebral Palsy 899
Muscular Dystrophies 901
Myelomeningocele 902
Arthritis 904

Summary of Considerations for Dental Hygiene Care 905
Documentation 907
References 908

CHAPTER 53
The Patient with an Endocrine Condition 911
Overview of the Endocrine System 912
Endocrine Gland Disorders 913
Pituitary Gland 913
Thyroid Gland 913
Parathyroid Glands 914
Adrenal Glands 915
Pancreas 916
Puberty 916
Women's Health 917
Documentation 919
References 920

CHAPTER 54
The Patient with Diabetes Mellitus 923
Diabetes Mellitus 924
Oral Health Implications of Diabetes Mellitus 924
Basics About Insulin 925
Identification of Individuals at Risk for Development of Diabetes 927
Classification of Diabetes Mellitus 928
Diagnosis of Diabetes 930
Standards of Medical Care for Diabetes Mellitus 930
Pharmacologic Therapy 933
Complications of Diabetes 934
Dental Hygiene Care Plan 935
Documentation 939
References 940

CHAPTER 55
The Patient with Cancer 943
Description 944
Surgery 945
Chemotherapy 945
Radiation Therapy 946
Hematopoietic Stem Cell Transplantation 947
Mucositis Management 948
Dental Hygiene Care Plan 949
Documentation 951
References 953

CHAPTER 56
The Oral and Maxillofacial Surgery Patient 955
Patient Preparation 956
Dental Hygiene Care 957
Patient with Intermaxillary Fixation 959
Fractured Jaw 960
Mandibular Fractures 962
Midfacial Fractures 964
Alveolar Process Fracture 964
Dental Hygiene Care 964
Dental Hygiene Care Before General Surgery 966
Documentation 967
References 968

CHAPTER 57
The Patient with a Seizure Disorder   **969**
Introduction   970
Seizures   970
Clinical Manifestations   972
Treatment   972
Oral Findings   973
Dental Hygiene Care Plan   975
Emergency Care   977
Documentation   978
References   979

CHAPTER 58
The Patient with a Mental Health Disorder   **981**
Overview of Mental Disorders   982
Anxiety Disorders   982
Depressive Disorders   984
Bipolar Disorder   986
Feeding and Eating Disorders   987
Schizophrenia   991
Mental Health Emergency   993
Documentation   994
References   995

CHAPTER 59
The Patient with a Substance-Related Disorder   **999**
Introduction   1000
Alcohol Consumption   1000
Metabolism of Alcohol   1001
Health Hazards of Alcohol   1002
Fetal Alcohol Spectrum Disorders (FASDs)   1003
Alcohol Withdrawal Syndrome   1005
Treatment for AUD   1005
Abuse of Prescription and Street Drugs   1005
Risk Management for Prescription Drugs of Abuse   1005
Most Common Drugs of Abuse   1006
Medical Effects of Drug Abuse   1012
Treatment Methods   1013
Dental Hygiene Process of Care   1015
Documentation   1019
References   1020

CHAPTER 60
The Patient with a Respiratory Disease   **1023**
The Respiratory System   1024
Upper Respiratory Tract Diseases   1026
Lower Respiratory Tract Diseases   1028
Acute Bronchitis   1028
Pneumonia   1028
Tuberculosis   1030
Asthma   1032
Chronic Obstructive Pulmonary Disease   1035
Cystic Fibrosis   1037
Sleep-Related Breathing Disorders   1039
Documentation   1039
References   1041

CHAPTER 61
The Patient with Cardiovascular Disease   **1043**
Introduction   1044
Classification   1044
Infective Endocarditis   1044
Congenital Heart Diseases   1045
Rheumatic Fever and Heart Disease   1047
Mitral Valve Prolapse   1048
Hypertension   1048
Ischemic Heart Disease   1049
Angina Pectoris   1051
Myocardial Infarction   1051
Heart Failure   1052
Cardiac Arrhythmias   1053
Lifestyle Management for the Patient with Cardiovascular Disease   1053
Surgical Treatment   1054
Antithrombotic Therapy   1056
Documentation   1057
References   1058

CHAPTER 62
The Patient with a Blood Disorder   **1061**
Normal Blood   1062
Plasma   1062
Red Blood Cells (Erythrocytes)   1062
White Blood Cells (Leukocytes)   1062
Platelets (Thrombocytes)   1065
Anemia   1065
Iron Deficiency Anemia   1066
Megaloblastic Anemia   1066
Sickle Cell Disease   1067
Polycythemias   1069
Disorders of White Blood Cells   1069
Platelet Disorders   1070
Bleeding or Coagulation Disorders   1070
Dental Hygiene Care Plan   1071
Documentation   1073
References   1075

CHAPTER 63
The Patient with an Autoimmune Disease   **1077**
Overview of Autoimmune Diseases   1078
Connective Tissue Autoimmune Diseases   1079
Oral Lichen Planus   1079
Rheumatoid Arthritis   1080
Scleroderma   1081
Gastrointestinal Tract Autoimmune Diseases   1083
Celiac Disease   1083
Crohn's Disease   1083
Ulcerative Colitis   1085
Neurologic System Autoimmune Diseases   1086
Multiple Sclerosis   1086
Myasthenia Gravis   1088
Systemic Autoimmune Diseases   1089
Sjögren's Syndrome   1089
Systemic Lupus Erythematosus   1090
Documentation   1091
References   1092

Glossary   *1095*
Index   *1133*

Preface

Dental hygienists are oral healthcare specialists with professional goals centered on the prevention and/or control of oral disease and the maintenance of oral and general health. As primary healthcare professionals, dental hygienists can apply their knowledge and skills in a wide variety of areas related to clinical practice, education, research, public health, and advocacy for health promotion and disease prevention. Dental hygienists collaborate with dentists and members of other health professions to provide oral healthcare that links with total body healthcare. New emphasis on the effect of oral health on systemic health challenges dental hygienists to widen their scope of practice.

OBJECTIVES

Objectives of the 13th edition include:
- To help prepare the beginning dental hygiene student to recognize the requirements of evidence-based dental hygiene practice.
- To develop skills and knowledge for entry into the profession.
- To help when studying for licensure board examinations; the condensed outline form aids in making review easier.
- To update professional hygienists already in practice to recognize changes in practice and the responsibility to apply evidence-based scientific approaches to patient care.

THE TEXTBOOK PLAN

Highlights

Highlights of *Wilkins' Clinical Practice of the Dental Hygienist*, 13th edition include the following:
- All chapters have been extensively updated with the best available evidence, edited, and reorganized to minimize redundancy.
- Key words are highlighted in each chapter and available in a comprehensive glossary at the end of the textbook.
- Chapter 4 Dental Hygiene Care in Alternative Settings has been updated from the 12th edition Homebound Patient and moved to Section I Orientation to Clinical Dental Hygiene Practice to better prepare students for patient care in alternative settings.

- Chapter 14 Family Violence was extensively updated based on consultation with a PANDA (Prevent Abuse and Neglect Through Dental Awareness) expert.
- Chapter 16 Hard Tissue Examination of the Dentition is a combination of the 12th edition Teeth, Occlusion, and Study Model chapters to be more concise and inclusive of information students require for the hard tissue examination.
- Chapter 17 Dental Soft Deposits, Biofilm, Calculus, and Stains is a combination of the 12th edition chapters on biofilm, calculus, and stains to offer information on deposits in one comprehensive chapter for students.
- Chapter 19 Periodontal Disease Development has been updated to include the new 2017 World Workshop on the Classification of Periodontal and Peri-Implant Diseases and Conditions. It also includes content from the 12th edition chapter on acute periodontal conditions.
- Chapter 25 Protocols for Prevention and Control of Caries has been updated to include the International Caries Classification and Management System as part of caries classification systems.
- Chapter 30 Care of Dental Prosthesis is a combination of the 12th edition chapters for the edentulous patient and care of the dental prosthesis.
- Chapter 31 The Patient with Dental Implants has been updated to include the 2017 World Workshop on the Classification of Periodontal and Peri-Implant Diseases and Conditions.
- Chapter 37 Instruments and Principles for Instrumentation and Chapter 39 Nonsurgical Periodontal Therapy and Adjunctive Therapy were reorganized to streamline content.
- Chapters in Section IX were reorganized by life cycle and then by conditions associated with body systems.
- Chapter 51 The Patient with a Disability now contains important content from the 12th edition chapter on the patient with sensory impairment, which has been eliminated.
- Chapter 63 The Patient with an Autoimmune Disease is new and addresses a rapidly emerging area in the medically complex patient. Some content from the 12th edition chapter on neurological disorders and stroke were relocated to Chapter 63.
- Additional color images have been added throughout.

Organization of the Textbook

As in past editions, sections of *Clinical Practice of the Dental Hygienist* are sequenced to conform to the Dental Hygiene Process of Care. There are nine sections in the 13th edition, six of which are specifically identified by name with the recognized components of the Process of Care. They are *assessment, dental hygiene diagnosis, care planning, implementation, evaluation,* and *documentation.*

The textbook opens with chapters devoted to an introduction to the profession of dental hygiene and chapters related to preparation for practice. They include infection control and ergonomic health for the clinical practitioner and patient. The final large section, Section IX, applies the process of care to patients with special needs.

The nine major sections are:

I. Orientation to Clinical Dental Hygiene Practice

II. Preparation for Dental Hygiene Practice

III. Documentation

IV. Assessment

V. Dental Hygiene Diagnosis and Care Planning

VI. Implementation: Prevention

VII. Implementation: Treatment

VIII. Evaluation

IX. Patients with Special Needs

Supplementary information is available online:

I. American Dental Hygienists' Association Code of Ethics for Dental Hygienists

II. National Dental Hygienists' Association Code of Ethics

III. Canadian Dental Hygienists Association Dental Hygienists' Code of Ethics

IV. International Federation of Dental Hygienists' Code of Ethics

V. Guidelines for Infection Control in Dental Health Care Settings

VI. Average Measurements of Human Teeth

VII. Prefixes, Suffixes, and Combining Forms

VIII. Charting Symbols and Standardized Abbreviations Useful for Documenting Dental Hygiene Care

FEATURES OF THIS EDITION

All chapters have been updated and many have been extensively revised. Each chapter includes the following features:

♦ Detailed **outline format** for the text makes it easier to study and locate information quickly. In this era of information, the condensation of printed material into outline form can provide busy, overloaded students with a new efficiency for learning.

♦ **Chapter Outlines** at the opening of each chapter provide a preliminary review for readers before they start to concentrate on the meat of the chapter; the outline can help readers locate material within the chapter at any time.

♦ **Learning Objectives** at the beginning of each chapter guide the student in studying the chapter.

♦ **Key Words** are bolded throughout the chapter to indicate these words are included in an alphabetized listing in the glossary.

♦ **Everyday Ethics** boxes ("EEs") provide students with the opportunity to become aware of and discuss clinical problems from real-life practice. Principles of ethical dental hygiene practice need to be brought into the curriculum at an early stage if students are to develop into ethical practitioners. This feature has been continued from previous editions because of the expressed appreciation of teachers and students.

♦ **Factors to Teach the Patient** boxes help students to select topics from the chapter that need special emphasis while teaching patients self-care and responsibility for oral health for their own lifetime, as well as that of their family and community.

♦ **Documentation** brings the clinical care of a patient full cycle. Example documentation for a variety of patients, written using the SOAP notes format outlined in Chapter 10, can increase students' awareness of the necessary components and significance of such notes in the permanent record of each patient.

STUDENT WORKBOOK

A unique study guide, *Active Learning Workbook for Wilkins' Clinical Practice of the Dental Hygienist,* prepared by Jane F. Halaris and Charlotte J. Wyche for previous editions, has been recognized as a major contribution to student learning. The 13th edition workbook, revised to highlight new chapters and updated information from the textbook, also contains revised crossword and word search puzzles.

Everyday Ethics boxes in the workbook include individual learning, cooperative learning, or discovery activities designed to help the student reflect on or apply ethical theory–related "Questions for Consideration" found in the textbook. Activities and questions related to patient case scenarios, patient assessment summaries, and documentation of patient care provide an emphasis on case-based application of knowledge. Boxes in each chapter contain Medical Subject Heading (MeSH) terms to help students develop effective and efficient PubMed literature searches.

ADDITIONAL RESOURCES

Digital Connections

Wilkins' Clinical Practice of the Dental Hygienist, 13th edition includes additional resources for both instructors and students that are available online.

Instructors

Approved adopting instructors will be given access to the following additional resources:

- Test bank
- Slides in PowerPoint format
- Lesson plans
- Image bank of images and tables from the book
- Answers to the exercises found in *Active Learning Workbook for Wilkins' Clinical Practice of the Dental Hygienist*, by Jane F. Halaris and Charlotte J. Wyche (book available for separate purchase)

Students

The following additional student resources are available online:

- Audio pronunciation glossary for select clinical terms
- Appendices
- Videos
- Flashcards
  See the inside front cover of this text for more details.

INDIVIDUALIZED REVIEW

Customized practice quizzing with Navigate 2 TestPrep for *Wilkins' Clinical Practice of the Dental Hygienist* remediates to the book. This powerful tool offers students practice tests, detailed rationales, and powerful data dashboards.

ACKNOWLEDGMENTS

A textbook of the size and scope of *Wilkins' Clinical Practice of the Dental Hygienist* shows the work of many contributors. Comments and suggestions come from teachers, students, and practitioners from around the world, as the book has been translated into a variety of languages. Any suggestion, whether for one word or whole chapters, is welcomed and considered. It is hoped that this new edition will bring comments and requests as in the past.

Recognition for Our Contributors

We start with expressed recognition and appreciation to our listed contributors for their new or revised chapters. Each has spent much time for selective revision and to survey the literature for new material and references.

Other Appreciation

Appreciation is expressed to the following:

Marcia Williams of Santa Fe, New Mexico. Many illustrations for this and previous editions have been the work of our talented artist. Her personal interest and patience in preparing new drawings, revising previous ones, and adding color to enhance the line drawings are acknowledged with sincere gratitude.

Our Readers. And, finally, an expression of appreciation goes to our readers over the years: students, teachers, and practicing dental hygienists. Send us your comments and suggestions. As stated in the first edition, it is hoped that through greater understanding of each patient's oral and general health needs, more complete and effective dental hygiene services can be rendered.

—*Linda Boyd, Lisa Mallonee, and Charlotte Wyche*

Contributors

Jessica August, RDH, MS
Assistant Professor
Department of Dental Hygiene
Idaho State University
Pocatello, Idaho

Lisa B. Johnson, RDH, MSDH
Adjunct Faculty, Master's Public Health Program
MCPHS University
Clinical Research Coordinator
Division of Oral Medicine & Dentistry
Brigham and Women's Hospital
Boston, Massachusetts

Sara L. Beres, RDH, BA, MS
Instructor and Dental Hygiene Program Manager
Department of Dental Hygiene
Sheridan College
Sheridan, Wyoming

Linda D. Boyd, RDH, RD, EdD
Professor and Associate Dean
Forsyth School of Dental Hygiene
MCPHS University
Boston, Massachusetts

Lisa M. Byrne, RDH, BS, MHSc
Instructor
Forsyth School of Dental Hygiene
MCPHS University
Boston, Massachusetts

Jennifer Cullen, RDH, MPH
Director, Dental Hygiene Degree Completion Program
Department of Periodontics and Oral Medicine
University of Michigan School of Dentistry
Ann Arbor, Michigan

Ernestine R. Daniels, RDH, BS
Adjunct Instructor, Dental Programs
Department of Dental Hygiene
Florida State College at Jacksonville
Jacksonville, Florida

Heather Doucette, DipDH, BSc, Med
Assistant Professor
School of Dental Hygiene
Dalhousie University
Halifax, Nova Scotia

Christine A. Fambely, DH, BA, MEd
Instructor
Dental Hygiene Department
John Abbott College
Sainte-Anne-de-Bellevue, Quebec, Canada

Lori J. Giblin-Scanlon, RDH, MS, DHSc
Associate Professor and Associate Dean, Clinical Programs
Forsyth School of Dental Hygiene
MCPHS University
Boston, Massachusetts

Sharon M. Grisanti, RDH, BA, MCOH
Assistant Professor
Dental Hygiene Program
St. Petersburg College
St. Petersburg, Florida

Janet M. Gruber, RDH, MS, MPA
Professor
Department of Dental Hygiene
Farmingdale State College of New York
Farmingdale, New York

S. Kim Haslam, DipDH, BA, MEd
Assistant Professor
School of Dental Hygiene
Dalhousie University
Halifax, Nova Scotia, Canada

Valerie G. Herring RDH, BsM, MEd
Educational Coordinator/Didactic & Clinical Educator
Vancouver, British Columbia, Canada

Heather Hessheimer, RDH, MSDH
Assistant Professor
Department Dental Hygiene
University of Nebraska Medical Center-College of Dentistry
Lincoln, Nebraska

Michelle Hurlbutt, RDH, MSDH, DHSc
Associate Professor and Dean
Dental Hygiene PROGRAM
West Coast University
Anaheim, California

Susan J. Jenkins, RDH, PhD
Associate Professor
Forsyth School of Dental Hygiene
MCPHS University
Boston, Massachusetts

Evie F. Jesin, RDH, BSc
Professor
School of Dental Health
George Brown College
Toronto, Ontario, Canada

Faizan Kabani, BSDH, MHA, MBA, PhD
Assistant Professor
Caruth School of Dental Hygiene
Texas A&M College of Dentistry
Dallas, Texas

Robin L. Kerkstra, RDH, MSDH
Assistant Professor
Dental Hygiene Program
University of New Haven
New Haven, Connecticut

Lisa M. LaSpina, RDH, MS, DHSc
Associate Professor
Forsyth School of Dental Hygiene
MCPHS University
Boston, Massachusetts

Lory A. Libby, RDH, MSDH
Assistant Professor
Forsyth School of Dental Hygiene
MCPHS University
Boston, Massachusetts

Christine R. Macarelli, RDH, MS
Assistant Professor
Dental Hygiene Program
New York City College of Technology
Brooklyn, New York

Wendy Male, MBA, BDSc, RDH
Clinical Assistant Professor
Dental Hygiene Program
University of Alberta
Edmonton, Alberta

Lisa F. Mallonee, RDH, RD, LD, MPH
Professor and Graduate Program Director
Caruth School of Dental Hygiene
Texas A&M College of Dentistry
Dallas, Texas

Deborah S. Manne, RDH, RN, MSN, OCN
Adjunct Instructor
Department of Otolaryngology—Head and Neck Surgery
St. Louis University School of Medicine
St. Louis, Missouri

Catherine A. McConnell, RDH, BDSc, MEd
Clinic Coordinator
Dental Hygiene Department
John Abbott College
Sainte-Anne-de-Bellevue, Quebec, Canada

Jill C. Moore, RDH, BSDH, MHA, EdD
Adjunct Faculty
Dental Hygiene Program
University of New Haven
New Haven, Connecticut

Lisa J. Moravec, RDH, MSDH
Assistant Professor, West Division Site Coordinator
Department Dental Hygiene
University of Nebraska Medical Center-College
of Dentistry
Gering, Nebraska

Janice L. Murray, DipDH, BDSc(DH), MSDH, RDH
Former Program Leader
Charles Sturt University
School of Dentistry & Health Sciences
Wagga Wagga, Australia

Debra November-Rider, RDH, MSDH
Adjunct Assistant Professor
Forsyth School of Dental Hygiene
MCPHS University
Boston, Massachusetts

Uhlee (Yuri) Oh, RDH, BS, MSDH
Assistant Professor
Forsyth School of Dental Hygiene
MCPHS University
Boston, Massachusetts

Kristeen Perry, RDH, MSDH
Assistant Professor
Forsyth School of Dental Hygiene
MCPHS University
Boston, Massachusetts

Karen M. Portillo, RDH, MSDH
Adjunct Faculty
Dental Hygiene Program
Columbia Basin College
Pasco, Washington

Betty Ann Pryzdial, BSc, RDH, PID
Instructor
Vancouver College of Dental Hygiene
Vancouver, British Columbia, Canada

Lori Rainchuso, RDH, MS, DHSc
Associate Professor, Doctor of Health Sciences Program
School of Healthcare Business
MCPHS University
Worcester, Massachusetts

Catherine G. Ranson, RDH BHA, MET
School of Dental Health
George Brown College
Toronto, Ontario

Erin E. Relich, RDH, BSDH, MSA
Associate Professor
Division of Dental Hygiene
University of Detroit Mercy School of Dentistry
Detroit, Michigan

Dianne Smallidge, RDH, BS, MDH, EdD

Associate Professor and Interim Dean
Forsyth School of Dental Hygiene
MCPHS University
Boston, Massachusetts

Irina Smilyanski, RDH, MS, MSDH
Assistant Professor
Forsyth School of Dental Hygiene
MCPH University
Worcester, Massachusetts

Amy N. Smith, RDH, MS, MPH
Assistant Professor
Department of Dental Hygiene
Northern Arizona University
Flagstaff, Arizona

Katherine Soal, RDH, MSDH
Assistant Professor
Department of Dental Hygiene
Quinsigamond Community College
Worcester, Massachusetts

Lorie Speer, RDH, MSDH
Assistant Professor
Department of Dental Hygiene
Eastern Washington State University
Spokane, Washington

Tammy K. Swecker, BSDH, MEd
Associate Professor
Division of Dental Hygiene
Virginia Commonwealth University
Richmond, Virginia

Salima Thawer, MPH, BSc, RDH
Assistant Clinical Professor, Dental Hygiene
School of Dentistry
University of Alberta
Edmonton, Alberta

Carol Tran, PhD, BOH
Oral Health Therapist, Private Practice
Queensland, Australia
School of Dentistry, University of Queensland
Brisbane, Australia

Marsha A. Voelker, CDA, RDH, MS
Associate Professor, Junior Clinic Coordinator
Division of Dental Hygiene
University of Missouri—Kansas City School of Dentistry
Kansas City, Missouri

Shannon K. Waldron, RDH, BSc(DH), MSc
Part-time Faculty
Vancouver College of Dental Hygiene
Vancouver, British Columbia

Dianna S. Weikel, RDH, MS
Clinical Associate Professor
Department of Oncology and Diagnostic Sciences
University of Maryland School of Dentistry
Baltimore, Maryland

Lisa Welch, RDH, BS, MSDH
Associate Professor
Department of Dental Hygiene
Dixie State College
St. George, Utah

Esther M. Wilkins, BS, RDH, DMD

Charlotte J. Wyche, BSDH, MS
Retired
Department of Periodontics and Oral Medicine
University of Michigan School of Dentistry
Ann Arbor, Michigan

Katherine A. Yee, RDH, BSDH, MPH

Carolynn A. Zeitz, RDH, BS, RDA, MA
Clinical Associate Professor
Pediatric Dentistry
University of Detroit Mercy School of Dentistry
Detroit, Michigan

Denise Zwicker, BDH, MEd
Faculty of Dentistry
School of Dental Hygiene
Dalhousie University
Halifax, Nova Scotia, Canada

Reviewers

Meg D. Atwood, RDH, MPS
Professor
Department of Dental Hygiene
Orange County Community College
Middletown, New York

Judy Danielson, BSDH, MDH
Clinical Professor
Division of Periodontology
University of Minnesota School of Dentistry
Minneapolis, Minnesota

Barbara R. Ellis, RDH, EdD
Dental Studies
Monroe Community College
Rochester, New York

Terry Larson, MA, RDH
Dental Hygiene Sciences
Sinclair Community College
Dayton, Ohio

Leah MacPherson RDH, BS, MHP
Professor
Department of Dental Hygiene
Middlesex Community College
Bedford, Massachusetts

Lynn Douglas Mouden, DDS, MPH
Vice President, Quality and Performance
Avēsis Incorporated | A Guardian Company
Key Biscayne, Florida

Lynn Noonan, CDA, RDH, MBA
Adjunct Faculty
Allied Dental Education
New Hampshire Technical Institute
Concord, New Hampshire

Margaret Six, RDH, MSDH
Professor
Sarah Whitaker Glass School of Dental Hygiene
West Liberty University
West Liberty, West Virginia

Becky Smith, CRDH, EdD
Professor
Dental Hygiene Program
Miami Dade College
Miami, Florida

Maureen Strauss, CDA, RDH, MS
Professor
Dental Hygiene
Middlesex Community College
Lowell, Massachusetts

Sherie L. Tynes, CDA, RDH, PHDHP, BS
Assistant Professor-Dental Hygiene
Dental Hygiene CE Coordinator
Harrisburg Area Community College
Harrisburg, Pennsylvania

Orientation to Clinical Dental Hygiene Practice

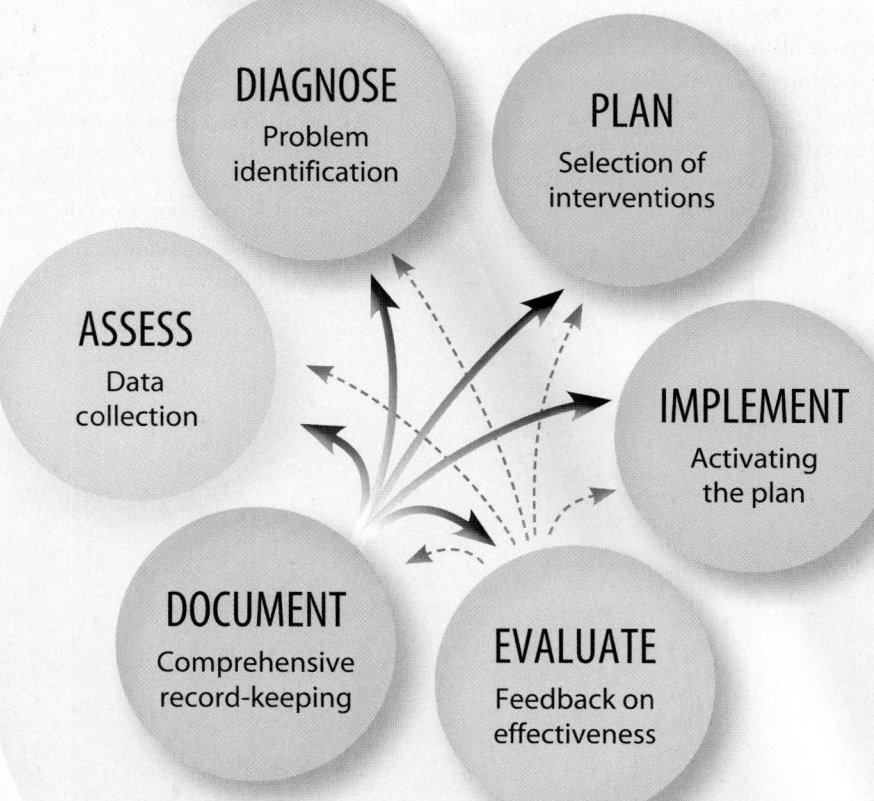

DIAGNOSE
Problem identification

PLAN
Selection of interventions

ASSESS
Data collection

IMPLEMENT
Activating the plan

DOCUMENT
Comprehensive record-keeping

EVALUATE
Feedback on effectiveness

FIGURE I-1 • The Dental Hygiene Process of Care.

INTRODUCTION FOR SECTION I

Professional dental hygiene practice is not defined solely by the clinical duties traditionally associated with private practice dental care settings. The professional roles, responsibilities, and ethical standards of the dental hygienist encompass both traditional clinical practice and alternative dental hygiene practice settings.

The dental hygienist is:

◆ An educated and licensed primary healthcare provider who fills numerous roles to contribute to better oral health.

◆ Concerned with the general health and well-being of both individual patients and population groups.

◆ Skilled in accessing, understanding, and analyzing the validity of current health information.

THE PROFESSIONAL DENTAL HYGIENIST

The professional dental hygienist is dedicated to:

◆ A dental hygiene process of care that meets standards for clinical dental hygiene practice.

◆ Ethical standards and core values outlined in professional Codes of Ethics to dental hygiene practice in every setting.

◆ Evidence-based, best-practice dental hygiene interventions.

◆ Communication approaches to build rapport with individuals and groups of all ages and across cultures.

◆ Patient education strategies to motivate positive health behavior changes.

◆ Healthcare interventions, supported by current research, which take into consideration the unique needs and requirements of each patient.

STANDARD OF CARE AND THE DENTAL HYGIENE PROCESS OF CARE

◆ The American Dental Hygienists' Association *Standards for Clinical Dental Hygiene Practice*[1] outlines criteria for competency in dental hygiene care, as illustrated by the components of the Dental Hygiene Process of Care.

◆ The Dental Hygiene Process of Care is the basis for providing preventive, educational, and therapeutic dental hygiene services that meet accepted standards of patient care.

◆ The process, illustrated in Figure I-1, as well as similar figures repeated on each section heading page, explains the series of interrelated steps the dental hygienist follows to provide clinical patient care.

◆ The overall process is explained in Chapter 1. Each step in the process is described more completely throughout the sections of the textbook.

ETHICAL APPLICATIONS

◆ Basic ethical concepts are described in the introduction to each section of the textbook.

◆ Reference charts are included to summarize ethical information.

◆ In each chapter, ethical decision making is illustrated in an Everyday Ethics scenario with questions that can be used to guide class discussions or individual reflection.

Reference

1. American Dental Hygienists' Association. *Standards for Clinical Dental Hygiene Practice*. Chicago, IL: American Dental Hygienists' Association; 2016. https://www.adha .org/resources-docs/2016-Revised-Standards-for-Clinical -Dental-Hygiene-Practice.pdf. Accessed March 3, 2019.

1

The Professional Dental Hygienist

Linda D. Boyd, RDH, RD, EdD, Lisa F. Mallonee, RDH, RD, LD, MPH,
Charlotte J. Wyche, BSDH, MS, and Esther M. Wilkins, BS, RDH, DMD

CHAPTER OUTLINE

HISTORY OF THE DENTAL HYGIENE PROFESSION

SCOPE OF DENTAL HYGIENE PRACTICE
- I. Roles of the Dental Hygienist
- II. Supervision and Scope of Practice
- III. Types of Clinical Services
- IV. Patient Education
- V. Dental Hygiene Specialties
- VI. Alternative Practice Settings
- VII. Advanced Practice Dental Hygiene
- VIII. Interprofessional Collaborative Patient Care
- IX. Advocacy for Oral Health

OBJECTIVES FOR PROFESSIONAL PRACTICE
- I. Overall Goals
- II. Personal Goals
- III. Clinical Practice Goals

STANDARDS FOR CLINICAL DENTAL HYGIENE PRACTICE

DENTAL HYGIENE PROCESS OF CARE
- I. Purposes of the Dental Hygiene Process of Care
- II. Assessment
- III. Dental Hygiene Diagnosis
- IV. The Dental Hygiene Care Plan
- V. Implementation
- VI. Evaluation
- VII. Documentation

DENTAL HYGIENE ETHICS

THE CODE OF ETHICS
- I. Purposes of the Code of Ethics
- II. Dental Hygiene Codes

CORE VALUES
- I. Core Values in Professional Practice
- II. Personal Values
- III. The Patient First
- IV. Lifelong Learning: An Ethical Duty

ETHICAL APPLICATIONS
- I. Ethical Issue
- II. Ethical Dilemma
- III. Models for Resolution of an Issue or a Dilemma
- IV. Summary: The Final Decision
- V. Applications: Everyday Ethics

LEGAL FACTORS IN PRACTICE

PROFESSIONALISM

EVERYDAY ETHICS

FACTORS TO TEACH THE PATIENT

REFERENCES

LEARNING OBJECTIVES

After studying this chapter, the student will be able to:

1. Identify and define key terms and concepts related to the professional dental hygienist.

2. Describe the scope of dental hygiene practice.

3. Identify and describe the components of the dental hygiene process of care.

4. Identify and apply components of the dental hygiene code of ethics.

5. Explain legal, ethical, and personal factors affecting dental hygiene practice.

6. Apply concepts in ethical decision making.

The American Dental Hygienists' Association (ADHA) defines the professional dental hygienist as *a primary care oral health professional* who[1]:

- Has graduated from an accredited dental hygiene program in an institution of higher education.
- Is licensed in dental hygiene to provide education, assessment, research, administrative, diagnostic, preventive, and therapeutic services.
- Supports overall health through the promotion of optimal oral health.

HISTORY OF THE DENTAL HYGIENE PROFESSION

- In the early part of the 20th century, Dr. Alfred C. Fones, a dentist in Bridgeport, Connecticut, realized that most children already had dental decay by the time they reached his dental chair.[2]
- He trained his assistant, Irene Newman, to demonstrate the value of education and prevention to reduce dental disease.[2]

- The name "dental hygienist" evolved because Fones felt that this term would create an association with the prevention, rather than the treatment of oral disease.[2]
- Box 1-1 provides a timeline of major events in the development of the profession of dental hygiene.
- Figure 1-1 illustrates how the appearance of the clinical dental hygienist has changed as the profession has changed and grown.

SCOPE OF DENTAL HYGIENE PRACTICE

- In the first textbook for dental hygienists, Dr. Alfred C. Fones, the "father of dental hygiene," emphasized education as the most important role in the practice of dental hygiene. He wrote: "It is primarily to this important work of public education that the dental hygienist is called. She must regard herself as the channel through which dentistry's knowledge of mouth hygiene is disseminated. The greatest service she can perform is

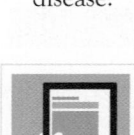

BOX 1-1
The Development of the Profession of Dental Hygiene: A Timeline

1910–1919	• Irene Newman, Dr. Fones' assistant, became:
	  • Licensed as the first dental hygienist.
	  • The first president of an organized dental hygiene society in Connecticut.
	• Graduates from the first dental hygiene school, created by Dr. Fones, began working in public schools.
	• A dental hygienist was employed outside of a public school setting, in New Haven Hospital.

1920–1929	• Licensed dental hygienists began to practice in numerous states, including Hawaii.
	• The American Dental Hygienists' Association (ADHA):
	  • Was incorporated in Detroit, Michigan, in 1927.
	  • Began publication of the *Journal of the ADHA*.

1930–1939	• Dental hygienists continued working in schools, began making home visits, and most found positions in private dental practices. • Transportation was provided to Forsyth Dental Infirmary from Boston schools and children visiting the clinic received oral prophylaxis and oral health instruction from dental hygiene students. • ADHA and American Dental Association recommended minimum high school graduation as one requirement for dental hygiene licensure. • University of Michigan offered the first baccalaureate degree in dental hygiene.

1940–1949	• ADHA recommended:
	  • Changing a 1-year program to a 2-year course of study for dental hygiene licensure.
	  • The term "registered dental hygienist" as the official credential for the profession.
	• Minimum standards for dental hygiene programs adopted.
	• Dr. Frank Lamons wrote the first dental hygienist oath, to be used in graduation exercises.
	• Grand Rapids, Michigan, became the first city to add fluoride to its drinking water.

1950–1959	• All states granted licensure for dental hygienists. • Minimum education standards for dental hygiene education set and the accreditation process for dental hygiene programs began. • Sigma Phi Alpha, the dental hygiene honor society, was founded. • ADHA membership restrictions based on race, creed, or color removed. • The first edition of the *Clinical Practice of the Dental Hygienist* textbook by Esther M. Wilkins, BS, RDH, DMD was published in 1959.

1960–1969	• The first National Dental Hygiene Board Examination implemented. • The first Regional Board Examination (North East) given. • The first dental hygiene master's degree program began at Columbia University in New York. • ADHA bylaws amended to allow for male dental hygienist members.
1970–1979	• The first International Symposium on Dental Hygiene, organized and funded by the ADHA, held in Italy. • The Forsyth Experiment, a groundbreaking investigation, proved conclusively that appropriately trained dental hygienists are safely and cost-effectively able to provide a defined set of restorative services. • Some state practice acts expand to include administration of local anesthesia by dental hygienists. • Continuing education guidelines drafted. • Dental hygienists began to serve on some state boards of dental examiners.
1980–1989	• Washington was the first state with unsupervised dental hygiene practice in hospitals, nursing homes, and other specified settings. • Colorado allowed unsupervised practice for dental hygienists in all settings. • ADHA advocated for baccalaureate as the minimum degree for entry into the dental hygiene profession. • On the basis of research about the transmission of blood-borne infectious diseases, dental hygiene clinicians began wearing gloves during all procedures.

1990–1999	• Occupational Safety and Health Administration's rules on occupational exposure to blood-borne pathogens implemented; use of gloves and face masks during dental hygiene procedures became standard practice.
	• The *Dental Hygiene Process: Diagnosis and Care Planning* textbook published, establishing a standard for clinical dental hygiene practice.
	• The National Center for Dental Hygiene Research established.
	• New Mexico became the first state to allow:
	  • Self-regulation of the profession by a dental hygiene committee.
	  • Dental hygiene practice under a collaborative agreement with a dentist rather than supervision.
	• California created the Registered Dental Hygienist in Alternative Practice, allowing dental hygienists to provide unsupervised oral care to special populations in alternative settings.

2000–2010	• The U.S. Department of Health and Human Services published *Oral Health in America: A Report of the Surgeon General*, which highlights the relevance of oral health to general health.
	• U.S. Centers for Disease Control and Prevention published *Guidelines for Infection Control in Dental Health Setting*.
	• Development of the mid-level oral health provider explored.
	  • The ADHA adopted policy to develop the Advanced Dental Hygiene Practitioner (**ADHP**).
	  • Dental Health Aide Therapists began providing dental care on tribal land in Alaska.
	  • Minnesota passed the first law in the United States, allowing dental hygienists to be further licensed as dental therapists using ADHP competencies.
	• Master-level dental hygiene programs increased in number.
	• Many states implemented "direct access" policies that allow dental hygienists in at least some settings to initiate dental hygiene care:
	  • Based on their assessment of the patient's needs.
	  • Without the specific authorization of a dentist.

2011–2020 and Beyond— Focus on the Future	• In 2013, ADHA celebrated 100 years of dental hygiene at the 90th ADHA Annual Session meeting in Boston.
	• Dental hygiene degree completion programs and online education opportunities expand.
	• Opportunities for alternative setting and autonomy in dental hygiene practice expand.
	• The dental hygiene profession affirms and pursues its commitment to:
	  • Optimal oral health as an essential component of general health.
	  • Access to safe, effective, oral health services for all people.
	  • Collaborative, interprofessional partnerships and coalitions for oral health.

Source: American Dental Hygienists' Association. *100: Celebrating a Century of Professional Prides.* Chicago, IL: ADHA; 2013:48.

the persistent education of the public in mouth hygiene and the allied branches of general hygiene."[3]

◆ While the role of education is still primary, dental hygiene has changed and the scope of practice has developed and broadened from Dr. Fones' original concept.

I. Roles of the Dental Hygienist

◆ Various roles of licensed dental hygienists include the following[4]:

• Education.

• Assessment.

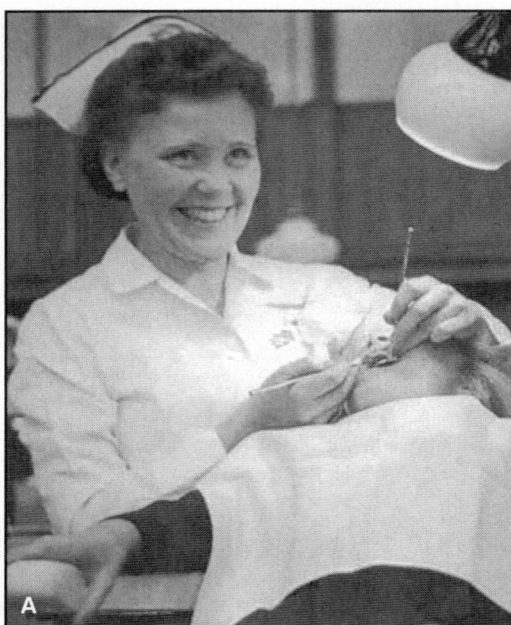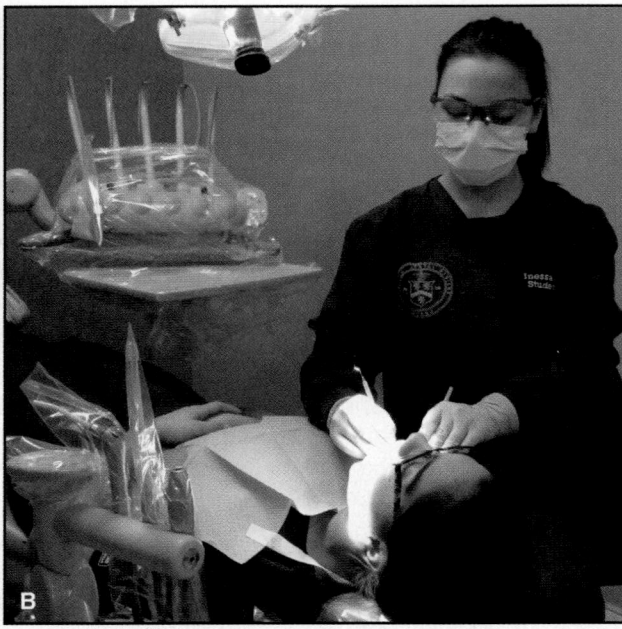

FIGURE 1-1 • There is More Difference Than Just a Uniform, but Over Time the Dental Hygienist's Commitment to Safe and Effective Patient Care Remains. A: The dental hygienist providing patient care in the 1930s dressed in a starched white uniform and cap (as nurses also did) to indicate their commitment to cleanliness and good care. **B:** The dental hygienist of today protects self and patient from cross-infection by donning personal protective equipment and surface barriers during patient care.

- Diagnosis.
- Prevention.
- Nonsurgical therapy.
- Research.
- Administration.
◆ Dental hygienists support oral health through their work in many settings including[4]:
  - General and specialty dental practices.
  - Public health programs.
  - Research centers.
  - Educational institutions.
  - Hospital and residential care facilities.
  - Federal programs, including the armed services.
  - Dental corporate industries.
◆ Within the wide span of dental hygiene practice areas, dental hygienists may serve in a variety of capacities.
◆ Areas of responsibility in this variety of roles are defined in Table 1-1.

II. Supervision and Scope of Practice

◆ The professional dental hygienist is responsible to provide only those services allowed within the scope of practice outlined within each state dental hygiene practice act.[5]
◆ The type of supervision by a dentist required for delivery of dental hygiene services is also determined by individual practice acts in each state.
◆ Types of supervision commonly used for dental hygiene practice are defined in Box 1-2.[6–8]

◆ Many states have enacted collaborative practice legislative initiatives and adopted practice rules that allow dental hygienists to provide care autonomously for underserved populations in specifically designated public health settings.[9]

III. Types of Clinical Services

The clinical responsibilities of the dental hygienist are divided into preventive, educational, and therapeutic services. Clinical and educational activities are inseparable and overlap as patient care is planned and accomplished.
◆ *Preventive services* are the methods employed by the clinician and/or patient to promote and maintain oral health.
  - Prevention is an essential component of dental hygiene practice.
  - The three categories of preventive services are defined in Box 1-3.
◆ *Educational services* are strategies developed for an individual or a group to elicit behaviors directed toward health.
  - Educational aspects of dental hygiene service permeate the entire patient care system.
  - Educate patients and the public about the growing body of evidence related to the association between oral and systemic disease to highlight the need to manage oral health for overall wellness.
  - Create a partnership with the patient that is essential for success of both preventive and therapeutic services.

TABLE 1-1 • Professional Roles of the Dental Hygienist

ROLE	DESCRIPTION	EXAMPLE EMPLOYMENT SETTINGS AND POSITIONS
Clinician	Provide direct patient care in collaboration with other health professionals	• Private dental practices and community-based clinics • Hospitals and long-term care facilities • Schools
Corporate	Employment in a company that supports oral health through promotion of oral health products and services	• Product sales and research • Corporate educator or administrator

Public health	Enhance access to care in community health programs funded by government or nonprofit organizations	• Clinician in:
		  • Community clinics
		  • Government health service
		  • School sealant programs
		• Oral health program administrator

Researcher	Conduct studies to test new procedures, products, or theories for accuracy and effectiveness	• Universities • Corporations • Government agencies
Educator	Use educational theory and methodology to educate competent oral health professionals or provide continuing education for licensed providers	• Dental hygiene program clinical or classroom instruction • Corporate educator
Administrator	Apply organizational skills, communicate objectives, identify and manage resources, evaluate and modify health or education programs	• Program director in clinical, educational, or corporate settings
Entrepreneur	Initiate or finance new oral health–related enterprises	• Practice management or product development • Consulting • Independent clinical practice • Professional speaker or writer

American Dental Hygienists' Association. Career Center: Career Paths. http://www.adha.org/professional-roles. Accessed February 16, 2019.

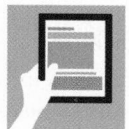

BOX 1-2
Types of Supervision in Dental Hygiene Practice

Direct supervision: the dentist needs to be present.

Personal supervision: the dentist needs to authorize, be present, and check work before dismissal of patient.

General supervision: the dentist has authorized the procedure for a patient of record but need not be present when the authorized procedure is carried out by a licensed dental hygienist. The procedure is carried out in accordance with the dentist's diagnosis and treatment plan.

Direct access supervision: the dental hygienist can provide services as determined appropriate during assessment without specific authorization. This type of supervision is usually limited to preventive services provided in specified public health settings.

Collaborative practice: the dental hygienist may practice without supervision with a collaborative agreement between a licensed dentist and a dental hygienist.

Indirect supervision: the dentist must authorize procedure and be in the office while the procedures are performed.

Remote supervision: the supervising dentist is not on-site. Communication between collaborating oral health practitioners is provided through use of current technologies. Sometimes referred to as teledentistry-assisted, affiliated dental hygiene practice.

Independent practice: the dental hygienist can provide services within the scope of dental hygiene practice in any setting and without authorization or supervision by a dentist.

Source: American Dental Hygienists' Association. Dental hygiene practice acts overview: permitted functions and supervision levels by state. Revised January 2019. http://www.adha.org/resources-docs/7511_Permitted_Services_Supervision_Levels_by_State.pdf. Accessed February 15, 2019.
Catlett A. A comparison of dental hygienists' salaries to state dental supervision levels. *J Dent Hyg*. 2014;88(6):380-385.
Summerfelt FF. Teledentistry-assisted, affiliated practice for dental hygienists: an innovative oral health workforce model. *J Dent Educ*. 2011;75(6):733-742.

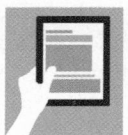

> **BOX 1-3**
> **Three Categories of Preventive Services**
>
> **Primary prevention:** measures carried out before disease occurs to prevent disease or injury.
> *Examples:* Sealants placed in deep grooves and pits to prevent caries; oral hygiene education; fluoridation of community water supplies; nutrition education on sugar-sweetened beverage consumption to reduce caries risk and obesity in children.
>
> **Secondary prevention:** treatment of early disease to prevent further progression of potentially irreversible conditions that, if not arrested, can lead eventually to extensive rehabilitative treatment or even loss of teeth.
> *Examples:* Removal of all calculus and dental biofilm while debriding a root surface in a relatively shallow periodontal pocket to prevent continued attachment loss and the formation of a deep pocket; remineralization therapy; sealants on noncavitated caries.
>
> **Tertiary prevention:** methods to replace lost tissues and to rehabilitate the oral cavity to a level where function is as near normal as possible after secondary prevention has not been successful.
> *Examples:* Replacement of a missing tooth using a fixed partial denture or implant and therefore restoring function; restorations; crowns; bone and tissue grafts.

- *Therapeutic services* are clinical treatments designed to arrest or control disease and maintain oral tissues in health.
  - Dental hygiene treatment services are an integral part of the patient's overall treatment plan.
  - Periodontal debridement, along with the steps in posttreatment care, is a part of the therapeutic phase in the treatment of periodontal infections.

IV. Patient Education

- Clinical services, both dental and dental hygiene, have limited long-range probability of success if the patient does not understand the need to take responsibility in daily oral self-care and regular appointments for professional care.
- Educational and clinical services, therefore, are mutually dependent and inseparable in the total dental hygiene care of the patient.
- Scientific information about the prevention of oral diseases has been advancing steadily.
- The public has become increasingly aware of the need for dental hygiene care and the value of oral health instruction provided by the dental hygienist.

V. Dental Hygiene Specialties

- Entry-level dental hygiene programs prepare students for basic clinical dental hygiene practice.[10]
- Continuing education can help build skills in advanced periodontal instrumentation.
- Private practice orthodontics, pediatric dentistry, and periodontics clinics particularly value dental hygienists as partners in prevention.
- Some educational institutions offer dental hygiene bachelor's degree, bachelor's degree completion programs, and master's degree programs.
- Bachelor and advanced degrees enhance the ability of dental hygienists to pursue opportunities outside of clinical practice.[10]
- Dental hygienists earn masters or doctoral degrees in a variety of areas such as:
  - Dental hygiene education.
  - Health behavior and education.
  - Public health and health policy.
  - Nutrition and dietetics.
  - Business and administration.
  - Law.
- A dental hygienist interested in specialty areas of practice can take advantage of many learning opportunities to enhance knowledge and skills.
  - Many continuing education opportunities exist for learning in all areas of dental hygiene practice.
  - In other special areas, short-term courses have been developed, such as instruction in the care of patients with disabilities.
- In-service training may be available in long-term care institutions, hospitals, and skilled nursing facilities.
- Other dental hygienists have learned to practice in a specialty through private study, special conferences, and personal experience.

VI. Alternative Practice Settings

- In 2018, 42 states allowed dental hygienists to provide direct access care (Figure 1-2) in a variety of community settings including, but not limited to[11]:
  - Schools.
  - Public health settings.
  - Headstart settings.
  - WIC (women, infants, and children) clinics.
  - Nursing home facilities.
  - Free clinics.
  - Community centers.
- *Direct access* means the dental hygienist can plan and initiate treatment based on patient assessment without specific authorization of the dentist.[11]
  - Each state practice act varies as to the scope of practice and level of supervision by a dentist.
- Dental hygiene care in alternative practice settings is further described in Chapter 4.

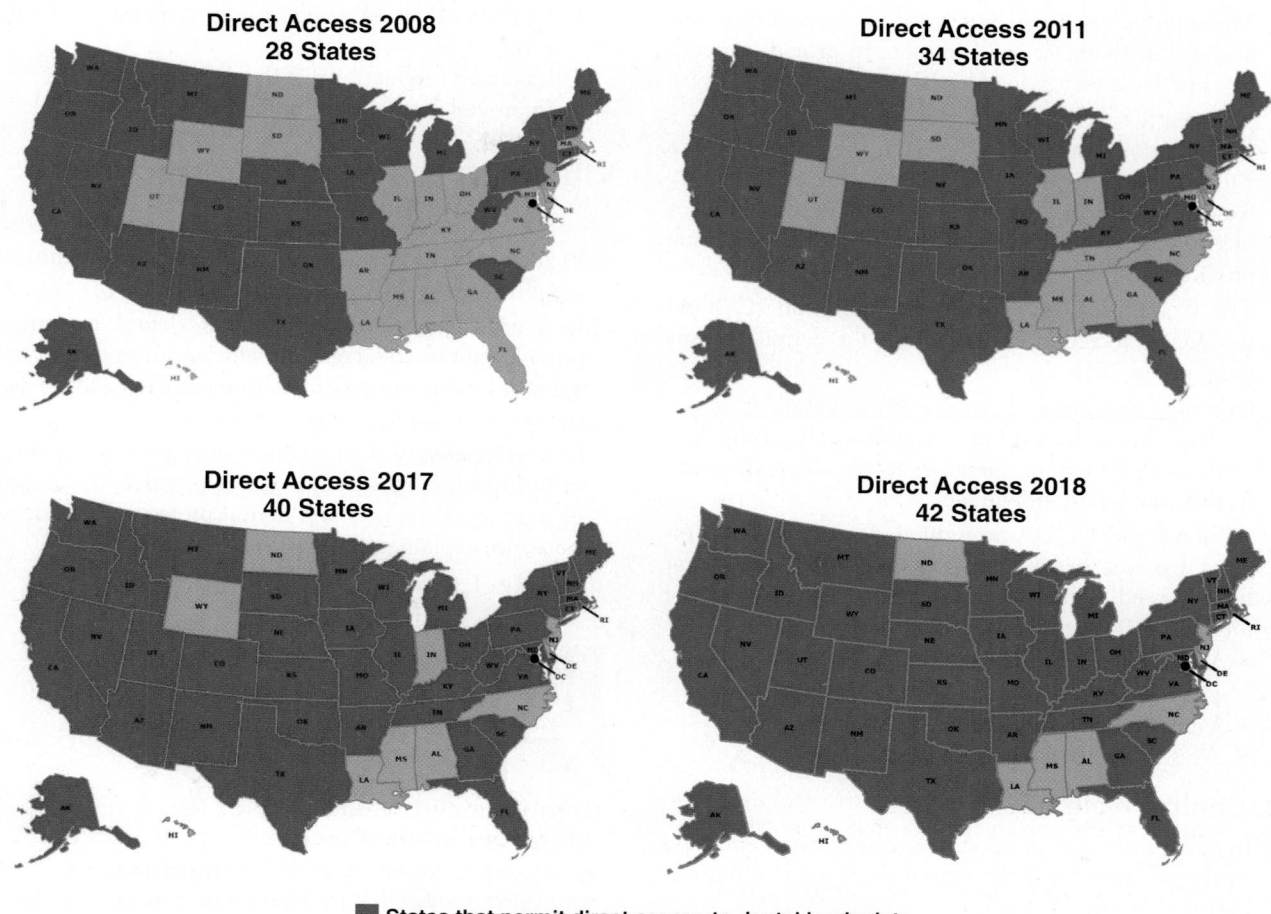

FIGURE 1-2 • American Dental Hygienists' Association (ADHA) Direct Access. Maps of the United States to show the changes in the number and location of states with direct access since 2008.

VII. Advanced Practice Dental Hygiene

◆ The current dental care model leaves many low-income individuals, at-risk populations, and those living in rural areas and inner cities without access to dental care.

◆ A number of mid-level dental provider models with a variety of names have emerged to address basic restorative and preventive care, particularly to children and in some states/countries to adults.

• Internationally, the dental therapist was first introduced in 1921 in New Zealand and is found in 54 countries.[12]

• In 1949, Forsyth Dental Infirmary began an experiment to train New Zealand–type dental nurses, but it was stopped because of pressure from the American Dental Association.[13]

• In 1971–1972, the Forsyth Experiment (more commonly known as the Rotunda Experiment) began training dental hygienists in basic restorative dentistry and local anesthesia.[14]

• From 1971 to 1976, the University of Iowa and the University of Kentucky both trained dental hygienists with advanced skills in restorative dentistry.[15,16]

• A Dental Health Aide Therapist (DHAT) was introduced in tribal villages in Alaska in 2006.[17] The DHAT model has also been authorized for pilots in Oregon and Washington tribal communities.

A. Advanced Dental Hygiene Practitioner or Advanced Dental Therapist

◆ A 2009 PEW Report[18] first recognized that creating new mid-level oral healthcare providers, such as the Advanced Dental Hygiene Practitioner proposed by the ADHA, could enhance access to oral health services for underserved populations.

◆ In 2009, the state of Minnesota approved the development of the master's-level degree program for advanced dental therapists (ADT), which requires applicants to be licensed dental hygienists holding a bachelor's degree.[19–21]

- These providers are dual licensed as a dental hygienist and dental therapist in Minnesota to provide preventive and basic restorative dental services[19–21]:
  - Directly to underserved populations.
  - Via a collaborative management agreement with a supervising dentist.
- Research findings suggest the safety and efficacy of restorative care provided by mid-level dental providers.[22–24]
- The Commission on Dental Accreditation (CODA) developed accreditation standards for dental therapy programs in 2015.[25]
- Currently, a variety of oral health stakeholder groups in many states are exploring legislation to create new workforce models to increase access to quality oral health care for all individuals.[26–29]
- Although no CODA-accredited dental therapy program has yet been approved, additional states that have passed dental therapy legislation include the following[26]:
  - Maine passed legislation for a dental hygiene therapist in 2014.
  - Vermont passed legislation in 2016.
  - Arizona and Michigan passed legislation in 2018.

B. Clinical Role of the ADT

- In addition to the traditional process of care performed by dental hygienists, the dental therapist has the following scope of practice[25]:
  - Caries removal, placement, and finishing of composite/resin and amalgam restorations.
  - Placement of space maintainers.
  - Fabrication and placement of stainless steel crowns and temporary crowns.
  - Pulpotomy.
  - Pulp vitality testing.
  - Simple extractions of erupted primary teeth.
  - Other duties may be specified in the state's scope of practice.
- ADT practice under a collaborative agreement with a dentist and patients who need more advanced care is referred.

C. Impact of ADT

- The first dental therapists graduated in Minnesota in 2011.
- Initial impacts of this provider as part of the dental team include the following[19]:
  - An increase in the number of patients served in mobile dental clinics and community health centers, particularly the underserved and special populations.
  - Reduction in waiting times for patients to receive services.
  - Decreased travel time for patients because preventive and restorative care can be provided during the same appointment.

- Possible reduction in emergency room use for dental care.
- Increased productivity of the dental team.
- Improved patient satisfaction.

VIII. Interprofessional Collaborative Patient Care

- In many situations, dental hygienists provide clinical patient care as a member of a dental team.
- In a growing number of facilities, dental hygienists provide care in collaboration with an interprofessional team of healthcare providers to meet the needs of patients with complex medical problems.
- Four competency domains necessary for participating in interprofessional collaborative practice, developed by a group of medical and dental professional associations, are explained in Box 1-4.[30]

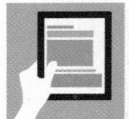

BOX 1-4
Four Competency Domains for Interprofessional Collaborative Practice

Competency 1: Values/Ethics for Interprofessional Practice:

Work with individuals of other professions to maintain a climate of mutual respect and shared values.

Competency 2: Roles/Responsibilities

Use the knowledge of one's own role and those of other professions to appropriately assess and address the healthcare needs of patients and to promote and advance the health of populations.

Competency 3: Interprofessional Communication

Communicate with patients, families, communities, and professionals in health and other fields in a responsive and responsible manner that supports a team approach to the promotion and maintenance of health and the prevention and treatment of disease.

Competency 4: Teams and Teamwork

Apply relationship-building values and the principles of team dynamics to perform effectively in different team roles to plan, deliver, and evaluate patient/population-centered care and population health programs and policies that are safe, timely, efficient, effective, and equitable.

Source: Interprofessional Education Collaborative Expert Panel. *Core Competencies for Interprofessional Collaborative Practice: 2016 Update.* Washington, DC: Interprofessional Education Collaborative; 2016. https://www.ipecollaborative.org/resources .html. Accessed February 15, 2019.

◆ Based on the work of the interprofessional education collaborative, most medical and dental accreditations standards contain a standard related to the competency domains.[30]

IX. Advocacy for Oral Health

◆ The professional dental hygienist is an active advocate for oral health in both personal and professional situations.

◆ The dental hygienist who is an advocate for oral health:
  • Influences legislators, health agencies, and other organizations to bring available resources together to improve access to care.
  • Analyzes barriers to change and helps develop mechanisms to effect change.
  • Implements and evaluates health policy and programs that promote health for individuals, families, or communities.
  • Promotes lifestyle changes that contribute to oral health.

◆ Examples of oral health advocacy activities include:
  • Joining other dental hygiene professionals to meet with legislators and public officials to encourage the inclusion of dental services in healthcare legislation.
  • Making public statements that support the oral health value of optimal fluoridation in community water systems when a community is considering defluoridation.

OBJECTIVES FOR PROFESSIONAL PRACTICE

I. Overall Goals

◆ Overall professional goals of the dental hygiene profession relate to health promotion and disease prevention.

◆ The goal of each dental hygienist is *to aid individuals and groups in attaining and maintaining optimum oral health.* Other professional objectives are related to this primary goal.

◆ A dental hygienist's self-assessment is essential to attain goals for service to each patient and community.

◆ Personal and professional goals are outlined and reviewed frequently in a plan for continued self-improvement.

II. Personal Goals

◆ Exemplify the highest degree of professional ethics and conduct.

◆ Demonstrate interpersonal relationships that assure oral health information is presented effectively.

◆ Apply a continuing process of self-evaluation throughout professional life.

◆ Recognize the need for lifelong learning to acquire updated knowledge through reading professional literature and enrolling in continuing education programs.

◆ Maintain membership and participate actively in the local, national, and international dental hygiene professional associations.

III. Clinical Practice Goals

◆ Practice safe and efficient clinical routines for the application of standard precautions for infection control.

◆ Apply evidence-based knowledge and understanding of the basic and clinical sciences to:
  • Associations between oral disease and a variety of systemic conditions.
  • Recognition of oral conditions.
  • Prevention of oral diseases.
  • Clinical and instructional procedures.

◆ Tailor care planning and interventions according to individual needs.

◆ Utilize motivational interviewing to engage the patient in becoming an active participant in their care to bring about lasting behavioral changes to support optimal oral health.

STANDARDS FOR CLINICAL DENTAL HYGIENE PRACTICE

◆ The primary purpose of standards for clinical practice is to guide dental hygiene practitioners in the development of a clinical relationship with their patients.[31]

◆ A secondary purpose is to educate the public, other healthcare providers, and policy makers about the profession of dental hygiene and the scope of dental hygiene practice.

◆ The six components of the dental hygiene process of care provide:
  • The foundation for clinical decision making and dental hygiene practice.
  • The framework for organizing the sections in this book.

DENTAL HYGIENE PROCESS OF CARE

◆ The dental hygiene process of care includes assessment, dental hygiene diagnosis, planning, implementation, evaluation, and documentation, as illustrated in Figure 1-3.[31,32]

◆ The procedures of evaluation and documentation are integrated within each of the other components in the process.

◆ As a process, the procedures performed are continual in nature and may overlap or occur simultaneously.

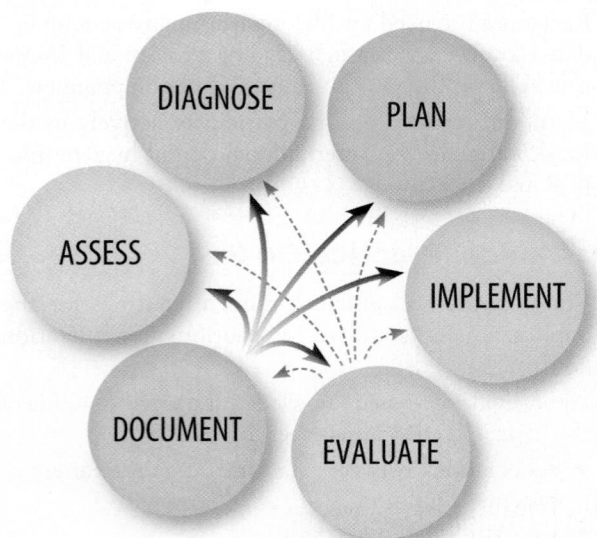

FIGURE 1-3 • The Six Interrelated Components of the Dental Hygiene Process of Care. The steps in the process are followed one after another in a cycle, beginning with assessment. Evaluation and documentation are each linked to all of the other steps.

I. Purposes of the Dental Hygiene Process of Care

◆ To provide a framework to individualize the process of care for each patient.

◆ To identify the risk factors to aid in prevention and/or management of oral disease through dental hygiene interventions.

II. Assessment

◆ The assessment phase is the first component of the dental hygiene process.

◆ This phase provides a foundation for patient care by collecting both subjective and objective data.

◆ Chapters 11–21 in this textbook are devoted to the assessment component of the dental hygiene process of care.

III. Dental Hygiene Diagnosis

◆ Dental hygiene diagnostic statements:
  • Employ the use of critical thinking to interpret assessment data, as indicated in Box 1-5.
  • Identify the health behaviors of each patient as well as the actual or potential oral health problems within the scope of practice for dental hygienists.
  • Provide the basis on which the dental hygiene care plan is designed, implemented, and evaluated.
  • Justify the treatment proposed to the patient.
◆ Chapter 22, Dental Hygiene Diagnosis, provides more information.

IV. The Dental Hygiene Care Plan

◆ Dental hygiene care planning is the selection of strategies and interventions that meet the needs of the patient in attaining oral health.

◆ The dental hygiene care plan is presented:
  • To the dentist for integration with the comprehensive dental care plan.
  • To the patient to develop understanding of the interventions needed and appointment requirements.
  • To the patient to obtain informed consent for treatment.
◆ Chapter 23 describes care planning and provides a template for the development of a written dental hygiene care plan.

V. Implementation

◆ The implementation phase in the dental hygiene process of care is the activation of the care plan.

◆ Further discussion of the concepts and procedures associated with implementation of dental hygiene preventive and treatment interventions is presented in Chapters 24–43.

VI. Evaluation

◆ The evaluation phase determines whether a specific area of a patient needs to be treated again, referred, or placed on a continuing care schedule.

◆ Evaluation of dental hygiene care is detailed in Chapter 44.

◆ Development of continuing care protocols is described in Chapter 45.

BOX 1-5
Critical Thinking Skills Used to Interpret Clinical Data

Information gathering: pertinent information is gathered from the clinical assessments as well as from the patient to identify individual characteristics.

Classification: involves sorting of information into specific categories such as general systemic, oral soft tissue, periodontal, dental, and oral hygiene.

Interpretation: relies upon critical thinking to identify significance. The cognitive processes of analysis, synthesis, inductive reasoning, and deductive reasoning are the basis for determining a diagnosis.

Validation: an attempt to verify the accuracy of data interpretation. Validation can assist in recognizing errors, isolating discrepancies, and identifying the need for additional information.

VII. Documentation

- ◆ The documentation of dental hygiene care:
  - Details all assessment data, diagnosis, care plan, treatments, patient education, and evaluation in a condensed, consistent format.
  - Represents a chronologic history of the patient's total care.
- ◆ Details for documentation are described in Chapter 10 and examples of documentation for a variety of dental hygiene interventions can be found at the end of each chapter.

DENTAL HYGIENE ETHICS

- ◆ The ethics of a profession provide the general standards of right and wrong that guide the behavior of the members in that profession.
- ◆ The members of a profession:
  - Have extensive specialized education.
  - Possess an intellectual body of knowledge from study and research.
  - Provide services important for the common good of society, for example, dental hygienists provide preventive, educational, and therapeutic services that protect and enhance the overall health of the public.
  - Maintain an organization of members that sets professional standards.
  - Exercise autonomy and judgment.
  - Adhere to their professional code of ethics.

THE CODE OF ETHICS

- ◆ Describes professional conduct.
- ◆ Outlines responsibilities and duties of each member toward patients, colleagues, and society in general.

I. Purposes of the Code of Ethics

- ◆ To increase the awareness of, and sensitivity to, ethical situations in practice.
- ◆ To define a standard of conduct that will give each individual a strong sense of ethical consciousness in professional practice as well as in all phases of life.

II. Dental Hygiene Codes

- ◆ The Codes of the ADHA, the National Dental Hygienists' Association, the Canadian Dental Hygienists' Association, and the International Federation of Dental Hygienists can be accessed online.
- ◆ Each dental hygienist is responsible for the study and application of the codes of the particular associations in which memberships are held.

CORE VALUES

Core values are selected principles of ethical behavior that are considered central to the code of a profession.

I. Core Values in Professional Practice

- ◆ The core values of the profession of dental hygiene are listed and defined in Box 1-6 and in the ADHA Code of Ethics.

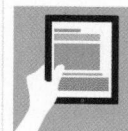

BOX 1-6
Core Values in Professional Dental Hygiene Practice

Individual autonomy and respect for human beings

People have the right to be treated with respect. They have the right to informed consent prior to treatment, and they have the right to full disclosure of all relevant information so that they can make informed choices about their care.

Confidentiality

We respect the confidentiality of patient information and relationships as a demonstration of the value we place on individual autonomy. We acknowledge our obligation to justify any violation of a confidence.

Societal trust

We value patient trust and understand that public trust in our profession is based on our actions and behavior.

Nonmaleficence

We accept our fundamental obligation to provide services in a manner that protects all patients and minimizes harm to them and others involved in their treatment.

Beneficence

We have a primary role in promoting the well-being of individuals and the public by engaging in health promotion/disease prevention activities.

Justice/fairness

We value justice and support the fair and equitable distribution of healthcare resources. We believe all people should have access to high-quality, affordable oral health care.

Veracity

We accept our obligation to tell the truth and expect that others will do the same. We value self-knowledge and seek truth and honesty in all relationships.

Source: American Dental Hygienists' Association. *Bylaws and Code of Ethics.* Chicago, IL: ADHA; Adopted June 25, 2018:32-33. http://www.adha.org/resources-docs/7611_Bylaws_and_Code_of_Ethics.pdf. Accessed February 16, 2019.

II. Personal Values

◆ Value development begins at an early age and is influenced by familial, social, and economic factors.

◆ Life experiences, grounded in previous successes and failures, serve as a foundation for professional virtues.

◆ Members of a health profession can benefit from periodic self-assessment of individual values, attitudes, and responsibilities.

III. The Patient First

◆ The responsibility to put the patient first is foremost.

◆ Dental hygienists are ethically, morally, and legally responsible to provide oral care for all patients without discrimination.

◆ Ethical decision making and professional behavior should be reflected in every aspect of dental hygiene practice.

IV. Lifelong Learning: An Ethical Duty

◆ To ensure optimal care for each patient.

◆ To maintain competency.

◆ To learn scientific advances from new research.

◆ To provide evidence-based patient care.

◆ To apply consistent ethical reasoning.

◆ To ensure fulfillment of each patient's rights.

ETHICAL APPLICATIONS

A dental hygienist may be involved in a variety of moral, ethical, and legal situations as part of the daily routine. In ethics, a problem situation is considered either an ethical issue or an ethical dilemma.

I. Ethical Issue

◆ More clearly defined than a dilemma.

◆ A common problem wherein a solution is grounded in the governing practice act, recognized laws, or accepted standards of care based on the standard rules of practice.

II. Ethical Dilemma

◆ A problem that may involve two morally correct choices or courses of action.

◆ May not have a single answer and, depending on the choice, the outcomes can differ.

III. Models for Resolution of an Issue or a Dilemma

◆ There are a number of models for resolution of an ethical issue or dilemma and all include elements of the following[33]:

• Identify the facts of the issue or dilemma.

• Identify who is involved in the issue or dilemma.

• List options or alternatives to resolve the dilemma.

• Rank and choose the best option or alternative to resolve the dilemma while trying to balance the various aspects of the ADHA Code of Ethics such as individual autonomy, beneficence, nonmaleficence, autonomy, and justice/fairness.[34]

◆ An ethical decision-making model that can be used by the dental hygienist to resolve an ethical issue or dilemma in a clinical setting is detailed in Box 1-7.[35]

IV. Summary: The Final Decision

◆ Many factors can be used to solve a dilemma.

◆ All dental healthcare providers involved in the decision process can participate in a follow-up evaluation of the action taken.

◆ Questions to ask once a decision has been made include:

• Is the decision/action that is selected morally defensible?

• Can the choice to solve the dilemma be defended?

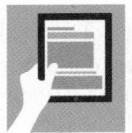

BOX 1-7

A Model for Resolution of an Ethical Issue or Dilemma

Step 1: Information	Gather information on the patient's medical, dental, and social history related to the situation.
Step 2: Identification	Assess whether this is an ethical issue or whether it is an issue best addressed by other resources.
Step 3: Clarification	Does the practitioner and patient understand the information relevant to the situation? What are the patient's rights? Is there a conflict of interest? Does an outside source need to be consulted?
Step 4: Assessment	Generate options or alternatives based on the patient situation and preferences. Consider the core values of the American Dental Hygienists' Association Code of Ethics to assess benefits and risks related to the alternatives. Collaboration with the patient and possibly other healthcare providers is part of the process of assessment of the alternatives.
Step 5: Recommendation	Choose the best alternative and obtain informed consent from the patient.
Step 6: Documentation	Document the recommendation in the patient record. Follow-up.

Source: Enck G. Six-step framework for ethical decision making. *J Health Serv Res Policy.* 2014;19(1):62-64.

◆ A professional dental hygienist may need to defend it to the patient, the dentist, members of the dental team, a state board, or even a court of law.

◆ Most importantly, the decision must be defensible based on standards of practice established for the dental and dental hygiene profession.

V. Applications: Everyday Ethics

◆ Various ethical issues and dilemmas are presented throughout this book for discussion and consideration.

◆ Examples are found in special boxes called "Everyday Ethics" and usually appear at the end of the chapter where the problem may apply.

LEGAL FACTORS IN PRACTICE

◆ The law must be studied and respected by each dental hygienist practicing within the state, province, or country.

◆ Although the various practice acts have certain basic similarities, differences in scope and definition exist.

◆ Terminology varies, but each practice act regulates the patient services delivered by the licensed dental hygienist.

  • It is the responsibility of each dental hygienist to stay current with changes to the practice act.

◆ Active engagement with the state dental hygiene association will aid in keeping the dental health professional up to date.

PROFESSIONALISM

◆ Each dental hygienist represents the entire profession to the patient, other healthcare professionals, and the community.

◆ Components of professionalism include[36]:

  • Competence: acquire and maintain a high level of knowledge through lifelong learning, clinical expertise, and professional behavior for provision of patient care.

  • Fairness: demonstrate consistency and equity when dealing with others. Promote equal access to care for the public.

  • Integrity: be honest, do the right thing, and demonstrate strong moral principles.

  • Responsibility: accountability for one's actions in accordance with the ADHA Code of Ethics.

  • Respect: value and honor others' feelings, rights, abilities, etc.

  • Service-mindedness: act for the benefit of the patients and public, and approach those served with compassion.

◆ The World Health Organization defines **health** as a state of physical, mental, and social well-being.[37] As healthcare providers, we must serve as a model for our patients.

◆ Basic components of self-care include a range of daily routine habits, health maintenance, and disease prevention behaviors. These components include the following:

  • *General physical needs* include personal hygiene, sleep, nutrition (Chapter 33), hydration, and disease prevention.

    • Routine examinations annually, including tests for hearing, sight, and certain communicable diseases.

    • Immunizations recommended for healthcare providers (Chapter 5).

    • The maintenance of a clean, healthy mouth demonstrates by example that the dental hygienist follows recommendations for prevention and control of oral disease.

  • *Physical activity* helps with weight control, maintaining mental health, prevention of chronic disease, strengthening bone and muscle, managing stress, and even improving daily activity performance.[38]

    • Recommendations for adults are for at least 150 min/wk of moderate-intensity aerobic activity in addition to muscle strengthening activities at least 2 d/wk.

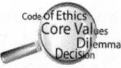

EVERYDAY ETHICS

The first term of the dental hygiene curriculum has just finished. The instructor asks for student volunteers to help at the college's health fair to provide basic routine brushing and flossing instructions for people who stop at the dental hygiene information table. Three students, Alice, Annette, and Josephine, sign up to volunteer for this community service. The day before the health fair, which takes place on a Saturday, Annette is asked to work in the dental office where she is employed part-time. Since she really needs the money, she decides not to attend the health fair and instead goes to work without telling anyone.

Questions for Consideration

1. In general, would this situation be described as a professionalism issue or an ethical dilemma? Explain.

2. Discuss Annette's actions in terms of the core ethical values.

3. What aspects of the dental hygiene code of ethics can support her student colleague's choice of action?

- *Mental health:* The mental health of the dental hygienist is reflected in interpersonal relationships and the ability to inspire confidence through a display of professional and emotional maturity.
  - Stress management helps to improve and manage mental health.[37]
- Avoid risky behaviors such as tobacco use, excessive alcohol use, illicit drug use, and risky sexual practices to prevent adverse effects and chronic diseases such as cardiovascular disease.[37]

Factors to Teach the Patient

▶ The role of the dental hygienist as a **cotherapist** with each patient, with the dentist, and with members of other health professions.

▶ The moral and ethical nature of being a dental hygiene professional.

▶ The scope of service of the dental hygienist as defined by the state practice act.

▶ The interrelationship of educational and clinical services in dental hygiene patient care.

▶ The shared responsibility of the patient for their oral health and how it can be improved and maintained.

ENHANCE YOUR UNDERSTANDING

ONLINE RESOURCES
(see the inside front cover for access information)

- Audio glossary
- Appendices

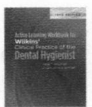

SUPPORT FOR LEARNING
(available separately)

- *Active Learning Workbook for Wilkins' Clinical Practice of the Dental Hygienist, 13th Edition*

INDIVIDUALIZED REVIEW

- Customized practice quizzing with Navigate 2 TestPrep for *Wilkins' Clinical Practice of the Dental Hygienist*

References

1. American Dental Hygienists' Association. *ADHA Policy Manual.* Chicago, IL: ADHA. https://www.adha.org/resources-docs/7614_Policy_Manual.pdf. Updated June 25, 2018. Accessed February 16, 2019.
2. American Dental Hygienists' Association. *100: Celebrating a Century of Professional Pride.* Chicago, IL: ADHA; 2013:48.
3. Fones AC, ed. *Mouth Hygiene.* 4th ed. Philadelphia, PA: Lea & Febiger; 1934:248.
4. American Dental Hygienists' Association. Career center: career paths. http://www.adha.org/professional-roles. Accessed February 16, 2019.
5. American Dental Hygienists' Association. Advocacy: scope of practice. http://www.adha.org/scope-of-practice. Accessed February 18, 2019.
6. American Dental Hygienists' Association. Dental hygiene practice acts overview: permitted functions and supervision levels by state. Revised January 2019. http://www.adha.org/resources-docs/7511_Permitted_Services_Supervision_Levels_by_State.pdf. Accessed February 15, 2019.
7. Catlett A. A comparison of dental hygienists' salaries to state dental supervision levels. *J Dent Hyg.* 2014;88(6):380-385.
8. Summerfelt FF. Teledentistry-assisted, affiliated practice for dental hygienists: an innovative oral health workforce model. *J Dent Educ.* 2011;75(6):733-742.
9. American Dental Hygienists' Association. Advocacy: direct access. http://www.adha.org/direct-access. Accessed February 18, 2019.
10. Battrell A, Lynch A, Steinbach P, Bessner S, Snyder J, Majeski J. Advancing education in dental hygiene. *J Evid Based Dent Pract.* 2014;14(suppl):209-221.
11. American Dental Hygienists' Association. Direct access states. https://www.adha.org/sites/default/files/7527_Changes_in_Direct_Access_Map.pdf. Accessed February 18, 2019.
12. Nash DA, Friedman JW, Mathu-Muju KR, et al. A review of the global literature on dental therapists. *Community Dent Oral Epidemiol.* 2014;42(1):1-10.
13. American Dental Association. Massachusetts dental nurse bill rescinded. *J Am Dent Assoc.* 1950;41:371.
14. Lobene RR. *The Forsyth Experiment: An Alternative System for Dental Care.* Cambridge MA: Harvard University Press; 1979.
15. Spohn EE, Chiswell LR, Davison DD. *The University of Kentucky Experimental Expanded Duties Dental Hygiene Project.* Lexington, KY: College of Dentistry, University of Kentucky; 1976:54.
16. Sisty NL, Henderson WG, Paule CL, Martin JF. Evaluation of student performance in the four-year study of expanded functions for dental hygienists at the University of Iowa. *J Amer Dent Assoc.* 1978;97:613-627.
17. Wetterhall S, Bader JD, Burrus BB, Lee JY, Shugars DA. Evaluation of the dental health aid therapist workforce model in Alaska. WK Kellogg Foundation, Rasmussen Foundation, Bethel Community Services Foundation. 2010. https://www.rti.org/publication/evaluation-dental-health-aide-therapist-workforce-model-alaska-final-report. Accessed February 18, 2019.
18. PEW Center on the States, National Academy for State Health Policy, WK Kellogg Foundation. Help wanted: a policy maker's guide to new dental providers. May 2009. https://www.wkkf.org/resource-directory/resource/2010/help-wanted-a-policy-makers-guide-to-new-dental-providers-issue-brief. Accessed February 18, 2019.
19. Minnesota Department of Health, Minnesota Board of Dentistry. *Early Impacts of Dental Therapists in Minnesota.* Minneapolis, MN: Minnesota Department of Health. https://mn.gov/boards/assets/2014DentalTherapistReport_tcm21-45970.pdf. Accessed February 18, 2019.
20. Gwozdek AE, Tetrick R, Shaefer HL. The origins of Minnesota's mid-level dental practitioner: alignment of problem, political and policy streams. *J Dent Hyg.* 2014;88(5):292-301.

21. American Dental Hygienists' Association. *The History of Introducing a New Provider in Minnesota.* Chicago, IL: American Dental Hygienists' Association; 2009:2. https://www.adha.org/resources-docs/75113_Minnesota_Story.pdf. Accessed February 18, 2019.

22. Mathu-Muju KR. Dental therapists provide technically competent clinical care when performing irreversible restorative procedures. *J Evid Based Dent Pract.* 2014;14(1):25-27.

23. Phillips E, Shaefer HL. Dental therapists: evidence of technical competence. *J Dent Res.* 2013;92(suppl 7):11S-15S.

24. Bailit HL, Beazoglou TJ, DeVitto J, McGowan T, Myne-Joslin V. Impact of dental therapists on productivity and finances: I. Literature review. *J Dent Educ.* 2012;76(8):1061-1067.

25. Commission on Dental Accreditation. *Accreditation Standards for Dental Therapy Education Programs.* Chicago, IL: ADA; 2014. https://www.ada.org/en/~/media/CODA/Files/dental_therapy_standards. Accessed February 18, 2019.

26. Koppelman J, Vitzthum K, Simon L. Expanding where dental therapists can practice could increase Americans' access to cost-efficient care. *Health Aff.* 2016;35(12):2200-2206.

27. PEW Charitable Trusts. *Expanding the Dental Team: Increasing Access to Care in Public Settings.* Philadelphia, PA: PEW Charitable Trusts; 2014. https://www.pewtrusts.org/en/research-and-analysis/reports/2014/06/30/expanding-the-dental-team. Accessed February 18, 2019.

28. American Association of Public Health Dentistry. Special issue: workforce development in dentistry: addressing access to care. *J Public Health Dent.* 2011:71(suppl 2):S1-S41.

29. Institute of Medicine. Board on Healthcare Services. *The U.S. Oral Health Workforce in the Coming Decade: Workshop Summary.* Washington DC: National Academic Press; 2009. http://www.nationalacademies.org/hmd/reports/2009/oralhealthworkforce.aspx. Accessed February 18, 2019.

30. Interprofessional Education Collaborative Expert Panel. *Core Competencies for Interprofessional Collaborative Practice: 2016 Update.* Washington, DC: Interprofessional Education Collaborative; 2016. https://www.ipecollaborative.org/resources.html. Accessed February 15, 2019.

31. American Dental Hygienists' Association. *Standards for Clinical Dental Hygiene Practice.* Chicago, IL: ADHA; 2008. http://www.adha.org/practice. Updated June 2016. Accessed February 19, 2019.

32. American Dental Hygienists' Association. *Dental Hygiene Diagnosis.* Chicago, IL: ADHA; 2008. http://www.adha.org/practice. Updated September 2015. Accessed February 19, 2019.

33. American College of Dentists. *Ethics Handbook for Dentists: An Introduction to Ethics, Professionalism, and Ethical Decision Making.* Gaithersburg, MD: American College of Dentists. Revised 2016. https://www.dentalethics.org/ethicshandbook.htm. Accessed February 24, 2019.

34. American Dental Hygienists' Association. *Bylaws and Code of Ethics.* Chicago, IL: ADHA; Adopted June 25, 2018:32-33. http://www.adha.org/resources-docs/7611_Bylaws_and_Code_of_Ethics.pdf. Accessed February 16, 2019.

35. Enck G. Six-step framework for ethical decision making. *J Health Serv Res Policy.* 2014;19(1):62-64.

36. American Dental Education Association. ADEA statement on professionalism in dental education. March 2009. https://www.adea.org/Pages/Professionalism.aspx. Accessed February 24, 2019.

37. World Health Organization, Regional Office for South-East Asia. 201. *Self Care for Health.* WHO Regional Office for South- East Asia. http://www.who.int/iris/handle/10665/205887. Accessed February 24, 2019.

38. U.S. Department of Health and Human Services (HHS). 2018. *Physical Activity Guidelines for Americans.* Washington, DC: U.S. Department of Health and Human Services. https://health.gov/paguidelines/second-edition/. Accessed March 3, 2019.

Evidence-Based Dental Hygiene Practice

Faizan Kabani, BSDH, MHA, MBA, PhD

CHAPTER OUTLINE

EVIDENCE-BASED PRACTICE
I. Definition
II. Purposes
III. The Need for EBP
IV. EBP Model for Dental Hygiene Practice
V. Skills Needed for Evidence-Based Dental Hygiene Practice

A SYSTEMATIC APPROACH
I. Assess: Determine the Clinical Issue
II. Ask: Develop a Research Question

III. Acquire: Search for Scientific Evidence
IV. Appraise: Clinically Evaluate Evidence
V. Apply: Integrate and Apply Evidence
VI. Audit: Evaluate Outcomes

APPROACHES TO RESEARCH
I. Research Designs
II. Research Types
III. Evidence Sources
IV. Levels of Evidence
V. Time Intervals

ETHICS IN RESEARCH
I. Ethical Standards
II. Ethical Research Involving Human Subjects
III. Informed Consent for Research
IV. Institutional Review Board

DOCUMENTATION

EVERYDAY ETHICS

FACTORS TO TEACH THE PATIENT

REFERENCES

LEARNING OBJECTIVES

After studying this chapter, the student will be able to:

1. Explain evidence-based practice and its importance in clinical dental hygiene care.

2. Discuss various approaches to research including the strength of evidence each provides.

3. Describe a systematic approach used to find credible scientific literature.

4. Describe skills needed for analyzing evidence-based health information.

One of the main goals of clinical dental hygiene practice is to improve and maintain the patient's oral health. Clinical problems occur daily and require interventions based on current, valid, and reliable evidence to improve the patient's overall well-being.

◆ The evidence-based clinician relies on established best practices to guide their decision-making processes.

◆ Evidence-based decision making (EBDM) is a process of making decisions that are grounded in the best available research, professional experience, and factors related to each patient's context, including needs and preferences.[1]

EVIDENCE-BASED PRACTICE

I. Definition

◆ An interprofessional approach to clinical care where the clinician, in consultation with the patient, uses the best scientific evidence available to make decisions about clinical interventions needed to promote health.[2]

◆ Evidence-based practice (EBP) is the practical application of EBDM across diverse clinical and nonclinical professions. In health care, an interprofessional EBP approach incorporates the knowledge and expertise from diverse professions (i.e., collaboration between medical, dental, and research) to provide the best quality of care to patients.

◆ EBP assists dental hygienists in formulating a plan for objective, effective, and scientifically sound interventions that meet patient needs and provide positive health outcomes.

◆ EBP involves three major elements[3] (Figure 2-1):
  • Clinically relevant scientific evidence.
  • Sensitivity to patient's needs and preferences.
  • Healthcare professional's clinical expertise.

II. Purposes

◆ To answer clinical questions quickly and efficiently.

◆ To resolve problems in patient care using current evidence.

◆ To improve patient's health outcomes and overall well-being.

III. The Need for EBP

A professional dental hygienist understands the following concepts and embraces the role of the evidence-based practitioner.

◆ Patients frequently search for health information on the Internet and other readily available sources. Patients:
  • Expect clinicians to be knowledgeable on the latest developments in health care.

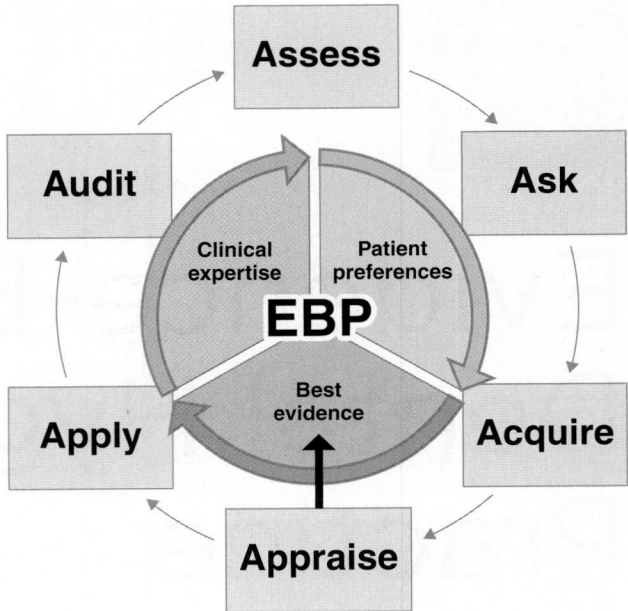

FIGURE 2-1 • Evidence-Based Practice (EBP) Model for Dental Hygiene. (Courtesy of Cathy J. Thompson PhD, RN, CCNS, CNE.)

  • Value practitioners who can discuss and help them evaluate the relevance, validity, and reliability of information obtained elsewhere.
  • Demand healthcare providers who remain current with evidence-based information on the most up-to-date oral health practices, techniques, technologies, and products.

◆ There are differences in practice procedures:
  • Clinicians are not consistently knowledgeable about all new and emerging therapies.
  • There may be inconsistencies between what is taught in dental hygiene schools and procedures tested by regional examination boards for licensure.

◆ Information management:
  • The amount of published evidence-based research continues to increase annually.
  • Clinicians need to be good consumers of current scientific literature and focus on higher levels of evidence to guide their decision making.

IV. EBP Model for Dental Hygiene Practice

The EBP model for dental hygiene care involves interaction between three primary components,[4] as illustrated in Figure 2-1.

◆ *Best available research evidence.* Review of relevant, current, and high-quality clinical research that identifies best-practice treatment choices.

◆ *Patient preferences or values.* Consider, respect, and evaluate the patient's needs, wants, expectations, and personal context (i.e., cultural, religious, capabilities, health status, and demographics).

◆ *Clinical expertise*. The dental hygienists' clinical skill and expertise enhance their ability to identify the patient's health, risks, needs, and potential for various interventions.

V. Skills Needed for Evidence-Based Dental Hygiene Practice

Implementing evidence-based dental hygiene (EBDH) practice into everyday clinical practice is an ethical responsibility for the dental hygienist. Identifying and using scientific evidence to support treatment and preventive interventions and recommendations require the dental hygienist to:

◆ *Understand EBDH practice*. Study a tutorial (examples listed in Box 2-1) to learn more about EBP.

◆ *Follow a systematic approach*. Develop a step-by-step approach by asking questions related to clinical practice to ensure success.

◆ *Read and understand research*. Recognize valid and reliable information. Determine strengths and limitations of publications, journal articles, research methods, study designs, and biostatistics.

◆ *Be computer literate*. Develop the skill to search for scientific literature in an effective and efficient manner. Practice critical thinking skills to evaluate information found online.

◆ *Embrace self-directed learning*. Develop a plan for continuing education and reading of professional literature that will help to maintain current knowledge.

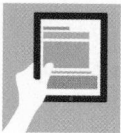

BOX 2-1
Evidence-Based Tutorials and Learning Opportunities

- Duke University: http://guides.mclibrary.duke.edu/c.php?g=158201&p=1036002
- Boston University Medical Campus: http://medlib.bu.edu/tutorials/ebm/
- University of Massachusetts Medical School: http://libraryguides.umassmed.edu/c.php?g=499783&p=3421956
- University of North Carolina at Chapel Hill: http://www.hsl.unc.edu/Services/Tutorials/EBM/welcome.htm
- University of Illinois at Chicago: http://researchguides.uic.edu/ebm
- The Cochrane Collaboration: http://www.cochrane.org/About%20us/Evidence-based%20health%20care/Webliography/Tutorials-tools
- PubMed Tutorial: http://www.nlm.nih.gov/bsd/disted/pubmedtutorial/cover.html

◆ *Be a resource for others*. Help patients and colleagues identify and value scientific support for clinical recommendations.

A SYSTEMATIC APPROACH

Dental hygienists should follow a systematic approach when identifying and selecting scientific evidence related to a particular patient's healthcare needs. The "6 A's" approach includes *Assess, Ask, Acquire, Appraise, Apply,* and *Audit*.[3] Figure 2-2 illustrates a step-by-step procedure that aids the dental hygienist in developing these crucial skills.

I. Assess: Determine the Clinical Issue

◆ The dental hygienist first completes an assessment of the patient or population.

◆ Identify what the clinical issue or problem is for the patient or population.

◆ Purpose is to clarify the clinical issue or problem.

II. Ask: Develop a Research Question

◆ Asking the right research question is fundamental and critical to the EBP model.

◆ Research questions should be focused and not be too broad or too narrow.

◆ A researchable question includes four parts, referred to as *PICO*. Examples of PICO questions related to dental hygiene practice can be found in Table 2-1.

◆ Good research questions should also adhere to the *FINER* criteria.

◆ Include important patient demographics (i.e., age, sex, race, and ethnicity).

A. PICO Criteria[5]

◆ *Patient problem or population (P)*: What are the most important issues the patient or population of interest is facing?

◆ *Intervention (I)*: What are you planning to do to address the patient's or population of interest's issues?

◆ *Comparison (C)*: What is the main alternative being suggested? Compare the alternative with the standard intervention for the patient or population of interest.

◆ *Outcome (O)*: What is the desired measurable outcome, accomplishment, improvement, or effect from the proposed intervention on the patient or the population of interest?

B. FINER Criteria[5]

◆ *Feasibility (F)*: Are the necessary resources available to conduct the research study?

◆ *Interesting (I)*: Is the research interesting, self-motivating, and/or intriguing?

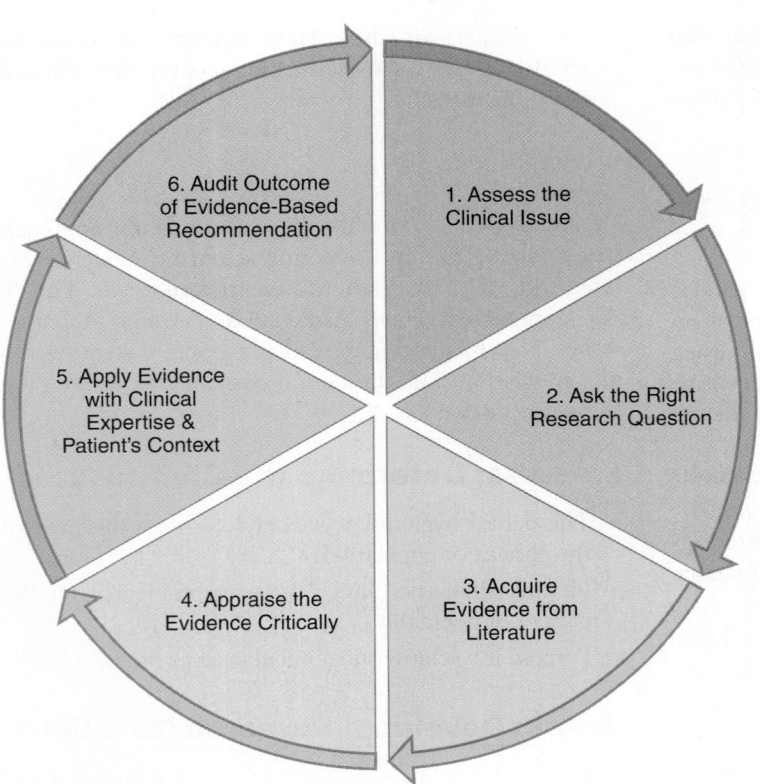

FIGURE 2-2 • Systematic Steps in Evidence-Based Dental Hygiene Practice. (Adapted by permission from BMJ Publishing Group Limited. [Evidence-Based Medicine, Alper BS and Haynes B, 214, 2016].)

TABLE 2-1 • Example of Clinical and Public Health–Related PICO Questions

SCENARIO	PICO QUESTION
Mr. Ali is a 65-year-old Asian American who presents for his periodontal maintenance appointment. He reports a chief complaint of dental hypersensitivity when drinking cold beverages. He currently uses a generic, over-the-counter fluoridated toothpaste. He is wondering if there is any particular active ingredient he should consider when purchasing a toothpaste.	For a patient with concerns of dental hypersensitivity, will a toothpaste with potassium nitrate be more effective at reducing hypersensitivity than a toothpaste with traditional fluoride? • **Patient/problem:** Patient reports chief complaint of dental hypersensitivity • **Intervention:** Toothpaste with potassium nitrate as active ingredient • **Comparison:** Traditional toothpaste with fluoride as active ingredient • **Outcome:** Reduction in dental hypersensitivity
Mrs. Sabzali is a 35-year-old African-American superintendent of a predominately Medicaid-based school district. She reports there is a dental caries epidemic in one of her elementary school's first-grade classrooms. Your dental office currently volunteers in an annual fluoride varnish program to help address dental caries. Mrs. Sabzali mentions that she has heard from one of her principals about placement of dental sealants as another way to address the dental caries epidemic. She is wondering which route, placement of fluoride varnish or dental sealants, best helps to address the dental caries epidemic in her school district.	For a population experiencing a dental caries epidemic, will placement of dental sealants be as effective (or more effective) as application of fluoride varnish to help reduce dental caries? • **Population/problem:** Dental caries epidemic in first-grade classroom of a predominately Medicaid-based school district • **Intervention:** Placement of dental sealants • **Comparison:** Application of fluoride varnish • **Outcome:** Reduction in dental caries epidemic

Research about comparative cost is in addition to the literature review.

- *Novel (N):* Is the research innovative? Does the research aim to address significant gaps in the literature?
- *Ethical (E):* Does the research align within ethical and legal standards/requirements?
- *Relevant (R):* Does the research advance the body of scientific knowledge in the particular healthcare field?

III. Acquire: Search for Scientific Evidence

- Select appropriate resources and conduct a thorough literature review. Scientific articles are available through library databases and by using appropriate search engines. Focus literature review toward current and higher level of evidence publications (Figure 2-3).

A. Types of Information Sources

- *Primary sources* are original accounts of events and/or publications. Primary sources are significant because they provide unfiltered access to an original record

of thought and/or achievement during a specific period in history. Examples of primary sources include narratives, speeches, autobiographies, government documents, patents, raw data sets, and experimental research reports.

- *Secondary sources* are published materials that synthesize and/or analyze original sources. Examples of secondary sources include biographies, literature reviews, and nonexperimental scholarly articles.
- *Tertiary sources* are published materials that provide overviews of particular topics with information gathered from multiple sources. Examples of tertiary sources include encyclopedias, textbooks, and websites.

B. Types of Publications

The sources for obtaining scientific information are growing daily. Knowing how to determine the validity and reliability of information is critical for selecting successful patient care strategies and interventions. Refer to Box 2-2 for a checklist of questions to ask when considering the validity and/or reliability of a publication.

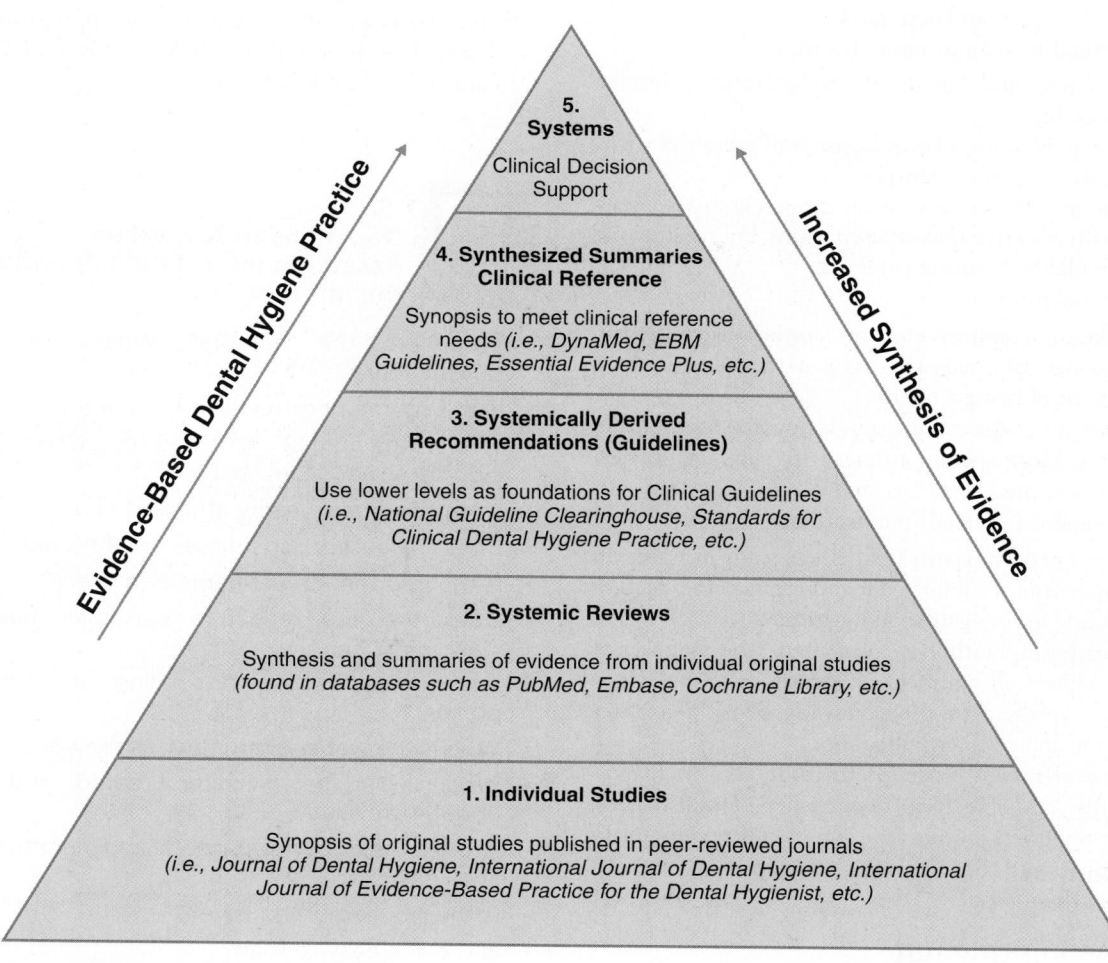

FIGURE 2-3 • Strength of Evidence Resources.

BOX 2-2

Questions to Ask When Considering the Validity of a Publication

- Who is sponsoring?
- Is there an editorial review board?
- Are the journal articles peer-reviewed?
- What are the credentials of the contributors?
- Are there advertisements? How many?
- Are there good-quality production standards?
- Is the manuscript preparation information included?
- What type of articles are included? (i.e., Informational? Opinion/Editorial? Case Reports? Scientific study?)

◆ Textbooks
  • Generally accepted as credible basic-level resources.
  • Drawn-out publication processes can make textbooks become outdated quickly.
◆ Commercial-based journals/magazines
  • Often free and based on product and/or service sponsorships.
  • Potentially written by in-house staff members without professional credentials.
  • Some articles summarize recent research that may contain selective reference citations, but not include all available scientific evidence.
◆ Professional journals
  • Produced by professional organizations. Membership dues payment is required, or receiving publications is a benefit of being a member.
  • Part or all of the publication is devoted to scientific studies. Most contain articles with supporting reference citations.
◆ Peer-reviewed (refereed) publications
  • Subject matter experts (SMEs) critically examine all components of submitted manuscripts before recommending for or against publication.
  • Contributing author(s) must revise the manuscript and address all significant concerns or answer questions expressed by the reviewing SMEs before receiving approval for publication.
  • The peer-review process helps assure the validity, reliability, and objectivity of published journal articles.
  • Peer-reviewed journals usually list all review board members and their respective credentials in each issue of the journal.

C. Online Information

◆ The Internet continues to evolve as an avenue for people to search for health-related information.

◆ American adults are increasingly using online resources to diagnose either themselves or others.[6]
◆ Many popular search engines lead to newspaper and magazine articles or websites that may not provide science-based and/or research-supported information.
  • Search engines cannot assure the validity, accuracy, and objectivity of information.
  • Search engines display only fractions of all available resources on a specific topic.
◆ Search engines can also provide access to more valid and reliable websites that offer a variety of health information. Be familiar with the credibility level of various domain names:
  • Highest credibility: Governmental sources (*.gov*) and educational sources (*.edu*).
  • Moderate credibility: Organizational sources (*.org*) and institutional sources (*.net*).
  • Lowest credibility: Commercial sources (*.com*).
◆ Refer to Box 2-3 for questions to ask when assessing information found on the Internet.
◆ Search engines and databases devoted to specific professional literature provide access to information from scholarly articles in biomedical and other health-related journals.
◆ Some governmental agencies and nongovernmental associations specifically help people find credible health-related information on the web. These include:

BOX 2-3

Questions to Ask When Assessing Information Found on the Internet

- Who are the authors? What are their qualifications?
- Is the source peer-reviewed or edited?
- What is the domain name and source? (i.e., .gov, .edu, .org, .net, .com, .mil)
- Does the site have any affiliated biases?
- Does the author list sources or citations?
- Is the information verifiable elsewhere?
- Does the site reflect a particular bias or viewpoint?
- Are obvious errors in spelling or grammar present?
- Who is the website targeting as their audience?
- When was the website created and last updated/revised?
- Are the links current, good, and helpful? Are any links dead?
- Is the site comprehensive?
- Is the site easy to read?
- Are the site and material well organized?

- HealthFinder.[7]
- MedlinePlus.[8]
- Medical Library Association.[9]
- ◆ Accrediting organizations provide certification aimed at assuring accurate and objective health information on the Internet.
  - Health on the Net Foundation.[10]
  - URAC Health Website Accreditation Program.[11]

Sites that display a symbol of accreditation from these organizations have met specific guidelines intended to assure the quality of health information they provide.

D. Biomedical Databases

- ◆ Refer to Box 2-4 for a list of some valid and reliable biomedical databases to use when searching for evidence-based information related to oral health and patient care.
- ◆ The *MEDLINE* database is the U.S. National Library of Medicine's (NLM) main scientific database.[12]
- ◆ MEDLINE provides access to articles from more than 5,600 scientific journals including PubMed and the Cochrane Collaboration database.
- ◆ MEDLINE indexes all published records using the NLM *Medical Subject Headings* (MeSH) format. MeSH enable researchers to connect search terms with keywords linked with each publication.[12]
- ◆ When journal articles or the abstract for a specific article is displayed, PubMed also provides:
  - The complete citation in NLM format.
  - In some cases, a link to the full text of the article.
  - Links to access "related citations."
- ◆ Systematic and effective MEDLINE searches include:
  - Use of the "related citations" link.
  - Checking the references listed in journal articles for additional relevant citations.
  - Using a combination of search techniques results in more efficient and effective searches.
  - Refer to Box 2-5 for basic MEDLINE literature searching techniques using the PubMed search engine.

E. The Cochrane Collaboration Database

- ◆ Global, independent, network working to promote access to credible and unbiased health information for both practitioners and patients.[13]
- ◆ Produces high-quality, systematic reviews and other synthesized research evidence to support clinical decision making.
- ◆ Each review article includes:
  - Complete scientifically written and well-supported analysis of search methods, data collection, and findings.
  - Plain language summary of results for nonhealthcare providers.
- ◆ Has a searchable database for a large number of health-related topics, including oral health.

BOX 2-4
Databases for Locating Biomedical Information

- MEDLINE (PubMed), http://www.ncbi.nlm.nih.gov/pubmed/: a service of the U.S. National Library of Medicine that includes over 16 million citations from MEDLINE and other life science journals for biomedical articles dating back to the 1950s; includes links to full-text articles and related resources.

- CINAHL (Cumulative Index to Nursing and Allied Health Literature), https://www.ebscohost.com/nursing/products/cinahl-databases/the-cinahl-database: a bibliographic database that includes abstracts of nursing and allied health articles.

- Cochrane Library (The Cochrane Collaboration), http://www.cochrane.org/: an international nonprofit and independent organization; produces and disseminates systematic reviews of healthcare interventions and promotes the search for evidence in the form of clinical trials and other studies of interventions.

- Database of Promoting Health Effectiveness Reviews (DoPHER), http://eppi.ioe.ac.uk/webdatabases4/Intro.aspx?ID=9: a database focused on covering systematic and nonsystematic reviews of effectiveness in health promotion and public health worldwide.

- ADA's EBD Website (The American Dental Association's Evidence-Based Dentistry), http://ebd.ada.org: a dental informatics resource; provides practitioners with access to current scientific information that is easy to comprehend and that can be quickly reviewed at the point of care.

- National Institutes of Health, http://health.nih.gov: an encyclopedia of health topics.

- Agency for Healthcare Research and Quality, https://www.ahrq.gov/: subsidiary of the U.S. Department of Health and Human Services; aims to produce evidence to make health care safer, higher quality, more accessible, equitable, and affordable.

IV. Appraise: Clinically Evaluate Evidence

Once literature on a particular topic is acquired, it is necessary for the dental hygienist to evaluate the validity, reliability, and overall credibility of the information before providing professional recommendations/interventions.

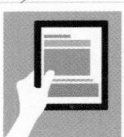

BOX 2-5
Basic MEDLINE Literature Search Techniques Using the PubMed Search Engine

- A text or key word search locates articles that have the relevant terms in the title, abstract, or body of an article.
- A medical subject heading search locates articles indexed in the database by specific headings.
- A clinical queries search locates articles related to three specific clinical research categories: clinical studies, systematic reviews, and medical genetics.

A. Critically Evaluate the Evidence for Validity

- Determine if the study logically follows all steps of the research process.
- Determine if the focus of the study relates to the patient or population's concerns.
- Determine if there are major concerns with internal validity.
- Determine if objectivity was maintained or if *bias* was introduced.
- Determine if the study has an adequate *sample size*.
- Determine if the most appropriate measurement scale and/or index was used.
- Determine if there are major concerns with external validity.
- Can the evidence be generalized to other similar patients or populations?

B. Critically Evaluate the Evidence for Clinical Value

- Analyze which specific variables the researchers used in their study.
  - *Dependent variable(s)*: Also termed as the *outcome variable*. A value that depends on other interventions and what researchers aim to predict or explain. For example, the amount of biofilm left on a tooth after brushing.
  - *Independent variable(s)*: Also termed as the *intervention variable*. Manipulating variable intended to create an effect on the dependent variable. For example, the different types of toothbrushes used to reduce biofilm left on a tooth.
  - *Extraneous variable(s)*: Factors not directly involved between the dependent and independent variable but having an altering effect on the overall relationship. Extraneous variables further subdivide into *control* and *confounding* variables. For example,

a person's age, sex, race, ethnicity, socioeconomic status, and/or the extent of oral hygiene instruction provided on proper brushing techniques can influence the overall relationship between the type of intervention used and observed outcome/result.

- Analyze both descriptive statistics and inferential statistics for significance and relevance to the current problem in question.[14]
- Analyze the difference between statistical significance and clinical significance.
  - Statistical significance refers to the likelihood that a relationship between two or more variables is due to something other than chance.
  - Clinical significance refers to the practical relevance and importance between multiple therapies. In other words, clinical significance focuses on whether the significant probability of a particular therapy has a noticeable effect on a patient or population.
  - Researchers typically use ≤ 0.05 as the prespecified probability value (p-value) to determine statistical significance. In this scenario, there is a less than 5% probability that the statistically significant difference between multiple variables occurred due to chance.
  - Researchers also report data using confidence intervals to identify minimum and maximum values for probability.
- Evaluate whether treatment outcomes are beneficial enough to justify treatment.
- Evaluate if researchers provide rational arguments for using results in clinical practice.
- Determine the availability and affordability of treatment to patients or populations.

V. Apply: Integrate and Apply Evidence

- Integrate and apply evidence with clinical expertise and the patient's preferences.
- Consider the patient or population's circumstances and the clinician's ability to help obtain potential results.
- Document interventions in the patient's chart as part of clinical progress notes.

VI. Audit: Evaluate Outcomes

- Determine whether:
  - Application of the EBP model successfully helped the patient.
  - There is a need for additional research strategies and information.
  - There is a need for a modification in the original outcome goal.
- Begin the EBP process again if patient outcome is not successful and/or when a new problem arises.

APPROACHES TO RESEARCH

◆ It is critical for dental hygienists to be aware of different approaches to and types of research designs, particularly when reading published literature to inform clinical EBP.[14]

◆ The dental hygienist can also conduct and/or participate in original research investigations.

◆ Depending on the clinical/public health problem and/or focused research question, dental hygienists can engage with research using a critical, objective, and methodical EBP approach.

I. Research Designs

◆ Qualitative Research
  • Purpose is to understand and subjectively interpret complex social interactions.
  • Sample sizes are typically smaller and not randomly selected.
  • Data are collected and reported through participant observations, interviews, open-ended questions, field notations, and narrative reflections.

◆ Quantitative Research
  • Purpose is to test hypotheses, view causal or correlational relationships, and make predictions.
  • Sample sizes are typically larger and randomly selected.
  • Data are collected and reported as quantifiable numbers and/or statistics.

◆ Mixed-Methods Research
  • Purpose is to combine the best of both qualitative and quantitative research approaches.
  • Sample sizes and random selection may vary.
  • Data are collected and reported as both qualitative insight and quantitative analysis.

II. Research Types

◆ Descriptive
  • Typically the first step in classifying and organizing information.
  • Focused on describing facts of people, places, and time.
  • Helps identify basic relationships that further studies need to examine.
  • Examples include case studies, natural observations, and population surveys.

◆ Correlational
  • Intended to predict and measure the relationship between multiple variables.
  • Determine the type and strength of relationships between multiple variables.
  • Focuses on preventing the post hoc fallacy (i.e., correlation does not mean causation).

  • Examples include case–control studies, cohort studies, observations, population surveys, cross-sectional and longitudinal studies.

◆ Quasi-experimental
  • Similar to the experimental approach minus the random assignment.
  • Researchers have lesser control than on true experimental designs.
  • Examples include correlational studies and results of case studies.

◆ Experimental
  • Intended to test cause and effect between variables.
  • Includes randomized assignment of study participants.
  • Experimental group receives intervention; control group does not receive intervention.
  • Examples include randomized controlled trials (RCTs).

◆ Review
  • Synthesizes relevant information on a particular research topic.
  • Intended to summarize and evaluate scientific literature.
  • Examples include critical review, narrative review, systematic review, and meta-analysis.

III. Evidence Sources

◆ *Primary research* refers to original studies including individual experimental and nonexperimental studies. Examples of primary research studies include RCTs, cohort studies, and case–control studies.

◆ *Secondary research* refers to existing studies used for purposes (i.e., reviews on previously conducted research). Examples of secondary research studies include systematic reviews, meta-analysis, and clinical practice guidelines.

IV. Levels of Evidence

The levels of evidence pyramid illustrates the hierarchy of research designs and strength of various scientific evidence.[15] The pyramid layout provides a visual representation of the number of studies published in literature; in particular, researchers conduct more lower-level than higher-level studies. Higher-level evidences provide the strongest basis for establishing clinical practice guidelines. Figure 2-4 organizes the levels of evidence as follows:

A. Meta-Analysis and Systematic Reviews

◆ Highest levels of evidence.

◆ *Meta-Analysis*, referred to as the *platinum standard*, is an advanced, analytical-based, literature review that follows a systematic process with explicit inclusion and exclusion criteria.

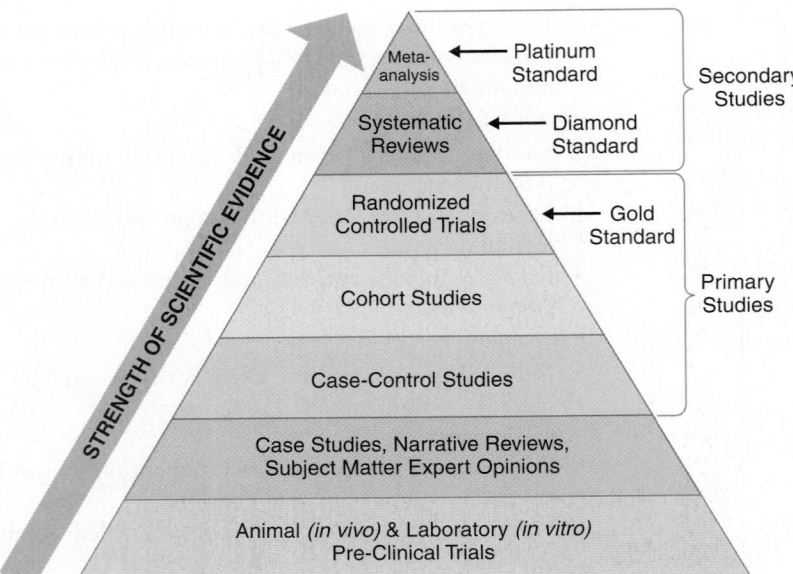

FIGURE 2-4 • Levels of Scientific Evidence Pyramid.

◆ Researchers perform statistical testing on all studies included in the final analysis.

◆ Through statistical testing, meta-analysis can potentially transform *gold-standard* randomized controlled studies into an even stronger "platinum standard" evidence base.

◆ *Systematic Reviews*, referenced to as the *diamond standard*, are advanced, descriptive-based, literature review that follows a methodological approach with explicit inclusion and exclusion criteria.

◆ Researchers produce a summary of all relevant studies based on preestablished criteria.

◆ Advantages of systematic reviews include:
  • Reduce bias.
  • Include only clinically relevant information.
  • Follow strict protocols.
  • Require prior determination of search methods.
  • Focus on specific clinical questions.
  • Have evaluation criteria.
  • Evaluate the strength of available evidence.

◆ A meta-synthesis best describes a systematic review of qualitative studies.

B. Randomized Controlled Clinical Trials: The "Gold-Standard" Clinical Study

◆ Randomized Controlled Clinical Trials are planned experiments that test the efficacy or effectiveness of an exposure.

◆ Random assignment/allocation of patients into one of at least two treatment groups.

◆ Researchers can reduce bias in RCTs by incorporating single-blinded, double-blinded, or triple-blinded protocols in their experiments.

◆ The double-blinded protocol in RCTs is the current gold-standard approach.

C. Cohort Studies and Case–Control Studies

◆ *Cohort Studies* follow the same subject group from the present to a specified point in the future. This research design compares a group with exposure against a group without an exposure.

◆ *Case–Control Studies* explore into the past to identify common factors between two groups, one with an exposure and the other without an exposure.
  • The *case group* refers to the treatment, intervention, or exposure group.
  • The *control group* refers to the group that either received the standard care (i.e., positive control group) or received no treatment/placebo (i.e., negative control group).

D. Case Studies, Case Reports, and Narrative Reviews

◆ *Case Reports* are professional articles that describe the diagnostic, preventive, and therapeutic services rendered to one patient with an unusual or complex condition.

◆ *Case Studies* are an in-depth analysis and description of a series of cases of an unusual or complex condition.

◆ *Narrative Reviews* are basic, descriptive-based literature reviews that synthesize information on a particular topic without a methodological approach.

E. Editorials and SME Opinions

◆ *Editorials* are articles in a newspaper or magazine that express the opinion of its editor or publisher.

◆ SME opinions are beliefs or conclusions held with confidence by experts in a particular field or topic but not substantiated by positive knowledge or proof.

F. Preclinical Trials (In Vitro and In Vivo)

◆ *Preclinical*, or *nonclinical*, research precedes trials involving human subjects.

◆ Purpose is to collect data to support safety of new treatment.

◆ In vitro trials refer to experimental testing completed through test tubes and other similar equipment in the laboratory.

◆ In vivo trials refer to experimental testing completed through the body of a nonhuman living organism (i.e., animal studies).

V. Time Intervals

◆ Prospective: A prospective study observes for outcomes, such as the development of a disease, between the present and some defined point in the future. These exposures are attributed as either risk or protective factors in the development of any given outcome.

◆ Retrospective: A retrospective study observes established outcomes, such as an existing disease, but examines by exploring potential risk or protective factors between a specified timeframe in the past.

◆ Cross-Sectional: Cross-sectional studies examine several different samples at one specified point in time (i.e., provide a snapshot). Can include annual surveys, single interventions, etc.

◆ Longitudinal: Longitudinal studies examine the same sample over an extended period (i.e., several points in time). Results from longitudinal studies can indicate potential causality claims.

ETHICS IN RESEARCH

◆ Research ethics focuses on the responsibility of researchers to conduct nonbiased research, report accurate results, and protect the rights of individuals participating as *research subjects*.[16]

◆ Bioethics is a subdivision concerned with the ethical implications of health-related research and its application on human health and well-being.[16]

  • Over the years, several unethical research studies (i.e., Tuskegee Syphilis Study) occurred due to unregulated policies.

  • The *Nuremberg Code (1947)*, *Declaration of Helsinki (1964)*, and the *Belmont Report (1979)* were substantial milestones in the field of bioethics.

◆ Although many dental hygienists may not actively fulfill the role of a researcher, each can look for evidence ensuring that researchers followed ethical principles when reading the report of a research study.

◆ Refer to Chapter 1 and Section Introductions throughout the book for basic ethical principles and decision-making guidelines.

I. Ethical Standards

The same ethical theories and ethical principles that guide professional interactions of the dental hygienist with patients, dental colleagues, other healthcare providers, and community members can apply when conducting research.[16] These include:

◆ *Respect for persons (autonomy)*: Obligation to respect others and that they should be able to make their own informed decisions.

◆ *Beneficence (protecting patients from harm)*: Obligation to "above all, do no harm." Focusing on maximizing benefits and minimizing harm.

◆ *Justice (integrity and fairness)*: Obligation to give each person his/her due.

II. Ethical Research Involving Human Subjects

The term human subjects refers to people who participate in clinical trials. Examples of dental hygiene–related human subjects research include studies on extracted teeth, discarded gingiva, other tissues, saliva, blood, urine, etc., as long as they are from living individuals.

Ethical standards in research protect individuals who participate as research subjects, with regard to their rights to:

◆ Self-determination.

◆ Privacy.

◆ Anonymity and confidentiality.

◆ Fair treatment.

◆ Protection from discomfort and harm.

◆ Understand the risks and benefits of participating in the study.

◆ Informed consent.

III. Informed Consent for Research

◆ Process of adequately explaining the research to prospective subjects and ensuring that they understand what will happen to them, especially the associated risks and benefits.

◆ All study participants need to volunteer and sign a standardized written consent form.

◆ Discussion of informed consent is included within the research proposal and includes:

  • A statement that the study involves research.

  • An explanation of the purposes of the research.

  • The expected duration of the subject's participation in the research.

  • A step-by-step description of the procedures.

- Identification of any procedures that are experimental.
- A confidentiality statement assuring the participant of anonymity.
- Refusal to participate will involve "no penalty or loss of benefits to which the subject is otherwise entitled."
- The subject may withdraw from the research at any time.

IV. Institutional Review Board

- Federal mandate requires that research proposals undergo evaluation by appropriately designated Institutional Review Boards (IRBs).
- The IRB is an *independent* board within the institution that reviews research proposals submitted by researchers. The group can require modifications before approving research or disapprove research based on its review.
- The purpose of IRB review is to protect the rights and welfare of human subject volunteers in research, in accordance with the policies of the Department of Health and Human Services.
- Published research articles often include an IRB preapproval statement before conducting the study.

DOCUMENTATION

Include the following factors in the patient's chart record when dental hygienists use current research findings from credible evidence sources to plan recommendations and/or interventions:

- Specify the issue that the patient inquired about during the appointment.
- List any limiting personal patient factors (i.e., disabilities, religious/cultural preferences).
- Articulate professional, evidence-based recommendations/interventions provided to the patient.
- Box 2-6 provides an example of a completed evidence-based patient progress note.

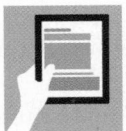

BOX 2-6
Example Documentation:
Providing an Evidence-Based Recommendation

S—A patient with a chief complaint of dental hypersensitivity when drinking cold beverages presents for routine periodontal maintenance appointment. He inquires about active ingredients he should consider when purchasing a toothpaste to help mitigate his dental hypersensitivity.

O—This patient's clinical attachment levels have decreased due to generalized gingival recession. Exposure of dentinal tubules places patient at higher risk for experiencing hypersensitivity.

A—Review of scientific literature (P = experiencing dental hypersensitivity, I = toothpaste with potassium nitrate, C = toothpaste with fluoride, O = reduction in experience of dental hypersensitivity). Evidence found that toothpaste with potassium nitrate has successful clinical outcomes of reduced dental hypersensitivity. (Kopycka-Kedzierawski DT, Meyerowitz C, Litaker MS, et al. Management of dentin hypersensitivity by practitioners in The National Dental Practice-Based Research Network. *J Am Dent Assoc.* 2017;148(10):728-736.)

P—Gave patient both verbal and written instructions on the importance of using toothpaste with potassium nitrate to reduce experience of dental hypersensitivity. American Dental Association's "Preventing and treating tooth sensitivity" educational pamphlet downloaded from the Internet and given to patient: http://www .ada.org/~/media/ADA/Publications/Files /FTDP_Sept2013_2.pdf?la=en

Next Step: Patient will bring new toothpaste at his next 3-month periodontal maintenance appointment. At next appointment, assess dental hypersensitivity.

Signed: _____, RDH

Date: _____

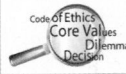

EVERYDAY ETHICS

Salim, a dental product representative, is trying to promote their company's newest desensitizing paste. After conducting a review of the literature related to the efficacy of the active ingredients in the new desensitizing paste, Sanya, the dental hygienist, informs Saira, the office manager, that there is not enough scientific evidence supporting the claim that this new paste is as good or superior to the current desensitizing paste used in their dental clinic. Saira, who has had a good working relationship with Salim and his company for several years, decides to order the new product anyways and tells Sanya that the newer product is considerably less expensive compared to the current product. Saira supports her decision by restating that Salim and his company claim that their desensitizing product is better.

Questions for Consideration

1. Why is this situation an ethical issue and dilemma for Sanya?

2. What is the chief concern/problem related to this situation? What are the long-term implications if Sanya is not able to resolve the situation?

3. What core values (Chapter 1, Box 1-6) apply as Sanya considers alternatives for resolving this situation? What personal values might Sanya review as she considers alternative actions to pursue?

Factors to Teach the Patient

▶ A result from one study does not necessarily provide the best answer. Take into consideration the type of study, patient's needs and preferences, and several other factors before making a decision about best-practice interventions.

▶ Research methods, study design, source of information, and many other factors can affect the validity, reliability, and usefulness of health-related information.

▶ A statistical significance cited in a study does not necessarily mean that it is the best clinical decision for a patient.

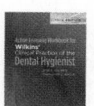

ENHANCE YOUR UNDERSTANDING

ONLINE RESOURCES
(see the inside front cover for access information)
- Audio glossary
- Appendices

SUPPORT FOR LEARNING
(available separately)
- *Active Learning Workbook for Wilkins' Clinical Practice of the Dental Hygienist, 13th Edition*

INDIVIDUALIZED REVIEW
- Customized practice quizzing with Navigate 2 TestPrep for *Wilkins' Clinical Practice of the Dental Hygienist*

References

1. Forrest J, Overman P. Keeping current: a commitment to patient care excellence through evidence based practice. *J Dent Hyg.* 2013;87(suppl 1):33-40.

2. Zimmerman K. Essentials of evidence based practice. *Int J Childbirth Educ.* 2017;32(2):37-43.

3. Duke University Medical Center Library. Introduction to evidence-based practice. http://guides.mclibrary.duke.edu/c.php?g=158201&p=1036021. Published 2014. Accessed September 15, 2017.

4. Frantsve-Hawley J, Clarkson J, Slot D. Using the best evidence to enhance dental hygiene decision making. *J Dent Hyg.* 2017;89(suppl 1):39-42.

5. O'Brien P, Broughton-Pipkin F. *Introduction to Research Methodology for Specialists and Trainees.* 3rd ed. Cambridge, England: Cambridge University Press; 2017.

6. Agency for Healthcare Research & Quality (ARHQ). Strategy 6D: internet access for health information and advice. https://www.ahrq.gov/cahps/quality-improvement/improvement-guide/6-strategies-for-improving/access/strategy6d-internet.html. Published 2017. Accessed November 1, 2017.

7. U.S. Department of Health and Human Services, National Health Information Center. Your source for reliable health information. Healthfinder.gov Web site. https://healthfinder.gov/. Published 2017. Accessed November 1, 2017.

8. National Library of Medicine. Health information. https://medlineplus.gov/. Published 2017. Accessed November 1, 2017.

9. Medical Library Association. For health consumers and patients. https://www.mlanet.org/p/cm/ld/fid=397. Published 2017. Accessed November 1, 2017.

10. Health on the Net Foundation. Our commitment to reliable health and medical information on the internet. http://www.hon.ch/home1.html. Published 2017. Accessed August 21, 2017.

11. URAC. Health web site. https://www.urac.org/. Published 2017. Accessed August 21, 2017.

12. U.S. National Library of Medicine. MEDLINE fact sheet. https://www.nlm.nih.gov/pubs/factsheets/medline.html. Published 2017. Accessed September 1, 2017.

13. Cochrane. What is Cochrane? http://www.cochrane.org/. Published 2017. Accessed August 21, 2017.

14. Hazra A, Gogtay N. Biostatistics series module 1: basics of biostatistics. *Indian J Dermatol.* 2016;61(1):10-20.

15. University of North Carolina Health Sciences Library. Evidence based dentistry. http://guides.lib.unc.edu/ebd. Published 2017. Accessed August 25, 2017.

16. Petersen S. Human subject review standards and procedures in international research: critical ethical and cultural issues and recommendations. *Int Perspect Psychol.* 2017;6(3):165-178.

3

Effective Health Communication

Salima Thawer, MPH, BSc, RDH

CHAPTER OUTLINE

TYPES OF COMMUNICATION
I. Verbal
II. Nonverbal
III. Media Communication

HEALTH COMMUNICATION
I. Skills and Attributes of Effective Health Communicators
II. Attributes of Effective Health Information
III. Barriers to Effective Health Communication
IV. Web-Based Health Messages
V. Factors That Influence Health Communication

HEALTH LITERACY
I. Health Learning Capacity
II. Assess and Address Health Literacy

COMMUNICATION ACROSS THE LIFE SPAN
I. Children and Adolescents
II. Older Adults

SOCIAL AND ECONOMIC ASPECTS OF HEALTH COMMUNICATION

CULTURAL CONSIDERATIONS
I. Culture and Health
II. Cross-Cultural Communication

III. Attaining Cultural Competence
IV. Cultural Competence and the Dental Hygiene Process of Care

INTERPROFESSIONAL COMMUNICATION

COMMUNICATION WITH CAREGIVERS

DOCUMENTATION

EVERYDAY ETHICS

FACTORS TO TEACH THE PATIENT

REFERENCES

LEARNING OBJECTIVES

After studying this chapter, the student will be able to:

1. Discuss the skills and attributes of effective health communication.

2. Identify factors that influence health communication.

3. Explain how the patient's age, culture, and health literacy level affect health communication strategies.

4. Identify communication theories relevant to effective health communication and motivational interviewing.

5. Health communication is the use of communication strategies to enhance the ability to provide patient-centered health information, motivate positive changes in health behaviors, and achieve improved health outcomes.

6. In the context of dental hygiene care, good communication skills help patients embrace healthy behaviors of all types that allow them to attain and maintain oral health.

TYPES OF COMMUNICATION

- ◆ Communication is a process that involves at least two, and sometimes multiple, individuals.
- ◆ The sender, who intends to communicate some specific concept, encodes and then transmits a message to at least one receiver who decodes the message.
- ◆ This process can then reverse itself and the receiver becomes the sender of a return message that may or may not provide direct feedback to the original message that was sent.
- ◆ The effectiveness of the communication depends on how closely the encoding and decoding match.
- ◆ All communication is either verbal or nonverbal. Each can be subdivided into vocal and nonvocal.

I. Verbal

- ◆ A form of communication based on language or words.
- ◆ Vocal communication is spoken language.
- ◆ Nonvocal communication is based on signs or signals that express language concepts, and include writing, Braille, and sign language.

II. Nonverbal

- ◆ Messages expressed by body language or affect can influence or interfere with a healthcare provider's ability to communicate, perhaps even more than the verbal method used.
- ◆ Nonverbal, vocal factors include:
  - • Vocal qualifiers (volume, pitch, tempo, and cadence).
  - • Vocal characterizers (crying, laughing).
- ◆ Nonverbal, nonvocal factors include:
  - • Body position (posture or use of social space).
  - • Movement of body parts such as hands or arms.
  - • Eye movements and facial expression.
  - • Appearance (grooming and dress).

III. Media Communication

- ◆ Media communication refers to the use of tools or technology to convey information.
- ◆ Media communication can be directed to:
  - • An individual recipient (written care plan provided for an individual patient).
  - • A wider, more diverse target audience (patient education brochures developed by a professional association or health information on the Internet).
- ◆ Public health efforts to enhance the health of populations are based on a community-based media approach to providing quality health information.
- ◆ Commercial media efforts, such as television commercials or magazine advertisements for various products, have an astonishing effect on the health-related choices made by targeted audiences.[1]

HEALTH COMMUNICATION

- ◆ The ultimate goal of health communication is to persuade behavior change that will support optimum health.
- ◆ Healthy People 2020 health communication objectives[2] related to direct patient care include:
  - • Shared decision making between patients and providers.
  - • Personalized, targeted, accurate, accessible, and actionable information, self-management tools, and resources.
  - • Increase of health literacy skills.

I. Skills and Attributes of Effective Health Communicators

- ◆ Healthcare providers who most effectively deliver preventive interventions demonstrate the following during patient interactions[3]:
  - • Expertise and knowledge in health and prevention.
  - • Understanding of learning/behavior change theories and principles of good communication.
  - • Relationship building skills.
  - • Interview and role modeling skills.
  - • Assessment for readiness to change behaviors.
  - • Attention to the patient's attitudes and beliefs.
  - • Personal attributes of confidence and flexibility.
- ◆ A motivational interviewing approach to patient counseling, based on development and use of those skills, is presented in Chapter 24.
- ◆ The use of "plain language" in both verbal and written health communication can improve patients' understanding of, and response to, health messages.[4]
- ◆ Plain language does not "dumb down" or "talk down" to the patient, but rather provides information in a clear and to the point manner, using words the patient can understand.

II. Attributes of Effective Health Information

Recommendations made by a health educator are more likely to be effective if the patient perceives the information to be[5]:

- ◆ Evidence-based, accurate, balanced, and reliable.
- ◆ Consistent with information from other sources.
- ◆ Culturally and linguistically appropriate.
- ◆ Delivered in an easily understood and accessible way.
- ◆ Provided when the patient is most ready to receive it.
- ◆ Repeated and reinforced over time.

Health information is often received from a variety of sources, some of which may be biased, incomplete, or conflicting.[6] Sources of health information may include:

- ◆ Mainstream media (e.g., TV, newspapers).
- ◆ Educational institutions (e.g., schools).

◆ Interactions with other people (e.g., family, friends, colleagues).

◆ Web-based resources.

◆ Social media.

◆ Health professionals.

◆ Product labels and pamphlets.

III. Barriers to Effective Health Communication

◆ It is rare that every message coded and transmitted by a sender is decoded and understood with complete accuracy by the receiver.

◆ Multiple factors that can affect the way health messages are understood are described in Table 3-1.

◆ Many of the factors listed in the table overlap in their description; more than one barrier may exist and have an effect on any attempt at communication.

◆ All of the factors listed can provide a barrier to communication in either direction between the clinician and the patient.

◆ Dental hygienists who strive to develop good listening skills, enhance their ability to assess a patient's needs, and approach each individual with empathy and respect can go far toward overcoming the barriers to effective health communication.

IV. Web-Based Health Messages

◆ There has been an explosion of health-related websites and an increasing number of patients of all ages who access Internet-based health information.

◆ Patients bring information they find on the Internet or via social media to the attention of their healthcare providers.

◆ Healthcare providers are responsible to keep up-to-date on Internet sources of information in order to respond to questions patients may bring to a health education discussion.

◆ Healthcare providers may also be the creators and distributors of web-based health information (e.g., websites, digital tools). Considerations should be made to ensure that information is easy for patients to access and understand.

◆ The U.S. Department of Health and Human Services, Office of Disease Prevention and Health Promotion offers a guide and tips to assist in creating user-friendly websites and digital tools (available from: https://health.gov/healthliteracyonline/).

◆ The dental hygienist can help patients determine reliability and credibility of websites as well as provide recommendations for high-quality resources for patients searching for additional information (see Chapter 2).

V. Factors That Influence Health Communication

◆ Communication skills of the caregiver and effectiveness of the health information can affect:

• The ability of healthcare providers to influence health behaviors.

• The ability of patients and populations to take advantage of new knowledge provided by the health messages.

TABLE 3-1 • Barriers to Effective Health Communication

BARRIER	DESCRIPTION
Cultural	Differences in social norms or perceptions related to differences in gender, age, language, economic, or ethnic background
Interpersonal	Discomfort related to perceptions about the individual; appearance causes distraction; individuals do not see "eye to eye" or relate well to each other
Attitudinal	Lack of sensitivity or respect; over- or underconfidence displayed by either patient or clinician
Physical	Distractions related to the physical environment; noise levels; face-to-face positioning not used
Physiologic	Inability to hear, see, touch, or vocalize as required to communicate
Psychosociologic	Emotional factors such as fear or pain cause distraction
Insufficient knowledge	Either the clinician is not well informed and cannot provide sufficient information or the patient has low health literacy and cannot understand the information provided
Lack of access to knowledge	Inability to access media or use technology to find information
Lack of interest	Patient is not ready to engage in health behavior change; clinician is experiencing "burn out" or disinterest in patient education
Information overload	Too much information on too many topics is provided at one time; no written reinforcement is provided
Poor communication skills	Either the patient or the clinician is not able to respond or provide feedback to messages received; clinician uses "jargon" or professional terminology that the patient does not understand

◆ Other factors that influence health communication include:
  • Health literacy of the patient or population receiving the health message.
  • The age and communication preferences of individuals receiving information.
  • The social and economic ability of the targeted individuals to take advantage of recommendations contained in the health messages.
  • The cultural background and health-related cultural norms of the individual receiving the message.
  • Cultural sensitivity and the ability to establish cultural rapport of individuals providing the health messages.

HEALTH LITERACY

◆ Health literacy is the ability of a patient to obtain, process, understand, and respond to health messages and be motivated to make health decisions that promote and maintain good health.[7]

◆ A large part of even an educated population may have low health literacy, and often, these are the patients with the highest treatment needs and the greatest barriers to receiving health information.

◆ Populations particularly vulnerable to low or limited health literacy include[6]:
  • Older adults.
  • Immigrant populations.
  • Minority populations.
  • People who speak little or no English.
  • People with low levels of education (i.e., less than high school).
  • Individuals living below the poverty level.

◆ Low health literacy is associated with less use of healthcare services and resources and ultimately with poorer health outcomes.[8]

I. Health Learning Capacity

◆ The level of a patient's health literacy depends on not only the reading level but also the complex interaction of cognitive and psychosocial skills.[9]

◆ Individuals faced with complex health information need to be able to or learn to[10]:
  • Access services and navigate complex healthcare facilities and systems.
  • Locate and be able to understand health information.
  • Evaluate information for credibility and quality.
  • Communicate with healthcare providers.
  • Analyze relative risks and benefits of treatment recommendations.
  • Evaluate test results.
  • Calculate medication dosages.

◆ Skills that support health learning capacity are listed in Table 3-2.

TABLE 3-2 • Skills and Attributes Necessary to Increase Health Literacy Capacity

DOMAIN	SKILLS AND ATTRIBUTES
Cognitive	• Knowledge and information (processing ability) • Reading and writing • Numeracy (mathematical ability) • Visual literacy (ability to understand graphs) • Comprehension and reasoning ability • Appraisal, evaluation, and critical thinking ability • Computer literacy (and access)
Behavioral	• Information seeking and obtaining ability • Communication ability • Application of information • Navigation ability (of the healthcare system) • Civic literacy (ethics and social responsibility)
Affective	• Self-control and regulation • Self-efficacy • Interest and motivation

Source: Bröder J, Okan O, Bauer U, et al. Health literacy in childhood and youth: a systematic review of definitions and models. *BMC Public Health.* 2017;17(1):361; National Network of Libraries of Medicine. Health literacy: skills needed for health literacy. http://nnlm.gov/outreach/consumer/hlthlit.html#A3. Accessed August 16, 2017.

II. Assess and Address Health Literacy

To enhance communication with all patients regardless of oral health literacy level[11,12]:

◆ Assess health literacy level and provide an individualized approach for every patient.

◆ Ensure a clinic environment that is helpful and user-friendly by providing clear directions, visible and clearly written signs or universal symbols, and color-coded maps where necessary.

◆ Encourage patients to write down and bring questions about their oral health to each appointment.

◆ Provide forms (e.g., health history, informed consent) that are written in plain language. Provide help if required in completing forms.

◆ Build on the patient's current knowledge base to encourage healthy decision making.

◆ Provide written patient education materials that use plain language and avoid materials that use professional jargon or provide complex explanations.

◆ Excellent "plain language" oral health patient education publications have been developed by the U.S. Department of Health and Human Services and are available for free on the National Institute of Dental and Craniofacial Research website (see Figure 3-1).

◆ Use visual aids such as drawings or photographs for education materials when appropriate (see Figure 3-2).

◆ Monitor to determine understanding of all forms and education materials. The "teach-back" method of asking patients to explain instructions to be followed is a helpful approach.

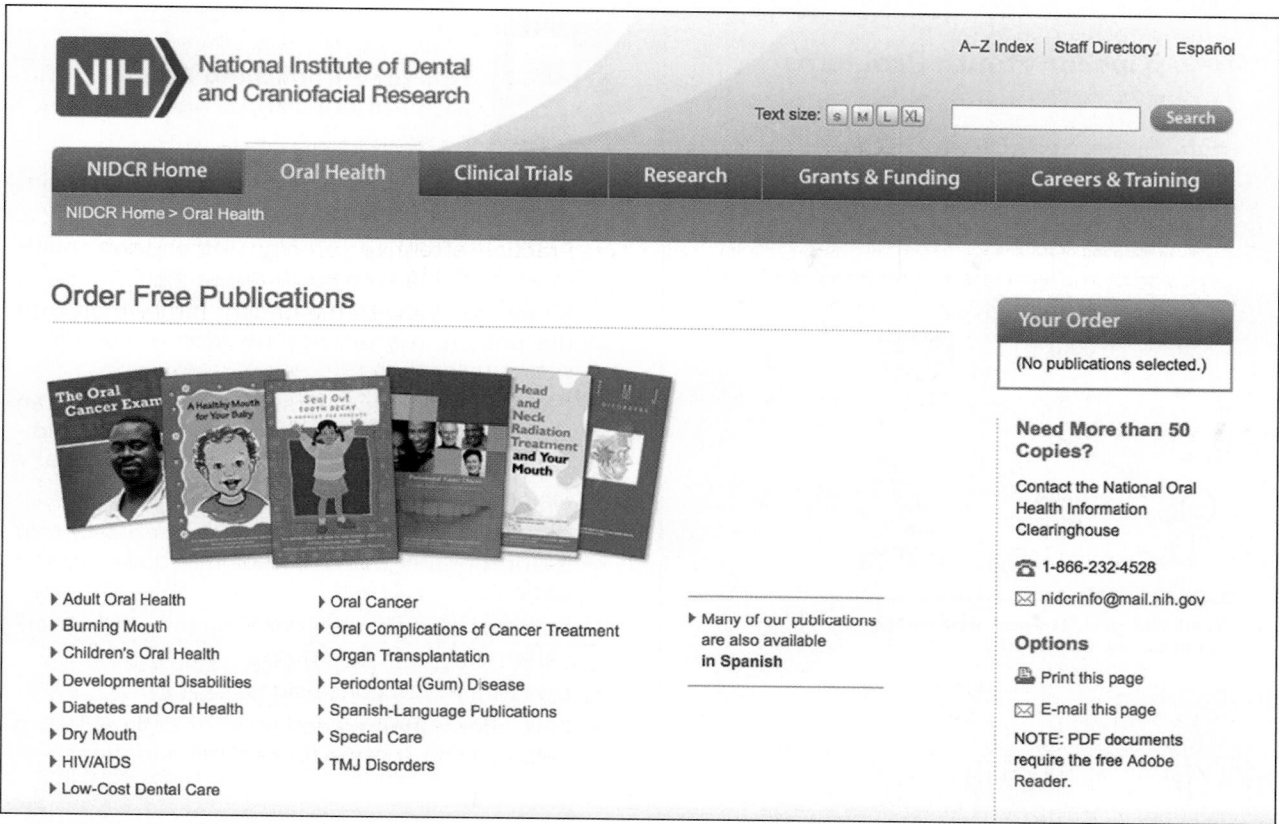

FIGURE 3-1 • A variety of excellent "plain language" oral health patient education publications have been developed by the U.S. Department of Health and Human Services, National Institutes of Health, and are available for free from the National Institute of Dental and Craniofacial Research website at: https://catalog.nidcr.nih.gov/OrderPublications/. Accessed September 2, 2017.

COMMUNICATION ACROSS THE LIFE SPAN

◆ Irrespective of the patient's age, building rapport is key to effective health communication.

◆ Tips for establishing rapport with patients of all ages are found in Box 3-1.

◆ Key points related to specific age groups are discussed in the subsequent sections.

I. Children and Adolescents

◆ Complete information about the oral health needs of children and adolescents is found in Chapter 47.

◆ Some age-appropriate communication strategies are listed below.[13]

A. Infants (Birth to 12 Months)

◆ Infants communicate primarily through their senses of touch, sight, and hearing.

◆ Techniques the clinician can use to communicate with an infant during a dental hygiene examination include:

• Interact playfully with a receptive infant by mimicking facial expressions, rocking, and talking softly or singing.

• Encourage an adult who is familiar with the infant to distract and comfort the child.

• Wait until the infant is calm to approach closely.

B. Toddlers and Preschoolers (Ages 1–2 and 3–5)

◆ Although dependent on adults for their care, most children appreciate and respond to being approached directly.

◆ Development of a sense of self enhances the need to assert independence and maintain control over any situation.

◆ Offer encouragement and gentle hints or engage in "parallel" actions to demonstrate, rather than directly assisting, to promote success in age-appropriate self-care tasks.

◆ Calmly distract or direct toward an alternative behavior to counter defiance or inappropriate behavior.

◆ To effectively control unwanted behavior, state specifically what the child is expected to do rather than criticize.

◆ Ask simple, specifically focused questions to help the child remember past experiences.

◆ To overcome the limited ability to process auditory information and short attention span, provide brief, truthful, and simple instructions and responses to questions.

Tips for Mouth Problems

Sore Mouth, Sore Throat

- Rinse often with
  - ¼ teaspoon of salt and
  - ¼ teaspoon of baking soda in 1 quart (4 cups) of warm water
  - Don't swallow.

- Ask your cancer care team about medicine that can help with the pain.

FIGURE 3-2 • **This example, which uses drawings to provide patient education, is taken from the illustrated booklet "Three Good Reasons to See a Dentist BEFORE Cancer Treatment."** Illustrated patient education materials are appropriate for adults with reading skills at the second grade level or below and for children. This entire publication can be downloaded or ordered from the NIDCR website at: https://catalog.nidcr.nih.gov/OrderPublications/. Accessed September 2, 2017.

- Toddlers are beginning to converse in short sentences, but if the adult becomes impatient or abrupt, the child may feel frustrated or ashamed and become unresponsive.
- Children of this age understand more than they are given credit for but often misinterpret language that is not familiar to them; therefore, serious discussions or use of certain words may distress them.

C. School-Age Children (6 Through 11)

- The ability to understand serious events logically and comprehend how it will impact themselves is developing.
- More aware of the needs of others but may be reluctant to state their own needs.
- Including the child as well as the parent/caregiver in the interaction is important; however, the level of involvement of each child will vary depending on individual factors.[14]

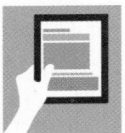

BOX 3-1

Tips for Establishing Rapport with Patients of All Ages

- Listen more than talk, especially at the beginning of a conversation.
- Practice attentive listening rather than multitasking during conversations.
- Sit eye to eye with the patient rather than with the patient in a reclined position or standing/sitting taller than the patient does.
- Convey a nonjudgmental attitude, reinforce an atmosphere of respect and valuing of the individual, even if the behavior is not acceptable.
- Maintain a calm, unhurried demeanor.
- Use a normal tone of voice and vocabulary that is appropriate, but does not talk down, to the patient.
- Look for clues, share your thoughts and observations, and ask questions.
- Do not jump to conclusions.
- Link information to activities of daily living to help provide context for recommendations.

- The ability and desire to respond to simple questions can allow the dental hygienist to assess knowledge and misconceptions.

D. Adolescents (12 Through 21)

- Marked by intense and often extreme feelings about situations and persons in their world.
- Strongly independent and desire to have their viewpoint considered with respect.
- Tendency to withdraw or become hostile if they feel they are misunderstood.
- A straightforward approach that explains and then solicits input into a discussion on topics that interest the adolescent is most effective to build rapport and establish trust.
- Confidentiality laws, which vary between jurisdictions, can help determine what behavior-related information the dental hygienist discusses with a parent or guardian. Anything that is an immediate safety issue (such as thoughts of suicide) is reported immediately.
- To develop a rapport and a trusting relationship with an adolescent patient:
  - Address the adolescent directly even when parent/guardian is present.
  - Ensure the adolescent has the opportunity to ask and answer questions independently (privately) as well as with parents/guardians.[15]

II. Older Adults[16,17]

- Oral health issues related to aging are discussed in Chapter 48.
- Providing effective health education for aging patients who are experiencing a communication difficulty requires respect for the needs of the individual and response to functional ability or limitations.
- Age-related communication difficulties can include:
  - Visual or hearing impairment.
  - Decreased ability to remember or formulate language.
  - Health conditions and related medications that may alter cognitive abilities.
- Strategies for communicating with older individuals experiencing communication difficulty are listed in Box 3-2.

A. Physical and Cognitive Changes

- Cognitive disabilities are more likely to be present as an individual ages and to interfere with understanding health-related information.
- Communication disorders such as dysarthria and aphasia are associated with conditions that are more common in an aging population.
- Sensory loss (particularly hearing loss) can provide challenges in interpersonal communication.
- Physiologic changes may occur in speech patterns, including voice tremor, pitch, loudness, and speaking rate.

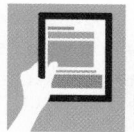

BOX 3-2
Strategies for Effective Communication with Older Adults

- Identify each individual's communication barriers (such as cognitive impairments) and modify communication approach appropriately.
- Avoid patronizing "elderspeak" and respect the patient's level of competence and independence.
- Suggest that the patient write down questions ahead of time.
- Practice attentive listening and avoid rushing the patient.
- Face the patient and maintain eye contact; remove masks during conversations.
- Speak slowly, clearly, and loud enough for the patient to hear.
- Use simple, patient-appropriate language.
- Present one idea at a time.
- Use visual aids, teach-back techniques, and repetition of key messages.
- Provide written summary or follow-up for key messages.

B. Communication Predicament[17-19]

- Healthcare providers often use an inappropriate over-modification of speech and language when addressing older patients.
- *Accommodative speech* refers to use of a high-pitched tone of voice, a "singsong" cadence, and relatively simplistic language when addressing an older adult.
- The use of *terms of endearment* (honey, sweetie, dearie) and *diminutive* forms of a patient's name can reflect a lack of respect for the individual as an adult person.
- The use of plural pronouns ("Are we ready for our appointment?") can imply that the patient cannot act alone or make independent decisions.
- This "baby talk" or "elderspeak" approach to communication does not enhance comprehension and can be perceived as patronizing or demeaning.

SOCIAL AND ECONOMIC ASPECTS OF HEALTH COMMUNICATION

- Social and economic factors, sometimes referred to as "social determinants of health," are the circumstances in which people are born, grow up, live, work, play, and age.[20]
- These factors:
  - Influence the ability of individuals and communities to receive and act upon health messages received from healthcare providers or public health media.
  - Are responsible for unfair and avoidable differences in health status seen within and between populations.[20,21]
- Oral health professionals have a responsibility to address the needs of individuals in the context of their environment and experience when providing oral health education.[21-23]

CULTURAL CONSIDERATIONS

- Sociocultural differences can impede communication between the dental hygienist and patient.[24]
- Culturally sensitive delivery of dental hygiene services can make a positive difference in oral health outcomes.[24]
- A cultural awareness checklist is found in Box 3-3.

I. Culture and Health

A. Effects of Culture on Health Status

- The increasing diversity of racial and ethnic communities and linguistic groups in North America influences the delivery of oral health services.
- Health disparities related to racial, ethnic, and socioeconomic background exist in the healthcare system.[25]

BOX 3-3
A Checklist to Enhance Cultural Awareness during Patient Care

- Examine and recognize any personal bias that may affect communication when working with patients from a different **culture**.
- Conduct all patient assessments with cultural sensitivity in mind.
- Assess to determine the patient's cultural identification and, if necessary, research to identify implications for dental hygiene practice.
- Determine language barriers, identify patient's preferred method of communication, and regularly double-check to assure comprehension.
- Identify religious and health-related beliefs, views, or misconceptions that may influence dental hygiene interventions.
- Identify and address cultural dietary considerations.
- Double-check verbal and nonverbal signs routinely to determine the level of the patient's trust of healthcare providers.

Source: Seibert PS, Stridh-Igo P, Zimmerman CG. A checklist to facilitate cultural awareness and sensitivity. *J Med Ethics.* 2002;28(3):143-146.

- Ignoring culture can lead to negative health consequences and/or poor clinical outcomes because culture and language can influence:
  - Beliefs and behaviors related to health, healing, and wellness.
  - Perceptions of illness, diseases, and their causes.
  - Attitudes of patients toward accessing health services or toward healthcare providers.
  - Attitudes and behaviors of providers who may have learned a set of values that are different from those of their patients.

B. Culturally Effective Oral Care[24]

- Culturally effective health care is patient centered and "responsive to diverse cultural health beliefs and practices, preferred languages, health literacy, and other communication needs."[26]
- Sensitivity to the effects of culture on healthcare delivery is "critical to reducing health disparities and improving access to high-quality health care."[27]
- Meeting each patient's individual oral care needs is the hallmark of dental hygiene practice.
- The ability to provide effective oral health education and dental hygiene services for culturally diverse patients requires assessing, being sensitive to, and respecting each patient's cultural differences.
- Culturally effective dental hygiene care respects each patient's health beliefs, practices, values, customs, and traditions in the plan for dental hygiene care.

II. Cross-Cultural Communication

- Communication with patients from other cultures is enhanced when the dental hygienist develops knowledge about and avoids stereotyping traditional behaviors and values of a patient's cultural group.
- Knowing general principles can enhance communication.

A. Nonverbal Communication

- Some culturally related differences in nonverbal communication are identified in Table 3-3.
- To communicate successfully, the dental hygienist will:
  - Follow the patient's lead for touching or personal space.
  - Use hand and arm gestures with caution.
  - Be careful interpreting facial expressions.
  - Follow the patient's lead for making eye contact.

B. Language Proficiency

- Simplify language as much as possible without speaking down to the patient.
- Eliminate professional jargon.
- Use pictures, diagrams, and demonstrations to help increase understanding.
- Provide "plain language" health information or publications in the patient's primary language to reinforce and support compliance with oral health recommendations.

C. Using an Interpreter

- When the patient's skills in the dominant language are not sufficient to assure informed consent or compliance with recommendations, a professional interpreter can be used to enhance communication.
- A professional interpreter will have proficiency in both languages as well as an ability to convey complex information completely and accurately.
- Family members or friends are not the same as a professional interpreter.
- Informal interpreters could hinder health communication[28] and are more likely to modify important information or interject their own opinions, beliefs, or prejudices.
- It is particularly inadvisable to ask children to interpret sensitive health information.
- Focus on and direct all communication to the patient, with pauses to allow the interpreter to translate.

D. Family Decision Making

- In many cultures, an individual's health problem is considered to be a family problem.
- Involvement of certain family members in the treatment planning process may be a key factor in determining recommendations and assuring compliance.
- Sensitivity is needed when family members or children, even older children, are involved in the discussion.

TABLE 3-3 • Nonverbal Communication and Cross-Cultural Considerations

ATTRIBUTE	EXPLANATION
Facial expressions	• Smiling, winking, and blinking may not signify the same intent in all cultures. • People from some cultures point at an object by shifting eyes or pursing lips because pointing with a hand or finger is inappropriate. • Expressions of pain and discomfort may differ among cultures or according to family experiences. Some cultures value stoicism, while others seem to emote effusively.
Gestures	• Hand signs can be interpreted in many ways among cultures. • Some commonly used gestures, such as the "OK" finger-thumb circle shape or the "thumbs-up" gesture, have vulgar connotations for members of some cultures.
Head movements and physical postures	• Head movement signs for "yes" and "no" vary greatly in some cultures. • Some cultures nod head (as in "yes") to indicate attention to or respect for the speaker—even if the answer to the question is not yes or if they do not understand what is being said. • Standing with hands on hips might indicate a challenge to members of some cultures. • Many cultures consider slouching or poor posture as a sign of disrespect. • Showing the bottom of the shoe (resting foot on top of knee while sitting) is considered impolite in some cultures.
Personal space and touching	• Individuals from some cultures are accustomed to standing or sitting very close and sometimes touching, even during casual interactions; others may express alarm if the provider stands or sits too close. • A light touch, a brief kiss on the cheek, or warm handshake is common in some cultures, even among people who have just met or individuals of the same gender. • In some cultures, such physical contact may be extremely inappropriate. • In some cultures, touching or accepting an article with the left hand is considered unclean.
Eye contact	• In some cultures, making direct eye-to-eye contact is a sign of respect; in others, it is a sign of disrespect especially if done by a child or toward an authority figure such as a healthcare provider. • The "languid" or half-closed eyes of individuals from some cultures is not necessarily a sign of disrespect or inattention.

Source: Management Sciences for Health Electronic Resource Center. The Provider's guide to quality & culture: non-verbal communication. https://www.innovations.ahrq.gov /qualitytools/providers-guide-quality-culture-0

III. Attaining Cultural Competence

◆ Achieving cultural competence in providing health care is a process[29] that requires a commitment to cultural awareness, a motivation to engage in cultural encounters, and an ongoing acquisition of cultural knowledge and communication skills.

◆ The dental hygienist who strives to become adept at providing culturally effective care:

- Values (and not simply tolerates) diversity.
- Conducts honest self-assessment to determine how personal health beliefs, traditions, and biases influence the ability to relate to culturally different individuals.
- Actively acquires knowledge about patients' health beliefs, behaviors, and cultural norms.
- Is nonjudgmental regarding cultural traditions and beliefs.
- Avoids stereotypes.
- Routinely adapts delivery of dental hygiene care in a way that reflects understanding of each patient's diversity and unique oral health needs.

IV. Cultural Competence and the Dental Hygiene Process of Care

◆ Respect for each patient's cultural differences, healthcare practices, health beliefs, and values can be integrated into all areas of the dental hygiene process of care.[30]

A. Assessment

◆ The ability to collect accurate, complete assessment data is key to providing dental hygiene interventions that meet patient needs.

◆ Culturally effective nonverbal communication and listening skills help build trust and patient rapport that can facilitate the transfer of essential personal health information.

◆ Skillful, nonjudgmental questioning can help elicit culture-specific data such as health beliefs and values, as well as avoid misunderstandings about a patient's culturally related health practices.

◆ Asking permission before touching a patient during the extra- and intraoral examination procedures can avoid problems with cultural differences in personal space.

B. Diagnosis

◆ A dental hygiene diagnosis is predicated on a clear understanding of the patient's history, medical status, symptoms, and current treatment modalities.

◆ The culturally competent dental hygienist will prepare diagnostic statements that take into consideration:

- Culture-specific health risks that are related to oral status.
- Cultural practices that may impact the patient's oral health status.

C. Planning

◆ The dental hygiene care plan formulates oral health goals that meet the needs of each individual patient realistically.

◆ The goals identified in the plan are based on a synthesis of needs determined by the dental hygienist and those expressed by the patient.

◆ A culturally sensitive dental hygiene care plan respects and takes into consideration the patient's current health practices and beliefs.

◆ With the patient's input, the plan may be devised to accept, modify, or eliminate current culturally relevant healthcare practices.

◆ The plan is sensitive to the practices, products, or substances that the patient's culture prohibits, such as mouth rinses containing alcohol for patients in some cultures.

◆ A culturally and linguistically sensitive approach to communicating the dental hygiene care plan can facilitate informed consent for dental hygiene interventions.

D. Implementation

◆ Culturally appropriate communication can enhance the patient's cooperation during treatment.

◆ Knowledge of culturally determined expressions of pain and discomfort during treatment can help the dental hygienist determine appropriate pain control measures during treatment.

◆ Language-appropriate instructions before, during, and after each procedure can enhance patient compliance with treatment.

◆ "Plain language" oral health materials can enhance patient compliance with recommendations.

E. Evaluation

◆ A dental hygienist who is sensitive to cultural differences evaluates treatment success on the basis of goals determined in a previously prepared culturally relevant care plan.

◆ Feedback provided for the patient respects culturally diverse beliefs and values related to oral health.

◆ Self-evaluation regarding the cultural effectiveness of the practitioner's approach can provide insight for planning modifications to the patient's continuing care plan.

INTERPROFESSIONAL COMMUNICATION

◆ Interprofessional collaboration is changing the way health care is delivered and resulting in positive health-care outcomes.[31,32]

◆ Teamwork is a vital skill that relies on collaboration between a variety of healthcare providers who have responsibility for the often complex aspects of an individual patient's care.

◆ Sufficient and ongoing communication is a major factor in developing a collaborative practice workforce that strengthens healthcare systems, provides high-quality care, and supports positive patient outcomes.[31,33,34]

◆ Continuous efforts to enhance interprofessional communication are necessary to improve the quality of patient care.[34,35]

◆ The ability to communicate with other health professionals in a manner that supports a team approach to patient care requires competency in the following skills[33]:

- Select effective communication tools and techniques, including information systems and communication technologies.
- Organize and express information in a form that is easily understood by providers in other health disciplines.
- Demonstrate active listening; encourage others to share ideas and opinions.
- Provide timely, sensitive, and instructive feedback to other members of the team.
- Be open to receiving feedback in a respectful and positive manner.
- Use respectful language when in a difficult situation or a professional conflict.
- Recognize how one's own communication style contributes to the interprofessional relationship.
- Consistently communicate the importance of teamwork in patient-centered care.

COMMUNICATION WITH CAREGIVERS

◆ Many patients with disabling conditions and also young children rely on someone else to help with or provide daily self-care regimens.

◆ In this situation, the dental hygienist communicates with the caregiver or parent as well as the patient.

◆ In a group conversation, keep the primary focus on the patient by maintaining eye contact and directing comments/questions to the patient, if appropriate, as well as the caregiver.

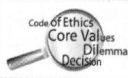

EVERYDAY ETHICS

Abelena Flores, a 65-year-old Mexican American female, presents to the clinic for the first time for her initial assessment appointment. Mrs. Flores speaks English moderately well, but Lisel, the dental hygienist, notices that she is not able to read the health history and seems to be confused during more complex explanations. Lisel offers to obtain a medical translator for the next appointment, but Mrs. Flores insists that her son, who speaks English, and her son's new wife, who does not speak English, will accompany her to help interpret and make decisions about the treatment plan that Lisel will present to her at that visit. Lisel is concerned that the family members will not be knowledgeable enough to be able to explain the needed treatment so that informed consent can be obtained.

Lisel considers arranging for a friend who is a medical translator to be present without telling Mrs. Flores beforehand. Lisel knows that her patient will not be charged for that service because the medical translator is a volunteer who has provided free translation services at the clinic in the past.

Questions for Consideration

1. Is this an ethical issue or an ethical dilemma for Lisel?

2. Explain which core values (Chapter 1, Box 1-6) Lisel will need to consider as she determines what action to take regarding the use of a translator during Mrs. Flores next appointment.

3. How might personal values related to Lisel's and Mrs. Flores' cultural differences affect Lisel's ethical duty in resolving this situation?

◆ Assess patient needs and caregiver relationships carefully to determine the extent of the caregiver's role in daily self-care.

◆ Encourage the caregiver to allow the patient to maintain as much independence as possible.

DOCUMENTATION

When documenting communication aspects of a patient visit, the following factors are included:

◆ Patient's age, gender, and ethnicity.

◆ Factors or observations related to health literacy level.

◆ Cultural characteristics that can affect communication or delivery of dental hygiene care.

◆ Significant factors such as patient hearing loss, need to communicate with caregiver, use of an interpreter, and description of specific modifications made to accommodate those factors.

◆ An example of documentation for communication aspects of a patient visit is found in Box 3-4.

Factors to Teach the Patient

▶ The dental hygienist's ability to provide good dental hygiene care is affected by the willingness and ability of the patient to communicate accurate and complete information about health status, needs, and concerns.

▶ The patient's motivation to follow oral health recommendations is affected by the rapport established and the trust developed between the patient and the clinician.

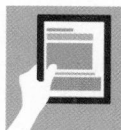

BOX 3-4

Example Documentation: Communication Aspects of a Patient Visit

S—Following an initial data collection appointment, a 65-year-old African-American male presents for a second appointment to receive and discuss his complex treatment plan. Patient has significant hearing loss and does not use a hearing aid but reads lips during casual conversation. He prefers to ask complex questions and receive answers by writing on a notepad.

O—Written dental hygiene care plan and dental treatment plans have been developed and are ready to be presented for patient consent.

A—Patient understanding is necessary for documenting informed consent.

P—Sequential presentation of each written component of the dental hygiene care plan and dental treatment plan. Additional appointment time scheduled so all questions can be answered in writing, as the patient prefers. Following the presentation of each component of the plan, the patient was asked to summarize or restate in writing to demonstrate that he understood what was discussed. At the end of the discussion, the patient wrote on his notepad that all of his questions were answered. Treatment Consent form was signed and dated.

Next Step: Begin implementation of phase 1 of dental hygiene care plan.

Signed: _____, RDH

Date: _____

ENHANCE YOUR UNDERSTANDING

ONLINE RESOURCES
(see the inside front cover for access information)
- Audio glossary
- Appendices

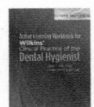

SUPPORT FOR LEARNING
(available separately)
- *Active Learning Workbook for Wilkins' Clinical Practice of the Dental Hygienist, 13th Edition*

INDIVIDUALIZED REVIEW
- Customized practice quizzing with Navigate 2 TestPrep for *Wilkins' Clinical Practice of the Dental Hygienist*

References

1. Boyland EJ, Nolan S, Kelly B, et al. Advertising as a cue to consume: a systematic review and meta-analysis of the effects of acute exposure to unhealthy food and nonalcoholic beverage advertising on intake in children and adults. *Am J Clin Nutr.* 2016;103(2):519-533.

2. Office of Disease Prevention and Health Promotion. Healthy People 2020 topics and objectives: health communication and health information technology [Web page]. Washington, DC: U.S. Department of Health and Human Services. https://www.healthypeople.gov/2020/topics-objectives/topic/health-communication-and-health-information-technology/objectives. Accessed September 17, 2017.

3. Burke LE, Fair J. Promoting prevention: skill sets and attributes of health care providers who deliver behavioral interventions. *J Cardiovasc Nurs.* 2003;18(4):256-266.

4. National Institutes of Health. Plain language [Web page]. http://www.nih.gov/clearcommunication/plainlanguage/index.htm. Accessed September 17, 2017.

5. U.S. Department of Health and Human Services. *Healthy People 2010: Objectives for Improving Health. Part A, Focus Area 11-Health communication:11.3–11.22.* Vol 1. 2nd ed. Washington, DC: U.S. Government Printing Office; 2000.

6. U.S. Department of Health and Human Services, Office of Disease Prevention and Health Promotion. *National Action Plan to Improve Health Literacy.* Washington, DC: U.S. Department of Health and Human Services; 2010. https://health.gov/communication/hlactionplan/pdf/Health_Literacy_Action_Plan.pdf. Accessed September 17, 2017.

7. Centers for Disease Control and Prevention. What is health literacy? [Web page] https://www.cdc.gov/healthliteracy/learn/index.html. Accessed September 17, 2017.

8. Berkman ND, Sheridan SL, Donahue KE, Halpern DJ, Crotty K. Low health literacy and health outcomes: an updated systematic review. *Ann Intern Med.* 2011;155(2):97-107.

9. Bröder J, Okan O, Bauer U, et al. Health literacy in childhood and youth: a systematic review of definitions and models. *BMC Public Health.* 2017;17(1):361.

10. National Network of Libraries of Medicine. Health literacy: skills needed for health literacy [Web page]. https://nnlm.gov/priorities/topics/health-literacy#toc-4. Accessed September 17, 2017.

11. Horowitz AM, Kleinman DV. Oral health literacy: the new imperative to better oral health. *Dent Clin North Am.* 2008;52(2):333-344, vi.

12. Horowitz AM, Kleinman DV. Creating a health literacy-based practice. *J Calif Dent Assoc.* 2012;40(4):331-340.

13. Deering C, Cody D. Communicating with children and adolescents. *Am J Nurs.* 2002;102(3):34-41.

14. Cahill P. *The Third Voice in the Consultation. Listening to Children and Young People in Healthcare Consultations.* Oxford, England: Radcliffe Publishing Ltd; 2010:31-43.

15. Mappa P, Baverstock A, Finlay F, Verling W. Current practice with regard to seeing adolescents on their own' during outpatient consultations. *Int J Adolesc Med Health.* 2010;22(2):301-305.

16. Yorkston KM, Bourgeois MS, Baylor CR. Communication and aging. *Phys Med Rehabil Clin N Am.* 2010;21(2):309-319.

17. Stein PS, Aalboe JA, Savage MW, Scott AM. Strategies for communicating with older dental patients. *J Am Dent Assoc.* 2014;145(2):159-164.

18. Brown A, Draper P. Accommodative speech and terms of endearment: elements of a language mode often experienced by older adults. *J Adv Nurs.* 2003;41(1):15-21.

19. Williams K, Kemper S, Hummert ML. Enhancing communication with older adults: overcoming elderspeak. *J Gerontol Nurs.* 2004;30(10):17-25.

20. World Health Organization. Social determinants of health: what are social determinants of health? [Web page]. http://www.who.int/social_determinants/sdh_definition/en/. Accessed September 17, 2017.

21. Williams DM, Sheiham A, Watt RG. Oral health professionals and social determinants. *Br Dent J.* 2013;214(9):427.

22. Lee JY, Divaris K. The ethical imperative of addressing oral health disparities: a unifying framework. *J Dent Res.* 2014;93(3):224-230.

23. Watt RG, Williams DM, Sheiham A. The role of the dental team in promoting health equity. *Br Dent J.* 2014;216(1):11.

24. Cadoret CA, Garcia RI. Health disparities and the multicultural imperative. *J Evid Based Dent Pract.* 2014;14:160-170.

25. Agency for Healthcare Research and Quality. *2016 National Healthcare Quality and Disparities Report.* Rockville, MD: U.S. Department of Health and Human Services. https://www.ahrq.gov/sites/default/files/wysiwyg/research/findings/nhqrdr/nhqdr16/2016qdr.pdf. Accessed September 17, 2017.

26. U.S. Department of Health and Human Services Office of Minority Health. *National Standards for Culturally and Linguistically Appropriate Services (CLAS) in Health and Health Care.* https://www.thinkculturalhealth.hhs.gov/assets/pdfs/EnhancedNationalCLASStandards.pdf. Accessed September 17, 2017.

27. National Institutes of Health. Clear communication: cultural respect [Web page]. https://www.nih.gov/institutes-nih/nih-office-director/office-communications-public-liaison/clear-communication/cultural-respect. Accessed September 17, 2017.

28. Au M, Taylor EF, Gold MR. *Improving Access to Language Services in Health Care: A Look at National and State Efforts.* Washington, DC: Mathematica Policy Research, Inc; 2009.

29. Campinha-Bacote J. The process of cultural competence in the delivery of healthcare services: a model of care. *J Transcult Nurs.* 2002;13(3):181-184.

30. Fitch P. Cultural competence and dental hygiene care delivery: integrating cultural care into the dental hygiene process of care. *J Dent Hyg.* 2004;78(1):11-21.

31. World Health Organization. *Framework for Action on Interprofessional Education & Collaborative Practice.* Geneva, Switzerland: World Health Organization; 2010. http://www.who.int/hrh/resources/framework_action/en/. Accessed September 17, 2017.

32. Reeves S, Pelone F, Harrison R, Goldman J, Zwarenstein M. Interprofessional collaboration to improve professional practice and healthcare outcomes. *Cochrane Database Syst Rev.* 2017;(6):CD000072.

33. Interprofessional Education Collaborative. *IPEC Core Competencies for Interprofessional Collaborative Practice: 2016 Update.* Washington, DC: Interprofessional Education Collaborative; 2016. http://www.asha.org/uploadedFiles/Interprofessional-Collaboration-Core-Competency.pdf. Accessed September 17, 2017.

34. Kishimoto M, Noda M. The difficulties of interprofessional teamwork in diabetes care: a questionnaire survey. *J Multidiscip Healthcare.* 2014;7:333-339.

35. Hepp SL, Suter E, Jackson K, et al. Using an interprofessional competency framework to examine collaborative practice. *J Interprof Care.* 2014;10:1-7.

4

Dental Hygiene Care in Alternative Settings

Jennifer Cullen, RDH, MPH, and Charlotte J. Wyche, BSDH, MS

CHAPTER OUTLINE

ALTERNATIVE PRACTICE SETTINGS
I. Barriers to Access
II. Eliminating Barriers
III. Portable Delivery of Care

RESIDENCE-BOUND PATIENTS
I. Private Homes
II. Residential Facilities
III. Community-Based Settings

DENTAL HYGIENE CARE
I. Common Oral Problems and Conditions
II. Significance of Oral Health to Overall Health

III. Objectives of Care
IV. Preparation for the Residential Visit
V. Approach to Patient
VI. Treatment Location
VII. Additional Considerations
VIII. Assessment and Care Planning
IX. Strategies for Prevention and Management

THE CRITICALLY ILL OR UNCONSCIOUS PATIENT
I. Instructions for Caregivers
II. Toothbrush with Suction Attachment

THE TERMINALLY ILL PATIENT
I. Objectives of Care
II. General Mouth Care Considerations

DOCUMENTATION
EVERYDAY ETHICS
FACTORS TO TEACH THE PATIENT
FACTORS TO TEACH THE CAREGIVER
REFERENCES

LEARNING OBJECTIVES

After studying this chapter, the student will be able to:

1. Identify and define key terms and concepts related to oral health care in alternative settings.

2. Identify materials necessary for providing dental hygiene care in alternative settings.

3. Plan and document adaptations to dental hygiene care plans and oral hygiene instructions for the patient who is residence-bound, bedridden, unconscious, or terminally ill.

◆ In recent years, increasing attention is being paid to the oral health needs of individuals who are not able to access oral health services in a traditional dental practice setting.[1]

◆ Individuals confined to hospitals, hospices, institutions, skilled nursing or long-term care facilities, or private homes:
   ● Experience barriers accessing routine dental services.
   ● Receive inadequate oral care from caregivers.
   ● Are likely to have poor oral health status and diminished quality of life.
   ● May need special adaptations for oral care.

◆ Most states now have laws that allow direct access to dental hygiene services through collaborative practice or varying levels of supervision in certain public health settings.[2]

◆ An important role for the dental hygienist is to triage and ensure optimum use of available dental care resources.
   ● Key words and definitions related to caring for patients in alternative settings are found in the glossary.

ALTERNATIVE PRACTICE SETTINGS

In recent years, increasing attention is being paid to the oral health needs of individuals who are not able to access oral health services in a traditional dental practice setting.
◆ Individuals confined to hospitals, hospices, institutions, skilled nursing or long-term care facilities, or private homes:
  • Experience barriers accessing routine dental services.
  • Receive inadequate oral care from caregivers.
  • Are likely to have poor oral health status and diminished quality of life.
  • May need special adaptations for oral care.
Most states now have laws that allow direct access to dental hygiene services through collaborative practice or varying levels of supervision in certain public health settings.
◆ An important role for the dental hygienist is to triage and ensure optimum use of available dental care resources.

I. Barriers to Access[3,4]

In addition to universal barriers such as cost and fear, providing care in alternative settings can also address unique barriers faced by this population.

Barriers to access for the residence-bound population may include:
◆ Limited mobility.
◆ Lack of suitable transportation.
◆ Often inaccessible physical environment of dental offices.
◆ Few on-site dental clinics in residential facilities.
◆ Limited availability of general and specialty practitioners who provide home-based services.
◆ Limited availability of direct access allied oral health providers.
◆ Limited or nonexistent federal/state insurance coverage for dental services for adults and older adults.[5]

II. Eliminating Barriers

Many services are delivered to residence-bound individuals by home health agencies.
◆ Certain allied health professionals, such as nurse practitioners, oversee programs that provide direct medical services for patients.
◆ New models of healthcare delivery, such as teledentistry, use Web-based communication tools to enhance potential for collaboration between on-site and supervising health team members.
◆ Current public health programs in numerous states allow dental hygienists to provide direct access care for certain underserved populations.
◆ Direct access care providers can address access issues related to shortage of dentists, limited availability of safety net options for low-income populations, and need for care in nontraditional settings.[6,7]
◆ Several direct access oral health provider models are currently being explored; some models are based on increased scope of practice for dental hygienists who have received additional education and certification.[8]

III. Portable Delivery of Care

For patients who cannot be transported to a dental treatment room, dental and dental hygiene services can be provided in a variety of surroundings using mobile equipment.
◆ Dental hygiene care:
  • Can be provided in any setting within the limits of state practice acts.
  • Particularly lends itself to care for residence-bound individuals because most dental hygiene treatments can be completed with manual instruments.

RESIDENCE-BOUND PATIENTS

◆ Potential residence-bound patients are listed in Box 4-1.
◆ The individual who is residence-bound may be:
  • Limited in one or more activities of daily living (see Chapter 22).
  • An American Society of Anesthesiologists' classification of III or higher (see Chapter 22).
  • Functionally dependent on caregivers.
◆ Instruction in personal oral preventive procedures has particular significance for comfort and quality of life, as well as the systemic health of these individuals.

I. Private Homes

Individuals who are residence-bound might live alone or with partner, spouse, friend, family members, or other caregivers.
◆ A private, traditional neighborhood residence.
◆ A variety of home-based healthcare and custodial care services are often utilized.

II. Residential Facilities

Studies indicate individuals residing in nursing homes generally have poor oral health status, do not receive adequate daily oral care, and cannot adequately access routine dental services.[3,9,10]
◆ Residential facilities can include:
  • Skilled nursing or long-term care including memory loss care.
  • Rehabilitation centers that provide temporary support for patients.
  • Independent and assisted living facilities for seniors or disabled individuals.

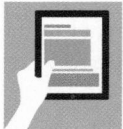

BOX 4-1
Potential Residence-Bound Patients

- **Frail elderly**
- Severely medically compromised
- **Critically** or **terminally ill**
- Physically or developmentally disabled
- **Chronically ill**
- **Cognitively impaired**

BOX 4-2
Services for Residents at Facilities That Receive Medicaid or Medicare Funding

Federal regulations require a facility receiving Medicaid or Medicare funding to help residents obtain the following services[11]:

- Comprehensive assessment of dental status
- Routine as well as emergency dental services
- Transportation to and from dental appointments
- Prompt referral to a dentist for lost or damaged dentures
- Supplies related to oral health (e.g., toothbrush, dental floss) at no cost to the individual

---

- Group homes that serve adults of all ages with physical, mental, or other medical disability.
- Federal regulations:
  - Require residential facilities that receive Medicaid or Medicare funding to contract with qualified dental personnel.
  - Do not require skilled nursing facilities to cover the costs of dental care.
  - Require facilities to assist residents in obtaining certain services (Box 4-2).
- State regulations vary significantly:
  - Regarding the provision of dental services for both Medicaid-eligible and -noneligible individuals.[12]
  - In terms of frequency of examinations or elements included in routine or emergency care.
  - In terms of requiring facilities contract with a dentist to advise on policies and education.

III. Community-Based Settings

Community-based settings for alternative dental hygiene practice may include:

- Senior/adult day programs and aggregate meal sites.
- Work/activity centers for disabled individuals.
- Medical practices.
- Homeless shelters and transitional housing programs.
- Churches.
- Elementary and secondary schools (some already provide school-based medical care) (Chapter 35).
- Head Start and day care centers.

DENTAL HYGIENE CARE

I. Common Oral Problems and Conditions

Residence-bound patients often experience compromised daily oral care and/or infrequent routine dental care.[9,10] Oral complications due to chronic disease, treatments, and medications can result in further pain and dysfunction.[13,14]

- Studies have found the following problems and conditions are frequently identified on clinical examination[9,10,13,14]:
  - Periodontal infections.
  - Difficulty biting and chewing.
  - Dental caries, especially root caries.
  - Toothache/pain and abscess/swelling.
  - Trauma, fractured/loose teeth, or dental restorations.
  - Lost fillings/crowns.
  - Angular cheilosis.
  - Clenching/bruxism.
  - Xerostomia.
  - Candidiasis infection.
  - General oral soreness (mucositis).
  - Denture problems.
- Table 4-1 identifies strategies for the prevention and management of select conditions.

II. Significance of Oral Health to Overall Health

A growing body of evidence supports the interdependent relationship between oral health and systemic conditions.[15] Residence-bound patients have additional challenges:

- Physical and cognitive limitations can compromise daily personal oral care abilities.
- Oral pain/discomfort/dysfunction can compromise nutritional status.
- Pain, including oral pain, can exacerbate negative behaviors in the cognitively impaired patient.
- Oral health status and oral cleanliness can affect patient self-esteem, quality of life, and ability to communicate with family and caregivers.

III. Objectives of Care

The objectives of dental hygiene care of residence-bound individuals will vary according to the patient's situation and needs. A dental hygienist providing care in a residential setting may:

- Provide intraoral/extraoral screening to triage and refer patients who need treatment by a dentist or specialist.
- Assist in preventing further complication of the patient's health status by identifying oral infections and other problems.
- Provide routine screening to detect lesions that may be pathologic, particularly those that may be early cancer.
- Provide dental hygiene treatment and education interventions to prevent dental caries and periodontal infections.
- Customize adaptive oral care practices that consider patients' and/or caregivers' unique needs (Section IX).
- Provide palliative care for the individual with a shortened life span.
- Participate in the patient's care as a member of the healthcare team.
- Contribute to the patient's general well-being and quality of life.

TABLE 4-1 • Strategies for Prevention and Management: Residence-Bound, Critically Ill, and Terminally Ill Patients

COMMON PROBLEMS	STRATEGIES FOR PLANNING DENTAL HYGIENE CARE (BASED ON ASSESSMENT OF INDIVIDUALIZED PATIENT NEEDS)
Barriers to professional oral care	• Assess and triage patient needs • Provide dental hygiene care • Refer/facilitate access for dental treatment
Inadequate biofilm removal	• Assess patient activities of daily living levels, emotional status, and knowledge related to ability to perform self-care regimens • Educate about the role of biofilm in oral and systemic disease • Provide oral hygiene aids or develop adaptive measures that facilitate self-care • Train caregivers, as necessary, to provide daily oral care
Increased risk for dental caries	• Identify/treat/prevent xerostomia • Provide professional and/or home fluoride application • Provide dietary analysis • Educate about reducing intake of fermentable carbohydrates • Educate about effective plaque removal • Engage caregivers, as necessary, to limit food/drink that promotes caries
Increased risk for periodontal infections	• Provide dental hygiene care • Educate about the relationship between oral disease and systemic health • Provide oral hygiene aids or develop adaptive measures that facilitate self-care • Train caregivers, as necessary, to provide daily oral care
Inadequate nutritional intake	• Assess for oral pain or inadequate chewing function that may be affecting the patient's nutritional intake • Severe weight loss can compromise denture fit • Consult with staff nutritionist, if available, in the patient's residential setting • Educate patient or caregivers, as necessary, regarding oral status and potential for compromised nutritional status
Oral pain/dysfunction	• Provide oral examination to identify oral/mucosal lesions • Document and follow-up on patient complaints of oral pain • Collaborate with patient's healthcare or palliative care team to advocate for dental needs • Train caregivers, as necessary, to provide regular oral inspection and record observations
Trauma	• Monitor patient for signs of abuse and neglect • Monitor/educate about potential for facial/oral trauma during a fall • Educate about protocols for oral injury emergency care
Xerostomia[25,27]	• Identify medications with a potential for causing xerostomia • Eliminate the use of oral products with alcohol, glycerin, or lemon • Educate about using sips of water or ice chips to relieve dryness • Use atomizer to help control the volume of water to avoid pooling or aspiration • Encourage use of over-the-counter saliva substitutes • Recommend use of nonsucrose-containing candies or gums • Train caregiver, as necessary, to identify/treat signs and symptoms
Candidiasis (and other oral infections)[25,27]	• Educate about increased risk with use of prolonged antibiotic therapy • Educate about signs and symptoms of infections • Recommend topical or systemic antifungal treatment • Educate about effect of oral infections on systemic health • Train caregivers, as necessary, to identify/treat signs and symptoms
General oral soreness (mucositis)[25,27]	• Monitor and document active lesions • Educate about daily inspection of tissues and need for immediate care to avoid secondary infections • Select saline mouth rinses, wax- or water-based lubricants, or topical anesthetics for comfort care
Denture problems[25,27]	• Inspect denture or prosthesis and adjacent soft tissue • Educate about exacerbation of oral problems/lesions due to ill-fitting denture • Educate about weight loss impact on fit of denture • Educate about accumulation of pathogenic biofilm on unclean denture • Soft reline material and proper daily care may address acute issues • Denture-induced lesions are described in Chapter 30

IV. Preparation for the Residential Visit

When providing patient care in any situation, the rule is "know before you go." The following steps will help prepare for a homebound patient visit.

A. Understanding the Patient

- Review the patient's medical history. (Hint: Provide the medical history form in advance for patient to complete and return.)
  - Monitor medication lists carefully, especially when the patient takes multiple prescription or over-the-counter preparations.
  - Telephone before visit to clarify responses or ask questions.
- Consider specific characteristics and problems associated with the patient's age, chronic medical condition, medications, mental health status, or physical/cognitive limitations.
  - Section IX reviews considerations for a variety of individuals with special needs.
- Determine precautions necessary for the individual patient's care and safety.
- Arrange with a dentist or attending physician when premedication or other prescription is required.
- Determine need for local anesthesia.

B. Instruments and Equipment

- Routine dental hygiene care can often be provided using manual instruments and without the need for powered equipment.
- Several dental equipment companies (listed in Box 4-3) manufacture portable dental delivery units, suctions, X-ray units, and autoclaves.

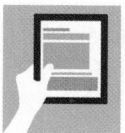

BOX 4-3
Commercial Sources for Portable Equipment

Dental Delivery Systems
A-Dec, Inc.
Website: www.a-dec.com
Toll-free phone: (800) 547-1883

Aseptico
Website: www.aseptico.com
Toll-free phone: (866) 244-2954

ASI Medical, Inc.
Website: www.asimedical.net
Toll-free phone: (800) 566-9953

Bell Dental
Website: www.belldental.com
Toll-free phone: (800) 920-4478

DNTLworks Equipment Corporation
Website: www.dntlworks.com
Toll-free phone: (800) 847-0694

Mobile Dental Systems
Website: www.mobiledentalsystems.com
Toll-free phone: (800) 321-6332

Safari Dental, Inc.
Website: www.safaridental.com
Toll-free phone: (800) 567-0013

Hand-Held X-Ray System
Aribex, Inc.
Website: www.aribex.com
Toll-free phone: (866) 340-5522

Autoclave
Alfa Medical
Website: www.statimsales.com
Toll-free phone: USA: (800) 839-0722

Illuminated Loupes
Orascoptic
Website: www.orascoptic.com
Toll-free phone: (800) 369-3698

PeriOptix, Inc.
Website: www.perioptix.com
Toll-free phone: (800) 445-0345

Suction Toothbrushes
Sage Products, Inc.
Website: www.sageproducts.com
Toll-free phone: (800) 323-2220

Trademark Medical
Website: www.trademarkmedical.com
Toll-free phone: (800) 325-9044

- Covered plastic tubs or boxes, labeled "clean" or "contaminated," are useful for carrying materials.
- The Organization for Safety, Asepsis, and Prevention provides infection control guidelines for safe delivery of oral care outside the dental office.[16]
- Additional equipment and supplies that can be transported by the clinician to the patient's residence are listed in Box 4-4.

C. Appointment Time

- Arrange the dental hygiene visit during a time when the patient is usually awake.
- Coordinate with patient or caregiver to assure visit is scheduled around nursing care and meals.

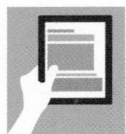

BOX 4-4

Instruments and Equipment to Provide Dental Hygiene Care for Residence-Bound Patients

Personal Protective Equipment

- See Chapter 6

Patient Education/Oral Hygiene Instruction Materials

- Toothbrushes, floss, interdental aids, tongue cleaner
- Denture brush, if needed
- Samples of adaptive aids for demonstration
- Hand mirror
- Written or printed patient education materials
- See Section IX for additional ideas on adaptive practices

Sterile Instruments

- Selection of hand instruments and other items required for patient care (i.e., mouth prop/bite block, sharpening stone, lip retractors)
- Are transported before treatment in the sealed packages in which they were sterilized
- Are transported after use in special plastic containers labeled for contaminated instruments

Disposable Items—Prepared in "Single Treatment" Packages That Are Convenient to Open and Use at Bedside

- Patient bib
- 2 × 2 gauze
- Cotton rolls/applicators
- Lubricant for patient lips

Additional Equipment

- Emesis basin (kidney-shaped basin facilitates the rinsing process)
- Portable headrest (attached to wheelchair or straight back chair to provide head support during treatment)
- A large plastic drape (helpful if patient's coordination is limited during rinsing)

Pharmaceuticals

- Pretreatment mouth rinse (only for patients who can spit)
- Disclosing agent
- Fluoride varnish topical fluoride preparation (varnish)
- **Silver diamine fluoride**[17]

Lighting

- Dental loupe systems with light-emitting diode (LED) headlight offer a direct light source and magnification (Figure 4-1A)

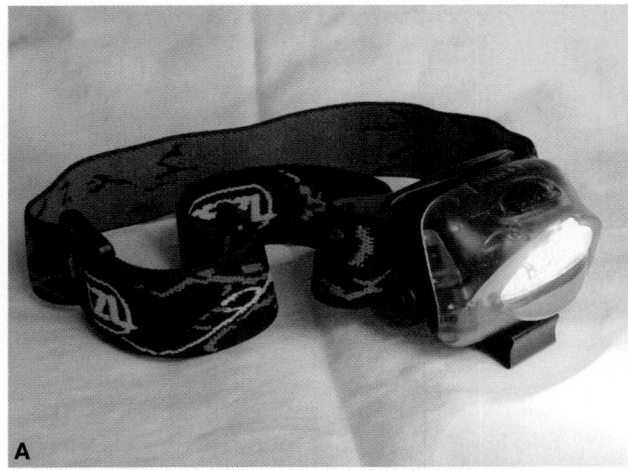

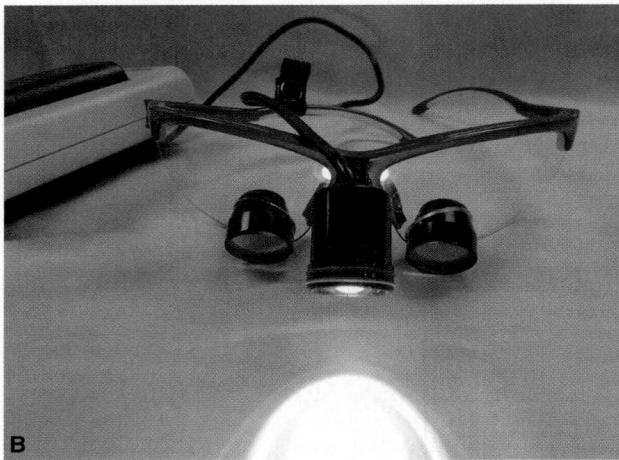

FIGURE 4-1 • Lighting. A: A small light-emitting diode (LED) light with an attached headband, sometimes called a "camping" headlamp. **B:** Safety glasses with loupes and an attached LED headlamp. With either lighting system, the beam can be adjusted so that it is focused directly into the patient's oral cavity.

- Alternatively, a common LED headlamp is a convenient and inexpensive form of light (Figure 4-1B)
- Lighted mouth mirror
- Photography spotlight or gooseneck lamp with narrow, concentrated beam and adequate wattage to facilitate visibility

Miscellaneous Items—Usually Available at the Patient's Home

- Large towels (for covering pillows)
- Pillows (firm enough to assist in maintaining patients' head in stationary position)
- Hospital bed (can be adjusted to position patient most effectively)
- Wheelchair or chair with high back for head support
- Container for prostheses
- Power toothbrush

D. Practice Management

◆ Dental hygienists providing direct access services in a residential setting may be working as a volunteer, employee, independent contractor, and/or business owner.[18] In these cases, the dental hygienist may need to consider the following factors:

- Individual state practice acts[19]; educational requirements, direct access scope of services; practice settings, referral methods
- Provider claim submission; procedures for billing for services provided by a dental hygienist (Health Insurance Portability and Accountability Act: National Provider Identifier number and Healthcare Provider Taxonomy code).
- Payment/reimbursement methods[20]; private insurance, state/federal programs, facility or agency funds, public/private grants
- Tax codes and policies; self-employed individuals, business owners

V. Approach to Patient

The dental hygienist may find approaching a relatively helpless, disabled, or ill person to be difficult. In addition, patients with cognitive disorders or impairments, such as dementia, can exhibit resistance to personal care.[21,22]

A. Communication

◆ Clinician empathy and understanding, as well as good interpersonal and communication skills, can help project a caring attitude toward the patient and put a vulnerable patient at ease.

◆ An oversolicitous attitude may not contribute to development of a cooperative patient relationship; a gentle but firm approach is most successful.

◆ Direct communication with the patient is most appropriate; however, communication with a caregiver may be necessary.

B. Personal Factors

◆ A patient who is comfortable with home-delivered care and aware of the difficulties under which the clinician is working may show significant appreciation.

◆ Establishment of rapport with the patient may depend on whether it was the patient or caregiver who requested/arranged for the appointment.

◆ Cooperation may depend on the patient's attitude toward the illness or disability.

◆ Residence-bound adults dependent on others for care can be at increased risk for abuse, neglect, and exploitation (see Chapter 14).

- Be alert to the signs and symptoms.
- Protocols for mandatory reporting vary by state.

◆ Prolonged illness, suffering, the effects of inactivity, and monotonous confinement can contribute to depression.

- A patient who is depressed may require extra attention to communication (see Chapter 58).

◆ Caring for the cognitively impaired or mentally ill patient can present unique challenges (see Chapters 48 and 58).

C. Suggestions for General Procedure

◆ Request the caregiver to be present to assist as needed and to demonstrate current method of personal daily oral care.

◆ For the safety of the patient, clinician, and others, ask that visitors remain out of the room during treatment.

◆ Introduce each step slowly to be sure patient knows what is being done. Do not make the patient feel rushed.

◆ Listen attentively; socializing is one of the best ways to establish rapport.

◆ Plan multiple appointments when extensive scaling is required to:

- Avoid tiring the patient.
- Observe tissue response.
- Provide encouragement in biofilm control procedures.

VI. Treatment Location

Ingenuity is needed to arrange patient position to provide access for treatment as well as maintain comfort for both the patient and the clinician (Figure 4-2).

A. Patient in Bed

◆ *Hospital bed:* Adjust to lift patient's head to desirable height.

◆ *Ordinary bed, sofa, or cushioned chair:* Use firm pillows to support and stabilize patient's head.

◆ *Small patient:* Positions for biofilm control described in Chapter 51 and shown in Figure 51-12 may be applicable during treatment.

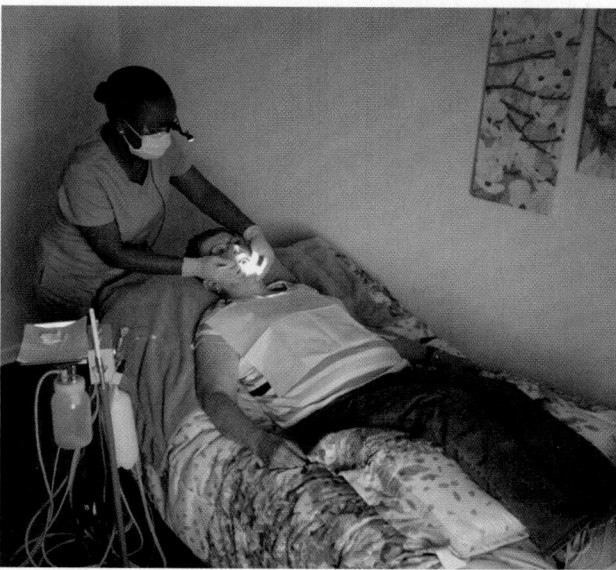

FIGURE 4-2 • A Dental Hygiene Student Provides Patient Care Using a Headlamp and a Portable Dental Unit.

B. Patient in Wheelchair

◆ Kitchen or a large bathroom can provide access to water and counter space.

◆ A portable headrest can be attached to the back of a straight chair or wheelchair (see Chapter 51).

◆ A straight chair or wheelchair can be backed against a wall to provide a stable headrest.

◆ Some wheelchairs tilt or slightly recline to facilitate patient positioning for care (Figure 4-3).

◆ A firm pillow can be inserted between the chair back and the patient's head to provide a cushioned resting surface.

VII. Additional Considerations

In addition to navigating patient treatment in an alternative setting, the unique needs of the residence-bound patient, and practice management matters, additional considerations may include:

◆ The role of the caregiver. Whether professional, family, or friend, the caregiver should be included in the care assessment, planning, and treatment according to the patient preferences and as much as they are able/willing.

◆ Pretreatment site visit. Schedule a time to visit the patient in their residence.

◆ Initial assessment of the environment, patient needs, and business agreement can be discussed before treatment is planned or rendered.

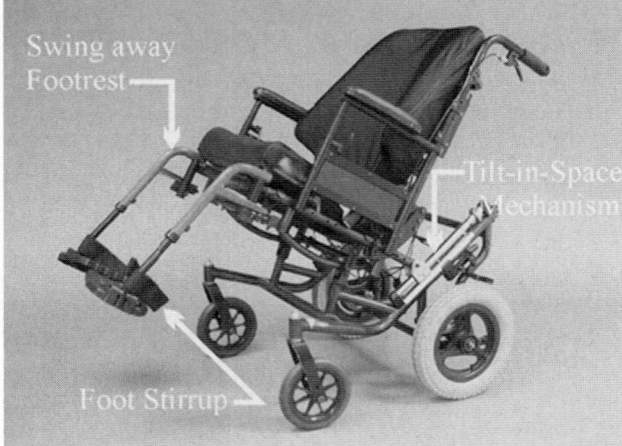

FIGURE 4-3 • A Wheelchair That Is Designed to Tilt Back, Providing Comfort and Easy Access for Dental Care. (From Frontera WR. *DeLisa's Physical Medicine and Rehabilitation.* 5th ed. Philadelphia, PA: Wolters Kluwer Health; 2010.)

VIII. Assessment and Care Planning

As in any patient care setting, dental hygiene interventions are provided using the dental hygiene process of care.

◆ Comprehensive patient *assessment* provides the basis for dental hygiene diagnoses.

◆ The dental hygiene *diagnosis* provides the foundation for planning *treatment* and prevention strategies that meet individualized patient needs.

◆ Follow-up appointments for maintenance and ongoing *evaluation* of the patient's oral condition determine whether treatment goals are met.

◆ Also, the direct access provider *refers* the patient to a dentist or specialist when warranted.

IX. Strategies for Prevention and Management

Table 4-1 identifies special considerations for developing a personalized prevention and management plan for residence-bound individuals.

◆ Additional strategies for preventing poor oral status can include:
  • Training caregivers.
  • Collaborating with members of interprofessional healthcare teams.

THE CRITICALLY ILL OR UNCONSCIOUS PATIENT

Maintenance of oral cleanliness for the acutely ill or unconscious patient requires special procedures and approaches.

◆ When the patient's illness or injury involves the oral cavity, the advice and recommendations of the attending physician and/or oral surgeon are followed.

◆ Effective oral care can reduce the risk of pneumonia by preventing debris and microorganisms in the mouth from being aspirated, particularly in patients who have received mechanical breathing assistance (see Chapter 60).[15,23,24]

The role of the dental hygienist is to evaluate and prioritize the patient's immediate oral care needs and provide appropriate curative or palliative oral care as needed.

◆ Be familiar with the nature of the patient's chronic condition.

◆ Observe the health status of the soft and hard oral tissues.

◆ Address oral pain and infection first.

◆ Determine what type of services will best improve or maintain patient's oral health status without putting undue stress on the patient.

I. Instructions for Caregivers

Personal oral care procedures for the unconscious or disabled patient can be accomplished by a caregiver.

◆ Assess caregiver's willingness and ability to provide daily oral care for the patient.

◆ Encourage and empower caregivers to provide daily oral care.

  • Include hands-on demonstration and practice.

  • For caregivers at a facility, this may include conducting an oral health in-service training program.

A. Patients Who Are Edentulous or Dentulous

◆ Use appropriate precautions when placing fingers in mouth to avoid injury from unintentional biting.

◆ A mouth prop can be placed in one side of the mouth while the other side is being retracted and cleaned.

◆ Gently brush or wipe all surfaces of the mouth (lips, teeth, gingiva, tongue, and oral mucosa) to remove biofilm at least twice a day. This will also prevent sordes.

  • A soft toothbrush or gauze-wrapped finger can be used to wipe the soft tissue.

  • A power toothbrush used with a very light touch or a suction toothbrush may be more efficient and thorough on the hard tissue.

B. Patients with Removable Prosthesis

◆ If dentures or other removable prostheses are present, remove before providing oral care.

  • Often hospital policy requires removal of dentures when a patient is unconscious.

◆ Procedure for removing dentures is described in Chapter 30.

◆ When the dentures are removed:

  • Instruct the caregiver to clean and mark them as described in Chapter 30.

  • Instruct the caregiver to change the water or liquid denture cleaner daily to prevent bacterial growth.

II. Toothbrush with Suction Attachment

A specialized, single-use toothbrush often used with patients who have difficulty swallowing or spitting.

◆ Tubing is connected from the end of a hollow toothbrush handle to an aspirator outlet or portable suction unit (Figure 4-4).

◆ During caregiver training, procedure for use is demonstrated and included in an oral care procedures manual.

◆ See Box 4-5 for instructions on how to use a suction toothbrush.

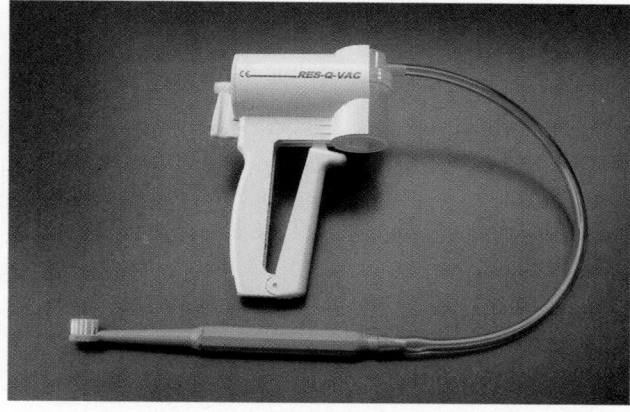

FIGURE 4-4 • **Commercial Suction Toothbrush.** Plak-Vac/Res-Q-Vac combination features the Plak-Vac oral suction evacuator brush with the Res-Q-Vac hand-powered suction system. (Trademark Medical, St. Louis, MO.)

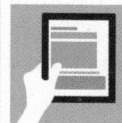

BOX 4-5
Procedure for Use of Suction Toothbrush

• Prepare the patient.

• Although not able to respond in a usual manner, the patient may be aware of what is going on.

• Tell patient that the teeth are going to be brushed, and thereafter maintain a one-way conversation despite patient's inability to respond verbally.

• Turn patient on the side and place a pillow at the back for support.

• Place a small towel behind the patient's head and an emesis basin under patient's chin.

• Follow routine infection control and personal protective equipment guidelines.

• Attach toothbrush to suction outlet and lay brush on towel near patient's mouth.

• Place a rubber bite block on one side of the patient's mouth between the posterior teeth. Floss tied to the bite block is fastened to patient's clothing with a safety pin.

• Dip brush in nonalcoholic, fluoridated mouth rinse or chlorhexidine; do not use toothpaste.

• Turn on suction.

• Gently retract lip and carefully apply the appropriate toothbrushing procedures; apply suction over each tooth surface with particular care at each interproximal area. Remoisten brush frequently.

• Move bite block to opposite side of mouth and continue brushing procedure.

• After brushing, place brush in a cup of clear water and allow water to be sucked through to clear and clean the tube.

• Remove bite block, wipe patient's lips, and apply a water-based lubricant.

• Rinse and disinfect toothbrush; sterilize bite block.

THE TERMINALLY ILL PATIENT

The major difference in providing dental hygiene care for a terminally ill patient is a focus on short-term palliative care rather than long-term preventive care.[25]

◆ Terminal illness is no excuse for neglect of oral cleanliness; daily personal oral hygiene care is essential.

◆ Emphasis is on symptom relief and a clean oral environment, which can:
  • Enhance the patient's sense of dignity.
  • Improve quality of life no matter how brief the life is to be.[13]

◆ The dental hygienist is in an ideal position to be a member of an interdisciplinary palliative care team.

I. Objectives of Care

The role of the dental hygienist is to provide oral care that emphasizes patient comfort more than preventive or restorative aspects of care. This may include:

◆ Providing relief of painful or aggravating symptoms of oral disease or lesions.

◆ Preventing aspiration of debris and oral microorganisms and reduce risk for pneumonia.

◆ Providing a "clean mouth" environment to reduce malodor and improve appearance and enhance personal interaction with caregivers and family members.

◆ Educating patients and caregivers about the importance of daily oral care.

◆ Helping develop standardized protocols for daily oral care as an integral part of the patient's overall palliative care treatment plan.

II. General Mouth Care Considerations

Poor oral hygiene is a common problem among terminally ill patients. Attention to mouth care and management of pain are essential components of providing end-of-life care.

A. Cleanliness

◆ Gentle but thorough daily cleaning of teeth, tongue, and oral mucosa is necessary.

◆ Provide oral care in any way the patient will allow, using soft toothbrush, gauze, or cloth.

◆ Dentifrice or other oral products are not necessary, but can add a refreshing flavor that the patient may like. Use caution as some products can cause irritation or create a burning sensation on already fragile tissues.

◆ Be mindful of the patient's limited swallow function or spitting ability.

B. Common Oral Conditions

◆ Xerostomia: Common among terminally ill individuals due to medications, dehydration, or mouth breathing.[26] Work with palliative care team to minimize medications that increase xerostomia.[27]

◆ Candidiasis infection: Oral cultures of *Candida albicans* were found in as many as 79% of terminally ill patients. In immunocompromised individuals, the infection can become life-threatening.[26]

◆ General oral soreness (mucositis): Approximately 75% of hospice patients examined in one study had evidence of pathologic changes in the oral mucosa, and 42% reported soreness of the oral mucosa.[26]

◆ Denture problems: More than 70% of hospice patients who wore dentures reported having some kind of difficulty wearing their dentures.[26]

C. Visual Inspection

◆ Frequent inspection of the patient's mouth is necessary to identify oral lesions that can cause discomfort or lead to serious infection.

◆ Use a pen light or small flashlight and soft handle of toothbrush to examine the oral cavity.

DOCUMENTATION

Key concepts for documenting dental hygiene care provided in alternative settings include:

◆ Description of location where treatment is provided.

◆ Description of the patient's current health status and functional ability, particularly related to ability to provide self-care.

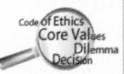

EVERYDAY ETHICS

Elena is 55 years old and is dying of esophageal cancer. She has been involved in an outpatient hospice program and receives all medical services in her home. Elena's daughter contacts the dental office of Dr. Gray and asks if someone can please come to the house and check her mother's teeth because they have not been able to help her brush every day and Elena's gums are bleeding.

Sandy, the dental hygienist in the practice, offers to go and provide whatever "comfort care" she can for Elena.

Questions for Consideration

1. What legal and ethical concerns need to be addressed before going to Elena's home since care will be limited?

2. Reviewing the principle of justice, if Elena's homebound status prevents her from accessing dental care, what options can the dental team offer to her at this time?

3. Describe several core values (Chapter 1, Box 1-6) that can be exhibited by the dental team to benefit this patient.

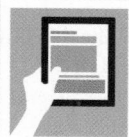

BOX 4-6

Example Documentation:
Bedside Oral Care for Patient in a Nursing Home

S—Routine nursing home visit for continuing care. The 89-year-old female patient is confined to a hospital bed, comfortable and alert; arm strength notably weakened since last visit and she is distressed that she can no longer support her own toothbrush for daily oral care. Nurse aide caregiver has been trying to assist but doesn't know how. Patient states: "Every time she tries to brush my teeth she chokes me or hurts my gums."

O—Excessive dental biofilm noted on facial surfaces of maxillary molars.

A—Patient can no longer engage independently, causing increased risk of oral infection and subsequent increased risk of systemic effects. Caregiver needs training to provide efficient, effective, and comfortable intraoral brushing.

P—Discussed benefits of daily oral biofilm removal. Demonstrated effective oral care. Assured both patient and caregiver that oral care can be provided without discomfort. Demonstrated and supervised caregiver providing bedside oral care and biofilm removal with soft child-sized toothbrush.

Next steps: Follow-up visit scheduled with patient and caregiver in 2 weeks.

Signed: _____, RDH

Date: _____

- Notation of whether or not caregiver assistance is needed/available for daily oral care.
- Summary of oral health assessment data.
- Specific recommendations/education for oral care techniques and adjunct oral hygiene aids.
- Details of dental hygiene interventions/services provided.
- Recommendations for follow-up care and referrals made.
- A sample documentation can be found in Box 4-6.

Factors to Teach the Patient

▶ Good oral health contributes to good general health and better quality of life.

▶ Dental caries is preventable through effective daily oral care and limited consumption of sugary food and drink, especially between meals.

▶ How to use customized adaptive oral care aids to facilitate patient's independence.

Factors to Teach the Caregiver

▶ Consider personal safety of caregiver and patient: environment, biting, infection control.

▶ Care for the patient's natural teeth and gums.

▶ Evaluate and address unique patient needs, adapt care as needed (Section IX).

▶ Care for the patient's removable and nonremovable prosthesis (Chapter 30).

▶ Offer food and drink that are not cariogenic.

▶ How to use a suction toothbrush, power brush, or other device that can mean better oral care for the patient.

ENHANCE YOUR UNDERSTANDING

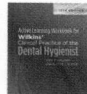

ONLINE RESOURCES
(see the inside front cover for access information)

- Audio glossary
- Appendices

SUPPORT FOR LEARNING
(available separately)

- *Active Learning Workbook for Wilkins' Clinical Practice of the Dental Hygienist, 13th Edition*

INDIVIDUALIZED REVIEW

- Customized practice quizzing with Navigate 2 TestPrep for *Wilkins' Clinical Practice of the Dental Hygienist*

References

1. Gluzman R, Meeker H, Agarwal P, et al. Oral health status and needs of homebound elderly in an urban home-based primary care service. *Spec Care Dentist.* 2013;33(5):218-226.

2. American Dental Hygienists' Association. Advocacy: practice issues: direct access. http://www.adha.org/direct-access. Accessed July 19, 2017.

3. Smith BJ, Ghezzi EM, Manz MC, et al. Perceptions of oral health adequacy and access in Michigan nursing facilities. *Gerodontology.* 2008;25(2):89-98.

4. Strayer MS. Perceived barriers to oral health care among the homebound. *Spec Care Dentist.* 1995;15(3):113-118.

5. Willink A, Schoen C, Davis K. Dental care and Medicare beneficiaries: access gaps, cost burdens, and policy options. *Health Affairs.* 2016;35(12):2241-2248.

6. Rodriguez TE, Galka AL, Lacy ES, et al. Can Midlevel dental providers be a benefit to the American public? *J Health Care Poor Underserved.* 2013;24(2):892-906.

7. Langelier M, Continelli T, Baker B, Surdu S. Expanded scopes of practice for dental hygienists associated with improved oral health outcomes for adults. *Health Affairs.* 2016;35(12):2207-2215.

8. Langelier M, Baker B, Continelli T. *Development of a New Dental Hygiene Professional Practice Index by State.* Rensselaer, NY: Oral Health Workforce Research Center, Center for Health Workforce Studies, School of Public Health, SUNY Albany; 2016:152.

9. Smith BJ, Ghezzi EM, Manz MC, et al. Oral healthcare access and adequacy in alternative long-term care facilities. *Spec Care Dentist.* 2010;30(3):85-94.

10. Chen X, Clark JJ, Naorungroj S. Oral health in nursing home residents with different cognitive statuses. *Gerodontology.* 2013;30(1):49-60.

11. U.S. Government Printing Office. Electronic code of federal regulations (Title 42: Public Health, Part 483—requirements for states and long term care facilities, Subpart B, Section 483.55, dental services). http://www.ecfr.gov/cgi-bin/text-idx?c=ecfr;sid=b97291f05d23f16ffa8e711922642bcc;rgn=div5;view=text;node=42%3A5.0.1.1.2;idno=42;cc=ecfr. Accessed July 14, 2017.

12. Medicaid.gov. Medicaid: dental care. https://www.medicaid.gov/medicaid/benefits/dental/index.html. Accessed July 14, 2017.

13. Fischer DJ, Epstein JB, Yao Y, et al. Oral health conditions affect functional and social activities of terminally ill cancer patients. *Support Care Cancer.* 2014;22(3):803-810.

14. Mercadante S, Aielli F, Adile C, et al. Prevalence of oral mucositis, dry mouth, and dysphagia in advanced cancer patients. *Support Care Cancer.* 2015;23(11):3249-3255.

15. Linden GJ, Lyons A, Scannapieco FA. Periodontal systemic associations: review of the evidence. *J Clin Periodontol.* 2013;84(40 suppl):S8-S19.

16. Organization for Safety, Asepsis and Prevention. Atlanta, GA: Organization for Safety, Asepsis and Prevention; Safe delivery of oral care outside the dental office. http://www.osap.org/?page=PortableMobile. Accessed July 14, 2017.

17. Horst J, Ellenikiotis H, Milgrom PM. UCSF protocol for caries arrest using silver diamine fluoride: rationale, indications, and consent. *J Calif Dent Assoc.* 2016;44(1):16-28.

18. Naughton D. Expanding oral care opportunities: direct access care provided by dental hygienists in the United States. *J Evid Based Dent Pract.* 2014;14 suppl:171-182.

19. American Dental Hygienists' Association. Scope of practice. http://www.adha.org/scope-of-practice. Accesses July 14, 2017.

20. American Dental Hygienists' Association. Reimbursement. https://www.adha.org/reimbursement. Accessed July 14, 2017.

21. Jablonski R, Therrien B, Mahoney EK, et al. An intervention to reduce care-resistant behaviors in persons with dementia during oral hygiene: a pilot study. *Spec Care Dentist.* 2011;31(3):77-88.

22. Ahn H, Horgas AL. Disruptive behaviors in nursing home residents with dementia: management approaches. *J Clin Outcomes Manag.* 2013;20(12):566-576.

23. Shi Z, Xie H, Wang P, et al. Oral Hygiene care for critically ill patients to prevent ventilator-associated pneumonia. *Cochrane Database Syst Rev.* 2013;(8):CD008367.

24. Quinn B, Baker DL, Cohen S, et al. Basic nursing care to prevent nonventilator hospital-acquired pneumonia. *J Nurs Scholarsh.* 2014;46(1):11-19.

25. Bhavana S, Lakshmi CR, Mpv P, et al. Palliative dental care. *J Clin Diagn Res.* 2014;8(6):1-6.

26. Aldred MJ, Addy M, Bagg J, et al. Oral health in the terminally ill: a cross-sectional pilot survey. *Spec Care Dentist.* 1991;11(2):59-62.

27. Jucan AC, Saunders RH. Maintaining oral health in palliative care patients. *Ann Longterm Care.* 2015;23(9):15-20.

Preparation for Dental Hygiene Practice

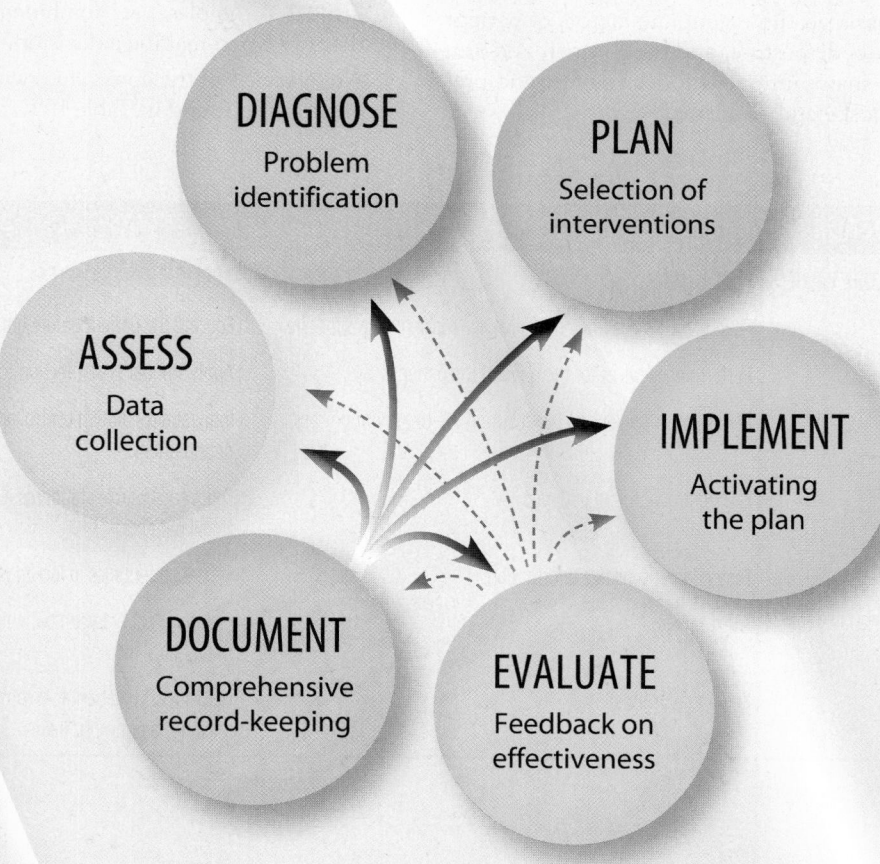

FIGURE II-1 • The Dental Hygiene Process of Care.

DIAGNOSE
Problem
identification

PLAN
Selection of
interventions

ASSESS
Data
collection

IMPLEMENT
Activating
the plan

DOCUMENT
Comprehensive
record-keeping

EVALUATE
Feedback on
effectiveness

INTRODUCTION FOR SECTION II

Preparation for dental hygiene care is centered on the use of standard precautions for infection control to ensure the comfort and safety of patients, dental personnel, and others who come in contact with the environment of the clinic or office.

◆ Health services facilities, including dental facilities, must be places for cure and prevention, not for increasing risk of disease or discomfort following inadequate precautionary measures and habits of the professional personnel.

◆ The responsibility of the entire team is to develop and maintain work practices for all appointments that will:
  • Prevent direct or indirect cross-infection between dental personnel and patients and from one patient to another.
  • Maintain comfort for both the patient and the oral health provider.

◆ Chapters in this section:
  • Provide specific information about the chain of infection and the microorganisms that can be transmitted in the dental setting when standard precautions are not observed.
  • Describe specific materials and procedures necessary for safe clinical practice. The Centers for Disease Control and Prevention Guidelines for *Infection Control in Dental Health-Care Settings* can be found on the online resource.
  • Place emphasis on the ergonomic factors of patient positioning; body posture; and hand, wrist, and arm positions to maintain practitioner comfort and prevent musculoskeletal problems.

THE DENTAL HYGIENE PROCESS OF CARE

Preparation for clinical practice does not form a specific step in the Dental Hygiene Process of Care (Figure II-1); however, practices described in this section protect the patient and the practitioner and are part of all the components of the process.

ETHICAL APPLICATIONS

◆ A dental hygienist may be involved in a variety of moral, ethical, and legal situations during all professional actions related to the process of care.

◆ A goal of preparation for dental hygiene practice is to increase awareness of, and sensitivity to, potential ethical situations.

◆ Basic core values and principles, as outlined in the various *Dental Hygiene Codes of Ethics* on the online resource, are applied in every phase of the dental hygiene appointment.

◆ Basic core values in dental hygiene are identified as selected principles of ethical behavior that can be considered integral to the code of the dental hygiene profession.

◆ Ethical principles contained in the codes clarify the standards of judgment that professionals will follow.

◆ Ethical principles are combined with philosophical theories when making a decision.

◆ An overview of the core values with definitions and applications is found in Table II-1.

TABLE II-1 • Dental Hygiene Core Values

ETHICAL PRINCIPLE/CORE VALUE	EXPLANATION	APPLICATION EXAMPLES
Autonomy	Patient's right to self-determination and making choices for care.	Educate the patient before obtaining informed consent.
Beneficence	Performing services for the good of the patient.	Apply standards of infection control for all patients.
Nonmaleficence	Removing or preventing harm during the treatment process.	Individualize biofilm control and perform subgingival debridement.
Justice	Fair treatment for all patients.	Follow acceptable standards and provide access to care for all patients.
Confidentiality	Protection of sensitive information.	Secure patient files in locked cabinets.
Veracity	Truth-telling.	Develop trust between patient and provider to obtain the medical history.
Fidelity	Keeping promises.	Help a fearful patient feel comfortable by using local anesthesia or nitrous oxide.

5

Infection Control: Transmissible Diseases

Katherine Soal, RDH, MSDH

CHAPTER OUTLINE

STANDARD PRECAUTIONS
I. Definition
II. Additional Transmission-Based Precautions

MICROORGANISMS OF THE ORAL CAVITY
I. Origin
II. Infection Potential
III. Cross-Contamination

THE INFECTIOUS PROCESS
I. Essential Features for Disease Transmission
II. Airborne Infection
III. Prevention of Transmission

PATHOGENS TRANSMISSIBLE FROM THE ORAL CAVITY

TUBERCULOSIS
I. Transmission
II. Clinical Management

VIRAL HEPATITIS
I. Hepatitis B
II. Hepatitis C
III. Hepatitis D Virus

HUMAN HERPESVIRUS DISEASES
I. General Characteristics
II. Relation to Periodontal Infections
III. Clinical Management for HHVs

HUMAN PAPILLOMAVIRUS

HIV/AIDS INFECTION
I. Transmission
II. HIV Testing for Diagnosis and Staging of Infection
III. Oral Manifestations of HIV Infection
IV. Prevention and Treatment of HIV Infection
V. Dental Hygiene Management

METHICILLIN-RESISTANT *STAPHYLOCOCCUS AUREUS*

DOCUMENTATION

EVERYDAY ETHICS

FACTORS TO TEACH THE PATIENT

REFERENCES

LEARNING OBJECTIVES

After studying this chapter, the student will be able to:

1. Apply the concept of standard precautions to the process of dental hygiene care.

2. Describe the infectious disease process and prevention of disease transmission.

3. Describe and identify transmissible diseases that may pose a risk to patients and dental healthcare personnel.

4. Evaluate the oral healthcare needs of each patient with transmissible disease(s).

For healthcare providers, infection and communicable disease can lead to illness, disability, and loss of work time. In addition, patients, family members, and community contacts can become exposed, may become ill, and lose productive time or suffer permanent aftereffects.

◆ In oral healthcare practice, the objective is to protect patients, dental healthcare personnel (DHCP), and others who may become exposed to infectious agents in the clinical environment.

◆ Health services facilities, including dental facilities, are places for cure and prevention, not for dissemination of disease due to inadequate precautionary measures and habits of the professional personnel.

◆ The first responsibility of the entire dental team is to organize and maintain a system for the disinfection, sterilization, and care of instruments and equipment.

◆ The second step is to develop and maintain work practices for all appointments that will prevent direct or indirect cross-infections between dental personnel and patients and from one patient to another.

STANDARD PRECAUTIONS

I. Definition[1,2]

◆ Standard precautions represent a standard of care to protect healthcare providers and their patients from pathogens spread by body fluids.

◆ Apply to all patients.

◆ Apply to contact with the following:
  • Blood.
  • Saliva.
  • All body fluids, secretions, and excretions (except sweat), regardless of whether they contain blood.
  • Nonintact (broken) skin.
  • Mucous membranes.

II. Additional Transmission-Based Precautions

◆ Droplet precautions
  • Respiratory or mucous membrane contact transmitted through airborne droplets (sneezing, coughing).
  • Examples: *Mycobacterium tuberculosis*, influenza virus, chickenpox virus.

◆ Contact precautions
  • Reduce risk of transmission of organisms and specific diseases by direct skin or indirect contact.
  • Examples: Vancomycin-resistant enterococci, methicillin-resistant *Staphylococcus aureus* (MRSA)

◆ Airborne precautions
  • Reduce risk of airborne transmission of infectious agents by droplet nuclei.

• Special air handling and ventilation required.
• Examples: *Legionella pneumophila*, M. *tuberculosis*.

◆ Sharps precautions
  • Reduce risk of bloodborne pathogen transmission and infection by percutaneous sharps injury.
  • Examples: Hepatitis B virus (HBV) and hepatitis C virus (HCV), human immunodeficiency virus (HIV)

MICROORGANISMS OF THE ORAL CAVITY

I. Origin

◆ In utero, the oral cavity is sterile, but after birth within a few hours to 1 day, a simple oral flora develops.[3,4]

◆ Microorganisms are transmitted to the infant from the mother and other family members or caretakers.

◆ As the infant grows, there is continuing introduction of microorganisms that are normal for an adult oral cavity. The microbiota of the adult is very complex.[5]

◆ Many of the salivary bacteria come from the dorsum of the tongue, but some are from mucous membranes and gingival/periodontal tissues.

◆ High counts of total microorganisms are found in dental biofilm, periodontal pockets, and carious lesions.

II. Infection Potential

◆ Intact mucous membranes of the oral cavity provide some protection against infection.
  • Pathogenic (disease-producing), potentially pathogenic, or nonpathogenic microorganisms may be present in the oral cavity of each patient.
  • Patients may be carriers of certain diseases but show no signs or symptoms (asymptomatic carrier).
  • Pathogenic organisms may be transient.

◆ Inadvertent transmission to subsequent susceptible patients or to dental personnel may occur because of inappropriate work practices, such as:
  • Careless handwashing.
  • Unhygienic personal habits.
  • Inadequate sterilization and handling of sterile instruments and materials.

III. Cross-Contamination

◆ Spread of microorganisms from one source to another: person to person, or person to an inanimate object and then to another person.

◆ Recognition of the possible transfer of infection in a dental practice or clinic provides a basis for planning the system of disinfection, sterilization, and management of instruments and equipment.

THE INFECTIOUS PROCESS

I. Essential Features for Disease Transmission

A chain of events is required for the spread of an infectious agent. The six essential links are shown in Figure 5-1 and described here.

◆ An *infectious agent* such as:
  • Bacteria, viruses, fungi, rickettsia, protozoa.
  • Each infectious agent has its own specific reaction in an infected host.

◆ A *reservoir* where the infectious agents are found in their own essential environment, which may be instruments, a dental unit waterline, or human cells or blood.
  • For example, a dental unit waterline is a potential reservoir for *L. pneumophila*, and humans are reservoirs for herpetic infections.

◆ A *port of exit* or mode of escape from the reservoir.
  • Infectious agents exit from their reservoir(s) through various modes, such as coughing, bleeding periodontium, dental needle use, or in water from a contaminated waterline.

◆ A *mode of transmission*
  • May be direct as in person to person, or indirect by contaminated hands or a dental needle.
  • Transmission by droplet may be direct from the respiratory tract of one person to the oral cavity of the receiving host by coughing or sneezing, or indirect by transfer to hands or instruments and then to the receiving host.

◆ A *port of entry* or mode of entry of the infectious agent into the new host.
  • Modes of entry may be similar to modes of escape.
  • Examples: the respiratory tract, eyes, mucous membranes, nonintact periodontium or skin, or needle stick.

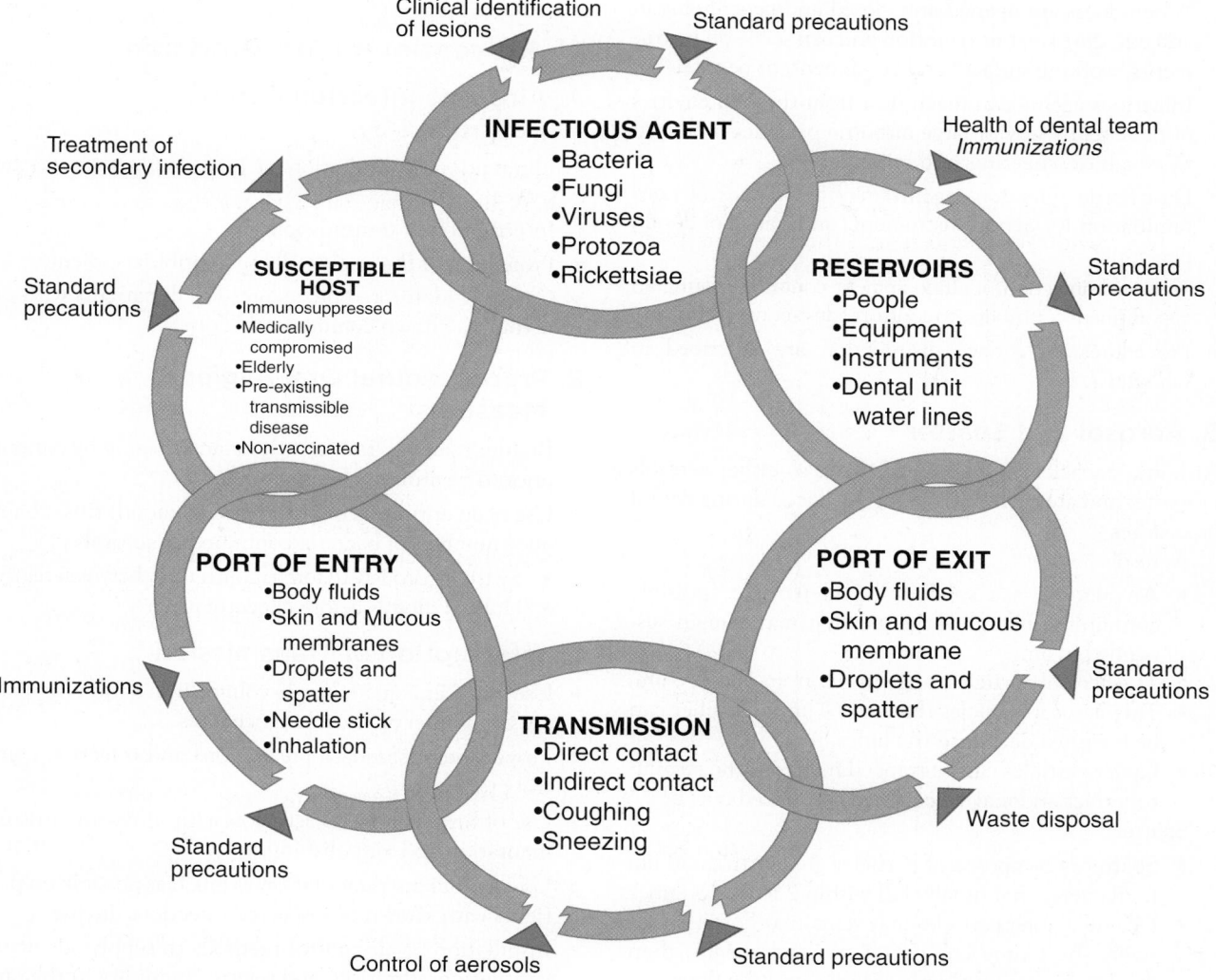

FIGURE 5-1 • Interventions to Break the Chain of Disease Transmission. A break in the chain of six major links is required to stop the spread of an infectious agent. Standard precautions are applied to interrupt the chain.

◆ A **susceptible host** that does not have **immunity** or defense to the invading infectious agent such as:
  • A patient taking an immunosuppressant drug to control autoimmune diseases such as psoriasis and rheumatoid arthritis, prevent solid organ transplant rejection, and cancer chemotherapy.
  • A patient who has not had or has not maintained recommended vaccinations or does not sero-convert after vaccination.
  • A patient who is medically compromised, elderly, or has a preexisting transmissible disease.

II. Airborne Infection

A. Dust-Borne Infectious Agents

◆ *Clostridium tetani* (tetanus bacillus) and enteric bacteria are among the infectious agents that may travel in dust brought in from outside and move in and about dental treatment areas.

◆ When doors are opened and closed and people pass in and out, dust is set into motion and can settle on instruments, working surfaces and equipment, or people.

◆ Infectious agents can reach dust from the oral cavities of patients by way of large airborne particles produced by coughing, sneezing, and talking.

◆ Dust-borne infectious agents may be sources of contamination for dental instruments and hands of dental personnel.

◆ Surface disinfection of all equipment contacted during an appointment contributes to control of dust-borne pathogens.

◆ Procedures for surface disinfection are described in Chapter 7.

B. Aerosol and Spatter[6,7]

Airborne particles are classified by size as either aerosols or spatter and are constantly being produced during dental procedures.

◆ Aerosols
  • An aerosol is a solid or liquid particle (possibly containing infectious agents) that may remain suspended in air.
  • The aerosol particles range in size from 1 to 100 μm.
  • Tiny aerosol particles that are 10 μm or smaller can be breathed deep into the lungs.
  • Larger particles can be trapped higher in the respiratory tract and may be coughed or sneezed out.

◆ Spatter
  • Spatter is composed of particles greater than 50 μm in diameter that usually fall within 2 feet of origin.[3]
  • Heavier, larger particles may remain airborne a relatively short time because of size and weight, then drop or spatter on objects, people, and the floor.
  • Spatter may be visible, particularly after it has landed on skin, hair, clothing, or environmental surfaces where gross contamination can result.
  • Spatter may come in direct contact with mucous membranes of the eyes, nose, and mouth.

◆ Origin of aerosols and spatter
  • Produced during all intraoral procedures, including examination and treatment.
  • Produced by air spray, air–water spray, hand piece activity, air polishing, and ultrasonic scaling.

◆ Aerosols and spatter may contain:
  • Single or clumps of infectious agents such as *Staphylococcus* and *Streptococcus* species, M. *tuberculosis*, and viruses.
  • Tooth and restoration fragments, tissue, saliva, biofilm, blood, sputum, oil from hand pieces, and water from dental unit waterlines.

◆ Concentration and distribution of aerosols and spatter:
  • Aerosols and spatter are in greater concentration close to the site of instrumentation.
  • Aerosols travel with air currents and may move from room to room.
  • Spatter may be distributed on clothing, equipment, instruments, and hands and may be transferred to all areas of the dental office.

III. Prevention of Transmission

A. Airborne Infection Can Be Controlled by:

◆ Elimination or limitation of infectious agents at the source.

◆ Interruption of transmission.

◆ Protection of the potentially susceptible recipient.

◆ Carefully monitored procedures for all patients with or without a known communicable disease.

B. Preprocedural Oral Hygiene Measures[7]

◆ Biofilm removal: toothbrushing and flossing by patient prior to beginning of appointment.

◆ Use of an antiseptic or antimicrobial mouth rinse to reduce numbers of bacteria contained in aerosols.
  • Swish vigorously to force mouth rinse between teeth.
  • Hold in mouth before expectorating.

C. Interruption of Transmission

◆ Use a rubber dam and high-volume evacuation for sealants and other applicable procedures.

◆ Proper use of standard precautions and infection control protocols.

◆ Use of high-volume evacuation with ultrasonic instrumentation and air polishing.

◆ Use manual instrumentation as much as possible on patients with known or suspected infectious disease.

◆ Installation of air-control methods to supply adequate ventilation, filtration, and relative humidity in the operatory area.

D. Clean Water[1,2,8]

◆ Use water that meets Environmental Protection Agency regulatory standards for drinking water (less than 500 CFU [colony-forming units]/mL of heterotrophic water bacteria).

◆ Waterlines must be flushed for at least 20–30 seconds between patients to reduce cross-contamination.[1,8]

◆ Flushing dental waterlines clears planktonic microorganisms; however, the effects are transient.

◆ Additional methods to prevent and treat dental waterline biofilm are needed to assure treatment water quality.[8]
  • Self-contained water systems.
  • Chemical treatments.
  • In-line water filters.
  • Antiretraction devices to prevent backflow.

E. Protection of Clinician

◆ Use personal protective equipment as described in Chapter 6.

◆ Check and maintain personal immunizations.

F. Protection of Patient

◆ Use protective eyewear to prevent direct spatter and aerosols to face and eyes.

G. Maintain and Review Infection Control Protocols

◆ Utilize recommendations described in Chapters 6 and 7

◆ The CDC Guidelines are available on the online resource.

PATHOGENS TRANSMISSIBLE FROM THE ORAL CAVITY

◆ Selected pathogens that may be transmitted by way of the oral cavity and their disease manifestations, mode of transfer, incubation periods, and communicability periods are provided in Table 5-1.

◆ Pathogens are often present within the oral cavity without producing oral signs or symptoms, a fact of particular importance to the total consideration of prevention of disease transmission.

◆ Tuberculosis (TB), viral hepatitis, herpetic infections, and acquired immunodeficiency syndrome (HIV/AIDS) are included in this chapter because of the special problems they create in personal and patient care.

TABLE 5-1 • Infectious Diseases Transmissible from the Oral Cavity

INFECTIOUS AGENT	DISEASE OR CONDITION	ROUTE OR MODE OF TRANSMISSION	INCUBATION PERIOD	COMMUNICABLE PERIOD	VACCINE
HIV	HIV infection (AIDS)	Blood and blood products (infected IV needles) Sexual contact Transplacental and perinatal	To detectable antibodies: <1 mo To disease diagnosis: <1–8 y or more	From asymptomatic through life	Vaccine in progress Pre- and postexposure medications available
HBV	Type B hepatitis "serum" hepatitis	Blood Saliva and all body fluids Sexual contact Perinatal	60–150 d (average 90 d)	Carrier state: indefinite	Yes
HCV	Type C hepatitis	Percutaneous exposure to blood and blood products (infected IV needles) Transplacental and perinatal	2 wk–6 mo (average 6–9 wk)	1 wk before onset of symptoms, persists in most persons indefinitely Carrier state: indefinite	Vaccine in progress
Delta hepatitis virus (HDV) Delta agent	Delta hepatitis	Coinfection with HBV Blood Sexual contacts Perinatal	2–8 wk	All phases of active infection	HBV vaccine
Hepatitis E virus (HEV) ET-NANB	Type E hepatitis Enterically transmitted non-A, non-B	Fecal–oral Contaminated water Consumption of infected animals	15–60 d (average 40 d)	Unknown	No
Herpes simplex virus Type 1 (HSV-1) Type 2 (HSV-2)	Acute herpetic gingivostomatitis Herpes labialis Ocular herpes Herpetic whitlow Genital herpes	Saliva Direct contact (lip, hand) Indirect contact (on objects, limited survival) Sexual contact	2–20 d (average 6 d)	Labialis: 1 d before lesions are crusted Acute stomatitis: 7 wk after recovery Viral shedding in saliva 1–4 d Asymptomatic infection: with viral shedding Reactivation period: with viral shedding	No

(Continues)

TABLE 5-1 • Infectious Diseases Transmissible from the Oral Cavity (*Continued*)

INFECTIOUS AGENT	DISEASE OR CONDITION	ROUTE OR MODE OF TRANSMISSION	INCUBATION PERIOD	COMMUNICABLE PERIOD	VACCINE
HPV	Genital warts Cervical cancer Anogenital cancer Oropharyngeal cancer Recurrent respiratory papillomatosis	Sexual contact	2–3 mo	Contagious for life	Vaccine available for types 6, 11, 16, 18
VZV (HHV-3)	Chicken pox (varicella) Shingles (zoster)	Chicken pox: direct and indirect contact, airborne droplet Shingles: reactivation of HHV-3	10–21 d Average 14–16 d	1–2 d prior to onset of rash until all vesicles are crusted of vesicles	Yes
EBV (HHV-4)	Infectious mononucleosis Oral hairy leukoplakia	Direct contact Saliva	4–6 wk	Prolonged Pharyngeal excretion up to 1 y after infection	No
CMV (HHV-5)	Neonatal CMV infection Cytomegaloviral disease	Perinatal Direct contact (most body secretions) Blood transfusion Organ transplantation Saliva	3–12 wk postpartum 2–4 wk after transfusion or transplant	Months to years	No
Mycobacterium tuberculosis	Tuberculosis	Droplet nuclei Sputum Saliva	3–8 wk, occasionally 12 wk Latency decades or indefinite	As long as viable bacilli are discharged in sputum	BCG (Bacille Calmette-Guérin) has limited efficacy approx. 15 y
Corynebacterium diphtheriae	Diphtheria	Direct and indirect	2–5 d	4 wk if no treatment; 3 d after antibiotic treatment started	Yes
Treponema pallidum	Syphilis Congenital syphilis	Direct contact Transplacental	10 d–3 mo (average 21 d)	Variable and indefinite 2–4 y	No
Neisseria gonorrhoeae	Gonorrhea Gonococcal pharyngitis	Direct contact Indirect (short survival of organisms)	2–5 d	May be subclinical and continue for months and years if untreated	No
Bordetella pertussis	Whooping cough Pertussis	Direct contact with discharges	up to 3 wk (average 7–10 d)	Untreated: 3 wk after paroxysmal cough Treated: 5 d after antibiotic started	Yes
Mumps virus (paramyxovirus)	Infectious parotitis (mumps)	Direct contact (saliva) Airborne droplet	14–25 d (average 18 d)	From 1 wk before parotid swelling until 5 d after swelling	Yes
Poliovirus types 1, 2, 3	Poliomyelitis	Direct contact (saliva) Droplet Fecal–oral	7–14 d	As long as virus is secreted, most infectious 7–10 d before and after onset of symptoms	Yes

TABLE 5-1 • Infectious Diseases Transmissible from the Oral Cavity (*Continued*)

INFECTIOUS AGENT	DISEASE OR CONDITION	ROUTE OR MODE OF TRANSMISSION	INCUBATION PERIOD	COMMUNICABLE PERIOD	VACCINE
Influenza viruses (A, B, C)	Influenza	Nasal discharge Respiratory droplets	Average 7–67 hr Type A average 34 hr Type B average 14 hr	1 d before symptoms Peaks 1–2 d after Can last for 7 d	Yes
Measles virus (Morbillivirus)	Rubeola (measles)	Direct contact Saliva Airborne droplet	7–18 d (average 10 d) to fever, 14 d to rash	Few days before fever to 4 d after rash appears	Yes
Rubella virus (Togavirus)	Rubella (German measles) Congenital rubella syndrome	Nasopharyngeal secretions Direct contact Airborne droplets Maternal infection first trimester	13–20 d	From 1 wk before to 5 d after rash appears Highly communicable Infants shed virus for months after birth	Yes
Group A streptococci (beta-hemolytic) Streptococcus pyogenes	Streptococcal sore throat Scarlet fever Impetigo Erysipelas Cellulitis Toxic shock syndrome Wound infections	Respiratory droplets Direct contact	1–5 d (average 2 d)	14–21 d, untreated Many nasal oropharyngeal carriers	No
Staphylococcus aureus Staphylococcus epidermidis	Abscesses Boils (furuncle) Cellulitis Impetigo Bacterial pneumonia	Saliva Exudates Respiratory droplets Nasal discharge	4–10 d Variable and indefinite	While lesions drain and carrier state persists	No
Candida albicans	Candidiasis	Secretions Excretions (oral, skin, vaginal)	Variable 2–5 d for "thrush" in children	While lesions are present	No
Streptococcus pneumoniae	Pneumonia Pneumococcal pneumonia	Droplet Direct contact Indirect	1–3 d Not well determined	While virulent organisms are discharged	Yes

TUBERCULOSIS[9]

M. *tuberculosis*, the etiologic agent in TB, is a resistant organism requiring special consideration when sterilization and disinfection methods are selected and administered. Clinical procedures are planned to prevent exposure and infection from this serious disease.

◆ Drug-resistant TB may occur when patients are noncompliant in their required extended drug therapy or if the medication is not available.

◆ Multidrug-resistant TB refers to resistance to at least two of the first-line drugs.

◆ Extensively drug-resistant TB refers to resistance to first-line drugs and at least one of three second-line drugs.

I. Transmission

◆ Inhalation

- TB is contracted when a vulnerable person inhales aerosolized droplet nuclei containing tubercle bacilli from sputum and saliva of an infected individual during coughing, sneezing, speaking, or singing (Figure 5-2).
- Use of ultrasonic, air polishing, air–water spray, and other hand pieces creates aerosols that can carry the tubercle bacilli.
- Droplet nuclei are small enough to pass through over 95% bacterial filtration efficiency required of standard surgical masks and may remain suspended in the air for hours. Standard precautions may be insufficient to protect the DHCP from transmission of TB in the healthcare setting.

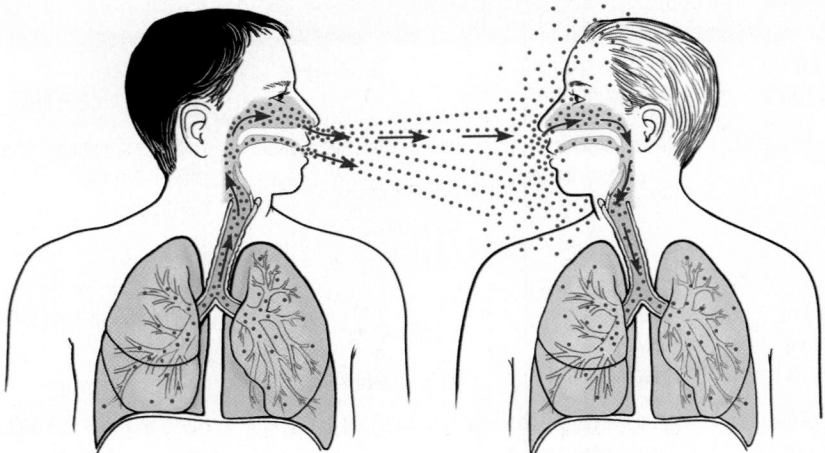

FIGURE 5-2 • Droplet Nuclei. Many potentially pathogenic microorganisms are disseminated by aerosols and spatter. The primary mode of transmission of tubercle bacilli is by droplet nuclei breathed directly into the lung.

- ◆ Factors affecting transmission of TB:
  - Degree to which the infected person produces infectious droplets.
  - Type and duration of exposure.
  - Susceptibility of recipient.
  - Some patients are more contagious than others.
  - Maximum communicability is usually just before the disease is diagnosed, when a person may have a severe cough and other respiratory symptoms.
- ◆ Areas of infection:
  - Infection primarily of the lungs.
  - Extrapulmonary TB: tubercle bacillus also infects lymph nodes, meninges (TB meningitis), kidneys, bone, skin, and the oral cavity.

II. Clinical Management

- ◆ Official recommendations from the Centers for Disease Control and Prevention (CDC) include the following[9]:
  - Risk assessment including community TB profile conducted annually.
  - DHCP: Screen all newly employed DHCP for latent TB infection and TB disease. A baseline two-step tuberculin skin test (TST), followed by annual TST is recommended.
  - DHCP with persistent cough (more than 3 weeks) or other suggestive symptoms are referred promptly for medical evaluation.
  - Medical history: Patients are routinely questioned about TB history and symptoms suggestive of TB infection; history is updated regularly.
  - Referral: Patients with symptoms or history suggestive of TB are referred immediately for medical evaluation.
  - Urgent dental care: Patients suspected of active TB infection are treated only in a facility with an airborne isolation room.

- Respiratory protection with a minimum N95 disposable filtration mask is used when caring for a patient with active (or suspected active) TB.
- Separation of suspected or confirmed TB patients; patients are isolated in a separate area until referral to the appropriate facility can be made.
- A patient management guide is available in Chapter 60.

VIRAL HEPATITIS

- ◆ Hepatitis is inflammation of the liver, which can be caused by virus(es).
- ◆ The most common viruses that cause hepatitis are HBV, HCV, and hepatitis D virus (HDV)
- ◆ Chronic or carrier disease state may occur with HBV, HCV, and HDV.
- ◆ Directly impacts the practice of dental hygiene and patient care.

I. Hepatitis B Virus[10]

- ◆ HBV is a serious, endemic, worldwide disease. Effective HBV vaccines are available for everyone (including neonates), and also for preexposure (PrEP) and postexposure prophylaxis (PEP).
- ◆ All vaccines act to stimulate antibodies and convey immunity.
  - Table 5-2 lists hepatitis B abbreviations and interpretation of serologic tests.

A. Transmission

- ◆ HBV is found in blood and body fluids including semen, tears, urine, and saliva.
- ◆ Transmission of HBV can occur from inanimate objects that have been exposed.
- ◆ Modes of transmission

TABLE 5-2 • Hepatitis B Abbreviations and Interpretation of Serologic Tests

TERM	TEST ABBREVIATION	SIGNIFICANCE
Hepatitis B surface antigen	HBsAg	Protein on surface of HBV. Presence indicates person is infectious, regardless of whether the infection is acute or chronic. HBsAg is used to make HBV vaccine.
Total hepatitis B core antibody	Anti-HBc	Indicates previous or ongoing infection in an undefined time frame. Does not develop in persons whose immunity to HBV is from vaccine. Anti-HBc generally persists for life and is not a serologic marker for acute infection.
Hepatitis B surface antibody	Anti-HBs	Presence indicates recovery and immunity against reinfection. Can occur in response to HBV vaccine.
IgM antibody to hepatitis B core antigen	IgM anti-HBc	Indicates recent (<6 mo) HBV infection and acute disease status.

Testing for HBV and disease status is determined by combining several of the above tests and interpreting the collective results.

TESTING GROUP	RESULTS	COLLECTIVE INTERPRETATION
HBsAg	Negative	Susceptible
Anti-HBc	Negative	
Anti-HBs	Negative	
HBsAg	Negative	Immune due to infection (not vaccination)
Anti-HBc	Positive	
Anti-HBs	Positive	
HBsAg	Negative	Immune due to vaccination
Anti-HBc	Negative	
Anti-HBs	Positive	
HBsAg	Positive	Acute infection
Anti-HBc	Positive	
IgM anti-HBc	Positive	
Anti-HBs	Negative	
HBsAg	Positive	Chronic infection
Anti-HBc	Positive	
IgM anti-HBc	Negative	
Anti-HBs	Negative	
HBsAg	Negative	Four possible interpretations:
Anti-HBc	Positive	1. Resolved infection
Anti-HBs	Negative	2. Resolving acute infection
		3. Low-level chronic infection
		4. False-positive anti-HBc therefore susceptible

- Hepatitis B is transmitted parenterally with a contaminated needle, accidental needlestick, sharps exposure including instruments, lancets used for glucose monitoring, or any object that can cause breaks in the skin even as minor as a scratch, burn, or abrasion.
- Sharing contaminated needles, syringes, and other intravenous drug paraphernalia.
- Contact with blood, wounds, open sores, or mucous membranes of infected person.
- Sexual exposure with an infected person.
- Sharing toothbrushes and razors with an infected person.
- HBV remains infectious for at least 7 days on inanimate surfaces and may be present and transmissible without visible blood.

◆ Perinatal transmission[11]

- Maternal HBV infection can be transmitted to the fetus in utero, during and after birth.

- Prevention of perinatal HBV infection involves screening of all pregnant women for HBV surface antigen (HBsAg) and vaccination of the pregnant mother if they are identified as high risk for infection and transmission such as:
  - Those who have had more than one sexual partner in the last 6 months or with a known infected sexual partner.
  - Those who have or are suspected of having a sexually transmitted disease.
  - Those who have current or recent injection drug use.

- Antiviral therapy (lamivudine, telbivudine, or tenovir) for infected mothers starting at weeks 28-32 of gestation along with vaccination of the infant at birth may reduce perinatal transmission.

B. Significance

◆ HBVs cause serious illnesses including acute and chronic hepatitis, cirrhosis, and liver cancer, sometimes leading to disability and death.

◆ Hepatitis B is a critical occupational hazard for DHCP because of their close association with potentially infected body fluids and sharps.

◆ Every healthcare individual requires immunization so that the possibilities of disease acquisition and transmission can be minimized.

C. Preventive Methods[11]

◆ Prenatal testing of all pregnant women for HBsAg and identification of household contacts that need to be vaccinated.

◆ Universal immunization of infants and children during routine healthcare visits.

◆ Immunization of adolescents and adults, particularly those at high risk.

◆ Enforce blood bank control measures.
  - Screening of donors and rejecting individuals with a history of viral hepatitis, drug addiction, recent transfusion, tattoo, and travelers from HBV-endemic areas.
  - Strict testing for all donated blood.

◆ Enforce strict sharps safety and use of disposable syringes and needles.
  - For acupuncture, skin testing, parenteral inoculations, body piercing, and tattoos.
  - Education of public to expect certain standards.

II. Hepatitis C[12]

A serologic test for antibody to HCV became available in 1991, and in 2013, the CDC recommended everyone born between 1945 and 1965 be tested for HCV.[13]

A. Transmission

◆ Hepatitis C is primarily transmitted parenterally and other modes similar to hepatitis B.

◆ Transmission rarely occurs from mucous membrane exposures to blood, and no transmission has been documented from intact or nonintact skin exposures to blood.

◆ Environmental contamination with blood containing HCV is not a significant risk for transmission in the healthcare setting.

◆ Although infrequent, sexual transmission of HCV can occur, especially among HIV-infected persons.

B. HCV Testing

◆ HCV testing is recommended for[12]:
  - Current and previous injection drug users.
  - Recipients of blood clotting factors before 1987.
  - Those who are or were long-term hemodialysis patients.
  - Those who have HIV.
  - Those with persistent elevated alanine aminotransferase levels (liver enzyme ALT).
  - Recipients of blood transfusions, blood components, organ transplants prior to 1992.
  - Anyone exposed to HCV-infected blood from needlestick, sharps injury, or had mucosal exposure.
  - Children born to HCV-infected mothers.

C. Prevention

◆ Education and behavior modification are essential since no vaccine is currently available for hepatitis C.

◆ Strict attention to standard infection control procedures for all healthcare personnel.

◆ Measures recommended for hepatitis B can be applied to hepatitis C.

III. Hepatitis D Virus[14]

HDV, also known as delta hepatitis, cannot cause infection except in the presence of HBV infection.

A. Transmission

◆ Delta infection is superimposed on HBsAg carriers.

◆ Occurs primarily in persons who have had multiple exposures to HBV; patients with hemophilia, HIV, and AIDS; and intravenous drug users.

◆ Transmission is similar to that of HBV; by direct exposure to contaminated blood and serous body fluids, contaminated needles and syringes, sexual contacts, and perinatal transfer.

B. Prevention

◆ All measures to prevent hepatitis B will prevent delta hepatitis because HDV is dependent on the presence of HBV.

◆ Immunization with hepatitis B vaccine also protects the recipient from HDV infection.

HUMAN HERPESVIRUS DISEASES

◆ Human herpesviruses (HHVs) are endemic worldwide, with over 95% of the adult population infected.

◆ Each virus causes a wide variety of highly infectious disease entities.

◆ HHV diseases are a significant public health problem due to lack of effective therapeutics and vaccines.

◆ There are nine major types of herpes viruses that are known to infect humans. These nine types are listed in Table 5-3 with abbreviations and some of the infections they cause.

I. General Characteristics

◆ HHVs produce diseases with latent, recurrent, and sometimes malignant tendencies.

- Herpes simplex virus type 2 (HSV-2) has been associated with cervical cancer.[15]
- Herpes simplex virus type 1 (HSV-1) has been implicated in oral cancer.[16]

- HSV-1 and HSV-2 have been implicated in aseptic encephalitis and an increased risk of transmitting and acquiring HIV.[17]
- Epstein–Barr virus (EBV; HHV-4) has been implicated in various types of cancer and increased risk of periodontitis.[18]

◆ HHVs travel along sensory nerve pathways to specific ganglia where they remain latent and become reactivated to produce recurrent infection after certain stimuli, or when the body's immunity is significantly lowered.

- HSV-1 travels to the trigeminal ganglion (Figure 5-3).
- HSV-2 goes to the thoracic, lumbar, and sacral dorsal root ganglia.
- Varicella–zoster virus (VZV) travels to the sensory ganglia of the vagal, spinal, or cranial nerves.

TABLE 5-3 • Herpes Viruses

HERPES VIRUS NUMBER	NAME OF VIRUS AND ABBREVIATION	INFECTIONS
HHV-1	Herpes simplex virus, type 1 HSV-1	Herpetic gingivostomatitis Herpes labialis Herpetic whitlow Herpetic conjunctivitis
HHV-2	Herpes simplex virus, type 2 HSV-2	Genital herpes
HHV-3	Varicella–Zoster virus VZV	Chicken pox Shingles
HHV-4	Epstein–Barr virus EBV	Infectious mononucleosis Oral hairy leukoplakia Burkitt's lymphoma Lymphoepithelial cysts of parotid gland Lymphatic cancers Nasopharyngeal cancers Periapical lesions Periodontal disease severity
HHV-5	Human cytomegalovirus CMV	Asymptomatic infections Associated with periapical pathosis and increased severity of periodontal diseases along with EBV and HSV Immunosuppressed persons: CMV retinitis, neurologic deficiencies, pneumonia, encephalitis Congenital infection: preterm and low birth weight (PLBW), microcephaly, seizures, intellectual and physical disabilities, vision and hearing loss
HHV-6A	Herpes lymphotropic virus (HLV-6A)	Associated with Hashimoto's thyroiditis and multiple sclerosis Immune system suppression
HHV-6B	Herpes lymphotropic virus (HLV-6B)	Roseola infantum (exanthema subitum or sixth disease) Associated with seizure disorders
HHV-7	Human herpes virus 7 HHV-7	Drug-induced hypersensitivity syndrome Encephalopathy Hepatitis Reactivation of HHV-4 and HHV-6B Lichen planus
HHV-8	Kaposi's sarcoma–related virus KSHV or KS	Kaposi's sarcoma Lymphoproliferative diseases Multicentric Castleman's disease

◆ Immunosuppressed patients have more frequent and severe HHV infections.

◆ HHVs are among the opportunistic infectious agents in HIV/AIDS, and several have been implicated as co-pathogens in HIV transmission and progression.[19]

II. Relation to Periodontal Infections

◆ HHVs have been detected in periodontitis pockets.

◆ Herpes virus–positive periodontitis lesions involving cytomegalovirus (CMV) and EBV have higher levels of major periodontal pathogenic bacteria.[20]

◆ A co-infection of CMV and EBV is associated with more severe chronic periodontitis.[20]

◆ CMV, EBV, and HSV-1 have a significant association with aggressive periodontitis.[21,22]

◆ Although other HHVs have been detected in periodontitis pockets, they have not shown any association with the initiation, progression, and severity of periodontal diseases.[20-22]

◆ The actual mechanisms surrounding the involvement of EBV and CMV in periodontitis are unclear and remain under investigation.[20-22]

III. Clinical Management for HHVs[23,24]

◆ Professional terminology may cause alarm with patients. Terms such as "fever blisters" or "cold sores" need to be used to ensure patient understanding.

◆ Postpone appointment if patient has an active lesion.

◆ Explain the contagious nature of the disease:
  • Limit personal contact with others while the lesion is active, especially saliva transfer and sharing of objects such as lip products, utensils, and drink containers.
  • Stress the importance of meticulous hygiene in limiting autoinfection through touching the lesion and then touching other susceptible body areas such as eyes and genitals. Auto-reinfection can also occur via lip moisturizing products and ointments used to treat the lesions.

◆ Prodromal stage can be the most transmissible to other patients and clinicians.
  • Autoinoculation possible from instrumentation that can splash viruses to the patient's eye or extend the lesion to the nose.
  • Irritation to the lesions can prolong the course and increase the severity of the infection.

A. HHV-1 (HSV-1)[24]

HHV-1 also known as HSV-1 is widespread, and it is estimated that between 50% and 90% of people worldwide are affected.

◆ Primary infection usually occurs in children but may occur at any age, especially in the immunocompromised.

◆ Antibodies (anti-HSV) are produced but do not guarantee immunity to recurrent herpes or to other herpesvirus infections.

◆ Sulcular epithelium can serve as a reservoir for the viruses. Anti-HSV is present in the gingival sulcus fluid. Trauma to the oral area during a dental or dental hygiene appointment may trigger a herpetic recurrence.

◆ Primary herpetic gingivostomatitis
  • Many cases of primary infection with HSV-1 are asymptomatic or mild and isolated to marginal and attached gingiva.
  • Acute herpetic gingivostomatitis is the most common pattern of symptomatic primary herpetic infection.
  • Full-blown herpetic gingivostomatitis presents with widespread oral ulcers that also may involve the pharyngeal areas.
  • When clinical disease is evident, gingivostomatitis and pharyngitis are the most frequent manifestations, with fever, malaise, severe pain often interfering with the ability to eat, and lymphadenopathy for 2–7 days.
  • Painful oral vesicular lesions may occur on the gingiva, mucosa, tongue, and lips.
  • Manifestations may vary from mild to severely debilitating.
  • A patient may be a subclinical carrier, and reactivation of a latent infection from the trigeminal ganglia (Figure 5-3) may be followed by asymptomatic excretion of the viruses in the saliva.
  • Reactivation may also lead to herpetic ulcerations of the lip, the typical "cold sore."

◆ Herpes labialis (cold sore, fever blister)[23-25]
  • Both HSV-1 and HSV-2 cause genital and oral facial infections that cannot be distinguished clinically, although they are antigenically different.
  • HSV-1 is spread predominantly through infected lesions in oral and ocular areas and is found in mucous membranes and skin above the waist.

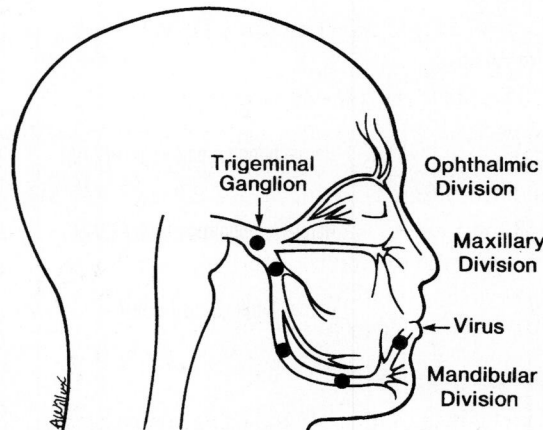

FIGURE 5-3 • Latent Infection of Herpes Simplex Virus. Path of the virus traced from point of viral penetration on lip to establishment of latent infection in the trigeminal ganglion.

- Recurrent HSV symptomatic lesions are common and may occur at or near the primary lesion at the vermillion border of the lower lip. Triggers include trauma, stress, sunlight, illness, or any conditions that deplete the patient's immune system.
  - Dental and dental hygiene appointments with associated emotional stress and oral trauma involved may be triggers of HSV lesions.
  - Six to 24 hours before the lesion appears, pain, burning, slight stinging, or sensations of localized warmth and erythema of the affected epithelium with slight swelling serve as a forewarning. A group of vesicles forms, eventually ruptures, and crusting follows; healing may take up to 10 days.
  - Lesions are infectious; the shedding virus may lead to autoinfection of the eye, mucous membranes, or fingers and infection of other people.
- Herpetic whitlow[26]
  - Herpetic whitlow is herpes simplex infection of the fingers resulting from HSV-1 or HSV-2 entering through skin abrasions around a fingernail.
  - Chronic herpetic whitlow may be a manifestation of HIV infection.[27]
  - Herpetic whitlow was once common among DHCP; standard precautions have almost eliminated the incidence among DHCP.
- Ocular/ophthalmic herpes[28]
  - Herpes simplex lesions in the eye can be a primary or recurrent infection of HSV-1 or HSV-2 and may lead to blindness.
  - Transmission can occur from splashing saliva or fluid from a vesicular lesion directly into an unprotected eye.
  - Prevent ocular herpetic infection by using standard precautions including eye protection for both clinician and patient.

B. HHV-2 (HSV-2)[25]

- HHV-2 also known as HSV-2 is commonly known as genital herpes, but it also occurs as oral and perioral infections.
- Genital herpes infection with HSV-1 is increasing in prevalence.[17]
- HSV-2 has been associated with cervical cancer.[15]
- *Neonatal herpes* is a serious disease that can cause delayed mental development, blindness, neurologic problems, and death to newborns infected during childbirth.[25]
  - Obstetricians may recommend delivery by cesarean section to women with active genital herpes to avoid transmission to the infant.
- Antiviral therapy can suppress HSV-2 lesions.

C. HHV-3 (VZV)[29]

- Chickenpox (varicella) and shingles (herpes zoster) are caused by VZV.
- Primary VZV infection causes varicella, and latency is established in dorsal root and cranial nerve ganglia.

- VZV reactivation may occur years later in the form of herpes zoster (shingles).
- Varicella (chickenpox) infection
  - Extremely contagious and primarily childhood disease transmitted via respiratory droplets and direct or indirect skin contact with discharge from vesicles and respiratory tract.
  - Can be life threatening to adults, immunocompromised patients, pregnant women, and newborns.
  - Varicella may lead to secondary bacterial skin infections, pneumonia, meningoencephalitis, kidney, liver, and bleeding complications.
  - Two doses of the varicella vaccine are recommended, with the first dose at 12–15 months old and the second between 4 and 6 years old.
- Zoster (shingles) infection
  - After primary infection, VZV remains latent in dorsal root and cranial ganglia.
  - After a few years to several decades later, VZV reactivates and spreads to skin along peripheral nerves, causing a painful vesicular rash lasting from 2 to 4 weeks.
  - Risk factors for zoster include: increasing age, HIV, physical trauma or surgery, cancer, transplants, and immunosuppressive medications.
  - Complications from zoster infection include postherpetic neuralgia, secondary skin infections and scarring, and ocular and neurologic conditions.
  - A zoster vaccine is available and is recommended for all adults 50 years and older.

D. HHV-4 (EBV)[30]

- HHV-4 also known as EBV is a common human virus with many cases remaining asymptomatic.
- No vaccine is available.
- EBV remains latent, may be reactivated in the immunocompromised, and has been associated with a variety of diseases including lymphomas and nasopharyngeal cancers (Table 5-3).
- Infectious mononucleosis
  - Mononucleosis is a symptomatic disease caused by infection with EBV and is common among teenagers and young adults.
  - Commonly spread through saliva even when the patient has no symptoms of disease.
  - May also be spread via sexual contact, organ transplants, and blood transfusions.
  - There may be a long period of communicability or a lasting carrier state.
  - Prevention: minimize contact with saliva by frequent handwashing, avoiding drinking from a common container; standard precautions by DHCP.
- Oral hairy leukoplakia[31]
  - EBV replicates within epithelial cells in oral hairy leukoplakia.

- Oral hairy leukoplakia once considered isolated to those with HIV has been found in HIV-negative patients with other immunosuppression risk factors such as long-term steroid use and anti-rejection drugs for solid organ transplants.

E. HHV-5 (CMV)[32]

HHV-5 also known as CMV infections are widespread, with the most severe disease developing in infants infected in utero and in immunocompromised patients, including HIV/AIDS. No vaccine is available.

- Transmission
  - Direct contact with infected bodily fluids including breast milk and respiratory droplets.
  - May also spread via sexual contact, solid organ and bone marrow transplants, and blood transfusions.
  - CMV can be spread among children attending day care and household members.
- Congenital CMV transmission
  - Virus from the mother's primary or recurrent infection can infect the infant in utero, in the birth canal, or through breast milk.
  - CMV infection in a fetus may lead to premature birth; low birth weight; lung, liver, and spleen disorders; microcephaly; intellectual and physical disabilities; seizures; vision and hearing loss.
- Prevention
  - Personal hygiene: handwashing.
  - Utilization of standard precautions by healthcare personnel.
  - Seropositivity of donor checked before organ transplant and other surgery.

F. HHV-6A and HHV-6B[33,34]

- HHV-6A and HHV-6B were previously known as herpes lymphotropic virus.
- As of 2012, HHV-6A and HHV-6B are considered to be distinct viral species rather than variants of the same species.[33]
  - Each has been implicated in a wide range of diseases, and both have been implicated in ocular inflammatory and neurologic diseases.
- HHV-6A
  - Found at low levels in saliva, which is thought to be the primary route of virus transmission, and in 54% of healthy adult lungs.
  - Acquired later in life, typically as an asymptomatic primary infection.
  - Possible risk factor in accelerating HIV infection.
  - Identified in 74% of pediatric glial tumors.
  - Associated with Hashimoto's thyroiditis and multiple sclerosis.
- HHV-6B
  - Primary infection with HHV-6B occurs in 100% of humans by the age of 3 and is known as roseola infantum, exanthem subitem, or sixth disease.

- Initial symptoms are fever, diarrhea, and rash, although more serious symptoms of seizures and encephalitis can occur.
- Reactivation of the virus occurs in those who are immunosuppressed, especially those with solid organ and stem cell transplants.
- HHV-6B has been found in endodontic abscesses and in the adenoids and tonsils of children with upper respiratory symptoms.
- Associated with mesial temporal lobe epilepsy and status epilepticus.
- HHV-6A, HHV-6B, HHV-7, and HHV-8 are considered lymphotropic.

G. Human Herpesvirus 7[34,35]

- A lymphotropic virus also found in saliva.
- Often found with HHV-6 and is implicated in a range of diseases and conditions.
- Along with HHV-6B it is a causative agent in roseola infantum.
- Symptoms associated with HHV-7 infection include acute febrile respiratory disease, low lymphocyte counts, fever, rash, vomiting, diarrhea, febrile seizures.
- Some persons infected with HHV-7 are asymptomatic.
- HHV-7 has been shown to cause or contribute to:
  - Drug-induced hypersensitivity syndrome (with HHV-6).
  - Encephalopathy.
  - Hepatitis.
  - Reactivation of HHV-4 (CMV) in transplant patients.
  - Reactivation of HHV-6B to cause febrile status epilepticus.
  - Lichen planus and multiple other cutaneous diseases.

H. Human Herpesvirus 8[36,37]

- HHV-8 is also known as Kaposi's sarcoma–associated herpesvirus and is associated with lymphoproliferative diseases and multicentric Castleman's disease
- Seroprevalence of HHV-8 varies tremendously throughout the globe and within certain populations. Some areas have endemic infection and others have rates below 6%.
- HHV-8 prevalence is high with men who have sex with men and in African migrants.
- HHV-8 is present in seminal fluid, nasal secretions, and saliva.
- Although HHV-8 is generally considered to be sexually transmitted, oral mucosa and saliva are the primary sites of viral shedding and infection transmission.
- Transplant transmission is also possible.
- Primary infection in the immunocompetent may be asymptomatic. Symptoms such as fever, rash, and upper respiratory infections can easily be attributed to other causes.

- In the immunocompromised, primary infection presents with lymphadenopathy, acute pancytopenia, and rapid progression to Karposi's sarcoma. Transplant patients are particularly susceptible, as are those with HIV infection.
- HIV increases the risk of HHV-8 infection.
- Those who are infected with HHV-8 after being infected with HIV are at significantly greater risk for rapid progression to Kaposi's sarcoma (KS).

HUMAN PAPILLOMAVIRUS[38,39]

- There are over 150 viruses considered to be human papillomaviruses (HPVs) and each is identified by a number.
- Almost all men and women will be infected by an HPV at some point in their lives.
- Most HPV infections are asymptomatic and are cleared by the immune system.
- Persistent HPV infections are known to cause cervical, oropharyngeal, vaginal, penile, anal, and rectal cancers.
- 13 types of HPV are oncogenic.
- 80% of HPV-associated cancers are attributed to types 16 and 18 and 12% to HPV types 31, 33, 45, 52, and 58.
- HPV-16 is the most likely oncogenic HPV to progress to cancer and is attributed to 95% of head and neck cancers.
- HPV-associated oropharyngeal cancer develops near the base of the tongue and in the tonsils.
- 63% of oropharyngeal cancers are associated with HPV infection.
- HPV testing is available for women undergoing cervical cancer screening.
- The CDC recommends HPV vaccination for:
  - All children aged 11–12.
  - All women through age 26 and all men through age 21.
  - Young men who have sex with men through age 26.
  - Transgender young adults through age 26.
  - Immunocompromised young adults through age 26.

HIV/AIDS INFECTION[40,41]

- HIV attacks the body's immune system, specifically the CD4+ T lymphocyte cells (T-cells).
- If untreated, HIV can destroy enough CD4+ T-cells to render the immune system unable to fight off infection, disease, and cancer.
- These infectious diseases are called opportunistic infections (OIs) because they take advantage of a weak immune system.
- There are numerous OIs such as: *Pneumocystis carinii* pneumonia, TB, KS, HIV wasting syndrome, toxoplasmosis, all HHVs, and candidiasis.

- A weakened immune system under attack from OIs signals the last stage of HIV infection known as AIDS.
- No cure currently exists but HIV can be controlled by highly active antiretroviral therapy (HAART), which was introduced in the mid-1990s.
- Before HAART, HIV could induce AIDS within a few years.
- With early diagnosis and treatment, HIV-infected individuals can have a near-normal life expectancy.
- Etiology and history of HIV
  - A type of chimpanzee in West Africa has been identified as the source of HIV.
  - The simian immunodeficiency virus was transmitted to humans through contact with infected blood as a result of hunting the chimpanzees for meat.
  - The virus may have jumped species as far back as the late 1800s and has been present in the United States since the mid- to late 1970s.
  - There are two types of HIV:
    - HIV-1 causes the majority of infections and is pandemic.
    - HIV-1 is more infectious and virulent than HIV-2.
    - HIV-2 is generally confined to West Africa.

I. Transmission[42]

- All bodily secretions of a patient with HIV infection contain HIV.
  - Only blood, semen, preseminal fluid, rectal fluids, vaginal fluids, and breast milk can transmit HIV.
- Common modes of HIV transmission include:
  - Parenteral:
    - Sharing needles or other injection equipment used to prepare and/or inject illicit drugs, hormones, silicone, and steroids.
  - Sexual:
    - All unprotected insertive and receptive oral, anal, penile, and vaginal contact.
    - Presence of other sexually transmitted diseases such as gonorrhea, syphilis, HPVs, HHVs, hepatitis, and chlamydia increase risk of contracting and transmitting HIV by about threefold.
- Less common and rare modes of HIV transmission:
  - Deep open-mouthed kissing with the presence of open sores and bleeding gingivae.
  - Although now rare and preventable due to HIV medications, the virus can be transmitted in utero across the placenta, during vaginal birth, and breastfeeding.
  - All forms of oral sex including fellatio, cunnilingus, and anal rimming.
  - Receiving contaminated blood transfusions, blood products along with organ and tissue transplants.
  - Contact with broken skin, wounds, and mucous membranes by blood and/or blood-contaminated body fluids.

- Prechewed food contaminated with infected blood.
- Human bites with severe skin damage.
- Breaches in or inadequate infection control.
- HIV is not transmitted by saliva, sweat, tears, insect bites, or social contact.

II. HIV Testing for Diagnosis and Staging of Infection[43]

◆ HIV tests are very accurate but cannot detect the virus immediately after infection.

◆ Laboratory tests to determine HIV infection include:
  - Nucleic acid test looks for the virus in the blood and is used for high-risk exposure or those who exhibit early signs of infection. It is not used for HIV screening.
  - Antigen/antibody tests look for HIV antibodies and antigens especially the p24 antigen that is produced before antibodies develop. Rapid antigen/antibody tests are available.
  - Antibody tests detect the presence of HIV antibodies.

◆ Rapid tests and home tests:
  - Most rapid and home tests look for HIV antibodies.
  - Home Access HIV-1 Test System® involves a finger stick to obtain a blood sample that is then sent anonymously to a licensed lab. Results can be obtained as fast as the next day.
  - OraQuick In-Home HIV Test® involves obtaining a swab of oral fluids and using the kit to perform the test at home. Results are available in 20 minutes; however, 1 in 12 test false-negative for HIV due to the lower levels of antibodies in oral fluids.

◆ CD4+ T lymphocyte and viral load counts
  - The CD4+ T lymphocyte counts and viral load counts are done to estimate, at one point in time, the health of the immune system and help evaluate a person's risk of serious illness from OIs.
  - The tests do not indicate health of the person, how they feel, or predict the future course of disease.
  - The tests evaluate the immune system by counting the CD4 cells and the virus by counting the viral load. If done frequently, the tests provide data to evaluate trends over time.
  - CD4+ T lymphocyte count:
    - A normal CD4+ T lymphocyte count is 500–1,500 cells/mm³ of blood in a non–HIV-infected adult.
    - CD4+ T-cells can also be represented as a percentage of all white blood cells, with 32%–68% considered normal in a non–HIV-infected adult.
    - A CD4+ T lymphocyte count below 200cells/mm³ or a CD4% of less than 14% indicates a person is at risk for OIs.
  - Viral load count:
    - A viral load count measures the amount of HIV in 1 mm³ of blood and only applies to those with HIV.

- The viral load count provides data to evaluate potential damage to the immune system, efficacy of HIV medications, and drug resistance of the virus.

◆ HAART drugs must be taken by strict regimen to achieve viral suppression. Viral suppression is when the viral load count is below 200 copies of HIV/mm³ and the virus can be suppressed to the point where it becomes undetectable in a blood test.

Stages of HIV Infection[40,41]

◆ Stage 1: Acute HIV Infection
  - Within 2–4 weeks after infection, the person may experience flu-like symptoms lasting a few weeks, some may be asymptomatic.
  - During this time, the viral load is very high and the person is highly infectious.
  - No AIDS defining OIs are present.
  - CD4+ T lymphocyte count ≥500 cells/mm³ or ≥29%.

◆ Stage 2: Clinical Latency
  - Also known as asymptomatic or chronic infection.
  - Can last 10 years or longer, although some infections will progress to stage 3 faster.
  - HIV medications can hold an infected person at this stage for decades.
  - HIV is active, replicating at a slow rate, and is still transmissible.
  - Those with a low viral load are less likely to transmit the virus.
  - No AIDS defining OIs are present.
  - CD4+ T lymphocyte counts are 200–499 cells/mm³ or 14%–28%.

◆ Stage 3: AIDS
  - Immune system is damaged and poorly functioning.
  - OIs can appear unchecked by the immune system.
  - Without treatment, people may only survive 3 years.
  - The viral load is extremely high and the person is very infectious.
  - Symptoms include: fever, sweats, chills, swollen lymph nodes, weight loss, muscle wasting, and weakness.
  - CD4+ T lymphocyte counts are below 200 cells/mm³ or 14%.

III. Oral Manifestations of HIV Infection[44-46]

◆ Oral lesions, conditions, and infections are significant indicators of HIV infection and markers of disease progression. The etiology of oral lesions associated with HIV/AIDS is listed in Table 5-4.

◆ Analysis of oral findings and patient provided information may provide insight into recognition and diagnosis of HIV infection and HIV/AIDS-related oral manifestations.

◆ HAART has changed the overall prevalence and pattern of HIV-related oral manifestations.

TABLE 5-4 • Etiology of Oral Lesions Associated with HIV/AIDS

FUNGAL INFECTIONS	VIRAL INFECTIONS	BACTERIAL INFECTIONS
Candida albicans	Herpes simplex 1 (HHV-1)	*Mycobacterium tuberculosis* (TB)
Candida glabrata	Herpes simplex 2 (HHV-2)	*Mycobacterium avium intracellulare*
Candida dubliniensis	Herpes zoster (HHV-3)	
Candida krusei	Epstein–Barr (HHV-4)	Periodontal infections
Cryptococcosis	CMV (HHV-5)	LGE
Histoplasmosis	KS (HHV-8)	Necrotizing ulcerative gingivitis (NUG)
Paracoccidioidomycosis	Human papillomavirus (HPV)	Necrotizing ulcerative periodontitis (NUP)
Penicilliosis		
Aspergillosis		

A. Oral Lesions Strongly Associated with HIV Infection

◆ HIV-Associated Oral Candidiasis (HIV-OC)

- Oral candidiasis is a fungal infection that is the most common oral lesion associated with HIV infection.
- HAART has reduced the prevalence of HIV-OC by 50%.
- Associated with CD4$^+$ T lymphocyte counts below 200 cells/mm^3 or 14%.
- *Candida albicans* is the most common pathogen.
- *Candida glabrata*, *Candida krusei*, and *Candida dubliniensis* are also associated with HIV-OC and demonstrate reduced azole drug susceptibility.
- HIV-OC can present as erythematous candidiasis, pseudomembranous candidiasis, and angular cheilitis.
- Candidiasis may be recognized by clinical examination or determined by the use of exfoliative cytology.

◆ HIV-Associated Oral Hairy Leukoplakia

- Caused by reactivation of latent HHV-4.
- Associated with CD4$^+$ T lymphocyte counts below 200 cells/mm^3 or 14%.
- More prevalent in males than females.

◆ Non-Hodgkin Lymphoma

- Associated with reactivation of HHV-4.
- 60 times more prevalent in HIV-infected persons.
- 25% of lesions are in the oral cavity.
- Lesions present as growths and ulcerations affecting gingiva, palatal tissues, and alveolar mucosa.
- Lesions can have a similar presentation to dental infections.

◆ Kaposi's Sarcoma

- KS is one of the main types of cancer to affect HIV patients and is the most common HIV-associated oral malignancy.
- KS is caused by HHV-8 (see prior section on HHV-8).
- Lesions are mostly found on the hard palate and gingivae and vary in color from purple to brown and black. They may be multifocal and progress rapidly with larger lesions, posing a risk of ulceration, secondary infection, and extensive periodontal destruction.
- Triggers for progression of HHV-8 to KS in HIV patients are unknown as KS can manifest independently of HIV viral load and CD4 count status.

◆ Gingival and Periodontal Infections[47-50]

- Atypical gingival changes may be an initial indicator of undiagnosed HIV infection.
- Patients with HIV infection who maintain a high level of personal and professional oral care may present with healthier periodontal tissues.
- Periodontal infections associated with HIV infection tend to show more severe symptoms and progress more rapidly.

◆ Necrotizing Periodontal Diseases (NPDs)[49,50]

- Necrotizing periodontal diseases are severe inflammatory diseases strongly associated with immune system impairment and are not isolated to those with HIV infection. Risk factors for NPDs include smoking, poor oral hygiene, stress, malnutrition, and immuno-compromise.
- NPDs are subcategorized and defined as:
  - Necrotizing Gingivitis (NG): No loss of attachment, necrosis of the interdental papillae, gingival bleeding, and pain.
  - Necrotizing Periodontitis (NP): Loss of attachment, necrosis of the interdental papillae, gingival bleeding, pain, halitosis, and rapid bone loss.
  - Necrotizing Stomatitis (NS): Lesions extending beyond the muco-gingival junction (MGJ), bone denudation, osteitis, and bone sequestrum.
- Other signs and symptoms may include pseudomembranous gingiva, regional lymphadenopathy, and fever.
- All NPDs are varying stages of the same disease with the same microflora.

B. Oral Lesions Less Commonly Associated with or Seen with HIV[44-46]

◆ HSV (HHV-1 and HHV-2) may present as recurrent herpes labialis; in patients with HIV/AIDS, painful, deep blistering lesions and fever may be manifest.

◆ Herpes zoster (HHV-3) or shingles lesions and blisters may appear on the head, face, and neck.

◆ CMV (HHV-5) causes ulceration of oral mucosa and spreads to the gastrointestinal tract. Thought to be a major cause of retinitis in HIV patients and may cause encephalitis.

◆ HPV lesions generally occur intraorally but may manifest in the HIV patient as papillomatous lesions or mucosal tags in the labial commissures.

◆ Cryptococcosis, histoplasmosis, Paracoccidioidomycosis, penicilliosis, and aspergillosis may be the primary etiology of oral fungal infections.

◆ M. *tuberculosis* is estimated to cause 13% of AIDS-related deaths and in advanced cases can manifest as oral lesions that may extend into paranasal sinuses.

◆ *Mycobacterium avium intracellulare* infection is rare but may cause oral lesions.

◆ Recurrent aphthous stomatitis.

◆ Intramucosal hemorrhages.

◆ Melanotic hyperpigmentation of oral mucosa.

◆ Salivary gland disease, swelling of salivary glands, and severe xerostomia.

C. Impact of HAART on HIV-Associated Oral Lesions[45,51,52]

◆ HAART has reduced the prevalence of HIV-associated oral lesions.

◆ KS, candidiasis, LGE, and oral hairy leukoplakia are the most responsive to HAART.

◆ As the viral load is reduced and the CD4$^+$ T lymphocyte counts improve, there is an improvement in immune system function. This improvement can prompt a strong inflammatory response resulting in immune reconstitution inflammatory syndrome (IRIS).

◆ Paradoxical IRIS is the worsening of an existing infection.

◆ Unmasking IRIS is the appearance of a new infection.

◆ Patients who are taking HAART may present with an exaggerated and atypical level of inflammation.

◆ The oral lesions most typically associated with IRIS are KS, oral candidiasis, HPV, salivary gland disease, ulcers, and oral hairy leukoplakia.

◆ Patients who are undergoing immune reconstitution may need more frequent care with a focus on prevention of oral candidiasis and HHVs.

IV. Prevention and Treatment of HIV Infection[40]

◆ PrEP with a combination of tenofovir disoproxil fumarate and emtricitabine has been shown to reduce the risk of infection in high-risk persons by up to 92%.

◆ PEP is the use of antiretroviral drugs within 72 hours of a high-risk exposure to stop HIV seroconversion.

◆ HIV treatment for prevention is the use of antiretroviral drugs to reduce the viral load to below 200 copies/mL of blood (viral suppression). Over time and with consistent use of the drug therapy, the viral load can be reduced to undetectable levels (undetectable viral load).

◆ A person with an undetectable viral load has effectively no risk of transmitting HIV to a noninfected sexual partner.

◆ Until a vaccine is available, prevention depends to a large degree on community education.

TABLE 5-5 • Commonly Prescribed HIV Medications	
DRUG CATEGORY AND ABBREVIATION	**GENERIC NAME(S) AND ABBREVIATION(S) (IF USED)**
Nucleoside Reverse Transcriptase Inhibitors (NRTIs)	Abacavir (ABC) Emtricitabine (FTC) Lamivudine (3TC) Tenofovir disoproxil fumarate (TDF or tenofovir DF) Tenofovir alafenamide (TAF) Zidovudine (AZT, ZDV)
Non-nucleoside Reverse Transcriptase Inhibitors (NNRTIs)	Efavirenz (EFV) Etravirine Nevirapine (NVP) Rilpivirine
Fusion Inhibitor	Enfuvirtide
CCR5 Antagonists	Maraviroc
Protease Inhibitors (PIs)	Atazanavir Nelfinavir Ritonavir Darunavir Fosamprenavir Saquinavir Tipranavir Lopinavir/Ritonavir
Integrase Strand Transfer Inhibitors (INSTIs)	Dolutegravir Elvitegravir Raltegravir
Pharmacokinetic Enhancer (PK)	Cobicistat

◆ Health education efforts need to be focused on awareness of risk, modes of transmission, and preventive measures necessary to halt HIV transmission, especially in high-risk groups.

◆ Dental personnel who are well informed with accurate, current information can provide care for HIV-infected patients and give support to community health programs.

◆ Antiretroviral medications do not cure HIV.

◆ Treatment usually requires a combination of several different medications sometimes combined into one pill.

◆ Medications must be taken on a strict regimen, and compliance may be problematic due to side effects, dose scheduling, illness, depression, fear of others finding out, and being unable to afford medications.

◆ Table 5-5 lists commonly prescribed Food and Drug Administration–approved medications to treat and manage HIV.

V. Dental Hygiene Management

◆ Legal and psychosocial considerations
  • DHCPs are ethically and legally obligated to treat HIV-positive or at-risk patients.

- All persons with HIV infection are protected by the Americans with Disabilities Act.
- Use language that does not stigmatize or judge the HIV-positive patient in regard to their sexual orientation, gender identity, sexual and/or drug behaviors, and other medical and/or social behaviors.
- Realize the patient may be infected through no fault of their own.
- Maintain strict patient confidentiality.
- The dental hygienist may be the first to suspect HIV infection when oral manifestations and symptoms are recognized.
- Encourage HIV testing for at-risk patients and adherence to HAART for those who are infected.
- Assisting HIV-infected patients in maintaining their oral health can significantly improve their quality of life by reducing pain and susceptibility to OIs.
- Pain and oral manifestations may be caused by the disease or medications.
- Adverse effects of HAART may include nausea and vomiting, which can be severe enough to contribute to dental caries and dental erosion.
- Emphasize on meticulous personal oral care and frequent professional periodontal therapy. Fluoride varnish needs to be included in the preventive oral hygiene program for all ages.

METHICILLIN-RESISTANT STAPHYLOCOCCUS AUREUS[47,48]

- *S. aureus* is a common cause of infection.
- MRSA is a strain of *S. aureus* resistant to many antibiotic therapies.
- MRSA infections are difficult to treat and can be endemic in hospitals and institutions.
- It is associated with acute osteomyelitis, bacteremia, septicemia, cellulitis, conjunctivitis, pneumonia, and toxic shock syndrome.
- Infections are spread by direct contact with an infected wound or from contaminated hands.
- The incubation period is 4–10 days, and the person remains infectious as long as the infection persists.
- Persons may be a carrier of MRSA and spread the infection to others even if they do not have signs or symptoms of infection.
- Risk factors for acquisition of MRSA include prolonged hospital stay, intensive care, prolonged antimicrobial therapy, and surgical procedures.

DOCUMENTATION

Suggested documentation for the patient with an infectious disease includes the following:

- If the patient is under treatment for an infectious condition, note the patient's medication, its purpose, adverse effects, effects on oral health, and patient adherence to medication(s).

- Record all consultations with specialists.
- When patient is not being treated, record referral and purpose.
- Record results of specific laboratory tests (CD4+ counts, viral load counts, antibody/antigen, biopsy results) that potentially affect dental hygiene treatment; note those values at each appointment.
- Box 5-1 provides a sample Progress Note.

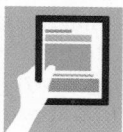

BOX 5-1
Example Documentation: Patient with Recurrent Aphthous Ulcers

S—28-year-old male presents for his regular periodontal maintenance appointment with chief complaint of large and frequently recurring aphthous ulcers. Medical history indicates patient has been under care of his physician for 2 years and is being treated for HIV. He is currently taking Combivir (zidovudine + lamivudine) and Invirase (saquinavir) and reports his condition is well controlled with a CD4+ count of 700 and a low viral load. Patient states he has been keeping up with his homecare.

O—Extraoral examination reveals bilateral slightly enlarged lymph nodes. No fever is evident. Intraoral examination reveals several ulcerations of the oral mucosa, ranging in size from 2 to 8 mm in diameter. The oropharynx is red with multiple white spots 2–3 mm in diameter. Saliva flow is difficult to stimulate. Oral hygiene: generalized light cervical biofilm. Gingival tissues: generally pink with isolated areas of slight marginal erythema around #6,7,26,27. Periodontal examination: slight bleeding on probing (BoP) #6,7,26,27, probing depths 2–4 mm, no furcation involvement, no pathologic mobility. Radiographic examination: stable bone heights when compared to previous radiographs.

A—The patient is at increased risk for oral and/or systemic complications such as candidiasis, recurrent aphthous ulcers, and moderate xerostomia.

P—Discussed etiology of candidiasis and aphthous ulcers. Referred patient to his physician for evaluation and treatment of candidiasis and aphthous ulcers. Discussed etiology and impacts of xerostomia. Advised patient to reduce frequency of sugar intake and take frequent sips of water. Oral hygiene reviewed and revised to address the areas of erythema and BoP #6,7,26,27. Regular periodontal maintenance was postponed until candidiasis and aphthous ulcers have resolved.

Signed: _____, RDH

Date: _____

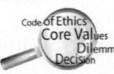

EVERYDAY ETHICS

Mr. Sands, a new patient to the dental hygiene clinic, had completed his admission history and basic examination at a previous appointment. He is assigned to Alison because she needs more credits for patients with heavy calculus. He is scheduled today for his personal instruction for home care and scaling for the first quadrant.

When Alison starts to read the record before clinic opened, she learns that Mr. Sands has a history of hepatitis C. She immediately makes up an excuse and asks Leah, her classmate in the clinic unit next to hers, to treat Mr. Sands, while she, Alison, attends to the two pediatric patients scheduled for sealants with Leah. Leah has already prepared for the appointment with the children and needs the four credits toward her sealants

requirement, although she also needs credits for a patient with heavy calculus.

Questions for Consideration

1. Which of the dental hygiene core values (Chapter 1, Box 1-6) is Alison violating by her actions to avoid caring for this patient?

2. Is this an ethical dilemma or an ethical issue for Leah? How can Leah resolve the problem? What might be the consequences for both if Leah reports Alison's action to the instructor in charge? What if Alison does a similar thing in the future?

3. Using the steps in the resolution of an ethical issue or dilemma listed in Chapter 1 (Box 1-7), determine a course of action that can help Leah resolve the problem.

Factors to Teach the Patient

▶ Reasons for postponing an appointment when a herpes lesion ("fever blister" or "cold sore") is present on the lip.

▶ Importance of not touching or scratching the herpetic lesion because of self-infection to fingers or eyes.

▶ How the viruses can survive on objects and transfer infection to other people.

▶ How to help by keeping the medical history up to date by informing of additional exposures and immunizations to communicable diseases for self and family members.

▶ Importance of oral health to overall systemic health.

▶ Preparation for a dental or dental hygiene appointment by thorough mouth cleaning with toothbrush and dental floss to lower the bacterial count and thus lessen aerosol contamination in the treatment room.

ENHANCE YOUR UNDERSTANDING

ONLINE RESOURCES
(see the inside front cover for access information)

• Audio glossary
• Appendices

SUPPORT FOR LEARNING
(available separately)

• *Active Learning Workbook for Wilkins' Clinical Practice of the Dental Hygienist, 13th Edition*

INDIVIDUALIZED REVIEW

• Customized practice quizzing with Navigate 2 TestPrep for *Wilkins' Clinical Practice of the Dental Hygienist*

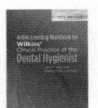

References

1. Centers for Disease Control and Prevention. *Summary of Infection Prevention Practices in Dental Settings: Basic Expectations for Safe Care.* Atlanta, GA: U.S. Department of Health and Human Services; 2016. https://www.cdc.gov/oralhealth/infectioncontrol/pdf/safe-care2.pdf. Accessed June 9, 2018.

2. Centers for Disease Control and Prevention. *Guidelines for Infection Control in Dental Health-Care Settings.* Atlanta, GA: U.S. Department of Health and Human Services; 2003. https://www.cdc.gov/mmwr/PDF/rr/rr5217.pdf. Accessed June 9, 2018.

3. Socransky SS, Manganiello SD. The oral microbiota of man from birth to senility. *J Periodontol.* 1971;42(8):485-494.

4. Gomez A, Nelson KE. The oral microbiome of children: development, disease, and implications beyond oral health. *Microb Ecol.* 2016;73(2):492-503.

5. Krishnan K, Chen T, Paster B. A practical guide to the oral microbiome and its relation to health and disease. *Oral Dis.* 2017;(3):276.

6. Abichandani S, Nadiger R. Cross contamination in dentistry: a comprehensive overview. *J Educ Ethics Dent.* 2012;2(1):3-9.

7. Singh A, Shiva Manjunath RG, Singla D, Bhattacharya HS, Sarkar A, Chandra N. Aerosol, a health hazard during ultrasonic scaling: a clinico-microbiological study. *Indian J Dent Res.* 2016;(27):160-162.

8. Wirthlin M, Roth M. Dental unit waterline contamination: a review of research and findings from a clinic setting. *Compend Contin Educ Dent.* 2015;36(3):216-219.

9. Centers for Disease Control and Prevention. *Guidelines for Preventing the Transmission of Mycobacterium tuberculosis in Health-Care Settings.* Atlanta, GA: Coordinating Center for Health Information and Service; 2005. https://www.cdc.gov/mmwr/pdf/rr/rr5417.pdf. Accessed June 9, 2018.

10. Centers for Disease Control and Prevention. *Epidemiology and Prevention of Vaccine-Preventable Diseases.* Washington, DC: Public Health Foundation; 2015:149-174.

11. Schillie S, Vellozzi C, Reingold A, et al. Prevention of hepatitis B virus infection in the United States: recommendations of the advisory committee on immunization

practices. *MMWR Recomm Rep.* 2018;67(No. RR-1):1-31. doi:10.15585/mmwr.rr6701a1.

12. Centers for Disease Control and Prevention. Recommendations for prevention and control of hepatitis C virus (HCV) infection and HCV-related chronic disease. *MMWR Recomm Rep.* 1998;47(No. RR-19):3-10. https://www.cdc.gov /mmwr/pdf/rr/rr4719.pdf. Accessed June 9, 2018.

13. Centers for Disease Control and Prevention. Recommendations for the identification of chronic hepatitis C virus infection among persons born during 1945–1965. *MMWR Recomm Rep.* 2012;61(No. RR-4). https://www.cdc.gov /mmwr/pdf/rr/rr6104.pdf. Accessed June 9, 2018.

14. Petersen J, Thompson A, Levrero M. Aiming for cure in HBV and HDV infection. *J Hepatol.* 2016;65(1):835-848.

15. Li S, Wen X. Seropositivity to herpes simplex virus type 2, but not type 1 is associated with cervical cancer: NHANES (1999-2014). *BMC Cancer.* 2017;17(1):726.

16. Jain M. Assessment of correlation of herpes simplex virus-1 with oral cancer and precancer—a comparative study. *J Clin Diagn Res.* 2016;10(8):ZC14-ZC17.

17. Bradley H, Markowitz LE, Gibson T, McQuillan GM. Seroprevalence of herpes simplex virus types 1 and 2—United States, 1999-2010. *J Infect Dis.* 2014;209(3):325-333.

18. Bilder L, Elimelech R, Machtei E. The prevalence of human herpes viruses in the saliva of chronic periodontitis patients compared to oral health providers and healthy controls. *Arch Virol.* 2013;158(6):1221-1226.

19. Munawwar A, Singh S. Human herpesviruses as copathogens of HIV infection, their role in HIV transmission, and disease progression. *J Lab Physicians.* 2016;8(1):5-18.

20. Zhu C, Li F, Wong MC, Feng XP, Lu HX, Xu W. Association between Herpesviruses and chronic periodontitis: a meta-analysis based on case-control studies. *PLos One.* 2015;10(12):e0144319.

21. Li F, Zhu C, Deng F, Wong M, Lu H, Feng X. Herpesviruses in etiopathogenesis of aggressive periodontitis: a meta-analysis based on case-control studies. *PLos One.* 2017;10(12):e0144319.

22. Aggarwal T, Lamba A, Faraz F, Tandon S. Viruses: bystanders of periodontal disease. *Microb Pathog.* 2017;102:54-58.

23. Clarkson E, Mashkoor F, Abdulateef S. Oral viral infections. *Dent Clin North Am.* 2017;61(2):351-363.

24. Stoopler E, Kuperstein A, Sollecito T. How do I manage a patient with recurrent herpes simplex? *J Can Dent Assoc.* 2012;78:c154.

25. Centers for Disease Control and Prevention. *Genital Herpes—CDC Fact Sheet (Detailed).* Atlanta, GA: Division of STD Prevention. https://www.cdc.gov/std/herpes/stdfact -herpes-detailed.htm. Accessed June 9, 2018.

26. Shoji K, Saitoh A. Herpetic whitlow. *N Engl J Med.* 2018;378(6):563-563.

27. Camasmie HR, Léda SB, Lupi O, Lima RB, D'Acri AM, Martins CJ. Chronic herpetic whitlow as the first manifestation of HIV infection. *AIDS.* 2016;30(14):2254-2256.

28. Abedi Kiasari B, Zare Tooranposhti Z. The changing epidemiology of Herpes Simplex Virus Type 1 infection: the associated effects on the incidence of ocular Herpes. *Arc Razi Inst.* 2016;71(2):125-134.

29. Centers for Disease Control and Prevention. *Epidemiology and Prevention of Vaccine-Preventable Diseases.* Washington, DC: Public Health Foundation; 2015:353-376.

30. Centers for Disease Control and Prevention. *Epstein-Barr Virus and Infectious Mononucleosis.* Atlanta, GA: National Center for Immunization and Respiratory Diseases; 2018. https://www.cdc.gov/epstein-barr/hcp.html. Accessed June 9, 2018.

31. Flores-Hidalgo A, Lim S, Curran A, Padilla R, Murrah V. Oral medicine: considerations in the diagnosis of oral hairy leukoplakia—an institutional experience. *Oral Surg Oral Med Oral Pathol Oral Radiol.* 2018;125(3):232-235.

32. Centers for Disease Control and Prevention. *Cytomegalovirus (CMV) and Congenital CMV Infection.* Atlanta, GA: National Center for Immunization and Respiratory Diseases, Division of Viral Diseases; 2017. https://www.cdc.gov/cmv /clinical/features.html. Accessed June 9, 2018.

33. Ablashi D, Agut H, Alvarez-Lafuente R, et al. Classification of HHV-6A and HHV-6B as distinct viruses. *Arch Virol.* 2014;159(5):863-870.

34. Komaroff AL, Boeckh M, Eliason E, Phan T, Kaufer BB. Summary of the 10th International Conference on Human Herpesviruses-6 and -7 (HHV-6A, -6B, and HHV-7). *J Med Virol.* 2018;90(4):625-630.

35. Wolz M, Sciallis G, Pittelkow M. Review: human herpesviruses 6, 7, and 8 from a dermatologic perspective. *Mayo Clin Proc.* 2012;87:1004-1014.

36. Dow D, Cunningham C, Buchanan A. A review of human herpesvirus 8, the Kaposi's sarcoma-associated herpesvirus, in the pediatric population. *J Pediatric Infect Dis Soc.* 2014;3(1):66.

37. Rohner E, Wyss N, Bohlius J, et al. HHV-8 seroprevalence: a global view. *Syst Rev.* 2014;3:11.

38. Centers for Disease Control and Prevention. Human papillomavirus–associated cancers—United States, 2008–2012. *MMWR Morb Mortal Wkly Rep.* 2016;65(26):661-666.

39. Bansal A, Singh M, Rai B. Human papillomavirus-associated cancers: a growing global problem. *Int J Appl Basic Med Res.* 2016;6(2):84.

40. Centers for Disease Control and Prevention. *Recommendations for HIV Prevention with Adults and Adolescents with HIV in the United States, 2014: summary for Clinical Providers.* Atlanta, GA: U.S. Department of Health and Human Services; 2014. https://stacks.cdc.gov/view/cdc/44065. Accessed June 9, 2018.

41. Centers for Disease Control and Prevention. *Division of HIV/AIDS Prevention, National Center for HIV/AIDS, Viral Hepatitis, STD, and TB Prevention, About HIV/AIDS.* Atlanta, GA: U.S. Department of Health and Human Services. https://www.cdc.gov/hiv/basics/whatishiv.html. Accessed June 9, 2018.

42. Centers for Disease Control and Prevention. *About HIV/ AIDS.* Atlanta, GA: Division of HIV/AIDS Prevention, National Center for HIV/AIDS, Viral Hepatitis, STD, and TB Prevention, HIV Transmission; 2018. https://www.cdc .gov/hiv/basics/transmission.html. Accessed June 9, 2018.

43. Centers for Disease Control and Prevention and Association of Public Health Laboratories. *Laboratory Testing for the Diagnosis of HIV Infection: Updated Recommendations.* Atlanta, GA: U.S. Department of Health and Human Services; 2018.

44. Coogan M, Greenspan J, Challacombe S. Oral lesions in infection with human immunodeficiency virus. *Bull World Health Organ.* 2005;83(9):700-706.

45. Patton LL. Current strategies for prevention of oral manifestations of human immunodeficiency virus. *Oral Surg Oral Med Oral Pathol Oral Radiol.* 2016;121(1):29-38.

46. Gnanasundaram N. Key to diagnose HIV/AIDS clinically through its oral manifestations. *J Indian Acad Oral Med Radiol.* 2010;22:119-125.

47. Malani PN. National burden of invasive methicillin-resistant *Staphylococcus aureus* infection. JAMA. 2014;311 (14):1438-1439.

48. Centers for Disease Control and Prevention. *Methicillin-Resistant Staphylococcus aureus (MRSA).* Atlanta, GA: U.S. Department of Health and Human Services; 2018. https://www.cdc.gov/mrsa/healthcare/index.html. Accessed June 8, 2018.

49. Caton J, Armitage G, Berglundh T, et al. A new classification scheme for periodontal and peri-implant diseases and conditions: introduction and key changes from the 1999 classification. *J Periodontol.* 2018;89(suppl 1):S1-S8. https://doi.org/10.1002/JPER.18-0157

50. Papapanou PN, Sanz M, et al. Periodontitis: consensus report of workgroup 2 of the 2017 world workshop on the classification of periodontal and peri-implant diseases and conditions. *J Periodontol.* 2018;89(suppl 1):S173-S182. https://doi.org/10.1002/JPER.17-0721

51. de Almeida V, Lima I, Ziegelmann P, Paranhos L, de Matos F. Impact of highly active antiretroviral therapy on the prevalence of oral lesions in HIV-positive patients: a systematic review and meta-analysis. *Int J Oral Maxillofac Surg.* 2017;11:1497-1504.

52. Shahani L, Hamill R. Therapeutics targeting inflammation in the immune reconstitution inflammatory syndrome. *Transl Res.* 2016;167(1):88-103.

Exposure Control: Barriers for Patient and Clinician

Lori J. Giblin-Scanlon, RDH, MS, DHSc

CHAPTER OUTLINE

INFECTION CONTROL
I. Standard Precautions

PERSONAL PROTECTION FOR THE DENTAL TEAM
I. Immunizations
II. Maintain Records

CLINICAL ATTIRE
I. Protective Clothing
II. Hair and Head Covering

USE OF FACE MASK: RESPIRATORY PROTECTION
I. Aerosols
II. Mask Efficiency
III. Use of a Mask
IV. Respiratory Hygiene

USE OF PROTECTIVE EYEWEAR
I. Indications for Use of Protective Eyewear
II. Suggestions for Clinical Application

HAND CARE
I. Bacteriology of the Skin
II. Hand Care

HAND-HYGIENE PRINCIPLES
I. Rationale
II. Purposes
III. Facilities

METHODS OF HAND HYGIENE
I. Indications
II. Descriptions

GLOVES AND GLOVING
I. Criteria for Selection of Treatment/Examination Gloves
II. Types of Gloves
III. Procedures for Use of Gloves
IV. Factors Affecting Glove Integrity

LATEX HYPERSENSITIVITY
I. Clinical Manifestations
II. Individuals at High Risk of Latex Sensitivity
III. Management

DOCUMENTATION

EVERYDAY ETHICS

FACTORS TO TEACH THE PATIENT

REFERENCES

LEARNING OBJECTIVES

After studying this chapter, the student will be able to:

1. Identify and define key terms and concepts related to exposure control, clinical barriers, and latex sensitivity.

2. Explain the rationale and techniques for exposure control.

3. Identify the criteria for selecting effective barriers.

4. Explain the rationale, mechanics, and guidelines for hand hygiene.

5. Identify and describe the clinical manifestations and management of latex sensitivity.

INFECTION CONTROL

- Exposure control refers to all procedures during clinical care necessary to provide top-level protection from exposure to infectious agents for members of the dental team and their patients.
- Dental healthcare personnel (DHCP) have a professional obligation to serve *all* patients with comprehensive oral care, including patients with known or unknown communicable diseases.

I. Standard Precautions

- The practice of *standard precautions* means that the body fluids of all patients are treated as if they were infectious.
  - An organized system for exposure control is needed.
  - A written exposure control plan is prepared to serve as a guide for the entire team.[1] The written plan can be the basis for training new personnel.
  - Consistency between DHCPs is necessary to maintain standards of asepsis and to prevent cross-contamination.
  - As new research and commercial products become available, and adopted for use, the written protocol is revised.
  - Using the protocol and transferring the objectives and overall aims to the clinical setting are the responsibilities of each member of the dental team.
  - Physical barriers and other requirements of the protocol provide safety for both the DHCP and the patients.
- Refer to review specific recommendations from the Centers for Disease Control and Prevention (CDC).

PERSONAL PROTECTION FOR THE DENTAL TEAM

The continuing health and productivity of DHCP depend to a large degree on individuals' efforts to maintain themselves in a high standard of good health. Resistance to disease, if exposed, is enhanced in a person with good health habits.

- Loss of work time, personal suffering, long-term systemic effects, and even exclusion from continued practice are possible results from communicable disease infection.
- The only safe procedure is to practice defensively at all times, with specific precautions for personal protection.
- All clinical staff members need to be aware of the signs and symptoms of diseases that are occupational hazards for clinical dental and dental hygiene practitioners.
- Seek early diagnosis and treatment of a seemingly minor condition that could be the initial symptom of a more serious communicable disease.

I. Immunizations

Dental personnel in a hospital setting are subject to the rules and regulations for all hospital employees. Policies often require certain immunizations for new employees or proof of antibodies.

- In private dental practices, individual initiative is required to maintain standards of safety for all dental team members relative to immunizations.
- Immunizations recommended for healthcare workers include[1]:
  - Hepatitis B.
  - Influenza.
  - MMR (measles, mumps, rubella).
  - Tetanus, diphtheria, pertussis.
  - Varicella–Zoster.
  - Meningococcal.
- General recommendations on immunizations are reviewed annually by the Advisory Committee on Immunization Practices.[2]
- At the time of employment, it is reasonable for a dentist employer to request a record of current immunizations, as well as specific tests, such as for tuberculosis.
- The needs differ in different climates, countries, and locations. Persons changing work location, or traveling for participation in dental hygiene programs, need to investigate specific precautions.

II. Maintain Records

- Records for personal immunizations are regularly updated.
- Obtain tests promptly when exposed to certain infectious diseases and seek prophylactic immunization as indicated and available.
- Keep confidential written records of immunizations, boosters, and reimmunizations; plan for regular follow-up.
- When the status of current immunizations is known, time is saved by not needing a susceptibility test before initiating passive immunizations when accidental exposure occurs.

CLINICAL ATTIRE

The clinical apparel of clinicians is vulnerable to contamination from splash, spatter, aerosols, and patient contact.

- Standard clothing, such as scrubs, and street clothes are not intended to protect against hazardous materials and are not considered protective clothing.[1]
- The recommended clinic attire is designed and cared for in a manner that protects exposure from infectious materials in splatter or aerosols and minimizes cross-contamination.
- Clinic attire and shoes are not to be worn outside the clinic practice setting.[1] When clinical attire is worn outside, contamination can be carried from, and brought into, the treatment area.

I. Protective Clothing

◆ Protective clothing, such as gowns or jackets, are designed to be worn over clinical attire to protect skin and prevent cross-contamination from blood and other potentially infectious materials (Figure 6-1).

◆ Gowns and jackets are expected to be clean and maintained as free as possible from contamination.

◆ The gown or jacket is closed at the neck and fastened in back.

◆ The fabric is disposable or reusable, stain and fluid resistant, can be washed commercially, and withstands washing with bleach.

◆ The garment must cover the knees when the clinician is seated during treatment.

◆ Long sleeves with fitted cuffs permit protective gloves to extend over the cuffs.

◆ Gloved hands, prepared for patient treatment, are kept from touching objects or being placed in pockets.

◆ In addition, a washable or a disposable apron may be used over the gown or laboratory coat when clinical procedures involving blood, spatter, or aerosols are performed.

◆ If soaked or soiled by infectious materials, change protective clothing immediately.

◆ When protective clothing is removed, turn inside out to prevent exposure to infectious material.

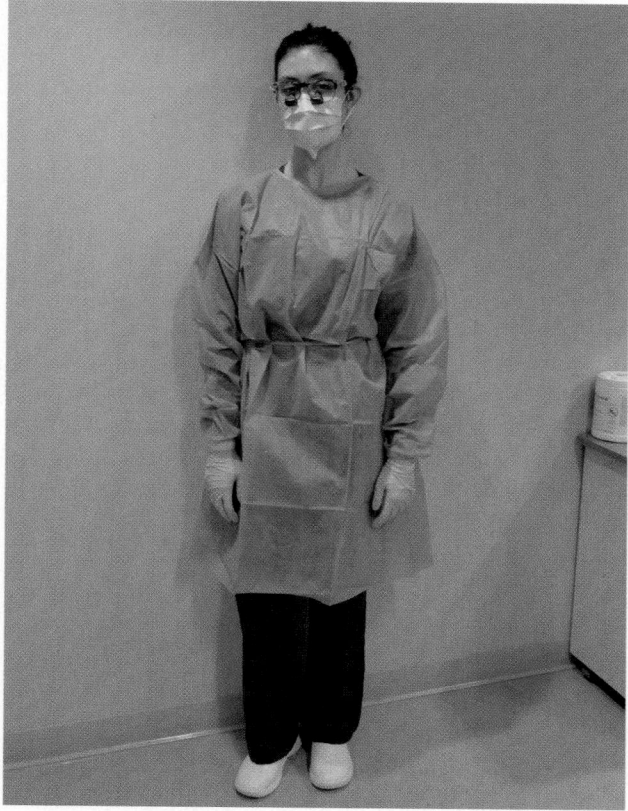

FIGURE 6-1 • Protective Clothing: Disposable Gown Worn Over Clinical Attire. (Courtesy of Susan Jenkins, RDH, MS.)

II. Hair and Head Covering

◆ Hair is worn off the shoulders and fastened back away from the face.
  • Because the hair is exposed to contamination, an appropriate head cover is advised when using handpieces and ultrasonic or air-powder polishing instruments that create aerosols.

◆ Facial hair needs to be covered with a face mask and face shield.

USE OF FACE MASK: RESPIRATORY PROTECTION

Basic personal barrier protection is composed of face mask, protective eyewear, and gloves.

◆ The use of the face mask is described first because it needs to be positioned first when preparing for clinical care procedures.

◆ The protective eyewear is placed second. After that, hand hygiene is performed before gloving.[3]

I. Aerosols

◆ Dispersion of particles of debris, polishing agents, calculus, and water, all of which are contaminated by the patient's oral flora, occurs regularly during treatment procedures.

◆ Aerosols are created following the use of a handpiece, prophylaxis angle, or a power-driven ultrasonic scaler.

◆ Particles can spread on the face, protective eyewear, uniform, and the barrier placed over the patient for protection from the spray.

II. Mask Efficiency

A. Criteria: Essential Characteristics (Box 6-1)

◆ *Filtration* (measured in bacterial filtration efficiency [BFE]):
  • The American Society for Testing and Materials uses a standard test method for evaluating the BFE of medical face masks. The BFE is a measurement of the masks resistant to bacteria.

BOX 6-1
Characteristics of an Ideal Mask

1. No contact with the wearer's nostrils or lips.
2. Has a high bacterial filtration efficiency rate.
3. Fits snugly around the entire edges of the mask.
4. No fogging of eyewear.
5. Convenient to put on and remove.
6. Made of material that does not irritate skin or induce allergic reaction.
7. Does not collapse during wear or when wet.

- Use a surgical mask that will cover the nose and mouth with >95% BFE.[3]
- Airborne droplets smaller than 3–5 μm in size can reach the alveoli of the lower respiratory tract and may potentially cause infection.[4]
- Droplet nuclei (*Mycobacterium tuberculosis*) range from 0.5 to 1 μm and are a risk in healthcare settings.[5]
- *Fit*: Proper fit over face is vital to protect against inhaling droplet nuclei from aerosols.
- *Moisture absorption*: Soak through is an important factor. Lining needs to be impervious.
- *Comfort*: Degree of comfort encourages compliance in wearing.

B. Materials

- Various materials have been used for masks, including:
  - Gauze and other cloth.
  - Plastic foam.
  - Fiberglass.
  - Synthetic fiber mat.
  - Paper.
- Foam, paper, and cloth have been shown to be the least adequate filters of aerosols, whereas glass fiber and synthetic fiber mat were shown to be the most effective.[6,7]
- Particulate respirator mask (PRM)
  - Use the National Institute for Occupational Safety and Health–certified PRM (e.g., N95, N99, or N100) for potentially infectious patient (active tuberculosis) when ventilation is poor, and procedures likely to produce droplet spatter or aerosols of oral or respiratory fluids.[5]
  - Heavy-duty mask designed with a tight fit.

III. Use of a Mask

- Adjust the mask and position eyewear before performing hand hygiene.
- Use a new mask for each patient.
  - Change mask each hour during routine procedures or more frequently when it becomes wet.
- Keep the mask on after completing a procedure while still in the presence of aerosols.
  - Particles 1–5 μm can remain suspended for hours and can be inhaled directly into terminal lung alveoli.[8]
  - Removal of a mask in the treatment room immediately following the use of aerosol-producing procedures permits direct exposure to airborne organisms.
- Mask removal
  - Grasp side elastic or tie strings to remove (Figure 6-2).
  - Never handle the outside of a contaminated mask with gloved or bare hands. Never place the mask under the chin.

IV. Respiratory Hygiene

- Implement respiratory hygiene protocols for patients or anyone who presents in a dental setting with signs or symptoms of a respiratory illness such as coughing,

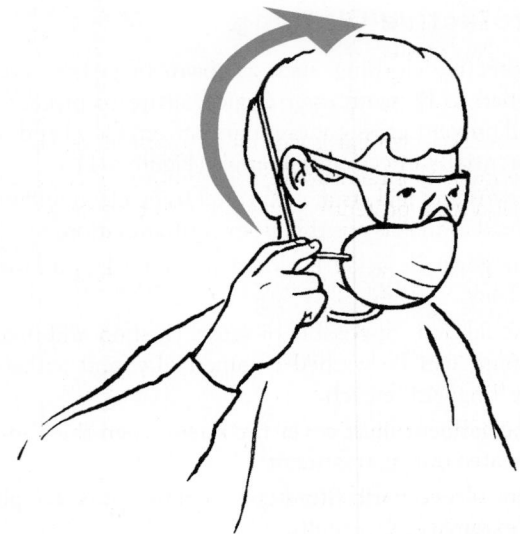

FIGURE 6-2 • Removal of Mask. Handle only by the elastic or tie strings, carefully avoiding the contaminated mask.

sneezing, or runny nose.[9] Signs are posted to inform patients with symptoms of respiratory illness to cover their mouth and nose when sneezing or coughing.[9]
- Tissues and receptacles with no touch technology for disposal are made available.[9]
- Offer methods for hand hygiene (sinks with soap and disposable towels or alcohol-based rub).[9]

USE OF PROTECTIVE EYEWEAR

Eye protection for the dental team members and patients is necessary to prevent physical injuries and infections of the eyes.
- Severe and disabling eye accidents and infections have been reported.[10-12]
- Eye involvement may lead to pain, discomfort, loss of work time, and, in certain instances, permanent injury.
- Accidents can occur at any time, and as with most accidents, they occur when least prepared for or expected.
- Eye infections can follow the accidental dropping of an instrument on the face or the splashing of various materials from a patient's oral cavity into the eye.
- Contamination can be introduced from saliva, biofilm, carious material, pieces of old restorative materials during cavity preparation, bacteria-laden calculus during scaling, and any other microorganisms contained in aerosols or spatter.
- Careful, deliberate techniques and instrument management, with evacuation and other procedures for the control of oral fluids, contribute to the prevention of accidents and infections of the eyes.
- All measures described for the prevention of airborne disease transmission by aerosols and spatter apply to eye protection.
- The most effective defense is the use of protective eyewear by all involved—dental team members and patients.

I. Indications for Use of Protective Eyewear

A. Dental Team Members

◆ Protective eyewear is worn for all procedures.

◆ Dental personnel who do not require corrective lens for vision wear protective eyewear with clear lens.

B. General Features of Acceptable Eyewear

◆ Sufficient eye coverage, with side shields, to protect around the eye.

◆ Shatterproof; made of strong, sturdy plastic.

◆ Lightweight.

◆ Flexible and with rounded smooth edges to prevent discomfort.

◆ Easily disinfected.
  • Smooth surface areas to prevent accumulation of infectious material.
  • Disinfectant used cannot damage or distort the frames or lens.

◆ A clear or lightly tinted lens, rather than a very dark lens, permits the dental team members to watch the patient's reactions and maintain contact and response.

◆ Desirable but not required: scratch-resistant, antifog, and antistatic.

C. Types of Eyewear

Many styles, including regular eyeglass shapes and those described as follows, have been used.

◆ *Goggles:* Shielding on all sides of the glasses may give the best protection, provided they fit closely around the edges. Goggle-style coverage is necessary for protection during laboratory work.

◆ *Eyewear with side shields* (Figure 6-3A): A side shield can provide added protection, but do not protect from splashes or droplets as well as goggles.[13] For the member of the dental team who depends on a prescription lens, separate side shields are available that can be connected to the bows.

◆ *Eyewear with curved frames* (Figure 6-3B): When the sides of the eyewear are curved back, they may provide a protection somewhat similar to that offered by those with the side shield.

◆ *Postmydriatic spectacles used by ophthalmologist:* Disposable glasses are available that are made of antiultraviolet flexible plastic (Figure 6-3C).

◆ *Dental loupes* (Figure 6-3D): Designed to protect the eyes and magnify the oral cavity. When they are designed with a light or flip-up, do not touch during clinical procedures.

◆ *Child-sized:* Child-sized sunglasses and children's play spectacles have been used.

D. Face Shield

◆ A clinician needs to wear a face shield over a regular mask when aerosol-producing handpiece, power scaler, or power polishing equipment is used.

E. Protective Eyewear for Patients

◆ Protective eyewear is essential for each patient at each appointment. A patient who has not been asked to wear protective eyewear at previous appointments will appreciate a simple explanation of the reasons for doing so.

◆ Patients with their own prescription lenses may prefer to wear them, but for the safety of the patient's glasses, the use of the protective eyewear provided in the office or clinic may be advisable.

◆ Protection against glare. Certain patients may request tinted lenses or prefer to wear their own sunglasses when their eyes are especially sensitive to the dental light.

II. Suggestions for Clinical Application

A. Contact Lenses

◆ Dental team members and patients who wear contact lenses always need to wear protective eyewear over them during dental and dental hygiene procedures.

B. Care of Protective Eyewear

◆ Rinse eyewear under running water to remove abrasive particles. Rubbing an abrasive agent over the plastic lens can create scratches.

◆ Materials used for protective lens may be damaged by some disinfectants. Clean with detergent and rinse thoroughly. Air-dry.

◆ Check periodically for scratches on the lens and replace appropriately.

C. Eye Wash Station

◆ Eye wash station equipment needs to be attached to a sink not used by clinicians for patient preparation.

◆ It must not be connected to the regular faucets unless the hot water source is turned off permanently.

HAND CARE

◆ In the infectious process of disease transmission, the hands may serve as a *means of transmission* of the blood, saliva, and dental biofilm from a patient.

◆ The hands, especially under the fingernails, may serve as a *reservoir* for microorganisms.

◆ *Skin breaks in the hands may serve as a port of entry* for potentially pathogenic microorganisms.

◆ By caring properly for the hands, using effective hand-hygiene procedures, and following the basic rules for gloving, primary cross-contamination can be controlled.

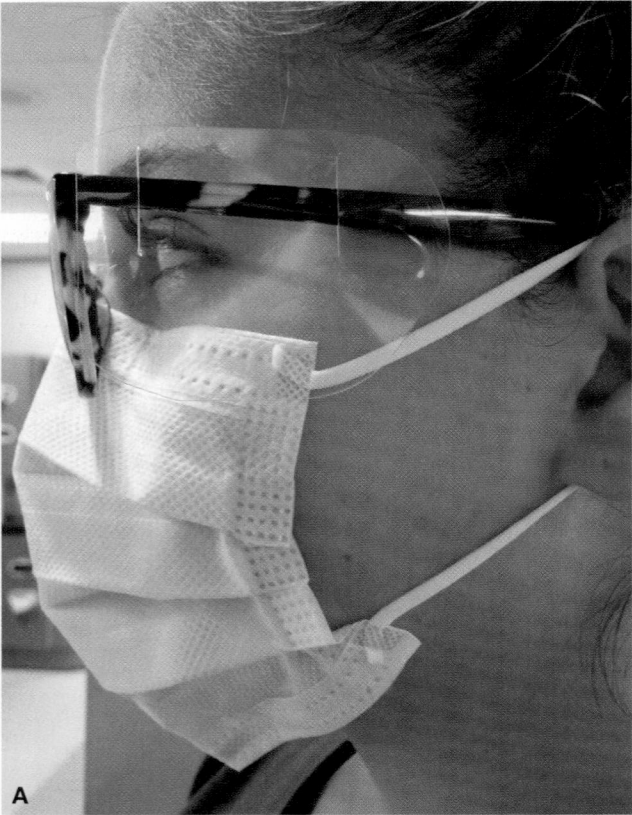

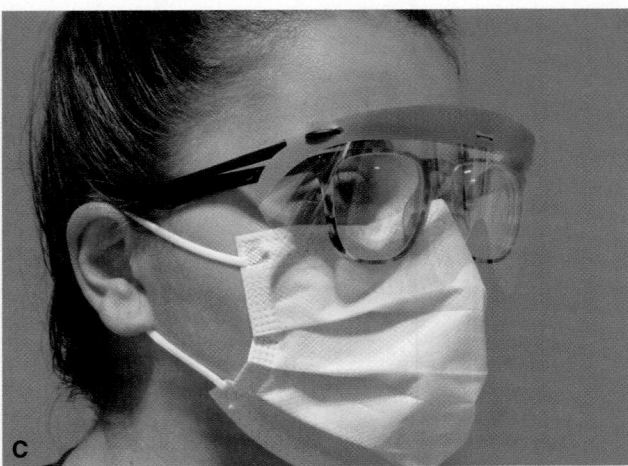

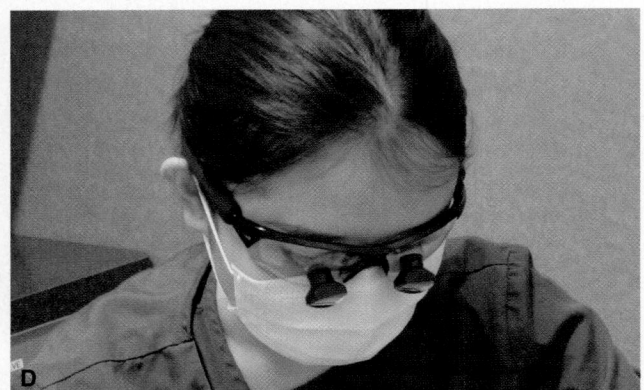

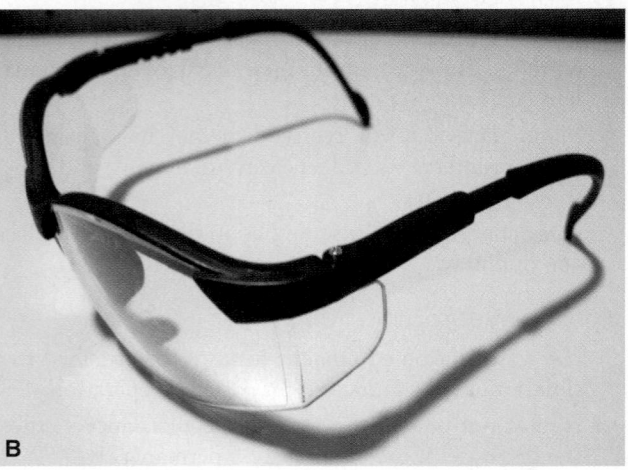

FIGURE 6-3 • Protective Eyewear. Protective cover for both patient and clinician may be goggles-style **(A)** glasses with side shields, **(B)** safety glasses, **(C)** disposable eyewear, and **(D)** loupes. (Courtesy of Susan Jenkins, RDH, MS.)

◆ A conscious effort is made to keep the gloved hands from touching objects other than the instruments and disinfected parts of the equipment prepared for the immediate patient.

I. Bacteriology of the Skin

◆ Resident bacteria
  • Many relatively stable bacteria inhabit the surface epithelium or deeper areas in the ducts of skin glands or depths of hair follicles; ultimately, they are shed with the exfoliated surface cells or with excretions of the skin glands.

  • Resident bacteria tend to be less susceptible to destruction by disinfection procedures.
◆ Transient bacteria
  • Transient bacteria reflect continuous contamination by routine contacts; some bacteria are pathogens.
  • They may be washed away or, in the event that a skin break exists, may cause an autogenous infection.
  • Most transients can be removed with soap and water by washing thoroughly or with 60%–95% ethanol or isopropanol-based hand rubs as directed by the manufacturer.

II. Hand Care

A. Fingernails

- Maintain clean, smoothly trimmed, short fingernails with well-cared-for cuticles to prevent breaks where microorganisms can enter.
- Effects of short nails:
  - Make handwashing more effective because of fewer microorganisms harbored under the nails.[14]
  - Prevent cuts from long nail in disposable gloves.
  - Permit selection of a closer fit of glove; longer glove fingers may be required to protect nails.
  - Allow greater dexterity during instrumentation.
  - Decrease chance of patient discomfort.

B. Artificial Nails

- Artificial nails or extenders are associated with fungal and bacterial pathogens in hospital settings and are not recommended for clinicians.[15-18]
- Wearing rings and nail polish is not recommended because chipped nail polish and skin under the ring may harbor bacteria.[3,19]

C. Wristwatch and Jewelry

- Remove hand and wrist jewelry at the beginning of the day.
- Microorganisms can become lodged in crevices of rings, watchbands, and watches.

D. Gloves

- After handwashing, put on gloves. Never expose open skin lesions or abrasions to a patient's oral tissues and fluids.
- After glove removal, wash hands to remove microorganisms.

HAND-HYGIENE PRINCIPLES

I. Rationale

- Effective and frequent hand hygiene can reduce the overall bacterial flora of the skin and prevent the organisms acquired from a patient from becoming skin residents.
- It is impossible to sterilize the skin, but every attempt is made to reduce the bacterial flora to a minimum.

II. Purposes

Hand hygiene, including handwashing, hand antisepsis, or surgical hand antisepsis, is critical for reducing the bacterial flora of the hands. The chosen method is dependent on the procedure and the degree of contamination. An effective hand-hygiene procedure can be expected to accomplish the following:
- Remove surface dirt and transient bacteria.
- Dissolve the normal greasy film on the skin.
- Rinse and remove all loosened debris and microorganisms.

III. Facilities

- Sink
  - Use a sink with a foot pedal or electronic control for water flow to avoid contamination to/from faucet handles.
  - For regular sink, turn on water at the beginning and leave on through the entire procedure. Turn faucets off with the towel after drying hands.
  - Clean around sink rim with disinfectant. The sink must be of sufficient size so that contact with the inside of the wash basin can be avoided. A sink cannot be sterilized and can become highly contaminated.
  - Prevent contamination of clothing by not leaning against the sink.
  - Use a separate area and sink reserved for instrument washing.
- Soap
  - Use a liquid or foam soap.
  - Apply from a foot- or knee-activated or electronically controlled dispenser to avoid contamination to and from a hand-operated dispenser or cake soap. Rinsing is a necessary part of the handwashing procedure.
- Scrub brushes
  - Avoid overvigorous use of a brush to minimize skin abrasion. Skin irritation and abrasion can leave openings for additional cross-contamination.
  - Disposable sponges are available commercially and may be preferred when a scrub brush is traumatic to the skin.
- Towels
  - Obtain disposable towel from a dispenser that requires no contact except with the towel itself, which hangs down, or a hands-free automatic dispenser.
  - Cloth towels are not recommended.

METHODS OF HAND HYGIENE

Hand hygiene is considered the most important single procedure for the prevention of cross-contamination (Box 6-2).

I. Indications

- Before and after treating each patient (before glove placement and after glove removal).
- Before regloving after removing gloves that are torn, cut, or punctured.
- After touching inanimate objects that may be contaminated with blood or saliva with ungloved hands.
- When hands are visibly soiled.
- Before leaving the treatment room.

BOX 6-2
Hand-Hygiene Methods and Indications

Method	Agent	Purpose	Duration (minimum)	Indication
Routine handwash	Water and nonantimicrobial soap (e.g., plain soap)	Remove soil and transient microorganisms	15 sec	Before and after treating each patient (e.g., before glove placement and after glove removal). After barehanded touching of inanimate objects likely to be contaminated by blood or saliva. Before leaving the dental operatory or the dental laboratory. When visibly soiled. Before regloving after removing gloves that are torn, cut, or punctured
Antiseptic handwash	Water and antimicrobial soap (e.g., chlorhexidine, iodine and iodophors, chloroxylenol [para-chloro-meta-xylenol, PCMX], triclosan)	Remove or destroy transient microorganisms and reduce resident flora	15 sec	
Antiseptic hand rub	Alcohol-based hand rub	Remove or destroy transient microorganisms and reduce resident flora	Rub hands until the agent is dry	
Surgical antisepsis	Water and antimicrobial soap (e.g., chlorhexidine, iodine and iodophors, chloroxylenol [PCMX], triclosan)	Remove or destroy transient microorganisms and reduce resident flora (persistent effect)	2–6 min	Before donning sterile surgeon's gloves for surgical procedures
	Water and nonantimicrobial soap (e.g., plain soap), followed by an alcohol-based surgical hand-scrub product with persistent activity		Follow manufacturer instructions for surgical hard-scrub product with persistent activity	

Source: U.S. Department of Health and Human Services, Centers for Disease Control and Prevention. Guidelines for infection control in dental health-care settings—2003. *MMWR Recomm Rep.* 2003;52(RR-17):15, 19.

II. Descriptions

A. Routine Handwash

Sufficient for routine dental examinations and nonsurgical dental procedures.[3]

◆ Wet hands with water, apply liquid, nonantimicrobial soap (plain soap); avoid hot water.

◆ Rub hands together for at least 15 seconds; cover all surfaces of fingers, hands, and wrists.

◆ Interlace fingers and rub to cover all sides.

◆ Rinse under running water; dry thoroughly with disposable towels.

◆ Turn off faucet with the towel.

B. Antiseptic Handwash

◆ Water and liquid antimicrobial soap (e.g., chlorhexidine, iodine and iodophors, chloroxylenol [para-chloro-meta-xylenol, PCMX], triclosan).[3]

◆ To remove or destroy transient microorganisms and reduce resident flora.[3]

1. Preliminary steps

• Remove watch and jewelry from hands.

• Fasten hair back securely.

• Put on protective eyewear and mask before handwashing to prevent contamination of washed hands ready for gloving.

• Use cool water.

2. Handwashing procedure
   - Lather hands, wrists, and forearms quickly with liquid antimicrobial soap.
   - Rub all surfaces vigorously; interlace fingers and rub back and forth with pressure.
   - Rinse thoroughly, running the water from fingertips down the hands. Keep water running.
   - Repeat two more times. One lathering for 3 minutes is less effective than are three short latherings and three rinses in 30 seconds.
   - The latherings serve to loosen the debris and microorganisms and the rinsings wash them away.
   - Use paper towels for drying, taking care not to recontaminate.

C. Antiseptic Hand Rub

An antiseptic hand rub is used to remove or destroy transient microorganisms and reduce resident flora.[3]
- ◆ Wash visibly soiled hands before use.
- ◆ Decontaminate hands with an (60%–95% ethanol or isopropanol) alcohol-based hand rub.
- ◆ Apply the product (follow manufacturer's directions for amount to use) to the palm of one hand, and vigorously rub hands together.
- ◆ If hands are dry after 10–15 seconds, the amount used may need to be increased.

D. Surgical Antisepsis[3] (Also Called Surgical Scrub[3])

- ◆ Water and antimicrobial liquid soap (e.g., chlorhexidine, iodine and iodophores, chloroxylenol [PCMX], triclosan).
- ◆ To remove or destroy transient microorganisms and reduce resident flora with a persistent or prolonged effect that inhibits proliferation or survival of microorganisms.
- ◆ Each hospital or oral surgery clinic has rules and regulations for surgical antisepsis. These will be posted over the scrub sinks.
- ◆ The minimum duration of a surgical antisepsis is 2–6 minutes.
- ◆ Following treatment of a contagious or isolated patient, the procedure will take at least 5 minutes.
   1. Preliminary steps
      - Remove watch and jewelry. Place hair and beard coverings and make sure hair is completely covered.
      - Put on protective eyewear and mask.
      - Open sterile brush package to have ready.
      - Wash hands and arms using surgical liquid antimicrobial soap to remove gross surface dirt before using the scrub brush.
      - Lather vigorously with strong rubbing motions, 10 on each side of hands, wrists, and arms.
      - Interlace the fingers and thumbs to clean the proximal surfaces.
      - Rinse thoroughly from fingertips across hands and wrists. Hold hands higher than elbows throughout the procedure. Leave water running.
      - Use orangewood stick from the sterile package to clean nails. Rinse.
   2. First hand
      - Lather the hands and arms and leave the lather on to increase the exposure time to the antimicrobial ingredient.
      - Apply surgical liquid antimicrobial soap and begin the brush procedure. Scrub in an orderly sequence without returning to areas previously scrubbed.
      - First hand and arm.
      - Brush back and forth across nails and fingertips, passing the brush under the nails.
      - Fingers and hand: use small circular strokes on all sides of the thumb and each finger, overlapping strokes for complete coverage.
      - Continue to wrist. Apply more soap to maintain a good lather.
      - When arm is completed, leave lather on.
   3. Second hand
      - Repeat on the other arm. Some systems require the use of a second sterile brush for the second hand. When this is so, discard the first brush into the proper container and obtain the second brush.
      - At one-half of scrub time, rinse hands and arms thoroughly, first one and then the other, starting at the fingertips and letting water pass down over the arm.
      - Lather and repeat.
      - At the end of time (or counts), rinse thoroughly, each arm separately, from fingertips. Apply towel from fingertips to elbow without reapplying to hand area.
      - Hold hands up and clasped together. Proceed to dressing area for gowning and gloving.

GLOVES AND GLOVING

Wearing gloves is a standard practice to protect both the patient and the clinician from cross-contamination.

I. Criteria for Selection of Treatment/Examination Gloves

A. Safety Factors
- ◆ Effective barrier; evidence from manufacturer of quality control standards.
- ◆ Impermeable to patient's saliva, blood, and bacteria.
- ◆ Strength and durability to resist tears and punctures.
- ◆ Impervious to materials routinely used during clinical procedures.
- ◆ Nonirritating or harmful to skin; use nonlatex gloves when the patient or clinician is allergic.
- ◆ Length: glove cuff extends to provide coverage over cuff of long sleeve.

B. Ergonomic Choice Factors

◆ Fit hand well; no interference with motion.

◆ Tactile sense not decreased.

◆ No tight pull over palm or between thumb and index finger.

II. Types of Gloves

◆ Material
  • Latex.
  • Nonlatex: neoprene, block copolymer, vinyl, *N*-nitrile.
◆ For patient care
  • Nonsterile single-use examination/treatment: latex, nonlatex.
  • Presterilized single-use surgical: latex, nonlatex.
◆ Utility gloves
  • Heavy duty: latex, nonlatex (puncture resistant for clinic cleanup).
  • Plastic: Food handler's glove to wear as overglove.

III. Procedures for Use of Gloves

◆ Mask and eyewear placement
  • Place mask and protective eyewear before performing hand hygiene and gloving.
  • Prevent the need for manipulating the mask around the face and hair after washing the hands.
◆ Pregloving hand hygiene
  • Use an antiseptic handwash or hand rub before gloving.
  • Hands must be dried thoroughly to control moisture inside glove and discourage growth of bacteria.
◆ Glove placement
  • Always glove and deglove in front of the patient; a patient may need assurance that gloves are new and used only for that appointment.
  • Place gloves over the cuff of long-sleeved clinic wear to provide complete protection of arms from exposure to contamination.
◆ Avoiding contamination
  • Keep gloved hands away from face, hair, clothing (pockets), telephone, patient records, clinician's stool, and all parts of the dental equipment that have not been predisinfected and covered with a barrier material.
◆ Torn, cut, or punctured glove
  • Remove immediately, wash hands thoroughly, and put on new gloves.
◆ Removal of gloves
  • Develop a procedure whereby gloves can be removed without contaminating the hands from the exposed external surfaces of the gloves.
  • Figure 6-4 illustrates one system for glove removal.
  • Wash hands promptly after glove removal. Organisms on the hands multiply rapidly inside the warm, moist environment of the glove, even when no external contamination has occurred.

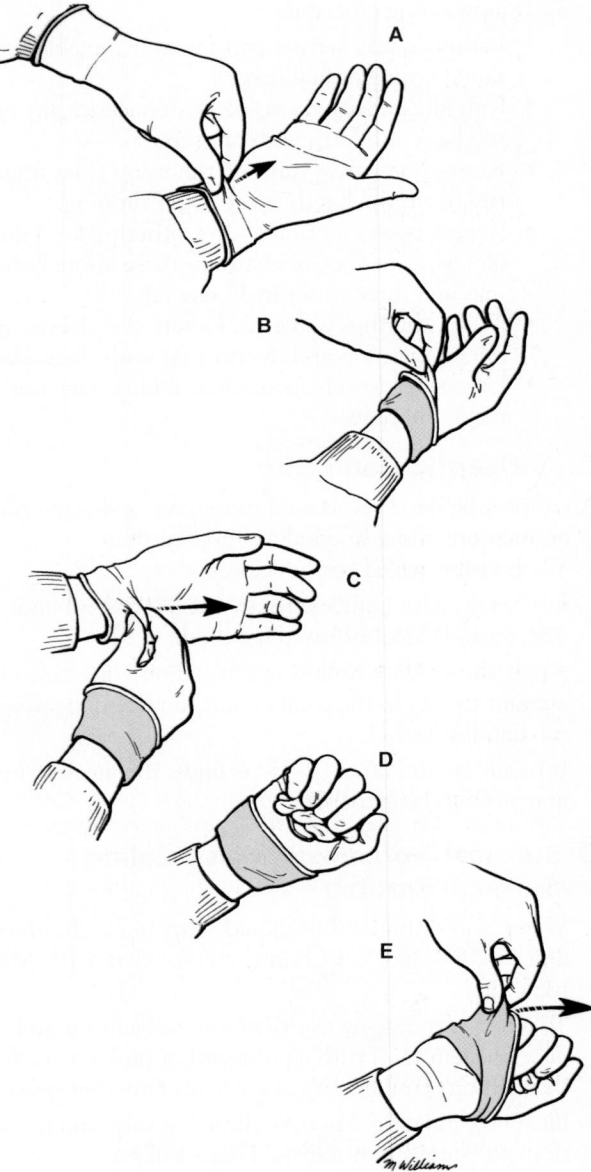

FIGURE 6-4 • Steps for Removal of Gloves. A: Use left fingers to pinch right glove near edge to fold back. **B:** Fold edge back without contact with clean inside surface. **C:** Use right fingers to contact outside of left glove at the wrist to invert and remove. **D:** Bunch glove into the palm. **E:** With ungloved left hand, grasp inner noncontaminated portion of the right glove to peel it off, enclosing the other glove as it is inverted.

IV. Factors Affecting Glove Integrity

◆ Length of time worn
  • New pair for each patient is the basic requirement.
  • Total time worn is no longer than 1 hour; when gloves develop a sticky surface, remove, wash hands, and reglove with a fresh pair.
◆ Complexity of the procedure
  • Certain procedures are more likely to promote perforations, especially when sharp instruments must be changed frequently.

◆ Packaging of the gloves
  • Gloves in a new package are tightly packed and can be torn when removed; must be handled carefully until pressure is relieved.
◆ Size of glove
  • When too long, the extra material at the fingertips can get caught, torn, or in the way; picking up small objects is difficult, especially sharp instruments.
◆ Pressure of time
  • Stress; working too fast increases the risk of glove damage.
◆ Storage of gloves
  • Keep in cool, dark place; exposure to heat, sun, or fluorescent light increases potential for deterioration and perforations.
◆ Agents used
  • Certain chemicals react with the glove material; for example, petroleum jelly, alcohol, and products made with alcohol tend to break down the glove integrity.
◆ Hazards from the hands
  • Long fingernails and rings worn inside gloves.

LATEX HYPERSENSITIVITY

Patients and clinicians may have or may develop sensitivity to natural rubber latex (NRL). Symptoms of a hypersensitive reaction range from a dermatitis to a life-threatening anaphylactic shock. The only available treatment for latex allergy is avoiding all contact.

◆ Latex sensitivity is due to the protein allergens and to additives used when the commercial latex is prepared.
◆ Latex allergens occur in any equipment or product used that contains NRL.
◆ Gloves are the most frequently used item that contains latex.
◆ Equipment listed in Box 6-3 may contain NRL. However, many of the items are also made of alternative materials. When the label on a product does not list the contents, the manufacturer can be contacted to identify latex-free items.

I. Clinical Manifestations

◆ Methods of exposure
  • Direct exposure to latex products.
  • Aeroallergen inhalation of the allergen when the powder (cornstarch) from the gloves becomes airborne.
  • Mucosal contact.
◆ Type I hypersensitivity (immediate reaction)
  • Urticaria: hives.
  • Dermatitis: rash, itching.
  • Nasal problems: sneezing, itchy nose, runny nose.
  • Eyes: watery, itchy watery, itchy.
  • Respiratory reaction: breathing difficulty, asthma-like wheezing, coughing.

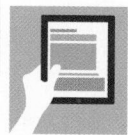

BOX 6-3
Equipment That May Contain Latex

Bite blocks
Blood pressure cuff
Gloves
Goggles
Lead apron cover
Masks (elastic head band)
Mixing bowl
Nitrous oxide nosepiece and tubing rubber dam
O ring (on ultrasonic insert)
Orthodontic elastics
Rubber polishing cup
Stethoscope
Stopper in anesthesia carpule
Suction adapter

  • Drop in blood pressure: shock.
  • Anaphylaxis.
◆ Type IV hypersensitivity (delayed reaction)
  • Contact dermatitis develops 8 hours to 5 days after contact.[20]

II. Individuals at High Risk for Latex Sensitivity

◆ Have had frequent exposure to latex products.
  • Occupational exposure: Healthcare personnel who wear latex gloves regularly for patient care or have worked in a rubber manufacturing plant.
  • Multiple medical surgeries or treatments requiring placement of rubber tubes or drains. Examples: genitourinary anomalies, spina bifida.
◆ Have other documented allergies
  • Examples: food allergies (avocado, banana, kiwi fruit, chestnuts, papaya, peanuts).

III. Management

A. Medical History

◆ Questions in history will reveal known allergies.
◆ Questions directed to latex may not suffice. Questions about other specific products need to be asked.
◆ Advise allergic patients to obtain and wear an alert badge (bracelet).

B. Document

◆ All information is carefully recorded for continuing reference.

C. Appointment Planning for Allergic Patient

◆ Treatment in a latex-free environment.

◆ Whenever possible, use nonlatex gloves and other non-latex products.[21]

◆ *Early in the day when powdered gloves are used:* Appointment before glove powder contaminates the air throughout the facility or outerwear of clinical attire becomes laden with airborne latex.

◆ Clean clinical areas:
  • Person preparing room must wear nonlatex gloves.
  • Wipe all surfaces to remove allergen.

◆ *No latex in the treatment room:* Use nonlatex products for high-risk patients (whether or not specific latex sensitivity has been known and reported in the history).

◆ *Prepare latex-free carts:* Materials and gloves, for use when seeing high-risk patients, can be readied in advance.[12]

D. Emergency Treatment Equipment and Drugs Ready

◆ Inform the entire dental team of appointment.

◆ Have a latex-free emergency cart available.[21]

◆ Alert for emergency.

DOCUMENTATION

Documentation needs to record the following:

◆ Irregularities related to personal protection that could have influenced the procedures of a routine appointment.

◆ How the special needs were taken care of for a patient with an allergy to latex.

◆ Information in medical alert that patient is sensitive to latex.

A sample progress note may be found in Box 6-4.

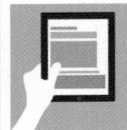

BOX 6-4

Example Documentation:
Patient with a Latex Sensitivity

S—Initial appointment for new patient to our practice. She reports sensitivity to latex gloves.

O—History form and questions completed. Informed patient that the office is latex free. Radiographs taken, risk assessment, caries examination, and periodontal assessment. Pocket depths 5–6 mm in the area of #30–31 with bleeding on probing, all other areas 3 mm or less. Plaque score 30%.

A—Patient has a history of skin reactions when latex gloves are used. Careful attention to avoiding use of products containing latex. Localized moderate chronic periodontitis between #30 and #31.

P—Review of oral self-care with attention to optimal biofilm removal #30–31. Localized nonsurgical periodontal therapy with local anesthetic with prophylaxis full mouth. About 5% sodium fluoride varnish due to moderate caries risk.

Signed: _____, RDH

Date: _____

Factors to Teach the Patient

▶ Need for the patient's complete history for the protection of both the patient and the professional person.

▶ Purposes for use of barriers (face mask, protective eyewear, and gloves) by the clinician for the benefit of the patient.

▶ Importance of eye protection.

▶ Significance of hand hygiene in the control of disease transmission (everywhere, not only dental office or clinic).

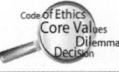

EVERYDAY ETHICS

After Mr. Green's dental hygiene treatment is completed, the dentist, Dr. Root, is notified so that the final examination can be made. Dr. Root comes in shortly and sits down next to the patient. He browses through the notations made in the patient's chart and then picks up the mirror and explorer to proceed with a clinical examination. It is apparent that he has not washed his hands and may not even have put on a new pair of gloves since he left the other treatment room. A similar situation has happened occasionally before.

Questions for Consideration

1. Mabel, the dental hygienist, notes the dentist did not change his gloves or wash his hands. Is Mable faced with an ethical dilemma or an ethical issue? Explain.

2. Read the nine "Standards of Professional Responsibility" in the American Dental Hygienists' Association Code of Ethics. Explain which of the standards are involved and how each is violated if Mable does not address this issue with Dr. Root.

3. Use the steps for making decisions in Chapter 1 Code of Ethics section to determine some actions that Mable might take to address this situation both immediately and long term.

ENHANCE YOUR UNDERSTANDING

ONLINE RESOURCES
(see the inside front cover for access information)
- Audio glossary
- Appendices

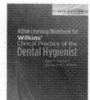

SUPPORT FOR LEARNING
(available separately)
- *Active Learning Workbook for Wilkins' Clinical Practice of the Dental Hygienist, 13th Edition*

INDIVIDUALIZED REVIEW
- Customized practice quizzing with Navigate 2 TestPrep for *Wilkins' Clinical Practice of the Dental Hygienist*

References

1. U.S. Department of Labor, Occupational Safety and Health Administration. 29 CFR Part 1910.1030. Occupational exposure to bloodborne pathogens; needlesticks and other sharps injuries; final rule. *Fed Regist.* 2001;66:5317-5325. As amended from and includes 29 CFR Part 1910.1030; Occupational exposure to bloodborne pathogens; final rule. *Fed Regist.* 1991;56:64174-64182.

2. U.S. Department of Health and Human Services, Centers for Disease Control and Prevention. Immunization of healthcare personnel. *MMWR Recomm Rep.* 2011;60(RR-07):1-45.

3. U.S. Department of Health and Human Services, Centers for Disease Control and Prevention. Guidelines for infection control in dental health-care settings—2003. *MMWR Recomm Rep.* 2003;52(RR-17):15, 19.

4. Gordon J, Ingalls T. Preventive medicine and epidemiology. *Prog Med Sci.* 1957;233:334-357.

5. U.S. Centers for Disease Control. Guidelines for preventing the transmission of Mycobacterium tuberculosis in health-care setting, 2005. *MMWR Recomm Rep.* 2005;54(RR-17):1-142.

6. Micik RE, Miller RL, Leong AC. Studies on dental aerobiology: III. Efficacy of surgical masks in protecting dental personnel from airborne bacterial particles. *J Dent Res.* 1971;50(3):626-630.

7. Miller RL, Micik RE. Air pollution and its control in the dental office. *Dent Clin North Am.* 1978;22(3):453-476.

8. Wells WF. Aerodynamics of droplet nuclei. In: Wells WF, ed. *Airborne Contagion and Air Hygiene: An Ecological Study of Droplet Infections.* Cambridge, MA: Harvard University Press; 1955:13-19.

9. Centers for Disease Control and Prevention. Respiratory hygiene/cough etiquette in healthcare settings. https://www.cdc.gov/flu/professionals/infectioncontrol/resphygiene.htm. Updated February 27, 2012. Accessed August 30, 2017.

10. Cooley RL, Cottingham AJ, Abrams H, et al. Ocular injuries sustained in the dental office: methods of detection, treatment, and prevention. *J Am Dent Assoc.* 1978;97(6):985-988.

11. Wesson MD, Thornton JB. Eye protection and ocular complications in the dental office. *Gen Dent.* 1989;37:19.

12. Roberts-Harry TJ, Cass AE, Jagger JD. Ocular injury and infection in dental practice: a survey and a review of the literature. *Br Dent J.* 1991;170(1):20-22.

13. Centers for Disease Control and Prevention. The National Institute for Occupational Safety and Health (NIOSH). Eye safety. https://www.cdc.gov/niosh/topics/eye/eye-infectious.html. Updated July 29, 2013. Accessed October 20, 2017.

14. Allen AL, Organ RJ. Occult blood accumulation under the fingernails: a mechanism for the spread of blood-borne infection. *J Am Dent Assoc.* 1982;105(3):455-459.

15. Foca M, Jakob K, Whittier S, et al. Endemic *Pseudomonas aeruginosa* infection in a neonatal intensive care unit. *N Engl J Med.* 2000;343(10):695-700.

16. Moolenaar RL, Crutcher JM, San Joaquin VH, et al. A prolonged outbreak of *Pseudomonas aeruginosa* in a neonatal intensive care unit: did staff fingernails play a role in disease transmission? *Infect Control Hosp Epidemiol.* 2000;21(2):80-85.

17. Parry MF, Grant B, Yukna M, et al. Candida osteomyelitis and diskitis after spinal surgery: an outbreak that implicates artificial nail use. *Clin Infect Dis.* 2001;32(3):352-357.

18. Passaro DJ, Waring L, Armstrong R, et al. Postoperative *Serratia marcescens* wound infections traced to an out-of-hospital source. *J Infect Dis.* 1997;175(4):992-995.

19. Arrowsmith VA, Taylor R. Removal of nail polish and finger rings to prevent surgical infection. *Cochrane Database Syst Rev.* 2012;5:CD003325.

20. Muller BA. Minimizing latex exposure and allergy: how to avoid or reduce sensitization in the healthcare setting. *Postgrad Med.* 2003;113(4):91-97.

21. Centers for Disease Control, National Institute for Occupational Safety and Health. *Alert: Preventing Allergic Reactions to Natural Rubber Latex in the Workplace.* Cincinnati, OH: Public Health Service, U.S. Department of Health and Human Services. June, 1997.

7

Infection Control: Clinical Procedures

Lory A. Libby, RDH, MSDH

CHAPTER OUTLINE

INFECTION CONTROL
I. Objectives
II. Basic Considerations for Safe Practice

TREATMENT ROOM FEATURES
I. Contact Surfaces
II. Housekeeping Surfaces

INSTRUMENT PROCESSING CENTER
I. Supplies

PRECLEANING PROCEDURES
I. Manual Scrubbing
II. Instrument Washer/Thermal Disinfector
III. Ultrasonic Processing

INSTRUMENT PACKING AND MANAGEMENT SYSTEM
I. Instrument Arrangement
II. Preparation

STERILIZATION
I. Approved Methods
II. Selection of Method
III. Tests for Sterilization

MOIST HEAT: STEAM UNDER PRESSURE
I. Autoclave Types
II. Use
III. Principles of Action
IV. Evaluation

DRY HEAT
I. Use
II. Principles of Action
III. Operation
IV. Evaluation

CHEMICAL VAPOR STERILIZER
I. Use
II. Principles of Action
III. Operation
IV. Care of Sterilizer
V. Evaluation

INTERMEDIATE-USE STEAM STERILIZATION

CHEMICAL LIQUID STERILIZATION

CARE OF STERILE INSTRUMENTS

CHEMICAL DISINFECTANTS
I. Manufacturer's Information
II. Categories
III. Uses
IV. Principles of Action
V. Criteria for Selection of a Chemical Agent

BARRIERS AND SURFACE COVERS
I. Benefits
II. Procedure

PREPARATION OF THE TREATMENT ROOM
I. Objective
II. Preliminary Planning
III. Surface Disinfection Procedure
IV. Clean and Disinfect Environmental Surfaces
V. Unit Water Lines

PATIENT PREPARATION
I. Preprocedural Oral Hygiene Measures
II. Application of a Surface Antiseptic

SUMMARY OF STANDARD PROCEDURES
I. Patient Factors
II. Clinic Preparation
III. Factors for the Dental Team
IV. Treatment Factors
V. Posttreatment

DISPOSAL OF WASTE
I. Regulations
II. Guidelines for Disposal of Waste

SUPPLEMENTAL RECOMMENDATIONS
I. Cleaning the Face
II. Smoking and Eating
III. Reception Area
IV. Sterilization Monitoring
V. Office Policy Manual

OCCUPATIONAL POSTEXPOSURE MANAGEMENT
I. Significant Exposures
II. Procedure Following Exposure
III. Follow-Up

DOCUMENTATION

EVERYDAY ETHICS

FACTORS TO TEACH THE PATIENT

REFERENCES

LEARNING OBJECTIVES

After studying this chapter, the student will be able to:

1. Describe the basic considerations for safe infection control practices.

2. Explain methods for cleaning and sterilizing instruments.

3. Describe procedures to prepare, clean, and disinfect the treatment area.

4. Explain process for managing hypodermic needles and occupational postexposure management.

5. List types of waste disposal and explain how each type is handled.

INFECTION CONTROL

The success of a planned system for control of disease transmission depends on the cooperative effort of each member of the dental team.

- The aim is to provide the highest level of infection control to ensure a safe environment for both patients and the clinical team.
- The presence of specific disease-producing organisms is rarely known; therefore, application of protective, preventive procedures is needed before, during, and following *all* patient appointments.

I. Objectives

The following are guidelines necessary to prevent the transmission of infectious agents and eliminate cross-contamination:

- Reduction of available pathogenic microorganisms to a level at which the normal resistance mechanisms of the body can prevent infection.
- Elimination of cross-contamination by breaking the chain of infection (see Chapter 5).
- Application of standard precautions by treating each patient as if all human blood and body fluids are infectious.

II. Basic Considerations for Safe Practice

When developing a safe practice routine, the sterilization and disinfection of patient care items are categorized into the following:

- *Critical items:* These items will come into contact with soft tissue and bone and run the highest risk of disease transition. These items should be disposable or sterilized using a heat sterilizer.[1] Examples of these are surgical instruments, scalers, probes, needles, and scalpel blades.
- *Semi-critical items:* These items come into contact with nonintact skin. Semi-critical items have a lower risk of transmitting disease than do critical items; however, these should also be disposable or be processed using heat sterilization.[2] If these items are heat sensitive, they should be processed using a high-level disinfectant.[3]

Examples of these include mouth mirrors and impression trays.

- *Noncritical items:* These items could potentially come into contact with intact skin and pose the lowest risk of disease transmission.[2]

TREATMENT ROOM FEATURES

A partial list of notable features is included here and illustrated in Figure 7-1. The objective is to have materials, shapes, and surface textures to facilitate the effective use of infection control measures.

I. Contact Surfaces

Contact surface can sometimes be referred to as noncritical items and consist of instruments and surfaces that may come into contact with intact skin.[1,2] These surfaces can potentially be contaminated by spray or splatter or by hand contact by a dental healthcare personnel. Contact surfaces can be disinfected using an Environmental Protection Agency (EPA)-registered hospital disinfectant but should be covered with a barrier whenever possible. Examples of these surfaces include light switches, draw handles, faucets, pens, pencils, doorknobs, telephones as well as the following standard features of a dental treatment room.[2]

A. The Unit

- Designed for easy cleaning and disinfection, with smooth, uncluttered surfaces.
- Removable hoses that can be cleaned, disinfected, and covered.
- Syringes with autoclavable tips or fitted with disposable tips.

B. Dental Chair

- Foot-operated controls.
- Surface and seamless finish of easily cleaned plastic material that withstands chemical disinfection without damage.
- Cloth upholstery to be avoided.

C. Light

- Removable handle for sterilization or disposable barrier cover.

TREATMENT ROOM FEATURES

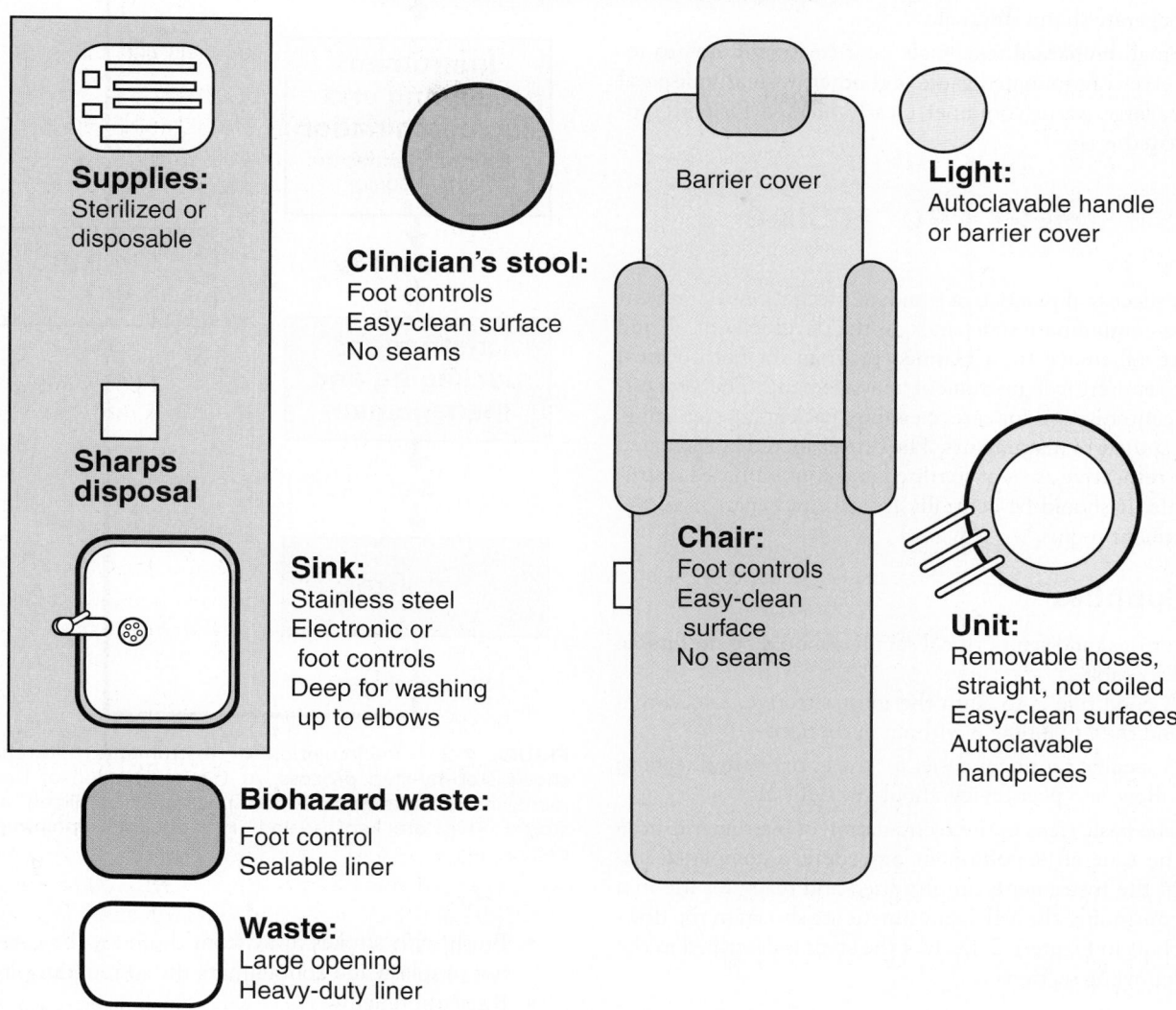

Supplies: Sterilized or disposable

Sharps disposal

Sink:
Stainless steel
Electronic or foot controls
Deep for washing up to elbows

Biohazard waste:
Foot control
Sealable liner

Waste:
Large opening
Heavy-duty liner

Clinician's stool:
Foot controls
Easy-clean surface
No seams

Barrier cover

Light:
Autoclavable handle or barrier cover

Chair:
Foot controls
Easy-clean surface
No seams

Unit:
Removable hoses, straight, not coiled
Easy-clean surfaces
Autoclavable handpieces

Floor: Smooth, easy clean, nonabsorbent, no carpeting

FIGURE 7-1 • Optimal Treatment Room Features.

D. Clinician's Chair

Smooth, plastic seat cover that is easily disinfected and has a minimum of seams and creases.

E. Radiographic Equipment

◆ Constructed of a smooth material for easily disinfection or disposable barrier cover.

II. Housekeeping Surfaces

Housekeeping surfaces consist of surfaces such as floors, wall, sinks, bathrooms, or any surface that poses no risk of disease transmission in dental care settings.[2] The Centers for Disease Control and Prevention (CDC) recommends these areas be cleaned using detergent and water or an EPA-registered hospital disinfectant/detergent.[2]

A. Floor

◆ No cloth carpeting.

◆ Smooth floor covering, easily cleaned, nonabsorbent.

B. Sink

◆ Smooth material (stainless steel).

◆ Wide and deep enough for effective handwashing without splashing or touching sides.

◆ Automatic water faucets and soap dispensers with electronic, "hand," "knee," or foot-operated controls.

C. Waste

◆ Most waste is disposed with usual waste.

◆ Receptacle with opening large enough to prevent contact with sides when material is deposited.

- ◆ Heavy-duty plastic bag liner to be sealed tightly for disposal.
- ◆ Separate sharps disposal.
- ◆ Small biohazard receptacle near treatment area to receive contaminated gauze and other waste, for disposal in large waste container clearly marked for contaminated waste.

INSTRUMENT PROCESSING CENTER

The successful practice of standard precautions to prevent cross-contamination depends on the development of, and strict adherence to, a planned program for both critical and semi-critical instrument management. The processing center is used for care, cleaning, packaging, sterilizing, and storage of instruments. The center should be separated into respective areas of sterilized and contaminated instruments. It should be centrally located and apart from the treatment rooms.[3]

I. Supplies

All critical and semi-critical supplies should be sterilizable or disposable.

- ◆ A good rule is to learn the most effective, safe system and then to follow it without exception.
- ◆ A specific routine is easier for the entire dental team to follow, and peer review should be built in.
- ◆ The basic steps in the recirculation of instruments from the time an appointment procedure is completed until the instruments are sterilized and ready for use in a continuing clinical appointment are shown in the flowchart in Figure 7-2. Each of the steps is described in the following sections.

PRECLEANING PROCEDURES

There are three basic methods for precleaning to remove any organic or inorganic debris from instruments before sterilization: manual scrubbing, washer/thermal disinfector, and ultrasonic processing.[1]

I. Manual Scrubbing

- ◆ The use of automated devices is the preferred method of instrument cleaning. Manual scrubbing is not a recommended cleaning method. However, if manual scrubbing is necessary, the following precautions are essential[3]:
  - • Wear heavy-duty gloves, protective eyewear, and mask.
  - • Dismantle instruments with detachable parts. Open jointed instruments.
  - • Use detergent and scrub with a long-handled brush under running water; hold the instruments low in the sink. Scrubbing one instrument at a time minimizes risk of puncture injury.

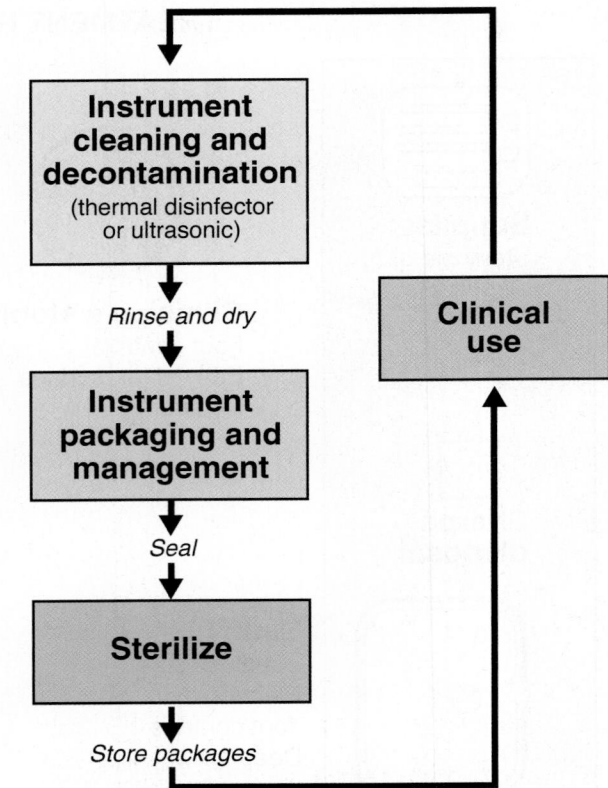

FIGURE 7-2 • Recirculation of Instruments. Flowchart shows step-by-step process. At the completion of treatment, instruments are cleaned, packaged, sterilized, and stored. They are kept sealed until patient appointment begins.

- • Brush with strokes away from the body; be careful not to splash and contaminate the surrounding area.
- • Rinse thoroughly.
- • Air-dry resting on paper towels to avoid saturation of the sterilization package.
- ◆ Care of Brushes
  - • Color code instrument brushes to distinguish from handwash brushes.
  - • Soak and wash contaminated brushes in detergent; rinse thoroughly and sterilize.

II. Instrument Washer/Thermal Disinfector

- ◆ The instrument washer uses high-velocity hot water and a detergent to clean instruments.
  - • Some models are equipped to dry the instruments.
  - • Household dishwashers may look similar to instrument washers but are different and not appropriate for dental instruments.[4]
- ◆ The instrument washer/thermal disinfector also differs from the plain washer by having a higher degree of temperature, so it disinfects as well as cleans the instruments[4] (Figure 7-3A). Benefits from the use of washer/

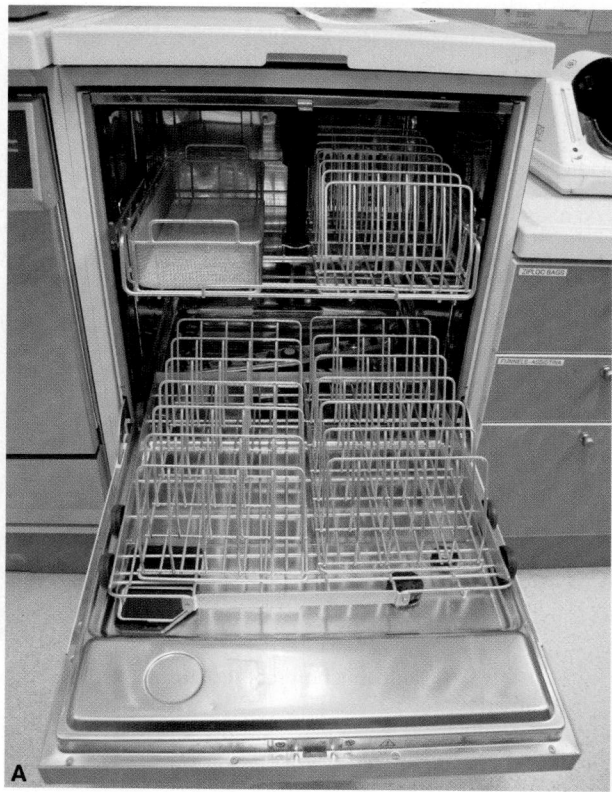

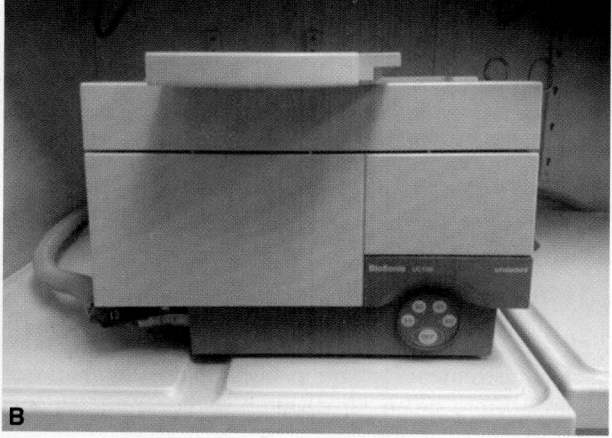

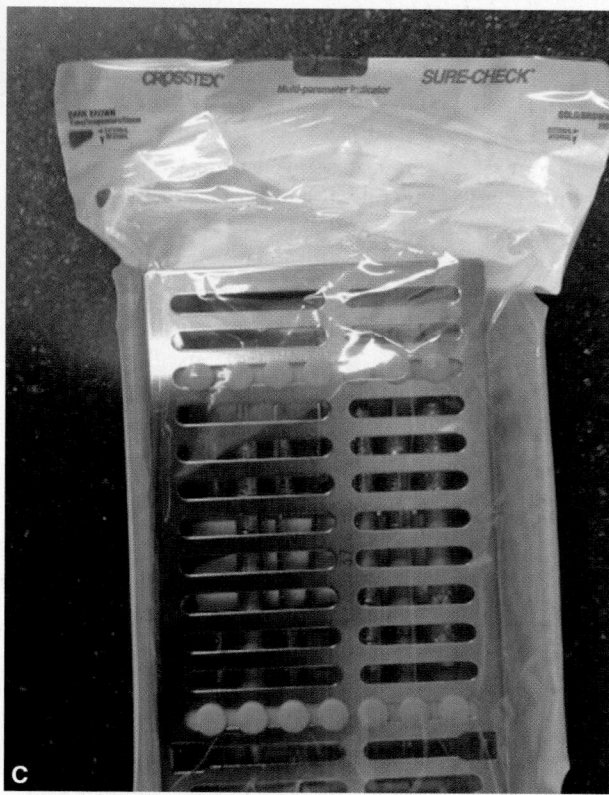

FIGURE 7-3 • **A:** Instrument washer. **B:** Ultrasonic processor. **C:** Instrument cassette in a sterilization pouch.

thermal disinfector and ultrasonic cleaning versus manual scrubbing include the following[5]:

- Increased efficiency in obtaining a high degree of cleanliness for improved disinfection.
- Reduced danger to clinician from direct contact with potentially pathogenic microorganisms.
- Elimination of possible dissemination of microorganisms through release of aerosols and droplets, which can occur during the scrubbing process.

◆ Disinfection allows the instruments in cassettes to be handled with gloves while packaging.

III. Ultrasonic Processing

An Ultrasonic Processor removes debris from instruments using acoustic energy waves transmitted in liquid disrupting the attachment of debris from an object.[1,5]

◆ Ultrasonic cleaning before sterilization is safer than manual cleaning. Manual cleaning of instruments is a dangerous, difficult, and time-consuming procedure.

◆ Ultrasonic equipment is maintained and used according to manufacturer's guidelines (Figure 7-3B).

◆ *Ultrasonic processing is not a substitute for sterilization; it is only a cleaning process to remove debris.*

A. Procedure

◆ Guard against overloading; the solution must contact all surfaces. Instruments need to be completely immersed.

◆ Dismantle instruments with detachable parts. Open jointed instruments.

◆ Time accurately by manufacturer's instructions.

◆ Drain, rinse, and air-dry.

B. Indications for Thorough Drying

When sterilizing by dry heat or chemical vapor, non–stainless steel instruments or carbon steel require predip in rust inhibitor before steam autoclaving; water on instruments dilutes the antirust solution.

INSTRUMENT PACKING AND MANAGEMENT SYSTEM

Instrument management systems are important to have in place in order to prevent contamination of newly sterilized instruments. The system should:

◆ Provide a means of organizing instrument packets for different procedures.

◆ Assure instruments are sterilized and ready for immediate use on opening.

◆ Provide a means of storing instruments packets.

I. Instrument Arrangement

◆ Each package is dated and marked for identification of contents: for example, *Adult Prophylaxis; Examination.*

◆ Clear packages that self-seal and permit instrument identification without special labeling are often used (Figure 7-3C).

◆ Instruments can be organized into tray systems, dental storage containers, or cassettes customized based on various dental hygiene procedures such as an initial exam of an adult patient, child patient, or periodontal maintenance patient.

◆ Instruments and accessories held in one unit provide a sterile environment for instruments during treatment.

◆ After the treatment, they serve as packaging for the process of cleaning, disinfection, and sterilization.

II. Preparation

◆ Cassettes can be wrapped or packaged, and single instruments are packaged.

  • Each method of sterilization has specific requirements, and the manufacturers' recommendations are followed.

  • The packaging material permits the steam or chemical vapor to pass through the contents and maintains sterility during transport and storage.

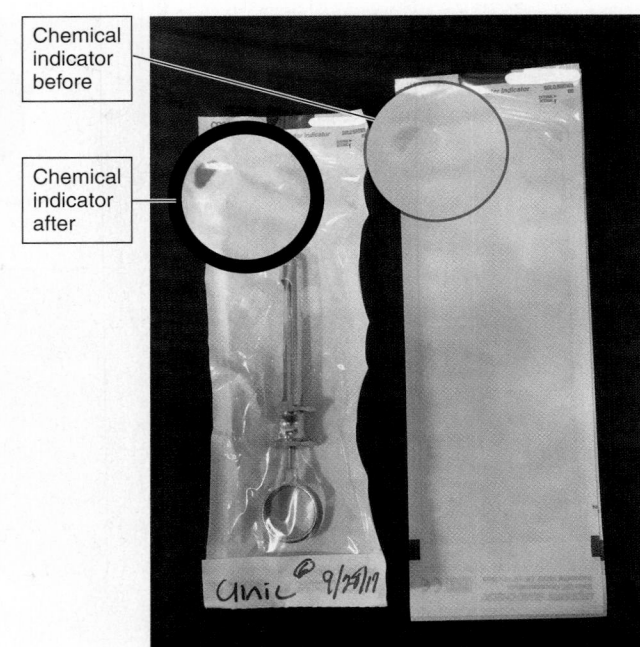

Chemical indicator before

Chemical indicator after

FIGURE 7-4 • Built-in Chemical Indicator Before and After Sterilization.

  • Sturdy wrapping is necessary to prevent punctures or tears that break the chain of asepsis and require a repeat of the process.

◆ Seal

  • Pins, paper clips, or other types of metal fasteners are not used to seal packages because they may create holes for the entry of microorganisms.

  • Chemical indicator tape is used unless the package is self-seal and the wrap has built-in indicators (Figure 7-4).

  • The change of color on the indicator confirms the autoclave reached a designated temperature required for penetration. This is not a conformation of sterilization but an indication the device is working properly.[3]

  • When using indicator tape, distinct black stripes will appear. A lighter color change may be a warning signal that the autoclave function needs to be checked.

  • The striped indicator tape is left on the sealed package and thereby serves to identify those packages ready for use. Packages are kept completely sealed until unwrapped in front of the patient.

STERILIZATION

Sterilization is accomplished with equipment cleared by the U.S. Food and Drug Administration (FDA). Sterilizing equipment should be used according to the manufacturer's specifications. Each of the methods listed here are described in the following sections. Table 7-1 summarizes the operating requirements of each.

TABLE 7-1 • Comparison of Methods for Sterilization

METHOD	STERILIZING REQUIREMENT	
	TIME (MIN)	TEMPERATURE
Steam under pressure (autoclave)		
1. Gravity displacement	15–30	250°F (121°C)
2. Prevacuum	3.5–10	270°F (132°C)
Dry heat oven	120	320°F (160°C)
Unsaturated chemical vapor	20	270°F (132°C)

I. Approved Methods

◆ Steam under pressure (autoclave).

◆ Dry heat.

◆ Chemical vapor.

◆ Immediate-use steam sterilization (flash).

◆ Chemical (cold) sterilization—not recommended.

II. Selection of Method

◆ All materials and items cannot be treated by the same system of sterilization.

◆ The method for sterilization selected provides complete destruction of all microorganisms, viruses, and spores and yet must not damage the instruments and other materials.

◆ Incomplete sterilization frequently results from inadequate preparation of the materials to be sterilized (cleaning all debris, packaging), misuse of the equipment (overloading, timing, temperature selection), or inadequate maintenance.[1]

III. Tests for Sterilization

◆ Sterilization is the process by which all forms of life are destroyed. That definition provides the rationale for testing whether a sterilizer is working properly.[1]

◆ Three tests are used: an external and an internal chemical indicator and a biologic monitor.

◆ Weekly testing is recommended or when changes such as repair or relocation of unit occur.[1,6]

◆ Equipment can be obtained for performing the testing, or commercial mail-in services are available.

◆ *External chemical indicator:* to seal the package and changes color to show the autoclave temperature has been reached.

◆ *Internal chemical indicator:* color change assesses instrument exposure to temperature and steam for the required time.

◆ Biologic monitor (*spore testing*): tests for proper functioning of the autoclave.

- The testing system requires use of selected test microorganisms put through a regular cycle of sterilization and then cultured. When no growth occurs, the sterilizer has performed with maximum efficiency.

- *Microorganisms used:*
  1. Steam autoclave: *Geobacillus stearothermophilus* (formerly *Bacillus stearothermophilus*) vials, ampules, or strips.[3]
  2. Dry heat oven: *Bacillus atrophaeus* (formerly *Bacillus subtilis*) strips.[3]
  3. Chemical vapor: *Geobacillus stearothermophilus* (formerly *Bacillus stearothermophilus*) strips.[3]

- *Procedures*
  1. Manufacturer's directions determine the placement and location of bacterial indicators.[4] If there are not any instructions, the ampule, vial, or strip is placed in the center of a package, which in turn is placed in the middle of the load of packages to be sterilized.
  2. After the cycle has been completed at the customary time and temperature, the ampule or strip is incubated. Ampules and vials show the color change associated with no living microorganisms, whereas the strip organisms are cultured and show no growth if the sterilizer has performed properly.
  3. Table 7-2 lists indications for performing spore tests in dental settings. Records or logs showing dates and outcomes of each test must be maintained.

TABLE 7-2 • Spore Testing

WHEN	WHY
Once per week	To verify proper use and functioning
Whenever a new type of packaging material or tray is used	To ensure that the sterilizing agent is getting inside to the surface of the instruments
After training of new sterilization personnel	To verify proper use of the sterilizer
New sterilizer	To make sure unfamiliar operating instructions are being followed
After repair of a sterilizer	To make sure that the sterilizer is functioning properly
With every implantable device and hold device until results of test are known	Extra precaution for sterilization of item to be implanted into tissues
After any other change in the sterilizing procedure	To make sure change does not prevent sterilization

Source: U.S. Department of Health and Human Services, Centers for Disease Control and Prevention. Guidelines for infection control in dental health-care settings—2003. *MMWR Morb Mortal Wkly Rep.* 2003;52(RR-17):27.

◆ Indications for spore testing[1,7,8]
  • Once per week to verify proper use and functioning.
  • Whenever a new type of packaging material or tray is used.
  • After training new personnel to ensure proper use.
  • During initial uses of a new sterilizer to make sure the directions are being followed.
  • After sterilizer repair to check functioning.
  • Any load containing an implantable device should be spore tested and device should remain out of service until results are known.

MOIST HEAT: STEAM UNDER PRESSURE

Destruction of microorganisms by heat takes place because of inactivation and coagulation of essential cellular proteins or enzymes.

I. Autoclave Types

Autoclaves use steam under pressure to achieve sterilization and are available in the prevacuum and gravity displacement models. The two types of autoclaves differ mostly in the manner in which the evacuation of steam occurs and the process length. A time/temperature comparison of sterilization systems is provided in Table 7-1.

◆ *Gravity displacement:* self-generation of steam forces out the air; steam enters to penetrate through the cassettes or packages.
◆ *High-speed prevacuum:* pump removes the air from the chamber and allows faster penetration of the steam for sterilizing.

II. Use

◆ Moist heat may be used for all materials except:
  • Oils, waxes, and powders that are impervious to steam.
  • Materials that cannot be subjected to high temperatures.

III. Principles of Action

◆ Sterilization is achieved by action of heat; pressure serves only to attain high temperature.
◆ Sterilization depends on the penetrating ability of steam.
◆ Air must be excluded; otherwise steam penetration and heat transfer are prevented.
◆ Space between objects is essential to ensure access for the steam.
◆ Air discharge occurs in a downward direction; load must be arranged for free passage of steam toward the bottom of autoclave.

IV. Evaluation

◆ Advantages
  • All microorganisms, spores, and viruses are destroyed quickly and efficiently.
  • Wide variety of materials may be treated; most economical method of sterilization.
◆ Disadvantages
  • If precautions are not taken, carbon steel instruments may corrode.

DRY HEAT

Dry heat sterilizers achieve sterilization by oxidation of molecules, resulting in death of the organism. The most common dry sterilizers include:

◆ *Static air sterilizers:* like an oven, the chamber is brought to temperature by heating coils located within the unit.
◆ *Forced air sterilizers:* heated forced air is circulated at a high velocity, rapidly bringing the sterilizer to the appropriate temperature.

I. Use

◆ Primarily for materials that cannot be safely sterilized with steam under pressure.
◆ For small metal instruments enclosed in special containers or that might be corroded or rusted by moisture.

II. Principles of Action

◆ Sterilization is achieved by heat conducted from the exterior surface to the interior of the object; the penetration time varies among materials.
◆ Sterilization can result when the material is treated for a sufficient length of time at the required temperature; therefore, timing for sterilization must start when the entire contents of the sterilizer have reached the peak temperature needed for the load.

III. Operation

◆ Temperature
  • A temperature of 160°C (320°F) maintained for 2 hours; 170°C (340°F) for 1 hour.[9] Timing starts after the desired temperature has been reached.
  • Penetration time: Heat penetration varies with different materials.
  • Nature and properties of various materials are considered.
◆ Care
  • Care is taken not to overheat because certain materials can be affected. Temperatures over 160°C (320°F) may destroy the sharp edges of cutting instruments.

IV. Evaluation

- Advantages
  - Useful for materials that cannot be subjected to steam under pressure, such as heat-sensitive handpieces, burs, or plastics.
  - When maintained at correct temperature, this method is well suited for sharp instruments.
  - No corrosion compared with steam under pressure.
- Disadvantages
  - Long exposure time required; penetration slow and uneven.
  - High temperature critical to certain materials.

CHEMICAL VAPOR STERILIZER

A combination of alcohols, formaldehyde, ketone, water, and acetone heated under pressure produces a gas that is effective as a sterilizing agent.

I. Use

Chemical vapor sterilization cannot be used for materials or objects that can be altered by the chemicals that make the vapor or that cannot withstand the high temperature. Examples are low-melting plastics, liquids, or heat-sensitive handpieces.

II. Principles of Action

Microbial and viral destruction results from the permeation of the heated formaldehyde and alcohol. Heavy, tightly wrapped, or sealed packages would not permit the penetration of the vapors.

III. Operation

- Temperature
  - From 132°C (270°F) with 20–40 pounds' pressure in accord with the manufacturer's directions.[9]
- Time
  - Minimum of 20 minutes after the correct temperature and pressure have been attained. Time is extended for a large load or a heavy wrap.
- Cooling at the completion of the cycle
  - Instruments are dry. Instruments need a short period for cooling.

IV. Care of Sterilizer

- Refilling depends on the amount of use and is needed at least every 30 cycles.
- In accord with manufacturer's instructions, the condensate tray is removed, the exhausted solution emptied, and the tray cleaned.

V. Evaluation

- Advantages
  - Corrosion- and rust-free operation for carbon steel instruments.
  - Ability to sterilize in a relatively short total cycle.
  - Ease of operation and care of the equipment.
- Disadvantages
  - Adequate ventilation is needed; cannot use in a small room.
  - Slight odor, which is rarely objectionable.

INTERMEDIATE-USE STEAM STERILIZATION

Sometimes called flash sterilization, this form of rapid steam heat sterilization is a method used to sterilize unwrapped instruments for immediate use. The rapid contact with steam allows for shorter sterilization times.[1]

- Use
  - Should only be used when there is urgent need to sterilize an item.
  - Not recommended for items that require biologic spore test results before use, that is, implantable items.[3]
- Care
  - Follow manufacturer's temperature and setting directions for immediate-use sterilizing.
  - Monitors and indicators should be used and checked for each cycle.
  - Items are to be used immediately after sterilizing.
  - Items are hot upon removal, so care must be used in handling.
  - Caution must be used in the transport of instruments to avoid contamination.
  - Items are meant for immediate use and should not be stored.

CHEMICAL LIQUID STERILIZATION

Chemical liquid sterilization is often referred to as "cold sterile." Many chemicals have been FDA approved for sterilization; however, biologic monitoring to verify sterility with this method is not possible. The CDC recommends this method of sterilization only when other methods of sterilization cannot be used.[9]

CARE OF STERILE INSTRUMENTS

- Instruments stored without sealed wrappers are only momentarily sterile because of airborne contamination.
- Labeled, sterilized, and sealed packages are stored unopened in clean, dry cabinets or drawers.

- All stored packages are dated and used in rotation.
- Paper-wrapped packages are handled carefully to prevent tearing.
- Packages wrapped and sealed in paper may not need resterilizing for several months to 1 year.
- Plastic or nylon wrap with a tape or heat seal may be expected to remain sterile longer.
- The expected shelf life before resterilizing depends on the area surrounding the stored packages. A closed, protected area without exposure, such as a cabinet or drawer that can be disinfected routinely, is preferred for storage.

CHEMICAL DISINFECTANTS

There is no evidence bloodborne infections can be transmitted through housekeeping surfaces; however, healthcare facilities are expected to be kept clean and have cleaning protocol and procedures in place for all surface types.[1]

- Chemical disinfectants are used in several forms, including:
  - Surface disinfectants.
  - Immersion disinfectants, immersion sterilants.
  - Hand antimicrobial agent.
- Each variety has specific chemicals, dilutions, and directions for application.

I. Manufacturer's Information

- All manufacturers of products should include or supply a Manufacturer's Safety Data Sheet (MSDS). An MSDS provides facts about the safety and effectiveness of the product including:
  - Effectiveness and stability expressed by:
    a. Shelf life: the expiration date indicating the termination of effectiveness of the unopened container.
    b. Use life: the life expectancy for the solution once it has been activated.
    c. Reuse life: the amount of time a solution can be used and reused while being challenged with instruments that are wet or coated with contaminants.
  - Directions for activation (mixing directions).
  - Type of container for use and storage.
  - Storage directions (light and temperature).
  - Directions for use:
    a. Precleaning and drying of items.
    b. Time/temperature ratio.
  - Instructions for disposal of used solution.
  - Warnings
    a. Toxic effects (eyes, skin).
    b. Directions for emergency care (e.g., splash in eye).

II. Categories

- Disinfectants are categorized by their biocidal activity as high level, intermediate level, or low level.
- Biocidal activity refers to the ability of the chemical disinfectant to destroy or inactivate living organisms.
  - *High-level disinfectants* inactivate spores and all forms of bacteria, fungi, and viruses. Applied at different time schedules, the high-level chemical is either a disinfectant or a sterilant.
  - *Intermediate-level disinfectants* inactivate all forms of microorganisms but do not destroy spores.
  - *Low-level disinfectants* inactivate vegetative bacteria and certain lipid-type viruses but do not destroy spores, tubercle bacilli, or nonlipid viruses.

III. Uses

- Environmental surfaces disinfection: Following each appointment, the treatment area is cleaned and disinfected.
- Dental laboratory impressions and prostheses:
  - Impressions can be carriers of infectious material to a dental laboratory.
  - Completed prostheses must be disinfected before delivery to a patient.

IV. Principles of Action

- Disinfection is achieved by:
  - Coagulation, precipitation, or oxidation of protein of microbial cells.
  - Denaturation of the enzymes of the cells.
- Disinfection depends on the contact of the solution at the known effective concentration for the optimum period of time.
- Items are thoroughly cleaned and dried because action of the agent is altered by foreign matter and dilution.
- A solution has a specific shelf life, use life, and reuse life.
  - Some may be altered by changes in pH, or the active ingredient may decrease in potency.
  - Check manufacturer's directions.

V. Criteria for Selection of a Chemical Agent

- Objective: To select a product that is effective in the control of microorganisms and practical to use. No one product is the best choice for all dental setting. Properties of an ideal disinfectant are shown in Box 7-1. When choosing a product, consider the level of contamination and surface type.
- Identify contamination type
  - Blood.
  - No blood.

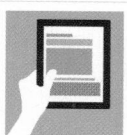

BOX 7-1
Properties of a Disinfectant

1	Broad spectrum	Wide antimicrobial spectrum
2	Fast acting	A rapid lethal action on all vegetative forms and spores of bacteria and fungi, protozoa, and viruses
3	Unaffected by physical factors	Active in the presence of organic matter, such as blood, sputum, and feces. Compatible with soaps, detergents, and other chemicals encountered in use
4	Nontoxic	
5	Surface compatibility	Will not corrode instruments and other metallic surfaces. Will not cause the disintegration of cloth, rubber, plastics, or other materials
6	Residual effect on treated surfaces	
7	Easy to use	
8	Odorless	Inoffensive odor to facilitate routine use
9	Economical	Reasonable cost

- Clinical contact surfaces
  - No blood: Use EPA-registered hospital-grade disinfectant plus hepatitis B virus (HBV) and human immunodeficiency virus (HIV) kill claim or tuberculocidal activity.
  - Blood: Use EPA-registered hospital disinfectant plus tuberculocidal activity.
- Housekeeping surfaces
  - No blood: Use EPA-registered hospital disinfectant or detergent and water.
  - Blood: Use EPA-registered hospital disinfectant plus tuberculocidal activity.

BARRIERS AND SURFACE COVERS

Barriers and surface covers are used to protect a surface from contaminants. They come in different sizes and shapes and are available in sheets, wrap, pre-cut, and fitted for different items, such as hoses, light handles, keyboards, and head rests. Covers should be moisture resistant, easily removable, and disposable (Figure 7-5).

I. Benefits

There are many benefits to using surface barriers not only on hard-to-clean surfaces but also on any contact surfaces.

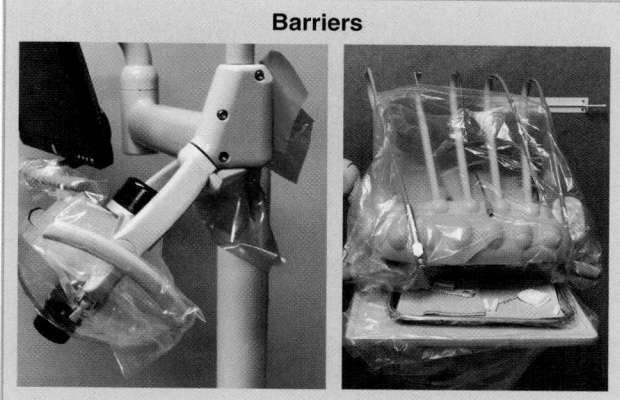

Barriers

FIGURE 7-5 • **Surface Covers and Barriers.**

Barriers and surface covers eliminate the contact time required by disinfectants and are chemical free, efficient, and safe. A comparison of barriers versus cleaning and disinfecting spray is shown in Figure 7-6.

II. Procedure

- Before treatment
  - Identify areas where barriers and covers can be used.
  - Apply the appropriate barrier prior to patient visit.
  - Be sure the barrier is secure and will not be dislodged during patient treatment.
- After treatment
  - Wear appropriate personal protective equipment (**PPE**) when removing contaminated barriers.
  - Be careful not to contaminate surfaces with gloves or unclean barriers.
  - If surfaces are contaminated, clean and disinfect surface.
  - Discard used barriers and covers in trash according to state law.
  - Remove contaminated gloves, perform hand hygiene, and apply fresh surface covers and barriers.

PREPARATION OF THE TREATMENT ROOM

- The cleanliness and neatness of the treatment room reflect the character and conscientiousness of the dental team.
- Patients may have limited knowledge of sterilization and infection control procedures and may request information.
- The continued orderliness and cleanliness of treatment rooms is necessary to create an environment to minimize cross-contamination.
- An excellent test for effectiveness is for dental personnel to occasionally view the operatory from the patient's vantage point by becoming the patient.

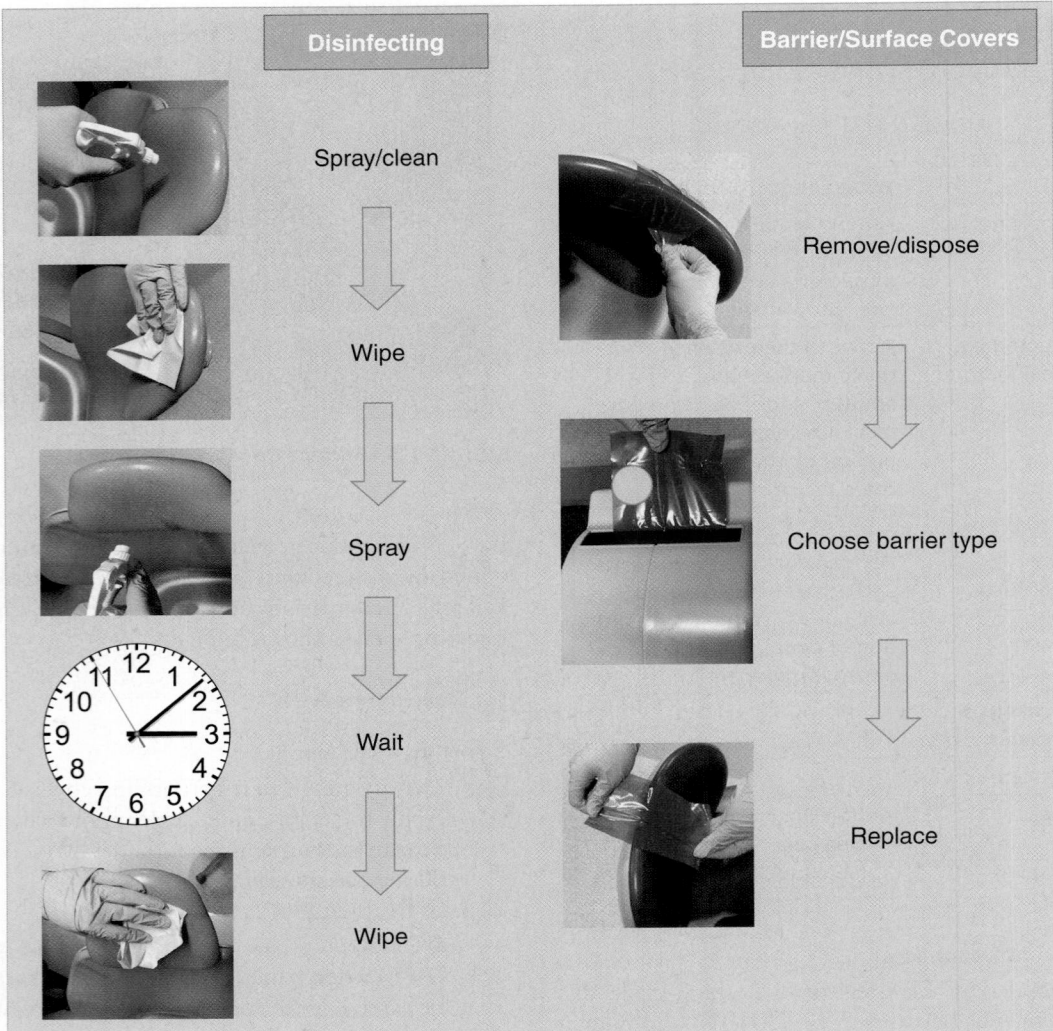

FIGURE 7-6 • Comparison of Disinfecting versus Barriers Diagram.

I. Objective

Effective care of instruments and equipment is essential in order to control disease transmission by way of environmental surfaces and maintenance of equipment and instruments.

II. Preliminary Planning

◆ All surfaces and items that will be used or contacted during the appointment can be categorized as critical, semi-critical, and noncritical.

◆ The classification of inanimate objects (Table 7-3) provides a guide for analysis.

◆ All surfaces should be cleaned at the end of every work day.

◆ Preparation of treatment room when time between appointments is limited requires an efficient procedural system.

III. Surface Disinfection Procedure

◆ The most logical and scientific sequence for preparation for the appointment can then be outlined.

◆ *Hand "Touch Contacts"*
  • Only contacts essential to the service to be performed are made.
  • Planning ahead to have materials ready so cabinet knobs or drawer handles do not have to be contacted is an example.

◆ *Sterilizable items*
  • Critical and semi-critical items are sterilized or are disposable.

◆ *Disposable items*
  • Disposable items are used wherever possible.

◆ *Items that may be covered*
  • Barrier coverings prevent contamination from reaching surfaces.

TABLE 7-3 • Classification of Inanimate Objects

SURFACE CATEGORY	DEFINITION	STERILIZATION/DISINFECTION	EXAMPLES
Critical	Penetrate soft tissue or bone	Sterilize or disposable	Needles Curets Explorers Probes
Semi-critical	Touch intact mucous membrane, oral fluids Does not penetrate	Sterilize after each use High-level disinfection when sterilization cannot be used	Radiographic bite block Ultrasonic handpiece Amalgam condenser Mirror
Noncritical	Do not touch mucous membranes (only contact unbroken epithelium)	Cleaning and tuberculocidal intermediate-level disinfection	Light handles Certain X-ray machine parts Safety eyewear
Environmental	No contact with patient surfaces (or only intact skin)	Cleaning and intermediate to low disinfection	Counter tops Equipment surfaces Housekeeping surface

- Covers for light handles, counter tops, X-ray machine parts, computer keyboard, and mouse are examples.
- Care is taken when removing the covers not to contaminate the object beneath.
◆ *Items that require chemical disinfection*
- Objects and surfaces that cannot be included in one of the preceding categories are treated with a chemical disinfectant.
- When the material is not compatible with the chemical action of the disinfectant, a disposable or coverable substitute is needed.

IV. Clean and Disinfect Environmental Surfaces[1,10]

A. Agent
◆ The effectiveness of the disinfection procedure is the result of two actions:
- The physical rubbing and removal of contaminated material.
- The chemical inactivation of the living microorganisms.
◆ Surface disinfectants are concentrated, premixed solutions, sprays, foams, impregnated wipes, and dissolved tablets.
- Do not store gauze sponges in the solution because cotton fibers contained in gauze may shorten the effectiveness of disinfectants when stored in containers.[10]

B. Procedure
1. Wear your PPE as needed including: protective eyewear, surgical mask, protective apparel, medical gloves, or chemical/puncture-resistant utility gloves.
2. Determine the degree of disinfection required.

3. Be sure the product has been prepared correctly and is not expired.
4. Check the label to be sure the disinfectant is compatible with the surface to be disinfected.
5. Clean blood or other potentially infectious material with a low-level or intermediate-level disinfectant effective against HBV and HIV.
6. Clean and scrub surfaces with soap and water, EPS-registered detergent, or low-level disinfectant.
7. Disinfectant must be followed by vigorous scrubbing in order to remove the film of microorganisms.
8. Once cleaned, spray surface again leaving the disinfectant on the surface for the recommended amount of time.
9. Scrub the disinfectant over the entire surface, with attention to irregularities where contaminated material can aggregate.
10. A disinfectant-soaked sponge or wipe in each hand can decrease the time of cleaning certain objects. Contaminated objects, such as tubings, can be held with one sponge while scrubbing with the other sponge.
11. Use a brush if surfaces do not become visibly clean from rubbing.
12. Used product according to manufacturer's directions leaving the surfaces wet for the recommended period of time.
13. Wipe surfaces dry.

V. Unit Water Lines
◆ A biofilm of microorganisms can form on the inside of the water-line tubing during overnight standing.
◆ Tests have been conducted on tubing to hand pieces, water syringes, and ultrasonic scalers. When the lines

were flushed for 2 minutes, the microbial counts were reduced.[1,3]

- Contaminated water cannot be used for surgical purposes or during the irrigation of pocket areas because infective microorganisms can be introduced.
- If contaminated water is directed forcefully into a pocket, microorganisms can enter the tissue and infection or bacteremia can result.
  - The procedure for clinical use is to flush all water lines at least 2 minutes at the beginning of each day.
  - Run water through water tubing for 30 seconds before and 30 seconds after each patient appointment.
- Refer to the CDC Infection Prevention and Control Guidelines and Recommendations.
- If dental unit is more than 20 years old, contact the manufacturer to determine if antiretraction valves are present.

PATIENT PREPARATION

- Oral procedures that penetrate tissue, such as giving anesthesia by injection or scaling subgingival pocket surfaces, can introduce bacteria into the tissues and hence into the bloodstream.
  - Organisms injected into the tissue could multiply and create an abscess. Natural resistance helps the body handle and destroy invading microorganisms, provided the numbers can be kept to a minimum.
  - Though clinical research has not proven this prevents or reduces the incidence of disease transmission, it has been shown to reduce the number of microorganisms in the oral cavity, aerosols or introduced into the patient's bloodstream.[1,3]
- Practical procedures for the preparation of a patient include preprocedural oral hygiene measures and rinsing with an antimicrobial mouthrinse.

I. Preprocedural Oral Hygiene Measures

- Toothbrushing
  - Demonstration of biofilm removal from the teeth, tongue, and gingiva contributes to lowering the microbial count before treatment procedures.
- Rinsing[11]
  - The numbers of bacteria on the gingival or mucosal surfaces can be reduced by the use of a preprocedural antiseptic mouthrinse.[11,12]
  - The substantivity of 0.2% chlorhexidine provides a lowered bacterial count for more than 60 minutes.
  - Preprocedural rinsing before injections is advised.

II. Application of a Surface Antiseptic

- *Before injection of anesthetic*[13]
  - As a needle is introduced into the mucosa for penetration to deeper tissues, microorganisms on the surface can be carried into the tissue.

- A topical antiseptic applied before the injection can decrease the risk of introducing septic material into the soft tissue.
- *Before scaling and other dental hygiene instrumentation*[12]
  - Instrumentation in a sulcus or pocket and around the gingival margin can create breaks in the tissue where bacteria can enter.
  - Subgingival instrumentation in a pocket with broken-down sulcular epithelium contributes to the entrance of bacteria into the underlying tissues and bacteremia.[13]
  - Evidence does not currently support use of subgingival irrigation with antiseptic solutions to reduce bacteremia posttreatment, but recommend the use of a preprocedural 2% chlorhexidine rinse.[14]

SUMMARY OF STANDARD PROCEDURES

Basic procedures for clinical management are listed here.

I. Patient Factors

- Prepare a comprehensive patient history and make necessary referrals.
- Ask the patient to rinse with an antimicrobial mouthrinse to reduce the numbers of oral microorganisms.
- Provide protective eyewear.
- Avoid elective procedures for a patient who is suffering from a communicable condition, such as a respiratory infection, or who has an open lesion on or about the lips or oral tissues.

II. Clinic Preparation

- Run water through all water lines, including the air–water syringe, hand pieces, and ultrasonic unit, for 2 minutes at the start of the day and for at least 30 seconds before and after each use during the day.
- Disinfect all environmental surfaces that may be "touch surfaces" during the appointment. Make an orderly sequence for surface cleaning and disinfection. Apply barrier covers as indicated.
- Sterilize instruments and all other equipment that can be sterilized by one of the methods for complete sterilization. Maintain closed sterilized packages until ready for use.

III. Factors for the Dental Team

- Have medical examinations; keep immunizations up to date; have appropriate testing on a periodic basis.
- Always use mask, protective eyewear, gloves, and a clean closed-front gown with fitted wrist cuffs.
- Utilize thorough hand hygiene and cleansing before putting on and after removing gloves.
- Develop habits to minimize contact with switches and other parts of the dental unit, dental chair, light, and clinician's stool, and avoid all environmental contacts unrelated to the procedure at hand.

IV. Treatment Factors

A. Syringe Needles

◆ Use a safe recapping and disposal methods (Chapter 36) to prevent accidental penetration or self-inoculation.

B. Removable Oral Prostheses

◆ Gloves are worn to receive a prosthesis from a patient.

◆ Place the prosthesis in a disposable cup or plastic resealable zipper bag and cover with a disinfectant.

◆ Use a fresh solution of 0.05% iodophor in water, or a 1:5 dilution of 5% sodium hypochlorite.

◆ Place cup or bag alone in an ultrasonic cleaner, making sure it does not tip and spill.

V. Posttreatment

◆ Use heavy puncture-resistant gloves to handle contaminated, unsterile instruments.

◆ Follow routines to disinfect, clean, and prepare the instruments for sterilization.

◆ Contaminated waste is secured in disposable plastic bag and infectious waste in a container with a secure lid.[1]

◆ Disinfect safety eyewear for patient and dental team members.

DISPOSAL OF WASTE

Wastes created in a dental setting can include contaminated, hazardous, or infectious/regulated waste.

I. Regulations

◆ Investigate the regulations of each town or city sanitation division (or health department) for rules concerning disposal of contaminated waste.

◆ Figure 7-7 illustrates the universal label required by the U.S. Occupational Safety and Health Administration (OHSA). The labels must be attached to containers used to store or transport hazardous waste materials.

II. Guidelines for Disposal of Waste

◆ Disposable materials, such as gloves, masks, wipes, paper drapes, or surface covers, that are contaminated with blood or body fluids but not saturated are carefully handled and discarded in sturdy, impervious plastic bags to minimize human contact.[1]

◆ Blood, suctioned fluids, or other liquid waste may be carefully poured into a drain connected to a sanitary sewer system in compliance with applicable local regulations.

◆ Sharp items, such as needles and scalpel blades, are placed intact into a puncture-resistant, leak-proof biohazard container (see Chapter 36).

◆ Human tissue, extracted teeth, and contaminated solid wastes can be disposed of according to the requirements

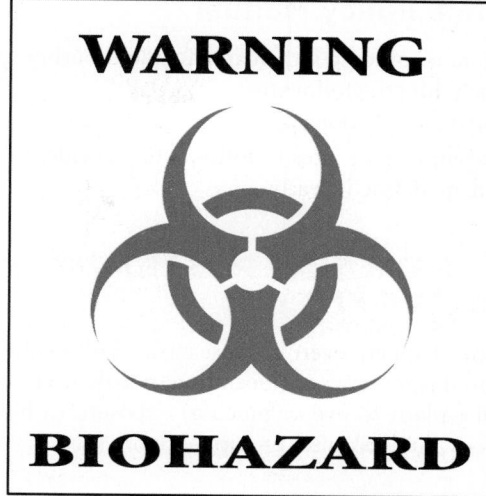

FIGURE 7-7 • Universal Label for Hazardous Material. A hazard-warning label is fluorescent orange or orange-red with lettering or a symbol in a contrasting color. The label must be attached to containers used to store or transport waste. A label is not required for regulated waste that has been decontaminated (such as dental waste that has been autoclaved).

established by local or state environmental regulatory agencies and published recommendations. Disposable bags need to be color coded or identified as biohazard.[1]

◆ Disposal methods for both liquid and solid chemicals vary with the type of chemical and local regulations governing waste-management practices.

SUPPLEMENTAL RECOMMENDATIONS

I. Cleaning the Face

◆ Check and clean the exposed parts of the face not covered by mask or protective eyewear, where spatter collects, as an aid to disease control as well as for general sanitation.

II. Smoking and Eating

◆ Smoking, drinking, and eating are banned in treatment areas.

III. Reception Area

◆ Select toys and other reception area items that can be cleaned and disinfected.

◆ Provide hand sanitizer gel in the reception area.

IV. Sterilization Monitoring

◆ Keep a written record of dates when processing tests and biologic monitor tests are performed for each sterilizer.

◆ Indicate advance dates for the next testing clearly on a calendar or other reference point.

◆ Perform tests made weekly on the same day to ensure compliance.

V. Office Policy Manual

The clinic or office policy manual should outline procedures including the following:

◆ Standard precautions.

◆ Emergency procedures to follow when accidentally exposed are defined clearly.

OCCUPATIONAL POSTEXPOSURE MANAGEMENT

Accidents happen even to the most skillful clinician. Accidental percutaneous (laceration, needle stick) or permucosal (splash to eye or mucosa) exposure to blood or other body fluids requires prompt action.

I. Significant Exposures

◆ Percutaneous or permucosal stick or wound with needle or sharp instrument contaminated with blood, saliva, or other body fluids.

◆ Contamination of any obviously open wound, nonintact skin, or mucous membrane with blood, saliva, or a combination.

◆ Exposure of patient's body fluids to unbroken skin is not considered a significant exposure.

II. Procedure Following Exposure

◆ Perform basic first aid to clean the area affected.
  • Immediately wash the wound with soap and water; rinse well.
  • Flush nose, mouth, eyes, or skin with clear water, saline, or a sterile irrigator.

◆ Report to designated official.

◆ Complete an incident report as required.

◆ Follow the required predetermined, posted procedures of the clinic, institution, or individual practice setting.

• The University of California, San Francisco maintains a Clinician Consultation Center with a *PEP (postexposure prophylaxis) Quick Guide for Occupational Exposures* based on the most current U.S. Public Health Services and CDC guidelines. Consultations can be obtained by calling the Clinicians' Post-Exposure PEPline (888-448-4911).[15]

◆ Immediately obtain medical evaluation so if treatment is recommended, it can be initiated quickly.

◆ If the source (patient) is present and agrees, the patient should accompany the dental provider for medical evaluation and testing.
  • If the source is not known or unwilling to go for medical evaluation, baseline testing would be performed on the dental provider.

◆ If baseline testing is negative, no other follow-up may be necessary, but often 6-week follow-up testing is recommended.

◆ Obtain counseling services if necessary.

III. Follow-Up

◆ Report signs and symptoms associated with infectious disease such as hepatitis or HIV.

◆ Obtain medical evaluation of any illness involving fever, rash, and lymphadenopathy.

◆ Pursue counseling and further testing.

DOCUMENTATION

Documentation for a patient with concerns about infection control procedures would include:

◆ Name, record number, address, telephone (home and cell), e-mail.

◆ Medical history for history of HBV, hepatitis C virus (HCV), or HIV; high-risk history associated with these diseases; patient consent to be tested for HBV, HCV, and HIV.

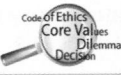

EVERYDAY ETHICS

Kimberly, the dental hygienist, is about to begin the patient examination when she notices that the indicator tape on the sterilizing cassette had not changed color. She excuses herself and finds out from the receptionist that a call to the repair service has been made because the autoclave has been shutting down before completion of the cycle. It is after 1:00 PM, and patients are scheduled all afternoon.

Questions for Consideration

1. When proper sterile technique is not followed, what ethical principles and core values are involved? Describe Kimberly's duty to her patients.

2. Use the steps to decision making in Chapter 1 to determine possible solutions for this situation. Describe how each could be defended to the patient, the dentist, and other dental team members.

3. Which American Dental Hygienists' Association professional roles (Chapter 1) does Kimberly serve in when she plans to make changes that ensure that this kind of situation does not happen again? Explain each role and how it applies for Kimberly.

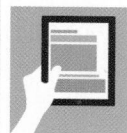

BOX 7-2
Example Documentation: Patient with Concerns About Infection Control

S—Patient presents for routine periodontal maintenance appointment. Patient asked how instruments were "cleaned" between patients.

O—Health history update indicates patient has been recently diagnosed as human immunodeficiency virus positive.

A—She was concerned about an increased risk for opportunistic infections as well as the fact that her condition might increase risk for other patients seen in the office.

P—Explained that standard precautions and infection control procedures used during all patient treatment are designed to protect all patients from cross-contamination. Explained each set of instruments is sterilized utilizing steam under pressure (autoclave). Tests for sterilization are done for each cycle of instruments, in addition to weekly and monthly tests to ensure the autoclave is functioning properly. Opened all sterilized instrument kits in her presence.

Signed: _____, RDH

Date: _____

◆ HIV-positive patient: current medications and previously taken, if they were ineffective; most recent viral load, current CD4 if known.

◆ A sample progress note for a patient with concerns about infection control procedures can be reviewed in Box 7-2.

Factors to Teach the Patient

▶ The meaning of "standard precautions" and what is included under the term; how these precautions protect the patient and the dental team members.

▶ The contribution of the accurately completed medical and dental personal history to the provision of the best, safest treatment possible.

▶ Methods for sterilization of instruments, including handpieces; how the autoclave or other sterilizer is tested daily or weekly.

▶ Facts about the normal oral flora and the factors that influence an increased number of bacteria on the tongue, mucosa, and in the dental biofilm on the teeth.

▶ Methods for personal daily control of the oral bacteria through biofilm control and tongue brushing.

▶ Reasons for preprocedural rinsing.

▶ Method for thorough rinsing.

ENHANCE YOUR UNDERSTANDING

ONLINE RESOURCES
(see the inside front cover for access information)
- Audio glossary
- Appendices

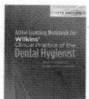

SUPPORT FOR LEARNING
(available separately)
- *Active Learning Workbook for Wilkins' Clinical Practice of the Dental Hygienist, 13th Edition*

INDIVIDUALIZED REVIEW
- Customized practice quizzing with Navigate 2 TestPrep for *Wilkins' Clinical Practice of the Dental Hygienist*

References

1. Organization for Safety & Asepsis Procedures, Centers for Disease Control and Prevention. *From Policy to Practice: OSAP's Guide to the CDC Guidelines: A Step-by-Step Implementation Workbook.* Atlanta, GA: OSAP; 2016. http://c.ymcdn.com/sites/www.osap.org/resource/resmgr/issues_files/Boilwater_2016.pdf. Accessed October 22, 2017.

2. Centers for Disease Control and Prevention, Division of Oral Health. *Guidelines and Recommendations: Infection Prevention & Control in Dental Settings.* Atlanta, GA: CDC; September, 2017. https://www.cdc.gov/oralhealth/infectioncontrol/guidelines/index.htm. Accessed September 21, 2017.

3. Centers for Disease Control and Prevention, Center for Chronic Disease Prevention and Health Promotion. *Recommendations from the Guidelines for Infection Control in Dental Health-Care Settings.* Atlanta, GA: CDC; 2003. https://www.cdc.gov/oralhealth/infectioncontrol/pdf/recommendations-excerpt.pdf. Accessed October 22, 2017.

4. Miller CH, Tan CM, Beiswanger MA, Gaines DJ, Setcos JC, Palenik CJ. Cleaning dental instruments: measuring the effectiveness of an instrument washer/disinfector. *Am J Dent.* 2000;13(1):39-43.

5. Centers for Disease Control and Prevention. *Summary of Infection Prevention Practices in Dental Settings: Basic Expectations for Safe Care.* Atlanta, GA: CCDC, USDHHS; October, 2016. https://www.cdc.gov/oralhealth/infectioncontrol/pdf/safe-care2.pdf. Accessed October 22, 2017.

6. Miller CH, Palenik CJ. *Infection Control and Management of Hazardous Materials for the Dental Team.* 4th ed. St Louis, MO: Mosby Elsevier; 2010.

7. Miller CH. Use of spore tests for quality assurance in infection control. *Am J Dent.* 2001;14(2):114.

8. Spry C. Understanding current steam sterilization recommendations and guidelines. *AORN J.* 2008;88(4):537-550; quiz 551-4.

9. Centers for Disease Control and Prevention. *Guidelines for Disinfection & Sterilization Guidelines in Healthcare Facilities.* Atlanta, GA: CDC; 2008. https://www.cdc.gov/infectioncontrol/pdf/guidelines/disinfection-guidelines-H.pdf. Accessed June 7, 2019.

10. Cottone J, Terezhalmy G, Molinari J. *Practical Infection Control in Dentistry.* 5th ed. Philadelphia, PA: Lippincott, Williams and Wilkins; 2009.

11. Gupta G, Mitra D, Ashok KP, et al. Efficacy of preprocedural mouth rinsing in reducing aerosol contamination produced by ultrasonic scaler: a pilot study. *J Periodontol.* 2014;85(4):562-568.

12. Reddy S, Prasad MGS, Kaul S, Satish K, Kakarala S, Bhowmik N. Efficacy of 0.2% tempered chlorhexidine as a pre-procedural mouth rinse: a clinical study. *J Indian Soc Periodontol.* 2012;16(2):213-217.

13. Johnson SM, Saint John BE, Dine AP. Local anesthetics as antimicrobial agents: a review. *Surg Infect.* 2008;9(2): 205-213.

14. Barbosa M, Prada-López I, Álvarez M, Amaral B, de los Angeles CD, Tomás I. Post-tooth extraction bacteraemia: a randomized clinical trial on the efficacy of chlorhexidine prophylaxis. *PLoS One.* 2015;10(5):e0124249.

15. UCSF, Clinician Care Center. PEP Quick guide for occupational exposures. June, 2017. http://nccc.ucsf.edu /clinical-resources/pep-resources/pep-quick-guide/. Accessed October 22, 2017.

8

Patient Reception and Ergonomic Practice

Irina Smilyanski, RDH, MS, MSDH

CHAPTER OUTLINE

PREPARATION FOR THE PATIENT
- I. Treatment Area
- II. Records

PATIENT RECEPTION
- I. Introduction
- II. Escort Patient to Dental Chair

POSITION OF THE PATIENT
- I. General Positions
- II. The Dental Chair
- III. Use of Dental Chair

POSITION OF THE CLINICIAN

NEUTRAL WORKING POSITION
- I. Objectives
- II. The Effects of NWP
- III. Description of Neutral Seated Position
- IV. Clinician–Patient Positioning

THE TREATMENT AREA
- I. The Clinician's Chair
- II. Vision: Lighting
- III. Vision: Magnification
- IV. Handpieces
- V. Cords

ERGONOMIC PRACTICE
- I. Scope of Ergonomic Dental Hygiene
- II. Related Occupational Problems
- III. Ergonomic Risk Factors

SELF-CARE FOR THE DENTAL HYGIENIST
- I. Daily Functional Movement Exercises

DOCUMENTATION

EVERYDAY ETHICS

FACTORS TO TEACH THE PATIENT

REFERENCES

LEARNING OBJECTIVES

After studying this chapter, the student will be able to:

1. Describe the rules of etiquette in relationship to patient reception and care.

2. Describe the components of ergonomic practice and relationship to career longevity.

3. Identify the range of working positions for a right-handed and left-handed clinician.

4. Describe the elements of a neutral working position.

5. Explain the musculoskeletal disorders and their causes and symptoms most often associated with the clinical practice of dental hygiene.

6. Explain the ergonomic risk factors of clinical dental hygiene practice.

The patient's presence in the office or clinic is an expression of confidence in the dentist and the dental hygienist. Confidence is inspired by the reputation for professional knowledge and skill, the appearance of the office, and the actions of the workers in it.

- The physical arrangement and interpersonal relationships provide the setting for specific services to be performed.
- The patient's well-being is the all-important consideration throughout the appointment.
- At the same time, the clinician must function effectively and efficiently in a manner that minimizes stress and fatigue to ensure personal health.
- Musculoskeletal disorders, repetitive stress injuries, and cumulative trauma disorders are common work-related conditions that require continuing preventive physical and mental energy on the part of each clinical dental hygienist.
- The science of ergonomics has provided information for the development of standards for human performance and workplace design that can maximize health, comfort, and efficiency for dental hygienists in clinical practice.

PREPARATION FOR THE PATIENT

I. Treatment Area

The requirements for preparation of the treatment area are standard precautions for all patients whether or not the presence of a communicable disease is known.

- *Environmental surfaces:* All clinical contact areas are thoroughly disinfected or covered to control cross-contamination.
- *Instruments:* Sterile packaged instruments remain sealed until the start of the actual treatment.
- *Equipment:* Prepare and make ready other materials that will be used, such as for the determination of blood pressure and patient instruction. Anticipate specific needs for procedures being delivered.
- *Patient's dental chair:* Upright for current patient reception; chair arm adjusted for ease of access.
- *Clinician's chair:* Set at proper height for the entire day.

II. Records

- For the patient of record, review the patient's medical and dental history for pertinent appointment information, updating, and assessment.
- Read previous appointment progress notes to focus the current treatment plan.
- Anticipate examination procedures and new record making for a new patient.

PATIENT RECEPTION

I. Introduction

- The dental assistant or the dentist may introduce the new patient to the dental hygienist, but more frequently, a self-introduction is in order.
- The patient is greeted by name, and the hygienist's name is clearly stated, for example, "Good morning, Mrs. Smith; I am Anna Jones, the dental hygienist."
- Procedure for introducing the patient to others:
  - A woman's name always precedes a gentleman's.
  - An older person's name precedes the younger person's (when of the same sex and when the difference in age is obvious).
  - In general, the patient's name precedes that of a member of the dental personnel.
  - An older patient is not called by the first name except at the patient's request.

II. Escort Patient to Dental Chair

- Invite patient to be seated and adjust the chair as needed.
- Assist the elderly, disabled, or very small children; guide into the chair (support the patient's arm when patient requests or accepts it).
- Assist with wheelchair. Bring wheelchair adjacent to the dental chair. Wheelchair procedures are described in the Wheelchair Transfer section in Chapter 51.
- Suggestions for helping the patient with a vision impairment may be found in Chapter 51.
- Place handbag in a safe place, if possible within the patient's view.
- Provide protective eyewear. When a patient removes personal corrective eyeglasses to substitute those provided, make sure the personal glasses are placed in their case in a safe place.

POSITION OF THE PATIENT

I. General Positions

Four body positions for delivery of care are shown in Figure 8-1.

A. Upright

- This is the initial position for patient reception from which chair adjustments are made.

B. Semi-Upright

- The back of the chair is reclined at approximately 45° angle.
- Patients with certain types of cardiovascular, respiratory, or vertigo problems may need this position.
- Figure 8-2 illustrates the patient and clinician using a semi-upright position during patient care.

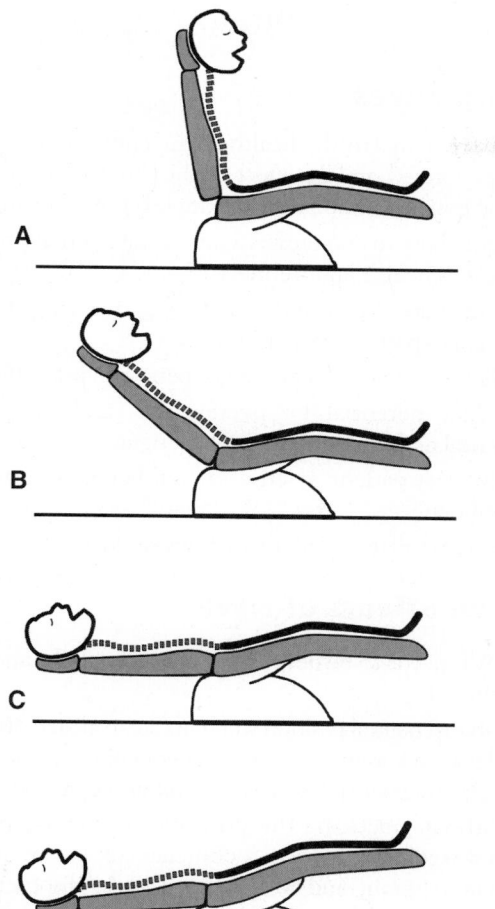

FIGURE 8-1 • Basic Patient Positions. A: Upright. **B:** Semi-upright. **C:** Supine or horizontal with the brain on the same level as the heart. **D:** Trendelenburg, with the brain lower than the heart and the feet slightly elevated.

C. Supine

◆ The chair is in a supine or flat position, the brain is at the same level as the heart.

◆ A patient is ideally situated for support of the circulation; rarely could a patient faint while lying in a supine position.

◆ The back of the chair is parallel to the floor.

◆ Position used most for treatment procedures.

◆ Figure 8-3 illustrates the patient and clinician while using the supine position.

D. Trendelenburg

◆ The person is said to be placed in the Trendelenburg position if they are in the supine position and tipped back and down 10°–15° so that the brain is lower than the heart.

◆ The back of the chair is less than parallel to the floor.

◆ The basic position in management of some medical emergencies.[1]

II. The Dental Chair

◆ A dental chair provides complete body support for the patient, which increases patient relaxation.

◆ A comfortable patient is more compliant and allows the procedure to be completed more efficiently.

◆ Seat and leg support move as a unit; back and headrest move as a unit; both are power controlled.

◆ Has a thin back so that the chair may be lowered close to the clinician's elbow height.

◆ Chair base permits the chair to be lowered as needed for appropriate treatment position.

◆ Chair controls need to be available to both the assistant and clinician.

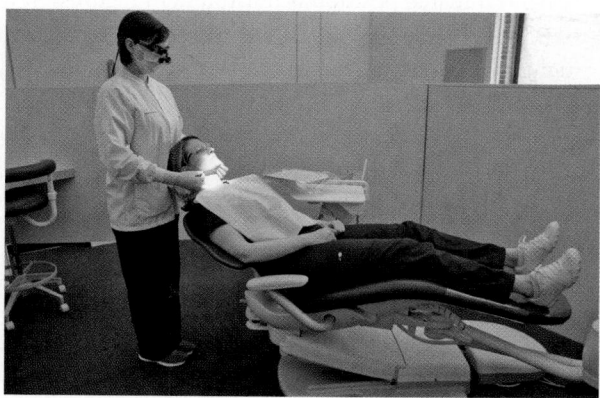

FIGURE 8-2 • Patient in a Semi-Upright Position. This photograph illustrates ergonomic patient and clinician position for patient care in a semi-upright position when the clinician stands to provide care for the patient who cannot be moved to the supine position.

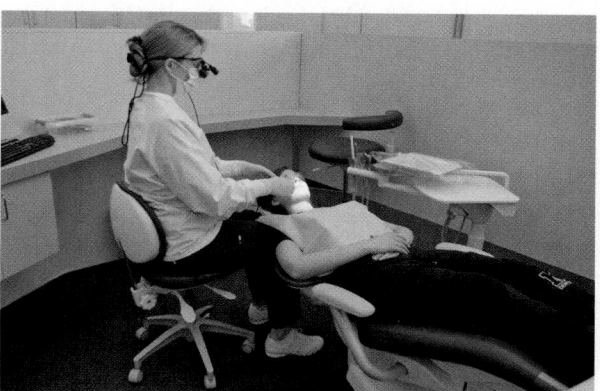

FIGURE 8-3 • Patient in a Supine Position. This photo illustrates ergonomic patient and clinician position for patient care in a supine position. Note the neutral seating position of the clinician and the use of loupes magnifying system with attached headlamp.

III. Use of Dental Chair

A. Prepositioning for Patient Reception

◆ Chair at low level; back upright.

◆ Chair arm is moved out of patient's way on side of approach.

B. Adjustment Steps

◆ Patient is seated with back upright.

◆ Chair seat and foot portion are raised first to help the patient settle back.

◆ Lower back to the supine position for maxillary instrumentation and to a 20° angle with the floor for mandibular treatment.

◆ Request patient to slide up to rest the head at upper edge of the headrest or backrest and turn head to left or right as needed for visibility and access.

◆ Adjust chair height until patient's mouth is at the clinician's elbow height with shoulder relaxed (Figure 8-3).

C. Conclusion of Appointment

◆ Secure instruments on the instrument tray.

◆ Move instrument tray away and turn off light.

◆ Slowly raise back of chair and tilt chair forward.

◆ Request patient to remain seated in an upright position briefly to avoid postural hypotension.

D. Contraindications for Supine Position

◆ Review patient history for indications of need for adaptation.

◆ Patient may request a position variation.

◆ Conditions that may contraindicate the supine position include congestive heart failure, vertigo, and respiratory conditions such as emphysema, severe asthma, or sinusitis.

◆ During the second and third trimester of pregnancy, supine position might need to be modified.[2] Chair positioning for the pregnant patient is described in Chapter 46.

POSITION OF THE CLINICIAN

◆ The clinician is in the neutral working position (NWP), with good access, light, and visibility, which in turn contribute to an efficient procedure.

◆ The patient is positioned so that a thorough, biologically oriented service may be performed conveniently and efficiently within a reasonable length of time.

◆ The positions of the patient and the clinician are interdependent.

◆ When clinician and patient positioning is considered, it is realistic to remember that the patient's position will be assumed for a relatively short time compared with that of the clinician.

NEUTRAL WORKING POSITION

I. Objectives

Objectives concern the health of the clinician, the service to be performed, and the effect on the patient. The preferred neutral position attempts to accomplish the following:

◆ Contribute to and preserve rather than detract from clinician's health and wellness.

◆ Contribute to ease and efficacy of performance that encourages patient cooperation.

◆ Allow endurance for prolonged periods of peak efficiency.

◆ Reduce potential for overexertion and injury from mental and physical stress and fatigue.

◆ Give the patient a sense of well-being, security, and confidence.

◆ Accommodate a patient with special needs.

II. The Effects of NWP

◆ NWP needs to be developed, practiced daily, and made habitual.

◆ Habitual neutral position will translate to all activities, outside of work as well. An internal environment can be created for ongoing physical ease, comfort, safety, and activity.

◆ Without practicing the principles of neutral position on a regular daily basis, a clinician can experience discomfort, pain, and work-related stress disorders. The long-term result can be shortened or compromised career longevity with changes in daily life activities.

◆ Analysis and assessment of posture can give direction to corrections for treatment. A posture assessment instrument is available.[3]

III. Description of Neutral Seated Position[4,5]

◆ A neutral seated position is illustrated in Figure 8-4A.

◆ *Back:* in neutral alignment with natural spinal curves, including cervical lordosis, thoracic kyphosis, and lumbar lordosis.

◆ *Head:* on top of neutral spine with forward neck flexion between 15° and 20° or less.

◆ *Eyes:* directed downward to prevent neck and eye strain.

◆ *Shoulders:* relaxed and parallel with the hips and floor.

◆ *Elbows:* close to the body.

◆ *Forearms:* parallel with the floor.

◆ *Wrist:* forearm and wrist are in a straight line.

◆ *Hips:* slightly higher than knees.

◆ *Thighs:* full body weight distributed evenly on seat; comfortable space (about 3 inches) between edge of seat and back of knee.

◆ *Knees:* slightly apart.

◆ *Feet:* flat on the floor.

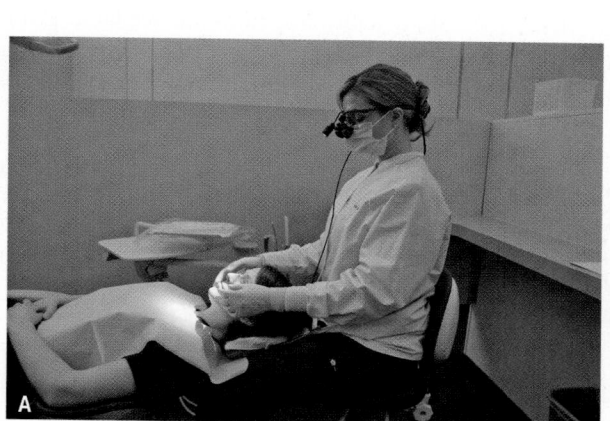
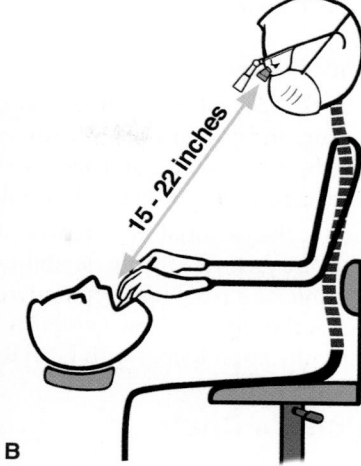

FIGURE 8-4 • Clinician's Working Distance. A: Clinician in 12:00 working position and drawing. **B:** Clinician in 8:00 working position. Both illustrate acceptable positioning, which shows the patient at the clinician's elbow level and the oral cavity of the patient between 15 and 22 inches from the clinician's eyes.

IV. Clinician–Patient Positioning

A. Distance

◆ Patient's oral cavity is adjusted to clinician's elbow height.

◆ Distance from clinician's eyes to the patient's oral cavity when the clinician is seated in neutral position will be within the range of 15–22 inches (Figure 8-4B).

◆ The distance is defined as the "working distance," which is a significant measurement when fitting magnification loupes for an individual clinician.

B. Selection

◆ NWP is combined with effective access to the patient for treatment procedures.

◆ Orientation of position of the clinician to patient can be compared to the hours of a clock around the patient's head with 12:00 at the top of the patient's head as shown in Figure 8-5.

◆ Clock hours correspond with clinician–patient relation associated with instrumentation in different areas of the patient's oral cavity.

C. Flexibility[4]

◆ Orientation for the right-handed clinician is associated with the 8–12 o'clock position; for the left-handed clinician, orientation is associated with the 12–4 o'clock position.[5]

◆ Access and visual adjustment determines which side the clinician will select for a given procedure.

◆ Movement of the clinician's chair freely on wheels and turning of the patient's head facilitate positioning and patient treatment from either side.

◆ Moving past 12 o'clock clockwise for right-handed clinicians and counterclockwise for left-handed clinicians improves access and visibility in certain areas.

◆ In treatment rooms with limited space, the dental chair may be swiveled to change the angle of the chair to allow the clinician space to move past 12 o'clock.

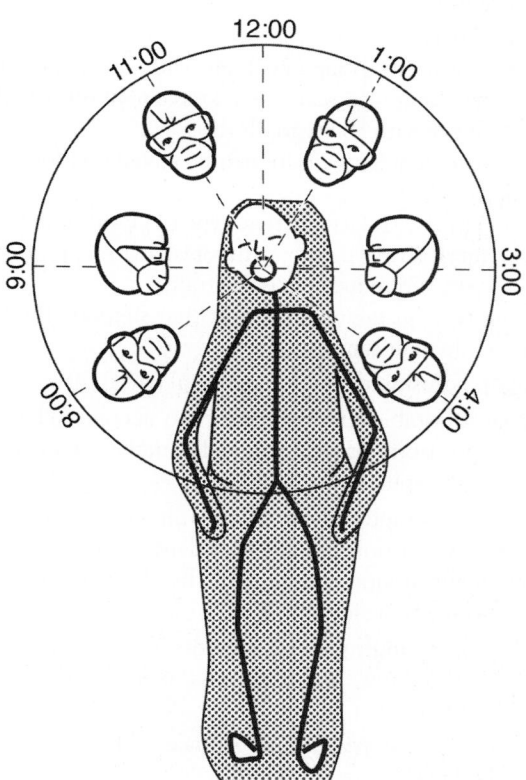

FIGURE 8-5 • Range of Positions for Clinician. The patient's head is placed at the upper edge of the backrest or headrest for convenient access by the clinician during treatment. The range of positions is compared with the numbers on a clock.

THE TREATMENT AREA

- The treatment area centers on the patient's oral cavity.
- The entire "work area" refers to the dental chair with patient, the unit, and the instrument tray as they are positioned for the convenience and accessibility of the clinician and assistant for four-handed dental hygiene.
- For the clinician, the essentials for access and visibility for patient care are provided by the flexibility of movement of the clinician's stool and appropriate lighting, supplemented by the clinician's own visibility enhanced by wearing magnification loupes with head light.

I. The Clinician's Chair

- The chair is a significant adjunct to implement ergonomic practice.
- Optimal design provides adequate support and the opportunity and means to change body posture frequently during the workday as clinicians, patients, and procedures change.
- The clinician adjusts the chair to personal specifications.

A. Characteristics of an Acceptable Chair[6,7]

- *Base:* broad and heavy with five casters; a chair with five casters provides greater stability.
- *Seat design:*
  - *Traditional:*
    - Size needs to support thighs without back of knees touching edge, seamless, textured upholstery, padded firmly, with ability to tilt the seat 5°–15°; accommodates requirements for neutral seated position.
  - *Saddle chair:*
    - This is a relatively new type of chair modeled after a riding saddle; promotes neutral spine position and reduces muscle strain.
- *Armrests:* adjustable at a height that supports the forearm while maintaining NWP.
- *Height:* adjustable for wide personal variability.
- *Back:* adjustable lumbar support to accommodate different positions, procedures, and clinicians while maintaining the spinal curve.
- *Mobility:* completely mobile; built with free-rolling casters; not connected to other dental equipment; free movement around the patient's head for instrumentation from either side.
- *Adjustment:* multiple adjustments for different positions, procedures, and clinicians; mechanisms easy to learn and use.
- *Infection control friendly:* all surfaces able to withstand standard precautions regimen.

II. Vision: Lighting

- During treatment, visibility in the oral cavity is prerequisite to thoroughness without undue trauma to the tissues.

- With adequate light, efficiency increases, treatment time is decreased, and patient cooperation increases.
- Many lighting options are available. All need to be directed properly to the oral cavity for adequate visualization, optimal patient care, and clinician comfort and safety.

A. Dental Light: Suggested Features

- Is readily adjustable both vertically and horizontally.
- Beam of light is capable of being focused.
- Set within a comfortable arm's reach.
- Does not require awkward or forceful movement to position it for visualization.

B. Dental Light: Location

- *Attachment*
  - Unit attachment.
  - Ceiling-mounted light on a track is most versatile.
  - Coaxial headlight can be added to improve visualization with targeted illumination.
- *Dual lighting*
  - Advantages of the use of two clinic lights have been demonstrated with a supine patient position in a contoured chair.
  - One light directed from the front of the patient may be attached to the dental unit; the other light is mounted on a ceiling track.
- *Dental light: adjustment principles*
  - Light allows clear illumination of entire treatment area.
  - Figure 8-6 shows position of light for maxillary and mandibular treatment.

III. Vision: Magnification[8-11]

Magnification is needed to improve visualization, support NWP, and enhance treatment procedures.

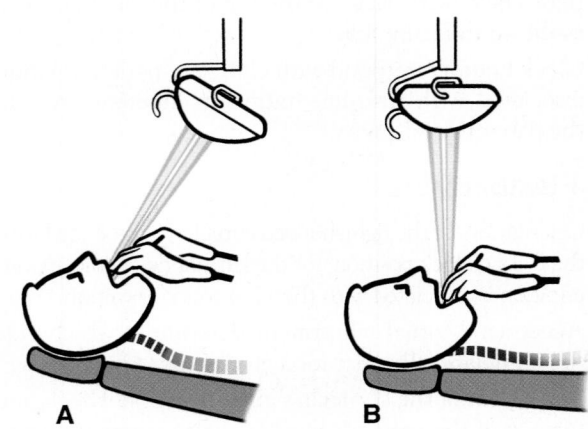

FIGURE 8-6 • Lighting. Light does not obstruct clinician, allows clear illumination of the treatment area. **A:** Maxillary arch; chin up position; beam of light often between 60° and 45° angle to floor. **B:** Mandibular arch; chin down position; beam of light nearly perpendicular to floor.

A. Choice of Loupe Systems

- Fixed through the lens: customized for individuals
  - Adjusted with the clinician's prescription as needed.
  - Magnifying lenses mounted directly into the lens.
  - Fixed interpupillary distance; angle of the lens not adjustable.
  - Not adjustable; enables the clinician to maintain correct posture.
- Front lens mounted without vertical adjustment
  - Prescription lenses are available.
  - Magnifying lenses mounted to a hinge on the frame; loupes can be adjusted up or down. Interpupillary distance can be adjusted; angle of lens not adjustable.
- Front lens mounted with vertical adjustment
  - Prescription lenses are available.
  - Magnifying lenses mounted to a hinge on the frame; loupes can be adjusted up or down.
  - Interpupillary distance can be adjusted; angle of lens can be adjusted.

B. Features

- Proper fit is essential to successful incorporation of magnification into the clinician's treatment environment.
- Proper fit is dependent on the clinician's working distance and neutral position.
- Clinicians need to research the differences to select best option.

IV. Handpieces

- Technology has provided handpieces that are ergonomically compatible with procedures clinicians provide.
- The best designs are small, light, and well-suited for the size of dental hygienist's hand.[12]
- Ergonomically designed handpieces are lightweight, decreasing stress on hand and wrist.
  - Fit in the contours of the clinician's hand and allow functional light grasp.
  - Reduce fatigue and strain.
  - Allow maneuverability.
  - Provide power assist without strain.
  - Produce less heat buildup.
  - Are available in a cordless option.

V. Cords

A. Management

- Managing cords is a significant aspect of ergonomic practice.
- Cords are part of most dental units and are an integral part of delivery of care for every patient.
- Ultrasonics, air/water syringes, slow-speed handpieces, and all power-driven equipment require cords connected to a power source.
- Improper management and inefficient design of the cords can increase drag on hand, wrist, and arm, increasing risk of repetitive injury.
- Cord design must allow for disinfection; cords should not interfere with functionality of other equipment.

B. Curly Cords

- Can cause excessive stretching and pulling by clinician.
- Associated with bending, reaching, and awkward postures to position for treatment.
- Increase the strain on hand, wrist, arm, and shoulder of clinician.
- Provide an ergonomic risk by increasing fatigue level and creating muscle imbalances.
- Straight cords may be generally easier to manage.

ERGONOMIC PRACTICE

I. Scope of Ergonomic Dental Hygiene

- Includes all practices that make work safe, decrease strain and fatigue, eliminate hazards, and improve work process affecting health and well-being of clinician and patient.
- Box 8-1 lists items of the equipment, work layout, and work process organization that need attention during practice if physical occupational disorders are to be prevented.

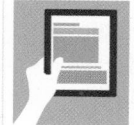

BOX 8-1
Factors to Consider for Ergonomic Practice

Equipment

- PPE (Personal Protective Equipment)
- Lighting (Figure 8-6)
- Magnification, coaxial headlight
- Properly fitted gloves
- Instruments balanced, sharp, of varied diameters, with knurling on handles
- Power instruments
- Handpiece lightweight and ergonomically designed
- Cords and cord management
- Foot pedals
- Suction
- Air/water syringe

Work Layout

- Uncluttered, easy access to patient, patient records, computer, radiographs
- Counters clear with designated area for documentation
- Instrument tray within arm's reach
- Light fixture within arm's length, easy to move and adjust

- Orderly tray setup with complete armamentarium for services to be delivered
- Convenient treatment room setup and design for patient chair, air/water syringe, suction, cords, foot pedals

Work Process Organization

- Clinician neutral working position (NWP)
- Use of magnification system supporting NWP
- CPP (Clinician–Patient Positioning)
- Light within easy arm's reach with clear illumination of treatment area
- Access and management of suction and air/water syringe
- Cords and cord maintenance

Instrumentation

- Reach of tray
- Order of instruments on tray
- Consistent instrumentation sequence for all surfaces of sextants
- Proper grasp and fulcrum technique for dominant hand
- Proper grasp and fulcrum technique for non-dominant hand
- Sharp instruments
- Correct working stroke for location and type of deposit
- Inclusion of power instrumentation
- Placement and access of foot pedals
- Selective polishing
- Placement and access to overgloves
- Documentation procedure

II. Related Occupational Problems

- The physical challenges inherent in dental hygiene practice place the clinicians at risk for developing work-related musculoskeletal disorders.[13]
- Table 8-1 lists a variety of disorders that can occur among clinicians.
- Prevention of the slow developing conditions is a daily responsibility.

III. Ergonomic Risk Factors

- Prevention begins with the recognition of the **risk factors** that can point to potential body injury and more serious permanent musculoskeletal disorders.[14]
- Table 8-2 lists and defines significant risk factors and provides examples of various practices that can lead to musculoskeletal disorders.

TABLE 8-1 • Musculoskeletal Disorders Affecting Dental Hygienists

With any symptoms or any ongoing discomfort, take action to find the source of the problem and how to relieve the symptom. Prevention is the best course of action. Early intervention will decrease the risk of a more involved condition or a more costly injury. If not addressed in a timely manner, any of these conditions could lead to a limited ability to practice or total disability.

CONDITION	CAUSES	SYMPTOMS
Carpal Tunnel Syndrome		
A symptomatic compression of the median nerve within the carpal tunnel (Figure 8-7)	Deviations of wrist from neutral Pinch grasp with insufficient rest	Numbness; tingling in the thumb, index, and middle fingers
Thoracic Outlet Syndrome		
Painful disorder of the fingers, hand, and/or wrist from compression of the brachial nerve plexus and vessels between the neck and shoulder	Tilting head forward Hunched and/or rounded forward shoulders Continuously reaching overhead	Numbness, tingling, and/or pain in the hand or wrist
Bursitis		
Inflammation of the bursa	Areas of friction or impingement anywhere in the body, usually the shoulder	Decreased range of motion. Aching
Tendonitis		
Painful inflammation of the wrist resulting in strain	Repeated wrist extension or palmar flexion	Pain in the wrist, especially along the outer edges of the hand rather than through the center of the wrist
Disk Herniation		
Displacement of the nucleus of the disk with resultant pressure on the spinal cord or peripheral nerves	Prolonged, static postures of forward flexion, hyperextension, lateral bending, or rotation of the spine Can present on cervical, thoracic, or lumbar areas of the spine	Pain, numbness, tingling of the arm, fingers, lower back, hip, or leg

TABLE 8-2 • Ergonomic Risk Factors

Intensity (strength or concentration of exposure), *frequency* (how often is the exposure), and *duration* (length of time of exposure) are related to the detrimental effects of the risk factor. A combination of risk factors intensifies risk and increases potential for injury.

RISK FACTOR	DEFINITION	EXAMPLE
Prolonged awkward position	Body postures that deviate from the normal resting or neutral positions	Twisting the torso during instrumentation Arm raised when scaling
Static positions long-term static load	Assuming and holding any position for a long period; stresses the body, accelerates fatigue and discomfort	Bending neck for long periods Retracting cheek with nondominant hand without stable fulcrum Prolonged seated posture
Repetition	Performing the same motion or series of motions continually or frequently	Scaling and root planing Probing Exposing radiographs Using computer keyboard Writing
Force/grasp	Physical effort needed to lift, push, pull, grasp, and pinch items in the work environment Often required to handle and control equipment and tools Force increases as contact area decreases	Manual instrumentation Exposing radiographs
Environmental	Can directly influence comfort and risk of injury	Cold Heat Poor lighting Noise
Vibration	The physical exposure to rapidly oscillating tools or machinery	Tools such as jackhammers Additional research is needed to demonstrate the effect power scaling and handpieces have on dental personnel
Insufficient rest	Performing the same motion or series of motions continually or frequently without sufficient recovery time for muscles	Scaling procedures Probing Exposing radiographs Unreasonable patient scheduling Insufficient breaks
Stress	A physical, chemical, or emotional factor that causes bodily or mental tension and may be a factor in disease causation or fatigue Involves clinician perception of control of work environment and psychosocial factors	Having no control over scheduling Delivering care when patient arrives late Poor team communication Insufficient input concerning workload at work
Poor physical fitness	Decreased capacity for body to resist the negative consequences of physical demands of dental hygiene practice	Demands of long periods of sitting Demands of repeated instrumentation

SELF-CARE FOR THE DENTAL HYGIENIST

- Responsible self-care and attention to the risk factors of musculoskeletal disorders are central to ergonomic practice.
- Self-care is built on but not limited to all safe work practices that incorporate ergonomic principles for health and well-being. Self-care includes but is not limited to:
  - *Physical fitness:* immunizations, healthy diet, adequate sleep, exercise.
  - *Standard precautions:* personal protective equipment.
  - *Clinical practice:* clinician–patient positioning (CPP), instrument selection and use, prevention of sharps injuries.
  - *NWP:* in all activities, not only clinical practice.
  - *Stress management:* reasonable patient scheduling; adequate breaks.

I. Daily Functional Movement Exercises

- In dental hygiene practice, it is necessary to give constant attention to maintaining a healthy spine.

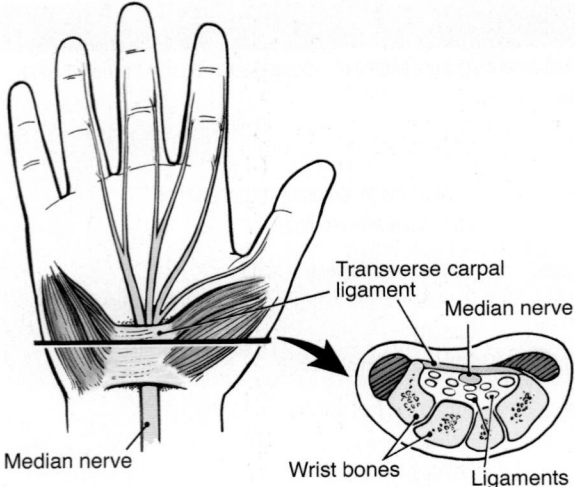

FIGURE 8-7 • Anatomy of the Wrist (Palmar View). Left, the median nerve passes through the transverse carpal tunnel of the wrist and branches to innervate the thumb, the index and middle fingers, and the medial aspect of the ring finger. Right, cross section of wrist shows the median nerve passing through the carpal tunnel. The tunnel is formed by the concave arch of the carpal (wrist) bones and roofed over by the transverse carpal ligament.

- Achieving neutral work posture throughout the work day.
- Performing effective CPP, and practicing daily functional movement exercises will protect and encourage a healthy spine.
◆ A healthy spine requires that it be flexible. To accomplish a flexible spine, encourage movement in all directions so that no one area of the spine becomes overused, limiting its movement potential and affecting other areas of the spine.

◆ With impingement of an area of the spine for any length of time, blood flow and oxygenation to the area are affected.
◆ Chronic poor postural habits can lead to nerve impingement, resulting in chronic pain and possible injury.
◆ Practicing daily functional movement exercises for the spine and other joints in the practice setting and at home is a preventive strategy for all dental personnel.

DOCUMENTATION

Documentation for a patient with requirements for a personalized dental chair positioning during instrumentation would include:

◆ Medical history notations indicating health history and current problem causing physical limitations or breathing difficulties.
◆ Potential emergency that could occur if patient is overstressed; need for preparation at future appointments.
◆ Notation for reference to length of appointment and time of day if needed.
◆ Example documentation using the SOAP format can be reviewed in Box 8-2.

Factors to Teach the Patient

▶ How certain positions of the clinician are necessary for safe ergonomic practice and patient care.
▶ How patient cooperation makes it possible for the dental hygienist to practice with less stress and strain to prevent musculoskeletal discomfort and pain and deliver better patient care.

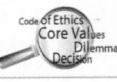

EVERYDAY ETHICS

After practicing for a few years as a dental hygienist, Delia has developed chronic pain in her neck, back, and hands. As a result, she knows that her instrumentation is affected and patients are not receiving definitive scaling at their appointments.

Questions for Consideration

1. What is Delia's ethical responsibility to herself in this situation? (Note: the *ADHA Code of Ethics for Dental Hygienists*, Section 7, Standards of Professional Responsibility.)

2. Explain which core values (Chapter 1, Box 1-6) apply to Delia's ethical responsibility to her patients if her ability to perform dental hygiene treatment is compromised?

3. Explain which of the questions (included in Chapter 1, Box 1-6) for making ethical decisions might help direct Delia in determining actions she can take now to assure that her patients continue to receive the best possible dental hygiene care.

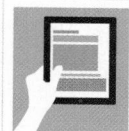

BOX 8-2

Example Documentation:
The Patient Who Is Unable to
Tolerate the Supine Position

S—Patient presents for routine 3-mo periodontal maintenance appointment; however, she came in on crutches due to a broken hip in a recent car accident. The patient provided a letter from her orthopedic surgeon clearing her for dental treatment. She is undergoing physical therapy twice a week for the next month or longer. The patient reports moderate soreness of back, arms, legs, and neck. Chief complaint is having a "dirty mouth" due to time spent in hospital and rehab, combined with inability to keep arms raised to clean teeth. She requests that the chair remain in the upright position during treatment.

O—Examination showed limited opening of mouth, plaque index (PI) score 72%, compared with PI of 12% from last visit. Noted: moderate biofilm on maxillary and mandibular posterior teeth, supragingival calculus in the mandibular anterior region; probing mostly within 3 mm range with a few bleeding spots.

A—The patient's current medical condition is preventing her from providing adequate self-care. Pain in arms and shoulders may be from use of crutches.

P—Adjusted chair per patient's request for most comfortable position. Limited opening and patient position caused difficulty in accessing dentition. Completed assessments only; patient requested appointment be stopped due to pain in back and legs. Advised patient to alert physician and physical therapist if increase in level, duration, or frequency of pain.

Next Step: Reappoint patient in 1 mo for periodontal maintenance completion pending improved physical condition.

Signed: _____, RDH

Date: _____

References

1. Prasad KD, Hegde C, Alva H, Shetty M. Medical and dental emergencies and complications in dental practice and its management. *J Educ Ethics Dent.* 2012;2(1):13.

2. Hemalatha VT, Manigandan T, Sarumathi T, Aarthi Nisha V, Amudhan A. Dental considerations in pregnancy—a critical review on the oral care. *J Clin Diagn Res.* 2013;7(5):948.

 ENHANCE YOUR UNDERSTANDING

ONLINE RESOURCES
(see the inside front cover for access information)
- Audio glossary
- Appendices

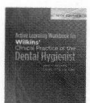

SUPPORT FOR LEARNING
(available separately)
- *Active Learning Workbook for Wilkins' Clinical Practice of the Dental Hygienist, 13th Edition*

INDIVIDUALIZED REVIEW
- Customized practice quizzing with Navigate 2 TestPrep for *Wilkins' Clinical Practice of the Dental Hygienist*

3. Branson BG, Williams KB, Bray KK, McIlnay SL, Dickey D. Validity and reliability of a dental operator posture assessment instrument (PAI). *J Dent Hyg.* 2002;76(4):255.

4. Sanders MJ, Turcotte CM. Posture makes perfect. *Dimens Dent Hyg.* 2011;9(11):30-32, 35.

5. Brame JL. Seating, positioning, and lighting. *Dimens Dent Hyg.* 2008;6(9):36-37.

6. Jordre BD, Bly J. Prevent pain with the right operator stool. *Dimens Dent Hyg.* 2014;12(1):16-18.

7. Valachi B. *Practice Dentistry Pain-free: Evidence-based Strategies to Prevent Pain and Extend Your Career.* Portland, OR: Posturedontics Press; 2008.

8. Shah MA, Pellegrini JM. Magnification basics. *Dimens Dent Hyg.* 2010;8(11):36-38.

9. Maillet JP, Millar AM, Burke JM, et al. Effect of magnification loupes on dental hygiene student posture. *J Dent Educ.* 2008;72(1):33-44.

10. Sunell S, Rucker L. Surgical magnification in dental hygiene practice. *Int J Dental Hyg.* 2004;2(1):26-35.

11. Chang BJ. Ergonomic benefits of surgical telescope systems: selection guidelines. *J Calif Dent Assoc.* 2002;30(2):161-169.

12. Dong H, Loomer P, Barr A, Laroche C, Young E, Rempel D. The effect of tool handle shape on hand muscle load and pinch force in a simulated dental scaling task. *Appl Ergon.* 2007;38(5):525-531.

13. Hayes MJ, Smith DR, Cockrell D. An international review of musculoskeletal disorders in the dental hygiene profession. *Int Dent J.* 2010;60(5):343-352.

14. Sanders MJ, Turcotte CM. Occupational stress in dental hygienists. *Work.* 2010;35(4):455-465.

9

Emergency Care

Wendy Male, MBA, BDSc, RDH

CHAPTER OUTLINE

EMERGENCY PREPAREDNESS

PREVENTION OF EMERGENCIES
I. Attention to Prevention
II. Factors Contributing to Emergencies

PATIENT ASSESSMENT
I. Assessment for Routine Treatment
II. The Patient's Medical History
III. Vital Signs
IV. Extraoral and Intraoral Examinations
V. Recognition of Increased Risk Factors

STRESS MINIMIZATION
I. Recognize the Patient with Stress Problems
II. Suggestions for Effective Communication
III. Reduction of Stress

EMERGENCY MATERIALS AND PREPARATION
I. Communication: Telephone Numbers for Medical Aid
II. Equipment for Use in an Emergency
III. Care of Drugs
IV. Medical Emergency Report Form
V. Practice and Drill

BLS CERTIFICATION

OXYGEN ADMINISTRATION
I. Equipment
II. Patient Breathing: Use Supplemental Oxygen
III. Patient Not Breathing: Use Positive Pressure

SPECIFIC EMERGENCIES

DOCUMENTATION
I. Comprehensive Record Keeping
II. Consults
III. New Entries

EVERYDAY ETHICS

FACTORS TO TEACH THE PATIENT

REFERENCES

LEARNING OBJECTIVES

After studying this chapter, the student will be able to:

1. Develop a plan to prevent and prepare for medical emergencies.

2. Identify signs and symptoms related to a possible emergency.

3. Define key words related to emergencies.

4. Describe stress minimization techniques.

5. Identify procedures for specific emergencies.

6. Incorporate documentation into the emergency plan.

EMERGENCY PREPAREDNESS

The public expects competence in emergency situations. This chapter is designed to help prevent emergencies from escalating into more serious conditions. Emergency drills can reveal weaknesses in team responses that may identify a need for further training or education for dental office personnel.[1,2] Emergencies in the dental office were reported by more than half of those surveyed,[3-5] but the following measures may increase emergency preparedness:

◆ Periodic review of the literature to update drills is necessary for evidence-based response to emergencies.

◆ Well-maintained emergency equipment stored in a convenient location.

◆ Post a *Quick Reference* with emergency equipment so it is readily available.

  • *Quick Reference* must include symptoms, equipment needed, and management of common emergencies.

◆ Box 9-1 contains abbreviations.

PREVENTION OF EMERGENCIES

I. Attention to Prevention

Prevention of emergencies requires preparedness, alertness, and anticipation. The following patient assessment procedures may reduce the occurrence of a medical emergency:

◆ Thorough medical history questionnaires updated at every appointment.[6-8]

◆ Documentation of baseline vital signs, updated at each appointment.[9]

◆ Documentation of findings on Medical Alert Tags; wrist or ankle bracelet or necklace that provides information on patient's medical condition.

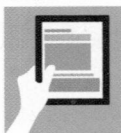

BOX 9-1
Emergency Care Abbreviations

• **ACLS:** advanced cardiac life support
• **AED:** automated external defibrillator
• **AHA:** American Heart Association
• **ALS:** advanced life support
• **BCLS:** basic cardiac life support
• **BLS:** basic life support
• **CAD:** coronary artery disease
• **CPR:** cardiopulmonary resuscitation
• **ECC:** emergency cardiac care
• **ECG:** electrocardiogram
• **EMD:** emergency medical dispatcher
• **EMS:** emergency medical service
• **EMT:** emergency medical technician
• **EMT-P:** emergency medical technician paramedic

BOX 9-2
Five-Point Plan to Prevent Emergencies

• Use careful, routine patient assessment procedures.
• Document and update accurate, comprehensive patient records.
• Implement stress reduction protocols.
• Recognize early signs of emergency distress.
• Organize team management plan for emergency preparedness.

◆ Physical assessment beginning with the first interaction with a patient.[10]

◆ Incorporation of proper risk management and stress reduction protocols into the patient care plan.[3,8]

◆ Implementation of preparatory steps when a careful review and update of the patient record identifies potential risks. Box 9-2 suggests a basic five-point plan for emergency prevention.

II. Factors Contributing to Emergencies

◆ Increased number of older and medically compromised patients in society with natural teeth and dental diseases that require invasive procedures.[6,11-13]

◆ Many patients, especially older adults, are taking medications that may interact adversely with drugs used in dentistry.[11,14]

◆ More complex dental procedures require longer appointments.[15]

◆ Increased use of drugs in dentistry.[15]

  • Anesthesia: local, general, conscious sedation.
  • Tranquilizers.
  • Pain medications (central nervous system depressants).
  • Antibiotics.

PATIENT ASSESSMENT

I. Assessment for Routine Treatment

A. First Contact

◆ Start with the first interaction with the patient.

◆ Note abnormalities of patient's voice on the telephone during appointment scheduling.

◆ Handwriting on medical history can indicate steadiness, ability to communicate, and education.

◆ Assess overall appearance and gait when patient enters the dental office or clinic.

◆ Document findings in the patient's record.

B. Parts of the Assessment

♦ Physical assessment (signs and symptoms).

♦ Comprehensive patient history to include medical, dental, and psychosocial history.

♦ Vital signs.

♦ Extraoral and intraoral examination.

♦ Comprehensive documentation of findings.

C. Emergency Indicators

Changes in a patient's appearance on the day of an appointment may suggest indicators that encourage preparation for emergencies.

II. The Patient's Medical History

A. Update and Document Changes

♦ Review at each appointment.[11]

♦ Discuss changes with dental team members who are providing treatment for the patient.

♦ A comprehensive medical history includes all the items found in Chapter 11.

B. Use of Medical Alert Box

♦ Many dental offices utilize computerized patient records but some are limited to paper records.

♦ If paper records are utilized, charts or folder are required for confidentiality and Health Insurance Portability and Accountability Act.

♦ Only the patient's name and/or record number may be included on the folder or chart.

♦ The "Medical Alert Box" is usually located on the front page of the medical history to alert the dental team of information that may predispose a patient to a medical emergency before, during, or postdental treatment. Significant items include:

• Physical conditions that may lead to an emergency.

• Diseases the patient has or previously had.

• Previous surgeries.

• Medical emergencies the patient experienced previously.

• Medications the patient has taken within the past 2 years.

• Allergies and adverse drug reactions.

• Previous adverse reactions to dental treatment.

III. Vital Signs

♦ Vital signs are essential to assess a patient's overall health status and to evaluate the severity of a medical emergency by comparison with baseline findings.

♦ A well-prepared dental team takes vital signs routinely to record baseline findings, not only during the earliest sign of emergency distress.[9]

A. The Vital Signs

Pulse, blood pressure, respirations, temperature, height, weight, and the information from the patient's personal Medical Alert Tag (bracelet, necklace, or anklet) provide essential information.

B. Baseline Vital Signs

The vital signs taken at the first appointment are considered baseline.[16] The ranges of vital signs are described in Chapter 12.

C. During Emergency

Compare vital signs to baseline findings during a medical emergency.

♦ *Compensating:* In most medical emergencies, patients will experience a "fight or flight" reaction, during which time they are said to be compensating. The vital signs are elevated above the baseline findings.[17]

♦ *Decompensating:* When vital signs have fallen below baseline, the patient could be going into a state of shock.[18]

♦ *Shock:* A state of lack of perfusion (saturation) of oxygenated blood to all cells of the brain and body. When brain cells are deprived of oxygenated blood, they cease to provide respiratory and circulatory function.

IV. Extraoral and Intraoral Examinations

Extraoral and intraoral examinations can provide significant clues to underlying disease processes that predispose a patient to a medical emergency. Thorough examinations are an integral part of the prevention of medical emergencies.[19,20]

A. Extraoral

Blood disorders, cancers, and endocrine disorders may be suspected or discovered from extraoral palpation, skin color changes, abnormalities of the eyes, and asymmetry of the face or neck.

B. Intraoral

Oral manifestations and lesions can be indications of many disease states, such as diabetes, anemia, leukemia, lupus erythematosus, or human immunodeficiency virus/acquired immune deficiency syndrome.

V. Recognition of Increased Risk Factors

The carefully prepared and regularly updated medical and personal history, with adequate follow-up consultation with the patient's physician for integration of dental and medical care, can prevent many emergencies by alerting dental personnel to the individual patient's needs and idiosyncrasies. Special needs may include:

◆ Specific physical conditions that may lead to an emergency, for example, genetic predispositions, seizures, diabetes.

◆ Diseases for which the patient is (or has been) under the care of a physician and the type of treatment, including medications.

◆ Allergies or drug reactions or interactions.[19]

STRESS MINIMIZATION

◆ Stress and anxiety are the basis for many of the common emergencies that occur in a dental office or clinic.

◆ The clinic atmosphere and the warmth and sincerity of the personnel can help a patient feel accepted and secure.

◆ The apprehension and anxiety associated with dental treatment compounds the risk factors for medical emergencies.[8,19]

I. Recognize the Patient with Stress Problems

◆ Apprehension or anxiety-related disorders related to dental procedure.

◆ Elderly patients are prone to medical emergencies, as they may have cardiovascular diseases or other undiagnosed conditions.[6,11]

◆ Essential medications: ensure certain prescriptions are taken on schedule to avoid risk of an emergency. The medications may cause adverse reactions that can lead to a medical emergency such as orthostatic hypotension.

II. Suggestions for Effective Communication

Provide a stress reduction plan to any patient who is apprehensive or medically predisposed to emergencies. Reduction of stress includes the development of patient rapport through effective communication between the dental team and the patient.

A. Actively Listen to a Patient's Fears

◆ Develop rapport so the patient senses the listener is empathetic and interested in alleviating the apprehension.

◆ Communicate with the patient about their fear of treatment. When a patient confides in a caregiver, trust is established and the patient is calmer.

◆ Patient trust in the care provider can be beneficial for emergency prevention.

B. Effects of Fear

Patients who try to repress their fears are more likely to hyperventilate or experience syncopal episodes.

III. Reduction of Stress

A. Appointment Scheduling

◆ *New patient*: Initial appointment for consultation and assessment provides an opportunity to build rapport and to evaluate the patient's level of anxiety. Stress reduction can be built into treatment appointments.[9]

◆ *Time of appointment*: Plan in accordance with personal health requirements.[8,9,19]

◆ *Waiting time minimized*: First appointment in the morning prevents building of anxiety by waiting all day for the appointment. In addition, anxiety can be decreased by taking the patient into the treatment room immediately and starting treatment promptly.[8,9]

◆ *Eating requirements*: Identify usual mealtime and ask about previous meal eaten to prevent hypoglycemia.[9,20]

◆ *Length of appointment*: Limited to the patient's tolerance.[9,19]

B. Medication

◆ Premedication when indicated and prescribed by the physician or dentist.[19]

◆ Pain control during treatment.[19]

◆ Patient's own prescriptions. Patients subject to emergencies are instructed to bring their own prescribed medicines, for example, the patient with asthma or one who is subject to attacks of angina pectoris.

C. Posttreatment Care

◆ Postcare instructions for prevention and/or relief of discomfort.

◆ Postcare pain control as needed. Analgesics may be prescribed.[8]

◆ Place a follow-up telephone call to an anxious patient to make certain there were no postoperative complications.

EMERGENCY MATERIALS AND PREPARATION

◆ Organization is a key concept in emergency preparedness.[21]

◆ The first steps in preparing for managing emergencies include setting up the emergency equipment and a systematic protocol.[21,22]

◆ Group planning and individual acceptance of responsibility can provide the team with efficiency, composure, and freedom from fear at the time of crisis.[23]

I. Communication: Telephone Numbers for Medical Aid

Postemergency telephone numbers near each extension that permits outside calls.

Rescue squads with paramedics (fire, police, flying squad, or 911 in many cities in the United States and Canada).

Ambulance service.

Nearest hospital emergency department.

Poison information center: 1-800-222-1222 in the United States. In Canada, visit SafeMedicationUse.ca for poison center telephone listings by province.

Physicians

Patient's physician is listed in the permanent record in a standard, convenient place.

Physicians available for emergency calls.

II. Equipment for Use in an Emergency

Every dental office or clinic should have an emergency kit or cart,[9,24] and everyone in the office must become familiar with its contents. Kits can be purchased commercially (Figure 9-1).

The kit is kept in order, its contents replenished, and outdated materials replaced as needed.

The emergency equipment is portable, well-maintained, and kept in a place readily accessible to all treatment rooms.

Materials are plainly marked and kept separate from other office supplies.

Materials included are selected to accomplish emergency treatment by current methods.

The items included in the kit imply proper training in their use.

Members of a team can add new items for the list in keeping with their training and abilities.

Table 9-1 provides a typical list of essential emergency equipment items.

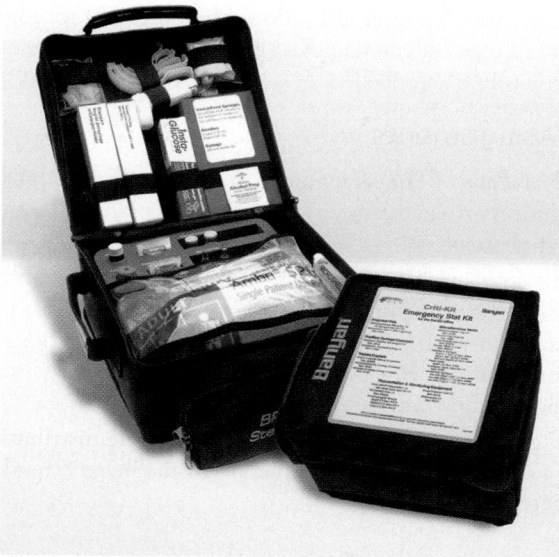

FIGURE 9-1 • Emergency Medical Kit for the Dental Office.

TABLE 9-1 • Equipment in an Emergency Kit or Cart

CATEGORY	ESSENTIAL ITEMS

Required equipment	• Series E portable oxygen tank
	  • Low-flow oxygen regulator
	  • Nasal cannula
	  • Simple face mask
	  • Nonrebreather mask
	  • Bag-valve masks (adult and pediatric)
	  • Demand valve resuscitator
	• Automated external defibrillator (AED)
	• Oro- and nasopharyngeal airways
	  • Sizes: pediatric to large adult
	  • Water-soluble lubricant
	• Sphygmomanometer
	  • Blood pressure cuffs: pediatric, adult regular, and large adult
	• Magill forceps
	• Syringes: 2–3 mL Luer-Lok tip 21-gauge needles
	• Medical Emergency Report Forms
	• Cricothyrotomy equipment[a]
	• Intravenous equipment[a]

Injectable drugs	• Epinephrine via autoinjector (EpiPen®) • Diphenhydramine (injectable antihistamine) • Cortisone[a] • Glucagon[a] • Midazolam[a] • Atropine[a]
Noninjectable drugs	• Antiplatelet: aspirin • Respiratory stimulant: ammonia vaporole or ammonia inhalant capsule • Bronchodilator: albuterol inhaler • Antihypoglycemic: glucose gel, glucagon paste • Vasodilator: nitroglycerin tablets, nitrolingual spray • Diphenhydramine tablets • Naloxone (Narcan): nasal spray

Supplementary equipment	• Thermometer
	• Blood glucose meter, lancets, and test strips
	• Pen flashlight
	• Stopwatch
	• Razor (for hair removal for AED pads)
	• Scissors
	• Cotton pliers
	• Emesis basin
	• Blanket
	• Pillow
	• Inflatable splints
	• Backboard (12 × 249 for patients who cannot be moved for cardiopulmonary resuscitation)
	• Quick-activated cold packs
	• Betadine wipes (Povidone-Iodine antiseptic wipes)
	• Sterile packages of gauze and adhesive tape
	  • 2 × 2 inches
	  • 4 × 4 inches
	  • Rolled gauze (2 × 5 inches)

[a]Administered only by personnel with advanced medical training.

III. Care of Drugs

◆ All dental personnel become familiar with the emergency drugs maintained in the particular office or clinic.[15]

◆ Only specially trained, experienced persons will administer injectable medications.[21]

◆ The only drugs kept in the dental office are those that the dentist or emergency team is trained to use.[15,21]

A. Identification

◆ The purpose and method of administration of each drug is clearly identified on the container.[15]

◆ A compartmentalized clear plastic cabinet or box can be useful for this purpose because the labels and instructions can be seen from the outside and efficient selection can be made.[15,25]

◆ The expiration date appears clearly on each item that has a limited shelf life.[15,25]

◆ When narcotics are included in the list of drugs available for emergencies, they are stored in a secured location other than the emergency kit, and typically purchased in predosed amounts for specific emergency situations.

B. Record of Drugs

◆ Label each with information about shelf life and due date for replacement. Example: Nitroglycerin is replaced at 6 months.[15]

◆ Check weekly to maintain emergency kit in workable order.[15]

◆ A complete record of each available drug is kept. The following are recorded:
  • Name of drug.
  • Dosage.
  • Date purchased.
  • Address of source if different from the usual local pharmacy.
  • Itemized record, signed by the staff member responsible.
  • Specific entry as each drug is used.
  • Expiration dates checked at routine intervals.
  • Instructions for disposal.

C. Disposal of Drugs

◆ Follow specific disposal instructions on the drug label or patient information sheet.

◆ Do not flush prescription drugs down the toilet.

◆ Take advantage of community drug take-back programs that allow the public to bring unused drugs to a central location for disposal.

IV. Medical Emergency Report Form

◆ Figure 9-2 shows an example of a form that can be used to record the essential information during an emergency.

◆ Such a form can be filed or scanned and stored in the computerized patient record control system to include in the patient's permanent record.

◆ The forms can be placed on a clipboard on the emergency cart.

◆ A copy of the emergency report is given to the emergency medical service (EMS) personnel to present to those in the emergency room at the hospital or other medical facility when the patient is admitted.[26]

A. Purposes

◆ Organize data collected during the emergency.

◆ Serve as a time reference during the monitoring of vital signs.

◆ Prepare a record from which the medical personnel can interpret the patient's condition at the time of transfer from the dental facility.[26]

B. Uses

◆ Evaluation for planning dental and dental hygiene appointments to avoid future emergencies for the patient.

◆ Provide a reference in the event legal questions arise. A well-kept record can be vital, and each emergency, however insignificant the incident may seem, is recorded.[15]

V. Practice and Drill

A. Staff Instruction

◆ In an emergency situation, seconds count and there is no time for fumbling or discussion.[23]

◆ Each member of the clinic and office staff is thoroughly familiar with the location, purpose, effect, and application of each item of equipment and its source.[25]

◆ Each staff member also knows the order of procedures in all types of emergencies (Figure 9-3) and can assume any role when needed.[15,25]

B. Assignments

◆ *Preparation:* The assignment of specific responsibilities during an emergency is the result of planning by the whole team.[3,4,23]

◆ *Substitutions:* Because a staff member may be absent from the scene at the time of an emergency, each person learns and practices the duties for all positions so substitutions can be made with a minimum of discussion and no confusion.[3,4,23]

◆ Figure 9-4 shows an example of a possible distribution of duties when three people are available to attend to the patient.

Medical Emergency Report

Patient's Name	Smith, Joe	Today's Date	10/27/20

Description of incident: Patient exhibited signs of anaphylaxis after exposure to latex gloves. Urticaria and pruritus were evident on arms, neck and chest. Signs of lip, tongue and laryngeal edema were exhibited with difficulty swallowing and breathing. Quickly explained to patient that he was having an allergic reaction. Patient was immediately given epinephrine (.3mg) via EpiPen autoinjector and EMS was summoned. 50mg of Benadryl and 100mg of Solu-Cortef were also administered IM. Oxygen was delivered by non-rebreather at 15 L/min. Within 5 minutes vital signs and symptoms improved. At 8 minutes vital signs were near baseline. Patient was released to EMS in 15 minutes and transported to the hospital.

Time of onset		Time EMS summoned		Time EMS arrived		Time patient was released	
Stopwatch	Clock time	Stopwatch	Clock time	Stopwatch	Clock time	Stopwatch	Clock time
0:00 minutes	10:30 am	0:10 minutes	10:30 am	13:00 minutes	10:43 am	15:00 minutes	10:45 am

Patient released to: EMS who transported patient to Tallahassee Memorial Regional Medical Center

Cessation of breathing: Ø		Cessation of pulse: Ø		CPR initiated: Ø	
Stopwatch	Clock time	Stopwatch	Clock time	Stopwatch	Clock time
N/A	N/A	N/A	N/A	N/A	N/A

	Initial findings	Stopwatch times	Followup finding	Stopwatch times	Followup finding	Stopwatch times
Blood pressure	90/60	2:15 minutes	110/80	5:15 minutes	120/80	8:15 minutes
Pulse	50 bpm	1:00 minutes	68 bpm	5:00 minutes	72 bpm	8:30 minutes
Respirations	10	1:30 minutes	12	5:30 minutes	16	8:00 minutes
O_2 delivery method	non-rebreather (15 L/min)	1:45 minutes	non-rebreather (15 L/min)	5:30 minutes	non-rebreather (15 L/min)	8:30 minutes

Drugs administered	Route	Dosage	Stopwatch times
Epinephrine via EpiPen ®	I.M. (Quad)	.3 mg	0:45
Benadryl ®	I.M. (Deltoid)	50 mg	1:15
Solu-Cortef ®	I.M. (Deltoid)	100 mg	1:30

FIGURE 9-2 • Sample Medical Emergency Report. The form is prepared in duplicate. One copy accompanies the patient to the emergency clinic, and the second copy is retained in the patient's dental record file.

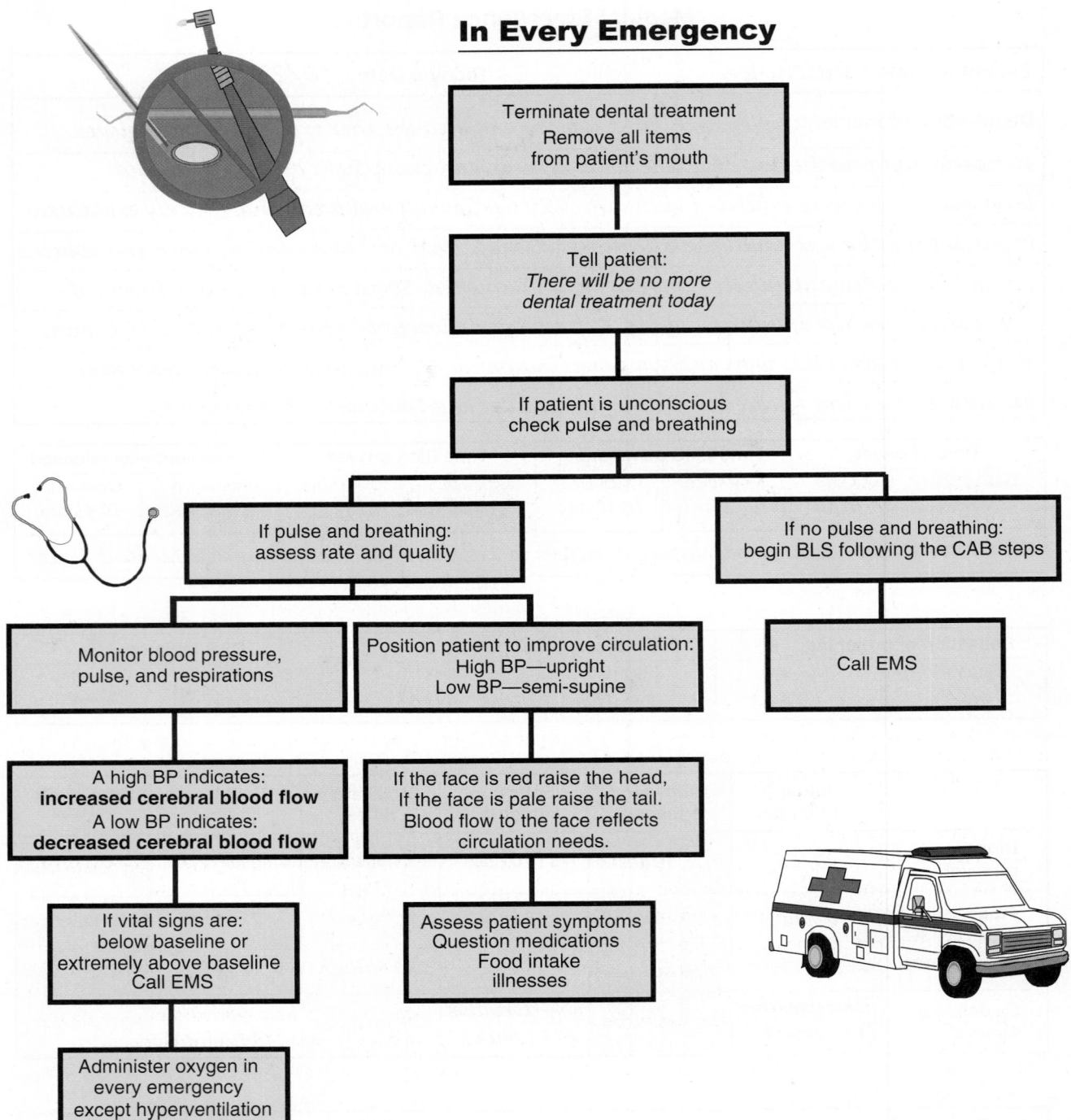

In Every Emergency

Terminate dental treatment
Remove all items
from patient's mouth

Tell patient:
*There will be no more
dental treatment today*

If patient is unconscious
check pulse and breathing

If pulse and breathing:
assess rate and quality

If no pulse and breathing:
begin BLS following the CAB steps

Monitor blood pressure,
pulse, and respirations

Position patient to improve circulation:
High BP—upright
Low BP—semi-supine

Call EMS

A high BP indicates:
increased cerebral blood flow
A low BP indicates:
decreased cerebral blood flow

If the face is red raise the head,
If the face is pale raise the tail.
Blood flow to the face reflects
circulation needs.

If vital signs are:
below baseline or
extremely above baseline
Call EMS

Assess patient symptoms
Question medications
Food intake
illnesses

Administer oxygen in
every emergency
except hyperventilation

FIGURE 9-3 • Flowchart: In Every Emergency. BLS, basic life support; EMS, emergency medical service.

◆ *Advantages of assignments*
- Organization efficiently uses personnel.
- Sharing responsibility relieves pressure.
- Duties can be carried out quietly, without excess discussion or attention from others in the clinic.
- Necessary work gets done without duplication and without omissions.

C. Drills

◆ Regular reviews and rehearsals for each type of emergency are conducted, preferably on a "surprise" basis, at least once a month.[23]

◆ A specific emergency code call can be used when an intercom or other message system is available. Mentioning "code" in front of a number or phrase may panic the

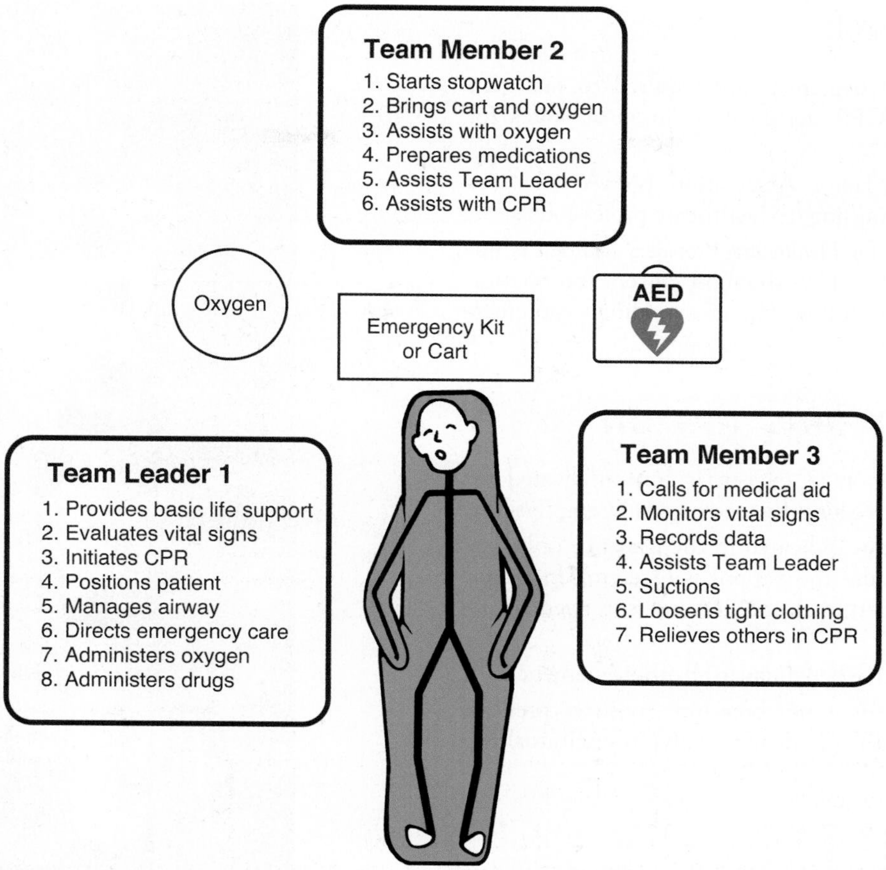

Team Member 2
1. Starts stopwatch
2. Brings cart and oxygen
3. Assists with oxygen
4. Prepares medications
5. Assists Team Leader
6. Assists with CPR

Oxygen

Emergency Kit or Cart

AED

Team Leader 1
1. Provides basic life support
2. Evaluates vital signs
3. Initiates CPR
4. Positions patient
5. Manages airway
6. Directs emergency care
7. Administers oxygen
8. Administers drugs

Team Member 3
1. Calls for medical aid
2. Monitors vital signs
3. Records data
4. Assists Team Leader
5. Suctions
6. Loosens tight clothing
7. Relieves others in CPR

FIGURE 9-4 • Division of Duties for Three-Person Emergency Team. Suggested distribution of responsibilities to be memorized and practiced by the dental personnel who form the emergency team. AED, automated external defibrillator; CPR, cardiopulmonary resuscitation.

other patients; therefore, it is best to use only a number like "17."

◆ For each type of emergency, practice in the use of procedures, including oxygen administration, resuscitation, and airway maneuvers, as well as specific positioning of a patient for all emergencies is indicated.[23]

◆ Equipment and materials can be checked at the time of the drill to ensure their availability and that each is in working order. Outdated supplies are replaced. One staff member is designated to be in charge of the emergency supplies.[25]

◆ A record of drills is kept with a diary of dates, procedures practiced, and names of those present.

D. New Staff Member

◆ Assignment of duties and practice for new members are a part of the first working day's orientation.

◆ New members are expected to renew basic life support (BLS)/cardiopulmonary resuscitation (CPR) certification by taking necessary refresher courses within a specified time. Most states and/or provinces require a renewal certificate for annual licensure.

◆ The Commission on Dental Accreditation has established standards requiring all clinic personnel to be healthcare provider BLS/CPR certified.

E. Procedures Manual

A paper manual is a valuable reference, but an electronic format is a currently accepted method of storing procedure manuals. They need to be accessible from a computer or mobile device readily available in the clinic.

◆ Reviewed and updated three or four times each year.

◆ Useful during the orientation of a new member.

◆ Contains work assignments and checklists for equipment and resources.

◆ Provides reference information concerning specific emergencies organized in color-coded sections and alphabetical order to outline signs, symptoms, and initial treatment.

◆ Members of the team are given assignments to update the manual by conducting a critical review of the scientific literature for quality assurance and evidence-based, patient-centered care.

◆ All updates are referenced in the index of the manual.

BLS CERTIFICATION

◆ Licensed dental hygienists are required to maintain a current BLS/CPR certification in most states for licensure.

◆ The American Heart Association (AHA) provides guidelines and training for healthcare professionals.

◆ The *AHA BLS for Healthcare Providers Manual* is updated regularly to reflect the most current information and procedures to follow when responding to an emergency situation.

OXYGEN ADMINISTRATION

◆ High concentration of oxygen is contraindicated for chronic obstructive lung diseases, especially emphysema.

◆ Oxygen is also not indicated in the presence of hyperventilation because the patient is receiving increased amounts of oxygen in air inhaled and is in need of carbon dioxide.[15,24]

◆ The use of oxygen is beneficial in all other emergencies.[15]

◆ When the patient is not breathing, positive pressure oxygen (also known as demand valve resuscitator) delivery is needed.[24]

I. Equipment

Oxygen delivery systems with indications, flow rate, and percentage of oxygen delivered are listed in Table 9-2. A portable oxygen delivery system is shown in Figure 9-5.

A. Parts

Oxygen resuscitation equipment consists of the following:

◆ An oxygen tank.

◆ A reducing valve.

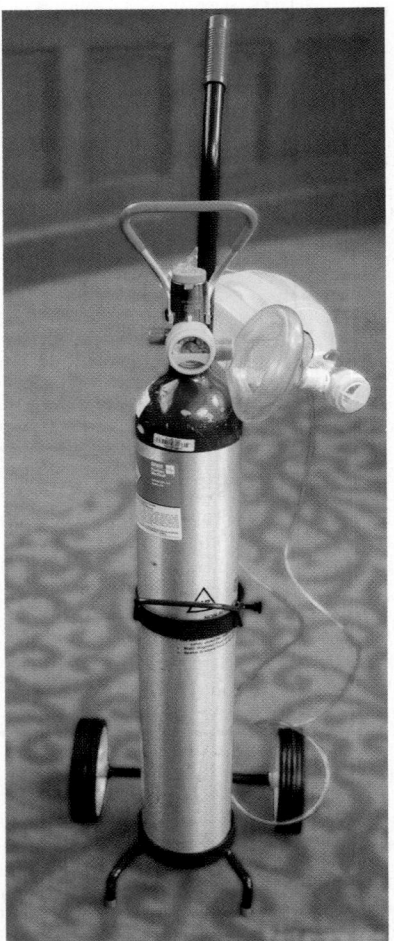

FIGURE 9-5 • Portable Oxygen Delivery System. The portable unit is stored in an area immediately accessible to all treatment areas in the dental clinic. If a fixed oxygen delivery system is available in the treatment area, it can be used in an emergency situation.

TABLE 9-2 • Oxygen Delivery Systems			
DEVICE	INDICATIONS	FLOW RATE (L/MIN)	OXYGEN DELIVERY (%)
Cannula	For patient who is breathing and needs low levels of oxygen	2–6	25–40
Face mask	For patient who is breathing and needs moderate levels of oxygen: • When cannula is not tolerated • When more oxygen is desired • Patient is in shock	8–12	60
Nonrebreather mask	For patient who is breathing and needs high levels of oxygen: • Patient is in shock • When more oxygen is desired	10–15	60–90
Bag mask	When patient has stopped breathing; bag mask is used instead of mouth-to-mouth resuscitation	10–15	90–100
Demand valve resuscitation	Positive pressure delivery of oxygen on demand	Used by emergency medical technicians or others professionally trained	100

Laminate and affix to the oxygen tank.

- ◆ A flow meter.
- ◆ Tubing.
- ◆ Mask.
- ◆ A positive pressure bag.

The *E* cylinder, which can provide oxygen for 30 minutes, is the minimum size recommended. Smaller tanks provide little oxygen for short periods only, and larger tanks are less portable.[24]

B. Directions

Box 9-3 outlines the steps for operation of an oxygen tank. Clear, readable directions are permanently attached to the tank's portable carriage. Practice is a definite part of team drills.

II. Patient Breathing: Use Supplemental Oxygen

- ◆ Apply a full-face clear mask or a nasal cannula.[24]
- ◆ Supplemental oxygen is started at 6–10 L/min.[24]
- ◆ Monitor breathing; if breathing stops, proceed with positive pressure oxygen.

III. Patient Not Breathing: Use Positive Pressure

For persons not trained in the use of the bag-valve mask or positive pressure delivery, a mouth-to-mask procedure is used.[27,28]

- ◆ Apply full-face clear mask so a tight seal is formed. One dental team member may need to apply pressure to the face mask to maintain a complete seal.
- ◆ Adjust oxygen flow so the positive pressure bag remains filled.
- ◆ Compress the bag manually, one ventilation every 5–6 seconds to provide 10–12 respirations/min for an adult. For a child, 1 ventilation every 3 seconds.
- ◆ Watch chest rise. When the chest does not rise, recheck airway for obstruction. Proceed with airway obstruction management.
- ◆ *Call EMS.*

SPECIFIC EMERGENCIES

- ◆ Certain systemic disease conditions and physical injuries require specific treatment during an emergency.
- ◆ In Tables 9-3 and 9-4, the *Emergency Reference Charts*, several conditions are listed with their symptoms and treatment procedures.
- ◆ Some of the same conditions have been described in detail in Section IX of this book.

DOCUMENTATION

All details about the patient, the treatments, reactions, healing, and comments by the patient provide crucial information in a medical emergency or posttreatment complication.

BOX 9-3
Operation of Oxygen Tank

Operation of Oxygen Tank
To turn on:
- Attach oxygen delivery system to tank.
- Turn **key** on top of tank in *counterclockwise direction* to open flow of oxygen.
- Adjust **low-flow regulator knob and turn in the direction the arrow indicates to increase or open**; many regulators are opposite of sink faucets and open clockwise instead of counterclockwise.
- Attach oxygen delivery system to patient.

To turn off:
- Remove oxygen delivery system from patient.
- Turn **key** on top of tank in *clockwise direction* to shut off flow of oxygen.
- Turn the **low-flow regulator knob** to the open position to bleed oxygen from the system.
- After bleeding, gently close the **low-flow regulator knob**.

Laminate and Affix to the Oxygen Tank
To turn on:
- Attach oxygen delivery system to tank.
- Turn **key** on top of tank in counterclockwise direction to open flow of oxygen.
- Adjust the **low-flow regulator knob**.
- **To increase O$_2$ flow: turn the knob in the direction the arrow indicates.** (Many regulators are the opposite of sink faucets and open clockwise instead of counterclockwise.)
- Attach oxygen delivery system from patient.

To turn off:
- Remove oxygen delivery system from patient.
- Turn **key** on top of tank in *clockwise direction* to shut off flow of oxygen.
- Turn the **low-flow regulator knob** to open position to bleed oxygen from the system.
- After bleeding, gently close the **low-flow regulator knob**.

I. Comprehensive Record Keeping

- ◆ All medical findings and changes.
- ◆ Treatments provided, including types and amounts of local anesthesia, general anesthesia, nitrous oxide, or other types of sedation.[15]
- ◆ Regimens of medications prescribed for patients are crucial information should a medical emergency or a posttreatment complication occur.

TABLE 9-3 • Emergency Reference Chart: Medical Emergencies

EMERGENCY	SIGNS/SYMPTOMS	PROCEDURE
All Cases Call Emergency Medical Service (EMS) immediately if problem with: Breathing Unconsciousness **Anaphylaxis** Bleeding Poisoning Chest pain		i. Determine consciousness (tap and shout): yell for help **If patient is unconscious: Call EMS and get automated external defibrillator (AED)** i. Conduct primary assessment: C—Circulation: check for pulse for 10 sec, if none: start compressions A—Airway: open with head tilt-chin lift B—Breathing: (look, listen, feel) if none: give 2 (1-sec) breaths D—Defibrillate: 1 shock: then 5 cycles of cardiopulmonary resuscitation (CPR) **If patient is conscious and breathing:** i. Conduct secondary assessment: a. Evaluate level of consciousness 1. Does patient know own name, location, date? 2. Use penlight to see if pupils react equally to light 3. If conscious: check for equal hand strength by asking patient to squeeze your hands 4. Position according to signs/symptoms 5. If face is red, raise the head 6. If face is pale, raise the tail 7. Evaluate heart rate, blood pressure, respirations b. Findings in patient record or medical alert bracelet 1. Disabilities, diseases, drugs, baseline vital signs: **Call EMS**
Respiratory failure	Labored or weak respirations or cessation of breathing **Cyanosis** or ashen-white with blood loss Pupils dilated Loss of consciousness	Position: semisupine if not breathing; upright if breathing Check for and remove foreign material from mouth Establish airway. **Begin CPR**. If patient does not spontaneously breathe: **Call EMS** Monitor vital signs: blood pressure, pulse, respirations Administer oxygen by nonrebreather mask if patient is already breathing
Mild airway obstruction	Good air exchange, coughing, wheezing (patient can speak)	Sit patient up Loosen tight collar, belt No treatment; let patient cough
Severe airway obstruction	Poor air exchange; noisy breathing; weak, ineffective cough; difficult respirations; gasping. Unable to speak, breathe, cough. Cyanosis, dilated pupils	Reassure patient Treat for complete obstruction **Conscious patient:** Perform Heimlich maneuver Patient becomes unconscious: **Begin CPR** **Unconscious patient:** **Call EMS**
Hyperventilation syndrome	Light-headedness, giddiness Anxiety, confusion Dizziness Overbreathing (25–30 respirations/min) Feelings of suffocation Deep respirations Palpitations (heart pounds) Tingling or numbness in the extremities	Terminate oral procedure Remove rubber dam and objects from mouth Position upright Immediately tell patient: "There will be no more dental treatment today" Loosen tight collar Reassure patient Explain overbreathing; request that each breath be held to a count of 10. Ask patient to breathe deeply (7–10/min) into a paper bag adapted closely over nose and mouth Never use a bag for a patient with diabetes or patients exhibiting signs of diabetic coma, e.g., fruity breath odor, **Kussmaul breathing**, lethargy, dry skin
Heart failure	Difficult or labored breathing Pulmonary congestion with cough and difficulty breathing May cough up pink sputum Rapid, weak pulse Dilated pupils May have chest pain	Place patient in upright position. **Call EMS**. Make patient comfortable: cover with blanket Administer oxygen by nonrebreather mask Reassure patient. Provide basic life support (BLS)

TABLE 9-3 • Emergency Reference Chart: Medical Emergencies (*Continued*)

EMERGENCY	SIGNS/SYMPTOMS	PROCEDURE
Cardiac arrest	Skin: ashen gray, cold, clammy No pulse No heart sounds No respirations Eyes fixed, with dilated pupils; no constriction with light Unconscious	**Call EMS**. Check oral cavity for debris or vomitus; leave dentures in place for a seal. **Begin CPR**[27]
Asthma attack	Difficulty breathing, wheezing (extreme cases—silence, indicating little to no air exchange) Cyanosis Dilated pupils Confusion due to lack of oxygen Chest pressure Sweating	Position patient upright with arms up and supported forward Assist with patient's own bronchodilator Administer supplemental oxygen by nasal cannula Epinephrine if patient decompensates Supplemental cortisone to patients on corticosteroid therapy BLS—may need demand valve resuscitator if patient experiences respiratory depression. **Call EMS**
Syncope (fainting)	Pale gray face, anxiety Dilated pupils Weakness, giddiness, dizziness, faintness, nausea Profuse cold perspiration Rapid pulse at first, followed by slow pulse Shallow breathing Drop in blood pressure Loss of consciousness	Position: **Trendelenburg** Open airway Loosen tight collar, belt Place cold, damp towel on forehead Crush ammonia vaporole and place under patient's nose Keep warm (blanket) Monitor vital signs: blood pressure, pulse, respirations Keep airway open Administer oxygen by nasal cannula Keep in supine position 10 min after recovery to prevent nausea and dizziness Reassure patient, especially during recovery
Shock	Skin: pale, moist, clammy Rapid, shallow breathing Low blood pressure Weakness and/or restlessness Nausea, vomiting Thirst, if shock is from bleeding Eventual unconsciousness if untreated	Position: Trendelenburg Open airway Keep quiet and warm Monitor vital signs: blood pressure, respirations, pulse Keep airway open Administer oxygen by nonrebreather bag If patient does not recover fully and/or vital signs not at baseline: **Call EMS**
Stroke (cerebrovascular accident)	*Premonitory* dizziness, vertigo Transient **paresthesia** or weakness Transient speech defects Serious headache (with cerebral hemorrhage) Breathing labored, deep, slow Chills Paralysis on one side of body Nausea, vomiting Convulsions Loss of consciousness (slow or sudden onset)	***Conscious patient:*** **Call EMS**. Turn patient on paralyzed side; semiupright Loosen clothing about the throat Reassure patient; keep calm, quiet Monitor vital signs: blood pressure, pulse, respirations Administer oxygen by nasal cannula Clear airway; suction vomitus because the throat muscles may be paralyzed ***Unconscious patient:*** Position: supine BLS CPR if indicated

(*Continues*)

TABLE 9-3 • Emergency Reference Chart: Medical Emergencies (*Continued*)

EMERGENCY	SIGNS/SYMPTOMS	PROCEDURE
Cardiovascular diseases	Symptoms vary depending on cause	***For all patients:*** **Call EMS** Be calm and reassure patient Keep patient warm and quiet; restrict effort Always administer oxygen when there is chest pain
Angina pectoris	Sudden crushing, **paroxysmal** pain in substernal area Pain may radiate to shoulder, neck, arms Pallor, faintness Shallow breathing Anxiety, fear	Position: upright, as patient requests, for comfortable breathing If patient has been diagnosed with angina and has own nitroglycerin: Place nitroglycerin sublingually only when the blood pressure is at or above baseline Administer oxygen by nasal cannula Reassure patient Without prompt relief from nitroglycerin: **Call EMS**. Treat as a **myocardial infarction**
Myocardial infarction (heart attack)	Sudden pain similar to angina pectoris, which may radiate, but of longer duration Pallor; cold, clammy skin Cyanosis Nausea Breathing difficulty Marked weakness Anxiety, fear Possible loss of consciousness	**Call EMS**. Position: with head up for comfortable breathing Symptoms are not relieved with nitroglycerin Encourage to chew 1 adult (not enteric coated) or 2 low-dose "baby" aspirin if the patient has no allergy to aspirin[29] Monitor vital signs: blood pressure, pulse, respirations Administer oxygen by nonrebreather bag Alleviate anxiety; reassure
Adrenal crisis (cortisol mental deficiency)	Anxious, stressed Confusion Pain in abdomen, back, legs Muscle weakness Extreme fatigue Nausea, vomiting Lowered blood pressure Elevated pulse Loss of consciousness Coma	***Conscious patient:*** Terminate oral procedure **Call EMS** Request telephone call for medical assistance Administer oxygen by nonrebreather mask Monitor blood pressure and pulse Place patient on stable side with legs slightly raised ***Unconscious patient:*** **Call EMS** BLS Try ammonia vaporole when cause is undecided Administer oxygen
Insulin reaction (hyperinsulinism, hypoglycemia)	Sudden onset Skin: moist, cold, pale Confused, nervous, anxious Bounding pulse Salivation Normal to shallow respirations Convulsions (late)	***Conscious patient:*** Administer glucose gel Observe patient for 1 hr before dismissal Determine time since previous meal, and arrange next appointment following food intake ***Unconscious patient:*** **Call EMS** BLS Position: supine Maintain airway Administer oxygen by nonrebreather bag Monitor vital signs Administer intramuscular glucagon or intravenous glucose

TABLE 9-3 • Emergency Reference Chart: Medical Emergencies (*Continued*)

EMERGENCY	SIGNS/SYMPTOMS	PROCEDURE
Diabetic coma (ketoacidosis) (hyperglycemia)	Slow onset Skin: flushed and dry Breath: fruity odor Dry mouth, thirst Low blood pressure Weak, rapid pulse Exaggerated respirations (Kussmaul breathing)	***Conscious patient:*** **Call EMS**. Keep patient warm Administer oxygen by nasal cannula ***Unconscious patient:*** BLS Position: supine
Seizure • Generalized **tonic-clonic** • Generalized absence	Coma Anxiety or depression Pale, may become cyanotic Muscular contractions Loss of consciousness Brief loss of consciousness Fixed posture Rhythmic twitching of eyelids, eyebrows, or head May be pale	**Call EMS**. Position supine: Do not attempt to move from dental chair Make safe by placing movable equipment out of reach Do not force anything between the teeth; a soft towel or large sponges may be placed while mouth is open Open airway; monitor vital signs Administer oxygen by nasal cannula or face mask Allow patient to sleep during postconvulsive stage EMS to determine need for transport to hospital Take objects from patient's hands to prevent their being dropped
Allergic reaction • Delayed (anaphylactic shock)	Skin **Erythema** (rash) **Urticaria** (wheals, itching) **Angioedema** (localized swelling of mucous membranes, lips, larynx, pharynx) Respiration Distress, **dyspnea** Wheezing Extension of angioedema to larynx: may have obstruction from swelling of vocal apparatus	Skin Administer antihistamine Respiration Position: upright Administer oxygen by nasal cannula Epinephrine may be needed if breathing difficulty If airway obstruction: Position: supine Airway maintenance Epinephrine (EpiPen®)
• Immediate anaphylaxis	Skin Urticaria (wheals, itching) Flushing Nausea, abdominal cramps, vomiting, diarrhea Angioedema Swelling of lips, membranes, eyelids Laryngeal edema with difficulty swallowing Respiration distress Cough, wheezing Dyspnea, airway obstruction Cyanosis Cardiovascular collapse Profound drop in blood pressure Rapid, weak pulse Palpitations Dilation of pupils Loss of consciousness (sudden) Cardiac arrest	Rapid treatment needed. Administer epinephrine via autoinjector (EpiPen®) **Call EMS** Position: supine (except when dyspnea predominates) Administer oxygen by nonrebreather mask BLS Monitor vital signs CPR if airway obstructed

(Continues)

TABLE 9-3 • Emergency Reference Chart: Medical Emergencies (Continued)

EMERGENCY	SIGNS/SYMPTOMS	PROCEDURE
Local anesthesia reactions • Psychogenic • Allergic (very rare) • Toxic overdose	Reaction to injection, not the anesthetic Syncope Hyperventilation syndrome Anaphylactic shock Allergic skin and mucous membrane reactions Bronchial asthma attack Effects of intravascular injection rather than increased quantity of drug more common Stimulation phase Anxious, restless, apprehensive, confused Rapid pulse and respirations Elevated blood pressure Tremors Convulsions Depressive phase follows stimulation phase Drowsiness, lethargy Shocklike symptoms: pallor, sweating Rapid, weak pulse and respirations Drop in blood pressure Respiratory depression or respiratory arrest Unconsciousness	Syncope Hyperventilation See earlier in this table Mild reaction Stop injection Position: supine Loosen tight clothing Reassure patient Monitor blood pressure, heart rate, respirations Administer oxygen by nasal cannula Severe reaction: **Call EMS** BLS: maintain airway Administer oxygen by nonrebreather mask Continue to monitor vital signs CPR Administration of anticonvulsant
Opioid overdose • Fentanyl overdose	Trouble breathing, very slow breathing, or not breathing Unresponsive Limp, immobile Snoring, gurgling sounds Cold, clammy skin Blue lips, fingernails Drowsiness, lethargy Tiny pupils[30]	Assess for unresponsiveness: **Call EMS** Observe breathing vs. no breathing or only gasping BLS: if unresponsive with no breathing or only gasping, begin CPR Administer Naloxone 2 mg intranasal (may repeat after 4 min) Assess response: if move purposefully, breathe regularly, moan, or otherwise respond—stimulate and reassess Continue to monitor responsiveness and breathing until EMS arrives. If person stops responding, begin CPR and repeat Naloxone Assess response: if no response, continue CPR and use AED if available[28]

TABLE 9-4 • Emergency Reference Chart: Traumatic Injuries

EMERGENCY	SIGNS/SYMPTOMS	PROCEDURE
Hemorrhage	Prolonged bleeding Spurting blood: artery Oozing blood: vein	Compression over bleeding area 1. Apply gauze pack with direct pressure 2. Bandage pack into place firmly where possible 3. Elevate injury above the heart if possible Severe bleeding: digital pressure on pressure point of supplying vessel If shock symptoms: **Call EMS**
	Bleeding from tooth socket	Pack with folded gauze; do not dab Have patient bite down firmly If bleeding does not stop, instruct patient to gently bite down on a damp tea bag and hold in place for 10 min

TABLE 9-4 • Emergency Reference Chart: Traumatic Injuries (*Continued*)

EMERGENCY	SIGNS/SYMPTOMS	PROCEDURE
	Nosebleed	Seat patient upright, head elevated Tell patient to breathe through mouth Apply cold application to nose Press nostril on bleeding side for a few minutes Advise patient not to blow the nose for an hour or more If bleeding does not stop, wet cotton rolls with water and lubricate with water-soluble lubricant Pack nostril Instruct patient to breathe through the mouth Leave packing in place until patient sees a physician
Chemical burn	Reddened, discolored	Immediate: copious irrigation with water for $1/2$ hr Check directions on chemical container for antidote or other advice Burn caused by acid: rinse with bicarbonate of soda; burn caused by alkali: rinse in weak acid (e.g., vinegar)
Internal poisoning	Signs of corrosive burn around or in oral cavity Evidence of empty container or information from patient Nausea, vomiting, cramps	Call Poison Control Center: 1-800-222-1222 in the United States. In Canada, visit SafeMedicationUse.ca for poison center telephone listings by province. Be calm and supportive Basic life support (BLS): airway maintenance Artificial ventilation (inhaled poison) Record vital signs Do *not* give water or milk or Ipecac unless instructed to do so by Poison Control Center Avoid nonspecific and questionably effective antidotes, stimulants, sedatives, or other agents, which may do more harm **Call EMS**
Foreign body in eye	Tears Blinking	Wash hands Ask patient to look down Bring upper lid down over lower lid for a moment; move it upward Turn down lower lid and examine: if particle is visible, remove with moistened cotton applicator Use eye cup: wash out eye with plain water When unsuccessful, seek medical attention: prevent patient from rubbing eye by placing gauze pack over eye and stabilizing with adhesive tape
Chemical solution in eye	Tears Stinging	Irrigate promptly with copious amounts of water Turn head so water flows away from inner aspect of the eye; continue for 15–20 min
Dislocated jaw	Mouth is open: patient is unable to close	Stand in front of seated patient Wrap thumbs in towels and place on occlusal surfaces of mandibular posterior teeth Curve fingers and place under body of the mandible Press down and back with thumbs, and at the same time pull up and forward with fingers (Figure 9-6) As joint slips into place, quickly move thumbs outward Place bandage around head to support under chin
Facial fracture	Pain, swelling **Ecchymoses** Deformity, limitation of movement **Crepitation** on manipulation Zygoma fracture: depression of cheek Mandibular fracture: abnormal occlusion	Place patient on side BLS Support with bandage around face, under chin, and tied on the top of the head **Call EMS**
Tooth forcibly displaced (avulsed tooth)	Swelling, bruises, or other signs of trauma depending on the type of accident	Instruct patient or parent to hold the tooth by the crown, and avoid touching the root(s) If the tooth is dirty, rinse it gently in cool water, but do not scrub it or remove tissue fragments from its root surface Keep the tooth moist by placing it in milk to transport to dentist Bring the tooth and the patient to dental office or clinic *immediately* The longer the time lapse between avulsion and replantation, the poorer the prognosis
Broken dental instrument during treatment	Instrument tip missing after use in patient's mouth	Examine carefully for broken piece A radiograph may assist in locating the broken segment of the instrument Gently sweep through the sulcus/pocket with a curet or periodontal probe to try to remove broken piece of the instrument Patient may need to be referred to an oral surgeon or periodontist for further evaluation

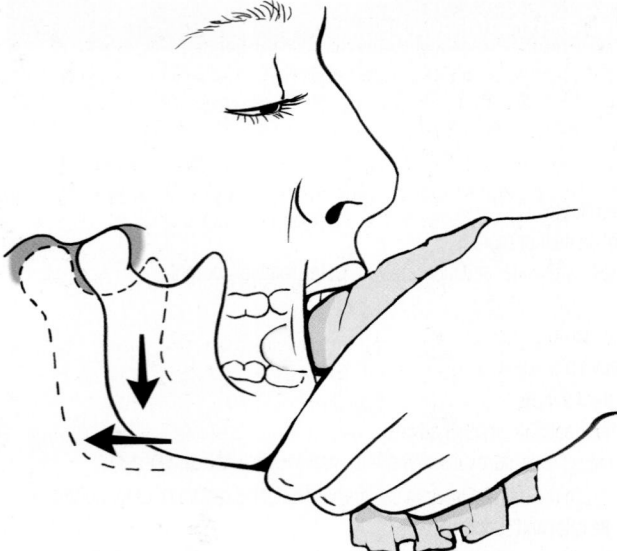

FIGURE 9-6 • Treatment for a Dislocated Mandible. With thumbs wrapped in toweling and placed on the buccal cusps of the mandibular teeth, the fingers are curved under the body of the mandible. The jaw is pressed down and back with the thumbs while pulling up and forward with the fingers to permit the condyle to pass over the articular eminence into its normal position in the glenoid fossa. As the jaw slips into place, the thumbs are moved quickly aside.

II. Consults

In the patient's record, document telephone and written responses of consultations with physicians or other healthcare providers.[15]

III. New Entries

◆ *Response to treatment:* Document a patient's reactions and responses to treatments, whether they are unremarkable or remarkable.

◆ *Previous appointment review:* Complete a comprehensive review of previous appointment documentation before providing additional treatment at sequential appointments.

◆ *Current information:* Update information about the patient's health status including vital signs as an integral part of the prevention of medical emergencies.[8]

◆ *Emergency documentation:* Include a copy of the Medical Emergency Report Form (Figure 9-2) in the patient's permanent record.[26]

◆ *Progress notes:* Box 9-4 contains an example progress note for an emergency that happens during an appointment.

Factors to Teach the Patient

▶ Stress minimization to prevent emergencies.

▶ If medications are prescribed by the dentist, review the instructions with the patient to ensure an understanding.

▶ Schedule appointments when there is no waiting, first appointment of the morning or afternoon.

▶ Eat breakfast before morning appointment, or lunch before afternoon appointment, unless instructed by the patient's physician not to eat before the appointment.

▶ If patient has prescription medications for emergency episodes, bring those medications to the appointment. Examples: nitroglycerin tablets for angina, asthma inhaler, glucagon for hypoglycemia.

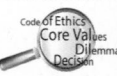

EVERYDAY ETHICS

A 12-year-old patient, Jonathan, had just received local anesthesia in Dr. Spar's treatment room in preparation for a restorative procedure. Suddenly Jonathan started to have a rhythmic twitching of the eyelids and appeared pale. Dr. Spar's assistant, Loraine, called the usual emergency alarm, and Elisa, the dental hygienist, joined in the team protocol for medical emergencies.

In a few minutes, the generalized absence (petit mal) seizure was over and the patient was conscious with no other symptoms evident. Dr. Spar went about the dental procedure as if nothing had happened. Neither Loraine nor Dr. Spar made an entry in the record at the time. Elisa glanced over the patient's record and nothing she could find in

the history showed that Jonathan had a susceptibility to seizures. As Elisa went back to her own treatment room, she wondered if she needed to record the emergency or ask Dr. Spar about it.

Questions for Consideration

1. Which of the dental hygiene core values (Chapter 1, Box 1-6) apply in this situation? Explain the relationship.

2. Who needs to be informed of the event, and what potential ethical responsibilities are related to the patient?

3. What considerations for future treatment appointments are needed? From an ethical point of view, in what way were the patient's best interests compromised?

BOX 9-4

Example Documentation:
Emergency during Patient Treatment

S—Patient experienced blatant signs of anaphylaxis after exposure to latex gloves during a routine scaling appointment.

O—Patient presented with urticaria and **pruritus** on the arms, neck, and chest. Signs of lip, tongue, and laryngeal edema were exhibited with difficulty swallowing and breathing. Quickly informed the patient that he was experiencing an allergic reaction and needed an injection of epinephrine.

A—Findings indicate need for nonlatex gloves and caution during dental appointments especially when using new materials. At 8 minutes, the patient's vital signs were near baseline. Patient was released to emergency medical service (EMS) after 15 min to determine the extent of anaphylaxis. Patient was in stable condition.

P—Epinephrine was administered via EpiPen® and EMS was summoned. About 50 mg of Benadryl and 100 mg of Solu-Cortef were also administered intramuscularly. Oxygen was delivered by nonrebreather mask at 15 L/min. A Medical Emergency Report Form (Figure 9-2) was completed and given to EMS with one copy included in the patient's chart and the other sent to the patient's physician.

Signed: _____, DDS or DMD Date: _____

Signed: _____, RDH Date: _____

 ENHANCE YOUR UNDERSTANDING

ONLINE RESOURCES
(see the inside front cover for access information)

- Audio glossary
- Appendices

SUPPORT FOR LEARNING
(available separately)

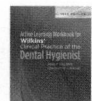

- *Active Learning Workbook for Wilkins' Clinical Practice of the Dental Hygienist, 13th Edition*

INDIVIDUALIZED REVIEW

- Customized practice quizzing with Navigate 2 TestPrep for *Wilkins' Clinical Practice of the Dental Hygienist*

References

1. Brooks-Buza H, Fernandez R, Stenger JP. The use of in situ simulation to evaluate teamwork and system organization during a pediatric dental clinic emergency. *Simul Healthc*. 2011;6(2):101-108.

2. Skryabina E, Reedy G, Amlot R, et al. What is the value of health emergency preparedness exercises? A scoping review study. *Int J Disaster Risk Reduct*. 2017;21:274-283.

3. Jevon P. Updated guidance on medical emergencies and resuscitation in the dental practice. *Br Dent J*. 2012;212(1):41-43.

4. Malamed SF. Medical emergencies in the dental surgery. Part 1: preparation of the office and basic management. *J Irish Dent Assoc*. 2015;61(6):302-308.

5. Muller MP, Hansel M, Stehr SN, et al. A state-wide survey of medical emergency management in dental practices: incidence of emergencies and training experience. *Emerg Med J*. 2008;25:296-300.

6. Abraham-Inpijn L, Russell G, Abraham DA, et al. A patient-administered Medical Risk Related History questionnaire (EMRRH) for use in 10 European countries (multicenter trial). *Oral Surg Oral Med Oral Pathol Oral Radiol Endod*. 2008;105(5):597-605.

7. de Jong KJM, Borgmeijer-Hoelen A, Abraham-Inpign L. Validity of a risk-related patient-administered medical questionnaire for dental patients. *Oral Surg Oral Med Oral Pathol*. 1991:527-533.

8. Malamed SF. Knowing your patients. *JADA*. 2010:3S-7S.

9. Meiller TF, Wynn RL, McMullin AM, et al. *Dental Office Medical Emergencies*. 5th ed. Hudson, OH: Lexi-Comp; 2012:9, 89.

10. Reed KL. Basic management of medical emergencies: recognizing a patient's distress. *JADA*. 2010;141:S20-S24.

11. Smeets EC, de Jong KJM, Abraham-Inpijn L. Detecting the medically compromised patient in dentistry by means of the medical risk-related history. *Prev Med*. 1998;27:530-535.

12. Anders PL, Comeau RL, Hatton M, et al. The nature and frequency of medical emergencies among patients in a dental school setting. *J Dent Educ*. 2010;74(4):392-396.

13. Tanzawa T, Futaki K, Kurabayashi H, et al. Medical emergency education using a robot patient in a dental setting. *Eur J Dent Educ*. 2013;17:e114-e119.

14. Dawoud BE, Roberts A, Yates JM. Drug interactions in general dental practice—considerations for the dental practitioner. *Br Dent J*. 2014;216(1):15-23.

15. Malamed SF. *Medical Emergencies in the Dental Office*. 7th ed. St. Louis, MO: Mosby; 2014:3.

16. Baseline. The free dictionary: medical dictionary. 2003-2017. http://medical-dictionary.thefreedictionary.com/baseline. Accessed August 24, 2017.

17. Compensation. The free dictionary: medical dictionary. 2003-2017. http://medical-dictionary.thefreedictionary.com/compensation. Accessed August 30, 2017.

18. Decompensation. The free dictionary: medical dictionary. 2003-2017. http://medical-dictionary.thefreedictionary.com/decompensation. Accessed August 30, 2017.

19. Patton LL. Medical history, physical evaluation, and risk assessment. In: *The ADA Practical Guide to Patients with Medical Conditions*. 2nd ed. Hoboken, NJ: John Wiley & Sons, Inc; 2016:1-24.

20. Little JW, Falace DA, Miller CS, et al. Patient evaluation and risk assessment. In: Little JW, Falace DA, eds. *Little and Falace's Dental Management of the Medically Compromised Patient*. 8th ed. St. Louis, MO: Elsevier Mosby; 2013:2-19.

21. Rosenberg M. Preparing for medical emergencies. The essential drugs and equipment for the dental office. *JADA*. 2010;141:S14-S19.

22. Chapman PJ. Medical emergencies in dental practice and choice of emergency drugs and equipment: a survey of Australian dentists. *Aust Dent J*. 1997;42(2):103-108.

23. Haas DA. Preparing dental office staff members for emergencies. Developing a basic action plan. *JADA*. 2010; 141:S8-S13.

24. Haas DA. Management of medical emergencies in the dental office: conditions in each country, the extent of treatment by the dentist. *Anesth Prog*. 2006;53:20-24.

25. Dym H, Barzani G, Mohan N. Emergency drugs for the dental office. *Dent Clin N Am*. 2016;60:287-294.

26. Bost N, Crilly J, Patterson E, et al. Clinical handover of patients arriving by ambulance to a hospital emergency department: a qualitative study. *Int Emerg Nurs*. 2012;20:133-141.

27. Berg RA, Hemphill R, Abella BS, et al. Adult basic life support: 2010 American Heart Association Guidelines for cardiopulmonary resuscitation and emergency cardiovascular care. *Circulation*. 2010;122(suppl 3):S685-S705.

28. Hazinski MF, Shuster M, Donnino MW, et al. Highlights of the 2015 American Heart Association. Guidelines update for CPR and ECC. Professional.heart.org. https://eccguidelines .heart.org/wp-content/themes/eccstaging/dompdf-master /pdffiles/part-5-adult-basic-life-support-and-cardiopulmonary -resuscitation-quality.pdf. Published October, 2015. Accessed August 31, 2017.

29. Markenson D, Ferguson JD, Chameides L, et al. Part 17: first aid: 2010 American Heart Association Guidelines for cardiopulmonary resuscitation and emergency cardiovascular care. *Circulation*. 2010;122(suppl 3):2685-2705.

30. Kingston, Frontenac and Lennox & Addington Public Health. Fentanyl. KFL & A Public Health. https://www .kflaph.ca/en/healthy-living/fentanyl.aspx. Published 2016. Accessed May 25, 2017.

Documentation

DIAGNOSE
Problem
identification

PLAN
Selection of
interventions

ASSESS
Data
collection

IMPLEMENT
Activating
the plan

DOCUMENT
Record findings in
permanent record
as well as progress
notes at each
patient visit

EVALUATE
Feedback on
effectiveness

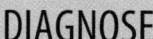

FIGURE III-1 • The Dental Hygiene Process of Care.

INTRODUCTION FOR SECTION III

Maintenance of complete records for every aspect of care provided for each patient is a key aspect of dental hygiene practice.

◆ Patient records may be kept in many different formats, both handwritten and electronic, in different dental practices.

◆ Essential factors for legal documentation of all aspects of dental hygiene care include record-keeping that is:
  • Chronological (each entry dated).
  • Systematic.
  • Comprehensive.
  • Accurate.
  • Unaltered.
  • Signed by the dental hygienist.

THE DENTAL HYGIENE PROCESS OF CARE

◆ Documenting patient care is an integral component of each step in the Dental Hygiene Process of Care, as illustrated in Figure III-1.

◆ Every step in the process is documented in each patient record at the initial appointment and at every continuing care or treatment appointment.

◆ Comprehensive, accurate, and concise documentation of each step forms a complete and chronologic record of the patient's oral health status and treatment over time.

ETHICAL APPLICATIONS

◆ A dental hygienist may be involved in a variety of moral, ethical, and legal situations related to documentation of patient information during practice.

◆ Understanding the patient record can be subpoenaed in the event of litigation is a basic tenant of ethical and legal risk management for professional practice.

◆ Knowledge of and adherence to Health Insurance Portability and Accountability Act (HIPAA) requirements for privacy and security of patient records is imperative.

◆ An overview of the key concepts in patient record-keeping, with explanations and examples of ethical applications is found in Table III-1.

TABLE III-1 • Essentials of Ethical Record-Keeping

CONCEPT	EXPLANATION	ETHICAL APPLICATION
Privacy	Patient's right to control access to identifiable personal health information.	Unless permission is given, a family member cannot receive information about the patient.
Confidentiality	The responsibility of the healthcare provider to protect patient's information.	HIPAA training is provided for new employees.
Security	Protection against unsecured patient data.	A secure computer network is used or paper records are kept in locked files.
Accuracy	Recorded information is not altered after the fact.	A new entry (dated and signed) is made in the patient's record to correct an error or omission in documentation during the patient appointment.
Authenticity	Only data actually obtained during the patient visit are recorded.	Completely document only what actually happened during a patient visit.
Impersonal/Objective	Personal opinion or negative social observations not pertinent to the patient's treatment are never placed in the patient record.	Uncooperative behavior or noncompliance are documented using subjective, factual statements.

Documentation for Dental Hygiene Care

Christine A. Fambely, DH, BA, MEd, and Charlotte J. Wyche, BSDH, MS

CHAPTER OUTLINE

THE PATIENT RECORD
I. Purposes and Characteristics
II. Components of a Patient Record
III. The Handwritten Record
IV. The Electronic Record

THE HEALTH INSURANCE PORTABILITY AND ACCOUNTABILITY ACT
I. The HIPAA Privacy Rule
II. The HIPAA Security Rule

DOCUMENTING THE EXTRA- AND INTRAORAL EXAMINATION

TOOTH NUMBERING SYSTEMS
I. Universal System

II. Fédération Dentaire Internationale Two Digit
III. Palmer Notation System

CHARTING OF HARD AND SOFT TISSUES
I. Purpose
II. Forms Used for Charting
III. Sequence for Charting

PERIODONTAL RECORDS
I. Clinical Observations of the Gingiva
II. Items to Be Charted
III. Deposits
IV. Factors Related to Occlusion
V. Radiographic Findings
VI. Severity of Periodontal Disease

DENTAL RECORDS
I. The Anatomic Tooth Chart Form
II. Items to Be Charted

CARE PLAN RECORDS

INFORMED CONSENT

DOCUMENTATION OF PATIENT VISITS
I. Purpose
II. Essentials of Good Progress Notes
III. Systematic Documentation: The SOAP Approach
IV. Risk Reduction and Legal Considerations

EVERYDAY ETHICS

FACTORS TO TEACH THE PATIENT

REFERENCES

LEARNING OBJECTIVES

After studying this chapter, the student will be able to:

1. Identify and define key terms and concepts related to written and computerized dental records and charting.

2. Describe concepts related to ensuring confidentiality and privacy of patient information.

3. Compare three tooth numbering systems.

4. Discuss the various components of a patient's permanent, comprehensive dental record.

5. Recognize and explain a systematic method for documenting patient visits.

THE PATIENT RECORD

I. Purposes and Characteristics

Accurate record keeping is essential to a safe, thorough, and caring dental hygiene practice as well as clinical and ethical risk management.[1]

◆ Complete and accurate documentation of patient information and treatment provided facilitates communication, coordinated planning, and continuity of care.

◆ Patient records serve as a basis for the evaluation of the quality of care and aid when a review is made of the effectiveness of patient care practices.

◆ Data from health records are utilized in research and education.

◆ Documentation in the patient's record is considered legal evidence in any legal or forensic situation.[2,3]

◆ Documentation in a patient record is[2]:
  • Authentic: genuine and undisputed reality.
  • Accurate and comprehensive.
  • Legible.
  • Objective.

◆ Patient record entries are:
  • Recorded promptly during or following treatment.
  • Recorded using clear, concise, objective statements. Subjective information is written using objective statements.
  • Dated.
  • Signed by the clinician.

II. Components of a Patient Record

The format of a patient record will vary among private dental practices and clinics; however, essential elements remain consistent regardless of the clinical environment.

◆ All information collected during the initial examination and during continuing patient appointments is an official part of the permanent records.[2,4,5]

◆ To meet the dental hygiene standard of care, all components of the dental hygiene process of care are addressed, including the dental hygiene care plan.[6]

◆ Required components of a complete and regularly updated patient record include[2]:
  • Medical history and vital signs.
  • Dental history.
  • Clinical assessment and diagnosis.
  • Treatment recommendations and written treatment plan.
  • Progress notes for each patient visit.
  • Signed acknowledgment of confidentiality measures (see HIPAA section in this chapter).

◆ Additional components, required when applicable, include[2]:
  • Informed consent forms.[7]
  • Radiographs and radiographic assessment.
  • Periodontal risk assessment.
  • Caries risk assessment.
  • Trauma and/or surgery anesthesia records.
  • Study models.
  • Oral photographs.[8]
  • Orthodontic records, if available.
  • Laboratory orders and test results.
  • Referral records and copies of consultation correspondence with dental specialists or medical practitioners.

◆ Each component of the patient record is marked with patient identification and/or demographic information.

III. The Handwritten Record

Historically, dental healthcare personnel have maintained handwritten documentation of patient records.

◆ Handwritten records are recorded legibly and written in ink.

◆ Records have also been dictated into a machine to be typewritten into the permanent record later.

◆ Mistakes are corrected by placing a single line through the error, writing the correct information immediately after, and signing the entry.

◆ If a late entry is necessary, the new information:
  • Follows the most recent entry in the patient record.
  • Is noted as a late entry.
  • Includes the date and time that the late entry was made.

◆ Systems may involve the completion of forms with topics and spaces to check off and spaces for writing descriptive information and/or prose-style summary.

◆ Strict infection control protocols are required to prevent contamination of paper records during patient care.

◆ For written records, a filing system is needed that provides accessibility to the health records by authorized personnel only.

IV. The Electronic Record

Computerized records have provided a faster, more convenient, and better organized mode of information gathering, preserving, and sharing patient information with other healthcare professionals or providers.

A. Characteristics[9]

◆ Data can be accessed from anywhere within the system by authorized personnel.

◆ A variety of custom software programs are available to include complete patient information, appointment schedules, medical alerts, and financial aspects of patient care.

◆ Systems may provide methods for documenting dental and periodontal assessments with automated, voice-activated recordings.

◆ Other systems permit printing hard copies for the patient when indicated.

◆ Computerized records require computer terminals where only authorized personnel can access required information.

◆ Computer monitors are directed away from the view of unauthorized persons.

◆ Infection control protocols include providing plastic barriers for computer keyboard and mouse, as well as disinfection of chairside monitors.

B. Features

Specially designed software and record storage systems can:

◆ Standardize terminology used for data entry.

◆ Improve efficiency and accountability; speed up entry of information and encourage entry of more comprehensive information.[10]

◆ Increase the legibility of information.

◆ Provide easier, faster access to clinical information.

◆ Enhance communication with patients and with consulting dental specialists or other multidisciplinary team members who may not be together at one clinical site.[10]

◆ Provide new ways of analyzing clinical information and outcomes of various clinical treatment approaches or treatment procedures.

◆ Maintain digital radiographs and photographs within the patient record.

THE HEALTH INSURANCE PORTABILITY AND ACCOUNTABILITY ACT

◆ The Health Insurance Portability and Accountability Act (HIPAA) of 1996 took effect for dental practices in the United States on April 14, 2003.

◆ The law provides federal privacy standards that protect patient records and other health-related information in an emerging electronic information environment.[11]

◆ The law applies to:
  • Healthcare facilities.
  • Healthcare insurance companies.
  • Healthcare providers.

◆ Some states may have stricter laws that take priority over the federal standards.

◆ The current law is divided into two separate components that address:
  • Privacy and the patient's ability to access their health information.
  • Security of patient information in healthcare settings.

◆ Legislation is in place in Canada and some European countries to protect the privacy of personal information.[12,13]

◆ In Canada, healthcare privacy legislation is largely a provincial responsibility.
  • The Personal Information Protection and Electronic Documents Act exists at the federal level.
  • There are also specific health privacy acts in most provinces.
  • Dental hygiene colleges/regulatory bodies have their own professional guidelines, which reinforce the jurisdictional acts.[14]

I. The HIPAA Privacy Rule

Establishes a national standard to protect individual's privacy and access to medical records and other health information.[15]

◆ Patients have the right to:
  • Receive a copy of personal health records.
  • Ask to change incorrect or incomplete information.
  • Receive reports on when, why, and with whom their health information is shared.
  • Decide, in some cases (such as marketing), whether health information can be shared.
  • Ask to be contacted regarding health information in a specific location or by a specific method such as telephone or mail.
  • File a complaint with the provider, health insurer, or the U.S. government regarding concerns about use of their health information.

◆ Healthcare facilities are responsible to:
  • Develop required privacy and confidentiality forms.
  • Adopt written privacy policies and educate staff about confidentiality of patient information.
  • Appoint staff privacy officers and privacy contact persons.
  • Provide patients with a Notice of Privacy Practices document at the beginning of their care and receive signed acknowledgment of receipt.
  • Implement security measures, policies, and formal protocols that protect patient information.
  • Conduct analysis of security risks and vulnerabilities.
  • Establish sanctions for workforce members who fail to comply with policies.

◆ Healthcare providers are responsible to:
  • Comply with protocols and practices that protect patient information and avoid inappropriate disclosure.

II. The HIPAA Security Rule

Updated in 2013 by establishing a national set of standards to strengthen digital security standards and enhance enforcement for protection of health information that is held or transferred in electronic form.[5,15]

◆ Comprises three separate standards[5]:
  • Administrative safeguards: limitation of access to appropriate members in the workforce.

- Physical safeguards: use of storage systems and procedures that prevent access for unauthorized individuals.
- Technical safeguards: use of technology, such as coding and encryption, to control access to patient information.

DOCUMENTING THE EXTRA- AND INTRAORAL EXAMINATION

- A specific objective of the extra- and intraoral examination as a part of the total patient assessment is the recognition of deviations from normal that may be **signs** and symptoms of disease (see Chapter 13).
- The need for careful, thorough documentation of hard and soft examination findings cannot be overemphasized.
- Concentration and attention to detail are necessary in order that each slight deviation from normal may be entered on the record.

TOOTH NUMBERING SYSTEMS

Different systems are used in the various dental offices and clinics worldwide. The three most commonly used tooth designation systems are described here:

I. Universal System

This tooth numbering method is referred to as the Continuous Numbers 1–32 or American Dental Association (*ADA*) system.[16] Figure 10-1 shows the crowns of the teeth with the corresponding numbers.

A. Permanent Teeth

- Start with the patient's right maxillary third molar (number 1).
- Follow around the arch to the left maxillary third molar (16).
- Descend to the left mandibular third molar (17).
- Follow around to the right mandibular third molar (32).

B. Primary or Deciduous Teeth

- Use continuous upper case letters A–T in the same order as described for the permanent teeth.
- Right maxillary second molar (A) around to left maxillary second molar (J).
- Descend to left mandibular second molar (K) and around to the right mandibular second molar (T).

II. Fédération Dentaire Internationale Two Digit

The Fédération Dentaire Internationale system (Figure 10-2) is also called the *International* system.[17,18]

A. Permanent Teeth

Each tooth is identified by the quadrant (1 through 4) represented by the first digit. The second digit will then identify the tooth within the quadrant (1 through 8).

- Quadrant numbers—FIRST digit
  1 = Patient's maxillary right
  2 = Maxillary left
  3 = Mandibular left
  4 = Mandibular right
- *Tooth numbers within each quadrant:* Start with number 1 at the midline (central incisor) to number 8, third

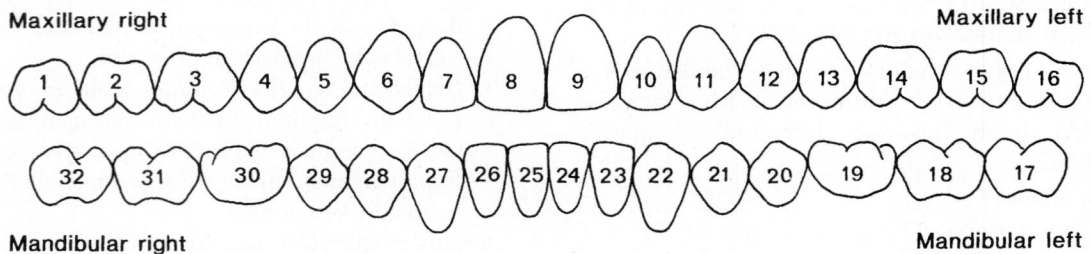

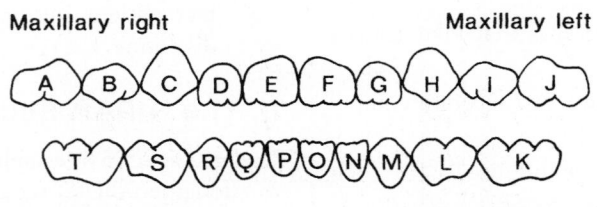

FIGURE 10-1 • Universal Tooth Numbering (American Dental Association). *Above,* permanent dentition designated by numbers 1–32, starting at the maxillary right with 1 and following around to the maxillary left third molar (number 16) to the left mandibular third molar (number 17) and around to the right mandibular third molar (number 32). *Below,* primary teeth are designated by letters in the same sequence.

PERMANENT TEETH

Q–1 Maxillary right								Q–2 Maxillary left							
18	17	16	15	14	13	12	11	21	22	23	24	25	26	27	28
48	47	46	45	44	43	42	41	31	32	33	34	35	36	37	38
Mandibular right Q–4								Mandibular left Q–3							

PRIMARY TEETH

Q–5 Maxillary right					Q–6 Maxillary left				
55	54	53	52	51	61	62	63	64	65
85	84	83	82	81	71	72	73	74	75
Mandibular right Q–8					Mandibular left Q–7				

FIGURE 10-2 • International Tooth Numbering—Fédération Dentaire Internationale. It is a two-digit system. The first digit indicates the quadrant; the second digit identifies the specific tooth. Each quadrant is numbered 1–4, with number 1 on the patient's maxillary right, number 2 on the maxillary left, number 3 on the mandibular left, and number 4 on the mandibular right. Each tooth in a quadrant is numbered 1–8 from the central incisor. Quadrants of the primary dentition are numbered from 5 through 8.

molar. Figure 10-2 shows each tooth number in the four quadrants.

◆ *Designation:* The digits are pronounced separately. For example, "two-five" (25) is the permanent maxillary left second premolar, and "four-two" (42) is the permanent mandibular right lateral incisor.

B. Primary or Deciduous Teeth

Each tooth is numbered by quadrant (5 through 8) to continue with the permanent quadrant numbers. The teeth are numbered within each quadrant (1 through 5).

◆ Quadrant numbers—FIRST digit
   5 = Maxillary right
   6 = Maxillary left
   7 = Mandibular left
   8 = Mandibular right

◆ *Tooth numbers within each quadrant:* Number 1 is the central incisor, and number 5 is the second primary molar.

◆ *Designation:* The digits are pronounced separately. For example, "eight-three" (83) is the primary mandibular right canine, and "six-five" (65) is the primary maxillary left second molar.

III. Palmer Notation System

Names to identify this method are the *Palmer System* or *Set-square*.[19]

A. Permanent Teeth

◆ Each tooth is designated using the numbers 1 (central incisor) through 8 (third molar) in each quadrant.

◆ The patient's right and left quadrants for each tooth are designated using a specific pattern of vertical and horizontal lines as shown in Figure 10-3.

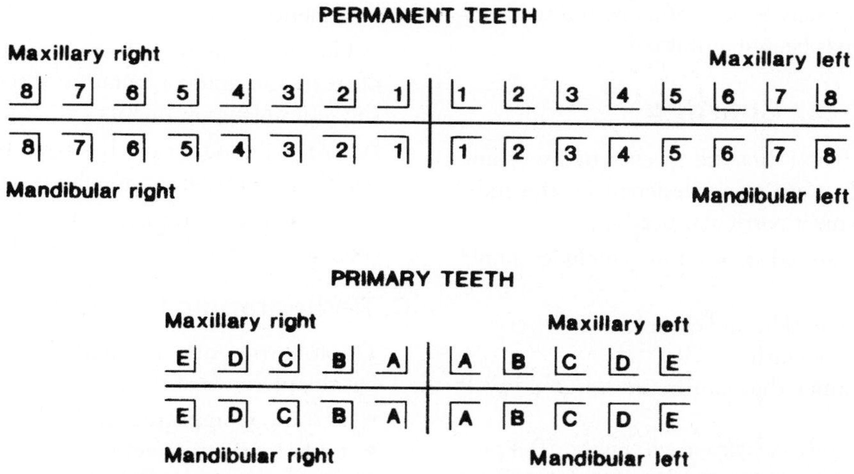

PERMANENT TEETH

Maxillary right   Maxillary left

8	7	6	5	4	3	2	1	1	2	3	4	5	6	7	8
8	7	6	5	4	3	2	1	1	2	3	4	5	6	7	8

Mandibular right   Mandibular left

PRIMARY TEETH

Maxillary right   Maxillary left

E	D	C	B	A	A	B	C	D	E
E	D	C	B	A	A	B	C	D	E

Mandibular right   Mandibular left

FIGURE 10-3 • Palmer System Tooth Numbering. Each permanent tooth is designated by numbers 1–8, starting at the central incisor of each quadrant. Quadrants are designated by horizontal and vertical lines. Primary teeth are identified by the letters A–E, starting at the central incisor.

B. Primary or Deciduous Teeth

◆ Upper case letters A–E are used instead of the numbers.

CHARTING OF HARD AND SOFT TISSUES

I. Purpose

The purpose of each type of charting is defined by its title. *Dental chart* (hard tissue) includes diagrammatic representation of existing conditions of the teeth. *Periodontal chart* (soft tissue) indicates clinical features of the periodontium.

◆ The use of separate chart forms to record the special features of periodontal and dental findings is preferable.

◆ Dental and periodontal charts are updated routinely on new forms with current dates to record changes in the patient's oral features over time.

◆ Neatness in the markings of symbols, drawings, and labels goes hand-in-hand with the accuracy of the examination itself.

◆ An accurate, detailed, and carefully recorded charting is used for:
  • *Care planning:* The charting is a graphic representation of the existing condition of the patient's teeth and periodontium from which needed treatment procedures can be organized into a treatment plan.
  • *Treatment:* During dental and dental hygiene appointments, the charting is useful for guiding specific procedures.
  • *Evaluation:* The outcome and degree of treatment effects are determined by comparing the findings of the initially recorded examination with periodic follow-up examinations.
  • *Protection:* In the event of misunderstanding by a patient, or if legal questions should arise, the records and chartings are evidence.
  • *Identification:* In the event of emergency, accident, or disaster, a patient may be identified by the teeth for which a record has been maintained.

II. Forms Used for Charting

Many variations of chart forms are in current use: some available commercially, and some designed by the individual practitioner to meet particular needs.

◆ Specifications for an adequate form include ample space to:
  • Chart neatly, accurately, and completely.
  • Label as needed for clarity.
  • Record in a manner that can be interpreted by all who use it.

◆ *Anatomic drawings of the complete teeth:* Figure 10-4 provides a typical example of a form that may be used for periodontal and/or dental charting.

◆ *Geometric:* A diagrammatic representation that provides space to record findings for each tooth. Examples

of geometric charting forms used to record a patient's disclosed biofilm for teaching personal disease control are shown in Figures 21-1 and 21-2 in Chapter 21.

III. Sequence for Charting

A. Basic Entries

◆ *Name, birth date.*

◆ *Date of examination:* Every entry is dated.

◆ *Missing teeth:* When radiographs are available in advance, missing teeth can be charted before the clinic appointment. Whether dental or periodontal charting is completed first, marking the missing teeth will be necessary.

B. Systematic Procedure

◆ An accurate odontogram is a systematic representation of both intraoral clinical findings and radiographic findings.

◆ The use of a set routine is essential to accomplishing a complete and accurate charting, not only for the tooth surface-to-surface pattern but also for the parts of the charting itself.

◆ Charting all of one item for the entire mouth, rather than complete charting of one tooth, helps to ensure accuracy.
  • For example, in the dental charting, record all the restorations first.
  • Then start again at the first tooth and chart all the deviations from normal.
  • Missing teeth.
  • Location of crowns, bridges, and implants.
  • Charting all restorations and deviations for each tooth separately is less efficient.

◆ The patient's permanent records include the itemized findings of all the clinical and radiographic examinations.

◆ Prepare entries that are clear and easily understood by all who read them and use them in continuing treatment.

◆ Additions to the records are made to show the progress of treatment and comparative observations throughout the series of appointments.

◆ After the periodontium has been brought to a state of health, a continuing care plan is outlined.

◆ At each succeeding appointment, new and comparative records and chartings are made.

C. Radiographic Charting

◆ The following may be charted from radiographs without the presence of the patient:
  • Missing or impacted teeth.
  • Endodontic treatment.
  • Overhanging margins of existing restorations.
  • Proximal surface carious lesions.
  • Other deviations from normal evident from the radiographs.

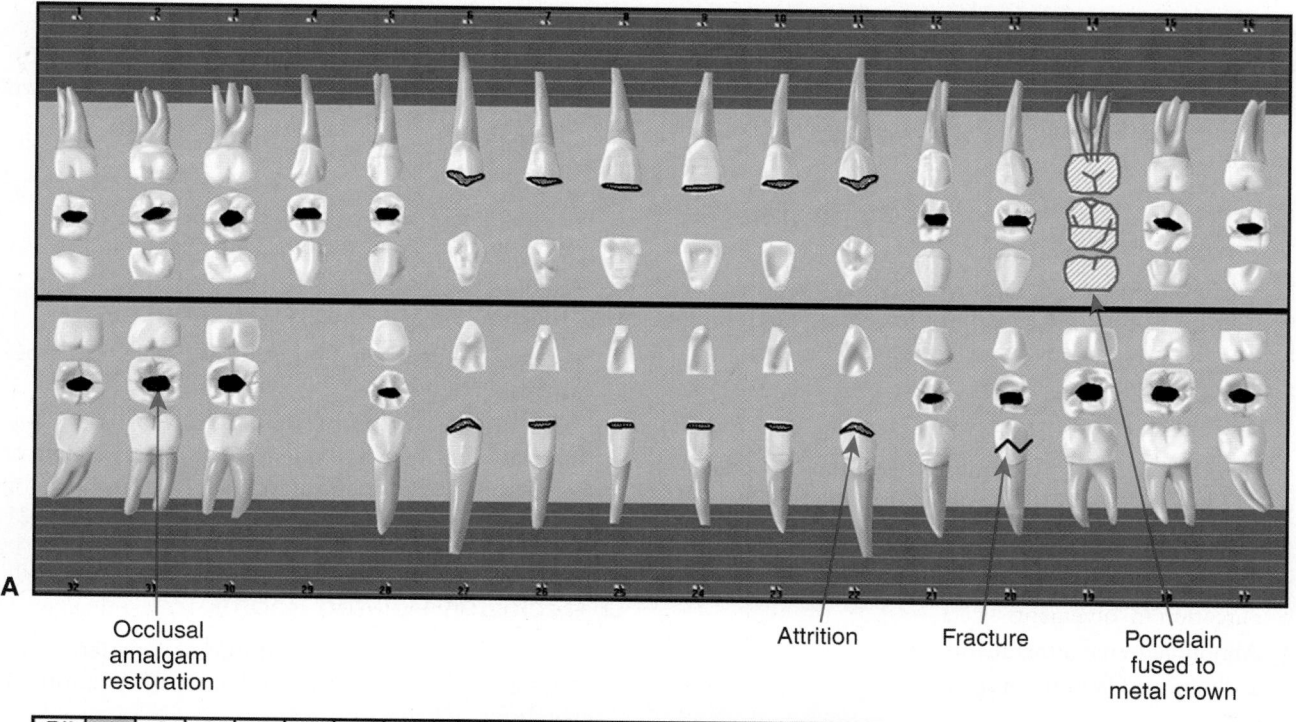

FIGURE 10-4 • Periodontal and Dental Charting. A: Example of dental charting notations. **B:** Example of computerized periodontal charting with key.

♦ Supplemental and confirmational observations and checks are made during the clinical examination with the patient. For example, when a carious lesion is suspected but not visible on the radiograph, clinical examination is required.

D. Study Models

Study models are useful to record details related to occlusion (see Chapter 16).

PERIODONTAL RECORDS

I. Clinical Observations of the Gingiva

Clinical observations are recorded either on the chart form or in the patient progress notes during each patient visit. Examine gingiva and record findings before disclosing agent is used for biofilm score.

A. Describe Gingiva

◆ Color, size, position, shape, consistency, and surface texture; extent of bleeding when probed; and areas where there is minimal attached gingiva (Table 18-1 in Chapter 18).

B. Describe Distribution of Gingival Changes

Localized or generalized; specify the areas with disease involvement as mild, moderate, or severe. Use tooth numbers to identify adjacent gingival tissue.

II. Items to Be Charted

◆ Gingival line (margin) and mucogingival lines (junctions).
◆ Probing depths (except around dental implants).
◆ Recession.
◆ Areas of suspected mucogingival involvement.
◆ Furcation involvement.
◆ Abnormal frenal attachments.
◆ Mobility and fremitus of teeth.

III. Deposits

Deposits can be recorded on forms such as the one illustrated in Figure 10-4 or on dental index forms, which are illustrated in Chapter 21.

A. Stains

◆ *Extrinsic:* Record type of stain, color, distribution; specific location by tooth number; whether slight, moderate, or heavy.
◆ *Intrinsic:* Record separately from extrinsic and identify by type when known.

B. Soft Deposits

◆ *Food debris:* Distribution and amount. Record location by teeth when the biofilm control instruction requires special emphasis on a particular area.
◆ *Dental biofilm:*
  • Record direct observations with or without disclosing agent; include distribution and degree or amount.
  • Record biofilm index or score as described in Chapter 21.

C. Calculus

◆ Record distribution and amount of supragingival and subgingival calculus separately for treatment planning purposes.
◆ Record subgingival calculus in periodontal pockets on the probing chart.

IV. Factors Related to Occlusion

Clinical signs of trauma from occlusion are described in Chapter 16. The following list is for consideration with other records for the treatment planning.

A. Mobility of Teeth

Record degree of mobility for each tooth (see Chapter 20). An example of a method for recording mobility is shown in Figure 10-4.

B. Fremitus

◆ Fremitus determination is described in Chapter 20.
◆ Record the significance in relation to mobility.

C. Possible Food Impaction Areas

◆ Ask the patient where fibrous foods usually catch between the teeth.
◆ Use dental floss to identify inadequate contact areas that may contribute to food impaction. An example of one method for recording an open contact is shown by the vertical parallel lines between teeth numbered 21 and 22 in Figure 10-4.

D. Occlusion-Related Habits

◆ Observe for evidence of, and question patient concerning, such parafunctional habits as bruxism or clenching.
◆ Note wear patterns and facets on study cast.
◆ Note attrition.

V. Radiographic Findings

Specific notes are made to correlate the radiographic findings with the clinical observations just listed.

◆ Details of radiographic findings in periodontal disease are described in Chapter 20.
◆ The following are recorded in relation to the specific teeth involved:
  • Height of bone as related to the cementoenamel junction.
  • Horizontal or angular shape of remaining interdental bone.
  • Intact, broken, or missing crestal lamina dura.
  • Furcation involvement.
  • Widening of periodontal ligament space.
  • Overhanging fillings, large carious lesions, and other dental biofilm–retention factors.

VI. Severity of Periodontal Disease

Determination of the severity of periodontal disease is based on analysis of gingival changes.

◆ Clinical assessment procedures include periodontal probing recordings, sites of bleeding on probing, clinical attachment level, tooth mobility and fremitus, and the radiographic findings.
◆ A dental or dental hygiene diagnosis statement can be developed using the disease classifications outlined in Chapter 19.

DENTAL RECORDS

- The patient's permanent records include the itemized clinical and radiographic findings related to the teeth, periodontal descriptors along with subjective symptoms reported by the patient.
- Information about conditions related to the teeth is included in Chapter 16.
- Occlusion and mobility of teeth are documented during the periodontal examination because the causes of mobility are related to the patient's periodontal status.
- After initial entries are recorded, new and comparative records and chartings are prepared at each periodic maintenance visit to show the progress of treatment.
- The need for meticulous examination and recording cannot be overemphasized.
  - Finding and recording a carious lesion may mean saving a tooth for the patient's lifetime.
  - Inadvertent neglect of a tooth may lead eventually to a need for endodontic therapy or even extraction.

I. The Anatomic Tooth Chart Form

Figure 10-4 is an example of a quadrant of dental charting using anatomic tooth drawings. When charting, clinical and radiographic findings are coordinated.

II. Items to Be Charted

A list of basic items to be charted includes:

- Missing teeth.
- Existing restorations. Note restorative materials so that the care plan can designate selective polishing agents that will not harm the surfaces of restorations.
- Fixed and removable prostheses.
- Dental sealants.
- Abrasion and erosion.
- Overhangs, open contacts, open margins, and other irregularities.
- Cavitated carious lesions and questionable demineralized noncavitated lesions.
- Inadequate contact areas and observed proximal surface roughness. Use dental floss. Fraying of dental floss as it is passed over a rough proximal surface may mean the defective margin of a restoration, a sharp cavity margin, or dental calculus.
- Pulp vitality. Record numbers in the permanent record. Chart forms sometimes include a specific place for the recording of such data.
- Tooth sensitivity. The patient may report hypersensitive areas. Record the tooth number and surface for reference during the treatment phase.

CARE PLAN RECORDS

- Along with a comprehensive dental treatment plan, a formal dental hygiene care plan that includes dental hygiene diagnostic statements and addresses the patient's risk factors is included in the patient's record.
- Chapter 23 provides more information about developing a written dental hygiene care plan.
- The initial care plan developed during an initial examination and copies of updated plans are included as part of the comprehensive, permanent patient record.

INFORMED CONSENT

- Documentation of informed consent obtained before initiating treatment is an essential component of each patient's record.
- Information about obtaining and documenting informed consent is found in Chapter 23.

DOCUMENTATION OF PATIENT VISITS

I. Purpose

Documentation completed during or immediately following a patient visit, sometimes referred to as a progress note, is a chronologic history of treatment received by the patient during each appointment.

II. Essentials of Good Progress Notes

- Dental hygiene progress notes document all aspects of the dental hygiene process of care and record all interactions between the patient and the practice.[4]
- In addition to documentation about treatment rendered, essential components of a patient progress note are listed in Box 10-1.
- Each entry in the patient record is dated and signed by the clinician.
- The use of unique abbreviations that are not easily understood by others can cause clinical or legal problems. A selected list of standard abbreviations and symbols developed by the ADA is found in Appendix VII.
- Information that is *never* in the patient record includes:
  - Speculation.
  - Derogatory statements.
  - Financial matters, professional disputes, legal actions, or risk-management protocol.

III. Systematic Documentation: The SOAP Approach

A systematic, standardized approach to writing patient progress notes assures that no details are missing from the patient's record.

BOX 10-1
Essential Components of a Patient Progress Note

- Purpose of the visit
- History review
- Assessment findings
- Description of treatment provided
- Drugs (including topical or local anesthetic) administered during treatment or prescribed by the dentist
- Self-care and other instructions provided
- Referrals, consultations with physician or dental specialist
- Laboratory tests ordered; results of laboratory tests
- Next visit appointments scheduled or recommended; appointment cancellations
- Details related to patient conversations, including telephone and e-mail
- Signature of clinician and date

TABLE 10-1 • Components of SOAP Documentation and Examples of Factors to Include in Progress Notes

	DESCRIPTION	EXAMPLES
S	Subjective Characteristics stated by the patient or perceived by the clinician	• Age and gender as stated by the patient • Type of appointment scheduled • Medical history findings provided by the patient • Patient's chief complaint • Patient's self-care regimen • Social history
O	Objective Characteristics observed during examination	• Head and neck examination findings • Periodontal examination findings, bleeding, soft tissue condition • Hard tissue examination findings; current cavitated carious lesions and demineralized noncavitated lesions • Radiographic findings • Comparison of current findings with previous findings
A	Assessment/ Analysis Identification of problems or patient needs	• Risk factors for oral disease • Caries risk level • Calculus level • Current periodontal diagnosis/case type and status • Periodontal disease risk level
P	Procedures Interventions performed or planned	• Dental hygiene interventions performed • Medicaments or local anesthesia applied and to which teeth • Consult with dentist or other health providers • Self-care instructions • Goals for patient improvement • Pending/planned dental hygiene interventions

Source: Jacks ME, Blue C, Murphy D. Short- and long-term effects of training on dental hygiene faculty members' capacity to write SOAP notes. *J Dent Educ.* 2008;72(6):719-724.

BOX 10-2
Example of Patient Care Documentation: Using the SOAP Format

S—Patient presents for reassessment of oral self-care 2 weeks following oral hygiene instruction. Patient states that he notices a reduction in biofilm following oral self-care instructions provided at the previous appointment.

O—Today's "Plaque-Free Score" = 89%; sulcus bleeding index (SBI) score = 2.

A—"Plaque-Free Score" compared with previous score of 22%; SBI score compared with previous score of 5. Significant improvement in biofilm control noted in all areas except buccal surfaces of maxillary molars.

P—Patient congratulated on areas of success. Additional instruction provided specifically related to biofilm removal on posterior buccal and proximal tooth surfaces. Patient observed while brushing and flossing maxillary molar areas using a mirror. Next visit: 3 months reevaluation.

Signed: _____, RDH

Date: _____

- Many clinicians and most electronic patient record systems have developed their own systematic approach to recording patient information.
- Several formalized documentation systems have been developed to make sure documentation is comprehensive.
- One approach, which uses the acronym *SOAP* as a guide, is well accepted for use in the medical and dental professions and is recommended for use by the American Pediatric Dentistry Association.[2,5,20]
  - **S** = Subjective.
  - **O** = Objective.
  - **A** = Assessment (or analysis).
  - **P** = Procedures (provided or planned).
- Table 10-1 further defines the components of the SOAP acronym and provides examples of factors that are included in patient progress notes.
- Box 10-2 provides an example of documentation for a patient visit written using the SOAP format.
- Additional documentation examples, each related to a clinical situation and formatted using the SOAP approach, can be reviewed near the end of each chapter of this book.

IV. Risk Reduction and Legal Considerations

- **Malpractice** allegations can, unfortunately, occur against even a dental hygienist who routinely meets every standard when providing dental hygiene care.

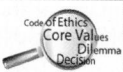

EVERYDAY ETHICS

Mrs. Belvedere, the office manager in Dr. Grain's office, has online access to all electronic patient records from her computer at home. With Dr. Grain's permission, she often uses her home e-mail to contact patients and insurance companies regarding treatment plans, insurance coverage, or financial records. Patients receive HIPAA information about confidentiality and security of their information, but are not told that Mrs. Belvedere has access to their records at her home. Hanna, who is a new dental hygienist in the office, inadvertently finds out that sensitive patient information is being sent out from the same home e-mail account that is used by both Mrs. Belvedere's husband and her adult son. When Hanna approaches Dr. Grain

about the potential breach in security of patient information, he seems unconcerned.

Questions for Consideration

1. What dental hygiene core values (Chapter 1, Box 1-6) are being compromised if Hanna decides not to follow through to try to change the situation?

2. What standards of professional responsibility, identified in the American Dental Hygienists' Association code of ethics, apply in this situation?

3. Which essential record keeping concepts, as described in Table III-1 (Section III Introduction), can support Hanna as she decides how to approach Mrs. Belvedere and Dr. Grain to make changes in the way patient records and information are handled?

◆ Because litigation can occur years after the patient visit when the details and even the patient may have been forgotten, excellent comprehensive documentation in each patient record entry is the best protection for the clinician against allegations of wrongdoing.

Factors to Teach the Patient

▶ Interpretation of all recordings; meaning of all numbers used, such as for probing depths.

▶ The importance of making a complete study of the patient's oral problems before beginning treatment.

▶ Advantages of cooperation and patience in furnishing information that will help dental personnel to interpret observations accurately so that the correct diagnosis and appropriate treatment plan can be made.

▶ Assurance that all information received is completely confidential.

ENHANCE YOUR UNDERSTANDING

ONLINE RESOURCES
(see the inside front cover for access information)

• Audio glossary
• Appendices

SUPPORT FOR LEARNING
(available separately)

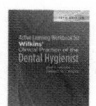

• *Active Learning Workbook for Wilkins' Clinical Practice of the Dental Hygienist, 13th Edition*

INDIVIDUALIZED REVIEW

• Customized practice quizzing with Navigate 2 TestPrep for *Wilkins' Clinical Practice of the Dental Hygienist*

References

1. Collier A. The management of risk, Part 3: recording your way out of trouble. *Dent Update*. 2014;41(4):338-340.

2. American Academy of Pediatric Dentistry, Council on Clinical Affairs. *Record-Keeping*. Chicago, IL: American Academy of Pediatric Dentistry; 2017. https://www.aapd.org/globalassets/media/policies_guidelines/bp_record keeping.pdf. Accessed June 2, 2019.

3. Dym H. Risk management techniques for the general dentist and specialist. *Dent Clin North Am*. 2008;52(3): 563-577, ix.

4. American Association of Dental Boards. *Guidelines on the Dental Patient Record*. Chicago, IL: American Association of Dental Boards; 2009:4-12.

5. Leeuw W. Maintaining proper dental records. *Dent Assist*. 2014;83(2):22-23, 26-30, 32-34.

6. American Dental Hygienists' Association. *Standards for Clinical Dental Hygiene Practice*. Chicago, IL: American Dental Hygienists' Association; 2008:9.

7. Collier A. The management of risk. Part 2: good consent and communication. *Dent Update*. 2014;41(3):236-238, 241.

8. Wander P, Ireland RS. Dental photography in record keeping and litigation. *Br Dent J*. 2014;217(3):133-137.

9. Emmott L. Electronic dental records in dentistry. *J Am Coll Dent*. 2010;77(1):10-12.

10. Hudis S. Converting to electronic dental records. *J Am Coll Dent*. 2010;77(1):13-15.

11. U.S. Department of Health and Human Services. Health information privacy. http://www.hhs.gov/ocr/privacy/hipaa/administrative/index.html. Accessed September 16, 2014.

12. Office of the Privacy Commissioner of Canada. Privacy legislation in Canada. https://www.priv.gc.ca/resource/fs-fi/02_05_d_15_e.asp. Accessed September 16, 2014.

13. European Commission. Data Protection in the EU. http://ec.europa.eu/health/data_collection/data_protection/in_eu/index_en.htm. Accessed September 16, 2014.

14. Genge A. Responsibility without power: the dilemma of privacy compliance for Canadian dental hygienists. *Oh Canada*. 2016, 35-37.

15. U.S. Department of Health and Human Services. Health information privacy: summary of the HIPAA security rule. http://www.hhs.gov/ocr/privacy/hipaa/understanding/srsummary.html. Accessed September 16, 2014.

16. American Dental Association. *System of Tooth Numbering and Radiograph Mounting*. Chicago, IL: American Dental Association; 1968.

17. Fédération Dentaire Internationale. Two-digit system of designating teeth. *Int Dent J*. 1971;21(1):104.

18. Türp JC, Alt KW. Designating teeth: the advantages of the FDI's two-digit system. *Quintessence Int*. 1995;26(7):501-504.

19. Palmer C. Palmer's dental notation. *Dent Cosmos*. 1891;33:194.

20. Rethman J. Clean up your records with SOAP. S (subjective findings), O (objective findings), A (assessment), P (plan). *Dent Today*. 1995;14(8):80.

Assessment

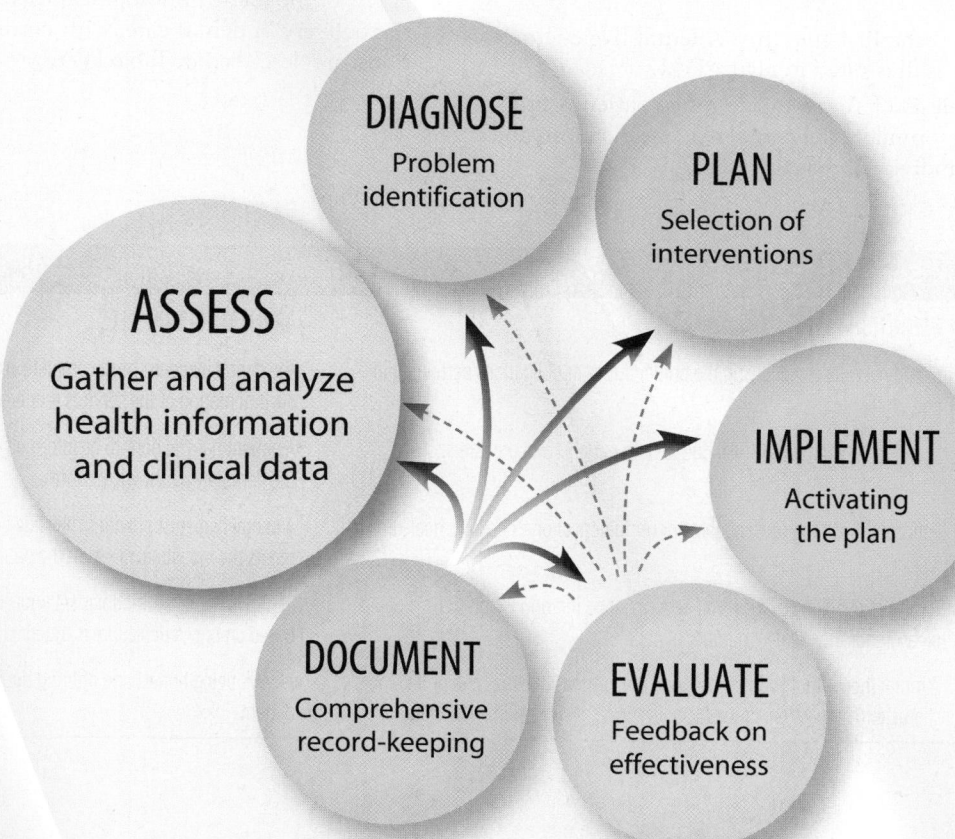

FIGURE IV-1 • The Dental Hygiene Process of Care.

INTRODUCTION FOR SECTION IV

Assessment in dental hygiene practice is the collection of pertinent facts, clinical data, and dental materials, such as radiographs and study models related to the patient's oral health and overall health status.

- Initial assessment data are used:
  - In planning care.
  - As a guide during all treatment.
- After care has been provided, assessment data must be gathered again to evaluate the outcomes of the dental hygiene interventions.
- An efficiently conducted assessment and critical analysis of assessment findings:
  - Provide a permanent, continuing, accurate, and complete record of the patient's oral and general health.
  - Help formulate dental hygiene diagnostic statements from which a patient-oriented dental hygiene care plan can be prepared to include individualized preventive and treatment interventions.
  - Guide instrumentation during dental hygiene treatment.
  - Provide the basis to correlate dental hygiene care with the comprehensive dental treatment plan.

THE DENTAL HYGIENE PROCESS OF CARE

- Assessment is the first step in the dental hygiene process of care, as illustrated in Figure IV-1.
- Critical analysis of the data identifies patient's problems used to formulate the dental hygiene diagnosis and develop an individualized care plan.

- Comprehensive and accurate assessment data aid the dental hygienist in identifying:
  - Health-related factors affecting the management of dental hygiene care.
  - Risk factors for oral or systemic disease.
  - Description of personal and culturally related habits affecting oral status.
  - Health-related attitudes of the patient and the value placed on maintenance of oral health and the prevention of disease.
  - Oral hygiene methods and communication strategies that meet the patient's needs.
- Built into the sequence of clinical procedures is the initiation of steps for arresting oral disease processes and controlling etiologic factors, and prevent episodes of recurrence of oral disease.

ETHICAL APPLICATIONS

- An ethical theory, often based on norms or rules that ask which type of action is morally correct, offers a general approach to an ethical problem.
- A dental professional may consider the most favorable outcome of a particular situation, what guidelines to follow, or whether to rely on personal and professional virtues when making a judgment.
- A few of the many philosophical theories that apply to the delivery of dental care, with corresponding definitions, are described in Table IV-1.

TABLE IV-1 • Some Ethical Theories		
THEORY	**DEFINITION**	**APPLICATION EXAMPLES**
Deontology	A study of rules by following the proper duties or obligations pertaining to one's role.	The dental hygienist must complete accurate and detailed documentation of the services rendered for every patient.
Rights theory	Focusing on what is rightfully due to both patients and providers.	A patient has the right to be informed of what treatment the dental hygienist will perform.
Teleology	Concerned with the consequences or usefulness of one's actions, goal-driven.	A dental hygienist provides chairside education that meets the individual needs of the patient.
Utilitarianism	A form of teleology that says an action is good if it brings about the greatest pleasure for the greatest number of people.	Dental insurance companies set limits of reimbursement based on how a procedure is coded.
Virtue ethics	A moral theory that is concerned with the virtuous qualities of a professional's character (compassion, empathy, honesty, respect, wisdom, patience).	Always being honest and offering the best care to every patient.

11

Medical, Dental, and Psychosocial Histories

Lisa Welch, RDH, BS, MSDH, and Linda D. Boyd, RDH, RD, EdD

CHAPTER OUTLINE

INTRODUCTION
I. Significance
II. Purpose of the History

HISTORY PREPARATION
I. Methods
II. Record Forms
III. Introduction to the Patient
IV. Limitations of a History

THE QUESTIONNAIRE
I. Types of Questions
II. Advantages of a Questionnaire
III. Disadvantages of a Questionnaire (If Used Alone without a Follow-up Interview)

THE INTERVIEW
I. Participants
II. Setting
III. Pointers for the Interview
IV. Interview Form
V. Advantages of the Interview
VI. Disadvantages of the Interview

ITEMS INCLUDED IN THE HISTORY
I. Dental History
II. Medical History
III. Psychosocial History

APPLICATION OF PATIENT HISTORIES
I. Medical Consultation
II. Radiation
III. Prophylactic Premedication

PRETREATMENT ANTIBIOTIC PROPHYLAXIS
I. American Heart Association Guidelines
II. Recommendations Based on Principles
III. Medical Conditions That Require Antibiotic Premedication before Invasive Dental and Dental Hygiene Procedures
IV. Recommended Antibiotic Protocol

AMERICAN SOCIETY OF ANESTHESIOLOGISTS DETERMINATION

REVIEW AND UPDATE OF HISTORY

DOCUMENTATION

EVERYDAY ETHICS

FACTORS TO TEACH THE PATIENT

REFERENCES

LEARNING OBJECTIVES

After studying this chapter, the student will be able to:

1. Relate and define key terms and concepts utilized in the creation of patient histories.

2. Explain the significance and purpose of accurate and complete patient medical, dental, and psychosocial histories.

3. Compare and contrast the different methods available for the compilation of patient histories and the advantages and disadvantages of each.

4. Discuss how the components of patient histories relate directly to the application of patient care.

INTRODUCTION

For safe, evidence-based dental and dental hygiene care, a thorough patient health history is an essential part of the complete assessment. The history directs and guides steps to be taken in preparation for, during, and following appointments. Some important points about the patient history are listed here.

◆ The history is needed before oral examination procedures with periodontal probe and explorer are carried out.

◆ The use of instruments that would manipulate the soft tissue around the teeth is contraindicated until it has been determined that antibiotic premedication is not indicated.

◆ When a question exists about the medical history as described by the patient, or when an unusual or abnormal condition is observed, consultation with the patient's primary care provider or referral for examination of the patient who does not have a primary care provider is required.

◆ Even emergency treatment must be postponed or kept to a minimum until the patient's medical status is determined.

I. Significance

The significance of taking a complete and accurate patient history cannot be overemphasized for the following reasons:

◆ Oral conditions reflect the general health of the patient; dental procedures may complicate or be complicated by existing pathologic or physiologic conditions elsewhere in the body.

◆ General health factors influence response to treatment, such as tissue healing, and thereby influence the outcomes that may be expected from oral care.

◆ The state of the patient's health is constantly changing. Therefore, the history must be updated continually.

II. Purpose of the History

Carefully prepared medical, dental, and psychosocial histories are used in comprehensive patient care to:

◆ Provide information pertinent to the etiology and diagnosis of oral conditions and the total patient care plan.

◆ Reveal conditions that necessitate precautions, modifications, or adaptations during appointments to ensure dental and dental hygiene procedures will not harm the patient and to prevent emergency situations.

◆ Aid in the identification of possible unrecognized conditions for which the patient will be referred for further diagnosis and treatment.

◆ Permit appraisal of the general health and nutritional status, which, in turn, contributes to the prognosis of success in patient care and instruction.

◆ Give insight into emotional and psychological factors, attitudes, and prejudices that may affect present appointments as well as continuing care.

◆ Document records for reference and comparison over a series of appointments for periodic follow-up.

◆ Furnish evidence in legal matters if questions arise.[1]

◆ Identify cultural beliefs and practices that affect risk for oral disease.

◆ Determine ethnic/racial influences on risk factors for oral disease.

HISTORY PREPARATION

The general methods in current use for obtaining a health history are the *interview*, the *questionnaire* (which may be paper or electronic), or a combination of the two. There are several methods for obtaining the history.

I. Methods

◆ Preappointment information
  • Basic information obtained before the initial assessment appointment can save time and facilitate the process.
  • A brief telephone screening interview or downloadable questionnaire can help determine potential medical problems, need for premedication or consultation with the patient's primary care provider, and identification of medically compromised or physically challenged patients for whom modifications in routine care may be needed.

◆ Self-history
  • Because a self-history can be prepared at home, the history form can be provided online for the patient to download and complete, sent via e-mail, or mailed to the patient in advance of the first appointment.
  • This kind of form might include some items that can be checked or circled, with space to allow the patient to provide additional information.

◆ Complete history
  • A complete patient history is gathered at the initial visit and is a combination of interview and questionnaire.
  • At successive appointments, the complete history is reviewed with the patient and changes are considered when planning patient care.

II. Record Forms

◆ Basic history forms
  • Forms are available commercially or from the American Dental Association (ADA) for a fee, but many dentists and dental hygienists prefer to develop their own and have a form printed to their specifications.
  • ADA and other organizations have basic history forms translated into a variety of languages. Many are available on the Internet.

◆ An adequate basic history form will:
- Enable the recording of important details in a logical sequence.
- Permit quick identification of special needs of a patient when the history is reviewed before each appointment.
- Allow ample space whenever possible to record the patient's own words in the interview method or for self-expression by the patient on a questionnaire.
- Have space for notes concerning attitudes and knowledge as stated or displayed by the patient during the history-taking or other later appointments.
- Be provided, when possible, in the patient's primary or dominant language.

◆ Supplementary forms
- A secondary, more detailed questionnaire can be used to determine additional information for specialized topics.
- The basic questionnaire reveals whether a topic applies to an individual. If the answer is positive, additional information is requested.
- *Example:* Simple questions on the basic questionnaire indicate the use of tobacco products. Completion of another questionnaire provides details about the type of tobacco used and frequency of use. Chapter 32 illustrates a tobacco use assessment form.

III. Introduction to the Patient

◆ Patient education about why the information requested in the history is essential before treatment can be undertaken.

◆ Convey the idea that oral health and general health are interrelated, without creating undue alarm concerning potential ill effects or harmful sequelae from required treatment.

◆ To build rapport, allow children to participate in their history preparation, but most of the information will need to be supplied by a parent or legal guardian. The signature of the responsible adult is required on the record.

IV. Limitations of a History

Many patients cannot or will not provide complete or, in certain cases, correct information when answering medical or dental history questions. Reasons for inaccuracy or incompleteness of information can include:

◆ Problems related to the method of obtaining the histories, how the questions are worded, or an inadvertent lack of neutrality in the attitude of the person gathering the history.

◆ Difficulty in comprehending a self-administered test because the patient cannot read or has a language barrier.

◆ The location in which the questionnaire is completed, such as a crowded reception area without sufficient privacy.

◆ The patient's limited knowledge and inability to understand the relationship between certain diseases or conditions and dental treatment. Information may seem irrelevant, so it is withheld.

◆ Reluctance to discuss a health condition that may be embarrassing, such as history of infectious or communicable disease. The patient may fear refusal of treatment.

THE QUESTIONNAIRE

Positive findings on a questionnaire are explained further in a personal interview. A questionnaire by itself cannot be expected to satisfy the overall purposes of the history, but it can provide some basic personal history, dental history, and factual information in the medical history.

I. Types of Questions

Figures 11-1 and 11-2 provide useful examples of questions necessary for a thorough patient evaluation.

◆ *System oriented*
- Direct questions to determine if the patient has had a disease. Often the questions are organized as a review of systems, for example, the digestive system, respiratory system, or urinary system.
- The questions may contain references to specific organs, for example, the stomach, lungs, or kidneys.

◆ *Disease oriented*
- A typical set of questions may start with "Do you have, or have you had, any of the following diseases or problems?"
- A listing under that question contains items such as diabetes, asthma, or hypertension arranged alphabetically or grouped by systems or body organs.
- Follow-up questions can determine dates of illness, severity, and outcome.

◆ *Symptom oriented*
- In the absence of previous or current disease states, questions may lead to a suspicion of a condition, which, in turn, can provide an opportunity to recommend and encourage the patient to schedule an examination by a primary care provider.
- Examples of the symptom-oriented questions are "Are you thirsty much of the time?" "Does your mouth frequently become dry?" or "Do you have to urinate more than six times a day?"
- Positive answers could lead to tests for diabetes detection.

◆ *Culture oriented*
- Identify ethnic or gender-related increase in risk for systematic or oral disease.
- Determine traditional, culturally related health beliefs that may influence dental hygiene interventions or recommendations.

MEDICAL INFORMATION

PLEASE PROVIDE THE NAME, ADDRESS, AND PHONE NUMBER OF YOUR PHYSICIAN   NONE [   ]

PHYSICIAN'S FIRST NAME   PHYSICIAN'S LAST NAME

ADDRESS   CITY   STATE   ZIP CODE

PHONE NUMBER: _____

Last physical exam: _____
                      Month   Year

Have you ever been hospitalized for any surgical operation or serious illness? YES ( )   NO ( )

Your Height: _____   Current Weight: _____
              Feet   Inches   lbs

Are you wearing contacts: YES ( )   NO ( )

DENTAL INFORMATION

PLEASE PROVIDE THE NAME, ADDRESS, AND PHONE NUMBER OF YOUR DENTIST   NONE [   ]

DENTIST'S FIRST NAME   DENTIST'S LAST NAME

ADDRESS   CITY   STATE   ZIP CODE

PHONE NUMBER: _____

Last dental visit: _____   Reason for the dental visit: _____

NAME OF YOUR DENTAL INSURANCE CO.: _____ GROUP & ID NUMBER: _____

Mark your answer with an (X)

1. Is it important for you to keep your teeth?   YES ( )   NO ( )
2. Do you need to take an antibiotic prior to dental treatment?   YES ( )   NO ( )
3. Do you become anxious about having dental treatment?   YES ( )   NO ( )
4. Do you have pain or sensitivity in your mouth or teeth?   YES ( )   NO ( )
5. Have you previously or do you currently have any mouth sores?   YES ( )   NO ( )
6. Have you ever had dental x-rays taken?   YES ( )   NO ( )
7. Have you ever had periodontal surgery?   YES ( )   NO ( )
8. Do your gums bleed?   YES ( )   NO ( )
9. Have you ever had any complications due to dental procedures?   YES ( )   NO ( )
10. Do you have any dental implants?   YES ( )   NO ( )
11. Have you ever had orthodontics/braces?   YES ( )   NO ( )
12. Do you have/wear full or removable/partial dentures?   YES ( )   NO ( )

Patient Name _____   Record # _____

FIGURE 11-1 • Medical History: General Medical/Dental History.

- Identify herbal preparations or other traditional medications used by the patient that may affect oral care or risk for disease.

II. Advantages of a Questionnaire

- Broad in scope; useful during the interview to identify positive answers needing additional clarification.
- Time saving.
- Consistent; all selected questions are included, and none is omitted because of time or other factors.
- Patient has time to think over the answers—not under pressure from the interviewer.
- Patient may write information that might not be expressed directly in an interview.
- Legal aspects of a written or an electronic record with the patient's signature.

DO YOU HAVE OR HAVE YOU EVER HAD ANY OF THE FOLLOWING CONDITIONS?
Mark your answer with an (X)

BLOOD DISORDERS			MENTAL HEALTH CONDITIONS		
Anemia (iron/folate deficiency or sickle cell)	YES ( )	NO ( )	Anxiety Disorder	YES ( )	NO ( )
Hemophilia or Von Willebrand disease	YES ( )	NO ( )	Bipolar Disorder (manic depressive)	YES ( )	NO ( )
Leukemia	YES ( )	NO ( )	Depression	YES ( )	NO ( )
CARDIOVASCULAR			Feeding or eating Disorder	YES ( )	NO ( )
Arrhythmia or atrial fibrillation	YES ( )	NO ( )	Post-traumatic stress disorder (PTSD)	YES ( )	NO ( )
Angina	YES ( )	NO ( )	Other mental health conditions	YES ( )	NO ( )
Coronary artery disease	YES ( )	NO ( )	**RESPIRATORY SYSTEM**		
Congenital heart condition	YES ( )	NO ( )	Asthma	YES ( )	NO ( )
Endocarditis	YES ( )	NO ( )	Emphysema	YES ( )	NO ( )
Heart attack, myocardial infarction (MI)	YES ( )	NO ( )	Chronic obstructive pulmonary disease	YES ( )	NO ( )
Heart failure	YES ( )	NO ( )	Sleep apnea	YES ( )	NO ( )
Heart murmur (mitral valve prolapse)	YES ( )	NO ( )	**SUBSTANCE USE DISORDERS**		
Heart transplant	YES ( )	NO ( )	Alcoholism	YES ( )	NO ( )
Heart valve disease, prosthetic heart valve	YES ( )	NO ( )	Prescription drug addiction	YES ( )	NO ( )
High or low blood pressure	YES ( )	NO ( )	Recreational drug addiction	YES ( )	NO ( )
Pacemaker	YES ( )	NO ( )	Tobacco addiction	YES ( )	NO ( )
ENDOCRINE SYSTEM			**TRANSMISSIBLE DISEASES**		
Borderline Diabetes	YES ( )	NO ( )	Hepatitis B or C virus	YES ( )	NO ( )
Diabetes Mellitus Type 1	YES ( )	NO ( )	Tuberculosis (TB)	YES ( )	NO ( )
Diabetes Mellitus Type 2	YES ( )	NO ( )	HIV/AIDS	YES ( )	NO ( )
Pre-diabetes	YES ( )	NO ( )	Mononucleosis	YES ( )	NO ( )
Hypothyroid or hyperthyroid	YES ( )	NO ( )	Herpes Simplex Virus (Type 1 or 2)	YES ( )	NO ( )
GASTROINTESTINAL SYSTEM			Sexually Transmitted Disease	YES ( )	NO ( )
Celiac disease	YES ( )	NO ( )	**WOMEN**		
IBD (Crohn's disease or ulcerative colitis)	YES ( )	NO ( )	Pregnancy	YES ( )	NO ( )
Lactose intolerance	YES ( )	NO ( )	Breastfeeding/Nursing	YES ( )	NO ( )
GERD (reflux disease, heartburn)	YES ( )	NO ( )	Menopause	YES ( )	NO ( )
Peptic ulcer disease	YES ( )	NO ( )	**OTHER CONDITIONS**		
IMMUNE SYSTEM			Attention deficit disorder	YES ( )	NO ( )
Allergies (hay fever, food, etc.)	YES ( )	NO ( )	Autism spectrum	YES ( )	NO ( )
Lupus	YES ( )	NO ( )	Cancer	YES ( )	NO ( )
Multiple sclerosis	YES ( )	NO ( )	Learning disability	YES ( )	NO ( )
Rheumatoid Arthritis	YES ( )	NO ( )	Physical limitation/disability	YES ( )	NO ( )
Other autoimmune disease	YES ( )	NO ( )	Traumatic brain injury	YES ( )	NO ( )
LIVER/KIDNEY SYSTEMS			**ADDITIONAL HEALTH RELATED QUESTIONS**		
Liver disease (cirrhosis, fatty liver, etc.)	YES ( )	NO ( )	Have you ever been hospitalized?	YES ( )	NO ( )
Chronic kidney disease or kidney failure	YES ( )	NO ( )	Have you had any of the following?	YES ( )	NO ( )
Kidney transplant	YES ( )	NO ( )	Surgery?	YES ( )	NO ( )
MUSCULOSKELETAL SYSTEM			Radiation therapy?	YES ( )	NO ( )
Fibromyalgia	YES ( )	NO ( )	Chemotherapy?	YES ( )	NO ( )
Osteoarthritis	YES ( )	NO ( )	Excessive bleeding or bruising?	YES ( )	NO ( )
Osteoporosis	YES ( )	NO ( )	Excessive thirst?	YES ( )	NO ( )
NEUROLOGICAL SYSTEM			Excessive urination?	YES ( )	NO ( )
Alzheimer's disease or other dementia	YES ( )	NO ( )	**OTHER CONDITION(S) NOT LISTED**		
Epilepsy or other seizure disorder	YES ( )	NO ( )			
Parkinson's disease or other movement disorder	YES ( )	NO ( )			
Stroke	YES ( )	NO ( )			

Patient Name _____ Record # _____

FIGURE 11-2 • Medical History: Medical Conditions.

III. Disadvantages of a Questionnaire (If Used Alone without a Follow-Up Interview)

◆ Impersonal; no opportunity to develop rapport.

◆ Inflexible; no provision for additional questioning in areas of specific importance to an individual patient.

THE INTERVIEW

In long-range planning for a patient's health, much more is involved than asking questions and receiving answers. The rapport established during the interview contributes to the continued cooperation of the patient.

I. Participants

◆ The interviewer is alone with the patient or parent of the child patient and, if necessary, a qualified professional translator/interpreter.

◆ The history is never to be taken in a reception area when other patients are present.

II. Setting

◆ A consultation room or office is preferred; if possible, move the patient away from the atmosphere of the treatment room, where thoughts may be on the services to be provided.

◆ The treatment room may be the only available place with privacy. If the treatment room is used for a patient interview:
  • Seat patient comfortably in upright position.
  • Turn off running water and dental light, and close the door (if possible).
  • Sit on clinician's stool to be at eye level and face-to-face with the patient.

III. Pointers for the Interview

Interviewing involves communication between individuals. Communication implies the transmission or interchange of facts, attitudes, opinions, or thoughts through words, gestures, or other means.

◆ Communication through tactful but direct questioning can elicit necessary information from the patient. Frequently, the patient is unaware of a health problem.

◆ The most effective attitude for the clinician to portray is one of friendly understanding, reassurance, and acceptance.

◆ Genuine interest and willingness to listen when a patient wishes to describe symptoms, complaints, or current health practices not only aids in establishing the rapport needed but also frequently provides insight into the patient's real attitudes and prejudices.

◆ By asking simple questions at first and more personal questions later after rapport has developed, the patient will be more relaxed and truthful in answering.

◆ Skill is required because tact, ingenuity, judgment, and cultural sensitivity are taxed to the fullest in the attempt to obtain accurate and complete information from the patient.

◆ The culturally sensitive dental hygienist will be aware of nonverbal communication issues when interviewing a patient from a different culture (see in Chapter 3).

IV. Interview Form

◆ The interviewer may use a structured form with places to check and fill in.

◆ Another method is to record on blank sheets from questions created from a guide or list of topics.

◆ Either type of form can involve reference to the positive or negative answers on a previously completed questionnaire.

◆ Familiarity with the items on the history permits the interviewer to be direct and informal without reading from a fixed list of topics, a method that may lack the personal touch necessary to gain the patient's confidence.

◆ When appropriate, the patient's own words are recorded.

V. Advantages of the Interview

◆ Personal contact contributes to development of rapport for future appointments.

◆ Flexibility for individual needs; details obtained can be adapted for supplementary questioning.

VI. Disadvantages of the Interview

◆ Time-consuming when not prefaced with questionnaire.

◆ Unless a list is consulted, items of importance may be omitted.

◆ Patient may be embarrassed to talk about personal conditions and may hold back significant information.

ITEMS INCLUDED IN THE HISTORY

Information obtained by means of the history is directly related to how the goals for patient care are established and will be accomplished. In Tables 11-1 through 11-3, items are listed with possible medications and other treatments the patient may have or has had, along with suggested considerations for appointment procedures.

◆ In specialized practices, objectives may require increased emphasis on certain aspects of the history.

◆ The age group most frequently served will influence the focus of the history. *Example:* parental history and prenatal and postnatal information may take on particular significance for the treatment of a small child; in a pediatric dentistry practice, a special form could be developed to include all essential items.
  • The American Academy of Pediatric Dentistry (www.aapd.org) also has a form that can be used, which includes medical conditions, medications, dental history, supplemental questions for infants/toddlers related to dietary habits, and supplemental questions for adolescents.

◆ Insight and awareness shown while preparing the patient history depend on background knowledge of the manifestations of systemic diseases and the medications for various conditions.

◆ Objectives for the items to include in the various parts of the history are listed here.

I. Dental History

The dental history (Table 11-1; sample form Figure 11-1) contributes to the care provider's knowledge of:

◆ The immediate problem, chief complaint, cause of present pain, or discomfort in the oral cavity.

◆ Risk assessment forms, such as the American Academy of Pediatric Dentistry Caries Risk Assessment Tool and the ADA Caries Risk Assessment forms, provide the information needed for planning individualized dental hygiene interventions based on the patient's risk factors.

◆ Previous dental hygiene and dental care, including preventive care, periodontal treatments, and the extent of restorative and prosthetic replacement, as well as any adverse effects.

◆ Personal daily oral self-care habits.

TABLE 11-1 • Items for the Dental History

ITEMS TO RECORD IN THE HISTORY	RECORD NOTES	CONSIDERATIONS FOR APPOINTMENT PROCEDURES
Reason for present appointment	Chief complaint in patient's own words Pain or discomfort Onset, symptoms, duration of an acute condition	Need for immediate treatment Attitude toward dentistry and preventive care
Previous dental appointments	Date of last treatment Services performed Regularity	Patient knowledge concerning regular dental care Cooperation anticipated
Anesthetics used	Local, general Adverse reactions	Choice of anesthetic
Radiation history	Type, number, dates of dental and medical radiographs Therapeutic radiation Availability of dental radiographs from previous dentist Amount of exposure considered with exposure for medical purposes	Amount of exposure; limitations Educate patient about value of radiographs in diagnosis
Family dental history	Parental tooth loss or maintenance	Attitude toward saving teeth and preventive dentistry Culturally related oral health beliefs and practices
Previous dental treatment	Type of treatment; frequency of maintenance appointments	Value for dental care Previous familiarity with role of dental hygienist
Periodontal	History of periodontal disease and treatment	Attitude toward oral self-care and disease control
Orthodontic	Age during treatment; completion date Previous problem Habit correction Compliance with wearing appliances	For current treatment, consultation with orthodontist
Endodontic	Dates, etiology	Determine if monitoring continues
Prosthodontic	Types of prostheses	Care of prostheses and abutment teeth
Other dental treatment	Extent of restorations Tooth loss Implants	Understanding prevention
Injuries to face or teeth	Causes and extent Fractured teeth or jaws	Limitation of opening Special care during healing
Temporomandibular joint	History of injury, discomfort, disease, dislocation Previous treatment	Effect on opening; accessibility during instrumentation
Oral habits	Clenching, bruxism Mouth breathing Biting objects; fingernails, pipe stem, thread, other Cheek or lip biting Patient awareness of habits	Stress level of patient Instruction relative to effects of habits

(Continues)

TABLE 11-1 • Items for the Dental History

ITEMS TO RECORD IN THE HISTORY	RECORD NOTES	CONSIDERATIONS FOR APPOINTMENT PROCEDURES
Piercing	Types and locations of piercings Date for piercing History of infection related to piercing	Evaluate for oral health changes related to piercing Educate patient on any risks the piercings may pose
Fluorides	Systemic, topical, dates Residence during tooth development years Amount of fluoride in drinking water	Current preventive procedures and need for reevaluation
Biofilm control procedures	Toothbrushing: current procedures, type of brush (manual or powered), texture of filaments, frequency of use, age of brush; frequency of having a new brush Dentifrice name how selected; reason Additional cleansing devices and frequency of use Mouthrinse or other agents: frequency, purpose Source of instruction in care of oral cavity	Ask about patient oral self-care routine Explore challenges encountered in changing habits Adapt education to patient needs, abilities, preferences, and disease state Educate about risk factors for oral disease For parents/caregivers of young children, educate on need to perform and supervise oral care

II. Medical History

Objectives of the medical history (Table 11-2) are to determine whether the patient has or has had any conditions. Samples of forms for the medical conditions and medications in Figures 11-2 and 11-3. The following are categories to be assessed in a medical history:

◆ Personal information (Figure 11-1)

Examples: age; address and contact information; dental insurance; physician's name and contact information; height/weight.

◆ Conditions that may complicate certain kinds of dental and dental hygiene treatment

TABLE 11-2 • Items for the Medical History

ITEM TO RECORD	RECORD NOTES	MEDICATIONS AND TREATMENT MODALITIES	CONSIDERATIONS FOR APPOINTMENT PROCEDURES
Personal or demographic information	Contact information Emergency contact Birthdate Ethnicity/race Gender Marital status Occupation Primary care provider (PCP) contact information	Age-related change Age-, ethnicity/race-, and gender-related risk for disease/conditions	Age may impact need for parental or guardian consent May impact choice of approaches to patient education
General health and appearance	Disabilities Overall impression of well-being Patient's appraisal of own health		Response, cooperation, and attitude to expect during appointments
Medical examination	Date of most recent examination Reason for the examination Tests performed; results Anticipated surgery	New prescriptions received Previous prescriptions continued	Verification with physician for added information Need for stable oral health prior to: • Any long recovery is expected when maintenance appointments may be delayed • Transplant, heart surgery, or prosthesis
Major illnesses, hospitalizations, surgeries	Causes of illness Type and duration of treatment Anesthetics used Convalescence Course of healing: normal, not normal	Medications, treatments	Influence of illnesses on health and care of the oral cavity Anesthetic choice Expected outcome from gingival treatment

TABLE 11-2 • Items for the Medical History (*Continued*)

ITEM TO RECORD	RECORD NOTES	MEDICATIONS AND TREATMENT MODALITIES	CONSIDERATIONS FOR APPOINTMENT PROCEDURES
Age factors	Problems of health in different age groups Elderly: multiple disease entities; patient may need to bring the containers for identification of medications	See individual medical problem Update drug regimen at each appointment	Effects on dental and dental hygiene procedures and personal care
Height and weight	Weight changes over past years or months Obesity Undernourishment Child growth pattern	Diet pills Substance use	Marked weight change may be a symptom of undiagnosed disease; suggest referral for medical examination Influence on dietary instructions for oral health
Medications prescribed by physician	Reasons: relation to dental care Frequency Patient's regularity of taking sugar containing of liquid medicines, effect on dental caries Previous history of bisphosphonate use	List all drugs by name Ask patient for drugs, medicine, injections, vitamins, patches, pills, and capsules Dosage; route of administration	Consultation with PCP concerning adjustments in dosage for dental appointments Indications for premedication Side effects of drugs (e.g., increased risk of gingival hyperplasia with history of dilantin use)
Self-medication	Type, frequency of over-the-counter medications, herbals, vitamins, other supplements Recreational substance use	Pain relievers Sleeping tablets Cough syrup Antacids Vitamins Diet pills	Information not revealed by patient could complicate treatment Lack of interest in oral health, only pain relief Drug side effects
Family medical history	Predisposition to certain diseases (e.g., diabetes) Family history of disease	Cultural beliefs about medications	May help patient seek medical examination when symptom suggests possible disease
Allergies	Determine substances to which the patient is allergic • Latex • Anesthetics • Penicillin • Medicaments • Foods • Iodine	Antihistamines Inhalers Decongestants Steroids	Preparation for emergency Xerostomia Avoid use of substances to which the patient is allergic
Arthritis	Joint pain Immobility Temporomandibular joint involvement	Aspirin Nonsteroidal anti-inflammatory drugs Corticosteroids Total joint replacements	Antibiotic premedication: consult physician if treated with chemotherapeutic agent Dental chair adjustment
Blood disorder	Type and duration of disease Leukemia: remission, thrombocytopenia	Vitamins Minerals: iron (iron deficiency anemia) Folic acid supplement (macrocytic anemia) Antineoplastic drugs	Consultation with PCP (primary care provider) Need for high level of oral health Antibiotic premedication Immunosuppression Increased bleeding Oral lesions

(*Continues*)

TABLE 11-2 • Items for the Medical History (*Continued*)

ITEM TO RECORD	RECORD NOTES	MEDICATIONS AND TREATMENT MODALITIES	CONSIDERATIONS FOR APPOINTMENT PROCEDURES
Bleeding	Bleeding associated with previous dental appointments History of coagulation disorder History of transfusions Regular use of aspirin and herbal supplements (relation to bleeding tendency)	Anticoagulant medication Hemophilia factor replacement	Emergency prevention Laboratory tests for bleeding time, coagulation may be needed Application of direct pressure or hemostatic agent after scaling Special measures for hemophilia
Cancer	Head and neck radiation effects on oral cavity, salivary glands Dental and dental hygiene therapy updated before start of surgery, radiation therapy, or immunosuppression Blood count before dental and dental hygiene therapy Previous history of bisphosphonate prescription	Radiation therapy Fluoride therapy: daily topical application Antineoplastic drugs, alkylating agents, antimetabolites, antibiotics, plant alkaloids, steroids	Bleeding; infection; poor healing response Avoid trauma to tissues Effect on oral radiographic survey: prevention of overexposure Dental caries: preventive measures Xerostomia: substitute saliva Increased risk of osteonecrosis with history of bisphosphonate use
Cardiovascular diseases	Consultation with PCP Refer for examination when patient unable to provide adequate information	Cardiac glycosides Antiarrhythmics Antianginals Antihypertensives Anticoagulants	Minimize stress Premedication for stress Ensure medications have been taken Monitor vital signs
Congenital heart disease	Risk factors for infective endocarditis (IE) Type of problem		Antibiotic premedication may be required
Previous history of IE	Susceptibility to recurrence of IE Type of problem; date		Consultation with PCP required to determine if antibiotic premedication is necessary
Hypertension	Symptom of associate disease states Monitor blood pressure for each appointment Anesthesia: consult with PCP about amount of epinephrine recommended	Diuretics Antiadrenergic agents Vasodilators Angiotensin-converting enzyme inhibitors Calcium channel blocking agent	Postural hypotension (raise back of dental chair slowly) Xerostomia: saliva substitute and fluoride rinse may be needed Gingival enlargement possible with calcium channel blockers
Angina pectoris	Prepare for symptoms; have ready amyl nitrite inhalant or nitroglycerin tablets or spray	Amyl nitrite, nitroglycerin, or other antianginal drugs	Allay fears and prevent stress Morning appointment
Heart diseases	History of disease, symptoms of fatigue, shortness of breath, or cough Consult with PCP	Glycosides (digitalis) Anticoagulants Antiarrhythmic drugs Pacemaker	Monitor vital signs Short, more frequent appointments Adjust dental chair slowly and may need semi-supine position Patient with breathing problem (sleeps with two + pillows) Bleeding tendency due to anticoagulant Check use of ultrasonic (unshielded pacemaker)
Surgically corrected cardiovascular lesions	Type, date of surgery Consultation with physician Before surgical procedure, when possible: the patient needs oral examination and dental work completed. Stress need for meticulous daily oral self-care	No tobacco use Anticoagulants Cyclosporine Nifedipine	Consult with PCP about antibiotic premedication Gingival bleeding may occur Gingival enlargement

TABLE 11-2 • Items for the Medical History (*Continued*)

ITEM TO RECORD	RECORD NOTES	MEDICATIONS AND TREATMENT MODALITIES	CONSIDERATIONS FOR APPOINTMENT PROCEDURES
Cerebrovascular accident (stroke)	Date of onset; residual disabilities Speech, vision, mental function	No tobacco; low-salt diet Anticoagulants Antihypertensives Vasodilator Steroid Anticonvulsant	Gingival bleeding likely when anticoagulants are used Adapt procedures for physical disability
Infectious diseases	History of diseases; immunizations Present disease; communicability Residence or extended trips in countries with high incidence of certain diseases Risk group factor	Immunizations Drug therapy for current infection	Appointment postponement
Hepatitis	Jaundice history Clarification of type of hepatitis Laboratory clearance	Prevention with Hepatitis B (HBV) vaccine series HBV antiviral medications, i.e., lamivudine, telbivudine Hepatitis C (HCV protease inhibitors): Daclatasvir Elbasvir-grazoprevir	Consultation with PCP may be needed to determine if patient can be treated Precautions against percutaneous injury
Tuberculosis	Active or passive Cough Duration of disease	Isoniazid Rifampin Pyrazinamide	Length of treatment; infectivity diminished after few months of treatment
Herpes simplex virus	Open lesions are transmissible	Palliative treatment: Acyclovir	Postpone routine care when active oral lesions are present
HIV AIDS	Oral manifestations	Possible opportunistic infections ART (antiretroviral treatment)	Viral load and CD4 count Oral lesions Universal precautions
Diabetes mellitus	Undiagnosed prediabetes/diabetes: excess thirst, appetite, and urination Family history Complications from poor control (vision problems, kidney failure, cardiovascular, nervous system)	Insulin (may use insulin pump) Diet control Biguanides, i.e., metformin Sulfonylureas, i.e., Glyburide Thiazolidinediones, i.e., Actos Dipeptidyl peptidase-4 inhibitors Alpha-glucosidase inhibitors, i.e., acarbose Combination therapies	Prepare for hypoglycemia Have glucose monitor nearby Plan appointment related to meals and medications, morning is usually best Frequent maintenance appointments More severe periodontal disease Referral to identify undiagnosed prediabetes/diabetes
Ears	Deafness or degree of hearing impairment Infections, ringing, dizziness, balance	Treatment for infection Hearing aid	Adaptations for patient education
Endocrine	Age group–related conditions: Puberty Pregnancy Menstruation Menopause	Thyroid hormone supplement Antithyroid Estrogen/progestin Oral contraceptives	Meticulous biofilm control Monitor blood pressure
Epilepsy	Type, frequency of seizures precipitating factors Preparation for emergency seizure	Anticonvulsant Sedative	Minimize stress Monitor medication side effects PCP consultation

(Continues)

TABLE 11-2 • Items for the Medical History (*Continued*)

ITEM TO RECORD	RECORD NOTES	MEDICATIONS AND TREATMENT MODALITIES	CONSIDERATIONS FOR APPOINTMENT PROCEDURES
Eyes	Disturbance of vision Purpose for corrective eyeglasses or contact lenses Manifestations of systemic disease	Eye drops (e.g., glaucoma)	Protective eyewear during appointment Adaptations for communication with limited sight
Gastrointestinal (Crohn disease, irritable bowel syndrome, celiac disease, lactose intolerance, gastroesophageal reflux)	Nature and treatment of disease Diet restriction prescribed by PCP/dietitian	Antacids H2 blockers Proton pump inhibitors Antidiarrheals Laxatives Antispasmodics Corticosteroids Wide variety of medications	Explore side effects of condition/medications, i.e., vomiting, acid reflux into oral cavity and esophagus Xerostomia Stress reduction protocol Steroid-induced osteoporosis Possible need for additional steroids and/or antibiotics
Kidney	Renal disease; kidney stones Hemodialysis: hypertension, anemia, hepatitis carrier Transplant: hypertension, hepatitis	Salt restrictions Posttransplant drugs may include cyclosporine, tacrolimus, steroids, antiproliferative agents Medications during dialysis may include erythropoietin, iron, vitamin D, E, B-complex, phosphorus binders	Monitor blood pressure Bleeding tendency Poor healing Consult with PCP about need for antibiotic prophylaxis due to susceptibility to infection Steroid-induced osteoporosis Stress reduction protocol
Liver (fatty liver, cirrhosis, etc.)	History of jaundice, hepatitis Impaired drug metabolism Cirrhosis	Nutritional emphasis Abstinence from alcohol	Consult with PCP before prescribing any medication Avoid acetaminophen Bruising and bleeding problems Cheilitis Xerostomia
Mental health issues	Depression and other mental health conditions may negatively impact care-seeking behavior and oral self-care	Antipsychotic drugs Antianxiety drugs Tranquilizers Antidepressants	Stress reduction protocol Xerostomia Nausea/vomiting
Physical disabilities	Extent, cause, duration Type of treatment related to individual condition Consultation with PCP or specialist	Pain reliever Muscle relaxant Anticonvulsant	Adjustment of physical arrangements Wheelchair accessibility and transfer Adaptations of techniques and patient education
Pregnancy	Month, parturition date Possible oral manifestations History of previous pregnancies Iron deficiency anemia	Iron Folic acid Multivitamins	Adjust physical position for comfort Frequent appointments for maintaining periodontal health Meticulous oral self-care
Respiratory (chronic obstructive pulmonary disease, asthma, emphysema)	Breathing problems Persistent cough or wheezing Chest tightness Precipitation of asthmatic attack	Antihistamine Inhalers (anticholinergic, beta-agonist, corticosteroids) Oral steroids Oxygen	Dental chair position Stress reduction protocol Oral candidiasis Nitrous oxide contraindicated Minimize aerosols Watch local anesthetics with sulfites for those with allergies Smoking cessation

Examples: Lowered resistance to infection; uncontrolled hypertension; uncontrolled diabetes; or systemic disease that requires treatment before stressful dental procedures, particularly surgery, can be carried out.

◆ Conditions or diseases that may require special precautions or premedication before treatment

Examples: Increased osteonecrosis risk related to previous treatment with bisphosphonates; or antibiotic coverage for the patient at risk for infective endocarditis (IE).

◆ Conditions under treatment by a physician that require medicating drugs that may influence or contraindicate certain procedures

Examples: Anticoagulant therapy requires consultation with physician; antihypertensive drugs may alter the amount and/or choice of local anesthetic used.

◆ Gender or ethnic/racial influences that increase risk for systemic and oral disease

Example: American Indians and African Americans have increased risk for diabetes and a related increased risk for periodontal disease.

◆ Allergic or adverse reactions

Examples: Latex hypersensitivity; medication or material for which there was a previous adverse reaction.

◆ Diseases and drugs with manifestations in the mouth

Examples: Hematologic disorders; phenytoin-induced gingival overgrowth; infectious diseases such as herpesvirus.

◆ Communicable diseases

Examples: Active tuberculosis; viral hepatitis; herpes.

◆ Physiologic state of the patient

Examples: Pregnancy and birth control pills.

III. Psychosocial History

◆ The psychosocial history (Table 11-3) gathers information about many aspect of the patient's life that may impact their oral and overall health in the following ways[2]:
   • Alter health behaviors such as smoking, drug use, and dietary intake.
   • These factors may also impact resistance to disease, that is, stress.

TABLE 11-3 • Items for the Psychosocial History

ITEMS TO RECORD	RECORD NOTES	MEDICATIONS AND TREATMENT MODALITIES	CONSIDERATIONS FOR APPOINTMENT PROCEDURES
Personal information	Living situation Source of food and food prep Health belief or practices	Herbal supplements should be considered when planning treatment	Try to incorporate health beliefs into education and recommendations
Daily diet	Primary care provider (PCP) recommendations Vitamin supplements Appetite Regularity of meals Types and frequency of snacking and beverage intake Food likes and dislikes	Vitamin supplements	Instructions to be given relative to oral health Prognosis for healing after treatment Need for dietary assessment and analysis
Physical activity	Overall health consciousness	Good health habits Regular exercise	Contribute to cooperative attitude in maintaining oral health
Alcohol consumption	Frequency Amount History of substance abuse	Recovering alcoholic: May be taking disulfiram, avoid all alcohol-containing preparations including mouthrinses	Excessive use: effect on anesthesia; increased healing time Poor nutritional state is common; lack of oral care Avoid alcohol-containing mouthrinse May result in poor patient cooperation
Tobacco use	Form of tobacco, amount used Frequency Knowledge of effects on oral tissues	Instruction concerning oral effects Tobacco cessation program Periodontal risk Dental stains; dentifrice selection	Tobacco use
Drug use	Type of drug Amount used Frequency Method of administration History of trying to stop use Overdose history Rehab history	Instructions regarding oral effects Interest in referral to addiction services	Avoid use of nitrous oxide and prescription pain medications May impact self-care, nutritional status, and healing ability

PLEASE NOTE ANY ALLERGIES

ALLERGIES		
Antibiotics (i.e., Penicillin)	YES ( )	NO ( )
Aspirin or other pain medications	YES ( )	NO ( )
Iodine	YES ( )	NO ( )
Latex products	YES ( )	NO ( )
Local anesthetic (i.e., Novocain)	YES ( )	NO ( )
Pine nuts	YES ( )	NO ( )
OTHER		

PLEASE LIST THE NAME OF ANY DRUGS YOU ARE CURRENTLY TAKING OR HAVE PREVIOUSLY TAKEN IN THE SPACE PROVIDED.

Place (X) in the box
If medication is current, list the dosage.

Antianxiety (i.e., xanax)	YES ( )	NO ( )	Dosage:
Antibiotics	YES ( )	NO ( )	Dosage:
Anticoagulants (i.e., warfarin, coumadin)	YES ( )	NO ( )	Dosage:
Depression medications (i.e., zoloft, celexa)	YES ( )	NO ( )	Dosage:
Anti-inflammatory	YES ( )	NO ( )	Dosage:
Blood pressure medications (i.e., norvasc, lisinopril, lopressor, hydrochlorothiazide)	YES ( )	NO ( )	Dosage:
Aspirin/Pain Medication	YES ( )	NO ( )	Dosage:
Anti-seizure (i.e., Dilantin)	YES ( )	NO ( )	Dosage:
Bisphosphonates (i.e., fosamax, boniva)	YES ( )	NO ( )	Dosage:
Codeine	YES ( )	NO ( )	Dosage:
Diabetes medications (i.e., metformin, glucophage)	YES ( )	NO ( )	Dosage:
Digitalis	YES ( )	NO ( )	Dosage:
Insulin	YES ( )	NO ( )	Dosage:
Steroid (i.e., prednisone)	YES ( )	NO ( )	Dosage:
Cholesterol medications (i.e., simvastatin, lipitor)	YES ( )	NO ( )	Dosage:
Nitroglycerin	YES ( )	NO ( )	Dosage:
Over-the-Counter Medication (i.e., zantac, prilosec, ibuprofen)	YES ( )	NO ( )	Dosage:
Vitamin supplements	YES ( )	NO ( )	Dosage:
Herbal supplements	YES ( )	NO ( )	Dosage:
Other	YES ( )	NO ( )	Dosage:

Please explain in detail all YES responses:

FIGURE 11-3 • Medical History: Medications.

◆ Areas to be assessed include (sample in Figure 11-4), but are not limited to:
  • Living situation and social support.
  • Education.
  • Employment situation.
  • Health literacy levels that may impact communication.
  • Beliefs and attitudes about health, illness, and oral health.
  • Culturally related health practices that may impact the patient's oral health.

APPLICATION OF PATIENT HISTORIES

◆ Information from the histories influences all aspects of total patient care and dental hygiene care planning.

◆ Immediate evaluation of the histories is necessary before proceeding to complete the assessment.

◆ Together with information from all other parts of the diagnostic workup, the patient histories are essential for the preparation of the dental hygiene care plan.

I. Medical Consultation

Dentist and primary care provider need to consult relative to the patient's current therapy and medications or to elements of the patient's past health status that could influence dental treatment needs.[3]

◆ *Telephone or personal contact*
  • Immediate consultation may be needed so that urgent treatment may proceed.
  • Follow-up in writing by electronic communication, fax, or mailed hard copy to provide a legal record of the advice or decision to avoid a misunderstanding.

◆ *Written request*
  • A formal letter is the preferred procedure for medical consultation. This may be e-mailed or faxed to the physician.

Please answer the following questions as accurately as possible.

PERSONAL INFORMATION			
Do you live alone?	YES ( )	NO ( )	If not, who lives in your household?
Do you shop for food in your household?	YES ( )	NO ( )	
Do you prepare the food in your household?	YES ( )	NO ( )	How often do you buy prepared meals?
Do you work outside the home?	YES ( )	NO ( )	What kind of work do you do?
Do you travel for your job?	YES ( )	NO ( )	
Are there any specific health beliefs or practices we should know about?	YES ( )	NO ( )	
Are you physically active daily?	YES ( )	NO ( )	
DIETARY INFORMATION			
Do you eat regular meals and snacks?	YES ( )	NO ( )	What types of snacks do you typically eat? What kinds of beverages do you drink? How often?
Have you had any large weight gains or losses?	YES ( )	NO ( )	How much did you gain or lose? What was the time period?
Do you follow a specific diet?	YES ( )	NO ( )	Who prescribed the diet?
Have you eliminated any types	YES ( )	NO ( )	What types of foods? For how long? Are you being monitored by a medical provider?
TOBACCO PRODUCTS			
Cigarettes	YES ( )	NO ( )	Number of cigarettes per day or week:
Cigars	YES ( )	NO ( )	Number of cigars per week:
E-cigarettes	YES ( )	NO ( )	Number of cartridges per day or week:
Waterpipe/hookah	YES ( )	NO ( )	Approximate amount of time per day or week:
Smokeless	YES ( )	NO ( )	Number of cans/pouches per day/week:
Dissolvable strips, sticks, orbs, etc.	YES ( )	NO ( )	Amount per day or week:
Other types of tobacco products	YES ( )	NO ( )	Amount per day or week:
Have you tried quitting tobacco use in the past?	YES ( )	NO ( )	If you have tried to quit: How long did you quit last time? What did you use to help you quit? What was the longest time you have quit? What has caused you to relapse?
ALCOHOL USE			
Do you drink alcohol?	YES ( )	NO ( )	What kind of alcohol? How often do you have a drink containing alcohol? How many drinks containing alcohol do you have on a typical day?
Have you ever felt you need to cut down?	YES ( )	NO ( )	
RECREATIONAL DRUGS			
Do you use any recreational drugs?	YES ( )	NO ( )	What type of drugs? When did this start? How often do you use drugs? What is the method of administration? Have you ever been in trouble because of your drug use? Have you ever tried to stop using drugs? Have you ever been in rehab?

FIGURE 11-4 • Medical History: Psychosocial.

- A prepared form can be developed with spaces for filling in the specific questions and with space in the lower half for the primary care provider to complete confidential information from the patient's medical record or to provide the necessary recommendations.

◆ Referrals
  - Referral for medical examination when signs of a possible disease condition are present.
  - Referral for laboratory tests may be necessary when recent test results are not available or follow-up tests are needed.

II. Radiation

◆ When a patient is receiving radiation therapy or has had recent radiation for other purposes, a conference with the primary care provider or oncologist is recommended regarding the need for dental radiographs.

◆ It is the dental practitioner's responsibility to utilize all available clinical, assessment, and health history information when contemplating the necessity of diagnostic radiographs in order to optimize care while minimizing radiation exposure.[4]

III. Prophylactic Premedication

◆ Selected patients at risk for IE receive antibiotic premedication before any oral tissue manipulation that could create a bacteremia.

◆ The patient history and the information in Box 11-1 are reviewed to identify a patient needing premedication in accordance with the recommendations of the American Heart Association (AHA) guidelines.

◆ Routine use of antibiotic premedication is never indicated. Overuse of antibiotics can induce microbial resistance and, rarely, allergy or toxicity to the drug used.[5]

◆ The subgingival use of instruments (e.g., periodontal probe or curet) is avoided until the level of risk has been assessed, the condition has been discussed with the patient's primary care provider, and the prescription has been obtained, and taken as directed.

◆ The oral antibiotic prescription is required 1 hour before instrumentation begins to assure adequate blood concentration during and immediately following instrumentation.

◆ At-risk patients already taking an antibiotic for other health conditions may require additional antibiotic prophylaxis before dental and dental hygiene instrumentation. A different class of antibiotic is prescribed rather than to increase the dose of the current drug being taken.[5]

BOX 11-1
Medical Conditions That Require Antibiotic Premedication before Dental and Dental Hygiene Treatment

Antibiotic prophylaxis with dental procedures is recommended only for patients with cardiac conditions associated with the highest risk of adverse outcomes from endocarditis, including:

• Prosthetic cardiac valve.

• Previous endocarditis.

• Congenital heart disease only in the following categories:

  ◆ Unrepaired cyanotic congenital heart disease, including those with palliative shunts and conduits.

  ◆ Completely repaired congenital heart disease with prosthetic material or device, whether placed by surgery or catheter intervention, during the first 6 months after the procedure. (*Prophylaxis is recommended because endothelialization of prosthetic material occurs within 6 months of the procedure.*)

  ◆ Repaired congenital heart disease with residual defects at the site or adjacent to the site of a prosthetic patch or prosthetic device (which inhibit endothelialization).

• Cardiac transplantation recipients with cardiac valvular disease.

Source: Wilson W, Taubert KA, Gewitz M, et al. Prevention of infective endocarditis: guidelines from the American Heart Association: a guideline from the American Heart Association Rheumatic Fever, Endocarditis, and Kawasaki Disease Committee, Council on Cardiovascular Disease in the Young, and the Council on Clinical Cardiology, Council on Cardiovascular Surgery and Anesthesia, and the Quality Care and Outcomes Research Interdisciplinary Working Group. *Circulation*. 2007;116(15):1736-1754.

PRETREATMENT ANTIBIOTIC PROPHYLAXIS

I. AHA Guidelines

A. Brief Historical Review

◆ The AHA has made recommendations for the prevention of IE for many years. The first document was published in 1955. There have been nine revisions since then including the latest one published in *Circulation* 2007 reviewed and updated on the AHA website in 2014.[6,7]

B. Rationale for 2007 Revision and 2014 Review[6,7]

◆ Former guidelines were based more on expert opinion or individual case studies; the 2007 guidelines, 2014 review, attempted to be more evidence based.

◆ Frequent exposure to random bacteremias resulting from daily activities are more likely to cause IE than are treatment procedures performed at dental and dental hygiene appointments.

◆ Antibiotic prophylaxis may prevent a very small number of cases of IE, if any, in patients receiving a dental or dental hygiene treatment procedure.

◆ There are risks of antibiotic-associated adverse events that may exceed the benefit, if any, of antibiotic therapy.

◆ Maintenance of optimal oral health with daily biofilm removal may reduce the incidence of IE due to bacteremias caused by daily activities. Such prevention can be more significant than prophylactic antibiotics given occasionally for a dental or dental hygiene invasive treatment procedure.

◆ Literature reviews found no evidence-based method to decide exactly which procedures require prophylactic antibiotic premedication and which do not need it.

◆ Other factors limiting conduct of controlled research trials are:

- Low incidence of IE.
- Wide variety of types of cardiac diseases.
- Wide variety of invasive dental procedures.
- Incidents when antibiotic premedication did not prevent IE following a dental invasive procedure.

II. Recommendations Based on Principles[5-7]

◆ Only an extremely small number of cases of IE might be prevented by antibiotic prophylaxis for dental procedures even if such prophylactic therapy were 100% effective.

◆ IE prophylaxis for dental procedures is recommended only for patients with underlying cardiac conditions associated with the highest risk of adverse outcomes from IE.

◆ For patients with these underlying cardiac conditions, prophylaxis is recommended for all dental procedures that involve manipulation of gingival tissue, the periapical region of teeth, or perforation of the oral mucosa.

◆ Patients requiring antibiotic prophylaxis may carry a wallet card documenting their need for premedication.

◆ Antibiotic prophylaxis is not recommended based solely on an increased lifetime risk of acquisition of IE.

III. Medical Conditions That Require Antibiotic Premedication before Invasive Dental and Dental Hygiene Procedures

◆ Box 11-2 lists the cardiac conditions for which antibiotic prophylaxis is recommended.

◆ Box 11-2 lists the following:

- Dental and dental hygiene procedures for which endocarditis prophylaxis is recommended.
- Procedures for which prophylaxis is *not* needed.
- A codeveloped evidence-based guideline for the prevention of orthopedic implant infection in patients undergoing dental procedures was released in 2012 by the ADA and the American Academy of Orthopaedic Surgeons.[8]
- A 2014 systematic review found no direct evidence that dental procedures cause prosthetic joint implant infections.[9] Evidence-based clinical practice guidelines for dental practitioners recommend against the routine use of antibiotics prior to dental procedures to prevent prosthetic joint infection[9]; however, premedication may be considered in the case of the high-risk medically complex or immunocompromised patient.[10] Consultation with the patient's primary care provider regarding the need for antibiotic prophylaxis for patients with prosthetic joints is recommended.[9,10]

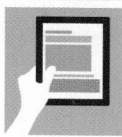

BOX 11-2
Dental and Dental Hygiene Procedures for Which Endocarditis Prophylaxis Is Recommended for Patients in Box 11-1

All dental and dental hygiene procedures that involve:

- Manipulation of gingival tissue.
- The periapical region of teeth.
- Perforation of the oral mucosa need antibiotic premedication (Table 11-4).

The following procedures and events do *not* need prophylaxis:

- Routine anesthetic injections through noninfected tissue.
- Taking dental radiographs.
- Placement of removable prosthodontic or orthodontic appliances.
- Adjustment of orthodontic appliances.
- Placement of orthodontic brackets.
- Shedding of primary teeth.
- Bleeding from trauma to the lips or oral mucosa.

Source: Wilson W, Taubert KA, Gewitz M, et al. Prevention of infective endocarditis: guidelines from the American Heart Association: a guideline from the American Heart Association Rheumatic Fever, Endocarditis, and Kawasaki Disease Committee, Council on Cardiovascular Disease in the Young, and the Council on Clinical Cardiology, Council on Cardiovascular Surgery and Anesthesia, and the Quality Care and Outcomes Research Interdisciplinary Working Group. *Circulation.* 2007;116(15):1736-1754.

IV. Recommended Antibiotic Protocol

◆ Table 11-4 provides the recommended antibiotic prescriptions for prevention of cardiac endocarditis.

AMERICAN SOCIETY OF ANESTHESIOLOGISTS DETERMINATION

With the completion of the patient histories, an overall estimate of medical risk of a patient can be made. American Society of Anesthesiologists (ASA) Physical Status Classification System[11] describes six categories of physical status and provides examples of adaptations necessary for providing dental hygiene care for a patient in each category.

◆ **ASA I:** a patient without apparent systemic disease: a normal healthy patient.

◆ **ASA II:** a patient with mild systemic disease.

◆ **ASA III:** a patient with severe systemic disease that limits activity but is not incapacitating.

◆ **ASA IV:** a patient with an incapacitating systemic disease that is a constant threat to life.

◆ **ASA V:** a moribund patient not expected to survive 24 hours with or without care.

TABLE 11-4 • Prophylactic Regimens for Dental, Oral, Respiratory Tract, or Esophageal Procedures

SITUATION	AGENT	REGIMEN—SINGLE DOSE; 30–60 min BEFORE PROCEDURE	
		ADULT	CHILD[a]
Standard general prophylaxis	Amoxicillin	2.0 g orally	50 mg/kg orally
Unable to take oral medications	Ampicillin or cefazolin or ceftriaxone	2.0 g IM or IV 1.0 g IM or IV	50 mg/kg IM or IV 50 mg/kg IM or IV
Allergic to penicillins or ampicillin—oral	Cephalexin[b] or clindamycin or azithromycin or clarithromycin	2.0 g orally 600 mg orally 500 mg orally	50 mg/kg orally 20 mg/kg orally 15 mg/kg orally
Allergic to penicillins and unable to take oral medications	Cefazolin or ceftriaxone[b] or clindamycin	1.0 g IM or IV 600 mg IM or IV	50 mg/kg IM or IV 25 mg/kg IM or IV

[a]Total child dose never exceeds adult dose.

[b]Cephalosporins are not prescribed for individuals with immediate-type hypersensitivity reaction (urticaria, angioedema, or anaphylaxis) to penicillins or ampicillin.

IM, intramuscularly; IV, intravenously.

Source: Nishimura RA, Carabello BA, Faxon DP, Freed MD, Lytle BW, O'Gara PT, American College of Cardiology/American Heart Association Task Force, et al. ACC/AHA 2008 guideline update on valvular heart disease: focused update on infective endocarditis: a report of the American College of Cardiology/American Heart Association Task Force on Practice Guidelines: endorsed by the Society of Cardiovascular Anesthesiologists, Society for Cardiovascular Angiography and Interventions, and Society of Thoracic Surgeons. *Circulation.* 2008 Aug 19;118(8):887-896.

REVIEW AND UPDATE OF HISTORY

◆ Updating the patient's health history at each appointment is essential.

◆ Changes in health status revealed by interim medical examinations or evidenced by reported illness or hospitalizations are recorded and considered during continuing treatment.

◆ Post a wall plaque that states *Please Advise Us of Any Change in Your Medical History Since Your Last Visit* in an appropriate place in a dental office or clinic to remind patients about the importance of updating information at each appointment.

◆ Following a review of the previously recorded history, questions can be directed to the patient to compare the present condition with the previous one and to determine at least the following:

• Interim illnesses; changes in health.
• Visits to physician; reasons and results.
• Laboratory tests performed and the results; blood, urine, or other analyses.
• Current medications.
• Changes in the oral soft tissues and the teeth observed by the patient.

DOCUMENTATION

◆ Date all records.
◆ All hard copy permanent records are written in ink.
◆ Electronic patient records are stored on a secure server on password-protected computers, with only office staff having access to the computers and passwords. All electronic charting documentation are signed electronically and saved in such a way that falsifications to patient records cannot be made.

◆ The patient signature must be recorded upon completion of the health history to verify the information.[1,3] The completed history for a minor is signed by a parent or guardian. A signature is also needed on the informed consent form. Signatures may be recorded or electronically dependent on the method in which the information is collected.

◆ All information obtained for a patient history should be maintained with the strictest privacy.

◆ For patients with special health problems that require premedication, coded tab systems on paper charts or pop-up alerts in electronic records should be used to notify all dental personnel to check the medical history before each appointment.

◆ Evaluate the usefulness of items on the patient history form periodically, and plan for revision as scientific evidence reveals new information.

◆ Progress notes document regular update of forms completed and changes in personal, dental, or health history since last appointment.

◆ Box 11-3 provides an example of a progress note related to completion of personal, dental, and medical histories.

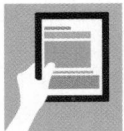

BOX 11-3

Example Documentation:
Updating a Patient's Medical History

S—Forty-five-year-old patient presents for routine 6-month maintenance appointment. She is new to the office and reports she has always taken penicillin prior to her "cleaning" appointments. She completed and signed a new health history form. Her medical history indicates she has a heart murmur, and she reports this is why she has been told to take penicillin before appointments. She became quite concerned about not premedicating with antibiotics.

O—The recommendations for antibiotic prophylaxis were reviewed with the patient and a consult with the primary care provider determined she was not a candidate for premedication. A full series of radiographs was taken and the clinical examination was completed. No dental caries noted. Pocket depths in the maxillary molar area range from 5 to 6 mm with bleeding on probing. No suppuration present. No mobility. Furcation involvement Grade II on ML and DL of #2, 3, 14, and 15. Plaque score 15%, primarily in maxillary molar areas.

A—Caries risk: low; periodontal risk: high; oral cancer risk: low. On the basis of the comprehensive periodontal examination and radiographic findings, she has localized Stage II, Grade A periodontitis.

P—Oral self-care review of interdental brush for maxillary molar areas. Full-mouth debridement with localized scaling and periodontal debridement on #2, 3, 14, and 15. One carpule: 2% lidocaine with 1:100,000 epinephrine for a posterior superior alveolar upper right and upper left. Selective polishing: 5% sodium fluoride varnish was applied. A 3-month periodontal maintenance interval was recommended.

Signed: _____, RDH

Date: _____

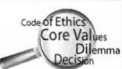

EVERYDAY ETHICS

Chris, the dental hygienist, was waiting for her new patient at 1:00 PM. All she knew was that Irina was 70 years old, from Russia, and could speak and understand English fairly well. Chris heard the front door to the office open and went out to greet her patient. The woman was on the arm of a teenage boy who quickly helped Irina to a chair and turned to leave after saying to Chris (pointing to the patient) "Just back from hospital. They fixed her heart and told her to get her teeth cleaned to keep her healthy. Car not parked." Then to his grandmother, "Back in an hour," before he rushed out.

Chris ushered Irina into the treatment room and helped her into the chair, then started the history questions with "What were you in the hospital for?" Irina grabs Chris's arm and firmly requests, "Want teeth cleaned." Chris attempts to explain why she is asking the questions about her health. Then she asks for her physician's name and permission to call the physician to obtain the information. Irina points to her heart, but just becomes more agitated and keeps repeating "Want teeth cleaned" and refuses to give approval to call her doctor. Chris is alarmed at the thought of providing

care for this patient without complete information about her health history, but hates to waste the scheduled appointment time, given how difficult it is for patients to get an appointment.

Questions for Consideration

1. Professionally and ethically, what are a dental hygienist's responsibilities to take time to help a patient understand the seriousness of an illness and the need for a complete personal, dental, and medical history before receiving dental treatment?

2. Provide an example of how each of the ethical theories (Table IV-1, Section IV Introduction) might apply as Chris determines how to resolve this issue?

3. Which of the dental hygiene core values (Chapter 1, Box 1-6) apply as Chris determines what action to take?

Factors to Teach the Patient

▶ The need for obtaining the personal, medical, and dental history before performance of dental and dental hygiene procedures and the need for keeping the histories up to date.

▶ The assurance that recorded histories are kept in strict professional confidence.

▶ The relationship between oral health and general physical health.

▶ The interrelationship of medical and dental care.

▶ All patients who require antibiotic premedication need special attention paid to (1) the importance of preventive dentistry, (2) the imperative need for regular dental care, and (3) the necessity for taking the prescribed prescription 1 hour before the appointment starts.

ENHANCE YOUR UNDERSTANDING

ONLINE RESOURCES
(see the inside front cover for access information)
· Audio glossary
· Appendices

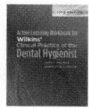

SUPPORT FOR LEARNING
(available separately)
· *Active Learning Workbook for Wilkins' Clinical Practice of the Dental Hygienist, 13th Edition*

INDIVIDUALIZED REVIEW
· Customized practice quizzing with Navigate 2 TestPrep for *Wilkins' Clinical Practice of the Dental Hygienist*

References

1. Collier A. The management of risk. Part 3: recording your way out of trouble. *Dent Update*. 2014;41(4):338-340.

2. Kye SY, Park K. Psychosocial factors and health behavior among Korean adults: a cross-sectional study. *Asian Pac J Cancer Prev*. 2012;13(1):49-56.

3. Chiodo GT, Rosenstein DI. Consultation between dentists and physicians. *Gen Dent*. 1984;32(1):19-22.

4. U.S. Department of Health and Human Services, U.S. Food and Drug Administration. ADA/FDA Guide to patient selection for dental radiographs. https://www.fda.gov/Radiation-EmittingProducts/RadiationEmittingProductsandProcedures/MedicalImaging/MedicalX-Rays/ucm116503.htm. Accessed August 30, 2017.

5. American Academy of Pediatric Dentistry. Guideline on antibiotic prophylaxis for dental patients at risk for infection (Originating Committee Clinical Affairs, Committee Review Council, Council on Clinical Affairs Adopted 1990 Revised 1991, 1997, 1999, 2002, 2005, 2007, 2008, 2011, 2014). http://www.aapd.org/media/Policies_Guidelines/G_AntibioticProphylaxis.pdf. Accessed August 30, 2017.

6. Wilson W, Taubert KA, Gewitz M, et al. Prevention of infective endocarditis: guidelines from the American Heart Association: a guideline from the American Heart Association Rheumatic Fever, Endocarditis, and Kawasaki Disease Committee, Council on Cardiovascular Disease in the Young, and the Council on Clinical Cardiology, Council on Cardiovascular Surgery and Anesthesia, and the Quality Care and Outcomes Research Interdisciplinary Working Group. *Circulation*. 2007;116(15):1736-1754.

7. American Heart Association. Infective endocarditis. http://www.heart.org/HEARTORG/Conditions/CongenitalHeartDefects/TheImpactofCongenitalHeartDefects/InfectiveEndocarditis_UCM_307108_Article.jsp#.Wadd4LKGPIX. Accessed August 30, 2017.

8. American Academy of Orthopaedic Surgeons, American Dental Association Clinical Practice Guideline Unit. Prevention of orthopaedic implant infection in patients undergoing dental procedures evidence-based guideline and evidence report. http://www.ada.org/~/media/ADA/Member%20Center/FIles/PUDP_guideline.ashx. Accessed August 30, 2017.

9. Sollecito T, Abt E, Lockhart P, et al. The use of prophylactic antibiotics prior to dental procedures in patients with prosthetic joints: evidence-based clinical practice guideline for dental practitioners—a report of the American Dental Association Council on Scientific Affairs. *JADA*. 2015;146(1):11-16.

10. Elliot A, Hellstein JW, Lockhart PB, et al. American Dental Association guidance for utilizing appropriate use criteria in the management of the care of patients with orthopedic implants undergoing dental procedures. *JADA*. 2017;148(2):57-59.

11. American Society of Anesthesiologists. New classification of physical status. *Anesthesiology*. 1963;24(1):111.

12

Vital Signs

Lisa B. Johnson, RDH, MSDH

CHAPTER OUTLINE

INTRODUCTION
I. Patient Preparation and Instruction
II. Dental Hygiene Care Planning

BODY TEMPERATURE
I. Indications for Taking the Temperature
II. Maintenance of Body Temperature
III. Methods of Determining Temperature
IV. Care of Patient with Temperature Elevation

PULSE
I. Maintenance of Normal Pulse
II. Procedure for Determining Pulse Rate

RESPIRATION
I. Maintenance of Normal Respirations
II. Procedures for Observing Respirations

BLOOD PRESSURE
I. Components of Blood Pressure
II. Factors That Influence Blood Pressure
III. Equipment for Determining Blood Pressure
IV. Procedure for Determining Blood Pressure
V. Hypertension (High Blood Pressure)
VI. Blood Pressure Follow-up Criteria

DOCUMENTATION
EVERYDAY ETHICS
FACTORS TO TEACH THE PATIENT
REFERENCES

LEARNING OBJECTIVES

After studying this chapter, the student will be able to:

1. List and explain the vital signs and why proper assessment is key to identifying the patient's health status.

2. Demonstrate and explain the correct procedures for assessing the vital signs: temperature, respiration, radial pulse, and blood pressure.

3. Recognize and explain factors that may affect temperature, respiration, pulse, and blood pressure.

4. Describe and evaluate equipment used for assessing temperature and blood pressure.

5. Recognize normal vital signs across varied age groups.

INTRODUCTION

Determination of four vital signs—*body temperature, pulse, respiratory rates,* and *blood pressure*—is considered standard procedure in patient care. Table 12-1 summarizes the normal values of the four basic vital signs for infant through older adults.

I. Patient Preparation and Instruction

◆ Seat patient in upright position, at eye level for instruction.

◆ Explain the vital signs and obtain consent.

◆ Explain how vital signs can affect dental hygiene and dental treatment.

◆ During the process, explain each step as needed by the individual patient (Box 12-1).

II. Dental Hygiene Care Planning

◆ Recording vital signs contributes to the proper systemic evaluation of a patient in conjunction with the complete medical history.

◆ Dental hygiene care planning and appointment sequencing are directly influenced by the findings.

TABLE 12-1 • Resting Vital Sign Ranges Infant through Older Adult[10,14,15]

AGE (RANGE)	TEMPERATURE (°F)	PULSE (BPM)	RESPIRATION (RPM)	BLOOD PRESSURE (mm Hg)	
				SYSTOLIC	DIASTOLIC
12 mo	99.4–99.7	80–160	30–60	80–89	34–42
1–2 y	99–99.7	80–130	24–40	84–91	39–47
4–5 y	98.6–99	80–120	22–34	88–96	47–56
6–11 y	98–98.6	75–110	18–30	91–107	53–63
≥13 y	97–99	60–90	12–20	104–120	60–80
Adult	97–99	60–100	12–20	90–120	60–80
Older adult (>60)	97–99	60–100	12–20	90–120	60–80

Children and adolescent blood pressure recommendations are based on recently revised guidelines from the USDHHS 4th Report on Diagnosis, Evaluation, and Treatment of Blood Pressure in Children and Adolescents.

◆ When vital signs are not within normal, advise the patient check with the primary care provider.

◆ Referral for medical evaluation and treatment is indicated.

BODY TEMPERATURE

While preparing the patient history and making the extraoral and intraoral examinations, the need for taking the temperature may become apparent, or the dentist may have requested the procedure in conjunction with current oral disease.

I. Indications for Taking the Temperature

◆ For the new patient's initial permanent record along with all vital signs.

◆ For complete examination during a continuing care appointment.

◆ When oral infection is known to be present.
  • Necrotizing ulcerative gingivitis or periodontitis.
  • Apical or periodontal abscess.
  • Acute pericoronitis.

◆ With other vital signs, prior to administration of local anesthetic.

◆ At any appointment when the patient reports illness or there is a suspected infection.
  • Protection of the health of the healthcare personnel and patients or families who may be exposed secondarily.
  • Special significance during epidemics when community exposures are at risk.
  • For patient's referral for medical care when indicated.

II. Maintenance of Body Temperature

◆ *Normal*
  • *Adults:* The normal average temperature is 98.6°F (37°C). The normal range is from 97 to 99°F (36.1–37.2°C).

  • *Older adults:* Over 70 years of age, the average temperature is slightly lower (96.8°F, 36°C).
  • *Children:* There is no appreciable difference between boys and girls. Average temperatures are as follows:
    • First year—99.1°F (37.3°C).
    • Fourth year—99.4°F (37.5°C).
    • Fifth year—98.6°F (37°C).
    • Twelfth year—98°F (36.7°C).

◆ *Temperature variations*
  • *Fever (pyrexia):* values over 99.5°F (37.5°C).
  • *Hyperthermia:* values over 104°F (40°C).
  • *Hypothermia:* values below 96°F (35.5°C).

◆ *Factors that alter body temperature*
  • *Time of day:* highest in late afternoon and early evening; lowest during sleep and early morning.
  • *Temporary increase:* exercise, hot drinks, smoking, or application of external heat.
  • *Pathologic states:* infection, dehydration, hyperthyroidism, myocardial infarction, or tissue injury from trauma.
  • *Decrease:* starvation, hemorrhage, or physiologic shock.

III. Methods of Determining Temperature

A. Locations for Measurement

◆ *Oral:* most common site due to ease of access.
  • Drinking hot or cold liquids just prior can affect results; wait at least 15 minutes before oral measurement is taken.
  • Not recommended for infants, young children, and unconscious or highly behavioral patients.

◆ *Temporal artery (forehead):* measurements taken with electronic device; easily tolerated and results comparable to oral thermometers.

◆ *Ear:* with a tympanic device.

◆ *Medical/hospital applications:* also use axilla or rectum for assessment.

B. Types of Thermometers

◆ *Electronic thermometer* (Figure 12-1A)
  • Cover with disposable protective sheath.
  • Place under tongue; short time required.
  • Read on the digital display.
◆ *Tympanic thermometer* (Figure 12-1B)
  • Cover with protective sheath.
  • Insert gently into ear canal.
  • Short exposure (2–5 seconds) before reading appears on digital unit.
◆ *Temporal artery thermometer* (Figure 12-1C)
  • Measures the temperature of the skin over the temporal artery on the head.
  • Place the scanner on the center of the forehead, midway between the eyebrow and hairline.
  • Slide the thermometer across the forehead until the hairline is reached.
  • Read the temperature on the display.
  • Replace the protective cap.
  • More accurate in infants than the tympanic thermometer.

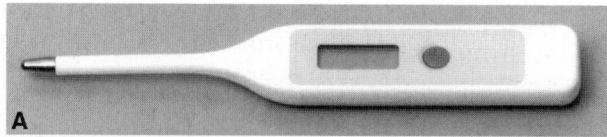

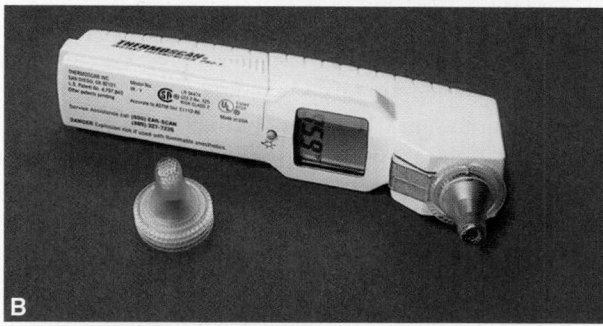

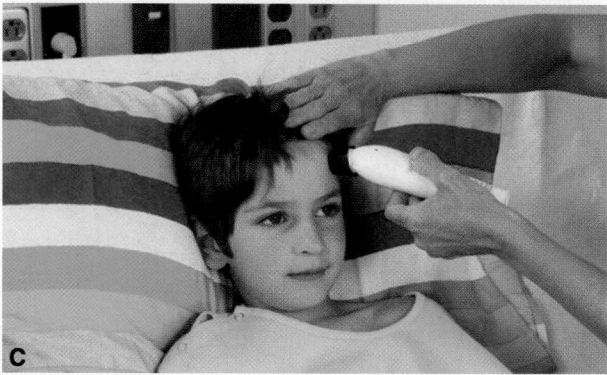

FIGURE 12-1 • **Types of Thermometers. A:** Electronic thermometer. **B:** Tympanic membrane thermometer. **C:** Temporal artery thermometer. (**A**, Reprinted from Springhouse. *Nursing Procedures.* 4th ed. Philadelphia, PA: Lippincott Williams & Wilkins; 2006; **B, C**, Reprinted from Lynn P. *Taylor's Clinical Nursing Skills.* 3rd ed. Philadelphia, PA: Lippincott Williams & Wilkins; 2010.)

IV. Care of Patient with Temperature Elevation

◆ *Temperature over 104°F (40°C)*[1,2]
  • Treat as a medical emergency.
  • Transport to a hospital for medical care.
◆ *Temperature 99.6–104°F (37.6–40°C)*[1]
  • Check possible temporary causes of pyrexia, such as hot beverage or smoking; observe patient while repeating the determination.
  • Review the dental and medical history.
  • Postpone elective oral care when there are signs of respiratory infection or other possible communicable disease.

PULSE

◆ The pulse is the intermittent throbbing sensation felt when the fingers are pressed against an artery.
◆ It is the result of the alternate expansion and contraction of an artery as a wave of blood is forced out from the heart.
◆ The pulse rate or heart rate is the count of the heartbeats.
◆ Irregularities of strength, rhythm, and quality of the pulse are noted while counting the pulse rate.

I. Maintenance of Normal Pulse

A. Normal Pulse Rates

◆ *Adults*: There is no absolute normal. The adult range is 60–100 beats per minute (BPM), slightly higher for women than for men.
◆ *Children*: The pulse or heart rate falls steadily during childhood.

B. Factors That Influence Pulse Rate

An unusually fast heartbeat (over 100 BPM in an adult) is called tachycardia; an unusually slow heartbeat (below 50 BPM) is bradycardia.

◆ *Increased pulse*: caused by exercise, stimulants, eating, strong emotions, extremes of heat and cold, and some forms of heart disease.
◆ *Decreased pulse*: caused by sleep, depressants, fasting, quiet emotions, and low vitality from prolonged illness.
◆ *Emergency situations*: listed in Tables 9-3 and 9-4 in Chapter 9.

II. Procedure for Determining Pulse Rate

◆ *Sequence*
  • The pulse rate is obtained following the body temperature.
◆ *Sites*
  • The pulse may be felt at several points over the body.
  • *Radial pulse*: at the wrist (Figure 12-2).

- Other sites convenient for use in a dental office or clinic are the *temporal* artery on the side of the head in front of the ear, or the *facial* artery at the border of the mandible.
- *Carotid pulse*: used during cardiopulmonary resuscitation for an adult.
- *Brachial pulse*: used for an infant (Figure 12-2).

◆ *Prepare the patient*

1. Tell the patient what is to be done.
2. Have the patient in a comfortable position with arm and hand supported, palm down.
3. Locate the radial pulse on the thumb side of the wrist with the tips of the first three fingers (Figure 12-3). Do not use the thumb because it contains a pulse that may be confused with the patient's pulse.

◆ *Count and record*

1. When the pulse is felt, exert light pressure and count for 1 clocked minute. Use the second hand of a watch or clock. Check with a repeat count when there is a question about rate or quality of pulse.
2. While taking the pulse, observe the following:
   - Rhythm: regular, regularly irregular, irregularly irregular.
   - Volume and strength: full, strong, poor, weak, thready.
3. Record the date, pulse rate as BPM, with other characteristics in patient's record. Document BPM

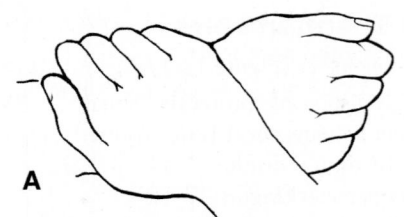
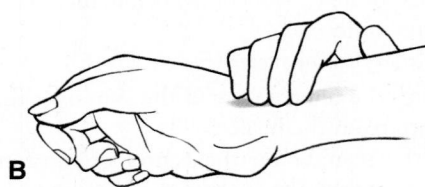

FIGURE 12-3 • Determination of Pulse Rate. A: Correct position of hands. **B:** The tips of the clinician's first three fingers are placed over the radial pulse located on the thumb side of the ventral surface of the wrist.

reading prior to administering local anesthesia (see Chapter 36) when included in the care plan.

- A pulse rate over 100 is considered abnormal for an adult and requires further investigation before proceeding with dental treatment.

RESPIRATION

◆ The function of respiration is to supply oxygen to the tissues and to eliminate carbon dioxide.

◆ Variations in normal respirations may be shown by such characteristics as the rate, rhythm, depth, and quality and may be symptomatic of disease or emergency states.

I. Maintenance of Normal Respirations

A respiration is one breath taken in and let out.

◆ *Normal respiratory rate*
   - *Children*: The respiratory rate decreases steadily during childhood.[3]
   - *Adults*: The adult range is from 12 to 20/min, slightly higher for women.
   - *Older Adults*: Respiratory rate has been shown to have a higher predictive value for serious adverse events and should be considered an important component of vital sign assessment.[4]

◆ *Factors that influence respirations.*

◆ Many of the same factors that influence pulse rate also influence the number of respirations. A rate below 12/min (bradypnea) is considered subnormal for an adult, rate over 28 is accelerated (tachypnea), and rates over 60 are extremely rapid and dangerous.

◆ *Increased respiration*: caused by work and exercise, excitement, nervousness, strong emotions, pain, hemorrhage, and shock.

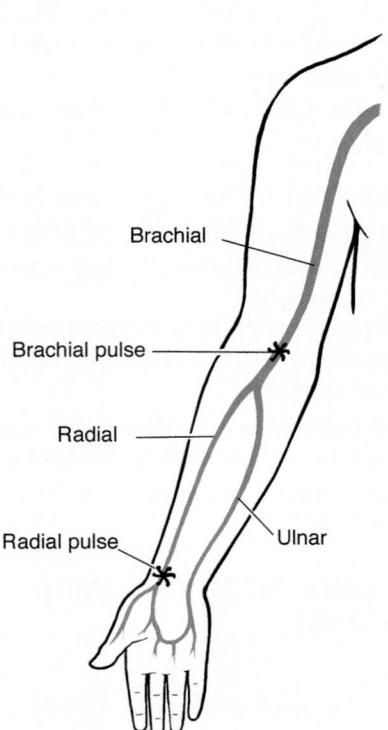

FIGURE 12-2 • Arteries of the Arm. Note the location of the radial pulse. The brachial pulse may be felt just before the brachial artery branches into the radial and ulnar arteries.

Brachial

Brachial pulse

Radial

Radial pulse

Ulnar

◆ *Decreased respiration*: caused by sleep, certain drugs, pulmonary insufficiency, apnea.

◆ *Emergency situations*: such as anoxia are included in Chapter 9.

II. Procedures for Observing Respirations

◆ *Determine rate*

1. Make the count of respirations immediately after counting the pulse.

2. Maintain the fingers over the radial pulse.

3. Respirations must be counted so that the patient is not aware, as the rate may be voluntarily altered.

4. Count the number of times the chest rises in 1 clocked minute. It is not necessary to count both inspirations and expirations.

◆ *Factors to observe*

• *Depth*: Describe as shallow, normal, or deep.

• *Rhythm*: Describe as regular (evenly spaced) or irregular (with pauses of irregular lengths between).

• *Quality*: Describe as strong, easy, weak, or labored (noisy). Poor quality may have an effect on body color; for example, a bluish tinge of the face or nail beds may mean an insufficiency of oxygen.

• *Sounds*: Describe deviant sounds made during inspiration, expiration, or both.

• *Position of patient*: When the patient assumes an unusual position to secure comfort during breathing or prefers to remain seated upright, mark records accordingly.

◆ *Record*

Record all findings in the patient's record.

BLOOD PRESSURE

I. Components of Blood Pressure

◆ *Blood pressure is the force exerted by the blood on the blood vessel walls.*

• When the left ventricle of the heart contracts, blood is forced out into the aorta and travels through the large arteries to the smaller arteries, arterioles, and capillaries. The vessels of the heart are shown in Chapter 61.

• The pulsations extend from the heart through the arteries and disappear in the arterioles.

• During the course of the cardiac cycle, the blood pressure is changing constantly.

◆ **Systole Phase**

• The systole phase occurs during ventricular contraction. It is measured as systolic pressure. It is the peak or the highest pressure exerted by the heart during contraction.

• The normal systolic pressure for an adult is less than 120 mm Hg.

◆ *Diastole* **Phase**

• Diastolic pressure is the lowest pressure. It is the effect of ventricular relaxation.

• The normal diastolic pressure for an adult is less than 80 mm Hg.

◆ **Pulse Pressure**

• The pulse pressure is the difference between the systolic and diastolic pressures.

II. Factors That Influence Blood Pressure

◆ Blood pressure depends on the following:

• Force of the heartbeat (energy of the heart).

• Peripheral resistance; condition of the arteries; changes in elasticity of vessels, which may occur with age and disease.

• Volume of blood in the circulatory system.

◆ *Factors that increase blood pressure*

• Exercise, eating, stimulants, and emotional disturbance.[5]

• Use of oral contraceptives; blood pressure increases with age and length of use.[6,7]

◆ *Factors that decrease blood pressure*

• Fasting, rest, depressants, and quiet emotions.

• Such emergencies as fainting, blood loss, shock (Tables 9-3 and 9-4, Chapter 9).

III. Equipment for Determining Blood Pressure

A sphygmomanometer is made up of a pressure-measuring device (manometer) and an inflatable cuff to wrap around the arm or under certain circumstances, the leg.

◆ *Mercury sphygmomanometer (analog)*

• Traditional system, but mercury is a potential health hazard because of mercury spillage and is less commonly used.[8,9]

• Has shown to be more accurate and consistent than other types.

◆ *Aneroid sphygmomanometer (analog)*

• Compact, portable glass-enclosed gauge with needle for registration of blood pressure.

• Requires regular calibration to keep accurate.

◆ *Electronic sphygmomanometer (digital)*

• Automatic determination of blood pressure without use of stethoscope.

• Size: Choosing the correct size cuff (see Figure 12-4) is critical to accurate blood pressure results.

• The cuff needs to be long enough to encircle 80% of the arm and wide enough to encircle 40% of the arm at its midpoint.[10] A longer, wider cuff is required for obese or muscular individuals and children require pediatric-sized cuffs.[11] Always refer to the recommended cuff sizes for accuracy of readings (Figure 12-5).

◆ *Wrist or finger devices*

• Considered to be less accurate.[8]

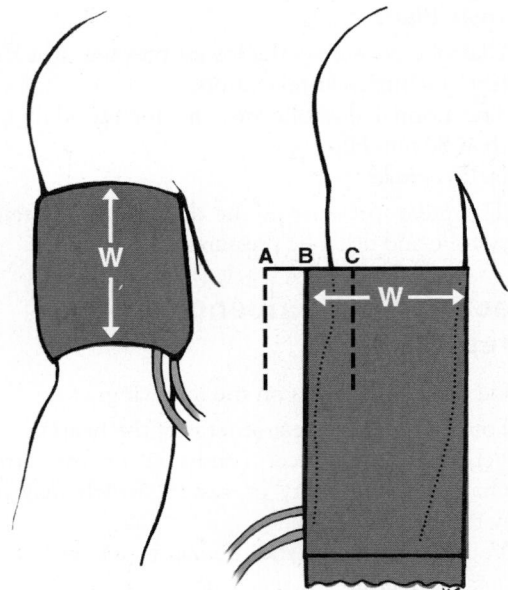

FIGURE 12-4 • Selection of Cuff Size. The correct width (W) is 20% greater than the diameter of the arm where applied. **A:** Too wide. **B:** Correct width. **C:** Too narrow.

◆ *Stethoscope*
   • Consists of an endpiece that has a flat diaphragm on one side and (may or may not have) a smaller, concave-shaped bell side. Both sides transmit and send sound through tubes to the earpieces.

IV. Procedure for Determining Blood Pressure

◆ *Prepare patient*
   1. Tell patient briefly what is to be done. Detailed explanations need to be avoided because they may excite the patient and change the blood pressure.
   2. Seat patient comfortably, with the arm slightly flexed, with palm up, and with the whole forearm supported on a *level surface at the level of the heart.*[10]
      • Arm above heart will result in a false low reading.[8]
      • Arm below heart level will result in false high reading.[8]
      • Improper cuff selection will result in false high or low depending on size.[8,10,12]
   3. Use either arm unless otherwise indicated, for example, handicap, history of vascular surgery or mastectomy would indicate arm on opposite side be used. Repeat blood pressure determinations need to be made on the same arm because a variation in pressure may exist between arms.[8,10,12]
   4. Take pressure on bare arm, not over clothing.[8,12] Loosen a tight sleeve.
   5. Select cuff size as described in Figure 12-5.
◆ *Apply cuff*
   1. Apply the completely deflated cuff to the patient's arm, supported at the level of the heart. If the arm rests on the arm of a dental chair, lower than the

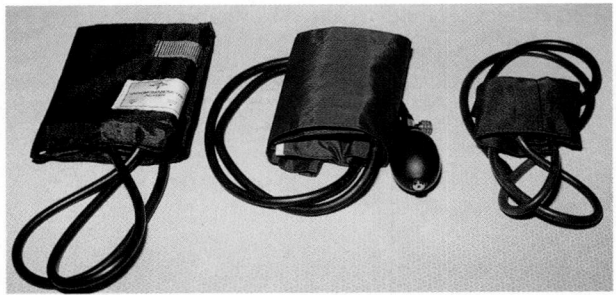

FIGURE 12-5 • Three Sizes of Blood Pressure Cuff. Extra-large, regular, and pediatric cuff.

heart, the diastolic pressure may show a small but significant increase.[8]
   2. Place the portion of the cuff that contains the inflatable bladder directly over the brachial artery. The cuff may have an arrow to show the point that is placed over the artery. The lower edge of the cuff is placed 1 inch above the antecubital fossa (Figure 12-6). Fasten the cuff evenly and snugly.[8]
   3. Adjust the position of the gauge/dial so that it is clearly visible and facing you.
◆ *Locate the radial pulse* (Figures 12-2 and 12-3).
   1. Palpate 1 inch below the antecubital fossa to locate the brachial artery pulse (Figure 12-6).
   2. Hold the fingers on the pulse.
◆ *Determine maximum inflation level (MIL) or estimated systolic* blood pressure.
   1. Close the needle valve (air lock) attached to the hand control bulb firmly but so it may be released readily.
   2. Pump to inflate the cuff until the radial pulse stops. Monitor the gauge to note the level at which the pulse disappears. This is the estimated systolic pressure.
   3. Continue to pump until the gauge reads 30 points beyond where the radial pulse was no longer felt. This is the MIL. It means that the brachial artery is collapsed by the pressure of the cuff and no blood is flowing through. *Unless the MIL is determined, the level to which the cuff is inflated will be arbitrary. Excess pressure can be very uncomfortable for the patient.*[8]
◆ *Position the stethoscope.*
◆ Place the endpiece over the palpated brachial artery, 1 inch below the antecubital fossa, and slightly toward the inner side of the arm (Figures 12-6 and 12-7). Hold lightly in place.
   • Earpieces should be angled forward into the ear canal for proper auscultation (Figure 12-8A and B).
   • Manual stethoscopes can be turned on/off by rotating the endpiece. Power stethoscopes can be turned on/off by the push of a button or tap of the diaphragm.
   • Tap gently and listen to confirm it is on (in active mode).

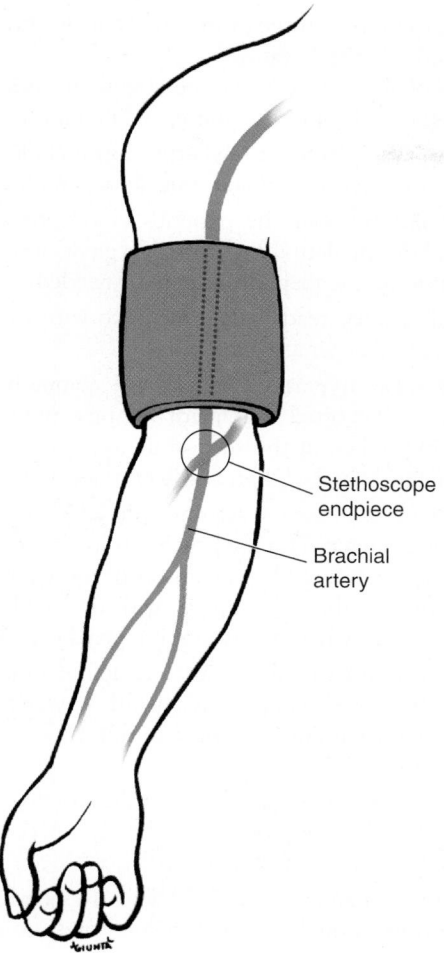

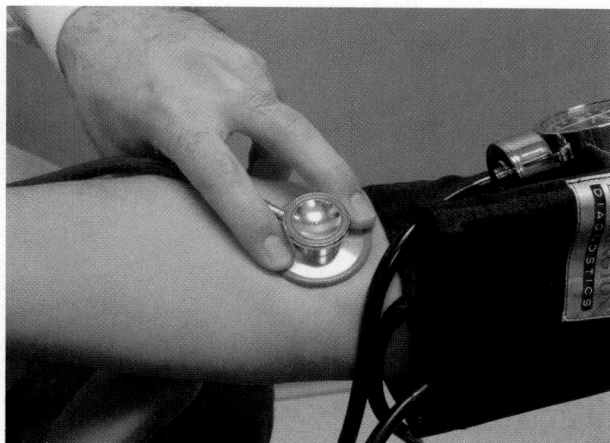

FIGURE 12-7 • **Forearm Properly Supported during Blood Pressure Assessment.**

FIGURE 12-6 • **Blood Pressure Cuff in Position.** The lower edge of the cuff is placed approximately 1 inch above the antecubital fossa. The stethoscope endpiece is placed over the palpated brachial artery pulse point approximately 1 inch below the antecubital fossa and slightly toward the inner side of the arm.

- Diaphragm or bell side of endpiece should be placed with light, steady, and complete contact with skin. Either side of the endpiece can be used for reliable measurement[13] (Figure 12-7).

- Avoid contact with cuff to prevent extraneous sounds that may distract from Korotkoff sounds.
- *Support patient's arm at heart level* (see Figure 12-9). The position of the arm is critical to accuracy and can greatly influence readings. The upper arm raised above the heart can produce a false low reading and when placed below heart level will result in a false high reading.[8,10]
- *Deflate the cuff gradually*
  1. Release the air lock slowly so that the dial drops very gradually and steadily, approximately two to three lines.
  2. Listen for the first Karotkoff sound ("tap tap"). This is the beginning of the flow of blood past the cuff. Note the number on the dial as the *systolic pressure*.
  3. Continue to release the pressure slowly. The sound will continue, first becoming louder, then diminishing and becoming muffled, until finally disappearing. Note the number on the dial where the last distinct tap was heard. That number is the *diastolic pressure*.

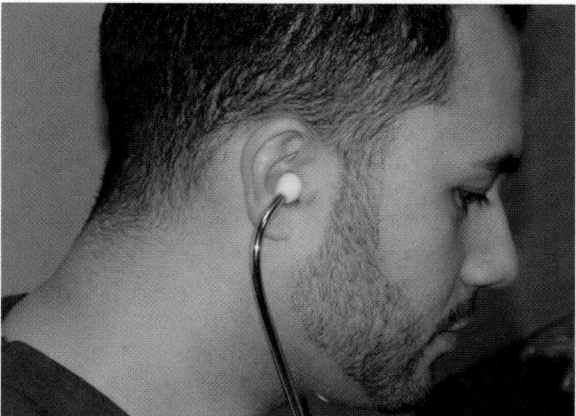

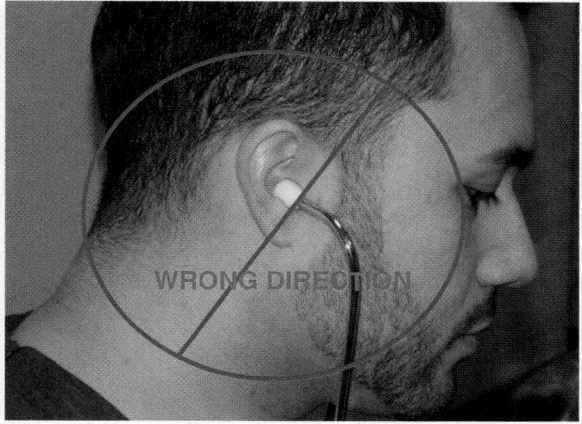

FIGURE 12-8 • **Placement of the Earpieces for the Stethoscope. A:** Proper placement of the earpieces for the stethoscope. **B:** Improper placement.

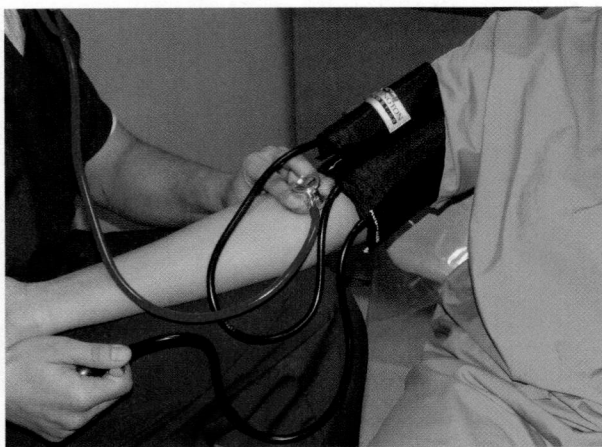

FIGURE 12-9 • Correct Stethoscope Endpiece Placement, Away from Cuff and in Contact with Skin.

4. Release further (about 10 points) until all sounds cease. That is the second diastolic point. In some clinics and hospitals, the last sound is taken as the diastolic pressure.

5. Let the rest of the air out rapidly.

◆ *Repeat for confirmation*
  • Wait 30 seconds before inflating the cuff again.
  • More than one reading is needed within a few minutes to determine an average and ensure a correct reading.

◆ *Record*
  • Write date, arm used, and seated or standing.
  • Record blood pressure as a fraction, for example, 120/80.

V. Hypertension (High Blood Pressure)

Hypertension (HTN) or high blood pressure (HBP) is a serious condition that affects nearly one out of every three individuals in the United States and is the leading cause of death in the United States.[5,8]

◆ HTN of above 140/90 is associated with cardiovascular diseases, stroke, kidney failure, and premature death.[8,10]

◆ Contributing factors to hypertension include smoking, stress, obesity, alcohol and drug abuse, and life style.[5]

◆ Information about the patient's blood pressure is essential during dental and dental hygiene appointments because special adaptations may be needed.

◆ Blood pressure readings are recorded with the medical history and other assessment data.

◆ White-coat hypertension is more common in older adults and reported as frequent among centenarians.[4,6,8] Readings taken at the start of an appointment can be significantly higher than at the end of treatment.[12]

◆ To establish a baseline reading and determine the need for patient referral for medical attention, more than one reading is advised. A comparison of the reading at the beginning of the appointment with one at the close of appointment when the patient is relaxed may be helpful.

◆ Screening for blood pressure in dental practices has been shown to be an effective health service for all ages since many patients are unaware that they have hypertension (see Table 12-2).

◆ Growing evidence indicates that primary hypertension is commonly asymptomatic and often unrecognized in young children and adolescents.[14]

  • Children above 3 years old who are seen in medical settings should have their blood pressure measured annually. Blood pressure should be measured at each dental encounter for children with obesity, renal disease, diabetes, aortic arch obstruction or coarctation or taking medications known to elevate blood pressure.[14]

TABLE 12-2 • Adult Blood Pressure Classifications[14]			
BLOOD PRESSURE CLASSIFICATION	SYSTOLIC (mm Hg)	DIASTOLIC (mm Hg)	RECOMMENDATIONS
Hypotension and Postural Hypotension	<90	<60	Observe for possible light-headedness and syncope. If persistent, referral for evaluation is indicated.
Normal/Normotensive	<120	<80	Proceed as planned.
Elevated Blood Pressure	120–129	<80	Retake after 5 min. If still elevated, inform patient of prehypertension status. Recommend primary care provider consult and encourage life style modifications.
Hypertension			
Stage 1	130–139	80–89	Retake after 5 min. If still elevated, inform patient of elevated blood pressure. Refer for primary care provider consult. Employ stress reduction to routine dental treatment. Modify local anesthetic to 1:100,000 vasoconstrictor.
Stage 2	≥140	≥90	Retake after 5 min. If still elevated, inform patient of elevated blood pressure and refer for primary care provider assessment. Delay dental treatment until hypertension is controlled.
Hypertensive Crisis	>180	>120	Discontinue care and retake BP after 5 min to confirm findings. Refer for immediate medical care/call 911 depending on your clinic protocol.

- Children and adolescent blood pressure should be matched to Guidelines in the *updated* (2017) U.S. Department of Health and Human Services (USDHHS) 4th Report on Diagnosis, Evaluation, and Treatment of Blood Pressure in Children and Adolescents.[14]
  - The USDHHS guidelines use age, sex, and height percentile data to more accurately determine the presence or absence of hypertension in children and adolescents. Updated guidelines of 2017 reflect normal blood pressure tables based on children with normal weight.[14]
- Cardiovascular diseases are described in Chapter 61. That information can be a helpful introduction and is recommended for reading in conjunction with this section on the techniques for obtaining blood pressure.

VI. Blood Pressure Follow-up Criteria

- Dental personnel have an obligation to advise and *refer for further evaluation*.
- Diagnosis of hypertension would never be made or treatment initiated based on an isolated reading.
- Vital signs should be recorded for all new patients, and pre- and postoperatively if medically compromised.
- Rechecking within 1 year is recommended for persons at increased risk for hypertension, such as family history, weight gain, obesity, African American, use of oral contraceptives, smoking, and excessive alcohol consumption (see Tables 12-1 and 12-2).[7,10,14]
- Lifestyle modifications are indicated for all levels of blood pressure classification[5,15] and HBP management should follow current evidence-based management guidelines through collaborative efforts with the patients primary care provider.[14,16] Immediate consultation with a patient's primary care provider is indicated prior to dental or dental hygiene treatment when either reading is more than or equal to 180/110 (Tables 12-2 and 12-3).

DOCUMENTATION[15]

Documentation in the permanent record of a patient with HBP would include the following:

- Carefully document medical history with regular updates at each maintenance appointment.
- Reminder to help patient realize the importance of regularly taking prescribed medication.
- Prepared and documented blood pressure reading at each appointment especially when anesthesia is included in the care plan.
- Box 12-1 contains a sample progress note.

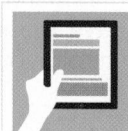

BOX 12-1

Example Documentation:
Vital Signs

S—Mrs. Patel apologized for arriving 5 minutes late and stated she had no concerns at the start of her dental appointment.

O—Vital signs at 9:00 AM; pulse 64; respirations 12; blood pressure (right arm) 190/88 seated.

A—Hypertension stage 3 range.

P—Advised Mrs. Patel her blood pressure is measuring at a high and an unsafe level for treatment. Blood pressure remained elevated when reassessed 10 minutes later. Discussed hypertension range with dentist and referred patient to primary care provider for urgent follow-up. Delay maintenance appointment until hypertension under control. Follow-up later today by phone.

Signed: _____, RDH

Date: _____

TABLE 12-3 • Lifestyle Modifications for Hypertension Management[10]		
MODIFICATION	RECOMMENDATION	APPROXIMATE REDUCTION IN SYSTOLIC BLOOD PRESSURE RANGE
Weight loss	Normal body weight maintenance based on average body mass index	5–20 mm Hg/10 kg weight loss
Dietary approaches to stop hypertension	A diet rich in fruits, vegetables, and low-fat dairy products with reduced saturated and total fat	8–14 mm Hg
Dietary sodium intake	Reduce Na intake to ≤100 mmol/d (2.4 g Na or 6 g NaCl)	2–8 mm Hg
Physical activity	Aerobic activity at least 30 min/d	4–9 mm Hg
Moderate alcohol consumption	Limit to no more than 2 drinks/d for most men and no more than 1 drink/d for women or lighter-weight individuals[a]	2–4 mm Hg

[a]1 oz or 20 mL ethanol, that is, 24 oz beer, 10 oz wine, or 2 oz 80 proof whiskey.

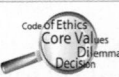

EVERYDAY ETHICS

Gracie was having a very busy day and at 10:15 AM was already late for the 10:00 AM patient, Mr. McElroy, who had arrived early and was waiting in the reception area. While completing his history, to save time, she copied over the blood pressure recording from his previous appointment just 2 weeks ago. It had been 130/83, only slightly into the prehypertension level.

The appointment was planned for the maxillary left quadrant with anesthesia. After the scaling was complete and Mr. McElroy was climbing out of the dental chair, looking a bit unsteady as he stood up, he casually remarked: "I just remembered while you were working that my Doc gave me a new prescription—I suppose I should have told you

before. But it is only one pill a day—for keeping the blood pressure down. I don't have any trouble anyway, he just wanted to be sure."

Questions for Consideration

1. Explain how the principles of beneficence and maleficence apply to Gracie's actions with Mr. McElroy's examination and charting procedures.

2. How has Gracie placed the office at risk for a possible medical emergency given Mr. McElroy's physical status? Answer by describing the rights and duties of both the hygienist and the patient.

3. Who is responsible for ensuring that accurate documentation has been completed on all patients, from an ethical and a quality assurance perspective?

Factors to Teach the Patient

▶ How vital signs can influence dental and dental hygiene appointments.

▶ The importance of having a blood pressure determination at regular intervals.

▶ For the patient diagnosed as hypertensive, encourage regular continuing use of prescription drugs for control of HBP.

▶ Encourage healthy lifestyle changes such as tobacco cessation, drug and/or alcohol counseling, exercise, and healthy dietary habits (see Table 12-3).

ENHANCE YOUR UNDERSTANDING

ONLINE RESOURCES
(see the inside front cover for access information)

· Audio glossary

· Appendices

SUPPORT FOR LEARNING
(available separately)

· *Active Learning Workbook for Wilkins' Clinical Practice of the Dental Hygienist, 13th Edition*

INDIVIDUALIZED REVIEW

· Customized practice quizzing with Navigate 2 TestPrep for *Wilkins' Clinical Practice of the Dental Hygienist*

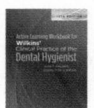

References

1. MayoClinic. Thermometers: understand the options. 2017. https://www.mayoclinic.org/diseases-conditions/fever/in-depth/thermometers/art-20046737. Accessed April 23, 2019.

2. MedlinePlus. Temperature measurement. 2017. https://medlineplus.gov/ency/article/003400.htm. Accessed April 23, 2019.

3. Fleming S, Thompson M, Stevens R, et al. Normal ranges of heart rate and respiratory rate in children from birth to 18 years of age: a systematic review of observational studies. *Lancet.* 2011;377:1011.

4. Chester JG, Rudolph JL. Vital signs in older patients: age-related changes. *J Am Med Dir Assoc.* 2011;12:337-343.

5. U.S. Preventive Services Task Force; Grossman DC, Bibbins-Domingo K, Curry SJ, et al. Behavioral counseling to promote a healthful diet and physical activity for cardiovascular disease prevention in adults without cardiovascular risk factors: U.S. Preventive Services Task Force recommendation statement. *JAMA.* 2017;318:167-174.

6. Aronow WS, Fleg JL, Pepine CJ, et al. ACCF/AHA 2011 expert consensus document on hypertension in the elderly: a Report of the American College of Cardiology Foundation Task Force on Clinical Expert Consensus Documents Developed in Collaboration with the American Academy of Neurology, American Geriatrics Society, American Society for Preventive Cardiology, American Society of Hypertension, American Society of Nephrology. *J Am Soc Hypertens.* 2011;5:259.

7. American Heart Association. High blood pressure and women. 2016. https://www.heart.org/en/health-topics/high-blood-pressure/why-high-blood-pressure-is-a-silent-killer/high-blood-pressure-and-women. Accessed April 23, 2019.

8. Pickering TG, Hall JE, Appel LJ, et al. Recommendations for blood pressure measurement in humans and experimental animals: part 1: blood pressure measurement in humans: a statement for professionals from the Subcommittee of

Professional and Public Education of the American Heart Association Council on High Blood Pressure Research. *Hypertension*. 2005;45:142.

9. Herman WW, Konzelman JL Jr, Prisant LM. New national guidelines on hypertension: a summary for dentistry. *J Am Dent Assoc*. 2004;135:576.

10. Chobanian AV, Bakris GL, Black HR, et al. Seventh report of the Joint National Committee on Prevention, Detection, Evaluation, and Treatment of High Blood Pressure. *Hypertension*. 2003;42:1206.

11. U.S. Department of Health and Human Services. The fourth report on the diagnosis, evaluation, and treatment of high blood pressure in children and adolescents. 2013:60. https://www.nhlbi.nih.gov/files/docs/resources/heart/hbp_ped.pdf. Accessed April 23, 2019.

12. Kallioinen N, Hill A, Horswill MS, Ward HE, Watson MO. Sources of inaccuracy in the measurement of adult patients' resting blood pressure in clinical settings: a systematic review. *J Hypertens*. 2017;35:421-441.

13. Kantola I, Vesalainen R, Kangassalo K, Kariluoto A. Bell or diaphragm in the measurement of blood pressure? *J Hypertens*. 2005;23:499-503.

14. Flynn JT, Kaelber DC, Baker-Smith CM, et al. Clinical practice guideline for screening and management of high blood pressure in children and adolescents. *Pediatrics*. 2017;140.

15. Centers for Disease Control and Prevention. High blood pressure fact sheet | Data & statistics | DHDSP | CDC. 2014. https://www.cdc.gov/dhdsp/data_statistics/fact_sheets/fs_bloodpressure.htm. Accessed April 23, 2019.

16. James PA, Oparil S, Carter BL, et al. 2014 Evidence-based guideline for the management of high blood pressure in adults: report from the panel members appointed to the eighth joint national committee (jnc 8). *JAMA*. 2014;311:507-520.

17. Bader JD, Bonito AJ, Shugars DA. A systematic review of cardiovascular effects of epinephrine on hypertensive dental patients. *Oral Surg Oral Med Oral Pathol Oral Radiol Endod*. 2002;93:647.

Extraoral and Intraoral Examination

Lisa B. Johnson, RDH, MSDH

CHAPTER OUTLINE

RATIONALE FOR THE EXTRAORAL AND INTRAORAL EXAMINATION

COMPONENTS OF EXAMINATION
   I. Types of Examinations
   II. Methods for Examination
   III. Signs and Symptoms
   IV. Preparation for Examination

ANATOMIC LANDMARKS OF THE ORAL CAVITY
   I. Oral Mucosa

SEQUENCE OF EXAMINATION
   I. Extraoral Examination
   II. Intraoral Examination
   III. Documentation of Findings

MORPHOLOGIC CATEGORIES
   I. Elevated Lesions
   II. Depressed Lesions
   III. Flat Lesions
   IV. Other Descriptive Terms

ORAL CANCER
   I. Location
   II. Appearance of Early Cancer

CLINICAL RECOMMENDATIONS FOR EVALUATION OF ORAL LESIONS
   I. Biopsy

DOCUMENTATION

EVERYDAY ETHICS

FACTORS TO TEACH THE PATIENT

REFERENCES

LEARNING OBJECTIVES

After studying this chapter, the student will be able to:

1. Explain the rationale for a comprehensive extra- and intraoral examination.

2. Explain the systematic sequence of the extra- and intraoral examination.

3. Identify normal hard and soft tissue anatomy of the head, neck, and oral cavity.

4. Describe and document physical characteristics (size, shape, color, texture, and consistency) and morphologic categories (elevated, flat, and depressed lesions) for notable findings.

5. Identify suspected conditions that require follow-up and referral for medical evaluation.

RATIONALE FOR THE EXTRAORAL AND INTRAORAL EXAMINATION

The extra- and intraoral examination is performed for early identification of abnormalities and pathologies, especially oral cancer.

Although an essential goal of the examination is to detect cancer of the mouth at the earliest possible stage, a thorough examination may also reveal signs of thyroid disorders, eating disorders, nutritional deficiencies, sexually transmitted diseases, and a host of systemic conditions.

COMPONENTS OF EXAMINATION

- The standard of patient care is that the total patient is being treated, not only the oral cavity, and particularly not just the teeth and immediate surrounding tissues.
- The examination is all-inclusive to detect possible physical or psychological influences on the patient's oral health.
- Thorough examination is essential for each continuing care appointment so that the treatment for the control and prevention of oral diseases will be effective.
- Assessment of health-related risk factors such as[1]:
  - History of previous cancer
  - Family history of squamous cell carcinoma (SCC)
  - Tobacco.
  - Alcohol use.
  - Cultural and genetic susceptibility.
  - Sun exposure and lack of use of sun protection.
  - Diet.
  - Certain surgeries such as organ or bone marrow transplant and subsequent long-term immunosuppressive medications.
  - Sexual behaviors involving orogenital contact may increase the risk of human papillomavirus (HPV) transmission.[2]

I. Types of Examinations

- *Complete*
  - A complete examination includes a thorough summary of all the components of the assessment.
  - The extra- and intraoral examination is a component of a patient's complete assessment and is performed for all new patients and at each routine continuing care visit.
- *Screening*
  - Screening implies a brief, preliminary examination, usually for a particular purpose such as pain relief or for initial patient assessment and triage to determine priorities for treatment.
- *Limited examination*
  - A type of brief examination made for an emergency situation. It may be used in the management of an acute condition.
- *Follow-up*
  - Brief follow-up examination to check healing following a treatment.

- *Continuing care/reevaluation*
  - After a specific period of time following the completion of the care plan and the anticipated restoration to health.
  - A continuing care examination is a complete reassessment from which a new dental hygiene diagnosis and care plan are derived.

II. Methods for Examination

The extra- and intraoral examination is accomplished by various visual and tactile, manual, and instrumental methods. Patient position, optimum lighting, and effective retraction for accessibility and visibility contribute to the accuracy and completeness of the examination.

- *Visual examination*
  - *Direct observation:* Visual observation is carried out in a systematic sequence to note surface appearance (color, contour, size) and to observe movement and other evidence of function.
  - *Radiographic examination:* The use of radiographs can reveal deviations from normal not observable by direct vision.
  - *Transillumination:* A strong light directed through a soft tissue or a tooth to enhance examination is useful for detecting irregularities of the teeth and locating calculus. Hold the mouth mirror to view from the lingual to see the translucency.
- *Palpation*
  - Palpation is examination using the sense of touch through tissue manipulation or pressure on an area with the gloved fingers of one hand or both.
  - *Digital:* The use of a single finger. Example: index finger applied to the lingual side of the mandible beneath the canine and premolar area to determine presence of a torus mandibularis.
  - *Bidigital:* The use of finger and thumb of same hand. Example: palpation of the lips (Figure 13-1).
  - *Bimanual:* The use of finger or fingers and thumb from each hand applied simultaneously in coordination.

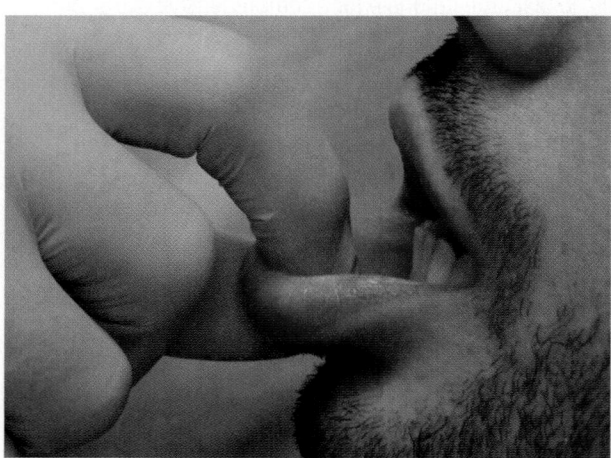

FIGURE 13-1 • Palpation of the Lip to Illustrate the Use of a Finger and Thumb of the Same Hand.

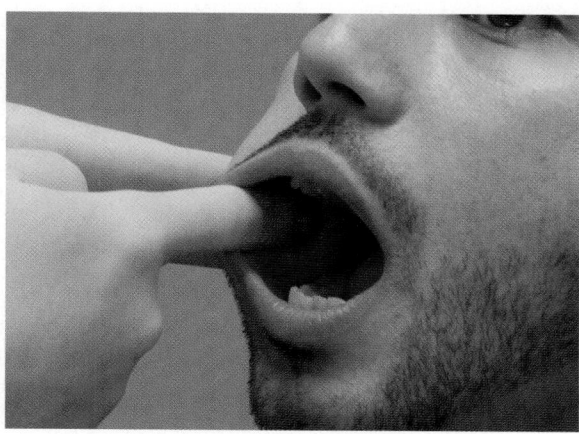
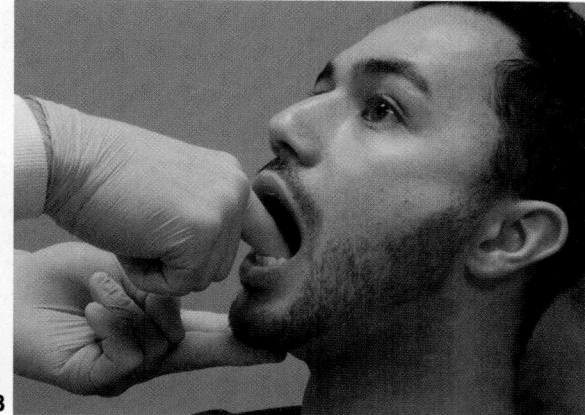

FIGURE 13-2 • Bimanual Palpation. A: Examination of the buccal mucosa by simultaneous palpation extraorally and intraorally. **B:** Examination of the floor of the mouth by simultaneous palpation with fingers of each hand in apposition.

Example: index finger of one hand palpates on the floor of the mouth inside, while a finger or fingers from the other hand press on the same area from under the chin externally (Figure 13-2A and B).
- *Bilateral:* Two hands are used at the same time to examine corresponding structures on opposite sides of the body. Comparisons can be made. Example: fingers placed beneath the chin to palpate the submandibular lymph nodes (Figure 13-3).
◆ *Instrumentation*
- Examination instruments, such as a periodontal probe and an explorer, are used for specific examination of the teeth and periodontal tissues.
◆ *Percussion*
- Percussion is the act of tapping a surface or tooth with the fingers or an instrument.
- Information about the status of health is determined either by the response of the patient or by the sound. When a tooth is known to be sensitive in any way, percussion needs to be avoided.

◆ *Electrical test*
- An electric pulp tester may be used to detect the presence or absence of vital pulp tissue.
- Methods for use of a pulp tester are described in Chapter 16.
◆ *Auscultation*
- Auscultation is the use of sound.
- Example: The sound of clicking of the temporomandibular joint when the jaw is opened and closed. Figure 13-4 shows examination of the temporomandibular joint.

III. Signs and Symptoms

◆ A specific objective for patient examination as a part of the complete assessment is the recognition of deviations from normal that may be signs or symptoms of disease.
◆ General signs and symptoms may occur in various disease conditions. Example: Fever, or increase in body temperature accompanies most infections.

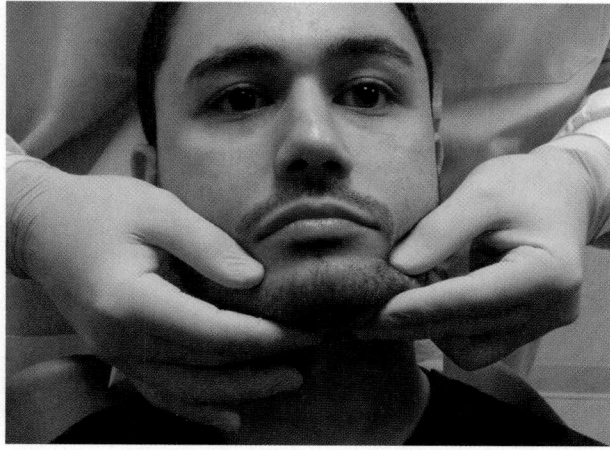

FIGURE 13-3 • Bilateral Palpation. Bilateral palpation is used to examine corresponding structures on opposite sides of the body.

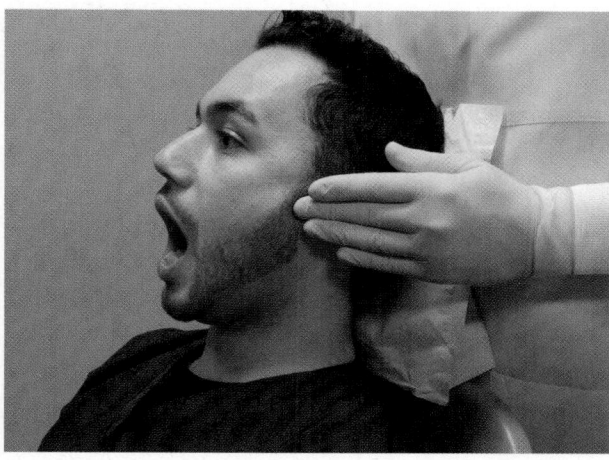

FIGURE 13-4 • Assessment of the Temporomandibular Joint. The joint is palpated as the patient opens and closes the mouth.

◆ A *pathognomonic* sign or symptom is unique to a disease and may be used to distinguish that condition from other diseases or conditions.

A. Signs

◆ A sign is any abnormality identified by a healthcare professional while examining a patient.

◆ A sign is an *objective symptom*. Examples of signs include observable changes such as color, shape, consistency, or abnormal findings revealed using a probe, explorer, radiograph, or other instrument for disease detection.

B. Symptoms

◆ A symptom is any departure from normal that may be indicative of disease.

◆ It is a subjective abnormality that can be observed by the patient.

◆ Examples are pain, tenderness, and bleeding when toothbrushing as described by the patient.

IV. Preparation for Examination

◆ Review the patient's health histories and dental/medical record, including risk factors, radiographs, dental caries, periodontal, and oral cancer risk assessments.

◆ Examine dental radiographs.

◆ Explain the procedures to be performed and relevance of the procedures.

- Example: "I am going to perform an extra-/intraoral examination to look for abnormalities that can affect your oral and overall health."

- Patients understanding the rationale for an extra- and intraoral examination is critical to acceptance and education.

- When a patient is wearing a scarf or other head/neck covering for cultural or religious purposes, the dental hygienist uses culturally sensitive communication skills (Chapter 3).

ANATOMIC LANDMARKS OF THE ORAL CAVITY

Familiarization with structures (Figures 13-5 through 13-7) and normal anatomy is a prerequisite to understanding abnormal presentations in the head and neck region.[1-3]

I. Oral Mucosa

The lining of the oral cavity, the oral mucosa, is a mucous membrane composed of connective tissue covered with stratified squamous epithelium. There are three divisions or categories of oral mucosa.

A. Masticatory Mucosa

◆ Covers the *gingiva* and *hard palate*, the areas most used during the mastication of food.

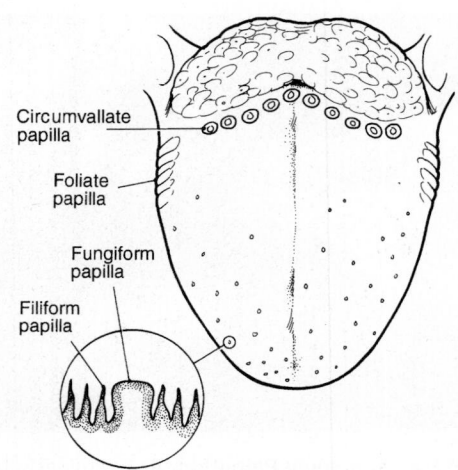

FIGURE 13-5 • Papillae of the Tongue.

◆ Except for the free margin of the gingiva, the masticatory mucosa is firmly attached to underlying tissues.

◆ The normal epithelial covering is keratinized.

B. Lining Mucosa

◆ Covers the inner surfaces of the lips and cheeks, floor of the mouth, underside of the tongue, soft palate, and alveolar mucosa.

◆ These tissues are not firmly attached to underlying tissue.

◆ The epithelial covering is not keratinized.

C. Specialized Mucosa

◆ Covers the dorsum (upper surface) of the tongue.

◆ Composed of many papillae; some contain taste buds.

◆ The distribution of the four types of papillae is shown in Figure 13-5.

- *Filiform:* threadlike keratinized elevations that cover the dorsal surface of the tongue; they are the most numerous of the papillae.

- *Fungiform:* mushroom-shaped papillae interspersed among the filiform papillae on the tip and sides of the tongue, appear redder than the filiform papillae and contain variable numbers of taste buds. The inset enlargement in Figure 13-5 shows the comparative shape and size of the filiform and fungiform papillae.

- *Circumvallate (vallate):* the 10–14 large round papillae arranged in a "V" between the body of the tongue and the base. Taste buds line the walls.

- *Foliate:* vertical grooves on the lateral posterior sides of the tongue; also contain taste buds.

SEQUENCE OF EXAMINATION

◆ Conducting an examination with routine order will minimize the possibility of excluding areas and overlooking details of importance. A systematic sequence improves efficiency, promotes professionalism, and inspires patient confidence.

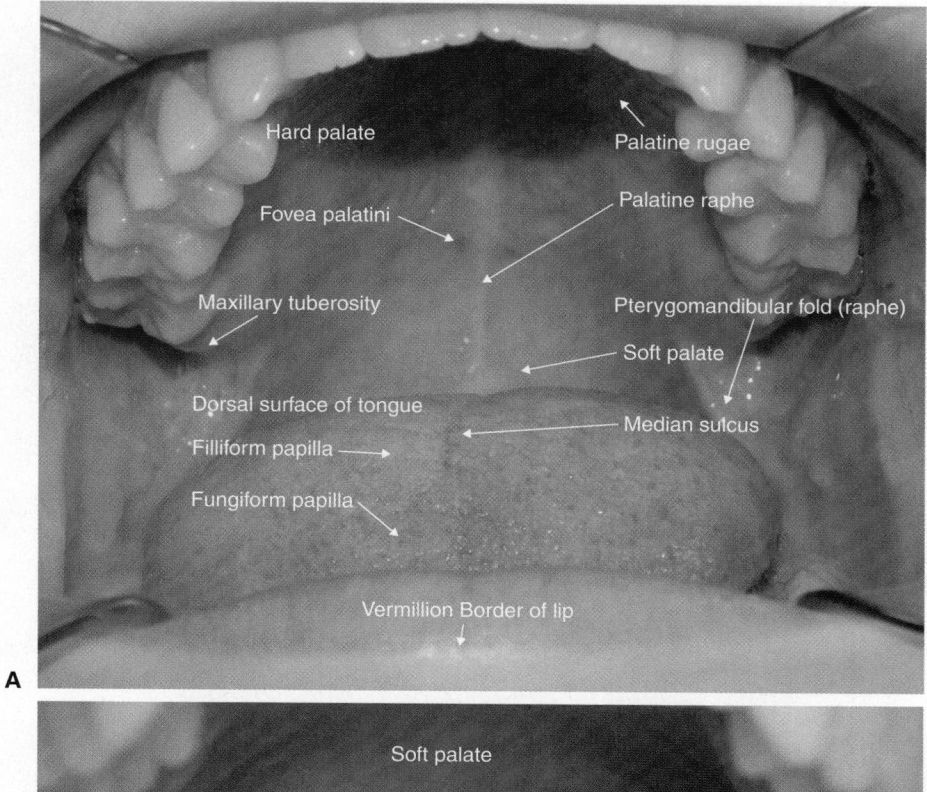

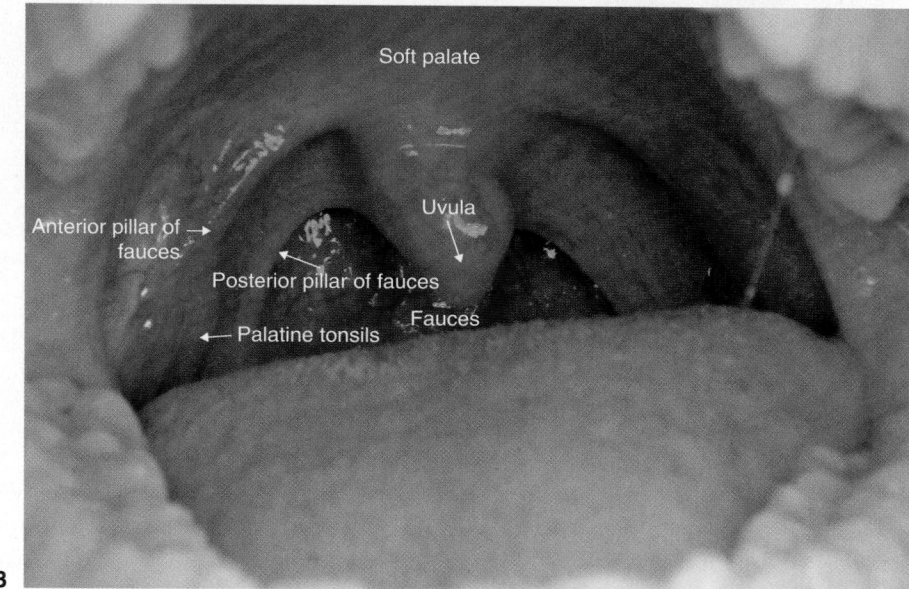

FIGURE 13-6 • Anatomic Landmarks of the Oral Cavity—Dorsal Tongue View. A: View of hard and soft palate. **B:** View of uvula and oropharynx.

◆ A recommended sequence for examination is outlined in Box 13-1 in which factors to consider during appointments are related to the actual observations made and recorded.

◆ This sequence is adapted from *Detecting Oral Cancer*, available from the National Institutes of Health and the National Cancer Institute.[3,4]

◆ In addition to proper sequence, familiarization of anatomic structures common to normal anatomy is critical to understanding abnormal findings (Table 13-1).[5]

I. Extraoral Examination

1. Observe patient during reception and seating to note physical characteristics and abnormalities, and make an overall appraisal.

2. Observe head, face, eyes, and neck and evaluate the skin of the face and neck.

3. Request the patient to remove prosthesis prior to performing the intraoral examination. Explain how this will improve the ability to inspect all areas of the mouth adequately.

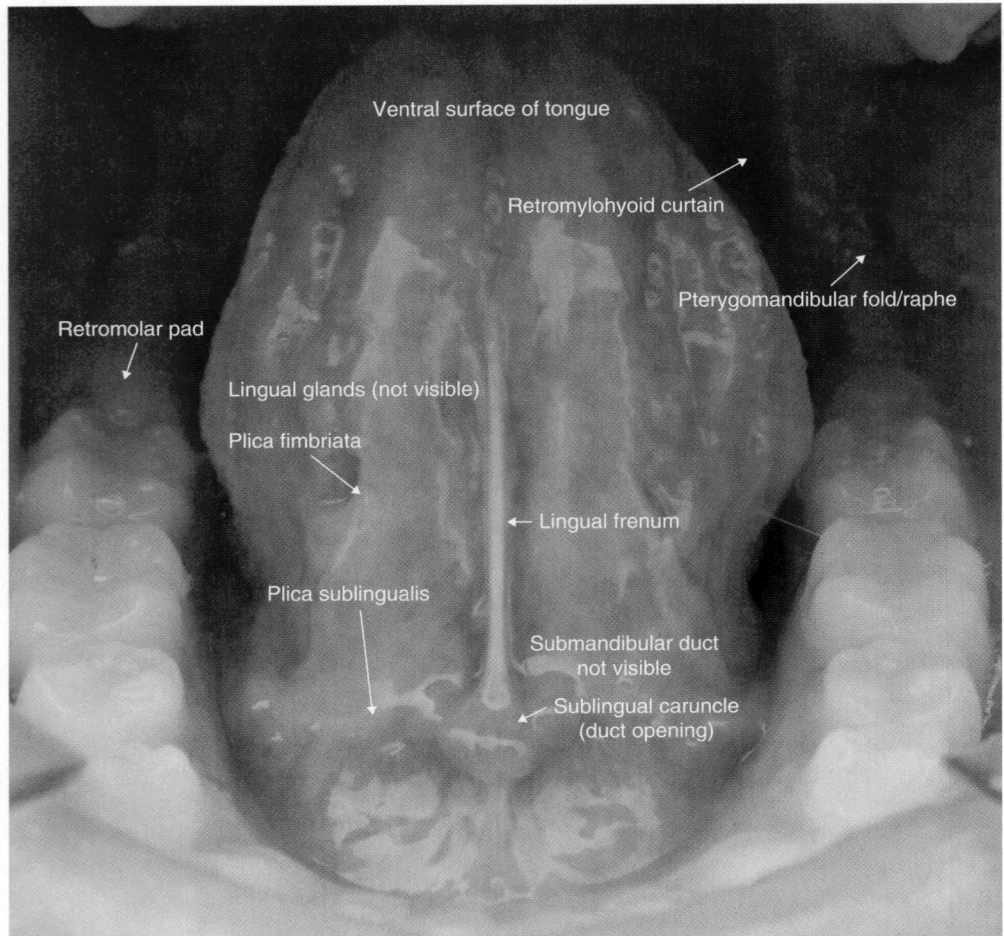

FIGURE 13-7 • Anatomic Landmarks of the Oral Cavity—Ventral Tongue View.

BOX 13-1
Anatomic Landmarks of the Oral Cavity

Lips
Vermillion border
Labial commissure
Labial mucosa
Buccal mucosa
Philtrum
Nasolabial groove
Fauces
Oral pharynx
Vestibule
Buccal vestibule
Buccinator muscle
Labial
Buccal
Mucobuccal fold
Buccal frenum
Labial frenum

Exostosis
Wharton's duct
Lingual vein
Sublingual fold
Plica fimbriata
Sublingual caruncle
Median sulcus
Lingual tonsils
Lingual frenum
Ankyloglossia
Marginal gingiva
Attached gingiva
Free gingival groove
Canine eminence
Pterygomandibular raphe
Parotid papilla

Midpalatine raphe
Palatine rugae
Fovea palatine
Torus palatinus
Incisive papilla
Uvula
Palatine tonsils
Pharyngeal adenoid tonsils
Tonsillar pillars
Tongue:
  Dorsal
  Ventral
  Lateral border
Filiform papilla
Fungiform papilla
Folate papillae

Circumvallate papilla
Lingual tonsils
Stensen's duct
Maxillary tuberosity
Retromolar pad
Ramus of mandible
Zygomatic arch
Mandibular tori (prevalence varies)
Alveolar mucosa
Mylohyoid muscle

Refer to Figures 13-6 and 13-7

TABLE 13-1 • Extraoral and Intraoral Examination

SEQUENCE OF EXAMINATION	OBSERVE	INDICATION AND INFLUENCES ON APPOINTMENTS
1. Overall appraisal of patient	Posture, gait General health status; size Hair; scalp Breathing; state of fatigue Voice, cough, hoarseness	Response, cooperation, attitude toward treatment Length of appointment
2. Face	Expression: evidence of fear or apprehension Shape: twitching; paralysis Jaw movements during speech Injuries; signs of abuse	Need for alleviation of fears Evidence of upper respiratory or other infections Enlarged masseter muscle (related to bruxism)
3. Skin	Color, texture, blemishes Traumatic lesions Eruptions, swellings Growths, scars, moles	Relation to possible systemic conditions Need for supplementary history Biopsy or other treatment to recommend Influences on instruction in diet
4. Eyes	Size of pupils Color of sclera Eyeglasses (corrective) Protruding eyeballs	Dilated pupils or pinpoint may result from drugs, emergency state Eyeglasses essential during instruction Hyperthyroidism

5. Nodes (palpate) (Figure 13-8)
  a. Pre- and postauricular
  b. Occipital
  c. Submental; submandibular
  d. Cervical chain (Figure 13-9)
  e. Supraclavicular
	Adenopathy; lymphadenopathy
	Induration or pain
		Need for referral
		Medical consultation
		Ear infection
		Coordinate with intraoral examination

6. Glands (palpate)
  a. Parotid
  b. Submental
  c. Submandibular (Figure 13-3)
	Enlargement or pain
	Induration longer than 2 wk
		Referral for medical consult

7. Temporomandibular joint (palpate) (Figure 13-4)	Limitations or deviations of movement Trismus Tenderness; sensitivity Noises: clicking, popping, grating	Disorder of joint; limitation of opening Discomfort during appointment and during personal biofilm control

8. Lips
  a. Observe closed, then open
  b. Palpate (Figure 13-1)
	Color, texture, size
	Cracks, angular cheilosis
	Blisters, ulcers
	Traumatic lesions
	Irritation from lip-biting
	Limitation of opening; muscle elasticity; muscle tone
	Evidences of mouth breathing
	Induration
		Need for further examination: referral
		Immediate need for postponement of appointment when a lesion may be communicable or could interfere with procedures
		Care during retraction
		Accessibility during intraoral procedures
		Patient instruction: dietary, special biofilm control for mouth breather

9. Breath odor	Severity Relation to oral hygiene, gingival health	Possible relation to systemic condition Alcohol use history; special needs

10. Labial and buccal mucosa, left and right examined systematically
  a. Vestibule
  b. Mucobuccal folds
  c. Frena
  d. Opening of Stensen duct
  e. Palpate cheeks (Figure 13-2A)
	Color, size, texture, contour
	Abrasions, traumatic lesions, cheek bite
	Effects of tobacco use
	Ulcers, growths
	Moistness of surfaces
	Relation of frena to free gingiva
	Induration
		Need for referral, biopsy, cytology
		Frena and other anatomic parts that need special adaptation for radiography or impression tray
		Avoid sensitive areas during retraction

(Continues)

TABLE 13-1 • Extraoral and Intraoral Examination (*Continued*)

SEQUENCE OF EXAMINATION	OBSERVE	INDICATION AND INFLUENCES ON APPOINTMENTS
11. Tongue a. Vestibule b. Dorsal (Figure 13-6A) c. Lateral borders d. Base of tongue (Figure 13-10) e. Deviation on extension	Shape: normal asymmetric Color, size, texture, consistency **Fissures**; papillae Coating Lesions: elevated, depressed, flat Induration	Need for referral, biopsy, cytology Need for instruction in tongue cleaning
12. Floor of mouth a. Ventral surface of tongue (Figure 13-7) b. Palpate (Figure 13-2B) c. Duct openings d. Mucosa, frena e. Tongue action	Varicosities Lesions: elevated, flat, depressed, traumatic Induration Limitation or freedom of movement of tongue Frena; tongue-tie	Large muscular tongue influences retraction, gag reflex, accessibility for instrumentation Film placement problems
13. Saliva	Quantity; quality (thick, ropy) Evidence of dry mouth; lip wetting Tongue coating	Reduced in certain diseases, by certain drugs Special dental caries control program Influence on instrumentation Need for saliva substitute
14. Hard palate (Figure 13-6A)	Height, contour, color Appearance of rugae Tori, growths, ulcers	Need for referral, biopsy, cytology Signs of tongue thrust, deviate swallow Influence on radiographic film placement
15. Soft palate, uvula (Figure 13-6B)	Color, size, shape Petechiae Ulcers, growths	Referral, biopsy, cytology Large uvula influences gag reflex
16. Tonsillar region, throat (Figure 13-6B)	Tonsils: size and shape Color, size, surface characteristics Lesions, trauma	Referral, biopsy, cytology Enlarged tonsils encourage gag reflex Throat infection, a sign for appointment postponement

4. Palpate the salivary glands and lymph nodes. Figure 13-8 shows the location of the major lymph nodes of the face, oral regions, and neck. Palpation is a significant component of the extra-/intraoral examination (Figure 13-9).

◆ Note any of the following symptoms or experiences:
 • Pain or discomfort upon palpation and/or upon swallowing.
 • Persistent difficulty swallowing in the absence of pain.

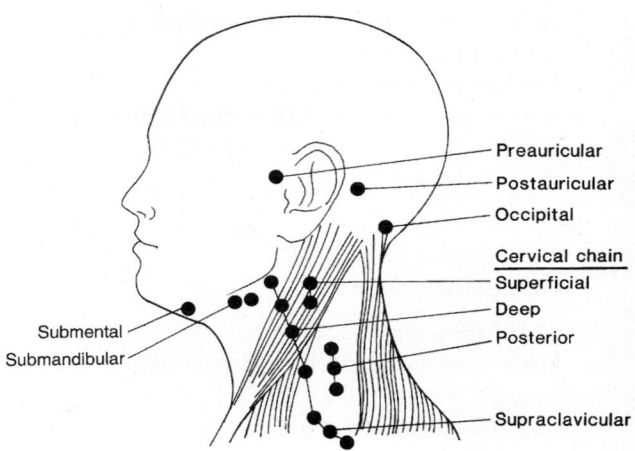

FIGURE 13-8 • Lymph Nodes. The locations of the major lymph nodes into which the vessels of the facial and oral regions drain.

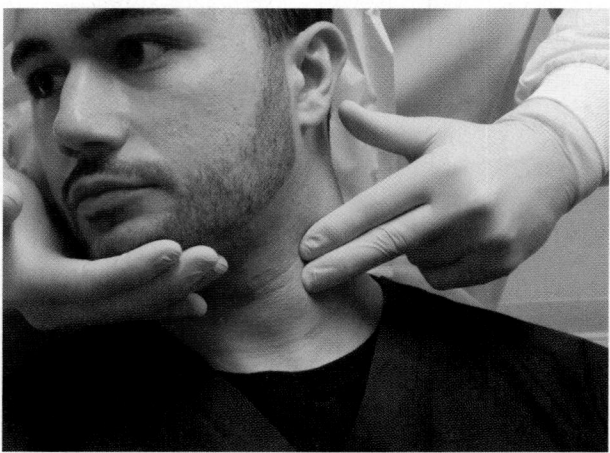

FIGURE 13-9 • Cervical Node Palpation. Left anterior cervical lymph node chain is examined. Finger tips gently press and roll nodes along the length of the sternocleidomastoid muscle.

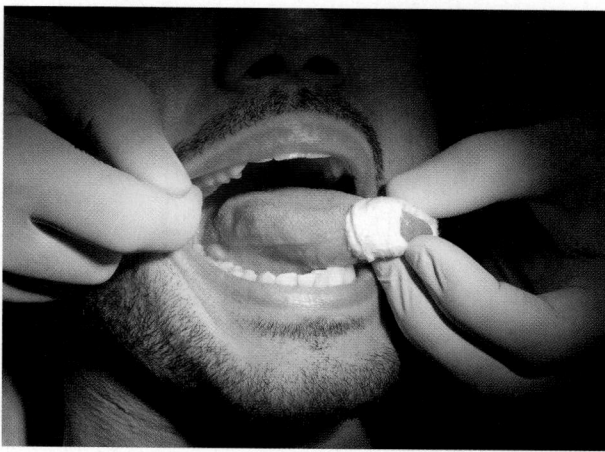

Figure 13-10 • Examination of the Tongue. To observe the posterior third of the tongue and the attachment to the floor of the mouth, hold the tongue with a gauze sponge, retract the cheek, and move the tongue out, first to one side and then the other, as each section of the mucosa is carefully examined.

- Any recent noticeable lumps the patient may have experienced without pain.
- Persistent earache or hoarseness of voice.[6]

5. Observe mandibular movement and palpate the temporomandibular joint (Figure 13-4). Relate to items from questions in the medical/dental history.[7,8]

II. Intraoral Examination

1. Make a preliminary examination of the lips and intraoral mucosa by using a mouth mirror or a tongue depressor.
2. View and palpate lips, labial and buccal mucosa, and mucobuccal folds (Figures 13-1 and 13-2A).
3. Examine and palpate the tongue, including the dorsal and ventral surfaces, lateral borders, and base. Retract to observe posterior third, first to one side and then the other (Figure 13-10).
4. Observe mucosa of the floor of the mouth. Palpate the floor of the mouth (Figure 13-2B).
5. Examine the hard and soft palates, tonsillar areas, and pharynx (Figure 13-6A and B). Use a mirror to observe the oropharynx, nasopharynx, and larynx.
6. Note amount and consistency of the saliva and evidence of dry mouth (xerostomia).

III. Documentation of Findings

A. History

Questions directed to the patient provide necessary information in the management of an oral lesion. Because alarming the patient must be avoided, judgment is needed for selecting the appropriate time to obtain the history of a lesion.

- Whether the lesion is known or not known to the patient; previous evaluation.

- If known, when first noticed; if recurrence, previous date when lesion was first noticed.
- Duration, symptoms, changes in size and appearance.

B. Location and Extent

- When a lesion is first seen, its location is noted in relation to adjacent structures.
- Document a complete description of each finding including the location, extent, size, color, surface texture or configurations, consistency, morphology, and history.
- Intraoral photography can be of value to record images of anatomical deviations, location, and proportions.[9]
- Descriptive words to define the location and extent include the following:
  - *Localized:* Lesion limited to a small focal area.
  - *Generalized:* Involves most of an area or segment.
  - *Single lesion:* One lesion of a particular type with a distinct margin.
  - *Multiple lesions:* More than one lesion of a particular type. Lesions may be:
    - Separate: discrete, not running together; may be arranged in clusters.
    - Coalescing: close to each other with margins that merge.

C. Physical Characteristics

- *Size and shape*
  - Record length and width in millimeters.
  - The height of an elevated lesion may be significant.
  - Use a probe to measure, as shown in Figure 13-11.

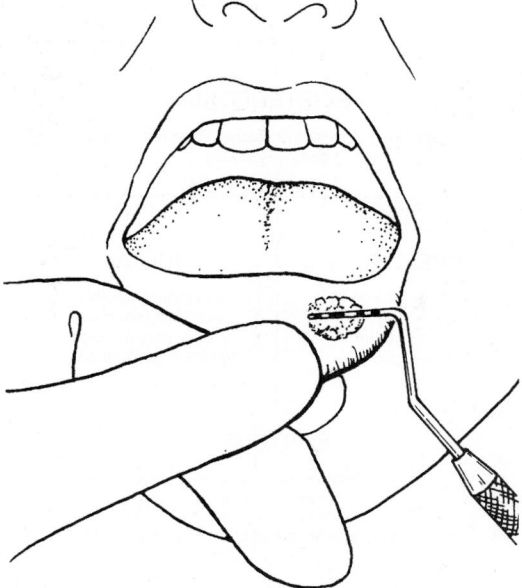

FIGURE 13-11 • Use of a Probe to Measure a Lesion. In addition to the exact location, the width and length of a lesion is recorded. Using the probe provides a convenient method.

◆ *Color*

  • Red, pink, white, and red and white are the most commonly seen.
  • Other more rare lesions may be blue, purple, gray, yellow, black, or brown.

◆ *Surface texture*

  • A lesion may have a smooth or an irregular surface.
  • The texture may be papillary, verrucous or wart-like, fissured, corrugated, or crusted.

◆ *Consistency*

  • Lesions may be soft, spongy, resilient, hard, or indurated.

MORPHOLOGIC CATEGORIES

◆ Most lesions can be classified readily as *elevated, depressed,* or *flat* as they relate to the normal level of the skin or mucosa.

◆ Flowcharts of elevated lesions (Figure 13-12A), depressed lesions (Figure 13-12B), and flat lesions (Figure 13-12C) break down the terms used for describing lesions in each category.[10]

I. Elevated Lesions

An elevated lesion (Figure 13-12A) is above the plane of the skin or mucosa. Elevated lesions are considered *blisterform* or *nonblisterform.*

◆ Blisterform

◆ Blisterform lesions contain fluid and are usually soft and translucent. They may be vesicles, pustules, or bullae.

  • *Vesicle:* A vesicle is a small (1 cm or less in diameter), circumscribed lesion with a thin surface covering. It may contain serum or mucin and appear white.
  • *Pustule:* A pustule may be more than or less than 5 mm in diameter and contain pus giving it a yellowish color.
  • *Bulla:* A bulla is large (>1 cm). It is filled with fluid, usually mucin or serum, but may contain blood. The color depends on the fluid content.

◆ Nonblisterform

◆ Nonblisterform lesions are solid and do not contain fluid. They may be papules, nodules, tumors, or plaques. Papules, nodules, and tumors are also characterized by

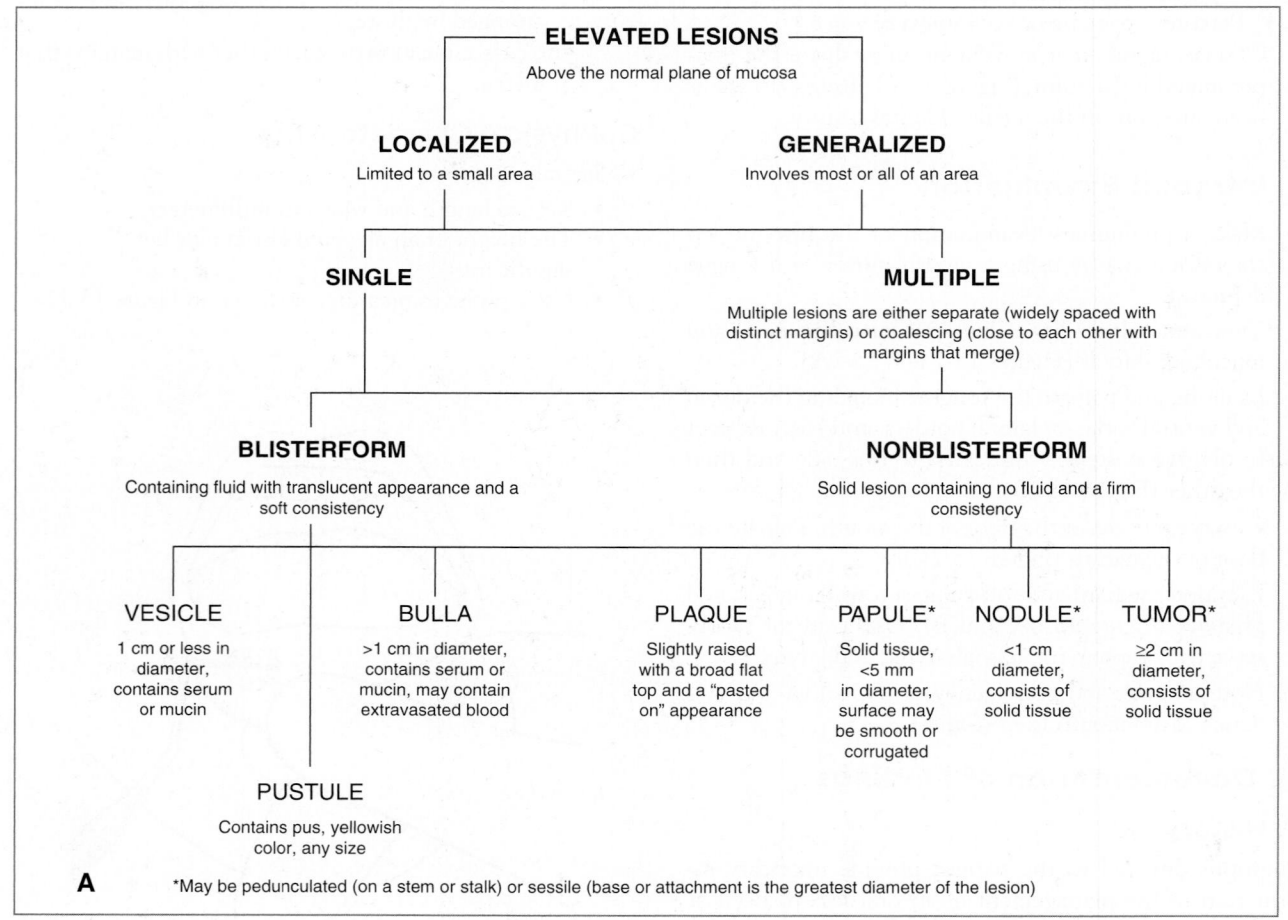

FIGURE 13-12 • Flowcharts. A: Description of elevated soft tissue lesions. Elevated lesions are blisterform or nonblisterform. **B:** Description of depressed soft tissue lesions. Depressed lesions are below the normal plane of the mucosa, usually an ulcer where there is a loss of continuity of epithelium. **C:** Description of flat soft tissue lesions. Flat lesions are on the level of normal plane of the mucosa. (**A–C** reprinted with permission from McCann A. Describing soft tissue lesions of the oral cavity. *Dent Hyg News.* 1992;5:9.)

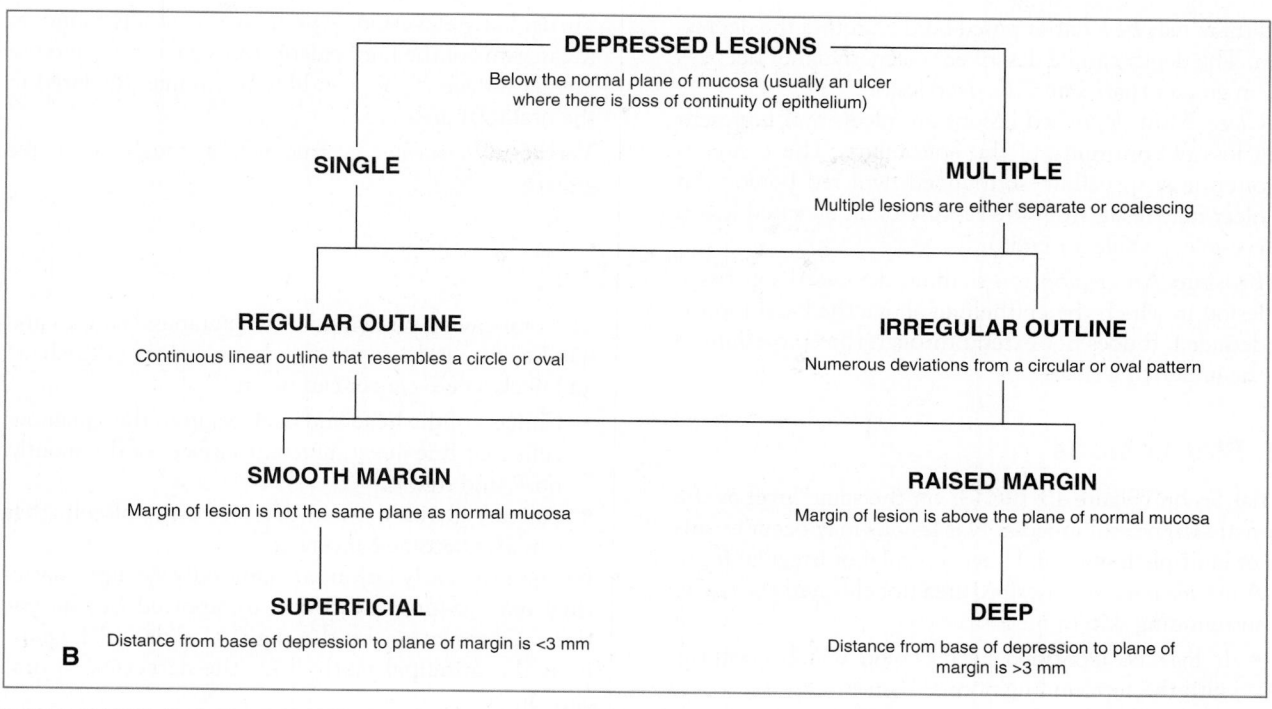

B

DEPRESSED LESIONS
Below the normal plane of mucosa (usually an ulcer
where there is loss of continuity of epithelium)

SINGLE

MULTIPLE
Multiple lesions are either separate or coalescing

REGULAR OUTLINE
Continuous linear outline that resembles a circle or oval

IRREGULAR OUTLINE
Numerous deviations from a circular or oval pattern

SMOOTH MARGIN
Margin of lesion is not the same plane as normal mucosa

RAISED MARGIN
Margin of lesion is above the plane of normal mucosa

SUPERFICIAL
Distance from base of depression to plane of margin is <3 mm

DEEP
Distance from base of depression to plane of
margin is >3 mm

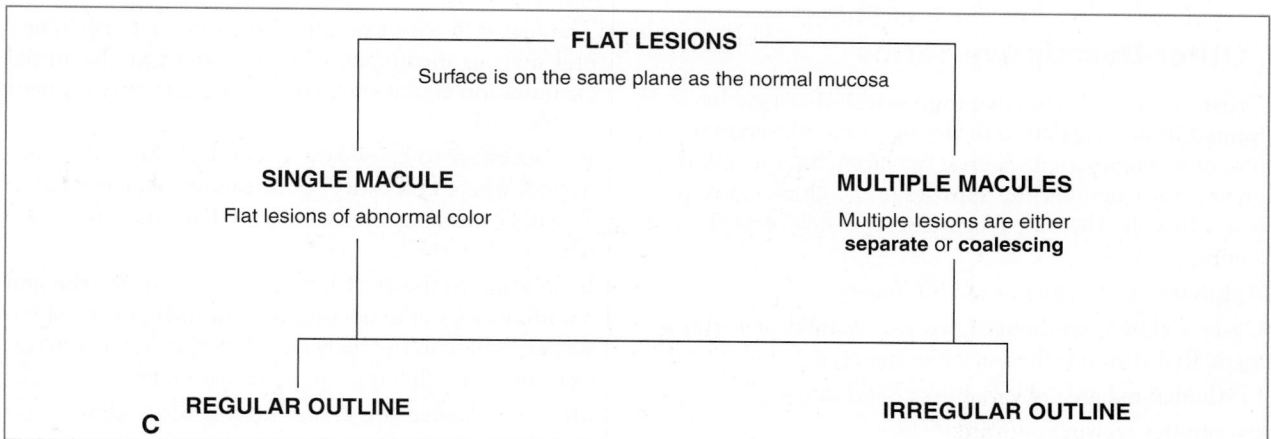

C

FLAT LESIONS
Surface is on the same plane as the normal mucosa

SINGLE MACULE
Flat lesions of abnormal color

MULTIPLE MACULES
Multiple lesions are either
separate or **coalescing**

REGULAR OUTLINE

IRREGULAR OUTLINE

FIGURE 13-12 • (*Continued*)

the base or attachment. As shown in Figure 13-13, the peduncalated lesion is attached by a narrow stalk or pedicle, whereas the sessile lesion has a base as wide as the lesion itself.

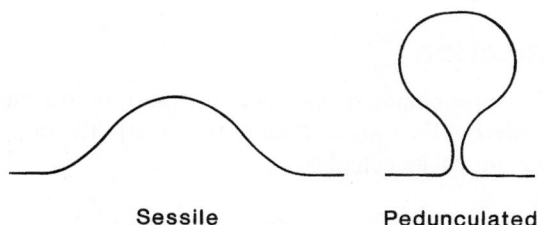

Sessile   Pedunculated

FIGURE 13-13 • Attachment of Nonblisterform Lesions. The *sessile lesion has a base as wide as the lesion itself*; the pedunculated lesion is attached by a narrow stalk or pedicle.

- *Papule:* A papule is a small (pinhead to 5 mm in diameter), solid lesion that may be pointed, rounded, or flat topped.
- *Nodule:* A nodule is larger than a papule (>5 mm but <2 cm).
- *Tumor:* A tumor is 2 cm or greater in width. In this context, "tumor" means a general swelling or enlargement and does not refer to neoplasm, either benign or malignant.
- *Plaque:* A plaque is a slightly raised lesion with a broad, flat top. It is usually larger than 5 mm in diameter, with a "pasted on" appearance.

II. Depressed Lesions

A depressed lesion (Figure 13-12B) is below the level of the skin or mucosa. The outline may be regular or irregular, and there may be a flat or raised border around the depression. The depth can be described as superficial or deep. A lesion greater than 3 mm is a deep lesion.

◆ *Ulcer:* Most depressed lesions are ulcers and represent a loss of continuity of the epithelium. The center is often gray to yellow, surrounded by a red border. An ulcer may result from the rupture of an elevated lesion (vesicle, pustule, or bulla).

◆ Erosion: An erosion is a shallow, depressed soft tissue lesion in which the epithelium above the basal layer is denuded. It does not extend through the epithelium to the underlying tissue.

III. Flat Lesions

A flat lesion (Figure 13-12C) is on the same level as the normal skin or oral mucosa. Flat lesions may occur as single or multiple lesions and have a regular or irregular form.

◆ A *macule* is a circumscribed area not elevated above the surrounding skin or mucosa.

  • It may be identified by its color, which contrasts with the surrounding normal tissues.

IV. Other Descriptive Terms

◆ Crust: an outer layer, covering, or scab that may have formed from coagulation or drying of blood, serum, or pus, or a combination. A crust may form after a vesicle breaks; for example, the skin lesion of chickenpox is first a macule, then a papule, then a vesicle, and then a crust.

◆ Aphtha: a small white or reddish ulcer.

◆ Cyst: a closed, epithelial-lined sac, normal or pathologic, that contains fluid or other material.

◆ Erythema: red area of variable size and shape.

◆ Exophytic: growing outward.

◆ Idiopathic: of unknown etiology.

◆ Indurated: hardened or abnormally hard.

◆ Papillary: resembling a small, nipple-shaped projection or elevation.

◆ Petechiae: minute hemorrhagic spots of pinhead to pinpoint size.

◆ Pseudomembrane: a loose membranous layer of exudate containing organisms, precipitated fibrin, necrotic cells, and inflammatory cells produced during an inflammatory reaction on the surface of a tissue.

◆ Polyp: any mass of tissue that projects outward or upward from the normal surface level.

◆ Punctate: marked with points or dots differentiated from the surrounding surface by color, elevation, or texture.

◆ Purulent: containing, forming, or discharging pus.

◆ Rubefacient: reddening of the skin.

◆ Torus: bony elevation or prominence usually found on the midline of the hard palate (torus palatinus) and the lingual surface of the mandible (torus mandibularis) in the premolar area.

◆ Verruca: *Verrucous* (verrucose): a rough, wart-like growth.

ORAL CANCER

◆ The oral cavity, pharynx, larynx, paranasal sinuses and nasal cavity, and salivary glands are regions of the head and neck where cancer can begin.[11]

  • Cancers of the head and neck begin in the squamous cells that line moist, mucosal surfaces of the mouth, nose, and throat.[12]

  • Salivary glands contain different types of cells that can also become cancerous.[12]

◆ Because the early lesions are generally asymptomatic, they may go unnoticed and unreported by the patient. Observation by the dentist or dental hygienist is the principal method for the detection of oral cancer.

◆ The first step is to examine the entire face, neck, and oral mucous membrane of each patient at the initial examination and at each continuing care appointment (Table 13-1).

◆ It is necessary to know how to conduct the oral examination, where oral cancer occurs most frequently, what an early cancerous lesion may look like, and what to do when such a lesion is found.

◆ In addition to the early lesions of oral cancers, the oral manifestations of neoplasms or abnormal growth of tissue, elsewhere in the body as well as the oral manifestations of chemotherapy, can be recognized.

◆ Most oral cancers are related to tobacco and/or excessive alcohol use.[2,12]

◆ Additional risk factors include infection with HPV-16 type, multiple sex partners, weakened immune system, age 40 years and more, and sun exposure to the lips.[1,2,12]

◆ Increasing incidence of oral cancers in adults younger than 40 years suggests all patients, regardless of age or risk factors, must be screened for oral cancer.[13]

I. Location

◆ The most common sites for oral cancer are the lateral borders of the tongue, floor of the mouth, the lips, and the soft palate complex.

II. Appearance of Early Cancer

Early oral cancer takes many forms and may resemble a variety of common oral lesions. All types need to be examined with suspicion. Five basic forms are listed here[1,12,14]:

- *White areas*
  - White areas vary from a filmy, barely visible change in the mucosa to heavy, thick, heaped-up areas of dry white keratinized tissue.
  - Fissures, ulcers, or areas of induration or sclerosis in a white area are most indicative of malignancy.
  - *Leukoplakia* is a white patch or plaque that cannot be scraped off or characterized as any other disease. It may be associated with physical or chemical agents and the use of tobacco.
- *Red areas*
  - *Erythroplakia* is a term used to designate lesions of the oral mucosa that appear as bright red patches or plaques.
  - Lesions appear red, of velvety consistency, and may coincide with small ulcers.
  - Erythroplakia is an oral lesion that cannot be characterized as any specific disease. It is less common than leukoplakia and more likely to manifest as dysplasia (precancerous) or malignancy.
- *Ulcers*
  - Ulcers may have flat or raised margins.
  - Palpation may reveal induration.
- *Masses*
  - Papillary masses, sometimes with ulcerated areas, occur as elevations above the surrounding tissues.
  - Other masses may occur below the normal mucosa and may be found only by palpation.
- *Pigmentation*
  - Brown or black pigmented areas may be located on mucosa where pigmentation does not normally occur.

CLINICAL RECOMMENDATIONS FOR EVALUATION OF ORAL LESIONS

- Updated medical, social, and dental history along with the extra- and intraoral examination is recommended for all adult patients.[2]
- Adult patients with lesions considered to be innocuous or nonsuspicious of malignancy should be followed to determine no further evaluation is needed.[2]
- Biopsy is indicated for adult patients with lesions considered to be suspicious of potential malignancy or malignant disorder or other symptoms.[2]
- Although not recommended for potential malignancy, cytologic adjuncts for minimally invasive detection of oral cancer can be performed when a patient refuses biopsy of the lesion or referral to a specialist. Cytologic adjuncts include brush cytology and toluidine blue, diffuse tissue reflectance, and laser-induced

autofluorescence.[15] The rationale for performing adjunctive cytologic testing is to reinforce the need for biopsy or referral.[15]

I. Biopsy

- Biopsy is the removal and microscopic examination of a section of tissue or other material from the body for the purposes of diagnosis.
  - A biopsy is either *excisional*, when the entire lesion is removed, or *incisional*, when a representative section from the lesion is taken.
  - Considered the "gold standard" in oral cancer diagnosis.[1,14]
- *Indications for biopsy*
  - Any unusual oral lesion that cannot be identified with clinical certainty must be biopsied.
  - Any lesion that has not healed in 2 weeks is considered suspicious for malignancy until proven otherwise.
  - A persistent, thick, white, hyperkeratotic lesion and any mass (elevated or not) that does not break through the surface epithelium.
- *Pathology report.*
- Diagnostic criteria may vary, but one of the most recent guidelines for oral cytology includes the following[16]:
  - NILM (negative for intraepithelial lesion or malignancy): normal, infection, inflammation, benign epithelial lesion, etc.
  - LSIL (low-grade squamous intraepithelial lesion): mild to moderate dysplasia (cell changes).
  - HSIL (high-grade squamous intraepithelial lesion): severe dysplasia.
  - SCC (squamous cell carcinoma).
  - Other malig (other malignancy).
  - IFN (indefinite for neoplasia or non-neoplasia).

DOCUMENTATION

Documentation in the permanent record of a patient who had a biopsy (or smear) because of a questionable cancerous lesion is needed and will contain a minimum of the following:

- Details of the oral examination and follow-up procedures with reports from consultants, laboratories, medical follow-up, and outcomes.
- Recommendations for the frequency of a complete oral examination at future dental hygiene maintenance appointments.
- Review of lifestyle habits that may be a risk factor for an oral lesion with recommendations for specific preventive methods.
- A progress note at the patient's maintenance appointment following the biopsy with the results may be reviewed in Box 13-2.

BOX 13-2

Example Documentation:
Patient with an Oral Lesion

S—50-year-old female presents for routine preventive maintenance with no current concerns at today's appointment. When questioned during intraoral examination, patient recalls recently accidently biting her tongue.

O—Patient smokes 1 pack cigarettes daily for the past 35 years and admits to drinking 1–2 beers nightly; left lateral border of tongue erythematous lesion 1 cm × 5 mm, flat.

A—High risk for oral cancer, erythematous lesion requires further evaluation.

P—Discuss concerns with patient regarding high-risk behaviors of tobacco use and alcohol. Recommend 2-week follow-up for reevaluation of lesion and further referral if no improvement. Recommended and offered tobacco cessation information.

Signed: _____, RDH

Date: _____

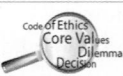

EVERYDAY ETHICS

Abby and Sylvia are the two part-time dental hygienists in Dr. Anthony's practice. They practice on different days at the office, so they rarely see each other except to attend local dental hygiene association meetings. Most patients know both hygienists and may be scheduled with either depending on available time.

Mr. Peters came in for his 3-month maintenance appointment carrying his unlit pipe as usual. This time his appointment was with Abby, and jokes were exchanged about the pipe. During the intraoral examination, Abby found a red lesion on the side of his tongue that was about 4 mm wide. She asked him if he had seen it and his answer was, "Oh yeah, Sylvia mentioned it when I was here last time." Abby glanced at the record and noted that his last date was over 4 months ago. There was no documentation in the patient's dental record that mentioned any oral lesions.

Questions for Consideration

1. Which of the dental hygiene code values (Table II-1, in Section II Introduction) are involved here? How?

2. Consider the questions in Table VI-1, Section VI Introduction to help Abby decide options help Mr. Peters and improve office policies.

3. Privately, Abby is upset, and she is determined that this needs to be discussed with both Sylvia and Dr. Anthony. Dr. Anthony has never specified a policy for this type of issue. Where and how can she approach them and what recommendations does she need to propose for an office policy?

Factors to Teach the Patient

► Reasons for a careful extra- and intraoral examination at each maintenance appointment.

► Guidance and support on tobacco cessation and provide appropriate referral.

► How to conduct self-examination monthly to watch for changes in oral tissues and identify lesions that last longer than 2 weeks. Examination includes the face, neck, lips, gingiva, cheeks, tongue, palate, and throat. Any changes are reported to the dentist and the dental hygienist.

► General dietary and nutritional influences on the health of the oral tissues.
  ▷ Benefits of diet rich in fruits and vegetables.

► How the oral cavity tends to reflect the general health.

► The warning signs of oral cancer from the American Cancer Society including the following[13]: a swelling, lump, or growth anywhere, with or without pain.
  ▷ White scaly patches or red velvety areas.
  ▷ Any sore that does not heal promptly (within 2 weeks).
  ▷ Numbness or tingling.
  ▷ Excessive dryness or wetness.
  ▷ Prolonged hoarseness, sore throats, persistent coughing, or the feeling of a "lump in the throat."
  ▷ Difficulty with swallowing.
  ▷ Difficulty in opening the mouth.

ENHANCE YOUR UNDERSTANDING

ONLINE RESOURCES
(see the inside front cover for access information)
- Audio glossary
- Appendices

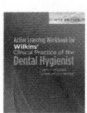

SUPPORT FOR LEARNING
(available separately)
- *Active Learning Workbook for Wilkins' Clinical Practice of the Dental Hygienist, 13th Edition*

INDIVIDUALIZED REVIEW
- Customized practice quizzing with Navigate 2 TestPrep for *Wilkins' Clinical Practice of the Dental Hygienist*

References

1. Rivera C. Essentials of oral cancer. *Int J Clin Exp Pathol.* 2015;8(9):11884-11894.

2. Lingen MW, Abt E, Agrawal N, et al. Evidence-based clinical practice guideline for the evaluation of potentially malignant disorders in the oral cavity. *J Am Dent Assoc.* 2017;148:712.e710-727.e710.

3. National Institute of Dental and Craniofacial Research, National Institutes of Health. Detecting oral cancer: a guide for health care professionals. https://www.nidcr.nih.gov /OralHealth/Topics/OralCancer/DetectingOralCancer.htm. Updated July, 2017. Accessed November 11, 2017.

4. National Cancer Institute, National Institute of Health. Head and neck cancer—health professional version. https://www .cancer.gov/types/head-and-neck/hp. Accessed November 11, 2017.

5. American Dental Education Association. Compendium of curriculum guidelines for allied dental education programs May 2015–2016. http://www.adea.org/cadpd/toolkit/. Updated 2016. Accessed November 11, 2017.

6. Soni S, Chouksey S. A study of clinicopathological profile of patients of hoarseness of voice presenting to tertiary care hospital. *Indian J Otolaryngol Head Neck Surg.* 2017;69(2):244-247.

7. Coakley MC. Temporomandibular joint dysfunction (TMJ): the role of the dental hygienist. *J Dent Hyg.* 1988;62:521-256.

8. Pupo YM, Pantoja LL, Veiga FF, et al. Diagnostic validity of clinical protocols to assess temporomandibular disk displacement disorders: a meta-analysis. *Oral Surg Oral Med Oral Pathol Oral Radiol.* 2016;122(5):572-586.

9. Oral Cancer Foundation. Referral-form. http://oralcancer foundation.org/resources/screening-event-downloads/referral -form/. Accessed November 11, 2017.

10. McCann AL, Wesley RK. A method for describing soft tissue lesions of the oral cavity. *Dent Hyg.* 1987;61(5):219-223.

11. National Institute of Dental and Craniofacial Research, National Institute of Health. Oral cancer. https://www.nidcr .nih.gov/OralHealth/Topics/OralCancer/OralCancer.htm. Updated September, 2016. Accessed November 11, 2017.

12. Rethman MP, Carpenter W, Cohen EE, et al. Evidence-based clinical recommendations regarding screening for oral squamous cell carcinomas. *Tex Dent J.* 2012;129(5):491-507.

13. American Cancer Society. What are the key statistics about oral cavity and oropharyngeal cancers? https://www.cancer .org/cancer/oral-cavity-and-oropharyngeal-cancer/about /key-statistics.html. Updated January 6, 2017. Accessed November 11, 2017.

14. Speight PM, Epstein J, Kujan O, et al. Screening for oral cancer—a perspective from the Global Oral Cancer Forum. *Oral Surg Oral Med Oral Pathol Oral Radiol.* 2017;123(6):680-687.

15. Lingen MW, Tampi MP, Urquhart O, et al. Adjuncts for the evaluation of potentially malignant disorders in the oral cavity: diagnostic test accuracy systematic review and meta-analysis—a report of the American Dental Association. *J Am Dent Assoc.* 2017;148(11):797.e52-813.e52.

16. Sekine J, Nakatani E, Hideshima K, Iwahashi T, Sasaki H. Diagnostic accuracy of oral cancer cytology in a pilot study. *Diagn Pathol.* 2017;12:27.

14

Family Violence

Janice L. Murray, DipDH, BDSc(DH), MSDH, RDH, Lisa F. Mallonee, RDH, RD, LD, MPH, and Linda D. Boyd, RDH, RD, EdD

CHAPTER OUTLINE

FAMILY VIOLENCE
- I. Categories of FV
- II. Types of FV

CHILD ABUSE AND NEGLECT
- I. Definitions
- II. Risk Factors
- III. Consequences of Child Abuse
- IV. General Signs of Child Abuse and Neglect
- V. Extraoral Wounds and Signs of Trauma
- VI. Intraoral Signs of Abuse and Neglect
- VII. Parental Attitude

Munchausen Syndrome By Proxy
- I. General Considerations

HUMAN TRAFFICKING
- I. General Considerations
- II. Indicators of a Patient Involved in Human Trafficking

ELDER ABUSE AND NEGLECT
- I. General Considerations
- II. Definitions
- III. General Signs of Elder Abuse and Neglect
- IV. Physical Signs of Elder Abuse and Neglect
- V. Orofacial Signs of Abuse and Neglect

INTIMATE PARTNER VIOLENCE
- I. Prevalence of IPV
- II. Physical Injury from IPV
- III. General Health Consequences of IPV
- IV. Orofacial Impact of IPV
- V. Role of the Dental Hygienist

REPORTING ABUSE AND/OR NEGLECT
- I. Proper Training
- II. Reporting Laws
- III. Reportable Required Information

FORENSIC DENTISTRY
- I. Use of Forensics in Abuse Cases
- II. Other Uses of Forensics

DOCUMENTATION
- I. Purposes of Thorough and Accurate Documentation
- II. Content of the Record

EVERYDAY ETHICS

FACTORS TO TEACH THE PATIENT

REFERENCES

LEARNING OBJECTIVES

After studying this chapter, the student will be able to:

1. Describe the general, extraoral, and intraoral signs of child abuse and neglect.

2. Describe the general, physical, extraoral, and intraoral signs of elder abuse and neglect.

3. Discuss the signs and attitudes of the abused in an intimate partner violence situation.

4. Discuss the role of the dental hygienist in reporting suspected abuse or neglect of children, elders, and intimate partners.

5. Discuss Munchausen syndrome by proxy and describe indicators associated with the syndrome.

6. Describe the general and behavioral indicators of human trafficking victims.

FAMILY VIOLENCE

Abuse is a global problem with no economic, geographic, or social boundaries. The entire dental team must advocate to support those who suffer from family violence (FV) and obtain the proper knowledge and skills required to identify and report suspected cases to authorities.[1,2]

I. Categories of FV

◆ FV is abusive behavior by one individual toward another in an intimate or family relationship.

◆ Those most at risk are children, the elderly, people with disabilities, and women.[1,3]

◆ Categories for FV may include[3]:
  • Child abuse and neglect.
  • Intimate partner violence (IPV) or domestic violence (DV).
  • Elder abuse and neglect.

II. Types of FV

◆ FV may include[3]:
  • Physical abuse.
  • Emotional, verbal, or psychological abuse.
  • Sexual abuse.
  • Neglect or abandonment.
  • Financial exploitation.

◆ Figure 14-1 summarizes the major types of FV.

CHILD ABUSE AND NEGLECT

According to the World Health Organization,

> "child maltreatment is the abuse and neglect that occurs to children under 18 years of age. It includes all forms of physical and/or emotional ill-treatment, sexual abuse, neglect, negligent treatment or commercial or other exploitation, resulting in actual or potential harm to the child's health, survival, development or dignity in the context of a relationship of responsibility, trust or power."[4]

I. Definitions

◆ *Child abuse*: The nonaccidental physical, emotional (psychological), or sexual acts against a child.[5]

◆ *Child neglect*: The intentional or unintentional failure to provide for a child's basic physical, emotional, educational, and medical/dental needs.[5]

◆ *Dental neglect*: The willful failure of a parent or guardian to seek and follow through with treatment necessary to ensure a level of oral health essential for adequate function and freedom from pain and infection.[6]

II. Risk Factors

◆ Those at greatest risk for abuse include:
  • Males.[3]
  • Younger children are most vulnerable to death as the result of child abuse and neglect.[3,7,8]
  • Children with special needs, persistent crying, or having abnormal physical features are more at risk for abuse.[3,9]

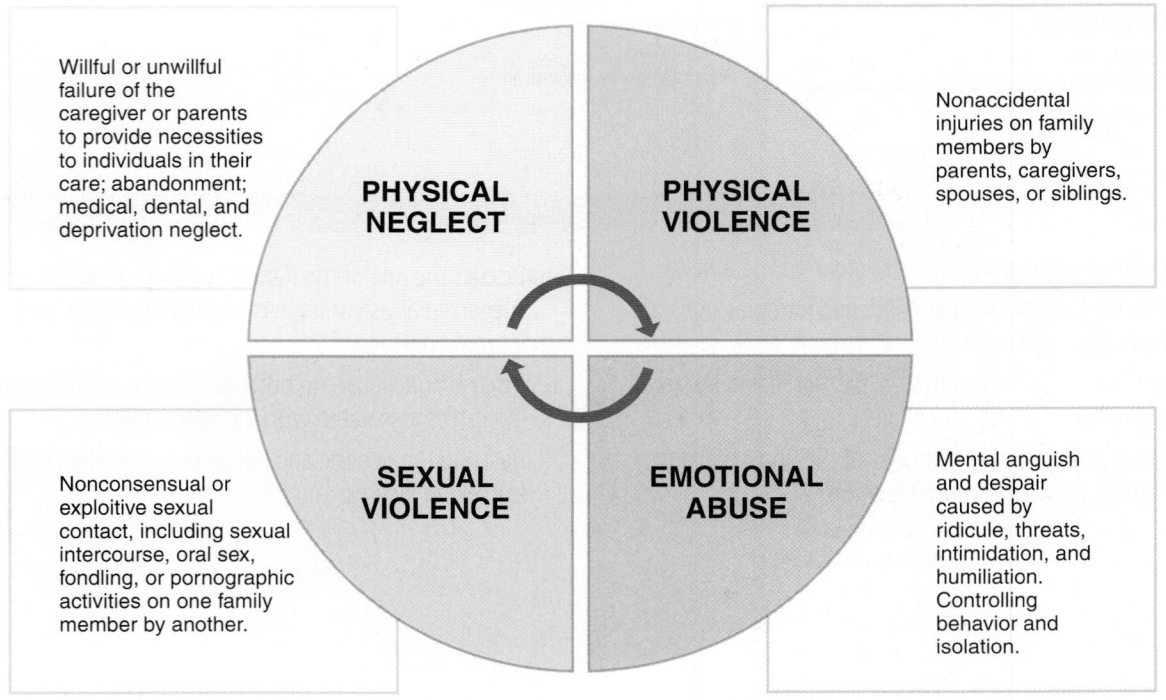

Willful or unwillful failure of the caregiver or parents to provide necessities to individuals in their care; abandonment; medical, dental, and deprivation neglect.

PHYSICAL NEGLECT

PHYSICAL VIOLENCE

Nonaccidental injuries on family members by parents, caregivers, spouses, or siblings.

Nonconsensual or exploitive sexual contact, including sexual intercourse, oral sex, fondling, or pornographic activities on one family member by another.

SEXUAL VIOLENCE

EMOTIONAL ABUSE

Mental anguish and despair caused by ridicule, threats, intimidation, and humiliation. Controlling behavior and isolation.

FIGURE 14-1 • Major Types of Family Maltreatment.

III. Consequences of Child Abuse

◆ Several thousands of children a year die as a result of severe physical damage and others suffer permanent brain damage or physical deformities as well as emotional trauma.[8]

◆ Craniofacial and head and neck injuries occur in more than half of child abuse cases.[10]

◆ Abuse should be considered in the differential diagnosis for any injury involving a child.

IV. General Signs of Child Abuse and Neglect

◆ The dental hygiene standards of practice framework promote comprehensive patient care through thorough assessments and identifying risk factors that impede the health and wellness of the patient.[11,12]

◆ Recognizing signs of suspected abuse and following proper reporting protocol will promote health and safety for all individuals.

◆ Categories of child abuse and neglect are distinguished into physical, behavioral, emotional, cognitive, and social indicators (Table 14-1).

A. Physical Indicators

◆ The child patient should be assessed for mannerisms, overall appearance, and indicators suggestive of abuse or neglect.

◆ Clothing with long sleeves, long pants, or hat, even in warm weather, may suggest that bruises and lacerations are being concealed from view.[10]

◆ Uncleanliness, body odor, and soiled garments may show a lack of care by the caregiver.[4,10]

◆ Infestation of lice. This can be in the form of live insects on the scalp, lice eggs on the shaft of the hair, or noticeable insect bite marks on the scalp.[13]

◆ Failure to thrive—malnutrition. Skin appears pale and may feel like parchment paper due to dehydration.[13]

◆ Body fat ratio low for child's age and height is not within normal developmental range.[4]

B. Behavioral Features

◆ Externalizing is common and may include aggressive, destructive, or antisocial behavior.[14]

◆ Internalizing is also frequent and includes withdrawn behavior.[14]

◆ Impulsivity, inattention, and hyperactivity.[14]

TABLE 14-1 • Indicators and Features of Child Abuse and Neglect

TYPE OF CHILD ABUSE AND NEGLECT	PHYSICAL INDICATORS	BEHAVIORAL INDICATORS	EMOTIONAL FEATURES	COGNITIVE FEATURES

Physical abuse	*Unexplained bruises and welts*
	• face, lips, mouth
	• torso, back, buttocks, thighs
	• various stages of healing
	• clustered, regular patterns
	• reflecting shape of article used to inflict (e.g., buckle)
	• on several different areas
	• regular appearance after absence, weekend, vacation
	Unexplained burns
	• cigarette, cigar burns, especially on soles, palms, back, buttocks
	• immersion burns (sock or glovelike, circular, on buttocks or genitalia)
	• patterned: electric burner, iron
	• rope burns on arms, legs, or torso
	• unexplained fractures
	• skull, nose, facial structures
	• in various stages of healing
	• multiple or spiral fractures
	Unexplained laceration or abrasion
	• to mouth, lips, gingiva, eyes
	• to external genitalia
	Malnutrition/underweight
		• Wary of adult contacts
		• Apprehensive when others cry
		• Behavioral extremes:
		  • Aggressive
		  • Withdrawn
		• Frightened of parents or caregiver
		• Afraid to go home
		• Reports injury by parents
		• Risky sexual behavior
			• Higher risk for mental health issues:
			  • Depression
			  • Anxiety
			  • Panic disorder
			  • PTSD
			  • Eating disorders
			  • Alcohol/drug abuse
			  • Suicide	

(Continues)

TABLE 14-1 • Indicators and Features of Child Abuse and Neglect (*Continued*)

TYPE OF CHILD ABUSE AND NEGLECT	PHYSICAL INDICATORS	BEHAVIORAL INDICATORS	EMOTIONAL FEATURES	COGNITIVE FEATURES

Physical neglect	• Constant hunger, poor hygiene, inappropriate dress
	• Consistent lack of supervision, especially in dangerous situations or for long periods
	• Unattended physical problems or medical/dental needs
	• Abandonment
		• Begging, stealing food
		• Extended stays at school, early arrival, late departure
		• Constant fatigue, falling asleep in class
		• Impulsivity
		• Alcohol or drug abuse
		• Externalizing
		  • Aggressive
		  • Destructive
		  • Antisocial/delinquency
		• Internalizing
		  • Withdrawn
		  • Says there is no caretaker
		  • Difficulty making friends
			• Low self-esteem
			• Difficulty regulating emotion
			• Fewer coping strategies
			• Depression
			• Lower levels of emotional understanding of peers
				• Lower general intelligence
				• Poorer executive functioning
				• Poorer manual dexterity, auditory
				• More problems with attention
				• Better problem-solving skills

Sexual abuse	• Difficulty in walking or sitting • Torn, stained, bloody underwear • Pain or itching in genital area • Bruises or bleeding on external genitalia, vaginal, or anal areas • Venereal disease, especially in preteen • Pregnancy	• Unwilling to change for physical education • Withdrawal, fantasy, or infantile behavior • Bizarre, sophisticated sexual knowledge, or behavior • Poor peer relationship • Delinquency; runaways • Reports sexual assault by caretaker	• Emotional dysregulation • Dissociation • Mental health issues, i.e., depression and compulsive behavior.	

Emotional maltreatment	• Speech disorders
	• Lags in physical development
	• Failure to thrive
		• Habit disorders (sucking, biting, rocking, etc.)
		• Conduct disorders (antisocial, destructive)
		• Neurotic traits (sleep disorders, inhibited play)
		• Psychoneurotic behaviors (hysteria, phobia, obsession, compulsion, hypochondria)
		• Impulsivity
		• Behavioral extremes:
		  • Compliant, passive
		  • Aggressive, demanding
		• Overly adaptive behavior:
		  • Inappropriately adult
		  • Inappropriately infantile
		• Attempted suicide
			• Poor social skills
			• Difficulty making friends
			• Low self-esteem
				• Lower general intelligence
				• Poorer executive functioning

Sources: Mouden LD, Lowe JW, Dixit UB. How to recognize situations that suggest abuse/neglect. *Missouri Dental J.* 1992 Nov-Dec; 26-29; Maguire SA, Williams B, Naughton AM, et al. A systematic review of the emotional, behavioural and cognitive features exhibited by school-aged children experiencing neglect or emotional abuse. *Child Care Health Dev.* 2015;41(5):641-653; Norman RE, Byambaa M, De R, Butchart A, Scott J, Vos T. The long-term health consequences of child physical abuse, emotional abuse, and neglect: a systematic review and meta-analysis. *PLoS Med.* 2012;9(11):e1001349; Hébert M, Langevin R, Oussaïd E. Cumulative childhood trauma, emotion regulation, dissociation, and behavior problems in school-aged sexual abuse victims. *J Affect Disord.* 2017;225:306-312.

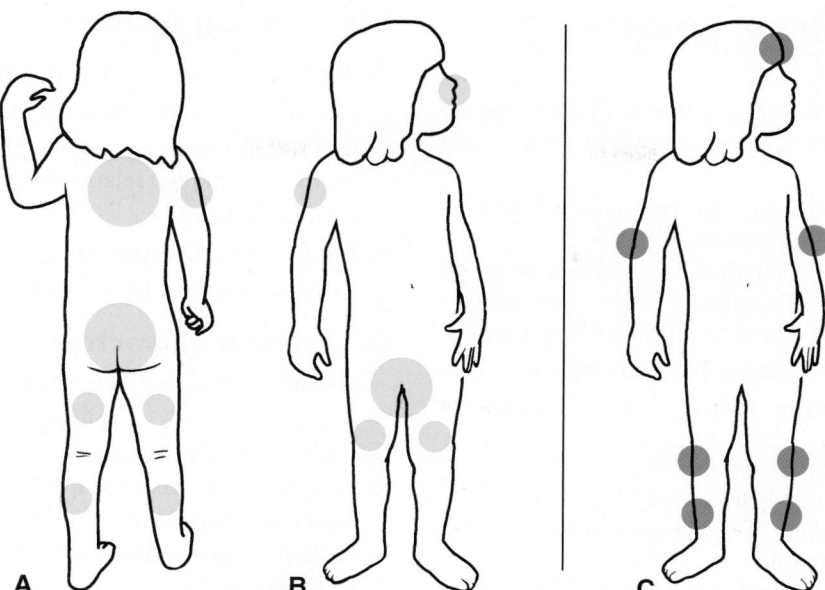

FIGURE 14-2 • Common Sites of Children's Injuries. A and B: Common sites of inflicted or deliberate injuries. **C:** Common sites of accidental injuries.

C. Social Behavior

◆ Observe the parent–child relationship. Child may act differently when the parent is present than when alone, which may provide clues to the type of relationship that exists.[13]

◆ Physically neglected children often have more difficulty with establishing and maintaining relationships.[14]

◆ A strong desire to please.[14]

◆ More likely to use compensation in social settings such as being the "class clown."[14]

D. Emotional Well-Being

◆ Neglected children have lower self-esteem.[14]

◆ Difficulty regulating emotions and may fail to understand negative emotions like anger and sadness.[14]

◆ Higher levels of depressive symptoms are seen in physical and emotionally maltreated children.[14]

E. Cognitive Features

◆ Neglected children may exhibit lower IQ along with less developed communication, reading, and math skills.[14]

◆ However, neglected children may exhibit well developed problem-solving skills.[14]

V. Extraoral Wounds and Signs of Trauma

◆ Abrasions and lacerations may be present at varying degrees of healing inconsistent with explanations given by the caregiver or child.[15]

◆ Recognizing injuries to the head and neck and connecting them to suspected child maltreatment can lead to early intervention and save the lives of the children involved.

◆ Accidental injuries usually occur only on one side. Accidental injuries that occur on both sides of the face are uncommon and may be pathognomonic of abuse.

◆ Common sites of deliberate injuries inflicted on children and accidental injuries on children are illustrated in Figure 14-2.
  • Skull injuries; edema, combined with ecchymosis of varying stages.[8,13]
  • Multicolor/fading bruises (indicating they were sustained over time).[16] Bald spots (traumatic alopecia) caused by pulling the hair out by the roots.
  • Raccoon sign: bilateral periorbital ecchymosis.
  • Nose fractures or displacements.
  • Lip bruises and lacerations; angular bruising, lichenification, or scarring, which can be caused from gags applied to the mouth.[6,15]
  • Marks on the skin that form a pattern of an object such as a belt buckle or handprint.[15]
  • Human bite marks.[6,13,15]

◆ Table 14-2 lists the possible conditions that can mimic lesions from child maltreatment.

TABLE 14-2 • Conditions That Can Mimic Abuse	
APPEARANCE	**POSSIBLE CONDITIONS**
Bruising	Accidental injuries
	Idiopathic thrombocytopenia purpura
	Hemophilia
Burns/red lesions	Port-wine stain
	Accidental burns
Skin lesions	Bullous impetigo
	Birthmarks

VI. Intraoral Signs of Abuse and Neglect

- A complete medical history followed by thorough intraoral/extraoral examinations are vital to assess traumatic injuries.
  - A sequential examination technique should be maintained on every patient.[11,12]
- Many injuries of the mouth in children can also be caused by accidental means. Therefore, it is important that the clinical presentation of the injuries match the explanation.
- Intraoral findings suggesting abuse may include:
  - Lacerations of the tongue, buccal mucosa, or palate.[6,15]
  - Lingual and labial frenal tears.
  - Discolored teeth (pulpal necrosis).[15]
  - Burns or lacerations of the gingiva, tongue, palate, or floor of the mouth.[15]
  - Teeth that are fractured, displaced, avulsed, or nonvital (may find multiple residual roots).[15]
  - Radiographic evidence of fractures in different degrees of healing.

A. Signs of Sexual Abuse

- Bruising or petechiae of the hard or soft palate can indicate forced oral sex.
- Sexually transmitted genital lesions found intraorally.
  - Sexually transmitted diseases suspected in prepubertal children should prompt an evaluation for sexual abuse.[16]
  - Condyloma acuminatum presents as a focal sessile-based lesion and also as a multiple papillary lesion (cauliflower). When present, it is necessary to look for other signs of oral sexual abuse because condyloma acuminatum can also occur with contact to verruca vulgaris or from self-inoculation.[17]
  - Primary herpetic gingivostomatitis can occur as a primary infection of herpes simplex virus type 2, which is a genital infection transmitted through oral sex. Presents as an oral or perioral painful, reddened area with a grapelike cluster of vesicles (blisters) that rupture to form lesions or sores.[17]
- Exhibits difficulty in walking or sitting.
- Extreme fear of the oral examination.

B. Intraoral Signs of Neglect

- Failure of the caregiver, who is responsible for the child, to seek dental care for that child can be considered intentional or unintentional neglect.
- Neglect becomes intentional when there is failure by the caregiver to follow through with treatment deemed necessary.
- Intraoral signs may include:
  - Signs of lack of personal daily care.[13]
  - Untreated disease, including rampant dental caries, pain, gingival inflammation, and bleeding.[6]
  - Lack of regularity of dental care; appointments made primarily for tooth or mouth pain only.[18,19]

VII. Parental Attitude

A. Reasons for Dental Neglect

- Oral health care may be considered a low priority.
- Lack of education concerning the significance of oral health care and the relation to general health.
- Limited finances.[20]
- Family isolation: access to care.[20]
- Religious and/or cultural beliefs.

B. Common Characteristics

- Disinterest or denial in relationship to the child.
- Critical, scolding, or belittling in front of others, including dental personnel.[20]
- Provides inconsistent information about the sources and causes of damaged teeth, bruises, or other signs of trauma.
- Lack of interest in proposed dental and dental hygiene treatment plan for significant oral disease, dental caries, or trauma.[20]
- Failure to complete a recommended course of treatment despite obvious need.[20]

C. Contributing Parental Factors for Abuse or Neglect

- Immature and unprepared for accepting the responsibilities of parenthood.[21]
- May have been maltreated themselves as a child.
- May have witnessed violence as a child.
- Unable to handle daily stresses of financial difficulties, work stress, job loss, and marital conflicts.[22]
- Drug use and alcoholism.
- Lacking a support network.[21]
- History of criminal activity.

D. Community and Social Factors

- Gender or social inequality.[21]
- Lack of adequate housing or services to support families.[7,21]
- High amounts of unemployment and/or poverty.[7,21]
- Availability of alcohol and drugs.
- Social, economic, and health and education policies that lead to poor living standards, or to socioeconomic inequality or instability.[21]
- Increased stress and community isolation.[22]

MUNCHAUSEN SYNDROME BY PROXY

I. General Considerations

- Munchausen Syndrome by Proxy (MSBP) is a type of abuse where a parent/caregiver fabricates or induces a disease on a child.[23]
- Difficult to diagnose: patient presents with a dramatic medical and/or dental history.[23]

- Disease does not follow the normal history of clinical presentation and is unsubstantiated.
- More commonly initiated by mother of child.[23]
- Over half of the mothers are found to be past victims of abuse.[23]
- Death of a child can occur.[23,24]
- Presented most often in young children 2 to 6 years of age.[24]
- Perpetrator wants to progress to more invasive diagnostic procedures for child.[23,24]
- Motive is attention and sympathy from healthcare professionals.[23,24]
- Child may grow to participate in the deception as they grow older.[24]

HUMAN TRAFFICKING

I. General Considerations

- *Trafficking in persons*, also known as human trafficking, is the recruitment, transportation, transfer, harboring, or receipt of persons by means of threat or use of force or other forms of coercion, abduction, fraud, deception, abuse of power or of a position of vulnerability, or the giving or receiving of payments or benefits to achieve the consent of a person having control over another person for the purpose of exploitation.
- Can include prostitution, sexual exploitation, forced labor or services, and slavery.[25]
- Occurs in the victim's own country or abroad.[26]
- Those most at risk are youth who are homeless, currently in foster system or previous history in the system, runaways, or those in juvenile detention centers.[25]
- Healthcare professionals may encounter a trafficking victim while they are still in captivity.
- Dental team may be first to render care to victim.[26]
- Similar universal signs of child abuse are observable.[27]
- Poor living conditions.[25]
- Victims comply and do not attempt escape for fear of retaliation on themselves or family.
- Can blame themselves for getting into situation (debt to trafficker).
- Dental staff must be aware of indicators of human trafficking and be able to provide resources to contact for assistance.[28]

II. Indicators of a Patient Involved in Human Trafficking

- Patient escorted by another person who seems controlling.[28]
- Accompanying person insists on speaking for the patient.[28]
- The escort does not know patient's medical details or is vague.[25,28]

- Patient seems submissive and fearful (avoids eye contact).[28]
- May have tattoos or other forms of branding of ownership (sexual exploitation).[27,28]
  - The tattoo may be a male name or nickname in an unusual place like the back of the neck, underarm, inner thigh, and so on.
- May show signs of malnutrition and poor oral hygiene.[28]
- May show serious dental disease from neglect (infections and tooth loss).[28]
- Treatment is usually cosmetic only and long-term maintenance or health is not a priority.

ELDER ABUSE AND NEGLECT

I. General Considerations

- Globally, one in six elders.[29]
- Estimated global population aged 60 years and older will be 2.1 billion by 2050.[29]
  - If the proportion of elder abuse remains constant, elder victims will increase to approximately 320 million by 2050.
- Elder abuse affects all socioeconomic groups, cultures, races, and ethnicities.
- Longitudinal study found victims of elder abuse are more likely to die prematurely.[29]
- Elderly women are at a higher risk of neglect and financial abuse.
- Widowed older adults who have poor physical health or cognitive impairments are also vulnerable to abuse.[29]
- Maltreatment occurs in institutional settings as well as in family home environments.
- Harm to the elder can occur through intentional (active) infliction or by unintentional (passive) neglect.
- Family members are the primary perpetrators of elder abuse.[29]
- Dental team must be vigilant in discerning the indicators of elder abuse and have the proper knowledge and resources to assist elderly patients.[29]
- The dental team, as in child abuse, can be a key source for the gathering of information to prove or disprove abuse of the elder patient.[30]

II. Definitions

- *Physical abuse*: the intentional use of force resulting in bodily injury, pain, or anguish.
- *Physical neglect*: the failure to provide basic necessities such as food, clothing, water, shelter, medicine, dental care, and personal hygiene.
  - This type of neglect can be intentional or unintentional due to the caregiver's lack of ability to provide such care.

◆ *Psychological abuse*: mental anguish and despair caused by ridicule, name-calling, humiliation, harassment, manipulation, threats, and controlling behavior.

◆ *Psychological neglect*: nonverbal anguish caused by the lack of communication and isolation.

◆ *Financial exploitation*: improper, illegal, or unethical exploitation of resources or assets.

◆ *Sexual abuse*: sexual contact with an older individual who is unable to consent or otherwise nonconsensual sexual contact or exploitation.

◆ *Self-neglect*: the behavior of an elderly person that threatens his or her own health or safety. This can occur owing to depression from a loss of a loved one. The elder may feel unable to continue living.

III. General Signs of Elder Abuse and Neglect

◆ When assessing for the possibility of abuse, it is necessary to have a working knowledge of lesions related to aging, health problems, or medications.

◆ Taking a thorough history and comparing it with lesions present will help determine an appropriate differential diagnosis.

◆ Signs of abuse or neglect may include, but not be limited to the following[31,32]:
  • May appear withdrawn, anxious, and shy; low self-esteem.
  • Provides an illogical explanation of how an injury occurred.
  • Depression or hostility may be exhibited.
  • May flinch at another person's movement as if expecting to be hit.
  • A sign of psychological abuse or intimidation can be deferral for response to questions to a caregiver or possible abuser.
  • May show signs of fear or apprehension if caregiver present.

IV. Physical Signs of Elder Abuse and Neglect

◆ Physical signs of abuse and neglect may include:
  • Bruises in various degrees of healing.
  • Human bite marks.
  • Contusions or abrasions exhibiting handprint or fingertip patterns.
  • Poor personal hygiene.
  • Inadequate clothing for the season.
  • Scratches or burns.
  • Traumatic alopecia.
  • *Wrapping bruises* (evidence of being restrained on the legs or wrists).
  • Patterned marks and bruising indicating object used to inflict injury such as belt buckle, ropes, or a hand (Figure 14-3).
  • Cachexia.

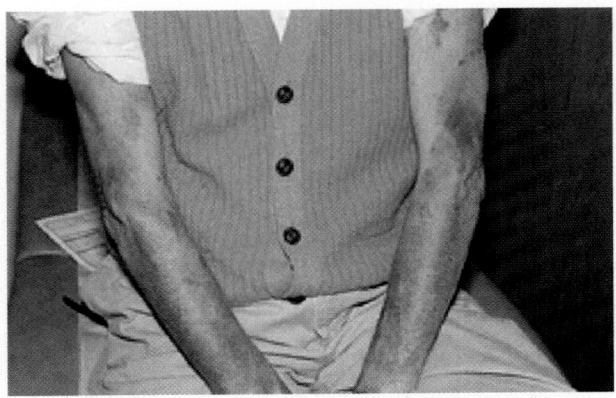

FIGURE 14-3 • Hand- and Finger-Shaped Bruises. Large and small bruises in various stages of healing on the upper arms of this elderly patient may trigger suspicions of abuse. (From Weber JR, Kelley JH. *Health Assessment in Nursing.* 2nd ed. Philadelphia, PA: Wolters Kluwer Health; 2006.)

V. Orofacial Signs of Abuse and Neglect

◆ Orofacial injuries are present in about 50% of those who have experienced elder abuse.

◆ Extraoral injuries may include[30,31]:
  • Lip trauma.
  • Bruising of facial tissues.
  • Eye injuries.
  • Broken eyeglasses or frames
  • Fractured or bruised mandible.
  • Temporomandibular joint pain.

◆ Intraoral injuries may include[17,31]:
  • Fractured, displaced, or avulsed teeth.
  • Sexually transmitted disease lesions such as condyloma acuminatum and primary herpetic gingivostomatitis.
  • Lesions or sore areas in the mouth from ill-fitting dentures: epulis fissuratum and atrophic candidiasis.
  • Fractured denture.
  • Poor oral hygiene.
  • Rampant dental caries.
  • Untreated periodontal disease.

INTIMATE PARTNER VIOLENCE

◆ IPV also known as domestic violence has been identified as global concern.[32]

◆ Many victims are hesitant to disclose the abuse due to emotional or familiar attachment (past or present).[32,33]

I. Prevalence of IPV

◆ IPV may include physical violence, psychological aggression, sexual violence, and stalking.[33]

◆ Severe physical violence by an intimate partner was experienced by 22.3% of women and 14% of men in the United States.[33]

◆ About 47% of women experience at least one act of psychological aggression by an intimate partner in their lifetime.[33]

◆ About 55.3% of all murders of women are committed by intimate partners.[34]
  • Black and American Indian/Alaska Native women have the highest rate of homicide in connection with partner violence.

II. Physical Injury from IPV

◆ Many of the same injuries listed for the elder abuse are also evident with partner violence.

◆ Injuries most frequently involve the face, eyes, and neck.[35]

◆ Physical injury may include[35,36]:
  • Scratches, bruises, contusions, and lacerations.
  • Fractured teeth.
  • Fractured bones, joint dislocations, strains, and sprains.
  • Abdominal and pelvic injuries.
  • Head injuries.
  • Strangulation-related injuries such as neck bruises, voice changes, swelling, and swallowing or breathing difficulties.

III. General Health Consequences of IPV

◆ In addition to acute injury from IPV, there are many long-term health impacts for victims of IPV.

◆ The health consequences reported include:
  • Chronic pain such as abdominal pain, pelvic pain, headache, and neck and low back pain.
  • Gastrointestinal disorders may include ulcers, irritable bowel syndrome, and gastroesophageal reflux.
  • Physical symptoms may include insomnia, fainting, and so on.
  • Increased risk for chronic disease such as high blood pressure, strokes, and cardiovascular system.
  • Increased rates of HIV and sexually transmitted diseases.
  • Increased risk for alcohol abuse and substance abuse.
  • Mental health consequences may include depression, posttraumatic stress disorder, and suicide.
  • Unintended pregnancy with increased risk of having a baby with low birth weight.[35]

IV. Orofacial Impact of IPV

◆ There is a correlation between IPV and oral health of the victim.[2]

◆ Head and neck injuries are common as previously noted.[2,35]
  • Chipped, cracked, or fractured teeth.
  • Avulsed teeth.
  • Fractured jaw.

◆ Poor oral health behaviors due to mental health consequences of IPV such as depression resulting in increased risk for caries and periodontal disease.[2]

◆ The psychological impact of IPV may result in fear of dental treatment due to loss of control.[2]

◆ Stress and anxiety can impact dental health (canker sores, cold sores, bruxism).[2]

V. Role of the Dental Hygienist

◆ IPV may be detected in the dental setting due the frequency of orofacial injuries, so it is essential for the dental team to properly identify and make appropriate referrals to support services if IPV is suspected or reported.

◆ Follow dental hygiene process or care protocol to perform thorough assessments and documentation of clinical findings.[11,12]

◆ Practice routine inquiry, especially for women.
  • General question: Do you feel safe at home?
  • Specific questions: "Have you ever been hit, kicked, punched, hurt, or frightened by someone important to you?" "How are things at home (HATAH)?" "Is it safe to go home?"

◆ Perform and document detailed extraoral/intraoral findings, including photographs of injuries.[11,12]

◆ Provide support; encourage open communication in a nonjudgmental manner.[11,12]

◆ Respect and maintain confidentiality; talk in a private setting (door closed to treatment room).

◆ Offer references for counseling; telephone numbers; community services.

◆ Respect patient's autonomy; ask about plans for future safety.

◆ Prepare to share your findings with authorities when called to provide evidence.

◆ When it is possible the interview will be used in a legal setting, a witness needs to be present.

REPORTING ABUSE AND/OR NEGLECT

◆ Dental professionals are ethically and legally mandated to report child and elder abuse and neglect.[37,38]

◆ Studies suggest both dentists and dental hygienists feel inadequately prepared to screen or report abuse.[39,40] Therefore, training is critical to meet the legal obligation to report abuse.

◆ Despite discomfort in asking questions to screen for abuse, research shows individuals experiencing abuse would have liked their dental provider to ask about their injuries and be given referral for assistance.[39,41]

I. Proper Training

- Training in the recognition and reporting of abuse and neglect needs to be implemented in every dental practice.
  - Many state governing boards require completion of continuing education courses on abuse and neglect before licensure and re-licensure to practice dentistry and dental hygiene.
- "Prevent Abuse and Neglect through Dental Awareness" (PANDA) is a program for training dental personnel and others interested in preventing FV.[37]
  - The coalition, founded in 1992 by the Missouri Bureau of Dental Health and Delta Dental of Missouri, is a public–private partnership committed to the education of all dental professionals in the recognition and reporting of suspected cases of child abuse and neglect.
  - Since its inception, nearly all of the United States and several international coalitions have replicated the program.
- "Ask, Validate, Document, Refer (AVDR) Tutorial for Dentists" is an interactive tutorial program that utilizes a case study to demonstrate the AVDR four-step process in response to DV.[42]
  - *Asking* the patient about the abuse.
  - *Validating* messages that acknowledge abuse is wrong.
  - *Documenting* the signs, symptoms, and disclosures.
  - *Referring* victims to specialists and community resources.
- Project RADAR is a provider-focused initiative in healthcare settings to promote assessment and prevention of IPV.[43]
  - **R**outinely ask about IPV.
  - **A**sk directly about violence, that is, "*Has a partner hit or otherwise frightened you?*"
  - **D**ocument findings in the patient chart.
  - **A**ssess safety by asking questions such as "*Do you feel safe to return home?*"
  - **R**eview options and referrals.
- Each office should have a list of resources to assist the patient in your community.

II. Reporting Laws

- Recognizing signs of suspected abuse and following proper reporting protocol will promote health and safety for all individuals.
- It is important for all healthcare providers (including dental providers) to be observant and knowledgeable about signs and symptoms of child abuse and neglect and to know how to respond.[6]
- Each state has laws regarding the reporting of abuse and neglect to the proper authorities. It is imperative to research the laws for the state and have them available for reference in the office.
- Each dental practice needs a written protocol for the documentation and reporting of abuse and neglect.[37,44]

III. Reportable Required Information

- All states mandate healthcare workers to report suspected abuse and neglect of children, disabled individuals, and the elderly.[37,38,44]
- Many states have hotlines for reporting child, disabled persons, and elder abuse.
  - A national hotline for child abuse is 800.4.A.CHILD (800.422.4453).
  - A national domestic violence hotline is 800.799.SAFE (800.799.7233).
  - State resources for elder abuse can be found on the National Center for Elder Abuse https://ncea.acl.gov/Resources/State.aspx. Accessed June 21, 2019.
  - A national adult abuse hotline for elder abuse is (800) 222-8000.
- When reporting suspected child maltreatment, it is necessary to have the following information available:
  - Name and address of the child and parents or other persons having custody of the child.
  - Child's age.
  - Names of siblings, if any.
  - Nature of the child's condition, including evidence of previous injuries.
  - Any information that might be helpful in establishing the cause of abuse or neglect and the identity of the person believed to have caused such abuse or neglect.
- The information needed for reporting suspected abuse/neglect of the elderly or a disabled individual would be similar to that needed for a child.
- Healthcare workers are required by law to report suspected IPV in some states.

FORENSIC DENTISTRY

Forensic dentistry is that aspect of dental science that relates and applies dental facts to legal problems.

- Forensic dentistry encompasses dental identification, malpractice litigation, legislation, peer review, and dental licensure.
- Forensics is a specialty and is not within the scope of practice of any dentist or auxiliary without proper advanced training and certification or recognition.

I. Use of Forensics in Abuse Cases

- There are instances when it becomes necessary to request the aid of a forensic odontologist to determine if a particular injury, usually a bite mark, is a result of trauma caused by a particular suspect.[45]
  - Many times, the abuser will state the bite mark occurred from a sibling squabble, an animal bite, or the child biting himself or herself.
  - Animal bite and human bites have distinctly different presentations on the skin surface.

- When photographs have been obtained and the history of the injury does not match the location of the marks, a bite mark analysis can be requested of the forensic odontologist.
  - An expert is required when a bite mark may be a relevant evidence in a case of abuse.[45,46]
- A forensic expert can take impressions and a bite registration from the suspect/caregiver.
  - Careful analysis will determine if the bite came from that suspect.[45]
  - Different teeth produce specific shape injuries that assist with analysis.[45]
- The information obtained can then be used in the prosecution of someone accused of abuse.

II. Other Uses of Forensics

- Forensic procedures are used primarily in the identification of victims of a disaster or suspicious death.[46]
- DNA extracted from dentition may be used in identification of victims.[45]
- Forensic teams include dentists, dental hygienists, and assistants with special training in the process of identifying remains by comparing the dentition of the remains with dental records.
- Team members are assigned a task, and the team works together to check and double-check results. Along with the legal implications, forensics may allow families of the victims to have closure regarding the loss of a loved one.

DOCUMENTATION

I. Purposes of Thorough and Accurate Documentation

- For future reference and comparison.
- To provide authorities meticulous information to support an investigation.
- To protect the abused patient from harmful circumstances or even death. A second person needs to be present to witness the examination and interview.

II. Content of the Record

- Obtain thorough histories of the injury from both the caregiver and the patient. Identify inconsistencies.
- Document the date, time, and place of the examination.
- Record all observable facts.
- Record questions asked of the abused patient and document all answers in the patient's exact words as closely as possible.
- Document all lesions, giving descriptive location, estimation of size, shape, and color. Pay close attention to ecchymosis of varying colors and bilateral injuries.

- Use diagrams showing the location, size, and description.[45]
- Photographs and radiographs can also be used to supplement findings.
  - Photographs can only be made with patient consent and could be released only with consent.
  - There may be special provisions by law that allow the taking and releasing of photographs without consent when the healthcare provider is required by law to report suspected abuse.
- Scale photography would be necessary for bite marks, so further analysis can be done.
- Use the words *suspected abuse* if the patient denies abuse.[45]
- Box 14-1 provides a sample of documenting suspected abuse noted during a patient visit.

BOX 14-1

Example Documentation: Patient Injury Related to Suspected Abuse

S—A 23-year-old female presents for an emergency visit because of pain in mandibular right second premolar area. Patient complains of recent headaches and pain in right temporomandibular joint area. She states "my boyfriend slapped me recently, but he has been under a lot of pressure lately and he didn't mean to bruise me." Patient seems nervous and agitated.

O—Patient presents with multiple contusions on right side of face above inferior border of mandible and right buccal mucosa. Bruises are in various stages of healing; red, purple, and greenish yellow. Bruises are oval shaped about 2 to 5 cm in size. Intraoral and extraoral photographs were taken.

A—Panoramic radiograph revealed a simple fracture on the body of the mandible below right second premolar area. Patient confirmed that injuries are likely related to partner abuse.

P—Reassured patient that she did not deserve the abuse and provided her with the national domestic violence hotline number. Patient was referred to oral surgeon for evaluation of fractured mandible.

Next step: Follow-up telephone call to patient after her scheduled appointment with the oral surgeon.

Signed: _____, RDH

Date: _____

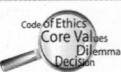

EVERYDAY ETHICS

Mrs. Kelly is an 82-year-old patient in Dr. Tyler's dental practice for 10 years. Mrs. Kelly's husband recently passed away 3 months ago. Today Mrs. Kelly has returned for her 6-month dental hygiene appointment with Tammy, the dental hygienist. Upon reviewing Mrs. Kelly's chart, a new address has been noted. Tammy has been informed by the office manager that Mrs. Kelly now resides with her adult son and his family since her husband's passing.

Today Mrs. Kelly's son Rick has accompanied her for the appointment. Upon entry to the treatment room, Rick asks Tammy in an annoyed tone, "How long is this going to take?" Tammy informs Rick that Mrs. Kelly's appointment is usually around 1 hour. Rick tells his mother he is going to grab a coffee at the shop across the street and motions Mrs. Kelly to give him some money. As Mrs. Kelly extends her forearm to reach for some cash in her wallet, it is then that Tammy notices a pattern of bruises of varying colors exposed on Mrs. Kelly's forearm. She hands Rick a 10-dollar bill and he reaches in and takes another 10 and quickly leaves the room. Mrs. Kelly smiles faintly as she pulls down her sleeve.

During her appointment, Tammy performs a routine oral tissue exam and notes a 4-mm scar on her left vermillion border of her upper lip that was not present 6 months ago. When she inquires about the cause, Mrs. Kelly tears up and says she fell in the shower. She said that is how she also got the bruises on her forearms too. Tammy suspects that Mrs. Kelly is not being truthful and that she is being abused. She asks if she feels safe in her new living arrangements and Mrs. Kelly shakes her head in a "no" motion. She tells Tammy she misses her husband. Just then Rick returns and says they have to go as he has been called to work. Mrs. Kelly is dismissed before any further discussion can occur.

Questions for Consideration

1. Which of the dental hygiene core values apply in this case? Explain the relationship of each dental hygiene Core Value you select?

2. Is this an ethical issue or an ethical dilemma for Tammy? Why? Using the four-step approach in making ethical decisions in Chapter 1, develop a course of action that would assist Tammy in resolving the issue.

3. How would Tammy incorporate her suspicions about Mrs. Kelly into her discussion of the assessment findings with Dr. Tyler?

Factors to Teach the Patient

Factors to Teach the Abused Elder or Intimate Partner

▶ Where help can be obtained: emergency assistance including phone numbers and referrals.

▶ The tendency for the maltreatment to increase in severity and frequency over time.

▶ Abuse can escalate and can be life-threatening.

▶ Maltreatment is a choice. It is used to gain power and control over another individual.

ENHANCE YOUR UNDERSTANDING

ONLINE RESOURCES
(see the inside front cover for access information)

• Audio glossary

• Appendices

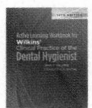

SUPPORT FOR LEARNING
(available separately)

• *Active Learning Workbook for Wilkins' Clinical Practice of the Dental Hygienist, 13th Edition*

INDIVIDUALIZED REVIEW

• Customized practice quizzing with Navigate 2 TestPrep for *Wilkins' Clinical Practice of the Dental Hygienist*

References

1. Sumner SA, Mercy JA, Dahlberg LL, et al. Violence in the United States: status, challenges, and opportunities. *JAMA.* 2015;314(5):478-488.

2. Kundu H, Basavaraj P, Singla A, et al. Domestic violence and its effect on oral health behaviour and oral health status. *J Clin Diagn Res.* 2014;8(11):ZC9-ZC12.

3. Tolan P, Gorman-Smith D, Henry D. Family violence. *Annu Rev Psychol.* 2006;57:557-583.

4. Krug EG, Dahlberg LL, Mercy JA, Zwi AB, Lozana R, eds. *Child Abuse and Neglect by Parents and Other Caregivers.* World Report on Violence and Health. Geneva, Switzerland: World Health Organization; 2002. http://www.who.int/violence_injury_prevention/violence/global_campaign/en/chap3.pdf. Assessed July 23, 2018.

5. Consultation on Child Abuse Prevention, World Health Organization, Violence and Injury Prevention Team & Global Forum for Health Research. *Report of the Consultation on Child Abuse Prevention.* March 29-31, 1999. Geneva, Switzerland: World Health Organization. http://www.who.int/iris/handle/10665/65900. Accessed January 29, 2019.

6. Leeb RT, Paulozzi L, Melanson C, Simon T, Arias I. *Child Maltreatment Surveillance: Uniform Definitions for Public Health and Recommended Data Elements, Version 1.0.* Atlanta, GA: Centers for Disease Control and Prevention, National Center for Injury Prevention and Control; 2008. https://www.cdc.gov/violenceprevention/pdf/cm_surveillance-a.pdf. Accessed February 3, 2019.

7. Fisher-Owens SA, Lukefahr JL, Tate AR, American Academy of Pediatric Dentistry, Council on Clinical Affairs, Council on Scientific Affairs, Ad Hoc Work Group on Child Abuse and Neglect, American Academy of Pediatrics, Section on Oral Health Committee on Child Abuse and Neglect. Oral and dental aspects of child abuse and neglect. *Pediatr Dent.* 2017;39(4):278-283.

8. Maclean MJ, Sims S, Bower C, Leonard H, Stanley FJ, O'Donnell M. Maltreatment risk among children with disabilities. *Pediatrics.* 2017;139(4):e20161817.

9. U.S. Department of Health & Human Services, Administration for Children and Families, Administration on Children, Youth and Families, Children's Bureau. Child maltreatment 2017. 2019. https://www.acf.hhs.gov/cb/research-data-technology/statistics-research/child-maltreatment. Accessed May 21, 2019.

10. Christian CW, Committee on Child Abuse and Neglect. The evaluation of suspected child abuse. *Pediatrics.* 2015;135(5):e1337-e1354.

11. American Dental Hygienists' Association. ADHA Standards for clinical dental hygiene practice. June 2016. https://www.adha.org/resources-docs/2016-Revised-Standards-for-Clinical-Dental-Hygiene-Practice.pdf. Accessed June 8, 2018.

12. Canadian Dental Hygienists' Association. Entry to practice competencies and standards for Canadian Dental Hygienist. 2010. https://www.cdha.ca/pdfs/Competencies_and_Standards.pdf. Accessed June 8, 2018.

13. Child Welfare Information Gateway. *What is Child Abuse and Neglect? Recognizing the Signs and Symptoms.* Washington, DC: U.S. Department of Health and Human Services, Children's Bureau. 2013. https://www.childwelfare.gov/pubs/factsheets/whatiscan/. Accessed June 8, 2018.

14. Maguire SA, Williams B, Naughton AM, et al. A systematic review of the emotional, behavioural and cognitive features exhibited by school-aged children experiencing neglect or emotional abuse. *Child Care Health Dev.* 2015;41(5):641-653.

15. Costacurta M, Benavoli D, Arcudi G, et al. Oral and dental signs of child abuse and neglect. *Oral Implantol.* 2016;8(2-3):68-73.

16. Adams JA, Kellogg ND, Farst KJ, et al. Updated guidelines for the medical assessment and care of children who have been sexually abused. *J Pediatric Adolesc Gynecol.* 2016;29(2):81-87.

17. Percinoto AC, Danelon M, Crivelini MM, Cunha RF, Percinoto C. Condyloma acuminata in the tongue and hard palate of a sexually abused child: a case report. *BMC Res Notes.* 2014;7:467.

18. Lourenco CB, Saintrain MV, De L, Vieira F. Child, neglect and oral health. *BMC Pediatrics.* 2013;13:188. doi:10.1186/1471-2431-13-188.

19. Harris JC. The mouth and maltreatment: safeguarding issues in child dental health. *Arch Dis Child.* 2018;103:722-729.

20. Bhatia SK, Maguire SA, Chadwick BL, et al. Characteristics of child dental neglect: a systematic review. *J Dent.* 2014;42(3):229-239.

21. Fortson BL, Klevens J, Merrick MT, Gilbert LK, Alexander SP. *Preventing Child Abuse and Neglect: A Technical Package for Policy, Norm, and Programmatic Activities.* 2016. Atlanta, GA: National Center for Injury Prevention and Control, Centers for Disease Control and Prevention. https://www.cdc.gov/violenceprevention/pdf/can-prevention-technical-package.pdf. Accessed January 16, 2018.

22. Tucker MC, Rodriguez CM. Family dysfunction and social isolation as moderators between stress and child physical abuse risk. *J Fam Violence.* 2014;29(2):175-186.

23. Olczak-Kowalczyk D, Wolska-Kusnierz B, Bernatowska E. Fabricated or induced illness in the oral cavity in children. A systematic review and personal experience. *Cent Eur J Immunol.* 2015;40:109-114.

24. Gehlawat P, Gehlawat VK, Singh P, Gupta R. Munchausen syndrome by proxy: an alarming face of child abuse. *Indian J Psychol Med.* 2015;37:90-92.

25. Greenbaum J, Bodrick N, AAP Committee on Child Abuse and Neglect, AAP Section on International Child Health. Global human trafficking and child victimization. *Pediatrics.* 2017;140(6):e20173138.

26. O'Callaghan MG. Human trafficking and the dental professional. *J Am Dent Assoc.* 2012;143:498-504.

27. Fang S, Coverdale J, Nguyen P, Gordon M. Tattoo recognition in screening for victims of human trafficking. *J Nerv Ment Dis.* 2018;206(10):824-827.

28. Shandro J, Chisolm-Straker M, Duber HC, et al. Human trafficking: a guide to identification and approach for the emergency physician. *Ann Emerg Med.* 2016;68(4):501-508.

29. Yon Y, Mikton CR, Gassoumis ZD, Wilber KH. Elder abuse prevalence in community settings: a systematic review and meta-analysis. *Lancet Glob Health.* 2017;5(2):e147-e156.

30. Furnari W. Oral health professional alert: elder abuse concern in the United States and Canada. *Can J Dent Hygiene.* 2011;45(2):98-102.

31. Petti S. Elder neglect—Oral diseases and injuries. *Oral Dis.* 2018;24:891-899.

32. Lachs MS, Pillemer KA. Elder abuse. *N Engl J Med.* 2015;373(20):1947-1956.

33. Breiding MJ, Smith SG, Basile KC, Walters ML, Chen J, Merrick MT. Prevalence and characteristics of sexual violence, stalking, and intimate partner violence victimization—national intimate partner and sexual violence survey, United States, 2011. *MMWR Surveill Summ.* 2014;63(8):1-18.

34. Petrosky E, Blair JM, Betz CJ, Fowler KA, Jack SP, Lyons BH. Racial and ethnic differences in homicides of adult women and the role of intimate partner violence—United States, 2003–2014. *MMWR Morb Mortal Wkly Rep.* 2017;66:741-746.

35. Sugg N. Intimate partner violence: prevalence, health consequences, and intervention. *Med Clin North Am.* 2015;99(3):629-649.

36. Pritchard AJ, Reckdenwald A, Nordham C. Nonfatal strangulation as part of domestic violence: a review of research. *Trauma Violence Abuse.* 2017;18(4):407-424.

37. Katner D, Brown C. Mandatory reporting of oral injuries indicating possible child abuse. *J Am Dent Assoc.* 2012;143(10):1087-1092.

38. U.S. Department of Justice. State elder abuse statutes. https://www.justice.gov/elderjustice/elder-justice-statutes-0. Accessed February 10, 2019.

39. Parish CL, Pereyra MR, Abel SN, Siegel K, Pollack HA, Metsch LR. Intimate partner violence screening in the dental setting: results of a nationally representative survey. *J Am Dent Assoc.* 2018;149(2):112-121.

40. Harris CM, Boyd L, Rainchuso L, et al. Oral healthcare providers' knowledge and attitudes about intimate partner violence. *J Dent Hyg.* 2016;90(5):283-296.

41. Nelms AP, Gutmann ME, Solomon ES, Dewald JP, Campbell PR. What victims of domestic violence need from the dental profession. *J Dent Educ.* 2009;73(4):490-498.

42. Kwon-Hsieh N, Herzig K, Gansky SA, Danley D, Gerbert B. Changing dentists' knowledge, attitudes, and behaviors regarding domestic violence through an interactive multimedia tutorial. *J Am Dent Assoc.* 2006;137:596-603.

43. Alpert EJ. *Intimate Partner Violence: The Clinician's Guide to Identification, Assessment, Intervention, and Prevention.* 6th ed. Waltham, MA: Massachusetts Medical Society Committee on Violence Intervention and Prevention. 2015. http://www.massmed.org/Patient-Care/Health-Topics/Violence-Prevention-and-Intervention/Intimate-Partner-Violence-(pdf). Accessed February 10, 2019.

44. Child Welfare Information Gateway. Mandatory reporters of child abuse and neglect. Children's Bureau. 2015. https://www.childwelfare.gov/pubPDFs/manda.pdf. Accessed May 21, 2019.

45. Sweet D, Pretty IA. A look at forensic dentistry—Part 2: teeth as weapons of violence—Identification of bitemark perpetrators. *Br Dent J.* 2001;190(8):415-418.

46. Gupta S, Agnihotri A, Chandra A, Gupta OP. Contemporary practice in forensic odontology. *J Oral Maxillofac Pathol.* 2014;18(2):233-250.

15

Dental Radiographic Imaging

Janet M. Gruber, RDH, MS, MPA

CHAPTER OUTLINE

INTRODUCTION

HOW X-RAYS ARE PRODUCED
I. The X-Ray Tube
II. Circuits
III. Transformers
IV. Machine Control Devices
V. Steps in the Production of X-Rays

DIGITAL RADIOGRAPHY
I. Digital Imaging Principles
II. Digital Imaging and Sensors
III. Steps in the Production of a Digital Radiograph
IV. Evaluation

CHARACTERISTICS OF AN ACCEPTABLE RADIOGRAPHIC IMAGE
I. Radiolucency and Radiopacity
II. Radiopacity
III. Radiolucency

FACTORS THAT INFLUENCE THE FINISHED RADIOGRAPH
I. Collimation
II. Filtration
III. Kilovoltage
IV. Milliampere Seconds
V. Distance
VI. Image Receptors

EXPOSURE TO RADIATION
I. Ionizing Radiation
II. Exposure
III. Sensitivity of Cells

RISK OF INJURY FROM RADIATION
I. Rules for Radiation Protection
II. Protection of Clinician
III. Protection of Patient
IV. Assessment
V. Risk Reduction

PROCEDURES FOR IMAGE RECEPTOR PLACEMENT AND ANGULATION OF CENTRAL RAY

IMAGE RECEPTOR SELECTION FOR INTRAORAL SURVEYS
I. Periapical Surveys
II. Bitewing (Interproximal) Surveys
III. Occlusal Surveys

PERIAPICAL SURVEY: PARALLELING TECHNIQUE
I. Patient Position
II. Image Receptor Placement and Central Ray Angulation
III. Paralleling Technique: Features

BITEWING SURVEY
I. Positioning
II. Image Receptor Placement: Horizontal Bitewing Survey
III. Image Receptor Placement: Vertical Bitewing Survey

PERIAPICAL SURVEY: BISECTING-ANGLE TECHNIQUE

OCCLUSAL SURVEY
I. Uses and Purposes
II. Maxillary Midline Topographic Projection
III. Mandibular Topographic and Cross-Sectional Projection

PANORAMIC RADIOGRAPHIC IMAGES
I. Technique
II. Uses
III. Limitations
IV. Procedures

INFECTION CONTROL
I. Practice Policy
II. Basic Procedures
III. No-Touch Method for Films and PSP Plates

TRADITIONAL FILM PROCESSING
I. Image Production
II. Darkroom Lighting
III. Automated Processing
IV. Manual Processing

HANDHELD X-RAY DEVICES

ANALYSIS OF COMPLETED RADIOGRAPHS
I. Mounting
II. Anatomic Landmarks
III. Identification of Errors in Radiographs
IV. Interpretation

OWNERSHIP

DOCUMENTATION
I. Radiation Exposure History
II. Patient Care Progress Notes

EVERYDAY ETHICS

FACTORS TO TEACH THE PATIENT

REFERENCES

LEARNING OBJECTIVES

After studying this chapter, the student will be able to:

1. Compare different imaging systems and describe the advantages and disadvantages of each.

2. Describe factors that influence the finished radiograph.

3. Identify electrical components located in an X-ray unit's tube head and describe how radiographs are produced.

4. Explain clinician and patient radiation protection guidelines and published recommendations for patient selection and exposure.

5. Assess need and justify radiographic exposure for each patient.

INTRODUCTION

Radiographic images are integral assessment components useful when planning comprehensive care for a patient. They provide the clinician with important diagnostic tools that can be used:

◆ To detect lesions, diseases, and other conditions of teeth and supporting structures.

◆ To localize foreign objects.

◆ To assess growth and development.

◆ To document changes in, and progress of, a condition over time.

The dentist is responsible for determining the need for radiographs.

◆ Designation of the number and types of dental exposures is made selectively only after a review of the patient's health history and a complete clinical examination.[1]

◆ A history of oral and body exposures to radiation is recommended.

◆ Excessive dental exposure to low levels of ionizing radiation cannot be justified.[2]

The objective in radiography is to use procedures that expose the patient to the least possible amount of radiation to produce radiographs of the greatest interpretive value. The first consideration is to limit the number of exposures to those that have been deemed necessary.

This chapter provides a summary of terminology and fundamentals of dental radiology, including:

◆ X-ray production.

◆ Procedures for all image receptor exposures and traditional film processing.

◆ Safety factors.

◆ Analysis of the completed radiographs.

◆ Suggestions for patient instruction.

HOW X-RAYS ARE PRODUCED

X-ray energy is electromagnetic ionizing radiation of very short wavelengths, resulting from the bombardment of a target made of tungsten by highly accelerated electrons in a vacuum. Electric and magnetic fields positioned at right angles to one another produce electromagnetic energy.

The various types of energy in the electromagnetic spectrum have similar attributes. The properties of X-rays are listed in Box 15-1.

Essential to X-ray production are:

◆ A source of electrons.

◆ A high voltage to accelerate the electrons.

◆ A target to stop the electrons.

The parts of the tube and the circuits within the machine are designed to provide these elements.

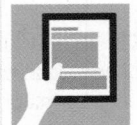

BOX 15-1
Properties of X-Rays

Characteristic
- Invisible
- No mass
- No weight

Travel
- In straight line; can be scattered
- At the speed of light

Wavelengths
- Have short wavelengths, high frequency
- Hard X-rays: short wavelengths, high penetration
- Soft X-rays: relatively longer wavelengths; relatively less penetrating; more likely to be absorbed into the tissue

Penetration
- Pass through matter, or
- Absorbed by matter, depending on atomic structure of matter

Causes
- Ionization
- Fluorescence of certain crystals
- Biologic changes in living cells

Produces
- A radiographic image

I. The X-Ray Tube

A. Protective Tube Housing

◆ A heavy metal enclosure houses the X-ray tube (Figure 15-1) and reduces primary radiation to permissible exposure levels and prevents leakage radiation.

B. X-Ray Tube

◆ A highly evacuated leaded glass tube composed of a cathode and an anode and surrounded by a specially refined oil with high insulating powers.

C. Cathode

◆ Tungsten filament, which is a coiled wire heated to generate a cloud of electrons. It is a component of the low-voltage circuit.

◆ Molybdenum cup around the filament to focus the electrons toward the anode.

D. Anode (+)

◆ A tungsten target embedded in a copper stem, positioned at an angle to the electron beam.

E. Aperture

◆ The window through which the useful beam emerges from the tube, covered with a permanent seal of glass.

F. Aluminum Disks

◆ Thin (0.5-mm) sheets of aluminum placed over the aperture to filter out longer-wavelength X-rays.

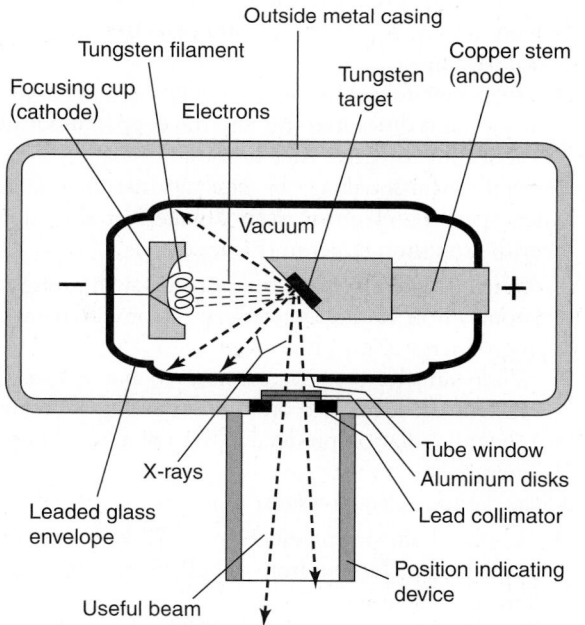

FIGURE 15-1 • X-Ray Tube. High-speed electrons flowing from cathode to anode hit the tungsten target and create X-ray photons. X-rays exit through the tube window and position-indicating device.

G. Lead Diaphragm

◆ A lead collimator with a hole to restrict the size of the X-ray beam.

H. Position-Indicating Device

◆ Open-ended cylinder, or rectangle, that shapes and aims the X-ray beam.

II. Circuits

A circuit is the complete path over which an electrical current may flow. Two circuits are used to produce X-rays. Refer to Figure 15-2 to examine the electrical circuits in a dental X-ray machine. Two circuits used to produce X-rays are:

◆ Low-voltage filament circuit
◆ High-voltage cathode–anode circuit.

III. Transformers

A transformer increases or decreases the incoming voltage.
◆ *Autotransformer*
  • A voltage compensator that corrects minor variations in line voltage.
◆ *Filament step-down transformer*
  • Decreases the line voltage to approximately 3 V to heat the filament and form the electron cloud.
◆ *High-voltage step-up transformer*
  • Increases the current from 110 V to 60 to 90 kVp (kilovoltage peak) to give electrons the energy required to produce X-ray photons.

IV. Machine Control Devices

Machines vary, but, in general, when operating an X-ray machine, there are four factors to control: the power switch (to the electrical outlet), the kilovoltage, the milliamperage, and the time.

A. Voltage Control

Voltage is the unit of measurement used to describe the force that pushes an electric current through a circuit.
◆ *Circuit voltmeter*: Registers line voltage before voltage is stepped up by the transformer (with alternating current [AC], this is 110 V) or may register the kilovoltage that results after step-up.
◆ *kVp (selector)*: Used to change the line voltage to a selected kilovoltage (60–90 kVp).

B. Milliamperage Control

◆ *Ampere*: The unit of intensity of an electrical current produced by 1 V acting through a resistance of 1 Ω. A milliampere (mA) is 1/1,000 of an ampere.
◆ *Milliammeter*: Instrument used to select the actual current through the tube circuit during the time of exposure.

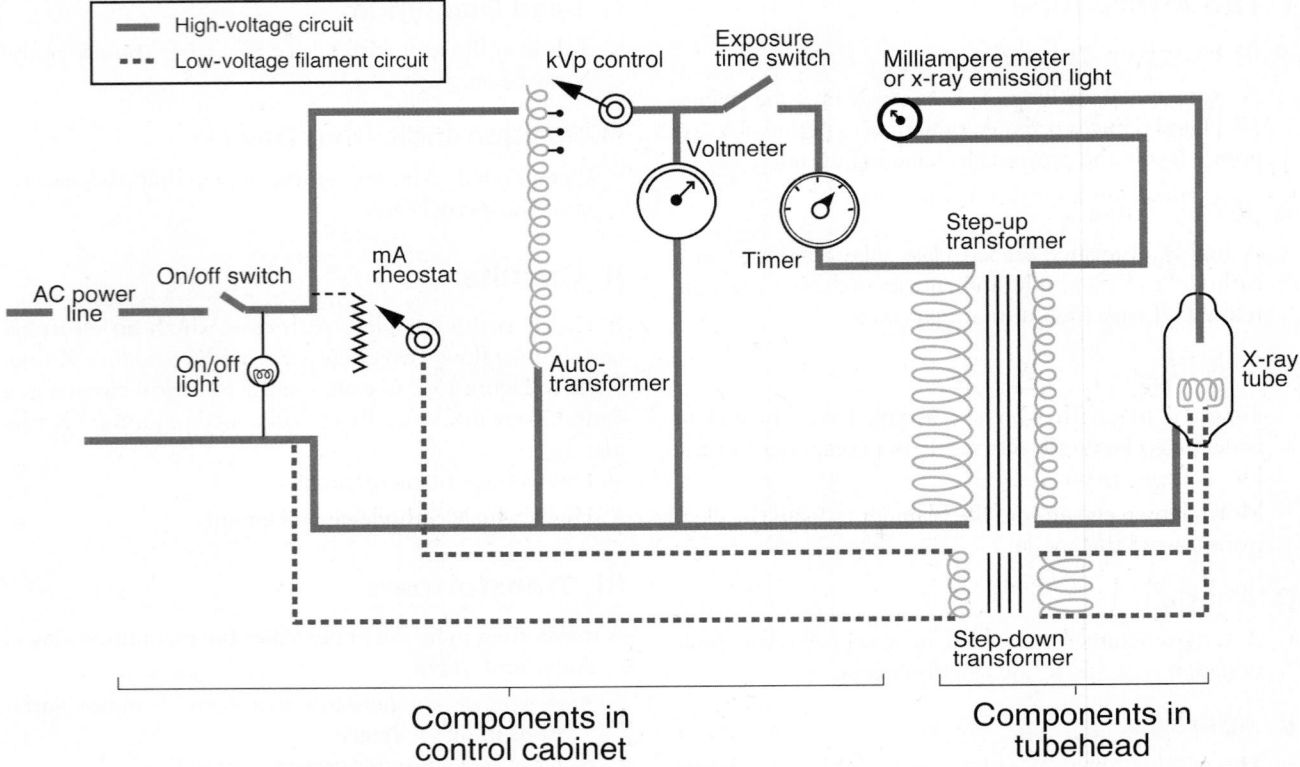

FIGURE 15-2 • Dental X-Ray Machine Circuits. High- and low-voltage circuits in a dental X-ray machine demonstrating flow of electricity from the on/off switch to the X-ray tube head. (Adapted with permission from Olson SS. *Dental Radiography Laboratory Manual.* Philadelphia, PA: W.B. Saunders; 1995:40.)

C. Time Control

- *X-ray timer:* A time switch mechanism used to control the length of the exposure time.
- *Time-delay switch:* Mechanism that applies power to the high-voltage circuit once the filament is heated.
- *Electronic timer:* Vacuum tube device; resets itself automatically to the last-used exposure time. The timer is calibrated in seconds or in impulses, with 60 *impulses* in each second (in a 60-cycle AC).

V. Steps in the Production of X-Rays

X-rays are produced when high-speed electrons are slowed down or stopped suddenly.

- Tungsten filament is heated, and a cloud of electrons is produced.
- Difference in electrical potential is developed between the anode and the cathode.
- Electrons traveling at a high speed are attracted to the anode from the cathode when the anode is charged positive and the cathode negative. When AC is used with a self-rectifying tube, the electrons are attracted back into the tungsten filament.
- Curvature of the molybdenum cup controls the direction of the electrons and causes them to be projected toward the focal spot.

- Reaction of the electrons as they strike the tungsten target results in loss of energy.
  - Approximately 1% of the energy of electrons is converted to X-ray energy (greater percentage at higher kilovoltages).
  - Approximately 99% of the energy is converted to heat and is dissipated through the copper anode and oil of the protective tube housing.
- *General (bremsstrahlung, or braking) radiation* occurs when speeding electrons stop, "brake," or slow down near the tungsten target in the anode.
  - When an electron hits the nucleus of the tungsten atom, all of its kinetic energy is converted into a high-energy X-ray photon.
  - When an electron comes close to but misses the nucleus, an X-ray photon of lower energy is created.
  - General radiation produces X-rays of many different energies.
- *Characteristic radiation results:*
  - When a bombarding electron, at 70 kVp or above, displaces an electron from a shell of the target atom, ionizing the atom.
  - Another electron in an outer shell replaces the missing electron, causing a cascading effect.
  - When the displaced electron is replaced, a photon is emitted, resulting in characteristic radiation.
  - Characteristic radiation contributes approximately 10% to the useful beam.

◆ *X-rays leave the tube through the aperture to form the useful beam.*

- *Useful beam:* The part of the primary radiation that is permitted to emerge from the tube head aperture and the accessory collimating devices.
- *Central beam* (central ray): The center of the beam of X-rays emitted from the tube.

DIGITAL RADIOGRAPHY

◆ Traditional film-based systems to record radiographic images have been in existence in dentistry since 1895.

◆ In the mid- to late 1980s, the first direct digital imaging system was introduced and adopted by dental professionals.

◆ Digital imaging is a method of imaging using a sensor, breaking it into small electronic pieces, and presenting and storing the image using a computer.

◆ Digital systems include intraoral, panoramic, and cephalometric imaging.

I. Digital Imaging Principles

◆ Digital radiography requires conventional equipment to generate X-rays.

◆ The image is captured on sensors or plates of varying sizes, similar to conventional film.

◆ The information is then recorded as a digital image and displayed as pixels representing multiple shades of gray.

◆ The image is subsequently displayed on a computer monitor.

◆ The image can be enhanced and manipulated, by changing factors such as density and contrast, stored on the hard drive for future reference, and/or electronically sent to other professionals.[3-5]

II. Digital Imaging and Sensors

A. Direct Digital Imaging

◆ A corded or cordless charge-coupled device (CCD) or complementary metal-oxide semiconductor (CMOS) sensor in a rigid case is used. Both convert X-radiation to electrons that are stored in electron wells and converted to visible images. With CMOS technology, individual pixels can be made smaller (Figure 15-3).

◆ Viewing of the image is possible on the computer screen, within seconds of exposure.

B. Indirect Digital Imaging

◆ A cordless photostimulable phosphor (PSP) plate is used that converts X-radiation into stored energy to record the image (Figure 15-4).

◆ Information on the PSP plate is then read by a laser scanner and converted to digital data.

◆ The digital image is displayed on a monitor.

◆ Traditional films can also be scanned as analog images and converted to digital.

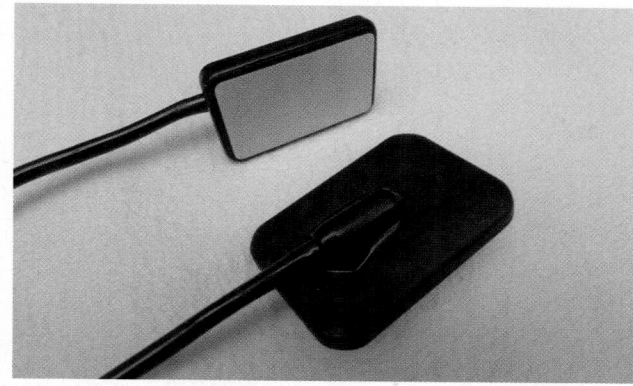

FIGURE 15-3 • Direct Digital Sensors. Two sensor sizes are shown. Charge-coupled device or complementary metal-oxide semiconductor sensors have integrated circuits made up of a grid of small transistor elements that convert X-rays to electrons in electron wells. Each element represents one pixel in the final image. This information is passed through a cable to the computer for processing.

III. Steps in the Production of a Digital Radiograph

◆ The sensor, direct or indirect (Figures 15-3 and 15-4), is encased in a plastic sleeve (Figure 15-5), held in a sensor holder, and placed in the patient's mouth.

◆ When exposed to radiation, an electronic charge is produced on the surface of the sensor.

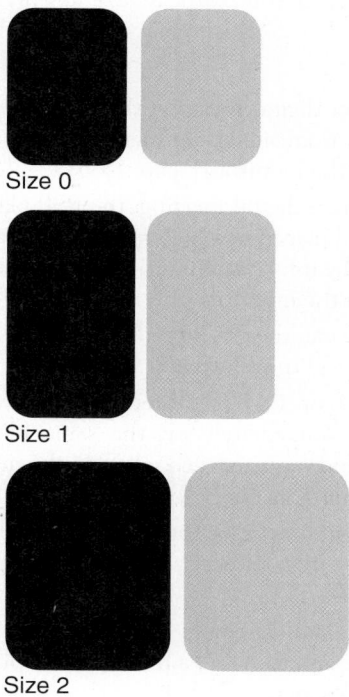

Size 0

Size 1

Size 2

FIGURE 15-4 • Indirect Digital Sensors. The light blue exposure and black nonexposure sides of three sizes of photostimulable phosphor (PSP) sensors are shown. PSP sensors are available in intraoral 0–4 sizes, as well as panoramic and cephalometric sizes. The light blue exposure side is covered with phosphor crystals that store X-ray exposure energy. When the sensor is placed in a laser scanner, the energy is released from the phosphor layer and converted to a digital image.

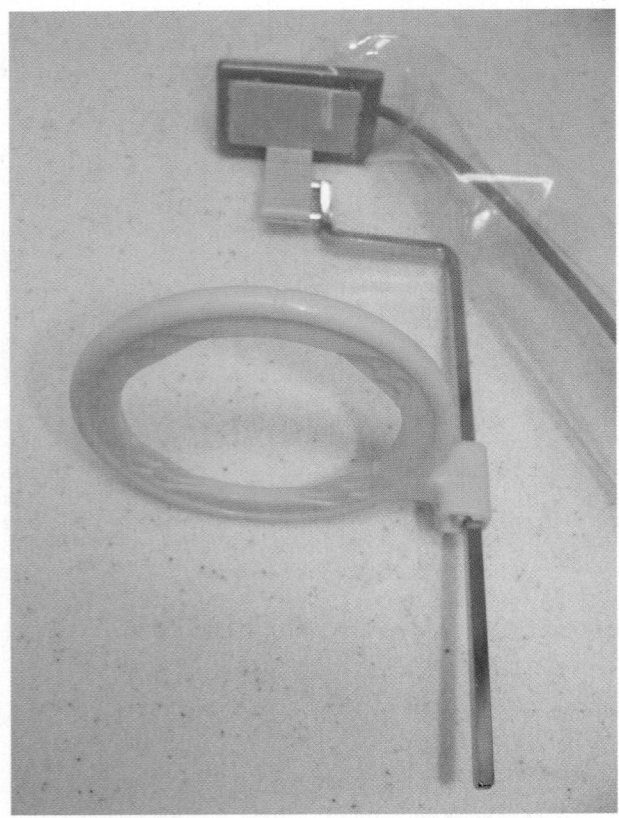

FIGURE 15-5 • Sensor Holder in Plastic Sleeve. The sensor holder is encased in a plastic sleeve for infection control purposes.

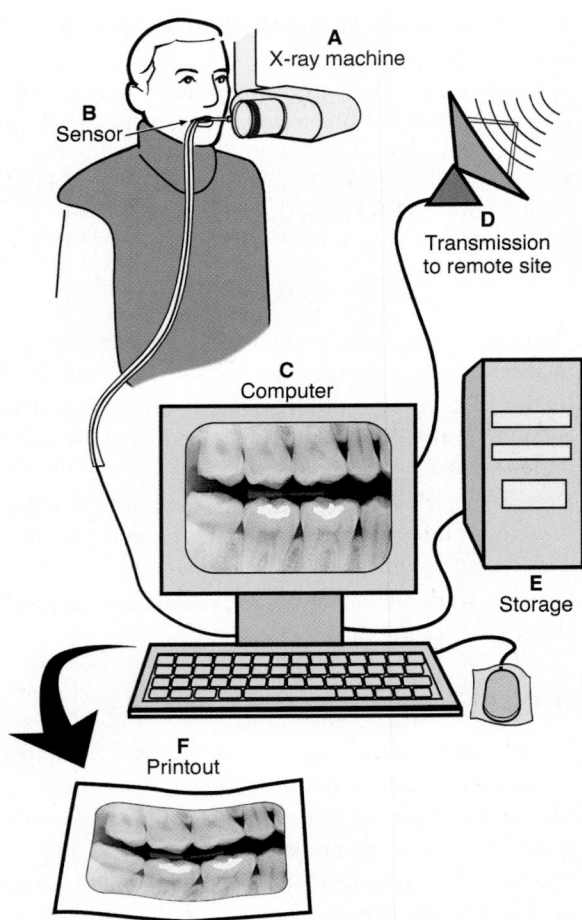

FIGURE 15-6 • Direct Digital Imaging System. The image is exposed by an X-ray machine **(A)**, captured on a charge-coupled device or complementary metal-oxide semiconductor sensor in the patient's mouth **(B)**. **C:** The signal is transmitted via a cable to the computer, where it is digitized into multiple gray levels. The image is displayed on the computer's monitor, transmitted electronically to a remote site **(D)**, stored on a file server **(E)**, or printed on paper **(F)**.

◆ With direct digital imaging: the image is immediately converted from analog form to digital form and displayed on the monitor (Figure 15-6).

◆ With indirect digital imaging: the PSP plates store the image until placed in a high-speed laser scanner, which converts the information into a digitized image and displays it on the monitor.

◆ The image can then be stored, manipulated, enhanced, retrieved, and transmitted.

◆ The CCD or CMOS (direct imaging) sensors can be reused immediately on the same patient or unwrapped and sanitized, according to the manufacturer's recommendations.

◆ The PSP (indirect imaging) plate is erased in the scanner or by a high-intensity light box for approximately 30 seconds.

◆ The PSP plates resemble traditional film in that they are pliable and thin and aid in operator placement and patient tolerance.

◆ The CCD/CMOS sensors are thick, rigid, and bulky and are associated with patient limitations. These sensors become more user friendly after a learning curve.

◆ A cross between paralleling and bisecting-angle techniques is required for CCD/CMOS sensor exposures. The clinician must be well versed in both to be successful.[6,7]

IV. Evaluation

A. Advantages of Digital Radiography

◆ Reduction of radiation dosage due to lower exposure time when compared to traditional film.

◆ Faster image acquisition.

◆ No darkroom or processing chemistry.

◆ Immediate feedback for diagnosis.

◆ Improved diagnostics through software tools.

◆ Effective patient education tool.

◆ Electronic record keeping.

◆ Reduced cross-contamination.

◆ Ability to send image electronically.

B. Disadvantages of Digital Radiography

◆ Initial setup expense.

◆ Bulky direct imaging sensors may increase film placement errors.

◆ Infection control of sensors: are covered by plastic sleeves as they cannot be heat sterilized.

◆ Direct imaging sensors are fragile and expensive.

CHARACTERISTICS OF AN ACCEPTABLE RADIOGRAPHIC IMAGE

A *radiographic image* is the visible image on a radiation-sensitive film or a digitized image created by the computer.

◆ The image is produced after exposure to ionizing radiation that has passed through an area or, specifically for dentistry, through teeth or a part of the oral cavity.

◆ A *radiographic survey* refers to a series of radiographic images.

◆ Before making a radiographic image, it is necessary to know the characteristics that are expected to result in a radiograph of maximum diagnostic value. The basic essentials are:

• The appearance of the image itself.
• The area covered.
• The quality of the processed radiograph.
• Table 15-1 provides a list of characteristics of an acceptable radiograph.

I. Radiolucency and Radiopacity

◆ A radiographic image has gradations from white to black that are referred to as radiopaque or radiolucent.

◆ For example, a dense material, such as a metallic restoration, prevents the passage of X-rays and appears white on the processed radiograph.

◆ Soft tissue does not resist passage of X-rays and, thus, appears black to gray.

II. Radiopacity

The appearance of light (white) images on a radiograph is a result of the lesser amount of radiation that penetrates the structures and reaches the image receptor.

◆ A radiopaque structure inhibits the passage of X-rays.

◆ Examples include:
• Enamel.
• Dentin.
• Metallic restorations.
• Implants.

III. Radiolucency

The appearance of dark images on a radiograph is a result of the greater amount of radiation that penetrates the structures and reaches the image receptor.

◆ A *radiolucent* structure permits the passage of radiation with relatively little attenuation by absorption.

◆ Examples include:
• Pulp.
• Cysts.
• Cavitated lesions.
• Periodontal ligament.

FACTORS THAT INFLUENCE THE FINISHED RADIOGRAPH

As the beam leaves the X-ray tube (Figure 15-1):

◆ It is collimated, filtered, and allowed to travel a designated source–image receptor (or focal spot–image receptor) distance before reaching the image receptor of a selected speed.

◆ The quality or diagnostic usefulness of the finished radiograph, as well as the total exposure of the patient and clinician, is influenced by the *kilovoltage, milliampere seconds, time, collimation, filtration, target–receptor distance, object–receptor distance,* and *film speed,* as outlined in Box 15-2.

TABLE 15-1 • Characteristics of an Acceptable Radiograph	
CHARACTERISTIC	APPEARANCE
Image	All parts of teeth of interest are shown close to natural size, with minimal overlap and minimal distortion
Area covered	Sufficient tissue surrounding tooth for diagnostic purposes
Density	Proper density for diagnosis
Contrast	Proper contrast for diagnosis
Definition and sharpness	Clear outline of objects; minimal **penumbra**

BOX 15-2
Factors That Influence the Radiographic Image

Kilovoltage Peak
• Affects contrast and density
• Low kVp yields high (short-scale) contrast
• High kVp yields low (long-scale) contrast

Milliamperage
• Affects density
• High mA yields high density
• Low mA yields low density

Time
- Affects density
- Long time yields high density
- Short time yields low density

Collimation
- Restricts and shapes the beam
- Not to exceed 2.75 inches or 7 cm at the patient's skin

Lead Diaphragm
- Position-indicating device (PID)
- Rectangular
- Cylindrical

Filtration
Types
- Aluminum filters remove low-energy X-rays
- Rare earth filters remove low- and high-energy X-rays
- Methods of filtration

Inherent
- Glass window
- Insulating oil
- Tube head seal

Added
- Aluminum disks
- 1.5 mm for 50–70 kVp
- 2.5 for above 70 kVp

Total Filtration
- Combination of inherent and added

Target–Film Distance
- Longer PID increases resolution of image
- Longer PID decreases scatter of radiation

Object–Film Distance
- Increased object–film distance achieves parallelism
- Decreased object–film distance decreases penumbra

Film Speed
- Faster speed film decreases definition; image is more grainy

◆ Traditional film processing also directly influences the quality of the radiograph and indirectly the total exposure. Re-exposure would be necessary should the film be rendered inadequate during processing.

I. Collimation

◆ Collimation is the technique for controlling the size and shape of the beam of radiation emitted.
◆ A *collimator* is a diaphragm or system of diaphragms made of an absorbing material designed to define the dimensions and direction of a beam of radiation.

A. Purposes
◆ Eliminate peripheral or divergent radiation.
◆ Minimize exposure to patient's face.
◆ Minimize secondary radiation, which can fog the film and expose the bodies of patient and clinician.

B. Methods
◆ Lead diaphragm
  - Made of lead with a central aperture of the smallest practical diameter for making radiographic exposure.
  - Located between the aluminum filters in the tube head and the position-indicating device (PID).
  - Recommended thickness of lead: 1/8 inch.
  - Recommended maximum size of aperture: to permit a diameter of the beam of radiation equal to 2.75 inches or 7 cm at the end of the PID next to the patient's face.
◆ Rectangular collimation
  - As shown in Figure 15-7.
  - When used, the size of the beam is greatly reduced and patient receives approximately 66% less radiation compared to round collimation.
  - The beam of radiation's diameter is approximately 1.5×2 inches at the skin.
  - The collimator is rotated to accommodate films positioned horizontally or vertically. A rectangular PID can be used or an external one can be added to the open end of a cylindrical PID.
◆ Lead-lined cylindrical or rectangular PID
  - The PID is an open-ended cylinder, or rectangle, lined with lead, to reduce secondary radiation.

C. Relation to Techniques
◆ Dimensions of a #2 size image receptor range in size and can be up to approximately 1.3×1.7 inches.
◆ Precise angulation techniques are required to eliminate "cone-cut" of image receptor, particularly when rectangular collimation is used.
◆ "Cone-cut" refers to an error of technique that results when the PID is not angled with the central ray centered on the image receptor being exposed.

II. Filtration

Filtration is the insertion of absorbers or filters for the preferential attenuation of radiation from a primary beam of X-radiation. Two different types of filters provide filtration in the dental X-ray machine.

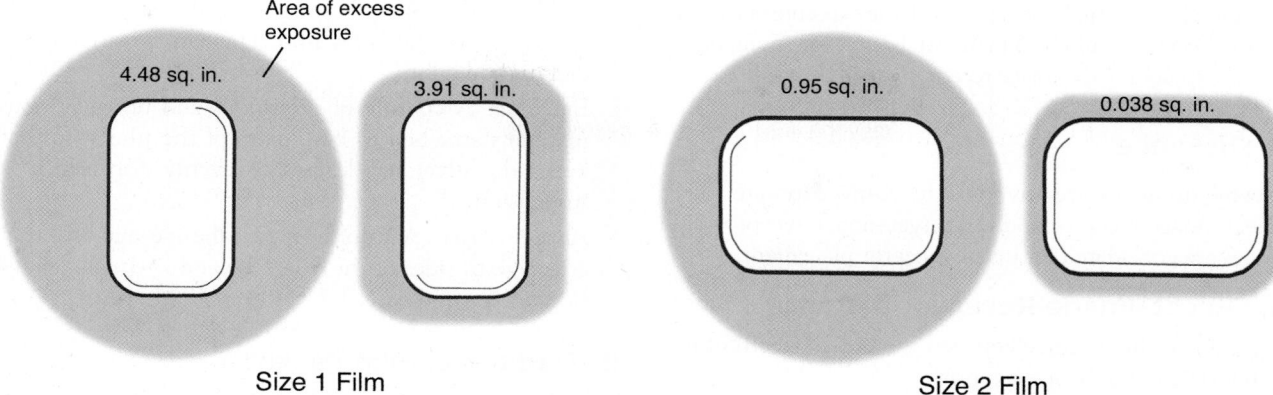

Size 1 Film   Size 2 Film

FIGURE 15-7 • Cylindrical and Rectangular Position-Indicating Device. The useless areas of radiation are greatly lessened when rectangular collimation is used. The patient can be spared exposure to excessive radiation. (Adapted from Shannon SA. Rectangular versus cylindrical collimation. *Dent Hyg.* 1987;61:173. Copyright 1987 by the American Dental Hygienists' Association.)

A. Types of Filters

◆ *Aluminum filters* remove low-energy X-ray photons from the X-ray beam.

B. Purpose

◆ To minimize exposure of the patient's skin to unnecessary radiation.

C. Methods

◆ *Inherent filtration:* Includes the glass envelope encasing the X-ray tube and the glass window in the tube housing (Figure 15-1).
◆ *Added filtration:* Thin, pure, aluminum disks inserted between the lead diaphragm and the X-ray tube.
◆ *Total filtration:* The sum of inherent and added filtration. The recommended total is the equivalent of 0.5 mm (below 50 kVp), 1.5 mm (50–70 kVp), and 2.5 mm (above 70 kVp) of aluminum.

III. Kilovoltage

Kilovoltage is the potential difference of force that moves electrons between the negative cathode and the positive anode of an X-ray tube.

◆ When the kilovoltage is increased, the speed of electrons is increased and the resulting X-rays have a shorter wavelength and more penetrating power.
◆ kVp refers to the crest value (in kilovolts) of the potential difference of a pulsating generator. When only one-half of the wave is used, the value refers to the useful half of the cycle.

A. How kVp Affects the Radiographic Image

◆ *Affects the contrast*
  • Low kilovoltage produces high contrast, with sharp black–white differences in densities between adjacent areas but a small range of distinction between subject thicknesses recorded.

  • High kilovoltage produces low contrast, with a wide range of subject thicknesses recorded; greater range of densities from black to white (more gray tones), which provide more interpretive details.
◆ *Affects the density*
  • Increased kilovoltage results in increased density (other factors remaining constant).
  • To maintain the same image *density*, the milliampere seconds is decreased as the kVp is increased.

B. Advantages of High kVp

◆ Permits shorter exposure time.
◆ Reduces exposure to tissues lying in front of the image receptor.
◆ Facilitates the detection of bone changes.

C. Disadvantages of High kVp

◆ Increased radiation to tissues outside the edges of the image receptor.
◆ More internal scattered radiation at 90 kVp than at 70 kVp.

IV. Milliampere Seconds

A. Milliamperage

◆ The measure of the electron current passing through the X-ray tube.
◆ Regulates the heat of the filament, which determines the number of electrons available to bombard the target.
◆ As the milliamperage is increased, the density of the image is increased.

B. Quantity of Radiation

◆ Quantity of radiation is expressed in milliampere seconds (mAs) or milliampere impulses (mAi).
◆ Definition: mAs is the milliamperes multiplied by the exposure time in seconds; mAi is the milliamperes multiplied by the exposure time in impulses.

◆ Example: At 10 mA for 1/2 second, the exposure of the image receptor would be 5 mAs. At 10 mA for 15 impulses, the exposure of the image receptor would be 150 mAi.

V. Distance

Several distances are involved in X-ray exposure. The object–image receptor and the target–image receptor distances are considered for image receptor placement.

A. Object–Image Receptor Distance

◆ Refers to the distance between the object (teeth of interest) and the image receptor.

◆ With the paralleling technique and the use of an image receptor holder, the object–image receptor distance is greater than it is for the bisecting-angle technique.

◆ A collimated beam and increased source–image receptor distance compensate to maximize definition and resolution.

B. Target–Image Receptor Distance

◆ The PID on the X-ray machine is designed to indicate the direction of the X-ray beam and to serve as a guide in establishing desired target–surface and target–image receptor distances.

◆ Techniques using 8-, 12-, and 16-inch target–image receptor distances are common.

◆ The *source* is the *tungsten target*. The target–image receptor distance (sometimes called the source–image receptor distance) is the sum total of the distance from the tungsten target to the film. The PID lightly touches the face.

◆ Principles related to target–image receptor distance are SmAs, kVp, and time.

C. Advantages in the Use of a Long PID

◆ Increased definition.

◆ Decreased magnification.

◆ Decreased skin exposure owing to decreased scatter.

VI. Image Receptors

◆ Image receptors refer to both traditional film and digital sensors used to capture a radiographic image.

◆ With optimum filtration, collimation, fast film, and digital sensors, the skin dose to the face can be reduced significantly.

◆ Very slow-speed films have been discontinued, and the speed of traditional films has been increased.

◆ Digital imaging also requires a low exposure time.

A. Traditional Film Composition

A film is a thin, transparent sheet of cellulose acetate coated on both sides with an emulsion of gelatin and silver halide crystals.

◆ *Film base:* A flexible piece of polyester plastic that is used to provide support for the emulsion.

◆ *Halide crystals:* Silver bromide and silver iodide crystals are used in dental X-ray film. They are sensitive to radiation and light.

◆ *Emulsion:* A coating of gelatinous and nongelatinous materials attached to both sides of the film base that keeps the silver halide crystals evenly dispersed in a suspension.

◆ *Adhesive layer:* A thin layer of adhesive material that covers both sides of the film base and keeps the emulsion on the film base.

B. Traditional Film Packet

Sealed paper or plastic envelope that is small, light proof, and moisture resistant, containing an X-ray film (or two), black paper, and a thin sheet of lead foil.

◆ Two-film packet: useful for processing one film differently from the other to make diagnostic comparisons; for sending to specialist to whom patient may be referred; and for legal evidence.

◆ Purpose of black paper: to protect against light.

◆ Purposes of lead foil backing: to prevent exposure of the film by scattered radiation that could enter from back of packet and to protect the patient's tissues lying in the path of the X-ray.

C. Traditional Film Speed

◆ Film speed or film emulsion speed refers to the sensitivity of the film to radiation exposure.

◆ The speed is the amount of exposure required to produce a certain image density.

◆ The smaller the grain size, the slower the film speed and the less grainy the image.

◆ *Classification:* Films have been classified by the American National Standards Institute (ANSI) in cooperation with the American Dental Association (ADA).

◆ The ANSI/ADA Specification No. 22 designates six groups:
  • **A–F** speed groups.
  • A, B, and C, the slowest, are associated with excess radiation exposure and are no longer used.
  • D and E are the slowest of those still in use.
  • *Choice:* F speed film is recommended for use with rectangular collimation for marked reduction in radiation exposure.

D. Digital Sensors

◆ In digital radiography, there are three types of receptors that replace traditional film:
  • CCD.
  • CMOS.
  • PSP plates.

◆ CCD and CMOS detectors are known as "direct imaging sensors." When exposed to X-ray energy, an image appears on a computer monitor within seconds.

◆ PSP plates are known as "indirect imaging sensors." When irradiated, an image is stored on them until scanned by a laser. The scanner then transmits the image to the computer.

- CCD and CMOS sensors require radiation exposure times approximately 10%–20% lower than "F"-speed film.
- PSP plate exposure times are similar to "F"-speed requirements.

EXPOSURE TO RADIATION

I. Ionizing Radiation

Ionizing radiation is electromagnetic radiation (e.g., *X-rays or gamma rays*) or particulate radiation (e.g., *electrons, neutrons, or protons*) capable of ionizing air directly or indirectly.

- The phenomenon of separation of electrons from molecules to change their chemical activity is called ionization.
- The organic and inorganic compounds that make up the human body may be altered by exposure to ionizing radiation.
- The biologic effects following irradiation are secondary effects in that they result from physical, chemical, and biologic action set in motion by the absorption of energy from radiation.
- Factors that would influence the biologic effects of radiation are outlined in Box 15-3.
- Radiation to *somatic* tissues will affect only the irradiated individual, whereas radiation to *genetic* tissues will affect offspring and possibly future generations.

II. Exposure

A. Types of Exposure

Exposure is a measure of the X-radiation to which a person or an object, or a part of either, is exposed at a certain place; this measure is based on its ability to produce ionization.

- *Threshold exposure:* The minimum exposure that produces a detectable degree of any given effect.

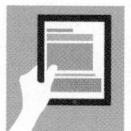

BOX 15-3
Factors That Influence the Biologic Effects of Radiation

- Quality of the radiation
- Chemical composition of the absorbing medium
- Sensitivity of tissues
- Total dose and dose rate
- Blood supply to the tissues
- Size of the area exposed
- Somatic versus genetic cells

- *Entrance or surface exposure:* Exposure measured at the surface of an irradiated body, part, or object. It includes primary radiation and backscatter from the irradiated underlying tissue.
- *Skin exposure:* Exposure measured at the center of an irradiated skin surface area.
- *Erythema exposure:* The radiation necessary to produce a temporary redness of the skin.

B. Exposure Units

- The units of absorbed dose are expressed in joules/kilogram (1 rad = 0.01 J/kg).
- The units shown in Table 15-2 are the recommendations of the International Commission on Radiation Units and Measurements.[8]
- The unit of measurement is the *gray* (Gy). An absorbed dose of 1 Gy is equal to 1 J/kg; therefore, an absorbed dose of 1 Gy is equal to 100 rad.
- The unit of biologic equivalence is the *Sievert* (Sv). 1 Sv = 100 rem.

C. Dose

- The radiation dose is the amount of energy absorbed per unit mass of tissue at a site of interest.
- A lethal dose is the amount of radiation that is, or could be, sufficient to cause death of an organism.

D. Permissible Dose

- The amount of radiation that may be received by an individual within a specified period without expectation of any significantly harmful result is called the permissible dose.
- Assumptions on which permissible doses are calculated include the following:
  - No irradiation is beneficial.
  - There is a dose below which no somatic cellular changes can be produced.
  - Children are more susceptible than are older people.
  - There is a dose below which, even though it is delivered before the end of the reproductive period, the probability of genetic effects is slight.

E. Maximum Permissible Dose

The maximum dose equivalent a person (or specified parts of that person) is allowed to receive in a stated period of time; the dose of radiation that would not be expected to produce any significant radiation effects in a lifetime.

F. Radiation Hazard

- A condition under which persons might receive radiation in excess of the maximum permissible dose is considered a hazard.
- Exposure would be a risk in an area where X-ray equipment is being used or where radioactive materials are stored.

TABLE 15-2 • Radiation Units

DEFINITION	S.I. UNIT	TRADITIONAL UNIT	EQUIVALENT
Unit of radiation exposure	Coulomb per kilogram (C/kg)	Roentgen (R)	-2.58×10^{-4} C/kg = 1 R
Unit of absorbed dose	Gray (Gy)	Rad	1 Gy = 100 rad
Unit of dose equivalent	Sievert (Sv)	Rem	1 Sv = 100 rem
Unit of radioactivity	Becquerel (Bq)	Curie (Ci)	3.7×10^{10} Bq = 1 Ci

S.I. (System International) is from the French Système International d'Unités.

G. National Council on Radiation Protection and Measurements

◆ Maximum permissible dose limits for dentists and dental personnel (see Table 15-3).

◆ Limits for patients: Exposure to radiation shall be kept to the minimum level consistent with clinical requirements for accurate diagnosis based on patient need.[8]

◆ Radiation exposures are kept as low as reasonably achievable (ALARA). This concept is accepted and enforced by all regulatory agencies.

III. Sensitivity of Cells

A. Factors Affecting Cell Sensitivity to Radiation

◆ *Cell differentiation:* Immature cells are most sensitive. Highly specialized cells are radioresistant.

◆ *Mitotic activity:* Rapidly reproducing cells are more sensitive; most sensitive when undergoing mitosis.

◆ *Cell metabolism:* Cells are more sensitive in periods of increased metabolism.

TABLE 15-3 • Maximum Permissible Dose Equivalent Values[a] to Whole Body, Gonads, Blood-Forming Organs, Lens of Eye

AVERAGE WEEKLY EXPOSURE[b]	MAXIMUM 13-WK EXPOSURE	MAXIMUM YEARLY EXPOSURE	MAXIMUM ACCUMULATED EXPOSURE[c]
0.001 Sv	0.03 Sv	0.05 Sv	0.05 (N − 18) Sv
0.1 R	3 R	5 R	5 (N − 18) R[d]

[a]Exposure of persons for dental or medical purposes is not counted against their maximum permissible exposure limits.
[b]Used only for the purpose of designating radiation barriers.
[c]When the previous occupational history of an individual is not definitely known, it shall be assumed that the full dose permitted by the formula 5 (N − 18) has already been received.
[d]N = Age in years and is greater than 18. The unit for exposure is the roentgen (R) or Sievert (Sv).

B. Radiosensitive and Radioresistant Tissues

◆ Radiosensitive: a cell that is sensitive to radiation.

◆ Radioresistant: a cell that is resistant to radiation.

◆ Radiation sensitivity of tissues and organs: the relative sensitivities are shown in Box 15-4.

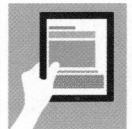

BOX 15-4
Radiation Sensitivity of Tissues and Organs

High
- Bone marrow
- Reproductive cells
- Intestines
- Lymphoid tissue

Moderately High
- Oral mucosa
- Skin

Moderate
- Growing bone
- Growing cartilage
- Small vasculature
- Connective tissue

Moderately Low
- Salivary glands
- Mature bone
- Mature cartilage
- Thyroid gland tissue

Low
- Liver
- Optic lens
- Kidneys
- Muscle
- Nerve

C. Tissue Reaction

◆ *Latent period:* Lapse between the time of exposure and the time when effects are observed. (May be as long as 25 years or relatively shorter, as in the case of the production of a skin erythema.)

◆ *Cumulative effect*
- Amount of reaction depends on dose; the reaction to radiation received in fractional doses is less than the reaction to one large dose.
- Partial or total repair occurs as long as destruction is not complete.
- Some irreparable damage may be cumulative as, little by little, more radiation is added (e.g., hair loss, skin lesions, falling blood cell count).

RISK OF INJURY FROM RADIATION

◆ The risk of injury from dental diagnostic radiation is extremely low; however, the more radiation received, the higher the chance of cellular injuries.

◆ With each exposure to radiation, cellular damage is followed by repair.

◆ The effects of radiation exposure are cumulative, and any cellular changes not repaired result in damaged tissues.

◆ Most of the damage caused by dental diagnostic low-level radiation is repaired within the body cells.

I. Rules for Radiation Protection

◆ *Dental X-ray protection,* prepared by the National Council on Radiation Protection and Measurements,[9] provides specific information about radiation barriers, film speed group rating, personal monitoring service sources, X-ray equipment data, and operating procedure regulations.

◆ To protect the clinician and patient from excessive radiation, attention is paid to unnecessary radiation that may result from retakes due to inadequate clinical procedures.

◆ Perfecting techniques contribute to the accomplishment of minimum exposure for maximum safety.

II. Protection of Clinician

A. Protection from Primary Radiation

◆ Stand behind a protective barrier.
◆ Avoid the useful beam of radiation.
◆ Never handhold the image receptor during exposure.

B. Protection from Leakage Radiation

◆ Do not handhold the tube housing or the PID of the machine during exposures.
◆ Test machine for leakage radiation.
◆ Wear monitoring device for testing exposure.

C. Protection from Secondary Radiation

The major sources of secondary radiation are the irradiated soft tissues of the patient. Other sources may be the leakage from the tube housing or scatter from furniture and walls contacted by the primary beam. Methods of protection are related to these sources.

Minimization of Total X-Radiation

◆ Use high-speed films and digital sensors.
◆ Have X-ray machines tested frequently for X-ray output and leakage.
◆ Replace older X-ray machines with modern equipment.

Collimation of Useful Beam

Use diaphragms and long PIDs to collimate the useful beam to an area no larger than 2.75 inches or 7 cm in diameter at the patient's skin. Rectangular collimation is shown to be more effective than round collimation (Figure 15-7).

Type of PID

Use a shielded cylinder that is rectangular, long, and open ended, or use some other form of rectangular collimation.

Position of Clinician While Making Exposures

◆ The correct position for the clinician is behind an appropriate radiation-resistant barrier wall, preferably with a leaded window to permit a view of the patient during exposures.

◆ When protective barrier shielding is not available, the clinician shall stand as far as practical from the patient, at least 6 feet (2 m) in the zone between 90° and 135° to the primary central ray, as shown in Figure 15-8.

◆ Safety increases with distance.

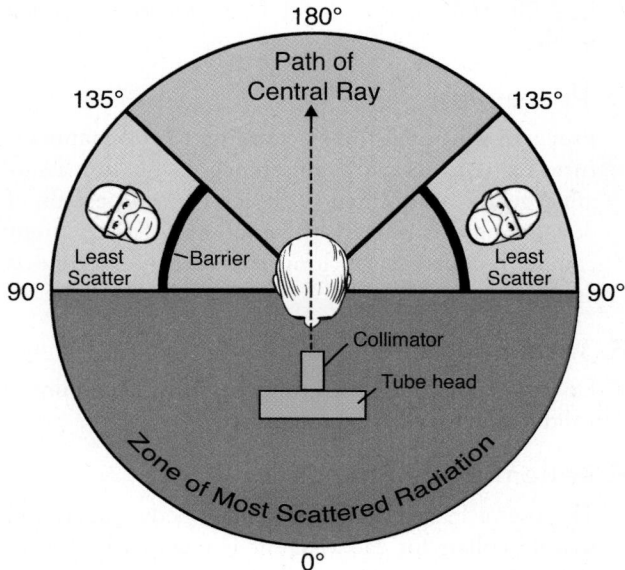

FIGURE 15-8 • Safe Position for Clinician. While making an exposure, the clinician stands behind the patient's head, between 90° and 135° from the primary beam.

◆ *Exposure of the region of the central incisors:* Stand at 45° to the path of the central ray. This position is approximately behind either the left or the right ear of the patient (Figure 15-8).

◆ *Exposure of other regions:* Stand behind the patient's head and at an angle of 45° to the path of the central ray of the X-ray beam.

D. Monitoring

The amount of X-radiation that reaches the dental personnel can be measured economically with a personal monitoring badge. Badges can be obtained from one of several laboratories. The monitoring badge is:

◆ Used to measure exposure of the wearer.

◆ Worn at waist level for 1, 2, or 4 weeks.

◆ Returned on a routine basis to the laboratory by mail and processed; its exposure is evaluated.

◆ Wearer is notified by mail of the exposure totals.

III. Protection of Patient

A. Image Receptors

◆ Use high-speed image receptors.

◆ Use the largest intraoral receptor that can be placed skillfully in the mouth. Maximum coverage is provided in this manner with one exposure.

◆ Two exposures may be required if smaller receptors are used to examine the same area.

B. Collimation

◆ Use diaphragms and an open-ended, shielded (lead lined), rectangular PID to collimate the useful beam.

C. Filtration

◆ Use filtration of the useful beam to recommended levels.

D. Processing

◆ Process traditional films according to the manufacturer's directions with adherence to quality assurance guidelines. When a choice of two periods of development is offered, the exposure of the patient can be reduced if the longer development time is employed.

E. Total Exposure

◆ Do not expose the patient unnecessarily. Determine a valid reason for each exposure.

F. Patient Body Shields

◆ The use of leaded or lead-free alloy body shields and thyroid collars for each patient is required by law in many states and countries. The purpose of the shield is to absorb scattered rays. An acceptable lead shield contains a minimum of 0.25 mm of lead thickness.

Protective Apron

◆ *Types*
  • General body coverage with extensions over the shoulders and down over the gonadal area.
  • Body coverage, with cervical thyroid collar attached.
  • Body coverage, with added coverage for the patient's upper back for wear during panoramic radiography.

◆ *Care*
  • Prevent cracks in leaded shields by hanging (Figure 15-9).
  • Disinfect the apron and collar before and after each use.

Thyroid Cervical Collar

◆ Thyroid cancer can result from long-term exposure of the gland to X-rays.[10,11]

◆ The gland is completely covered during exposure to X-rays. Figure 15-10 shows the position of a thyroid collar over the neckline of a body apron.

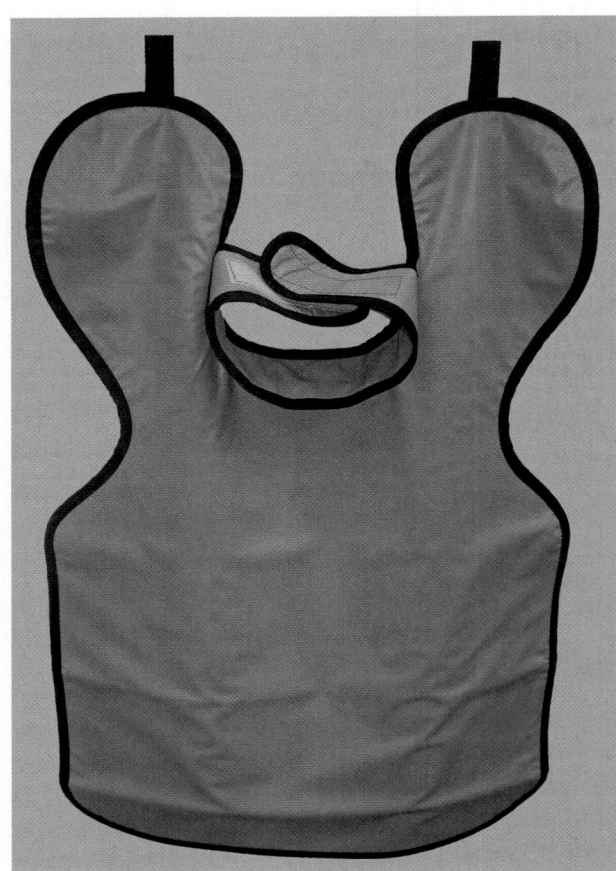

FIGURE 15-9 • Care of Leaded Apron. The apron can be kept on hooks or a hanging device near the X-ray machine to prevent cracks and prolong the usefulness of the apron. The thyroid collar may be attached on a separate shield.

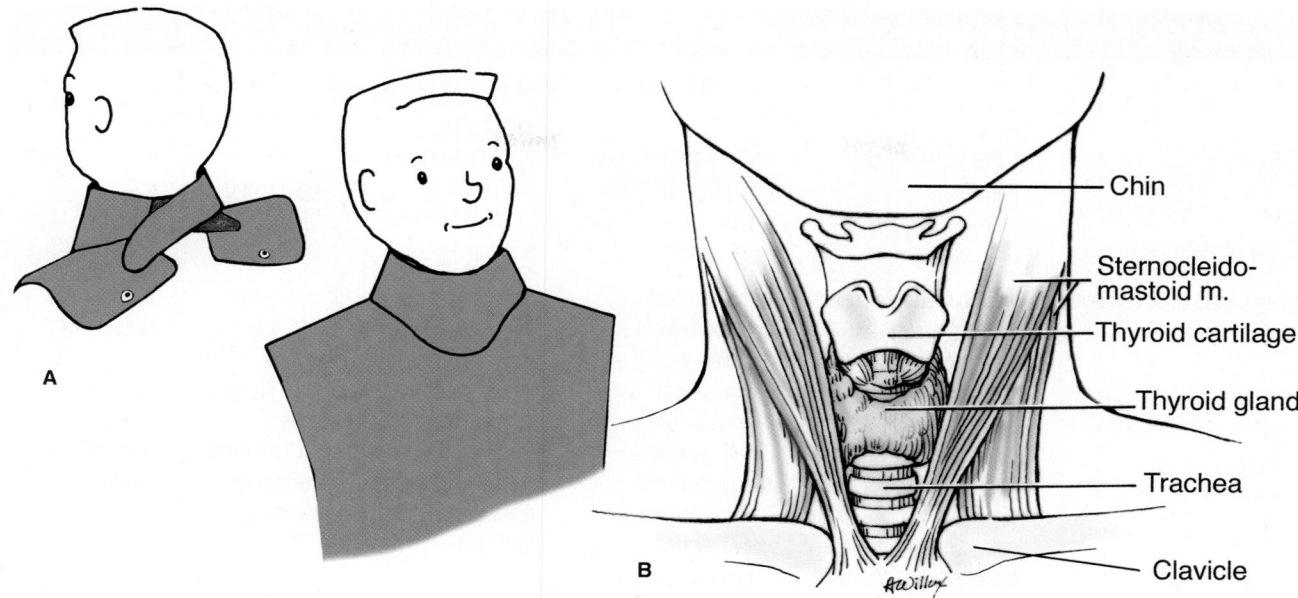

FIGURE 15-10 • Thyroid Cervical Collar. A: Thyroid collar in position, covering the neck and overlapping the leaded apron used for general body coverage. Velcro tabs facilitate overlap fastening at back of neck. Collars are available in child and adult sizes. **B:** The thyroid gland is located over the trachea approximately halfway between the chin and the clavicles. Drawing shows anatomic relationship to the sternocleidomastoid muscle.

IV. Assessment

An assessment regarding the need for radiographic exposure must be made for each patient based on:

◆ Review of health history.
◆ Preparation or review of radiation exposure history.
◆ Review of medical diagnostic or therapeutic radiation.
◆ Review of dates of dental surveys and availability of previous radiographs.
◆ Review of clinical examination.
◆ Assessment of Caries Management by Risk Assessment (CAMBRA) score.
◆ After assessment, consult with dentist and obtain dentist's prescription for number and type of radiographs. The ALARA concept should guide practice principles as radiation is damaging and cumulative and is to be kept to the minimum necessary to meet diagnostic requirements. Refer to the *Guidelines for Prescribing Dental Radiographs* in Tables 15-4 and 15-5.

V. Risk Reduction

A. Preparation of Clinic Facility: Infection Control Routine

◆ Standard precautions are followed for all radiographic equipment and materials.
◆ Use single-use plastic barriers for all surfaces to be contacted, including X-ray machine controls.
◆ Use disposable materials wherever possible.
◆ Wear gloves or overgloves for handling of all radiographic materials.

B. Preparation of Clinician

◆ Use full barrier protection that includes a cover-up gown, a mask, protective eyewear, and gloves.
◆ Apply standard precautions throughout the radiographic procedure.

C. Preparation of Patient

◆ Provide cup for holding removable dental prostheses.
◆ For panoramic radiographs, request patient to remove oral and/or facial piercings and all other jewelry worn above the shoulders.
◆ Provide antiseptic mouthrinse to lower bacterial contamination of radiographs and aerosols.

D. Intraoral Examination

◆ To determine necessary adaptations during film placement.

Factors of Particular Interest

◆ Accessibility, determined by height and shape of palate, flexibility of muscles of orifice, floor of the mouth, possible gag reflex, and size of tongue.
◆ Position of teeth and edentulous areas.
◆ Apparent size of teeth.
◆ Unusual features, such as tori, sensitive areas of the mucous membranes.

E. Patient Cooperation: Prevention of Gagging

◆ Gagging may be the result of psychological or physiologic factors.

TABLE 15-4 • Recommendations for Prescribing Dental Radiographs

TYPE OF ENCOUNTER	PATIENT AGE AND DENTAL DEVELOPMENTAL STAGE				
	CHILD WITH PRIMARY DENTITION (prior to eruption of first permanent tooth)	**CHILD WITH TRANSITIONAL DENTITION** (after eruption of first permanent tooth)	**ADOLESCENT WITH PERMANENT DENTITION** (prior to eruption of third molars)	**ADULT, DENTATE OR PARTIALLY EDENTULOUS**	**ADULT, EDENTULOUS**
New patient being evaluated for oral diseases	Individualized radiographic examination consisting of selected periapical/occlusal views and/or posterior bitewings if proximal surfaces cannot be visualized or probed. Patients without evidence of disease and with open proximal contacts may not require a radiographic examination at this time	Individualized radiographic examination consisting of posterior bitewings with panoramic examination or posterior bitewings and selected periapical images	Individualized radiographic examination consisting of posterior bitewings with panoramic examination or posterior bitewings and selected periapical images. A full mouth intraoral radiographic examination is preferred when the patient has clinical evidence of generalized oral disease or a history of extensive dental treatment		Individualized radiographic examination, based on clinical signs and symptoms
Recall patient with clinical caries or at increased risk for caries[a]	Posterior bitewing examination at 6- to 12-mo intervals if proximal surfaces cannot be examined visually or with a probe			Posterior bitewing examination at 6- to 18-mo intervals	Not applicable
Recall patient with no clinical caries and not at increased risk for caries[a]	Posterior bitewing examination at 12- to 24-mo intervals if proximal surfaces cannot be examined visually or with a probe		Posterior bitewing examination at 18- to 36-mo intervals	Posterior bitewing examination at 24- to 36-mo intervals	Not applicable
Recall patient with periodontal disease	Clinical judgment as to the need for and type of radiographic images for the evaluation of periodontal disease. Imaging may consist of, but is not limited to, selected bitewing and/or periapical images of areas where periodontal disease (other than nonspecific gingivitis) can be demonstrated clinically.				Not applicable
Patient (new and recall) for monitoring of dentofacial growth and development and/or assessment of dental/skeletal relationships	Clinical judgment as to need for and type of radiographic images for evaluation and/or monitoring of dentofacial growth and development or assessment of dental and skeletal relationships	Clinical judgment as to need for and type of radiographic images for evaluation and/or monitoring of dentofacial growth and development, or assessment of dental and skeletal relationships. Panoramic or periapical examination to assess developing third molars		Usually not indicated for monitoring of growth and development. Clinical judgment as to the need for and type of radiographic image for evaluation of dental and skeletal relationships	
Patient with other circumstances including, but not limited to, proposed or existing implants, other dental and craniofacial pathoses, restorative/endodontic needs, treated periodontal disease, and caries remineralization	Clinical judgment as to need for and type of radiographic images for evaluation and/or monitoring of these conditions				

These recommendations are subject to clinical judgment and may not apply to every patient. They are to be used by dentists only after reviewing the patient's health history and completing a clinical examination. Even though radiation exposure from dental radiographs is low, once a decision to obtain radiographs is made, it is the dentist's responsibility to follow the ALARA principle to minimize the patient's exposure.

[a]Factors increasing risk for caries may be assessed using the ADA Caries Risk Assessment forms (0–6 years of age and over 6 years of age).

ADA, American Dental Association; ALARA, as low as reasonably achievable.

Source: From American Dental Association Council on Scientific Affairs, U.S. Department of Health and Human Services, U.S. Food and Drug Administration. Dental radiographic examinations: recommendations for patient selection and limiting radiation exposure. http://www.fda.gov/Radiation-EmittingProducts/RadiationEmittingProductsandProcedures/MedicalImaging/MedicalX-Rays/ucm116504.htm. Accessed April 17, 2018.

TABLE 15-5 • Clinical Situations for Which Radiographs May Be Indicated

A. POSITIVE HISTORICAL FINDINGS	B. POSITIVE CLINICAL SIGNS/SYMPTOMS
1. Previous periodontal or endodontic treatment	1. Clinical evidence of periodontal disease
2. History of pain or trauma	2. Large or deep restorations
3. Familial history of dental anomalies	3. Deep carious lesions
4. Postoperative evaluation of healing	4. Malposed or clinically impacted teeth
5. Remineralization monitoring	5. Swelling
6. Presence of implants, previous implant-related pathosis, or evaluation for implant placement	6. Evidence of dental/facial trauma
	7. Mobility of teeth
	8. Sinus tract ("fistula")
	9. Clinically suspected sinus pathosis
	10. Growth abnormalities
	11. Oral involvement in known or suspected systemic disease
	12. Positive neurologic findings in the head and neck
	13. Evidence of foreign objects
	14. Pain and/or dysfunction of the temporomandibular joint
	15. Facial asymmetry
	16. Abutment teeth for fixed or removable partial prosthesis
	17. Unexplained bleeding
	18. Unexplained sensitivity of teeth
	19. Unusual eruption, spacing, or migration of teeth
	20. Unusual tooth morphology, calcification, or color
	21. Unexplained absence of teeth
	22. Clinical tooth erosion
	23. Peri-implantitis

This list is not comprehensive.

Source: From American Dental Association Council on Scientific Affairs, U.S. Department of Health and Human Services, U.S. Food and Drug Administration. Dental radiographic examinations: recommendations for patient selection and limiting radiation exposure. http://www.fda.gov/Radiation-EmittingProducts/RadiationEmittingProductsandProcedures/MedicalImaging/MedicalX-Rays/ucm116504.htm. Accessed April 17, 2018.

◆ May present some problem in the placement of all films for molar radiographs.

◆ May be initiated in the patient who ordinarily does not gag when techniques are carried out efficiently.

Causes of Gagging

◆ *Hypersensitive oral tissues:* Particularly common in posterior region of oral cavity.

◆ *Techniques:* Image receptor moved over the oral tissues or retained in the mouth longer than is necessary.

◆ *Anxiety and apprehension*

- Fear of unknown and of the image receptor touching a sensitive area.
- Previous unpleasant experiences with radiographic techniques.
- Failure to comprehend the clinician's instructions.
- Lack of confidence in the clinician.

Preventive Procedures

◆ Inspire confidence in ability to perform the service.

◆ Alleviate anxiety; explain procedures carefully. Smile and display a positive attitude.

◆ Minimize tissue irritation.

- Ask patient to swallow before each image receptor placement.

- Expose anterior image receptors before posterior as placement is easier to tolerate.
- Place image receptor firmly and positively without sliding the film over the tissue, especially the palate.
- Rub a finger over the tissues where the image receptor placement is intended to desensitize the tissues.
- Instruct patient to breathe through nose with quick breaths.
- Use stick-on film cushions to make image receptor placement more comfortable.

◆ Use a premedicating agent prescribed by the dentist.

◆ Use a topical anesthetic.

PROCEDURES FOR IMAGE RECEPTOR PLACEMENT AND ANGULATION OF CENTRAL RAY

The image projected onto the radiograph is a shadow of the teeth and the surrounding structures. The dental radiographer follows as closely as possible the five principles of shadow casting, listed in Box 15-5, when exposing radiographs.

Two fundamental periapical procedures are used in practice: the *paralleling* or right angle and the *bisecting angle*. The principles for image receptor placement are shown in Figure 15-11.

BOX 15-5
Principles of Shadow Casting

1. Place the image receptor as parallel as possible to the object.
2. Use as small an effective focal spot as practical.
3. Use as long a target–object distance as possible.
4. Use as short an object–image receptor distance as possible.
5. Aim the X-ray beam perpendicular to the image receptor.

Clinicians vary in their application of the principles of the two techniques. Basic to both the paralleling technique and the bisecting-angle technique are:

◆ The primary beam passes through the teeth of interest.
◆ The image receptor is placed in relation to the teeth so that all parts of the image are shown as close to their natural size and shape as possible.
◆ Dimensional distortion is minimized.
◆ The development of a systematic, comfortable, smooth procedure saves time and energy for both patient and clinician, and the clinician is able to:
  • Increase the confidence of the patient.
  • Allow for consistency in technique.
  • Produce good-quality radiographs.
  • Minimize the length of time the image receptor remains in the patient's mouth.

IMAGE RECEPTOR SELECTION FOR INTRAORAL SURVEYS

I. Periapical Surveys

A. Area Covered

◆ To obtain a view of the entire tooth and its periodontal supporting structures.

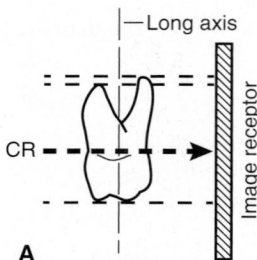
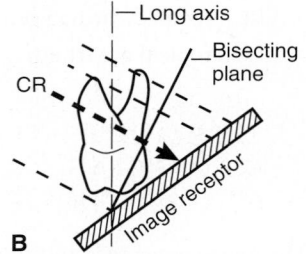

FIGURE 15-11 • Comparison of Paralleling and Bisecting-Angle Techniques. A: Paralleling technique. The image receptor is parallel with the long axis of the tooth and the central ray (CR) is directed perpendicularly both to the image receptor and to the long axis of the tooth. **B:** Bisecting-angle technique. The CR is directed perpendicularly to an imaginary line that bisects the angle formed by the image receptor and the long axis of the tooth.

B. Traditional Film Sizes

◆ *Child size:* No. 0 (22 × 35 mm) for primary teeth and small mouths.
◆ *Anterior:* No. 1 (24 × 40 mm) for anterior regions where width of arch makes positioning of standard film difficult or impossible.
◆ *Standard:* No. 2 (31 × 41 mm) may be used for all positions.
◆ *Long bitewing:* No. 3 (27 × 54 mm) infrequently used as periapical film.

C. Digital Sensor Sizes

◆ No. 0 for primary teeth and small mouths.
◆ No. 1 for anterior teeth where the width of the arch makes positioning of the size 2 sensor difficult or impossible.
◆ No. 2 may be used for all positions.
◆ No. 3 may be used for a long bitewing or periapical.

D. Number of Image Receptors Used in a Complete Survey

◆ Fourteen to 16 projections plus bitewings depending on:
  • The clinician's preferences.
  • The anatomy of the patient's mouth.
  • The size of the image receptors used.

II. Bitewing (Interproximal) Surveys

A. Area Covered

◆ *Horizontal bitewing radiographic images. To show:*
  • The crowns of the teeth and the alveolar crest in a dentition with normal to slight bone loss.
  • Proximal surface root caries.
  • Overhanging restorations.
◆ *Vertical bitewing radiographic images. To show:*
  • The crowns of the teeth and the alveolar bone level with moderate-to-severe bone loss.
  • Proximal surface root caries.
  • Overhanging restorations.

B. Image Receptors

◆ Sizes of image receptors are shown in Figures 15-3 and 15-4.
◆ The number and size of image receptors used for bitewing surveys are determined by:
  • The size of the dental arch.
  • The number of teeth present.
  • Patient tolerance. Use largest size sensor the patient will tolerate.

III. Occlusal Surveys

A. Purpose

◆ To show large areas of the maxilla, mandible, or floor of the mouth.

B. Image Receptors

◆ No. 4 for use in self-contained packet or in intraoral cassette.

◆ No. 2 for child or individual areas of adult.

PERIAPICAL SURVEY: PARALLELING TECHNIQUE

The paralleling technique is based on the principles that the image receptor is placed as parallel to the long axis of the tooth as the anatomy of the oral cavity permits, and the central ray is directed at right angles to the image receptor. Figure 15-11A shows the parallel relationship of the film or sensor with the long axis of the tooth and the right-angle direction of the central ray.

◆ *Maxillary projections:* The image receptor is placed toward the midline of the palate. Apices missing due to shallow palate may require an increase in vertical angulation.

◆ *Mandibular projections:* The image receptor is placed close to the teeth of interest as long as parallelism is maintained.

◆ *Premolar projections:* The image receptor is placed toward the midline, as far forward as possible and closer to the opposite arch canine to capture the distal surface of the canine.[12]

I. Patient Position

◆ As long as the image receptor is parallel to the long axis of the tooth, which is represented by an imaginary line passing longitudinally through the center of the tooth, and the central ray is directed at right angles to the image receptor, the head may be in any position convenient to the clinician and comfortable for the patient.

◆ Slight modification of positioning may be needed for making radiographs in a supine position.

II. Image Receptor Placement and Central Ray Angulation

A. Image Receptor Position and Angulation of the Central Ray

The image receptor is centered over the teeth to be examined.

◆ *Horizontal angulation* is the angle at which the central ray of the useful beam is directed within a horizontal plane. The central ray is directed at the center of the image receptor and through the interproximal area in order to eliminate overlapping or superimposition of parts of the adjacent teeth in the radiograph and cone-cutting.

◆ *Vertical angulation* is the plane at which the central ray of the useful beam is directed within a vertical plane. The central ray is directed at a right angle to the image receptor to eliminate elongation where there is inadequate vertical angulation and foreshortening where there is excessive vertical angulation.

B. Image Receptor Positioning Holders

◆ The use of an image receptor holder (film-positioning device) facilitates obtaining the correct angulation of the central ray.

◆ Lining up the PID with coordinating parts of the image receptor holder sets the correct vertical and horizontal angulation so that the central ray is perpendicular to the image receptor.

◆ Figure 15-12 shows an example of a disposable image receptor positioning device.

◆ *Purposes:* The use of a beam-guiding, field size–limiting, image receptor holding instrument provides:

● Dose reduction.

● Improved image quality.

● Diagnostic radiographs without frequent retakes.

● Improved infection control.

◆ *Characteristics:* An effective image receptor positioning device has characteristics such as the following:

● Simple and adaptable to all positions.

● Aids in reducing radiation exposure to patient.

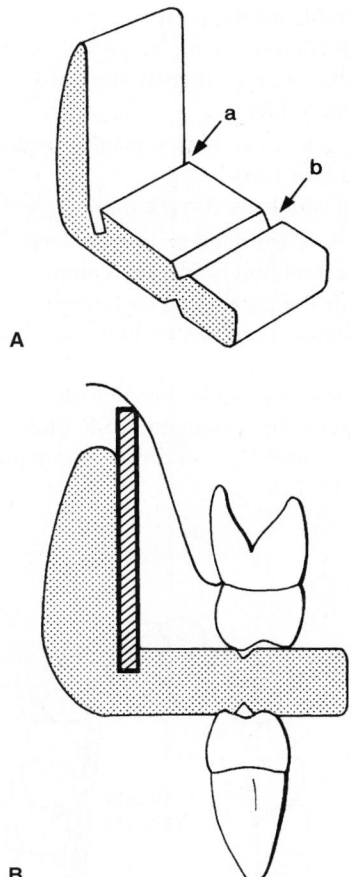

FIGURE 15-12 • Styrofoam Disposable Film/Photostimulable Phosphor (PSP) Holder. A: Empty holder to show: a, slot for insertion of the traditional film or PSP plate, and b, break-off point to shorten the bite surface for use in the mandibular posterior positions. **B:** Film/PSP plate placement for maxillary molar radiograph for patient with a high palatal vault.

BOX 15-6
Image Receptor Positioning Devices

Bite blocks, plastic or foam

Stabe (Styrofoam disposable film/photostimulable phosphor plate holder)

Snap-a-ray

X-C-P (extension cone paralleling)

B-A-I (bisecting-angle instrument)

V.I.P. (versatile intraoral positioner)

Hemostat with rubber bite block

Supplements

Removable denture for stabilization of film holder

Cotton roll to achieve parallelism

- Aids in alignment of X-ray beam.
- Comfortable for the patient.
- Minimal complexity for learning.
- Disposable or conveniently sterilized.
- Types of film holders
  - Several types of common image receptor holders are listed in Box 15-6.
- *Examples* of widely used types include the following:
  - Rinn X-C-P film and sensor holders. A plastic and stainless steel film holder with aiming devices that is used with the paralleling technique.
  - Bite blocks vary depending on selected image receptor.
  - Styrofoam disposable bite block for use with a traditional film or digital PSP plate when utilizing the paralleling or bisecting-angle techniques (Figure 15-12).

III. Paralleling Technique: Features

A. Accuracy

The paralleling technique gives a more accurate size and shape of dental structures with less distortion and superimposition of other anatomic structures than when the bisecting-angle technique is used.

B. Horizontal Ray Direction

No rays are directed toward the thyroid, whereas with the bisecting-angle technique, several maxillary radiographs require a relatively steep vertical angulation.

BITEWING SURVEY

Figure 15-13 shows in diagram form:

- The position of the horizontal molar bitewing image receptor in relation to the teeth.
- The horizontal and vertical angulation.
- The image objective for both the premolar and the molar completed radiographs when standard image receptor is used.

I. Positioning

A. Patient Position

- *Patient in upright position:*
  - Sagittal plane that divides the midline into right and left is perpendicular to the floor.
  - Occlusal plane, represented by a curve from the incisal edges of the central incisors to the tips of the occluding surfaces of the third molars, is parallel with the floor.
- *Patient in supine position:* The planes are reversed in their relation to the floor.

B. Vertical Angulation of Central Ray

- Set at +8° to +10° for horizontal or vertical bitewings (Figure 15-13B).

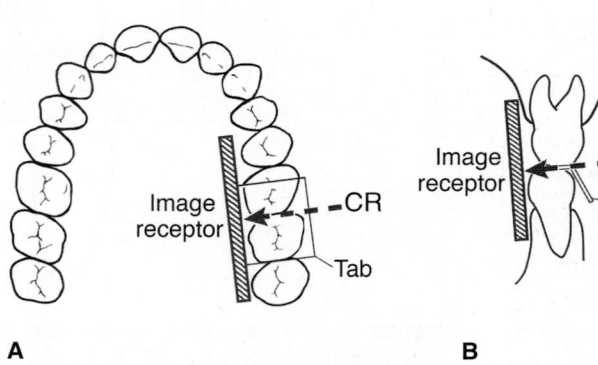
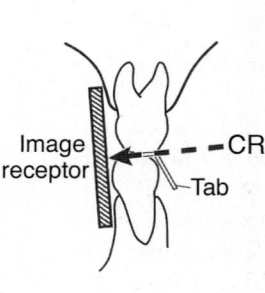
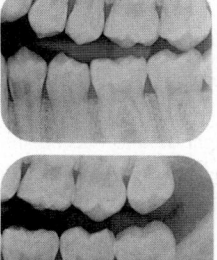

A   B   C

FIGURE 15-13 • Horizontal Bitewing Radiograph. A: Image receptor position showing horizontal angulation for molar viewing, with central ray (CR) directed through the interproximal space to the center of the image receptor. Image receptor is centered over the second molar. **B:** Vertical angulation set at +8° to +10°. **C:** Image objective for molar (*above*) and premolar (*below*) regions.

C. Horizontal Angulation of Central Ray

◆ The horizontal angulation is adjusted to direct the central ray perpendicular to the center of the image receptor.

◆ The central ray passes through the interproximal space or parallel to a line through the interproximal spaces of the teeth of interest (Figure 15-13A).

II. Image Receptor Placement: Horizontal Bitewing Survey

◆ *Molar*
- Standard image receptor in horizontal position.
- Center the image receptor on the second molar to ensure capturing the first and third molars on the radiograph (see Figure 15-13A).

◆ *Premolar*
- Standard image receptor in horizontal position.
- Center the film/sensor over the second premolar.
- Place the mesial border of image receptor at midline of the mandibular canine to include the distal surfaces of maxillary and mandibular canines and a clear view of both the first and second premolars.
- If using rigid sensors, move mesial portion of image receptor closer to the opposite arch canine to ensure canine visibility.

III. Image Receptor Placement: Vertical Bitewing Survey

◆ *Molar*
- Standard image receptor in vertical position.
- Center of the image receptor positioned over the middle of the second molar.
- Include at least the distal portion of both the maxillary and mandibular first molars and the mesial portion of the third molars, as illustrated in Figure 15-14.

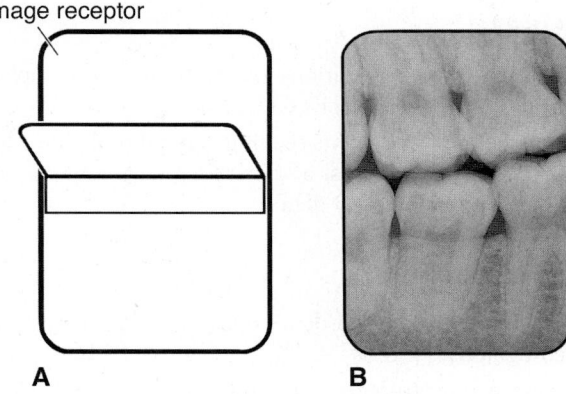

Image receptor

A   **B**

FIGURE 15-14 • **Vertical Bitewing Radiograph. A:** Vertical bitewing image receptor with the tab positioned vertically over the center of the image receptor. **B:** Image objective of maxillary and mandibular molar regions. Image receptor is placed centered over the mandibular second molar.

◆ *Premolar*
- Standard image receptor in vertical position.
- Position the mesial border of image receptor at midline of the mandibular canine.
- Include the distal portion of maxillary and mandibular canines and a clear view of the first and second premolars.

◆ *Anterior*
- Center of image receptor at proximal space between the lateral and canine for the two canine/lateral bitewings.
- Center of image receptor at midline for central bitewing.

PERIAPICAL SURVEY: BISECTING-ANGLE TECHNIQUE

The bisecting-angle technique is based on the geometric principle that the central ray is directed perpendicularly to an imaginary line that is the bisector of the angle formed by the long axis of the tooth and the plane of the image receptor.

◆ Figure 15-11B illustrates in diagram form the relationship of the long axis of the tooth, the image receptor, and the bisector of the angle formed by these two.

◆ Types of image receptor holders:
- *Rinn snap-a-ray:* A rigid plastic image receptor holder without a backing plate to prevent receptor bending, used in both posterior and anterior regions of the mouth. Useful in patients who cannot tolerate the receptor backing devices of a bite block.
- *Rinn B-A-I film and sensor holders:* A plastic and stainless steel image receptor holder with an aiming device that is used with the bisecting-angle technique.
- *Styrofoam disposable holder:* A disposable bite block used with the bisecting-angle or paralleling technique.

OCCLUSAL SURVEY

The central midline films for maxillary and mandibular arches are described in this section. A variety of positions for the occlusal survey are possible, depending on the area to be examined.

I. Uses and Purposes

◆ To observe areas not shown on other image projections.

◆ To position image receptor when obtaining periapical image projections is impossible.

◆ To supplement the angulation provided by other image receptors for such conditions as fractures, impacted teeth, or salivary duct calculi.

II. Maxillary Midline Topographic Projection

A. Position of Patient's Head

◆ The line from the tragus of the ear to the ala of the nose is parallel with the floor.

B. Position of Film

◆ The exposure side of the image receptor is toward the palate.

◆ Posterior border of image receptor is brought back close to the third molar region. Image receptor is held between the teeth with edge-to-edge closure.

C. Angulation

◆ The PID is directed toward the bridge of the nose at a +65° angle.

III. Mandibular Topographic and Cross-Sectional Projection

A. Position of Patient's Head

◆ The head is tilted directly back.

B. Position of Image Receptor

◆ The exposure side is toward the floor of the mouth.

◆ The posterior border of the image receptor is in contact with the soft tissues of the retromolar area.

◆ The image receptor is held between the teeth in an edge-to-edge bite.

C. Angulation

◆ Topographical: Point PID at chin for incisal region: −55° angle.

◆ Cross-sectional: Direct PID under the chin for the floor of the mouth, perpendicular to the image receptor.

PANORAMIC RADIOGRAPHIC IMAGES

Panoramic radiography, or pantomography, refers to methods that produce continuous radiographs showing the maxillary and mandibular arches with adjacent structures on a single radiograph.

The panoramic radiograph is an option to a periapical survey, but it is not a substitute because of the loss of sharpness and detail. The principal advantages of panoramic images are:

◆ Broad coverage of facial bones and teeth.

◆ Low patient radiation dose.

◆ Convenience of the examination for the patient.

◆ Short time required to expose a panoramic image.

◆ Useful for patients who cannot open their mouths.

◆ Visibility for patient education.

I. Technique

A panoramic radiograph is a radiographic projection that is positioned outside the mouth during X-ray exposure and is used to examine the maxillary and mandibular jaws on a single image.

◆ The movement of the image receptor and tube head produces an image through the process known as tomography.

◆ The prefix tomo means section; tomography is a radiographic technique that depicts one layer or section of the body in focus while surrounding structures in other planes are blurred.

◆ In a panoramic tomograph, the attempt is to radiograph the maxillary and mandibular dentitions in focus on one image receptor.

◆ The image receptor and tube head rotate around the patient's head in opposite directions.

◆ The focal trough refers to a plane of tissue in focus during the exposure.

A. Patient Position

◆ Patient positioning depends on the panoramic unit and the patient's height, as they can be standing or sitting.

• Stabilize the head with a chin support or one of several types of head holders characteristic of each machine.

• Position the patient to ensure that the Frankfort plane (orbital to tragus of the ear) is parallel to the floor and the midsagittal plane perpendicular to the floor.

• Close the anterior teeth on the intraoral bite block using the machine guide to ensure that the arch is not positioned too far back or forward.

B. Cassette

◆ Curved or flat.

◆ Rigid or flexible.

◆ Marked to denote left or right side of the patient.

◆ Contains calcium tungstate or preferably rare earth intensifying screens that provide for reduced radiation exposure to the patient.

II. Uses

◆ The numerous applications for panoramic radiographic images are outlined in Box 15-7.

◆ Routine use for patients seeking general oral care cannot be recommended as a substitute for a periapical survey as there is a loss of detail.

III. Limitations

◆ Loss of definition and detail compared with periapical radiographs.

◆ Distortion of structures and findings.

◆ Proximal caries is usually not evident on radiographs, except for large cavitated lesions that can be seen by direct examination.

◆ Inadequate for examination of periodontal structures.

BOX 15-7
Uses for Panoramic Images

- Detection and diagnosis of oral pathologic lesions
- Evaluation of impacted teeth
- Examination of the extent of large lesions
- Survey for edentulous patients
- Detection of calcified carotid arteries: potential stroke victims
- Evaluation of growth and development for pedodontic patients
- Evaluation of teeth and jaw position for orthodontic patients
- Detection of fractured jaws and traumatic injuries
- When intraoral films are impossible
  Trismus
  Parkinson's disease
  Cerebral palsy
  Hyperactive gag reflex

A. Inferiority of Definition and Detail

Causes of poor definition are:
◆ Use of intensifying screens.
◆ Increased object–image receptor distance.
◆ Movement of X-ray tube and image receptor.

B. Distortion

◆ Magnified images are produced because of increased distance between the image receptor and object.
◆ Overlapping
  • In periapical techniques, each image receptor is angulated with the central ray so that when a tooth is out of line, adjustment is made to prevent overlapping.
  • With panoramic technique, the head and teeth remain fixed, and the ray and image receptor are positioned only for the average.

IV. Procedures

Learning to use panoramic equipment is not difficult. Each machine has its own characteristics that can be learned readily from the manufacturer's instructions.

A. Patient Preparation

◆ Thyroid shield
  • Cannot be used because of superimposition on the image.
  • A special shield for panoramic radiography is available with coverage over the shoulders and partway or fully down the back.

B. Image Receptor

◆ Image receptor sizes are usually either 5 × 12 or 6 × 12 inches. Fast-speed film or digital sensors are used to minimize radiation.

C. Processing

◆ Regular processing solutions are used for traditional panoramic film. Special film holders for panoramic films are used during manual processing.

INFECTION CONTROL

I. Practice Policy

◆ Personnel of each office or clinic can determine a specific protocol appropriate to their facility and the type of processing used.
◆ A written policy is necessary for infection control during image receptor exposure, processing, and mounting and during management of the completed radiographs throughout clinical treatment appointments.[13]

II. Basic Procedures

Basic procedures are followed to prevent cross-contamination during transport to the digital laser scanner or darkroom and during use of manual and automatic processing equipment.[13] Steps are outlined in Box 15-8.

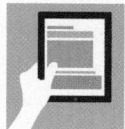

BOX 15-8
Basic Infection Control Procedures

- Digital photostimulable phosphor (PSP) plates and traditional films covered with contaminated saliva are confined to a disposable cup after exposure.
- Gloved hands fresh from contamination from the patient's mouth do not come in contact with walls, doors, light switches, and other environmental surfaces when transporting a cup of contaminated exposed PSP plates to the scanner or traditional films to the dark room.
- The darkroom or computer monitor/keyboard work area is prepared by the disinfection of all touch surfaces, and the counter is covered with clean paper.
- Traditional processing procedures may reduce the bacterial counts, but the potential for cross-contamination still exists.
- Dispose of PSP plate and traditional film wrappers, cups, and contaminated gloves with contaminated waste. Lead foil is disposed of according to environmental waste guidelines.

III. No-Touch Method for Films and PSP Plates

◆ With gloved hands and under appropriate safelight, pull open packets by their tabs or from their barrier envelopes as shown in Figure 15-15.

◆ Allow films/PSP plates to drop out into a cup, transport box, or the clean barrier-covered surface.

◆ Take care not to touch the films/PSP plates. Remove gloves, wash hands, and place films on hangers or into the automatic processor, being careful to touch the films by the edges only. Place PSP plates into the laser scanner.

◆ Dispose of waste properly.

◆ Alternative no-touch method.

    • Wear overgloves over powder-free treatment gloves and remove them after dropping film/PSP plates into the cup.

    • Films/PSP plates are then processed while wearing powder-free treatment gloves.

TRADITIONAL FILM PROCESSING

Film processing is the chemical transformation of the latent image, produced in a traditional film emulsion by exposure to radiation, into a stable image visible by transmitted light.

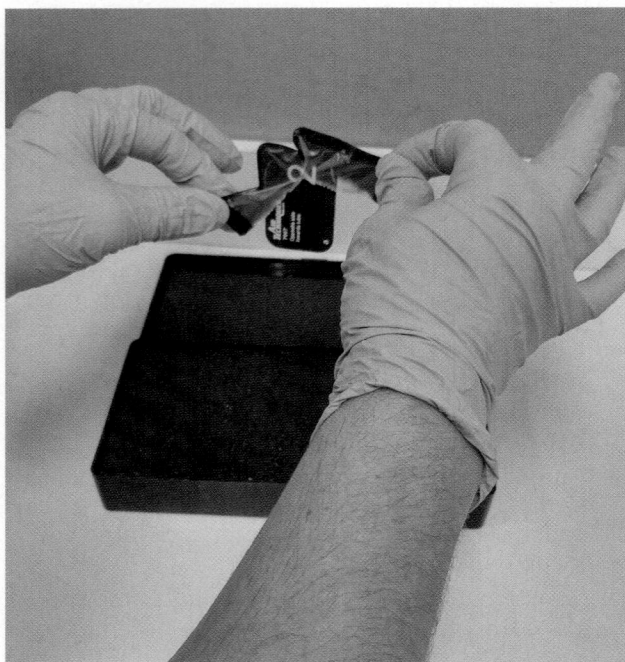

FIGURE 15-15 • Photostimulable Phosphor (PSP) Plate Barrier. Opening PSP plate barrier over a transport box using the no-touch method. Plastic barriers placed over intraoral image receptors are used to protect image receptors from salivary contamination.

I. Image Production

◆ Film emulsion contains crystals of silver halides (bromide and iodide).

◆ Development consists of selective reduction of affected silver halide salts to metallic silver grains.

◆ X-ray exposure changes the silver halides to silver and halide ions.

◆ Developer reacts with the halide ions, leaving only the metallic silver in an arrangement corresponding with the radiolucency and radiopacity of the tissue being exposed.

◆ Fixation consists of selective removal of unaffected silver halide crystals.

◆ Fixer removes only those crystals of silver halide that were not exposed to radiation.

◆ Washing removes processing chemicals.

◆ End result is a *negative*, showing various degrees of lightness and darkness (microscopic grains of black metallic silver).

II. Darkroom Lighting

◆ Find and eliminate all possible light leaks.

◆ Safelighting:

    • 15-watt bulb or less.

    • Light-emitting diode safelight can be used.

    • Positioned a minimum of 4 feet above the working surface.

    • Filter is selected according to film type.

III. Automated Processing

Automatic film processing refers to the use of equipment designed to transport film mechanically through a series of solutions under controlled conditions. The film is transported from the entry slot to the developer, fixer, water bath, dryer, and exit slot.

A. Advantages of Automated Processing

◆ Consistency of results.

◆ Conservation of time by dental personnel.

◆ Finished radiographs in 4–6 minutes.

B. Principles of Operation

◆ Rollers or tracks are used to carry traditional film through developing, fixing, washing, and drying. Some machines may process only standard intraoral films, whereas others may also accommodate extraoral sizes.

◆ Increased temperature decreases processing time.

IV. Manual Processing

The darkroom has three tanks of chemicals and water for processing by hand: the developing tank, fixing tank, and water bath. In most darkrooms, the developer is in the left tank, the water bath is in the center tank, and the fixer is in the right tank.

A. Processing Temperature and Times

◆ The quality of the radiographic image depends greatly on the processing time and temperature. Optimal developing condition for manual processing is 68°F for 5 minutes.

◆ Higher temperatures would produce films with excessive density; cooler temperatures, too little density. Follow manufacturer's directions for proper time and temperature.

B. Equipment and Steps for Manual Processing

◆ Check level and temperature of solutions with processing thermometer; stir solutions with stirring rods.

◆ Turn on safelights and turn off the white lights.

◆ Load films from the film packet or cassette onto hangers.

◆ Immerse film in the developer; activate timer.

◆ When timer buzzes, rinse films in circulating water for 30 seconds.

◆ Immerse the films in the fixer for twice the clearing time.

◆ Wash the films in circulating water for 10 minutes.

◆ Dry films until they are no longer tacky.

C. Disposal of Liquid Chemicals

Fixer and developer are considered environmentally hazardous waste material and are disposed of according to governmental regulations.

HANDHELD X-RAY DEVICES

X-ray devices held by the operator are now used in dentistry. They provide a way to bring radiographic diagnostic examinations into such places as outreach, temporary, and emergency clinics (Figure 15-16).

◆ Use only Food and Drug Administration–approved devices.

◆ Units are safe if tube head shielding and backscatter ring shield are in place.

◆ Institute proper position of the handheld unit relative to the operator to keep operator exposure levels low.

◆ Use of personal monitoring is recommended when using handheld X-ray units.

◆ Training and usage protocols must be in place to ensure compliance.[14]

ANALYSIS OF COMPLETED RADIOGRAPHS

The completed radiographs are mounted and examined on a computer monitor or at a viewbox. Interpretation of radiographs is difficult, and the determination of a pathologic condition requires keen evaluation. Attempting to

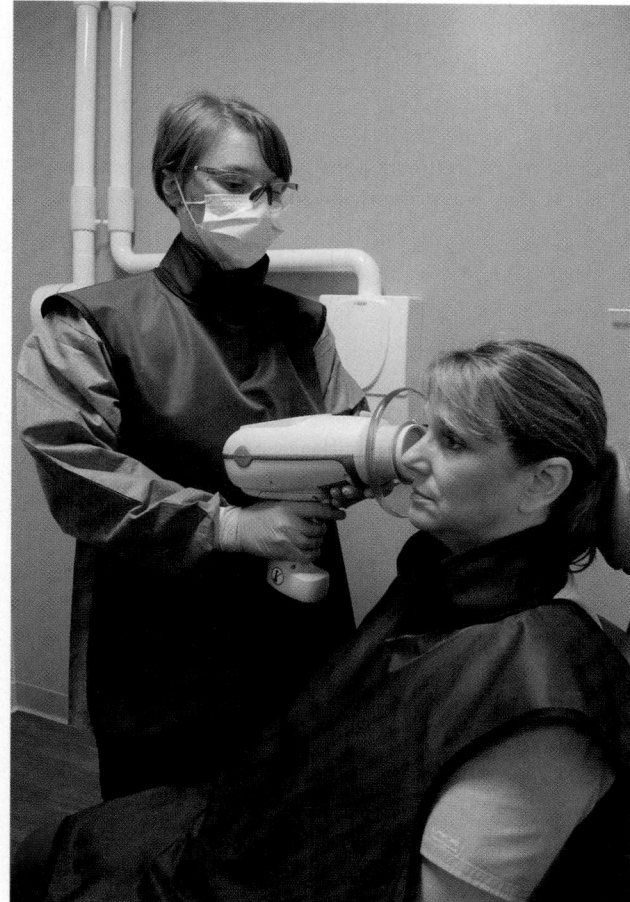

FIGURE 15-16 • Handheld X-Ray Device. The position of the operator in relation to the handheld X-ray device affects the radiation exposure received by the operator.

base interpretation on inadequate, insufficient radiographs will result in guesswork rather than in an accurate, timely diagnosis.

I. Mounting

◆ If using traditional film, legibly mark the mount with the name of patient, age, date, name of dentist; printing is preferred.

◆ Handle radiographs only by the edges with clean, dry hands.

◆ Arrange radiographs in front of the viewbox on clean, dry paper.

◆ The embossed dot near the edge of the radiograph is the guide to mounting; the raised side of the dot is on the facial side.

◆ Identify individual radiographs by teeth and other anatomic landmarks.

◆ Approved mounting system is as follows: Looking at the teeth from outside the mouth, the teeth are viewed and mounted in the same manner as the approved tooth numbering system.

II. Anatomic Landmarks

A. Definition

An anatomic landmark is an anatomic structure, the image of which may serve as an aid in the localization and identification of the regions portrayed by a radiograph. The teeth are the primary landmarks.

B. Landmarks That May Be Seen in Individual Radiographs

◆ *Maxillary molar:* Maxillary sinus, zygomatic process, zygomatic (malar) bone, hamular process, coronoid process of the mandible, maxillary tuberosity, lateral pterygoid plate.

◆ *Maxillary premolar:* Maxillary sinus.

◆ *Maxillary canine:* Maxillary sinus, junction of the maxillary sinus and nasal fossa (Y-shaped, radiopaque).

◆ *Maxillary incisors:* Incisive foramen, nasal septum and fossae, anterior nasal spine (V-shaped), median palatine suture, symphysis of the maxillae.

◆ *Mandibular molar:* Mandibular canal, internal oblique line, external oblique ridge, mylohyoid ridge, submandibular gland fossa.

◆ *Mandibular premolar:* Mental foramen.

◆ *Mandibular incisors:* Lingual foramen, mental ridge, genial tubercles, symphysis of the mandible. Nutrient canals are seen most frequently in this radiograph.

III. Identification of Errors in Radiographs

Table 15-6 outlines the more common errors, their causes, and the keys to correction.

A. Causes

Errors may be related to any step in the entire procedure, including image receptor placement, angulation, exposure, processing if using traditional film, and care and handling of the image receptors.

B. Error Types

◆ *Distortion:* An inaccuracy in the size or shape of an object in the radiograph. Distortion is brought about by misalignment of the PID relative to the object. Vertical distortion produces elongation or foreshortening of the object.

◆ *Fog:* A darkening of the whole or part of a radiograph by sources other than the radiation of the primary beam to which the image receptor was exposed. Types of fog include chemical, light, and radiation.

◆ *Artifact:* A blemish or an unintended radiographic image that can result from faulty manufacture, manipulation, exposure, or processing of an image receptor.

IV. Interpretation

◆ Radiographs are used in conjunction with clinical assessment for a complete care program. Periodic radiographs permit continuing evaluation.

◆ As part of the permanent record, radiographs help to document the oral condition for comparison as well as for legal and forensic purposes.

◆ The quality of the radiographs determines their value for diagnostic interpretation.

◆ Procedures for the preparation of radiographs are perfected so that the radiographs have maximum interpretability with minimum radiation exposure of the patient.

A. Prerequisites for Interpretation

◆ *Mounting:* Mount traditional radiographs in an opaque mount to prevent light between each radiograph from creating glare.

◆ *Viewbox:* Use an adequately lighted viewbox for traditional films. Holding the radiographs up to view by window, room, or unit light is inadequate, and only gross interpretation can be accomplished.

◆ *Digital software tools:* Use magnifiers or a magnifying glass for traditional film to examine films, manipulate brightness and contrast, invert image densities, etc., to enhance diagnostic capabilities.

B. Systematic Examination

◆ Observe one radiographic feature at a time. Examine all of the radiographs in a survey for that feature, rather than taking each radiograph separately to find everything. It is important to note comparisons for each change over the entire survey, and comparisons to past surveys if available.

◆ When examining a particular tooth, compare the appearance of that tooth in each radiograph in which it appears, including bitewings. At different angulations, different findings may become apparent.

C. Correlation with Clinical Examination

◆ A description of examination of the teeth is found in Chapter 16 and of the periodontal tissues in Chapter 20.

◆ Correlation of radiographic findings with the clinical examination, using probe and explorer, is basic to an understanding of the true oral condition of the patient.

OWNERSHIP

◆ Radiographs belong to the dental practice, even though they were paid for by the patient.

◆ Patient has a right to a copy of their records and their radiographs.

◆ If using traditional films, originals are kept by the dental practice and a duplicate series is to be given to the patient.

TABLE 15-6 • Analysis of Radiographs: Causes of Errors

	ERROR	CAUSE: FACTORS IN CORRECTION
Image	Elongation	Insufficient vertical angulation
	Foreshortening	Excessive vertical angulation
	Superimposition (overlapping)	Incorrect horizontal angulation (central ray not directed through interproximal space)
	Partial image	Cone-cut (incorrect direction of central ray or incorrect image receptor placement) Incompletely immersed in processing tank Traditional film touched other film or side of tank during processing
	Blurred or double image	Patient, tube, or image receptor movement during exposure Image receptor exposed twice
	Stretched appearance of trabeculae or apices	Bent traditional film or PSP plate
	No image	Machine malfunction from time switch to wall plug Failure to turn on the machine Traditional film placed in fixer before developer
Density	Too dark	Excessive exposure for all image receptors For traditional film: excessive developing Developer too warm Unsafe safelight Accidental exposure to white light
	Too light	Insufficient exposure for all image receptors For traditional film: insufficient development or excessive fixation Solutions too cool Use of old, contaminated, or poorly mixed solutions Film placement: tube side not placed toward teeth Film used beyond expiration date
Fog	Chemical fog	For traditional film: an imbalance or deterioration of processing solutions
	Light fog	For traditional film: an unintentional exposure to light to which the emulsion is sensitive, either before or during processing Unsafe safelight Darkroom leak Holding unprocessed films too close to the safelight too long Improper storage of unused traditional film
	Radiation fog	Traditional film exposed to scatter radiation before processing
Reticulation	Puckered or pebbly surface	For traditional film: sudden temperature changes during traditional film processing, particularly from warm solutions to very cold water
Artifacts	Dark lines	Bent or creased film or PSP plate Fingernail used to grasp traditional film or PSP plate For traditional film: static electricity when removed from wrapper with excessive force
	Herringbone pattern (light film)	Traditional film packet placed in mouth backward with foil next to teeth
Discoloration	Stains and spots	For traditional film: unclean film hanger Spattering of developer, fixer, dust Insufficient rinsing after developing before fixing Splashing dry negatives with water or solutions Air bubbles adhering to surface during processing (insufficient agitation) Overlap of film on film in tanks or while drying Paper wrapper stuck to film (film not dried when removed from patient's mouth)
	Stains at later date after storage of completed radiographs	For traditional film: Incomplete processing or rinsing Storage in too warm a place Storage near chemicals

PSP, photostimulable phosphor.

DOCUMENTATION

I. Radiation Exposure History

◆ Inquire whether the patient is receiving or has recently received radiation therapy. It may be necessary to minimize the number of exposures. A consultation with the patient's physician is recommended.

◆ Maintain an exposure log for each patient that indicates the date, number of exposures, kVp, mA, time, and area exposed.

II. Patient Care Progress Notes

Patient care progress notes include the following components:

◆ Patient complaint, if applicable, including:
  • Location of symptomatic area.
  • Duration and severity of symptoms.
◆ Clinical findings.
◆ Recommended diagnostic procedures.
  • Explain to patient necessity of radiographs for accurate diagnosis and treatment.
  • Patient has the right to refuse radiographs.
  • Obtain the patient's signature to a statement of refusal in the event a legal issue should arise.
◆ Type of radiographs (periapical or bitewing), number of exposures, and area(s) exposed.
◆ Box 15-9 provides example documentation for the patient who has received dental radiographs.

BOX 15-9

Example Documentation: Assessment for Dental Radiographic Examination

S—Patient presents for routine maintenance appointment and complains about heat sensitivity related to tooth #10. The patient stated that he was hit in the mouth with a soccer ball approximately a year ago.

O—Last radiographs consisted of four bitewings exposed 2 years ago. The most recent periapical radiograph of tooth #10, dated 3 years ago, reveals a healthy lamina dura and periodontal ligament space. The patient has several porcelain-fused-to-metal crowns and large amalgam restorations in the posterior sextants. Teeth in the anterior sextants are natural and contain no restorative materials.

A—Discussed with the patient that #10 may have been traumatized and that a periapical pathology may exist. He has recently undergone numerous medical radiographs and requests minimal radiation exposure today.

P—After a complete clinical examination, and consultation with the patient, two premolar and two molar bitewing radiographs, along with one periapical film of #10 were exposed.

Next steps: Tooth #10 revealed a periapical pathology. The patient was referred to an endodontist for care.

Signed: _____, RDH

Date: _____

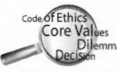

EVERYDAY ETHICS

Kathy, a dental hygienist with 10 years' experience, has been employed by a new practitioner for 1 month. A 25-year-old patient of record arrives at the office for a routine hygiene appointment. The patient had four bitewing radiographs exposed 6 months ago, has a negative medical history, a low CAMBRA score, a negative intra- and extraoral examination, and has had 10 occlusal fillings done when he was between the ages of 10 and 16. Kathy was asked to take a new set of bitewings on this patient as it is routine in this office and the insurance that this patient has will pay for it.

Questions for Consideration

1. List ethical concerns Kathy has for actions that take both patient safety and employer concerns into consideration.

2. Which core values are involved as Kathy discussed those alternatives with her employer? Explain why the core values were chosen.

3. What ethical theory and recommendations can provide guidance as Kathy tries to resolve this issue? Explain the reason for your choice.

Factors to Teach the Patient

When the Patient Asks about the Safety of Radiation

▶ Patients ask questions about safety factors, and occasionally a patient may refuse to have any radiographs exposed. The patient can be reassured with confidence, instructed as to why radiographs are necessary at this time, and informed about how modern equipment and techniques are in accord with radiation standards.

▶ Adapt the answer to the patient. Certain patients have more fear; others have more knowledge about X-rays. The clinician who expresses confidence aids in allaying fears. Hesitation increases the patient's doubt.

▶ Radiographs are essential to diagnosis and treatment. Without the information provided, the clinician can only guess at conditions not visible clinically.

▶ The benefits resulting from the intelligent use of X-rays outweigh any possible negative effects.

▶ Modern X-ray machines are equipped for safety. Simple details about filtration, collimation, film speed, use of protective shields, and short exposure times can be explained.

Educational Features in Dental Radiographs

▶ Position of unerupted permanent teeth in relation to primary teeth.

▶ Detection of early cavitated carious lesions not visible by clinical examination.

▶ Effects of loss of teeth and the importance of having replacements.

▶ Periodontal changes and other pathologic conditions appropriate to an individual patient.

 ENHANCE YOUR UNDERSTANDING

ONLINE RESOURCES
(see the inside front cover for access information)
- Audio glossary
- Appendices

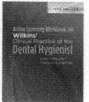

SUPPORT FOR LEARNING
(available separately)
- *Active Learning Workbook for Wilkins' Clinical Practice of the Dental Hygienist, 13th Edition*

INDIVIDUALIZED REVIEW
- Customized practice quizzing with Navigate 2 TestPrep for *Wilkins' Clinical Practice of the Dental Hygienist*

References

1. American Dental Association Council on Scientific Affairs, U.S. Department of Health and Human Services, U.S. Food and Drug Administration. The selection of patients for dental radiographic examinations. https://www.fda.gov/radiation-emitting-products/medical-x-ray-imaging/selection-patients-dental-radiographic-examinations. Accessed June 20, 2019.
2. National Research Council, (BEIR-VII Phase 2). Health Risks of Exposure to Low Levels of National Academies Press. *Ionizing Radiation*. Washington, DC: National Academies Press; 2006. https://www.nap.edu/catalog/11340/health-risks-from-exposure-to-low-levels-of-ionizing-radiation. Accessed June 20, 2019.
3. Parks ET. Digital radiographic imaging: is the dental practice ready? *JADA*. 2008;139(4):477-481.
4. van der Stelt PF. Better imaging: the advances of digital radiography. *JADA*. 2008;139(suppl 3):7S-13S.
5. Gart C, Zamanian K. Global trends in dental imaging: the rise of digital. Dental Tribune. July 27, 2010. https://us.dental-tribune.com/news/global-trends-in-dental-imaging-the-rise-of-digital/. Accessed April 17, 2018.
6. Matzen LH, Christensen J, Wenzel A. Patient discomfort and retakes in periapical examination of mandibular third molars using digital receptors. *Oral Surg Oral Med Oral Pathol Oral Radiol Endod*. 2009;107(4):566-572.
7. Williamson GF. Intraoral imaging: basic principles, techniques and error correction, March, 2018. Dentalcare.com Professional Education. https://www.dentalcare.com/en-us/professional-education/ce-courses/ce559. Accessed June 20, 2019.
8. International Commission on Radiation Units and Measurements. Radiation Quantities and Units. ICRU Report No. 33. Washington, DC: ICRU; 1980. https://onlinelibrary.wiley.com/doi/abs/10.1002/jlcr.2580180918. Accessed April 17, 2018.
9. National Council on Radiation Protection and Measurements. Radiation Protection in Dentistry. NCRP Report No. 145. Washington, DC: NCRP; 2003. https://ncrponline.org/publications/reports/ncrp-reports-145/. Accessed June 20, 2019.
10. White SC, Mallya SM. Update on the biological effects of ionizing radiation, relative dose factors and radiation hygiene. *Aust Dent J*. 2012;57(suppl 1):2-8.
11. Anjum M, Godward S, Williams D, et al. Dental x-rays and the risk of thyroid cancer: a case-control study. *Acta Oncol*. 2010;49(4):447-453.
12. Thomson EM. Reduce retakes. *Dimens Dent Hyg*. 2011;9(10):58-61.
13. Frommer HH, Stabulas-Savage JJ. *Radiology for the Dental Professional*. 9th ed. St. Louis, MO: Mosby; 2011.
14. Makdissi J, Pawar RR, Johnson B, Chong BS. The effects of device position on the operator's radiations dose when using a handheld portable x-ray device. *Dentomaxillofac Radiol*. 2016;45(3):20150245. doi:10.1259/dmfr.20150245.

16

Hard Tissue Examination of the Dentition

Lorie Speer, RDH, MSDH, and Linda D. Boyd, RDH, RD, EdD

CHAPTER OUTLINE

THE DENTITIONS
I. Primary (Deciduous) Dentition
II. Mixed or Transitional Dentition
III. Permanent Dentition
IV. The Teeth

HARD TISSUE EXAMINATION PROCEDURE
I. Dental Charting of Existing Restorations
II. Assessment of Noncarious and Carious Lesions
III. Occlusion
IV. Study Models

DEVELOPMENTAL ENAMEL LESIONS
I. Enamel Hypoplasia
II. Hypomineralization
III. Hypomaturation

DEVELOPMENTAL DEFECTS OF DENTIN
I. Types and Etiology

NONCARIOUS DENTAL LESIONS
I. Attrition

NONCARIOUS CERVICAL LESIONS
I. Erosion
II. Abrasion
III. Abfraction

FRACTURES OF THE TEETH
I. Causes of Tooth Fractures
II. Description

III. Classification of Dental Injuries
IV. Recommendations for Treatment

DENTAL CARIES
I. Development of Dental Caries
II. Classification of Carious Lesions

ENAMEL CARIES
I. Stages in the Formation of a Carious Lesion
II. Nomenclature by Surfaces
III. Types of Dental Caries

EARLY CHILDHOOD CARIES
I. Microbiology
II. Clinical Appearance

ROOT CARIES
I. Stages in the Formation of a Root Surface Lesion
II. Risk Factors for Root Caries

TESTING FOR PULP VITALITY
I. Causes of Loss of Vitality
II. Indications for Pulp Vitality Testing
III. Response to Pulp Testing
IV. Thermal Pulp Testing
V. Electrical Pulp Tester

OCCLUSION
I. Normal Occlusion
II. Malocclusion
III. Malrelations of Groups of Teeth

IV. Terminology for Malposition of Individual Teeth

OCCLUSION OF THE PRIMARY TEETH
I. Normal Occlusion
II. Malocclusion of the Primary Teeth

DYNAMIC OR FUNCTIONAL OCCLUSION
I. Types of Occlusal Contacts
II. Proximal Contacts

TRAUMA FROM OCCLUSION
I. Types of Occlusal Trauma
II. Effects of Trauma from Occlusion
III. Recognition of Signs of Occlusal Trauma

STUDY MODELS
I. Purposes and Uses of Study Models

THE INTEROCCLUSAL RECORD
I. Purposes

DOCUMENTATION

EVERYDAY ETHICS

FACTORS TO TEACH THE PATIENT

REFERENCES

LEARNING OBJECTIVES

After studying this chapter, the student will be able to:

1. Identify the three divisions of the human dentition: primary teeth, mixed (transitional) dentition, and permanent teeth.

2. Recognize and explain the various developmental and noncarious dental lesions.

3. Describe types of dental injuries and tooth fractures that may occur.

4. List the G.V. Black, American Dental Association Caries Classification, and International Caries Detection and Assessment System classification of dental carious lesions used for diagnosis, treatment planning, management, cavity preparations, and finished restorations.

5. Explain the initiation and development of early childhood caries.

6. Compare methods for determining the vitality of the pulp of a tooth.

7. Provide a list of the factors to be observed and recorded during a complete dental charting with a new patient.

8. Explain the basic principles of occlusion.

9. Classify occlusion on a patient or case study according to Angle's classification and describe facial profile associated with each classification.

10. Describe functional and parafunctional contacts.

11. Give examples of parafunctional habits.

12. Discuss types of occlusal trauma and explain the effects on the oral structures.

13. List the purposes and uses of study models.

14. Identify and explain the purposes and uses of study models in the clinical practice of dental hygiene.

Clinical examination and assessment of the teeth are essential before treatment to provide guidelines for treatment planning, instrumentation, instruction, and follow-up evaluation.

◆ Background study of dental anatomy, oral histology, and oral pathology is essential to the examination of the hard tissues of the oral cavity.

THE DENTITIONS

The three divisions are the primary (deciduous) dentition, mixed (transitional) dentition, and permanent dentition. Refer to the online resource for the average measurement of primary and permanent teeth.

I. Primary (Deciduous) Dentition

◆ Formation of the primary teeth begins in utero.

◆ The weeks in utero when each primary tooth begins to mineralize. Average age after birth when the enamel is completely formed before the date of eruption is found in Chapter 47.

II. Mixed or Transitional Dentition

◆ Mixed or transitional dentition occurs between the ages of 6 and 12 years when primary teeth are being exfoliated and permanent teeth erupt.

◆ Succedaneous teeth are permanent teeth that erupt into the positions of exfoliated primary teeth.

◆ Figure 16-1 illustrates the mixed dentition of a child approximately 6 years of age just as the first permanent molars are erupting.

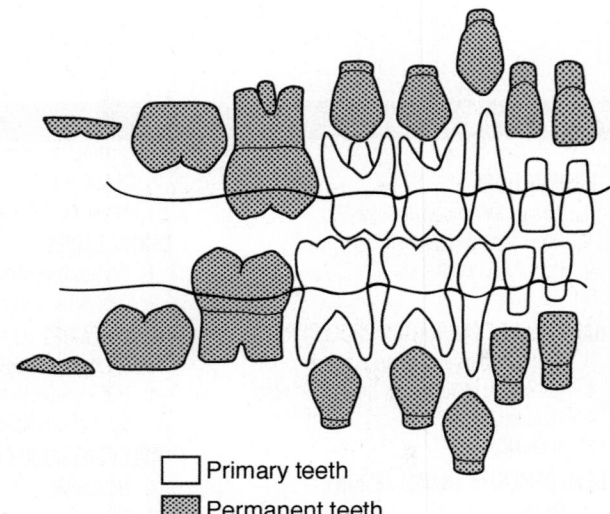

☐ Primary teeth
▨ Permanent teeth

FIGURE 16-1 • Mixed Dentition at Approximately Age 6 Years. The average child has 20 primary teeth in place, and root resorption of the incisors has started as the developing permanent incisors move into position. The first permanent molars are partially erupted.

III. Permanent Dentition

◆ Consists of 32 teeth that replace the primary teeth and serve throughout life.

◆ Mineralization of the permanent teeth starts at birth and continues into adolescence. The chronology of development and eruption of the permanent teeth is listed in Table 16-1.

◆ Roots are completely formed about 3 years after eruption into the oral cavity.

TABLE 16-1 • Tooth Development and Eruption: Permanent Teeth

		HARD TISSUE FORMATION BEGINS	ENAMEL COMPLETED (YEARS)	ERUPTION (YEARS)	ROOT COMPLETED (YEARS)
Maxillary	Central incisor	3–4 mo	4–5	7–8	10
	Lateral incisor	10 mo	4–5	8–9	11
	Canine	4–5 mo	6–7	11–12	13–15
	First premolar	$1^1/_2$–$1^3/_4$ y	5–6	10–11	12–13
	Second premolar	2–$2^1/_4$ y	6–7	10–12	12–14
	First molar	At birth	$2^1/_2$–3	6–7	9–10
	Second molar	$2^1/_2$–3 y	7–8	12–13	14–16
	Third molar	7–9 y	12–16	17–21	18–25
Mandibular	Central incisor	3–4 mo	4–5	6–7	9
	Lateral incisor	3–4 mo	4–5	7–8	10
	Canine	4–5 mo	6–7	9–10	12–14
	First premolar	$1^3/_4$–2 y	5–6	10–12	12–13
	Second premolar	$2^1/_4$–$2^1/_2$ y	6–7	11–12	13–14
	First molar	At birth	$2^1/_2$–3	6–7	9–10
	Second molar	$2^1/_2$–3 y	7–8	11–13	14–15
	Third molar	8–10 y	12–16	17–21	18–25

Source: Logan WH, Kronfield R. Development of the human jaws and surrounding structures from birth to age fifteen. *JADA.* 1933;35(20):379-424; Orban B. *Oral Histology and Embryology.* St. Louis, MO: Mosby; 1944. Schour I, McCall JO. Chronology of the human dentition. In: Orban B, ed. *Oral Histology and Embryology.* St Louis, MA: Mosby; 1944:240.

IV. The Teeth

◆ Clinical crown is the part of the tooth above the attached periodontal tissues. It can be considered the part of the tooth that is visible (not covered with gingiva) when in the mouth and where restorative treatment procedures are performed (Figure 16-2).

◆ Clinical root is the part of the tooth not visible because it is below the base of the gingival sulcus or periodontal pocket (is not visible when in the mouth). It is the part of the root to which periodontal fibers are attached.

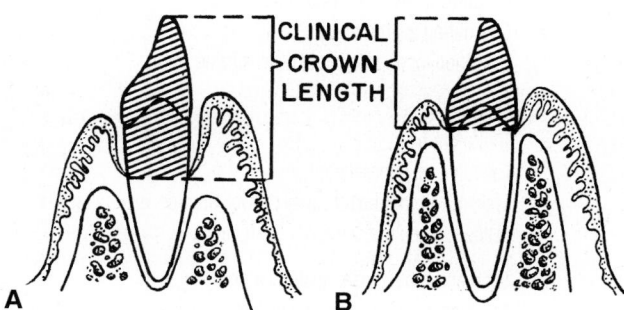

FIGURE 16-2 • Clinical Crown. The part of the tooth that is above the attached periodontal tissue. **A:** When the periodontal pocket depth is increased, the clinical crown extends to a position at which the clinical crown length is greater than the clinical root length. The clinical root is the part of the tooth with attached periodontal tissues. **B:** When the clinical attachment level is at the cementoenamel junction, the clinical crown and the anatomic crown are the same.

◆ Anatomic crown is the part of the tooth covered by enamel.

◆ Anatomic root is the part of the tooth covered by cementum.

HARD TISSUE EXAMINATION PROCEDURE

The hard tissue examination includes dental charting of the existing restorations along with carious lesions and noncarious lesions. Radiographs are utilized to aid in identification of carious lesions and other pathologies. Documentation of occlusion and preparation of study models to aid with treatment planning are also part of the hard tissue examination. Table 16-2 lists factors to observe during the hard tissue examination.

I. Dental Charting of Existing Restorations

◆ Missing, supernumerary, or unerupted teeth are recorded.

◆ A systematic approach to charting restorations should be utilized to avoid errors, for example, start with tooth #1.

II. Assessment of Noncarious and Carious Lesions

A. Visual Examination Procedure

◆ Carefully visually inspect each surface, use air to clean and dry tooth surface, and utilize adequate lighting.[1,2]

TABLE 16-2 • Examination of the Teeth

FEATURE	TO OBSERVE	DENTAL HYGIENE IMPLICATION
Morphology	Number of teeth (missing teeth verified by radiographic examination) Size, shape Arch form Position of individual teeth (**diastema**) Injuries: fractures of the crown (root fractures observed in radiographs)	Selection and adaptation of instruments Areas prone to dental caries initiation, particularly difficult-to-reach areas during biofilm control Pulp test for vitality may be indicated
Development	Anomalies and developmental defects Pits and white spots	Distinguish **hypoplasia** and dental fluorosis from demineralization Identify pits for sealants
Eruption (Table 16-1)	Sequence of eruption: normal, irregular Unerupted teeth observed in radiographs	Care in using floss in the col area where the epithelium is usually less mature in young children Orthodontic needs Procedures for preservation of primary teeth
Deposits (Table 17-1) Food debris Biofilm Calculus Supragingival Subgingival	Overall evaluation of oral self-care and biofilm control measures Relation of appearance of teeth to gingival health Extent and location of biofilm, debris, and calculus Calculus and the tooth surface pocket wall	Need for instruction and guidance Frequency of follow-up and maintenance appointments
Stains (see Chapter 17) Extrinsic Intrinsic	Extrinsic: colors relate to causes Intrinsic: dark, grayish Tobacco stain	Need for test for pulp vitality Stain removal procedures; selection of polishing agent Dentifrice recommendation Biofilm control emphasis for biofilm-related stains Provide information concerning oral effects of tobacco use Tobacco cessation program (see Chapter 32)
Noncarious lesions	Attrition: primary and permanent Abrasion: physical agents that may be a cause Erosion	Evaluate causes and treat or counsel for prevention Dietary analysis Selection of nonabrasive dentifrice Habit evaluation
Exposed cementum	Relation to gingival recession, pocket formation Areas of narrow attached gingiva Hypersensitivity	Special care areas such as narrow attached gingiva Nonabrasive dentifrice advised Measures to prevent root surface caries Care during instrumentation Indication for application of desensitizing agent
Dental caries	Areas of demineralization Stages of carious lesions Proximal lesions observed in radiographs **Arrested caries** Root caries	Charting Treatment plan Cavitated vs. noncavitated Preventive program for caries control, fluoride, dietary factors Follow-up and frequency of maintenance
Restorations	Contour of restorations, overhangs Proximal contact Surface smoothness Staining	Chart and correct inadequate margins Selection of instruments and polishing agents Dentifrice selection to prevent discoloration
Factors related to occlusion	Health of supporting structures; observation of radiographs for signs of trauma from occlusion	Need for study of bruxism and other parafunctional habits
Tooth wear	Facets; worn-down cusp tips	Chart inadequate contacts for corrective measures

TABLE 16-2 • Examination of the Teeth (Continued)

FEATURE	TO OBSERVE	DENTAL HYGIENE IMPLICATION
Proximal contacts	Use of floss to find open contact areas Areas of food retention	Use of floss by patient
Mobility	Degree; comparison of chartings Possible causes	Need for reduction of related inflammatory factors Dentist will identify and treat factors related to occlusal trauma
Classification	Position of teeth Angle's classification	Relationship to orthodontic treatment needs
Habits	Nail or object biting; lip or cheek biting Observe effects on lip, cheek, teeth **Tongue thrust**; reverse swallow	Guidance for habit correction when indicated
Edentulous areas	Radiographic evaluation for impacted, unerupted teeth, supernumerary teeth, retained root tips, other deviations from normal	Alternative fulcrum selection during instrumentation Applied biofilm control procedures for abutment teeth
Replacement for missing teeth Dentures Partial dentures Implants	Teeth and tissue that support a prosthesis Cleanliness of a prosthesis Factors that contribute to food and debris retention	Instruction in personal care of fixed and removable dentures; use of floss under fixed partial denture; other appropriate care
Saliva	Amount and consistency Dryness of mouth	Instruction for prevention of dental caries: more caries can be expected in a dry mouth Use of saliva substitute; fluoride

- ◆ Observe changes in the color and translucency of tooth structure.
- ◆ Changes noted can then be studied in the radiograph or documented for future review.
- ◆ Variations in color and translucency include the following:
  - • Chalky white areas of demineralization.
  - • Grayish-white discoloration of marginal ridges caused by dental caries of the proximal surface underneath.
  - • Grayish-white color spreading from margins of restorations.
- ◆ Transillumination is especially useful for anterior teeth and unrestored posterior teeth.

B. Radiographic Examination

- ◆ Carefully review and interpret radiographic findings to identify areas to investigate during the clinical examination. Neither radiographic nor clinical examination is complete without the other.
- ◆ In addition to possible caries lesions, other important areas to investigate in the radiographic examination include: anomalies, impactions, fractures, internal and root resorption, and periapical radiolucencies.
- ◆ Panoramic, extraoral, or occlusal radiographs are needed for detecting or defining anomalies and pathologic lesions outside the scope of periapical radiographs.

C. Clinical Examination Procedure

- ◆ If caries cannot be confirmed visually or radiographically, gently use a rounded or ball-end explorer to confirm visual findings.
- ◆ It is essential not to break through a tooth surface that may be remineralizing with a sharp explorer.
- ◆ Intraoral images can also document the existing oral condition and provide visual representation of treatment needs both for documentation in the patient record and to educate the patient.

D. Document the Following:

- ◆ Existing restorations.
- ◆ Developmental enamel lesions.
- ◆ Noncarious cervical lesions (NCCLs).
- ◆ Carious lesions using a recognized classification system described later in the chapter.
- ◆ Any other pathology noted during the radiographic or clinical examination.

III. Occlusion

Assessment of occlusion will include:
- ◆ Normal occlusion.
- ◆ Malocclusion.
- ◆ Malrelations of groups of teeth.

◆ Malpositions of individual teeth.

◆ Dynamic (or functional) occlusion.

◆ Traumatic occlusion.

IV. Study Models

Study models may be taken to assess and document occlusal relationships.

DEVELOPMENTAL ENAMEL LESIONS

I. Enamel Hypoplasia

Enamel hypoplasia is a defect that occurs as a result of a disturbance during formation of the enamel matrix.

A. Types and Etiology

◆ Genetic.[3]

- Amelogenesis imperfecta is a hereditary enamel defect in which the enamel is either thin or absent. The enamel may also have surface pitting or vertical grooves.
- Other inherited syndromes associated with enamel defects may be associated with dermatologic conditions or defects in mineralization such as hypoparathyroidism.

◆ Systemic conditions contributing to enamel hypoplasia during tooth development may include[3]:

- Metabolic disturbances such as celiac disease and chronic renal or liver disease.
- Infections causing fever such as chicken pox, rubella, measles, or congenital syphilis.
- Chemicals and drugs such as fluoride and tetracycline.
- Nutritional deficiencies like rickets.
- Preterm birth.

◆ Local insults to developing tooth may include:

- Trauma.
- Periapical inflammation of a primary tooth may injure the developing permanent tooth.

B. Appearance

◆ Genetic

- The teeth may appear yellow or brown.

◆ Systemic

Also called "chronologic hypoplasia" because the lesions are found in areas of the teeth where the enamel was forming during the systemic disturbance.

- *Single narrow zone* (smooth or pitted): Disturbance lasted a short period of time.
- *Multiple*: Disturbance to the ameloblast occurred over a period of time or several times (Figure 16-3).
- *Teeth most frequently affected*: First molars, incisors, canines, because the disturbances generally occur during the first year when those teeth are mineralizing.

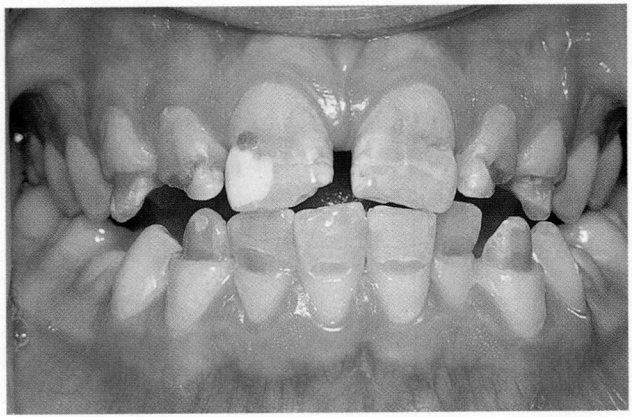

FIGURE 16-3 • Enamel Hypoplasia. Enamel hypoplasia, usually in the form of white or brown grooves or pits, at a level corresponding with the stage of development of the teeth.

◆ Hypoplasia of Congenital Syphilis

- Transmission of syphilis from mother to fetus after the 16th week of pregnancy may alter the development of the tooth germs.
- Figure 16-4 illustrates tooth forms that may result, including the mulberry molar. The mesiodistal width may be reduced, and incisors are frequently narrowed at the incisal third, as shown by the Hutchinson's incisors and the peg lateral incisor.

◆ Local Enamel Hypoplasia

- A single tooth with a yellow or brown intrinsic stain.

II. Hypomineralization

Hypomineralization occurs during the mineralization stage of the enamel.

A. Etiology[3]

◆ Children with celiac disease are at risk for hypomineralization because of malabsorption and potential for mineral deficiencies.

◆ Chronic liver or kidney disease may impact mineralization during tooth development.

◆ Acquired infection such as chicken pox and respiratory and urinary tract infections.

◆ Chemicals and drugs such as fluoride and tetracycline.

B. Types[3]

◆ Molar incisor hypomineralization appears as yellow or brownish demarcated areas on permanent molars and incisors.

- Prevalence tends to be highest in Australia, some areas of Europe, Brazil, and Iraq.

III. Hypomaturation

Hypomaturation occurs during the last stages of mineralization and results in the enamel fracturing easily. It may appear as opaque or discolored enamel.

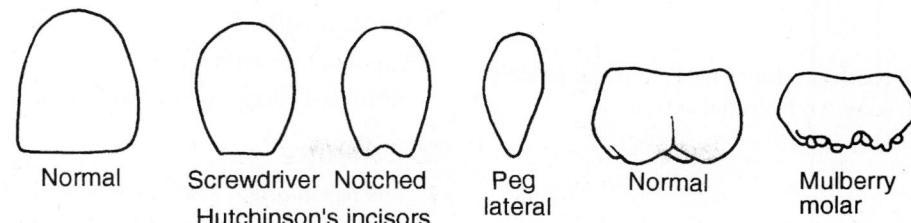

FIGURE 16-4 • Crown Forms of Enamel Hypoplasia. Hutchinson's incisors and mulberry molars are typical crown forms that result from congenital syphilis. The central incisors are narrowed at the incisal third, and the lateral incisors may be conical or peg shaped.

DEVELOPMENTAL DEFECTS OF DENTIN

I. Types and Etiology

A. Genetic[3]

◆ Dentinogenesis imperfecta is the most common type resulting in rapid wear and attrition of the teeth.

◆ Dentine dysplasia.

◆ A familial or inherited form of rickets.

B. Appearance

◆ Opalescent brown discoloration.

◆ Progressive pulp obliteration.

NONCARIOUS DENTAL LESIONS

I. Attrition

Attrition is the wearing away of a tooth as a result of tooth-to-tooth contact (Figure 16-5).

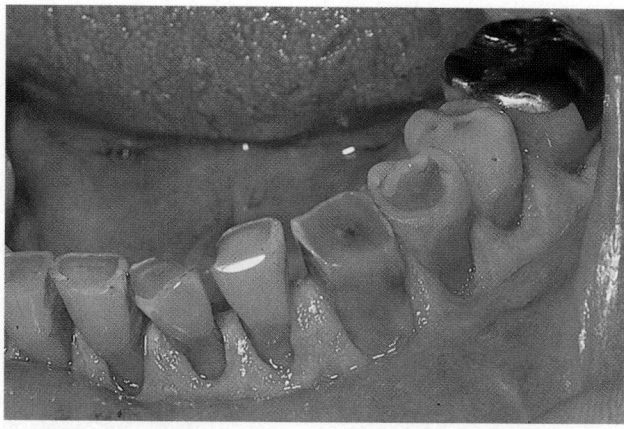

FIGURE 16-5 • Attrition. The incisal surfaces of mandibular anterior teeth have been worn to expose the dentin. Dentin usually appears as a yellow-brown line or ring. (From Langlais RP, Miller CS. *Color Atlas of Common Oral Diseases.* Philadelphia, PA: Lea & Febiger; 1992. Used with permission.)

A. Occurrence

◆ Location

• May be found on occlusal, incisal, and proximal surfaces.

◆ Impact of age and gender

• Effects of attrition are cumulative over time so an increase in attrition is often associated with increasing age.[4]

• More attrition is seen in men than in women of comparable age.

B. Etiology

◆ Bruxism[5]

• There are two main types of bruxism: sleep and awake bruxism.

• Predisposing factors may be psychological, stress, or occlusal interferences.

• Sleep bruxism in children may be related to sleep disturbances and secondhand smoke.[6]

◆ Environmental factors

• Coarse foods, chewing tobacco, culturally related chewing habits, or abrasive dusts associated with certain occupations.

C. Appearance

◆ Initial lesion

• Small shiny, flat, worn spot on the surface of a tooth known as a facet is found on a cusp tip or ridge, or slight flattening of an incisal edge.

◆ Advanced

• Gradual reduction in cusp height; flattening of incisal or occlusal plane as shown in Figure 16-5.

• Staining of exposed dentin.

• Radiographically the pulp chamber and canals may be narrowed and sometimes obliterated as a result of formation of secondary dentin.

NONCARIOUS CERVICAL LESIONS

NCCLs are lesions resulting from loss of tooth structure near the cementoenamel junction and include erosion, abrasion, and abfraction.[7] NCCLs impact the structural integrity of the tooth, esthetics, and may retain dental biofilm and exhibit dentin sensitivity.[7]

I. Erosion

Erosion is the loss of tooth substance by a chemical process that does not involve known bacterial action.

A. Occurrence

◆ Location
  • Facial or lingual surfaces are mostly commonly affected (Figure 16-6).
  • Two types of erosion can occur: endogenous and exogenous.
◆ Usually involves multiple teeth.

B. Etiology

◆ Extrinsic acids[8]
  • *Occupational acid exposure:* battery, ammunition, or galvanizing factory workers; wine tasters; and professional swimmers.
  • *Acidic food:* acidic soft drinks, sports drinks, citrus fruits or drinks, vinegar, wine.
  • *Acidic drugs:* aspirin, iron tablets, vitamin C supplements.
◆ Intrinsic acids[8]
  • *Eating disorders:* bulimia.
  • Gastroesophageal reflux disease.
  • Alcohol abuse.

C. Appearance

◆ Smooth, shallow, hard, shiny (in contrast to dental caries, in which appearance is soft and discolored).
◆ Shape varies from shallow saucer-like depressions of the cusps to deep wedge-shaped grooves; margins are not sharply demarcated.
◆ May progress to involve the dentin and stimulate secondary dentin.
◆ May occur in combination with dental caries, calculus, or dental restorations.[1]

II. Abrasion

Abrasion is the mechanical wearing away of tooth substance by forces other than mastication.

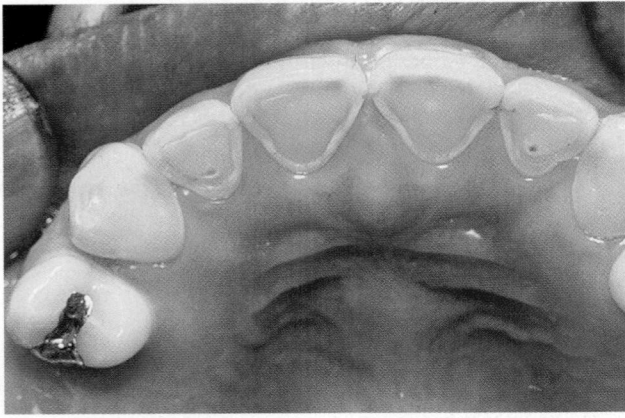

FIGURE 16-6 • Erosion. Enamel erosion on the lingual of mandibular anterior teeth caused by chronic vomiting in bulimia.

A. Occurrence

◆ Exposed root surfaces.
◆ At incisal edge or on occlusal surface.

B. Etiology

◆ The lesion originates from mechanical abrasion and the cervical areas are the most commonly affected tooth surface (Figure 16-7).[9]
◆ The action of microorganisms is not implicated in the development of abrasion. Dental caries may occur in the abraded area as a secondary lesion.
◆ Primary factors impacting development of cervical abrasion include the abrasiveness of the dentifrice, stiffness of the toothbrush bristles, and the area where the patient first begins brushing.[9,10] Figure 16-7 shows the effect on the root surface.
◆ *Occupational causes:* cement factories and granite workers along with iron miners.[9]
◆ Habits putting the patient at risk for abrasion include: pipe smoking, chewing pens, betel nut chewing, and pica (eating nonfood items).[9]

C. Appearance

◆ V- or wedge-shaped with hard, smooth, shiny surface and clearly defined margins.
◆ Except for occlusal or incisal abrasion, the lesions occur initially on exposed cementum, then extend into the dentin.

III. Abfraction[7]

Abfraction means to break away and results from microfractures in the hydroxyapatite crystals of enamel and dentin.

A. Occurrence

◆ Primarily occurs on buccal surfaces.
◆ Wedge- or V-shaped lesions with relatively sharp angles.

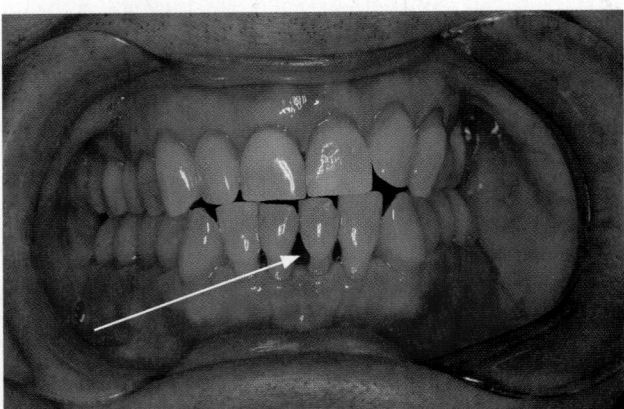

FIGURE 16-7 • Abrasion. The lower anterior teeth exhibit areas of abrasion. Note that the area of abrasion on the root surface undermines the enamel. (Photograph courtesy of Dr. Paul Epstein, DMD.)

B. Etiology

◆ Multifactorial.

◆ Research has not confirmed that traumatic occlusion is the cause.

◆ Dentin demineralization may increase the risk of abfraction, and occlusal forces may increase progression of the lesion.

C. Appearance

◆ V- or wedge shaped with hard, smooth, shiny surface and clearly defined margins.

◆ Except for incisal biting habits, the lesions occur initially on exposed cementum, then extend into the dentin.

FRACTURES OF THE TEETH

◆ Trauma to the face may involve fractured bones and teeth in addition to soft tissue injuries. Fractured jaw and methods of treatment were described in Chapter 9.

◆ Emergency care for a forcibly displaced tooth is found in Chapter 9.

I. Causes of Tooth Fractures

◆ Automobile, bicycle, and diving accidents.

◆ Contact sports when mouth protectors are not worn.

◆ Blows to the face.

◆ Falls.

II. Description

A. Line of Fracture

◆ May be horizontal, diagonal, or vertical.

◆ Figure 16-8 illustrates fractures of a central incisor.

B. Radiographic Signs of Trauma

◆ Widened periodontal ligament (PDL) space.

◆ Radiolucent fracture line.

◆ Radiopaque areas where fracture segments overlap.

◆ Tooth displacement.

III. Classification of Dental Injuries[11]

Both primary and permanent dentitions are included.

◆ Fracture of enamel of tooth such as chipping and incomplete fractures (cracks).

◆ Fracture of crown of tooth without pulpal involvement.

◆ Fracture of crown with pulpal involvement.

◆ Fracture of root of tooth.

◆ Fracture of crown and root of tooth with or without pulpal involvement.

◆ Luxation (dislocation) of tooth: This category may involve concussion, subluxation, and luxation. Concussion means the tooth is sensitive to percussion but is not loosened or displaced. Loosening without displacement is subluxation, and loosening with displacement is luxation.

◆ Intrusion or extrusion of tooth: Intrusion into the alveolar bone is usually accompanied by fracture of the alveolar socket. Extrusion from the socket is a partial displacement.

◆ Avulsion of tooth: Avulsion is the complete displacement of the tooth out of its socket due to forcible trauma.

IV. Recommendations for Treatment

◆ Diagnosis and planning are necessary for satisfactory healing.

◆ Guidelines for treatment planning have been prepared by the *International Association of Dental Traumatology* and include:

  • Clinical diagnosis and immediate emergency treatment.
  • Radiographs to detect root fracture.
  • Location of tooth fragments.
  • Pulp testing.
  • Mobility; tenderness.
  • Follow-up for additional requirements.

DENTAL CARIES

The World Health Organization has defined dental caries as a "localized, posteruptive, pathologic process of external origin involving softening of the hard tooth tissue and

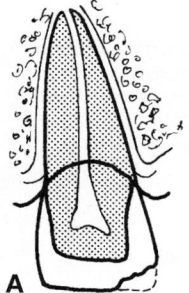 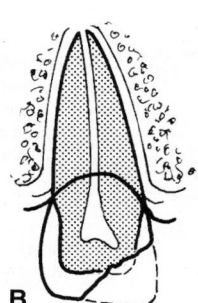 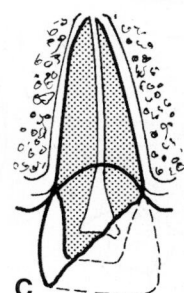 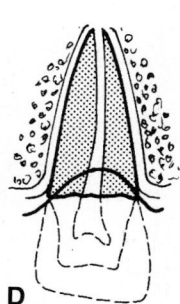 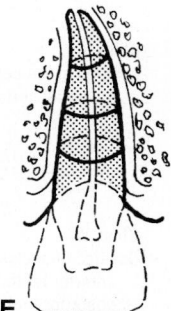

FIGURE 16-8 • Fractures of Teeth. A: Enamel fracture. **B:** Crown fracture without pulpal involvement. **C:** Crown fracture with pulpal involvement. **D:** Fracture of crown and root near neck of tooth. **E:** Root fractures involving cementum, dentin, and the pulp may occur in the apical, middle, or coronal third of the root.

proceeding to the formation of a cavity."[12] Dental caries, a preventable disease, is characterized by demineralization of the hard components and dissolution of the organic matrix.

I. Development of Dental Caries

Requirements for the development of a carious lesion are microorganisms, fermentable carbohydrate, and a susceptible tooth surface. Chapter 33 shows four overlapping circles to illustrate the essential factors in dental caries initiation.

◆ Dental biofilm contains many types of bacteria. Classic theory is that *Streptococcus mutans* and *Lactobacillus* are primarily responsible for dental caries; however, research suggests the oral microbiome is much more complex than originally thought and caries results from an imbalance in the oral microbes.[13]

The role of oral microbiome, dental biofilm, and other factors involved in dental caries development is described in Chapter 17.

II. Classification of Carious Lesions

A. G.V. Black's Classification[14]

◆ The standard method for classifying dental caries was developed by Dr. G.V. Black, a noted dental educator who divided the categories into classes according to surfaces of the teeth; each class is represented by a Roman numeral.

◆ The G.V. Black classification was associated with a surgical approach where diseased portions of the tooth were removed with placement of restorations.[15] Figure 16-9 defines and illustrates the classifications.

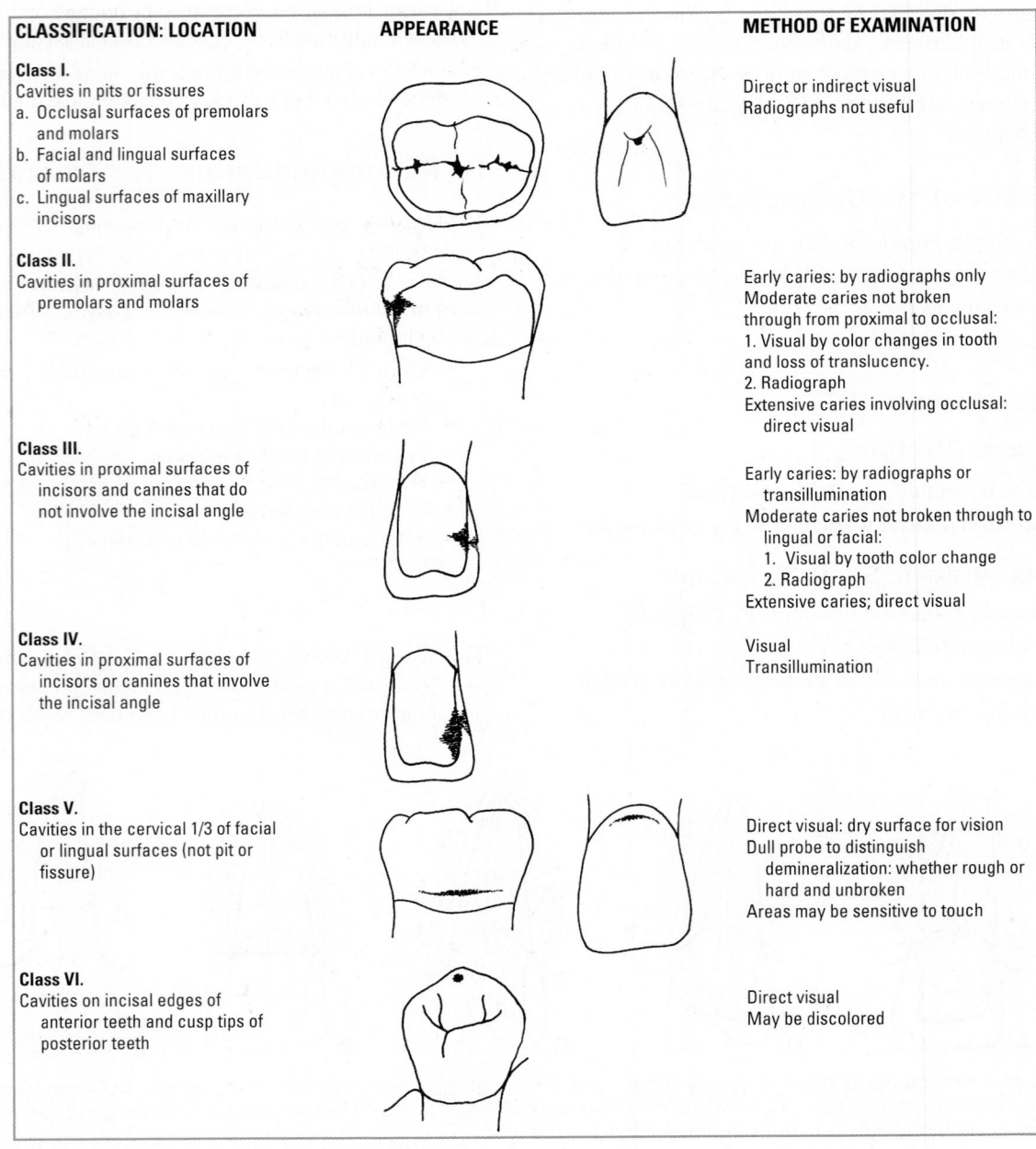

CLASSIFICATION: LOCATION	APPEARANCE	METHOD OF EXAMINATION
Class I. Cavities in pits or fissures a. Occlusal surfaces of premolars and molars b. Facial and lingual surfaces of molars c. Lingual surfaces of maxillary incisors		Direct or indirect visual Radiographs not useful
Class II. Cavities in proximal surfaces of premolars and molars		Early caries: by radiographs only Moderate caries not broken through from proximal to occlusal: 1. Visual by color changes in tooth and loss of translucency. 2. Radiograph Extensive caries involving occlusal: direct visual
Class III. Cavities in proximal surfaces of incisors and canines that do not involve the incisal angle		Early caries: by radiographs or transillumination Moderate caries not broken through to lingual or facial: 1. Visual by tooth color change 2. Radiograph Extensive caries; direct visual
Class IV. Cavities in proximal surfaces of incisors or canines that involve the incisal angle		Visual Transillumination
Class V. Cavities in the cervical 1/3 of facial or lingual surfaces (not pit or fissure)		Direct visual: dry surface for vision Dull probe to distinguish demineralization: whether rough or hard and unbroken Areas may be sensitive to touch
Class VI. Cavities on incisal edges of anterior teeth and cusp tips of posterior teeth		Direct visual May be discolored

FIGURE 16-9 • G.V. Black's Classification of Carious Lesions.

◆ This classification system applies when completing the dental charting of existing restorations.

B. International Caries Classification and Management System[16]

◆ The International Caries Classification and Management System (ICCMS) approach classifies the tooth surface from healthy to severe decay and allows for early detection of enamel changes that will benefit from remineralization.

◆ The goal of this standardized system is for early detection in order to make informed decisions about caries management. Figure 16-10 describes and illustrates the International Caries Detection and Assessment System. More information can be found at www.icdas.org.

		Definition of ICCMS™ Caries Merged categories	
Caries categories	**Sound surfaces** (ICDAS™ code 0)	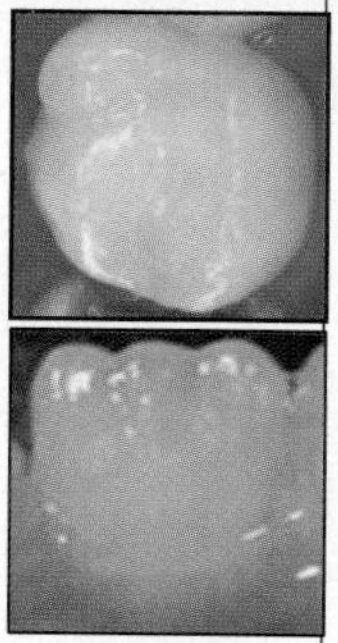	**Sound tooth surfaces** show no evidence of visible caries (no or questionable change in enamel translucency) when viewed clean and after prolonged air-drying (5 seconds).[8-9] (*Surfaces with developmental defects such as enamel hypomineralization (including fluorosis), tooth wear (attrition, abrasion and erosion), and extrinsic or intrinsic stains will be recorded as sound*).
	Initial stage caries (ICDAS™ codes 1 and 2)	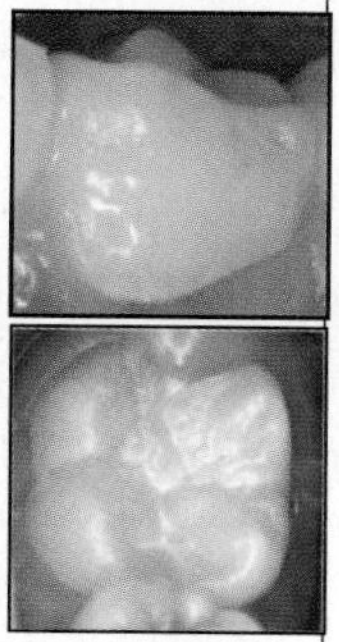	**First or distinct visual changes in enamel** seen as a carious opacity or visible discoloration (white spot lesion and/or brown carious discoloration) not consistent with clinical appearance of sound enamel (ICDAS™ code 1 or 2) and which show no evidence of surface breakdown or underlying dentine shadowing.
	Moderate stage caries (ICDAS™ codes 3 and 4)	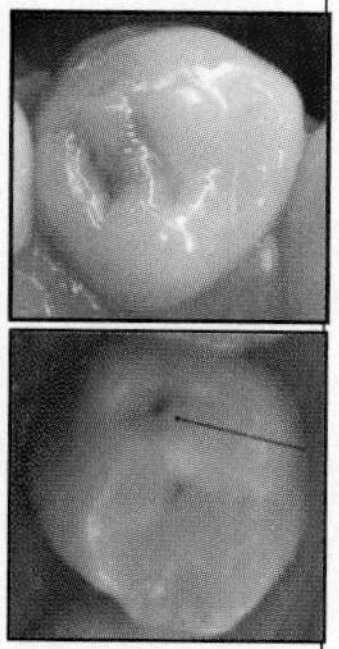	A white or brown spot lesion with **Localized enamel breakdown,** without visible dentine exposure (ICDAS™ code 3), **or an Underlying dentine shadow** (ICDAS™ code 4), which obviously originated on the surface being evaluated. (*To confirm enamel breakdown, a WHO/CPI/PSR ball-end probe can be used gently across the tooth area—a limited discontinuity is detected if the ball drops into the enamel micro-cavity/discontinuity*).
	Extensive stage caries (ICDAS™ codes 5 and 6)	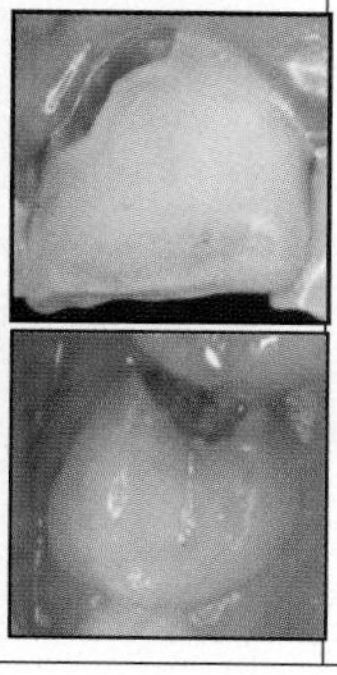	A **distinct cavity** in opaque or discolored enamel **with visible dentine** (ICDAS™ code 5 or 6). (*A WHO/CPI/PSR probe can confirm the cavity extends into dentine*).

FIGURE 16-10 • Definition of International Caries Classification and Management System (ICCMS™) Caries Categories. (Pitts NB, Ismail AI, Martignon S, Ekstrand K, Douglas GVA, Longbottom C; ICDAS Foundation. ICCMS International Caries Classification and Management System (ICCMS) Guide for Practitioners and Educators. 2014; https://iccms-web.com /uploads/asset/592845add7ac8756944059.pdf. Accessed July 2, 2019.)

C. American Dental Association Caries Classification System[1]

◆ The Caries Classification System (CCS) ranges from a healthy or sound tooth to noncavitated lesions to advanced carious lesions.

◆ Each tooth surface is scored according to the presence or absence of a carious lesion, severity of the change, and estimation of activity or progression. This information is then used to determine management or treatment options.

ENAMEL CARIES

I. Stages in the Formation of a Carious Lesion[1,2,16,17]

A. ICCMS Initial Stage Caries or CCS Initial Caries Lesion

In this stage, there is demineralization of the enamel. This may also be called early caries or an incipient lesion.

◆ *Subsurface demineralization:* Acid products from cariogenic dental biofilm pass through microchannels (pores) from the surface of the enamel to the subsurface area in the dentin.

◆ *First clinical evidence:* First visual changes in enamel may appear whitish/yellowish (white spot lesion); when dried, the surface may be opaque or dull rather than shiny as in health.

  • There is no breakthrough or cavitation of the enamel surface.
  • Surface may become brownish over time or in pits and fissures.

◆ *Remineralization:* At this stage, the dental hygienist is central to preventing progression of the lesion with meticulous oral biofilm removal and remineralization. Approaches to control and management of caries are discussed in more detail in Chapter 25.

◆ Chapter 34 shows examples of levels of concentration of fluoride in surface enamel and in a white demineralized area.

B. ICCMS Moderate Stage Caries or CCS Moderate Caries Lesion

◆ *Breakdown of enamel over the demineralized area:* Visible to observation with localized breakdown of enamel or an underlying dark shadow with transillumination. Radiographically, the radiolucency extends into the dentin.

◆ *Progression of carious lesion:* Follows general direction of enamel rods.

◆ *Spread of carious lesion:* Spreads at dentinoenamel junction; continues along the dentinal tubules (Figure 16-11).

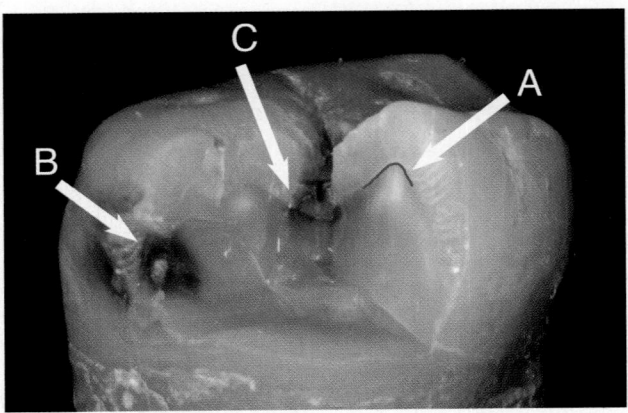

FIGURE 16-11 • Dental Caries. The red line labeled **(A)** follows the dentinoenamel junction (DEJ) of one cusp. The arrow labeled **(B)** points to caries that began on the smooth proximal surface of the tooth enamel showing that when it reaches dentin, it spreads out along the DEJ. The arrow labeled **(C)** points to pit and fissure caries, which began in the occlusal pit (almost hidden from view clinically) showing that once it reaches dentin, it also spreads out at the DEJ. (Scheid RC. *Woelfel's Dental Anatomy Its Relevance to Dentistry.* 7th ed. Philadelphia, PA: Lippincott Williams & Wilkins; 2007.)

C. ICCMS Extensive Stage Caries or CCS Advanced Caries Lesion

◆ Cavitation exposing dentin.

◆ Radiographically, the radiolucency extends into the inner half of dentin or into the pulp.

II. Nomenclature by Surfaces

◆ *Simple cavity:* involves one tooth surface. Example: occlusal cavity.

◆ *Compound cavity:* involves two tooth surfaces. Example: mesio-occlusal cavity, referred to as an "M-O" cavity.

◆ *Complex cavity:* involves more than two tooth surfaces. Example: mesio-occlusal-distal, referred to as an "M-O-D" cavity.

III. Types of Dental Caries

A. Pit and Fissure

◆ Caries begins in a minute fault in the enamel.

◆ Pit or fissure irregularity occurs where three or more lobes of the developing tooth join; closure of the enamel plates is imperfect. Examples: occlusal pits of molars and premolars.

B. Smooth Surface

◆ Caries begins in smooth surfaces where there is no pit, groove, or other defect.

◆ It occurs in areas where dental biofilm is protected from removal, such as proximal tooth surfaces, protected area near a contact, cervical thirds of teeth, and other difficult-to-clean areas.

C. Primary

◆ Occurs on a surface not previously affected.
◆ Also called initial caries.
◆ Early lesion may be referred to as incipient caries.

D. Recurrent

◆ Occurs on a surface adjacent to a restoration.
◆ Recurrent caries may become very involved because it can be difficult to detect radiographically and clinically.

E. Arrested

◆ Carious lesion that has become stationary and does not show a tendency to progress further.
◆ Frequently has a hard surface and takes on a dark brown or reddish-brown color.

F. Rampant Caries

◆ Sudden, rapidly spreading caries resulting in early pulp involvement in which typically 10 or more new lesions occur each year on tooth surfaces not typically affected.
◆ The three types include: early childhood, adolescent, and xerostomia-induced rampant caries.
◆ Restoration is often challenging due to the deep, burrowing nature of the decay.

EARLY CHILDHOOD CARIES[18,19]

◆ Early childhood caries (ECC) is a form of caries found in very young children. Common causes are the routine use of a nursing bottle (with milk or sweetened beverage) when going to sleep or prolonged at-will breast-feeding. ECC is discussed in more detail in Chapter 47.
  • Other names for the condition include: nursing bottle mouth, baby bottle syndrome, baby bottle caries, and prolonged nursing habit.

I. Microbiology[20]

◆ High levels of S. mutans is a strong risk indicator for the initiation of ECC.
◆ Lactobacilli and Candida may also be associated with the progression of the disease.

II. Clinical Appearance[18]

◆ Demineralization begins along the cervical third of the maxillary anterior teeth as white spot lesions (Figure 16-10).

◆ As the lesions progress, the caries spreads to the maxillary and mandibular molars.
◆ Eventually, the crown of the tooth may be destroyed to the gingival margin, abscesses may develop, and the child may suffer severe pain and discomfort.

ROOT CARIES

◆ Root caries is a soft, progressive lesion of cementum and dentin that involves bacterial infection, tends to be shallow, and spreads laterally (Figure 16-12).[21] It is also called cemental caries, cervical caries, or radicular caries.
◆ Typically occurs on exposed root surfaces.

I. Stages in the Formation of a Root Surface Lesion

The ICCMS provides criteria for the stages and activity of root caries.[2,17] The American Dental Association CCS uses the same criteria for root caries as for other caries.

A. Initial Lesion

◆ A clearly demarcated discoloration (light/dark brown or black) below the cementoenamel junction with no cavitation.

B. Moderate/Extensive Lesion

◆ Discolored (light/dark brown or black) area on the root surface with cavitation. May have a leathery texture.

II. Risk Factors for Root Caries[22]

◆ Age: people are retaining their teeth longer and root surfaces become physiologically (aging) or pathologically exposed due to periodontal disease, providing a susceptible root surface.

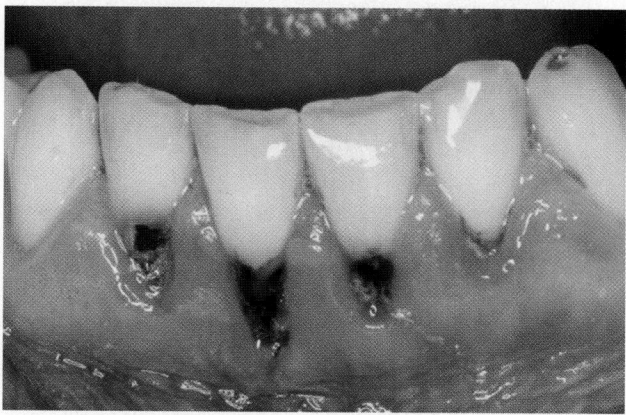

FIGURE 16-12 • Root Caries. A root surface lesion starts near the cementoenamel junction after gingival recession has exposed the root surface. The lesion is progressive, undermining the enamel. (Courtesy of Dr. Richard J. Foster, Guilford Technical Community College, Jamestown, NC.)

◆ History of root caries.

◆ Number of teeth present is also associated with a greater incidence of root caries.

◆ Poor oral biofilm removal.

TESTING FOR PULP VITALITY

Diagnosis of vitality is made with the patient history, clinical and radiographic examinations, and diagnostic testing. Pulp vitality testing (Figure 16-13) may or may

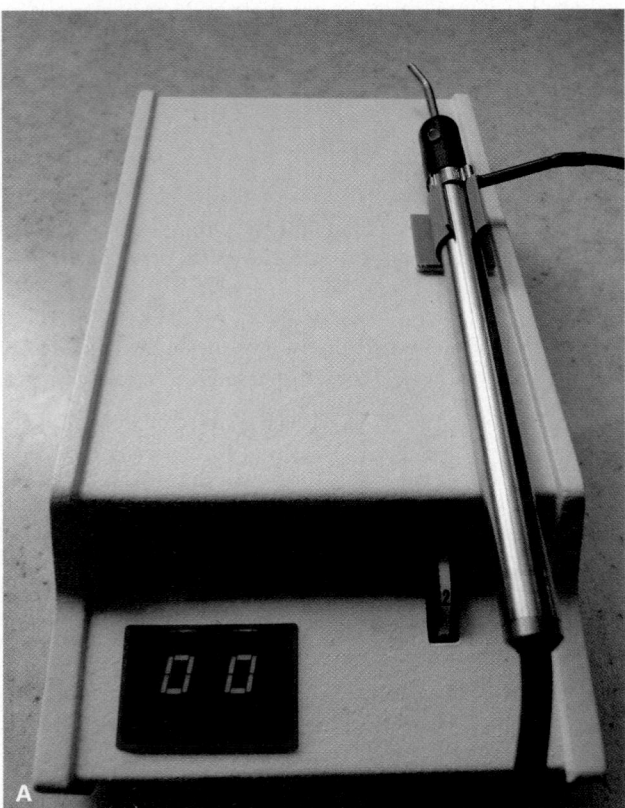

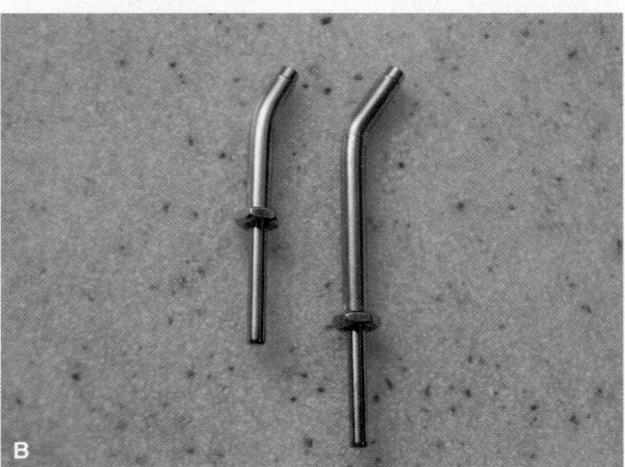

FIGURE 16-13 • A: This is a sample electrical pulp vitality testing machine. **B:** The tips used for the vitality testing. (Courtesy of Susan Jenkins, MCPHS University Forsyth School of Dental Hygiene.)

not be in the scope of practice for the dental hygienist within your state.

◆ Any tooth suspected of being nonvital needs to be tested for pulpal vitality or degree of vitality.

◆ The two basic types of pulp testing are thermal and electric.

I. Causes of Loss of Vitality

◆ A tooth may become nonvital from bacterial causes, particularly invasion of the pulp from dental caries or periodontal diseases.

◆ Physical causes may be mechanical or thermal injuries. Examples of mechanical injuries are trauma, such as a blow, or iatrogenic dental procedures, such as cavity preparation or too-rapid orthodontic movement.

II. Indications for Pulp Vitality Testing[23]

◆ Diagnosis to assess origin of oral pain.

◆ Evaluation of apical radiolucency.

◆ Prior to dental procedures when pulp health may be questionable, that is, advanced dental caries.

◆ Assessment following trauma.

III. Response to Pulp Testing

◆ Pulp testing is based on the knowledge that a stimulus can create pain to which a patient will react. The pulp tester, therefore, determines the conduction of stimuli to the sensory receptors.

◆ The vitality of the pulp depends on the density of the nerve fibers.

◆ Outcomes for pulp testing[24]:
  • Pulp is normal in response to stimuli of pulp testing.
  • Pulpitis is present as indicated by an exaggerated response to pain. Pulpitis can be reversible or irreversible.
  • There is no response because the pulp is necrotic.

IV. Thermal Pulp Testing[23,24]

Cold or hot stimuli may be used. For all methods, a control test is performed on a healthy tooth on the opposite side of the arch. A positive response indicates some nerve fibers are functioning. Cold testing has been shown to be more accurate than heat testing.

◆ Cold testing may be accomplished with an ice, ethyl chloride on a cotton pellet, carbon dioxide, or dry ice. Isolate the test teeth and dry with gauze.

◆ Heat testing is done with gutta-percha or compound material heated to melting and applied directly to the tooth. This technique is sensitive and may result in overheating the pulp.

V. Electrical Pulp Tester[23,24]

Electric stimuli are used to stimulate intact nerves in the pulp (Figure 16-13A and B). This will feel like a tingling sensation to the patient.

◆ The pulp tester probe is applied to the tooth in question and the intensity of the electric stimuli is gradually increased to a preselected value.

◆ The tooth in question is isolated to prevent spread of the stimuli to nearby teeth.

◆ A digital display provides values for when the patient first feels the stimuli.

◆ *Note:* Studies show the use of electrical devices (e.g., ultrasonic scalers, pulp testers) in patients with cardiac implantable devices such as pacemakers produced only slight interference, but did not interfere with overall function.[25,26]

OCCLUSION

Static occlusal relationships are seen when the jaws are closed in centric occlusion, that is, the maximum intercuspation or contact of the teeth of the opposing arches. There are a number of occlusion classification systems, but Dr. Edward Hartley Angle is credited with first describing an occlusal classification system in 1900.[27] Dr. Angle based his classification on the relationship of the first molars.

I. Normal Occlusion

Normal occlusion is the ideal mechanical relationship between the teeth of the maxillary arch and teeth of the mandibular arch with an even bilateral distribution of occlusal forces between maxillary and mandibular arches that is symmetrical (Figure 16-14).[27,28]

A. Facial Profile

◆ Mesognathic: slightly protruded jaws, which give the facial outline a relatively flat appearance (straight profile) (Figure 16-15).

B. Molar Relation

◆ The mesiobuccal cusp of the maxillary first permanent molar occludes with the buccal groove of the mandibular first permanent molar.

◆ Occlusal force is greater on the posterior teeth than on the anterior teeth.

C. Canine Relation

◆ The maxillary permanent canine occludes with the distal half of the mandibular canine and the mesial half of the mandibular first premolar.

II. Malocclusion

Malocclusion is any deviation from the physiologically acceptable relationship of the maxillary arch and/or teeth to the mandibular arch and/or teeth. Because the mandible is

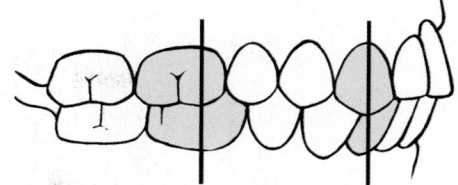

Normal (Ideal) Occlusion
Molar relationship: mesiobuccal cusp of maxillary first permanent molar occludes with the buccal groove of the mandibular first permanent molar.

Malocclusion
Class I: Neutrocclusion
Molar relationship: same as Normal, with malposition of individual teeth or groups of teeth.

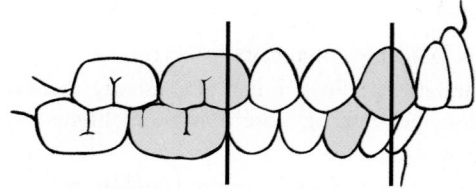

Class II: Distocclusion
Molar relationship: buccal groove of the mandibular first permanent molar is distal to the mesiobuccal cusp of the maxillary first permanent molar by at least the width of a premolar.
Division 1: mandible is retruded and all maxillary incisors are protruded.

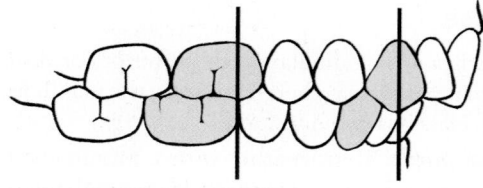

Class II: Distocclusion
Division 2: mandible is retruded and one or more maxillary incisors are retruded.

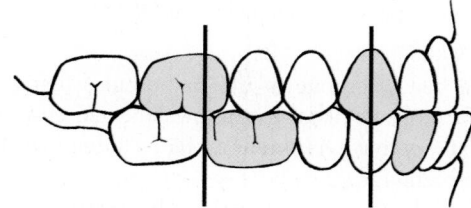

Class III: Mesiocclusion
Molar relationship: buccal groove of the mandibular first permanent molar is mesial to the mesiobuccal cusp of the maxillary first permanent molar by at least the width of a premolar.

FIGURE 16-14 • Normal Occlusion and Classification of Malocclusion.

movable and the maxilla is stationary, the classes describe the relationship of the mandible to the maxilla. Three general classes of malocclusion are described in the following sections. These classes are designated by Roman numerals (Figure 16-14).

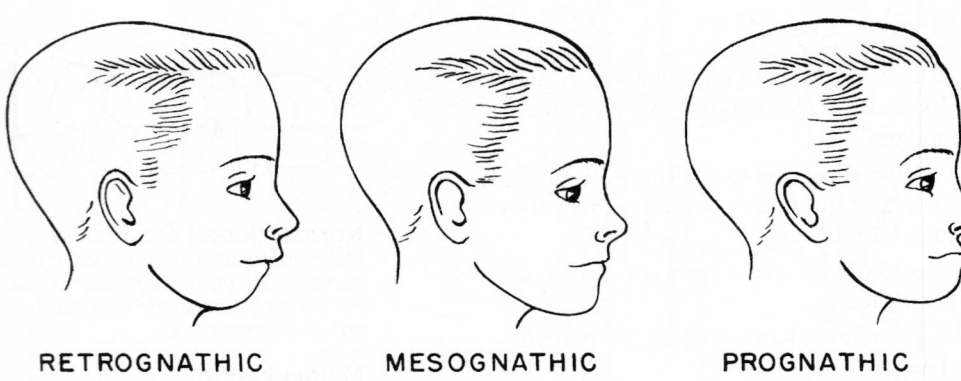

RETROGNATHIC   MESOGNATHIC   PROGNATHIC

FIGURE 16-15 • Types of Facial Profiles.

A. Class I

◆ *Facial profile:* Mesognathic.

◆ *Molar relation:* First molars are usually in normal occlusion, but one or more may be in lingual or buccal occlusion.[27]

◆ *Canine relation:* Same as normal occlusion.

◆ *Malposition of individual teeth or groups of teeth.*

- Crowded maxillary or mandibular anterior teeth.
- Protruded or retruded maxillary incisors.
- Anterior or posterior crossbite.
- Mesial drift of molars resulting from premature loss of teeth.

B. Class II

◆ *Description:* mandibular teeth posterior (or distally) to normal position in their relation to the maxillary teeth. This class has two divisions.

◆ *Facial profile:* Retrognathic with a prominent maxilla and a mandible posterior to its normal relationship (convex profile). Lower lip is full and often rests between the maxillary and mandibular incisors and the mandible appears retruded (Figure 16-15).

◆ *Molar relation*

- The buccal groove of the mandibular first permanent molar is distal to the mesiobuccal cusp of the maxillary first permanent molar by at least the width of a premolar.
- When the distance is less than the width of a premolar, the relation can be classified as *tendency toward Class II.*

◆ *Canine relation*

- The distal surface of the mandibular canine is distal to the mesial surface of the maxillary canine by at least the width of a premolar.
- When the distance is less than the width of a premolar, the relation can be classified as *tendency toward Class II.*

◆ *Class II, Division 1*

- Description: The maxillary arch is narrow and lengthened with protruding maxillary incisors.[27]

- General types of conditions that frequently occur in Class II, Division 1 malocclusion: deep overbite, excessive overjet, abnormal muscle function (lips), short mandible, or short upper lip.

◆ *Class II, Division 2*

- Description: Less narrowing of the maxillary arch, and the mandible is retruded with one or more maxillary incisors are retruded.
- General types of conditions that frequently occur in Class II, Division 2 malocclusion: Maxillary lateral incisors protrude while both central incisors retrude, crowded maxillary anterior teeth, or deep overbite.

C. Class III

◆ *Description:* Mandibular teeth are anterior to normal position in relation to maxillary teeth.

◆ *Facial profile:* Prognathic with a prominent, protruded mandible and lower lip and normal (usually) maxilla (concave profile) (Figure 16-15).

◆ *Molar relation*

- The buccal groove of the mandibular first permanent molar is mesial to the mesiobuccal cusp of the maxillary first permanent molar by at least the width of a premolar.
- When the distance is less than the width of a premolar, the relation can be classified as *tendency toward Class III.*

◆ *Canine relation*

- The distal surface of the mandibular canine is mesial to the mesial surface of the maxillary canine by at least the width of a premolar.
- When the distance is less than the width of a premolar, the relation can be classified as *tendency toward Class III.*

◆ *General types of conditions that occur in Class III malocclusion*

- True Class III: Maxillary incisors are lingual to mandibular incisors in an anterior crossbite (Figure 16-16).
- Maxillary and mandibular incisors are in edge-to-edge occlusion.
- Mandibular incisors are very crowded but lingual to maxillary incisors.

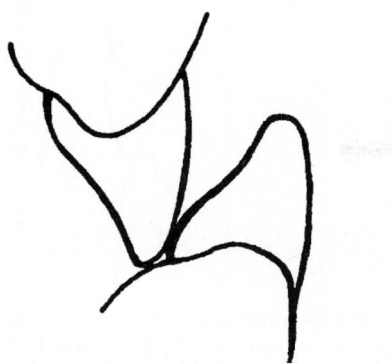

FIGURE 16-16 • Anterior Crossbite. Maxillary anterior teeth are lingual to mandibular anterior teeth. Anterior crossbite occurs in Angle's Class III malocclusion.

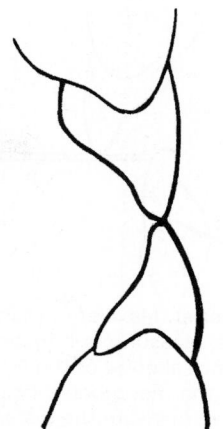

FIGURE 16-18 • Edge-to-Edge Bite. Incisal surfaces occlude.

III. Malrelations of Groups of Teeth

A. Crossbites

◆ *Posterior:* Maxillary or mandibular posterior teeth are either facial or lingual to their normal position. This condition may occur bilaterally or unilaterally (Figure 16-17).

◆ *Anterior:* Maxillary incisors are lingual to the mandibular incisors (see Figure 16-16).

B. Edge-to-Edge Bite

Incisal surfaces of maxillary anterior teeth occlude with incisal surfaces of mandibular teeth instead of overlapping as in normal occlusion (Figure 16-18).

C. End-to-End Bite

Molars and premolars occlude cusp-to-cusp as viewed mesiodistally (Figure 16-19).

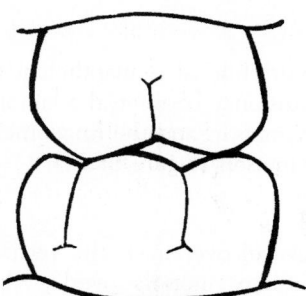

FIGURE 16-19 • End-to-End Bite. Molars in cusp-to-cusp occlusion as viewed from the facial.

D. Open Bite

Lack of occlusal or incisal contact between certain maxillary and mandibular teeth because either or both have failed to reach the line of occlusion. The teeth cannot be brought together, and a space remains as a result of the arching of the line of occlusion (Figure 16-20).

E. Overjet

The horizontal distance between the labioincisal surfaces of the mandibular incisors and the linguoincisal surfaces of the maxillary incisors (Figure 16-21).

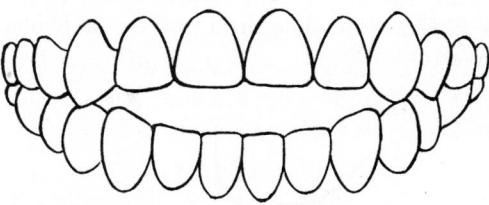

FIGURE 16-20 • Open Bite. Lack of incisal contact. Posterior teeth in normal occlusion.

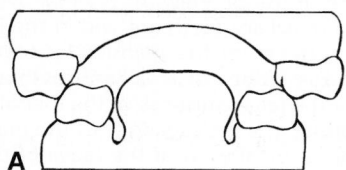 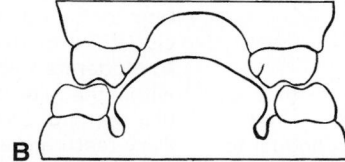 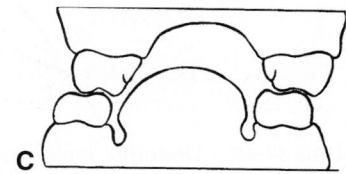

FIGURE 16-17 • Posterior Crossbite. A: Mandibular teeth lingual to normal position. **B:** Mandibular teeth facial to normal position. **C:** Unilateral crossbite: right side, normal; left side, mandibular teeth facial to normal position.

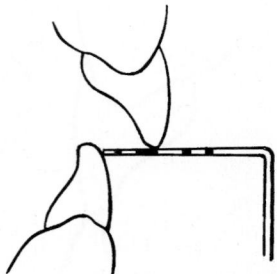

FIGURE 16-21 • Overjet. Maxillary incisors are labial to the mandibular incisors. Measurable horizontal distance is evident between the incisal edge of the maxillary incisors and the incisal edge of the mandibular incisors. A periodontal probe can be used to measure the distance.

◆ One way to measure the amount of overjet is to place the tip of a probe on the labial surface of the mandibular incisor and, holding it horizontally against the incisal edge of the maxillary tooth, read the distance in millimeters.

F. Underjet

Maxillary teeth are lingual to mandibular teeth. Measurable horizontal distance between the labioincisal surfaces of the maxillary incisors and the linguoincisal surfaces of the mandibular incisors (Figure 16-22).

G. Overbite

Overbite, or vertical overlap, is the vertical distance by which the maxillary incisors overlap the mandibular incisors.

◆ *Normal overbite:* An overbite is considered normal when the incisal edges of the maxillary teeth are within the incisal third of the mandibular teeth, as shown in Figure 16-23 in side view and in Figure 16-24A in anterior view.

◆ *Moderate overbite:* An overbite is considered moderate when the incisal edges of the maxillary teeth appear within the middle third of the mandibular teeth (Figure 16-24B).

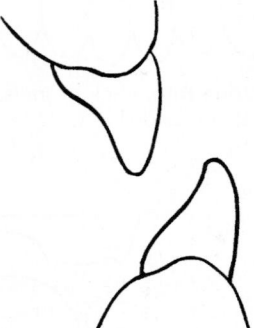

FIGURE 16-22 • Underjet. Maxillary incisors are lingual to the mandibular incisors. Measurable horizontal distance is evident between the incisal edges of the maxillary incisors and the incisal edges of the mandibular incisors.

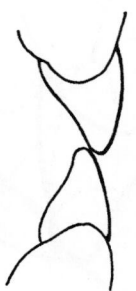

FIGURE 16-23 • Normal Overbite. Profile view to show the position of the incisal edge of the maxillary tooth within the incisal third of the facial surface of the mandibular incisor.

◆ *Deep (severe) overbite*
  • Deep (severe): When the incisal edges of the maxillary teeth are within the cervical third of the mandibular teeth (Figure 16-24C).
  • Very deep: When, in addition, the incisal edges of the mandibular teeth are in contact with the maxillary lingual gingival tissue. A side view of very deep overbite is shown in Figure 16-25.
◆ *Clinical examination of overbite*
  • Direct observation: With the posterior teeth closed together, the lips can be retracted and the teeth observed, as in Figure 16-25. The degree of anterior overbite is judged by the position of the incisal edge of the maxillary teeth:

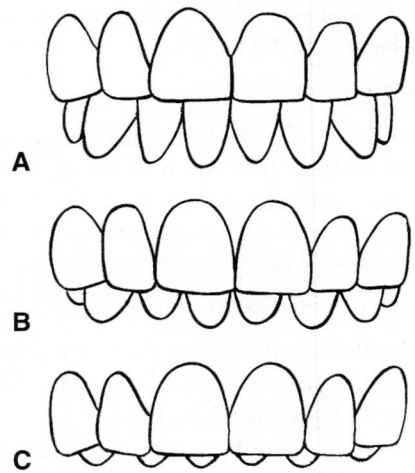

FIGURE 16-24 • Overbite, Anterior View. A: Normal overbite: incisal edges of the maxillary teeth are within the incisal third of the facial surfaces of the mandibular teeth. **B:** Moderate overbite: incisal edges of maxillary teeth are within the middle third of the facial surfaces of the mandibular teeth. **C:** Severe overbite: the incisal edges of the maxillary teeth are within the cervical third of the facial of the mandibular teeth. When the incisal edges of the mandibular teeth are in contact with the maxillary lingual gingival tissue, the overbite is considered very severe.

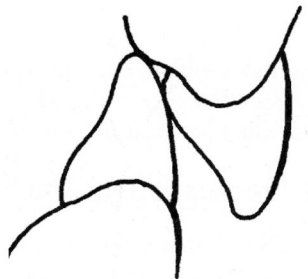

FIGURE 16-25 • Deep (Severe) Anterior Overbite. Incisal edge of the maxillary tooth is at the level of the cervical third of the facial surface of the mandibular anterior tooth. See the facial view in Figure 16-24C.

- Mirror view: By placing a mouth mirror under the incisal edge of the maxillary teeth, one can sometimes see the mandibular teeth in contact with the maxillary palatal gingiva. When contact is not visible, an examination of the lingual gingiva may reveal teeth prints or at least enlargement and redness from the contact.

IV. Terminology for Malposition of Individual Teeth

- Labioversion: A tooth that has assumed a position labial to normal.
- Linguoversion: Tooth position is lingual to normal.
- Buccoversion: Tooth position is buccal to normal.
- Supraversion: Elongated above the line of occlusion.
- Torsiversion: Tooth is turned or rotated.
- Infraversion: Tooth is depressed below the line of occlusion, for example, primary tooth that is submerged or ankylosed.

OCCLUSION OF THE PRIMARY TEETH

I. Normal Occlusion

A. Primary Canine Relation

Same as permanent dentition.

- With primate space[29,30]:
  - Mandibular: between mandibular canine and first molar (Figure 16-26A).
  - Maxillary: between maxillary lateral incisor and canine (Figure 16-26B).
- Without primate spaces: closed arches put the child at risk for crowding of the permanent dentition.

B. Second Primary Molar Relation

The mesiobuccal cusp of the maxillary second primary molar occludes with the buccal groove of the mandibular second primary molar.

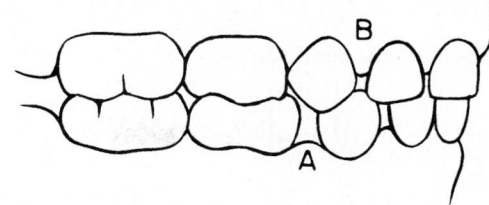

FIGURE 16-26 • Primary Teeth with Primate Spaces. A: Mandibular primate space between the canine and the first molar. **B:** Maxillary primate space between the lateral incisor and the canine.

- *Variations in distal surface relationships:* terminal step.
  - The distal surface of the mandibular primary molar is mesial to that of the maxillary, thereby forming a mesial step (Figure 16-27A).
  - Morphologic variation in molar size; maxillary and mandibular primary molars have approximately the same mesiodistal width.
- *Variation:* terminal plane.
  - The distal surfaces of the maxillary and mandibular primary molars are on the same vertical plane (Figure 16-27B).
  - The maxillary molar is narrower mesiodistally than the mandibular molar (occurs in many patients).
- *Effects on occlusion of first permanent molars*
  - Terminal step: First permanent molar erupts directly into proper occlusion (Figure 16-27A).
  - Terminal plane: First permanent molars erupt end to end. With mandibular primate space, early mesial shift of primary molars into the primate space occurs, and the permanent mandibular molar shifts into proper occlusion. Without primate spaces, late mesial shift of permanent mandibular molar into proper occlusion occurs, following exfoliation of second primary molar (Figure 16-27B).

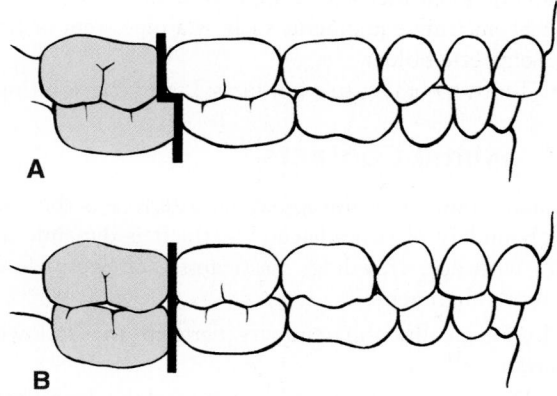

FIGURE 16-27 • Eruption Patterns of the First Permanent Molars. A: Terminal step. The distal surface of the mandibular second primary molar is mesial to the distal surface of the maxillary primary molar. **B:** Terminal plane. The distal surfaces of the mandibular and maxillary second primary molars are on the same vertical plane; permanent molars erupt in end-to-end occlusion.

II. Malocclusion of the Primary Teeth

Same as permanent dentition.

DYNAMIC OR FUNCTIONAL OCCLUSION

In contrast to static occlusion, which pertains to the relationship of the teeth when the jaws are closed, dynamic (or functional) occlusion consists of all contacts during chewing, swallowing, or other normal action.

◆ Dynamic occlusion has two guidance systems[31]:
  • The posterior guidance system of the mandible is the temporomandibular joint.
  • The anterior guidance is provided by the canines during lateral excursion of the mandible.
◆ Masticatory (chewing) performance or efficiency depends on the type and severity of malocclusion as well as the number and location of teeth.[32]

I. Types of Occlusal Contacts

A. Functional Contacts

Functional contacts are the normal contacts that are made between the maxillary teeth and the mandibular teeth during chewing and swallowing.

B. Parafunctional Contacts

Parafunctional describes abnormal or deviated function.

◆ Pathologic wear occurs as a result of parafunctional activity and may result in[33]:
  • Accelerated tooth wear creating facets and attrition.
  • Pulpal involvement.
  • Tooth movement changing interocclusal relationships.
◆ Etiology may include:
  • Tooth-to-tooth contact: Clenching and bruxism.
  • Tooth-to-hard-object contacts: Nail biting; occupational use of such objects as tacks or pins; use of smoking equipment, such as a pipe stem or hard cigarette holder.
  • Tooth-to-oral-tissues contacts: Lip or cheek biting.

II. Proximal Contacts

Proximal contacts or interproximal interface is the common boundary of two adjacent teeth. It is dynamic and varies with age, crowding, masticatory (chewing) force, and tooth alignment.

◆ Physiologically, the contacts perform the following functions[34]:
  • Dissipates masticatory forces around the dental arch.
  • Prevents mesial migration or drifting of teeth.
  • Protects the arch integrity.
  • Prevents food impaction.
  • Aberration in proximal contacts can ultimately impact bone health and result in interdental crestal bone loss.

TRAUMA FROM OCCLUSION

Trauma to the periodontium by dynamic (or functional) or parafunctional forces that exceed the adaptive and reparative capacities is called occlusal trauma.

I. Types of Occlusal Trauma[35]

◆ Historically occlusal trauma has been classified as:
  • *Primary occlusal trauma* results from excessive occlusal force on a tooth with normal bone support.
  • *Secondary occlusal trauma* results when normal or abnormal occlusal forces are placed on a tooth with bone loss and inadequate alveolar bone support.
◆ There has been controversy that the effects on the periodontium are similar with primary and secondary occlusal trauma and the following types are more descriptive:
  • Acute trauma from occlusion happens unexpectedly as a result of biting on a hard object.
  • Chronic trauma from occlusion is an ongoing, long-term pathology.

II. Effects of Trauma from Occlusion

The main purpose of the oral attachment apparatus (PDL, cementum, and alveolar bone) is to keep the tooth in the socket in a functional state. In a healthy situation, occlusal pressures and forces during chewing and swallowing are readily dispersed or absorbed and no unusual effects are produced.

◆ However, secondary occlusal trauma may be a factor in the rate of progression of existing periodontal disease.[35]

III. Recognition of Signs of Occlusal Trauma

No one clinical or radiographic finding clearly defines the presence of trauma from occlusion. Diagnosis of the condition is complex. Clinical findings listed below are recorded for evaluation and correlation with the patient history and all other clinical determinations.

A. Clinical Findings Associated with Occlusal Trauma[35]

◆ Clinical signs of occlusal trauma:
  • Progressive change in tooth mobility.
  • Fremitus is movement of the teeth subjected to dynamic or functional occlusion. It can be assessed by gently palpating the buccal aspect of the teeth as the patient taps up and down.
  • Discomfort or sensitivity of teeth to pressure, chewing, and/or percussion.
  • Tooth drifting or pathologic migration.
◆ Radiographic signs of occlusal trauma:
  • Thickening of the lamina dura. Note: thickened lamina dura is frequently associated with teeth that have undergone orthodontic treatment and may not be associated with occlusal trauma.

- Widening of PDL space, particularly angular thickening (triangulation).
- Root resorption.

STUDY MODELS

A study model provides a life-size reproduction of the teeth, gingiva, and adjacent structures, which can be used in the assessment and care of a patient (Figure 16-28).

- The study models, radiographs, and clinical examination with recordings and chartings, together with the medical and dental histories, are utilized in the diagnosis, comprehensive care planning, and treatment.

I. Purposes and Uses of Study Models

- Serve as a permanent record of the patient's present condition including:
  - Existing and missing teeth.
  - Tooth position and tooth anatomy.
  - Position, size, and shape of the gingiva and interdental papillae.
  - Position of frena.
- During examination of the occlusion, to observe the static relations (Angle's classification, malrelations of groups of teeth, and malpositions of individual teeth) and other features, such as wear patterns and the effects of premature loss of teeth.
- An effective visual aid to use when the oral conditions are explained and the dental and dental hygiene care plans are presented; to enable the patient to visualize and understand the need for the specific care outlined.
- Provide assistance during forensic examination along with dental charting and radiographs.

THE INTEROCCLUSAL RECORD

I. Purposes

- Interocclusal record or *bite registration* relates the maxillary and mandibular models correctly (Figure 16-29).
- Many, if not most, models orient to each other readily in only one position.
- When such problems as open bite, crossbite, edentulous areas, or end-to-end (or edge-to-edge) relations interfere with direct occlusion of the models, a bite registration is needed.
- Placed between the models during trimming and storage to prevent breakage of the model teeth.

DOCUMENTATION

Documentation of the findings from the hard tissue examination includes existing and missing teeth; existing restorations; white spot and cavitated carious lesions; noncarious lesions; NCCLs; and fractures (see Figure 16-30). In addition, occlusal findings are also recorded in the patient dental chart. In addition to charting conditions, the following should be documented in the clinical notes:

- If study models and interocclusal record are indicated, this should also be documented in the chart notes.
- Record occlusal habits including bruxism, clenching, or other parafunctional habits along with any patient reports of discomfort associated with these habits.
- Previous orthodontic treatment; dates, patient report of satisfaction.
- Sample progress notes are included in Boxes 16-1 and 16-2.

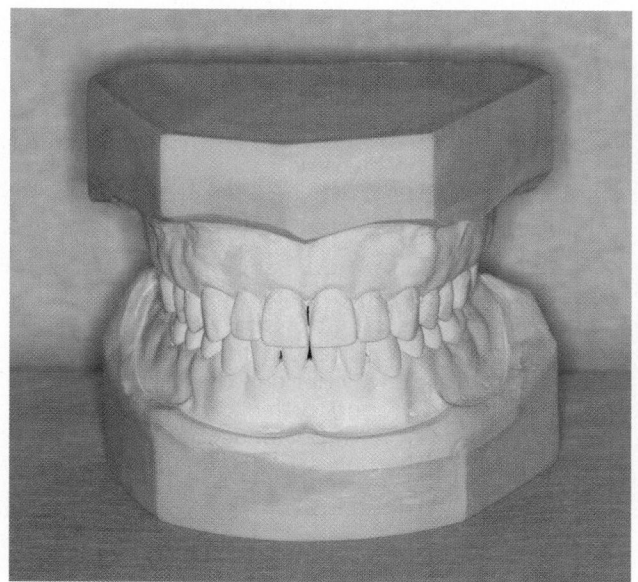

FIGURE 16-28 • Trimmed and Finished Study Models.

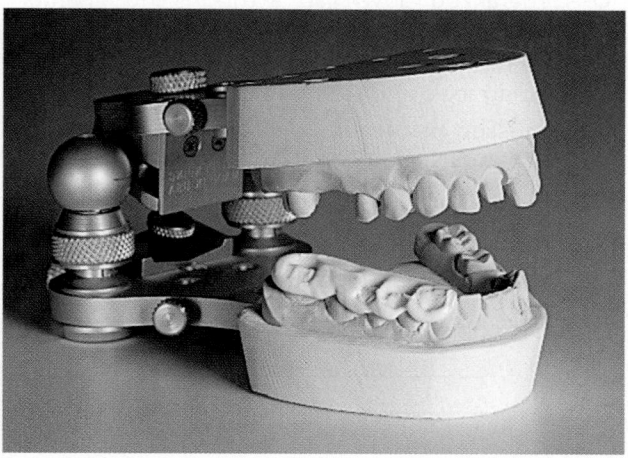

FIGURE 16-29 • Models Mounted on a Simple Articulator with a Bite Registration on the Mandibular Right Quadrant Made of Impression Material. (Courtesy of GC America, Inc., Alsip, IL.)

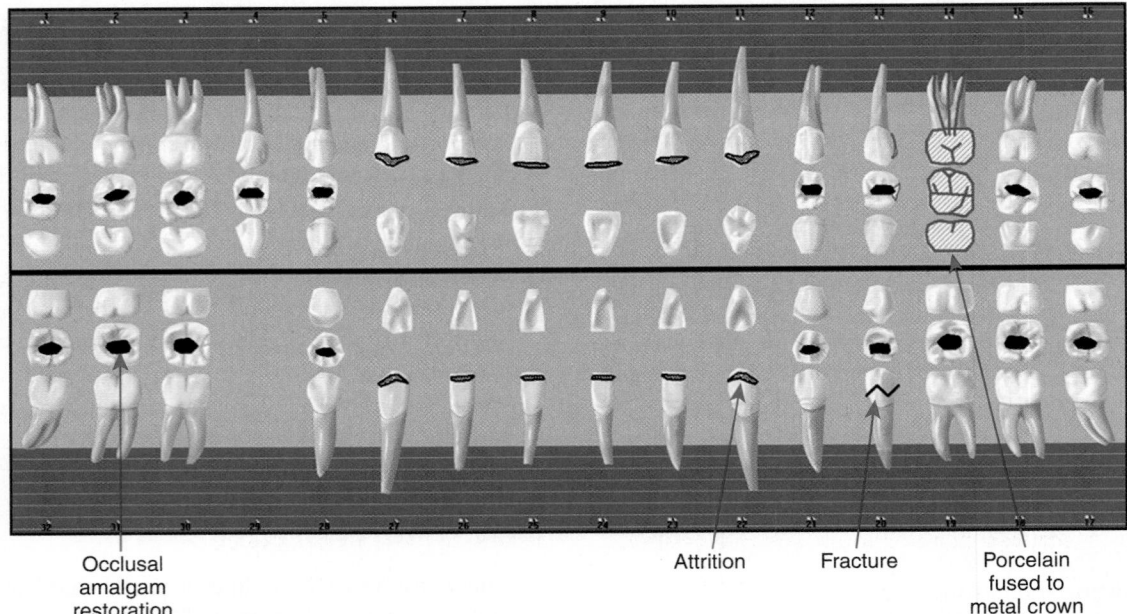

Occlusal
amalgam
restoration

Attrition   Fracture   Porcelain
fused to
metal crown

FIGURE 16-30 • Sample Dental Charting. This is an example of dental charting. Symbols and colors used for various conditions will vary between offices/clinics.

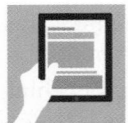

BOX 16-1
Example Documentation: The Patient with Noncarious Tooth Lesions

S—An 87-year-old male patient presents for new patient examination. He states, "My lower front teeth seem to be wearing away. About a month or so ago, I noticed some pieces chipped off my upper front tooth. In fact two of them are feeling kind of sharp." Further questioning revealed his wife reported he grinds his teeth at night and he states he often chews on a pencil while working on his daily crossword puzzle.

O—Generalized advanced attrition and enamel fractures on 7, 8, and 9.

A—Patient needs referral for comprehensive dental diagnosis and treatment plan.

P—Discussed risk to oral health status related to oral habits such as grinding and biting on hard objects. Answered patient questions about potential treatment options. Provided assurance that the dentist would thoroughly discuss the specific options best for the patient's particular circumstances. Referred to attending dentist for diagnosis and treatment planning.

Signed: _____, RDH

Date: _____

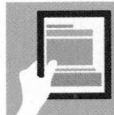

BOX 16-2
Example Documentation: Patient Needing Orthodontic Referral

S—A 9-year-old female patient, accompanied by her mother, presents for routine continuing care and oral examination. Chief complaint: Mother states, "Since the last time we saw you, I notice her teeth are all coming in crooked and her smile seems lopsided to me. Does she need to see an orthodontist?"

O—No changes in health history, no significant extraoral, intraoral, or radiographic findings. Good tissue health and low caries risk. Occlusion classification: Class II, Division 2 with retruded maxillary incisors, maxillary left lateral incisor, and canine in buccoversion and rotated. Facial profile is normal.

A—Referral for orthodontic assessment is indicated.

P—Prophylaxis completed. Panoramic radiograph taken and a copy provided to the mother along with contact information for two local orthodontists who have treated our patients in the past. Discussed why her child's caries risk may be increased during orthodontic procedures and stressed the importance of maintaining the regular schedule of continuing care and dental hygiene appointments.

Signed: _____, RDH

Date: _____

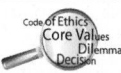

EVERYDAY ETHICS

Many of the first-year dental hygiene students struggled to learn the classifications of malocclusion and how to recognize them in their patients. The problem was often a locker room discussion item, and it was agreed that they noticed that the instructors did not always look for the details of a patient's occlusion when the record was checked.

One clinic day Roxanne was confused, and she decided to write just anything down on the patient's chart. When the instructor came to check the oral examination, she questioned why Roxanne had the classification of the occlusion documented as a Class II Disto-occlusion. Roxanne just shrugged her shoulders and said, "I don't know."

Questions for Consideration

1. Summarize the ethical concerns related to Roxanne's deciding to "just write down anything" rather than look up the information she needs to provide an accurate assessment of the patient's condition.

2. What legal issues might be connected with inaccurate documentation of information in the patient's permanent record? For an example, use a forensic examination team seeking help from a dental office record.

3. Discuss why this situation can be regarded as both an ethical issue and an ethical dilemma.

ENHANCE YOUR UNDERSTANDING

ONLINE RESOURCES
(see the inside front cover for access information)
- Audio glossary
- Appendices

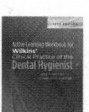

SUPPORT FOR LEARNING
(available separately)
- *Active Learning Workbook for Wilkins' Clinical Practice of the Dental Hygienist, 13th Edition*

INDIVIDUALIZED REVIEW
- Customized practice quizzing with Navigate 2 TestPrep for *Wilkins' Clinical Practice of the Dental Hygienist*

Factors to Teach the Patient

- Education on the benefits (function and esthetics) of orthodontic care to patients referred by the dentist to an orthodontist.
- Impact of chewing (masticatory) efficiency on food selection in the diet, which impact nutritional status and health.
- Education on the need to correct oral habits with negative impacts on oral health.
- The space-maintaining function of the primary teeth in prevention of malocclusion of the emerging permanent teeth in children.
- The role of malocclusion as a predisposing factor for dental biofilm retention increasing the risk of dental caries and periodontal infections.
- Dental biofilm removal methods for reducing dental calculus and soft deposit retention in areas where teeth are crowded, displaced, or otherwise not in normal occlusion.
- The relation of the occlusion and the position of the teeth to the patient's selection of oral self-care products such as interdental aids.
- Need for continuing care appointments related to malocclusion and while in the process of having orthodontic therapy.

References

1. Young DA, Novy BB, Zeller GG, Hale R, Hart TC, Truelove EL. The American Dental Association Caries Classification System for clinical practice: a report of the American Dental Association Council on Scientific Affairs. *J Am Dent Assoc.* 2015;146(2):79-86.
2. ICDAS Foundation; Pitts NB, Ismail AI, Martignon S, Ekstrand K, Douglas GVA, Longbottom C. International Caries Classification and Management System (ICCAM) Guide for Practitioners and Educators. 2014; https://www.icdas.org. Accessed November 24, 2017.
3. Seow WK. Developmental defects of enamel and dentine: challenges for basic science research and clinical management. *Aust Dent J.* 2014;59 suppl 1:143-154.
4. Sarig R, Hershkovitz I, Shpack N, May H, Vardimon AD. Rate and pattern of interproximal dental attrition. *Eur J Oral Sci.* 2015;123(4):276-281.
5. Castrillon EE, Ou KL, Wang K, Zhang J, Zhou X, Svensson P. Sleep bruxism: an updated review of an old problem. *Acta Odontol Scand.* 2016;74(5):328-334.
6. Castroflorio T, Bargellini A, Rossini G, Cugliari G, Rainoldi A, Deregibus A. Risk factors related to sleep bruxism in children: a systematic literature review. *Arch Oral Biol.* 2015;60(11):1618-1624.
7. Nascimento MM, Dilbone DA, Pereira PN, Duarte WR, Geraldeli S, Delgado AJ. Abfraction lesions: etiology, diagnosis, and treatment options. *Clin Cosmet Investig Dent.* 2016;8:79-87.

8. Kanzow P, Wegehaupt FJ, Attin T, Wiegand A. Etiology and pathogenesis of dental erosion. *Quintessence Int.* 2016;47(4):275-278.

9. Milosevic A. Abrasion: a common dental problem revisited. *Prim Dent J.* 2017;6(1):32-36.

10. Wiegand A, Schwerzmann M, Sener B, et al. Impact of toothpaste slurry abrasivity and toothbrush filament stiffness on abrasion of eroded enamel—an in vitro study. *Acta Odontol Scand.* 2008;66(4):231-235.

11. DiAngelis AJ, Andreasen JO, Ebeleseder KA, et al. Guidelines for the management of traumatic dental injuries: 1. Fractures and luxations of permanent teeth. *Pediatr Dent.* 2016;38(6):358-368.

12. World Health Organization. The World Oral Health Report. 2003; http://www.who.int/oral_health/publications/report03/en/. Accessed November 20, 2017.

13. Yang F, Zeng X, Ning K, et al. Saliva microbiomes distinguish caries-active from healthy human populations. *ISME J.* 2012;6(1):1-10.

14. Blackwell RR. G.V. *Black's Operative Dentistry.* 9th ed. Milwaukie, WI: Medico-Dental Publishing Co; 1955.

15. Tyas MJ, Anusavice KJ, Frencken JE, Mount GJ. Minimal intervention dentistry—a review. FDI Commission Project 1-97. *Int Dent J.* 2000;50(1):1-12.

16. International Caries Detection and Assessment System Foundation. International caries detection and assessment system. 2017; https://www.iccms-web.com/content/iccms-learn-more. Accessed July 2, 2019.

17. Ismail AI, Pitts NB, Tellez M. The International Caries Classification and Management System (ICCMS™): an example of a caries management pathway. *BMC Oral Health.* 2015;15(suppl 1):S9-S9.

18. Anil S, Anand PS. Early childhood caries: prevalence, risk factors, and prevention. *Front Pediatr.* 2017;5:157.

19. Leong PM, Gussy MG, Barrow SY, de Silva-Sanigorski A, Waters E. A systematic review of risk factors during first year of life for early childhood caries. *Int J Paediatr Dent.* 2013;23(4):235-250.

20. Hemadi AS, Huang R, Zhou Y, Zou J. Salivary proteins and microbiota as biomarkers for early childhood caries risk assessment. *Int J Oral Sci.* 2017;9(11):e1.

21. Takahashi N, Nyvad B. Ecological hypothesis of dentin and root caries. *Caries Res.* 2016;50(4):422-431.

22. Ritter AV, Shugars DA, Bader JD. Root caries risk indicators: a systematic review of risk models. *Community Dent Oral Epidemiol.* 2010;38(5):383-397.

23. Gopikrishna V, Pradeep G, Venkateshbabu N. Assessment of pulp vitality: a review. *Int J Paediatr Dent.* 2009;19(1):3-15.

24. Chen E, Abbott PV. Dental pulp testing: a review. *Int J Dent.* 2009;2009.

25. Elayi CS, Lusher S, Meeks Nyquist JL, Darrat Y, Morales GX, Miller CS. Interference between dental electrical devices and pacemakers or defibrillators. *J Am Dent Assoc.* 146(2):121-128.

26. Lahor-Soler E, Miranda-Rius J, Brunet-Llobet L, Sabate de la Cruz X. Capacity of dental equipment to interfere with cardiac implantable electrical devices. *Eur J Oral Sci.* 2015;123(3):194-201.

27. Angle EH. *Classification of Malocclusion.* 6th ed. Philadelphia, PA: SS White Dental Manufacturing Company; 1900.

28. Watanabe M, Hattori Y, Satoh C. Biological and biomechanical perspectives of normal dental occlusion. *Int Congr Ser.* 2005;1284(suppl C):21-27.

29. Ngan P, Alkire RG, Fields H. Management of space problems in the primary and mixed dentitions. *J Am Dent Assoc.* 1999;130(9):1330-1339.

30. Vegesna M, Chandrasekhar R, Chandrappa V. Occlusal characteristics and spacing in primary dentition: a gender comparative cross-sectional study. *Int Sch Res Notices.* 2014;2014:7.

31. Davies S, Gray RM. What is occlusion? *Br Dent J.* 2001;191(5):235-238, 241-235.

32. Magalhaes IB, Pereira LJ, Marques LS, Gameiro GH. The influence of malocclusion on masticatory performance. A systematic review. *Angle Orthod.* 2010;80(5):981-987.

33. Alani A, Patel M. Clinical issues in occlusion—part I. *Singapore Dent J.* 2014;35(suppl C):31-38.

34. Sarig R, Lianopoulos NV, Hershkovitz I, Vardimon AD. The arrangement of the interproximal interfaces in the human permanent dentition. *Clin Oral Investig.* 2013;17(3):731-738.

35. Davies SJ, Gray RJ, Linden GJ, James JA. Occlusal considerations in periodontics. *Br Dent J.* 2001;191(11):597-604.

17

Dental Soft Deposits, Biofilm, Calculus, and Stains

Catherine A. McConnell, RDH, BDSc, MEd

CHAPTER OUTLINE

DENTAL BIOFILM AND OTHER SOFT DEPOSITS

ACQUIRED PELLICLE
I. Pellicle Formation
II. Types of Pellicle
III. Significance of Pellicle
IV. Removal of Pellicle

DENTAL BIOFILM
I. Stages in the Formation of Biofilm
II. Changes in Biofilm Microorganisms

SUPRAGINGIVAL AND SUBGINGIVAL DENTAL BIOFILM
I. Supragingival Biofilm
II. Subgingival Biofilm

COMPOSITION OF DENTAL BIOFILM
I. Inorganic Elements
II. Organic Elements

CLINICAL ASPECTS OF DENTAL BIOFILM
I. Distribution of Biofilm
II. Detection of Biofilm

SIGNIFICANCE OF DENTAL BIOFILM
I. Dental Caries

MATERIA ALBA
I. Clinical Appearance and Content
II. Prevention

FOOD DEBRIS

CALCULUS
I. Supragingival Calculus
II. Subgingival Calculus

CALCULUS COMPOSITION
I. Inorganic Content
II. Organic Content

CALCULUS FORMATION
I. Mineralization
II. Structure of Calculus
III. Formation Time

ATTACHMENT OF CALCULUS
I. Attachment by Means of an Acquired Pellicle
II. Attachment to Minute Irregularities in the Tooth Surface by Mechanical Locking into Undercuts
III. Attachment by Direct Contact between Calcified Intercellular Matrix and the Tooth Surface

SIGNIFICANCE OF DENTAL CALCULUS

CLINICAL CHARACTERISTICS
I. Supragingival Examination
II. Subgingival Examination

PREVENTION OF CALCULUS
I. Personal Dental Biofilm Control
II. Regular Professional Continuing Care
III. Anticalculus Dentifrice and Mouthrinse

DENTAL STAINS AND DISCOLORATIONS

SIGNIFICANCE OF DENTAL STAINS
I. Classification of Stains
II. Recognition and Identification
III. Application of Procedures for Stain Removal

EXTRINSIC STAINS
I. Yellow Stain
II. Green Stain
III. Black-Line Stain
IV. Tobacco Stain
V. Brown Stains
VI. Orange and Red Stains
VII. Metallic Stains

ENDOGENOUS INTRINSIC STAINS
I. Pulpless or Traumatized Teeth
II. Disturbances in Tooth Development
III. Drug-Induced Stains and Discolorations

EXOGENOUS INTRINSIC STAINS
I. Restorative Materials
II. Stain in Dentin
III. Other Local Causes

DOCUMENTATION

EVERYDAY ETHICS

FACTORS TO TEACH THE PATIENT

REFERENCES

LEARNING OBJECTIVES

After studying this chapter, the student will be able to:

1. Define acquired pellicle and discuss the significance and role of the pellicle in the maintenance of oral health.

2. Describe the different stages in biofilm formation and identify the changes in biofilm microorganisms as biofilm matures.

3. Differentiate between the types of soft and hard deposits.

4. Recognize the factors that influence the accumulation of biofilm, calculus, and stain.

5. Explain the location, composition, and properties of dental biofilm, calculus, and stain.

6. Identify the modes of attachment of supra- and subgingival calculus to dental structure.

7. Describe the clinical and radiographic characteristics of supra- and subgingival calculus and its detection.

8. Educate patients regarding the etiology and prevention of dental biofilm, calculus, and stain.

9. Differentiate between exogenous and endogenous stains and identify extrinsic and intrinsic dental stains and discolorations.

10. Determine the appropriate clinical approaches for stain removal and maintenance.

11. Design biofilm, calculus, and stain management strategies to meet each patient's individual needs.

DENTAL BIOFILM AND OTHER SOFT DEPOSITS

During clinical examination of the teeth and surrounding soft tissues, soft and hard deposits are assessed. The presence of dental biofilm is a primary risk factor for gingivitis, inflammatory periodontal diseases, and dental caries.[1]

◆ The soft deposits are referred to as acquired pellicle, dental biofilm, materia alba, and food debris.

◆ A comparison of the types of dental deposits with descriptions is found in Table 17-1.

TABLE 17-1 • Tooth Deposits

TOOTH DEPOSIT	DESCRIPTION	DERIVATION	REMOVAL METHOD
Acquired enamel pellicle	Translucent, homogeneous, thin, unstructured film covering and adherent to the surfaces of the teeth, restorations, calculus, and other surfaces.	Supragingival: saliva, oral mucosa, microorganism Subgingival: gingival crevicular fluid	Toothbrush and appropriate interdental aid such as floss.
Microbial (bacterial) biofilm Nonmineralized	Dense, organized bacterial communities embedded in EPS matrix adheres tenaciously to the teeth, calculus, prostheses, and other surfaces in the oral cavity.	Colonization of oral microorganisms	Toothbrush and appropriate interdental aid such as floss.
Materia alba Nonmineralized	Loosely adherent, unstructured, white or grayish-white mass of oral debris and bacteria that lies over dental biofilm	Incidental accumulation	Vigorous rinsing and water irrigation can remove materia alba.
Food debris Nonmineralized	Unstructured, loosely attached particulate matter	Food retention following eating	Self-cleansing activity of tongue and saliva. Rinsing vigorously removes debris. Toothbrushing, flossing, and other aids.
Calculus Mineralized	Calcified dental biofilm; hard, tenacious mass that forms on the clinical crowns of the natural teeth and on dentures and other oral appliances.	Biofilm mineralization	
a. Supragingival	Occurs coronal to the margin of the gingiva; is covered with dental biofilm.	Source of minerals is saliva	Manual instrumentation. Ultrasonic instrumentation.
b. Subgingival	Occurs apical to the margin of the gingiva; is covered with dental biofilm.	Source of minerals is gingival crevicular fluid	Manual instrumentation. Ultrasonic instrumentation.

ACQUIRED PELLICLE

- The acquired pellicle is a thin, acellular tenacious film formed of proteins, carbohydrates, and lipids.[2]
- Pellicle is uniquely positioned at the interface between the tooth surfaces and the oral environment. It forms over exposed tooth surfaces and prostheses.
- The thickness of the pellicle varies from 100 to 1,000 nm, depending on its location in the mouth; it is thickest near the gingival margin and areas undisturbed by the activities of chewing, swallowing, and speaking.[3]

I. Pellicle Formation

- Immediately upon exposure to saliva after eruption or after all soft and hard deposits have been removed from the tooth surfaces (such as by rubber cup or air polishing), the pellicle begins to form and is fully formed within 30 to 90 minutes.[2,3]
- Composition: primarily glycoproteins, selectively adsorbed by the hydroxyapatite of the tooth surface.
  - Protein components are derived from the saliva, oral mucosal cells, gingival crevicular fluid (GCF), and microorganisms.[4]
- Initial attachment of bacteria to the pellicle is by selective adherence of microorganisms originating from the oral mucosa.
  - Innate characteristics of the pellicle determine the adhesive interactions that cause planktonic bacteria to aggregate, forming clusters to initiate biofilm formation.
  - Salivary proteins have a high affinity for the hydroxyapatite tooth surface and initiate the process of pellicle formation.[4]
- The adsorbed material becomes a highly insoluble coating on teeth, existing calculus deposits, restorations, and removable dental prostheses such as dentures, orthodontic appliances, and athletic mouth guards.

II. Types of Pellicle

A. Supragingival Pellicle

- Supragingival pellicle is clear, translucent, insoluble, and not readily visible until application of a disclosing agent.[5]
  - Pellicle can take on extrinsic stain and become gradations of brown, gray, or other colors.
  - When stained with a disclosing agent, pellicle appears thin, with a pale staining that contrasts with the thicker, darker staining of dental biofilm.

B. Subgingival Pellicle

- Subgingival pellicle is continuous with the supragingival pellicle and can become embedded in tooth structure, particularly where the tooth surface is partially demineralized or rough due to abrasion.[5]

III. Significance of Pellicle

The pellicle plays an important role in the maintenance of oral health as it protects, lubricates, and acts as a nidus of attachment for the bacteria and subsequent calculus on the tooth surfaces.[2] The various roles the pellicle plays include[2]:

- Protective
  - Pellicle appears to provide a barrier against acids, impacting remineralization and demineralization.
- Lubrication
  - Pellicle keeps surfaces moist and prevents drying, which in turn enhances the efficiency of speech and mastication.
- Nidus for bacteria
  - Pellicle participates in biofilm formation by aiding the adherence of microorganisms.
- Attachment of calculus
  - One mode of calculus attachment is to the pellicle.

IV. Removal of Pellicle

- Pellicle is not resilient enough to withstand rigorous patient oral self-care.[6]
- Extrinsic factors that may interfere with pellicle formation and maturation include[7]:
  - Abrasive toothpastes.
  - Whitening products.
  - Intake of acidic foods and beverages.

DENTAL BIOFILM

The oral microbiome is composed of microorganisms, their genetic make-up, and the environments found in the oral cavity.[8]

- The mouth has a number of environments, including the teeth, gingival sulcus, attached gingiva, tongue, oral mucosa, lips, and hard and soft palates with their own microbial inhabitants.[8]
- The permanent teeth as the only nonshedding surface in the body serve as a unique environment for biofilm formation and maturation.[8]
- The microorganisms in the oral cavity perform both pro- and anti-inflammatory activities, which maintains homeostasis in health.[8]
- Dental biofilm is a dynamic, structured community of microorganisms, encapsulated in a self-produced extracellular polymeric substance (EPS) forming a matrix around microcolonies.
- The matrix is composed of polysaccharides, proteins, and other compounds; it acts to protect the biofilm from the host's immune system and antimicrobial agents.
- The microcolonies are separated by a network of open water channels that supply nutrients deep within the biofilm community.

◆ The three-dimensional structure of biofilms enhances their ability to communicate with each other, adapt, and respond to their environment.

◆ Adheres to the pellicle coating on all hard and soft oral structures, including teeth, existing calculus, and fixed and removable restorations.

◆ There are over 700 distinct microorganisms in the oral cavity, including bacteria, viruses, protozoa, and yeast.[8] Morphologic forms of bacteria that are found within biofilms are shown in Figure 17-1.

I. Stages in the Formation of Biofilm

◆ Biofilm formation involves a series of complex interactions specific to oral biofilm development.

◆ Gene expression controls many of the growth and attachment capabilities and varies depending on the variety of microbial species within a biofilm community.[9]

A. Stage 1—Formation

◆ Biofilm formation begins with initial attachment of planktonic bacterial cells to the pellicle on the tooth surface (physicochemical).

◆ Initially, the adherent cells are not "committed" to this process, and during this stage of adhesion, the process is reversible. When cells are disrupted (with oral self-care activities), they may dislodge from the surface to resume planktonic life and either be eliminated or begin the formation process elsewhere in the oral cavity.

Bacilli (rod shaped)

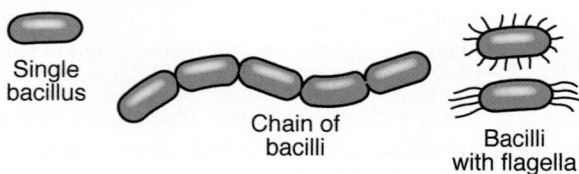

Single bacillus — Chain of bacilli — Bacilli with flagella

Cocci (spherical)

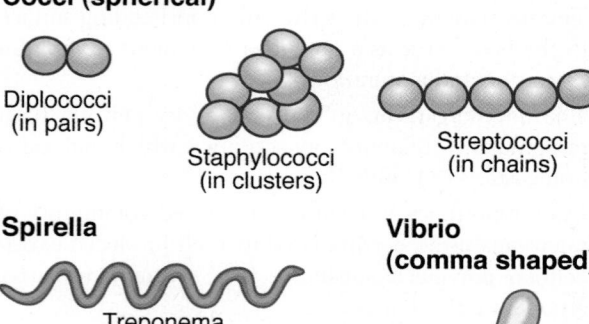

Diplococci (in pairs) — Staphylococci (in clusters) — Streptococci (in chains)

Spirella — Treponema — Borrelia

Vibrio (comma shaped)

FIGURE 17-1 • Bacteria Shapes: Cocci, Bacilli, Spiral. (Adapted from Sakai J. *Practical Pharmacology for the Pharmacy Technician.* Baltimore, MD: Lippincott Williams & Wilkins; 2008.)

B. Stage 2—Bacterial Multiplication and Colonization

◆ Planktonic microorganisms attach themselves using cell adhesion structures such as fimbriae, pili, flagella, and adhesion proteins.

◆ Microcolonies multiply in layers growing upward and outward, creating the three-dimensional aspect of biofilm structures.

◆ With growth, colonies produce EPS to firmly attach in an irreversible manner; rough surfaces will result in more rapid irreversible attachment.

◆ Organisms colonizing the biofilm in the first few hours are primarily gram-positive cocci and rods.

C. Stage 3—Matrix Formation

◆ Bacteria within the aggregate of cells continue to secrete EPS as bacteria multiply to form a matrix.

◆ Components of the EPS are:
  • Polysaccharides, glucans, and fructans or levans produced by certain bacteria within the community and from dietary sucrose.
  • EPS provides a scaffold to anchor the bacteria together increasing adherence to dental and other structures and provide protection as the bacterial community continues to grow.[1]
  • EPS contains components such as antimicrobial enzymes to protect the biofilm.[1]

◆ The adaptive characteristics, structure, and EPS of the biofilm result in higher antimicrobial resistance limiting effectiveness of common antimicrobial agents.[1,9]

D. Stage 4—Biofilm Growth

◆ This stage is characterized by further development of the biofilm architecture to enhance the cell-to-cell communication process, also known as quorum sensing[1]:
  • Quorum sensing controls the growth of the microbial community and signals microorganisms when to leave the biofilm to find new sites.[1]
  • Activated by specific genes located on the surface of the bacterial cells within the biofilm.

◆ The mass and thickness of biofilm increase as the bacteria multiply; if left undisturbed, bacteria continuously adhere to the biofilm community and surrounding surface area.

E. Stage 5—Maturation

◆ Bacterial colonies mature and release planktonic cells to spread and colonize other areas within the oral cavity.

◆ Bacteria can disperse as single cells or in clumps.

II. Changes in Biofilm Microorganisms

◆ Dental biofilm consists of a complex mixture of microorganisms in microcolonies. The microbial density is very high and increases as biofilm ages and matures.

◆ The potential for the development of dental caries and/or gingivitis increases with more microorganisms, especially as the numbers of pathogenic microorganisms outnumber the nonpathogenic microorganisms.[1]

◆ With undisrupted biofilm for approximately 7 days, negative anaerobic bacteria growth is favored, which increased risk for dental caries and gingivitis, and eventually other inflammatory periodontal diseases increases.[1]

◆ Although there is significant variability between individuals in the pattern of dental biofilm development, the changes in oral flora follow a general pattern. The formation of dental biofilm may vary by days of accumulation (Figure 17-2):

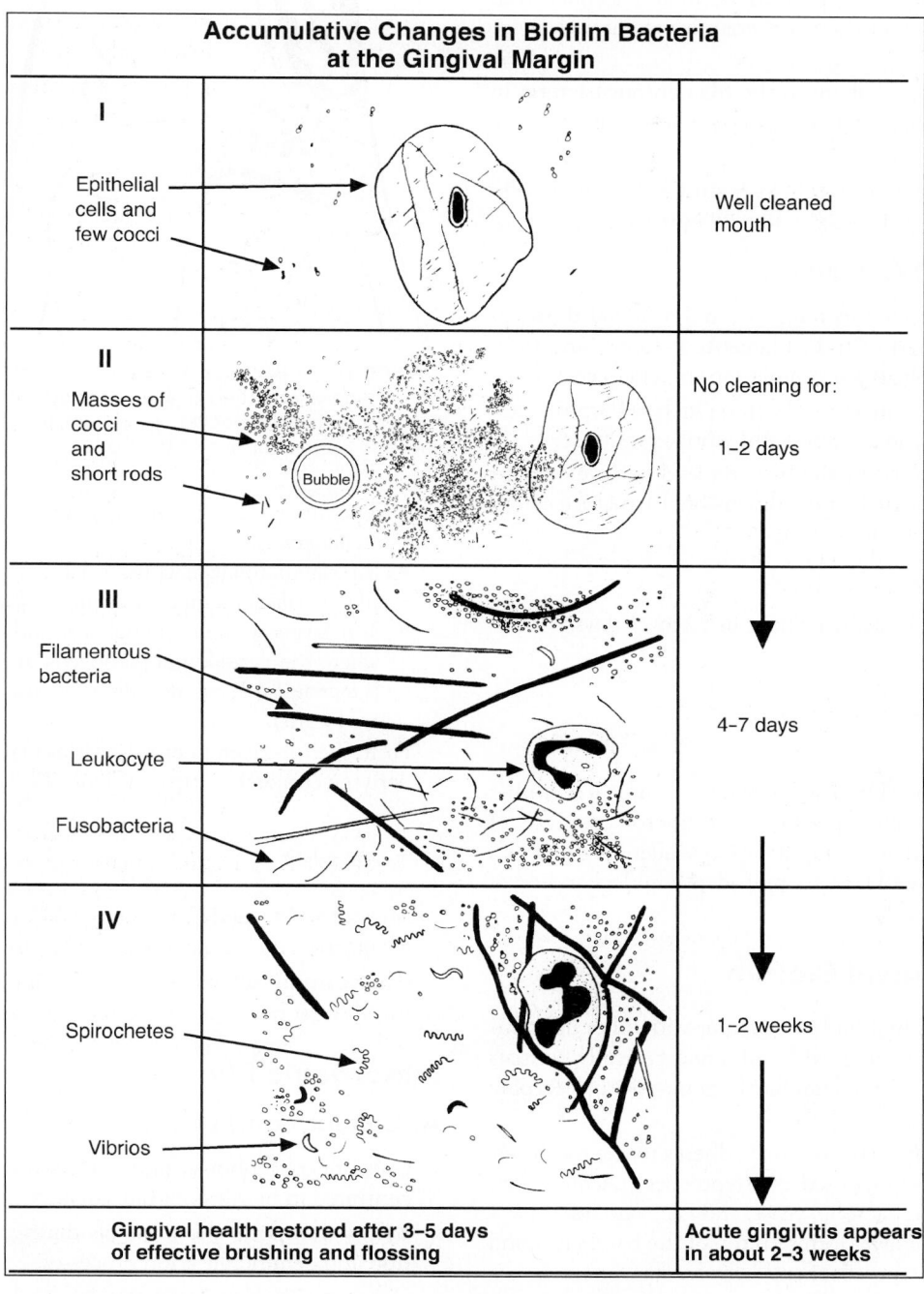

Accumulative Changes in Biofilm Bacteria at the Gingival Margin

I — Epithelial cells and few cocci		Well cleaned mouth
II — Masses of cocci and short rods (Bubble)		No cleaning for: 1–2 days
III — Filamentous bacteria, Leukocyte, Fusobacteria		4–7 days
IV — Spirochetes, Vibrios		1–2 weeks
Gingival health restored after 3–5 days of effective brushing and flossing		**Acute gingivitis appears in about 2–3 weeks**

FIGURE 17-2 • Biofilm Microorganisms. On the right are the time intervals from 1 day to 3 weeks. On the left are the changes in the biofilm content that take place as biofilm ages. As the numbers of microorganisms increase, the numbers of defense cells (leukocytes) also increase. (From Crawford JJ. Microbiology. In: Barton RE, Matteson SR, Richardson RE, eds. *The Dental Assistant*. 6th ed. Philadelphia, PA: Lea & Febiger; 1988.)

A. Days 1–2

◆ Early biofilm consists primarily of gram-positive cocci.[10]

◆ Streptococci, which dominate the bacterial population, include *Streptococcus mutans* and *Streptococcus sanguinis*.[1]

B. Days 2–4

◆ The cocci still dominate while increasing numbers of gram-positive filamentous form and slender rods join the surface of the cocci colonies along with more leukocytes.[10]

◆ Gradually, cocci adhere to the filamentous bacteria in a "corn cob" appearance and this is when the bacteria secrete EPS.[1]

◆ Dental biofilm is said to have matured by 72 hours and is capable of initiating the inflammatory process.[1]

C. Days 6–10 (on average)

◆ Filaments increase in numbers, and a mixed flora appears comprised of rods, filamentous forms, and fusobacteria with heavy accumulations of leukocytes.[10]

◆ Gram-negative anaerobic bacteria such as Porphyromonas gingivalis, spirochetes, and vibrios proliferate.[1,10]

◆ The EPS secreted by the bacteria lead to development of a well-organized three-dimensional structure of the biofilm.[1]

D. Days 10–21

◆ Gingivitis is clinically evident in 10 to 21 days.[10]

SUPRAGINGIVAL AND SUBGINGIVAL DENTAL BIOFILM

Recent technology innovations such as confocal scanning electron microscopy, epifluorescent microscopy, use of DNA probes, and gene amplification sequencing research studies have allowed for a more in-depth understanding of the science of biofilms.

I. Supragingival Biofilm

◆ Supragingival biofilm has a greater variability in architecture than subgingival biofilm and typically consists of two layers of predominantly gram-positive aerobic bacteria[11]:

• The first layer (basal layer) adheres to the tooth surface and is composed of streptococci, *Actinomyces*, filamentous bacteria, yeast, and *Lactobacillus*.

• The second layer forms on top of the basal layer and includes streptococci and *Lactobacillus*.

II. Subgingival Biofilm

◆ Subgingival biofilm is made up of four layers, which includes predominantly gram-negative anaerobic and motile organisms[11]:

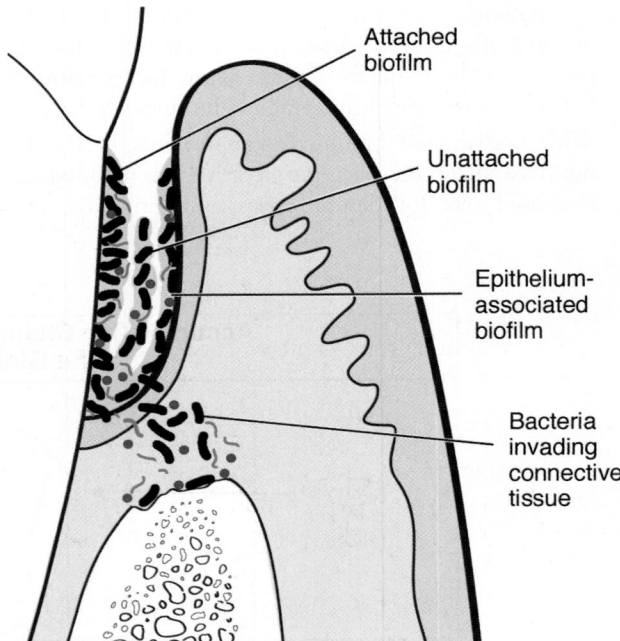

FIGURE 17-3 • Bacterial Invasion. Diagram of a periodontal pocket shows attached and unattached biofilm (planktonic) bacteria within the pocket epithelium, in the connective tissue, and on the surface of the bone.

• The first layer (basal layer) contains bacteria such as *Actinomyces*.

• Intermediate layers contain bacteria such as *Tannerella forsythia* and *Fusobacterium nucleatum*.

• Top layers contain spirochetes and this is typically where the periodontal pathogens such as *P. gingivalis*, *P. intermedia*, *P. endodontalis*, *P. gingivalis*, *or P. nigrescens* are located.

◆ From the top layer, microorganisms may invade the underlying connective tissue (Figure 17-3).[1]

COMPOSITION OF DENTAL BIOFILM

◆ Microorganisms and EPS comprise 20% of the biofilm that are organic and inorganic solids. The other 80% is water.

◆ Composition differs among individuals and among tooth surfaces.

I. Inorganic Elements

A. Calcium and Phosphorus

◆ Calcium, phosphorus, and magnesium are more concentrated in biofilm than in saliva.[12]

◆ Saliva transports the minerals during the mineralization and demineralization processes.

B. Fluoride

◆ Fluoride concentration in biofilm is higher in the presence of fluoridated water, following professional topical fluoride applications and with the use of fluoride-containing dentifrices and oral rinses.[13]

II. Organic Elements

The organic EPS forms a scaffold for biofilm development and contains primarily carbohydrates and proteins, with small amounts of lipids.[14]

A. Carbohydrates

◆ Carbohydrates include glucans such as dextran and fructans or levans formed by bacterial metabolism of dietary sucrose and starch.[1,14]

◆ The glucans contribute to the adherence of microorganisms to each other and to the tooth, adding to biofilm's tenacious adherence to tooth surfaces.[14]

B. Proteins

◆ The proteins of supragingival biofilm originate from the gingival sulcus fluid (crevicular fluid) and bind with glucans leading to further growth of biofilm.[14]

CLINICAL ASPECTS OF DENTAL BIOFILM

I. Distribution of Biofilm

A. Location

◆ *Supragingival biofilm:* coronal to the gingival margin.

◆ *Gingival biofilm:* forms on the external surfaces of the oral epithelium and attached gingiva.

◆ *Subgingival biofilm:* located between the epithelial attachment and the gingival margin, within the sulcus or pocket.

◆ *Fissure biofilm:* develops in pits and fissures of the teeth.

B. By Surfaces

◆ *During formation*
   • Supragingival biofilm formation begins at the gingival margin, particularly on proximal surfaces, and extends coronally when left undisturbed.
   • It spreads over the gingival third and on toward the middle third of the crown.
◆ *Tooth surfaces involved*
   • Biofilm is heaviest on lingual, posterior, and proximal surfaces.[15]
   • Anterior surfaces have the least biofilm.[15]

C. Factors Influencing Biofilm Accumulation

◆ Dental biofilm accumulates readily around crowded teeth as shown in Figure 17-4. With effective biofilm control, biofilm accumulation around crowded teeth is not greater than that around well aligned teeth.
   • Special accommodations such as using a toothbrush placed in a vertical position can remove thick biofilm on the lingual of the crowded mandibular anterior.
◆ *Rough surfaces:* Biofilm develops more rapidly on rough tooth surfaces, existing calculus, poorly contoured restorations, and removable appliances; thick, dense deposits can be difficult to remove.

◆ *Occlusion:* Deposits may extend over an entire crown of a tooth that is unopposed, out of occlusion, or not actively used during mastication.

D. Removal of Biofilm

◆ Toothbrushing and interdental cleaning are the most universal daily mechanical disruption method.

II. Detection of Biofilm

A. Direct Vision

◆ *Thin biofilm:* May be translucent and therefore not visible without a disclosing agent.

◆ *Stained biofilm:* Extrinsic stains may make biofilm more visible, for example, yellow, green, tobacco stains.

◆ *Thick biofilm:* The tooth may appear dull and dingy, with a matted furlike surface. Materia alba or food debris may collect over the biofilm.

B. Use of Explorer or Probe

◆ *Biofilm disruption:* Biofilm may be disturbed by passing the side of a probe over the suspected tooth surface.

C. Use of Disclosing Agent

◆ When a disclosing agent is applied, biofilm takes on the color and becomes readily visible (Figure 17-4).

D. Clinical Record

◆ A Biofilm Control record should be used to document initial biofilm accumulation, followed by continuing changes over the treatment and follow-up appointments.

◆ Record biofilm by location and thickness (slight, moderate, or heavy). For objective evaluations, an index or a biofilm score is recommended (see Chapter 21).

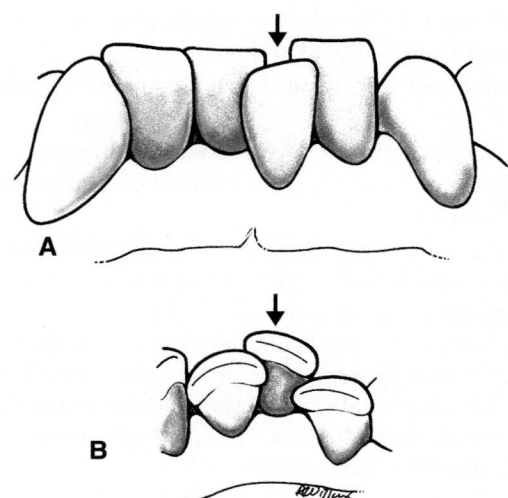

FIGURE 17-4 • Biofilm Accumulation in Protected Areas. A: Crowded mandibular anterior teeth demonstrate dental biofilm after use of a disclosing agent. Thickest biofilm is on proximal surfaces and at cervical thirds of teeth. **B:** Note central incisors with thick extensive biofilm on the less accessible protected surfaces.

SIGNIFICANCE OF DENTAL BIOFILM

- Biofilm plays a major role in the initiation and progression of dental caries and periodontal diseases, caused by pathogenic microorganisms found in oral biofilms.[1]
- Biofilm is significant in the formation of dental calculus, which is essentially mineralized dental biofilm.

I. Dental Caries

- Dental caries is a disease of the dental calcified structures (enamel, dentin, and cementum) characterized by demineralization of the mineral components and dissolution of the organic matrix (see Chapter 16).
- The sequence of events leading to demineralization and dental caries is shown in Figure 17-5.

A. Cariogenic Microorganisms in Biofilm

- In severe and long-term acidic environments, Mutans streptococci (*Streptococcus mutans* and *Streptococcus sobrinus*, predominantly) and Lactobacilli dominate are thought to be involved in the initiation and progression of a carious lesion.[16]
- Xerostomia (decreased salivary flow) and frequent fermentable carbohydrate exposure results in growth of nonmutans streptococci, which created a more acidic environment in the biofilm favoring demineralization of the tooth surface.[16]

B. The pH of Biofilm

- Acid formation begins *immediately* once a cariogenic substance is taken into the biofilm, resulting in a rapid drop in the pH of the biofilm.[16]
- Critical pH for enamel demineralization averages 5.5.[17–20]
- The critical pH for root surface demineralization is higher because of the lower mineral content of dentin and cementum.[19]
  - The critical pH for dentin is approximately 6.2 to 6.4, which is especially relevant for patients with multiple areas of recession and xerostomia.[21]
- The extent of demineralization depends on the length of time and frequency the pH is below critical level; biofilm composition, pH-lowering ability of the microorganisms, and action of saliva are additional factors that affect the caries process.[17]

C. Effect of Diet on Biofilm

- Cariogenic Foods
  - In a highly cariogenic diet, biofilm gradually increases its pH-lowering ability.[17,22]

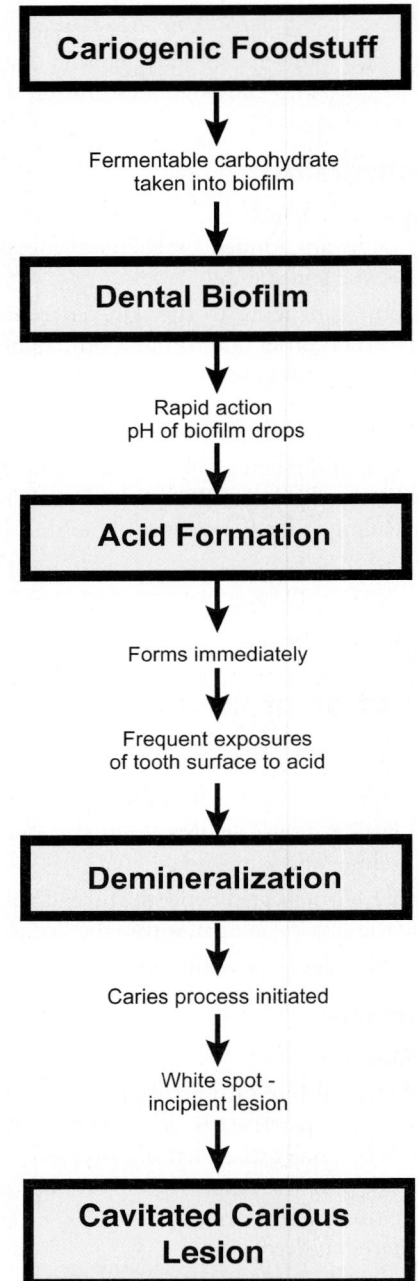

FIGURE 17-5 • Development of Dental Caries. Flowchart shows the step-by-step action within the microbial biofilm on the tooth surface.

MATERIA ALBA

I. Clinical Appearance and Content

- Materia alba is a soft, whitish tooth deposit that is clinically visible without application of a disclosing agent. It may have a cottage cheese-like texture and appearance.
- Materia alba is an unorganized accumulation of living and dead bacteria, desquamated epithelial cells, disintegrating leukocytes, salivary proteins, and food debris. This differentiates it from organized oral biofilms.

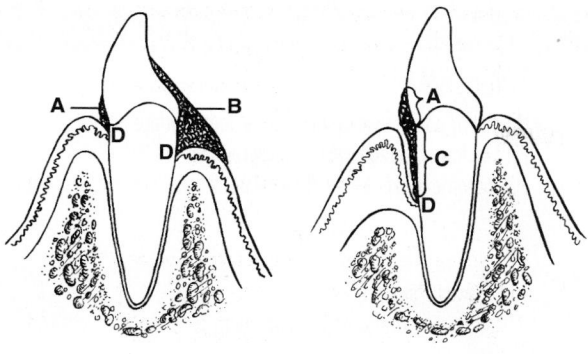

FIGURE 17-6 • Dental Calculus. A: Supragingival calculus on cervical third of a mandibular anterior tooth extends slightly subgingivally. **B:** Supragingival calculus over crown, exposed root surface, and the margin of the gingiva. **C:** Subgingival calculus along root to the base of a periodontal pocket. **D:** Base of pocket.

II. Prevention

- Materia alba can be removed with a water spray, oral irrigator, or tongue action, whereas only the surface organisms of biofilm can be removed.
- Removal of materia alba requires the same basic biofilm control procedures (see Chapters 26 and 27).

FOOD DEBRIS

- After food consumption, food remnants may collect about the cervical third and proximal embrasures of the teeth.

- Vertical food impaction results during mastication as food is forced into open contact areas due to mobility of teeth or occlusal irregularities such as plunger cusps.[22]
- Left unattended, the accumulation of food debris adds to a general unsanitary condition of the mouth and may contribute to the initiation of dental caries and oral malodor.[23]

CALCULUS

Dental calculus is dental biofilm mineralized by crystals of calcium phosphate mineral salts between previously living microorganisms.

- The calculus is covered with a layer of nonmineralized dental biofilm containing live bacteria.
- The hard, tenacious mass forms on the clinical crowns of natural teeth, dental implants, dentures, and other dental prostheses.
- Dental calculus is classified by its location on a tooth surface as related to the adjacent free gingival margin, that is, *supragingival* and *subgingival* calculus as shown in Figure 17-6.
- A comparison of supragingival and subgingival calculus is presented in Table 17-2.

I. Supragingival Calculus

A. Location

- On clinical crowns coronal to the margin of the gingiva.
- On implants, complete and partial dentures.

TABLE 17-2 • Characteristics of Supragingival and Subgingival Biofilm		
CHARACTERISTIC	**SUPRAGINGIVAL BIOFILM**	**SUBGINGIVAL BIOFILM**
Location	Coronal to the margin of the free gingiva	Apical to the margin of the free gingiva
Origin	Salivary glycoprotein forms acquired enamel pellicle Microorganisms from saliva are selectively attracted to pellicle	Down growth of bacteria from supragingival biofilm
Distribution	Starts on proximal surfaces and other protected areas Heaviest collection on areas not cleaned daily by patient Cervical third, especially facial Lingual mandibular molars Proximal surfaces Pit and fissure biofilm	Shallow pocket: similar to supragingival biofilm Undisturbed; held by pocket wall Attached biofilm covers calculus Unattached biofilm extends to the periodontal attachment
Adhesion	Firmly attached to acquired enamel pellicle, other bacteria, and tooth surfaces	Adheres to tooth surface, subgingival pellicle, and calculus
	Surface bacteria (unattached): loose; washed away by saliva or swallowed	Subgingival flora: loose, floating, motile organisms in deep pocket do not adhere; they are between adherent biofilm on tooth and the pocket epithelium
Retention	Rough surfaces of teeth, existing calculus, or restorations Malpositioned teeth Carious lesions	Pocket holds biofilm against tooth Overhanging margins of fillings that extend into pockets hold biofilm

(Continues)

TABLE 17-2 • Characteristics of Supragingival and Subgingival Biofilm (*Continued*)

CHARACTERISTIC	SUPRAGINGIVAL BIOFILM	SUBGINGIVAL BIOFILM
Shape and size	Friction of tongue, cheeks, lips, limits shape and size Thickness: thicker at the cervical third and on proximal surfaces Healthy gingiva: thin biofilm, 15–20 cells thick Chronic gingivitis: thick biofilm, 100–300 cells thick	Molded by pocket wall to shape of the tooth surface Follows form created by subgingival calculus May become thicker as the diseased pocket wall becomes less tight
Structure	Adherent, densely packed microbial layer over acquired enamel pellicle on tooth surface Intermicrobial matrix Onset: small isolated colonies 2–5 d; colonies merge to form a covering of biofilm	Three layers (Figure 17-3) 1. Tooth-surface-attached biofilm: many gram-positive rods and cocci 2. Unattached biofilm in middle: many gram-negative, motile forms; spirochetes; leukocytes 3. Epithelium-attached biofilm: gram-negative, motile forms predominate; many leukocytes migrate through epithelium
Microorganisms	Early biofilm: primarily gram-positive cocci Older biofilm (3–4 d): increased numbers of filaments and fusiforms 4–9 d undisturbed: more complex flora with rods, filamentous forms 7–14 d: vibrios, spirochetes, more gram-negative organisms	Environment conducive to growth of anaerobic population Diseased pocket: primarily gram-negative, motile, spirochetes, rods
Sources of nutrients for bacterial proliferation	Saliva Ingested food Microorganisms metabolites	Tissue fluid (gingival crevicular fluid) Exudate Leukocytes
Significance	Etiology of gingivitis Supragingival calculus Dental caries (Figure 17-5)	Etiology of gingivitis Periodontal infections subgingival calculus

B. Distribution: Most Frequent Sites

- On the lingual surfaces of mandibular anterior teeth and the facial surfaces of maxillary first and second molars, opposite the openings of the ducts of the submandibular and parotid salivary glands.
  - Figure 17-7 shows heavy supragingival calculus forming a continuous "bridge" across several teeth.
- On the crowns of teeth out of occlusion; nonfunctioning teeth; or teeth that are neglected during daily biofilm removal (toothbrushing, flossing, or other personal care).
- On surfaces of dentures, dental prostheses, and oral piercings.

II. Subgingival Calculus

A. Location

- On the clinical crown apical to the margin of the gingiva and extending toward the clinical attachment on the root surface.
- On dental implants.

B. Distribution

- May be generalized or localized on single teeth or a group of teeth.

- Heaviest deposits are related to areas most difficult for the patient to access during personal oral biofilm removal procedures.
- Figure 17-8 illustrates subgingival calculus on an extracted molar and premolar. In Figure 17-9A and B, ledges of interproximal calculus can be seen radiographically.

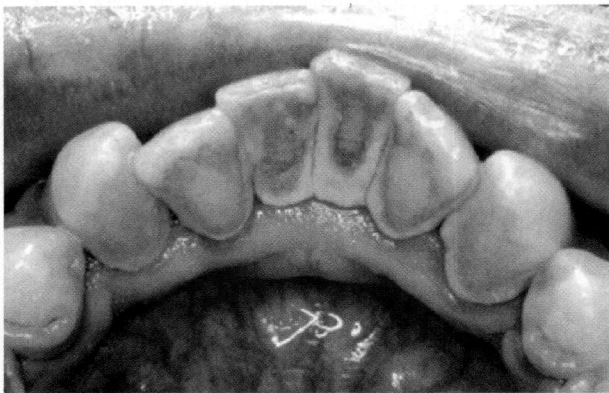

FIGURE 17-7 • Supragingival Calculus. Heavy calculus deposits on the lingual surfaces of the mandibular anterior teeth. These deposits are so large that they interfere with the patient's oral self-care efforts. In addition, calculus deposits harbor living bacteria that are in constant contact with the gingival tissue. (Reprinted from Nield-Gehrig J, Willmann D. *Foundations of Periodontics for the Dental Hygienist.* 3rd ed. Philadelphia, PA: Lippincott Williams & Wilkins; 2011.)

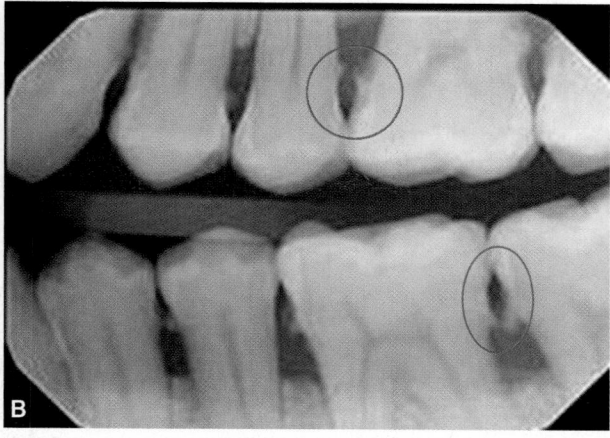

FIGURE 17-9 • **Subgingival Calculus in Radiographs. A:** Heavy supra- and subgingival proximal calculus is shown on the mandibular anterior teeth (#24–25). **B:** The bitewing radiographs show heavy ledges or spines of subgingival calculus in the proximal areas of premolar and molar areas.

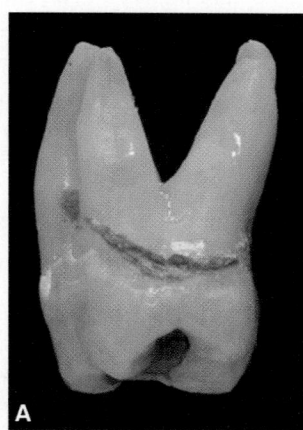
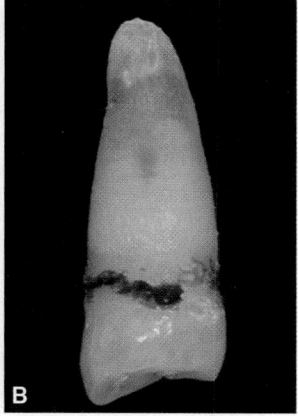

FIGURE 17-8 • **Subgingival Calculus on Extracted Teeth. A:** On a maxillary first molar, calculus that formed in the subgingival environment is dark brown because elements of blood were incorporated during calcification. Additionally, some of the bacteria that are formed in calculus produce pigment. It can be seen here on surfaces where it most commonly forms and is often missed during periodontal instrumentation: near the cementoenamel junction (CEJ), at line angles, in grooves (the concavity just coronal to the buccal furcation), and furcations. **B:** Calculus at and apical to the CEJ on a premolar. (Reprinted from Weiss G, Scheid R. *Woelfel's Dental Anatomy.* 9th ed. Philadelphia, PA: Lippincott Williams & Wilkins; 2016.)

- The calculus typically will form at the cementoenamel junction as recession and pocket formation continue.
- The color of subgingival calculus comes from exposure to the products of blood and blood breakdown products.

CALCULUS COMPOSITION

- Calculus is composed of inorganic and organic components and water.

- The percentages vary depending on the age, hardness of a deposit, and location of the calculus, that is, supragingival calculus in maxillary molar areas tends to be high in calcium, phosphorus, and ash content than on the lingual of mandibular anterior teeth.[24]
- Mature calculus usually contains inorganic components; the rest is organic components and water.

I. Inorganic Content

A. Major Inorganic Components

- The main components are calcium (Ca), phosphorus (P), carbonate (CO_3), sodium (Na), and magnesium (Mg).[24]

B. Trace Elements

- Trace elements include zinc (Zn), strontium (Sr), manganese (Mn), silicon (Si), fluorine (F), iron (Fe), and potassium (K).[25]

C. Fluoride in Calculus

- Fluoride is present in dental calculus and tends to be higher in subgingival than supragingival calculus.[26]
- Fluoride selectively binds to the hydroxyapatite crystal resulting in a lowering of the solubility of the fluorapatite crystal reducing demineralization.[27]
  - The concentration of fluoride in calculus varies depending on the patient's exposure to fluoridated drinking water, topical applications, dentifrices, or any form in contact with the external surface of the calculus.

D. Crystals

- At least two-thirds of the inorganic content of calculus is crystalline, principally apatite.
- The predominant form is hydroxyapatite, which is the same crystal present in enamel, dentin, cementum, and bone.

◆ The mineral par to dental calculus also contains varying amounts of brushite, whitlockite, and octacalcium phosphate.[27]

E. Calculus Compared with Teeth and Bone

◆ Dental enamel is the most highly mineralized tissue in the body and contains 95% to 97% inorganic salts; dentin contains 65% and cementum and bone contain 45% to 70%.[28]

◆ Mature calculus has approximately 70% to 80% inorganic content.[29]

◆ A comparison of calculus with the tooth parts provides insight into the effects of instrumentation, the difficulty of distinguishing calculus from cementum or dentin when scaling subgingivally, and the modes of attachment of calculus to the tooth surface.

II. Organic Content

◆ The organic proportion of calculus consists of various types of microorganisms, desquamated epithelial cells, leukocytes, and mucin from the saliva.

◆ Substances identified in the organic matrix include lipids such as free fatty acids and phospholipids and a protein portion.[27]

CALCULUS FORMATION

◆ Calculus results from the deposition of minerals into a biofilm organic matrix.

◆ Calculus formation occurs in three basic steps: *pellicle formation*, *biofilm formation*, and *mineralization*.

◆ Mineralization of supragingival and subgingival calculus is essentially the same, although the source of the elements for mineralization is not the same.

I. Mineralization

A. Early Calculus Formation

◆ Microorganisms adhere to the pellicle layer-coated tooth surface.

◆ Colonies are formed. In early calculus, the colonies consist primarily of cocci and rod-shaped organisms. By the fifth day, the biofilm is mostly made up of filamentous organisms.[27]

  • The filamentous microorganisms provide the matrix for the deposition of minerals.

◆ Underneath the layer of microorganisms, areas of mineralization foci (centers) form.[27]

◆ Undisturbed, within 24 to 72 hours, more and more mineralization centers develop close to the underlying tooth surface. With time, the centers grow and expand to touch and unite.

  • As the deposit ages, some microorganisms become calcified.

◆ The calcium phosphate crystals of calculus directly bond to the enamel and cementum apatite crystals, which explains why clinical calculus removal is difficult.[30]

B. Sources of Minerals

◆ *Supragingival calculus*: The source of elements for supragingival calculus is the saliva.

◆ *Subgingival calculus*: The GCF and inflammatory exudate supply minerals for the subgingival deposits. As the amount of GCF and exudate increases with inflammation, more minerals are available for mineralization of subgingival biofilm.

C. Crystal Formation

◆ Mineralization consists of crystal formation, namely, hydroxyapatite, octacalcium phosphate, whitlockite, and brushite, each with a characteristic developmental pattern.[27]

◆ The crystals form in the intercellular matrix and on the surface of bacteria and finally within the bacteria.[33,34]

D. Mechanism of Mineralization

◆ Calculus formation is affected by factors such as salivary flow, salivary supersaturation with calcium phosphate salts, and inhibitors and promoters of calculus formation.[27]

  • Supersaturation of saliva and plaque biofilm is the driving force for mineralization.

  • Calculus inhibitors for supragingival calculus include pyrophosphate and zinc salts.[27]

  • Calculus promoters include urea and silicon. Rice-based diets can be higher in silicon and contribute to greater calculus formation.[27]

◆ The difference between supragingival and subgingival calculus crystal is the calcium-to-phosphorus ratio is lower in supragingival calculus.[27]

◆ Heavy calculus formers have higher salivary levels of calcium and phosphorus than do light calculus formers.

II. Structure of Calculus

A. Layers

◆ Calculus forms in layers, parallel with the tooth surface.

◆ The layers are separated by lines that appear to be pellicle deposited over the previously formed calculus, and as mineralization progressed, the pellicle became imbedded.

◆ The lines between the layers of calculus are called *incremental lines*. They form around the tooth in supragingival calculus, but they form irregularly from crown to apex on the root surface in subgingival calculus. The lines are evidence calculus grows or increases by apposition of new layers.

B. Surface

◆ The surface of a calculus mass is typically rough and detectable with the use of an explorer or probe.

C. Outer Layer

◆ The outer layer of subgingival calculus is partly calcified.

◆ The surface is a thick, matlike, soft layer of dental biofilm.

◆ The outer surface of the biofilm on the subgingival calculus is in contact with the diseased pocket epithelial lining where it is inaccessible to daily oral self-care.

D. Types of calculus deposits

◆ Crusty, spiny, or nodular deposits.

◆ Ledge or ring formation.

◆ Thin, smooth veneers.

◆ Finger- and fernlike formations.

◆ Individual calculus islands or spots.

◆ Supragingival on subgingival deposits.

III. Formation Time

◆ The average time required for the primary soft deposit to change to the mature mineralized stage is about 12 days.[31]

  • Mineralization can begin as early as 24 to 48 hours when a patient's personal daily oral hygiene is inadequate.

◆ Formation time depends on individual factors such as genetic variation, diet, bacterial load, and so on.[31]

◆ Estimation of the approximate formation time for an individual is helpful when planning oral self-care instruction as well as treatment planning for professional care and frequency of maintenance appointments.

ATTACHMENT OF CALCULUS

◆ The ease or difficulty of calculus removal is related to the manner of attachment of the calculus to the tooth surface.

◆ Several modes of attachment have been observed by conventional histologic techniques and electron microscopy. On any one tooth and in any one area, more than one mode of attachment may be found.

◆ When studying the attachment types, the character of the hard, smooth enamel surface and that of the rough, porous, cemental surface can be compared.

I. Attachment by Means of an Acquired Pellicle

◆ Calculus attachment is superficial because no interlocking or penetration occurs and calculus can be easily removed.[32]

II. Attachment to Minute Irregularities in the Tooth Surface by Mechanical Locking into Undercuts

◆ Dentin irregularities include cracks, lamellae, and carious defects.[32]

• Cemental irregularities include tiny spaces left at previous locations of Sharpey's fibers, resorption lacunae, root gouging from improper scaling, and cemental tears.

◆ Difficult to be certain all calculus is removed when it is attached by this method because calculus becomes locked into the irregularities.

III. Attachment by Direct Contact between Calcified Intercellular Matrix and the Tooth Surface

◆ Interlocking of inorganic apatite crystals of the enamel and cementum with the mineralizing dental biofilm (calculus).[30]

◆ Research suggests this mode of attachment results in a portion of the calculus that is prone to fracture during removal, but it may leave calculus crystals attached to the tooth surface.[30]

  • The remaining calculus calcium phosphate crystals may serve as a nidus for biofilm formation.

SIGNIFICANCE OF DENTAL CALCULUS

◆ There has been a long-standing debate over whether subgingival calculus has a role in periodontal disease.[31]

◆ Despite the debate, the microorganisms in the biofilm layer covering calculus perpetuate the inflammatory state supragingivally and subgingivally.[27,31]

  • With its rough surface, permeable structure, and porosity, calculus acts as a reservoir for endotoxins and tissue breakdown products.

  • The biofilm in contact with the diseased pocket epithelium promotes gingivitis and periodontitis.

  • Irritation to the pocket lining stimulates greater flow of gingival sulcus fluid, which contains minerals for subgingival calculus formation.

◆ The cornerstone of nonsurgical periodontal therapy is the daily control of biofilm by the patient, supplemented by definitive professional calculus removal, to reduce or eliminate gingival inflammation and bleeding on probing.

CLINICAL CHARACTERISTICS

◆ Identification of calculus prior to removal depends on knowledge of its appearance, consistency, and distribution.

◆ Appointment planning, selection of instruments, and techniques depend on understanding the texture, morphology, and mode of attachment of calculus. Table 17-3 lists a summary of clinical characteristics.

I. Supragingival Examination

A. Direct Examination

Supragingival deposits may be seen directly or indirectly, using a mouth mirror.

TABLE 17-3 • Clinical Characteristics of Dental Calculus

CHARACTERISTIC	SUPRAGINGIVAL CALCULUS	SUBGINGIVAL CALCULUS
Color	White, creamy yellow, or gray May be stained by tobacco, food, tea, or coffee Slight deposits may be invisible until dried with compressed air	Light to dark brown, dark green, or black Stains derived from blood pigments from diseased pocket
Shape	**Amorphous**, bulky Gross deposits may • form interproximal bridge between adjacent teeth (Figure 17-7) • extend over the margin of the gingiva • Shape of calculus mass is determined by the anatomy of the teeth, contour of gingival margin, and pressure of the tongue, lips, cheeks	Flattened to conform with pressure from the pocket wall Combination of the following calculus formations occur • Crusty, spiny, or nodular • Ledge or ringlike • Thin, smooth veneers • Finger- and fernlike • Individual calculus islands
Consistency and texture	Moderately hard Newer deposits less dense and hard Porous surface covered with nonmineralized biofilm	Brittle, flintlike Harder and more dense than supragingival calculus Newest deposits near bottom of pocket are less dense and hard Surface covered with dental biofilm
Size and quantity	Quantity has direct relationship to • Personal oral care procedures and biofilm control measures • Physical character of diet • Individual tendencies • Function and use of the teeth • Increased amount in tobacco smokers	Related to pocket depth Increased amount with age because of accumulation Quantity is related to personal care, diet, and individual tendency as it is with supragingival Subgingival is primarily related to the development and progression of periodontal infection
Distribution on individual tooth	Coronal to margin of gingiva May cover a large portion of the visible clinical crown, or may form fine thin line near gingival margin	Apical to margin of gingiva Extends to bottom of the pocket and follows contour of soft-tissue attachment With gingival recession, subgingival calculus may become supragingival and become covered with typical supragingival calculus
Distribution on teeth	Symmetrical arrangement on teeth except when influenced by • Malpositioned teeth • Unilateral hypofunction • Inconsistent personal care Abrasion from food occurs with or without associated subgingival deposits. Location related to openings of the salivary gland ducts: • Facial surface of maxillary molars • Lingual surface of mandibular anterior teeth	Heaviest on proximal surfaces, lightest on facial surfaces Occurs with or without associated supragingival deposits

Source: Everett FG, Potter GR. Morphology of submarginal calculus. *J Periodontol.* 1959;30(1):27-31.

B. Use of Compressed Air

◆ Small amounts of calculus may be invisible when they are wet with saliva.

◆ With adequate light and drying with air, small deposits usually become visible.

II. Subgingival Examination

A. Visual Examination

◆ Dark edges of calculus may be seen at or just beneath the gingival margin.

◆ Gentle air blast can deflect the gingival margin from the tooth to gain some visibility into the coronal portion of the pocket.

◆ Using transillumination, a dark, opaque, shadowlike may be visible on a proximal tooth surface to suggest the presence of subgingival calculus.

B. Gingival Tissue Color Change

◆ Dark calculus may be visible as a dark shadow along the gingival margin and suggest the presence of subgingival calculus.

C. Tactile Examination

◆ *Probe*: While probing for sulcus/pocket characteristics, a rough subgingival tooth surface may be felt when calculus is present.

◆ *Explorer*: With a subgingival explorer like an ODU 11/12, each tooth is explored carefully to the base of the pocket to detect any calculus deposits.

D. Radiographic Examination

◆ Radiographic examination may detect large calculus deposits on proximal surfaces (see Figure 17-9A and B).

E. Dental Endoscopy

◆ The use of the dental endoscope in deep pockets and furcations can detect otherwise undetectable calculus, especially burnished or veneer-type calculus.[33]

PREVENTION OF CALCULUS

◆ Risk factors related to calculus formation are similar to those for dental biofilm formation and relate to the patient's daily biofilm removal regime.

◆ There are several methods for managing and minimizing calculus formation, including effective daily biofilm removal, professional clinical nonsurgical periodontal therapy, and chemotherapeutic agents such as pyrophosphates (antitartar) and triclosan (antimicrobial).[27]

I. Personal Dental Biofilm Control

A. Objective

◆ Removal of dental biofilm by appropriately selected brushing, interdental care, and supplementary methods is a major factor in the control of dental calculus reformation.

B. Oral Self-Care Education

◆ Patient education includes
  • Identification and hands-on demonstration of the oral hygiene aids appropriate for the patient's needs.
  • Follow-up at continuing care appointments to commend the patient's successes and review and refine techniques as necessary.
  • Identification of dietary behaviors that may be enhancing biofilm growth such as sugar-sweetened beverages and sugary snacks between meals.

II. Regular Professional Continuing Care

◆ Professional maintenance appointments on a regular basis supplements daily oral self-care.

◆ With emphasis on good oral hygiene and routine professional removal, low levels of supragingival and subgingival calculus can be maintained.[35]

III. Anticalculus Dentifrice and Mouthrinse

A. Objective

◆ Calculus-control dentifrices aim to inhibit calculus crystal growth, which may lessen the amount of calculus formation (see Chapter 28).

◆ Dentifrices do not have an effect on existing calculus deposits; however, they may prevent formation of new supragingival calculus.

◆ For a patient who cannot control supragingival calculus, and hence cannot achieve optimum gingival tissue health, an anticalculus dentifrice may provide motivation, as well as be a supplement to mechanical biofilm removal efforts.

B. Chemotherapeutic Anticalculus Agents

◆ Agents used in "tartar-control" mouthrinses or dentifrices are mineralization inhibitors.
  • Examples include pyrophosphates, zinc citrate, and pyrophosphates plus triclosan.[35,36]

DENTAL STAINS AND DISCOLORATIONS

◆ Discolorations of the teeth and restorations occur in three general ways:[37]
  • Adheres directly to the surfaces.
  • Contained within calculus and soft deposits.
  • Incorporated within the tooth structure or the restorative material.

SIGNIFICANCE OF DENTAL STAINS

◆ The significance of stain is primarily the appearance or cosmetic effect.

◆ In general, any detrimental effect on the teeth or gingival tissues is related to the dental biofilm or calculus in which the stain occurs.

◆ Thick deposits of stain conceivably can provide a rough surface on which dental biofilm can collect and irritate the adjacent gingiva.

◆ Certain stains provide a means of evaluating oral cleanliness and the patient's habits of personal care.

I. Classification of Stains

A. Classified by Location

◆ *Extrinsic*: Extrinsic stains occur on the external surface of the tooth and may be removed by procedures of toothbrushing, scaling, and/or polishing.
  • Origins are metallic and nonmetallic.[37]

◆ *Intrinsic*: Intrinsic stains occur within the tooth surface and cannot be removed by scaling or polishing. Intrinsic stains may be improved by certain whitening procedures.

B. Classified by Source

◆ *Exogenous*: Exogenous stains develop or originate from sources outside the tooth. Exogenous stains may be extrinsic and stay on the outer surface of the tooth or intrinsic and become incorporated within the tooth structure.

◆ *Endogenous*: Endogenous stains develop or originate from within the tooth. Endogenous stains are always intrinsic and usually are discolorations of the dentin reflected through the enamel.

II. Recognition and Identification

More than one type of stain may occur and more than one etiologic factor may cause the stains and discolorations of an individual's dentition. A differential diagnosis may be needed in order to plan whether an appropriate intervention is indicated.

A. Medical and Dental History

◆ Developmental complications, medications, use of tobacco, marijuana, or betel or areca nut, and fluoride histories all contribute necessary information.

◆ Accurately prepared medical, dental, and social histories and ethnic practices can provide information to supplement clinical observations.

B. Food Diary

◆ Assessment of a patient's food diary may aid in identifying certain contributing factors.
  • Examples of staining from beverages include tea, coffee, dark-colored juices, and wine.

C. Oral Hygiene Habits

◆ The history of personal biofilm removal routines may help explain the presence of certain stains.

◆ The state of oral hygiene and oral cleanliness impacts the occurrence of dental stains.

III. Application of Procedures for Stain Removal

A. Stains Occurring Directly on the Tooth Surface

◆ Stains directly associated with the biofilm or pellicle on the surface of the enamel or exposed cementum are removed as much as possible during toothbrushing or interdental cleaning.

◆ Certain stains can be removed with debridement and/or polishing (see Chapter 42).

◆ When stains are tenacious, avoid excessive polishing. Use of the least abrasive polishing agent is recommended to prevent the following:
  • Abrasion of the tooth surface or gingival margin.
  • Removal of a layer of fluoride-rich tooth surface.
  • Overheating of the dental structure with a power-driven polisher.

B. Stains Incorporated within Tooth Deposits

◆ When stain is included within the substance of a soft deposit or calculus, it can be removed with the deposit.

C. Stains Incorporated within the Tooth

◆ When stain is intrinsic, whether exogenous or endogenous, it cannot be removed by scaling or polishing. Evaluation for possible whitening procedures may be considered (see Chapter 43).

EXTRINSIC STAINS

There are two broad categories for extrinsic stains[37]:

◆ *Directed extrinsic stains* caused by compounds, organic chromogens, attached to the pellicle producing a stain.

◆ *Indirect extrinsic stains* result from chemical interaction with the tooth surface that create a colored stain.

The most frequently observed stains, yellow, green, black line, and tobacco, are described first; descriptions of the less common orange, red, and metallic stains follow.

I. Yellow Stain

A. Clinical Features

◆ Dull, yellowish discoloration of dental biofilm is illustrated in Figure 17-10.

B. Distribution on Tooth Surfaces

◆ Yellow stain can be generalized or localized.

C. Occurrence

◆ Common to all ages.

◆ More evident when personal oral care procedures are neglected.

D. Etiology

◆ Usually dietary sources.

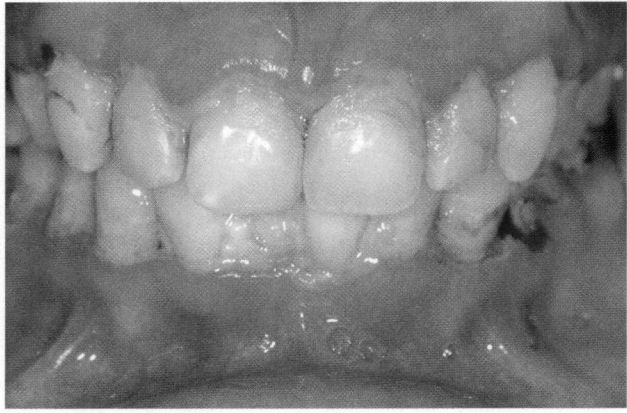

FIGURE 17-10 • Yellow Stain. Generalized, dull, yellowish discoloration of dental biofilm. (Photograph used by permission of Dr. Ali Seyedain, University of Pittsburgh.)

II. Green Stain

A. Clinical Features

◆ Light or yellowish green to very dark green.

◆ Embedded in dental biofilm.[38]

  • The stain is frequently superimposed by soft yellow or gray debris (materia alba and food debris).

◆ Occurs in three general forms[38]:

  • Small curved line following contour of facial gingival margin.

  • Irregular coverage of flat tooth surfaces.

  • Streaked, following grooves or lines in enamel.

◆ Dark green may become embedded in surface enamel and be observed as an exogenous intrinsic stain when superficial layers of deposit are removed.[38]

  • Enamel under stain may be demineralized due to cariogenic biofilm. The rough demineralized surface encourages biofilm retention, demineralization, and recurrence of green stain.

B. Distribution on Tooth Surfaces

◆ Primarily facial; often extends to proximal and lingual surfaces.

◆ Most frequently facial gingival third of maxillary anterior teeth.

C. Composition

◆ Chromogenic bacteria.

◆ Decomposed hemoglobin.

◆ Inorganic elements include calcium, potassium, sodium, silicon, magnesium, phosphorus, and other elements in small amounts.[38]

D. Occurrence

◆ May occur at any age; primarily found in childhood.

◆ Collects on both permanent and primary teeth.

E. Recurrence

◆ Recurrence depends on thoroughness of personal oral care.

F. Etiology

◆ Green stain results from poor oral hygiene, dental biofilm retention, chromogenic bacteria, and gingival hemorrhage.[37]

◆ Chromogenic bacteria are retained and nourished in dental biofilm where the green stain is produced.[37]

◆ Blood pigments from hemoglobin are decomposed by bacteria.

G. Clinical Approach

◆ Often, an area of demineralized tooth structure underlies the stain and soft deposits so care should be taken in scaling the area.

◆ The patient may be able to remove the soft deposits with a toothbrush during oral self-care education.

◆ Dependent on caries risk and presence of demineralization, consider appropriate fluoride recommendations (see Chapter 34).

H. Other Green Stains

◆ In addition to the clinical entity known as "green stain" that was just described, dental biofilm and acquired pellicle may become stained a green color by a variety of substances.

◆ Differential distinction may be determined by questioning the patient or from items in the medical or dental histories. Green discoloration may result from the following:

  • Chlorophyll preparations.

  • Metallic dusts of industry.

  • Green tea.

  • Certain drugs, such as smoking marijuana.

III. Black-Line Stain

◆ Black-line stain is a highly retentive black or dark brown calculuslike stain that forms along the gingival third near the gingival margin. It may occur on primary or permanent teeth.

A. Other Names

◆ Pigmented dental biofilm, brown stain, black stain.

B. Clinical Features

◆ Continuous or interrupted fine line formed by pigmented spots, 1 mm wide (average), no appreciable thickness.[39]

  • May be a wider band or even occupy entire gingival third in severe cases (rare).

◆ Follows contour of gingival margin about 1 mm from margin.

  • Usually separated from gingival margin by clear white line of unstained enamel.

◆ Appears black at bases of pits and fissures.

◆ Lower numbers of cariogenic microorganisms compared to dental biofilm that is not discolored.[39]

C. Distribution on Tooth Surfaces

◆ Facial and lingual surfaces; follows contour of gingival margin onto proximal surfaces.

◆ Rarely on facial surface of maxillary anterior teeth.

◆ Most frequently: lingual and proximal surfaces of maxillary posterior teeth and occlusal pits.

D. Composition and Formation

◆ Black-line stain is composed of microorganisms embedded in a ferric sulfide–phosphorus–calcium matrix.[39]

  • The microorganisms are primarily gram-positive rods, with smaller percentages of cocci.

- The composition of black-line stain is different from the composition of supragingival calculus, in which cocci predominate.
- Attachment of black-line stain to the tooth is by a pelliclelike structure.
- Mineralization in black-line stain is similar to the formation of calculus.

E. Occurrence

- Occurrence increases with age, although most research has been done with children.[39]

F. Recurrence

- Black-line stain tends to form again despite regular personal care.
- Quantity may be less when biofilm control procedures are meticulous.

G. Predisposing Factors

- No definitive etiology, but several have been proposed including[39,40]:
  - *Actinomyces* may be involved in growth of the black pigmentation.
  - Dietary habits.
  - Conflicting data exists about a connection between black line stain and poor oral hygiene.
  - Iron supplements may promote development.

IV. Tobacco Stain

A. Clinical Features

- Light brown to dark leathery brown or black (see Figure 17-11).
- Shape.
  - Diffuse staining of dental biofilm.
  - Narrow band that follows contour of gingival crest, slightly above the crest.
  - Wide, firm, tarlike band may cover cervical third and extend to central third of crown.

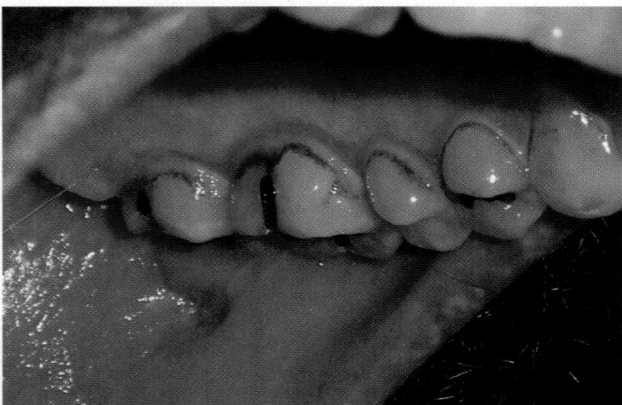

FIGURE 17-11 • Tobacco Stain. Dark brown band following contour of gingival crest. (Photograph used by permission of Dr. Julius Manz, San Juan College, NM.)

- Incorporated in calculus deposit.
- Heavy deposits (particularly from smokeless tobacco) may penetrate the enamel and become exogenous intrinsic.[41]

B. Distribution on Tooth Surface

- Cervical third, primarily lingual surfaces.
- Any surface, including pits and fissures.

C. Composition

- Tar and products of combustion.[41]
- Brown pigment from smokeless tobacco.

D. Predisposing Factors

- Smoking or chewing tobacco or use of hookah to inhale tobacco. The quantity of stain is not necessarily proportional to the amount of tobacco used.
- Personal oral care procedures: increased deposits occur with neglect.
- Extent of dental biofilm and calculus available for adherence.

V. Brown Stains

A. Brown Pellicle

- The pellicle can take on stains of various colors that result from chemical alteration of the pellicle.[41]
  - Found primarily on buccal of maxillary molars and lingual of mandibular anterior surfaces.
  - Poor oral hygiene may be associated with it.
  - Tannins in tea, coffee, soy sauce, and other foods may also deposit in the pellicle resulting in brown stain (Figure 17-12).

B. Stannous Fluoride

- Light brown, sometimes yellowish, stain forms on the teeth in the pellicle.[42]
  - Studies suggest minimal stain accumulation after 6 months with twice daily use, so it is important to weigh the risk of stain with the benefits of use in reducing gingivitis and as an anti-plaque agent.[43,44]
- The brown stain results from the formation of stannous sulfide or brown tin oxide from the reaction of the tin ion in the fluoride compound.[43]

D. Antimicrobial Agents

- Chlorhexidine, alexidine, essential oil/phenol, and cetylpyridinium chloride are used in mouthrinses and are effective against biofilm formation.[37,45]
- Chromogenic polyphenols in the diet such as coffee, tea, and wine may interact with chlorhexidine and worsen the staining.[37]
- A brownish stain on the tongue and tooth surfaces may result, usually more pronounced on proximal and

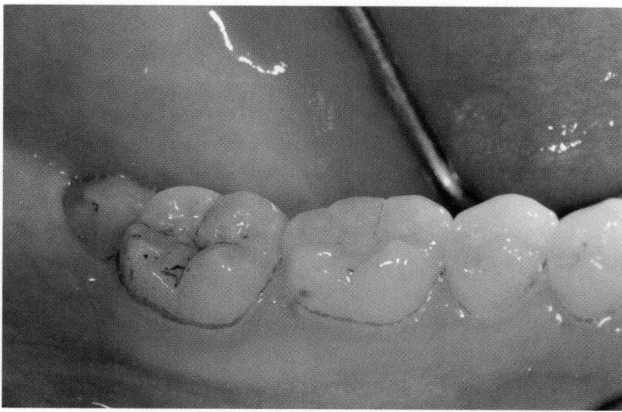

FIGURE 17-12 • Brown Stain. Most likely caused by pigmented foods or drinks. (Photograph used by permission of Dr. Ali Seyedain, University of Pittsburgh.)

other surfaces less accessible to routine biofilm control procedures.[37]

- The stain also tends to form more rapidly on exposed roots than on enamel. Tooth staining is considered a significant side effect.
- Clinical implications
  - Stain may not be removable from enamel defects, anterior composite, crown- or veneer-type restorations.
  - Careful consideration of risk versus benefit of use as an antimicrobial agent is needed by the patient and clinician.[45]

E. Betel/Areca

- The betel nut is a seed of the Areca catechu, a type of palm tree.
  - The nut is ground and other ingredients such as flavoring and tobacco may be added to create a "chew" or "quid." Betel chewing is common among people of all ages in Micronesian islands, such as Guam, and Asian countries, particularly China.[46]
  - In the Polynesian islands, the use has cultural connections and is used in religious ceremonies.
- The discoloration imparted to the teeth is a dark mahogany brown, sometimes almost black. It may become thick and hard, with partly smooth and partly rough surfaces.
- Microscopically, the black deposit consists of microorganisms and mineralized material with a laminated pattern characteristic of subgingival calculus.[47]
- Some research has suggested betel nut has a caries-inhibiting effect, but the oral cancer risk far outweighs any potential benefit.[47,48,49]

F. Swimmer Stain

- Frequent exposure to pools disinfected with chlorine or bromine can cause yellowish or dark brown stains on the facial surfaces of maxillary and mandibular incisor teeth.[50]

VI. Orange and Red Stains

A. Clinical Appearance

- Orange or red stains appear at the cervical third.

B. Distribution on Tooth Surfaces

- More frequently on anterior than on posterior teeth.

C. Occurrence

- Rare (red more rare than orange).

D. Etiology

- Possibly chromogenic bacteria.[37]

VII. Metallic Stains

A. Metals or Metallic Salts from Metal-Containing Dust of Industry

- Clinical appearance/examples of colors on teeth[37]:
  - Copper or brass: green or bluish-green.
  - Iron: brown to greenish-brown.
  - Nickel: green.
  - Cadmium: yellow or golden brown.
- Distribution on tooth surfaces
  - Primarily anterior; may occur on any teeth.
  - Cervical third more commonly affected.
- Manner of formation
  - Industrial worker inhales dust through mouth, bringing metallic substance in contact with teeth.
  - Metal imparts color to pellicle.
  - Occasionally, stain may penetrate tooth substance and become exogenous intrinsic stain.
- Prevention
  - Workers need to be advised to wear a mask while working.

B. Metallic Substances Contained in Drugs

- Clinical appearance/examples of colors on teeth[37]:
  - Iron: black (iron sulfide) or brown.
  - Manganese (from potassium permanganate): black.
- Distribution on tooth surfaces
  - Generalized, may occur everywhere.
- Manner of formation
  - Drug enters biofilm substance, imparts color to biofilm and calculus.
  - Pigment from drug may attach directly to tooth enamel.
- Prevention
  - Take medication through a straw or in tablet or capsule form to prevent direct contact with the teeth.

ENDOGENOUS INTRINSIC STAINS

I. Pulpless or Traumatized Teeth

Not all pulpless teeth discolor. However, traumatized teeth that have not been treated endodontically often discolor.

A. Clinical Appearance

◆ A wide range of colors exists; stains may be light yellow-brown, slate gray, reddish-brown, dark brown, bluish-black, or black. Others have an orange or greenish tinge.

B. Etiology

◆ Blood and other pulp tissue elements may be available for breakdown as a result of hemorrhages in the pulp chamber, root canal treatment, or necrosis and decomposition of the pulp tissue.[37]

◆ Pigments from the decomposed hemoglobin and pulp tissue penetrate and discolor the dentinal tubules.

II. Disturbances in Tooth Development

◆ Stains incorporated within the tooth structure may be related to the period of tooth development.[37]

◆ Defective tooth development may result from factors of genetic abnormality or environmental influences during tooth development.

A. Hereditary: Genetic

◆ *Amelogenesis imperfecta:* The enamel is partially or completely missing due to a generalized disturbance of the ameloblasts. Teeth are yellow to yellowish-brown.[37]

◆ *Dentinogenesis imperfecta (Opalescent dentin):* The dentin is abnormal as a result of disturbances in the odontoblastic layer during development. The teeth appear translucent or opalescent and vary in color from gray to bluish-brown.[37]

B. Enamel Hypoplasia

◆ Enamel hypoplasia results from damage to the tooth germ during development and the location of the defect(s) is typically related to the timing of the injury during development.[37]

• *Generalized hypoplasia* (chronologic hypoplasia resulting from ameloblastic disturbance of short duration) may extend across multiple teeth.

• *Local hypoplasia* affects a single tooth. For example, individual white spots, caused by trauma to a primary tooth that interferes with development of permanent tooth, results in "Turner tooth."

◆ Clinical appearance[37]:

• Teeth erupt with white spots, pits, or grooves depending on the severity of the injury to the tooth germ.

• Over time, the enamel hypoplasia defects are prone to extrinsic stain.

◆ Etiology[37]

• Trauma or infection of an individual tooth.

• Rubella infection or disease causing a high fever.

• Drug intake during pregnancy.

• Hypocalcemia (low calcium) levels such as in premature infants.

C. Dental Fluorosis

◆ Dental fluorosis was originally called "brown stain." Later, Dr. Frederick S. McKay studied the condition and described it in the dental literature as "mottled enamel."

◆ Etiology

• Enamel hypomineralization results from ingestion of excessive fluoride ion from any source during the period of mineralization. The enamel alterations are a result of toxic damage to the ameloblasts.

• Severity is related to the age and dose of fluoride exposure.[37]

◆ Fluorosis classification

• Dean provided the original definitions for five grades of fluorosis (Chapter 34). They ranged from "questionable" (a few white flecks or spots) to "severe" (marked brown staining and pitting of the enamel surfaces).[51]

• More specific classifications have been developed for clinical and research purposes, such as the tooth surface index of fluorosis.[51]

◆ Clinical appearance

• When the teeth erupt, the color of the enamel ranges from chalky white spots to brown. Depending on the severity of the enamel defect(s), discoloration may occur over time.

• Severe effects of excess fluoride during development may produce cracks or pitting. This condition and appearance led to the name *mottled enamel.*

III. Drug-Induced Stains and Discolorations

A. Tetracycline

◆ Tetracycline antibiotics have an affinity for mineralized tissues (Figure 17-13).[52]

• Are absorbed by the bones and teeth.

• Can be transferred through the placenta and enter fetal circulation.

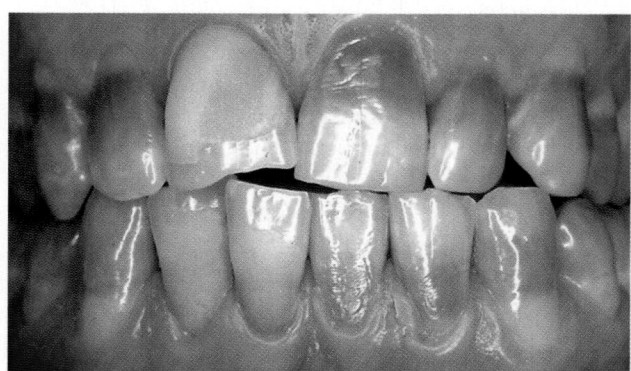

FIGURE 17-13 • Tetracycline Stain. Tetracycline staining in this permanent dentition resulted from the administration of tetracycline antibiotic during the time that crowns formed. Teeth have the appearance of yellow to gray-brown horizontal bands across the crowns. (The staining on tooth no. 8 has been covered with a tooth-colored restorative material such as composite resin.) (Courtesy of Carl Allen, DDS, MSD.)

◆ Discoloration of a child's teeth may result when the drug is administered to the mother during the third trimester of pregnancy or to the child in infancy and early childhood.[52]

◆ Etiology
  • The discoloration depends on the dosage, length of time used, and type of tetracycline prescribed.
  • The mechanism for staining is not fully understood, but is believed to be the tetracycline binding with the calcified tooth structure during development.[52]

◆ Clinical appearance[52]
  • Discoloration may be generalized or localized to individual teeth that were developing at the time of administration of the antibiotic.
  • Color of teeth may be light green to dark yellow, or a gray-brown, with or without banding and approximate age when the antibiotic was taken.
  • The patient's medical history may reveal the illness for which the antibiotic was prescribed.

B. Minocycline

◆ Unlike tetracycline, minocycline has been reported to cause generalized intrinsic staining posteruption.[52]

◆ Clinical appearance
  • Use of minocycline can result in a blue-gray to gray darkening of the crowns of permanent teeth.[53]

◆ Etiology
  • The mechanism is unknown but may result from calcium-minocycline compounds deposited in dentin.[37]

EXOGENOUS INTRINSIC STAINS

◆ When intrinsic stains come from an outside source, not from within the tooth, the stain is called exogenous intrinsic.

◆ Extrinsic stains result from stain in the tooth following development and may occur when the stain penetrates enamel defects and exposed dentin to become intrinsic (Figure 17-14).

◆ The sources of these stains may include[37]:
  • Developmental defects.
  • Acquired defects such as tooth wear and gingival recession.
  • Dental caries.
  • Restorative materials.

I. Restorative Materials

A. Silver Amalgam

◆ Silver amalgam can impart a gray to black discoloration to the tooth structure around a restoration.

◆ Tin migrates from the amalgam restoration into the enamel and dentin.[37]

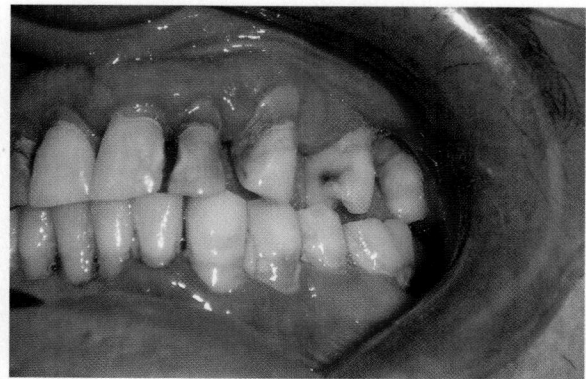

FIGURE 17-14 • Intrinsic Stain. Most likely exogenous; likely from an outside source such as tobacco or food and becomes intrinsic over time. Areas of cervical erosion and recession allow yellow color of underlying dentin to be exposed and become further stained. (Photograph used by permission of Dr. Julius Manz, San Juan College, NM.)

B. Endodontic Therapy

◆ Discoloration tends to be most evident on the cervical third of the crown and root surface.[54]

◆ Materials used during endodontic therapy can cause intrinsic staining.[54]
  • Endodontic sealers may cause stain ranging in color from orange-red to gray.
  • Endodontic medicaments, which may include tetracycline, may cause a dark brown intrinsic stain.
  • Portland cement-based materials may cause a gray intrinsic stain.
  • Antibiotic pastes used in regenerative endodontic procedures may also contain tetracycline, but also ciprofloxacin, metronidazole, or minocycline and result in a green-brown staining.

II. Stain in Dentin

◆ Discoloration resulting from a carious lesion is an example.

◆ Arrested decay or secondary dentin can present as black stain on severely decayed teeth. The surface is hard and glossy, and stain cannot be removed.

III. Other Local Causes

◆ Enamel erosion is the loss of hard tissue by chemical means such as acidic foods (including carbonated drinks), eating disorders (bulimia), and gastroesophageal reflux disease.[37]
  • Resulting thinner enamel allows the yellow color of the underlying dentin to show through and cause the teeth to appear duller gray or yellow (Figure 17-15).

◆ Attrition of occlusal surfaces can result in loss of enamel, allowing a yellow or brown outline of dentin to show through (Figure 17-16).

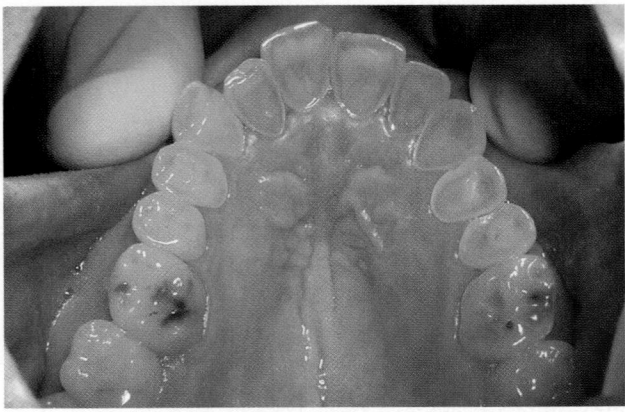

FIGURE 17-15 • Enamel Erosion. This extensive enamel erosion revealing the yellow color of the dentin on the lingual of anterior teeth and premolars. This was an individual with chronic severe gastroesophageal reflux disease (GERD) of more than 10 years' duration.

DOCUMENTATION

The permanent records for each patient should include information relating to the soft deposits, calculus, and stain including:

◆ Clinical description of appearance of the teeth relative to the biofilm, materia alba, or food debris as indications of the personal oral care on a daily basis.

◆ The extent of supragingival and subgingival deposits (slight, moderate, or heavy) should be described in the initial examination record: charted to show location for reference during the clinical removal and during teaching personal care for prevention.

◆ Record color, type, extent, and location of stains with the patient's examination and assessment.

◆ Personal patient care procedures demonstrated; preventive measures discussed; and frequency of continuing care appointments recommended.

See Box 17-1 for a sample documentation note.

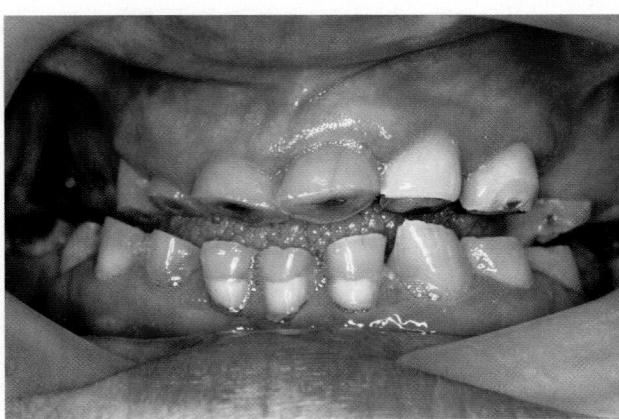

FIGURE 17-16 • Attrition: Pronounced Attrition of the Maxillary Teeth Exposing the Yellow Dentin and Brown of the Pulp Chamber. (Courtesy of Dr. Richard Foster, Guilford Technical Community College, Jamestown, NC.)

BOX 17-1
Example Documentation: Patient with Calculus and Stain

S—Male patient, aged 35 years, medical history indicates no medication, no health compromise. Cigarette smoker, $\frac{1}{2}$ pack per day. Patient presents for new patient exam. His last dental cleaning was 2 years ago. Chief complaint: Oral malodor, bleeding gums when brushing and he would like whiter teeth.

O—Generalized pocket depths of lesser than 3 mm with bleeding on probing, Light-localized subgingival calculus. Light generalized supragingival calculus with generalized moderate tobacco stain.

A—Poor oral self-care with generalized moderate gingivitis and coated tongue. Discuss and demonstrate proper oral self-care instruction. Bass method brushing, daily interdental flossing, oral rinsing, and tongue cleaning. Evaluate patient's readiness for smoking cessation plan.

P—Medical/dental history, intra–extra oral examination performed, completed new patient periodontal chart-odontogram, panoramic film, full mouth series, caries assessment, and consultation with dentist. Oral self-care instruction along with smoking cessation counselling. Prophylaxis completed with subgingival debridement mandible only. Educated patient regarding the etiology and significance of dental biofilm, calculus, tongue coating, and stain accumulation. Patient advised to return for one completion debridement appointment following with a 3-month preventive maintenance appointment to monitor patient's oral self-care and offer smoking cessation support.

Next step: Reappoint in 1 week to complete debridement and follow-up soft-tissue evaluation.

Reappoint in 3 months for preventive maintenance appointment.

Signed: _____, RDH

Date: _____

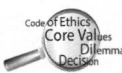

EVERYDAY ETHICS

Robert returned to the dental office of Dr. Taylor after 3 years of working in Northern Quebec, Canada. At the age of 30, Robert was exhibiting signs of early periodontitis with gingival inflammation and moderate subgingival calculus. Susan, the dental hygienist, educated Daniel about biofilm and suggested improvements for his personal daily brushing and flossing regimen. After debriding two quadrants with local anesthesia, Susan suggested that rinsing with chlorhexidine after brushing before going to bed would help the healing.

Dr. Taylor agreed with Susan's recommendation and wrote the prescription. A few days later Robert called to complain about the "awful brown stain on his teeth and horrible taste of the mouthrinse." He further indicated that he had stopped using the product and wanted to come in and have the stain removed immediately.

Questions for Consideration

1. Which of the dental hygiene core values might apply in this scenario? How does each core value selected enter the picture?

2. Robert seems more concerned about the tooth staining and flavor of the chlorhexidine rinse than about the health of his gingival tissues while Susan's concerns are for improving his gingival health. What ethical principles may be in effect here?

3. Using the questions in Table VI-1 (in Section VI, Introduction), help Susan develop a favorable response explaining her choice of therapy for her patient's poor gingival health.

Factors to Teach the Patient

▶ Location, composition, and properties of dental biofilm and calculus with emphasis on its role in dental caries and periodontal infections.

▶ Effects of personal oral care procedures in the prevention of dental biofilm, calculus, and stain.

▶ Biofilm control procedures with special adaptations for individual needs.

▶ Sources of cariogenic foodstuff in the diet and frequency of consumption in relation to dental caries formation.

▶ What calculus is and how it forms from dental biofilm.

▶ Etiology of individual's dental stains and discolorations with suggestions for modification of sources of extrinsic stain.

▶ Advantages of a smoking cessation program.

▶ Effect of tetracyclines on developing teeth. Need to avoid use during pregnancy and by children to age 12.

▶ Select products with an American Dental Association or Canadian Dental Association Seal of Acceptance.

ENHANCE YOUR UNDERSTANDING

ONLINE RESOURCES
(see the inside front cover for access information)

- Audio glossary
- Appendices

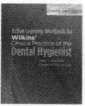

SUPPORT FOR LEARNING
(available separately)

- *Active Learning Workbook for Wilkins' Clinical Practice of the Dental Hygienist, 13th Edition*

INDIVIDUALIZED REVIEW

- Customized practice quizzing with Navigate 2 TestPrep for *Wilkins' Clinical Practice of the Dental Hygienist*

References

1. Seneviratne CJ, Zhang CF, Samaranayake LP. Dental plaque biofilm in oral health and disease. *Chin J Dent Res.* 2011;14(2):87-94.

2. Siqueira WL, Custodio W, McDonald EE. New insights into the composition and functions of the acquired enamel pellicle. *J Dent Res.* 2012;91(12):1110-1118.

3. Hanning M. Ultrastructural investigation of pellicle morphogenesis at two different intraoral sites during a 24-h period. *Clin Oral Investig.* 1999;3:88-95.

4. Hanning M, Joiner A. The structure, function and properties of the acquired pellicle. *Monogr Oral Sci.* 2006;19:26-64.

5. Meckel AH. Formation and properties of organic films on teeth. *Arch Oral Biol.* 1965;10(4):585-598.

6. Kuroiwa M, Kodaka T, Kuroiwa M, et al. Acid resistance of human enamel by brushing with and without abrasive dentifrice. *J Biol Buccale.* 1992;20:175-180.

7. Hara AT, Zero DT. The caries environment: saliva, pellicle, diet, and hard tissue ultrastructure. *Dent Clin North Am.* 2010;54(3):455-467.

8. Kilian M, Chapple IL, Hannig M, et al. The oral microbiome—An update for oral healthcare professionals. *Br Dent J.* 2016;221(10):657-666.

9. Stoodley P, Sauer K, Davies DG, et al. Biofilms as complex differentiated communities. *Annu Rev Microbiol.* 2002;56:187-209.

10. Löe H, Theilade E, Jensen SB. Experimental gingivitis in man. *J Periodontol.* 1965;36:177-187.

11. Zijnge V, van Leeuwen M, Degener J, et al. Oral biofilm architecture on natural teeth. *PLoS One.* 2010;5(2):e9321.

12. Tanaka M, Matsunaga K, Kadoma Y. Correlation in inorganic ion concentration between saliva and plaque fluid. *J Med Dent Sci.* 2000;47(1):55-59.

13. Ekstrand J, Oliveby A. Fluoride in the oral environment. *Acta Odontol Scand.* 1999;57(6):330-333.

14. Koo H, Falsetta ML, Klein MI. The exopolysaccharide matrix: a virulence determinant of cariogenic biofilm. *J Dent Res.* 2013;92(12):1065-1073.

15. Sreenivasan PK, Prasad KVV. Distribution of dental plaque and gingivitis within the dental arches. *J Int Med Res.* 2017;45(5):1585-1596.

16. Struzycka I. The oral microbiome in dental caries. *Pol J Microbiol.* 2014;63(2):127-135.

17. Lingström P, van Ruyven FO, van Houte J, Kent R. The pH of dental plaque in its relation to early enamel caries and dental plaque flora in humans. *J Dent Res.* 2000;79(2):770-777.

18. Hicks J, Garcia-Godoy F, Flaitz C. Biological factors in dental caries enamel structure and the caries process in the dynamic process of demineralization and remineralization (part 2). *J Clin Pediatric Dent.* 2005;28(2):119-124.

19. Bowen WH. The Stephan Curve revisited. *Odontology.* 2013;101(1):2-8.

20. Sung YH, Son HH, Yi K, Chang J. Elemental analysis of caries-affected root dentin and artificially demineralized dentin. *Restor Dent Endod.* 2016;41(4):255-261.

21. Gustafsson BE, Quensel CE, Lanke LS, et al. The Vipeholm dental caries study: the effect of different levels of carbohydrate intake on caries activity in 436 individuals observed for five years. *Acta Odontol Scand.* 1954;11(34):232-264.

22. Li QL, Ying Cao C, Xu QJ, Xu XH, Yin JL. Atraumatic restoration of vertical food impaction with an open contact using flowable composite resin aided by Cerclage wire under tension. *Scientifica.* 2016;2016:4127472.

23. Aylıkcı BU, Colak H. Halitosis: From diagnosis to management. *J Nat Sci Biol Med.* 2013;4(1):14-23.

24. Little MF, Casciani CA, Rowley J. Dental calculus composition. 1. Supragingival calculus: ash, calcium, phosphorus, sodium, and density. *J Dent Res.* 1963;42(1):78-86.

25. Perez CA, Sanchez HJ, Barrea RA, Grenon M, Abraham J. Microscopic x-ray fluorescence analysis of human dental calculus using synchrotron radiation. *J Anal Atom Spectrom.* 2004;19:392-397.

26. Okumura H, Nakagaki H, Kato K, Ito F, Weatherell JA, Robinson C. Distribution of fluoride in human dental calculus. *Caries Res.* 1993;27(4):271-276.

27. Jin Y, Yip HK. Supragingival calculus: formation and control. *Crit Rev Oral Biol Med.* 2002;13(5):426-441.

28. Palmer LC, Newcomb CJ, Kaltz SR, et al. Biomimetic systems for hydroxyapatite mineralization inspired by bone and enamel. *Chem Rev.* 2008;108(11):4754-4783.

29. Roberts-Harry EA, Clerehugh V. Subgingival calculus: where are we now? A comparative review. *J Dent.* 2000;28(2):93-102.

30. Rohanizadeh R, Legeros RZ. Ultrastructural study of calculus-enamel and calculus-root interfaces. *Arch Oral Biol.* 2005;50(1):89-96.

31. Akcalı A, Lang NP. Dental calculus: the calcified biofilm and its role in disease development. *Periodontol 2000.* 2018;76(1):109-115.

32. Zander HA, Hazen SP, Scott DB. Mineralization of dental calculus. *Proc Soc Exp Biol Med.* 1960;103:257-260.

33. Osborn JB, Lenton PA, Lunos SA, et al. Endoscopic vs. tactile evaluation of subgingival calculus. *J Dent Hyg.* 2014;88(4):229-236.

34. Schätzle M, Faddy MJ, Cullinan MP, et al. The clinical course of chronic periodontitis. V. Predictive factors in periodontal disease. *J Clin Periodontol.* 2009;36(5):365-371.

35. Netuveli GS, Sheiham A. A systematic review of the effectiveness of anticalculus dentifrices. *Oral Health Prev Dent.* 2004;2(1):49-58.

36. Riley P, Lamont T. Triclosan/copolymer containing toothpastes for oral health. *Cochrane Database Syst Rev.* 2013;12:CD010514.

37. Watts A, Addy M. Tooth discoloration and staining: a review of the literature. *Br Dent J.* 2001;190:309-316.

38. Shay DE, Haddox JH, Richmond JL. An inorganic qualitative and quantitative analysis of green stain. *J Am Dent Assoc.* 1955;50(2):156-160.

39. Zyła T, Kawala B, Antoszewska-Smith J, et al. Black stain and dental caries: a review of the literature. *Biomed Res Int.* 2015;2015:469392.

40. Saba C, Solidani M, Berlutti F, Vestri A, Ottolenghi L, Polimeni A. Black stains in the mixed dentition: a PCR microbiological study of the etiopathogenic bacteria. *J Clin Pediatr Dent.* 2006;30(3):219-224.

41. Hattab FN, Qudeimat MA, Al Rimawi HS. Dental discoloration: an overview. *J Esthet Restor Dent.* 1999;11(6):291-310.

42. Ellingsen JE, Eriksen HM, Rolla G. Extrinsic dental stain caused by stannous fluoride. *Eur J Oral Sci.* 1982;90(1):9-13.

43. Milleman KR, Patil A, Ling MR, Mason S, Milleman JL. An exploratory study to investigate stain build-up with long term use of a stannous fluoride dentifrice. *Am J Dent.* 2018;31(2):71-75.

44. Sälzer S, Slot DE, Dörfer CE, Van der Weijden GA. Comparison of triclosan and stannous fluoride dentifrices on parameters of gingival inflammation and plaque scores: a systematic review and meta-analysis. *Int J Dent Hyg.* 2015;13(1):1-17.

45. Van Strydonck DA, Slot DE, Van der Velden U, Van der Weijden F. Effect of a chlorhexidine mouthrinse on plaque, gingival inflammation and staining in gingivitis patients: a systematic review. *J Clin Periodontol.* 2012;39(11):1042-1055.

46. Warnakulasuriya S, Trivedy C, Peters TJ. Areca nut use: an independent risk factor for oral cancer. *BMJ.* 2002;324(7341):799-800.

47. Reichart PA, Lenz H, König H, et al. The black layer on the teeth of betel chewers: a light microscopic, microradiographic, and electronmicroscopic study. *J Oral Pathol.* 1985;14(6):466-475.

48. Howden GF. The cariostatic effect of betel nut chewing. *P N G Med J.* 1984;27(3-4):123-131.

49. Hu YJ, Chen J, Zhong WS, et al. Trend analysis of betel nut-associated oral cancer and health burden in China. *Chin J Dent Res.* 2017;20(2):69-78.

50. Escartin J, Arnedo A, Pinto V, et al. A study of dental staining among competitive swimmers. *Community Dent Oral Epidemiol.* 2000;28:10-17.

51. Rozier RG. Epidemiologic indices for measuring the clinical manifestations of dental fluorosis: overview and critique. *Adv Dent Res.* 1994;8(1):39.

52. Kumar A, Kumar V, Singh J, et al. Drug-induced discoloration of teeth: an updated review. *Clin Pediatr.* 2012;51(2):181-185.

53. Raymond J, Cook D. Still leaving stains on teeth-the legacy of minocycline? *Australas Med J.* 2015;8(4):139-142.

54. Krastl G, Allgayer N, Lenherr P, Filippi A, Taneja P, Weiger R. Tooth discoloration induced by endodontic materials: a literature review. *Dent Traumatol.* 2013;29(1):2-7.

The Periodontium

Linda D. Boyd, RDH, RD, EdD, and Esther M. Wilkins, BS, RDH, DMD

CHAPTER OUTLINE

THE NORMAL PERIODONTIUM
   I. Gingiva
   II. Periodontal Ligament
   III. Cementum
   IV. Alveolar Bone

THE GINGIVAL DESCRIPTION
   I. Color
   II. Size
   III. Shape (Form or Contour)

   IV. Consistency
   V. Surface Texture
   VI. Position
   VII. Bleeding
   VIII. Exudate

THE GINGIVA OF YOUNG CHILDREN
   I. Signs of Health
   II. Changes in Disease

THE GINGIVA AFTER PERIODONTAL SURGERY
   I. Pocket Reduction Surgery
   II. Gingival Grafting Surgery
   III. Implant Surgery

DOCUMENTATION

EVERYDAY ETHICS

FACTORS TO TEACH THE PATIENT

REFERENCES

LEARNING OBJECTIVES

After studying this chapter, the student will be able to:

1. Recognize normal tissues of the periodontium.
2. Know the clinical features of the periodontium.
3. Describe the characteristics of healthy gingiva.

4. Compare and contrast the characteristics of gingiva in health and disease.
5. Describe the characteristics of healthy gingiva following periodontal surgery.

THE NORMAL PERIODONTIUM

The periodontium is the functional unit of tissues surrounding and supporting the tooth. It is made up of two parts: the *gingiva*, which protects the underlying tissues, and the attachment apparatus, which consists of the *periodontal ligament (PDL)*, *cementum*, and *alveolar bone*.[1] Recognizing normal, healthy periodontium by clinical observation and periodontal assessment is an essential component of accurate diagnosis and treatment planning.

I. Gingiva

The gingiva surrounds the roots of the teeth, alveolar bone, and underlying connective tissue.

Anatomically the gingiva is made up of the free gingiva, interdental gingiva (interdental papilla), and attached gingiva.[2]

A. Free Gingiva (Marginal Gingiva)

In health, the free gingiva surrounds the tooth, but is not attached to the tooth or alveolar bone. It connects with the attached gingiva at the free gingival groove and attaches to the tooth at the coronal portion of the junctional epithelium (JE) as shown in Figures 18-1 and 18-2 to form the gingival sulcus.

- Gingival margin (gingival crest, margin of the gingiva, or free margin, Figures 18-1 and 18-2)
  - *Location:* This is the edge of the gingiva, nearest to the incisal or occlusal surface.
  - The gingival margin is 0.08–2.1 mm coronal to the cementoenamel junction (CEJ) in health.[3]
  - Marks the opening of the gingival sulcus.
- Free gingival groove
  - *Location:* The free gingival groove is a shallow, linear groove demarcating the free from the attached

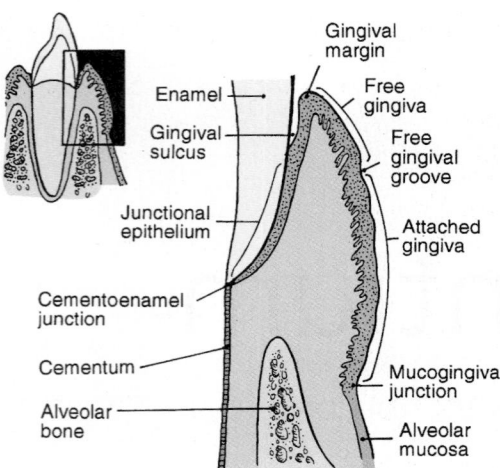

FIGURE 18-1 • Parts of the Gingiva. Cross-sectional diagram shows the parts of the gingiva and adjacent tissues of a partially erupted tooth. Note that the junctional epithelium is on the enamel.

gingiva. In health, there may be a free gingival groove visible in about one-third of adults.[4]

- In the absence of inflammation and pocket formation, the gingival groove runs parallel with and about 0.5–1.5 mm from the gingival margin.[5]
- The gingival groove is approximately at the level of the bottom of the gingival sulcus.

◆ Oral epithelium (outer gingival epithelium, Figure 18-3)

- *Location:* Covers the free gingiva from the gingival groove over the gingival margin.
- Composed of keratinized stratified squamous epithelium.
- Cells turnover every 9–12 days.[4]

B. Gingival Sulcus

◆ *Location:* The gingival sulcus is the crevice or space between the free gingiva and the tooth extending from the free gingival margin to the JE (Figures 18-1 and 18-3).

◆ *Sulcular epithelium*

- The continuation of the oral epithelium from the free gingiva.
- Non-keratinized.[1]
- Plays a crucial role in sealing off the oral environment from the periodontal tissues.

◆ *Depth of sulcus*

- Average histologic depth of the healthy sulcus is about 0.8–2.1 mm with no bleeding on probing.[3]
- Average clinical probing depth of the normal gingival sulcus is 1.3–2.7 mm.[3]

◆ *Gingival crevicular fluid or sulcular fluid*

- The gingival crevicular fluid (GCF) is a serum-like fluid that seeps from the connective tissue through the epithelial lining of the sulcus or pocket.
- Flow rate is slight to none in a normal sulcus; GCF flow rate reflects changes in permeability of the tissue due to inflammation.[6]
- It is part of the local defense mechanism and is able to transport many substances, including endotoxins, enzymes, antibodies, and certain systemically administered drugs.
- Possible use as a diagnostic aid for periodontal disease activity because the composition changes in the presence of inflammation.[6]

C. Interdental Gingiva (Interdental Papilla)

◆ *Location*

- In health, the interdental gingiva or interdental papilla occupies the interproximal area between two adjacent teeth that are in contact (see Figure 18-2).
- The tip and lateral borders are continuous with the free gingiva, whereas other parts of the papilla are attached gingiva.
- An interproximal area is also called an embrasure.

◆ *Shape*

- *Varies with spacing or overlapping of the teeth:* The interdental gingiva may be flat or saddle shaped when there are wide spaces between teeth, or it may be

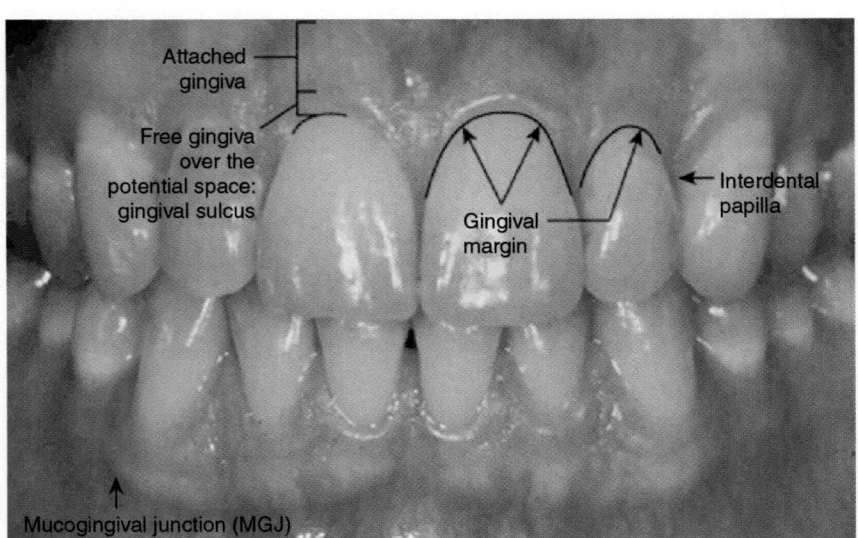

FIGURE 18-2 • Picture of Gingival Tissues. Gingiva surrounds each tooth forming a characteristic scalloped shape gingival margin. Interproximal papillae fill the spaces between most teeth. The potential space between the free gingiva and the tooth can be accessed with a periodontal probe. The attached gingiva is the gingiva that is firmly attached to the underlying bone. The mucogingival junction (MGJ) where the attached gingiva and alveolar mucosa meet. (Reprinted from Scheid R, Weiss G. *Woelfel's Dental Anatomy: Its Relevance to Dentistry.* 8th ed. Philadelphia, PA: Lippincott Williams & Wilkins; 2011.)

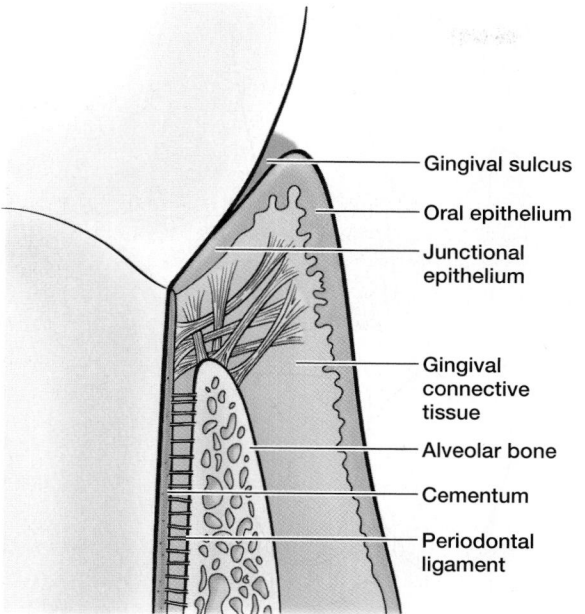

FIGURE 18-3 • **The Gingival Tissues.** Cross-sectional diagram shows the relationships of the oral, sulcular, and junctional epithelia and the connective tissue.

tapered and narrow when teeth are crowded or overlapped.

* *Between anterior teeth*: pointed, pyramidal.
* *Between posterior teeth*
    * Flatter than anterior papillae because of wider teeth, wider contact areas, and flattened interdental bone.
    * Two papillae, one facial and one lingual, connected by a col, are found when teeth are in contact.
* *Col*
    * A col is the depression under the contact area between a lingual or palatal and facial papilla that

conforms to the proximal contact area as shown in Figure 18-4A and B.

* The width of the col from buccal to lingual ranges from 2 to 6 mm and the depth ranges from 0.3 to 1.5 mm.[7]
* The center of the col area is not usually keratinized and thus is more susceptible to infection.[7]

* A *classification system for papillary height*[8] *is as follows* (Figure 18-5A–D):
    * Normal: The interdental papilla fills the space between teeth.
    * Class I embrasure: The tip of the interdental papilla is apical to the contact point of adjacent teeth, but the interproximal CEJ is not visible.
    * Class II embrasure: The tip of the interdental papilla is at or apical to the interproximal CEJ, but coronal to the height of the facial CEJ.
    * Class III embrasure: Complete loss of the interdental papilla due to extensive gingival recession.

D. Junctional Epithelium

* *Description*
    * The junctional epithelium (JE) is a stratified squamous non-keratinized mucosa made up of two strata (layers), one adjacent to the connective tissue and the other facing the tooth surface.
    * The JE is continuous with the sulcular epithelium and completely encircles the tooth to form a tight seal.
    * JE cells have wider fluid-filled intercellular spaces that contain polymorphonuclear leukocytes and monocytes that pass into the gingival sulcus to manage the constant microbial challenge.[9]
    * JE cells turnover rapidly in about 5 days.[7]
* *Size*
    * The JE may be up to 15 or 30 cells in thickness where it joins the sulcular epithelium and tapers down to 1 or 3 cells in thickness at the apical end.[9]
    * The length ranges from 0.25 to 1.35 mm.[9]

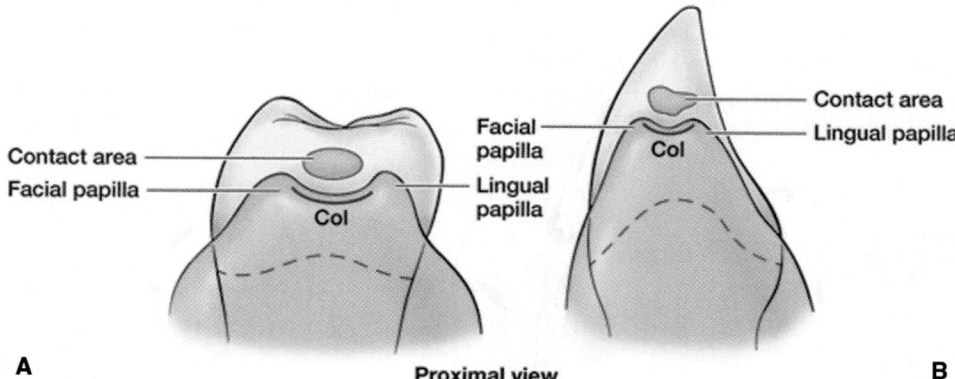

FIGURE 18-4 • **Col.** A col is the depression between the lingual or palatal and the facial papillae under the contact area. **A:** Mesial of mandibular molar to show wide col area. **B:** Mesial of mandibular incisor to show a narrow col. The col deepens when gingival enlargement occurs. (Reprinted from Nield-Gehrig J, Willmann D. *Foundations of Periodontics for the Dental Hygienist*. Philadelphia, PA: Lippincott Williams & Wilkins; 2011.)

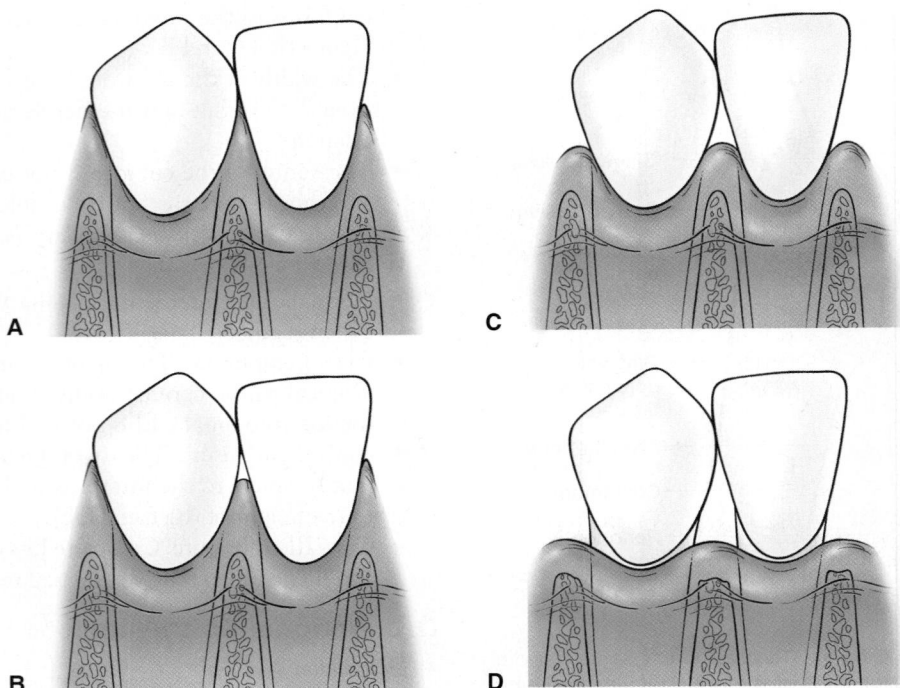

FIGURE 18-5 • Interdental Embrasure Classifications. A: Normal papilla: fills the space between teeth. **B:** Class I embrasure—tip of interdental papilla is apical to the contact point, but the interproximal cementoenamel junction (CEJ) is not visible. **C:** Class II embrasure—tip of interdental papilla is at or apical to the interproximal CEJ, but coronal to the facial CEJ. **D:** Class III embrasure—the interdental papilla is at or apical to the level of the facial CEJ.

◆ *Position*
  • As the tooth erupts, the attachment is on the enamel; during eruption, the epithelium migrates toward the CEJ (Figure 18-6A–C).
  • At full eruption, the attachment is usually on the cementum, where it becomes firmly attached (Figure 18-6D).
  • With wear of the tooth on the incisal or occlusal surface and with periodontal infections, the attachment migrates along the root surface (Figure 18-6E).
◆ *Relation of crest of alveolar bone to the attached gingival tissue*
  • The distance between the epithelial attachment and the crest of the alveolar bone is approximately 2.04 mm.[10] This is also referred to as the biologic width.
  • This distance is maintained in disease when the epithelium moves along the root surface and bone loss occurs.

◆ *Epithelial attachment to the tooth surface*
  • The JE attaches gingiva to the tooth and tissue by a basal lamina and hemidesmosomes.[7]

E. Attached Gingiva

◆ *Extent*
  • The attached gingiva is continuous with the oral epithelium of the free gingiva and is covered with keratinized stratified squamous epithelium.
  • Maxillary palatal gingiva is continuous with the palatal mucosa.
  • Attached gingiva of the mandibular facial and lingual gingiva and maxillary facial gingiva is demarcated from the alveolar mucosa by the mucogingival junction (MGJ) (Figures 18-1, 18-2, and 18-7).

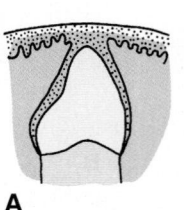 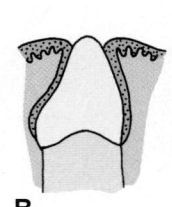 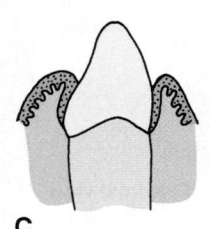 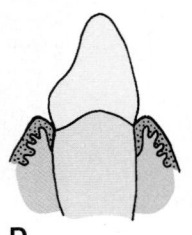 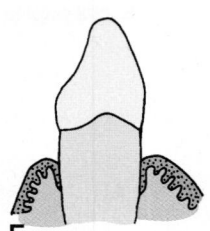

FIGURE 18-6 • Tooth Eruption and the Gingiva. A: Before eruption, the oral epithelium covers the tooth. **B:** As the tooth emerges, the reduced epithelium joins the oral epithelium as the gingival sulcus is formed. **C:** Partial eruption with the junctional epithelium (JE) along the enamel. **D:** Eruption complete, with JE at the cementoenamel junction. **E:** From disease or other cause, the attachment migrates along the root surface, exposing the cementum.

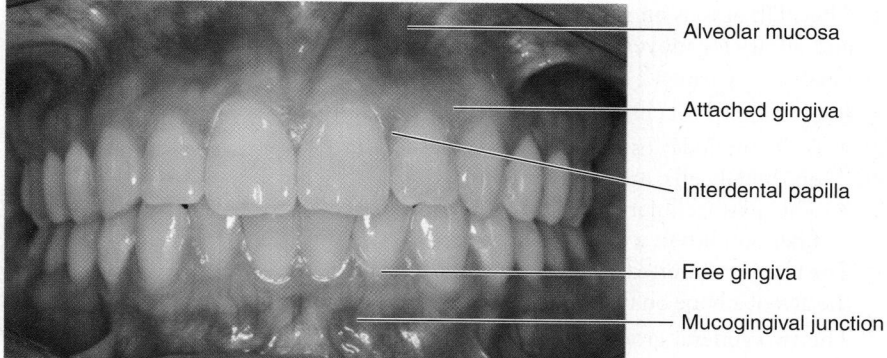

Alveolar mucosa

Attached gingiva

Interdental papilla

Free gingiva

Mucogingival junction

FIGURE 18-7 • Parts of the Gingiva.

◆ *Attachment*
  • Firmly bound to the underlying alveolar bone.
◆ *Shape*
  • Follows the depressions between the eminences of the roots of the teeth.

F. Mucogingival Junction

◆ *Location*
  • The MGJ is where the attached gingiva and the alveolar mucosa meet (Figures 18-1, 18-2, and 18-7).
  • A mucogingival line is found on the facial surface of both arches and on the lingual surface of the mandibular arch.
  • There is no alveolar mucosa on the palate. The palatal tissue is firmly attached to the bone of the roof of the mouth.
◆ *Appearance*
  • The MGJ appears as a line, a contrast can be seen between the pink of the keratinized, stippled, attached gingiva, and more vascular alveolar mucosa that is a deeper reddish-pink.
  • In the anterior area the MGJ is scalloped, but it is fairly straight in posterior areas.

G. Alveolar Mucosa

◆ *Description*
  • Movable tissue loosely attached to the underlying bone.

  • It has a smooth, shiny surface with non-keratinized, thin epithelium. Underlying capillaries may be seen through the epithelium.
◆ *Frena (singular: Frenum or Frenulum)*
  • *Description:* A frenum is a narrow fold of mucous membrane connecting more fixed tissue to movable mucosa, for example, from the attached gingiva at the MGJ to the lip, cheek, or undersurface of the tongue. A frenum serves to restrict movement.
  • *Locations*
    • Maxillary and mandibular anterior frena: At midlines between central incisors. Figure 18-7 shows the location of the maxillary anterior frena.
    • Lingual frenum: Connects undersurface of the tongue to the floor of the mouth.
    • Buccal frena: In the canine–premolar areas, both maxillary and mandibular.
  • *Attachment of frena in relation to the attached gingiva*
  • Closely associated with the MGJ.
  • When the attached gingiva is narrow or missing, the frena may pull on the free gingiva and displace it laterally. A "tension test" is used to locate frenal attachments and check the adequacy of the attached gingiva (Chapter 20).

II. Periodontal Ligament

The periodontal ligament (PDL) is the fibrous connective tissue that surrounds and attaches the alveolar bone to the cementum (Figure 18-8).

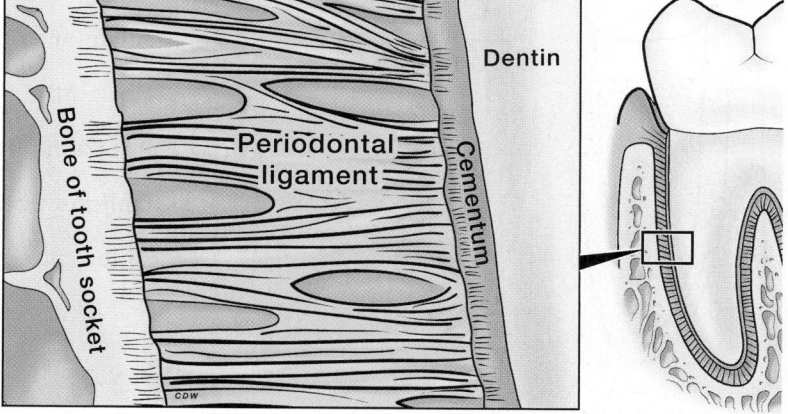

Dentin

Bone of tooth socket

Periodontal ligament

Cementum

FIGURE 18-8 • Periodontal Ligament. On tooth side, the ends of the periodontal ligament fibers are anchored in the cementum of the root. On the bone side, the ends of the periodontal ligament fibers are anchored in the alveolar bone of the tooth socket.

- The PDL acts as an interface between bone and tooth and allows for movement to distribute the chewing or masticatory forces.[11]
- It is composed of cells and an extracellular compartment.[1]
  - Cells include osteoblasts, osteoclasts, fibroblasts, epithelial cells, and cementoblasts.
  - The extracellular compartment contains collagen fiber bundles in a ground substance.
- The fibers are inserted into the cementum on one side and the alveolar bone on the other are called Sharpey's fibers.
- The two general groups of fibers are the *gingival groups* (Figure 18-9) (around the cervical area within the gingival tissues) and the *principal fiber groups* (surrounding the root).[1]

A. Gingival Fiber Groups

- *Dentogingival fibers* (free gingiva): from the cementum in the cervical region into the free gingiva to give support to the gingiva.
- *Alveologingival fibers* (attached gingiva): from the alveolar crest into the free and attached gingiva to provide support.
- *Circumferential fibers* (circular): continuous around the neck of the tooth to help to maintain the tooth in position.
- *Dentoperiosteal fibers* (alveolar crest): from the cervical cementum over the alveolar crest to blend with fibers of the periosteum of the bone.
- *Transseptal fibers*: from the cervical area of one tooth across to an adjacent tooth (on the mesial or distal only) to provide resistance to separation of teeth.

B. Principal Fiber Groups

The five principal groups of collagen fibers (Figure 18-10) are named for their location on the root and for their direction. They are also called the dentoalveolar fiber groups.

- *Apical fibers*: extend from the root apex to adjacent surrounding bone to resist vertical forces.

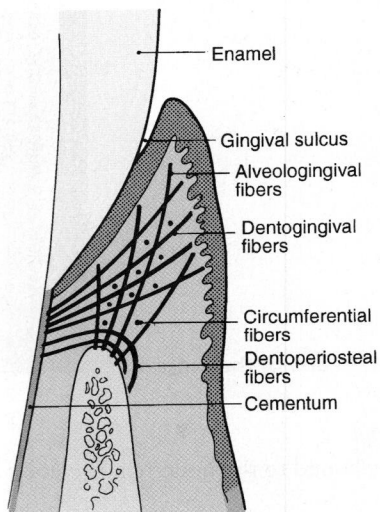

FIGURE 18-9 • Gingival Fiber Groups. Cross section of the gingiva shows the relation of the gingival fiber groups to the gingival sulcus, free gingiva, cementum, and alveolar bone.

- *Oblique fibers*: extend obliquely from the cementum to bone in a coronal direction and are the majority of the principal fibers. They help the tooth to resist vertical and unexpected strong forces.[12]
- *Horizontal fibers*: from the cementum in the middle of each root to adjacent alveolar bone to resist tipping of the tooth.
- *Alveolar crest fibers*: from the alveolar crest to the cementum just below the CEJ to resist intrusive forces.
- *Interradicular fibers*: from cementum between the roots of multi-rooted teeth to the adjacent bone to resist vertical and lateral forces.

III. Cementum

The cementum is a thin layer of calcified connective tissue that covers the tooth from the CEJ to, and around, the apical foramen.

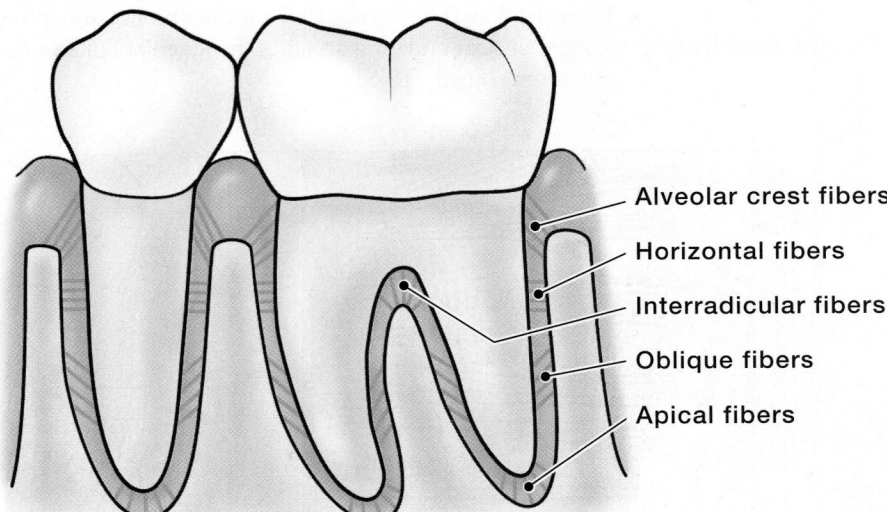

Alveolar crest fibers

Horizontal fibers

Interradicular fibers

Oblique fibers

Apical fibers

FIGURE 18-10 • Principal Fiber Groups of the Periodontium. The five principal groups (apical, oblique, horizontal, alveolar crest, and interradicular) are shown. The transseptal fibers of the gingival fiber groups are also shown as they span across from the cervical area of one tooth to the neighboring tooth.

A. Functions

◆ Supports the tooth along with the alveolar bone by serving as the attachment for periodontal fiber groups of the PDL.[13]
◆ Seals the tubules of the root dentin.

B. Characteristics

◆ Thickness is 50–200 μm.[13]
◆ Thickness of cementum increases with age.
◆ Two types of cementum:[12]
  • Acellular cementum is on the cervical half to two-thirds of the root and serves as a place for attachment of the PDL fibers.
  • Cellular cementum is found primarily on the apical half or third of the root and serves as a repair tissue to fill defects.
◆ Relationship of enamel and cementum at the cervical area is shown in Figure 18-11. Estimates for the relationship of enamel to cementum are as follows:
  • A gap between cementum and enamel exposing dentin in 10–40% of teeth.
  • Enamel and cementum meet edge-to-edge in 50–70% of the teeth.
  • The cementum overlaps the enamel in approximately 7–14%.[14]

IV. Alveolar Bone

The alveolar bone is a specialized part of the mandibular and maxillary bones with a primary function to support the teeth.
◆ *Description*
  • Alveolar bone undergoes rapid and continual remodeling due to the demands of tooth eruption, orthodontic tooth movement, and occlusal forces.[15]

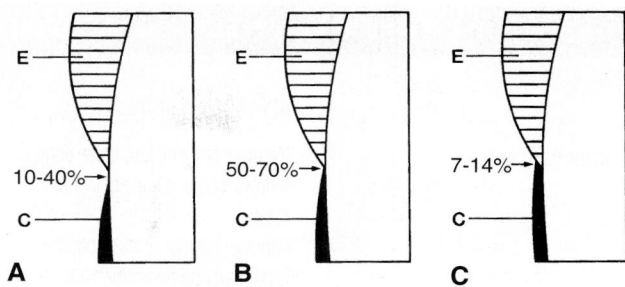

FIGURE 18-11 • Relationship of Enamel and Cementum. The possible relationships of the enamel and the cementum of the cementoenamel junction. **A:** The cementum and the enamel do not meet, and there is a small zone of dentin exposed in 10%–40% of teeth. **B:** The cementum meets the enamel in approximately 50%–70% of teeth. **C:** The cementum overlaps the enamel in 7%–14% of teeth.

  • The architecture is similar to other bone tissues, but the rate of bone remodeling is unique to alveolar bone.[15]
  • When teeth are lost, the alveolar bone is progressively resorbed.

THE GINGIVAL DESCRIPTION

The examination of the gingiva includes evaluation of color, size, shape, consistency, surface texture, position, MGJs, bleeding, and exudate. These are summarized in Table 18-1, which can be used as a clinical reference chart. Figure 18-12A and B show an image of healthy gingiva, and Figure 18-12C shows gingiva exhibiting signs of disease (gingivitis).

TABLE 18-1 • Examination of the Gingival Clinical Markers

	APPEARANCE IN HEALTH	CHANGES IN DISEASE CLINICAL APPEARANCE	CAUSES FOR CHANGES
Color	Uniformly pale pink or coral pink Variations in pigmentation related to complexion, race	Acute: bright red Chronic: bluish pink, bluish red Attached gingiva: color change may extend to the mucogingival line	Inflammation Capillary dilation Increased blood flow Vessels engorged Blood flow sluggish Venous return impaired Anoxemia Increased fibrosis Deepening of pocket, mucogingival involvement
Size	Not enlarged Fits snugly around the tooth	Enlarged	Edematous: inflammatory fluid, cellular exudate, vascular engorgement, hemorrhage Fibrotic: new collagen fibers

(Continues)

TABLE 18-1 • Examination of the Gingival Clinical Markers (*Continued*)

	APPEARANCE IN HEALTH	CHANGES IN DISEASE CLINICAL APPEARANCE	CAUSES FOR CHANGES
Shape (contour)	Marginal gingiva: flat, knife-edged, follows a curved line about the tooth Papillae: normal contact: papilla is pointed and pyramidal; fills the interproximal area space (diastema) between teeth; gingiva is flat or saddle shaped	Marginal gingiva: rounded rolled Papillae: bulbous, flattened, blunted cratered	Inflammatory changes: edematous or fibrous **Bulbous** with gingival enlargement Cratered in necrotizing ulcerative gingivitis
Consistency	Firm Attached gingiva firmly bound down	Soft, spongy: dents readily when pressed with probe Associated with red color, smooth shiny surface, loss of stippling, bleeding on probing	Edematous: fluid between cells in connective tissue Fibrotic: collagen fibers
Surface texture	Free gingiva: smooth Attached gingiva: stippled	Acute condition: smooth, shiny gingiva Chronic: hard, firm, with stippling, sometimes heavier than normal	Inflammatory changes in the connective tissue; edema, cellular infiltration Fibrosis
Position of gingival margin	Fully erupted tooth: margin is 1–2 mm above CEJ, at or slightly below the enamel contour	Enlarged gingiva: margin is higher on the tooth, above normal, pocket deepened Recession: margin is more apical; root surface is exposed	Edematous or fibrotic JE has migrated along the root; gingival margin follows
Position of JE	During eruption along the enamel surface (Figure 18-6) Fully erupted tooth: the JE is at the CEJ	Position determined by the use of probe, is on the root surface	Apical migration of the epithelium along the root
Mucogingival junctions	Make clear demarcation between the pink, stippled, attached gingiva and the darker alveolar mucosa with smooth shiny surface	No attached gingiva: Color changes may extend full height of the gingiva; mucogingival line obliterated Probing reveals that the bottom of the pocket extends into the alveolar mucosa Frenal pull may displace the gingival margin from the tooth	Apical migration of the JE Attached gingiva decreases with pocket deepening Inflammation extends into alveolar mucosa
Bleeding	No spontaneous bleeding or upon probing	Spontaneous bleeding Bleeding on probing: bleeding near margin in acute condition; bleeding deep in pocket in chronic condition	Degeneration of the sulcular epithelium with the formation of pocket epithelium Blood vessels engorged Tissue edematous
Exudate	No exudate expressed on pressure or during probing	White, yellow, or green suppuration, visible on digital pressure or during probing Amount not related to pocket depth	Inflammation in the connective tissue Excessive accumulation of white blood cells with serum and tissue makes up the exudate (suppuration or pus)

CEJ, cementoenamel junction; JE, junctional epithelium.

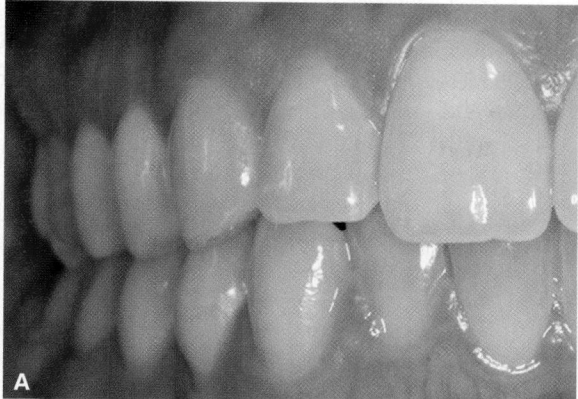

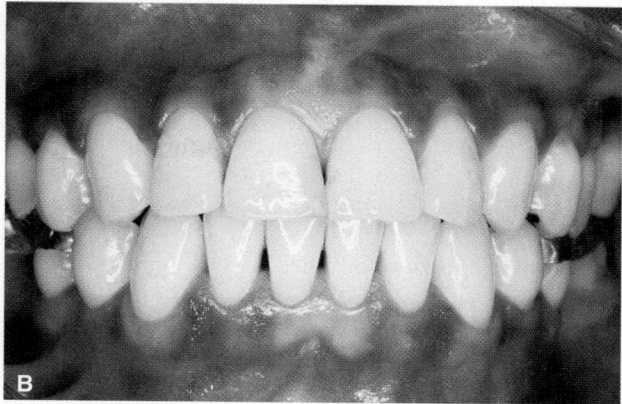

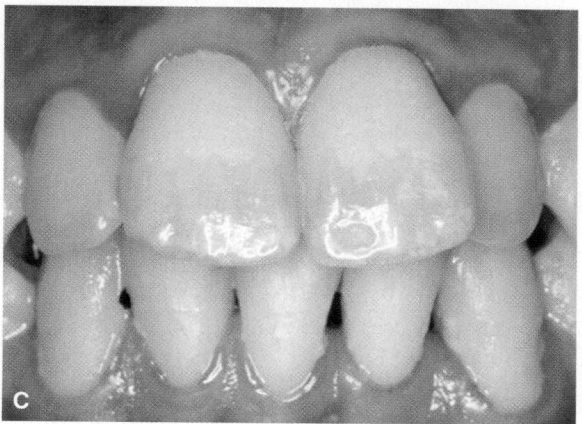

FIGURE 18-12 • Signs of Health. A: Health: Coral pink color, stippling is evident, gingival margins are knife-edged, and interdental papilla are pointed. **B:** Pigmentation of the gingiva showing how the gingiva can vary in color in some patients. Signs of disease. **C:** Pinkish-red color, loss of stippling, redness and enlargement of gingival margin, and interdental papilla are slightly bulbous in maxillary areas. (**A** and **C:** Reprinted from Nield-Gehrig J, Weiss G. *Fundamentals of Periodontal Instrumentation and Advanced Root Instrumentation.* 7th ed. Philadelphia, PA: Lippincott Williams & Wilkins; 2012.)

I. Color

A. Signs of Health

◆ *Pale pink:* Darker in people with darker complexions due to melanin pigmentation (Figure 18-12B).

◆ *Factors influencing color*
  • Vascular supply.
  • Thickness of epithelium.
  • Degree of keratinization.
  • Physiologic pigmentation: Melanin pigmentation frequently occurs in African Americans, Asians, Indians, and Caucasians of Mediterranean countries.

B. Changes in Disease

◆ *In chronic inflammation:* dark red, bluish red, magenta, or deep blue.

◆ *In acute inflammation:* bright red.

◆ *Extent:* Deep involvement can be expected when diffuse color changes extend into the attached gingiva, or from the marginal gingiva to the MGJ, or through into alveolar mucosa.

II. Size

A. Signs of Health

◆ *Free gingiva:* flat, not enlarged; fits snugly around the tooth.

◆ *Attached gingiva*

• Width of attached gingiva varies among patients and among teeth for an individual from 1–9 mm.[16]
• Wider in maxilla than mandible; broadest zone related to incisors, narrowest at the canine and premolar regions.

B. Changes in Disease

◆ *Free gingiva and papillae*
  • Become enlarged.
  • May be localized or limited to specific areas or generalized throughout the gingiva.
  • The col deepens as the papillae increase in size.

◆ *Attached gingiva:* decreases in amount as the pocket deepens.

C. Enlargement from Drug Therapy

◆ Certain drugs used for specific systemic therapy cause gingival enlargement as a side effect such as phenytoin, cyclosporine, and nifedipine.[17]

III. Shape (Form or Contour)

A. Signs of Health

◆ *Free gingiva*
  • Follows a curved line around each tooth; may be straighter along wide molar surfaces.
  • The margin is knife-edged or slightly rounded on facial and lingual gingiva; closely adapted to the tooth surface.

◆ *Papillae*
  • Facial and lingual gingiva are pointed or pyramidal papillae with a col area under the contact between adjacent teeth.
  • Spaced teeth (with diastemata). Interdental gingiva is flat or saddle shaped.

B. Changes in Disease

◆ *Free gingiva*: rounded or rolled.
◆ *Papillae*: blunted, flattened, bulbous, cratered (Figure 18-13A–C).
◆ "McCall's festoon": An enlargement of the marginal gingiva with the formation of a lifesaver-like gingival prominence. Frequently, the total gingiva is very narrow, with associated apparent recession, as shown in Figure 18-13D.

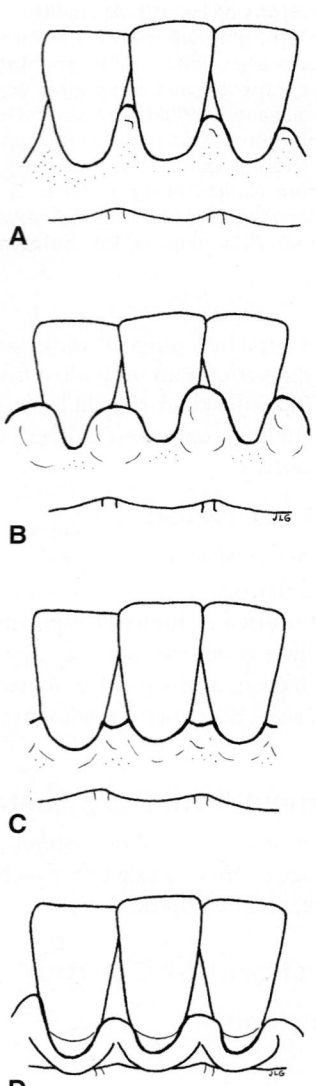

FIGURE 18-13 • Gingival Shape or Contour. A: Blunted papillae. **B:** Bulbous papillae. **C:** Cratered papillae. **D:** Rolled, lifesaver-shaped "McCall's festoons."

◆ "Stillman's cleft" (Figure 18-14A and B).
  • A localized recession may be V-shaped, apostrophe shaped, or form a slitlike indentation. It may extend several millimeters toward the MGJ or even to or through the junction.
◆ Floss cleft: A cleft created by incorrect floss positioning appears as a vertical linear or V-shaped fissure in the marginal gingiva and can result in bone loss if not corrected.[18]
  • Usually occurs at one side of an interdental papilla.
  • The injury can develop when dental floss is curved repeatedly in an incomplete "C" around the line angle so the floss is pressed across the gingiva.

IV. Consistency

A. Signs of Health

◆ Firm when palpated with the side of a blunt instrument (probe).
◆ Attached gingiva is bound down firmly to the underlying bone.

B. Changes in Disease

◆ *To determine consistency*: Gently press side of probe on free gingiva. Soft, spongy gingiva dents readily; firm, hard tissue resists.
◆ *Soft, spongy gingiva*: Related to acute stages of inflammation with increased infiltration of fluid and inflammatory elements.
  • The tissue appears red, may be smooth and shiny with loss of stippling.
  • Tissue may be **friable** or thin and fragile.
  • Has marginal enlargement and bleeds readily on probing.

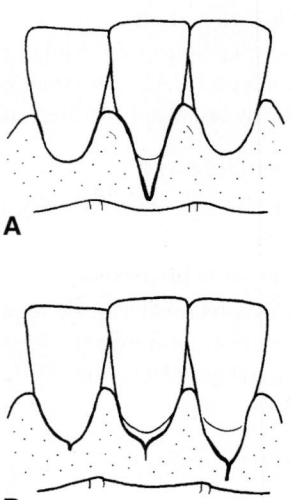

FIGURE 18-14 • Gingival Clefts. A: V-shaped Stillman's cleft. **B:** Slitlike Stillman's clefts of varying degrees of severity in relation to the mucogingival junction.

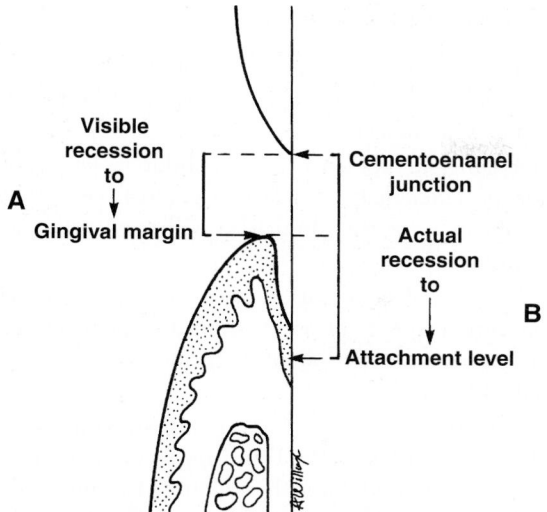

FIGURE 18-15 • **Gingival Recession. A:** Clinically visible recession of the gingival margin with root surface apparent to the eye. **B:** The actual recession exposes the root surface as the periodontal attachment migrates along the root surface.

◆ *Firm, hard gingiva*: Related to chronic inflammation with increased fibrosis.
  • The tissue may appear pink and well stippled.
  • Bleeding, when probed, usually occurs only in the deeper part of a pocket, not near the margin.
◆ *Retraction of the margin away from the tooth*: Normally, the free gingiva fits snugly about the tooth.
  • When the margin tends to hang slightly away or is readily displaced with a light air blast.
  • The gingival fibers that support the margin have been destroyed (Figure 18-15).

V. Surface Texture

A. Signs of Health

◆ *Free gingiva*: smooth.
  • *Attached gingiva*: stippled (minutely "pebbled" or "orange peel" surface).
  • *Interdental gingiva*: The free gingiva is smooth; the center portion of each papilla is stippled.

B. Changes in Disease

◆ *Inflammatory changes*: may be loss of stippling, with smooth, shiny surface.
◆ Hyperkeratosis: may result in a leathery, hard, or nodular surface.
◆ *Chronic disease*: Tissue may be hard and fibrotic, with a normal pink color and normal or deep stippling.

VI. Position

◆ The *actual* position of the gingiva is the level of the epithelial attachment. It is not directly visible but can be determined through periodontal probing.
◆ The *apparent* position of the gingiva is the level of the gingival margin or crest of the free gingiva that is seen by direct observation.

A. Signs of Health

For the fully erupted tooth in an adult, the apparent position of the gingival margin is at the level of, or slightly below, the enamel contour or prominence of the cervical third of a tooth.

B. Changes in Disease

◆ *Effect of gingival enlargement*: When the gingiva is enlarged, the gingival margin is coronal to the CEJ, partly or nearly covering the anatomic crown.
◆ *Effect of gingival recession*
  • Definition: Recession is the exposure of root surface resulting from the apical migration of the JE exposing the CEJ (Figure 18-15).
  • Actual recession: The actual recession is measured from the CEJ to the gingival margin.
  • Visible recession: Exposed root surface visible on clinical examination from the gingival margin to the CEJ.
  • Localized recession (Figure 18-16): A localized recession may be narrow or wide and deep or shallow. The root surface is denuded, and the visible recession may extend to or through the MGJ.
  • Measurement: Both actual and visible recession can be measured with a probe from the CEJ. Total recession is the distance from the CEJ to the bottom of the sulcus.

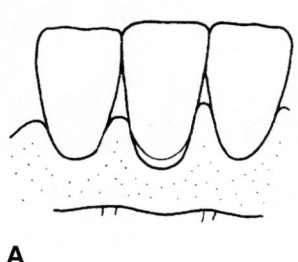
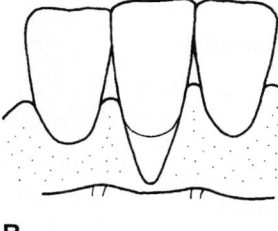
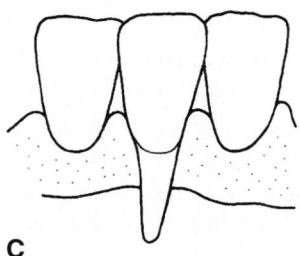

A   B   C

FIGURE 18-16 • **Localized Recession.** A single tooth may show narrow or wide, deep or shallow recession. **A:** Wide, shallow. **B:** Wide, deep, with narrow attached gingiva. **C:** Narrow, deep, with missing attached gingiva.

VII. Bleeding

A. Signs of Health

◆ Healthy gingival tissue does not bleed during periodontal probing.[19]

B. Changes in Disease

◆ Sulcular epithelium becomes a diseased *pocket epithelium*.

◆ The ulcerated pocket wall bleeds spontaneously or during periodontal probing.

VIII. Exudate

A. Signs of Health

There is no exudate in health.[7]

B. Changes in Disease

◆ Increased GCF in presence of inflammation with flow rate increasing as periodontal disease progresses.[7,20]

◆ Suppuration (or pus) is another indicator of active periodontal breakdown and may be seen in about 25% of patients with chronic periodontitis.[21]

THE GINGIVA OF YOUNG CHILDREN

I. Signs of Health

A. Primary Dentition

◆ *Color*: pink.

◆ *Shape*: thick, rounded, or rolled.

◆ *Consistency*: less fibrous than adult gingiva; not as tightly adapted to the teeth.

◆ *Surface texture*: may or may not have stippling; in children with healthy gingiva, stippling may be present in less than 50%.[22]

◆ *Attached gingiva*: width of attached gingiva in children is typically between 4 and 5 mm.[23]

◆ *Interdental gingiva*
  • Anterior: The maxillary midline diastema is present in the primary dentition in 97% of cases[24] and is considered normal; the papillae in areas of diastemas are flat or saddle shaped.
  • Posterior: Col between facial and lingual papillae when teeth are in contact (Figure 18-4A).

B. Mixed Dentition

◆ Constant state of change with periods of inflammation related to exfoliation and eruption.[25]

◆ Free gingiva may appear rolled or rounded, slightly reddened, shiny, and with a lack of firmness.

◆ The gingiva covers a varying portion of the anatomic crown, depending on the stage of eruption (Figure 18-6).

◆ Alveolar bone height varies during exfoliation and eruption and should be monitored until the dentition is fully erupted.[25]

◆ The attached gingiva width gradually increases as the crowns of the teeth erupt.[25]

II. Changes in Disease

◆ Gingivitis occurs frequently in children but is usually reversible with improved oral self-care without leaving permanent damage.

◆ Mucogingival problems occur in children. The recognition of deficiencies of attached gingiva has particular significance for the child who will need orthodontic treatment.[23]

◆ A periodontal examination is conducted at dental visits for early diagnosis of periodontal disease according to the Academy of Periodontology and American Academy of Pediatric Dentistry.[25–27]

◆ The British Society of Periodontology and the British Society of Paediatric Dentistry recommend the use of the Simplified Basic Periodontal Examination for screening of children and adolescents.[28]

THE GINGIVA AFTER PERIODONTAL SURGERY

I. Pocket Reduction Surgery

◆ The characteristics of "normal healthy gingiva" take on different dimensions for the patient who has completed treatment for pockets, bone loss, and other signs of a periodontal infection.

◆ The JE may be apical to the CEJ (see Figure 18-17).

◆ After healing, the sulcus depths may be within normal range and no bleeding occurs when probed.

◆ With each periodontal maintenance appointment, a thorough, careful examination is necessary to control factors that may permit recurrence of disease.

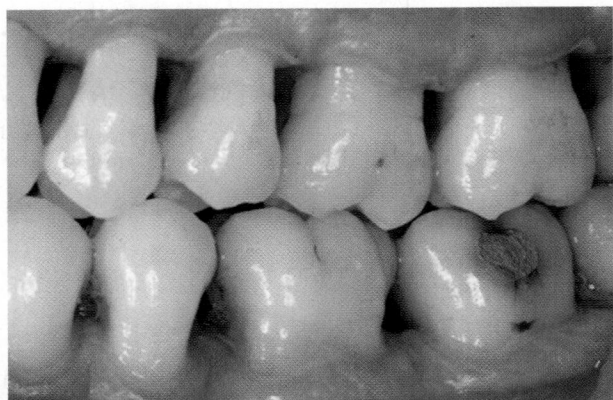

FIGURE 18-17 • Gingiva after Pocket Reduction Periodontal Surgery. The gingival margin is significantly apical to cementoenamel junction leading to exposure of the root surface and root concavities. The embrasures (space) between teeth is no longer filled by the papillae. (Reprinted from Nield-Gehrig J. *Fundamentals of Periodontal Instrumentation and Advanced Root Instrumentation.* 7th ed. Philadelphia, PA: Lippincott Williams & Wilkins; 2012.)

II. Gingival Grafting Surgery

◆ Depending on the exact type of gingival or connective tissue grafting surgery performed, examination shows changes from the initial evaluation.

  • For example, where the initial examination showed a deficiency of attached gingiva with frenal pull, mucogingival surgery may have created new attached gingiva.

III. Implant Surgery

◆ Gingiva around the implant should have the same color and consistency as gingiva surrounding a natural tooth (see Chapter 31).

◆ Contour of the gingiva will depend on the placement of the implant, but may result in open embrasures interproximally like those seen after pocket reduction surgery.

DOCUMENTATION

The permanent records of a patient who received treatment for a gingival or periodontal condition would have a minimum of the following:

◆ Health history with routine follow-up recorded for each visit.

◆ Initial charting and descriptive material to show disease symptoms with information to show need for and actual treatment carried out by a series of progress notes defining each appointment with changes identified resulting from specific treatment.

◆ Individual oral self-care instruction with biofilm scores to monitor progress. Any personal care products recommended, their demonstration, and report of use by the patient. Record of improvements in gingival health noted over the series of appointments.

◆ Patient's own comments related to oral health change, habit changes, dietary changes, all successes, along with an agreement to a recommended plan for a periodontal maintenance program.

◆ A progress note for an individual patient appointment may be read in Box 18-1.

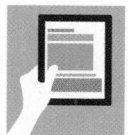

BOX 18-1

Example Documentation:
Description of the Periodontium

S—55-year-old Hispanic female presents for continuing care appointment with chief complaint of bleeding when she brushes her teeth.

O—Gingival description: color: normal pigmentation, generalized dark reddish inflammation of free gingival margin. Size: general slight enlargement of interdental papilla. Shape: bulbous areas in maxillary anterior. Consistency: generally soft and spongy, shiny surface, generalized bleeding on probing. Probing depths generally 3–4 mm. Biofilm score: 50%.

A—Diagnosis is plaque-induced gingivitis.

P—Oral biofilm was disclosed and patient demonstrated toothbrushing and flossing technique. Review of modified Bass technique was provided to assist in accessing biofilm along gingival margins. Floss technique was good, but the patient needs to be more consistent flossing daily. Treatment goals: (1) brush 2×/day, (2) flossing daily, and (3) reduce bleeding on probing by 20%. Subgingival debridement and prophylaxis completed. Five percent sodium fluoride varnish applied because of moderate caries risk. Next visit: 6 month continuing care.

Signed: _____, RDH

Date: _____

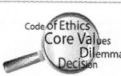

EVERYDAY ETHICS

Britain and Nicholas were first-year dental hygiene students just beginning to practice on each other as student partners in the preclinical program. Today their clinical practice was to provide the description of each other's gingiva; the next session would be learning to use the probe for the periodontal examination. Nicholas told her his "gums bled when he brushed." As she began, the gingiva seemed soft and loose, but Britain was not sure she understood what is "normal" when she remembered that her instructor had referred to a "range" of normal.

Britain decided to focus on and document the areas that looked pink with pointed papillae in the interproximal areas. She carefully recorded this information with great detail and then signaled for her instructor to verify the findings. When the instructor reviewed the examination, she was pleased with Britain's thoroughness. The instructor provided positive feedback and quickly moved on to the next pair of students. Britain began to feel uneasy that she had not described the characteristics of the gingival tissues that she thought were not normal.

Questions for Consideration

1. Which of the core values have application in this scenario? How and why?

2. Describe the instructor's role in guiding Britain to help her identify signs of disease along with the areas of normal tissue.

3. Ethically, what alternatives or actions can Britain take at this time to address the "uneasy" feeling she has about Nicholas' gingival status?

Factors to Teach the Patient

▶ Role and responsibility for self-management of periodontal disease.

▶ Characteristics of normal healthy gingiva.

▶ The significance of bleeding; healthy tissue does not bleed.

▶ Relationship of findings during a gingival examination to the daily oral self-care procedures for infection control.

▶ The special attention needed for an area of gingival recession to prevent abrasion, inflammation, and further involvement.

▶ How the brushing method, stiffness of toothbrush filaments, abrasiveness of a dentifrice, and pressure applied during brushing can be factors in gingival recession.

ENHANCE YOUR UNDERSTANDING

ONLINE RESOURCES
(see the inside front cover for access information)

- Audio glossary
- Appendices

SUPPORT FOR LEARNING
(available separately)

- *Active Learning Workbook for Wilkins' Clinical Practice of the Dental Hygienist, 13th Edition*

INDIVIDUALIZED REVIEW

- Customized practice quizzing with Navigate 2 TestPrep for *Wilkins' Clinical Practice of the Dental Hygienist*

References

1. Nanci A, Bosshardt DD. Structure of periodontal tissues in health and disease. *Periodontol 2000*. 2006;40:11-28.

2. Bartold PM, Walsh LJ, Narayanan AS. Molecular and cell biology of the gingiva. *Periodontol 2000*. 2000;24(1):28-55.

3. Ainamo J, Loe H. Anatomical characteristics of gingiva. A clinical and microscopic study of the free and attached gingiva. *J Periodontol*. 1966;37(1):5-13.

4. Leblevicioglu B, Claman, L. Periodontal anatomy. In: Scheid RC, Weiss, G, eds. *Dental Anatomy*. 9th ed. Philadelphia, PA: Wolters Kluwer; 2016:215-248.

5. Orban B. Clinical and histologic study of the surface characteristics of the gingiva. *Oral Surg Oral Med Oral Pathol*. 1948;1(9):827-841.

6. Gupta G. Gingival crevicular fluid as a periodontal diagnostic indicator. II: Inflammatory mediators, host-response modifiers and chair side diagnostic aids. *J Med Life*. 2013;6(1):7-13.

7. Schroeder HE, Listgarten MA. The gingival tissues: the architecture of periodontal protection. *Periodontol 2000*. 1997;13(1):91-120.

8. Nordland WP, Tarnow DP. A classification system for loss of papillary height. *J Periodontol*. 1998;69(10):1124-1126.

9. Bosshardt DD, Lang NP. The junctional epithelium: from health to disease. *J Dent Res*. 2005;84(1):9-20.

10. Nugala B, Kumar BS, Sahitya S, Krishna PM. Biologic width and its importance in periodontal and restorative dentistry. *J Conserv Dent*. 2012;15(1):12-17.

11. Ho SP, Kurylo MP, Fong T, et al. The biomechanical characteristics of the bone-periodontal ligament-cementum complex. *Biomaterials*. 2010;31(25):6635-6646.

12. Cho MI, Garant PR. Development and general structure of the periodontium. *Periodontol 2000*. 2000;24:9-27.

13. Yamamoto T, Hasegawa. T, Yamamoto T, Hongo H, Amizuka, N. Histology of human cementum: Its structure, function, and development. *Jpn Dent Sci Rev*. 2016;52(3):63-74.

14. Astekar M, Kaur P, Dhakar N, Singh J. Comparison of hard tissue interrelationships at the cervical region of teeth based on tooth type and gender difference. *J Forensic Dent Sci*. 2014;6(2):86-91.

15. Sodek J, McKee MD. Molecular and cellular biology of alveolar bone. *Periodontol 2000*. 2000;24(1):99-126.

16. Lang NP, Loe, H. The relationship between the width of keratinized gingiva and gingival health. *J Periodontol*. 1972;43(10):623-627.

17. Trackman PC, Kantarci A. Molecular and clinical aspects of drug-induced gingival overgrowth. *J Dent Res*. 2015;94(4):540-546.

18. Hallmon WW, Waldrop TC, Houston GD, Hawkins BF. Flossing clefts. Clinical and histologic observations. *J Periodontol*. 1986;57(8):501-504.

19. Meitner SW, Zander HA, Iker HP, Polson AM. Identification of inflamed gingival surfaces. *J Clin Periodontol*. 1979;6(2):93-97.

20. Goodson JM. Gingival crevice fluid flow. *Periodontol 2000*. 2003;31:43-54.

21. Silva-Boghossian CM, Neves AB, Resende FA, Colombo AP. Suppuration-associated bacteria in patients with chronic and aggressive periodontitis. *J Periodontol*. 2013;84(9):e9-e16.

22. Bimstein E, Peretz B, Holan G. Prevalence of gingival stippling in children. *J Clin Pediatr Dent*. 2003;27(2):163-165.

23. Maynard JG, Jr., Ochsenbein C. Mucogingival problems, prevalence and therapy in children. *J Periodontol*. 1975;46(9):543-552.

24. Gkantidis N, Kolokitha OE, Topouzelis N. Management of maxillary midline diastema with emphasis on etiology. *J Clin Pediatr Dent*. 2008;32(4):265-272.

25. Drummond BK, Brosnan MG, Leichter JW. Management of periodontal health in children: pediatric dentistry and periodontology interface. *Periodontol 2000*. 2017;74(1):158-167.

26. Califano JV; Research, Science and Therapy Committee American Academy of Periodontology. Position paper: periodontal diseases of children and adolescents. *J Periodontol*. 2003;74(11):1696-1704.

27. AAPD. Guideline on periodicity of examination, preventive dental services, anticipatory guidance/counseling, and oral treatment for infants, children, and adolescents. *Pediatr Dent*. 2016;38(6):133-141.

28. Cole E, Ray-Chaudhuri A, Vaidyanathan M, Johnson J, Sood S. Simplified basic periodontal examination (BPE) in children and adolescents: a guide for general dental practitioners. *Dental Update*. 2014;41(4):328-337.

19

Periodontal Disease Development

Linda D. Boyd, RDH, RD, EdD, and Esther M. Wilkins, BS, RDH, DMD

CHAPTER OUTLINE

PERIODONTAL-SYSTEMIC DISEASE CONNECTION

RISK ASSESSMENT
I. Types of Factors Involved
II. Risk Assessment Tools

ETIOLOGY OF PERIODONTAL DISEASE

RISK FACTORS FOR PERIODONTAL DISEASES
I. Modifiable Risk Factors
II. Nonmodifiable Risk Factors
III. Local Factors

PATHOGENESIS OF PERIODONTAL DISEASES
I. Acute Inflammatory Response
II. Development of Gingival and Periodontal Infection

GINGIVAL AND PERIODONTAL POCKETS
I. Gingival Pocket or Pseudopocket
II. Periodontal Pocket
III. Tooth Surface Irregularities

COMPLICATIONS RESULTING FROM PERIODONTAL DISEASE PROGRESSION
I. Furcation Involvement
II. Mucogingival Involvement

THE RECOGNITION OF GINGIVAL AND PERIODONTAL INFECTIONS
I. The Clinical Examination
II. Signs and Symptoms
III. Causes of Tissue Changes

CLASSIFICATION OF PERIODONTAL HEALTH
I. Pristine Periodontal Health
II. Clinical Periodontal Health (Intact Periodontium)
III. Periodontal Disease Stability (Reduced Periodontium)
IV. Periodontal Disease Remission/Control (Reduced Periodontium)

CLASSIFICATION OF GINGIVITIS
I. Plaque (Biofilm)-Induced Gingivitis
II. Non-Plaque (Biofilm)-Induced Gingivitis

CLASSIFICATION OF PERIODONTITIS
I. Periodontal Classifications
II. Terminology for Staging Periodontitis
III. Terminology for Grading Periodontitis
IV. Steps to Staging and Grading the Periodontal Classification

ACUTE PERIODONTAL LESIONS
I. Periodontal Abscess
II. Necrotizing Periodontal Disease
III. Endo-Periodontal Lesions

DOCUMENTATION

EVERYDAY ETHICS

FACTORS TO TEACH THE PATIENT

REFERENCES

LEARNING OBJECTIVES

After studying this chapter, the student will be able to:

1. List and describe the modifiable and nonmodifiable risk factors for periodontal disease.

2. Explain the signs and symptoms of periodontal disease.

3. Define the stages of development for periodontal lesions.

4. Compare and contrast the staging and grading of periodontal disease in the current classification system.

5. Describe the dental hygienist's role in educating the patient about management of modifiable risk factors for periodontal disease.

The periodontium gives the support needed to maintain the teeth in function (Figure 19-1).

◆ Periodontal diseases are chronic diseases initiated by microorganisms in the dental biofilm, which collects on the teeth when oral self-care is inadequate.

PERIODONTAL-SYSTEMIC DISEASE CONNECTION

◆ There has been significant research on the association between periodontal infections and a number of systemic diseases and conditions including[1,2]:

- Cardiovascular disease.
- Adverse pregnancy outcomes, including premature low birth weight babies.
- Respiratory disease.
- Chronic kidney disease.
- Rheumatoid arthritis.
- Obesity.
- Cognitive impairment.
- Osteoporosis.
- Inflammatory bowel disease.
- Some cancers.

◆ Despite the association, periodontal disease has not been shown to *cause* systemic disease.

◆ The mechanism for the association is not yet clear, but infection and inflammation are common elements of all the diseases and conditions.[3]

◆ The association between periodontal infection and various systemic diseases/conditions makes it critical for early identification, treatment, and management of periodontal disease (infection) by dental and dental hygiene professionals as part of the interprofessional healthcare team.

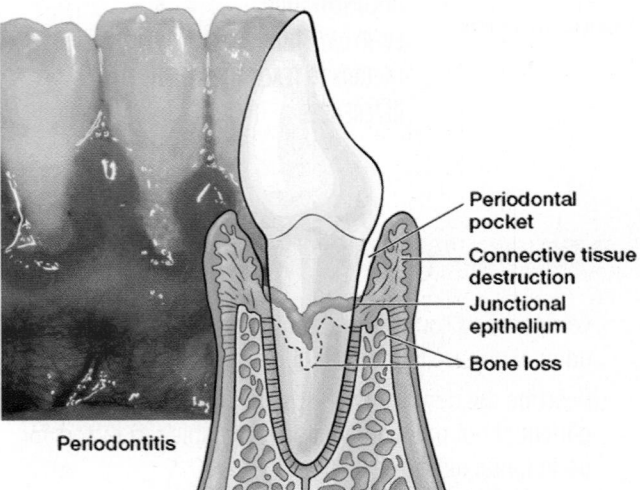

Periodontitis

Periodontal pocket
Connective tissue destruction
Junctional epithelium
Bone loss

FIGURE 19-1 • Clinical Changes in Periodontitis. Periodontitis is characterized by inflammation within the supporting tissues of the teeth, progressive destruction of the periodontal ligament, and loss of supporting alveolar bone.

RISK ASSESSMENT

I. Types of Factors Involved

Complicating and risk factors for disease development may be etiologic, predisposing, or contributing. They are delineated as follows:

◆ *Etiologic factor:* the actual cause of a disease or condition.

◆ *Predisposing factor:* renders a person susceptible to a disease or condition.

◆ *Contributing factor:* lends assistance to, supplements, or adds to a condition or disease.

◆ *Risk factor:* increases the probability that disease will occur.

◆ Etiologic, predisposing, and contributing factors may be local or systemic, defined as follows:

- *Local factor:* a factor in the immediate environment of the oral cavity or specifically in the environment of the teeth and periodontium.
- *Systemic factor:* a factor that results from or is influenced by a general physical or mental disease or condition.

II. Risk Assessment Tools

◆ Risk assessment identifies the level of likelihood for developing and progression of periodontal disease and is an integral part of individualizing preventive strategies and periodontal treatment.[4,5]

◆ Risk assessment may reduce the need for more advanced periodontal therapy and improve patient outcomes to reduce oral healthcare costs.[4]

◆ Examples of periodontal risk assessment (PRA) tools:

- Periodontal risk calculator (PRC) is a Web-based risk assessment tool that uses known factors such as smoking history, diagnosis of diabetes, and periodontal history and status to predict risk for periodontal disease and has shown a high level of accuracy in a 15-year study.[4,6,7]
- A Periodontal Risk Assessment (PRA) tool based on tooth loss, genetic, and systemic conditions and periodontal status can also be located on the Internet at www.perio-tools.com/pra/en/ and has been shown to predict the progression of periodontal disease.[4,8]

◆ Risk assessment can be used to educate the patient about the level of risk and the factors that can be modified. The patient can use the tools to manage their personal disease risk.

◆ The clinician uses the risk assessment information to identify the modifiable risk factors to be addressed in the treatment plan.

ETIOLOGY OF PERIODONTAL DISEASE

◆ Microorganisms in the form of subgingival biofilms forming communities called microbiomes are the primary etiologic agents of periodontal disease/infection.[4,9]

- The microbiome complexity and diversity increases in periodontitis when compared to health.[9]
- The microbiome of gingivitis is not the same as in periodontitis.[9]
- The type of organisms shifts to gram-negative anaerobic species including *Porphyromonas gingivalis* and *Tannerella forsythia* (previously known as *Bacteroides forsythus*), *Treponema denticola*, and *Fretibacterium* species.[9]

RISK FACTORS FOR PERIODONTAL DISEASES

- Identification of risk factors for periodontal diseases can provide significant insight into assessment and care planning for an individual patient.
- The various periodontal pathogenic microorganisms do not affect all people with the same degree of severity. It is clear that host factors play a significant role.[2]

I. Modifiable Risk Factors

- The common risk factors for periodontal disease and systemic disease include tobacco exposure, diabetes, metabolic syndrome (MetS), obesity, diet, and excess alcohol intake.[3]
  - These are all modifiable risk factors; however, most require a interprofessional collaboration with medical providers.

A. Tobacco Use

- The evidence provides strong that support smoking as an independent risk factor for periodontal disease (see Figure 19-2).[3,10]
  - Evidence is emerging to show that cannabis or marijuana use is associated with more severe periodontitis.[11]
- The odds for developing periodontal disease in people who smoke range from three to seven times higher than in nonsmokers.[10]

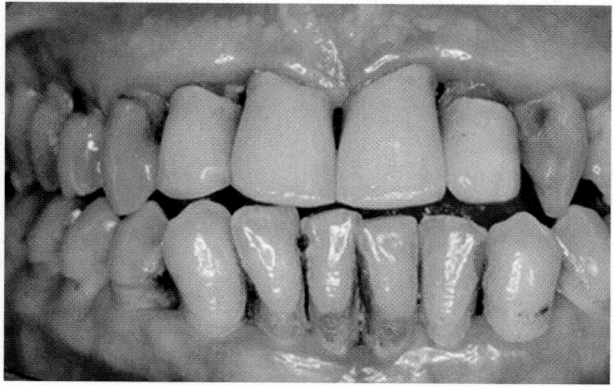

FIGURE 19-2 • Attachment (Bone Loss) in Smoker. A 58-year-old female, cigarette smoker of 20 pack years with advanced periodontitis. Note that clinical signs of inflammation, such as marginal redness, are minimal. The teeth are discolored due to nicotine deposits.

- More than 40% of cases of periodontitis are a result of cigarette smoking.[10]
- Periodontal treatment may be less effective in smokers than in those who do not smoke.
- Users of smokeless tobacco products experience oral effects, including predisposition to oral cancer. Periodontal lesions with severe recession and clinical attachment loss (CAL) occur where the quid is held.[12]

B. Diabetes Mellitus

- Periodontal disease and diabetes mellitus have a bidirectional relationship, meaning a patient who does not control blood glucose is more likely to have more severe periodontal disease.[13]
- Poor control of blood glucose (glycemic control) increases the risk of developing periodontal disease and results in poor outcomes to treatment.[3,13,14]
- As a result of the increase in diabetes in the U.S. population, there is an increase in prevalence of periodontitis in children and adolescents with type 1 diabetes mellitus.[15]
- Although diabetes is a chronic disease, research suggests management of periodontal infection results in improvement in control of blood glucose.[3,16]

C. Metabolic Syndrome

- MetS is a group of risk factors for heart disease and diabetes that includes hypertension, hyperglycemia, excess abdominal fat, and high cholesterol/triglycerides.
- A systematic review and meta-analysis found individuals with MetS are 38% more likely to have periodontitis.[3,17]
- MetS increases risk of periodontal disease.[3,17]

D. Obesity

- Obesity prevalence is about 40% in the United States and continues to increase resulting in a major public health problem.[18]
- Obesity, overweight, weight gain, and increased waist circumference are emerging as risk factors for periodontal disease in adults, adolescents, and children.[3,19,20]
- The odds of having periodontal disease in obese and overweight individuals is doubled.[3]

E. Alcohol Consumption

- Alcohol intake is associated with an increased risk for periodontal disease.[21]
- The risk in women was doubled and for men the risk was 25% greater for periodontal disease with heavy alcohol (>30 grams/day or >2 standard drinks) consumption.[22]

F. Diet

- Macronutrient and micronutrient intake may be modifying factors in periodontal disease.[3,23]
  - Macronutrient intake such as high carbohydrate intake impacts glycemic control and may be involved

in initiation of the inflammatory state in periodontal disease.[23]

- Micronutrient deficiencies, such as vitamin C, vitamin D or vitamin B12, may impact onset, healing, and progression of periodontal disease.[23]

G. Psychosocial Factors

- Some research suggests individuals under psychological stress, anxiety, or depression are more likely to have periodontal disease.[3,24]
  - The association may be related to the impact on the immune response as well as behavior changes.

H. Medications

- Medications for specific systemic conditions can lead to gingival enlargement.[10] The enlarged tissue encourages dental biofilm retention and complicate removal, thus increasing the potential for periodontal infections. These medications may or may not be modifiable in discussion with the medical provider.
  - *Phenytoin-induced gingival enlargement:* Phenytoin is a drug used to control seizures (see Figure 19-3).
  - *Cyclosporine-induced gingival enlargement:* Cyclosporine is an immunosuppressant drug used for patients with organ transplants to prevent rejection.
  - *Nifedipine-induced gingival enlargement:* Nifedipine is a calcium-channel blocker used in the treatment of angina and ventricular arrhythmias.
- Oral contraceptives with high doses of estrogen, progestin, or both.[10]

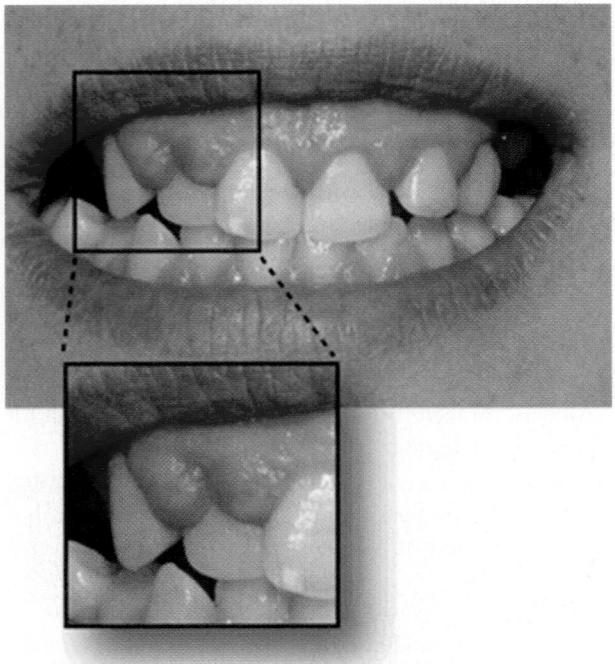

FIGURE 19-3 • Gingival Hyperplasia in Patient Treated with Phenytoin. (From Science Source, New York, NY.)

II. Nonmodifiable Risk Factors

A. Genetic Predisposition

- From 33 to 39% of the risk for periodontal disease is related to genetic factors.[10]
- Genetic testing is likely to become more cost effective and will benefit patients and dental providers in targeting those at risk for enhanced prevention.

B. Host Response

- Host response refers to the way an individual's immune response interacts with bacteria to resolve inflammation.
- Bacteria initiate an inflammatory response in periodontal disease and in susceptible individuals the body's immune response becomes chronic resulting in tissue destruction.[25]
- In addition to chronic diseases that impair the immune response, such as diabetes, genetic disorders associated with deficiencies in the immune system, such as Down syndrome, also result in a higher prevalence and severity of periodontal disease.[2,14]

C. Osteoporosis

- Research suggests an association between osteoporosis and periodontal disease with three times the risk of greater than 4 mm of CAL.[2,26]
- There was a five times greater risk of CAL greater than or equal to 6 mm.[26]
- In osteopenia, there was nearly a two times greater risk of greater than 4 mm of CAL.[26]

D. Age

- Age also is factored into the 2017 Periodontal grading system to take into consideration more severe periodontal disease at an earlier age.[14]
  - The grading of periodontitis is related to the potential for disease progression and will be described later in this chapter.

III. Local Factors

- Although dental biofilm is the primary etiologic factor in the development of inflammatory gingival and periodontal diseases, a variety of other factors predispose some patients to the retention of bacterial deposits and to the development of periodontal disease.[27]
  - Retentive areas may be associated with rough surfaces of teeth and restorations; tooth contour and position; and gingival size, shape, and position.
  - Iatrogenic causes, that is, factors created by professionals during patient treatment or neglect of proper treatment and can impact development and progression of periodontal disease.
  - Factors, such as mastication (chewing), saliva, the tongue, cheeks, lips, oral habits, and personal biofilm control procedures, contribute to retention.

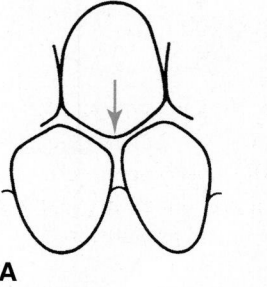 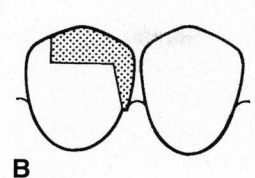 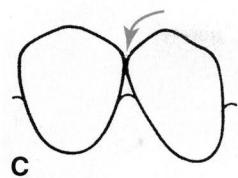 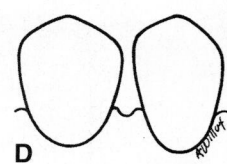

FIGURE 19-4 • Effect of Tooth Position. A: Food impaction area, shown by plunger cusp (with arrow) directing pressure between lower teeth with open contact area. **B:** Inadequate restoration without proximal contact and with overhang. **C:** Tipped tooth leaving irregular marginal ridge relation. **D:** Natural open contact (diastema) with saddle-shaped gingival margin.

A. Dental Factors

◆ Tooth surface irregularities: Pellicle and biofilm microorganisms attach to defective or rough surfaces include the following:

- Pits, grooves, cracks.
- Calculus.
- Exposed altered cementum with irregularities.
- Demineralization and cavitated dental caries.
- Iatrogenic factors such as rough or grooved surfaces left after scaling or inadequately contoured and polished dental restorations (Figure 19-4B).

◆ Tooth contour: Altered shape may interfere with oral self-cleansing mechanisms (see Chapters 16 and 27).

- *Congenital abnormalities*: extra or missing cusps or bell-shaped crown with prominent facial and lingual contours that tend to provide deeper retentive areas in the cervical third.
- Teeth with flattened proximal surfaces have faulty contact with adjacent teeth, thus permitting debris to wedge between the teeth.
- Occlusal and incisal surfaces altered by attrition interrupt normal excursion of food during chewing. Marginal ridges have worn down.
- Areas of erosion and abrasion.
- Carious lesions.
- Heavy calculus deposits; biofilm retained on rough surface.
- Overcontoured, undercontoured, or overhanging restorations (see Figure 19-5).

◆ Tooth position

1. *Malocclusion*: Irregular alignment of a single tooth or groups of teeth leaves areas prone to collection of biofilm formation.

- Crowded or overlapped.
- Rotated.
- Deep anterior overbite (Chapter 16).
- Mandibular teeth force food particles against maxillary lingual surface.
- Lingual inclination of mandibular teeth allows maxillary teeth to force food particles against mandibular facial gingiva.

2. Tooth adjacent to edentulous area may be inclined or migrated; contact missing.

3. When an opposing tooth is missing, the tooth may extrude beyond the line of occlusion.

4. *Related to eruption*

- Incomplete eruption: the teeth do not erupt into the line of occlusion.
- Partially erupted impacted third molar.

5. Lack of function or the use of teeth eliminates or decreases effectiveness of natural cleansing:

- Lack of opposing teeth.
- Open bite (Figure 19-6).
- Marked maxillary anterior protrusion.
- Crossbite with limited lateral excursion.
- Unilateral chewing.

6. *Food impaction*

- Created by the combined effect of tooth contour, missing proximal contact, proximal carious lesions, and irregular marginal ridge relationship.
- Inclination related to loss of adjacent tooth and a plunger cusp from the opposite arch (Figure 19-4A).

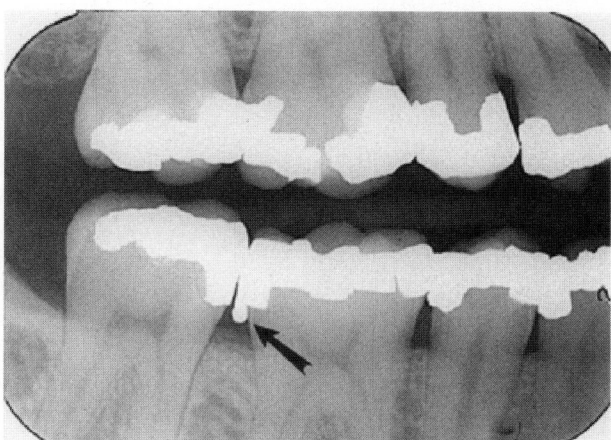

FIGURE 19-5 • Restoration with an Overhang. The distal surface of the mandibular first molar in this radiograph has a faulty restoration that creates a food trap and harbors biofilm.

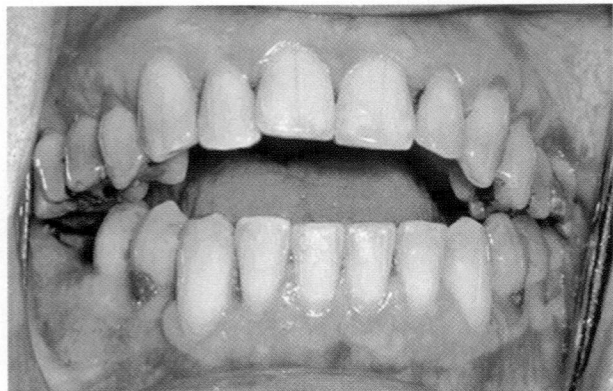

FIGURE 19-6 • **Anterior Open Bite.**

7. *Defective contact area*
- Restoration margin is faulty, and the contact area is missing, improperly located, or unnaturally wide (Figure 19-4B).
- Inclined tooth with irregular marginal ridge relation (Figure 19-4C).
- Dental appliances and prostheses
- Orthodontic appliances provide retentive areas (see Figure 19-7).
- Fixed partial denture with deficient margin on an abutment tooth or an unusually shaped pontic.
- Removable partial denture with poorly fitting clasps.

B. Gingival Factors

- *Position*
- Deviations from normal provide retentive areas for biofilm.
- *Gingival recession*: may expose root irregularities that serve as areas for biofilm retention.
- *Enlarged gingival margin or papillae*: extended to or over the height of contour.

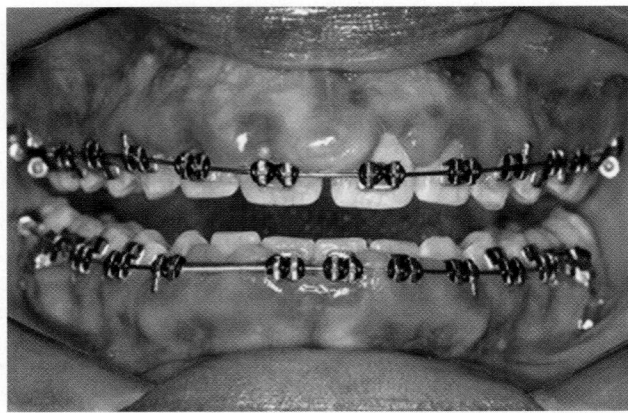

FIGURE 19-7 • **Orthodontic Appliances as a Predisposing Factor for Periodontal Disease.** Infrequent oral self-care and biofilm accumulation resulted in periodontitis in this individual with orthodontic appliances. (Courtesy of Dr. Richard Foster, Guilford Technical Community College, Jamestown, NC.)

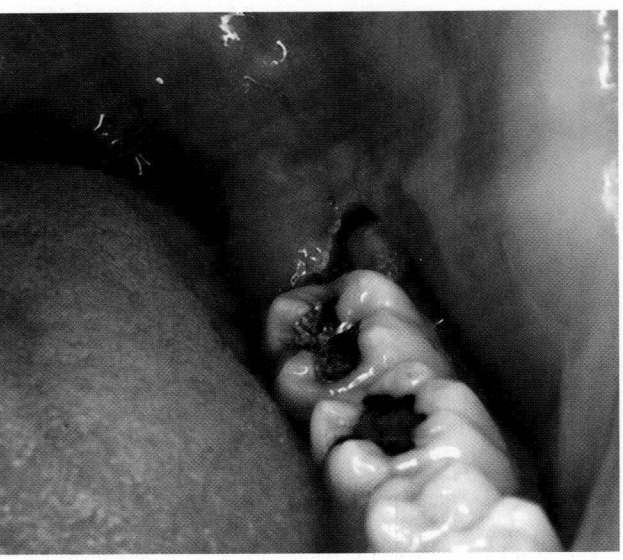

FIGURE 19-8 • **Operculum Is a Flap of Tissue over a Partially Erupted Third Mandibular Molar.** This flap makes removal of biofilm difficult and may lead to inflammation and infection. (Courtesy of Dr. Carl Allen.)

- Reduced height of interdental papilla creating an open interdental area.
- Operculum: Tissue flap over occlusal surface of an erupting tooth (Figure 19-8).
- *Periodontal pocket*: Depth and shape can make biofilm removal difficult.
- Calculus creating a rough retentive surface.
- *Size and contour*
- Deviation of shape of enlarged gingiva: rolled, bulbous, and cratered.
- Combination with presence of irregular restorations or dental prosthesis can result in marked biofilm retention.
- *Effect of Mouth Breathing*
- Dehydration of oral tissues in the anterior region leads to changes in size, shape, surface texture, and consistency.

C. Other Factors

A variety of factors may predispose or contribute to the progression of periodontal infections. Some of the items listed here may have an indirect effect, whereas others have a direct effect on the oral tissues.
- Personal oral self-care[28]
- *Neglect*: This can lead to generalized dental biofilm accumulation and disease promotion.
- *Inadequate biofilm control techniques*: Incorrect use of brush and interdental cleaning aids.
- *Awareness of oral cleanliness*: Cleansing habits, including both self-cleansing mechanisms and mechanical biofilm removal, depend in part on an individual's perception and feeling of debris through taste and tongue activity. This can become impaired in individuals with some conditions like poststroke.

◆ Diet and eating habits.[29]

- Soft foods tend to be less nutrient dense and more retentive than fibrous, firm foods.
- Masticatory deficiencies limit diet selection. Missing teeth, ill-fitting partial dentures, and various occlusal deficiencies alter diet selection and eating habits.

PATHOGENESIS OF PERIODONTAL DISEASES

Pathogenesis refers to the process by which a disease develops and progresses. The primary etiology of periodontal disease is bacteria that initiate an inflammatory process.

◆ The inflammatory process is very complex and influenced by patient and environmental factors and progression of disease is impacted by the individual's response to the bacterial challenge.[30–32]

I. Acute Inflammatory Response

◆ When the immune response is working effectively with no disease modifiers, that is, diabetes or smoking, the presence of biofilm results in gingival inflammation with no breakdown of tissue.[30–32]

◆ Activation of the local acute inflammatory response begins the process of lesion development.

II. Development of Gingival and Periodontal Infection

The stages of development of gingivitis and periodontitis are divided into the *initial lesion*, *early lesion*, *established lesion*, and *advanced lesion*.[30,32] With an accumulation of dental biofilm on the cervical tooth surface adjacent to the gingival margin, an inflammatory reaction is initiated, and the immune system responds.

A. The Initial Lesion

◆ Inflammatory response to dental biofilm[30,32]

- Occurs within 2–4 days in response to bacterial accumulation.
- Migration and infiltration of white blood cells (neutrophils) into the junctional epithelium and gingival sulcus result from the natural body response to infectious agents.
- Increased flow of gingival crevicular fluid.
- Early breakdown of collagen of the supporting gingival fiber groups (Chapter 18).
- Fluid fills the spaces in the connective tissue.

◆ Clinical appearance

- No clinical evidence of change may appear in the earliest phases.
- Marginal redness with enlargement due to the fluid collection follows as the infection develops.

B. The Early Lesion

◆ Increased inflammatory response[30,32]

- Dental biofilm becomes older and thicker (7–14 days; time reflects individual differences).
- Infiltration of fluid, macrophages, T-cells, and neutrophils with a few plasma cells migrating into the connective tissue.
- Breakdown of collagen fiber support to the gingival margin.
- *Epithelium proliferates*: Epithelial extensions and rete ridges are formed.

◆ Clinical appearance

- Early signs of gingivitis become apparent with slight gingival enlargement; will become an established lesion if undisturbed.
- Early gingivitis is reversible when biofilm is controlled and inflammation is reduced. Healthy tissue may be restored.
- Susceptibility of individuals varies; time before lesion becomes established varies.

C. The Established Lesion

◆ Progression from the early lesion

- Migration of B-lymphocytes and plasma cells within connective tissue are characteristics of the established lesion.[30,32]
- Formation of *pocket epithelium*.
  1. Proliferation of the junctional and sulcular epithelium continues in an attempt to wall out the inflammation.
  2. Pocket epithelium is more permeable; areas of ulceration of the lining epithelium develop.
  3. Early pocket formation with bleeding on probing.
- Collagen destruction continues; connective tissue fiber support is lost.
- Progression to early periodontal lesion may occur or the established lesion may remain stable for extended periods of time.

◆ Clinical appearance

- Clear evidence of inflammation is present with marginal redness, bleeding on probing, and spongy marginal gingiva.
- This is followed by chronic fibrosis development.

D. The Advanced Lesion

◆ *Extension of inflammation*

- The two hallmarks of the advanced lesion include: alveolar bone resorption and collagen breakdown.[30,32] B-lymphocytes and plasma cells are thought to influence both these processes due to the cytokines released.[32]

◆ *Progressive destruction of connective tissue*

- Connective tissue fibers below the junctional epithelium are destroyed; the epithelium migrates along the root surface.

- Coronal portion of junctional epithelium becomes detached.
- Exposed cementum where Sharpey's fibers were attached becomes altered by the host response to the bacterial challenge.
- Diseased cementum contains a thin superficial layer of endotoxins from the bacterial breakdown.
- Without treatment, loss of attachment results with an increase in pocket depth.
- *Characteristics of the advanced lesion*
  - Pocket formation, bleeding, inflammation, and bone loss are all signs of periodontitis.
  - Persistence of the chronic inflammatory process; plasma cells predominate.
  - Junctional epithelium continues to migrate; lesion extends through connective tissue.
  - Periods of disease inactivity alternating with periods of activity.

GINGIVAL AND PERIODONTAL POCKETS

- The presence or absence of infection distinguishes a pocket from a sulcus and the level of attachment on the tooth distinguishes a gingival pocket from a periodontal pocket.
- A pocket has an *inner wall (the tooth surface)* and an *outer wall (the sulcular epithelium or pocket epithelium)* of the free gingiva. The two walls meet at the base of the pocket.
  - The base of the pocket is the coronal margin of the attached periodontal tissues.
  - Histologically, the base of a healthy sulcus is the coronal border of the junctional epithelium, whereas the base of a pocket (diseased sulcus) may be at the coronal border of the connective tissue attachment.
- *Substances found in a pocket*
  - Communication of the opening of the pocket with the oral cavity provides an opportunity for dental biofilm to collect.
  - The deeper the pocket, the more difficult it is to clean by toothbrushing or other biofilm control devices.
- The following may be found in a pocket:
  - *Microorganisms and their products*: enzymes, endotoxins, and other metabolic products.
  - Gingival crevicular fluid.
  - Desquamated epithelial cells.
  - Leukocytes, the numbers of which increase with increased inflammation in the tissues.
  - Purulent exudate made up of living and broken down leukocytes, living and dead microorganisms, and serum.
- Pockets are divided into *gingival* and *periodontal* types to clarify the degree of anatomic involvement.

- Periodontal pockets are further categorized by their position in relation to the alveolar bone, that is, whether their pocket base is suprabony or intrabony (Figure 19-9).

I. Gingival Pocket or Pseudopocket

- *Definition*: A pocket formed by gingival enlargement without apical migration of the junctional epithelium (Figure 19-9B).
- The margin of the gingiva has moved toward the incisal or occlusal without the deeper periodontal structures becoming involved.
- The tooth wall of the pocket is enamel.
- During eruption, the base of the sulcus is at various levels along the enamel. The base of the sulcus of a fully erupted tooth is near the cementoenamel junction.
- All gingival pockets are suprabony, that is, the base of the pocket is coronal to the crest of the alveolar bone.

II. Periodontal Pocket

- *Definition*: A pocket formed as a result of disease or degeneration causing apical migration of the junctional epithelium along the cementum.
- The periodontal deeper structures (attachment apparatus) are involved, that is, the cementum, periodontal ligament, and bone.
- The tooth wall of the pocket is cementum or partly cementum and partly enamel.
- The base of the pocket is on cementum at the level of attached periodontal tissue.
- Periodontal pockets may be suprabony or intrabony.
  - *Suprabony*: Pocket in which the base of the pocket is coronal to the crest of the alveolar bone (Figure 19-9A–C).
  - *Intrabony*: Pocket in which the base of the pocket is below or apical to the crest of the alveolar bone (Figure 19-9D). "Intra" means located within the bone. The term "infrabony" is used in some texts. "Infra" means under or beneath.

III. Tooth Surface Irregularities

- Supragingival tooth surface irregularities are detected by drying the surface and observing under adequate direct or indirect light; limited use of the sharp tip of an explorer is recommended.
- Subgingival examination is dependent, for the most part, on tactile and auditory sensitivity transmitted by a probe or an explorer.
- Causes of surface roughness on the enamel surface include the following:
  - Structural defects: cracks and grooves.
  - Demineralization; cavitated dental caries.
  - Calculus deposits and heavy stain deposits.

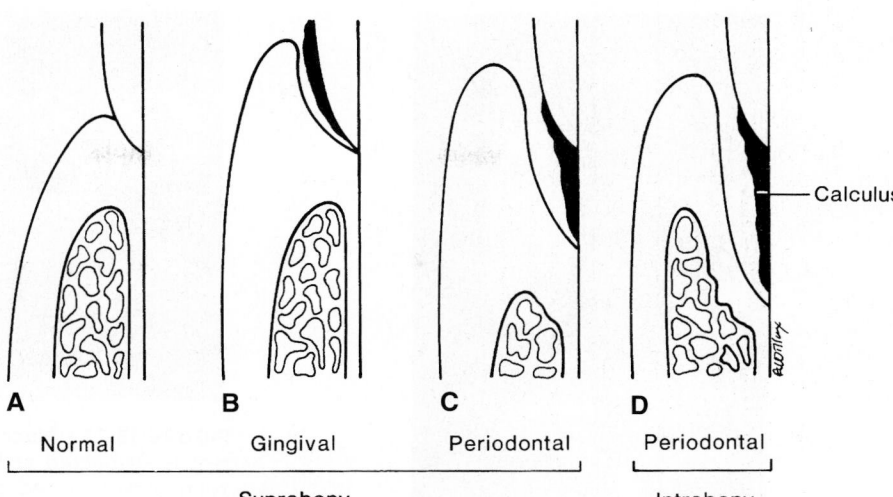

FIGURE 19-9 • **Types of Periodontal Pockets. A:** Normal relationship of the gingival tissue and the cementoenamel junction in a fully erupted tooth. **B:** Gingival pocket showing attachment at the cementoenamel junction and the pocket formed by enlarged gingival tissue. There is no bone loss. **C:** Periodontal pocket showing attachment on cementum with root surface exposed. Gingival tissue has enlarged. **D:** Periodontal intrabony pocket with the bottom of the pocket within the bone. See the text for further description of each type of pocket.

- Erosion, abrasion.
- Pits and irregularities from hypoplasia.
◆ *Root surface* irregularities
  - Diseased cementum.
  - Cemental resorption.
  - Root caries.
  - Abrasion.
  - Calculus.
  - Deficient or overhanging filling (see Figure 19-5).
  - Grooves from improper instrumentation.
◆ Irregularities at the *cementoenamel junction*
  - The relationships of enamel and cementum at the cementoenamel junction are shown in Chapter 18.

COMPLICATIONS RESULTING FROM PERIODONTAL DISEASE PROGRESSION

I. Furcation Involvement

Furcation involvement means the clinical attachment level and bone loss have extended into the furcation area between the roots of a multirooted tooth (see the Glickman furcation grades in Chapter 20 and Figure 19-10).

◆ Presence of furcation involvement increases the risk of tooth loss.[33]
  - It is difficult to adequately remove biofilm and calculus from the furcation area (see Figure 19-11) for both the dental hygienist and the patient who makes it challenging to manage the inflammation and infection in this area.

A. Clinical Observations

◆ When the gingiva over the furcation has not receded, the following may be seen:
  - The furcation is covered by the periodontal pocket wall.
  - No differences in color, size, or other tissue changes may exist to differentiate the area from adjacent gingiva, but when color changes do exist, they provide clues to guide further examination.
  - A radiolucency in the furcation area (sometimes called a furcation arrow) may be noted on the radiographs (Figure 19-12).
◆ When the gingiva over a molar furcation is receded, the root division may be seen directly (Figure 19-10).

B. Detection

A suggested procedure for probing furcation areas is described in Chapter 20.

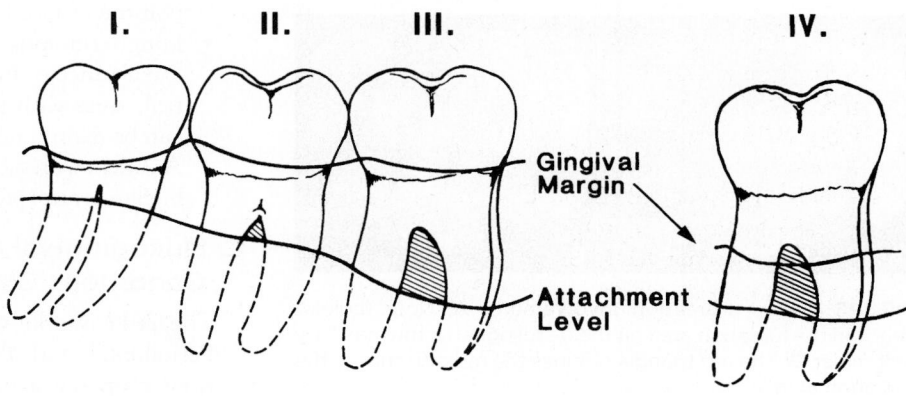

FIGURE 19-10 • **Classification of Furcations.** I: Early, beginning involvement. II: Moderate involvement, in which the furcation can be probed but not through and through. III: Severe involvement, when the bone between the roots is destroyed and a probe can be passed through. IV: Same as III, with clinical exposure resulting from gingival recession.

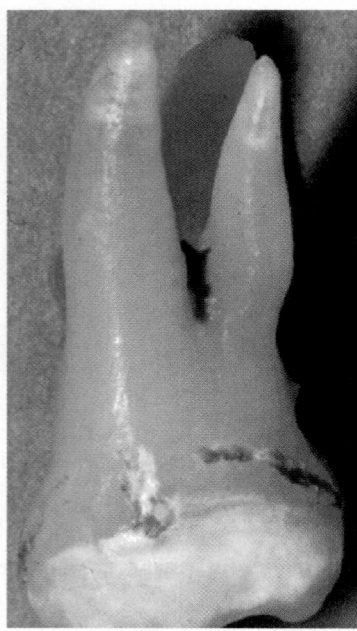

FIGURE 19-11 • Calculus in the Furcation Area and Root Depressions. This extracted molar has mineralized deposits (calculus) in the furcation. Once disease progresses into the furcation area, access for removal becomes difficult.

II. Mucogingival Involvement

A pocket that extends to or beyond the mucogingival junction and into the alveolar mucosa is described as *mucogingival involvement* (Figure 19-13). There is no attached gingiva in the area, and a probe can pass through the pocket and beyond the mucogingival junction into the alveolar mucosa.

A. Significance of Attached Gingiva

◆ Functions of attached gingiva
  • Give support to the marginal gingiva.
  • Withstand the frictional stresses of mastication and toothbrushing.
  • Provide attachment or a solid base for the movable alveolar mucosa for the action of the cheeks, lips, and tongue.
◆ Barrier to passage of inflammation

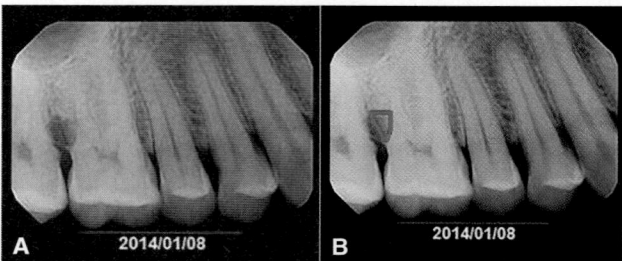

FIGURE 19-12 • Furcation Involvement. A: Note radiolucency in the furcation area on the distolingual of the maxillary first molar. **B:** The red triangle outlines the radiolucency in the furcation area.

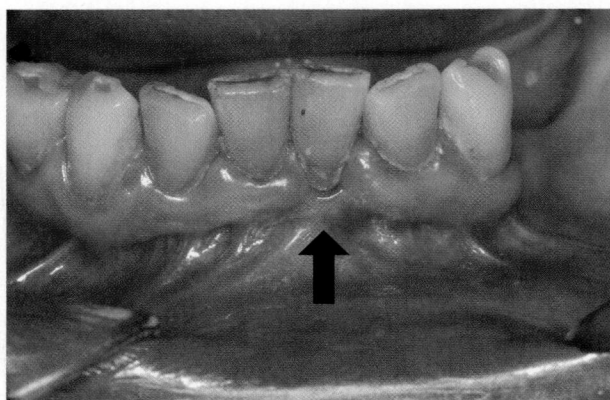

FIGURE 19-13 • Mucogingival Defect. A mucogingival defect is suspected at tooth #24, which has a very narrow zone of keratinized gingiva. (From Scheid RC. *Woelfel's Dental Anatomy: Its Relevance to Dentistry.* 7th ed. Philadelphia, PA: Lippincott Williams & Wilkins; 2007.)

  • The junctional epithelium (epithelial attachment) acts as a barrier to keep infection outside the body.
  • With destruction of the connective tissue and periodontal ligament fibers under the junctional epithelium, the epithelium migrates along the root.
  • In a patient with poor oral hygiene, lack of attached gingiva or keratinized tissue is a predisposing factor for inflammation and possible further gingival recession.[34,35]

B. Clinical Observations

◆ Color changes, tension test, and probe measurements are used during assessment of the mucogingival areas (see Chapter 20).
◆ *Thickness of attached gingiva:* In patients with a thin type of gingiva, the periodontal probe will be visible through the gingiva when probing and these individuals are at greater risk for gingival recession.[35]
◆ *Width of keratinized or attached gingiva:* current evidence suggests 1–2 mm of attached gingiva is desirable, although a minimal amount is not needed if the patient can execute optimal biofilm control at the site(s).[35]
  • When the attached gingiva measures 1–2 mm and there is no bleeding on probing or marginal inflammation, it is recorded and reevaluated at each continuing care or periodontal maintenance appointment (see Figure 19-14A and B).
  • Long-term, longitudinal studies have shown that in the absence of inflammation and good biofilm control, areas with a narrow band of attached gingiva can be maintained for long periods.[34]
  • A patient with such an area needs specific instruction in biofilm control procedures for preventive maintenance.

C. Mucogingival Deformities and Conditions Classification

◆ The 2017 World Workshop on the Classification of Periodontal and Peri-Implant Diseases and Conditions proposed a new classification for mucogingival

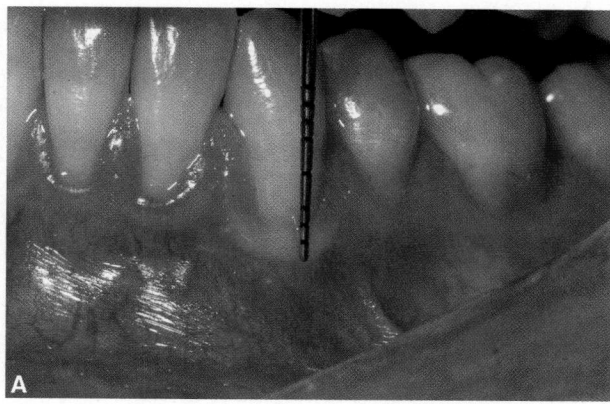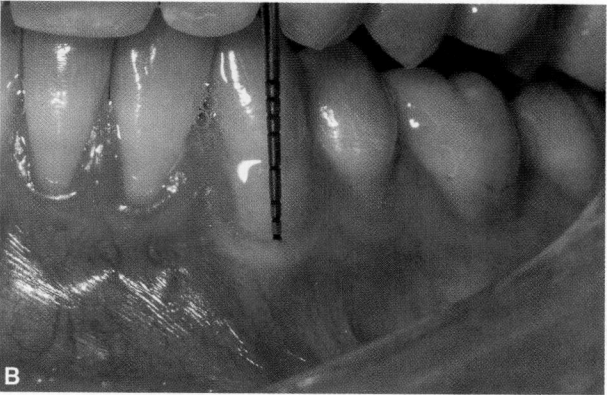

FIGURE 19-14 • Measuring for a Mucogingival Defect. A: The width of keratinized gingival is measured at 2 mm. **B:** The probe depth is measured at less than 2 mm (only 1 mm), indicating no mucogingival defect. If the probe depth reached or exceeded the mucogingival junction (exceeded the width of keratinized gingiva), there would be no attached gingiva, and a mucogingival defect would be present. (From Scheid RC. *Woelfel's Dental Anatomy: Its Relevance to Dentistry.* 7th ed. Philadelphia, PA: Lippincott Williams & Wilkins; 2007.)

conditions based more on treatment and potential for root coverage. It is quite complex and includes the following components[35]:

- Periodontal biotype related to the thickness of the gingiva, width of keratinized tissue, tooth dimension, and bone thickness.
- Gingival recession related to interdental CAL, facial/lingual attachment loss, severity, gingival thickness and width, cervical carious or non-carious lesions, hypersensitivity, and esthetic concerns.
- Lack of keratinized gingiva.
- Frenum position.
- Gingival excess.
- Abnormal color.

THE RECOGNITION OF GINGIVAL AND PERIODONTAL INFECTIONS

I. The Clinical Examination

The recognition of normal gingiva, gingival infections, and deeper periodontal involvement depends on a systematic, step-by-step examination.

- ◆ It is necessary to know the *extent* of the disease:
  - *Gingival infections* are confined to the gingiva.
  - *Periodontal infections* include all parts of the periodontium, namely, the gingiva, periodontal ligament, bone, and cementum.
- ◆ A comprehensive periodontal examination to gather assessment information and identify the signs of inflammation include the following:
  - Gingival tissue changes (color, size, shape, surface texture, position).
  - Mucogingival involvement (width of attached gingiva).
  - Probing depths.
  - Clinical attachment levels.
  - Bleeding on probing.

- Exudate or suppuration.
- Furcation involvement.
- Dental biofilm and calculus distribution.
- Tooth mobility.
- Fremitus.
- Radiographic evaluation.

II. Signs and Symptoms

- ◆ Patients may or may not have specific symptoms to report because periodontal infections may be painless.
- ◆ Symptoms the patient reports may include:
  - Bleeding gingiva while brushing or flossing.
  - On occasion, spontaneous bleeding of the gingiva.
- ◆ Other possible symptoms the patient may notice include:
  - Sensitivity to hot and cold.
  - Tenderness or discomfort while eating or pain after eating.
  - Food retained between the teeth.
  - Unpleasant mouth odors.
  - Chronic bad taste.
  - A feeling that the teeth are loose.

III. Causes of Tissue Changes

- ◆ Disease changes produce alterations in color, size, position, shape, consistency, surface texture, bleeding readiness, and exudate production.
- ◆ To understand the changes that take place in the gingival tissues during the transition from health to disease, the clinician must understand:
  - The role of biofilm in the development of disease.
  - The inflammatory response initiated by the body.
- ◆ When the products of the biofilm microorganisms cause breakdown of the intercellular substances of the sulcular epithelium, injurious agents can pass into the connective tissue, where an inflammatory response is initiated.

◆ An inflammatory response means there is increased blood flow, increased permeability of capillaries, and increased collection of defense cells and tissue fluid.

◆ The changes produce tissue alterations, such as in color, size, shape, and consistency.

CLASSIFICATION OF PERIODONTAL HEALTH

Before reviewing the classification of gingival and periodontal conditions, it is important to first define the classifications of periodontal health.[28]

I. Pristine Periodontal Health

◆ Signs associated with pristine periodontal health[28]:
  • No attachment loss.
  • No bleeding on probing.
  • No pocket depths greater than 3 mm.
  • No gingival redness, swelling, edema, or suppuration.

II. Clinical Periodontal Health (Intact Periodontium)

◆ Signs of clinical periodontal health classification[28]:
  • Absence or minimal levels of clinical inflammation.
  • No or minimal bleeding on probing.
  • No attachment loss.
  • No pocket depths greater than 3 mm.

III. Periodontal Disease Stability (Reduced Periodontium)

◆ Signs of periodontal disease stability[28]:
  • No or minimal bleeding on probing.
  • Optimal reduction in pocket depths.
  • Control of modifying factors such as optimal control of diabetes and reduction or cessation of smoking.

IV. Periodontal Disease Remission/ Control (Reduced Periodontium)

◆ The periodontal disease remission/control classification is characterized by[28]:
  • Reduction in inflammation, bleeding on probing, and pocket depth.
  • May not have optimal control of modifying factors, that is, diabetes.

CLASSIFICATION OF GINGIVITIS

Gingivitis continues to be designated into plaque-induced and non-plaque-induced gingivitis classifications. An overview is shared here, but there are many complexities to the classifications so the original 2017 World Workshop articles should be reviewed or a current periodontology textbook.

I. Plaque (Biofilm)-Induced Gingivitis

Common clinical signs of gingivitis include inflammation, erythema, bleeding, swelling (enlargement), and possible tenderness.[27]

A. Dental Biofilm–Associated Gingivitis

◆ Dental biofilm is the primary etiology, but the severity may be impacted by tooth and root anatomy, restorative factors, and other tooth-related factors.[27]

◆ No loss of attachment; however, gingivitis can also occur on a reduced periodontium and appears as inflammation of the gingival margin with no progression of attachment loss.[27]

B. Modifying Factors for Plaque-Induced Gingivitis

◆ Sex steroid hormones occur at various points in the life cycle can exacerbate gingivitis and include[27]:
  • Puberty.
  • Menstruation.
  • Pregnancy.
  • Oral contraceptives.

◆ Systemic conditions may also modify plaque-induced gingivitis and include[27]:
  • Hyperglycemia is often seen in poorly controlled diabetes.
  • Leukemia: enlarged, glazed, spongy gingiva that is red to deep purple in color.
  • Smoking.
  • Malnutrition.

◆ Local risk factors (predisposing factors) include[27]:
  • Poorly contoured restorations.
  • Hyposalivation or xerostomia: Sjogren's syndrome, medication-induced, anxiety, etc. may result in xerostomia.

C. Drug-Induced Gingival Enlargement

◆ A number of drugs such as antiepileptic drugs (e.g., dilantin and valproate), calcium-channel blockers (e.g., nifedipine, verapamil, diltiazem), and immunosuppressants (e.g., cyclosporine), and high-dose oral contraceptives.[27]

◆ Occurs most commonly in the anterior areas and usually seen earliest in the papilla.

II. Non-Plaque (Biofilm)-Induced Gingivitis

Plaque-induced gingivitis is one of the most common inflammatory diseases and although less common, non-plaque-induced gingivitis may be of importance for some patients.[36]

A. Genetic/Developmental Disorders

◆ Genetic causes of gingivitis are rare, an example is hereditary gingival fibromatosis.[36]

B. Specific Infections

- Bacterial origin[36]
  - Necrotizing gingivitis and stomatitis are due to underlying risk factors such as poor oral hygiene, stress, and compromised immunity with no loss of attachment.
  - Sexually transmitted disease such as gonorrhea and syphilis.
  - Tuberculosis.
- Viral origin[36]
  - Herpes simplex, that is, primary herpetic infection or gingivostomatitis resulting in many vesicles that rupture leaving irregular mucosal ulcers.
  - Human papilloma virus.
  - Varicella-zoster virus.
- Fungal infections such as candidosis.[36]

C. Inflammatory and Immune Conditions

- Autoimmune diseases, that is, lupus erythematosus, lichen planus.
- Hypersensitivity reactions that is, contact allergies.
- Granulomatous inflammatory conditions, that is, Crohn's disease.

D. Reactive Processes

- Lesions are thought to be due to a response to local irritation or trauma and may include pyogenic granuloma (pregnancy), fibrous epulis, etc.[36]

E. Neoplasms

- Premalignant lesions such as leukoplakia and erythroplakia.
- Malignant conditions such as leukemia and lymphoma.

F. Endocrine, Nutritional, and Metabolic Diseases

- Vitamin deficiencies like scurvy (vitamin C).[36]

G. Traumatic Lesions

- Physical/mechanical insults, that is, toothbrush abrasion, habits causing self-injury.
- Chemical insults, that is, etching, cocaine, dentifrice ingredients.
- Thermal insults, that is, mucosal burns.

H. Gingival Pigmentation

- Gingival pigmentation may be the result of smoker's melanosis, amalgam tattoo, or drug induced (minocycline), etc.[36]

CLASSIFICATION OF PERIODONTITIS

The classification of periodontitis focuses on detectable interdental CAL.[14]

I. Periodontitis Classifications

A. Necrotizing Periodontitis

- Necrotizing periodontal disease (NPD) begins as an acute condition with rapid tissue destruction, but NPD may also become chronic.
- Characterized by a history of pain, ulceration of the gingival margin, and punched out papillae.[14]
- A major predisposing factor is a compromised host immune response. Factors associated with host response include[37]:
  - HIV/AIDS: CD4 counts less than 200 and detectable viral load.
  - Immunosuppression.
  - Severe malnutrition.
  - Psychological stress and insufficient sleep.
  - History of NPD and poor oral self-care.

B. Periodontitis as a Manifestation of Systemic Disease

- Genetic disorders are rare, but may be significantly impact periodontal status. These include immunologic, metabolic, and endocrine disorders; and connective tissue, oral mucosa, and gingival tissue diseases.[38]
- Systemic diseases have a variable effect on the course of periodontitis, but can influence the occurrence and severity. These include[38]:
  - Diabetes mellitus.
  - Obesity.
  - Osteoporosis.
  - Arthritis (rheumatoid and osteoarthritis).
  - Emotional stress and depression.
  - Smoking.
  - Medications.
- Systemic disorders associated with loss of periodontal tissue independent of periodontitis include:
  - Neoplasms, that is, odontogenic tumors and squamous cell carcinoma.
  - Other disorders such as hyperparathyroidism and scleroderma.

C. Periodontitis

The periodontitis case definition or classification system aids in identification of disease, risk factors for progression of disease, and aid in identifying individualized approaches to management and treatment of the disease. The 2017 World Workshop on the Classification of Periodontal and Peri-Implant Diseases and Conditions system for classification of periodontitis takes into account the following elements[14]:

- *Severity* relates to the periodontal attachment loss at diagnosis and affects the complexity of management and treatment.
- *Complexity of management* includes factors such as probing depths, type of bone loss (vertical vs. horizontal), furcation involvement, occlusal issues.

♦ *Extent* refers to the number of teeth and distribution of the periodontitis and uses the terminology localized (<30% of teeth affected), generalized (>30% of teeth affected), and molar–incisor involvement only.

♦ *Rate of progression* is primarily dependent on radiographic evidence over time of attachment loss, but other methods to assess progression are under investigation.

♦ *Risk factors.*

II. Terminology for Staging Periodontitis

As previously noted, the staging of periodontitis includes: severity, complexity, and extent and distribution (Figure 19-15).[14]

♦ Stage I is mild periodontitis.

♦ Stage II is moderate periodontitis.

♦ Stage III is severe periodontitis.

♦ Stage IV is very severe or advanced periodontitis.

A. Severity

1. Interdental CAL at site of greatest loss[14]:
   • Slight or mild = 1–2 mm CAL.
   • Moderate = 3–4 mm CAL.
   • Severe or advanced = >5 mm CAL.
2. Radiographic bone loss (RBL)[14]
   • Coronal third (<15%).
   • Coronal third (15–33%).
   • Extends beyond mid-third of root apically.

3. Tooth loss
   • No tooth loss due to periodontitis.
   • Loss of four or lesser teeth due to periodontitis.
   • Loss of five or more teeth due to periodontitis.

B. Complexity

1. Pocket depth
   • Maximum pocket depth less than 4 mm.
   • Pocket depths greater than 5 mm.
   • Pocket depths greater than 6 mm.
2. Type of bone loss
   • Horizontal bone loss.
   • Vertical bone loss greater than or equal to 3 mm.
3. Furcation involvement.
4. Occlusal issues.

C. Extent and Distribution

♦ *Localized*: The gingiva is involved about a single tooth or a specific group of teeth (<30% of teeth involved).

♦ *Generalized*: The gingiva is involved about all or nearly all of the teeth throughout the mouth (>30% of teeth involved).

♦ *Molar/incisor pattern*: Bone loss limited to molar and incisor areas may suggest a more aggressive or rapid progression of disease (formerly called juvenile periodontitis).

Although not included in the staging of periodontitis, the following terminology may also be used when describing the extent and distribution of gingival inflammation.

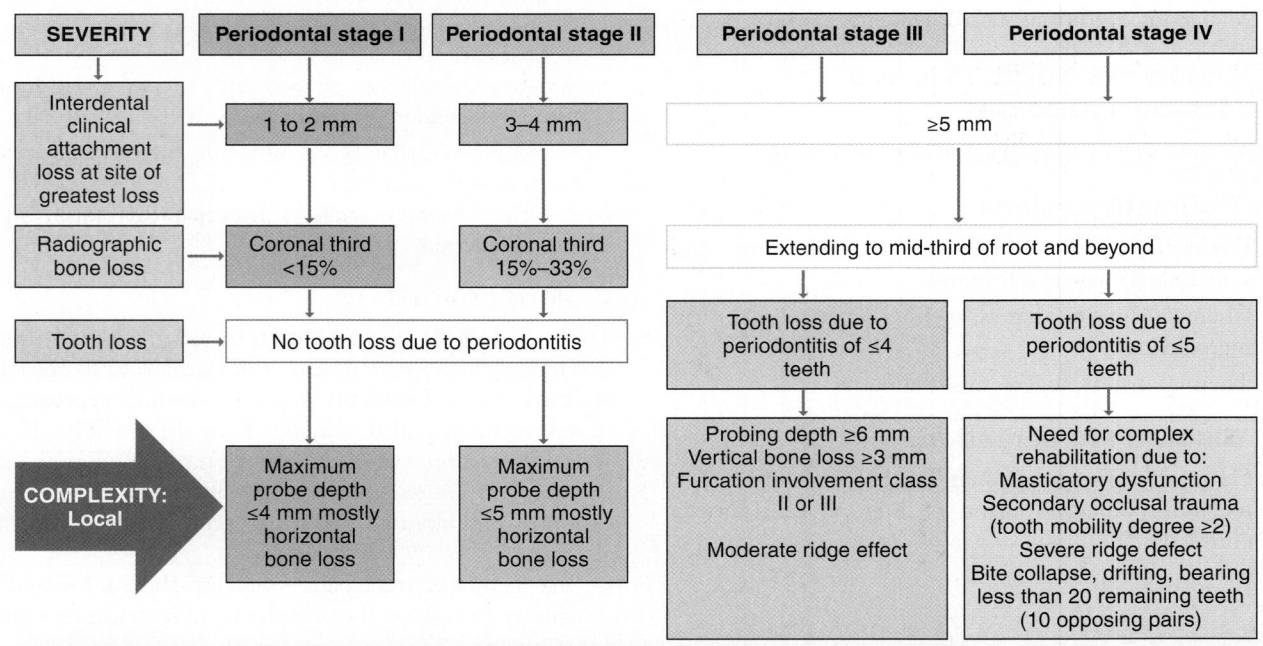

SEVERITY	Periodontal stage I	Periodontal stage II	Periodontal stage III	Periodontal stage IV
Interdental clinical attachment loss at site of greatest loss	1 to 2 mm	3–4 mm	≥5 mm	
Radiographic bone loss	Coronal third <15%	Coronal third 15%–33%	Extending to mid-third of root and beyond	
Tooth loss	No tooth loss due to periodontitis		Tooth loss due to periodontitis of ≤4 teeth	Tooth loss due to periodontitis of ≤5 teeth
COMPLEXITY: Local	Maximum probe depth ≤4 mm mostly horizontal bone loss	Maximum probe depth ≤5 mm mostly horizontal bone loss	Probing depth ≥6 mm Vertical bone loss ≥3 mm Furcation involvement class II or III Moderate ridge effect	Need for complex rehabilitation due to: Masticatory dysfunction Secondary occlusal trauma (tooth mobility degree ≥2) Severe ridge defect Bite collapse, drifting, bearing less than 20 remaining teeth (10 opposing pairs)

Extent and Distribution: Add to stage as a descriptor. For each stage, describe extent as localized (<30% of teeth involved), generalized, or molar/incisor pattern.

FIGURE 19-15 • Periodontitis Stage Flow chart. (Credit: Lori J. Giblin-Scanlon, RDH, DHSc, Forsyth School of Dental Hygiene.)

◆ *Marginal*: A change that is confined to the free or marginal gingiva. This is specified as either localized or generalized.

◆ *Papillary*: A change that involves a papilla but not the rest of the free gingiva around a tooth. A papillary change may be localized or generalized.

◆ *Diffuse*: Spread out, dispersed; affects gingival margin, attached gingiva, and interdental papillae; may extend into alveolar mucosa.

III. Terminology for Grading Periodontitis

Grading of periodontitis allows for recognition of factors that may impact the progression and management of the disease and includes: primary criteria, grade modifiers, risk of systemic impact of periodontitis, and biomarkers (Figure 19-16).[14]

◆ *Grade A* denotes a slow rate of progression.

◆ *Grade B* is potential for a moderate rate of progression.

◆ *Grade C* is suggestive of a rapid rate of progression.

A. Primary Criteria

◆ Direct evidence of progression[14]

  • No evidence of bone loss over 5 years (radiographic or CAL).

  • Less than 2 mm over 5 years
  • Greater than or equal to 2 mm over 5 years

◆ Percent bone loss divided by age.[14] For example: RBL is 30% and age is 60 = 0.5. If the RBL is 30% and the age is 25, then the result is 1.2. This accounts for more severe bone loss at an early age.

  • Less than 0.25.
  • 0.25–1.0.
  • Greater than 1.0.

◆ Case phenotype[14]

  • Heavy biofilm with low levels of destruction.
  • Destruction consistent with biofilm.
  • Destruction in excess of expectations given biofilm present and evidence of rapid progression.

B. Grade Modifiers (Risk Factors)

◆ Smoking

  • Nonsmoker.
  • Smokes less than 10 cigarettes/day.
  • Smokes greater than 10 cigarettes/day.

◆ Diabetes

  • No diabetes.
  • Hemoglobin A1c (HbA1c) less than 7.0 in patient with diabetes.
  • HbA1c greater than or equal to 7.0 in patients with diabetes.

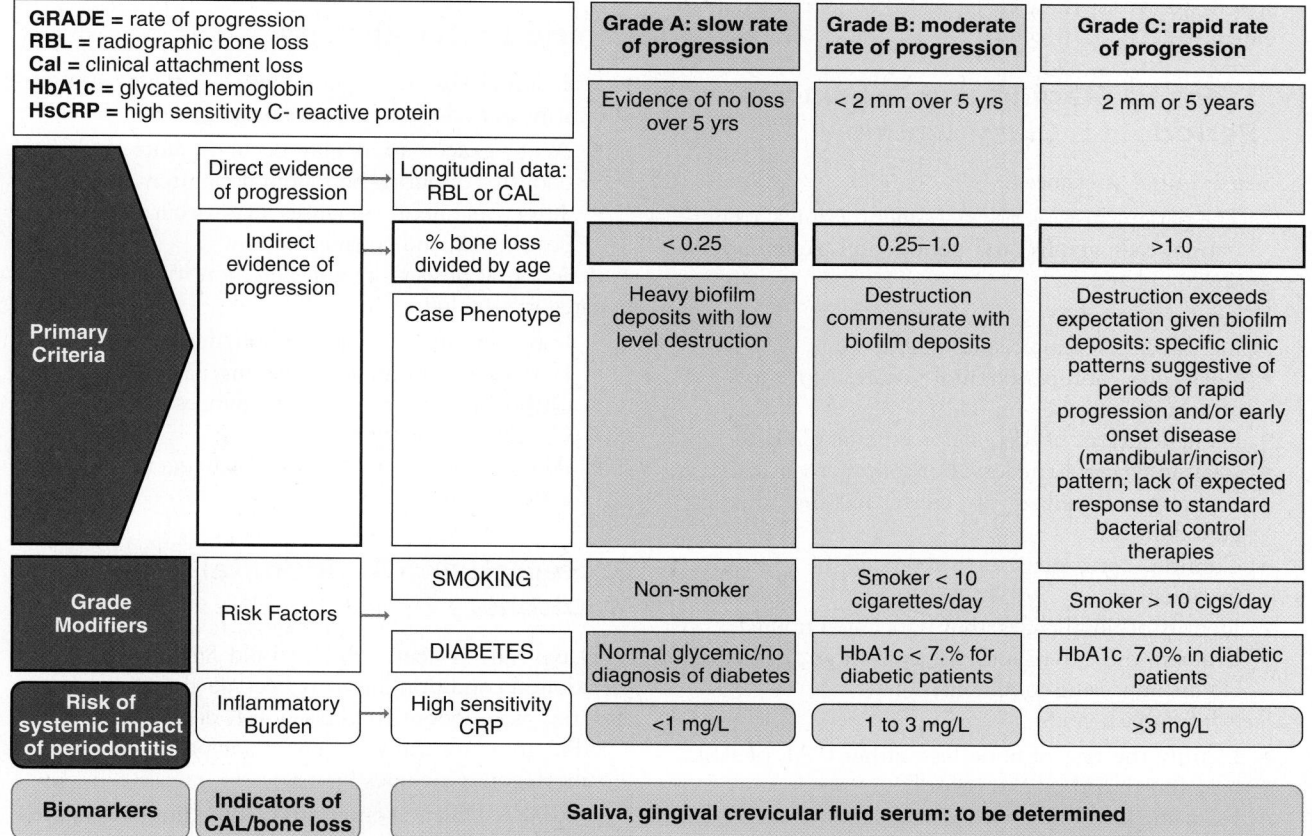

GRADE = rate of progression RBL = radiographic bone loss Cal = clinical attachment loss HbA1c = glycated hemoglobin HsCRP = high sensitivity C- reactive protein			Grade A: slow rate of progression	Grade B: moderate rate of progression	Grade C: rapid rate of progression
Primary Criteria	Direct evidence of progression	Longitudinal data: RBL or CAL	Evidence of no loss over 5 yrs	< 2 mm over 5 yrs	2 mm or 5 years
	Indirect evidence of progression	% bone loss divided by age	< 0.25	0.25–1.0	>1.0
		Case Phenotype	Heavy biofilm deposits with low level destruction	Destruction commensurate with biofilm deposits	Destruction exceeds expectation given biofilm deposits: specific clinic patterns suggestive of periods of rapid progression and/or early onset disease (mandibular/incisor) pattern; lack of expected response to standard bacterial control therapies
Grade Modifiers	Risk Factors	SMOKING	Non-smoker	Smoker < 10 cigarettes/day	Smoker > 10 cigs/day
		DIABETES	Normal glycemic/no diagnosis of diabetes	HbA1c < 7.% for diabetic patients	HbA1c 7.0% in diabetic patients
Risk of systemic impact of periodontitis	Inflammatory Burden	High sensitivity CRP	<1 mg/L	1 to 3 mg/L	>3 mg/L
Biomarkers	Indicators of CAL/bone loss		Saliva, gingival crevicular fluid serum: to be determined		

FIGURE 19-16 • **Periodontitis Grade Flow chart.** (Credit: Lori J. Giblin-Scanlon, RDH, DHSc, Forsyth School of Dental Hygiene.)

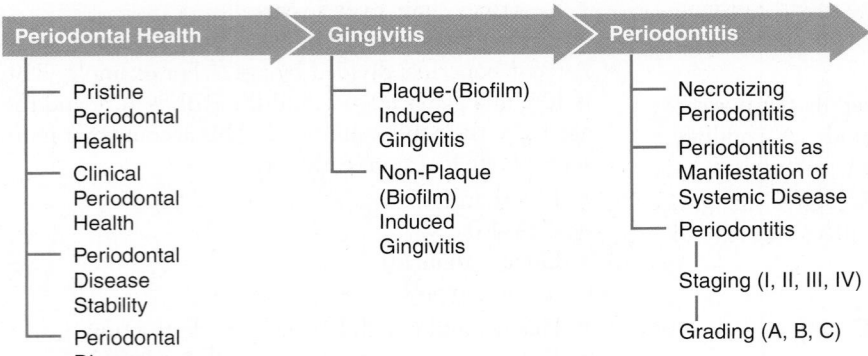

FIGURE 19-17 • **Classifications of Periodontal Health, Gingivitis, and Periodontitis.**

C. Risk of Systemic Impact of Periodontitis

◆ If laboratory values are available, a measure of inflammation is C-reactive protein. This can also be used as part of the grading when available.
  • Less than 1 mg/L.
  • 1–3 mg/L.
  • Greater than 3 mg/L.

D. Biomarkers

◆ Biomarkers that serve as indicators of bone loss or CAL have not been definitively identified, but the grading system allows for these to be added as more evidence emerges.

IV. Steps to Staging and Grading the Periodontal Classification

◆ *Step 1*: Initial assessment
  • The patient history, risk assessment, clinical examination, radiographs, and periodontal examinations are completed.
◆ *Step 2*: Establish stage
  • Identify areas of interdental CAL.
  • Rule out non-periodontal causes for loss of attachment.
  • Evaluate extent of RBL and maximum CAL.
  • Identify type of bone loss (horizontal or vertical).
  • Determine number of teeth missing due to periodontitis.
  • Confirm presence or absence of furcation involvement.
  • Identify occlusal issues, that is, occlusal trauma.
  • Evaluate the extent and distribution of disease and factors impacting complexity.
◆ *Step 3*: Establish grade
  • Identify the rate of bone loss, either CAL or RBL, over time based on past records.
  • From medical and psychosocial history, assess risk facts such as smoking and diabetes control.

• Evaluate attachment loss in relationship to the amount of biofilm present.
• Assess rate of progress by dividing RBL (% bone loss) by age.
◆ A simplified diagram of the classifications for periodontal health, gingival, and periodontal diseases is provided in Figure 19-17.

ACUTE PERIODONTAL LESIONS

The acute periodontal lesions are classified according to the etiology.[37]

I. Periodontal Abscess

◆ Periodontal abscess in periodontitis patient (in a preexisting periodontal pocket) subcategories includes[37]:
  • Acute exacerbation may occur in untreated periodontitis or during periodontal maintenance.
  • After treatment, abscesses may occur postscaling, postsurgery, and postmedication.
◆ Periodontal abscess in non-periodontitis patient subcategories includes[37]:
  • Impaction such as popcorn hull, dental floss.
  • Harmful habit such as nail biting.
  • Orthodontic treatment with changes in occlusion.
  • Gingival overgrowth.
  • Alteration of the root surface such as a root fracture, enamel pearl.

II. Necrotizing Periodontal Diseases

NPD typically is acute which would fall into the acute periodontal condition, but may become chronic and then classified as periodontitis as previously described.[37]
◆ NPD in chronically, severely compromised patients subcategories includes[37]:
  • HIV/AIDS and conditions causing immunosuppression in adults.

- In children, NPD may occur in severe malnutrition, severe viral infections, or extreme living conditions (such as lack of living situations).
- NPD in temporarily and/or moderately compromised patients subcategories includes[37]:
  - Gingivitis or periodontal patients with predisposing factors such as uncontrolled factors such as stress, nutrition, smoking; previous NPD; and predisposing factors for NPD.

III. Endo-Periodontal Lesions

This classification was updated from the 1999 classifications to focus on the current clinical condition and lesions in those with and without periodontitis to cover a broader range of situations.[37]
- Endo-periodontal lesion with root damage.[37]
  - This subclassification includes root fracture or crack, root canal perforation, and external root resorption.

- Endo-periodontal lesions without root damage.[37]
  - This includes lesions in patients with and without periodontitis uses a grading system (1–3) which is beyond the scope of dental hygiene care.

DOCUMENTATION

Documentation for a patient to determine periodontal classification includes:
- Initially a complete history and assessment is documented to include:
  - Medical, dental, and psychosocial history.
  - Chief complaint or problem.
  - Consultation with primary care providers for additional information, that is, history and current HbA1c for a patient with diabetes.
  - Risk assessment and identification of modifiable risk factors.
  - Comprehensive periodontal examination.
  - Periodontal classification.
- A sample progress note may be reviewed in Box 19-1.

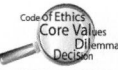

EVERYDAY ETHICS

Gloria is new to the office. The dental hygienist, Tina seats her in the operatory and begins the initial appointment with review of Gloria's medical history. On her medical history form, Gloria had written *borderline diabetes*. Upon further questioning, she says she does not check her blood sugar (glucose) and does not remember her HbA1c (hemoglobin A1c). Gloria reports taking metformin and "watching" her diet for her *borderline diabetes*. She is asked for the name and phone number of her primary care providers for follow-up on her medical history related to the *borderline diabetes*. She does not remember and says she will call the office with the information when she gets home. Gloria also states her previous dental office has a full set of x-rays taken less than a year ago and she would request them. The periodontal examination identifies generalized bleeding on probing, exudate on several teeth, and 4–6 mm pocket depths with Class II furcation involvement on #2, 3, and 14.

A tentative treatment plan for the dental hygiene care was developed in collaboration with the dentist, Dr. Nedham, with the understanding it would be finalized once the medical consultation and radiographs were received. As she rushed out of the office, Gloria made her appointment for 1 week later during her work lunch hour to finalize

the treatment plan and begin **NSPT (nonsurgical periodontal therapy)**. Tina arrives the following week late to her appointment and has not requested her radiographs or called the dental office with the name and contact information for her medical provider.

In Tina's judgment, treatment cannot be provided for the following reasons: (1) the radiographs had not yet arrived from the other dentist; (2) the dental office has not been able to request a medical consultation related to her diabetes; and (3) the treatment plan has not been finalized. Tina told Gloria that the appointment needed to be rescheduled for another day, but Gloria insisted the NSPT be started at this appointment. Gloria becomes upset and says she does not understand why Tina cannot "just clean her teeth."

Questions for Consideration

1. Which of the dental hygiene core values have application in this scenario? Explain how each of the ones selected apply.
2. Is this situation either an ethical issue or a dilemma for Tina? Explain your answer.
3. What options does Tina have at this appointment for Gloria's care?

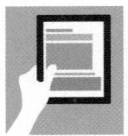

BOX 19-1

Example Documentation:
Patient with Periodontal Disease

S—A 58-year-old male presents with chief complaint of painful bleeding gums. On the medical history the patient reports having type 2 diabetes and hypertension. He reports his A1c was 8.2 at his last appointment. The patient takes Metformin and Cardizem. Patient indicates he smokes 1 pack/day and has smoked since he was 13 years old. He reports both his mother and father lost all their teeth because of gum disease.

O—Extraoral/intraoral findings were normal. Blood pressure: 120/80. Full mouth series of radiographs taken and reviewed. No new dental caries. A comprehensive periodontal examination reveals generalized 5-6 mm pocket depths with localized bleeding on probing. Radiograph reveals 4-5 mm of CAL with approximately 20-33% bone horizontal loss. No mobility was noted. Grade I furcations' involvement on the meso-lingual and disto-lingual of the maxillary molars. The gingiva is pink and fibrotic with bulbous interdental papillae throughout. Generalized heavy supragingival and subgingival calculus. Dental biofilm score 40%.

A—The periodontal classification is generalized Stage III, Grade C periodontitis. Recommended patient return for four appointments of NSPT using local anesthesia followed by a re-evaluation in 4-6 weeks.

P—Patient education about the risk factors for periodontal disease present including biofilm, genetic history of periodontal disease, lack of diabetes control, and tobacco use. The patient is interested in tobacco cessation and was referred to the state quit line and his primary care provider. Oral self-care was reviewed with a soft toothbrush and interdental brush and the patient demonstrated good technique. Patient referred to his primary care provider for follow-up on his diabetes control prior to beginning NSPT to facilitate healing. Next visit: Begin NSPT maxillary right quadrant and review oral self-care. Follow-up about progress on tobacco cessation and diabetes management.

Signed: _____, RDH

Date: _____

References

1. Linden GJ, Lyons A, Scannapieco FA. Periodontal systemic associations: review of the evidence. *J Periodontol.* 2013;84(suppl 4):S8-S19.
2. Albandar JM, Susin C, Hughes FJ. Manifestations of systemic diseases and conditions that affect the periodontal attachment apparatus: case definitions and diagnostic considerations. *J Periodontol.* 2018;89(suppl 1):S183-S203.

Factors to Teach the Patient

► Educate the patient about the connections between periodontal disease and systemic disease related to the patient's medical history.
► Describe the risk factors that put the patient at risk for periodontal disease and assist the patient in identifying ways to manage the modifiable risk factors.
► Explain a normal sulcus versus a diseased periodontal pocket.
► Explain the need for a comprehensive periodontal examination to assess the extent and severity of disease.
► Clarify the need for adequate oral self-care and continuing care to prevent or manage periodontal disease (infection).

ENHANCE YOUR UNDERSTANDING

ONLINE RESOURCES
(see the inside front cover for access information)
• Audio glossary
• Appendices

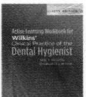

SUPPORT FOR LEARNING
(available separately)
• *Active Learning Workbook for Wilkins' Clinical Practice of the Dental Hygienist, 13th Edition*

INDIVIDUALIZED REVIEW
• Customized practice quizzing with Navigate 2 TestPrep for *Wilkins' Clinical Practice of the Dental Hygienist*

3. Genco RJ, Genco FD. Common risk factors in the management of periodontal and associated systemic diseases: the dental setting and interprofessional collaboration. *J Evid Based Dent Pract.* 2014;14(suppl):4-16.
4. Lang NP, Suvan JE, Tonetti MS. Risk factor assessment tools for the prevention of periodontitis progression a systematic review. *J Clin Periodontol.* 2015;42(suppl 16):S59-S70.
5. Ferraiolo DM. Predicting periodontitis progression? *Evid Based Dent.* 2016;17(1):19-20.
6. Page RC, Krall EA, Martin J, Mancl L, Garcia RI. Validity and accuracy of a risk calculator in predicting periodontal disease. *J Am Dent Assoc.* 2002;133(5):569-576.
7. Page RC, Martin J, Krall EA, Mancl L, Garcia R. Longitudinal validation of a risk calculator for periodontal disease. *J Clin Periodontol.* 2003;30(9):819-827.
8. Lang NP, Tonetti MS. Periodontal risk assessment (PRA) for patients in supportive periodontal therapy (SPT). *Oral Health Prev Dent.* 2003;1(1):7-16.

9. Diaz PI, Hoare A, Hong BY. Subgingival microbiome shifts and community dynamics in periodontal diseases. *J Calif Dent Assoc.* 2016;44(7):421-435.

10. Dentino A, Lee S, Mailhot J, Hefti AF. Principles of periodontology. *Periodontol 2000.* 2013;61(1):16-53.

11. Shariff JA, Ahluwalia KP, Papapanou PN. Relationship between frequent recreational cannabis (marijuana and hashish) use and periodontitis in adults in the United States: National Health and Nutrition Examination Survey 2011 to 2012. *J Periodontol.* 2017;88(3):273-280.

12. Kamath KP, Mishra S, Anand PS. Smokeless tobacco use as a risk factor for periodontal disease. *Front Public Health.* 2014;2:195.

13. Sanz M, Ceriello A, Buysschaert M, et al. Scientific evidence on the links between periodontal diseases and diabetes: consensus report and guidelines of the joint workshop on periodontal diseases and diabetes by the International Diabetes Federation and the European Federation of Periodontology. *Diabetes Res Clin Pract.* 2018;137:231-241.

14. Tonetti MS, Greenwell H, Kornman KS. Staging and grading of periodontitis: framework and proposal of a new classification and case definition. *J Periodontol.* 2018;89(suppl 1): S159-S172.

15. Ismail AF, McGrath CP, Yiu CK. Oral health of children with type 1 diabetes mellitus: a systematic review. *Diabetes Res Clin Pract.* 2015;108(3):369-381.

16. Teshome A, Yitayeh A. The effect of periodontal therapy on glycemic control and fasting plasma glucose level in type 2 diabetic patients: systematic review and meta-analysis. *BMC Oral Health.* 2016;17(1):31.

17. Daudt LD, Musskopf ML, Mendez M, et al. Association between metabolic syndrome and periodontitis: a systematic review and meta-analysis. *Braz Oral Res.* 2018;32:e35.

18. Hales CM, Carroll MD, Fryar CD, Ogden CL. Prevalence of obesity among adults and youth: United States, 2015–2016. NCHS Data Brief, No. 288. Hyattsville, MD: National Center for Health Statistics; 2017.

19. Keller A, Rohde JF, Raymond K, Heitmann BL. Association between periodontal disease and overweight and obesity: a systematic review. *J Periodontol.* 2015;86(6):766-776.

20. Martens L, De Smet S, Yusof MY, Rajasekharan S. Association between overweight/obesity and periodontal disease in children and adolescents: a systematic review and meta-analysis. *Eur Arch Paediatr Dent.* 2017;18(2):69-82.

21. Wang J, Lv J, Wang W, Jiang X. Alcohol consumption and risk of periodontitis: a meta-analysis. *J Clin Periodontol.* 2016;43(7):572-583.

22. Alsharief M, Kaye EK. Alcohol consumption may increase the risk for periodontal disease in some adult populations. *J Evid Based Dent Pract.* 2017;17(1):59-61.

23. Chapple IL, Bouchard P, Cagetti MG, et al. Interaction of lifestyle, behaviour or systemic diseases with dental caries and periodontal diseases: consensus report of group 2 of the joint EFP/ORCA workshop on the boundaries between caries and periodontal diseases. *J Clin Periodontol.* 2017;44(suppl 18):S39-S51.

24. Preeja C, Ambili R, Nisha KJ, Seba A, Archana V. Unveiling the role of stress in periodontal etiopathogenesis: an evidence-based review. *J Investig Clin Dent.* 2013;4(2):78-83.

25. Cekici A, Kantarci A, Hasturk H, Van Dyke TE. Inflammatory and immune pathways in the pathogenesis of periodontal disease. *Periodontol 2000.* 2014;64(1):57-80.

26. Penoni DC, Fidalgo TK, Torres SR, et al. Bone density and clinical periodontal attachment in postmenopausal women: a systematic review and meta-analysis. *J Dent Res.* 2017;96(3):261-269.

27. Murakami S, Mealey BL, Mariotti A, Chapple ILC. Dental plaque-induced gingival conditions. *J Periodontol.* 2018; 89(suppl 1):S17-S27.

28. Lang NP, Bartold PM. Periodontal health. *J Periodontol.* 2018;89(suppl 1):S9-S16.

29. Choi YK, Park DY, Kim Y. Relationship between prosthodontic status and nutritional intake in the elderly in Korea: National Health and Nutrition Examination Survey (NHANES IV). *Int J Dent Hyg.* 2014;12(4):285-290.

30. Page RC, Schroeder HE. Pathogenesis of inflammatory periodontal disease. A summary of current work. *Lab Invest.* 1976;34(3):235-249.

31. Kornman KS. Mapping the pathogenesis of periodontitis: a new look. *J Periodontol.* 2008; 79(suppl 8):1560-1568.

32. Hajishengallis G, Korostoff JM. Revisiting the Page & Schroeder model: the good, the bad, and the unknowns in periodontal host response forty years later. *Periodontol 2000.* 2017;75(1):116-151. doi:10.1111/prd.12181.

33. Huynh-Ba G, Kuonen P, Hofer D, Schmid J, Lang NP, Salvi GE. The effect of periodontal therapy on the survival rate and incidence of complications of multirooted teeth with furcation involvement after an observation period of at least 5 years: a systematic review. *J Clin Periodontol.* 2009;36(2):164-176.

34. Kim DM, Neiva R. Periodontal soft tissue non-root coverage procedures: a systematic review from the AAP regeneration workshop. *J Periodontol.* 2015;86(suppl 2):S56-S72.

35. Cortellini P, Bissada NF. Mucogingival conditions in the natural dentition: narrative review, case definitions, and diagnostic considerations. *J Periodontol.* 2018; 89(suppl 1): S204-S213.

36. Holmstrup P, Plemons J, Meyle J. Non-plaque-induced gingival diseases. *J Clin Periodontol.* 2018; 45(suppl 20): S28-S43.

37. Herrera D, Retamal-Valdes B, Alonso B, Feres M. Acute periodontal lesions (periodontal abscesses and necrotizing periodontal diseases) and endo-periodontal lesions. *J Periodontol.* 2018;89(suppl 1):S85-S102.

38. Jepsen S, Caton JG, Albandar JM, et al. Periodontal manifestations of systemic diseases and developmental and acquired conditions: consensus report of workgroup 3 of the 2017 World Workshop on the Classification of Periodontal and Peri-Implant Diseases and Conditions. *J Periodontol.* 2018;89(suppl 1):S237-S248.

20

Periodontal Examination

Linda D. Boyd, RDH, RD, EdD, and Esther M. Wilkins, BS, RDH, DMD

CHAPTER OUTLINE

BASIC INSTRUMENTS FOR EXAMINATION

THE MOUTH MIRROR
I. Purposes and Uses
II. Procedure for Use

AIR–WATER SYRINGE
I. Purposes and Uses

EXPLORERS
I. General Purposes and Uses
II. Specific Explorers and Their Uses

BASIC PROCEDURES FOR USE OF EXPLORERS
I. Use of Sensory Stimuli
II. Tooth Surface Irregularities
III. Types of Stimuli

EXPLORERS: SUPRAGINGIVAL PROCEDURES
I. Use of Vision
II. Facial and Lingual Surfaces
III. Proximal Surfaces

EXPLORERS: SUBGINGIVAL PROCEDURES
I. Essentials for Detection of Tooth Surface Irregularities

PERIODONTAL PROBE
I. Types of Probes
II. Purposes and Uses
III. Description of Manual Periodontal Probes

GUIDE TO PERIODONTAL PROBING
I. Pocket Characteristics
II. Evaluation of Tooth Surface
III. Factors Affecting Probe Accuracy

PRELIMINARY ASSESSMENT PRIOR TO PERIODONTAL EXAMINATION
I. Medical History
II. Dental and Psychosocial History
III. Vital Signs
IV. Extraoral/Intraoral Examination
V. Risk Assessment
VI. Radiographic Examination
VII. Dental Examination
VIII. Hard and Soft Deposits

PARAMETERS OF CARE FOR THE PERIODONTAL EXAMINATION
I. Periodontal Probing Procedure
II. Clinical Attachment Level

III. Mucogingival Examination
IV. Mobility Examination
V. Fremitus
VI. Furcation Examination

RADIOGRAPHIC CHANGES IN PERIODONTAL DISEASE
I. Bone Level
II. Shape of Remaining Bone
III. Crestal Lamina Dura
IV. Furcation Involvement
V. Periodontal Ligament Space

OTHER RADIOGRAPHIC FINDINGS
I. Calculus
II. Overhanging Restorations
III. Dental Caries

DOCUMENTATION

EVERYDAY ETHICS

FACTORS TO TEACH THE PATIENT

REFERENCES

LEARNING OBJECTIVES

After studying this chapter, the student will be able to:

1. Describe the components of a comprehensive periodontal examination.

2. List the instruments used for a periodontal examination.

3. Explain the technique for use of the periodontal probe and explorers.

4. Explain how procedure for the comprehensive examination will be described to the patient.

BASIC INSTRUMENTS FOR EXAMINATION

◆ Parts of the dental and periodontal clinical examinations are made by direct visual observation, whereas other parts require tactile examination using a periodontal probe and/or an explorer.

◆ Basic cassette setups for all patients with permanent teeth should include at least a mouth mirror, probes including a furcation probe, a plastic probe when dental implants are present, and a subgingival explorer.

◆ The general principles of instrumentation are described in Chapter 37.

THE MOUTH MIRROR

I. Purposes and Uses

A. Indirect Vision

◆ Indirect vision is used for all surfaces where direct vision is not possible.

◆ Examples are the distal surfaces of posterior teeth and lingual surfaces of anterior teeth.

B. Indirect Illumination

◆ The mirror is used to reflect the light from the dental overhead light or headlamp worn by the clinician to any area of the oral cavity.

C. Transillumination

◆ Transillumination refers to reflection of light through the teeth.
  • Mirror is used to reflect light from the lingual aspect of the teeth while examined from the facial.
  • Mirror is used for indirect vision on the lingual while light from the overhead dental light passes through the teeth. Dental caries or calculus deposits appear opaque.

D. Retraction

◆ The mirror is used to protect or prevent interference by the cheeks, tongue, or lips.

II. Procedure for Use

A. Grasp and Rest

◆ Use modified pen grasp with finger rest on a tooth surface near the working area.

◆ Provides stability and control.

◆ Assists in retraction of lips and cheek.

◆ Exercises for gaining skill in control of instruments are described in Chapter 37.

B. Retraction

◆ Use a thin layer of water-based lubricant on dry or cracked lips and corners of mouth.

◆ Adjust the mirror position so the angles of the mouth are protected from undue pressure by the shank of the mirror.

◆ Insert and remove mirror carefully to avoid hitting the teeth because this can be uncomfortable for the patient.

C. Maintain Clear Vision

◆ Warm the mirror with water or rub the surface of the mirror along the buccal mucosa to coat mirror with thin transparent film of saliva.

◆ Request patient breathe through the nose to prevent condensation of moisture on the mirror.

AIR–WATER SYRINGE

I. Purposes and Uses

A. Procedure for Use

◆ Grasp around the handle of the air–water syringe with palm; place thumb on button to activate air.

◆ Test the air flow before using in the mouth so the strength of flow can be controlled.

◆ Apply a controlled, steady stream of air directly to the area being assessed. The clinician needs to thoroughly dry the area to increase visibility.

◆ Supplement air drying with use of saliva ejector and folded gauze sponge placed in vestibule to maintain dry field.

B. To Improve and Facilitate Examination Procedures

◆ Make a thorough and more accurate examination.

◆ Dry supragingival calculus to facilitate identification.
  • Small deposits may be light in color and not visible until they are dried.
  • Dried calculus appears chalky and presents a contrast to tooth color.

◆ Deflect the free gingival margin (GM) for observation into the subgingival area. Subgingival calculus usually appears darker than supragingival calculus.

◆ Identify areas of demineralization and carious lesions.

◆ Recognize location and condition of restorations, particularly composite or tooth-colored restorations.

C. To Improve Visibility of the Treatment Area during Instrumentation

◆ Provide dry area for finger rest for stability during instrumentation.

◆ Facilitate effective scaling techniques.

◆ Minimize appointment time.

◆ Evaluate complete removal of supragingival calculus.

D. To Prepare Teeth and/or Gingiva for Certain Procedures

◆ Examples are to dry surfaces for:
  • Application of caries-preventive agents when indicated.

- Preparation to make impression for study model.
- Application of topical anesthetic.

E. Precautions

- Avoid sharp blasts of air on cervical areas of teeth or open carious lesions due to possible sensitivity of these areas. Such areas may be dried by blotting with a gauze sponge or cotton roll to avoid patient discomfort.
- Avoid forceful application of air, which can direct saliva and debris out of the oral cavity, contaminate the working area and clinician, and create aerosols.
- Avoid directing air toward the posterior region of the patient's mouth as it may cause coughing.
- Avoid startling the patient; give a warning when air is to be applied.

EXPLORERS

I. General Purposes and Uses

A. To Detect, by Tactile Sense, the Texture and Character of the Tooth Surfaces

- For calculus detection, irregularities in the tooth surface, defects in margins of restorations, and other irregularities not apparent to direct visual observation.
- An explorer is used to confirm direct observation. Avoid use of a sharp explorer on white spot lesions (demineralized tooth surfaces with potential to be remineralized).[1-3]

B. To Define the Extent of Instrumentation Needed and Guide Techniques

- For nonsurgical periodontal instrumentation (scaling and root planing).
- Removing an overhanging filling.

C. To Evaluate the Completeness of Treatment

II. Specific Explorers and Their Uses

- A variety of explorers are available, as shown by the examples in Figure 20-1.
- Explorer design impacts accessibility to proximal and root surfaces along with flexibility and tactile sensitivity.

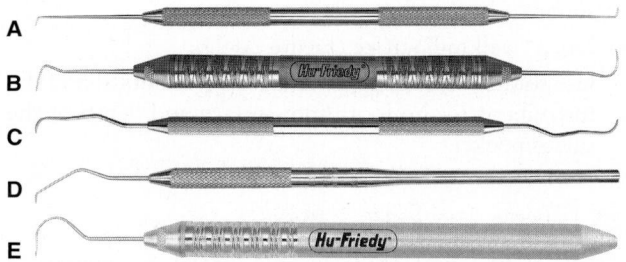

FIGURE 20-1 • Explorers. A: Pigtail. **B:** Cowhorn. **C:** ODU 11/12. **D:** TU 17. **E:** Shepherd hook/no. 23.

A. Subgingival Explorers

- *Use*:
  - Subgingival use of explorers such as the ODU 11/12 is facilitated by an angulated shank with a short tip (Figure 20-1C).
  - Supragingival use of TU-17 (Figure 20-1D): It may be adapted to all surfaces of anterior teeth, but is especially useful for proximal surface examination.
- *Features for subgingival examination*:
  - Back of tip can be applied directly to the base of the pocket without trauma or laceration.
  - The short tip can be adapted to rounded tooth surfaces and line angles.
  - Narrow short tip can be adapted at the base where the pocket narrows without undue displacement of the pocket soft tissue wall.

B. Supragingival Explorers

- Shepherd hook explorer (Figure 20-1E):
  - *Use*: examining pits and fissures and supragingival smooth surfaces; examining surfaces and margins of restorations and sealants.
- Pigtail or Cowhorn (Figure 20-1A and B):
  - *Use*: proximal surfaces for calculus, dental caries, or margins of restorations.
  - *Adaptability*: as paired, curved tips, they are applied to opposite tooth surfaces.

BASIC PROCEDURES FOR USE OF EXPLORERS

- Development of ability to use an explorer and a probe is achieved first by learning the anatomic features of each tooth surface and the types of irregularities that may be encountered on the surfaces.
- The second step is repeated practice of techniques for application of the instruments.
- The objective is to adapt the instruments in a routine manner that relays consistent comparative information about the nature of the tooth surface.
- Concentration, patience, attention to detail, and being alert to irregularities, however small it may seem, are necessary.

I. Use of Sensory Stimuli

- A slender, wirelike explorer such as the ODU 11/12 has a greater degree of flexibility that contributes to increased tactile sensitivity for the clinician when a light grasp is used than a thicker explorer.

II. Tooth Surface Irregularities

- Three basic tactile sensations can be distinguished when probing or exploring.
- These may be grouped as:
  - Normal tooth surface.

- Irregularities created by excess or elevations in the surface.
- Irregularities caused by depressions in the tooth surface.

Examples of these are listed next.

A. Normal

- *Tooth structure*: the smooth surface of enamel and root surface; anatomic configurations, such as cingula or furcations.
- *Restored surfaces*: smooth surfaces of metal (gold, amalgam) versus the feeling of composite; smooth margin of a restoration.

B. Irregularities: Elevations on Tooth Surface

- *Deposits*: calculus.
- *Anomalies*: enamel pearl.
- *Restorations*: overcontoured, irregular margins (overhangs).

C. Irregularities: Depressions and Grooves

- *Tooth surface*: demineralized or carious lesion, abrasion, erosion, pits such as those caused by enamel hypoplasia, areas of cemental resorption on the root surface.
- *Restorations*: deficient margin, rough surface.

III. Types of Stimuli

During exploring and probing, recognition of irregularities can be made through auditory and tactile means.

A. Tactile

- Tactile sensitivity is a very complex neurologic process with stimuli from vibrations created from the instrument passing over the tooth surface to the fingers and ultimately to the brain.[4]
- Tactile sensations, for example, may be the result of the explorer catching on an overcontoured restoration, soft, sticky surface of a carious lesion, encountering an elevated calculus deposit, or simply passing over a rough tooth surface.

B. Auditory

- As an explorer or a probe moves over the surface of enamel, cementum, a metallic restoration, a plastic restoration, or any irregularity of tooth structure or restoration, or a difference in texture is apparent. With each contact, sound may be created.
- The clean smooth enamel is quiet; the rough cementum or calculus is scratchy or noisy. Sometimes, a metallic restoration may "squeak" or have a metallic "ring." With experience, differentiations can be detected.

EXPLORERS: SUPRAGINGIVAL PROCEDURES

I. Use of Vision

- Visual examination of coronal tooth surfaces is most effective in combination with tactile examination with an explorer.[5]

- Visual examination can minimize unnecessary exploration with adequate light and air, proper retraction, and use of a mouth mirror.
- Limitations to visual examination include subgingival areas and the proximal areas of adjacent teeth.
- Visual examination can be quite effective for identification of supragingival calculus because when the tooth is dried, it can generally be seen as either chalky white or brownish-yellow in contrast to tooth color.

II. Facial and Lingual Surfaces

- Adapt the tip so the side of the point is always on the tooth surface.
- Move the instrument in short walking strokes over the surface being examined or direct the side of the tip gently over a suspected carious lesion.
- Careful noninvasive examination can be made using the side of the tip of a probe gently to test whether the demineralized area has slight roughness. Applying pressure to puncture or scratch the surface can result in cavitation that requires restoration.[1]

III. Proximal Surfaces

- Lead with the tip onto a proximal surface, rolling the handle between the fingers to ensure adaptation around the line angle. Keep the side of the point of the explorer in contact with the tooth surface at all times.
- Explore under the proximal contact area when there is recession of the papilla and the area is exposed. Overlap strokes from facial and lingual surfaces to ensure full coverage.

EXPLORERS: SUBGINGIVAL PROCEDURES

I. Essentials for Detection of Tooth Surface Irregularities

- Light grasp.
- Consistent finger rest with light pressure.
- Keep the side of the explorer tip in contact with the tooth and do not remove from the pocket for each stroke to avoid tissue trauma.
- Light touch as the instrument is moved over the tooth surface.
- Use a "walking" stroke (Figure 20-2).
- Use short, controlled strokes to allow adaptation of the instrument to the tooth/root surface and depth of the sulcus/pocket.

PERIODONTAL PROBE

- The periodontal probe is an essential component of assessment and diagnosis of the patient's periodontal disease status.

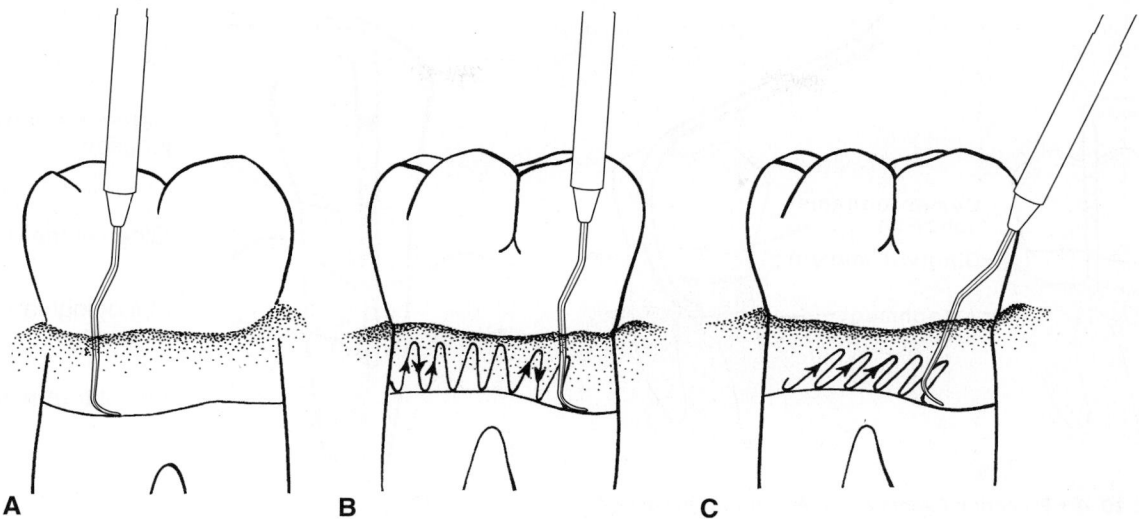

FIGURE 20-2 • Use of Subgingival Explorer. A: The lower shank (next to tip) is held parallel with the long axis of the tooth. The explorer is passed into the pocket and lowered until the back of the working tip meets resistance from the attached periodontal tissue at the base of the pocket. **B:** Vertical walking stroke. With the side of the tip in contact with the tooth surface at all times, the explorer is moved over the surface. **C:** Diagonal walking stroke. Complete exploration of the surface is needed; therefore, groups of strokes are overlapped.

◆ Treatment planning varies depending on whether the condition is gingivitis, which may be reversible, or periodontitis, which requires more extensive periodontal therapy.

I. Types of Probes

◆ Two general types of probes available are the traditional or standard manual probes and the controlled force or automated probes.

◆ Standard or traditional probes include the following:
  • Probes with colored markings in millimeter increments from 1 to 3 (see Figure 20-3).
  • Plastic probes for assessing the health of dental implants.
  • Probes specifically designed to assess furcation areas with and without colored millimeter markings, such as the Nabers probe (see Figure 20-4).

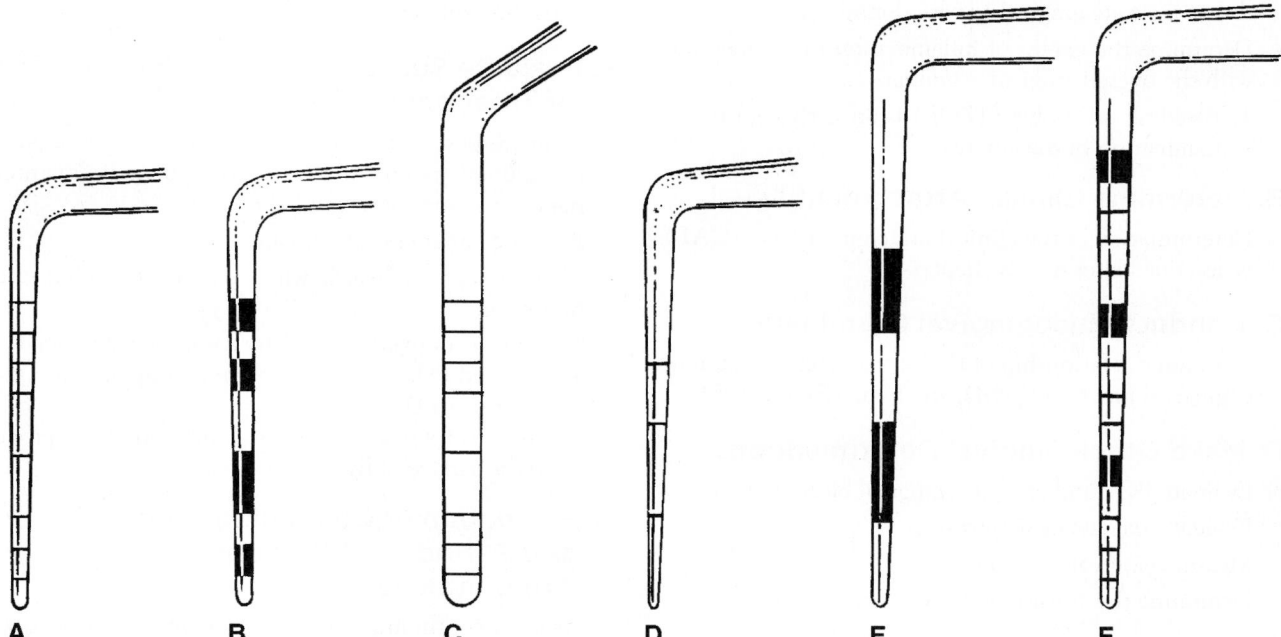

FIGURE 20-3 • Examples of Probes. Names and calibrated markings shown are **A:** Williams (1-1-1-2-2-1-1-1), **B:** Williams, color-coded, **C:** Goldman-Fox (1-1-1-2-2-1-1-1), **D:** Michigan O (3-3-2), **E:** Hu-Friedy or Marquis color-coded (3-3-3-3 or 3-3-2-3), and **F:** Hu-Friedy UNC 15 (each millimeter to 15), color-coded at 5-10-15. See Table 20-1 for additional data on probes.

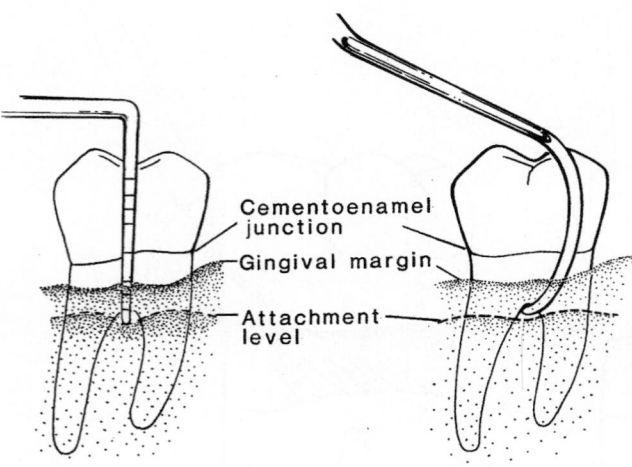

Cementoenamel
junction

Gingival margin

Attachment
level

FIGURE 20-4 • Furcation Examination. A: Limited access of a straight probe to examine a furcation. Williams probe inserted into bifurcation in area of gingival recession shows probing depth of 3 mm. **B:** Nabers furcation probe used to examine the topography of the furcation area.

♦ Automated probes were developed and researched in an attempt to overcome the problems in obtaining consistent readings with traditional probes and used primarily in clinical research.

II. Purposes and Uses

A probe is used for the following purposes.

A. Assess the Periodontal Status for Preparation of a Treatment Plan

♦ Classify the disease as gingivitis or periodontitis by determining whether bone loss has occurred and whether the pockets are gingival or periodontal.

♦ Determine the extent of inflammation in conjunction with the overall gingival examination.
  • Bleeding on probing (BOP) is an early sign of inflammation in the gingiva.

B. Determine Clinical Attachment Level

♦ Determination of the clinical attachment level (CAL) is described later in this chapter.

C. Conduct Mucogingival Examination

♦ Determine relationship of GM, attachment level, mucogingival junction (MGJ), and frena (Figure 20-5).

D. Make Other Gingival Determinations

♦ Evaluate BOP and prepare a gingival bleeding index.

♦ Evaluate exudate or suppuration.

♦ Measure gingival recession.

♦ Determine the consistency of the gingival tissue.

E. Guide Treatment

♦ Summarize gingival characteristics, including probing depth (PD), bleeding, and consistency (all determined

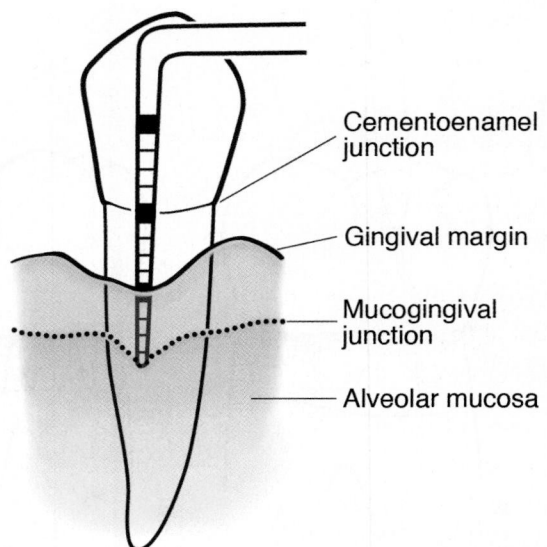

Cementoenamel
junction

Gingival margin

Mucogingival
junction

Alveolar mucosa

FIGURE 20-5 • Mucogingival Examination. Probe in position for measuring probing depth where attached gingiva is missing. The absence of attached gingiva permits the probe to pass through the mucogingival junction into the alveolar mucosa.

using a probe) to provide a basis for diagnosis and treatment planning.

♦ Define PD of sulcus or pocket for application of instruments for scaling, root planing, and maintenance debridement, as well as for use of an explorer for evaluation of these procedures.

♦ Detect anatomic configuration of roots, subgingival deposits, and root irregularities that complicate instrumentation. For this, the probe is used in conjunction with the explorer.

F. Evaluate Success and Completeness of Treatment

♦ Evaluate posttreatment tissue response to nonsurgical periodontal treatment as well as at periodic maintenance examinations.

♦ Evaluate patient's oral self-care.

♦ Identify signs of health when probing including the following:
  • No BOP or exudate; healthy tissue does not bleed.
  • Reduced PD; comparison of pretreatment and posttreatment PD.
  • Tissue is firm, as shown by application of the probe to the surface of the free gingiva.

G. Evaluation at Continuing Care and Periodontal Maintenance Appointments

♦ At each continuing care appointment, a reevaluation is needed.

♦ To identify early disease changes that require additional professional treatment.

III. Description of Manual Periodontal Probes

◆ A probe is a slender instrument with a smooth, rounded tip designed for examination of the depth and topography of a gingival sulcus or periodontal pocket.

◆ A probe has three parts: the handle, angled shank, and working end, which is the probe itself.

A. Materials

◆ Stainless steel.

◆ Plastic: for screenings and titanium implant probing.

B. Characteristics

◆ *Straight working end:*
  • Tapered, round, flat, or rectangular in cross section with a smooth, rounded end.
  • Calibrated in millimeters at intervals specific for each kind of probe; some have color coding. Figure 20-3 shows a comparison of a few typical markings; Table 20-1 lists probe markings with examples.

◆ *Curved working end:* Paired furcation probes have a smooth, rounded end for investigation of the topography and anatomy around roots in a furcation. Examples are the Nabers 1N and 2N probes (Figure 20-4B).

C. Selection

◆ Regular use of the same type of periodontal probe results in greater consistency of readings.

◆ Analysis of a periodontal probe and comparison with other probes are recommended. Following are the important features to be considered in probe selection:
  • *Adaptability:* The probe needs to be adaptable around the complete circumference of each tooth, both posterior and anterior, so that no millimeter area of the sulcus can be neglected. Flat probes require more attention to adaptation and are useful primarily on facial and lingual surfaces.
  • *Markings:* Markings need to be easy to read so PD can be readily identified and measured, and no disease area is overlooked. Color coding contributes to readability.

TABLE 20-1 • Types of Probes		
PROBE MARKINGS (mm)	**EXAMPLES**	**DESCRIPTION**
Marks at 1-2-3-5-7-8-9-10	Williams	Round, tapered (available with color code)
	Glickman	Round, narrow diameter, fine
	Merritt B	Round, with longer lower shank Round, single bend to shank
Marks at 3-3-2	Michigan O Marquis M-1	Round, fine, tapered, narrow diameter
Marks at 3-6-9-12 3-6-8-11 (and other variations)	Michigan O Marquis Nordent	Round, tapered, fine Color-coded
Marks at each mm to 15	UNC 12 or 15	Round Color-coded at 5-10-15
Marks at 3-5-7-10	Perioscreen®	Round Color-coded with green and red to indicate the absence and presence of periodontal disease
Marks at 3.5-5.5-8.5-11.5	WHO Probe (World Health Organization) (Figure 21-7)	Round, tapered, fine, with ball end Color-coded
Marks at 3-5-9-12 No marks	Nabers 1N, 2N	Curved, with curved shank for furcation examination

GUIDE TO PERIODONTAL PROBING

A pocket is a diseased gingival sulcus. The use of a probe is the only accurate, dependable method to locate, assess, and measure sulci and pockets.

I. Pocket Characteristics

◆ A pocket is measured from the base of the pocket (top of attached periodontal tissue) to the GM. Figure 20-6 shows GMs at the same level on two teeth with measurement of pocket depths.

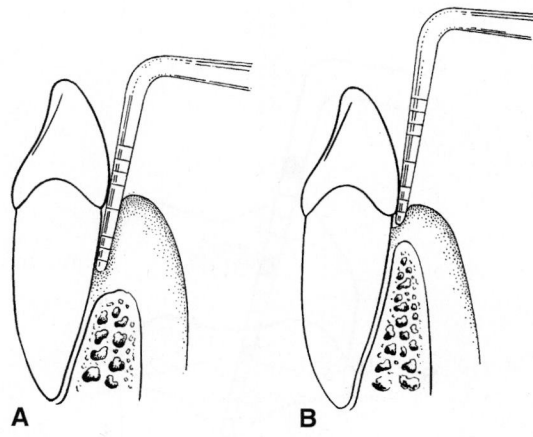

FIGURE 20-6 • Pocket Depth (PD). A pocket is measured from the gingival margin (GM) to the attached periodontal tissue. Shown is the contrast of probe measurements with GMs at the same level. **A:** Deep periodontal pocket (7 mm) with apical migration of attachment. **B:** Shallow sulcus (2 mm) with the attachment near the cementoenamel junction.

- The pocket (or sulcus) is continuous around the tooth and the entire sulcus needs to be measured. "Spot" probing is inadequate for a thorough assessment for diagnosis and treatment planning.
- The depth varies around an individual tooth; PD rarely measures the same all around a tooth or even around one surface of a tooth.
  - The level of attached tissue assumes a varying position around the tooth.
  - The GM varies in its position on the tooth.
- Proximal surfaces are approached by entering from both the facial and lingual aspects of a tooth.
  - Gingival and periodontal infections begin in the col area more frequently than in other areas (Chapter 19).
  - PD may be deepest directly under the contact area because of crater formation in the alveolar bone (Figure 20-7).
- Anatomic features of the tooth surface wall of the pocket influence the direction of probing. Examples are concave surfaces, anomalies, shape of cervical third, and position of furcations.

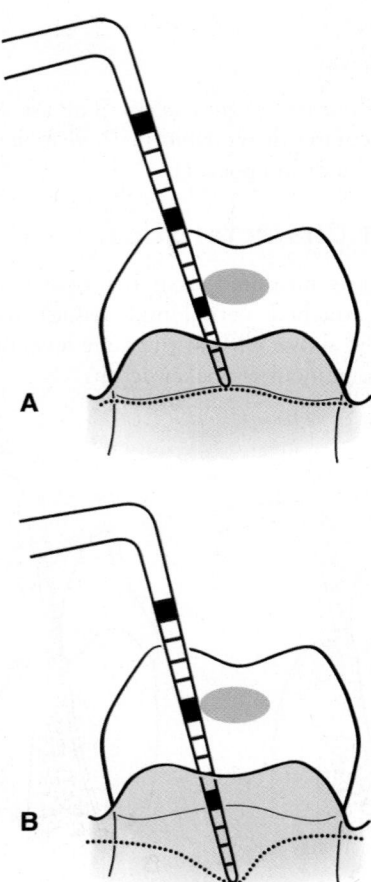

FIGURE 20-7 • Proximal Surface Probing. A: Probe must be applied more than half way across from facial to overlap with probing from the lingual. **B:** Probe in area of crater formation. Probing is often deeper on the proximal surface under the contact area than on the facial or lingual surfaces.

II. Evaluation of Tooth Surface

- During the movement of the probe, calculus, and tooth surface, irregularities can be felt and evaluated.
- The information obtained is used to plan the scaling and root planing appointments.

III. Factors Affecting Probe Accuracy

- The general objectives of probing are accuracy and consistency so recordings can be used for comparison with future probings as well as with colleagues in practice together.
- At the same time, patient discomfort and trauma to the tissues must be minimized.
- Probing is influenced by many factors, such as those described in the following topics.

A. Severity and Extent of Periodontal Disease

- Diseased tissue offers less resistance, so that with increased severity of inflammation, the probe inserts to a deeper level.[1]
  - *Normal healthy tissue*: The probe is at the base of the sulcus or crevice, at the coronal end of the junctional epithelium.
  - *Gingivitis and early periodontitis*: The probe tip is within the junctional epithelium.
  - *Advanced periodontitis*: The probe tip passes through the junctional epithelium to reach attached connective tissue fibers.

B. The Periodontal Probe

- *Calibration*: Must be accurately marked.
- *Thickness*: The recommended probe tip diameter is 0.6 mm.[1]
- *Readability*: Markings and color coding are easy to read.

C. Placement Problems

- *Anatomic variations*: tooth contours, furcations, contact areas, anomalies.
- *Interferences*: calculus, irregular margins of restorations, fixed dental prostheses.
- *Accessibility and visibility*: obstructed by tissue bleeding, limited opening by patient, macroglossia.

PRELIMINARY ASSESSMENT PRIOR TO PERIODONTAL EXAMINATION

The American Academy of Periodontology's Parameter on the Comprehensive Periodontal Examination includes the following[2]:

I. Medical History

◆ A thorough medical history is taken and reviewed to identify issues that may affect treatment and outcomes.

◆ Patients at risk of bacteremia may need prophylactic antibiotic premedication before examination or instrumentation (see Chapter 11).

II. Dental and Psychosocial History

◆ Document the dental history including oral self-care habits, previous dental history, and chief complaint (see Chapter 11).

◆ Psychosocial history may include information such as marital status, living situation, financial situation, work habits, diet, substance use, stress, and oral health literacy (Chapter 11).

  • Psychosocial factors are taken into consideration when planning treatment and setting treatment goals.

III. Vital Signs

◆ Vital signs are taken at each new patient appointment, at follow-up appointments for those with hypertension, and for treatment requiring local anesthesia (see Chapter 12).

IV. Extraoral/Intraoral Examination

◆ An extraoral/intraoral examination should be done at each examination appointment (see Chapter 13).

V. Risk Assessment

◆ The American Academy of Periodontology suggests risk assessment is becoming increasingly important in treatment planning and needs to be included in comprehensive dental and periodontal examinations.[3]

◆ Risk assessment for dental caries, periodontal disease, and oral cancer are conducted (see Chapters 19 and 25 for information on risk assessment tools).

◆ Additional risk assessment for factors such as diabetes (see Chapter 54) or tobacco use (Chapter 32) may be performed based on individual needs of the patient.

VI. Radiographic Examination

◆ Radiographs provide essential information to aid and supplement clinical findings to develop the diagnosis, prognosis, and treatment plan.[4]

◆ The need for radiographs is based on the needs of the patient and current guidelines (see Chapter 15).

◆ During the examination, and especially during the periodontal examination, the radiographs must be available for viewing.

  • When the radiographs are not available at the time of the initial examination, a definitive diagnosis and treatment plan cannot be completed.

  • The need for radiographs free from errors in technique and viewed with magnification on an adequately lighted viewbox or on the computer is essential.

◆ Selection of radiographs: For observing evidence of periodontal involvement, *periapical* radiographs are needed.

  • *Horizontal bitewing* radiographs do not show the complete periodontal tissues that extend around the roots. When bone loss is moderate to severe, the crest of the bone may be seen in a *vertical bitewing* survey (see Chapter 15), which is necessary during the periodontal maintenance phase.

VII. Dental Examination

◆ The dental examination includes documentation of missing teeth, caries, restorations, tooth position, parafunctional habits, and occlusion (see Chapter 16).

VIII. Hard and Soft Deposits

The location of dental biofilm and calculus is documented (see Chapter 17).

A. Supragingival Calculus

◆ *Distribution*

  Supragingival calculus is generally localized and commonly found on the lingual surfaces of the mandibular anterior teeth and the facial surfaces of the maxillary first and second molars, opposite the openings to the salivary ducts.

◆ *Amount*

  Indicate a subjective description of the amount using terms such as slight, moderate, and heavy.

B. Subgingival Calculus

◆ *Distribution*

  Subgingival calculus can be either localized or generalized. Record in relation to pocket PD on a chart or form to show exact locations.

◆ *Amount*

  Indicate a subjective description of the amount using terms such as slight, moderate, and heavy.

◆ *Type*

  • Include descriptive terminology for the type of calculus deposits (see Chapter 17).

PARAMETERS OF CARE FOR THE PERIODONTAL EXAMINATION

I. Periodontal Probing Procedure

A. Periodontal Probe Insertion

◆ Grasp probe with modified pen grasp.

◆ Establish finger rest on a neighboring tooth, preferably in the same dental arch.

◆ Hold side of instrument tip flat against the tooth near the GM. The cervical third of a primary tooth is more convex (Figure 20-8).

◆ Gently slide the tip under the GM.

- *Healthy or firm fibrotic tissue*: Insertion is more difficult because of the close adaptation of the tissue to the tooth surface; underlying gingival fibers are strong and tight.

- *Spongy, soft tissue*: GM is loose and flabby because of the destruction of underlying gingival fibers. Probe inserts readily, and bleeding can be expected on gentle probing.

B. Advance Probe to Base of Pocket

◆ Hold side of probe tip flat against the tooth surface; probe is parallel with long axis of the tooth for vertical insertion. The shape of the crown can make it difficult to maintain this angulation (Figure 20-8).

◆ Slide the probe along the tooth surface vertically down to the base of the sulcus or pocket.

- Maintain contact of the side of the tip of the probe with the tooth.

- *Gingival pocket*: Side of probe is on enamel.

- *Periodontal pocket*: Side of probe is on the cemental or dentinal surface when inserted to a level below the cementoenamel junction (CEJ).

- As the probe is passed down the side of the tooth, roughness may be felt, which may be calculus. Evaluation of the topography and nature of the tooth surface is essential to instrumentation.

- When obstruction by a hard bulky calculus deposit is encountered, lift the probe away from the tooth and follow over the edge of the calculus until the probe can move vertically into the pocket again.

- The base of the sulcus or pocket feels soft and elastic (compared with the hard tooth surface and calculus deposits).

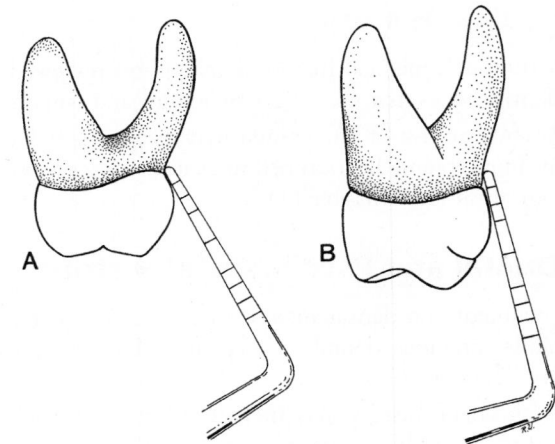

FIGURE 20-8 • Primary and Permanent Maxillary Molars. A: Accentuated convexity of the cervical third and widespread roots of the primary molar complicate probe placement. Probe may encounter the root. **B:** Permanent tooth with less convexity of the cervical third and roots that are less widely spread.

- The force used is approximately 0.20 g (50 N/cm^2) once the tension of the attached periodontal tissue at the base of the pocket is felt.[1,5]

◆ Position the probe for reading.

- Bring the probe to position as nearly parallel with the long axis of the tooth as possible for reading the depth.

- Interference of the contact area does not permit placing the probe parallel for the measurement directly beneath the contact area. Hold the side of the shank of the probe against the contact to minimize the angle (Figure 20-7).

C. Reading the Probe Measurement

◆ Measurement for a PD is made from the GM to the attached periodontal tissue or base of the sulcus or pocket.

◆ A comparison of pocket measurement using probes with different calibrations is shown in Figure 20-9.

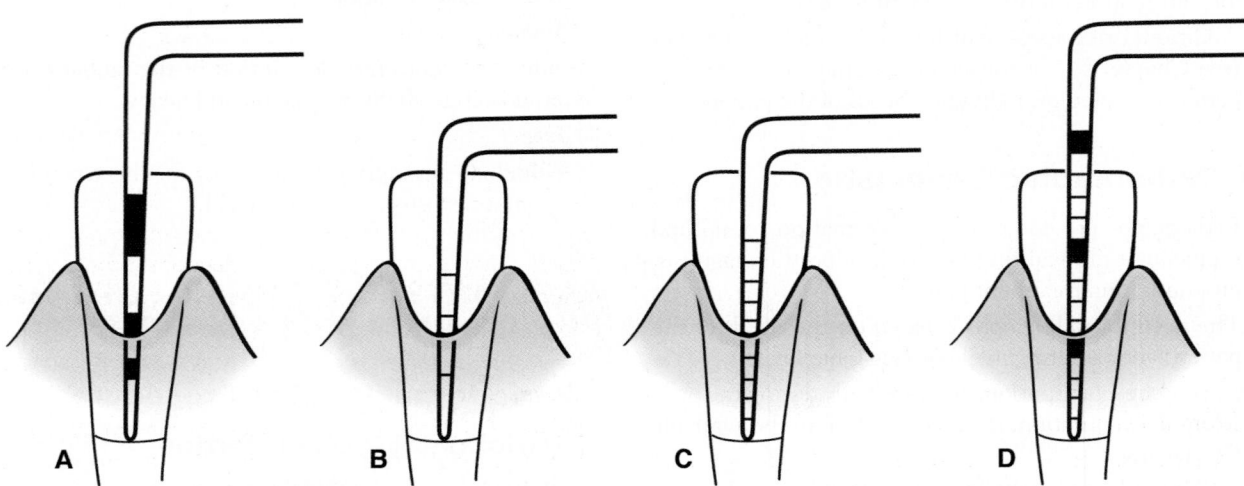

FIGURE 20-9 • Comparison of Probe Readings. Measurement of same 5-mm pocket with four different probes. **A:** Color-coded. **B:** Michigan O. **C:** Williams. **D:** Hu-Friedy UNC 15.

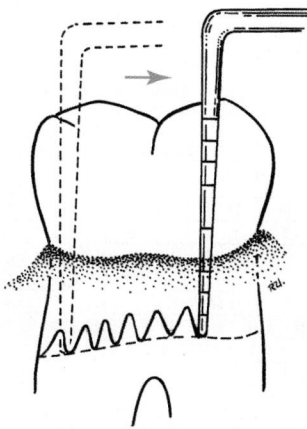

FIGURE 20-10 • Probe Walking Stroke. The side of the tip of the probe is held in contact with the tooth. From the base of the pocket, the probe is moved up and down in 1- to 2-mm strokes as it is advanced in the direction indicated by the blue arrow in 1-mm steps. The attached periodontal tissue at the base of the pocket is contacted on each down stroke to identify probing depth in each area.

◆ When the GM appears at a level between probe marks, round up to the higher marking on the probe for the final measurement.

◆ Dry the area being probed to improve visibility.

D. Circumferential Probing

◆ *Probe stroke*

Maintain the probe in the sulcus or pocket of each tooth as the probe is moved in a walking stroke in the direction of the blue arrow in Figure 20-10.

• It is not necessary to remove the probe and reinsert it to make individual readings. Use a continuous walking stroke to avoid missing a deep pocket area.

• Repeated withdrawal and reinsertion cause unnecessary trauma to the GM and increases posttreatment discomfort.

◆ *Walking stroke*

• Keep the side of the tip in contact with the tooth at the base of the pocket.

• Slide the probe up (coronally) about 1–2 mm and back to the attachment in a "touch . . . touch . . . touch . . ." rhythm (Figure 20-10).

• Observe and record probe measurement at the GM at each location as noted in Figure 20-11.

• Advance millimeter-by-millimeter along the facial and lingual surfaces into the proximal areas of each tooth.

E. Adaptation of Probe for Individual Teeth

◆ *Molars and premolars*

• Orient the probe at the distal line angle for both facial and lingual application.

• Insert the probe at the distal line angle and probe in a distal direction.

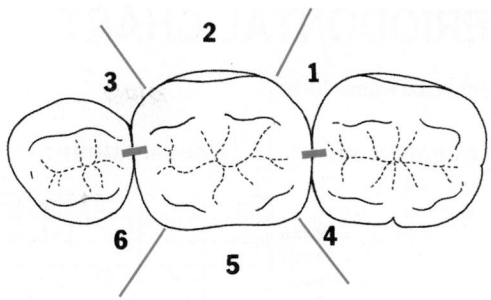

FIGURE 20-11 • Recording Periodontal Probing Depths. The pocket/sulcus is measured completely around each tooth. Record the deepest measurement for each of the six areas around the tooth. Areas 1, 3, 4, and 6 extend from the line angle to under the contact area.

• As the distal proximal area is probed, the probe should touch the contact area and be slanted toward the midline of the proximal surface in the col area (Figure 20-7).

• Note the PD and slide the probe back to the distal line angle. Proceed in the mesial direction around the mesial line angle and across the mesial surface.

• The pocket depth on the mesial is measured in the same manner as the distal proximal surface, and the probe should touch the contact area and be slanted to the midline of the col area where the proximal measurement is read.

• Overlap strokes from facial surface with strokes from lingual surface to ensure full coverage of the proximal area.

◆ *Anterior teeth*

• Initial insertion may be at the distal line angle or from the midline of the facial or lingual surfaces.

• Proceed around the distal line angle and across the distal surface; reinsert and probe the other half of the tooth.

F. Recording of Probing Measurements

◆ Six measurements are recorded for each tooth: three from the facial and three from the lingual or palatal as shown in Figure 20-11.

◆ For each of the six areas, the deepest probing measurement is recorded.

◆ Two recordings each are made for proximal areas: Numbers 3 and 6 for the mesial and numbers 1 and 4 for the distal in Figure 20-11. Frequently the deepest probing will be in the col, directly under the contact area.

◆ Recordings of PDs are part of the total periodontal charting.

◆ Figure 20-12 illustrates a typical chart form in which boxes are provided for recording PD, furcations, and mobility for each tooth (this chart form is missing the MGJ measurements). Many electronic charts also provide an area to calculate the CAL.

PERIODONTAL CHART

Date 3/4/2019

Patient Last Name **Does**   First Name **Jane**   Date Of Birth

☑ **Initial Exam**   ☐ **Reevaluation**   Clinician **Wilkins**

	1	2	3	4	5	6	7	8	9	10	11	12	13	14	15	16
Mobility		0	0	0	0	0	0	0	0	0	0	0	0	0	0	
Implant								■								
Furcation		◑	○											○	○	
Bleeding on Probing																
Plaque																
Gingival Margin		2 0	1 0 0	1 -2 0	0 -2 0	1 -3 1	1 0 1	1 0 1	0 0 0	0 0 0	0 -2 0	0 0 0	0 0 0	1 0 1	1 0 2	
Probing Depth		5 6 7	6 4 6	5 2 5	4 3 4	3 2 3	2 2 2	2 2 2	3 2 2	2 1 2	2 1 2	3 2 3	3 3 4	4 2 7	5 5 6	

Buccal

Lingual

	1	2	3	4	5	6	7	8	9	10	11	12	13	14	15	16
Gingival Margin		2 1 1	1 0 0	1 0 1	1 0 1	0 0 0	0 0 0	0 0 0	0 0 0	0 0 0	0 0 0	0 0 0	0 0 0	0 0 1	1 0 1	
Probing Depth		6 4 6	6 3 6	4 3 4	3 2 3	2 1 1	2 1 1	2 1 2	2 1 2	2 1 1	2 1 1	3 2 2	3 2 3	4 4 6	6 3 6	
Plaque																
Bleeding on Probing																
Furcation	│	○ ◑	○ ○			│						│		◑ ○	○ │	
Note																

Mean Probing Depth = **3** mm   Mean Attachment Level = **-2.7** mm   **48%** Plaque   **42%** Bleeding on Probing

	1	2	3	4	5	6	7	8	9	10	11	12	13	14	15	16
Note																
Furcation		○	○											○		
Bleeding on Probing																
Plaque																
Gingival Margin		2 1 1	1 1 1	1 1 1	1 1 1	0 0 0	0 0 0	0 0 0	0 0 0	0 0 1	1 0 1	1 1 1	2 3 2	2 2 3		
Probing Depth		6 5 5	4 5 5	3 2 3	3 2 3	3 2 2	2 1 2	2 1 2	2 1 2	2 1 2	2 2 3	3 2 2	3 2 3	5 4 6	7 6 8	

Lingual

Buccal

	32	31	30	29	28	27	26	25	24	23	22	21	20	19	18	17
Gingival Margin		2 1 1	1 -1 1	0 -2 0	0 -2 0	0 0 0	0 -1 0	0 -1 0	0 -1 0	0 -1 0	0 0 0	1 -2 1	1 -2 1	1 0 1	1 0 2	
Probing Depth		6 4 5	4 3 4	4 2 3	3 1 2	3 1 2	2 2 2	2 1 2	2 1 2	2 1 2	2 2 3	3 2 3	3 2 3	3 2 2	3 2 4	
Plaque																
Bleeding on Probing																
Furcation			○													
Implant																
Mobility		0	0	0	0	0	0	0	0	0	0	0	0	0	0	

FIGURE 20-12 • Sample Periodontal Chart Form. There are boxes to record the gingival margin, probing depth, plaque, bleeding on probing, furcations, and mobility. The form is missing boxes to record the mucogingival junction and boxes to calculate the clinical attachment level (CAL). The CAL is however graphically displayed by the blue band. (The blank form is available on perio-tools.com.)

G. Sources of Error in Periodontal Probing[6]

- Resistance of tissues that is affected by the level of inflammation in the tissues.
- Calculus.
- Diameter and/or variations in standardization of the probe marks.
- Clinician errors in angulation and/or insertion.
- Probing pressure or force.

II. Clinical Attachment Level

- Attachment level refers to the position of the periodontal attached tissues at the base of a sulcus or pocket.
- CAL is measured from a fixed point to the attachment, whereas the PD is measured from a changeable point (the crest of the free gingiva) to the attachment (Figure 20-13A).

A. Rationale

- Stability of attachment is a characteristic of health.
- A loss of clinical attachment is a primary clinical feature of periodontitis as the junctional epithelium migrates toward the apex.[7]
- When periodontal disease is active, pocket formation and migration of the attachment along the cemental surface continue.
- Evaluation can be made of the outcome of periodontal treatment and the stability of the attachment during maintenance examinations.

B. Procedure

- *Selecting a fixed point*
  - CEJ is used unless it cannot be detected because of abrasion or a restoration.
  - Margin of a permanent restoration.

- *Measuring in the presence of visible recession*
  - CEJ is visible directly.
  - Measure from the CEJ to the GM (Figure 20-13B).
  - The CAL is calculated by *addition* of the pocket depth to the GM to CEJ distance (PD + GM = CAL).
- *Measuring when the CEJ is covered by the gingiva margin*
  - Slide the probe along the tooth surface into the pocket until the CEJ is felt (Figure 20-13C). This is the CEJ to GM measurement.
  - *Subtract* the distance from the CEJ to GM from the total PD to the attachment (PD − GM = CAL).
- *Measuring when the GM is level with the CEJ*
  - With the GM at the CEJ, that measurement is the same as the PD.
  - The PD *equals* the CAL when the GM is level with the CEJ (Figure 20-13D).

III. Mucogingival Examination

A. Methods for Identifying MGJ

- *Purposes*
  - To detect adequacy of the width of the attached gingiva.
  - To locate frenal attachments and their proximity to the free gingiva.
- *Tension test procedure*
  - Retract cheeks and lips laterally by grasping the lips with the thumbs and index fingers.
  - Move the lips and cheeks up and down and back and forth, creating tension between the attached gingiva and mucosa to make the MGJ visible (Figure 20-14).
  - Follow around from the molar areas on the right to molar areas on the left, both maxillary and mandibular. Observe frenal attachments.

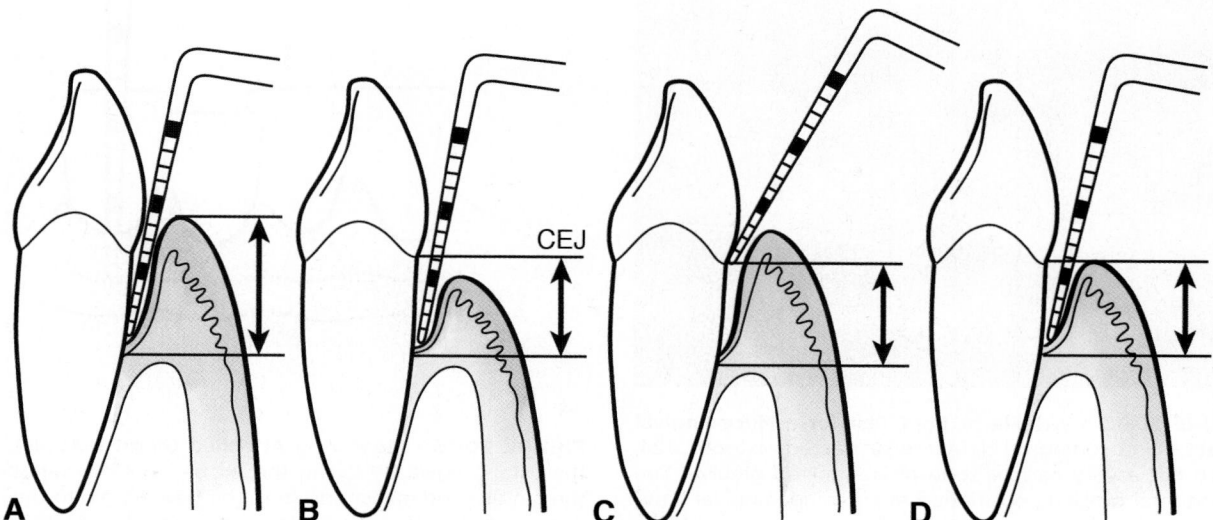

FIGURE 20-13 • Clinical Attachment Level (CAL). A: Pocket depth is measured from the gingival margin (GM) to the attached periodontal tissue. **B:** CAL in the presence of gingival recession is measured directly from the cementoenamel junction (CEJ) to the attached tissue. **C:** CAL when the GM covers the CEJ: first the CEJ is located as shown, and then the distance to the CEJ is measured and subtracted from the probing depth (PD). **D:** The CAL is equal to the PD when the GM is at the level of the CEJ.

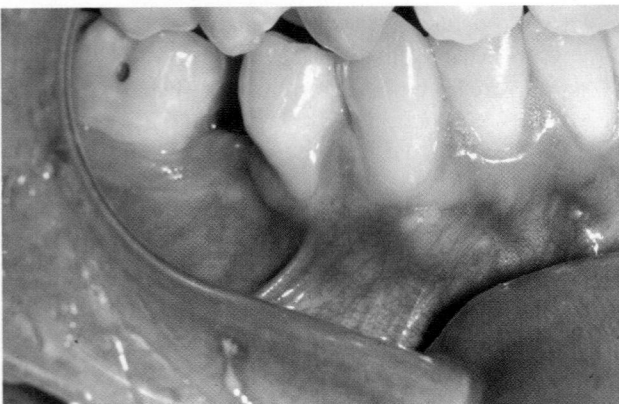

FIGURE 20-14 • Tension test. The tension test can be used to differentiate unattached mucosa and attached gingiva to aid in identifying the location of the MGJ to more accurately calculate the quantity of attached gingiva. (Credit: Dr. Ralph Arnold.)

- *Lingual (mandible)*
  - Hold a mouth mirror to tense the mucosa of the floor of the mouth, gently retracting the side of the tongue, so that the MGJ is clearly visible.
  - Request patient move the tongue to the left, to the right, and up to touch the palate.
- *Fold (or wrinkle) test procedure*
  - Retract the lip gently, but not to the point of tension between the attached gingiva and buccal mucosa.
  - The periodontal probe is oriented horizontal to the MGJ and very gentle pressure is used to fold or wrinkle the mucosa toward the GM (see Figure 20-15).[8]
  - This test can be used if the MGJ cannot be easily visualized with the tension test method.

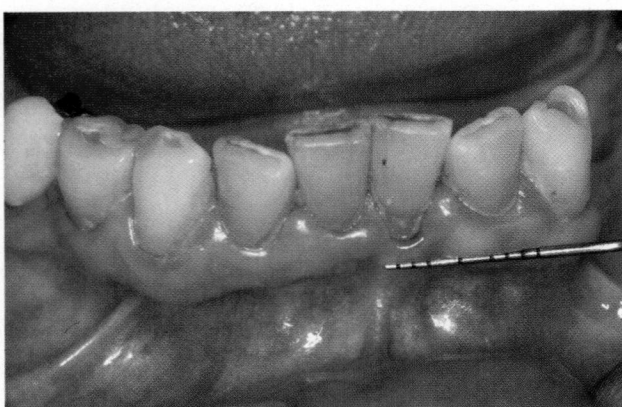

FIGURE 20-15 • Wrinkle or Fold Test for a Mucogingival Defect. A mucogingival defect is suspected at tooth #24, which has a very narrow zone of keratinized gingiva. The periodontal probe is positioned at the mucogingival junction and gently moved coronally against the mucosa. Blanching or wrinkling of the mucosa at the gingival margin indicates no attached gingiva. (Reprinted from Scheid R. *Woelfel's Dental Anatomy.* 7th ed. Philadelphia, PA: Lippincott Williams & Wilkins; 2007.)

B. Measurement of Width of Attached Gingiva

- Place the probe (no pressure) on the external surface of the gingiva and measure from the MGJ to the GM to determine the total width of the gingiva (Figure 20-16A).
- Measure PD (Figure 20-16B).
- Calculate the width of attached gingiva by *subtracting* the PD from the total width of the gingiva.
- Record findings.

C. Areas at Risk for Mucogingival Conditions[9]

- Area(s) of recession with little keratinized gingiva and the base of the sulcus or pocket is near the MGJ.
- When a pocket extends to or beyond the MGJ, the probe may pass through into the alveolar mucosa when probing the pocket (Figure 20-5).

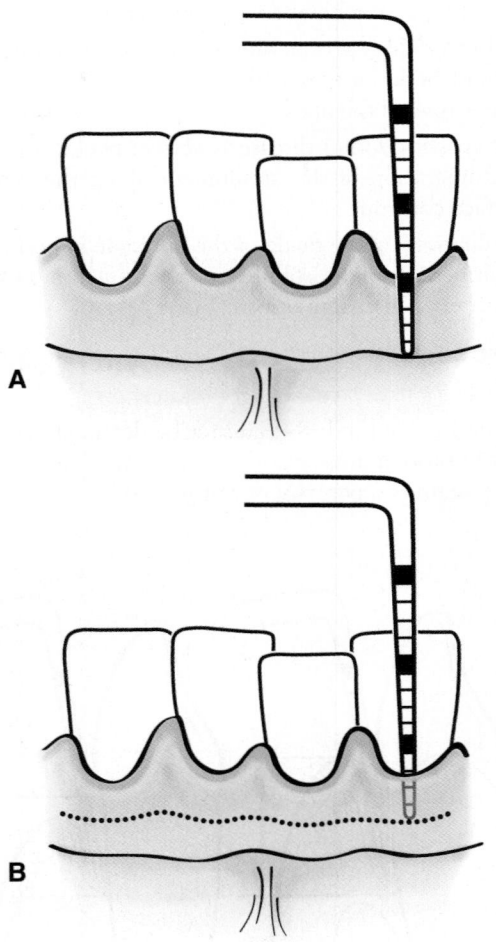

FIGURE 20-16 • Measuring Attached Gingiva. A: Measure the total gingiva by laying the probe over the surface of the gingiva and measuring from the free margin to the mucogingival junction. **B:** Measure the probing depth (PD). Dotted line represents the base of the pocket. Subtract the PD **(B)** from the total gingiva **(A)** to obtain the width of attached gingiva. The area illustrated shows 2 mm of attached gingiva.

♦ Absent or narrow attached (keratinized) gingiva.

♦ Anatomic differences such as tooth position and frenum insertions.

IV. Mobility Examination

♦ Because of the nature and function of the periodontal ligament, teeth have a slight normal mobility.

♦ Mobility can be considered abnormal or pathologic when it exceeds normal.

♦ Increased mobility can be a clinical sign of trauma from occlusion.

A. Procedure for Determination of Mobility

1. Position the patient for clear visibility with good light.

2. Stabilize the head: Motion of the head, lips, or cheek can interfere with an accurate evaluation of tooth movement.

3. Use two single-ended metal instruments with wide blunt ends, held with a modified pen grasp (Figure 20-17).

   • The use of wooden tongue depressors or plastic mirror handles is not recommended because of their flexibility.

   • Testing with the fingers without the metal instruments can be misleading because the soft tissue of the fingertips can move and give an illusion of tooth movement.

4. Apply specific, firm finger rests (fulcrums): A standardized finger rest pressure contributes increased consistency to the determinations. The teeth may be dried with air or gauze to prevent slipping of the instruments or the finger on the finger rest.

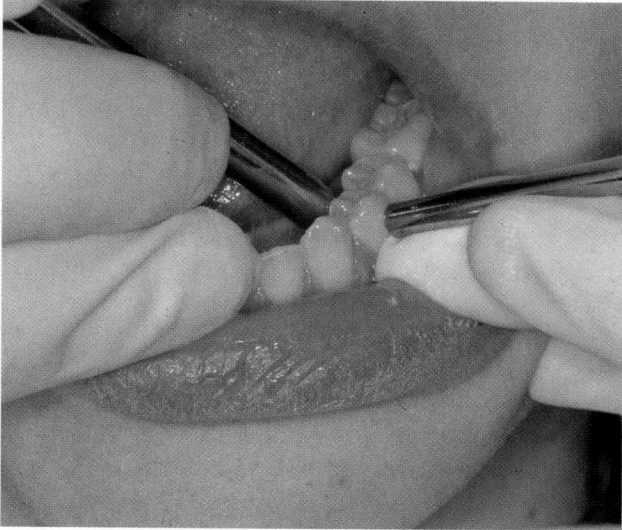

FIGURE 20-17 • Method for Determining Tooth Mobility. A: Two rigid instrument handles are applied to the tooth to see if it can be displaced either buccolingually or mesiodistally. For teeth with severe mobility, the tooth can be depressed or rotated (which is category 3 mobility). **B:** Technique for determining buccolingual mobility. Light, alternating (reciprocating) buccolingual forces are applied and movement observed relative to adjacent teeth.

5. Apply the blunt ends of the instruments to opposite sides of a tooth, and rock the tooth to test horizontal mobility. Keep both instrument ends on the tooth as pressure is applied first from one side and then the other.

6. Test vertical mobility (depression of the tooth into its socket) by applying pressure with one of the mirror handles to the occlusal or incisal surface.

7. Move from tooth to tooth in a systematic order.

B. Record Degree of Movement

The most widely used method to assess tooth mobility is the Miller Index first described in 1938.[10]

♦ *Scale*

The N, 1, 2, 3 or I, II, III are frequently used, sometimes with a plus sign (+) to indicate mobility between numbers.

♦ *Recording*

Although subjective, interpretation may be considered as follows[10]:

N = normal, physiologic.

1 = slight mobility, greater than normal.

2 = moderate mobility, greater than 1 mm displacement.

3 = severe mobility, moves vertically and is depressible in the tooth socket.

♦ *The letter N means normal mobility*

All teeth that have a periodontal ligament have normal mobility. No tooth has zero mobility, except in a condition such as ankylosis in which there is no periodontal ligament.

♦ *Chart form*

A chart form such as Figure 20-12 can provide for a place to record mobility. Preferably more than one space can be available, so comparative readings can be recorded at successive maintenance appointments.

V. Fremitus

A. Definition

♦ Fremitus means palpable vibration or movement.

♦ In dentistry, fremitus refers to the vibratory patterns of the teeth. A tooth with fremitus has excess contact, possibly related to a premature contact. Usually, the tooth also demonstrates some degree of mobility because the excess contact forces the tooth to move.

♦ The test is used in conjunction with occlusal analysis and adjustment.

♦ Because fremitus depends on tooth contact, determination is made only on the maxillary teeth.

B. Procedure for Determination of Fremitus

1. Seat the patient upright with the head stabilized against the headrest; the occlusal biting plane is parallel with the floor.

2. Gently place the index finger on each maxillary tooth at about the cervical third (Figure 20-18).

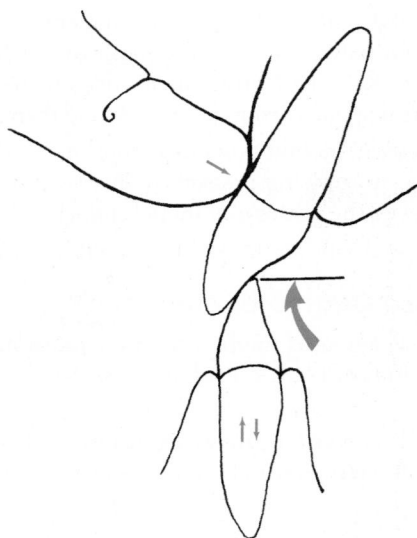

FIGURE 20-18 • Fremitus. With the patient seated upright and the head stabilized against the headrest, an index finger is placed firmly over the cervical third of each maxillary tooth in succession starting with the most posterior tooth on one side and moving around the arch. The patient is asked to click the posterior teeth.

3. Request the patient to close the back teeth together in a functional occlusion and tap up and down repeatedly.[11]

4. Start with the most posterior maxillary tooth on one side and move the index finger tooth by tooth around the arch.

5. Record by tooth number the teeth where vibration is felt and the teeth where actual movement is noted. The degree recorded may be subjective, but the following range has been suggested:
   - N = normal (without vibration or movement).
   - + = One-degree fremitus; only slight vibration can be felt.
   - + + = Two-degree fremitus; the tooth is clearly palpable but movement is barely visible.
   - + + + = Three-degree fremitus; movement is clearly observed visually.

VI. Furcation Examination

When a pocket extends into a furcation area, special adaptation of the probe must be made to determine the extent and topography of the furcation involvement.

A. Anatomic Features

◆ *Bifurcation (teeth with two roots)*
   1. *Mandibular molars:* The furcation area is accessible for probing from the facial and lingual surfaces (Figure 20-4).
   2. *Maxillary first premolars:* The furcation area is accessible from the mesial and distal aspects, under the contact area.
   3. *Primary mandibular molar:* Widespread roots.

◆ *Trifurcation (teeth with three roots)*
   1. *Maxillary molars:* A palatal root and two buccal roots, the mesiobuccal and the distobuccal roots. Access for probing is from the buccal (Figure 20-19A), mesiolingual, buccal (Figure 20-19B), and distolingual surfaces (Figure 20-19C).
   2. *Maxillary primary molars:* Widespread roots (Figure 20-8).

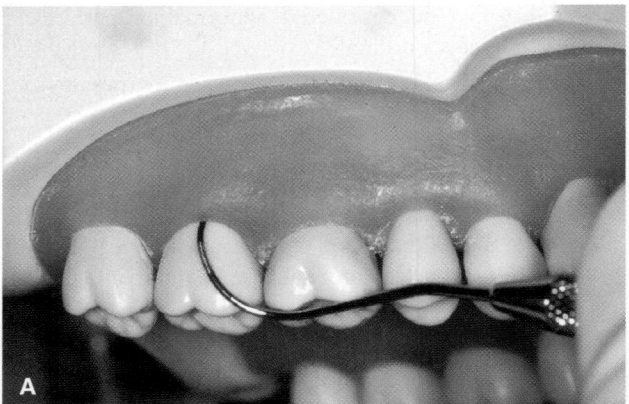

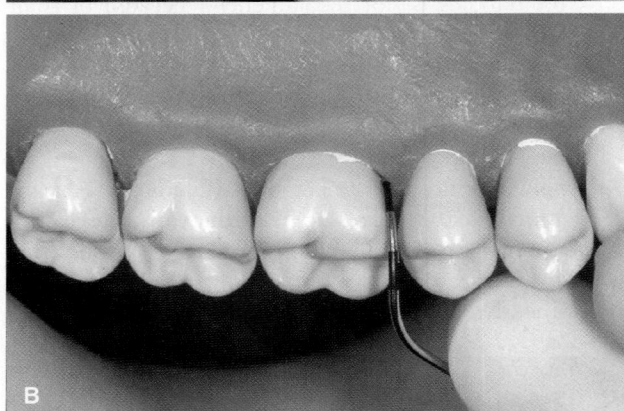

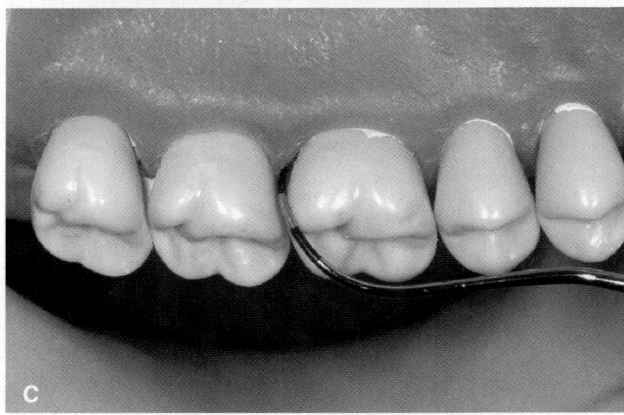

FIGURE 20-19 • Three Locations Used to Confirm Maxillary Molar Furcation Involvement. A: Buccal view: Buccal furcation is probed midbuccal. The furcation probe is shown as it enters the potential furcation near the middle of the facial surface of this maxillary molar. **B:** Palatal view: The mesial furcation on a maxillary molar is accessed through the palatal embrasure since the mesiobuccal root is wider than the palatal root. **C:** Palatal view: The distal furcation on a maxillary molar is probed through the palatal embrasure here, although the distobuccal root is about as wide as the palatal root.

B. Examination Methods

◆ *Furcation measurement procedure*[12]:

- Review the radiograph for signs of furcation involvement or radiolucency (Figure 20-20).
- Using knowledge of the anatomy of the multi-rooted teeth, use a furcation probe, such as the Nabers 1N or 2N probe, to walk around the area sulcus to identify the entrance to the furcation (Figure 20-4B).[13]
- If the Nabers probe enters the furcation, note the distance from the entrance to the furcation until resistance is felt, which provides the vertical depth of the furcation.

◆ *Furcation grades*

Furcation involvement is usually classified by the amount of bone destroyed in the furcation area. The most common classification is the Glickman furcation grades and include[14]:

- *Grade I*: early, beginning involvement. A probe can enter the concavity of the furcation but the bone between the roots (interradicular) is intact.
- *Grade II*: moderate involvement. Bone has been destroyed to an extent that permits Nabers probe to enter the furcation area between the roots but not extend all the way through to the opposite side.
- *Grade III*: severe involvement. A probe can be passed between the roots through the entire furcation.
- *Grade IV*: Same as grade III, with exposure resulting from gingival recession, especially after periodontal therapy.

◆ *Difficulties encountered in measurement of the furcation*[12]

- Anatomic variations that complicate furcation examination are fused roots, anomalies such as extra roots, or low or high furcations.
- Force, tip diameter, angulation, and type of probe used.
- Tissue quality variation.
- Interference by calculus, crown contour, or overhanging restorations.

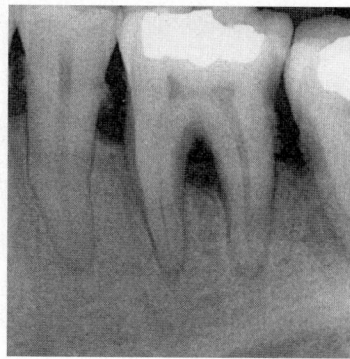

FIGURE 20-20 • Furcation Involvement. The furcation involvement (radiolucency) is easily visible on the mandibular first molar in this radiographic.

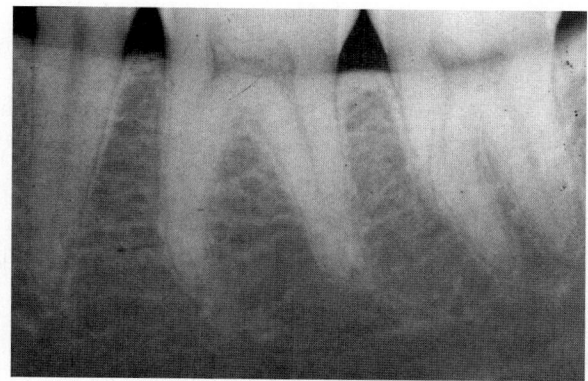

FIGURE 20-21 • Normal Bone Level. Drawing of a radiograph to show normal bone level, 1–1.5 mm from the cementoenamel junction.

RADIOGRAPHIC CHANGES IN PERIODONTAL DISEASE

I. Bone Level

A. Normal Bone Level

The crest of the interdental bone appears from 1.0 to 1.5 mm from the CEJ and is horizontal from the CEJ of one tooth to the adjacent tooth (Figure 20-21).

B. Bone Level in Periodontal Disease

The height of the bone is lowered progressively as the inflammation is extended and bone is destroyed.

II. Shape of Remaining Bone

A. Horizontal Bone Loss

◆ When the crest of the bone is parallel with a line between the CEJs of two adjacent teeth, the term *horizontal bone loss* is used (Figure 20-22).

◆ When inflammation is the sole destructive factor, the bone loss usually appears horizontal.

◆ When the amount of remaining bone is fairly evenly distributed throughout the dentition, the condition may be described as *generalized horizontal bone loss*. It may be designated either by millimeters from the position of the normal bone level or by percentage.

◆ When bone loss is confined to specific areas, the condition is described as *localized* horizontal bone loss.

B. Angular or Vertical Bone Loss

◆ Reduction in height of crestal bone that is irregular; the bone level is not parallel with a line joining the adjacent CEJs (Figure 20-23).

◆ Angular bone loss is more commonly *localized*; rarely generalized.

◆ When inflammation and trauma from occlusion are combined in causing the destruction and irregular shape of the bone, the bone may appear with "angular defects" or with "vertical bone loss."

III. Crestal Lamina Dura

A. Normal

White, radiopaque; continuous with and connects the lamina dura about the roots of two adjacent teeth; covers the interdental bone of the two molars in Figure 20-21.

B. Evidence of Disease

The crestal lamina dura is indistinct, irregular, radiolucent, and fuzzy (Figures 20-22 and 20-23).

IV. Furcation Involvement

A. Normal

Bone fills the area between the roots (Figure 20-21).

B. Evidence of Disease

◆ Radiolucent area in the furcation (Figure 20-20).

◆ Early furcation involvement shown in the mandibular second molar in Figure 20-23 may appear as a small radiolucent black area or as a slight thickening of the periodontal ligament space. It can be confirmed by clinical assessment with a Nabers probe.

◆ Furcation involvement of maxillary molars may become more advanced before radiographic evidence is seen. Superimposition of the palatal root may mask a small area of involvement.

◆ When the height of the interdental bone in the radiograph is at the level of the furcation, it can be used as an approximate guide to possible furcation involvement.[15]

◆ Maxillary first premolar furcation involvement cannot be seen in a radiograph with correct vertical and horizontal angulation because the roots are superimposed.

V. Periodontal Ligament Space

A. Normal

◆ The periodontal ligament is connective tissue and, hence, appears as a fine black radiolucent line next to the root surface.

◆ On its outer side is the lamina dura—the bone that lines the tooth socket and appears radiopaque.

B. Evidence of Disease

Widening or thickening.

◆ *Angular thickening or triangulation*: Widened only near the coronal third, near the crest of the interdental bone.

◆ *Periodontal ligament space widening may occur along an entire side of a root to the apex or around the root* (Figure 20-20): When viewed at different angulations (in the various radiographs of a complete survey), the

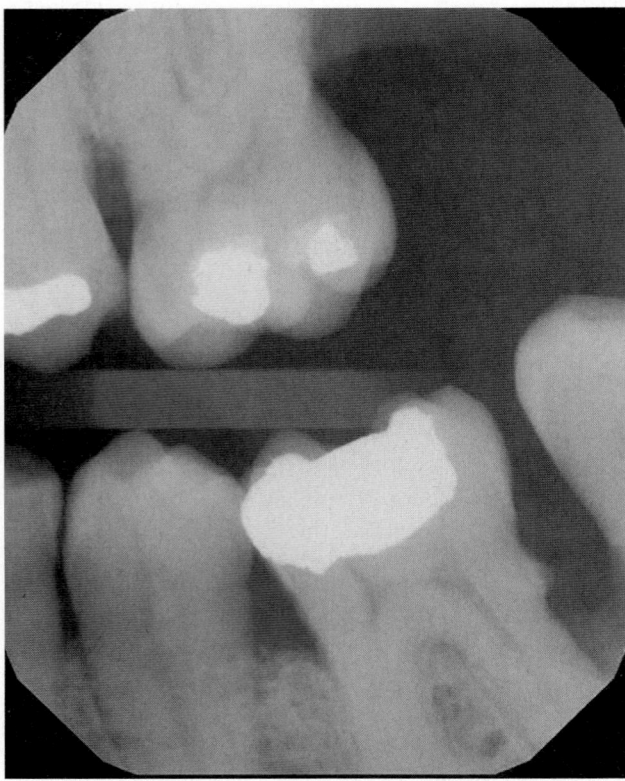

FIGURE 20-22 • Horizontal Bone Loss. Note that the level of the crestal bone is parallel with a line between the cementoenamel junctions of the mandibular second premolar and the mesially tipped first molar (also note calculus on the distal of the mandibular first molar).

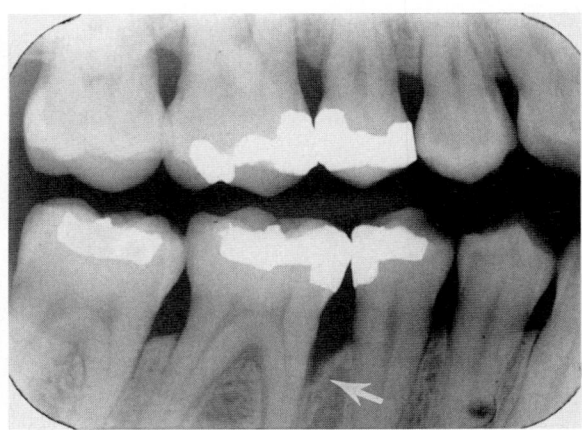

FIGURE 20-23 • Vertical Bone Loss. The *arrow* points to vertical bone loss on the mesial surface of the mandibular first molar.

ligament space may reveal varying thicknesses, thus showing the disease involvement is not consistent around the entire root or that other structures are superimposed.

OTHER RADIOGRAPHIC FINDINGS

◆ Any other radiographic findings related directly or indirectly to periodontal involvement and contributing factors are noted in the record.

◆ Certain findings have a direct relation to dental hygiene care and instruction, particularly local factors that contribute to food impaction or biofilm retention.

I. Calculus

◆ Gross deposits, primarily those on proximal surfaces, may be seen in radiographs (Figure 20-22).

◆ Radiographs have very limited value for calculus detection, so clinical assessment with an explorer is needed to determine the location and extent of the deposit.

II. Overhanging Restorations

◆ Some proximal overhanging margins may be seen on radiographs.

◆ The use of an explorer is necessary to detect irregular margins and to examine all proximal margins that do not reveal irregularities in the radiographs.

III. Dental Caries

◆ See Chapter 16.

DOCUMENTATION

Documentation in the permanent record for a patient with a gingival or periodontal condition needs to include a minimum of the following:

◆ Findings by clinical observation and comprehensive periodontal examination leading to the dental hygiene diagnosis.

◆ Mobility, fremitus, occlusal problems, and other findings that will tie the complete oral plan for dental hygiene care into the overall major treatment plan for dental care by a dentist.

◆ A sample progress note documenting a dental hygiene appointment is found in Box 20-1.

BOX 20-1

Example Documentation: Periodontal Examination Findings

S—Mr. Jones presents to the dental office for his first visit. He just moved to Boston a few months ago and needs a routine examination and "cleaning." He does not report any concerns about his mouth at this time. Mr. Jones reports he just had a physical examination with his new physician and was diagnosed with prediabetes and was put on metformin. His A1c was 6.5. He lives alone and eats out once or twice a day. He reports brushing daily, but he says he will not floss so don't lecture him about it.

O—His vital signs are normal, with a BP of 120/79. Extraoral examination/intraoral examination were normal. No full mouth series of radiographs in 5 years and his risk assessment indicated he was at high caries and periodontal risk. Comprehensive examination findings included a broken filling DO-#30 and a broken mesiolingual (ML) cusp on #31. He has generalized 5–6 mm pocket depths with BOP in all posterior areas with marginal inflammation. Grade I furcations noted ML and DL of #2, 3, 14, and 15. No mobility. Adequate attached gingiva in all areas.

A—The periodontal diagnosis is generalized moderate chronic periodontitis. High caries and periodontal risk. Slight-to-moderate localized subgingival calculus. Plaque score 60%.

P—Patient education for oral self-care included refinement of modified Bass brushing technique in posterior areas along with introduction of floss picks for interdental care. Patient demonstrated both home care aids and liked the floss picks. Education about periodontal disease and association with diabetes was discussed along with his diagnosis and need for nonsurgical periodontal therapy (NSPT) by quadrant with local anesthesia in posterior areas. The patient was shocked by the findings because he has been having "cleanings" every 6 months at his previous dental office, but he indicated he had never had all the "measuring" done before. He was very thankful to learn about the association between diabetes and periodontal disease. He seemed highly motivated to improve his oral health. The dentist also discussed the need for a crown on #31 and replacement of the filling on #30 once the NSPT was complete. Next visit: NSPT maxillary right quadrant with local anesthesia and review of oral self-care.

Signed: _____, RDH

Date: _____

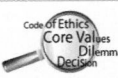

EVERYDAY ETHICS

Mrs. Claren, a neat-appearing lady in her 50s, was new to the practice. After a careful review of the medical history, Brittany, the dental hygienist, completed the comprehensive periodontal examination. The PDs were generally 5–6 mm with CAL of 4–5 mm. Brittany noted BOP in posterior areas with moderate subgingival calculus.

When Brittany finished the examination and sat the patient upright to discuss the findings, the patient said, "You aren't cleaning my teeth. What is it you are doing?" Brittany realized the patient may never have had a complete periodontal examination and was unaware of her generalized moderate chronic periodontitis.

Questions for Consideration

1. Which of the dental hygiene core values should be considered in this scenario with Brittany and Mrs. Claren? Think of each of the core values in relation to a first-time patient compared with a long-time patient.

2. Review the legal and ethical concepts to consider how they may be of help to Brittany as she thinks over how to answer Mrs. Claren. Make a list of explanations Brittany might use.

3. Is Brittany's role simply to explain office policy to a new patient or is informed consent the priority here?

Factors to Teach the Patient

▶ The need for a comprehensive examination to ensure treatment is planned to meet all of the patient's needs.

▶ The value of the various components of the comprehensive examination in assessing the patient's oral health. Examples are the complete radiographic survey and comprehensive periodontal examination.

▶ Why bleeding can occur when probing. Healthy tissue does not bleed.

▶ Relation of PD measurements to normal sulci.

▶ Significance of the periodontal findings such as mobility, furcation involvement, or inadequate attached gingiva.

ENHANCE YOUR UNDERSTANDING

ONLINE RESOURCES
(see the inside front cover for access information)
- Audio glossary
- Appendices

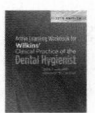

SUPPORT FOR LEARNING
(available separately)
- *Active Learning Workbook for Wilkins' Clinical Practice of the Dental Hygienist, 13th Edition*

INDIVIDUALIZED REVIEW
- Customized practice quizzing with Navigate 2 TestPrep for *Wilkins' Clinical Practice of the Dental Hygienist*

References

1. Garnick JJ, Silverstein L. Periodontal probing: probe tip diameter. *J Periodontol.* 2000;71(1):96-103.

2. American Academy of Periodontology. Parameter on comprehensive periodontal examination. *J Periodontol.* 2000;71(5)(suppl):847-848.

3. American Academy of Periodontology. American Academy of Periodontology statement on risk assessment. *J Periodontol.* 2008;79(2):202.

4. Corbet EF, Ho DK, Lai SM. Radiographs in periodontal disease diagnosis and management. *Aust Dent J.* 2009;(54)(suppl 1):S27-S43.

5. Larsen C, Barendregt DS, Slot DE, Van der Velden U, Van der Weijden F. Probing pressure, a highly undervalued unit of measure in periodontal probing: a systematic review on its effect on probing pocket depth. *J Clin Periodontol.* 2009;36(4):315-322.

6. Andrade R, Espinoza M, Gómez EM, Espinoza JR, Cruz E. Intra- and inter-examiner reproducibility of manual probing depth. *Braz Oral Res.* 2012;26(1):57-63.

7. Flemmig TF. Periodontitis. *Ann Periodontol.* 1999;4(1):32-38.

8. Guglielmoni P, Promsudthi A, Tatakis DN, Trombelli L. Intra- and inter-examiner reproducibility in keratinized tissue width assessment with 3 methods for mucogingival junction determination. *J Periodontol.* 2001;72(2):134-139.

9. American Academy of Periodontology. Parameters of mucogingival conditions. *J Periodontol.* 2000;71(suppl):861-862.

10. Laster L, Laudenbach KW, Stoller NH. An evaluation of clinical tooth mobility measurements. *J Periodontol.* 1975;46(10):603-607.

11. Davies SJ, Gray RJ, Linden GJ, James JA. Occlusal considerations in periodontics. *Br Dent J.* 2001;191(11):597-604.

12. Karthikeyan BV, Sujatha V, Prabhuji ML. Furcation measurements: realities and limitations. *J Int Acad Periodontol.* 2015;17(4):103-115.

13. Eickholz P, Kim TS. Reproducibility and validity of the assessment of clinical furcation parameters as related to different probes. *J Periodontol.* 1998;69(3):328-336.

14. Al-Shammari KF, Kazor CE, Wang HL. Molar root anatomy and management of furcation defects. *J Clin Periodontol.* 2001;28(8):730-740.

15. Grover V, Malhotra R, Kapoor A, et al. Correlation of the interdental and the interradicular bone loss: a radiovisuographic analysis. *J Indian Soc Periodontol.* 2014;18(4):482-487.

21

Indices and Scoring Methods

Charlotte J. Wyche, BSDH, MS

CHAPTER OUTLINE

TYPES OF SCORING METHODS
  I. Individual Assessment Score
  II. Clinical Trial
  III. Epidemiologic Survey
  IV. Community Surveillance

INDICES
  I. Descriptive Categories of Indices
  II. Selection Criteria

ORAL HYGIENE STATUS (BIOFILM, DEBRIS, AND CALCULUS)
  I. Biofilm Index
  II. Biofilm Control Record
  III. Biofilm-Free Score
  IV. Patient Hygiene Performance
  V. Simplified Oral Hygiene Index

GINGIVAL AND PERIODONTAL HEALTH
  I. Periodontal Screening and Recording
  II. Community Periodontal Index
  III. Sulcus Bleeding Index
  IV. Gingival Bleeding Index
  V. Eastman Interdental Bleeding Index
  VI. Gingival Index

DENTAL CARIES EXPERIENCE
  I. Permanent Dentition: Decayed, Missing, and Filled Teeth or Surfaces
  II. Primary Dentition: Decayed, Indicated for Extraction, and Filled (df and def)
  III. Primary Dentition: Decayed, Missing, and Filled (dmf)
  IV. Early Childhood Caries
  V. Root Caries Index

DENTAL FLUOROSIS
  I. Dean's Fluorosis Index
  II. Tooth Surface Index of Fluorosis

COMMUNITY-BASED ORAL HEALTH SURVEILLANCE
  I. WHO Basic Screening Survey
  II. Association of State and Territorial Dental Directors' Basic Screening Survey

DOCUMENTATION

EVERYDAY ETHICS

FACTORS TO TEACH THE PATIENT

REFERENCES

LEARNING OBJECTIVES

After studying this chapter, the student will be able to:

1. Identify and define key terms and concepts related to dental indices and scoring methods.

2. Identify the purpose, criteria for measurement, scoring methods, range of scores, and reference or interpretation scales for a variety of dental indices.

3. Select and calculate dental indices for a use in a specific patient or community situation.

This chapter provides an introduction to scoring methods used by clinicians, researchers, and community practitioners to evaluate indicators of oral health status. It is not possible to explain all of the many dental indices that have been used in a variety of settings, but several well-known and widely used indices and scoring methods are described in this chapter.

TYPES OF SCORING METHODS

Indices and scoring methods are used in clinical practice and by community programs to determine and record the oral health status of individuals and groups.

I. Individual Assessment Score

A. Purpose

In clinical practice, an index, a biofilm record, or a scoring system for an individual patient can be used for education, motivation, and evaluation.

- The effects of personal disease control efforts, the progress of healing following professional treatments, and the maintenance of health over time can be monitored.
- An example is the biofilm-free score, in which the dental hygienist is able to measure the effects of a patient's personal daily care efforts.

B. Uses

- To provide individual assessment to help a patient recognize an oral problem.
- To reveal the degree of effectiveness of oral hygiene practices.
- To motivate the patient during preventive and professional care for the elimination and control of oral disease.
- To evaluate the success of individual oral self-care and professional treatment over a period of time by comparing index scores.

II. Clinical Trial

A. Purpose

A clinical trial is planned to determine the effect of an agent or a procedure on the prevention, progression, or control of a disease.

- The trial is conducted by comparing an experimental group with a control group that is similar to the experimental group in every way, except for the variable being studied.
- Examiners who collect dental index data for research are calibrated or trained to measure the index in exactly the same way each time.
- Examples of indices used for clinical trials are the biofilm index[1] and the patient hygiene performance (PHP).[2]

B. Uses

- To determine baseline data before experimental factors are introduced.
- To measure the effectiveness of specific agents for the prevention, control, or treatment of oral conditions.
- To measure the effectiveness of mechanical devices for personal care, such as toothbrushes, interdental cleaning devices, or irrigators.

III. Epidemiologic Survey

A. Purpose

The word epidemiology denotes the study of disease characteristics of populations rather than individuals. Epidemiologic surveys provide information on the trends and patterns of oral health and disease in populations.

- An example is the decayed, missing, and filled teeth (DMFT) index[3] to determine the extent of dental caries.

B. Uses

- To determine the prevalence and incidence of a particular condition occurring within a given population.
- To provide baseline data on indicators that show existing dental health status in populations.
  - The Surgeon General's Report on *Oral Health in America* used epidemiologic data to identify oral health disparities in certain populations.[4]
- To provide data to support recommendations for public health interventions to improve the health status of populations, such as those provided in the U.S. *Healthy People 2020* document.[5]

IV. Community Surveillance

A. Purpose

Community oral health assessment is a multifaceted process of identifying factors that affect the oral health status of a selected population. Community surveillance of oral health indicators and determinants can be accomplished at many levels.

- Government agencies, local community-based service-providing agencies, and professional associations are examples of groups that collect data to determine oral health status by conducting oral health screenings.
- Information from community-wide oral screenings can be used when planning local community-based oral health services or education.
- An example of a system designed to be used by a community-based group is the Association of State and Territorial Dental Directors' (ASTDD) Basic Screening Survey.[6]

B. Uses

- To assess the needs of a community.
- To help plan community-based health promotion/disease prevention programs.
- To compare the effects or evaluate the results of community-based programs.

INDICES

An index is a way of expressing clinical observations by using numbers. The use of numbers can provide standardized information to make observations of a health condition consistent and less subjective than a word description of that condition.

I. Descriptive Categories of Indices

A. General Categories

- *Simple index:* measures the presence or absence of a condition. An example is the biofilm index that measures the presence of dental biofilm without evaluating its effect on the gingiva.

- *Cumulative index:* measures all the evidence of a condition, past and present. An example is the DMFT index for dental caries.

B. Types of Simple and Cumulative Indices

- *Irreversible Index:* measures conditions that will not change. An example is an index that measures dental caries experience.
- *Reversible Index:* measures conditions that can be changed. Examples are indices that measure dental biofilm.

II. Selection Criteria

A useful and effective index:

- is simple to use and calculate.
- requires minimal equipment and expense.
- uses a minimal amount of time to complete.
- does neither cause patient discomfort nor is otherwise unacceptable to a patient.
- has clear-cut criteria that are readily understandable.
- is as free as possible from subjective interpretation.
- is reproducible by the same examiner or different examiners.
- is amenable to statistical analysis; has validity and reliability.

ORAL HYGIENE STATUS (BIOFILM, DEBRIS, AND CALCULUS)

Indices that measure oral hygiene status can be used in a clinical setting to educate and motivate an individual patient. When data are collected in a community setting, such as a nursing home, the findings can help determine how daily oral care is being provided and monitor the results of oral hygiene education programs.

I. Biofilm Index

This index was historically known as plaque index (Pl I).[1,7]

A. Purpose

To assess the thickness of biofilm at the gingival area.

B. Selection of Teeth

The entire dentition or selected teeth can be evaluated.

- *Areas examined:* Examine four gingival areas (distal, facial, mesial, and lingual) systematically for each tooth.
- *Modified procedures:* Examine only the facial, mesial, and lingual areas. Assign double score to the mesial reading and divide the total by 4.

C. Procedure

- Dry the teeth and examine visually using adequate light, mouth mirror, and probe or explorer.
- Evaluate dental biofilm on the cervical third; pay no attention to biofilm that has extended to the middle or incisal thirds of the tooth.

- Use probe to test the surface when no biofilm is visible. Pass the probe or explorer across the tooth surface in the cervical third and near the entrance to the sulcus. When no biofilm adheres to the probe tip, the area is scored 0. When biofilm adheres, a score of 1 is assigned.
- Use a disclosing agent, if necessary, to assist evaluation for the 0–1 scores. When the Pl I is used in conjunction with the gingival index (GI), the GI is completed first because the disclosing agent masks the gingival characteristics.
- Include biofilm on the surface of calculus and on dental restorations in the cervical third in the evaluation.
- *Criteria*

BIOFILM INDEX	
SCORE	**CRITERIA**
0	No biofilm.
1	A film of biofilm adhering to the free gingival margin and adjacent area of the tooth. The biofilm may be recognized only after application of disclosing agent or by running the explorer across the tooth surface.
2	Moderate accumulation of soft deposits within the gingival pocket that can be seen with the naked eye or on the tooth and gingival margin.
3	Abundance of soft matter within the gingival pocket and/or on the tooth and gingival margin.

D. Scoring

- *Pl I for area*
  - Each area of a tooth (distal, facial, mesial, lingual, or palatal) is assigned a score from 0 to 3.
- *Pl I for a tooth*
  - Scores for each area are totaled and divided by 4.
- *Pl I for groups of teeth*
  - Scores for individual teeth may be grouped and totaled and divided by the number of teeth. For instance, a Pl I may be determined for specific teeth or groups of teeth. The right side of the dentition may be compared with the left.
- *Pl I for the individual*
  - Add the scores for each tooth and divide by the number of teeth examined. The Pl I score ranges from 0 to 3.
- *Suggested range of scores for patient reference*

RATING	SCORES
Excellent	0
Good	0.1–0.9
Fair	1.0–1.9
Poor	2.0–3.0

- *Pl I for a group*
  - Add the scores for each member of a group and divide by the number of individuals.

II. Biofilm Control Record

This index was previously known as the plaque control record.[8]

A. Purpose

To record the presence of dental biofilm on individual tooth surfaces to permit the patient to visualize progress while learning biofilm control.

B. Selection of Teeth and Surfaces

- All teeth are included. Missing teeth are identified on the record form by a single, thick horizontal line.
- Four surfaces are recorded: facial, lingual, mesial, and distal.
- Six areas may be recorded. The mesial and distal segments of the diagram may be divided to provide space to record proximal surfaces from the facial separately from the lingual or palatal surfaces (Figure 21-1).[9]

C. Procedure

- Apply disclosing agent or give a chewable tablet. Instruct patient to swish and rub the solution over the tooth surfaces with the tongue before rinsing.

- Examine each tooth surface for dental biofilm at the gingival margin. No attempt is made to differentiate the quantity of biofilm.
- Record by making a dash or coloring in the appropriate spaces on the diagram (Figure 21-1) to indicate biofilm on facial, lingual, palatal, mesial, and/or distal surfaces.

D. Scoring

- Total the number of teeth present and multiply by 4 to obtain the number of available surfaces. Count the number of surfaces with biofilm.
- Multiply the number of biofilm-stained surfaces by 100 and divide by the total number of available surfaces to derive the percentage of surfaces with biofilm.
- Compare scores over subsequent appointments as the patient learns and practices biofilm control. Ten percent or less biofilm-stained surfaces can be considered a good goal, but if the biofilm is regularly left in the same areas, special instruction is indicated.

Calculation: Example for Biofilm Control Record
Individual findings: 26 teeth scored; 8 surfaces with biofilm.
Multiply the number of teeth by 4: $26 \times 4 = 104$ surfaces.
Percent with biofilm =

$$\frac{\text{Number of surfaces with biofilm} \times 100}{\text{Number of available tooth surfaces}} = \frac{8 \times 100}{104}$$
$$= \frac{800}{104}$$
$$= 7.7\%$$

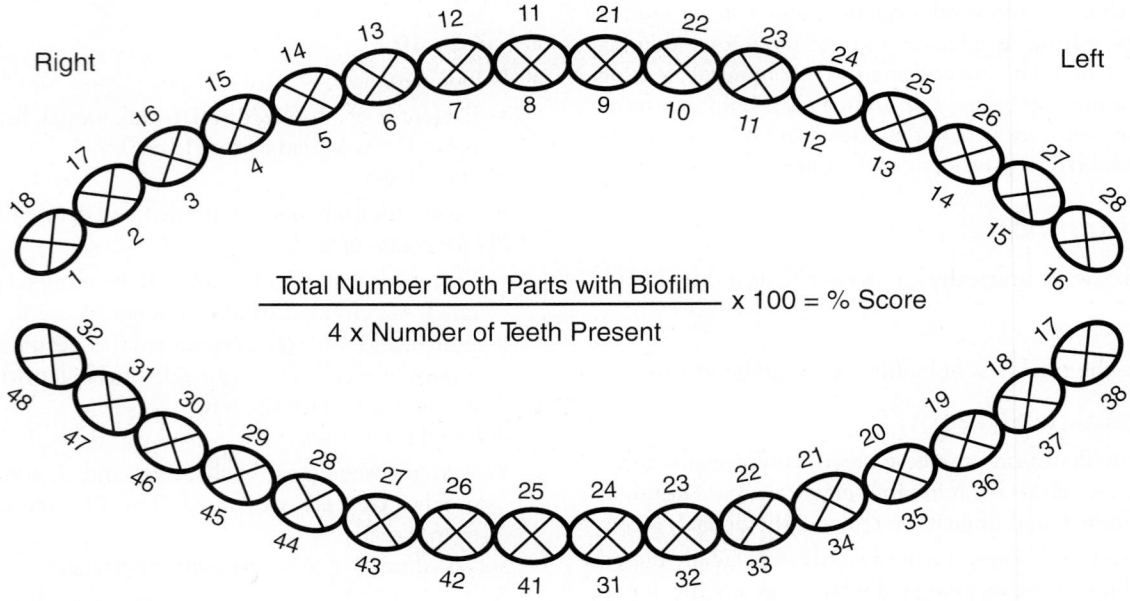

Total Number Tooth Parts with Biofilm ÷ (4 x Number of Teeth Present) x 100 = % Score

FIGURE 21-1 • Biofilm Control Record. Diagrammatic representation of the teeth includes spaces to record biofilm on six areas of each tooth. The facial surfaces are on the outer portion and the lingual and palatal surfaces are on the inner portion of the arches. Teeth are numbered by the American Dental Association system on the inside and by the Fédération Dentaire Internationale system on the outside. (Adapted with permission from Ramfjord SP, Ash MM. *Periodontology and Periodontics*. Philadelphia, PA: WB Saunders Co; 1979:273; from O'Leary TJ, Drake RB, Naylor JE. The plaque control record. *J Periodontol*. 1972;43:38.)

Interpretation

Although 0% is ideal, less than 10% biofilm-stained surfaces has been suggested as a guideline in periodontal therapy. After initial therapy and when the patient has reached a 10% level of biofilm control or better, necessary additional periodontal and restorative procedures may be initiated.[8] In comparison, a similar evaluation using a biofilm-free score would mean that a goal of 90% or better biofilm-free surfaces would have to be reached before the surgical phase of treatment could be undertaken.

III. Biofilm-Free Score

This index was historically called the plaque-free score.[10]

A. Purpose

To determine the location, number, and percentage of biofilm-free surfaces for individual motivation and instruction. Interdental bleeding can also be documented.

B. Selection of Teeth and Surfaces

◆ All erupted teeth are included. Missing teeth are identified on the record form by a single, thick horizontal line through the box in the chart form.

◆ Four surfaces are recorded for each tooth: facial, lingual or palatal, mesial, and distal.

C. Procedure

◆ *Biofilm-free score*

• Apply disclosing agent or give chewable tablet. Instruct patient to swish and rub the solution over the tooth surfaces with the tongue before rinsing.

• Examine each tooth surface for evidence of biofilm using adequate light and a mouth mirror.

• The patient needs a hand mirror to see the location of the biofilm missed during personal hygiene procedures.

• Use an appropriate tooth chart form or a diagrammatic form, such as that shown in Figure 21-2. Red ink for recording the biofilm is suggested when a red disclosing agent is used to help the patient associate

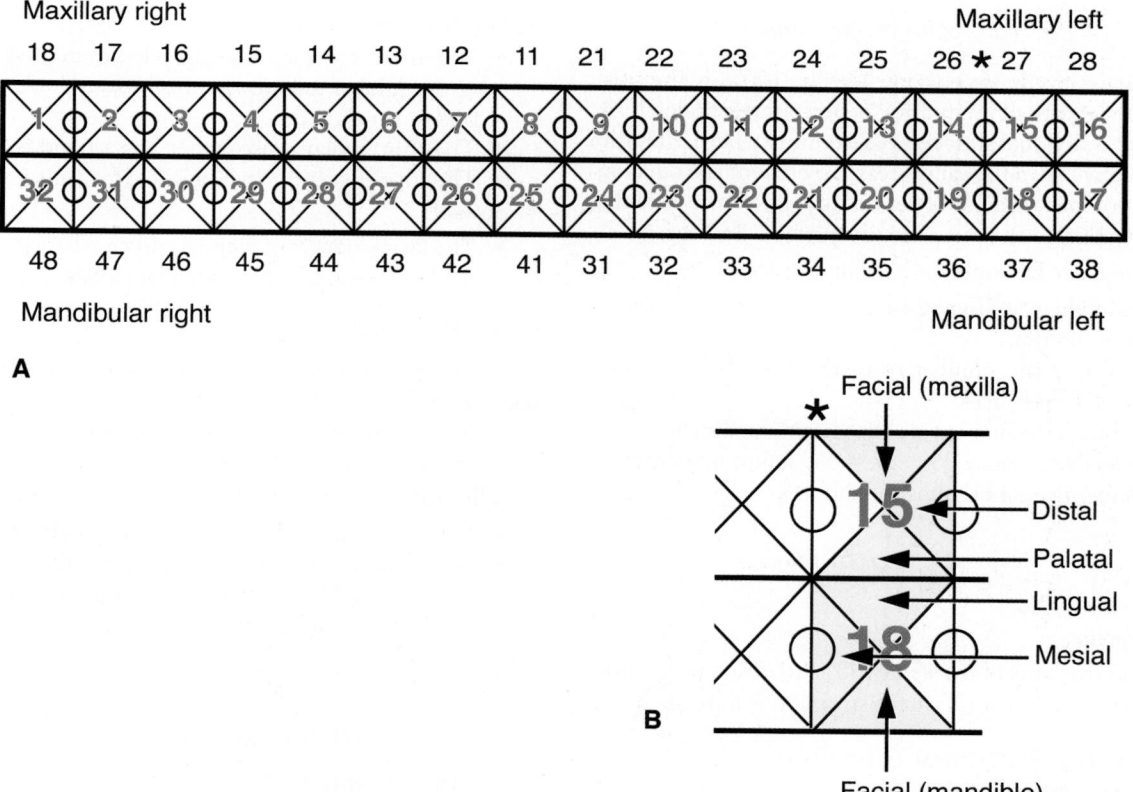

FIGURE 21-2 • Biofilm-Free Score. A: Diagrammatic representation of the teeth used to record biofilm and papillary bleeding. **B:** Enlargement of one section of the diagram shows tooth surfaces. Teeth are numbered by the American Dental Association system inside each block and by the Fédération Dentaire Internationale system outside each block. (Adapted with permission from Grant DA, Stern IB, Listgarten MA. *Periodontics.* 6th ed. St. Louis, MO: Mosby; 1988:613.)

the location of the biofilm in the mouth with the recording.

- *Papillary bleeding on probing*
  - The small circles between the diagrammatic tooth blocks in Figure 21-2 are used to record proximal bleeding on probing.
  - Improvement in the gingival tissue health will be demonstrated over a period of time as fewer bleeding areas are noted.

D. Scoring: Biofilm-Free Score

- Total the number of teeth present.
- Total the number of surfaces with biofilm that appear in red on the tooth diagram.
- To calculate the biofilm-free score
  - Multiply the number of teeth by 4 to determine the number of available surfaces.
  - Subtract the number of surfaces with biofilm from the total available surfaces to find the number of biofilm-free surfaces.
  - Biofilm-free score =

$$\frac{\text{Number of biofilm-free surface} \times 100}{\text{Number of available surfaces}}$$

$$= \text{Percentage of biofilm-free surfaces}$$

- Evaluate biofilm-free score: Ideally, 100% is the goal. When a patient maintains a percentage under 85%, check individual surfaces to determine whether biofilm is usually left in the same areas. To prevent the development of specific areas of periodontal infection, remedial instruction in the areas usually missed is indicated.
- *Calculation*: Example for biofilm-free score
  - Individual findings: 24 teeth scored and 37 surfaces with biofilm.
  - Multiply the number of teeth by 4: 24 × 4 = 96 available surfaces.
  - Subtract the number of surfaces with biofilm from total available surfaces: 96 − 37 = 59 biofilm-free surfaces.
  - Percentage of biofilm-free surfaces

$$\frac{59 \times 100}{96} = 61.5\%$$

- *Interpretation*
  - On the basis of the ideal 100%, 61.5% is poor. More personal daily oral care instruction is indicated.

E. Scoring: Papillary Bleeding on Probing

- Total the number of small circles marked for bleeding. A patient with 32 teeth has 30 interdental areas. The mesial or distal surface of a tooth adjacent to an edentulous area is probed and counted.
- Evaluate total interdental bleeding. In health, bleeding on probing does not occur.

IV. Patient Hygiene Performance[2]

A. Purpose

To assess the extent of biofilm and debris over a tooth surface. Debris is defined for the PHP as a soft foreign material consisting of dental biofilm, materia alba, and food debris loosely attached to tooth surfaces.

B. Selection of Teeth and Surfaces

- Teeth examined

MAXILLARY	MANDIBULAR
No. 3 (16)[a]	No. 19 (36)
Right first molar	Left first molar
No. 8 (11)	No. 24 (31)
Right central incisor	Left central incisor
No. 14 (26)	No. 30 (46)
Left first molar	Right first molar

[a]Fédération Dentaire Internationale system tooth numbers are in parentheses.

- Substitutions
  - When a first molar is missing, is less than three-fourths erupted, has a full crown, or is broken down, the second molar is used.
  - The third molar is used when the second is missing.
  - The adjacent central incisor is used for a missing incisor.
- Surfaces
  - The facial surfaces of incisors and maxillary molars and the lingual surfaces of mandibular molars are examined.

C. Procedure

Apply disclosing agent. Instruct the patient to swish for 30 seconds and expectorate, but not rinse.

- Examination is made using a mouth mirror.
- Each tooth surface to be evaluated is subdivided (mentally) into five sections (Figure 21-3A) as follows:
  - Vertically: Three divisions—mesial, middle, and distal.
  - Horizontally: The middle third is subdivided into gingival, middle, and occlusal or incisal thirds.
- Each of the five subdivisions is scored for the presence of stained debris as follows:

PATIENT HYGIENE PERFORMANCE	
SCORE	CRITERIA
0	No debris (or questionable).
1	Debris definitely present.
M	When all three molars or both incisors are missing.
S	When a substitute tooth is used.

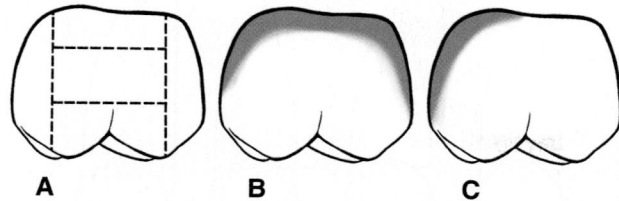

FIGURE 21-3 • Patient Hygiene Performance. A: Oral debris is assessed by dividing a tooth into five subdivisions, each of which is scored 1 when debris is shown to be present after use of a disclosing agent. **B:** Example of debris score of 3. Shaded portion represents debris stained by disclosing agent. **C:** Example of debris score of 1. (From Podshadley AG, Haley JV. A method for evaluating oral hygiene performance. *Public Health Rep.* 1968;83(3):259-264.)

D. Scoring

- *Debris score for individual tooth*
  - Add the scores for each of the five subdivisions. The scores range from 0 to 5. Examples are shown in Figure 21-3B and C.
- *PHP for the individual*
  - Total the scores for the individual teeth and divide by the number of teeth examined. The PHP ranges from 0 to 5.
- *Suggested range of scores for evaluation*

RATING	SCORES
Excellent	0 (no debris)
Good	0.1–1.7
Fair	1.8–3.4
Poor	3.5–5.0

Calculation: Example for an Individual

TOOTH	DEBRIS SCORE
No. 3 (16)	5
No. 8 (11)	3
No. 14 (26)	4
No. 19 (36)	5
No. 24 (31)	2
No. 30 (46)	3
Total	22

$$\frac{\text{Total debris score}}{\text{Number of teeth scored}} = \frac{22}{6} = 3.67$$

- *Interpretation*
  - According to the suggested range of scores, this patient with a PHP of 3.66 would be classified as exhibiting poor hygiene performance.

- *PHP for a group*
  - To obtain the average PHP score for a group or population, total the individual scores and divide by the number of people examined.

V. Simplified Oral Hygiene Index[11,12]

A. Purpose

To assess oral cleanliness by estimating the tooth surfaces covered with debris and/or calculus.

B. Components

The simplified oral hygiene index (OHI-S) has two components: the simplified debris index (DI-S) and the simplified calculus index (CI-S). The two scores may be used separately or may be combined for the OHI-S.

C. Selection of Teeth and Surfaces

- *Identify the six specific teeth* (see Figure 21-4)

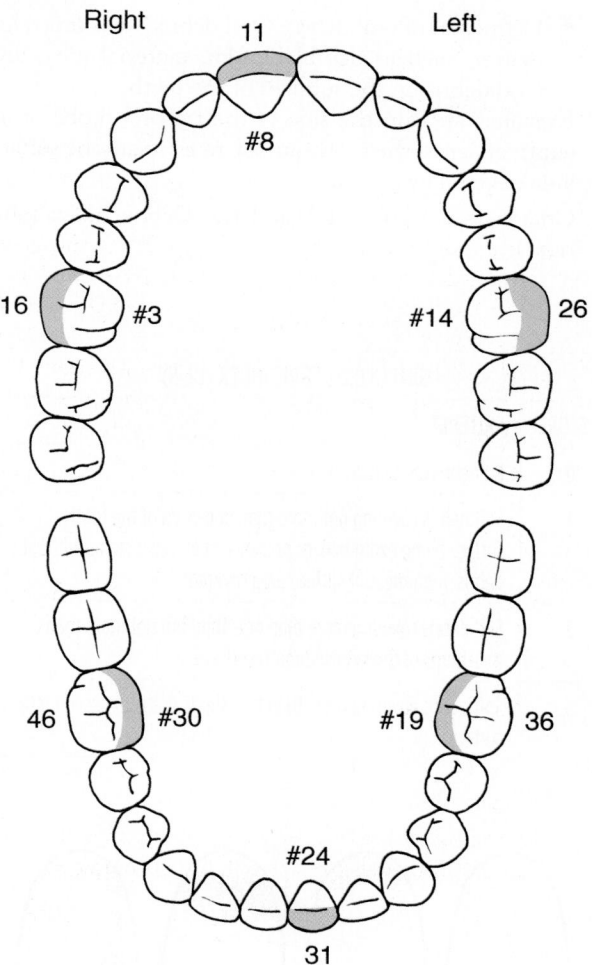

FIGURE 21-4 • Simplified Oral Hygiene Index. Six tooth surfaces are scored as follows: facial surfaces of maxillary molars and of the maxillary right and mandibular left central incisors, and the lingual surfaces of mandibular molars. Teeth are numbered by the American Dental Association system on the lingual surface and by the Fédération Dentaire Internationale system on the facial surface.

- *Posterior:* The facial surfaces of the maxillary molars and the lingual surfaces of the mandibular molars are scored. Although usually the first molars are examined, the first fully erupted molar distal to each second premolar is used if the first molar is missing.
- *Anterior:* The facial surfaces of the maxillary right and the mandibular left central incisors are scored. When either is missing, the adjacent central incisor is scored.
- ◆ *Extent*
  - Either the facial or lingual surfaces of the selected teeth are scored, including the proximal surfaces to the contact areas.

D. Procedure

- ◆ *Qualification:* At least two of the six possible surfaces are examined to calculate an individual score.
- ◆ *Record six debris scores*
  - Definition of oral debris: Oral debris is a soft foreign matter, such as dental biofilm, material alba, and food debris on the surfaces of the teeth.
- ◆ *Examination:* Run the side of the tip of a probe or an explorer across the tooth surface to estimate the surface area covered by debris.
- ◆ *Criteria* (see Figure 21-5 and the Debris Index table next).

SIMPLIFIED DEBRIS INDEX (DI-S)	
SCORE	CRITERIA
0	No debris or stain present.
1	Soft debris covering not more than one-third of the tooth surface being examined, or presence of extrinsic stains without debris, regardless of surface area covered.
2	Soft debris covering more than one-third but not more than two-thirds of the exposed tooth surface.
3	Soft debris covering more than two-thirds of the exposed tooth surface.

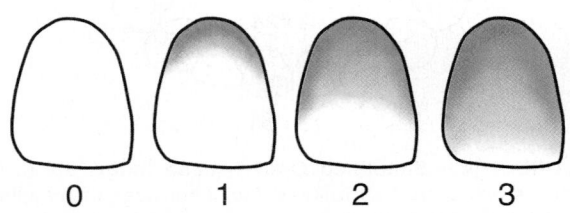

FIGURE 21-5 • Simplified Oral Hygiene Index. For the debris index, six teeth (Figure 21-3) are scored. Scoring of 0–3 is based on tooth surfaces covered by debris as shown.

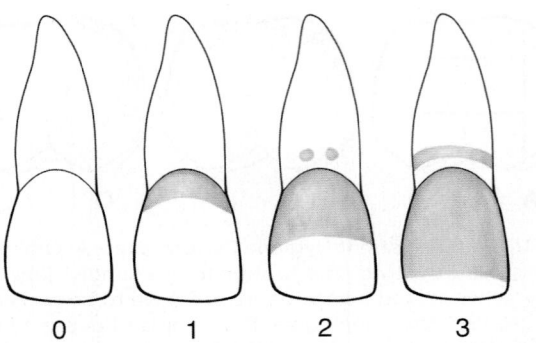

FIGURE 21-6 • Simplified Oral Hygiene Index. For the calculus index, six teeth (Figure 21-3) are scored. Scoring of 0–3 is based on location and tooth surface area with calculus as shown. Note slight subgingival calculus recorded as 2 and more extensive subgingival calculus as 3.

- ◆ *Record six calculus scores*
  - *Definition of calculus:* Dental calculus is a hard deposit of inorganic salts comprised primarily of calcium carbonate and phosphate mixed with debris, microorganisms, and desquamated epithelial cells.
- ◆ *Examination:* Use an explorer to estimate surface area covered by supragingival calculus deposits. Identify subgingival deposits by exploring and/or probing. Record only definite deposits of hard calculus.
  - *Criteria:* Location and tooth surface areas scored are illustrated in Figure 21-6.

SIMPLIFIED CALCULUS INDEX (CI-S)	
SCORE	CRITERIA
0	No calculus present.
1	Supragingival calculus covering not more than one-third of the exposed tooth surface being examined.
2	Supragingival calculus covering more than one-third but not more than two-thirds of the exposed tooth surface, or the presence of individual flecks of subgingival calculus around the cervical portion of the tooth.
3	Supragingival calculus covering more than two-thirds of the exposed tooth surface or a continuous heavy band of subgingival calculus around the cervical portion of the tooth.

E. Scoring

- ◆ *OHI-S individual score.*
- ◆ Determine separate DI-S and CI-S.
  - Divide each total score by the number of teeth scored (6).
  - DI-S and CI-S values range from 0 to 3.
- ◆ Calculate the OHI-S.

- Combine the DI-S and CI-S.
- OHI-S value ranges from 0 to 6.
◆ *Suggested range of scores for evaluation*[12]

RATING	SCORES
Individual simplified debris index (DI-S) and the simplified calculus index (CI-S)	
Excellent	0
Good	0.1–0.6
Fair	0.7–1.8
Poor	1.9–3.0
OHI-S (combined DI-S and CI-S)	
Excellent	0
Good	0.1–1.2
Fair	1.3–3.0
Poor	3.1–6.0

Calculation: Example for an Individual

TOOTH	SIMPLIFIED DEBRIS INDEX SCORE	SIMPLIFIED CALCULUS INDEX SCORE
No. 3 (16)	2	2
No. 8 (11)	1	0
No. 14 (26)	3	2
No. 19 (36)	3	2
No. 24 (31)	2	1
No. 30 (46)	2	2
Total	13	9

$$DI\text{-}S = \frac{\text{Total debris score}}{\text{Number of teeth scored}} = \frac{13}{6} = 2.17$$

$$CI\text{-}S = \frac{\text{Total calculus scores}}{\text{Number of teeth scored}} = \frac{9}{6} = 1.50$$

$$OHI\text{-}S = DI\text{-}S + CI\text{-}S = 2.17 + 1.50 = 3.67$$

◆ *Interpretation*
- According to the suggested range of scores, the score for this individual (3.67) indicates a poor oral hygiene status.
◆ *OHI-S group score*
- Compute the average of the individual scores by totaling the scores and dividing by the number of individuals.

GINGIVAL AND PERIODONTAL HEALTH

Measurements for gingival and periodontal indices have varied over the years. Two indices, not completely described here, are of historic interest.

◆ The papillary-marginal-attached index, attributed to Schour and Massler[13] and later revised by Massler,[14] was used to assess the extent of gingival changes in large groups for epidemiologic studies.

◆ The periodontal index of Russell,[15] another acclaimed contribution to the study of disease incidence, was a complex index that accounts for both gingival and periodontal changes. Its aim was to survey large populations.

◆ For patient instruction and motivation, several bleeding indices and scoring methods have been developed.

◆ Bleeding on gentle probing or flossing is an early sign of gingival inflammation and precedes color changes and enlargement of gingival tissues.[16,17]

◆ Bleeding on probing is an indicator of the progression of periodontal disease, so testing for bleeding has become a significant procedure for assessment prior to treatment planning, after therapy to show the effects of treatment, and at maintenance appointments to determine continued control of gingival inflammation.

I. Periodontal Screening and Recording[18,19]

A. Purpose

To assess the state of periodontal health of an individual patient.

◆ A modified form of the original community periodontal index of treatment needs (CPITN) index.[20]

◆ Designed to indicate periodontal status in a rapid and effective manner and motivate the patient to seek necessary complete periodontal assessment and treatment.

◆ Used as a screening procedure to determine the need for comprehensive periodontal evaluation.

B. Selection of Teeth

The dentition is divided into sextants. Each tooth is examined. Posterior sextants begin distal to the canines.

C. Procedure

◆ *Instrument:* Probe originally designed for World Health Organization (WHO) surveys (Figure 21-7), with markings at intervals from tip: 3.5, 5.5, 8.5, and 11.5 mm.

◆ Color coded between 3.5 and 5.5 mm.

◆ *Working tip:* A ball 0.5 mm in diameter. The functions of the ball are to aid in the detection of calculus, rough overhanging margins of restorations, and other tooth surface irregularities, and also to facilitate assessment at the probing depth and reduce risk of overmeasurement.

◆ *Probe application*

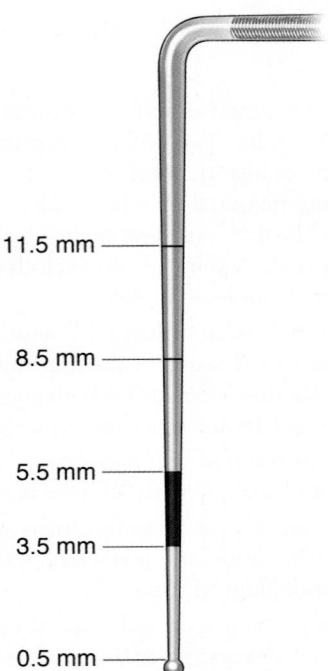

11.5 mm

8.5 mm

5.5 mm

3.5 mm

0.5 mm

FIGURE 21-7 • World Health Organization (WHO) Periodontal Probe. The specially designed WHO probe measures 3.5-, 5.5-, 8.5-, and 11.5-mm intervals. This probe is used to make determinations for the periodontal screening and recording and the community periodontal index. (Fédération Dentaire Internationale. A simplified periodontal examination for dental practices. Based on the Community Periodontal Index of Treatment Needs—CPITN. *Aust Dent J.* 1985;30(5):368-370.)

- Insert probe gently into a sulcus until resistance is felt.
- Apply a circumferential walking step to probe systematically about each tooth through each sextant.
- Observe color-coded area of the probe for prompt identification of probing depths.
- Each sextant receives one code number corresponding to the deepest position of the color-coded portion of the probe.

◆ *Criteria*
- Five codes and an asterisk are used. Figure 21-8 shows the clinical findings, code significance, and patient management guidelines.
- Each code may include conditions identified with the preceding codes; for example, Code 3 with probing depth from 3.5 to 5.5 mm may also include calculus, an overhanging restoration, and bleeding on probing.
- One need not probe the remaining teeth in a sextant when a Code 4 is found. For Codes 0, 1, 2, and 3, the sextant is completely probed.

◆ *Recording*
- Use a simple six-box form to provide a space for each sextant. The form can be made into peel-off stickers or a rubber stamp to facilitate recording in the patient's permanent record.

- One score is marked for each sextant; the highest code observed is recorded. When indicated, an asterisk is added to the score in the individual space with the sextant code number.

D. Scoring

◆ *Follow-up patient management*

Patients are classified into assessment and treatment planning needs by the highest coded score of their periodontal screening and recording (PSR).

Calculation: Example 1: PSR Sextant Score

4.	2	3
3	2.	4.

◆ *Interpretation*
- With Codes 3 and 4, a comprehensive periodontal examination is indicated. The asterisks indicate furcation involvement in two sextants and a mucogingival involvement in the mandibular anterior sextant. When the patient is not aware of the periodontal involvement, counseling is important if cooperation and compliance are to be obtained.

◆ *Calculation:* Example 2: PSR Sextant Score

2	1	2
2	1.	2.

◆ *Interpretation*
- An overall Code 2 can indicate calculus and overhanging restorations that can be removed. All restorations are checked for recurrent dental caries. Appointments for instruction in dental biofilm control are of primary concern.
  - In this example, the asterisks in two sextants indicate a notable clinical feature such as minimal attached gingiva.

II. Community Periodontal Index[21]

A. Purpose

To screen and monitor the periodontal status of populations.
◆ Originally developed as the CPITN index that included a code to indicate an individual and group-summary recording of treatment needs. However, because of changes in management of periodontal disease, the treatment needs portion of the index has been eliminated.
◆ One component of a complete oral health survey[21] designed by the WHO that includes the assessment of many oral health indicators, including mucosal lesions, dental caries, fluorosis, prosthetic status, and dentofacial anomalies.

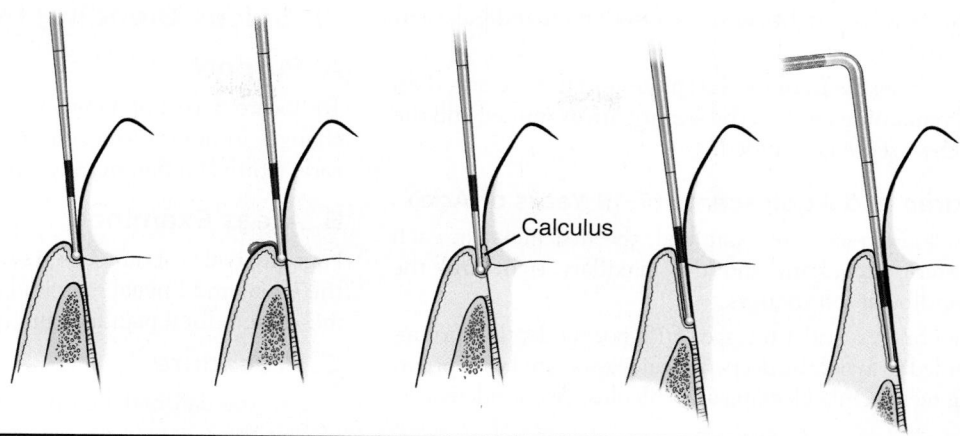

Calculus

PSR and CPI sextant scores	Code 0	Code 1	Code 2	Code 3	Code 4
CPI description	• Entire black band of the probe is visible.	• Entire black band of the probe is visible, but bleeding is present after gentle probin.	• Entire black band is visible, but calculus is present. • Bleeding may or may not be present.	• 4 to 5 mm pocket depth. • Black band on probe partially hidden by gingival margin.	• 6 mm or greater pocket depth. • Black band of probe completely hidden by gingival margin.
PSR sextant code description	• Colored area of probe completely visible. • No calculus, defective restoration margins, or bleeding.	• Colored area of probe completely visible. • No calculus or defective restoration margins. • Bleeding after gentle probing.	• Colored area of probe completely visible. • Supra-or subgingival rough surface or calculus. • Defective restoration margins.	• Colored area of probe only partially visible. • Calculus, defective restorations, and bleeding may or may not be present.	• Colored area of probe completely disappears (probing depth of 5.5 mm or greater).
PSR management guidelines	• Biofilm control instruction. • Preventive care.	• Biofilm control instruction. • Preventive care.	• Biofilm control instruction. • Complete preventive care. • Calculus removal. • Correction of defective restoration margins.	• Comprehensive periodontal assessment and treatment plan is indicated.	• Comprehensive periodontal assessment and treatment plan is indicated.

FIGURE 21-8 • Community Periodontal Index (CPI) and Periodontal Screening and Recording (PSR) Codes. (World Health Organization. *Oral Health Surveys: Basic Methods.* 4th ed. Geneva, Switzerland: WHO; 1997:27, 38 and the American Academy of Periodontology. Parameter on comprehensive periodontal examination. *J Periodontol.* 2000;71(5 suppl):847-848.)

◆ Later modified to form the PSR index for scoring individual patients.

B. Selection of Teeth

◆ The dentition is divided into sextants for recording on the assessment form.

◆ Posterior sextants begin distal to canines.

Adults (20 Years and Older)

◆ A sextant is examined only if there are two or more teeth present that are not indicated for extraction.

◆ Ten index teeth are examined.

◆ The first and second molars in each posterior sextant. If one is missing, no replacement is selected and the score for the remaining molar is recorded.

- The maxillary right central incisor and mandibular left central incisor.
- If no index teeth or tooth is present in the sextant, then all remaining teeth in the sextant are examined and the highest score is recorded.

Children and Adolescents (7–19 Years of Age)

- Six index teeth are examined; the first molar in each posterior quadrant and the maxillary right and the mandibular left incisors.
- For children under the age of 15, pocket depth is not recorded to avoid the deepened sulci associated with erupting teeth. Only bleeding and calculus are considered.

C. Procedure

- *Instrument:* A specially designed probe is used to record both the community periodontal index (CPI) and PSR. The probe is described in Figure 21-7.
- *Criteria:* CPI score.
  - Five codes are used to record bleeding, calculus, and pocket depth. Criteria for the CPI codes are similar to the criteria for the PSR, as illustrated in Figure 21-8 and the Community Periodontal Index table next.

COMMUNITY PERIODONTAL INDEX	
CODE	**CRITERIA**
0	Healthy periodontal tissues.
1	Bleeding after gentle probing; entire colored band of probe is visible.
2	Supragingival or subgingival calculus present; entire colored band of probe is visible.
3	4- to 5-mm pocket; colored band of probe is partially obscured.
4	6 mm or deeper; colored band on the probe is not visible.

- *Criteria:* Loss of attachment (LOA) code.
  - In conjunction with the CPI, the WHO probe is also used to record LOA. The five LOA codes used are illustrated in Figure 21-9. LOA is not recorded for individuals less than 15 years of age.

LOSS OF ATTACHMENT (LOA) CODE	CRITERIA
0	0–3 mm LOA
1	4–5 mm LOA
2	6–8 mm LOA
3	9–11 mm LOA
4	12 mm or greater LOA

III. Sulcus Bleeding Index[16]

A. Purpose

To locate areas of gingival sulcus bleeding and color changes in order to recognize and record the presence of early (initial) inflammatory gingival disease.

B. Areas Examined

Four gingival units are scored systematically for each tooth: the labial and lingual marginal gingiva (M units) and the mesial and distal papillary gingiva (P units).

C. Procedure

- Use standardized lighting while probing each of the four areas.
- Walk the probe to the base of the sulcus, holding it parallel with the long axis of the tooth for M units, and directed toward the col area for P units.
- Wait 30 seconds after probing before scoring apparently healthy gingival units.
- Dry the gingiva gently if necessary to observe color changes clearly.
- *Criteria*

SULCULAR BLEEDING INDEX	
CODE	**CRITERIA**
0	Healthy appearance of P and M, no bleeding on sulcus probing.
1	Apparently healthy P and M showing no change in color and no swelling, but bleeding from sulcus on probing.
2	Bleeding on probing and change of color caused by inflammation. No swelling or macroscopic edema.
3	Bleeding on probing and change in color and slight edematous swelling.
4	Bleeding on probing and change in color and obvious swelling or Bleeding on probing and obvious swelling.
5	Bleeding on probing and spontaneous bleeding and change in color, marked swelling with or without ulceration.

D. Scoring

- *Sulcus bleeding index (SBI) for area*
  - Score each of the four gingival units (M and P) from 0 to 5.
- *SBI for tooth*
  - Total scores for the four units and divide by 4.
- *SBI for individual*
  - Total the scores for individual teeth and divide by the number of teeth. SBI scores range from 0 to 5.

IV. Gingival Bleeding Index[22]

A. Purpose

To record the presence or absence of gingival inflammation as determined by bleeding from interproximal gingival sulci.

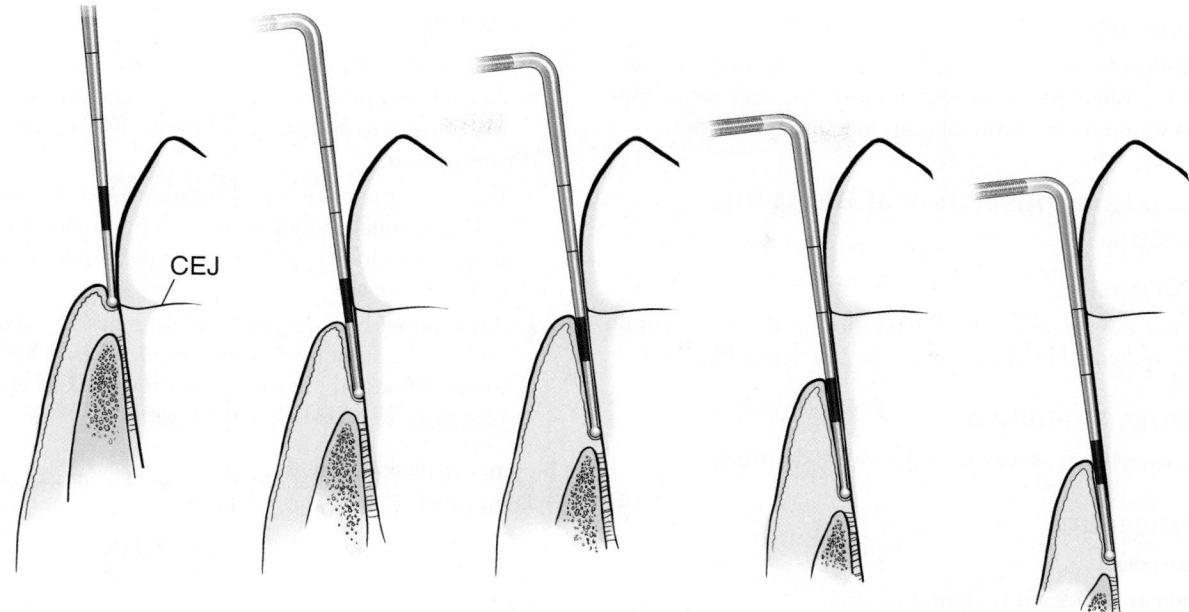

Code 0	Code 1	Code 2	Code 3	Code 4
• 0 to 3 mm loss of attachment. • Cementoenamel junction (CEJ) is covered by gingival margin and CPI score is 0 to 3. If CEJ is visible, or if CPI score is 4, LOA codes 1 to 4 are used.	• 3.5 to 5.5 mm loss of attachment. • CEJ is within the black band on the probe.	• 6 to 8 mm loss of attachment CEJ is between the top of the black band and the 8.5 mm mark on the probe.	• 9 to 11 mm loss of attachment. • CEJ is between the 8.5 mm and 11.5 mm marks on the probe.	• 12 mm or greater loss of attachment. • CEJ is beyond the highest (11.5 mm) marks on the probe.

FIGURE 21-9 • Loss of Attachment (LOA) Codes. (World Health Organization. *Oral Health Surveys: Basic Methods.* 4th ed. Geneva, Switzerland: WHO; 1997:27, 39.)

B. Areas Examined

Each interproximal area has two sulci, which can be scored as one interdental unit or scored separately.

◆ Certain areas may be excluded from scoring because of accessibility, tooth position, diastemata, or other factors, and if exclusions are made, a consistent procedure is followed for an individual and for a group if a study is to be made.

◆ A full complement of teeth has 30 proximal areas. In the original studies, third molars were excluded, and 26 interdental units were recorded.[23]

C. Procedure

◆ *Instrument*

• Unwaxed dental floss is used. Floss has the advantages of being readily available and disposable.

◆ *Steps*

1. Pass the floss interproximally first on one side of the papilla and then on the other.

2. Curve the floss around the adjacent tooth and bring the floss below the gingival margin.

3. Move the floss up and down for one stroke, with care not to lacerate the gingiva. Adapt finger rests to provide controlled, consistent pressure.

4. Use a new length of clean floss for each area.

5. Retract for visibility of bleeding from both facial and lingual aspects.

6. Allow 30 seconds for reinspection of an area that does not show blood immediately either in the area or on the floss.

◆ *Criteria*

• Bleeding indicates the presence of disease. No attempt is made to quantify the severity of bleeding.

D. Scoring

The numbers of bleeding areas and scorable units are recorded. Patient participation in observing and recording over a series of appointments can increase motivation.

V. Eastman Interdental Bleeding Index[23,24]

A. Purpose

To assess the presence of inflammation in the interdental area as indicated by the presence or absence of bleeding.

B. Areas Examined

Each interdental area around the entire dentition.

C. Procedure

- ◆ *Instrument*

Triangular wooden interdental cleaner.

- ◆ *Steps*
  1. Insert gently, then immediately remove, a wooden cleaner into each interdental area in such a way as to depress the papilla 1–2 mm (Figure 21-10).
  2. Make the path of insertion horizontal (parallel to the occlusal surface), taking care not to angle the point in an apical direction.
  3. Insert and remove four times; move to next interproximal area.
  4. Record the presence or absence of bleeding within 15 seconds for each area.

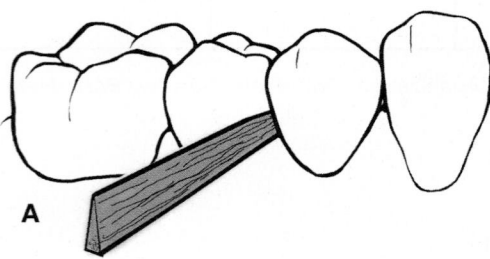

A

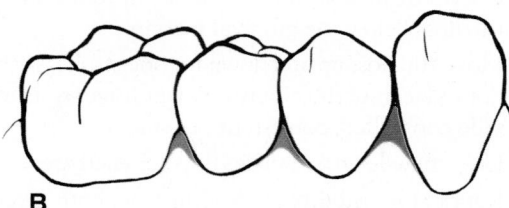

B

FIGURE 21-10 • Eastman Interdental Bleeding Index. The test for interdental bleeding is made by inserting a wooden interdental cleaner into each interdental space. **A:** Wooden interdental cleaner inserted in a horizontal path, parallel with the occlusal surfaces. **B:** The presence or absence of bleeding is noted within a quadrant 15 seconds after final insertion. Bleeding indicates the presence of inflammation.

D. Scoring

- ◆ *Number of bleeding sites*
  - • The number may be totaled for an individual score for comparison with scores over a series of appointments.
- ◆ *Percentage scores*
  - • Index is expressed as a percentage of the total number of sites evaluated. Calculations can be made for total mouth, quadrants, or maxillary versus mandibular.
- ◆ *Calculation example*
  - • An adult with a complete dentition has 15 maxillary and 15 mandibular interproximal areas. The Eastman interdental bleeding index revealed 13 areas of bleeding. To calculate percentage:

$$\frac{\text{Number of bleeding areas}}{\text{Total number of areas}} \times 100 = \text{Percent bleeding area}$$

$$\frac{13}{30} \times 100 = 43\%$$

VI. Gingival Index[7]

A. Purpose

To assess the severity of gingivitis based on color, consistency, and bleeding on probing.

B. Selection of Teeth and Gingival Areas

A GI may be determined for selected teeth or for the entire dentition.

- ◆ *Areas examined*
  - • Four gingival areas (distal, facial, mesial, and lingual) are examined systematically for each tooth.
- ◆ *Modified procedure*
  - • The distal examination for each tooth can be omitted. The score for the mesial area is doubled and the total score for each tooth is divided by 4.

C. Procedure

- ◆ Dry the teeth and gingiva; under adequate light, use a mouth mirror and probe.
- ◆ Use the probe to press on the gingiva to determine the degree of firmness.
- ◆ Slide the probe along the soft-tissue wall near the entrance to the gingival sulcus to evaluate bleeding (Figure 21-11).
- ◆ *Criteria*

GINGIVAL INDEX CODE	CRITERIA
0	Normal gingiva.
1	Mild inflammation--slight change in color, slight edema. *No bleeding* on probing.
2	Moderate inflammation--redness, edema, and glazing. *Bleeding* on probing.
3	Severe inflammation--marked redness and edema. Ulceration. Tendency to *spontaneous bleeding*.

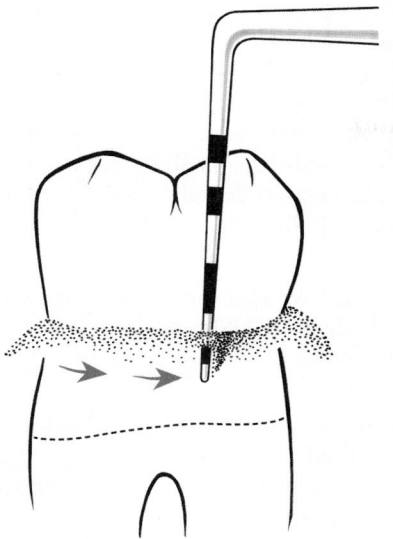

TOOTH NO.	M	F	D	L	
3 (16)	3	1	3	1	
9 (21)	1	0	1	1	
12 (24)	2	1	2	0	
19 (36)	3	1	3	3	
25 (41)	1	1	1	1	
28 (44)	2	1	2	0	
Total	12	5	12	6	= 35

$$\text{Gingival index} = \frac{\text{Total score}}{\text{Number of surfaces}} = \frac{35}{24} = 1.46$$

FIGURE 21-11 • Gingival Index. Probe stroke for bleeding evaluation. The broken line represents the level of attachment of the periodontal tissues. The probe is inserted a few millimeters and moved along the soft-tissue pocket wall with light pressure in a circumferential direction. The stroke shown here is in contrast with the walking stroke used for probing depth evaluation and measurement.

D. Scoring

- *GI for area*
  - Each of the four gingival surfaces (distal, facial, mesial, and lingual) is given a score of 0–3.
- *GI for a tooth*
  - Scores for each area are totaled and divided by 4.
- *GI for groups of teeth*
  - Scores for individual teeth may be grouped and totaled and divided by the number of teeth. A GI may be determined for specific teeth, group of teeth, quadrant, or side of mouth.
- *GI for the individual*
  - Scores for each tooth are added up and divided by the number of teeth examined. Scores range from 0 to 3.

Suggested range of scores for patient reference

RATING	SCORES
Excellent (healthy tissue)	0
Good	0.1–1.0
Fair	1.1–2.0
Poor	2.1–3.0

- *Calculation:* Example for an Individual
  - Using six teeth for an example of screening; teeth selected are known as the Ramfjord index teeth.[25]

- *Interpretation*
  - According to the suggested range of scores, the score for this individual (1.45) indicates only fair gingival health (moderate inflammation).
  - The ratings for each gingival area or surface can be used to help the patient compare gingival changes and improve oral hygiene procedures.
- *GI for a group*
  - Add the individual GI scores and divide by the number of individuals examined.

DENTAL CARIES EXPERIENCE

Dental caries experience data are most useful when measuring the prevalence of dental disease in groups rather than individuals. The population scores can document such information as the number of persons in any age group who are affected by dental caries, the number of teeth that need treatment, or the proportion of teeth that have been treated.

I. Permanent Dentition: Decayed, Missing, and Filled Teeth or Surfaces [3,26]

A. Purpose

To determine total dental caries experience, past and present, by recording either the number of affected teeth or tooth surfaces.

B. Selection of Teeth and Surfaces

- The DMFT is based on 28 teeth.
- The decayed, missing, and filled surfaces (DMFS) is based on surfaces of 28 teeth; 128 surfaces.
  - 16 posterior teeth × 5 surfaces (facial, lingual, mesial, distal, and occlusal) = 80 surfaces.
  - 12 anterior teeth × 4 surfaces (facial, lingual, mesial, and distal) = 48 surfaces.

- Teeth missing due to dental caries are recorded using 5 surfaces for posterior and 4 surfaces for anterior teeth.
- ◆ Teeth not counted.
  - Third molars.
  - Unerupted teeth. A tooth is considered erupted when any part projects through the gingiva. Certain types of research may require differentiation between clinical emergence, partial eruption, and full eruption.
  - Congenitally missing and supernumerary teeth.
  - Teeth removed for reasons other than dental caries, such as an impaction or during orthodontic treatment.
  - Teeth restored for reasons other than dental caries, such as trauma (fracture), cosmetic purposes, or use as a bridge abutment.
  - Primary tooth retained with the permanent successor erupted. The permanent tooth is evaluated because a primary tooth is never included in this index.

C. Procedures

- ◆ *Examination*
  - Examine each tooth in a systematic sequence.
  - Observe teeth by visual means as much as possible.
  - Use adequate light.
  - Review the stages of dental caries in Chapter 25.
- ◆ *Criteria for recording*[26]
  - Each tooth is recorded once when using the DMFT index.
  - Five surfaces for posterior teeth and 4 surfaces for anterior teeth are recorded when using the DMFS index.
  - DMF indices use a dichotomous scale (present or absent) to record decay.

DMF RATING	CRITERIA
Decayed (D)	Visible dental caries is present or both dental caries and a restoration are present.
Missing (M)	A tooth extracted because of dental caries or when it is carious, nonrestorable, and indicated for extraction.
Filled (F)	Any permanent or temporary restoration is present or a defective restoration without evidence of dental caries is present.

D. Scoring

- ◆ *Individual DMF*
  - Total each component separately.
    Total D + M + F = DMF
  - *Example:* An individual presents with dental caries on the mesial and occlusal surfaces of a posterior tooth and caries on the mesial surface of an anterior tooth. A molar tooth and an anterior tooth are missing because of dental caries and there is an amalgam

restoration on the mesial–distal–occlusal surfaces of a posterior tooth.
DMFT = 2 + 2 + 1 = 5
DMFS = 3 + 9 + 3 = 15

- ◆ A DMF score may have different interpretations. For example, an individual with a DMF score of 15 who has experienced regular dental care may have a distribution such as D = 0, M = 0, F = 15.
- ◆ *Group DMF*
  - Total the DMFs for each individual examined.
  - Divide the total DMFs by the number of individuals in the group.
- ◆ *Calculation:*
  - *Example:* A population of 20 individuals with individual DMF scores of 0, 0, 0, 0, 2, 2, 3, 3, 3, 4, 9, 9, 9, 10, 10, 10, 11, 11, 12, and 16 equals a group total DMF of 124.

$$\frac{124}{20} = 6.2 = \text{the average DMF for the group}$$

  - This DMF average represents accumulated dental caries experience for the group.
- ◆ The differences in caries experience between two groups of individuals within this population are notable and influence interpretation of the results. For the first 10 individuals, the group average is 17/10 = 1.7 and for the second 10 individuals the average DMF is 107/10 = 10.7.
- ◆ Scores for these two groups can be presented separately because of the wide difference.
- ◆ Average DMF scores can also be presented by age group.
- ◆ *Specific treatment needs of a group*
  - To calculate the percentage of DMF teeth that need to be restored, divide the total D component by the total DMF.
- ◆ *Calculation:*
  - *Example 1:* To calculate the *percent of DMF teeth* that need to be restored, divide the total D component by the total number of DMF teeth.
    D = 175, M = 55, F = 18
    Total DMFT = 248

$$\frac{D}{DMF} = \frac{175}{248} = 0.71 \text{ or } 71\% \text{ of the teeth need restorations}$$

  - *Example 2:* The same type of calculations can be used to determine the *percent of all teeth* missing in a group of individuals.
    20 individuals have 28 × 20 = 560 permanent teeth.
    D = 175, M = 55, F = 18 or nearly 10% of all their teeth lost because of dental caries.

$$\frac{M}{\text{Total \# of teeth}} = \frac{55}{560} = 0.098$$

II. Primary Dentition: Decayed, Indicated for Extraction, and Filled (df and def)[27]

A. Purpose

To determine the dental caries experience for the primary teeth present in the oral cavity by evaluating teeth or surfaces.

B. Selection of Teeth or Surfaces

◆ deft or dft: 20 teeth evaluated.

◆ defs or dfs: 88 surfaces evaluated.

  • *Posterior teeth:* Each has five surfaces: facial, lingual or palatal, mesial, distal, and occlusal. (8 teeth × 5 surfaces = 40 surfaces.)

  • *Anterior teeth:* Each has four surfaces: facial, lingual or palatal, mesial, and distal (12 teeth × 4 surfaces = 48 surfaces).

◆ Teeth not counted

  • Missing teeth, including unerupted and congenitally missing.

  • Supernumerary teeth.

  • Teeth restored for reasons other than dental caries are not counted as f.

C. Procedure

◆ *Instruments and examination*
  Same as for DMF.

◆ *Criteria*

DECAYED, INDICATED FOR EXTRACTION, FILLED (df AND def)	
RATING	**CRITERIA**
d	Primary teeth (or surfaces) with dental caries but not restored.
e	Primary teeth (or number of surfaces) that are *indicated for extraction* because of dental caries.
f	Primary teeth (or surfaces) restored with an amalgam, composite, or temporary filling. Each tooth (or surface) is scored only once. A tooth with recurrent caries around a restoration receives a "d" score.

◆ *Difference between deft/defs and dft/dfs*

  • In the deft and defs, both "d" and "e" are used to describe teeth with dental caries. Thus, d and e are sometimes combined, and the index becomes the dft or dfs.

D. Scoring

◆ *Calculation:*

  • *Example 1:* Individual def: A 2½-year-old child has 18 teeth. Teeth A (55) and J (65) are unerupted. There is no sign of dental caries in teeth M (73),

N (72), O (71), P (81), Q (82), and R (83). All other teeth have two carious surfaces each, except tooth B (54), which is broken down to the gum line.

  Summary:
  Total number of teeth = 18
  Number of "d" teeth = 11
  Number of "e" teeth = 1
  Number of "f" teeth = 0
  def = d + e + f = 11 + 1 + 0 = 12

◆ *Interpretation*

  • Twelve of 18 teeth (67%) with carious lesions indicates a serious need for dental treatment and a caries management program for the child.

◆ *Calculation:* Example 2: Individual dfs

  • Using the same 2½-year-old child to calculate dfs: Eleven teeth each have two carious surfaces: 11 × 2 = 22 carious surfaces
  Tooth B has 1 × 5 = 5 carious surfaces
  Total dfs: d + f = 27 + 0 = 27

◆ *Interpretation*

  • The child has 48 total anterior surfaces (12 teeth × 4 surfaces) and 30 total posterior surfaces (6 teeth × 5 surfaces) to total 78 surfaces.

$$\frac{dfs}{\text{Number of surfaces}} = \frac{27}{78}$$
$$= 0.35 \text{ or } 35\% \text{ of the surfaces in need of dental treatment}$$

E. Mixed Dentition

A DMFT or DMFS and a deft or defs are never combined or added together.

III. Primary Dentition: Decayed, Missing, and Filled (dmf)[27]

A. Purpose

To determine dental caries experience for children. Only primary teeth are evaluated.

B. Selection of Teeth or Surfaces

◆ dmft: 12 teeth evaluated (8 primary molars; 4 primary canines).

◆ dmfs: 56 surfaces evaluated.

  • *Primary molars:* 8 × 5 surfaces each = 40

  • *Primary canines:* 4 × 4 surfaces each = 16

◆ Each tooth is counted only once. When both dental caries and a restoration are present, the tooth or surface is scored as "d."

C. Procedure

◆ Instruments and examination are the same as for DMF.

◆ Criteria for dmft or dmfs

dmf RATING	CRITERIA
d	Primary molars and canines (or surfaces) that are carious.
m	Primary molars and canines (or surfaces) that are missing. A primary molar or canine is presumed missing because of dental caries when it has been lost before normal exfoliation.
f	Primary molars and canines (or surfaces) that have a restoration but are without caries.

D. Scoring

◆ *Calculation:* Example 1: Individual dmf
  • A 7-year-old boy has all primary molars and canines present. Examination reveals two carious surfaces on one molar tooth, one missing canine tooth, and one two-surface amalgam filling on a molar tooth:
  $$dmft = 1 + 1 + 1 = 3$$
  $$dmfs = 2 + 4 + 2 = 8$$

E. Mixed Dentition

Permanent and primary teeth are evaluated separately. A DMFT or DMFS and a dmft or dmfs are never added together.

IV. Early Childhood Caries[28]

A. Purpose

To provide case definitions that determine dental caries experience of children 5 years of age or younger.

B. Selection of Teeth or Surfaces

Each surface (mesial, distal, facial, lingual, and occlusal) of each tooth visible in the child's mouth is evaluated. Only primary teeth are scored.

C. Procedure

◆ Visual examination of all surfaces of each erupted tooth.
◆ Criteria for case definition are included in Table 21-1.

D. Scoring

◆ A designation of early childhood caries (ECC) or severe early childhood caries (S-ECC) for a particular individual relates the age of the child with the status of DMFT surfaces observed.

◆ Community-based surveys identify the percentage of a population with ECC and/or S-ECC.

V. Root Caries Index[29]

A. Purpose

To determine total root caries experience for individuals and groups and provide a direct, simple method for recording and making comparisons.

B. Selection of Teeth

◆ Up to four surfaces (mesial, distal, facial, and lingual/palatal) are counted for each tooth.
◆ Only surfaces with visible gingival recession are counted.
◆ Teeth with multiple roots and extreme recession, though rare, could present with two or three lesions on the same surface. In this case, the most severe lesion is selected for recording and each surface is counted only once.

C. Procedure

◆ *Examination*
  • Use adequate retraction and light to examine each tooth. Visible recession is shown in Figure 18-15, Chapter 18. An example of root caries is shown in Figure 16-12 in Chapter 16.
  • Apply current knowledge of the stages of dental caries to prevent damage to remineralizing areas during examination. Only cavitated lesions are recorded.
◆ *Record a rating for each root surface.*

ROOT CARIES INDEX RATING	CRITERIA
No R	Root surface with a covered cementoenamel junction and no visible recession (R = recession).
R − D	Root surface with recession present and root caries present (D = decay).
R − F	Root surface with recession present and the surface is restored (F = filled).
R − N	Root surface with recession, but no caries or restoration is present.
M	The tooth is missing.

TABLE 21-1 • ECC Case Definition				
AGE	BIRTH TO 3 YEARS (0–35 MONTHS)	3–4 YEARS (36–47 MONTHS)	4–5 YEARS (48–59 MONTHS)	5–6 YEARS (60–71 MONTHS)
ECC	One or more teeth with decayed (either cavitated or noncavitated), missing, or filled surfaces			
S-ECC	• One or more teeth with decay (either cavitated or noncavitated) or fillings present on smooth surface enamel OR one or more teeth missing due to caries	• One or more cavitated or filled smooth surfaces in primary maxillary anterior teeth • One or more missing teeth due to caries OR dmfs score ≥4	• One or more cavitated or filled smooth surfaces in primary maxillary anterior teeth • One or more missing teeth due to caries OR dmfs score ≥5	• One or more cavitated or filled smooth surfaces in primary maxillary anterior teeth • One or more missing teeth due to caries OR dmfs score ≥6

dmfs, total number of decayed missing and filled surfaces; ECC, early childhood caries; S-ECC, severe early childhood caries.
Source: Drury TF, Horowitz AM, Ismail AI, et al. Diagnosing and reporting early childhood caries for research purposes. *J Public Health Dent.* 1999;59(3):192-197.

D. Scoring

◆ *Calculation:* Formula

$$\frac{[R - D] + [R - F]}{[R - D] + [R - F] + [R - N]} \times 100 = RCI$$

◆ *Calculation:* Example individual root caries index (RCI)
  • A man, aged 70, presents with 23 natural teeth (23 × 4 = 92 surfaces). Clinical examination reveals:
    R − D = 26
    R − F = 8
    R − N = 58

$$RCI = \frac{26 + 8}{26 + 8 + 58} = \frac{37}{92} \times 100 = 36.9\%$$

◆ *Interpretation*
  • A score of 36.9% means that of all tooth surfaces with visible gingival recession, 36.9% have a history of root caries (cavitated or restored) carious lesions.
◆ *Group or community RCI*
  • The R − D, R − F, and R − N scores for all individuals in the group are added together and the RCI formula is calculated using the total scores.

DENTAL FLUOROSIS

Dental indices such as the Thylstrup–Fejerskov index,[30] the fluorosis risk index,[31] and the developmental defects of dental enamel index[32,33] have been used to investigate the effects of fluoride concentration on dental enamel. The two indices described here are the most commonly used for community-based assessment.

I. Dean's Fluorosis Index[34]

A. Purpose

To measure the prevalence and severity of dental fluorosis.
◆ Originally developed in the 1930s and refined in 1942 to relate the severity of hypomineralization of dental enamel to concentration of fluoride in the water supply.
◆ Considered less sensitive than some other measures of fluorosis, but still recommended for use in community studies.

B. Selection of Teeth

The smooth surface enamel of all teeth is examined.

C. Procedure

Each tooth is visually examined for signs of fluorosis and assigned a numerical score using the descriptive categories listed in Table 21-2.

TABLE 21-2 • Scoring System for Dean's Fluorosis Index

CATEGORY	DESCRIPTION	NUMERICAL SCORE
Normal	Smooth, creamy white tooth surface	0
Questionable	Slight changes from normal transparency	1
Very mild	Small, scattered opaque areas; less than 25% of tooth surface	2
Mild	Opaque areas; less than 50% of tooth surface	3
Moderate	Significant opaque and/or worn areas; may have brown stains	4
Severe	Widespread, significant hypoplasia, pitting, brown staining, worn areas, and/or a corroded appearance	5

Source: Dean HT. The investigation of physiological effect by the epidemiological method. In: Moulton FR, ed. *Fluorine and Dental Health.* Washington, DC: American Association for the Advancement of Science; 1942:23-71.

D. Scoring

◆ An individual fluorosis score is assigned using the highest numerical score recorded for two or more teeth.
◆ Community levels of fluorosis are indicated by the percentage of individuals in the sample or population that receive scores in each category.

II. Tooth Surface Index of Fluorosis [35]

A. Purpose

◆ To measure the prevalence and severity of dental fluorosis.
◆ More sensitive than Dean's index in identifying the mildest signs of fluorosis.

B. Selection of Teeth

The smooth surface enamel, cusp tips, and incisal edges of all teeth are examined.

C. Procedure

Each tooth is examined visually and assigned a numerical score using the criteria in Table 21-3.

D. Scoring

Tooth surface index of fluorosis (TSIF) data are presented as a distribution citing the percent of the population with each numerical score, rather than as mean scores for the entire group.

TABLE 21-3 • Scoring System for Tooth Surface Index of Fluorosis

DESCRIPTION	NUMERICAL SCORE
No evidence of fluorosis	0
Areas with parchment-white color; less than one-third of visible tooth surface; includes fluorosis confined to anterior incisal edges and posterior cusp tips	1
Parchment-white color on at least one-third but less than two-thirds of visible tooth surface	2
Parchment-white color on at least two-thirds of visible tooth surface	3
Staining (from light to very dark brown) in conjunction with parchment-white areas as described above in levels 1, 2, or 3	4
Discrete stained and rough pitted areas, but no staining on intact enamel surfaces	5
Discrete pitting plus staining of intact enamel surfaces	6
Confluent pitting over large areas of tooth surface; anatomy of tooth may be altered; dark-brown stain usually present	7

Source: Horowitz HS, Driscoll WS, Meyers RJ, et al. A new method for assessing the prevalence of dental fluorosis—the tooth surface index of Fluorosis. *J Am Dent Assoc.* 1984;109(1):37-41.

COMMUNITY-BASED ORAL HEALTH SURVEILLANCE

Community oral health screenings can be performed at every level: local, national, and worldwide. Data collected by such screenings are useful for monitoring health status and determining population access to or need for oral health services.

I. WHO Basic Screening Survey[21]

The WHO screening survey includes the CPI and the LOA indices described earlier.

A. Purpose

To collect comprehensive data on oral health status and dental treatment needs of a population. This system is suitable for surveying both adults and children.

B. Tissues/Areas Examined

Survey categories include the following:
- Orofacial (intraoral and extraoral) lesions and anomalies.

- Temporomandibular joint status.
- Periodontal status.
- Dentition status and treatment need.
- Prosthetic status and need.
- Need for immediate care/referral.

C. Procedures

- Standardized assessment form with boxes for data entry identifies the codes and descriptive criteria for each data collection category.
- Standardized codes facilitate computerized data entry and analysis.
- Photographs in the training manual provide examples of criteria for each code.

D. Scoring

- Data can be analyzed by survey team or arrangements can be made for data entry forms to be analyzed by the WHO.

II. ASTDD Basic Screening Survey[6]

A. Purpose

- *Developed by the ASTDD to provide oral screening for adult, school age, and/or preschool populations.*
  - Data levels are consistent with monitoring the U.S. Public Health Service national health objectives.
  - Data collected can easily be compared with data collected by other communities and states using the data collection techniques.
- *The system was designed to be used by screeners with or without dental background because:*
  - Sometimes nondental personnel have better access to some population groups.
  - Some communities have little access to dental public health professionals.

B. Selection of Teeth

All teeth are examined, but each individual patient receives one score for each category.

C. Procedure

- Oral screening can be combined with an optional questionnaire that collects additional data on demographics and access to dental care.
- Screeners are trained and calibrated. They record oral findings using photographs and detailed descriptions of associated criteria.

D. Scoring

- Table 21-4 outlines the scoring criteria and categories recorded for preschool and school children.

TABLE 21-4 • Association of State and Territorial Dental Directors' Basic Screening Survey Scoring Criteria: Preschool and School Children

CRITERIA	SCORE	PRESCHOOLERS	SCHOOL CHILDREN
Untreated caries (≥ 1/2 mm discontinuity in tooth surface)	0 = No untreated caries 1 = Untreated caries	✓	✓
Treated decay (amalgam, composite, or temporary filling)	0 = No treated decay 1 = Treated decay	✓	✓
Sealants on permanent molars	0 = No sealants 1 = Sealants		✓
Treatment urgency	0 = No obvious problem (routine dental care indicated) 1 = Early dental care (within 2 wk) 2 = Urgent care (as soon as possible—presents with pain, swelling, etc.)	✓	✓

A ✓ mark indicates that the oral condition category is scored in that particular age group. Some categories (i.e., sealants) are not scored in all age groups.

Source: ASTDD Basic Screening Surveys. Association of State and Territorial Dental Director Web Site. http://www.astdd.org/basic-screening-survey-tool. Accessed November 12, 2017.

◆ Table 21-5 lists the scoring criteria and categories recorded for older adults.

◆ Data from each indicator can be compiled and expressed in frequency graphs or tables as a percentage of the population that exhibits a specific category trait.

DOCUMENTATION

Factors related to dental indices to document in the patient records include:

◆ Name of the index or indices used.

◆ Score calculated for the index.

◆ Objective statement that provides an interpretation of the index score.

◆ Follow-up instructions provided to the patient.

◆ An example of documentation for use of a dental index appears in Box 21-1.

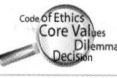

EVERYDAY ETHICS

Susanna began practicing in the team clinic at the dental school and found the work to be very challenging. As a hygienist, she was not only providing preventive treatment for patients but also responsible for data collection for several research projects. Suddenly, the importance of understanding and calculating the various indices became critical. In particular, Susanna found herself reviewing the procedures for the OHI-S, bleeding indices, and the DMFT.

Susanna had always enjoyed her clinical interactions with patients, but now scoring and recording information on each and every tooth was beginning to cause her some stress. Generally Susanna practiced without an assistant and found it difficult to do both examining and recording. Near the end of one day when she was organizing the day's work

for Dr. Lowe's caries study, she discovered that she had omitted several surfaces in one quadrant. This was the patient's final visit to the dental school. Susanna contemplated what to do when she realized the data were missing.

Questions for Consideration

1. Discuss how American Dental Hygienists' Association's roles for dental hygienists (Chapter 1) apply to Suzanna's daily duties.

2. Can Susanna "defend" her actions to Dr. Lowe by submitting the data she does have on the patient? Explain your rationale.

3. Which of the core values (Table II-1, Section II Introduction) or principles of ethical behavior come into play in collecting research data such as described in this scenario?

TABLE 21-5 • Association of State and Territorial Dental Directors' Basic Screening Survey Scoring Criteria: Older Adults

CRITERIA	SCORE
Removable upper denture	0 = No 1 = Yes
If yes: Do you wear upper denture when eating?	0 = No 1 = Yes
Removable lower denture	0 = No 1 = Yes
If yes: Do you wear lower denture when eating?	0 = No 1 = Yes
Number of upper natural teeth (include root fragments)	Range 0–16
Number of lower natural teeth (include root fragments)	Range 0–16
Root fragments	0 = No 1 = Yes 9 = Edentulous
Untreated decay	0 = No 1 = Yes 9 = Edentulous
Need for periodontal care	0 = No 1 = Yes 9 = Edentulous
Suspicious soft-tissue lesions	0 = No 1 = Yes 9 = Edentulous
Treatment urgency	0 = no obvious problem—next scheduled visit 1 = Early care—within next several weeks 2 = Urgent care—within next week—pain or infection
Obvious tooth mobility (optional indicator)	0 = No 1 = Yes 0 = Edentulous
Severe dry mouth (optional indicator)	0 = No 1 = Yes

Source: ASTDD Basic Screening Surveys. Association of State and Territorial Dental Director Web Site. http://www.astdd.org/basic-screening-survey-tool. Accessed November 12, 2017.

BOX 21-1

Example Documentation:
Use of a Dental Index during Patient Assessment

S—Patient presents for reassessment of biofilm and bleeding levels 14 days following oral hygiene instructions that were provided during the previous appointment.

O—Biofilm-free score = 89% compared with previous score of 22%; SBI score = 2 compared to previous score of 5.

A—Significant improvement noted in scores except on maxillary facial surfaces.

P—Patient congratulated on areas of success. Additional instruction provided specifically related to biofilm removal on posterior facial and proximal tooth surfaces. Patient observed while brushing and flossing maxillary molar areas using a mirror.

Next Step: 3 months re-evaluation.

Signed: _____, RDH

Date: _____

Factors to Teach Patient or Members of the Community

► How an index is used and calculated, and what the scores mean.
► Purpose for the selection of the particular index being used.
► Correlation of index scores with current oral health practices and procedures.
► Procedures to follow to improve index scores and bring the oral tissues to health.

ENHANCE YOUR UNDERSTANDING

ONLINE RESOURCES
(see the inside front cover for access information)
• Audio glossary
• Appendices

SUPPORT FOR LEARNING
(available separately)
• *Active Learning Workbook for Wilkins' Clinical Practice of the Dental Hygienist, 13th Edition*

INDIVIDUALIZED REVIEW
• Customized practice quizzing with Navigate 2 TestPrep for *Wilkins' Clinical Practice of the Dental Hygienist*

References

NOTE: Many of the citations below may seem not to be current or even seem completely out-of-date; however, the reader will note that most are "classic" references, which refer to the development and first use of the index.

1. Silness J, Loe H. Periodontal disease in pregnancy. II. Correlation between oral hygiene and periodontal condition. *Acta Odontol Scand.* 1964;22:121-135.

2. Podshadley AG, Haley JV. A method for evaluating oral hygiene performance. *Public Health Rep.* 1968;83(3):259-264.

3. Klein H, Palmer CE, Knutson JW. Studies on dental caries. I. Dental status and dental needs of elementary school children. *Public Health Rep.* 1938;53(19):751-765.

4. U.S. Department of Health and Human Services. *Oral Health in America: A Report of the Surgeon General.* Rockville, MD: U.S. Department of Health and Human Services, National Institute of Dental and Craniofacial Research, National Institutes of Health; 2000:63-89.

5. Healthy People 2020. Topics and objectives: oral health. Office of Disease Prevention and Health Promotion Web site. https://www.healthypeople.gov/2020/topics-objectives/topic/oral-health. Updated November 13, 2017. Accessed November 12, 2017.

6. Association of State and Territorial Dental Directors. *Basic Screening Surveys.* Reno, NV: ASTDD; 2014. http://www.astdd.org/basic-screening-survey-tool/. Accessed October 16, 2017.

7. Löe H. The gingival index, the plaque index and the retention index systems. *J Periodontol.* 1967;38(6 suppl):610-616.

8. O'Leary TJ, Drake RB, Naylor JE. The plaque control record. *J Periodontol.* 1972;43(1):38.

9. Ramfjord SP, Ash MM. *Periodontology and Periodontics.* Philadelphia, PA: WB Saunders Co; 1979:273.

10. Grant DA, Stern IB, Everett FG. *Periodontics.* 5th ed. St. Louis, MO: Mosby; 1979:529-531.

11. Greene JC, Vermillion JR. The simplified oral hygiene index. *J Am Dent Assoc.* 1964;68:7-13.

12. Greene JC. The Oral Hygiene Index—development and uses. *J Periodontol.* 1967;38(6 suppl):625-637.

13. Schour I, Massler M. Prevalence of gingivitis in young adults. *J Dent Res.* 1948;27(6):733.

14. Massler M. The P-M-A index for the assessment of gingivitis. *J Periodontol.* 1967;38(6 suppl):592-601.

15. Russell AL. A system of classification and scoring for prevalence surveys of periodontal disease. *J Dent Res.* 1956;35(3):350-359.

16. Mühlemann HR, Son S. Gingival sulcus bleeding—a leading symptom in initial gingivitis. *Helv Odontol Acta.* 1971;15(2):107-113.

17. Meitner SW, Zander HA, Iker HP, et al. Identification of inflamed gingival surfaces. *J Clin Periodontol.* 1979;6(2):93-97.

18. American Academy of Periodontology. Parameter on comprehensive periodontal examination. *J Periodontol.* 2000;71(5 suppl):847-848.

19. Khocht A, Zohn H, Deasy M, et al. Assessment of periodontal status with PSR and traditional clinical periodontal examination. *J Am Dent Assoc.* 1995;126(12):1658-1665.

20. Ainamo J, Barmes D, Beagrie G, et al. Development of the World Health Organization (WHO) community periodontal index of treatment needs (CPITN). *Int Dent J.* 1982;32(3):281-291.

21. World Health Organization. *Oral Health Surveys: Basic Methods.* Geneva, Switzerland: WHO; 1997:26-39.

22. Carter HG, Barnes GP. The gingival bleeding index. *J Periodontol.* 1974;45(11):801-805.

23. Abrams K, Caton J, Polson A. Histologic comparisons of interproximal gingival tissues related to the presence or absence of bleeding. *J Periodontol.* 1984;55(11):629-632.

24. Caton JG, Polson AM. The interdental bleeding index: a simplified procedure for monitoring gingival health. *Compend Contin Educ Dent.* 1985;6(2):88, 90-92.

25. Ramfjord SP. Indices for prevalence and incidence of periodontal disease. *J Periodontol.* 1959;30:51-59.

26. U.S. Department of Health and Human Services, Public Health Service, National Institutes of Health. *Oral Health Surveys of the National Institute of Dental Research, Diagnostic Criteria and Procedures.* Bethesda, MD: National Institute of Dental Research; 1991.

27. Gruebbel AO. A measurement of dental caries prevalence and treatment service for deciduous teeth. *J Dent Res.* 1944;23:163-168.

28. Drury TF, Horowitz AM, Ismail AI, et al. Diagnosing and reporting early childhood caries for research purposes. *J Public Health Dent.* 1999;59(3):192-197.

29. Katz RV. Assessing root caries in populations: the evolution of the root caries index. *J Public Health Dent.* 1980;40(1):7-16.

30. Thylstrup A, Fejerskov O. Clinical appearance of dental fluorosis in permanent teeth in relation to histologic changes. *Community Dent Oral Epidemiol.* 1978;6(6):315-328.

31. Pendrys DG. The fluorosis risk index: a method for investigating risk factors. *J Public Health Dent.* 1990;50(5):291-298.

32. Fédération Dentaire Internationale. An epidemiological index of developmental defects of dental enamel (DDE Index). Commission on Oral Health, Research and Epidemiology. *Int Dent J.* 1982;32(2):159-167.

33. Clarkson J, O'Mullane, D. A modified DDE index for use in epidemiological studies of enamel defects. *J Dent Res.* 1989;68(3):445-450.

34. Dean HT. The investigation of physiological effect by the epidemiological method. In: Moulton FR, ed. *Fluorine and Dental Health.* Washington, DC: American Association for the Advancement of Science; 1942:23-71.

35. Horowitz HS, Driscoll WS, Meyers RJ, et al. A new method for assessing the prevalence of dental fluorosis—the tooth surface index of fluorosis. *J Am Dent Assoc.* 1984;109(1):37-41.

Dental Hygiene Diagnosis and Care Planning

DIAGNOSE
Identify problems based on assessment data

PLAN
Select, prioritize, and sequence dental hygiene interventions

ASSESS
Data Collection

IMPLEMENT
Activating the plan

DOCUMENT
Comprehensive record-keeping

EVALUATE
Feedback on effectiveness

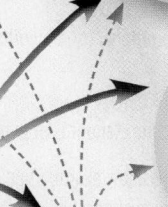

FIGURE V-1 • The Dental Hygiene Process of Care.

INTRODUCTION FOR SECTION V

After the initial assessment is completed, as described in Section IV, the data are assembled, sequenced, and analyzed in preparation for planning dental hygiene treatment and education interventions that help the patient acquire and maintain optimum oral health.

THE DENTAL HYGIENE PROCESS OF CARE

Figure V-1 shows the position of diagnosis and care planning in the total Dental Hygiene Process of Care.

◆ Dental hygiene diagnosis statements:
  • Analyze patient assessment data to identify significant oral hygiene problems.
  • Focus attention on behavioral aspects as well as deviations from normal oral health.
◆ The formal, written dental hygiene care plan, integrated with the total treatment plan for the patient, is used to:
  • Identify dental hygiene interventions based on diagnostic statements that define patient needs.
  • Educate the patient.
  • Secure informed consent for treatment.
  • Communicate planned dental hygiene interventions with other oral care team members.

ETHICAL APPLICATIONS

◆ Basic concepts of healthcare law apply to all dental hygiene professionals.
◆ The dental hygiene practice acts of each state or province govern the scope of dental hygiene functions and the criteria for licensure.
◆ The potential for an ethical situation arises anytime a dental hygienist interacts with:
  • A patient.
  • Members of the dental or interprofessional healthcare team.
  • Other individuals involved in the special needs of the patient, such as family and caregivers.
◆ A dental hygienist who provides ethical patient care:
  • Is cognizant of the respect each patient deserves.
  • Maintains communication among all parties responsible for dental and dental hygiene treatment.
  • Attains knowledge of current standards of care and legal scope of practice.
  • Possesses the ability to assess and justify the reporting of unacceptable practices.
  • Selected legal concepts and suggestions for application are described in Table V-1.

TABLE V-1 • Legal and Ethical Concepts

LEGAL CONCEPT	EXPLANATION	APPLICATION EXAMPLES
Professional liability	A licensed professional is legally accountable for all actions; bound by the law.	Responsibility for actions and decisions made during patient care.
Scope of practice	A dental hygienist is legally bound to provide care within the dental hygiene scope of practice.	Adherence to dental hygiene licensure requirements and performance of functions defined as legal within each state's Dental Hygiene Practice Act.
Standard of care	A professional uses: • Ordinary and reasonable skill commonly used by other dental professionals. • Prudent judgment. • All available resources to determine standards of practice.	Analyzing the patient's assessment data before selecting dental hygiene interventions.
Informed consent	Voluntary affirmation by a patient to allow examination or treatment by authorized dental hygienist or other member of the dental team.	An ongoing process of communication and education about oral health treatment options, not merely a printed form to sign.
Negligence/malpractice	Failure to perform professional duties according to the accepted standard of care.	Failure to inform and refer a patient when concerns outside the scope of dental hygiene practice exist.

Dental Hygiene Diagnosis

Catherine G. Ranson, RDH BHA, MET, Linda D. Boyd, RDH, RD, EdD, and
Charlotte J. Wyche, BSDH, MS

CHAPTER OUTLINE

INTRODUCTION
ASSESSMENT FINDINGS
  I. The Chief Complaint
  II. Risk Factors
  III. Patient's Overall Health Status
  IV. Oral Healthcare Literacy Level of the Patient
  V. The Patient's Self-Care Ability

THE PERIODONTAL DIAGNOSIS AND RISK LEVEL
  I. Current Periodontal Status
  II. Classification of Periodontal Disease
  III. Parameters of Care
DENTAL CARIES RISK LEVEL
THE DENTAL HYGIENE DIAGNOSIS
  I. Basis for Diagnosis
  II. Diagnostic Statements

THE DENTAL HYGIENE PROGNOSIS
  I. Criteria for Various Prognoses
  II. Factors in Assigning a Prognosis
DOCUMENTATION
EVERYDAY ETHICS
FACTORS TO TEACH THE PATIENT
REFERENCES

LEARNING OBJECTIVES

After studying this chapter, the student will be able to:

1. Explain the significance of developing a dental hygiene diagnosis as a component of the dental hygiene process of care.

2. Formulate a dental hygiene diagnosis based on the assessment findings.

3. Identify and define key terms and concepts related to planning dental hygiene care.

4. Identify and explain assessment findings and individual patient factors that affect patient care.

5. Identify additional factors that can influence planning for dental hygiene care.

INTRODUCTION

- Four basic steps to be considered when planning patient care are as follows[1]:
  1. Collect and analyze assessment information.
  2. Establish the diagnosis.
  3. Select treatment and education interventions based on the diagnostic findings.
  4. Develop a formal plan for care.
- In the dental hygiene process of care (Chapter 1), the dental hygiene diagnosis is the result of analysis and synthesis of assessment data and the application of clinical judgment and critical thinking skills.
- Then, using an evidence-based approach, a dental hygiene care plan and appointment sequence are formalized.

ASSESSMENT FINDINGS

Clinical assessment findings play a key role in the development of the dental hygiene diagnosis and dental hygiene care plan.

I. The Chief Complaint

- The chief complaint is the patient's statement regarding the reason for seeking dental and dental hygiene care.
- A significant concern expressed by the patient, such as pain, is addressed before initiating dental hygiene treatment.

II. Risk Factors

- Risk factors increase the patient's potential for diminished oral health status.
  - Modifiable risks factors are determinants that can be modified by intervention, thereby reducing the probability of disease.
- Anticipatory guidance through preventive education and counseling is an essential component of the care plan for a patient exhibiting one or more risk factors.

A. Individual Risk Factors for Periodontal Diseases[2]

- Stress.
- Lifestyle choices (e.g., tobacco, alcohol).
- Gender (more prevalent in male gender).
- Cultural, ethnicity.
- Systemic conditions (e.g., prediabetes, diabetes, obesity, metabolic syndrome, osteoporosis).
- Genetic factors.
- Nutritional status (e.g., dietary calcium, vitamin D).

B. Periodontal Disease Association with Systemic Conditions

Current research suggests the presence of periodontal infection is associated with a variety of systemic conditions, including:

- Cardiovascular disease.[3,4]
- Diabetes mellitus.[4]
- Metabolic syndrome (a cluster of health conditions that increase risk for heart disease and diabetes).[4]
- Obesity.[4]
- Respiratory disease (especially pneumonia).[5,6]
- Adverse pregnancy outcome.[7]
- Osteoporosis.[8]

C. Risk Factors for Dental Caries

- The current best practice, evidence-based approach for management of dental caries is by identifying and managing risk factors.[9]
- Risk factors for dental caries include[9–14]:
  - Behavioral factors (inadequate biofilm removal).
  - Dietary factors (frequent use of cariogenic foods/beverages).
  - Low fluoride.
  - Tooth morphology and position (deep occlusal pits and fissures, exposed root surfaces, rotated positioning).
  - Xerostomia.
  - Personal and family history of dental caries/restorative dentistry.
  - Developmental factors (modifications of dental enamel).
  - Genetic factors (immune response).

C. Risk Factors for Oral Cancer[13,14]

- Tobacco use of any kind.
- Heavy alcohol use.
- Excessive sun exposure (lips and face).
- Exposure to the human papillomavirus.
- Genetic susceptibility.

III. Patient's Overall Health Status

A. Physical Status

- The extent of the patient's medical, physical, and psychological risk determines modifications necessary during treatment.
- Examples of systematic approaches used to assess physical status include:
  - The American Society of Anesthesiologists' (ASA) classification system (Table 22-1).[15]
  - The Oral, Systemic, Capability, Autonomy, and Reality (OSCAR) Planning Guide (Table 22-2).[16]

TABLE 22-1 • ASA Physical Status Classification System

	ASA CLASSIFICATION	EXAMPLES OF PHYSICAL OR PSYCHOSOCIAL MANIFESTATIONS	DENTAL HYGIENE TREATMENT CONSIDERATIONS
ASA I	Without systemic disease; a normal, healthy patient with little or no dental anxiety	Able to walk one flight of stairs with no distress ADL/IADL level = 0	No modifications necessary
ASA II	Mild systemic disease or extreme dental anxiety	Needs to stop after walking one flight of stairs because of distress Well-controlled chronic conditions Upper respiratory infections Healthy pregnant woman Allergies ADL/IADL level = 1	Minimal risk; minor modifications to treatment and/or patient education may be necessary
ASA III	Systemic disease that limits activity but is not incapacitating	Needs to stop en route walking one flight of stairs Chronic cardiovascular conditions Controlled insulin-dependent diabetes Chronic pulmonary diseases Elevated blood pressure ADL/IADL level = 2 or 3	Elective treatment is not contraindicated, but serious consideration of treatment and/or patient/caregiver education modifications may be necessary
ASA IV	Incapacitating disease that is a constant threat to life	Unable to walk up one flight of stairs Unstable cardiovascular conditions Extremely elevated blood pressure Uncontrolled epilepsy Uncontrolled insulin-dependent diabetes	Conservative, noninvasive management of emergency dental conditions; more complex dental intervention may require hospitalization during treatment; caregiver training for daily oral care may be necessary
ASA V	Patient is moribund and not expected to survive	End-stage renal, hepatic, infectious disease, or terminal cancer	Only palliative treatment is delivered; caregiver training for daily oral care may be necessary

ADL, activities of daily living; ASA, American Society of Anesthesiologists; IADL, instrumental activities of daily living.
Source: American Society of Anesthesiologists. ASA physical status classification system. http://www.asahq.org/resources/clinical-information/asa-physical-status-classification-system.

TABLE 22-2 • The Oral, Systemic, Capability, Autonomy, and Reality Planning Guide

ISSUE	FACTORS OF CONCERN
A systematic approach to identifying factors to evaluate when planning dental hygiene care	
Oral	Teeth, restorations, prostheses, periodontium, pulpal status, oral mucosa, occlusion, saliva, tongue, alveolar bone
Systemic	Normative age changes, medical diagnoses, pharmacologic agents, interdisciplinary communication
Capability	Functional ability, self-care, caregivers, oral hygiene, transportation to appointments, mobility within the dental office
Autonomy	Decision-making ability, dependence on alternative, or supplemental decision makers
Reality	Prioritization of oral health, financial ability or limitations, significance of anticipated life span

Source: Reprinted with permission from Ship JA, Mohammad AR, eds. *Clinician's Guide to Oral Health in Geriatric Patients.* Baltimore, MD: American Academy of Oral Medicine; 1999:21.

B. Tobacco Use

◆ Tobacco in all forms affects oral status and dental hygiene treatment outcomes.

Information on planning dental hygiene interventions for the patient who uses tobacco is discussed in Chapter 32.

IV. Oral Healthcare Literacy Level of the Patient

◆ Before planning individualized patient care, the patient's oral health literacy is assessed.

◆ From that baseline, planned educational interventions can build on current knowledge rather than provide information too far above or below the patient's current literacy.

V. The Patient's Self-Care Ability

◆ The patient's ability to manipulate a toothbrush and interdental aid in order to comply with suggested oral care regimens will determine the success of planned interventions.

◆ Patients with disabilities or physical limitations will require modification to ensure adequate daily oral biofilm removal.

◆ An activities of daily living (ADL/IADL) classification level, described in Table 22-3, provides a guide to determine whether adaptive or assistive aids or caregiver training for personal oral care procedures are necessary.

THE PERIODONTAL DIAGNOSIS AND RISK LEVEL

Planning for the number and length of appointments in a treatment sequence is influenced by:

◆ Both the dental and dental hygiene periodontal diagnosis.[17–19]

◆ The patient's periodontal risk factors (see "Risk Factor" section).[18,20]

I. Current Periodontal Status

A description of past and current periodontal conditions, as well as risk factors affecting the progress of disease, determine a patient's current periodontal status (Chapter 19).

II. Classification of Periodontal Disease

◆ The extent, severity, and chronic or aggressive nature of the patient's periodontal disease can be characterized as listed in Table 22-4.

◆ For purpose of determining the sequences and number of appointments required for initial nonsurgical periodontal therapy, it is useful to divide the periodontal diagnosis into the following classifications (Chapter 19 for more information)[21]:

A. Gingivitis

Inflammation of the gingiva is characterized by changes in color, form, size, position of margin, with bleeding on probing, and no attachment loss.

TABLE 22-3 • Measures of Patient Functioning[a]

EXAMPLES OF ADL	EXAMPLES OF IADL	LEVELS
Brushing	Maintaining self-care regimens	*Level 0* Ability to perform the task without assistance
Flossing	Ability to make and keep dental appointments	
Applying interdental aids	Writing	*Level 1* Ability to perform the task with some human assistance; may need a device or mechanical aid but or still independent
Feeding	Cooking	
Ambulation (walking)	Shopping	
Bathing	Climbing stairs	*Level 2* Ability to perform the task with partial assistance
Continence	Managing medication	
Communication	Reading	*Level 3* Requires full assistance to perform the task; totally dependent
Dressing	Cleaning	
Toileting	Using telephone	
Transfer (from bed to toilet)		
Grooming		

[a]This scale provides a simple means of summarizing a person's ability to carry out the basic tasks needed for self-care.
ADL, activities of daily living; IADL, instrumental activities of daily living.

TABLE 22-4 • Parameters of Care

CLINICAL DIAGNOSIS	THERAPEUTIC GOALS	TREATMENT CONSIDERATIONS	
Biofilm-induced gingivitis	• To establish gingival health through elimination of etiologic factors	*Dental treatment plan* • The dental treatment plan may indicate surgical correction of gingival deformities	*Dental hygiene care plan* • Customized patient education • Supra- and subgingival debridement • Antimicrobial agents, and correction of biofilm-retentive factors
Stage I or II Periodontitis • With slight to moderate loss of periodontal support	• To arrest progression of disease and prevent recurrence • To preserve health, comfort, and function	*Dental treatment plan* • If resolution of the condition does not occur, consider periodontal surgery	*Dental hygiene care plan* • Elimination and control of systemic and local risk factors • Biofilm control • Supra- and subgingival scaling and root debridement • Adjunctive antimicrobial agents
Stage III or IV Periodontitis • With advanced loss of periodontal support	• To alter or eliminate microbial etiology and contributing risk factors • To arrest the progression of disease	*Dental treatment plan* • May include regeneration of periodontal attachment following the completion and evaluation of initial therapy	*Dental hygiene care plan* • Initial therapy as described above *Compromised therapy* • Severity/extent of disease, or the age/health of the patient preclude optimal results • Initial therapy and continued periodontal maintenance become the endpoint
Periodontal maintenance	• To minimize the recurrence and progression of the disease • To reduce the incidence of tooth loss		*Dental hygiene care plan* • Comparison of clinical data to previous baseline measurements • Assessment of personal oral hygiene status and compliance with maintenance intervals • Oral hygiene reinstruction or modification • Counseling on control of risk factors
Acute periodontal diseases include • Gingival abscess Periodontal abscess • Necrotizing diseases • Endo-Periodontal lesions	• To eliminate acute signs and symptoms of the condition as soon as possible	*Dental treatment plan* • Treatment considerations depend on the presenting condition	*Dental hygiene care plan* • Collaborate with the attending dentist to prioritize treatment for the immediate need
Mucogingival conditions • Deviations from normal anatomic relationship between gingival margin and mucogingival junction	• To maintain and restore function and esthetics	*Dental treatment plan* • May include surgical treatment	*Dental hygiene care plan* • Careful comparison of baseline and follow-up findings, control of inflammation through biofilm control, scaling and root debridement, and/or antimicrobial agents

Source: American Academy of Periodontology. Parameters of care. *J Periodontol.* 2000;71(suppl 5):i–ii, 847-883. Tonetti MS, Greenwell H, Kornman KS. Staging and grading of periodontitis: Framework and proposal of a new classification and case definition. *J Periodontol.* 2018;89(Suppl 1):S159-S172.

B. Stage I Periodontitis

Mild periodontitis with progression of inflammation into the deeper periodontal structures with slight bone loss and connective tissue attachment; subgingival calculus and measurable pocket depth with bleeding on probing.

C. Stage II Periodontitis

Moderate periodontitis, with increased destruction of the periodontal structures, increased probing depths with bleeding, noticeable loss of interdental bony support with early to moderate furcation invasions; mobility and fremitus.

D. Stage III or Stage IV Periodontitis

Further progression of periodontal inflammation with increased probing depths with bleeding, major loss of bony support, furcation invasions, and possible evidence of trauma from occlusion with increased tooth mobility and fremitus, and other signs and symptoms.

III. Parameters of Care

- Clinical diagnosis, therapeutic goals, treatment considerations, and outcomes assessment for periodontal disease are outlined in the periodontal American Academy of Periodontology Parameters of Care.[21]
- Planning considerations are determined by the severity of infection. Examples are listed in Table 22-4.

DENTAL CARIES RISK LEVEL

- Restorative treatment for dental caries is provided by the dentist or dental therapist; however, the plan for dental hygiene care includes interventions aimed at managing risk factors for dental caries.[22]
- Protocols and treatment guidelines for caries management based on risk factors are found in:
  - Chapter 25 for adults.
  - Chapter 47 for children 0–5.

THE DENTAL HYGIENE DIAGNOSIS

The diagnosis is a fundamental component of medical and dental care.
- The dental hygiene diagnosis is part of the process of care, involving the use of evidenced-based analysis of the assessment findings to determine the patient's or community's dental hygiene needs.[20]
- The dental hygiene diagnosis provides a basis for the dental hygiene care plan (therapeutic and preventive).[20]

I. Basis for Diagnosis[1,18-20]

- Patient interview data (chief complaint, identification of oral problems, and comprehensive personal/social, medical, and dental health histories).
- Physical assessment data (vital signs, extraoral and intraoral tissue examination, and dental and periodontal chartings).
- Radiographic series.

II. Diagnostic Statements

- Provide the basis for development of the care plan that focuses on education, oral self-care, prevention, dental hygiene treatment within the scope of dental hygiene practice and referral.[19,21]
- Examples of dental hygiene diagnostic statements are listed in Table 22-5.

THE DENTAL HYGIENE PROGNOSIS

The dental hygiene prognosis is a component of medical and dental care. Prognosis is a forecast of the outcome of a disease or condition. In the dental hygiene process of care, prognosis refers to the following[19,23]:
- A look ahead to an anticipated outcome or end point expected from the dental hygiene intervention selected for an individual patient.

TABLE 22-5 • Examples of Dental Hygiene Diagnostic Statements

PROBLEM	RISK FACTORS AND ETIOLOGY
Hypersensitivity	Related to: gingival recession resulting in exposed root surfaces
Gingival bleeding	Related to: biofilm accumulation causing inflammation
Increased caries risk (caries management by risk assessment [CAMBRA] level = extreme)	Related to: previous history of dental caries and consumption of sugar-sweetened beverages frequently throughout each day
Biofilm control record score = fair to poor score	Related to: limited ability to perform oral self-care tasks (activities of daily living Level 3)
Inflamed tissue distal to 47/operculum	Related to: biofilm accumulation causing inflammation
Decreased saliva flow/xerostomia	Related to: side effect of medication
Red patchy tissue on palate appears to be nicotine stomatitis	Related to: regular tobacco use
Generalized Stage II periodontitis	Related to: inadequate biofilm control, lack of regular professional dental care, radiographic evidenced of interdental clinical attachment loss, etc.

◆ Expressed in general terms for either an individual tooth or the overall prognosis for the patient's teeth. Typically, the overall prognosis will be determined in consultation with the dentist.

◆ Based on treatment and self-care behavior goals set by the clinician with the patient during the planning phase of care.

I. Criteria for Various Prognoses

The criteria for various prognoses are listed in Box 22-1.

II. Factors in Assigning Prognosis[24]

◆ Individual tooth prognosis:
  • Percentage of bone loss.
  • Clinical attachment loss.
  • Extent and type of bone loss (vertical vs. horizontal).

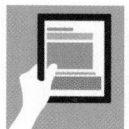

BOX 22-1
Criteria for Various Prognoses

Prognosis following periodontal therapy is determined by the following factors:

Good
• Adequate control of etiologic factors
• Adequate patient self-care ability
• Adequate periodontal support

Fair
• Adequate control of etiologic factors
• Adequate patient self-care ability
• Less than 25% attachment loss
• Class I or less furcation involvement

Poor
• Greater than 50% attachment loss with Class II furcation
• Patient self-care difficult due to location and depth of furcation

Questionable
• Greater than 50% attachment loss with poor crown-to-root ratio
• Poor root form: instrumentation access
• Inaccessible Class II furcation or Class III furcation
• Greater than 2+ mobility
• Significant root proximity

Hopeless
• Inadequate attachment to maintain the tooth

Source: McGuire, MK. Prognosis vs outcome: predicting tooth survival. *Compend Contin Educ Dent.* 2000;21:217-220, 222, 224.

• Presence and severity of furcation involvement.
• Mobility.
• Caries.
• Tooth position.
• Occlusal trauma.
• Crown-to-root ratio.
• Root form such as fused roots.

◆ Overall Prognosis
  • Age.
  • Medical status.
  • Rate of disease progression.
  • Patient cooperation and compliance with recommendations.
  • Financial constraints of the patient.
  • Oral habits and behaviors.
  • Oral health literacy

PUTTING IT ALL TOGETHER

The dental hygiene student is often challenged to put together all the assessment information they have gathered to develop the diagnosis and prognosis in preparation for development of the care plan (also referred to as a treatment plan).

I. Evaluation of Assessment Data

All the assessment information provided is analyzed and interpreted in order to determine interventions for the care plan.

◆ The Comprehensive Patient Assessment and Diagnosis Worksheet (see Figure 22-1) provides an approach to gather information together in one document to assist in the development of the diagnosis, prognosis, and care or treatment plan. The form includes the following components:
  • Summary of significant medical and dental history.
  • Chief complaint.
  • Risk factors.
  • Summary of periodontal examination findings.
  • Summary of radiographic interpretation.
  • Periodontal classification.
  • Diagnosis.
  • Prognosis.

II. Selection of Dental Hygiene Interventions

Dental hygiene interventions are planned based on the following:
◆ Evaluation of individual patients needs to develop personal goals and the interventions to aid the patient in achieving optimal oral health.[19,20]
◆ Clinical findings.
◆ Evidence-based interventions to prevent or manage oral disease.

Comprehensive Patient Assessment and Diagnosis Worksheet

Student Name _____ Patient Name _____ Patient Record# _____ Date _____

Medical History (significant findings):

Relevant Dental History (dental knowledge and behaviors):

History of NSPT: Yes/No If yes, when and what?

| Chief Complaint (reason for visit) | Plaque Score _____% | *Gingival Description:* | Periodontal Diagnosis: |
| | | | Caries Diagnosis: |

Local Risk Factors:
- ☐ Poor OH
- ☐ Calculus level (1, 2, 3, 4)
- ☐ Defective Restoration/Caries
- ☐ Orthodontics
- ☐ Malocclusion/Trauma
- ☐ Open Contact/Foot Retention
- ☐ Root Morphology/concavities
- ☐ Toothbrush Trauma
- ☐ Missing Teeth
- ☐ Previous HS of Perio/Reduced periodontium

Acquired Risk Factors:
- ☐ Genetics ☐ Cardio Disease
- ☐ Stress ☐ Obesity
- ☐ Endocrine Disorder
- ☐ Prediabetes/Diabetes
- ☐ Cancer
- ☐ Hormones
- ☐ Osteoporosis
- ☐ Hematologic Disorder
- ☐ Immuno-Compromised Host
- ☐ Nutritional Status
- ☐ Smoking
- ☐ Xerostomia
- ☐ Medication

Risk Factors/Indicators:
- ☐ Age, Ethnicity Gender
- ☐ Infrequent maintenance
- ☐ Knowledge level
- ☐ Psychological Factors
- ☐ Cultural Influence
- ☐ History of periodontal disease

Periodontal Assessment # of teeth/#of sites

	Total Teeth		
Bleeding		____	____
Furcation		____	____
Mobility		____	____
Probe depth			
1–3mm		____	____
4–5mm		____	____
6 or more		____	____
CAL:			
1–3mm		____	____
4–5mm		____	____
6 or more		____	____

RADIOGRAPHIC INTERPRETATION/EVALUATION

Alveolar Bone Loss/crestal irregularities: List Tooth #s

- Slight (10–20%) _____
- Moderate (20–40%) _____
- Severe (>40%) _____
- Horizontal _____
- Vertical _____
- Increased PDL Width _____
- Periapical Pathology _____
- Close Root Proximity _____
- Furcation Radiolucency's _____
- Caries _____

PROGNOSIS: *Prognosis following periodontal therapy is determined by the present of one or more of the following factors.*

GOOD = Adequate control of etiologic factors, patient self-care ability, and periodontal support.

FAIR = Adequate control of etiologic factors and patient self-care ability & less than 25% attachment loss, class I or less furcation involvement.

POOR = Greater than 50% attachment loss with class II furcation & patient self-care difficult due to location and depth of furcation.

QUESTIONABLE = Greater than 50% attachment loss with poor crown to root ration; poor root form: instrumentation access; inaccessible Class II/II furcation; > than 2+ mobility; significant root proximity.

HOPELESS = Inadequate attachment to maintain the tooth.

Source: McGuire, MK. Prognosis vs outcome: predicting tooth survival. *Compend Contin Educ* Dent. 2000; 21:217-220,222,224

PERIODONTAL CLASSIFICATION: EXTENT, SEVERITY AND STAGING/TREATMENT

	Gen. >30%	Local <30%	Grade A	Grade B	Grade C	Pro	Scaling in presence of mod-sev. inflamm.	Perio. Main.	NSPT	NSPT
HEALTH										
Gingivitis Plaque Induced										
Gingivitis Non-Plaque Induced										
Stage I Periodontitis										
Stage II Periodontitis										
Stage III Periodontitis										
Stage IV Periodontitis										
Acute Periodontal Lesions (Periodontal Abscess/ Necrotizing Periodontal Disease)										
Periodontal-Endo Lesions										
Mucogingival Conditions										
Other										

Date/Faculty/What was reviewed? _____/_____/_____.
_____/_____/_____.

References

American Academy of Periodontics. (2002). All Parameters of Care. Retrieved from http://www.joponline.org/toc/jop/71/5-s
Armitage, G.C. (1999). Development of a classification system for periodontal diseases and conditions. *Ann Periodontology*, 1 (4), 1-6. Retrieved from http://www.joponline.org/doi/pdf/10.1902/annals.1999.4.1.1
Genco, R. J., & Borgnakke, W. S. (2013). Risk factors for periodontal disease. *Periodontology 2000*, 62(1), 59-94. doi:10.1111/j.1600-0757.2012.00457.x [doi]
Genco, R. J., & Genco, F. D. (2014). Common risk factors in the management of periodontal and associated systemic diseases: The dental setting and interprofessional collaboration. *The Journal of Evidence-Based Dental Practice*, 14 Suppl, 4-16. doi:10.1016/j.jebdp.2014.03.003 [doi]

FIGURE 22-1 • Comprehensive Patient Assessment and Diagnosis Worksheet. The comprehensive assessment form includes a summary of significant medical and dental history findings, client's chief complaint, periodontal and caries diagnosis, local and acquired risk factors, radiographic findings, and treatment prognosis. The form can be utilized as a worksheet for the clinician to develop the dental hygiene care plan.

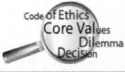

EVERYDAY ETHICS

Victoria, the dental hygienist, is discussing the assessment findings for her patient, Mr. Rush, with the rest of the dental team. Mr. Rush has reports he has been told by his general dental practice that he has extensive active periodontal disease. He was referred to this practice because he wants all of the most compromised teeth extracted and dental implants placed.

Mr. Rush has a number of risk factors, including poorly controlled diabetes and smoking. Because his dental insurance is running out in 3 months, everyone is in a hurry to get the treatment started, and the potential for a poor prognosis has not been discussed. In fact, Victoria's concerns about the patient's risk factors are being pushed aside.

Questions for Consideration

1. Is this an ethical issue or an ethical dilemma?

2. What is Victoria's obligation (duty) to make sure that Mr. Rush understands how his risk factors compromise the prognosis of his treatment plan? What action can Victoria take if her concerns continue to be ignored and treatment progresses without interventions that address the risk factors involved in Mr. Rush's case?

3. How can Victoria proceed to obtain informed consent from Mr. Rush and ensure that his rights to optimal care are maintained?

- Selecting interventions based on evidence from the professional literature can improve opportunities for achieving successful outcomes from dental hygiene treatment.
- The patient can benefit when the dental hygienist has developed skills in accessing and evaluating the scientific literature.

III. Dental Hygiene Care Plan

◆ Chapter 23 outlines specific procedures for preparation and documentation of a formal written dental hygiene care plan.

DOCUMENTATION

◆ All assessment findings are documented in preparation for development of a dental hygiene care plan.

◆ When patient treatment records are not computerized, all entries are recorded in ink.

◆ All entries are dated and signed by the dental hygiene clinician.

BOX 22-2

Example Documentation:
Assessment before Developing a Dental Hygiene Care Plan

S—A 35-year-old Asian female patient presents for initial new patient visit. Patient states no dental concerns.

O—Completed assessment data collected and documented, including vital signs, medical, social and dental histories, intraoral and extraoral examination findings, and dental radiographs, in preparation for developing a formal written dental hygiene care plan. All findings documented on the appropriate assessment forms.

A—Analysis of assessment findings and risk factors will be prepared prior to development of a final care plan.

P—Briefly discussed assessment findings and their relevance to the care plan that will be prepared. Told patient the dentist and dental hygienist together would complete both a comprehensive dental hygiene care plan and dental treatment plan. Explained that the plan would take into consideration all of the examination findings and assessment of risk factors for oral disease identified during this assessment appointment. Patient had no questions at this point. Appointment scheduled in 2 weeks.

Next steps: completed plan for both dental and dental hygiene treatment will be presented to patient at next appointment, scheduled in 2 weeks.

Signed: _____, RDH

Date: _____

- Standardized abbreviations are used to document all information; misunderstandings can lead to legal involvement.

◆ A suggested format for documenting a dental hygiene care plan is found in Chapter 23.

◆ Example documentation for an assessment appointment prior to development of a dental hygiene care plan is found in Box 22-2.

Factors to Teach the Patient

▶ A clear explanation of how assessment data are used in planning dental hygiene care.

▶ The importance of using scientific evidence of success in the selection of patient-specific therapeutic and preventive interventions.

▶ Why disease control measures are learned before and monitored throughout dental hygiene care.

▶ Facts of oral disease prevention and oral health promotion relevant to the patient's current level of healthcare literacy and individual risk factors.

▶ The long-term positive effects of comprehensive continuing care.

ENHANCE YOUR UNDERSTANDING

ONLINE RESOURCES
(see the inside front cover for access information)
- Audio glossary
- Appendices

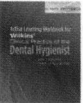

SUPPORT FOR LEARNING
(available separately)
- *Active Learning Workbook for Wilkins' Clinical Practice of the Dental Hygienist, 13th Edition*

INDIVIDUALIZED REVIEW
- Customized practice quizzing with Navigate 2 TestPrep for *Wilkins' Clinical Practice of the Dental Hygienist*

References

1. Newsome P, Smales R, Yip K. Oral diagnosis and treatment planning: part 1. Introduction. *Br Dent J.* 2012;213(1):15-19.
2. Genco RJ, Borgnakke WS. Risk factors for periodontal disease. *Periodontol 2000.* 2013;62(1):59-94.
3. Lockhart PB, Bolger AF, Papapanou PN, et al. Periodontal disease and atherosclerotic vascular disease: does the evidence support an independent association?: A scientific statement from the American Heart Association. *Circulation.* 2012;125(20):2520-2544.

4. Winning L, Linden GJ. Periodontitis and systemic disease: association or causality? *Curr Oral Health Rep.* 2017;4(1):1-7.

5. Chrysanthakopoulos NA, Chrysanthakopoulos PA. Association of periodontal disease with self-reported systemic disorders in Greece. *Oral Health Prev Dent.* 2013;11(3):251-260.

6. Linden GJ, Lyons A, Scannapieco FA. Periodontal systemic associations: review of the evidence. *J Periodontol.* 2013;84(suppl 4):S8-S19.

7. Usin MM, Menso J, Rodriguez VI, et al. Association between maternal periodontitis and preterm and/or low birth weight infants in normal pregnancies. *J Matern Fetal Neonatal Med.* 2016;29(1):115-119.

8. Pereira FM, Rodrigues VP, de Oliveira AE, Brito LM, Lopes FF. Association between periodontal changes and osteoporosis in postmenopausal women. *Climacteric.* 2015;18(2):311-315.

9. Hurlbutt M, Young DA. A best practices approach to caries management. *J Evid Based Dent Pract.* 2014;14(suppl):77-86.

10. Kutsch VK. Dental caries: an updated medical model of risk assessment. *J Prosthet Dent.* 2014;111(4):280-285.

11. Jenson L, Budenz AW, Featherstone JD, Ramos-Gomez FJ, Spolsky VW, Young DA. Clinical protocols for caries management by risk assessment. *J Calif Dent Assoc.* 2007;35(10):714-723.

12. Ram H, Sarkar J, Kumar H, Konwar R, Bhatt ML, Mohammad S. Oral cancer: risk factors and molecular pathogenesis. *J Maxillofacial Oral Surg.* 2011;10(2):132-137.

13. Yip K, Smales R. Oral diagnosis and treatment planning: part 2. Dental caries and assessment of risk. *Br Dent J.* 2012;213(2):59-66.

14. Mayo Clinic. Mouth cancer: risk factors. https://www.mayoclinic.org/diseases-conditions/mouth cancer/diagnosis-treatment/drc-20351002. Accessed January 13, 2018.

15. American Society of Anesthesiologists. ASA physical status classification system. 2014; http://www.asahq.org/resources/clinical-information/asa-physical-status-classification-system. Accessed January 13, 2018.

16. Ship JA, Mohammed AR, eds. *The Clinician's Guide to Oral Health in Geriatric Patients.* Baltimore, MD: American Academy of Oral Medicine; 1999.

17. Corbet EF. Oral diagnosis and treatment planning: part 3. Periodontal disease and assessment of risk. *Br Dent J.* 2012;213(3):111-121.

18. American Dental Hygienists' Association. Dental hygiene diagnosis position paper. 2015; http://www.adha.org/adha-position-papers. Accessed January 13, 2018.

19. American Dental Hygienists' Association. *Standards for Clinical Dental Hygiene Practice.* Chicago, IL: ADHA; 2016.

20. Canadian Dental Hygienists Association. *Entry-to-Practice Competencies and Standards for Canadian Dental Hygienists.* Ottawa, ON: CDHA; 2010.

21. American Academy of Periodontology. Parameters of care. *J Periodontol.* 2000;71(suppl 5):i-ii, 847-883.

22. Yip K, Smales R. Oral diagnosis and treatment planning: part 5. Preventive and treatment planning for dental caries. *Br Dent J.* 2012;213(5):211-220.

23. Miller PD Jr, McEntire ML, Marlow NM, Gellin RG. An evidenced-based scoring index to determine the periodontal prognosis on molars. *J Periodontol.* 2014;85(2):214-225.

24. McGuire MK, Nunn ME. Prognosis versus actual outcome. III. The effectiveness of clinical parameters in accurately predicting tooth survival. *J Periodontol.* 1996;67(7):666-674.

23

The Dental Hygiene Care Plan

Catherine G. Ranson, RDH BHA, MET, Linda D. Boyd, RDH, RD, EdD, and
Charlotte J. Wyche, BSDH, MS

CHAPTER OUTLINE

PREPARATION OF A DENTAL HYGIENE CARE PLAN
I. Description
II. Rationale
III. Objectives
IV. Parts of a Care Plan

COMPONENTS OF A WRITTEN CARE PLAN
I. Demographic Data
II. Assessment Findings and Risk Factors
III. Periodontal Diagnosis and Status
IV. Caries Risk Status
V. Diagnostic Statements
VI. Patient-Centered Oral Health Goals

VII. Planned Interventions
VIII. Expected Outcomes
IX. Evaluation Methods
X. The Appointment Plan
XI. Re-evaluation

ADDITIONAL CONSIDERATIONS
I. Role of the Patient
II. Pain and Anxiety Control

SEQUENCING AND PRIORITIZING PATIENT CARE
I. Objectives
II. Factors Affecting Sequence of Care

PRESENTING THE DENTAL HYGIENE CARE PLAN
I. Presenting the Plan to the Collaborating Dentist
II. Explaining the Plan to the Patient

INFORMED CONSENT
I. Informed Consent Procedures
II. Informed Refusal
III. Additional Considerations

DOCUMENTATION

EVERYDAY ETHICS

FACTORS TO TEACH THE PATIENT

REFERENCES

LEARNING OBJECTIVES

After studying this chapter, the student will be able to:

1. Discuss rationale and objectives for developing a dental hygiene care plan.

2. Identify the components of a dental hygiene care plan.

3. Prepare a written dental hygiene care plan from a dental hygiene diagnosis.

4. Apply procedures for discussing a care plan with the dentist and the patient.

5. Identify and apply measures for obtaining informed consent and informed refusal.

PREPARATION OF A DENTAL HYGIENE CARE PLAN

◆ A formal written dental hygiene care plan is an essential component of the dental hygiene process of care.

◆ Dental hygiene care is planned to address the needs of the entire oral cavity.

◆ The care plan is based on assessment of factors that influence the oral environment, including the:
  • Extraoral features.
  • Oral mucosa.
  • Teeth.
  • Periodontal supporting structures.

◆ Patient's individual health factors.

◆ A care plan that integrates a basic three-part plan to care for all of the patient's dental hygiene needs has a major influence on the future oral health of the patient.

I. Description

The written care plan is a prioritized sequence of evidence-based dental hygiene interventions that are:

◆ Predicated on the dental hygiene diagnosis.

◆ Composed of integrated plans for the care and control of periodontal disease, dental caries control, management of modifiable risk factors, and other preventive interventions.

◆ Integrated into a comprehensive treatment plan that encompasses the patient's preventive, restorative, and surgical needs (Table 23-1).

◆ Identifies treatment referrals to other healthcare providers.

◆ Contained within the scope of dental hygiene practice as defined by each state or province practice act.

II. Rationale

A written dental hygiene care plan will help to:

◆ Focus on individualized patient needs and risk factors when selecting dental hygiene interventions.

◆ Prioritize the sequence of planned preventive, education, and treatment.

◆ Serve as a checklist to ensure all planned interventions are accomplished.

III. Objectives

A well-prepared dental hygiene care plan includes the following:

◆ Addresses patient needs identified from assessment data.

◆ Is flexible and realistic.

TABLE 23-1 • Components of a Master Treatment Plan		
PHASE	**PROCEDURES**	**INCLUDED IN THE DENTAL HYGIENE CARE PLAN**
Preliminary phase	• Summary of information from assessment	✓
	• Develop dental hygiene diagnostic statements	✓
	• Establish patient-centered oral health goals	✓
	• Emergency care (pain, biopsy)	✓
Phase I therapy	• Dental biofilm control	✓
	• Introduction of additional preventive measures (diet changes, fluorides, mouthguard)	✓
		✓
	• Calculus removal	✓
	• Correction of restorative and prosthetic irritants (biofilm traps, overhangs)	
	• Restorative caries control	
Outcomes evaluation of phase I	• Periodontal assessment data	✓
	• Clinical signs of inflammation	✓
	• Dental biofilm control	✓
	• Evaluation of oral health goals	✓
	• Patient's participation	✓
Phase II surgical	• Periodontal	
	• Endodontic	
	• Implant placement	
Phase III restorative	• Final restorations	
	• Fixed/removable prostheses	
Evaluation of overall outcomes	• Periodontal response to restorations/implants	✓
	• Other response to restorations	✓
Phase IV maintenance	• Appointments for continuing care and re-evaluation	✓
	• Refining biofilm control techniques	✓

◆ Contains treatment and oral health goals in collaboration with the patient to address problems and risk factors identified in diagnostic statements.

◆ Assesses whether previous treatment goals have been met.
  • If goals have not met, identify barriers to assist in determining alternative treatment goals and/or strategies for successful goal attainment.

◆ Includes referrals to other healthcare providers.

◆ Provides interventions and recommendations based on current scientific evidence.

IV. Parts of a Care Plan

A. Periodontal/Gingival Health

◆ The primary objective of the dental hygiene plan for periodontal therapy is to restore and maintain health of the periodontal tissues.

◆ Attention is paid to interventions to address:
  • Modifiable risk factors for development and progression of periodontal disease.
  • Complications related to associations between systemic disease and periodontal disease.

B. Dental Caries Control

◆ The plan for caries control, based on an individualized assessment of caries risk, includes:
  • Identification of modifiable risk factors.
  • Evidence-based approaches to remineralization.
  • Fluorides.
  • Dental sealants.
  • Dietary control of fermentable carbohydrates.

◆ Even when the patient's caries risk level is low, the plan includes:
  • A minimum frequency of professional oral examinations to monitor risk factors.
  • Preventive recommendations such as daily use of fluoridated toothpaste.

C. Other

A plan for preventive care starts with the patient's personal daily oral biofilm control.

Additional interventions in an individual care plan may include:

◆ Interventions to eliminate modifiable risk factors for oral disease, such as tobacco cessation counseling.

◆ Desensitizing exposed dentin.

◆ Resolving halitosis.

◆ Nutritional counseling.

COMPONENTS OF A WRITTEN CARE PLAN

◆ A dental hygiene care plan may be written using a variety of formats.

◆ Software for electronic patient records includes a treatment plan template that can be used to develop a dental hygiene care plan.

◆ Figure 23-1 is a suggested template for a patient-specific care plan that follows the dental hygiene process of care.

◆ The recommended components of a written care plan are described in this section.

I. Demographic Data

◆ Patient name, date of birth (age), and gender.

◆ The date of the written plan was prepared.

◆ Notation of the patient's chief complaint or statement indicating the patient's reason for presenting for treatment.

◆ A designation of initial or maintenance therapy.

◆ The name of the student or clinician who prepared the written plan.

II. Assessment Findings and Risk Factors

This section of the plan contains a summarized description of significant findings.

A. Medical, Social, and Dental History

◆ ASA classification.

◆ Systemic diseases and conditions: current and past.

◆ Medications.

◆ Health behaviors.

◆ Cultural factors.

◆ Functional assessment.

B. Modifiable Risk Factors

◆ Risk for increased oral disease.

◆ Increased risk of systemic disease due to oral infection.

◆ Potential for compromised treatment outcomes.

III. Periodontal Diagnosis and Status

◆ Guidelines for noting the periodontal diagnosis and parameters of care, useful for planning dental hygiene treatment interventions, are found in Chapters 19 and 22.

IV. Caries Risk Status

◆ A caries risk assessment tool such as Caries Management by Risk Assessment, which provides guidelines for identifying caries risk status and selecting dental hygiene interventions based on risk factor assessment, is detailed in Chapters 25 and 47 for children and adult.

◆ Understanding of a patient's individualized modifiable risks for dental caries guide the plan for:
  • Oral health education and counseling.
  • Selection of treatment interventions, such as dental sealants or fluoride recommendations to enhance remineralization.

PATIENT SPECIFIC DENTAL HYGIENE CARE PLAN

Patient Name: Age: Gender: Record #:   Date:

Initial Therapy   Maintenance   Re-evaluation

Health /Social History findings impacting treatment:

ASA Classification: _____

Systemic disease: _____

Medications: _____

Health behaviors/Cultural factors: _____

Modifiable Risk Factors:

Related to Dental Hygiene Diagnosis: _____

_____

Related to Periodontal Diagnosis: _____

_____

Dental Hygiene Diagnosis (Related to Risk Factors and Etiology):

Periodontal Diagnosis and Status (Active or Stable, Classification, Extent, Stage, Grade):

Caries Management Risk Assessment (CAMBRA) level: ☐ Low   ☐ Moderate   ☐ High   ☐ Extreme

Medical and Dental Referrals Required:

Radiographic Exposures Completed/Interpreted: (identify film or digital)

☐ PAN   ☐ FMX   ☐ 2 BWX   ☐ 4/6 BWX

Initial Biofilm Score:

Planned Interventions (to arrest or control disease and regenerate, restore or maintain health)		
Clinical/Addresses DH Diagnosis and Periodontal Diagnosis	**Education/Counseling**	**Oral Hygiene Instruction/ Oral Self - Care (evidence-based & patient centered rationale)**
1) 2)		

Recommended Oral Self-Care Aids:

Recommended Preventive Agents and Chemotherapeutics (include type and percentage) (home use)

☐ Dentifrices: ☐ Mouth rinses: ☐ Fluoride:

Expected Outcomes		
Patient - Centered Goals	**Evaluation Methods**	**Time Frame**
1)		
2)		

FIGURE 23-1 • Patient-Specific Dental Hygiene Care Plan. The written care plan includes a summary of assessment findings and modifiable risk factors, the dental hygiene diagnosis, planned dental hygiene interventions, expected outcomes based on patient-centered goals, an appointment plan that sequences treatment procedures and education interventions for each appointment, and a section for patient signature indicating informed consent for the planned care.

Previous Treatment Goals Met/Not Met:

Recommended Dental Hygiene Treatment:

☐ Prophylaxis

☐ Periodontal Maintenance

☐ Non-Surgical Periodontal Therapy:

   Quadrant(s): _____

☐ Non-Surgical Periodontal Therapy 1-3 teeth

   _____

☐ Scaling in the presence of inflammation

☐ Local Anesthesia:

☐ Power Scaling

☐ Selective Polish Agent:

☐ Topical Fluoride: Agent:

☐ Sealants: Tooth #(s)

☐ Custom Tray: Type

☐ Education

☐ Nutritional Analysis

☐ Other:

Estimated Number of Treatment Appointments:

Recommended Maintenance or Continuing Care Interval with Rationale:

Appointment Plan (sequence of planned interventions)	
Appt#	**Plan for Treatment, Services** **Plan for Education, Counseling and Oral Hygiene Instruction**

FIGURE 23-1 • (*Continued*)

V. Diagnostic Statements

◆ Based on interpretation and analysis of the assessment data.

◆ Provides the basis for the treatment or care plan.

◆ Examples of dental hygiene diagnostic statements can be found in Chapter 22.

VI. Patient-Centered Oral Health Goals

◆ Diagnostic statements based on assessment findings require the creation of patient-specific goals linked to dental hygiene disease status and modifiable risk factors.

◆ The establishment of patient-centered goals are designed to accomplish the following:

  • Prioritize the modifiable risk factors for oral health disease.

  • Reflect priorities for the patient.

  • Address cognitive, psychomotor, affective aspects of the patient-specific oral health needs.

  • Describe observable behaviors with measurable outcomes.

  • Have a defined time frame.

VII. Planned Interventions

Dental hygiene interventions are measures applied to prevent, regenerate, restore, or maintain oral health and are specific to the individual patient's assessment findings and patient-centered goals. The interventions may include:

◆ Clinical treatments, such as nonsurgical periodontal therapy (scaling and root planing) and debridement, selected for the purpose of arresting or controlling existing disease.

◆ Preventive measures, such as dental sealants, to maintain tooth integrity.

◆ Education and counseling in topics such as etiology and progression of oral disease and elimination of risk factors.

◆ Individualized oral hygiene instructions and personal daily oral self-care regimens based on patient needs and abilities.

VIII. Expected Outcomes

A plan for treatment or personal oral care outcomes, created in consultation with the patient, contains:

◆ One or more measureable short-term goals and planning for long-term goals (see Chapter 24).

◆ A realistic time frame for measuring success of treatment goal outcomes.

IX. Evaluation Methods

◆ Evaluation of clinical outcomes is discussed more completely in Chapter 44.

◆ Evaluation methods identified in the dental hygiene care plan:

• Include assessment data collection at a subsequent appointment and comparison with initial assessment findings.

• Clearly define how progress toward each goal will be measured.

• Identify a short-term goal as the patient moves toward the long-term goal to allow for patient to be successful.

• An example of an evaluation method for the expected outcome is reduction of plaque score from 50% to 40%.

X. The Appointment Plan

An appointment plan for multiple appointments:

◆ Outlines a sequence of interventions.

◆ Can be modified at each appointment to respond to new information or an immediate need of the patient.

◆ Properly prioritized and sequenced treatment and education interventions will be:

• More comfortable for the patient.

• More effective in reaching planned oral health goals.

XI. Re-evaluation

At the re-evaluation appointment[1]:

◆ New assessment data are collected and analyzed.

◆ A determination is made regarding whether expected outcomes expressed in the oral health goals of the care plan have been met or not met.

◆ Continuing care appointment interval is determined.

ADDITIONAL CONSIDERATIONS

I. Role of the Patient

A. Purpose

The willingness and/or ability of the patient to participate in reducing risk factors and changing oral health behaviors will be the key to reaching goals set during planning.

B. Procedure

◆ Determine the patient's level of understanding of dental diseases, risk factors, and oral health behaviors.

◆ Determine the patient's physical ability to manipulate recommended oral care aids.

◆ Determine lifestyle factors that impact the patient's ability to comply with oral health recommendations.

◆ Educate patients regarding the importance of their role in eliminating modifiable risk factors, setting oral health goals, and complying with recommendations.

II. Pain and Anxiety Control

A. Purpose

◆ Control of discomfort during treatment procedures.

◆ More consistent patient compliance with recommended interventions and need to return for additional scheduled appointments.

B. Procedures

◆ When there is a patient complaint of pain or discomfort, treat those areas first.

◆ For a patient with dental anxiety, the clinician may choose to treat either the quadrant with the fewest teeth or the least severe periodontal infection first to ensure the following:

• Make the first scaling less complicated.

• Help orient an anxious patient to clinical procedures.

◆ If there is no dental anxiety, treat the quadrant with more severe disease first so that healing can be monitored at the following appointments.

◆ When two quadrants are to be treated at the same appointment, selecting a maxillary and mandibular quadrant on the same side minimizes the patient's posttreatment discomfort.

◆ The need for local anesthesia is determined by:

• Depth, bleeding, and severity of inflammation of periodontal pockets and furcation involvement.

• The patient's previous pain control experiences.

• Consistency and distribution of calculus.

• Potential patient discomfort during scaling.

• Sensitivity of the patient's tissues during instrumentation.

SEQUENCING AND PRIORITIZING PATIENT CARE

I. Objectives

Reasons for preparing a well-sequenced dental hygiene care plan are:

A. To Provide Evidence-Based, Individualized Patient Care

◆ Determined by analysis of assessment data.

◆ Based on evidence-based approaches to care.

◆ Enhanced by the clinician's clinical judgment in applying evidence-based care.

B. To Eliminate or Control Etiologic and Predisposing Disease Factors and Prevent Recurrence of Disease

◆ Educate patient on etiologic agents in both dental caries and periodontal and gingival diseases.

◆ Dental hygiene interventions can address modifiable risk factors that predispose the patient to oral disease.
  • Counseling on prevention measures and elimination of modifiable risk factors.
  • Instruction in daily oral self-care techniques.
  • Encouragement of regularly scheduled maintenance follow-up for dental hygiene care.

C. To Eliminate the Signs and Symptoms of Disease

Measures to eliminate signs of infection such as gingival bleeding and probing depths are included in the care plan.

II. Factors Affecting Sequence of Care

Treatment sequence defines the order in which the parts of an individual appointment are to be carried out. Sequence planning involves:

◆ Identification of overall treatment and education patterns appropriate for an individual patient's needs.

◆ Outline of a series of appointments, with specific services, treatment procedures, and educational interventions included.

◆ The sequence of care for an individual patient is determined by numerous factors.

A. Urgency

Discomfort or pain that requires urgent care could apply to:

◆ An area with an abscess or with necrotizing ulcerative gingivitis.

◆ Severe carious lesion(s).

◆ Mucositis or other mucosal lesions.

B. Existing Etiologic Factors

◆ In patients with gingival or periodontal infection or risk for dental caries, success of the treatment depends on thorough, daily biofilm removal.
  • Biofilm control measures are introduced, and success is evaluated before additional dental hygiene interventions are introduced so the patient does not become overwhelmed.

C. Severity and Extent of the Condition

◆ The number and length of appointments and the sequencing of procedures planned are affected by the severity of the condition.

◆ Findings that indicate the severity of gingival or periodontal infection include:
  • Changes in color, size, shape, or consistency of the gingiva.
  • Probing depths.
  • Bleeding on probing.
  • Suppuration or exudate.
  • Mobility of the teeth.
  • Clinical and radiographic signs of attachment or bone loss.

D. Individual Patient Requirements

Items from a patient's history that may require adaptation in appointment length, spacing, or sequencing when planning dental hygiene care include:

◆ Antibiotic premedication
  • Current recommended standard prophylactic regimens and a list of conditions that require antibiotic premedication are found in Chapter 11.
  • Because bacteremia can occur, initial instruction and practice of biofilm-removing procedures are carried out while the patient is premedicated.
  • Efficient use of appointment time and/or spacing of appointment dates will avoid unnecessary extra antibiotic coverage.

◆ Systemic diseases
  • Chronic disease will influence the content and length of appointments.
  • The associations between periodontitis and systemic conditions influence patient counseling.

◆ Physical disability
  • Physical limitations, such as those described in Chapter 51, will require adaptation of the appointment plan.

◆ Other considerations
  • An outline for continuing care appointments can be found in Chapter 45.
  • A suggested approach for motivating patient health behavior change is found in Chapter 24.

PRESENTING THE DENTAL HYGIENE CARE PLAN

Before treatment is begun, the care plan is coordinated with comprehensive care and explained to the patient.

I. Presenting the Plan to the Collaborating Dentist

A. Purpose

◆ To integrate the dental hygiene care plan into the patient's comprehensive treatment plan.

◆ To provide a coordinated dental and dental hygiene statement to the patient regarding oral health needs.

B. Procedure

◆ Follow sequence on the patient's written care plan.

◆ Summarize demographic data.

◆ Summarize major systemic and dental health assessment findings.

◆ Summarize risk factors.

◆ Indicate suggested intervention strategies, goals, expected outcomes, and referrals to other healthcare providers.

◆ Outline suggested appointment sequence and services to be provided.

◆ Be prepared to give detail and answer questions.

II. Explaining the Plan to the Patient

◆ Good communication skills are essential to build a trusting relationship with the patient.

◆ Use of radiographs and an intraoral camera during presentation of the plan for care provides visual documentation of need for oral health interventions.

◆ Using a motivational interviewing approach (Chapter 24) while discussing the plan can help determine and respond to the patient's readiness to change health behaviors that increase risk for oral disease.

A. Purpose

◆ To provide the patient with information needed to give informed consent for treatment.

◆ To reinforce the patient's role in setting and reaching oral health goals outlined in the plan.

B. Procedure

◆ Position the patient in an upright position, face-to-face with clinician.

◆ Use terminology appropriate to the patient's level of health literacy.

◆ Educate the patient regarding link between systemic and their oral disease.

◆ Educate the patient regarding recommended dental hygiene services, appointment sequence, expected outcomes, and referrals to other healthcare providers.

◆ Present information using visual aids such as the patient's own radiographs, dental models, drawings or pictures, videotapes, brochures, or an intraoral camera.

◆ Engage the patient in planning and setting goals.

◆ Be prepared to give detail and answer questions.

◆ Obtained signed informed consent.

INFORMED CONSENT

◆ Obtaining consent is about providing relevant information so that an educated decision about treatment can be made by the patient.[2]

◆ It is every patient's right to possess knowledge that will:
  • Aid the patient in making optimal decisions for their oral health.
  • Allow shared decision making with the oral care provider while treatment is being planned.

◆ Adequate documentation of informed consent in the patient's record includes evidence that the patient has received the information listed in Box 23-1.[2,3]

BOX 23-1
Criteria for Adequate Content in Informed Consent

• Complete description of the procedure including:
  • The patient's diagnosis
  • Nature and purpose of proposed treatment
  • Rationale for treatment
  • Duration of treatment
  • Effects of patient's current medical status on treatment.
• Risks and limitations of the proposed treatment including probability of risk occurring.
• Benefits of the treatment including prognosis.
• Alternative treatments available, including no treatment and the consequences of no treatment.
• Purpose of treatment.
• Demonstration of the opportunity to ask questions.
• Permission to deliberate if needed.
• Demonstration of consent (patient signature).

Sources: American Academy of Pediatric Dentistry. Guideline on informed consent. Revised 2015. https://www.aapd.org/globalassets/media/policies_guidelines/bp_informedconsent.pdf. Accessed July 4, 2019. Glick A, Taylor D, Valenza JA, Walji MF. Assessing the content, presentation, and readability of dental informed consents. *J Dent Educ.* 2010;74(8):849-861.

◆ Informed consent is a legal concept that can exist even without a written document.

◆ Informed consent can be lacking even when a document has been signed if the patient has not had the opportunity to comprehend and evaluate the risks and benefits of the suggested treatment.

◆ Implied consent granted by the patient's presence in the dental chair, only applies to nontreatment procedures, such as data collection, and treatment planning.

I. Informed Consent Procedures

◆ Box 23-2 provides information for obtaining informed consent.

◆ The patient is informed of all treatment options available, chooses the treatment option, and consents to follow the recommendations in the agreed-upon care plan.

◆ Patients do not always remember the information they received during informed consent; therefore, written documentation of all information provided for the patient is essential.[4]

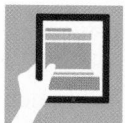

BOX 23-2
Informed Consent

Information to Disclose

- *Diagnosis*: description of patient's problem(s)
- *Treatment*: nature and rationale for the proposed treatment(s)
- *Alternatives*: viable alternatives to the proposed treatment(s)
- *Consequences*: risks and benefits of all proposed treatment alternatives, including physical and psychological effects, costs, and potential resulting problems
- *Prognosis*: expected outcome with treatment(s), with alternative treatment(s), and without treatment

Principles of Informing

- Assess the patient's ability to give informed consent.
- Simplify the terminology so the patient can understand.
- Encourage the patient and family to ask questions.
- Continue to assess the patient's understanding and reeducate as often as necessary.
- Document all relevant factors and include the signed form in patient record.

Source: Greco PM. Informed consent or informed refusal? *Am J Orthod Dentofacial Orthop.* 2013;143(5):598.

- When potential risks, complications, or failure are associated with therapy, it is necessary to obtain consent in writing prior to beginning treatment.
- Informed consent includes recommendations for referral to other healthcare providers as necessary.[5]
- If necessary, use forms written in simpler terms, larger print, or the patient's primary language.

II. Informed Refusal

- The patient's right to autonomy in making decisions regarding oral treatment requires that practitioners respect a patient's decision to refuse treatment.[6]
- Informed refusal of care as well as any recommended treatment options are documented in the patient's permanent record.
- Depending on the state or province practice act, this may or may not protect clinicians who provide treatment that does not meet the standard of care from legal action.

III. Additional Considerations

- Cultural differences of individual patients require special effort to obtain informed consent. Careful exploration of language skills, and potentially conflicting health beliefs and values can enhance communication.[7,8]
- Age or disability-related cognitive impairment may require consultation with a caregiver or legal guardian as well as the patient.[9]

DOCUMENTATION

- A written dental hygiene care plan documents all information related to each component of the formal plan as described in this chapter and illustrated in Figure 23-1.
- Example documentation for a patient appointment to explain the dental hygiene care plan and obtain informed consent is found in Box 23-3.

BOX 23-3
Example Documentation:
Presentation of Care Plan and Informed Consent for Dental Hygiene Care

S—A 35-year-old female patient presents 2 weeks following assessment data collection appointment. Patient expects to discuss the formal written dental hygiene care plan related to periodontal therapy and quadrant debridement.

O—No changes in patient's health history or other relevant assessment findings since previous appointment for data collection. Written care plan and treatment plan completed and available.

A—Patient appeared engaged in the discussion and eager to begin treatment.

P—Explained all assessment findings and risk factors, discussed dental hygiene diagnosis statement and patient-centered oral health goals, planned interventions expected outcomes of treatment, and referrals to other healthcare providers. Responded to numerous questions related to the rationale for scheduling multiple treatment appointments. Patient stated that all questions had been answered, then signed/dated the informed consent form. Copy of signed care plan was given to patient and a copy was placed in the patient record.

Next step: Begin treatment as described for appointment #1 on the care plan form.

Signed: _____, RDH

Date: _____

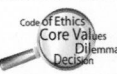

EVERYDAY ETHICS

Ellen is responsible for explaining two alternative treatment plans to Mrs. Kwan, who is new to the practice. Mrs. Kwan needs to decide between several extractions, which would require crown and bridge or implant replacement, or the treatment of periodontally involved teeth with poor prognosis. The decision must be made today if she is to begin treatment early next week, when there are several open appointments available.

English is not Mrs. Kwan's first language, and no one in the practice speaks her language. Ellen has explained the information carefully, using pictures and patient-appropriate words, and she has gone over both treatment alternatives several times. When Ellen asks Mrs. Kwan to summarize her understanding of the care plan she just nods her head, smiles, and says, "I'll sign whatever you say."

Questions for Consideration

1. Does it appear that Mrs. Kwan understands her treatment alternatives and is informed sufficiently to give consent? What alternatives can Ellen consider so that informed consent is ensured?

2. Does Ellen have an ethical responsibility, as the knowledgeable professional, to select the choice of treatments as Mrs. Kwan requests? Why or why not?

3. In what ways does the pressure of making a timely decision reflect an inappropriate approach to meeting Mrs. Kwan's needs?

Factors to Teach the Patient

▶ Why a dental hygiene care plan is made.

▶ Why patient input into the final care plan is important.

▶ Which parts of the plan are to be carried out by the patient.

▶ How the roles of patient and members of the dental team are interrelated in eliminating the patient's oral problems.

▶ The patient's rights and responsibilities regarding informed consent.

ENHANCE YOUR UNDERSTANDING

ONLINE RESOURCES
(see the inside front cover for access information)

· Audio glossary
· Appendices

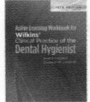

SUPPORT FOR LEARNING
(available separately)

· *Active Learning Workbook for Wilkins' Clinical Practice of the Dental Hygienist, 13th Edition*

INDIVIDUALIZED REVIEW

· Customized practice quizzing with Navigate 2 TestPrep for *Wilkins' Clinical Practice of the Dental Hygienist*

References

1. American Academy of Periodontology. Parameter of chronic periodontitis with slight to moderate loss of periodontal support. *J Periodontol.* 2000;71:853-855.

2. American Academy of Pediatric Dentistry. Guideline on informed consent. Revised 2015. https://www.aapd.org/globalassets/media/policies_guidelines/bp_informedconsent.pdf. Accessed July 4, 2019.

3. Glick A, Taylor D, Valenza JA, Walji MF. Assessing the content, presentation, and readability of dental informed consents. *J Dent Educ.* 2010;74(8):849-861.

4. Ferrús-Torres E, Valmaseda-Castellón E, Berini-Aytés L, Gay-Escoda C. Informed consent in oral surgery: the value of written information. *J Oral Maxillofac Surg.* 2011;69(1):54-58.

5. Greenwell H; Committee on Research, Science, and Therapy, The American Academy of Periodontology. Position paper: guidelines for periodontal therapy. *J Periodontol.* 2001;72(11):1624-1628.

6. Greco PM. Informed consent or informed refusal? *Am J Orthod Dentofacial Orthop.* 2013;143(5):598.

7. Chettih M. Turning the lens inward: cultural competence and providers' values in health care decision making. *Gerontologist.* 2012;52(6):739-747.

8. Fitch P. Cultural competence and dental hygiene care delivery: integrating cultural care into the dental hygiene process of care. *J Dent Hyg.* 2004;78(1):11-21.

9. Conti A, Delbon P, Laffranchi L, Paganelli C. Consent in dentistry: ethical and deontological issues. *J Med Ethics.* 2013;39(1):59-61.

Implementation: Prevention

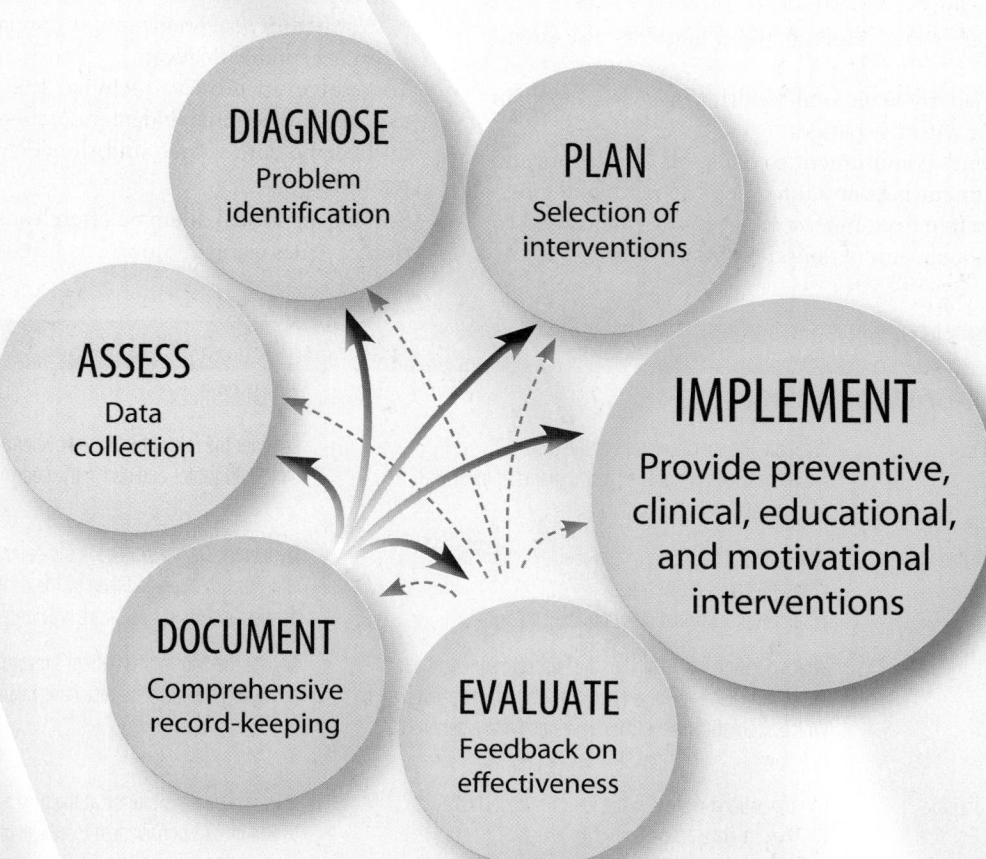

DIAGNOSE
Problem
identification

PLAN
Selection of
interventions

ASSESS
Data
collection

IMPLEMENT
Provide preventive,
clinical, educational,
and motivational
interventions

DOCUMENT
Comprehensive
record-keeping

EVALUATE
Feedback on
effectiveness

FIGURE VI-1 • The Dental Hygiene Process of Care.

INTRODUCTION FOR SECTION VI

The aim of health promotion and disease prevention is to help each patient accept responsibility for lifelong health practices and daily oral self-care regimens that prevent oral disease.

◆ Implementation of the prevention care plan is a significant component of both the dental hygiene care plan and the total treatment plan.

◆ The influence of oral health on total body health may be a new concept for many patients.

◆ In the sequence of patient treatment, introduction to preventive measures occurs first, before treatment interventions are implemented.

THE DENTAL HYGIENE PROCESS OF CARE

◆ The implementation phase of the Dental Hygiene Process of Care, illustrated in Figure VI-1, provides the dental hygiene interventions identified in a patient's dental hygiene care plan.

◆ Dental hygiene patient education and counseling interventions are:
  • The basis for oral health promotion and disease prevention.
  • Selected using individualized patient assessment data.
  • Designed to meet oral health goals developed in concert with the patient.

◆ The patient's commitment to daily self-care before and after treatment is essential to keep the teeth and gingival tissues free from new or recurrent disease caused by the microorganisms of dental biofilm.

◆ The dental hygienist has the responsibility to:
  • Consider each patient's current oral health practices, cultural factors, physical abilities, and life circumstances when implementing the preventive care plan.
  • Implement dental hygiene interventions for each patient that attain and maintain oral health and contribute to systemic health.
  • Educate about oral disease and prevention modalities based on individualized patient needs.
  • Identify an approach that will motivate each patient to accept and adhere to recommended preventive procedures and self-care protocols.

ETHICAL APPLICATIONS

◆ When complex ethical issues and dilemmas arise in the dental setting, the ethically competent dental hygienist can:
  • Understand the patient perspective.
  • View a concern from various perspectives.
  • Determine who is responsible.
  • Document and share clear, concise, and objective evidence.
  • Communicate clearly with all parties involved in the situation.
  • Act within acceptable moral standards to determine an acceptable decision.

◆ To resolve an ethical dilemma, the dental hygienist can use professional judgment, reflection about dental hygiene core values, and the components of moral reasoning.

◆ Solving an ethical dilemma often leads to the examination of issues using questions, as listed in Table VI-1.

TABLE VI-1 • Decision Alternatives through Questioning		
ETHICAL DECISION CONCEPT	QUESTIONS TO ASK	APPLICATION EXAMPLES
Recognize conflict	What are the specific details of the case? Are there issues of rights or moral character involved? At what level does the conflict exist?	Consider the role of the dental hygienist for each of the ethical principles outlined in the Code of Ethics.
Accumulate possible options	What alternative actions are available? Whose interests are at stake? What resources would other professionals use?	Review the Dental Practice Act to determine limitations of actions that can be taken by the dental hygienist, the dentist, and other healthcare providers.
Evaluate the alternatives	Which decision would lead to the best consequences overall? Are all individuals involved being respected and treated fairly? Which alternative(s) could be developed into a general rule to follow?	Review the entries in a patient's record to determine if all points of view from the case have been included.
Reflect on the decision	Can the action taken be justified as the best choice? What alternative actions could be selected?	Discuss a similar situation at the next office/staff meeting to enhance responsiveness to ethical protocols and evaluate the course of action.

Preventive Counseling and Behavior Change

Marsha A. Voelker, CDA, RDH, MS

CHAPTER OUTLINE

STEPS IN A PREVENTIVE PROGRAM
- I. Assess the Patient's Needs
- II. Plan for Interventions
- III. Implement the Plan
- IV. Perform Clinical Preventive Services
- V. Evaluate Progressive Changes
- VI. Plan Short- and Long-term Continuing Care

PATIENT COUNSELING
- I. When to Conduct
- II. The Setting for Preventive Counseling

PATIENT MOTIVATION AND BEHAVIOR CHANGE
- I. Health Behavior Change Model
- II. Transtheoretical Model
- III. Motivation for Health Behavior Change

MOTIVATIONAL INTERVIEWING
- I. Elements of the MI Spirit
- II. Guiding Principles
- III. Processes of MI

MI IMPLEMENTATION
- I. Information Exchange
- II. Agenda Setting
- III. Core Skills

EXPLORING AMBIVALENCE
- I. Sustain Talk versus Change Talk
- II. Decisional Balance
- III. Readiness Ruler

ELICITING AND RECOGNIZING CHANGE TALK
- I. Preparatory Change Talk
- II. Mobilizing Change Talk

STRENGTHENING COMMITMENT (THE PLAN)
- I. Clear Plan
- II. Several Clear Options
- III. Brainstorming

MI WITH PEDIATRIC PATIENTS AND CAREGIVERS

MOTIVATIONAL TRAINING AND COACHING

DOCUMENTATION

EVERYDAY ETHICS

FACTORS TO TEACH THE PATIENT

REFERENCES

LEARNING OBJECTIVES

After studying this chapter, the student will be able to:

1. Explain the steps in a preventive program, identify the need to conduct preventive counseling and describe the proper setting.

2. Describe the importance of partnering with the patient to come up with a plan for change.

3. Describe and explain the methods of motivational interviewing.

4. Describe how to recognize and explore the patient's ambivalence and describe techniques to elicit and recognize change talk.

5. Understand and explain various plans to strengthen the patient's commitment for change.

The dental hygienist is a primary care provider of preventive services. A specialist in oral health care, the dental hygienist is involved at all levels of prevention.

◆ Within the process of dental hygiene care, the needs of a patient are assessed from the histories and clinical findings. Then a dental hygiene diagnosis is made, and the care plan is outlined.

◆ When planning the sequence of treatment for the patient, initiation of preventive measures precedes clinical services except in an emergency.

◆ Oral health can only be attained and maintained if the patient learns and practices proper daily self-care.

STEPS IN A PREVENTIVE PROGRAM

Each patient needs a preventive care plan. To plan and carry out a program takes a collaborative effort by the patient and members of the dental team.

I. Assess the Patient's Needs

◆ Review all information from the histories, radiographic data, clinical examinations, and chartings.

◆ Identify the presence and severity of infection and the risk factors for systemic and oral disease.

◆ Utilize indices to rate the extent of the need and provide a baseline for continuing comparisons.

◆ For most patients, a dental biofilm score can be helpful to show the patient the extent of bacterial accumulation.

◆ A discussion of caries and periodontal risk factors will illustrate the dental concerns to the patient.

◆ The patient's use of oral aids (toothbrushing, flossing, interproximal aids) is assessed for proper technique.

◆ Factors to consider during assessment:
  • Explore what will work for the patient to make the needed changes.
  • Determine the patient's motivation and confidence to make changes.
  • Consider what the patient values. The cultural values and beliefs can either promote or block the patient's efforts to make an oral health change.

II. Plan for Interventions

◆ Apply information about the patient, such as educational level, occupation, socioeconomic background, cultural influences, and attitudes regarding oral care.

◆ Determine the current personal oral care procedures carried out by the patient and the frequency.

◆ Note factors that may affect the patient's dexterity when using oral cleaning devices. This information is helpful when the clinician is determining the appropriate oral health aid options to provide the patient.

◆ Recognize the influence of age, physical limitations, and cognitive disabilities. Determine whether another person (parent or other caregiver) is needed to carry out the necessary procedures.

◆ Discuss procedures needed and develop goals, both short- and long-term goals, with the patient.

◆ Discuss with the patient the expected oral health clinical outcomes.

III. Implement the Plan

◆ Initiate preventive counseling to help the patient become aware of oral health problems. This includes learning and practicing more effective health behaviors.

◆ Explore what oral aids and preventive measures the patient utilizes daily and motivation for oral self-care.

◆ Show methods for self-evaluation.

◆ Explore the patient's diet in relation to caries risk or periodontal conditions.

◆ Introduce tobacco cessation when indicated.

◆ Change takes time and preventive counseling needs to be revisited at each appointment.

IV. Perform Clinical Preventive Services

◆ Scaling for complete calculus and biofilm removal.

◆ Application of caries-preventive agents: such as fluoride (Chapter 34) and/or dental sealants (Chapter 35).

V. Evaluate Progressive Changes

◆ Have the patient demonstrate procedures for oral self-care to determine a need for modifications in technique.

◆ Record a dental biofilm score at each appointment and compare previous recordings with the patient.

◆ At appropriate intervals, perform periodontal probe to note improvement in tissue quality, bleeding on probing, and probing depths.

◆ For goals that have not been met, collaborate with the patient to revise them.

VI. Plan Short- and Long-term Continuing Care

◆ Determine appropriate maintenance intervals.

◆ Re-evaluate to monitor continuance of preventive practices.

◆ Provide supplemental care for the patient who does not respond to initial therapy.

PATIENT COUNSELING

◆ Personalized preventive counseling contributes to the knowledge, values, and practices of the individual. Then through the individual, these ideas can be passed on to the family and the community.

- Periodontal infections and dental caries can be prevented or controlled, and, therefore, teeth preserved throughout the lifetime of the individual.

- First, attention is given to the intra- and extraoral examination to recognize possible pathology requiring exfoliative cytology and/or biopsy.

- For most patients, major attention is placed on prevention and control of dental caries and/or periodontal infection.

- Other preventive measures involving oral trauma need to be brought to the patient's attention, such as mouth protectors for contact sports and accidents that lead to fractured anterior teeth in children.

- Knowledge and belief in health facts are not enough. Benefits result only when a partnership between the clinician and patient is established and patient autonomy is taken into consideration.

I. When to Conduct

- Preventive counseling is conducted after the clinician has completed the patient assessment.

- When having a conversation regarding preventive strategies, clinicians need to remember the patient is the decision maker and is key to making a sustainable behavior change.

- Preventive counseling is provided at each appointment to follow-up on the goals, both short- and long-term, established at the previous appointment.

- By revisiting goals at each appointment, the clinician is aware of how the patient is progressing toward the established oral health change. An example is provided in Box 24-1.

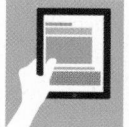

BOX 24-1

Example of Revisiting Patient Progress at Subsequent Appointments

- The patient's long-term goal is to floss 7 days a week and short-term goal is to begin flossing at least 3 days a week. The patient shows up for the 3-month continuing care appointment and has only begun flossing two times a week.

- Clinician provides affirmation about the progress the patient has made by flossing twice a week.

  - The clinician elicits to explore the possible obstacles the patient may have encountered and what ideas the patient has to overcome those obstacles.

  - The clinician may find out that the type of floss is breaking a lot when flossing or not getting into the embrasure space well.

- Therefore, the clinician will need to explore and elicit from the patient what other options may work to be successful.

- Clinicians need to recognize that health behavior changes do not happen at one preventive counseling session.

- Patient education may take multiple sessions before progress is made toward change. An example would be patients who are smokers due to the addictive nature of nicotine.

II. The Setting for Preventive Counseling

- Usually preventive counseling will take place in the dental hygiene treatment room with the patient placed in an upright position in the dental chair.

- The most effective counseling approach is with the clinician sitting face-to-face with the patient in a neutral position and maintaining eye contact.

- Face-to-face positioning style allows the patient to recognize the clinician is attentive, focused, and listening as well as builds a trusting relationship.

- Providing the appropriate setting for the clinician to explore the patient's ideas and thoughts toward an oral health behavior change is needed to maintain patient autonomy.

PATIENT MOTIVATION AND BEHAVIOR CHANGE

- Control and management of oral health conditions are dependent upon the self-care and compliance of the patient.[1]

- Traditionally, behavior change in the dental field has been approached in a prescriptive, authoritative manner where the clinician provides the information and shows the patient what to do.[2]

- However, research has concluded changes needed to prevent further disease do not happen only by providing knowledge or information to a patient.[2–7]

- Many health behavior change theories (Health Belief Model and Transtheoretical Model) have provided important perspectives on the factors to promote change and maintenance.

I. Health Behavior Change Model

- Developed in 1950s in an effort to explain unsuccessful attempt of patients to participate in programs to prevent or detect disease.[8,9]

- Later the model expanded to include patients' responses to symptoms and behavior response to diagnose illness and compliance with medical regimens.[8,9]

- The model is utilized to explain change and maintenance of health behavior and a guiding framework for health behavior interventions.

- Table 24-1 provides the key concepts of the health behavior model.

TABLE 24-1 • Key Concepts of the Health Behavior Model

PERCEIVED SUSCEPTIBILITY	CHANCES OF GETTING A CONDITION
Perceived severity	Seriousness of the disease and the effects
Perceived benefits	Effectiveness of the recommend action to reduce risk
Perceived barriers	Tangible and psychological costs of the recommend action
Cues to action	Strategies to motivate readiness
Self-efficacy	Confidence in the ability to take action

II. Transtheoretical Model

◆ The transtheoretical model suggests health behavior change involves progress through six stages of change.[9–12]

◆ Table 24-2 provides the six stages of change.

III. Motivation for Health Behavior Change

◆ Different theories have identified the following as important for clinicians to understand regarding behavioral change: various signs to change, six stages of change, self-efficacy, social support, and decisional processes.[9,10]

◆ All the various theories focus attention on the need to enhance a patient's motivation toward change. Therefore, the development of an effective approach for overcoming resistance to change was established, which is motivational interviewing (MI).[11]

MOTIVATIONAL INTERVIEWING[13]

◆ MI and brief motivational interviewing are person-centered, goal-directed methods of communication for eliciting and strengthening intrinsic motivation for positive change.

TABLE 24-2 • Transtheoretical Model—The Six Stages of Change

Precontemplation	Patient not intending to take action in future
Contemplation	Patient intends to change in next 6 mo
Preparation	Patient intends to take action in immediate future
Action	Patient made modifications to life style within the past 6 mo
Maintenance	Patient working to prevent relapse
Termination	Patient has no temptation and 100% self-efficacy

TABLE 24-3 • Basic Components of Motivational Interview (MI)

SPIRIT OF MI ELEMENTS (PACE)	GUIDING PRINCIPLES (RULE)	IMPLEMENTATION PROCESS

• Partnership acceptance
  • Absolute worth
  • Accurate empathy
  • Autonomy support
  • Affirmation
• Compassion evocation
	• Resist righting reflex
	• Understand the patient's motivation
	• Listen to the patient
	• Empower the patient
		• Engaging
		• Focusing
		• Evoking
		• Planning

◆ MI has been applied successfully within many health professions. This includes tobacco cessation, diabetic control, and eating behavior control, which all impact oral health.[2,14–21]

◆ Brief motivational interviewing[13,22] during a dental hygiene appointment assists the clinician to:
  • Effectively elicit the patient's own understanding of current oral health status and ideas about needed behavior change.
  • Avoid pushing the clinician's own ideals for behavior change onto the patient.

◆ Brief motivational interviewing is utilized in a healthcare or dental setting when MI is conducted in a brief amount of time, such as 5–10 minutes.[2,14,15,19,22]

◆ Table 24-3 lists the basic components of the MI approach to changing a patient's health behaviors.

I. Elements of the "MI Spirit"

◆ The "spirit of MI" is how a clinician relates to the patient through communication and interactions.

◆ Four interrelated elements of the spirit of MI can be easily remembered using the acronym PACE: partnership, acceptance, compassion, and evocation.

A. Partnership[23]

◆ Establish a positive interpersonal environment that encourages change but is not intimidating.

◆ Avoid the trap of communicating based entirely on professional expertise.

◆ Understand patients as individuals and attempt to see the world from their perspective.

◆ Patients are experts on themselves; it is more effective to elicit the patient's own ideas for change than to impose personal ideals or push expertise and knowledge.

B. Acceptance[23]

◆ The spirit of MI is an attitude of acceptance of what the patient brings.

- However, to accept a person does not mean to approve of the patient's actions and maintaining the status quo.
- There are four patient-centered conditions that convey acceptance.
  1. *Absolute worth*[23]
     - Honor the patient's worth and potential as a human being.
     - Respect the patient as an individual who has worth in their own right.
  2. *Accurate empathy*[23]
     - Empathy is not sympathy. The empathetic clinician demonstrates an active interest in understanding the patient's perspective.
  3. *Autonomy support*[13,23]
     - Autonomy is the patient's irrevocable right to choose and make an educated decision without being coerced, persuaded, or pressured.
     - The spirit of MI honors, respects, and provides support for a patient's autonomy.
     - Allows for patients to have complete independence to choose for themselves.
  4. *Affirmation*[13,23]
     - Affirmation instills hope and belief that the patient can indeed change and the recognition provides support and encouragement to the patient.

C. Compassion[23]

- Compassion is commitment to promoting the welfare and prioritizing the needs of the patient.
- The clinician is addressing the patient's best interest and needs and not the clinician's agenda.
- A compassionate spirit can assist with establishing trust with the patient.

D. Evocation[13,23]

- Commitment to elicit patients' assessment of their own strengths, thoughts, ideas, and resources is necessary for successful preventive counseling and behavior change.
- Patients provide a lot of information to the clinician about what will work for them in order to achieve their oral health goals through evocation.
- The overall spirit of MI begins with the premise that patients already have within them much of what is needed.
- The task of the clinician is to elicit and draw the motivation for change out of the patient.

II. Guiding Principles[13]

- MI has four guiding principles that assist the clinician in maintaining a rapport with the patient.
- The four principles can be remembered with the acronym RULE: resist–understand–listen–empower.

A. Resist Righting Reflex[13]

- Clinicians often have a desire to help and fix what is wrong and take the "expert role."
- This approach loses focus on the patient's ideas, experiences, and obstacles to overcome due to the clinician who is busy pouring knowledge out onto the patient.
- This urge to correct the patient's problem is often an automatic or reflexive habit.
- The reflexive nature of the clinician response can create a negative effect because patients tend to resist persuasion, especially when they are ambivalent about change.
- Instead, to establish and maintain the MI spirit of partnership, it is necessary to explore by eliciting the patient's own motivation and ideas for change.

B. Understand the Patient's Motivation[13]

- Determine the patient's own reasons for change rather than focusing on the clinician's perspective about why the patient needs to make the change.
- Be interested in the patient's own concerns, values, and motivations.
- Utilize MI to evoke and explore the patient's own perception about their current situation and motivations for change.
- Help the patient voice their own arguments for behavior change.

C. Listen to the Patient[13]

- All patients love a good listener and a truly good listener will forgo their own agenda in the interest of giving full attention to understanding the patient.
- The expectation of a clinician typically has been to know all the answers and give them to the patient.
- Patients have ideas about how to make the change.
- Active listening requires more than the clinician asking questions.
- Listening involves the clinician demonstrating an empathetic interest in making sure to understand the patient.
- A good listener does not direct or instruct, agree or disagree, persuade or advise, or warn or analyze what a patient says. There is no agenda to achieve other than understanding the world of the patient.

D. Empower the Patient[13]

- Patient empowerment is about supporting the patient's right to autonomy.
- Outcomes of behavior change increase when patients take an active interest and role in their own health care.
- Encourage patients by exploring how they can make a difference in their oral health and by listening and understanding the patient's own ideas for change.
- Patients are more likely to take steps toward change when they are included in the discussion and take an active role in the decision making.

III. Processes of MI[23]

- ◆ The four processes of MI form the flow of how clinicians use MI to direct patient behavior change.
- ◆ The flow of the four processes throughout a conversation with a patient will overlap and repeat. These processes are like stair steps illustrated in Figure 24-1 in which each process builds upon the other yet continues as the foundation.
- ◆ Box 24-2 provides a checklist of questions to help the clinician gauge the success of their MI approach at each step.

MI IMPLEMENTATION

I. Information Exchange[13]

- ◆ To provide information to a patient, begin by asking permission.
- ◆ Asking permission to provide information indicates respect and increases the willingness of the patient to hear what the clinician has to say.

A. Ask Permission[13,23]

- ◆ There are two approaches a clinician utilizes to ask the patient's permission to provide further detail or additional information.
- ◆ The clinician can:
  - • Relay information when a patient asks the clinician for that information.
  - • Directly ask permission to provide information even when the patient has not directly requested the information.
- ◆ For example, "I would like to discuss with you the assessment pertaining to your oral health; do you mind if I take a few minutes to go over my findings and address any concerns you may have?"
- ◆ Box 24-3 provides an example of information exchange utilizing asking permission.

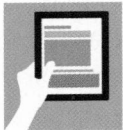

BOX 24-2

Clinician Checklist of the Four Processes of Motivational Interview[23]

Engaging
- • How comfortable is the patient in talking to me (clinician)?
- • Do I understand the patient's perspective and concerns?
- • Does this feel like a collaborative partnership?

Focusing
- • Are we (clinician and patient) working together for a common purpose?
- • What goals for change does the patient have?
- • Does this conversation feel more like dancing or a wrestling match?

Evoking
- • What are the patient's own reasons for change?
- • Is the reluctance for change about confidence or importance?
- • What change talk am I hearing?
- • Is the righting reflex pulling me (the clinician) to be the one arguing for change, instead of the patient?

Planning
- • What would be a reasonable next step toward change?
- • Am I remembering to evoke rather than prescribe a plan for the patient?
- • Am I offering needed information or advice with permission when appropriate?
- • Am I eliciting the patient's ideas for making the change?

Planning
Process encompasses both developing commitment to change and formulating a concrete plan of action

Evoking
Process involves eliciting the patient's own motivations for change and lies at the heart of MI

Focusing
Process by which you develop and maintain a specific direction in the conversation about change

Engaging
Process of establishing a helpful connection and working relationship

FIGURE 24-1 • Four Processes of Motivational Interview.

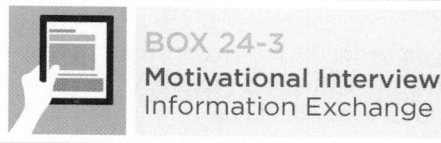

BOX 24-3
Motivational Interview:
Information Exchange

Clinician: Mrs. Poe do you mind if I discuss your oral assessment findings? (Ask permission)

Patient: Sure, that is fine.

Clinician: Great, we can discuss three areas of the assessment: Extra/intraoral findings, dental evaluation, or periodontal evaluation. Which would you like to begin with first? (Agenda setting)

Patient: Since I have a family history of gum disease, let's begin with the periodontal evaluation.

Clinician: Since you have a family history of gum disease, tell me what you know about gum disease? (Elicit)

Patient: My grandparents both wear dentures and father has a couple of missing teeth due to losing teeth to bone loss. Gum disease involves the loss of bone.

Clinician: Yes, that is correct. Gum disease, also known as periodontal disease, involves the loss of bone. What do you know about the various types of periodontal disease? (Elicit)

Patient: Nothing, I didn't realize there were different types. Can you tell me more about the kinds and how they relate to my current oral health?

Clinician: Sure, I will be happy to elaborate (pulls out a chart illustrating the various stages). Gingivitis is reversible and inflammation of the gums, slight periodontitis includes slight bone loss and recession, moderate periodontitis (beginning of bone loss between the roots of the teeth and mobility), and severe periodontitis. Currently you have slight periodontitis due to the recession and slight bone loss revealed in the radiographs in conjunction with the probe readings taken today. (Provide) What are your thoughts about the information provided? (Elicit)

B. Elicit Provide Elicit[13]

A strategy for easy exchange of information that maintains patient autonomy is the elicit-provide-elicit (EPE) approach.

◆ Three general functions of eliciting are:
  • Asking permission.
  • Exploring the patient's prior knowledge.
  • Determining the patient's interest in the information that may be provided by the clinician.
◆ An exploration of the patient's prior knowledge is necessary.
  • This avoids the "expert trap" so patients are not told things they already know.
  • It also allows the clinician to fill in any variances or gaps in the patient's knowledge.

◆ Querying interest allows the clinician to determine:
  • What the patient would like to know most.
  • Provide the information that increases attention and receptiveness.
  • Increase patient compliance.[10]
◆ Box 24-3 also provides an example utilizing the EPE strategy of information change.

II. Agenda Setting[13,23]

◆ Agenda setting (agenda mapping) is a brief discussion in which the patient is given as much decision-making freedom as possible to set the agenda for what information and recommendations the clinician provides and for when the information is provided.

◆ An agenda setting approach provides the patient with a list of topics regarding the oral health and choose which topic to discuss first.

◆ For example, "Mrs. Smith there are three areas we can discuss regarding the assessment findings, which are extraoral/intraoral evaluation, dental evaluation, and periodontal evaluation. Which area would you like to discuss first?"

◆ There may be areas the dental hygienist is concerned about; however, if the clinician decides the topic of conversation without consulting the patient, an opportunity to learn what behavior change the patient may be most ready to discuss is lost.

◆ Respect for the patient's autonomy to choose what topics to discuss will increase the patient's willingness to listen.

III. Core Skills[13,23]

◆ The core skills for MI are better known by the acronym OARS:
  • **O**pen-ended questions.
  • **A**ffirmations.
  • **R**eflective listening.
  • **S**ummary.
◆ Box 24-4 provides an example of a brief patient conversation that illustrate MI core skills.

A. Open-Ended versus Closed Questions[13,23]

◆ A skillful blend of open-ended questions and reflective listening is essential in the MI approach to patient counseling.

◆ Open-ended questions permit the patient to think about the response. This may yield information and insight about topics the clinician may have missed.

◆ This style of questioning invites conversation focused in a particular direction and provides insight into the patient's values, understanding of the oral health status, as well as the ability to change.

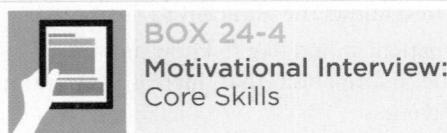

BOX 24-4
Motivational Interview:
Core Skills

Clinician: Mr. Brooks I notice you are a smoker from your chart. Please tell me what you know about smoking cessation? (Open question)

Patient: Yes, I do smoke and have for several years. I have been lectured in the past about smoking by previous healthcare providers and they mentioned something regarding smoking cessation. I think smoking cessation is guidance to quit smoking.

Clinician: I am not here to lecture you at all about smoking Mr. Brooks, but I am here to assist you with ways to quit when you are ready. Seems you have tried to quit before since you are familiar with the smoking cessation program to guide smokers on alternatives ways to quit. (Reflection) What further information have you received regarding smoking cessation? (Open question)

Patient: Well they told me there are medications and patches that could be used to assist with quitting. I have tried going cold turkey in the past. I need something to assist me with decreasing the number of cigarettes per day. Cold turkey does not work because it was just too much to handle with all the stress and I need something that will help me quit but slowly.

Clinician: I commend you on your efforts in the past to quit smoking and it seems you have really given thought to quitting based on what you are telling me your past experience. (Affirmation) You realize going cold turkey was not the best route and you need a way to decrease the amount of nicotine daily. More of a gradual way to quit smoking. (Summary)

- Examples of open-ended questions include:
  - "What brings you here today?"
  - "How do you hope your life might be like in 5 years?"
  - "What do you know about cavities?"
- Box 24-4 provides an example of a patient conversation that begins with an open-ended question.
- Closed questions, while good for gathering specific types of information, tend to limit the person's options for responding. An example: "Do you smoke?"
- Closed questions can disguise themselves as an open question.
  - An example would be "So what are you hoping to do: quit or cut down?"
  - This type is termed a "leading" question and does not allow the patient the option to elaborate nor provide patient autonomy.

B. Affirmations[23]

- Affirmations emphasize the positive attributes, particularly concerning strengths the patient has expressed in regard to making a behavior change.
- Affirmations help encourage and support a patient.
- Affirmations are genuine and contain a reflection of what is true regarding the patient.
- Patients are more likely to spend time with, trust, listen to, and be open with a healthcare provider who they perceive recognizes and affirms their strengths.
- Affirmations decrease or reduce defensiveness.
- Encourage self-affirmation by asking the patient to describe strengths and past successes. This type of self-affirming has shown to facilitate openness.[24,25]
- Good affirmations center on the word "you." Using statements beginning with "I" will focus more on the clinician than on the patient.
- Example of an affirmation statement: "Your intention was good even though it didn't turn out as you would like."
- An example of a patient conversation that includes affirmation is found in Box 24-4.

C. Reflective Listening[13,23]

- Reflective listening (reflection) is a response to what the patient is conveying with a statement or summary that is more than repeating verbatim what the patient has said.
- This allows the patient to know the clinician is hearing and understanding.
- Two categories for reflections are simple reflection and complex reflection.
- Simple reflection is slightly rephrasing the content that was relayed to you by the patient.
- Box 24-5 provides an example of a simple reflection.
- Complex reflection:
  - Adds meaning or emphasis to what the patient said.
  - Makes a guess about the unspoken content or what might come next.
  - Tend to move the conversation forward.
  - Box 24-6 provides an example of a complex reflection.

BOX 24-5
Motivational Interview:
Reflective Listening—Simple Reflection

Patient: I know that what you're trying to do is help me, but I'm just not going to do that!

Clinician: On the one hand, you know that there are some real problems here, and on the other, what I suggested is just not acceptable to you.

BOX 24-6

Motivational Interview: Reflective Listening—Complex Reflection

Patient: You're probably going to give me a laundry list of ways to take care of my mouth that I need to stick to, and tell me I have to get some of these interproximal brushes, superfloss, power toothbrush, and a bunch of other products. I don't have time for all that!

Clinician: If I were to tell you a whole lot of things that you have to do, it would immobilize you even further. It's ironic, isn't it? When you feel like you are being forced to do something, it actually prevents you from doing what you want to do.

D. Summarizing[13,23]

Summarizing information provided by the patient:
- Pulls together several items or ideas that a patient has provided.
- Is affirming because it implies the clinician remembers what the patient said and wants to understand.
- Assists the patient to reflect and think about the various experiences they communicated.

EXPLORING AMBIVALENCE[13,23]

- Patients often experience very divided feelings about changing health behaviors.
- On one hand, they may appreciate and value knowledge and recommendations the dental hygienist provides about how to attain and maintain their oral health.
- On the other hand, they often have very mixed feelings about how successful they could be at implementing the recommendations the care provider has suggested.
- The most effective way to explore and respond to a patient's ambivalence is by using the OARS core skills discussed in the previous section of this chapter.

I. Sustain Talk versus Change Talk[13,23]

- Listening carefully to the patient and responding appropriately is an important MI skill.
- Conversations with a patient may balance between sustain talk and change talk.
- A patient who is happy about current health-related behaviors will exhibit more discussion about maintaining the status quo (sustain talk) than someone who is ready to change.
- The skillful clinician who hears only sustain talk can use MI techniques to determine what information the patient is interested in receiving about oral health status and explore ambivalence.

- During patient conversations, the clinician may hear change talk, through patient statements that seem preparatory or mobilizing toward changing behaviors.
- When this occurs, the clinician can move to reflecting the change talk and eliciting a plan for change.
- Responding to both sustain talk and change talk, a clinician can use the MI process (OARS) to explore the patient's ambivalence toward change and to understand the issues that may be inhibiting their desire, motivation, or ability to change behaviors.

II. Decisional Balance[23]

A. The Balancing Act

- Decisional balance is the point at which a patient is determining whether the benefits outweigh the risks of the current behavior.
- The clinician can use this as an opportunity to explore and elicit more information from the patient about the pros and cons for making or not making the change.
- The key to success in this process is for the clinician to take a neutral position and provide a balanced way for the patient to explore the pros and cons of a behavior change.[25]
- The clinician's role is to elicit the patient's perception of:
  - Advantages of maintaining current behavior.
  - Disadvantages of maintaining the current behavior.
  - Advantages of making the change.
  - Disadvantages of making the change.
- The approach is very helpful when a patient seems to be uncertain about making a change.

B. Pro–Con Matrix

- Use of a pro–con matrix, illustrated in Figure 24-2, can also be beneficial in exploring decisional balance.
- The clinician can reflect and ask "What else?" at each interval during the patient's listing of pros and cons of making the change.
- When the decisional balance matrix has been completed, the clinician will focus on key items regarding the change of the behavior and provide a summary.
- Box 24-7 provides an example of the pro–con matrix in a conversation with a patient.

Pro–Con Matrix	Pros	Cons
If I don't change	A	B
If I do change	D	C

FIGURE 24-2 • Decisional Balance: Pro and Con Matrix.

MOTIVATIONAL TRAINING AND COACHING

- MI workshops alone will usually have little effect on the clinician's proficiency or changing practice.[15,22]
- In order to become proficient with MI, it is recommended to take introductory and advanced MI courses or workshops where feedback is provided through MI practice and coaching.[23,29]
- Ultimately, the skills of MI are learned through the feedback and coaching that is rendered and this can only be done by observed practice.
- Therefore, skill development is an ongoing process and MI must coincide with classroom, practice, and coaching in order to be properly trained.[23,29]
- There is additional information located on the MI Network of Trainers website (www.motivationalinterviewing.org), with additional information regarding trainings across the nation clinicians may attend as well as many other resources pertaining to MI.[30]

DOCUMENTATION

Routine documentation for a MI session includes a minimum of the following information.

- Assessment findings and areas of concern (disease status and risk).
- Patient's stage of readiness for making a change.
- Patient's motivation for change.
- The outcome of the conversation with the patient regarding the area(s) of concern such as:
  - Knowledge and understanding of their disease status and risk.
  - What the patient would like to address first.
  - What has worked in the past or what has not worked in the past.
  - How they plan to make the change.
  - Short- and long-term goals for making the change.
  - When they plan to begin to make the change.
- A documentation example is found in Box 24-13.

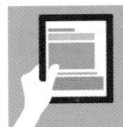

BOX 24-13

Example Documentation:
Motivational Interview (MI) Session during a Patient Appointment

S—A 30-year-old Caucasian male presents for 3-month continuing care visit. Previous assessment indicates high intake of sugar sweetened beverages. Previous entries in patient record indicate ongoing recommendations for limiting intake of sugar sweetened beverages. Patient states today that he sips three to five cans of cola-type beverage during the day and evening. He indicates he knows the beverages are what "cause my cavities" and that he would like to change his behavior so he wouldn't "get any more cavities," but that his motivation for behavior change on the readiness ruler is "about a 2."

O—Previous history of significant smooth surface decay, and today's examination indicates two new cavitated lesions on anterior facial surfaces, which were documented on the patient's dental chart.

A—Patient has knowledge of the cause of dental decay but expresses ambivalence to change that can correct the problem.

P—Used MI approach and the pro–con matrix to help the patient explore his ambivalence to behavior change and to explore factors that might affect his ability to change behavior and stop continually drinking sugar sweetened beverages. He will continue to explore other ways he can cut down and might begin drinking bottle water with sugar-free flavoring.

Next Steps: Continue to use MI approach to provide follow-up discussion and encouragement during patient's visit for restorative treatment in 2 weeks and at his next dental hygiene appointment in 3 months.

Signed: _____, RDH

Date: _____

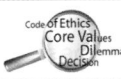

EVERYDAY ETHICS

Jeremy, now 15 years old, has been a patient of Tressa, the dental hygienist, since he was 3 years old. Jeremy had undergone extensive restorative work as a young child. He had collided on a swing set with an older sibling, which resulted in trauma to both maxillary and mandibular incisors and permanent tooth buds. Jeremy had received a "fair plus" on his oral homecare report card at the last few visits. However, this time when Tressa went to greet him in the waiting room, Jeremy's mother asked her to "really get on him" about brushing his teeth every day.

During her oral assessment, Tressa noted extremely heavy biofilm on all teeth, generalized bleeding on probing, staining on the anterior restorations, and a distinctly unpleasant odor. "Jeremy," she lectured, "you must take better care of your teeth! Your breath smells really bad. And you are jeopardizing all of that expensive dental work your parents have paid for." Turning very red, Jeremy

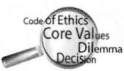

EVERYDAY ETHICS (*Continued*)

pulled his cap over his eyes, crossed his arms, and refused to reply. As she continued to provide preventive counseling, Jeremy was clearly not paying attention and Tressa became annoyed. She commented that she was going to speak to his mother about his poor attitude.

In a final attempt to turn his attention to prevention, Tressa showed Jeremy intraoral photographs she taken that morning of a patient with extreme periodontal disease. "Is that what you want to look like?" she asked.

Questions for Consideration

1. Describe how Tressa's approach to prevention violates Jeremy's autonomy, even though he is technically still a child and in spite of his mother's request.

2. Explain why showing Jeremy another patient's intraoral photographs violates the ethical standards of dental hygiene practice.

3. What core values and ethical principles can guide Tressa as she reflects on her **communication style** and develops an alternative approach to prevention that is both ethical and effective?

Factors to Teach the Patient

▶ Discuss the relationship between preventive measures and clinical services.

▶ Discuss preventive measures and suggested care plan options pertaining to the clinical assessment findings.

▶ Elicit what the patient knows about periodontal disease or their risk for caries and have a discussion utilizing the MI methods regarding possible changes the patient can pursue.

▶ Discuss self-assessment and alternative methods (disclosing agent) for determining the health of gingiva.

▶ Determine the patient's self-care technique (e.g., toothbrushing power or manual, flossing) and provide suggestions if need to modified technique to be effective.

▶ Provide the patient with various options regarding preventive measures for the disease status to choose that will be effective.

▶ Elicit from the patient's short- and long-term goals pertaining to what the patient would like to achieve regarding disease status and overall self-care.

ENHANCE YOUR UNDERSTANDING

ONLINE RESOURCES
(see the inside front cover for access information)

• Audio glossary
• Appendices

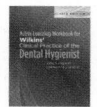

SUPPORT FOR LEARNING
(available separately)

• *Active Learning Workbook for Wilkins' Clinical Practice of the Dental Hygienist*, 13th Edition

INDIVIDUALIZED REVIEW

• Customized practice quizzing with Navigate 2 TestPrep for *Wilkins' Clinical Practice of the Dental Hygienist*

References

1. Gao X, Lo EC, Kot SC, Chan KC. Motivational interviewing in improving oral health: a systemic review of randomized controlled trials. *J Periodontol.* 2014;85(3):426-437. doi:10.1902/jop.2013.130205.

2. Bray KK, Catley D, Voelker MA, Liston R, Williams KB. Motivational interviewing in dental hygiene education: curriculum modification and evaluation. *J Dent Educ.* 2013;77(12):1662-1669.

3. Croffoot C, Krust Bray K, Black MA, Koerber A. Evaluating the effects of coaching to improve motivational interviewing skills of dental hygiene students. *J Dent Hyg.* 2010;84(2):57-64.

4. Kalsbeek H, Truin GJ, Poorterman JH, van Rossum GM, vam Rijkom HM, Verrips GH. Trends in periodontal status and oral hygiene habits in Dutch adults between 1983 and 1995. *Community Dent Oral Epidemiol.* 2000;28(2):112-118.

5. Ronis DL, Lang WP, Farghaly MM, Passow E. Tooth brushing, flossing, and preventive dental visits by Detroit-area residents in relation to demographic and socioeconomic factors. *J Public Health Dent.* 1993;53(3):138-145.

6. Smedslund G, Berg RC, Hammerstrøm KT, et al. Motivational interviewing for substance abuse. *Cochrane Database Syst Rev.* 2011;(5):CD008063.

7. Yevlahova D, Satur J. Models for individual oral health promotion and their effectiveness: a systematic review. *Aust Dent J.* 2009;54(3):190-197. doi:10.1111/j.1834-7819.2009.01118.x.

8. Glanz K, Lewis FM, Rimer BK. *Health Behavior and Health Education.* 2nd ed. San Francisco, CA: Jossey-Bass; 1997:41-59.

9. Emmons KM, Rollnick S. Motivational interviewing in health care settings: opportunities and limitations. *Am J Prev Med.* 2001;20(1):68-74.

10. Prochaska JO, Velicer WF. The transtheoretical model of health behavior change. *Am J Health Promot.* 1997;12(1):38-48.

11. Wilson GT, Schlam TR. The transtheoretical model and motivational interviewing in the treatment of eating and weight disorders. *Clin Psychol Rev.* 2004;24(3):361-378.

12. Bundy C. Changing behaviour: using motivational interviewing techniques. *J R Soc Med.* 2004;97(suppl 44):43-47.

13. Rollnick S, Miller WR, Butler CC. *Motivational Interviewing in Health Care: Helping Patients Change Behavior.* New York, NY: The Guilford Press; 2008:3-107.

14. Rubak S, Sandbaek A, Lauritzen T, Christensen B. Motivational interviewing: a systematic review and meta-analysis. *Br J Gen Pract.* 2005;55(513):305-312.

15. Lundahl BW, Kunz C, Brownell C, Tollefson D, Burke BL. A meta-analysis of motivational interviewing: twenty-five years of empirical studies. *Res Social Work Prac.* 2010; 20(2):137-159.

16. Lundahl B, Moleni T, Burke BL, et al. Motivational interviewing in medical care settings: a systematic review and meta-analysis of randomized controlled trials. *Patient Educ Couns.* 2013;93(2):157-168.

17. Hettema J, Steele J, Miller WR. Motivational interviewing. *Annu Rev Clin Psychol.* 2005;1:91-111.

18. Soria R, Legido A, Escolano C, Yeste AL, Montoya J. A randomised controlled trial of motivational interviewing for smoking cessation. *Br J Gen Pract.* 2006;56(531):768-774.

19. Koeber A, Crawford J, O'Connell K. The effects of teaching dental students brief motivational interviewing for smoking cessation counseling: a pilot study. *J Dent Educ.* 2003;67(4):439-447.

20. Hettema JE, Hendricks PS. Motivational interviewing for smoking cessation: a meta-analytic review. *J Consult Clin Psychol.* 2010;78(6):868-884.

21. Martins RK, McNeil DW. Review of motivational interviewing in promoting health behaviors. *Clin Psychol Rev.* 2009;29:283-293.

22. Rollnick S, Heather N. Negotiating behavior change in medical settings: the development of brief motivational interviewing. *J Mental Health.* 1992;1(1):25-38.

23. Miller WR, Rollnick S. *Motivational Interviewing: Helping People Change.* 3rd ed. New York, NY: The Guilford Press; 2013:3-292.

24. Critcher CR, Dunning D, Armor DA. When self-affirmations reduce defensiveness: timing is key. *Pers Soc Psychol Bull.* 2010;36(7):947-959.

25. Janis IL, Mann L. *Decision Making: A Psychological Analysis of Conflict, Choice and Commitment.* New York, NY: Free Press; 1977.

26. Skaret E, Weinstein P, Kvale G, Raadal M. An intervention program to reduce dental avoidance behaviour among adolescents: a pilot study. *Eur J Paediatr Dent.* 2003;4: 191-196.

27. Weinstein P, Harrison R, Benton T. Motivating parents to prevent caries in their young children: one-year findings. *J Am Dent Assoc.* 2004;135(6):731-738.

28. Weinstein P, Harrison R, Benton T. Motivating mothers to prevent caries: confirming the beneficial effect of counseling. *J Am Dent Assoc.* 2006;137:789-793.

29. Miller WR, Yahne CE, Moyers TB, Martinez J, Pirritano M. A randomized trial of methods to help clinicians learn motivational interviewing. *J Consult Clin Psychol.* 2004;72: 1050-1062.

30. Motivational Interviewing Network of Trainers. MINT excellence in motivational interviewing: MI Training and Resources. http://www.motivationalinterviewing.org/. Accessed September 2, 2017.

25

Protocols for Prevention and Control of Dental Caries

Michelle Hurlbutt, RDH, MSDH, DHSc, and Linda D. Boyd, RDH, RD, EdD

CHAPTER OUTLINE

HISTORY OF DENTAL CARIES MANAGEMENT

THE DENTAL CARIES PROCESS
  I. Acidogenic and Aciduric Bacteria
  II. Role of Fermentable Carbohydrates
  III. Acid Production
  IV. Demineralization
  V. Remineralization

DENTAL CARIES CLASSIFICATIONS
  I. Reversible Stages of Dental Carious Lesion

CARIES RISK ASSESSMENT SYSTEMS
  I. ADA Caries Risk Assessment
  II. American Academy of Pediatric Dentistry (AAPD) Caries-Risk Assessment Tool (CAT)

  III. Cariogram
  IV. Caries Management by Risk Assessment (CAMBRA®)
  V. International Caries Classification and Management System (ICCMS™)

IMPLEMENTATION OF CRA IN THE PROCESS OF CARE

CARIES RISK MANAGEMENT SYSTEMS
  I. AAPD Caries Risk Management Protocol
  II. Caries Management by Risk Assessment (CAMBRA®)
  III. International Caries Classification and Management System (ICCMS™)

PLANNING CARE FOR THE PATIENT'S CARIES RISK LEVEL
  I. The Patient with Low Caries Risk

  II. The Patient with Moderate Caries Risk
  III. The Patient with High and Extreme Caries Risk

CONTINUING CARE

DOCUMENTATION

EVERYDAY ETHICS

FACTORS TO TEACH THE PATIENT

REFERENCES

LEARNING OBJECTIVES

After studying this chapter, the student will be able to:

1. Describe the dental caries disease process.
2. Identify factors contributing to demineralization and remineralization.
3. Distinguish each step in caries management.
4. Evaluate each patient for individual risk for caries disease.
5. Apply caries risk status in developing individualized caries management protocols and carefully document.

HISTORY OF DENTAL CARIES MANAGEMENT

- In the early half of the 20th century, the history of dental caries management included placing restorations, removing diseased teeth, and providing prosthetic replacements.
- Reductions in caries incidence of 40%–60% since 1945 in the United States were observed for those fortunate enough to live in communities with community water fluoridation.[1]
- As the 20th century progressed, a drop in dental caries prevalence was generally related to the widespread home use of fluoride dentifrices and mouthrinses as well as professional topical applications of solutions, gels, and varnishes.
- In the early 21st century, studies revealed dental caries prevalence has remained the same and even increased in some populations in the United States as a result of lack of access to care.[2]
- Recent evidence suggests the prevalence of untreated dental caries decreased among preschoolers during 2011–2014 but the prevalence of having no dental caries in permanent teeth in children and adolescents has remained unchanged.[3]
- Dental caries remains a major problem in the health and welfare of adults, adolescents, and children.

THE DENTAL CARIES PROCESS

Dental caries is an infectious, transmissible disease. It is also preventable. When a caries infection occurs in the oral cavity, strategies exist to control the disease, reverse it in its early stages, and prevent further infection. Dental hygienists have new information from current research to share with their patients to increase their understanding of the dental caries process and disease prevention.

- The extended ecological plaque hypothesis proposes that dental caries is the result of a shift in the ecological balance of dental plaque toward a more cariogenic flora.[4]
- The basic caries process starts with certain acidogenic and aciduric bacteria in dental biofilm acting to metabolize the fermentable carbohydrates ingested by the patient.[5]
- Acids are formed that demineralize the enamel, cementum, and/or dentin and lead to cavity formation.
- On the tooth surface, a continuous process of demineralization and remineralization is occurring.
- This process is ongoing and takes place throughout the life of the tooth.
- Protocols exist to address caries disease prevention and management at the various stages of lesion

development; the goal being to halt and control the disease process.
- The interrelation of the microorganisms, tooth, salivary factors, and cariogenic foods in the caries process is shown in Chapter 33.

I. Acidogenic and Aciduric Bacteria

- Acidogenic and aciduric bacteria produce acid as a result of metabolizing fermentable carbohydrates consumed by the individual.
- When acidogenic and aciduric bacteria predominate the oral flora, the risk for dental caries disease increases.
- Although there are many acid-forming and acid-tolerant bacteria present, two groups of bacteria predominate in the caries process: the mutans streptococci (*Streptococcus mutans* and *Streptococcus sobrinus* are two most prevalent bacteria in the group) as well as *Lactobacillus* and *Actinomyces* and non-*Actinomyces* species.[4] *Bifidobacteria* are also associated with childhood caries.[6]
- Mutans streptococci are infectious organisms that colonize the teeth and help to form the dental biofilm because they create a sticky environment for survival and multiplication.
- Mutans streptococci and *Bifidobacteria* are most active during the initial stages of demineralization and cavity formation, whereas the lactobacilli are more active during the progression of the cavity.
- Permanent colonization of a child's teeth with the mutans streptococci group can take place soon after tooth eruption. Transmission of the acid-forming organisms is usually from close family members, particularly the mother.[7]

II. Role of Fermentable Carbohydrates

- Commonly consumed fermentable carbohydrates include all sugars (sucrose, glucose, fructose) and cooked starches.
- Acids produced during the metabolic processes include acetic, lactic, formic, and propionic.
- *Frequency* and *form* of fermentable carbohydrates enhance the amount of biofilm and acid produced and results in increased demineralization.[8,9]

III. Acid Production

- The acid formed passes freely into the tiny diffusion channels between the enamel rods or into the exposed root surfaces.
- Acids can dissolve the enamel crystals into calcium and phosphate ions.
- The subsurface initial carious lesion is formed as discussed in Chapter 16 and appears clinically as a white spot lesion.

IV. Demineralization

Demineralization and remineralization are natural processes as the fluids in the oral cavity constantly strive to maintain equilibrium.[10]

- Demineralization is the process by which the minerals of the tooth structure are dissolved into solution by organic acids produced from acidogenic bacteria that metabolize fermentable carbohydrates.

- With repeated bathing of the tooth surface with the acids, the tooth demineralization can outpace the remineralization process. The end product of this activity is the cavitated carious lesion.

- Smooth surface and pit and fissure carious lesions can result when cariogenic nutrients are available.

V. Remineralization

Remineralization is the natural repair process of moving minerals back into the subsurface of the intact enamel. Saliva provides protective factors to promote remineralization.[10]

A. Saliva

- Protective factors of healthy saliva can balance or reverse the destruction of the tooth structure.

- The functions of saliva related to caries management include[11]:
  - Buffering of acids and clearance of bacteria and food debris.
  - Supply minerals to replace calcium and phosphate ions dissolved from the tooth during demineralization.

- Low saliva flow (hyposalivation or xerostomia) reduces buffering capacity and aids in the demineralization process.

- Maintaining a neutral or basic saliva pH of 7 is necessary to maximize remineralization. After an exposure to fermentable carbohydrate, the pH drops to the critical pH of 5.5 (Figure 25-1) at which point demineralization occurs.[4]

- Exposure to topical fluoride can increase available salivary levels of fluoride.
  - Saliva is a reservoir for fluoride to aid in remineralization.
  - Fluoride accumulation in saliva comes from many sources, including water, dentifrice, mouthrinse, and professionally applied therapies.[12]

B. Fluoride Mechanisms of Action

- *Inhibits demineralization:* Fluoride available in biofilm and saliva can flow into the enamel diffusion channels and root surface and attach in the form of hydrogen fluoride (HF) as the oral environment attempts to achieve equilibrium.[5]

- *Enhances remineralization:* Sufficient saliva is integral in this process.
  - The buffering properties of saliva can neutralize acid pH.
  - This change in pH can reverse the equilibrium, driving calcium, phosphate, and fluoride ions into the tooth surface.[5]
  - The resulting fluorapatite bond is stronger less acid soluble than the hydroxyapatite bond, resulting in a stronger tooth surface.

- Inhibits bacterial growth:
  - In the biofilm, the HF diffuses through the cell membrane of acidogenic bacteria.
  - Fluoride ions interfere with the essential enzyme activity within the bacterial cell wall.[12]

DENTAL CARIES CLASSIFICATIONS

- As discussed in Chapter 16, there are several stages of caries development from noncavitated to cavitated carious lesion using either the American Dental Association (ADA) Caries Classification System (CCS) or International Caries Classification and Management System (ICCMS).

- Early diagnosis and detection of carious lesions still in the subsurface, incipient, or noncavitated state allows

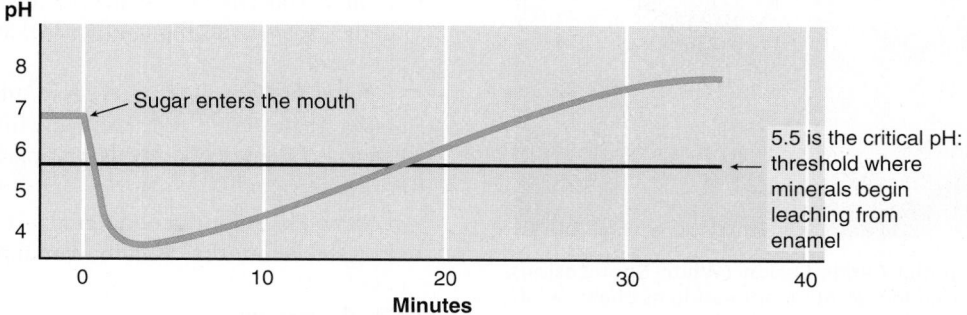

FIGURE 25-1 • The Stephan Curve Shows the Way the Saliva pH Changes from a Neutral pH of 7 Once Fermentable Carbohydrates Are Consumed to a Critical pH of 5.5 or Less at Which Point Demineralization Occurs.

the clinician to educate the patient, provide strategies to manage risk of further progression of the lesion, and provide preventive treatments to reverse the lesion.

◆ Examination for caries detection clinically and radiographically are reviewed in Chapter 16.

I. Reversible Stages of Dental Carious Lesion

Chapter 16 reviews the stages of caries lesion development.
◆ The stages when caries development is still reversible include the following[13,14]:
  • ICCMS Initial Stage Caries or CCS Initial Caries Lesion when there is no cavitation of the lesion (see Figure 25-2).
◆ The stages when caries development is irreversible include the following[13,14]:
  • ICCMS Moderate Stage Caries or CCS Moderate Caries Lesion where there is cavitation of the enamel.
  • ICCMS Extensive Stage Caries or CCS Advanced Caries Lesion where the lesion extends into the dentin.

CARIES RISK ASSESSMENT SYSTEMS

Risk assessment is commonly used to assess the risk factors for disease so that individualized prevention and management plans can be developed and implemented.
◆ Caries risk assessment (CRA) is an essential component of patient-centered caries management.[15]
  • The ideal CRA will be evidence-based, inexpensive, and easy to use in the process of patient care.
  • Identifying the validity of a CRA system long term in prevention of caries and stopping progression of early lesions is still undergoing further research.

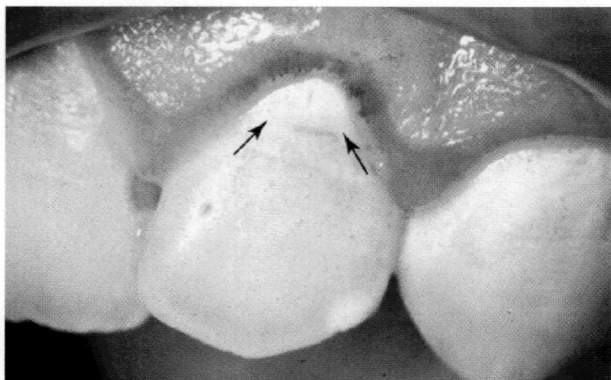

FIGURE 25-2 • Initial Caries Lesion (White Spot Lesion). Smooth surface demineralization appearing as chalky white area (at *arrows*) seen in the cervical third of a maxillary lateral incisor is evidence of the first stages of dental caries. If this demineralization continues, this area could develop a cavitation that would need to be restored.

◆ Risk factors fall into two categories:
  • Modifiable risk factors.
  • Nonmodifiable risk factors.

I. ADA Caries Risk Assessment

◆ This tool was developed based on expert opinion and available evidence.
◆ This CRA has assessment forms for age 0–6 and those over age 6.
◆ The assessment includes the following factors:
  • *Contributing conditions* such as fluoride exposure, consumption of sugary foods/drinks, and eligibility for government programs, dental home, and family caries experience (ages 0–6).
  • *General health conditions* such as special healthcare needs, eating disorders, medication-induced xerostomia, drug/alcohol abuse, and chemo/radiation therapy.
  • *Clinical conditions* such as radiographic caries lesions, missing teeth due to caries, noncavitated lesions, visible plaque biofilm, interproximal restorations, exposed root surfaces, fixed or removable prosthetic/orthodontic appliances, and salivary flow.
◆ Risk levels include low, moderate, and high risk.

II. American Academy of Pediatric Dentistry (AAPD) Caries-Risk Assessment Tool (CAT)

◆ The AAPD used a systematic review process to update the CAT tool in 2014.[16]
◆ The CAT is for infants, children, and adolescents.
  • 0–3 year olds for nondental providers such as physicians.
  • 0–5 year olds for dental providers.
  • Greater than 6 year olds for dental providers.
◆ The assessment includes the following factors:
  • *Biological factors* such as sugar containing snacks or beverages, special healthcare needs, recent immigrant, low socioeconomic status, and active caries in primary caregiver.
  • *Protective factors* such as fluoride exposure, brushing daily, professional topical fluoride, and regular dental care.
  • *Clinical findings* such as decayed/missing/filled surfaces or defective restorations, white spot lesions, elevated streptococci levels, and plaque.
◆ Risk levels include:
  • Low and high for the nondental providers.
  • Low, moderate, and high for dental providers.

III. Cariogram

◆ The Cariogram is a visual representation of the interaction of caries with various etiologic factors to predict future risk. Originally developed in 1976, decades of trials were conducted to validate it before it was launched online in 1997.[17]

- The Cariogram is the only system with data showing validity at this time.[15]

◆ The assessment includes the following factors:

- *Bacteria* including dental plaque amount and mutans streptococci count.
- *Diet* including fermentable carbohydrates and frequency.
- *Susceptibility* such as fluoride exposure and use, saliva secretion, and buffering capacity.
- *Circumstances* such as past caries experience, related diseases.

◆ Risk is displayed as a pie chart and the percentage of chance to avoid new caries is displayed as well as the contribution of each of the factors on the risk of new caries.

IV. Caries Management by Risk Assessment (CAMBRA®)

◆ CAMBRA® was developed following two consensus conferences beginning in 2003 in California. Large-scale pilot tests were conducted and the assessment form was modified and disseminated in 2007.[18]

◆ CAMBRA® has assessment forms for age 0–5 (see Chapter 47 for risk factors) and those age 6 through adult.

◆ The assessment includes the following categories of factors for ages 6 through adult (Table 25-1):

- *Disease indicators* (clinical observations) such as visible or radiographic caries, white spot lesions, restorations in last 3 years.
- *Risk factors* (biological predisposing factors) such as streptococci mutans and lactobacilli levels, visible

---

TABLE 25-1 • Caries Management by Risk Assessment (CAMBRA®)

RISK FACTORS AND MANAGEMENT GUIDELINES FOR PATIENTS AGE 6 AND OLDER

MANAGEMENT GUIDELINES	CAMBRA RISK LEVEL			
	LOW RISK	MODERATE RISK	HIGH RISK[a]	EXTREME RISK[b]
Risk factors	The number and extent or severity of risk factors are taken into consideration to determine an individual caries risk level for each patient.			
Social history	Dentally aware. Regularly scheduled dental visits. Low caries rate in family members.	Low knowledge of dental disease. Irregular or nonexistent dental visits. Family history of caries and generally poor oral health. Personal history of recreational drug use.		
Medical history	No serious medical problems. No or few medications. Normal salivary flow. No physical problems or handicaps.	Medically compromised. Disabled/handicapped. Xerostomia (side effect of medications or systemic disease). Radiation therapy.		
Use of fluoride	Drinks/cooks with fluoridated water. Lived in a fluoridated community as a child. Uses fluoride dentifrice and/or fluoride mouthrinse regularly.	Does not drink fluoridated water. Did not live in a fluoridated community as a child. Irregular or nonexistent use of fluoridated dentifrice or fluoride rinses. Irregular personal oral care habits.		
Dietary habits	Infrequent fermentable carbohydrate intake. Rarely snacks between meals. Avoids acidic beverages between meals. Uses xylitol gum or mints between meals	Frequent sugar intake. Snacks frequently. Not familiar with USDA MyPlate. Uses chewing tobacco frequently.		
Clinical/oral	Regular brushing at least 2× daily. Daily interdental cleansing. No prostheses, orthodontics, or other special care requirement. Good hand dexterity; no handicap. Low biofilm scores.	History of previous caries experience. Current cavitated lesions. Noncavitated (white) lesions. Multiple restorations. Unsealed deep pits and fissures. Exposed root surfaces; previously restored root surfaces.		

(Continues)

TABLE 25-1 • Caries Management by Risk Assessment (CAMBRA®) *(Continued)*

RISK FACTORS AND MANAGEMENT GUIDELINES FOR PATIENTS AGE 6 AND OLDER

MANAGEMENT GUIDELINES	CAMBRA RISK LEVEL			
	LOW RISK	MODERATE RISK	HIGH RISK[a]	EXTREME RISK[b]
Bitewing radiographs vertical bitewings for root caries	Every 24–36 mo	Every 18–24 mo	Every 6–18 mo	Every 6 mo until no cavitated lesions are observed.
Frequency of caries recall examination	Every 6 mo	Every 4–6 mo	Every 3–4 mo	Every 3 mo
Chemotherapeutic management	OTC (over the counter) fluoride dentifrice Optional NaF (sodium fluoride) varnish if root exposure or sensitivity	OTC fluoride toothpaste 0.05% NaF rinse daily Initial 1–2 application of NaF varnish, plus application at 4–6 mo recall	Fluoride varnish every 3–4 mo 1.1% NaF toothpaste used 2× daily 0.05% NaF rinse 2× daily	Fluoride varnish every 3 mo 1.1% NaF toothpaste used 2× daily 0.05% NaF rinse 2× daily
		Xylitol gum or candy 4× daily Optional: calcium phosphate topical paste if excessive root exposure	Initial 1–3 applications of NaF varnish, plus application at 3–4 mo recall Chlorhexidine rinse 1 min daily for 1 wk each mo Xylitol gum or candy 4× daily Optional: calcium phosphate topical paste	Initial 1–3 applications of NaF varnish, plus application at 3 mo recall Chlorhexidine rinse 1 min daily for 1 wk each mo Xylitol gum or candy 4× daily Acid-neutralizing rinses as needed if mouth feels dry Required: calcium phosphate topical paste 2× daily
Sealants	Optional	Recommended	Recommended	Recommended

[a]Patients with one or more cavitated lesions are assigned a *high* risk level.
[b]When xerostomia is present in addition to cavitated lesions, the *extreme* risk level is assigned.
Naf, sodium fluoride.
Source: Adapted with permission from Jenson L, Budnez AW, Featherstone JD, Ramos-Gomez FJ, Spolsky VW, Young DA. Clinical protocols for caries management by risk assessment. *J Calif Dent Assoc.* 2007;35(10):714-723.

plaque, frequent snacks, deep pits and fissures, recreational drug use, inadequate saliva flow, factors reducing saliva flow, exposed roots, and orthodontic appliances.
- *Protective factors* such as fluoridated water, toothpaste, mouthrinse, and topical fluoride application, chlorhexidine use, xylitol use, calcium and phosphate paste use, and adequate saliva flow.
◆ Risk levels were low, moderate, high, or extreme.

V. International Caries Classification and Management System (ICCMS™)

◆ ICCMS™ was developed through a consensus process by an international group of experts after review of the evidence.[19]

◆ The assessment includes the following factors:
  - Medical history such as prescribed and recreational drugs and conditions resulting in hyposalivation.
  - Head and neck radiation.
  - Sugary foods and beverages.
  - Low fluoride exposure.
  - Primary caregiver caries experience.
  - Oral hygiene behaviors and heavy plaque biofilm.
  - Socioeconomic status.
  - Caries experience and presence of active carious lesions.
  - Exposed root surfaces.
  - Oral appliances such as orthodontic retainers and partial dentures.
◆ The risk levels utilized by this system include low, medium, or high risk categories.

IMPLEMENTATION OF CRA IN THE PROCESS OF CARE

- The clinic or office must first identify which risk assessment system will be implemented.
- During review of the medical, dental, and psychosocial history (see Chapter 11), identify risk factors for caries such as medical conditions or medications that cause xerostomia.
  - Complete the portion of the risk assessment related to the medical, dental, and psychosocial history which should include diet assessment.
- The radiographic and clinical examination (see Chapters 13, 15–17 and 20) are used to assess some of the risk factors.
  - Some risk assessment systems require assessment of saliva and bacteria so this needs to be implemented at this point in the care process.
- Once the risk assessment is complete, using clinical judgment and the results of the risk assessment, the clinician needs to identify risk level and which risk factors are modifiable.
  - The modifiable risk factors are the ones to target for management when developing the treatment plan to reduce the risk of caries progression or development.

CARIES RISK MANAGEMENT SYSTEMS

Just as there are a number of CRA systems available, there are several caries risk management systems and a brief overview will be provided.

I. AAPD Caries Risk Management Protocol

- The AAPD protocol is based on evidence-based literature and judgment of an expert panel.[16]
- The protocol is based on risk and takes into account the level of patient/parent cooperation.
- The protocols are based on the age category of the child/adolescent and include the following:
  - Diagnostics: recommended frequency for radiographs and professional dental care.
  - Interventions: brushing frequency with fluoridated toothpaste, frequency of professional application of fluoride, use of fluoride supplements when appropriate, diet counseling, use of xylitol containing products, and sealants.
  - Restorative: active surveillance for progression of incipient lesions, restoration of cavitated lesions, and interim therapeutic restorations (when possible for very young children 1–3 years old).

II. Caries Management by Risk Assessment (CAMBRA®)

- The CAMBRA® recommendations were based on available evidence and developed by consensus of the Western CAMBRA Coalition.[20]

- The management protocol is based on risk level and clinical judgment of the clinician.
- The protocols vary based on risk level and may include the following (Table 25-1)[20]:
  - Diagnostics: frequency of radiographs, examinations, and preventive care.
  - Interventions: diet counseling, oral hygiene instruction, and use of fluoride rinses, sealants, bacterial testing, antimicrobial treatments such as chlorhexidine rinse, calcium phosphate paste, prescription fluorides, baking soda rinses, and xylitol products.
  - Restorative: glass ionomer resins, early minimally invasive for those at high risk to delay invasive restorative treatment.
- Research suggests patients who are compliant with recommendations based on their level of risk show a statistically significant reduction in caries.[18]

III. International Caries Classification and Management System (ICCMS™)

- The International Caries Detection and Assessment System (ICDAS™) and ICCMS™ systems are based on extensive critical analyses of the literature and consensus from a global group of experts.[19]
- The ICCMS is a systematic guide for the critical decisions clinicians need to make to develop a management plan based on caries risk.[20]
- The protocols vary by risk level and may include the following (see Figure 25-3)[20]:
  - Diagnostics: frequency of exams and professional preventive care.
  - Interventions: oral self-care, dietary counseling to reduce frequency of intake of fermentable carbohydrates, fluoridated toothpaste, fluoride varnish, high-dose fluoride pastes, that is, 5,000 ppm F, sealants, glass ionomer resins, and chlorhexidine.
  - Restorative: POP (tooth preserving operative procedures).

PLANNING CARE FOR THE PATIENT'S CARIES RISK LEVEL

- The dental hygienist is challenged to select a caries management strategy to meet the needs of each individual patient.
- The care plan will not only need to provide for treatment of existing nonreversible carious lesions but also provide a framework for changes in personal care previously unrecognized by the patient to prevent development of new lesions.
  - Dental carious lesions contain large numbers of acidogenic and aciduric bacteria, especially mutans streptococci and lactobacilli. Cavitated carious lesions need to be restored or bacteria from within the lesion will remain a source of infection.

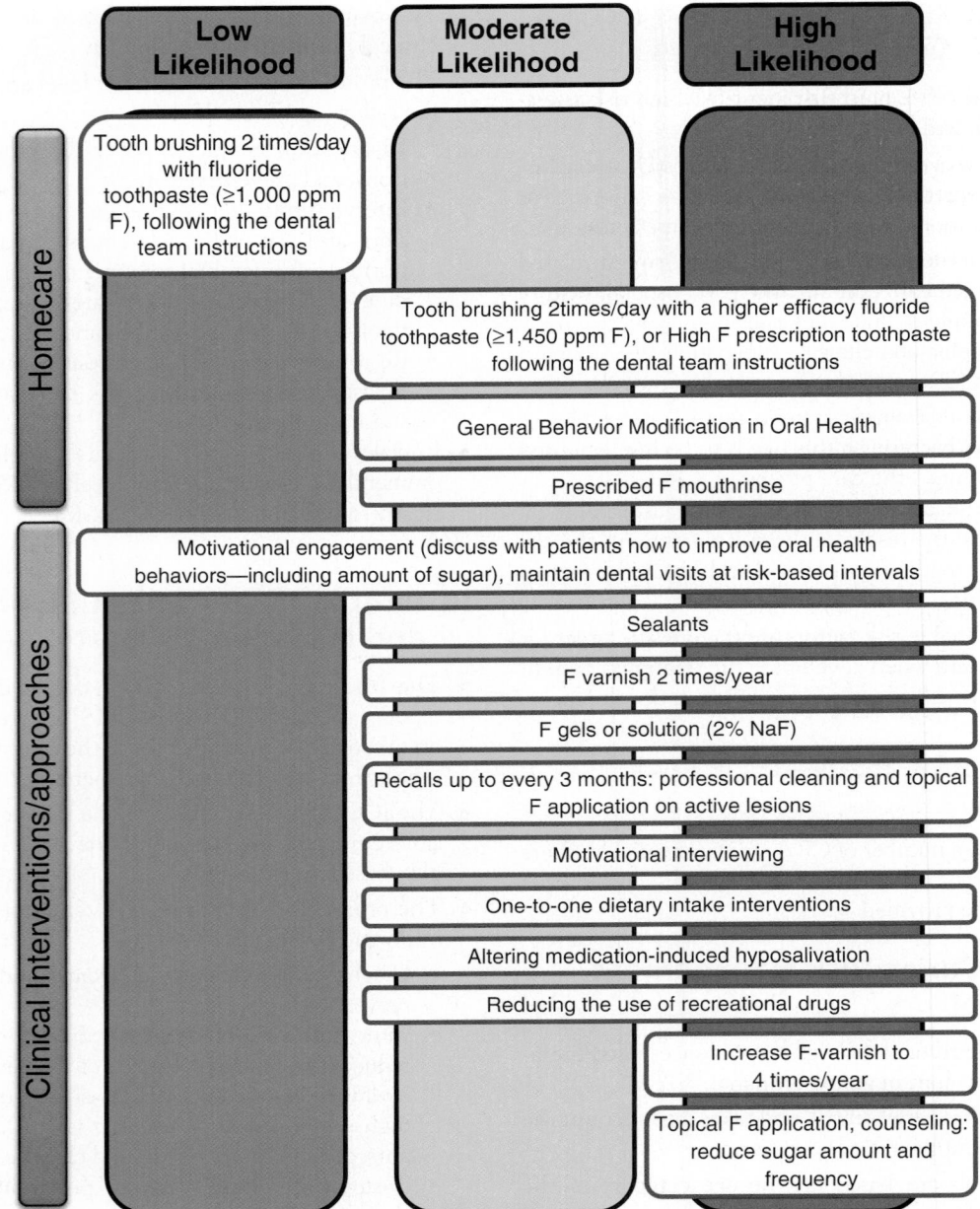

FIGURE 25-3 • ICCMS™ Caries Management System. Provides caries management strategy by risk level. (Adapted from Pitts NB, Ismail AI, Martignon S, Ekstrand K, Douglas GVA, Longbottom C; and ICDAS Foundation. ICCMS International Caries Classification and Management System (ICCMS) guide for practitioners and educators. https://www.iccms-web.com /uploads/asset/59284654c0a6f822230100.pdf. Published December 2014. Accessed July 4, 2019).

- Restorative materials containing fluoride are recommended wherever possible.
- Family members can continue to harbor cariogenic microorganisms so having close family members address carious lesions will further reduce individual exposure to these pathogens.[21]
- A plan for care is individualized depending on the disease risk level, physical and cognitive abilities, and patient or parent desire to change.
- It is essential to partner with the patient in setting goals and planning care as discussed in Chapter 24 in order to create a successful caries management plan.

I. The Patient with Low Caries Risk

- Primary prevention remains a top priority, as changes in habits may increase caries risk.
- Provide the patient with positive feedback and education so oral, periodontal, and dental health can be maintained.
- Review with the patient the existing habits that categorize them at *low caries risk*, such as good oral daily biofilm removal, healthy snacking habits, normal salivary flow, and daily exposure to fluoridated toothpaste and/or fluoridated water supply.
- Recommend routine continuing care appointments.

II. The Patient with Moderate Caries Risk

- This patient exhibits factors increasing their risk for developing dental carious lesions.
- Provide the patient with positive feedback and support for the protective factors they currently exhibit, such as fluoride use, healthy snacking habits, or sugar-free chewing gum use.[19,20]
- Motivational interviewing engages the patient in choosing behavior changes to increase compliance and success in reducing caries.[18,19]
- Work with the patient to guide them to reduce risk factors, such as acidic beverages, frequent fermentable carbohydrate snacks, and improved daily biofilm removal.
- Increase protective factors such as use of xylitol gum or mints, calcium phosphate paste, prescription fluoride rinse or gel.[18,19]
- Discuss addition of caries-preventive foods to diet, such as nuts, sugar-free yogurt, cheese.[22]
- Increasing protective factors can be accomplished by the dental hygienist especially application of fluoride varnish and sealant placement.[19,20]
  - Properly placed sealants close off the pits and fissures where microorganisms can live, multiply, and contribute to carious lesion development. Microorganisms cannot survive under a properly placed sealant.
- Recommend appropriate continuing care schedule.

III. The Patient with High and Extreme Caries Risk

The patient at high risk for caries displays *active carious* lesions, has a *recent history of restoration* to repair carious lesions, or may have *medications or systemic factors* that cause severe dry mouth (patients who are at high risk and also suffer from dry mouth are categorized as extreme risk).

- Improved biofilm removal.
- Dietary counseling to reduce intake of acidic foods and fermentable carbohydrates.
- Xylitol products such as gum, mints, or candy.[20,23,24]
  - Xylitol reduces levels of mutans streptococci and promotes remineralization.[24]
- Bacterial infection can be reduced and controlled with daily biofilm removal and antimicrobial therapy such as chlorhexidine mouthrinse 1 week each month.[20]
- Initial one to three fluoride varnish application followed by application once every 3–4 months.[19,20]

CONTINUING CARE

Continuing care appointments include the following:
- Biofilm control assessment: Use disclosing agent and record the biofilm score. Address oral self-care issues.
- Reassess caries risk.
- Clinical detection for demineralization areas, need for sealants, and poor margins on restorations.
- Radiographs prescribed as indicated by level of risk and clinical findings.
- Assess patient compliance with caries management recommendations.
- Determine changes needed in caries management protocol.

DOCUMENTATION

CRA, risk level, and compliance with management protocols are documented at each continuing care visit.

Thorough documentation includes assessment results, collaboration with the patient, health promotion education, and evaluation of patient attainment of goals at each appointment.

- Initial planning: Record all instructions and survey report from the analysis of risk factors.
- Note specific oral self-care and dietary changes recommended and progress in meeting goals.
- Note any phone or e-mail follow-up messages.
- At continuing care, note patient comments on individual efforts, likes and dislikes, successes, and changes that can be made to improve success.
- Set new goals.
- A sample of documentation can be found in Box 25-1.

BOX 25-1
Example Documentation: Patient with High Caries Risk

S—Admits drinking in the afternoon while studying. Chews lots of gum containing sugar. Brushes twice daily, but admits to flossing only a couple of times a week. Snacks frequently.

O—Resting pH—7.2; CRA—moderate. Moderate generalized biofilm in embrasures on disclosing with plaque-free score of 50%.

A—Increased risk for dental caries.

P—Recommended patient drink soda only during meals and sip fluoridated water while studying, chew sugar-free or xylitol gum, and use 1.1% sodium fluoride gel or paste daily. Discussed alternatives to flossing. Demonstrated interdental brushes. Pt. liked interdental brushes and said he would try to use them daily while studying. Reassess at 6 month continuing care visit.

Signed: _____, RDH

Date: _____

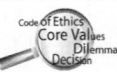

EVERYDAY ETHICS

Sophie and Helen were two sisters who had been Dr. Newbury's patients for the past 30 years. Now in their seventies, they were experiencing new concerns with restorations and crowns that showed signs of occlusal wear and recurrent caries. Many margins of amalgam restorations had catches with the explorer upon examination.

Ken, the dental hygienist, continued to stress the importance of more frequent continuing care visits, but Sophie curtly reminded him that she "has been coming to the dentist since before he was born!" Ken suspected they did not want to hear about crowns that should be replaced or make decisions about the restorations that needed replacement.

A progress note in Helen's chart read, "the patient was not open to new homecare education techniques or interested in a proposed treatment plan to replace amalgam restorations in teeth 15, 18, 19, 30, and 31."

Questions for Consideration

1. What ethical principles and dental hygiene Core Values are involved as Ken thinks about how to help these patients understand the need for treatment that they have stated they do not want?

2. Does the entry in the patient's chart provide sufficient information to document informed refusal? Why or why not? Explain your rationale using legal and ethical concepts.

3. Consult the Decision Alternatives through Questioning steps in Section VI to determine at least two alternative approaches Ken might pursue in order to deliver a professional standard of care for these patients without compromising their rights.

Factors to Teach the Patient

▶ What causes and process of caries development.

▶ Explain to the patient what demineralization means and how they can prevent it from progressing to a cavity that needs restoration.

▶ How remineralization can be helped by using fluoride toothpaste and drinking fluoridated water daily.

▶ Use of appropriate fluoride based on risk for dental caries is necessary throughout life.

ENHANCE YOUR UNDERSTANDING

ONLINE RESOURCES
(see the inside front cover for access information)

• Audio glossary
• Appendices

SUPPORT FOR LEARNING
(available separately)

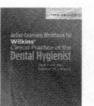

• *Active Learning Workbook for Wilkins' Clinical Practice of the Dental Hygienist, 13th Edition*

INDIVIDUALIZED REVIEW

• Customized practice quizzing with Navigate 2 TestPrep for *Wilkins' Clinical Practice of the Dental Hygienist*

References

1. Chankanka O, Cavanaugh JE, Levy SM, et al. Longitudinal associations between children's dental caries and risk factors. *J Public Health Dent.* 2011;71(4):289-300.

2. Beltrán-Aguilar ED, Barker L, Dye BA. Prevalence and severity of dental fluorosis in the United States, 1999–2004. *NCHS Data Brief.* 2010;(53):1-8.

3. Dye BA, Mitnik GL, Iafolla TJ, Vargas CM. Trends in dental caries in children and adolescents according to poverty status in the United States from 1999 through 2004 and from 2011 through 2014. *J Am Dent Assoc.* 2017;148(8):550-565.

4. Takahashi N, Nyvad, B. Caries ecology revisited: microbial dynamics and the caries process. *Caries Res.* 2008;42:409-418.

5. Featherstone JD. The science and practice of caries prevention. *J Am Dent Assoc.* 2000;131(7):887-899.

6. Palmer CA, Kent R Jr, Loo CY, et al. Diet and caries-associated bacteria in severe early childhood caries. *J Dent Res.* 2010;89(11):1224-1229.

7. Caufield PW, Cutter GR, Dasanayake AP. Initial acquisition of mutans streptococci by infants: evidence for a discrete window of infectivity. *J Dent Res.* 1993;72(1):37-45.

8. Lee JG, Messer LB. Intake of sweet drinks and sweet treats versus reported and observed caries experience. *Eur Arch Paediatr Dent.* 2010;11(1):5-17.

9. Marshall TA, Broffitt B, Eichenberger-Gilmore J, Warren JJ, Cunningham MA, Levy SM. The roles of meal, snack, and daily total food and beverage exposures on caries experience in young children. *J Public Health Dent.* 2005;65(3):166-173.

10. González-Cabezas C. The chemistry of caries: remineralization and demineralization events with direct clinical relevance. *Dent Clin North Am.* 2010;54:469-478.

11. Carpenter GH. The secretion, components, and properties of saliva. *Annu Rev Food Sci Technol.* 2013;4:267-276.

12. Featherstone JD. Prevention and reversal of dental caries: role of low level fluoride. *Community Dent Oral Epidemiol.* 1999;27(1):31-40.

13. International Caries Detection and Assessment System Foundation. International Caries Detection and Assessment System. 2017. https://www.iccms-web.com/content/icdas. Accessed July 4, 2019.

14. Young DA, Novy BB, Zeller GG, Hale R, Hart TC, Truelove EL; American Dental Association Council on Scientific Affairs. The American Dental Association Caries Classification System for clinical practice: a report of the American Dental Association Council on Scientific Affairs. *J Am Dent Assoc.* 2015;146(2):79-86.

15. Tellez M, Gomez J, Pretty I, Ellwood R, Ismail AI. Evidence on existing caries risk assessment systems: are they predictive of future caries? *Community Dent Oral Epidemiol.* 2013;41(1):67-78.

16. AAPD, Council of Clinical Affairs. Guideline on caries-risk assessment and management for infants, children, and adolescents. Reference Manual. 2014;37(6):15-16. http://www.aapd.org/media/Policies_Guidelines/G_CariesRisk Assessment.pdf. Accessed April 7, 2018.

17. Bratthall D, Petersson, GH, Stjernsward JR. Cariogram manual. 2014. https://www.mah.se/upload/FAKULTETER /OD/cariogram%20program%20caries/cariogmanual201net .pdf. Accessed April 8, 2018.

18. Featherstone JDB, Chaffee BW. The evidence for caries management by risk assessment (CAMBRA®). *Adv Dent Res.* 2018;29(1):9-14.

19. Ismail AI, Pitts NB, Tellez M, et al. The International Caries Classification and Management System (ICCMS™) An example of a caries management pathway. *BMC Oral Health.* 2015;15(suppl 1):S9.

20. Jenson L, Budenz AW, Featherstsone JD, Ramos-Gomez FJ, Spolsky VW, Young DA. Clinical protocols for caries management by risk assessment. *J Calif Dent Assoc.* 2007;35(10):714-723.

21. Childers NK, Momeni SS, Whiddon J, et al. Association between early childhood caries and colonization with *Streptococcus mutans* genotypes from mothers. *Pediatr Dent.* 2017;39(2):130-135.

22. Sönmez IS, Aras S. Effects of white cheese and sugarless yoghurt on dental plaque acidogenicity. *Caries Res.* 2007;41:208-211.

23. Hayes C. The effect of non-cariogenic sweeteners on the prevention of dental caries: a review of the evidence. *J Dent Educ.* 2001;65(10):1106-1109.

24. Janakiram C, Deepan Kumar CV, Joseph J. Xylitol in preventing dental caries: a systematic review and meta-analyses. *J Nat Sci Biol Med.* 2017;8(1):16-21.

26

Oral Infection Control: Toothbrushes and Toothbrushing

Christine R. Macarelli, RDH, MS, and Linda D. Boyd, RDH, RD, EdD

CHAPTER OUTLINE

DEVELOPMENT OF TOOTHBRUSHES
I. Origins of the Toothbrush
II. Early Toothbrushes

MANUAL TOOTHBRUSHES
I. Characteristics of an Effective Manual Toothbrush
II. General Description
III. Handle
IV. Brush Head
V. Filaments (or Bristles)

POWER TOOTHBRUSHES
I. Effectiveness
II. Purposes and Indications
III. Description

TOOTHBRUSH SELECTION FOR THE PATIENT
I. Influencing Factors
II. Toothbrush Characteristics
III. Stiffness of Filaments or Bristles

METHODS FOR MANUAL TOOTHBRUSHING

THE BASS AND MODIFIED BASS METHODS
I. Purposes and Indications
II. Procedure
III. Limitations

THE STILLMAN AND MODIFIED STILLMAN METHODS
I. Purposes and Indications
II. Procedure
III. Limitations

THE ROLL OR ROLLING STROKE METHOD
I. Purposes and Indications
II. Procedure
III. Limitations

CHARTERS METHOD
I. Purposes and Indications
II. Procedure
III. Limitations

THE HORIZONTAL (OR SCRUB) METHOD
I. Purposes and Indications
II. Procedure
III. Limitations

THE FONES (OR CIRCULAR) METHOD
I. Purposes and Indications
II. Procedure
III. Limitations

LEONARD'S (OR VERTICAL) METHOD
I. Purposes and Indications
II. Procedure
III. Limitations

METHOD FOR POWER TOOTHBRUSHING
I. Procedure
II. Limitations

SUPPLEMENTAL BRUSHING METHODS
I. Occlusal Brushing
II. Brushing Difficult-to-Reach Areas
III. Tongue Cleaning

GUIDELINES FOR TOOTHBRUSHING INSTRUCTIONS
I. Toothbrush Grasp
II. Brushing Sequence
III. Frequency of Brushing
IV. Duration of Brushing
V. Toothbrushing Force
VI. General Toothbrush Instruction

TOOTHBRUSHING FOR SPECIAL CONDITIONS
I. Acute Oral Inflammatory or Traumatic Lesions
II. Following Periodontal Surgery
III. Following Dental Extraction
IV. Oral Self-Care for the Neutropenic Patient

ADVERSE EFFECTS OF TOOTHBRUSHING
I. Soft Tissue Lesions
II. Hard Tissue Lesions
III. Bacteremia

CARE OF TOOTHBRUSHES
I. Supply of Brushes
II. Brush Replacement
III. Cleaning Toothbrushes
IV. Brush Storage

DOCUMENTATION

EVERYDAY ETHICS

FACTORS TO TEACH THE PATIENT

REFERENCES

LEARNING OBJECTIVES

After studying this chapter, the student will be able to:

1. Identify the characteristics of effective manual and power toothbrushes.
2. Differentiate between manual toothbrushing methods, including limitations and benefits of each.
3. Describe the different modes of action of power toothbrushes.
4. Identify the basis for power toothbrush selection.
5. Describe tongue cleaning and its effect on reducing dental biofilm.
6. Identify adverse effects of improper toothbrushing on hard and soft tissues.

The toothbrush has been the principal instrument in general use for oral care and is a necessary part of oral disease control.[1-4] There is a long history of development of toothbrushes since ancient times.

DEVELOPMENT OF TOOTHBRUSHES

I. Origins of the Toothbrush

- Evidence of toothbrushes has its origins in the Babylonian chew sticks in early 3500 BC.[5]
- The "chew stick," which has been considered the primitive toothbrush, appears in the Chinese literature around 1600 BC.[5]
  - Care of the mouth was associated with religious training and ritual: the Buddhists had a "toothstick," and the Mohammedans used the "miswak" or "siwak."
  - Chew sticks are made from various types of woods by crushing the end of a twig or root and spreading the fibers in a brushlike manner.
  - Miswaks are used in many African and Middle Eastern countries and evidence suggests[4] there are antimicrobial properties.[6]

II. Early Toothbrushes

- It is believed that the first toothbrush made of horse hair bristles was mentioned in the early Chinese literature around 1000 AD.[5]
- Pierre Fauchard in 1728 in *Le Chirurgien Dentiste* described many aspects of oral health. He was critical of the toothbrush made of horse's hair because it was too soft and advised the use of sponges to vigorously rub the teeth.[7]
- One of the earlier toothbrushes made in England was produced by William Addis about 1780.[8]
  - By the early 19th century, craftsmen in various European countries constructed handles of gold, ivory, or ebony in which replaceable brush heads could be fitted.
  - The first patent for a toothbrush in the United States was issued to HN Wadsworth in 1860.[9]
- In the early 1900s, celluloid began to replace bone handles.
- Nylon bristles were introduced by Dupont De Nemours in 1938.[10]

- World War II prevented Chinese export of wild boar bristles so synthetic materials were substituted for natural bristles.
- Since then, synthetic materials have improved and manufacturers' specifications standardized.
- Most toothbrushes are made exclusively of synthetic materials.
- The first power toothbrush to appear in the American market was a Broxodent in 1960.[10]

BOX 26-1

Historical Perspective on Proper Toothbrushing Instruction

Koecker, in 1842, wrote that after the dentist has scaled off the tartar, the patient will clean the teeth every morning and after every meal with a hard brush and an astringent powder. For the inner surfaces, he recommended a conical-shaped brush of fine hog's bristles. For the outer surfaces, he believed in an oblong brush made of the "best white horse-hair." He instructed the patient to press hard against the gums so the bristles go between the teeth and "between the edges of the gums and the roots of the teeth. The pressure of the brush is to be applied in the direction from the crowns of the teeth toward the roots, so that the mucus, which adheres to the roots under the edges of the gums, may be completely detached, and after that removed by friction in a direction toward the grinding surfaces."

Koecker L. Exhibiting a new method of treating the diseases of the teeth and gums. In: *Principles of Dental Surgery*. Baltimore, MD: American Society of Dental Surgeons; 1842:155-156.

MANUAL TOOTHBRUSHES

Little evidence exists related to the most effective characteristics of a toothbrush and other aspects of toothbrushing; so clinical experience and individual patient needs will guide recommendations.[11]

I. Characteristics of an Effective Manual Toothbrush

- Conforms to individual patient requirements in size, shape, and texture.
- Easily and efficiently manipulated.

◆ Readily cleaned and aerated; impervious to moisture.

◆ Durable and inexpensive.

◆ Soft bristles.[12]

◆ End-rounded filaments free of sharp or jagged edges.[12]

◆ Designed for utility, efficiency, and cleanliness.

◆ In the United States, look for the ADA (American Dental Association) Seal of Acceptance.[12]

II. General Description

A. Parts (Figure 26-1)

◆ *Handle*: the part grasped in the hand during toothbrushing.

◆ *Head*: the working end; consists of tufts of bristles or filaments.

◆ *Shank*: the section that connects the head and the handle.

B. Dimensions

◆ Recommendations in the literature and in different countries seem to vary.

◆ Generally the following should be considered in recommending a toothbrush to a patient[13]:

• Length of the brush head should cover two to three posterior teeth.

• Width of the toothbrush head should cover the intercuspal distance of the first molar.

◆ General recommendations from the ADA for dimensions include:

• *Total brush length*: about 15–19 cm (6–7.5 inches); junior and child sizes are shorter.

• *Head*: length of brushing plane, 25.4–31.8 mm (1–1.25 inches); width, 7.9–9.5 mm (5/16–3/8 inch).

• Bristle or filament height, 11 mm (7/16 inch).

III. Handle

A. Composition

◆ *Manufacturing specifications*: Most often a single type of plastic, or a combination of polymers.

◆ *Properties*: Combines durability, imperviousness to moisture, pleasing appearance, low cost, and sufficient maneuverability.

B. Shape

◆ Preferred characteristics

• Easy to grasp.

• Does not slip or rotate during use.

• No sharp corners or projections.

• Lightweight, consistent with strength.

◆ Variations

• A twist, curve, offset, or angle in the shank with or without thumb rests may assist the patient in adaptation of the brush to difficult-to-reach areas.

• A handle of larger diameter may be useful for patients with limited dexterity, such as children, aging patients, and those with a disability.

IV. Brush Head

A. Design

◆ *Length*: May be 5–12 tufts long and 3–4 rows wide.

◆ *Shape and size*: A variety of brush head shapes and sizes from rounded to tapered to angled are available.

◆ Arrangement of bristle tufts varies in configuration and angulation as shown in Figure 26-2.

B. Brushing Plane (Lateral Profile)

◆ *Length*: Range from filaments of equal lengths (flat planes) to those with variable lengths, such as rippled, scalloped, tapered, bi-level, multilevel, and angled (Figure 26-2).

◆ *Efficiency in biofilm removal*:

• Research results have been inconsistent on which type of bristle design is most effective at plaque removal, with some suggesting angled tufted designs remove more plaque than a conventional flat trim toothbrush design; however, some studies failed to find a significant difference between designs.[11,14]

• Ultimately, efficiency in cleaning the hard-to-reach areas, such as extension onto proximal surfaces, malpositioned teeth, or exposed root surfaces, depends on individual patient abilities and understanding.

V. Filaments (or Bristles)

◆ Most current toothbrushes have nylon filaments.

• The physical properties of natural bristles cannot be standardized.

• A comparison of natural bristles and synthetic filaments is reviewed in Table 26-1.

◆ Many manufacturers of synthetic filaments refer to filaments as "bristles" when communicating with consumers on the toothbrush package and in advertising.

• Dental professionals need to be aware that most manufacturers of toothbrushes today produce brushes using "synthetic filaments" but still refer to these as "bristles."

◆ Companies that produce a toothbrush with "natural bristles" may distinguish themselves by using the word "natural" in the product description.

◆ The bristle stiffness depends on the diameter and length of the filament.[4] Brushes designated as soft, medium, or hard may not be consistent between manufacturers.

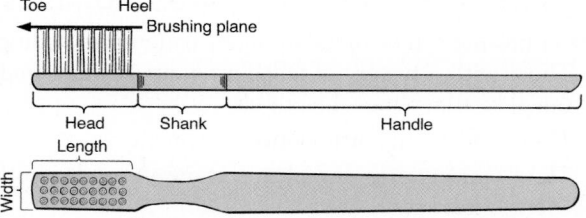

FIGURE 26-1 • Parts of a Toothbrush.

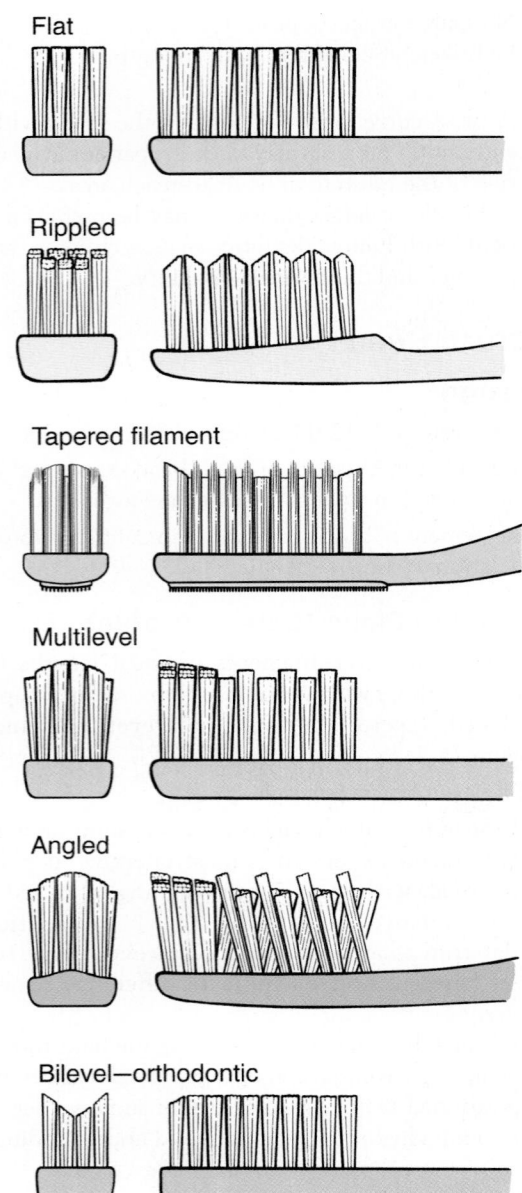

Flat

Rippled

Tapered filament

Multilevel

Angled

Bilevel—orthodontic

FIGURE 26-2 • Manual Brush Trim Profiles. A variety of filament profiles are available. In addition to the classic flat planed brush, other trims include the rippled, tapered filaments, bilevel, multilevel, and angled brushes. Brushes for use over orthodontic appliances are made with various bi-level shapes.

A. Filament or Bristle Design

◆ A variety of filament designs are available and may include, but are not limited to, end-rounded, feathered, and microfine, conical shaped.

◆ Another factor to keep in mind is that the quality of end-rounding varies in both adult and children's toothbrushes depending on the manufacturer.[15] Natural bristles cannot be end-rounded.

◆ Some evidence suggests end-rounded bristles are less abrasive to gingival damage than bristles that are non-end-rounded; however, the overall conclusion by a systematic review found the association of rounding of filaments (or bristles) to gingival recession to be inconclusive.[16]

◆ *Examples:* Figure 26-3 shows examples of non-rounded and end-rounded filaments.

POWER TOOTHBRUSHES

Power brushes are also known as power-assisted, automatic, mechanical, or electric brushes. The ADA Council on Scientific Affairs evaluates power brushes for the reduction of dental biofilm and gingivitis.[17]

I. Effectiveness

A. Evolution

◆ Current power brushes move at speeds and motions that cannot be duplicated by manual brushes.

◆ Power toothbrushes have evolved through time due to improved designs and features.

◆ Power toothbrushes of the 1960–1980 era mimicked the motions of manual brushing.

B. Power Toothbrushes versus Manual Toothbrushes

◆ There is moderate evidence that power toothbrushes result in a 10%–20% reduction in plaque and about a 10% reduction in gingivitis when compared to manual toothbrushes.[18]

◆ Rotating oscillating action power toothbrushes have been shown to be most effective than side-to-side power brushes for reducing plaque and gingivitis.[19,20]

◆ Sonic power toothbrushes have not been shown to be more effective over other types of power toothbrushes.[19,21,22]

◆ Power toothbrushes, as compared to their manual counterparts, do not damage gingival tissues as much; they may be less damaging because they have mechanisms to alert the patient when they apply excessive force.[4,11]

◆ Ultimately, recommendations are based on patient needs and preference.

II. Purposes and Indications

A. Purpose

◆ Recommended for physically able patients with ineffective manual biofilm removal techniques.

◆ To facilitate mechanical dental biofilm control or removal of food debris from the teeth and the gingiva.

◆ Reduce calculus and stain buildup.[23]

B. Indications for Use of Power Toothbrush

Power brushes can be useful for many patients, including:

◆ Those with a history of failed attempts at more traditional biofilm removal methods.

◆ Those undergoing orthodontic treatment.

◆ Those undergoing complex restorative and prosthodontic treatment.

TABLE 26-1 • Comparison of Natural Bristles and Synthetic Bristles or Filaments		
	NATURAL BRISTLES	BRISTLES/FILAMENTS
Source	Historically made from hair of hog or wild boar.	Synthetic, plastic materials, primarily nylon.
Uniformity	No uniformity of texture. Diameter or wearing properties depending upon the breed of the animal, geographical location, and season in which the bristles were gathered.	Uniformity controlled during manufacturing.
Diameter	Varies depending on portion of the bristle taken, age, and life of animal.	Ranges from extra soft at 0.075 mm (0.003 inch) to hard at 0.3 mm (0.012 inch).
End shape	Deficient, irregular, frequently open ended.	End-rounded.
Advantages and disadvantages	Cannot be standardized. Wears rapidly and irregularly. Hollow ends allow microorganisms and debris to collect inside.	• Rinse clean, dry rapidly. Durable and maintained longer. End-rounded and closed, repel debris and water. • More resistant to accumulation of microorganisms.

◆ Aggressive brushers: tendency to use less force or pressure when using a power brush than with a manual brush.
  • Many models of power toothbrushes will shut off automatically if too much pressure is applied during brushing, which can be a benefit for those who have a tendency to apply too much pressure.[4,11]
◆ Patients with disabilities or limited dexterity.
  • The large handle of a power brush can be of benefit.
  • Handle weight needs to be considered for these patients.
◆ When a parent or caregiver must brush for the patient.

III. Description

A. Motion

The motion of the head of power toothbrushes varies between models and may include one or more of the following (Table 26-2)[12]:

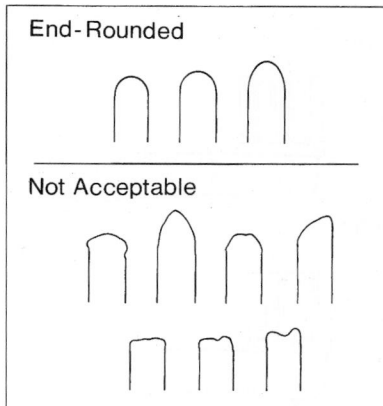

FIGURE 26-3 • **End-Rounded Filaments.** Examples of the shape of acceptable end-rounding and of those that are not acceptable are shown. (Adapted from Silverstone LM, Featherstone MJ. A scanning electron microscope study of the end rounding of bristles in eight toothbrush types. *Quintessence Int.* 1988;19(2):87-107 and Checchi L, Minguzzi S, Franchi M, et al. Toothbrush filaments end-rounding: stereomicroscope analysis. *J Clin Periodontol.* 2001;28(4):360-364.)

◆ Rotation oscillation.
◆ Counter oscillation.
◆ Sonic or ultrasonic motion.
◆ Side to side.
◆ Circular.

B. Speeds

◆ Vary from low to high.
◆ Generally, power brushes with replaceable batteries move slower than those with rechargeable batteries and have been shown to be less effective in plaque biofilm removal.[22]
◆ Movement per minute varies from 3,800 to over 48,000 depending on the manufacturer and type (battery, sonic, or ultrasonic).

TABLE 26-2 • Power Toothbrush Motions	
MOTION	DESCRIPTION
Rotational	Moves in a 360° circular motion.
Counterrotational	Each tuft of filaments moves in rotational motion; each tuft moves counter-directional to the adjacent tuft.
Oscillating	Rotates from center to the left, then to the right; degree of rotation varies from 25° to 55°.
Pulsating	When brush head is on the tooth, direct pulsations toward the interproximal.
Cradle or twist	Side to side with an arc.
Side to side	Side to side perpendicular to the long axis of the brush handle.
Translating	Up and down parallel to the long axis of the brush handle.
Combination	Combination of simultaneous yet different type of movement.
Ultrasonic	Brush head vibrates at ultrasonic frequency (>250 kHz).

C. Brush Head Design

◆ *Adult*: The variety of shapes continues to evolve, but a few examples are illustrated in Figure 26-4. They may be small and round, or like traditional manual heads. Trim profiles include flat, bi-level, rippled, or angled.

◆ *Child*: A child's power brush head should be specially designed to accommodate a smaller mouth, as shown in Figure 26-5.

D. Filaments or Bristles

◆ Made of soft, end-rounded nylon.

◆ Diameters: from extra soft, 0.075 mm (0.003 inch), to soft, 0.15 mm (0.006 inch).

E. Types of Power Source

◆ *Direct*

• Utilize an electrical outlet.

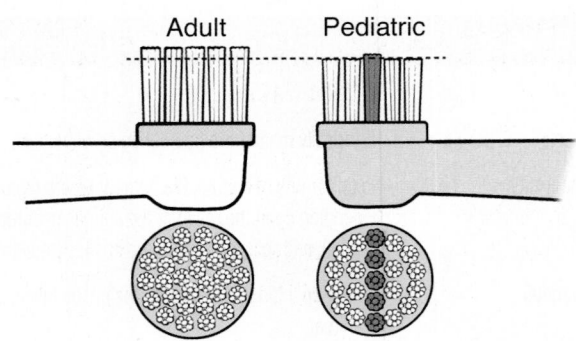

FIGURE 26-5 • Child Power Brush Profile. Power brushes for children could necessitate smaller head sizes and shorter filaments to allow for distal reach in tight posterior areas. Raised blue filaments allow for better access to occlusal pits and fissures.

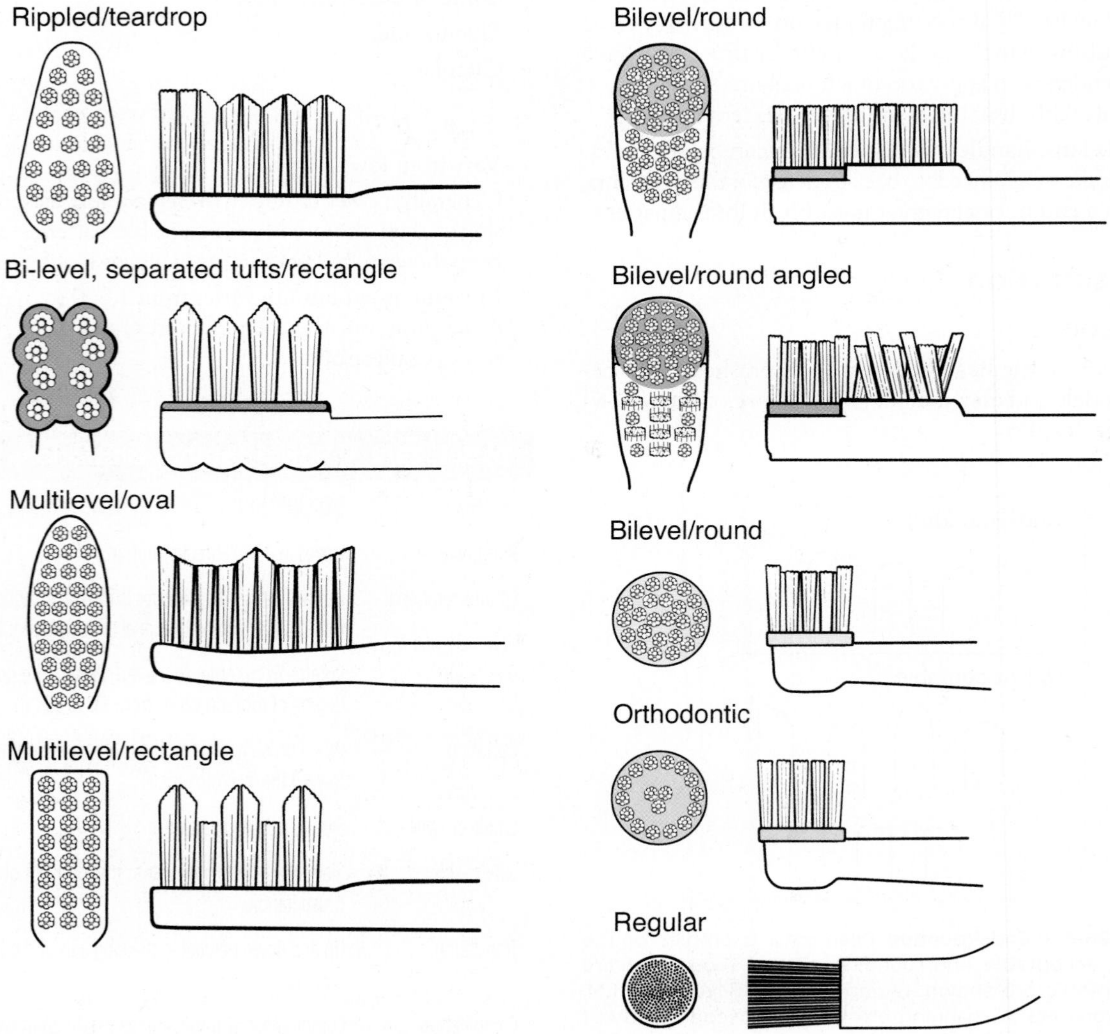

Rippled/teardrop

Bi-level, separated tufts/rectangle

Multilevel/oval

Multilevel/rectangle

Bilevel/round

Bilevel/round angled

Bilevel/round

Orthodontic

Regular

FIGURE 26-4 • Power Brush Trim Profiles. Power brushes are made in a variety of brush head shapes, such as oval, teardrop, rectangular, and round. Some power brushes have two different-shaped heads on the same brush. In addition, there are a variety of brush head trims on power brushes, including flat, bi-level, and multilevel.

◆ *Replaceable batteries*
  • Relatively inexpensive and convenient.
  • As most batteries lose their power, brush speed is reduced.
  • Advise patients to select a brush that has a water-tight handle to avoid corrosion of batteries.
◆ *Rechargeable*
  • Rechargeable, non-replaceable battery.
  • Recharges via a stand connected to an electrical outlet.
◆ *Disposable*
  • Batteries cannot be replaced or recharged.

TOOTHBRUSH SELECTION FOR THE PATIENT

Overarching factors in toothbrush selection include the quality of clinical research supporting the efficacy and safety of the brush and the ADA Seal of Approval along with the clinical decision making of the clinician regarding what is best for an individual patient.

I. Influencing Factors

Factors influencing the selection of a proper manual or power toothbrush for an individual patient include the following:

A. Patient
◆ Ability of the patient to use the brush and remove dental biofilm from tooth surfaces without damage to the soft tissue or tooth structure.
◆ Manual dexterity of the patient.
◆ The age of the patient and the differences in dentition and dexterity.

B. Gingiva
◆ Status of gingival and periodontal health.
◆ Anatomic configurations of the gingiva.

C. Position of Teeth
◆ Crowded teeth.
◆ Open contacts.

D. Compliance
◆ Patient preference may dictate which brush is recommended.
◆ Patient may have preferences and may resist change.
◆ Patient may lack motivation, ability, or willingness to follow the prescribed procedure.

E. Specific Factors to Consider for Selection of Power Toothbrush
◆ Replaceable brush head.
◆ Features that include a timer and pressure sensor.
◆ Patient affordability.

◆ Battery-operated models are often less expensive and may be a good way for the patient to try out a power toothbrush before investing in a more expensive rechargeable model.

II. Toothbrush Characteristics

◆ Brush head selection is dependent on the patient's ability to maneuver and adapt the brush correctly to all facial, lingual, palatal, and occlusal surfaces for dental biofilm removal.
◆ Some research suggests angled tufted designs of manual toothbrush heads and rotating, oscillating round power brush heads are most effective.[14,19]

III. Stiffness of Filaments or Bristles

◆ Toothbrush bristles are typically classified as hard, medium, soft, or extra soft.
  • The same classification for stiffness, that is, soft, may vary between manufacturers.[24]
◆ Filaments must have adequate stiffness to remove plaque biofilm and do no harm to oral soft and hard tissues.
◆ Despite beliefs that a soft toothbrush is more effective, more recent research suggests plaque biofilm removal may be significantly better with a medium toothbrush.[25] However, the ADA recommends a soft bristle toothbrush.[12]
◆ Tooth abrasion and/or gingival abrasion and gingival recession are multifactorial even though they are often attributed solely to the failure to use a soft toothbrush.[11]
  • Factors include anatomical features (e.g., tooth position and crowding), toothbrushing technique, frequency, duration, force (pressure), and self-inflicted gingival trauma, which points to the need to individualize recommendations.[26]
◆ An extra soft toothbrush may be indicated in conditions such as necrotizing ulcerative or following periodontal surgery.

METHODS FOR MANUAL TOOTHBRUSHING

The ideal toothbrushing technique is one that the patient can perform effectively to remove plaque biofilm while avoiding any damage to hard and soft oral tissues. Research on which method is better remains limited (see Box 26-1 for a historical perspective on proper toothbrushing instruction). However, hands-on instruction with the patient leads to improvement in their brushing methods.[27,28]
◆ Without instruction, normal brushing may consist of vigorous horizontal, vertical, and/or circular strokes.[28]
◆ Manual toothbrushing methods include the following:
  • Sulcular: modified Bass.
  • Roll: rolling stroke, modified Stillman.
  • Vibratory: Stillman, Charters, Bass.
  • Horizontal (or scrub).
  • Circular: Fones.
  • Vertical: Leonard.

THE BASS AND MODIFIED BASS METHODS

The Bass and modified Bass methods are widely accepted as an effective method for dental biofilm removal adjacent to and directly beneath the gingival margin (sulcus) despite conflicting evidence.[11,28,29] It is considered to be a type of sulcular brushing. The areas at the gingival margin and in the col are the most significant in the control of gingival and periodontal infections.

I. Purposes and Indications

◆ Dental biofilm removal adjacent to and directly beneath the gingival margin.

◆ Open embrasures, cervical areas beneath the height of contour of the enamel, and exposed root surfaces.

◆ Adaptation to abutment teeth or implants, under the gingival border of a fixed partial denture.

II. Procedure

A. Position the Brush[30]

◆ Direct the filaments apically (up for maxillary, down for mandibular teeth).

◆ First, position the sides of the filaments parallel with the long axis of the tooth (Figure 26-6A).

◆ From that position, turn the brush head toward the gingival margin to make approximately a 45° angle to the long axis of the tooth (Figure 26-6B).

◆ Direct the filament tips into the gingival sulcus (Figure 26-6A and B).

B. Strokes[24,30]

◆ Press lightly so the filament tips enter the gingival sulci and embrasures and cover the gingival margin. Do not bend the filaments with excess pressure.

◆ Vibrate the brush back and forth with very short strokes without disengaging the tips of the filaments from the sulci.

◆ Count at least 10 vibrations.

◆ In the modified Bass method, the vibratory, sulcular brush stroke is followed by rolling the toothbrush down over the crown of the tooth to clean the rest of the tooth surface.

C. Reposition the Brush

Apply the brush to the next group of two or three teeth. Take care to overlap placement, as shown in Figure 26-7.

D. Repeat Stroke

The entire stroke (steps A–C) is repeated at each position around the maxillary and mandibular arches, on both facial and lingual tooth surfaces.

E. Position Brush for Lingual and Palatal Anterior Surfaces

Tilt the brush handle somewhat vertically for the anterior components (Figure 26-6D).[12] The bristles are directed into the sulci.

III. Limitations

◆ The toothbrush bristles extend only 0.9 mm below the gingival margin so plaque removal in the sulcus is limited.[31]

◆ An individual who is an aggressive brusher may interpret "very short strokes" into a vigorous horizontal

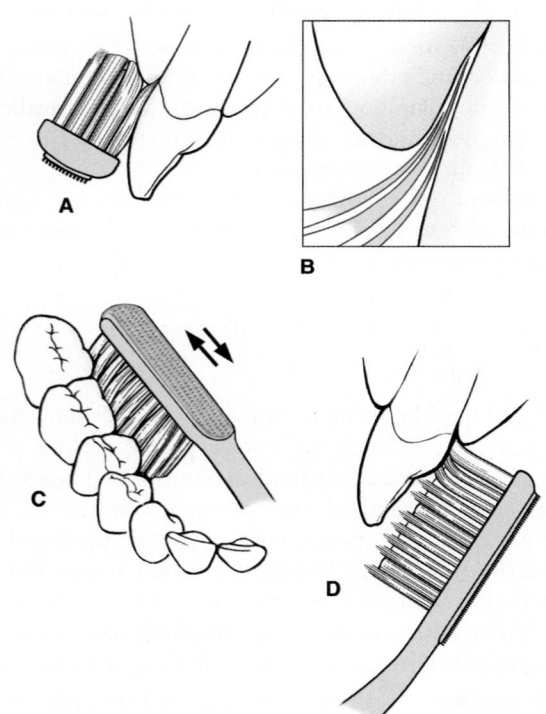

FIGURE 26-6 • Bass/Modified Bass Method of Brushing. A: Filament tips are directed into the gingival sulcus at approximately 45° to the long axis of the tooth. **B:** Brushes designed with tapered filaments reach below the gingival margin with ease. **C:** Brush in position for lingual surfaces of mandibular posterior teeth. **D:** Position for palatal surface of maxillary anterior teeth.

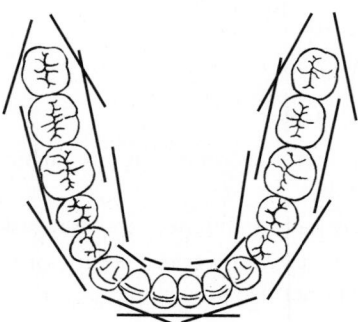

FIGURE 26-7 • Brushing Positions. Each brush position, as represented by a black line, will overlap the previous position. Note placement at canines, where the distal aspect of the canine is brushed with the premolars and the mesial aspect is brushed with the incisors. Short lines on the lingual anterior aspect indicate a brush placed vertically. The maxillary teeth require a similar number of brushing positions.

scrubbing motion causing injury to the gingival margin.

♦ Dexterity requirement for the vibratory stroke may be difficult for certain patients.

THE STILLMAN AND MODIFIED STILLMAN METHODS

The modified Stillman method is considered a sulcular brushing technique along with the modified Bass method.

I. Purposes and Indications

♦ As originally described by Stillman,[32] the method is designed for massage and stimulation, as well as for cleaning the cervical areas. The modified Stillman method adds a rolling stroke to the vibratory stroke to clean the crown of the tooth.[33]

♦ Dental biofilm removal from cervical areas below the height of contour of the crown and from exposed proximal surfaces.

♦ General application for cleaning tooth surfaces and massage of the gingiva.

II. Procedure[32]

A. Position the Brush

♦ *Place side of brush on the attached gingiva*: The filaments are directed apically (up for maxillary, down for mandibular teeth) in Figure 26-8A. When the plastic portion of the brush head is in level with the occlusal or incisal plane, generally the brush is at the proper height, as shown in Figure 26-7A.

♦ The brush ends are placed partly on the gingiva and partly on the cervical areas of the tooth and directed slightly apically.

B. Strokes

♦ *Press to flex the filaments*: The sides of the filaments are pressed lightly against the gingiva, blanching of the tissue occurs (Figure 26-8B).

♦ *Angle the filaments*: Turn the handle by rotating the wrist so that the filaments are directed at an angle of approximately 45° with the long axis of the tooth.

♦ *Activate the brush*: Use a slight rotary motion. Maintain light pressure on the filaments, and keep the tips of the filaments in position on the tooth surface. Count to 10 slowly as the brush is vibrated by a rotary motion of the handle.

♦ *Roll and vibrate the brush*: Turn the wrist and work the vibrating brush slowly down over the gingiva and tooth. Make some of the filaments reach interdentally (Figure 26-8C).

C. Replace Brush for Repeat Stroke

Reposition the brush by rotating the wrist. Avoid dragging the filaments back over the free gingival margin by holding the brush out, slightly away from the tooth.

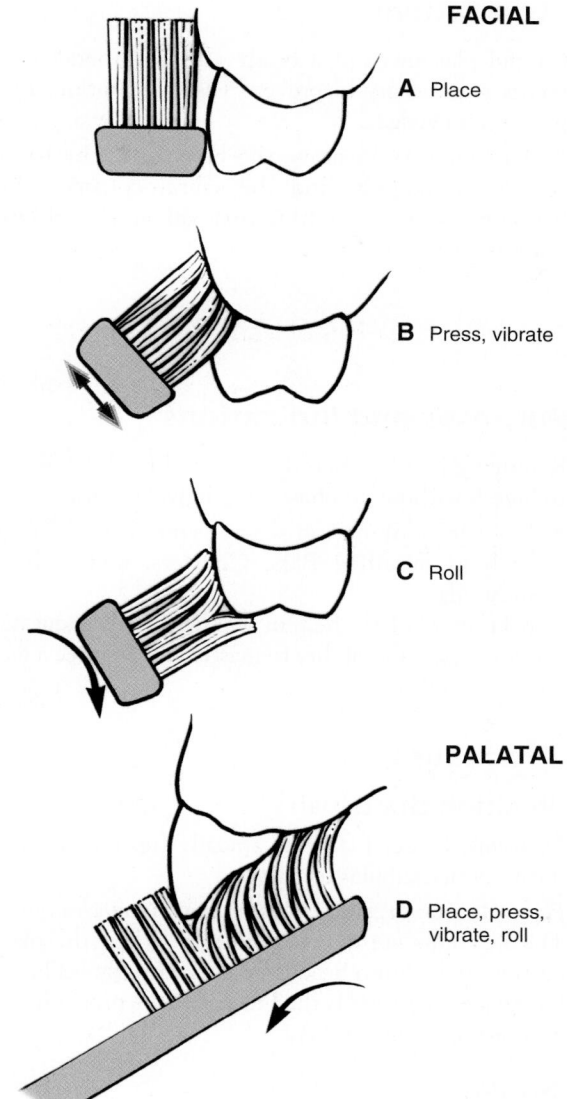

FACIAL

A Place

B Press, vibrate

C Roll

PALATAL

D Place, press, vibrate, roll

FIGURE 26-8 • Modified Stillman Method of Brushing. A: Initial brush placement with sides of bristles or filaments against the attached gingiva. **B:** The brush is pressed and angled, then vibrated. **C:** Vibrating is continued as the brush is rolled slowly over the crown. **D:** Using the toe of the brush, place the bristles into the gingival sulcus of the maxillary anterior teeth, press lightly, vibrate the bristles, and use a rolling stroke to clean the remainder of the lingual surface. Repeat for each anterior tooth and for the mandibular teeth.

D. Repeat Stroke Five Times or More

The entire stroke (steps A–C) is repeated at least five times for each tooth or group of teeth. When moving the brush to an adjacent position, overlap the brush position.

E. Position Brush for Anterior Lingual and Palatal Surfaces

♦ Position the brush somewhat vertically using the toe of the brush head for the anterior components (Figure 26-8D).

♦ Press and vibrate, roll, and repeat.

III. Limitations

- Careful placement of a brush with end-rounded filaments is necessary to prevent tissue laceration. Light pressure is needed.
- Patient may try to move the brush into the rolling stroke too quickly, and the vibratory aspect may be ineffective for biofilm removal at the gingival margin.

THE ROLL OR ROLLING STROKE METHOD

I. Purposes and Indications

- Removing biofilm, materia alba, and food debris from the teeth without emphasis on gingival sulcus.
  - Used in conjunction with a vibratory technique such as modified Bass, Charters, and Stillman methods.
- Can be particularly helpful when there is a question about the patient's ability to master and practice a more complex method.

II. Procedure[34]

A. Position the Brush

- *Filaments:* Direct filaments apically (up for maxillary, down for mandibular teeth).
- *Place side of brush parallel to and against the attached gingiva:* The filaments are directed apically. When the plastic portion of the brush head is in level with the occlusal or incisal plane, generally the brush is at the proper height, as shown in Figure 26-8A.

B. Strokes

- *Press to flex the filaments:* The sides of the filaments are pressed lightly against the gingiva. The gingiva will blanch.
- *Roll the brush slowly over the teeth:* As the brush is rolled, the wrist is turned slightly. The filaments remain flexed and follow the contours of the teeth, thereby permitting cleaning of the cervical areas. Some filaments may reach interdentally.

C. Replace and Repeat Five Times or More

- *Repeat the entire stroke:* The entire stroke (steps A and B) is repeated at least five times for each tooth or group of teeth.
- *Rotate the wrist:* When the brush is removed and repositioned, the wrist is rotated.
- *Stretch the cheek:* The brush is moved away from the teeth, and the cheek is stretched facially with the back of the brush head. Be careful not to drag the filament tips over the gingival margin when the brush is returned to the initial position.

D. Overlap Strokes

When moving the brush to an adjacent position, overlap the brush position, as shown in Figure 26-8.

E. Position Brush for Anterior Lingual or Palatal Surfaces

- Tilt the brush slightly vertically and use the toe of the brush head to access the lingual surfaces of the anterior teeth.
- Press (down for maxillary, up for mandibular) until the filaments lie flat against the teeth and gingiva.
- Press and roll (curve up for mandibular, down for maxillary teeth).
- Replace and repeat five times for each brush width.

III. Limitations

- Brushing too high during initial placement can lacerate the alveolar mucosa.
- Minimal plaque removal interproximally or in sulcular areas.
- Tendency to use quick, sweeping strokes results in failure to adequately remove plaque biofilm from the cervical third of the tooth because the brush tips pass over rather than into the area; likewise for the interproximal areas.

CHARTERS METHOD

Charters strongly believed in prevention and felt dentists were not doing their "full duty" if they were not taking the time to teach patients a system of home care.[35] He advocated for personal demonstration of techniques by the patient. Charters felt particularly strongly about teaching children proper home care and even went so far as to recommend it to be a part of the curriculum in schools.[35]

I. Purposes and Indications

- Loosen debris and dental biofilm.[35]
- Stimulate marginal and interdental gingiva.[35]
- Aid in biofilm removal from proximal tooth surfaces when interproximal tissue is missing creating open embrasures, for example, following periodontal surgery.[35]
- Remove dental biofilm from abutment teeth and under the gingival border of a fixed partial denture (bridge) or implant-supported bridge or partial denture.

II. Procedure[35]

A. Position the Brush

- *Filaments:* Direct bristles at 90° angle to the teeth.
- *Place side of brush at right angles* (90°) to the long axis of the teeth (Figure 26-9B).
- Note the contrast with position for the Stillman method (Figure 26-9A).

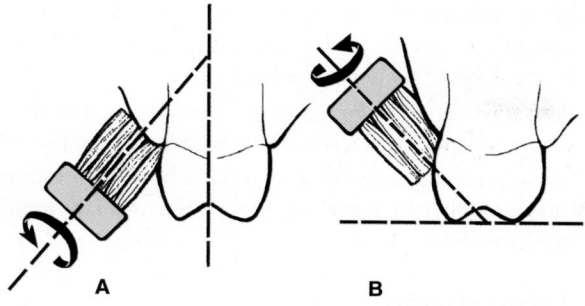

FIGURE 26-9 • Stillman and Charters Methods Compared.
A: Stillman: The brush is angled at approximately 45° to the long axis of the tooth. **B:** Charters: The brush is angled at approximately 45° to the occlusal plane, with brush tips directed toward the occlusal or incisal surfaces.

B. Strokes

◆ *Press the bristles gently between the teeth* being careful not to injure the gingiva.
◆ With the bristles between the teeth, use as little pressure as possible and *make three to four small rotary movements with the bristles.*
   • The sides of the bristles should come into contact with the gingival margin to massage or stimulate them.
◆ Remove the brush from the interproximal area and move to the next area.

C. Reposition the Brush and Repeat

Repeat steps A and B, as described, three to four times in each area on the maxillary and mandibular arches.

D. Overlap Strokes

Move the distance of one embrasure and repeat the process to overlap strokes.

III. Limitations

◆ Brush ends do not engage the gingival sulcus to disturb subgingival bacterial accumulations.
◆ In some areas, the correct brush placement is limited or impossible; modifications become necessary, consequently adding to the complexity of the procedure.

THE HORIZONTAL (OR SCRUB) METHOD

I. Purposes and Indications

◆ A systematic review suggested the most effective method for toothbrushing in children is the horizontal method up to the age of 6 or 7 years.[36]
◆ Once the child reaches the late mixed dentition stage, modification to another technique can be initiated as the horizontal method has limitations in terms of thorough plaque biofilm removal.

II. Procedure

A. Position the Toothbrush

◆ *Filaments:* Direct bristles at right angle to the tooth.
◆ *Place toothbrush head at a 90° angle to the long axis of the teeth* on both buccal and lingual posterior surfaces.
◆ For anterior teeth, the head of the *toothbrush is held parallel to the long axis of the tooth* and the toe of the brush is used.

B. Stroke

◆ *Bristles are moved in gentle back and forth motion on the posterior surfaces,* buccal, lingual, and occlusal.
◆ *Bristles are moved in an up and down motion on the anterior teeth* using the toe of the toothbrush.

III. Limitations

◆ Although this method can remove plaque biofilm on buccal and lingual surfaces, it does not reach interproximal areas.[29]
◆ There are also concerns about this method resulting in cervical abrasion if excessive pressure along with an abrasive toothpaste is used in adults.[11]

THE FONES (OR CIRCULAR) METHOD

I. Purpose and Indications

◆ This method is easy for children to learn.

II. Procedure

◆ *Place toothbrush at 90° to the long axis of the teeth,* buccal and lingual, and press bristles gently against the teeth.

A. Stroke

◆ *Bristles are moved in a circular motion* several times in each area and then the brush is moved to a new area (Figure 26-10).

III. Limitations

◆ Efficiency of plaque removal was the lowest as compared to sulcular and horizontal brushing methods.[37]

LEONARD'S (OR VERTICAL) METHOD

I. Purpose and Indication

◆ May work well for small children.

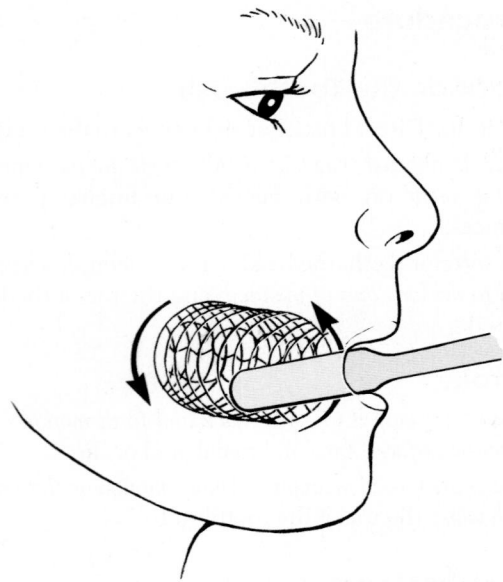

FIGURE 26-10 • Fones Method of Brushing. With the teeth closed, a circular motion extends from the maxillary gingiva to the mandibular gingiva using light pressure.

II. Procedure

◆ *Place toothbrush at 90° to the long axis of the teeth*, buccal and lingual, and press bristles gently against the teeth.
◆ *The teeth are edge to edge.*

A. Stroke

◆ *Bristles move in an up and down motion* with light pressure on the tooth surfaces. Move systematically from area to area around the mouth.

III. Limitations

◆ Much like the rolling stroke, there is minimal plaque removal interproximally and in the sulcular areas.[38]

METHOD FOR POWER TOOTHBRUSHING

As previously noted, a systematic review found powered toothbrushes reduced plaque biofilm and gingivitis better than a manual toothbrush and may be of benefit for some individuals.[18] However, the type of power supply, mode of action of the powered toothbrush, brushing duration, and method of instruction are factors impacting the effectiveness of biofilm removal.[22]

I. Procedure

Although no clearly defined brushing method has been evaluated, the following was developed by the Swiss Dental Society[24]:
◆ *Place bristles at a 45° to 90° angle to the long axis of the tooth*, then turn the brush *on*.

◆ *Move the brush over the buccal (or lingual) and interproximal surfaces of each tooth (or area depending on the size of the brush head) for about 5 seconds.*
◆ *Reposition the brush on the next tooth and repeat* both on the buccal and lingual surfaces in a systematic approach.
◆ Many powered toothbrushes have a built-in 2 minute timer which can signal to the patient the minimum brushing time.

II. Limitations

◆ Cost for the rechargeable models can be an economic hardship for some patients.
◆ Some people may not like the sound or vibration of the powered toothbrushes, especially those with oral hyposensitivity. However, desensitization may allow for power toothbrushes to be used and they have been shown to be effective in those with autism.[39]

SUPPLEMENTAL BRUSHING METHODS

I. Occlusal Brushing

A. Purpose

◆ Loosen food debris and biofilm microorganisms in pits and fissures.
◆ Remove biofilm from the margins of occlusal restorations.
◆ Clean pits and fissures to prepare for sealants.

B. Procedure

◆ *Place brush head on the occlusal surfaces* of molar teeth with filament tips pointed into the occlusal pits at a right angle.
◆ *Position the handle parallel* with the occlusal surface.
◆ Extend the toe of the brush to cover the distal grooves of the most posterior tooth (Figure 26-11A).
◆ *Strokes:* The two acceptable strokes include:
  • Vibrate the brush in a slight circular movement while maintaining the filament tips on the occlusal

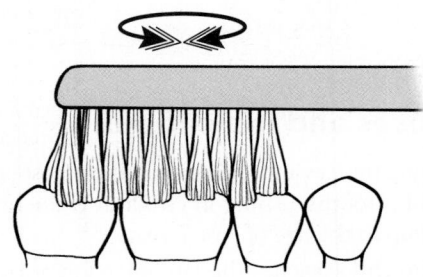

FIGURE 26-11 • Occlusal Brushing. Small circular or vibrating strokes with light pressure while maintaining filament tips on the occlusal surface permit tips to work their way into pits and fissures.

surface throughout a count of 10. Press moderately so filaments do not bend but go straight into the pits and fissures.

- Force the filaments against the occlusal surface with sharp, quick strokes; lift the brush off each time to dislodge debris; repeat 10 times.

◆ Overlap previous stroke by moving the brush to the premolar area. Gradually progress around each maxillary and mandibular arch until all occlusal surfaces have been thoroughly debrided.

II. Brushing Difficult-to-Reach Areas

A. Adaptations

◆ Hands-on demonstration by the patient is essential so the clinician can assess dexterity and ability of the patient to reach difficult areas. This also allows the clinician to determine if a different oral hygiene aid may be more effective.

◆ Use of disclosing solution to provide the patient and clinician with visibility of difficult-to-reach areas may be useful in order to work with the patient to modify the technique for effective plaque biofilm removal.

◆ At successive appointments, the difficult-to-reach areas should be monitored with continued refinement of oral self-care techniques.

B. Areas for Special Attention

◆ Distal surfaces of most posterior teeth (Figure 26-12). At best, the brush may reach only the distal line angles and a single- or end-tufted brush may be necessary (see Chapter 27).

◆ Facially displaced teeth, especially canines and premolars, where the zone of attached gingiva and buccal alveolar bone on the facial surface may be minimal. These areas are at risk for gingival recession and toothbrush abrasion.

◆ Lingually inclined teeth such as the maxillary anterior teeth.

◆ Exposed root surfaces: cemental and dentinal surfaces.

◆ Overlapped teeth or wide embrasures, which may require use of vertical brush position (Figure 26-13).

◆ Surfaces of teeth next to edentulous areas.

III. Tongue Cleaning

The dorsum of the tongue is an ideal environment for harboring bacteria and is a key component of the overall oral self-care process.[40]

A. Anatomic Features of the Tongue Conducive to Debris Retention[40]

◆ *Surface papillae:* Numerous filiform papillae extend as minute projections, whereas fungiform papillae are not as high and create elevations and depressions that entrap debris and microorganisms. These papillae provide a large surface area for the microflora of the tongue.

◆ *Fissures* may be several millimeters deep and also provide a surface for bacterial growth.

B. Microorganisms of the Tongue

◆ Anaerobic bacteria involved in the production of volatile sulfur compounds related to oral malodor (bad breath) or halitosis reside on the tongue.[40]

◆ Periodontal pathogens such as *Porphyromonas gingivalis*, *Prevotella intermedia*, and *Aggregatibacter actinomycetemcomitans* are also found on the dorsum of the tongue.[40,41]

◆ Microorganisms in saliva are typically the same as those found on the tongue.

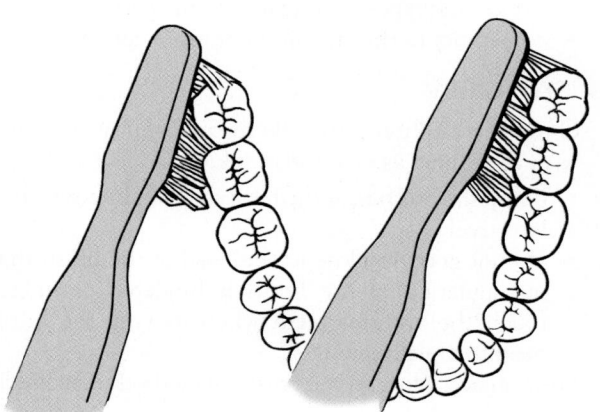

FIGURE 26-12 • Brushing Problems. Brush placement to remove biofilm from the distal surfaces of the most posterior teeth. The distobuccal surface is approached by stretching the cheek; the distolingual surface is approached by directing the brush across from the canine of the opposite side.

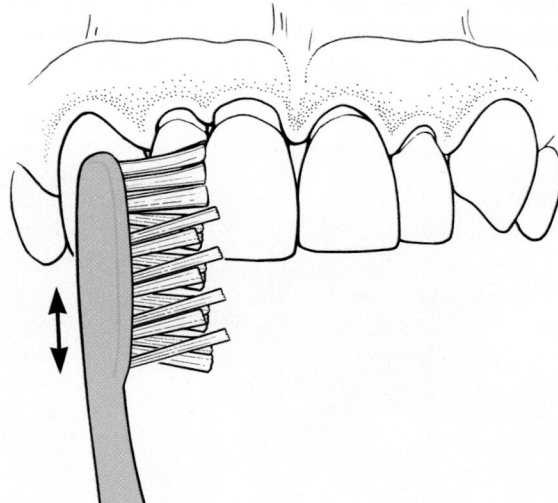

FIGURE 26-13 • Brush in Vertical Position. For overlapped teeth, open embrasures, and selected areas of recession, the dental biofilm on proximal tooth surfaces can be removed with the brush held in a vertical position.

C. Purposes and Indications

◆ Remove or reduce tongue coating.
  • Tongue coating is a white-brownish layer on the dorsum of the tongue and is made up of desquamated epithelial cells, blood cells and metabolites, food debris, and bacteria.[40]
  • The composition of the coating is affected by factors including periodontal status, salivary flow, age, tobacco use, and oral hygiene.[40]
  • The tongue coating is implicated in halitosis.
◆ Reduces bacterial load. However, research has not indicated that this reduces the periodontal pathogens on the dorsum of the tongue or in the saliva so the effect may be primarily on the bacteria producing halitosis.[41]
◆ Reduces potential for halitosis.[42] Tongue brushing and scraping can be effective in reducing halitosis. According to some research findings, the effect is unclear or may only provide short-term benefit.[3,40]

D. Brushing Procedure

◆ Hold the brush handle at a right angle to the midline of the tongue and direct the brush tips toward the throat.
◆ With the tongue extruded, the sides of the filaments are placed on the posterior part of the tongue surface.
◆ With light pressure, draw the brush forward and over the tip of the tongue. Repeat three or four times.
◆ A power brush can only be used for tongue cleaning when the switch is in the "off" position.

E. Types of Tongue Cleaners and Scrapers

As an alternative to brushing the tongue, a tongue cleaner or scraper can be used.
◆ Tongue cleaners or scrapers are typically made of plastic or a flexible metal strip. A variety of tongue cleaners and scrapers are available and may include the following:
  • Loop with a single handle (Figure 26-14).

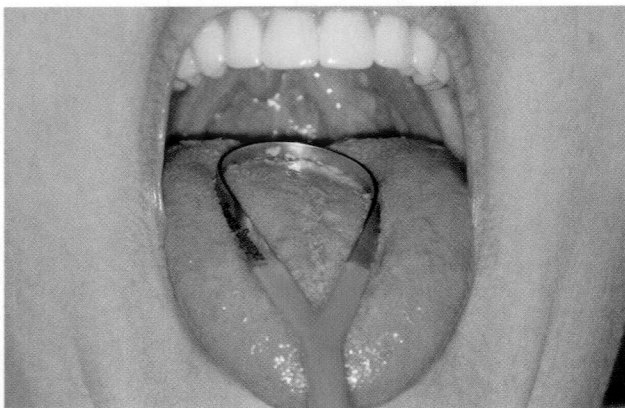

FIGURE 26-14 • Tongue Cleaners or Scrapers. A variety of plastic or flexible metal cleaners are available to clean the dorsal surface of the tongue.

  • Curved with two ends to hold.
  • Raised, textured rubber pad on the back side of the toothbrush head.
◆ *Procedure*
  • Place the cleaner toward the most posterior area of the dorsal surface (Figure 26-14).
  • Press with a light but firm stroke, and pull forward.
  • Repeat several times, covering the entire surface of the tongue.
  • Wash the tongue cleaner under running water to remove debris.

GUIDELINES FOR TOOTHBRUSHING INSTRUCTIONS

◆ Comprehensive toothbrushing instruction for a patient involves teaching what, when, where, and how (see Chapter 24 for guidance effectively educating the patient). Hands-on demonstration by the patient is essential.
◆ In addition to a description of specific toothbrushing methods, the following sections address the grasp, sequence, frequency, duration, and force for toothbrushing.
◆ Possible detrimental effects from improper toothbrushing and variations for special conditions are described.

I. Toothbrush Grasp

A. Objectives of Instruction on Grasp

◆ Ability to manipulate the brush for successful removal of dental biofilm.
◆ A light, but controlled grasp also accomplishes the following:
  • Control of the brush during all movements.
  • Effective positioning at the beginning of each brushing stroke, follow-through during the complete stroke, and repositioning for the next stroke.
  • Sensitivity to the amount of pressure applied.

B. Procedure

◆ Grasp the toothbrush handle in the palm of the hand with the thumb against the shank.
  • Grasp the brush near the head so it can be controlled effectively.
  • Do not grasp so close to the head of the brush that manipulation of the brush is hindered or fingers touch the anterior teeth when moving the brush head to molar regions.
◆ Position according to the brushing method to be used.
◆ Adapt grasp for the various positions of the brush head on the teeth throughout the procedure; adjust to permit unrestricted movement of the wrist and arm.
◆ Apply appropriate pressure for removal of the dental biofilm avoiding excessive pressure that results in soft tissue trauma.

II. Brushing Sequence

◆ There is no one recommended sequence for brushing. Research suggests similar results irrespective of whether patients begin on the buccal or lingual surfaces.[43]

◆ The brushing process should be approached in a systematic way to ensure complete coverage for each tooth surface.

◆ Divide the mouth into sextants or quadrants.

◆ Start brushing from a molar region of one arch around to the midline facial then lingual followed by brushing the occlusal surfaces.

◆ Repeat in the opposing arch.

◆ Each brush placement should overlap the previous one for thorough coverage as shown in Figure 26-7.

◆ Approaches to address areas where patients may have more difficulty removing plaque biofilm may include:

  • Changing the sequence and starting with areas where the patient misses plaque biofilm such as the lingual of the mandibular right for a right-handed patient and mandibular left for a left-handed patient.

  • Specific areas with active periodontal disease.

III. Frequency of Brushing

◆ Brushing a *minimum* of 2 times/day has been shown to reduce caries incidence and severity of periodontal disease.[44,45]

◆ Regular daily oral self-care is most effective at reducing risk and severity of oral disease. Infrequent brushing results in higher odds for dental caries and more severe periodontal disease.[44,45]

◆ Failure to adequate disturb plaque biofilm allows for continued maturation which increases the pathogenic potential of the biofilm (see Chapter 17).

◆ Quality of brushing technique for plaque biofilm removal is equally important as the frequency.

IV. Duration of Brushing

◆ The average times for brushing range from 60 to 80 minutes in the literature.[46]

◆ Several factors impact the time required for each individual including tendency to accumulate plaque, psychomotor skills, position of the teeth, orthodontics, etc.

◆ Research suggests an increase in plaque removal with increased brushing time.[47] However, more recent research with power toothbrushes suggests that there is no additional benefit beyond 120 seconds or 2 minutes for brushing duration.[48]

A. The Count System

To ensure thorough coverage with an even distribution of effort in all areas, a system of counting can be useful.

◆ Count the number of strokes in each area (or 5 or 10, whichever is most appropriate for the particular patient) for modified Stillman or other methods in which a stroke is used.

◆ Count slowly to 10 for each brush position while the brush is vibrated and filament ends are held in position for the Bass, Charters, or other vibratory method.

B. The Clock System

◆ Some patients brush thoroughly while watching a clock or an egg timer for 3 or 4 minutes.

◆ Timed procedures cannot guarantee thorough coverage, because the easily accessible areas may get more brushing time.

C. Combination

For many patients, the use of the "count" system in combination with the "clock" system may be most effective.

D. Built-in Timers

◆ Many power toothbrushes have built-in timers that signal lapsed time.

◆ Signals may be set for 30 seconds, 1 or 2 minutes.

◆ Timers can motivate patients to increase the total time spent brushing.

E. Oral Hygiene Mobile Applications

There are a variety of mobile toothbrushing applications (also known as apps) available for download on a variety of electronic devices including cell phones and tablets which provide an interactive brushing experience and reminders, thus enhancing patient oral hygiene.[49–51]

◆ These applications may include the following features[51]:

  • Educational videos and texts.

  • Goal setting with reminders such as "Time to brush!" set to times designated by the patient.

  • Monitoring of oral hygiene behaviors through reports and graphs of how often a patient brushes or flosses and the duration.

  • Feedback on progress toward goals such as badges for children.

  • Peer support through sharing of progress with friends.

◆ Research suggests these mobile applications hold promise in terms of improving oral hygiene.

  • In adolescents, use of a mobile app resulted in reductions in gingivitis and plaque compared to verbal oral hygiene instructions.[50]

  • In another study, the majority (>90%) of participants said the app motivated them to brush their teeth longer.[49]

V. Toothbrushing Force

◆ Toothbrushing force has been evaluated in terms of the impact on gingival recession and tooth abrasion as well as on effectiveness of plaque removal.[48,52,53]

  • Most research suggests that plaque removal is improved with force up to a point beyond which there is no benefit and potential harm.[53]

- Suggested optimal brushing force for plaque removal:
  - Manual toothbrushing: 400 g.[53]
  - Power toothbrushing: 150 g.[48]
- Although force alone does not cause soft and hard tissue injury, that is, gingival recession and tooth abrasion, it is important to provide patient education to avoid aggressive brushing techniques while effectively removing plaque biofilm.[54]
  - Many power toothbrushes have a mechanism to alert the user to excessive force which may help them to adjust the force applied in those who brush aggressively and are unable to modify their manual toothbrushing technique.[55,56]

VI. General Toothbrushing Instruction

A. Preparation for Instructing Patient

- The dental hygienist must become familiar with an oral self-care product before providing patient education.
- For power toothbrushes, review manufacturer instructions and practice with a toothbrush model, if available, prior to instructing the patient on using it effectively.

B. Patient Education

- Research suggests the most effective teaching strategies for patient education include computer technology, audio and videotapes, written materials, and demonstrations.[57]
  - Verbal instructions alone had only a small effect on patient outcomes, that is, plaque biofilm removal, and should not be used as a stand-alone educational strategy.
  - Demonstrations had the largest effect on patient outcomes and are an essential component of educating the patient.
  - Multiple educational strategies lead to further improvement in patient outcomes.
- When initially introducing a new power toothbrush or oral self-care aid, a demonstration model and/or video can be helpful to introduce the new product to the patient.
  - Adult learning theory suggests patients come to us with experience so it is important to understand what the patient already knows prior to beginning patient education.[58]
  - Like motivational interviewing (see Chapter 24), adult learning theory stresses the importance of the adult patient establishing the learning goals.
  - If a patient is familiar with an oral self-care tool such as a toothbrush, allow the patient to demonstrate their technique and help refine it as needed to be effective.
- Disclosing the plaque biofilm in the patient's mouth can be very useful to provide the patient with a way to visualize the biofilm and its removal when practicing brushing and other oral self-care aid techniques. Do not forget to provide the patient with a hand mirror.
  - Disclosing plaque biofilm makes it easy for the patient and clinician to assess whether the techniques have been effective in biofilm removal.

- In subsequent follow-up appointments, disclosing the plaque biofilm is also a way for the patient and clinical to assess progress toward plaque biofilm removal goals and to identify problem areas requiring further modification of techniques or a different oral self-care aid.
- Observe the patient's technique and refine as needed to show the patient how to adapt the brush head to reach difficult areas.

C. Toothbrushing Procedure

- Select a brush size and shape appropriate for the individual patient.
- Select a dentifrice with minimum abrasivity.
- Place a small amount of fluoride dentifrice on the brush and spread the dentifrice over the teeth.
- For a manual toothbrush:
  - Place the brush on the most posterior maxillary molar and begin moving around each arch on the buccal and then lingual surfaces using the chosen toothbrushing method until all surfaces are completed.
  - Move the brush to the mandibular teeth and repeat. This sequence may vary depending on the preferences of the patient.
  - Brush the occlusal surfaces of first the maxillary and then the mandibular teeth.
- For a power toothbrush, place the brush in the mouth before turning the power on to prevent splatter.
  - Place the brush on the most posterior maxillary molar and move the brush around all surfaces including angling into interproximal areas of each tooth if using a small circular brush.
  - If using a more typical rectangular brush head, start in the posterior and work on each area individually before moving to the next.
  - Carefully angle the brush head to access rotated, crowded, or otherwise displaced teeth.

TOOTHBRUSHING FOR SPECIAL CONDITIONS

Prolonged omission of biofilm removal is not indicated because of the association between oral infection and inflammation and many systemic diseases/conditions.[59] Examples of conditions that may require a temporary modification of oral self-care routines may include, but are not limited, to the following conditions.

I. Acute Oral Inflammatory or Traumatic Lesions

When an acute oral condition precludes normal oral self-care, instruct the patient to:
- Brush all areas of the mouth not affected and if tolerable clean the affected area with an extra soft toothbrush. Reducing the bacterial load is essential to aid in healing.

◆ Rinse with a warm, mild saline solution to encourage healing and debris removal.

◆ Consider prescribing an antimicrobial rinse like chlorhexidine to aid in the reduction of bacterial load until normal oral self-care can resume.

◆ Resume regular biofilm control measures on the affected area as soon as possible.

II. Following Periodontal Surgery

Provide specific instructions concerning brushing while sutures and/or a dressing are in place.

◆ Perform oral self-care in the areas not involved in the surgery as usual.

◆ Follow directions provided by the periodontal office for care of the surgical area.

◆ Rinsing and brushing the surgical area may not be recommended until at least 24 hours after surgery at which time care should be taken to avoid the gingival areas when brushing.

  • If gingival grafting was done, no brushing may be allowed until the postoperative follow-up appointment.

◆ An antimicrobial rinse like chlorhexidine may be prescribed to aid with reducing the bacterial load and to aid in healing while the oral self-care process is modified.

III. Following Dental Extraction

◆ Clean the teeth adjacent to the extraction site the day following surgery.

◆ Brush areas not involved in the surgery as usual to reduce biofilm and promote healing.

◆ Beginning 24 hours after surgery, rinse the mouth with a warm, mild saline solution after each meal or snack to help remove food debris from the extraction site.

◆ Detailed instructions for pre- and post-surgery are found in Chapter 56.

IV. Oral Self-Care of the Neutropenic Patient

Neutropenia or a low white blood cell count (<500 absolute neutrophil count) (see Chapter 62) occurs during treatment such as chemotherapy, radiotherapy, and bone marrow transplant associated with many cancers. Neutropenia puts the patient at increased risk for life-threatening infection. Oral complications can significantly impact the patient's quality of life and ability to recover primarily due to the impact on adequate nutrient intake.[60]

A. Oral Complications[60]

◆ Mucositis (inflammation and ulceration of the mucous membranes of the mouth and throat).

◆ Xerostomia (dry mouth).

◆ Dysgeusia (changes in taste).

◆ Fungal and viral infections such as Candida and herpetic lesions.

◆ Trismus (reduce opening of the mouth).

◆ Diffuse pain.

◆ Aggravation of existing periodontal diseases.

B. Oral Care Recommendations

◆ The Joint Task Force of the Multinational Association of Supportive Cancer Care in Cancer/International Society of Oral Oncology (MASCC/ISSOO) and European Society for Blood and Marrow Transplantation developed a protocol for basic oral care for before, during, and after treatment.[60]

◆ Ongoing interprofessional collaboration with the oncology team by the dental team is essential to maintain the patient's oral health.

◆ Prevention of infection in the oral cavity is needed to minimize the risk of systemic infection during this immune-compromised state. The following recommendations have been made by the MASCC/ISSOO guidelines:

  • Brush a minimum of 2 times/day with an extra soft or soft toothbrush with the bristles softened in hot water.

  • If mucositis is present, a topical anesthetic mouth rinse may be necessary for brushing to help minimize oral pain.

  • Replace the toothbrush regularly. It is suggested to replace the brush prior to each *neutropenic cycle*, meaning it should be replaced prior to the beginning of each chemotherapy or radiotherapy treatment cycle.

  • Use a fluoride toothpaste, non-mint flavored may be more comfortable if the patient is experiencing mucositis. A prescription fluoride gel, toothpaste, or rinse may also be recommended depending on the patient's caries risk and ability to be compliant with oral self-care.

  • A non-alcohol containing chlorhexidine rinse may also be helpful to reduce the bacterial load especially if brushing is compromised by mouth soreness.

  • Interproximal cleaning (see Chapter 27) should be done regularly using aids the patient is familiar with to avoid self-injury.

  • Clean the tongue by either brushing or using a tongue cleaner/scraper.

  • Any dental prostheses should be cleaned according to instructions found in Chapter 30.

ADVERSE EFFECTS OF TOOTHBRUSHING

I. Soft Tissue Lesions

◆ Gingival abrasion

  • Evidence of toothbrushing alone resulting in gingival recession is unclear.[16] However, frequency, duration, force, abrasivity of the dentifrice, and technique may be implicated in recession.[11]

- Localized gingival abrasion or trauma may occur with vigorous toothbrushing and is most common on the mid-facial aspect on canines, first premolars, or teeth in labioversion or buccoversion.
- The appearance may be a distinct surface wound where the epithelial tissue has been denuded or it may be punctate lesions that appear as red pinpoint spots.
- To prevent further gingival abrasion, recommend use of a soft toothbrush with end-rounded filaments and observe the patient's toothbrushing technique and modify it as needed.

II. Hard Tissue Lesions

- Dental Abrasion
  - These lesions result from mechanical abrasion and typically appear as wedge-shaped indentations in cervical areas with a smooth, shiny surface (see Chapter 16).
  - These lesions are multifactorial and include use of an abrasive dentifrice, stiffness of toothbrush bristles, occupational causes, and habits such as chewing on pens.[61]
  - Primarily on facial surfaces, especially of canines, premolars, and sometimes first molars, or on any tooth in buccoversion or labioversion, because typically more force is applied to these areas during toothbrushing.
  - When adjacent teeth are involved, the lesions appear in a linear pattern across the quadrant or sextant.
  - Educate the patient about the presence of the abrasion and advise use of a soft toothbrush with end-rounded bristles along with use of a less abrasive dentifrice. The patient should then demonstrate their brushing technique to determine what modifications are necessary.
  - A power toothbrush that alerts the user when too much pressure is applied may be helpful to train the patient not to use excessive force when brushing.

III. Bacteremia

- Evidence suggests that daily oral activities including chewing, toothbrushing, and flossing can produce transient bacteremia.[62]
  - The incidence and magnitude of bacteremia are significantly higher in patients with more dental biofilm accumulation and gingival inflammation following toothbrushing.
  - Power toothbrushes cause more bacteremia than manual toothbrushes.[63,64]
- Despite these findings, there is no clear association of transient bacteremia and infective endocarditis.
- However, it suggests the need for patients, especially those who are medically compromised, to maintain meticulous removal of dental biofilm on a daily basis to minimize the magnitude of bacteremia.

CARE OF TOOTHBRUSHES

When discussing the type and features of the toothbrush selected for an individual patient, the number of brushes needed and the frequency of replacement should be included.

I. Supply of Brushes

- Recommend at least two brushes for home use so they can be rotated to ensure they dry thoroughly between brushings. Most people will also want a third toothbrush in a portable container for use at work, school, or travel.
- Purchase of brushes needs to be staggered so that all brushes are not new at the same time and, more importantly, so that they are all not old at the same time, thereby resulting in less than optimum maintenance of the gingival condition.

II. Brush Replacement

- There is no ideal timeframe for toothbrush replacement, but a general recommendation is at least every 2–3 months.
- Brushes need to be replaced before filaments become splayed or frayed or lose resiliency.
- The point at which a toothbrush needs replacement is influenced by many factors, including frequency and method of use.

III. Cleaning Toothbrushes

- Clean the toothbrush thoroughly after each use.
- Rinse the brush head with tap water until completely clean of visible debris, dentifrice, and bacteria from between the filaments.[65]
- Allow to dry thoroughly.

A. Toothbrush Contamination

- Toothbrush contamination has been explored in the literature.[66,67] Transmission of bacteria to others in the household has also been suggested, but little evidence exists to support it at this time.
- Toothbrushes become contaminated with pathogenic microorganisms during use as well as depending on the design and the way in which they are stored.[66–68]

B. Toothbrush Disinfection

- The ADA does not support routine use of disinfection methods beyond rinsing and drying the toothbrush.
- The exception to this recommendation applies to those with a higher risk for systemic infection, such as those with compromised immune systems. In these situations, the following may be prudent[65]:
  - Rinse with an antimicrobial mouthrinse prior to brushing to reduce bacterial load.
  - Use of a toothpaste may also reduce bacterial load over not using toothpaste.[69]

- Soak the toothbrush in an antimicrobial rinse such as essential oil mouthwash, cetylpyridinium chloride, or chlorhexidine after brushing.[66]
- Toothbrush sanitizers have limited evidence of benefit.[65,70]

IV. Brush Storage

- Brushes need to be kept in open air with the head in an upright position, apart from contact with other brushes, particularly those of another person to avoid cross contamination.[65]
- Do not store in closed containers. If a portable brush container is used, try to dry the toothbrush prior to putting it in the container. A closed container encourages bacterial growth.[65,66]

DOCUMENTATION

In the dental chart or record, the documentation for initial toothbrush instruction will include the following:

- Type of toothbrush patient has used to date: manual versus power.
- Recommended changes in type of brush or method of use.
- Description of soft tissue health and/or plaque score with goal(s) for improvement.
- Description of toothbrush education and areas patient has difficulty reaching.
- Tongue cleaning method education provided.
- Box 26-2 shows a sample documentation for toothbrush selection and toothbrushing method.

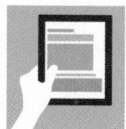

BOX 26-2
Example Documentation:
Toothbrush Selection and Toothbrushing Method

S—A 30-year-old male presents for his 6-month preventive appointment with a chief complaint of gums bleeding during toothbrushing. Patient has a negative medical history and reports taking no medications. Patient reports brushing 1× day with a hard manual toothbrush and uses a back and forth "scrubbing" method.

O—Intraoral assessment reveals generalized moderate edema, marginal erythema, and moderate bleeding on probing. Moderate plaque is noted along the gingival margin of posterior teeth. Ulcerations and denuded gingiva noted, particularly on the left side maxillary facial and mandibular molar lingual surfaces. Biofilm-free score 63%.

A—Acute tissue trauma related to the use of hard toothbrush and scrubbing method.

P—Oral self-care instructions given using a soft toothbrush, recommended twice daily using the modified Stillman method. Flossers were

introduced to the patient for removal of interdental plaque biofilm. Patient demonstrated modified Stillman method intraorally with some challenges on the lingual of mandibular molars. Patient demonstrated successfully the use of flossers. Patient committed to try the following behavior modifications: increase frequency of brushing from 1 to 2× a day, and floss at least 4× a week. Increase biofilm-free score to 85% at re-evaluation appointment. Next visit—6–8 weeks re-evaluation of gingival condition, plaque-free score, evaluate biofilm removal, and assess patient's toothbrushing and flossing technique. Modify as needed. Determine appropriate continue care visit for the patient.

Signed: _____, RDH

Date: _____

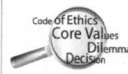

EVERYDAY ETHICS

Audra is a 40-year-old mother of four. In addition to her full-time job as a mother, she cares for her elderly parents. While she is fairly consistent with maintaining her 6-month preventive appointments, she admits to not being consistent with her oral hygiene routine. She uses a manual toothbrush and admits to buying "whatever" toothbrush is on sale. She reports brushing once a day in the morning. She rarely brushes her tongue. She presents with a chief complaint to Jean, the dental hygienist, of bleeding around the lower front teeth and "bad breath." The oral examination indicates 2 mm of recession on the facials of #6 and #11 and generalized marginal biofilm especially in sextant 5 where there is moderate crowding.

Audra is interested in an electric toothbrush and asks Jean about her opinion. Jean states, "Anything works if you use it properly. You don't need an electric toothbrush. Besides, I don't use one and my gums are healthy."

Questions for Consideration

1. Which core ethical values did Jean violate with regard to patient education? Explain how each applies to this scenario.

2. How could the information on the patient's social history be used to provide a patient-centered approach to oral self-care?

3. Given the patient's chief complaints and oral findings, identify intervention strategies that could have been recommended to assist Audra with maintaining optimal oral health (e.g., toothbrush, interdental aids). Explain the rationale for each.

4. What would be the best continuing care interval for Audra (2, 3, 6 months, or yearly)? What is your rationale for your recommendation?

Factors to Teach the Patient

► The effect of dental biofilm formation on the teeth and gingiva.

► Rationale for thorough daily removal of dental biofilm from the teeth, especially before going to sleep.

► The type of brush: manual, power, or both, recommended to maintain optimal oral health for a particular patient.

► Individualized hands-on instruction using an appropriate manual or power brushing method.

► Proper care and maintenance of manual and power brushes.

► Indications for and use of a tongue cleaner.

ENHANCE YOUR UNDERSTANDING

ONLINE RESOURCES
(see the inside front cover for access information)
- Audio glossary
- Appendices

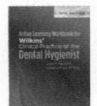

SUPPORT FOR LEARNING
(available separately)
- *Active Learning Workbook for Wilkins' Clinical Practice of the Dental Hygienist, 13th Edition*

INDIVIDUALIZED REVIEW
- Customized practice quizzing with Navigate 2 TestPrep for *Wilkins' Clinical Practice of the Dental Hygienist*

References

1. Arweiler NB, Auschill TM, Sculean A. Patient self-care of periodontal pocket infections. *Periodontol 2000*. 2018;76(1):164-179.

2. Berchier CE, Slot DE, Haps S, Van der Weijden GA. The efficacy of dental floss in addition to a toothbrush on plaque and parameters of gingival inflammation: a systematic review. *Int J Dent Hyg*. 2008;6(4):265-279.

3. Slot DE, De Geest S, van der Weijden FA, Quirynen M. Treatment of oral malodour. Medium-term efficacy of mechanical and/or chemical agents: a systematic review. *J Clin Periodontol*. 2015;42(suppl 16):S303-S316.

4. Van der Weijden FA, Slot DE. Efficacy of homecare regimens for mechanical plaque removal in managing gingivitis a meta review. *J Clin Periodontol*. 2015;42(suppl 16):S77-S91.

5. Gurudath G, Vijayakumar K, Arun R. Oral hygiene practices: ancient historical review. *J Orofac Res*. 2012;2:225-227.

6. Aumeeruddy MZ, Zengin G, Mahomoodally MF. A review of the traditional and modern uses of *Salvadora persica* L.

(Miswak): toothbrush tree of Prophet Muhammad. *J Ethnopharmacol*. 2018;213:409-444.

7. Guerini V. *A History of Dentistry from the Most Ancient Times Until the End of the Eighteenth Century*. Philadelphia, PA: Lea & Febiger; 1909.

8. McCauley HB. Toothbrushes, toothbrush materials and design. *J Am Dent Assoc*. 1946;33(5):283-293.

9. Wadsworth HN. Toothbrush. U.S. Patent US 28,794 A. 1860.

10. Library of Congress SRS. Everyday mysteries: who invented the toothbrush and when was it invented? 2017; https://www.loc.gov/rr/scitech/mysteries/tooth.html. Accessed December 16, 2017.

11. Asadoorian J. Canadian Dental Hygienists Association position paper: tooth brushing. *CJDH*. 2006;40(5):232-248.

12. Association AD. Oral health topics: toothbrushes. 2017; http://www.ada.org/en/member-center/oral-health-topics/toothbrushes. Accessed December 16, 2017.

13. Chun JA, Cho, MJ. The standardization of toothbrush form in Korean adult. *Int J Clin Prev Dent*. 2014;10(4):227-236.

14. Slot DE, Wiggelinkhuizen L, Rosema NA, Van der Weijden GA. The efficacy of manual toothbrushes following a brushing exercise: a systematic review. *Int J Dent Hyg*. 2012;10(3):187-197.

15. Turgut MD, Keceli TI, Tezel B, Cehreli ZC, Dolgun A, Tekcicek M. Number, length and end-rounding quality of bristles in manual child and adult toothbrushes. *Int J Paediatr Dent*. 2011;21(3):232-239.

16. Rajapakse PS, McCracken GI, Gwynnett E, Steen ND, Guentsch A, Heasman PA. Does tooth brushing influence the development and progression of non-inflammatory gingival recession? A systematic review. *J Periodontol*. 2007;34:1046-1061.

17. American Dental Association CoSA. Acceptance program: guidelines for toothbrushes. 1996; http://www.ada.org/en/science-research/ada-seal-of-acceptance/how-to-earn-the-ada-seal/guidelines-for-product-acceptance. Accessed December 21, 2017.

18. Yaacob M, Worthington HV, Deacon SA, et al. Powered versus manual toothbrushing for oral health. *Cochrane Database Syst Rev*. 2014(6):Cd002281.

19. Deacon SA, Glenny AM, Deery C, et al. Different powered toothbrushes for plaque control and gingival health. *Cochrane Database Syst Rev*. 2010;8:CD004971.

20. Nash DA, Friedman JW, Mathu-Muju KR, et al. A review of the global literature on dental therapists. *Community Dent Oral Epidemiol*. 2014;42(1):1-10.

21. Schmickler J, Wurbs S, Wurbs S, et al. The influence of the utilization time of brush heads from different types of power toothbrushes on oral hygiene assessed over a 6-month observation period: a randomized clinical trial. *Am J Dent*. 2016;29(6):307-314.

22. Rosema N, Slot DE, van Palenstein Helderman WH, Wiggelinkhuizen L, Van der Weijden GA. The efficacy of powered toothbrushes following a brushing exercise: a systematic review. *Int J Dent Hyg*. 2016;14(1):29-41.

23. Sharma NC, Galustians HJ, Qaqish J, Cugini M, Warren PR. The effect of two power toothbrushes on calculus and stain formation. *Am J Dent*. 2002;15(2):71-76.

24. Baruah K, Thumpala VK, Khetani P, Baruah Q, Tiwari RV, Dixit H. A review of toothbrushes and toothbrushing methods. *Int J Pharm Sci Invention*. 2017;6(5):29-38.

25. Versteeg PA, Rosema NA, Timmerman MF, Van der Velden U, Van der Weijden GA. Evaluation of two soft manual toothbrushes with different filament designs in relation to gingival abrasion and plaque removing efficacy. *Int J Dent Hyg*. 2008;6:166-173.

26. Litonjua LA, Andreana S, Bush PJ, Cohen RE. Toothbrushing and gingival recession. *Int Dent J*. 2003;53(2):67-72.

27. Brothwell DJ, Jutai DKG, Hawkins RJ. An update of mechanical oral hygiene practices: evidence-based recommendations for disease prevention. *J Can Dent Assoc*. 1998;64(4):295-306.

28. Poyato-Ferrera M, Segura-Egea JJ, Bullon-Fernandez P. Comparison of modified Bass technique with normal toothbrushing practices for efficacy in supragingival plaque removal. *Int J Dent Hyg*. 2003;1(2):110-114.

29. Smutkeeree A, Rojlakkanawong N, Yimcharoen V. A 6-month comparison of toothbrushing efficacy between the horizontal Scrub and modified Bass methods in visually impaired students. *Int J Paediatr Dent*. 2011;21(4):278-283.

30. Bass CC. An effective method of personal oral hygiene, Part II. *J Louisiana State Med Soc*. 1854;106:100-102.

31. Waerhaug J. Effect of toothbrushing on subgingival plaque formation. *J Periodontol*. 1981;52(1):30-34.

32. Stillman PR. A philosophy of the treatment of periodontal disease. *Dent Digest*. 1932;38(9):314.

33. Hirschfeld I. *The Toothbrush: Its Use and Abuse*. Brooklyn, NY: Dental Items of Interest Pubs; 1939.

34. Gibson JA, Wade AB. Plaque removal by the Bass and roll brushing techniques. *J Periodontol*. 1977;48:456-459.

35. Charters W. Home care of the mouth. I. Proper home care of the mouth. *J Periodontol*. 1948;19(4):136-137.

36. Muller-Bolla M, Courson F. Toothbrushing methods to use in children: a systematic review. *Oral Health Prev Dent*. 2013;11(4):341-347.

37. Patil SP, Patil PB, Kashetty MV. Effectiveness of different tooth brushing techniques on the removal of dental plaque in 6–8 year old children of Gulbarga. *J Int Soc Prev Community Dent*. 2014;4(2):113-116.

38. Shick RA, Ash MM. Evaluation of the vertical method of toothbrushing. *J Periodontol*. 1961;32(4):346-353.

39. Vajawat M, Deepika PC, Kumar V, Rajeshwari P. A clinico-microbiological study to evaluate the efficacy of manual and powered toothbrushes among autistic patients. *Contemp Clin Dent*. 2015;6(4):500-504.

40. Roldan S, Herrera D, Sanz M. Biofilms and the tongue: therapeutical approaches for the control of halitosis. *Clin Oral Investig*. 2003;7(4):189-197.

41. Laleman I, Koop R, Teughels W, Dekeyser C, Quirynen M. Influence of tongue brushing and scraping on the oral microflora of periodontitis patients. *J Periodontal Res*. 2018;53(1):73-79.

42. Van der Sleen MI, Slot DE, Van Trijffel E, Winkel EG, Van der Weijden GA. Effectiveness of mechanical tongue cleaning on breath odour and tongue coating: a systematic review. *Int J Dent Hyg*. 2010;8(4):258-268.

43. Van der Sluijs E, Slot DE, Hennequin-Hoenderdos NL, Van der Weijden GA. A specific brushing sequence and plaque removal efficacy: a randomized split-mouth design. *Int J Dent Hyg*. 2018;16(1):85-91.

44. Kumar S, Tadakamadla J, Johnson NW. Effect of toothbrushing frequency on incidence and increment of dental caries: a systematic review and meta-analysis. *J Dent Res*. 2016;95(11):1230-1236.

45. Zimmermann H, Zimmermann N, Hagenfeld D, Veile A, Kim TS, Becher H. Is frequency of tooth brushing a risk factor for periodontitis? A systematic review and meta-analysis. *Community Dent Oral Epidemiol*. 2015;43(2):116-127.

46. Gunjalli G, Kumar KN, Jain SK, Reddy SK, Shavi GR, Ajagannanavar SL. Total salivary anti-oxidant levels, dental development and oral health status in childhood obesity. *J Int Oral Health*. 2014;6(4):63-67.

47. Van der Weijden G, Timmerman M, Nijboer A, Lie M, Van der Velden U. A comparative study of electric toothbrushes for the effectiveness of plaque removal in relation to toothbrushing duration. Timerstudy. *J Clin Periodontol*. 1993;20(7):476-481.

48. McCracken GI, Janssen J, Swan M, Steen N, de Jager M, Heasman PA. Effect of brushing force and time on plaque removal using a powered toothbrush. *J Clin Periodontol*. 2003;30(5):409-413.

49. Underwood B, Birdsall J, Kay E. The use of a mobile app to motivate evidence-based oral hygiene behaviour. *Br Dent J*. 2015;219(4):E2.

50. Alkadhi OH, Zahid MN, Almanea RS, Althaqeb HK, Alharbi TH, Ajwa NM. The effect of using mobile applications for improving oral hygiene in patients with orthodontic fixed appliances: a randomised controlled trial. *J Orthod*. 2017;44(3):157-163.

51. Nolan SL, Giblin-Scanlon LJ, Boyd LD, Rainchuso L. Theory based development and Beta testing of a smartphone prototype developed as an oral health promotion tool to influence ECC. *J Dent Hyg*. 2018;92(2):6-14.

52. Van der Weijden GA, Timmerman MF, Reijerse E, Snoek CM, van der Velden U. Toothbrushing force in relation to plaque removal. *J Clin Periodontol*. 1996;23(8):724-729.

53. Van der Weijden GA, Timmerman MF, Danser MM, Van der Velden U. Relationship between the plaque removal efficacy of a manual toothbrush and brushing force. *J Clin Periodontol*. 1998;25(5):413-416.

54. Wiegand A, Schlueter N. The role of oral hygiene: does toothbrushing harm? *Monogr Oral Sci*. 2014;25:215-219.

55. Janusz K, Nelson B, Bartizek RD, Walters PA, Biesbrock AR. Impact of a novel power toothbrush with SmartGuide technology on brushing pressure and thoroughness. *J Contemp Dent Pract*. 2008;9(7):1-8.

56. Van der Weijden FA, Campbell SL, Dorfer CE, Gonzalez-Cabezas C, Slot DE. Safety of oscillating-rotating powered brushes compared to manual toothbrushes: a systematic review. *J Periodontol*. 2011;82(1):5-24.

57. Friedman AJ, Cosby R, Boyko S, Hatton-Bauer J, Turnbull G. Effective teaching strategies and methods of delivery for patient education: a systematic review and practice guideline recommendations. *J Cancer Educ*. 2011;26(1):12-21.

58. Papadakos CT, Papadakos J, Catton P, Houston P, McKernan P, Jusko Friedman A. From theory to pamphlet: the 3Ws and an H process for the development of meaningful patient education resources. *J Cancer Educ*. 2014;29(2):304-310.

59. Linden GJ, Herzberg MC. Periodontitis and systemic diseases: a record of discussions of working group 4 of the Joint EFP/AAP Workshop on Periodontitis and Systemic Diseases. *J Periodontol.* 2013;84(4 suppl):S20-S23.

60. Elad S, Raber-Durlacher JE, Brennan MT, et al. Basic oral care for hematology-oncology patients and hematopoietic stem cell transplantation recipients: a position paper from the joint task force of the Multinational Association of Supportive Care in Cancer/International Society of Oral Oncology (MASCC/ISOO) and the European Society for Blood and Marrow Transplantation (EBMT). *Support Care Cancer.* 2015;23(1):223-236.

61. Milosevic A. Abrasion: a common dental problem revisited. *Prim Dent J.* 2017;6(1):32-36.

62. Tomas I, Diz P, Tobias A, Scully C, Donos N. Periodontal health status and bacteraemia from daily oral activities: systematic review/meta-analysis. *J Clin Periodontol.* 2012;39(3):213-228.

63. Misra S, Percival R, Devine D, Duggal M. A pilot study to assess bacteraemia associated with tooth brushing using conventional, electric or ultrasonic toothbrushes. *Eur Arch Paediatr Dent.* 2007;8(1):42-45.

64. Bhanji S, Williams B, Sheller B, Elwood T, Mancl L. Transient bacteremia induced by toothbrushing a comparison of the Sonicare toothbrush with a conventional toothbrush. *Pediatr Dent.* 2002;24(4):295-299.

65. American Dental Association CoSA. Toothbrush care: cleaning, storing and replacement. 2011; http://www.ada.org/en/about-the-ada/ada-positions-policies-and-statements/statement-on-toothbrush-care-cleaning-storage-and-. Accessed January 7, 2017.

66. Frazelle MR, Munro CL. Toothbrush contamination: a review of the literature. *Nurs Res Pract.* 2012;2012:420630.

67. Ankola AV, Hebbal M, Eshwar S. How clean is the toothbrush that cleans your tooth? *Int J Dent Hyg.* 2009;7(4):237-240.

68. Wetzel WE, Schaumburg C, Ansari F, Kroeger T, Sziegoleit A. Microbial contamination of toothbrushes with different principles of filament anchoring. *J Am Dent Assoc.* 2005;136(6):758-765; quiz 806.

69. Warren DP, Goldschmidt MC, Thompson MB, Adler-Storthz K, Keene HJ. The effects of toothpastes on the residual microbial contamination of toothbrushes. *J Am Dent Assoc.* 2001;132(9):1241-1245.

70. Chandrdas D, Jayakumar HL, Chandra M, Katodia L, Sreedevi A. Evaluation of antimicrobial efficacy of garlic, tea tree oil, cetylpyridinium chloride, chlorhexidine, and ultraviolet sanitizing device in the decontamination of toothbrush. *Indian J Dent.* 2014;5(4):183-189.

27

Oral Infection Control: Interdental Care

Lisa J. Moravec, RDH, MSDH, and Linda D. Boyd, RDH, RD, EdD

CHAPTER OUTLINE

THE INTERDENTAL AREA
I.   Anatomy of the Interdental Area
II. Proximal Tooth Surfaces

PLANNING INTERDENTAL CARE
I.   Patient Assessment
II. Dental Hygiene Care Plan

SELECTIVE INTERDENTAL BIOFILM REMOVAL
I.   Relation to Toothbrushing
II. Selection of Interdental Aids

INTERDENTAL BRUSHES
I.   Types
II. Indications for Use
III. Procedure
IV. Care of Brushes

DENTAL FLOSS AND TAPE
I.   Types of Floss
II. Procedure
III. Prevention of Flossing Injuries

AIDS FOR FLOSSING
I.   Floss Threader
II. Tufted Dental Floss
III. Floss Holder
IV. Gauze Strip

POWER FLOSSERS
I.   Description
II. Indications for Use
III. Procedure

SINGLE-TUFT BRUSH (END-TUFT BRUSH)
I.   Description
II. Indications for Use
III. Procedure

INTERDENTAL TIP
I.   Composition and Design
II. Indications for Use
III. Procedure

TOOTHPICK IN HOLDER
I.   Description
II. Indications for Use
III. Procedure

WOODEN INTERDENTAL CLEANER
I.   Description
II. Indications for Use
III. Procedure

ORAL IRRIGATION
I.   Description
II. Types of Devices
III. Delivery Tips
IV. Procedure
V.   Application for Practice

DOCUMENTATION

EVERYDAY ETHICS

FACTORS TO TEACH THE PATIENT

REFERENCES

LEARNING OBJECTIVES

After studying this chapter, the student will be able to:

1. Review the anatomy of the interdental area and explain why toothbrushing alone cannot remove biofilm adequately for prevention of periodontal infection.

2. Describe the types of interdental brushes and explain why they may be more effective than floss for some patients.

3. Describe the types of dental floss and outline the steps for use of floss or floss loops for biofilm removal from proximal tooth surfaces.

4. Develop a list of the types and purposes of various floss aids, including floss holders and power flossing devices, and provide a rationale for the choice of the best ones to meet a specific patient's needs.

5. Demonstrate and recommend other devices for biofilm removal, including toothpick in holder, wooden interdental cleaner, interdental rubber tip, and oral irrigation.

Toothbrushing alone cannot accomplish biofilm removal from proximal tooth surfaces and adjacent gingiva to the same degree that it does for the facial, lingual, and palatal aspects. Therefore, interdental biofilm control is essential to complete the patient's oral self-care program.

Objectives and procedures for removal of dental biofilm from proximal tooth surfaces are included in this chapter. When the preventive treatment plan is outlined for an individual, assessment is made of the oral condition, the problem areas, and the overall prognosis for improvement or maintenance of gingival health.

◆ Measures for interdental biofilm control are selected to complement biofilm control by toothbrushing.[1]

◆ Daily interdental cleaning is necessary for plaque removal and to reduce gingival inflammation.[1]

THE INTERDENTAL AREA

◆ In health, the interdental gingiva fills the interproximal space and under the contact of the adjacent teeth.

◆ When the interdental papilla is missing or reduced in height, the shape of the interdental gingiva changes.

◆ Factors impacting the papilla height include[2]:
  • Shape of the tooth.
  • Interproximal bone height.
  • Thickness of the gingiva.

◆ The classification system on papillary height is illustrated in Chapter 18.

◆ Figure 27-1 shows a Class II embrasure from the proximal surface with the col and from the facial surface.

I. Anatomy of the Interdental Area

A review of the gingival and dental anatomy of the interdental area can give meaning to and clarify the role and purpose of the various devices available for interdental care.

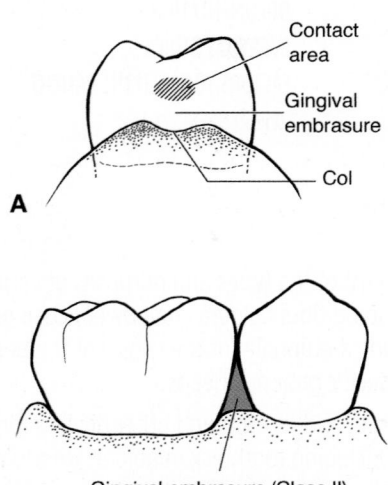

FIGURE 27-1 • Class II Gingival Embrasure. A: Embrasure shown from the proximal surface with the col. **B:** Facial view, with gingival embrasure shown in blue.

A. Posterior Teeth

◆ Between adjacent posterior teeth are two papillae, one facial and one lingual or palatal.

◆ The papillae are connected by a col, a depressed concave area that follows the shape of the apical border of the contact area (Figure 27-1).

B. Anterior Teeth

◆ Between anterior teeth in contact is a single papilla with a pyramidal shape.

◆ Tip of the papilla may form a small col under the contact area.

C. Epithelium

◆ The epithelium covering a col is usually thin and not keratinized epithelium.

◆ Col epithelium is less resistant to infection than keratinized surfaces.

◆ Inflammation in the papilla leads to enlargement; with increased inflammatory cells and edema, the col becomes deeper.

◆ The col area is inaccessible for ordinary toothbrushing and microorganisms may be harbored in the concave center.

◆ The incidence of gingivitis is greatest in the interdental tissues.[3]

II. Proximal Tooth Surfaces

◆ With bacterial infection and loss of attachment, the interdental papillae height is reduced, exposing the proximal tooth surfaces.

◆ As periodontitis progresses, concavities, grooves, and furcation areas become exposed, resulting in bacterial accumulations.[4,5]

◆ Irregularities of tooth position, such as rotation or overlapping, and deviations related to malocclusion or tooth loss may also be present.

◆ The increased root surface and complexity of the root morphology may make removal of bacterial deposits more difficult.

PLANNING INTERDENTAL CARE

I. Patient Assessment

A. History of Personal Oral Care

◆ Self-care history includes type of toothbrush, dentifrice, and adjunct interdental aids currently used (i.e., dental floss, interdental brush, oral irrigation device).[6]

◆ Frequency and time spent.

◆ Assess barriers to effective interdental care, including efficacy and patient compliance.

B. Dental and Gingival Anatomy

- Position of teeth.
- Types and shapes of embrasures: variation throughout the dentition (i.e., may recommend floss for anterior teeth with tight embrasures and interdental brush for posterior teeth with larger spaces).
- Clinical attachment level: classification of the periodontal condition.
- Prostheses present: special interdental care required for fixed and removable prostheses.
- Areas where toothbrush cannot reach.

C. Extent and Location of Dental Biofilm

- Preparation of a *plaque score* (see Chapter 21) to show the patient the extent of biofilm needing removal on a daily basis.
- Use of a disclosing agent to show specific sites where biofilms accumulate.
- Evidence of the patient's ability to care for difficult-to-access areas.

D. Personal Factors

- Disability that limits one's ability to carry out needed personal oral hygiene.
- Oral health literacy about and appreciation for interdental oral care.

II. Dental Hygiene Care Plan

A. Objectives

- Utilize motivational interviewing (see Chapter 24) to select appropriate interdental aids to help the patient reach optimum oral health.
- Determine if challenges with compliance exist, including lack of motivation to adhere or patient not remembering instructions for self-care.[6]
- Educate the patient on the oral care aids selected.
- The patient must accept responsibility for daily personal care and work as a partner with the oral health team.

B. Initial Care Plan

- Assess oral health behavior to create an individualized care plan that is sustainable and requires minimal reinforcement.[7]
- At first, the simplest procedures are selected for the patient's convenience and ease of learning based on the patient's current knowledge, preferences, and oral self-care habits.
- Minimum frequency: twice daily.
- Keep the daily oral self-care regimen at a realistic level with respect to the time the patient is able or willing to spend.

SELECTIVE INTERDENTAL BIOFILM REMOVAL

I. Relation to Toothbrushing

- Vibratory and sulcular toothbrushing, such as that performed with the Charters, Stillman, and Bass methods, can be successful to some degree in removing dental biofilm near the line angles of the facial and lingual or palatal embrasures.
- Brushing in vertical position is effective for additional access around line angles onto the proximal surfaces (see Chapter 26).

II. Selection of Interdental Aids

- The ideal interdental cleaning aid needs to be user-friendly, remove plaque effectively, and cause no damage to soft tissues or hard tissues.[8]
- Choices are dependent on oral self-care abilities, disease status, and the risk for future recurrence.
- A patient working to control or arrest disease may need more frequent oral self-care than a patient in the maintenance phase.
- With the judicious selection and use of the various methods for interdental care, the dedicated patient can accomplish disease control.

INTERDENTAL BRUSHES

I. Types

A. Small Insert Brushes with Reusable Handle

- Soft nylon filaments are twisted into a fine stainless steel plastic-coated wire. This brush is disposable and inserted into a plastic handle with an angulated shank (Figure 27-2A).
- The small tapered or cylindrical brush heads are of varying sizes, approximately 12–15 mm (1/2 inch) in length and 3–5 mm (1/8–1/4 inch) in diameter.

B. Travel Interdental Brush

- Soft nylon filaments are twisted into a fine stainless steel plastic-coated wire.
  - The wire is continuous with the handle, which is approximately 35–45 mm (1½–1¾ inches) in length (Figure 27-2B).
  - Travel brushes are also available (Figure 27-2B) and may be more convenient for patients.
- The very short, soft filaments form a narrow brush approximately 30–35 mm (1¼–1½ inches) in length and 5–8 mm (1/4–5/16 inches) in diameter (Figure 27-2 B).

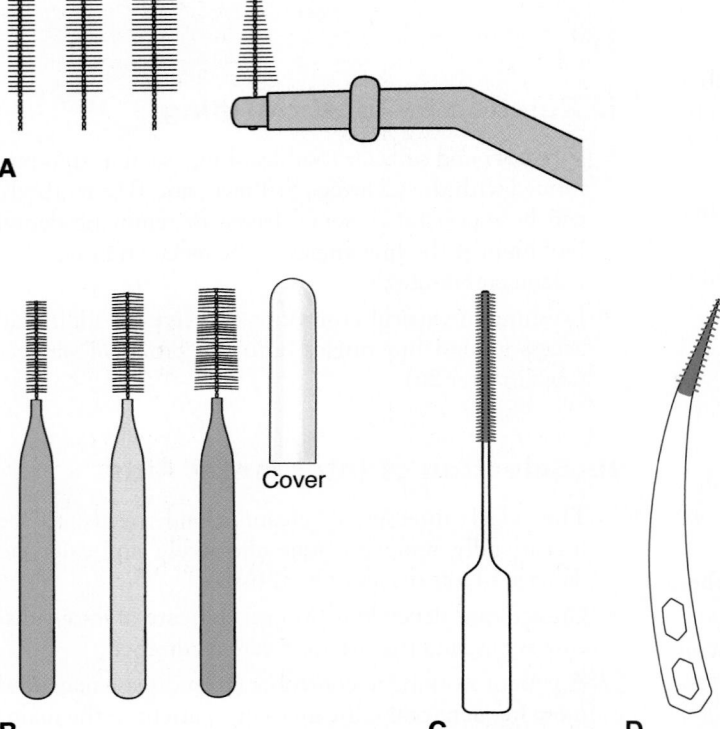

FIGURE 27-2 • Interdental Brushes and Cleaners. **A:** Insert brushes for a reusable handle with an angulated shank. **B:** Reusable interdental brush with filaments twisted onto a fine plastic-coated wire that ends in a handle and cover. **C:** Disposable interdental cleaner. **D:** Disposable curved interdental cleaner.

C. Rubber Interdental Cleaners

- Similar to an interdental brush, but do not have a wire. The rubber interdental cleaner or "soft-pick" has small elastomeric fingers that are perpendicular to a plastic core (Figure 27-2C).[9]
- The soft-pick is effective at biofilm removal and reducing gingival bleeding.[10,11]

II. Indications for Use

- It is suggested that interdental brushes should be the first choice for interproximal cleaning.[1]
- Patient preference and anatomy need to be considered when selecting size and style.
  - Interdental brushes have been shown to be easier to use and preferred by patients.[12]
- Size of the interdental embrasure also determines the choice of interdental brush or cleaner.
  - Interdental brushes are more effective in plaque removal than floss when the brush fills the embrasure.[1,12]

A. For Removal of Dental Biofilm and Debris

- Proximal tooth surfaces adjacent to open embrasures, orthodontic appliances, fixed prostheses, dental implants, periodontal splints, and space maintainers are well suited to interdental brushes and cleaners.

- Concave proximal surfaces are used where dental floss and other interdental aids cannot reach (Figure 27-3A). Floss will not access a concave surface, whereas the interproximal brush can reach and cleanse (Figure 27-3B).[6,8,9,13–15]
  - In patients with open embrasures and moderate to severe attachment loss, the interdental brush is often more effective than floss. However, it is important to choose an interdental brush that fills the embrasure to effectively clean concavities (Figure 27-3C).
  - Interdental brushes are a great choice for periodontal patients with larger interdental spaces with recession or root exposure.[1]
- Exposed Class IV furcations (see Chapter 20).

B. For Application of Chemotherapeutic Agents

- Fluoride dentifrice, gel, and/or mouthrinse for prevention of dental caries, particularly root surface caries, and for surfaces adjacent to any prosthesis.
- Antimicrobial agents for control of dental biofilm and the prevention of gingivitis.
- Desensitizing agents.

III. Procedure

- Select brush of appropriate diameter to fill the embrasure.
- Insert at an angle in keeping with gingival form; brush in and out.

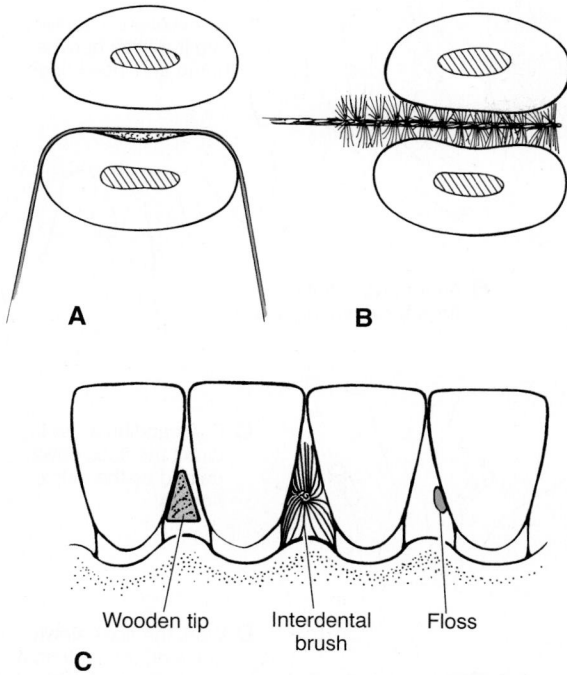

FIGURE 27-3 • Interdental Care. A: Floss positioned on the mesial surface of a maxillary first premolar shows the inability of the floss to remove dental biofilm on a concave proximal tooth surface. **B:** The use of an interdental brush in the same interproximal area to show how the proximal surfaces can be cleaned free of dental biofilm. **C:** Comparison of the access of a wooden tip, an interdental brush, and a piece of dental floss to an open interdental area.

- For wide embrasures, it is important to remember to apply pressure against the proximal root surfaces to remove the biofilm thoroughly.
  - Insert the interdental brush as shown in Figure 27-3B and C.
  - Apply pressure toward the mesial proximal surface to remove biofilm.
  - Then apply pressure toward the distal proximal surface and remove the surface biofilm.

IV. Care of Brushes

- Clean the brush during use to remove debris and biofilm by holding under actively running water.
- Clean thoroughly after use and dry in open air.
- Discard before the filaments become deformed or loosened.

DENTAL FLOSS AND TAPE

Despite daily dental floss along with toothbrushing being recommended to a majority of patients, effectiveness, compliance, and patient dexterity are limitations.[12]

- Recent studies show only a small reduction in interproximal bleeding in most patients due to low compliance and technique challenges with flossing.[1,8,12]

- Dental professionals need to determine whether high-quality flossing is an achievable goal when making individualized self-care plans for patients and effectiveness of plaque removal.

I. Types of Floss

- Research has shown no difference in the effectiveness of waxed or unwaxed floss for biofilm removal.[16]

A. Materials

- *Silk*: Historically, floss was made of silk fibers loosely twisted together to form a strand and waxed for proximal surface cleaning.
- *Nylon*: Nylon multifilaments, waxed or unwaxed, have been widely used in circular (floss) or flat (tape) form for biofilm removal from proximal tooth surfaces.
- *Polytetrafluoroethylene (PTFE)*: Monofilament PTFE is used for biofilm removal from proximal tooth surface.

B. Features of Waxed Floss

- Smooth surface provided by the wax coating helps the floss slide through the contact area.
- Easing the floss between the teeth may minimize tissue trauma.
- Wax gives strength and durability during application to minimize breakage.

C. Features of Unwaxed Floss

- Added color and flavor.
- Thinner floss may be helpful when contact areas are tight.
- Care must be taken to avoid injury when guiding floss through a tight contact area or when moving floss on the tooth surface in an apical direction.
- Unwaxed floss may become frayed due to irregular tooth surface, rough surface of a restoration, or calculus deposit and cause the patient to become frustrated, thereby resulting in lost motivation to floss regularly.

D. Features of PTFE

- Monofilament type resists breakage or shredding when passed over irregular tooth surface, restoration, or calculus deposit.
- Reduces the force required to pass the floss through the contact, which may improve patient compliance with regular flossing and reduce tissue injury or trauma.[17]

E. Enhancements

- Color and flavor have been added to dental floss.
- Therapeutic agents added include fluoride and whitening agents; however, limited research has been published relative to their effectiveness.

II. Procedure

- When dental floss is applied with good technique to a flat or convex proximal tooth surface, biofilm can be removed.
- Older biofilm is tenacious and may require more strokes for removal.
- When floss is placed over a concave surface, contact is not possible (Figure 27-3A), and supplementary devices are needed to remove a bacterial deposit completely.

A. Sequence of Flossing

There is no ideal time to perform the oral self-care procedure to floss, but it may be helpful to floss before brushing to help dislodge food debris and plaque biofilm.

B. Floss Preparation

- Figure 27-4 outlines the flossing steps described in detail here in this section.
- Hold a 12- to 15-inch length of floss with the thumb and index finger of each hand; grasp firmly with only half inch of floss between the fingertips. The ends of the floss may be tucked into the palm and held by the ring and little finger, or the floss may be wrapped around the middle fingers (Figure 27-4A and B).
- A circle of floss or "floss loop" may be made by tying the ends together; the circle may be rotated as the floss is used (Figure 27-5).
  - Advantages of creating a floss circle include improved user compliance and easier handling, lower string waste and improvement of string length, and increased string hygiene and plaque removal efficacy.[18]

C. Application

- *Maxillary teeth*: Direct the floss upward by holding the floss over two thumbs or a thumb and an index finger as shown in Figure 27-4C. Rest a side of a finger on the teeth of the opposite side of the maxillary arch to provide balance and a fulcrum.
- *Mandibular teeth*: Direct the floss down by holding the two index fingers on top of the strand. One index finger holds the floss on the lingual aspect and the other on the facial aspect. The side of the finger on the lingual side is held on the teeth of the opposite side of the mouth to serve as a fulcrum or rest.

D. Insertion

- Hold floss firmly in a diagonal or oblique position.
- Guide the floss past each contact area with a gentle back and forth or sawing motion (Figure 27-4D).
- Control floss to prevent snapping through the contact area into the gingival tissue.

E. Cleaning Stroke

- Clean proximal tooth surface separately; for the distal aspect, curve the floss mesially, and for the mesial aspect, curve the floss distally, around the tooth (Figure 27-4E and F).

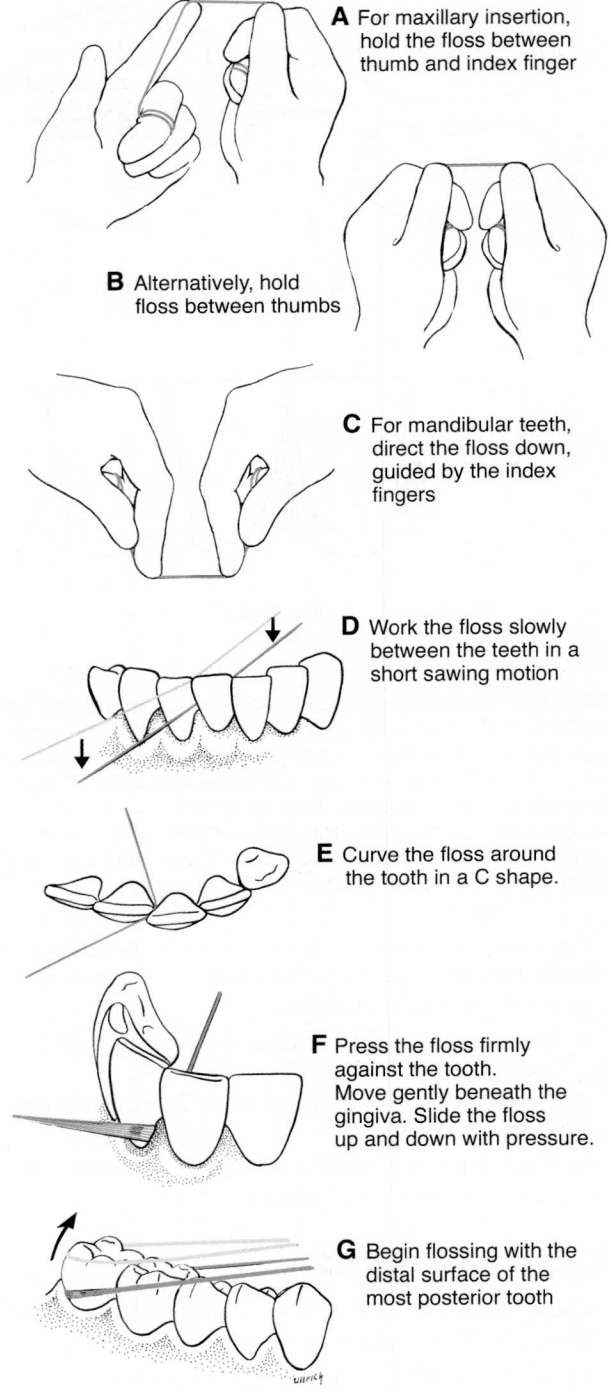

A For maxillary insertion, hold the floss between thumb and index finger

B Alternatively, hold floss between thumbs

C For mandibular teeth, direct the floss down, guided by the index fingers

D Work the floss slowly between the teeth in a short sawing motion

E Curve the floss around the tooth in a C shape.

F Press the floss firmly against the tooth. Move gently beneath the gingiva. Slide the floss up and down with pressure.

G Begin flossing with the distal surface of the most posterior tooth

FIGURE 27-4 • Use of Dental Floss. A: For maxillary insertion, hold the floss between the thumb and index finger. **B:** Grasp the floss firmly. Allow only 1/2-inch length between fingers. **C:** For the mandibular teeth, direct the floss down, guided by the index fingers. **D:** Curve the floss around the tooth in a C-shape and slowly move the floss back and forth in short motions to avoid snapping through the contact area. **E:** Curve the floss around the tooth in a C-shape. Hold the floss toward the mesial for cleaning the distal surfaces and toward the distal for cleaning the mesial surfaces. **F:** Press the floss firmly against the tooth. Move gently beneath the gingiva until tissue resistance is felt. The floss is moved in an up-and-down motion putting pressure against the tooth surface to disturb the biofilm. **G:** Begin flossing with the distal surface of the most posterior tooth, and work systematically around the arch.

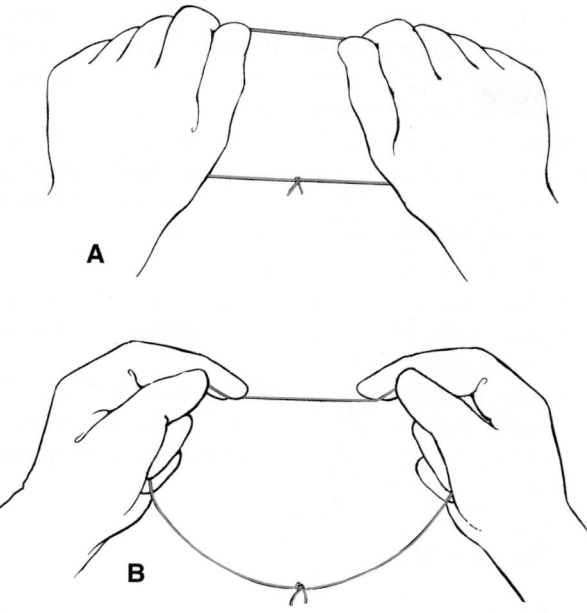

FIGURE 27-5 • Circle of Floss. The ends of the floss can be tied together for convenient holding. A child may be able to manage floss better with this technique. **A:** Floss held for maxillary teeth. **B:** Floss held for mandibular teeth.

◆ Pass the floss below the gingival margin, curve to adapt the floss around the tooth, press against the tooth, and slide up and down over the tooth surface several times.

◆ Move the floss to a new, unused portion for each proximal tooth surfaces.

◆ Loop the floss over the distal surfaces of the most posterior teeth in each quadrant and the teeth next to edentulous areas (Figure 27-4G). Hold firmly against the tooth and move the floss in an up-and-down motion.

III. Prevention of Flossing Injuries

◆ *Location:* Floss cuts or clefts occur primarily on facial and lingual or palatal surfaces directly beside or in the middle of an interdental papilla. They appear as straight-line cuts beginning at the gingival margin and may result in a floss cleft if the tissue is repeatedly injured.[19]

◆ *Causes*
  • Using a piece of floss that is too long between the fingers when held for insertion.
  • Snapping the floss through the contact area.
  • Not curving the floss about the tooth adequately and cutting into the gingival margin.

AIDS FOR FLOSSING

I. Floss Threader

A floss threader is used for biofilm and debris removal around orthodontic appliances or under fixed partial dentures (Figure 27-6).

A. Description

◆ Floss threaders are flexible plastic and looks like a needle with a very large loop at the end through which regular floss is placed.

B. Indication for Use

◆ Biofilm removal from mesial and distal abutments and under pontic of a fixed partial denture, implant, orthodontic arch wire, or other fixed prosthesis.

C. Procedure

◆ Individual Surface of Tooth or Implant
  • Take a 12- to 18-inch piece of floss and thread it through the loop on the threader.
  • Put the floss threader under the appliance and pull the floss under the fixed appliance (Figure 27-6A).
  • Then curve the floss in a "C" shape around the proximal surface to remove dental biofilm (Figure 27-6B and D).

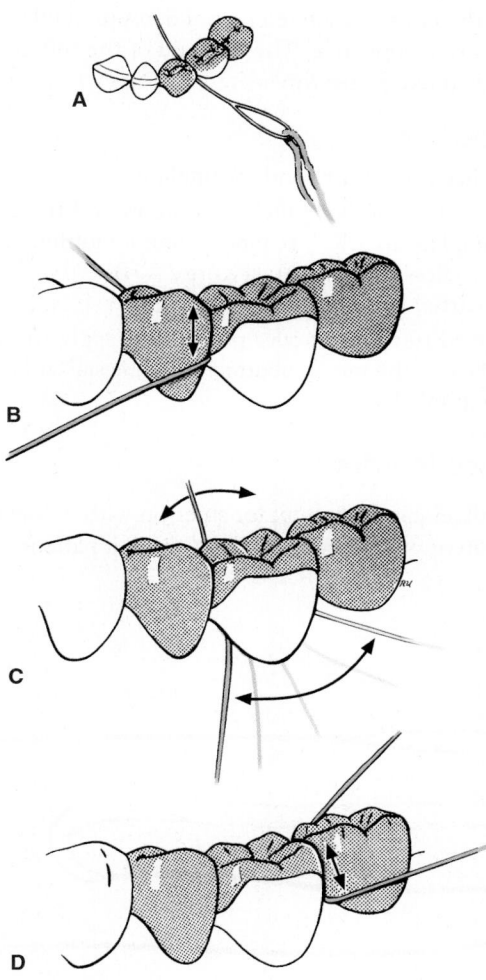

FIGURE 27-6 • Use of Floss Threader. A: Use floss threader to draw the floss between abutment and pontic. **B:** Apply floss to the distal surface of the mesial abutment; pull through 1 or 2 inches. **C:** Slide floss under pontic. Move back and forth several times, as shown by the arrows, to remove dental biofilm from the gingival surface of the pontic. **D:** Apply new section of floss to the mesial surface of the distal abutment.

◆ Fixed Partial Denture
- Thread floss over pontic and apply to distal surface of the mesial abutment and mesial surface of the distal abutment (Figure 27-6B–D).

II. Tufted Dental Floss

A. Description

Tufted dental floss is regular dental floss alternated with a thickened tufted portion. This type of floss is commercially available.

◆ *Single, precut lengths*
- Available in 2-feet length composed of a 5-inch tufted portion adjacent to a 3-inch stiffened end for inserting under a fixed appliance or orthodontic attachment (Figure 27-7A).
- Example: Super Floss®.

B. Indication for Use

◆ Biofilm removal from mesial and distal abutments and under the pontic of a fixed partial denture, implant, or orthodontic appliance. The stiff end of the tufted floss is inserted like a floss threader.

C. Procedure

◆ Individual Surface of Tooth or Implant
- Curve floss and/or tufted portion around the tooth or implant in a "C" to remove dental biofilm.
- Move floss horizontally (Figure 27-7B).
◆ Fixed Partial Denture
- Thread tufted floss over pontic and apply to distal surface of the mesial abutment and mesial surface of the distal abutment.

III. Floss Holder

A floss holder can be helpful for a person with a disability or for a parent or caregiver serving a child or patient.

◆ *Types*

- Multiuse: using 12–15 inches of floss, wrapping end around button and threading up across slot on prongs and back down toward button on the other side to keep floss taut (Figure 27-8A).
- Single-use: disposable floss holder that is for single use only (Figure 27-9). These disposable flossers go by many names, which include, but are not limited to sword floss, floss picks, or easy flossers.

◆ *Indications for use*
- The mechanical properties, including floss tension and angle, are important considerations when selecting a floss holder.[20]
- The effectiveness of holders maintaining adequate tension of floss through proximal contacts while not displacing the tissue is crucial for proper use.[20]

IV. Gauze Strip

◆ *Uses*
- For proximal surfaces of widely spaced teeth.
- For surfaces of teeth next to edentulous areas.
- For outer mesial and distal surfaces of abutment teeth of a fixed partial denture.
- For areas under posterior cantilevered section of a fixed appliance, such as the distal portion of a denture supported by implants.

◆ *Procedure*
- Cut 1-inch gauze bandage into a 6- to 8-inch length, and fold in thirds or down the center.
- Position the fold of the gauze on the cervical area next to the gingival crest and work back and forth several times; hold ends in a distal direction to clean a mesial surface, and in a mesial direction to clean a distal surface (Figure 27-10).

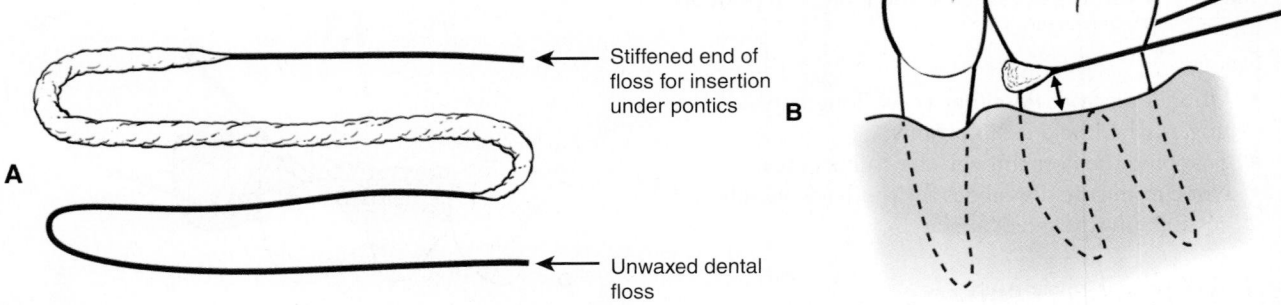

A

Stiffened end of floss for insertion under pontics

B

Unwaxed dental floss

FIGURE 27-7 • Tufted Dental Floss. A common brand is called Super Floss **(A)** in a precut length with a tufted portion and a 3-inch stiffened end for insertion under a fixed prosthesis. **B:** How the tufted part of the floss might be used interproximally to remove biofilm is shown.

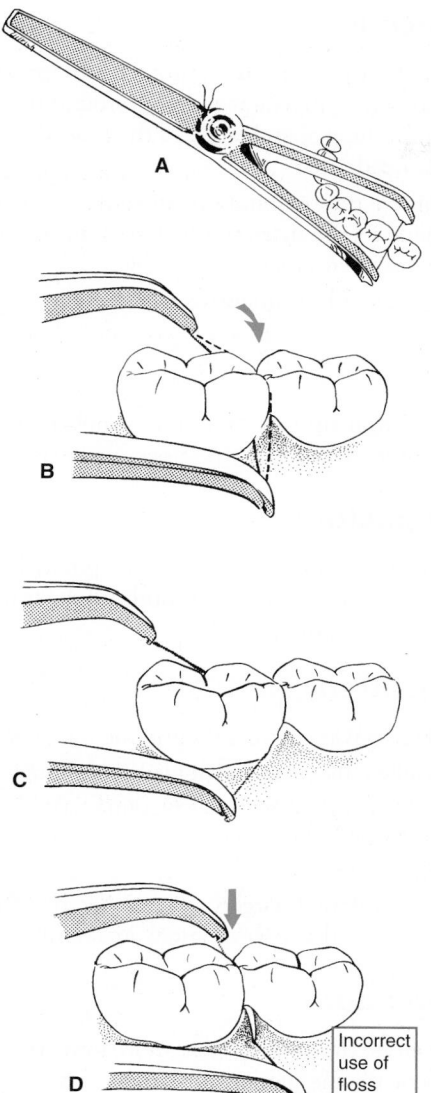

FIGURE 27-8 • Use of a Floss Holder. A: The floss is held over the proximal contact for insertion. A hand rest is maintained on the chin to prevent excess pressure. **B:** As the floss is lowered gently and drawn through the contact area, the holder is pulled mesially when the floss is applied to the distal surface and pushed distally when the floss is applied to the mesial surface. **C:** Floss is lowered slightly below the gingival margin. **D:** Floss cut in the papilla when used incorrectly.

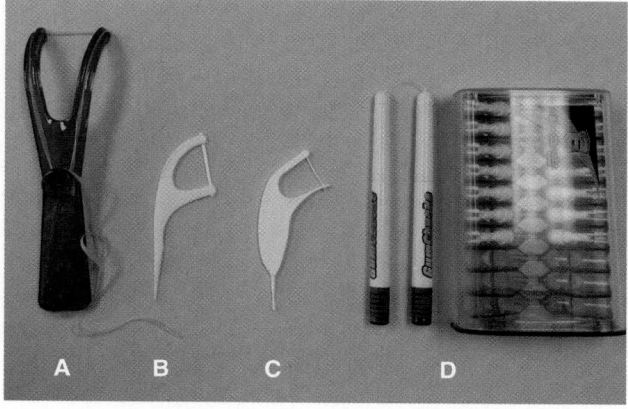

FIGURE 27-9 • Disposable Single-Use Floss Holders. A: Reusable floss holder device. **B:** Disposable floss holder. **C:** Ortho floss holder. **D:** Flossing aid with two handle aid and disposable tips.

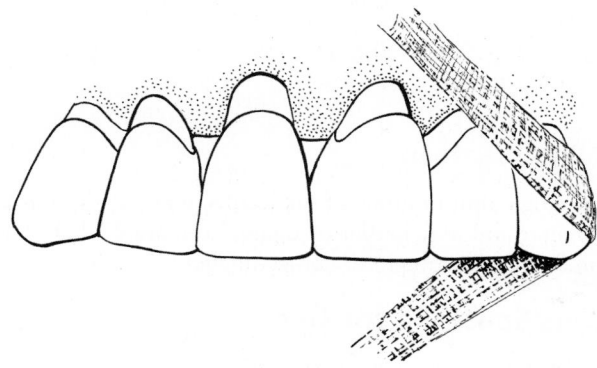

FIGURE 27-10 • Gauze Strip. A 6- or 8-inch length of 1-inch bandage is folded in thirds and placed around a tooth adjacent to an edentulous area, a tooth with interdental spacing, or the distal surface of the most posterior tooth. A back and forth motion is used to clean the dental biofilm from the surface.

POWER FLOSSERS

I. Description

◆ Several types of power flossers are available.

   • One type of power flosser is battery-operated and uses a disposable flexible nylon tip for interproximal care (Figure 27-11).

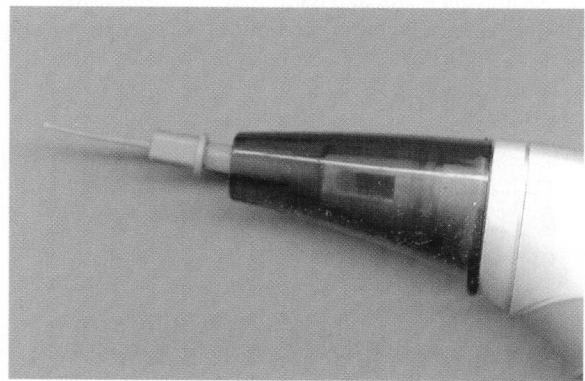

FIGURE 27-11 • Power Dental Flossing Device. An example of a powered dental flossing device.

- Another type of power flosser is an air flosser, which uses burst of air and water droplets to disrupt dental biofilm.
- Power flossers have not been found to be as effective as other interproximal aids, with one study finding the air flosser removed only 48% of interproximal biofilm.[21]

II. Indications for Use

- May be helpful for patients who are unable to use regular floss or those with manual dexterity issues.
- A power flosser can also be helpful for those who do not clean interproximally regularly and want to try this tool.

III. Procedure

- If the device has a reservoir, fill it with water.
- Standing near the sink, point the flosser interproximally and activate the device.
- Move systematically through the mouth on the facial and lingual interproximal areas.

SINGLE-TUFT BRUSH (END-TUFT BRUSH)

I. Description

The single tuft, or group of small tufts, may be 3–6 mm in diameter and may be flat or tapered (Figure 27-12). The handle may be straight or contra-angled.

II. Indications for Use

- *For open interproximal areas*
- *For fixed dental prostheses*
  - The single-tuft brush may be adaptable around and under a fixed partial denture, pontic, orthodontic appliance, precision attachment, or implant abutment.
- *For difficult-to-reach areas*
  - The lingual surfaces of the mandibular molars, abutment teeth, distal surfaces of the terminal molars, areas of missing teeth, and teeth that are crowded are examples of areas where an end-tuft brush may be of value.

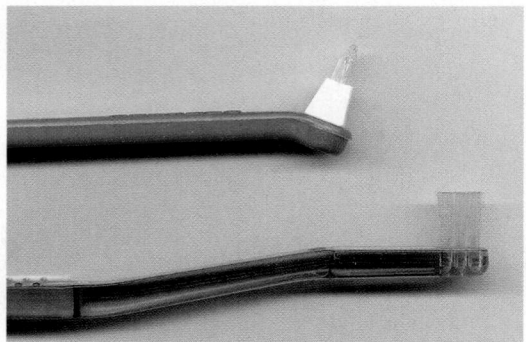

FIGURE 27-12 • **End-Tuft Brushes.** End-tuft brushes come in flat and tapered shapes and can be used to clean areas that are difficult to access with a standard toothbrush.

III. Procedure

- Direct the tip of the tuft into the interproximal area and along the gingival margin; go around the distal surfaces from lingual and facial of the most distal teeth in all four quadrants.
- Combine a rotating motion with intermittent pressure especially in the interproximal areas to reach as much of the proximal surfaces as possible.
- Use a sulcular brushing stroke.

INTERDENTAL TIP

The interdental tip may be called a rubber tip or rubber tip stimulator.

I. Composition and Design

Conical or pyramidal flexible rubber tip may be attached to the end of the handle of a toothbrush or is on a single plastic handle (Figure 27-13).

II. Indications for Use

- For cleaning debris from the interdental area.
- For biofilm removal at and just below the gingival margin.
- The rubber tip is sometimes recommended for stimulation of gingival blood flow, although literature to support this is absent.
- After periodontal surgery, the rubber tip may also be used to shape the interproximal area during healing.

III. Procedure

- Trace along the gingival margin with the tip positioned just beneath the margin (1–2 mm). The adaptation is similar to the toothpick in holder (Figure 27-14).
- Rinse the tip as indicated during use to remove debris, and wash thoroughly at the finish.

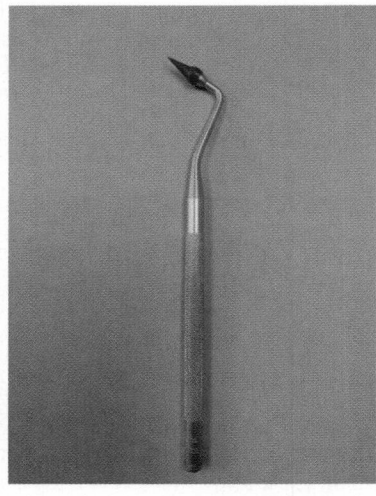

FIGURE 27-13 • **Rubber Tip (Also Called a Rubber Tip Stimulator) with Handle.**

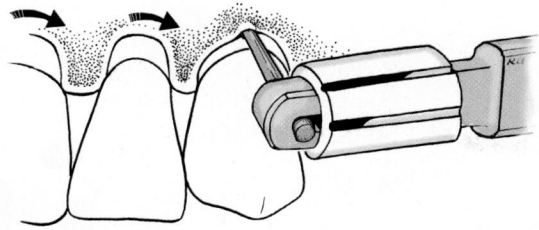

FIGURE 27-14 • Toothpick in Holder for Dental Biofilm at Gingival Margin. The tip is placed at or just below the gingival margin. Gently trace the gingival margin of each tooth.

TOOTHPICK IN HOLDER

I. Description

A round toothpick is inserted into a plastic handle with contra-angled ends for adaptation to the tooth surface at the gingival margin for biofilm removal. The device is also called a Perio-Aid®.

II. Indications for Use

◆ Patient with periodontitis
  • For biofilm removal at and just under the gingival margin, for interdental cleaning, particularly for concave proximal tooth surfaces, and for exposed furcation area.[22]
◆ Orthodontic patient
  • For biofilm removal at gingival margin above bands.

III. Procedure

A. Prepare Instrument

◆ Insert round, tapered toothpick into the end of the holder. One type of holder has angulated ends for use in various positions.
◆ Twist the toothpick firmly into place. Break off the long end so that sharp edges do not scratch the inner cheek or the tongue during use.

B. Application

◆ Apply toothpick at the gingival margin.
  • To remove biofilm just below the gingival margin, position the toothpick tip to a 70° angle to the long axis of the tooth and gently trace slightly subgingivally along the gingival margin from one interproximal space to the next[22] (Figure 27-14).
◆ For hypersensitive spots, usually at the cervical third of a tooth, the patient can use the tip daily to massage dentifrice for desensitization on the sensitive area.

WOODEN INTERDENTAL CLEANER

I. Description

The wooden cleaner is a 2-inch-long device made of soft basswood. It is triangular in cross section, as shown in Figure 27-15.
◆ A common brand is Stimudent®.

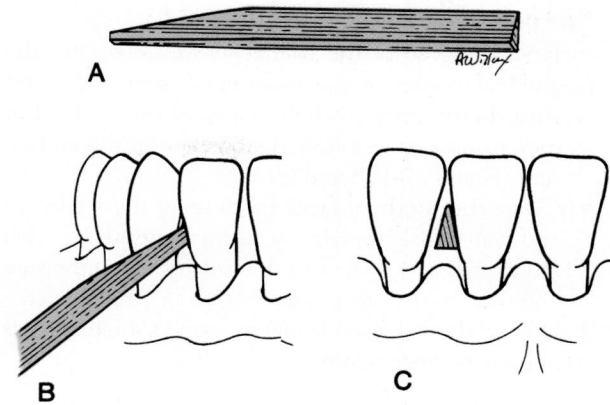

FIGURE 27-15 • Wooden Interdental Cleaner. A: The 2-inch wooden triangular cleaner. **B:** Application on the proximal surface of a tooth with a type III embrasure. The base of the triangle is on the gingival side. **C:** The side of the triangle is rubbed in and out against the proximal surface to remove dental biofilm.

II. Indications for Use

◆ *Application*
  • For cleaning proximal tooth surfaces where the tooth surfaces are exposed and interdental gingivae are missing. Space must be adequate, otherwise the gingival tissue can be traumatized.[23]
◆ *Advantages*
  • Ease of use.
  • Transported easily and can be used throughout the day.
  • Patients use woodsticks more frequently than dental floss.[23]
  • Although woodsticks do not remove plaque as effectively as dental floss, research suggests that they significantly reduce bleeding and interdental inflammation.[23]
◆ *Limitations*
  • As with most interdental devices, the wooden cleaner is advised only for patients who follow instructions carefully.
  • The wooden interdental cleaner cannot access root concavities and irregularities in proximal areas to adequately remove dental biofilm.
  • Difficult to use in posterior areas and from the lingual aspect of the teeth.[23]

III. Procedure

◆ Fulcrum
  • Teach the patient to use a fulcrum by placing the hand on the cheek or chin or by placing a finger on the gingiva convenient to the place where the tip will be applied.
◆ Preparation
  • Soften the wood by placing the pointed end in the mouth and moistening with saliva.

◆ Patient Instructions
  • Hold the base of the triangular wedge toward the gingival border of the interdental area and insert with the tip pointed slightly toward the occlusal or incisal surfaces to follow the contour of the embrasure (Figure 27-15B and C).
  • Clean the tooth surfaces by moving the wedge in and out while applying a burnishing stroke with moderate pressure first to one side of the embrasure and then to the other side, about four strokes each.
  • Discard the wooden cleaner as soon as the first signs of splaying are evident.

ORAL IRRIGATION

I. Description

◆ The oral irrigator was introduced in 1962 and may also be called a water flosser.[24]
◆ Irrigation is the targeted application of a pulsated or steady stream of water or other irrigant for preventive or therapeutic purposes.
  • The purpose of irrigation is to reduce the bacteria and inflammatory mediators that lead to the initiation or progression of periodontal infections.
  • For the patient, irrigation can be a part of routine self-care.
◆ Water flossers use pulsated stream of water under pressure.[25]
  • The water flossers have been shown to remove supragingival interproximal plaque and reduce gingival inflammation.[25-30] However, the research has been funded by a single manufacturer, so there is a risk of bias and more research is needed.
◆ The research on the benefits of subgingival irrigation with or without antimicrobial agents in managing microbial and clinical signs of periodontal disease remains inconsistent and more study is needed.[24,31]
  • The oral irrigator does not appear to reduce visible dental biofilm; however, it may have positive effects on gingival health over toothbrushing alone.[24]
  • In addition, some research suggests reduced counts of periodontal pathogens.[32]

II. Types of Devices

◆ Countertop power-driven model has a large reservoir for liquid (Figure 27-16A).
◆ Cordless model has a large base to serve as a reservoir for liquid and is good for travel (Figure 27-16B).
  • The handle is bulky because of the reservoir and may be too heavy for some patients.
◆ The shower model attaches to the showerhead or faucet and uses the pressure of the shower water, which may be somewhat lower than the irrigation delivered by the countertop model.

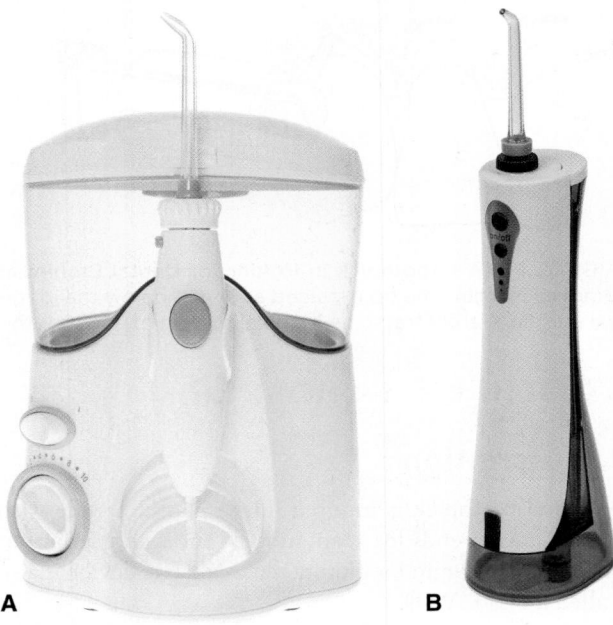

FIGURE 27-16 • Water Flossers. A: A countertop dental water jet that plugs into an electrical outlet. **B:** A portable dental water jet with a rechargeable battery. (A: © olegganko/Shutterstock; B: © addillum/Shutterstock)

III. Delivery Tips

◆ Standard jet tip delivers a steady flow of irrigant (Figure 27-17A).
◆ The subgingival tip is designed for subgingival irrigation with a soft rubber tip (Figure 27-17B) to be placed below the gingival margin.
◆ An orthodontic tip is available to remove debris and loose dental biofilm from brackets, wires, and bands (Figure 27-17C).
◆ A filament-type tip (Figure 27-17D).

IV. Procedure

These are general instructions for use of an oral irrigator:
◆ Fill the reservoir with water or other irrigant.
◆ Choose the appropriate tip.
◆ Direct the jet tip toward the interdental area until almost touching the tooth surface.
◆ Hold the tip at a right angle (90°) to the long axis of the tooth supragingival irrigation to remove food debris and loose dental biofilm.
◆ Lean over the sink to minimize splatter and splashing water on the mirror, countertop, and floor.
◆ Turn the unit on using low power and increase the water pressure to a rate that is comfortable.
◆ Use a systematic approach for moving through the mouth, that is, maxillary arch first, then the mandibular, facial, palatal, and lingual.
◆ When done, empty the reservoir to prevent bacterial growth.

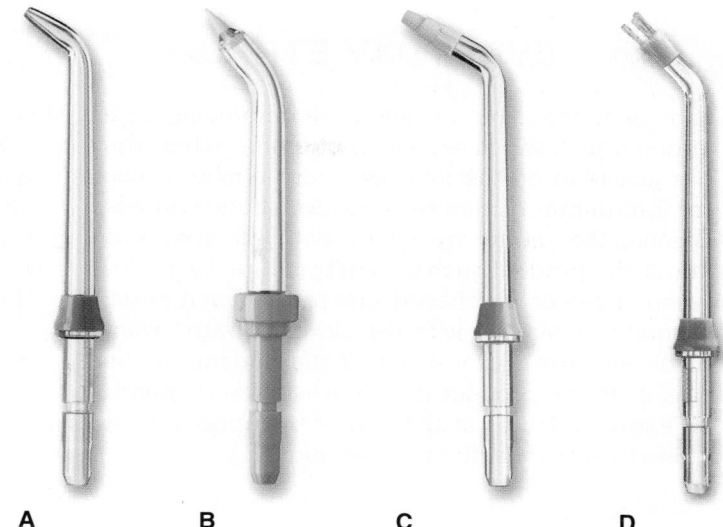

FIGURE 27-17 • Irrigation Tips. Four examples of irrigation tip designs. **A:** Standard irrigation tip. **B:** Subgingival tip. **C:** Orthodontic tip. **D:** Filament-type tip.

A   **B**   **C**   **D**

V. Applications for Practice

Regular use of daily personal oral irrigation is beneficial.[24] Use a patient-centered approach to evaluate each patient's needs individually to determine which techniques, products, or devices are appropriate.

A. Reduction of Gingival Inflammation

◆ The evidence is inconsistent on improving parameters of periodontal health, but there was a positive trend toward improving gingival health.[24] More research is needed.

B. Problem Areas

◆ Areas that are difficult to access with traditional mechanical methods:
  • Open interdental areas.
  • Malpositioned teeth.
  • Exposed furcations.

C. Special Needs Areas

◆ Prosthetic replacements such as a bridge with a pontic for a missing tooth and fixed partial dentures.
◆ Orthodontic appliances.
◆ Intermaxillary fixation appliances for orthognathic surgery and fractured jaw.
◆ Complex restorations and other extensive rehabilitation.
◆ Implant maintenance.
◆ Ineffective interdental technique due to physical ability or lack of compliance.

DOCUMENTATION

Documentation for a patient's interdental care progress needs to include a minimum of the following:

◆ Includes all interdental aid recommendations and demonstrations with the patient.
◆ A sample documentation can be found in Box 27-1.

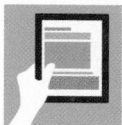

BOX 27-1

Example Documentation:
Recommendations for Daily Interdental Care

S—A 46-year-old female patient presents for routine 3-month continuing care appointment. Patient states, "I floss regularly, and have even tried using the 'fuzzy floss' that you gave me last time, but it almost seems as though the floss doesn't do a good job. Is there another way to clean that area?"

O—Generalized recession and extensive loss of interdental papilla on the upper right quadrant. Observed patient flossing area and found she uses good flossing technique.

A—Interdental brush may be a better choice than tufted floss for more thorough cleaning of the wide embrasure spaces in that area of her mouth.

P—Provided instructions for use of a travel interdental brush with a tapered or cone shape as well as an interdental brush handle with replaceable inserts. Observed patient use of the interdental brushes and worked with her to refine her technique. The patient felt these would do a better job of removing the debris and biofilm and will use these in every space where they fit and floss the remaining areas. Samples of two types of interdental brushes were provided and suggestions where she can purchase replacements.

Signed: _____, RDH

Date: _____

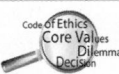

EVERYDAY ETHICS

Jane is at the clinic for a routine continuing care appointment and is excited about information she has just read on the Internet about a new device for interdental biofilm removal. She begins to ask Glenna, the dental hygienist, detailed questions about the product such as whether it really works, where it can be purchased, and how much it costs. Glenna is unfamiliar with the aid but doesn't want to be embarrassed in front of the patient so she tells Jane the product does not work and spends an extra 5 minutes at the end of the appointment going over manual flossing techniques.

Questions for Consideration

1. Which of the dental hygiene core values have application in this scenario? Also consider the ethical duty for lifelong learning.

2. From the patient's perspective, what is the role of the dental hygienist in this situation? Consider the roles of dental hygiene in Chapter 1.

3. Is it unethical to mislead the patient about a product when the value is unknown or the dental hygienist prefers the benefits of another (perhaps rival) product? Why or why not?

Factors To Teach The Patient

► Use of disclosing solution will provide the patient with a visual understanding of the limitation of the toothbrush in accessing and cleaning the interdental area thoroughly.

► Discuss dental biofilm and how it collects on the proximal tooth surfaces when left undisturbed.

► Educate the patient on the reason why the interdental area is more vulnerable to infection.

► Use hands-on demonstrations to show how interdental aids are used to clean the proximal tooth surfaces. It is essential the patient also demonstrates the use of the interdental aids.

► Ensure the patient understands the need to ask the dental professional about new products they see advertised and whether the product meets the patient's individual oral self-care needs.

ENHANCE YOUR UNDERSTANDING

ONLINE RESOURCES
(see the inside front cover for access information)
- Audio glossary
- Appendices

SUPPORT FOR LEARNING
(available separately)

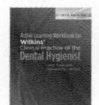

- *Active Learning Workbook for Wilkins' Clinical Practice of the Dental Hygienist, 13th Edition*

INDIVIDUALIZED REVIEW
- Customized practice quizzing with Navigate 2 TestPrep for *Wilkins' Clinical Practice of the Dental Hygienist*

References

1. Chapple IL, Van der Weijden F, Doerfer C, et al. Primary prevention of periodontitis: managing gingivitis. *J Clin Periodontol.* 2015;42(suppl 16):S71-S76.

2. Joshi K, Baiju CS, Khashu H, Bansal S, Maheswari IB. Clinical assessment of interdental papilla competency parameters in the esthetic zone. *J Esthetic Rest Dent.* 2017;29(4):270-275.

3. Smukler H, Nager MC, Tolmie PC. Interproximal tooth morphology and its effect on plaque removal. *Quintessence Int.* 1989;20(4):249-255.

4. Roussa E. Anatomic characteristics of the furcation and root surfaces of molar teeth and their significance in the clinical management of marginal periodontitis. *Clin Anat.* 1998;11(3):177-186.

5. Fox SC, Bosworth BL. A morphological survey of proximal root concavities: a consideration in periodontal therapy. *J Am Dent Assoc.* 1987;114(6):811-814.

6. Drisko CL. Periodontal self-care: evidence-based support. *Periodontol 2000.* 2013;62(1):243-255.

7. Wilder RS, Bray KS. Improving periodontal outcomes: merging clinical and behavioral science. *Periodontol 2000.* 2016;71(1):65-81.

8. Salzer S, Slot DE, Van der Weijden FA, Dorfer CE. Efficacy of inter-dental mechanical plaque control in managing gingivitis—a meta-review. *J Clin Periodontol.* 2015;42(suppl 16):S92-S105.

9. Graziani F, Palazzolo A, Gennai S, et al. Interdental plaque reduction after use of different devices in young subjects with intact papilla: a randomized clinical trial. *Int J Dent Hyg.* 2017;16(3):389-396.

10. Abouassi T, Woelber JP, Holst K, et al. Clinical efficacy and patients' acceptance of a rubber interdental bristle. A randomized controlled trial. *Clin Oral Investig.* 2014;18(7):1873-1880.

11. Hennequin-Hoenderdos NL, van der Sluijs E, van der Weijden GA, Slot DE. Efficacy of a rubber bristles interdental cleaner compared to an interdental brush on dental plaque, gingival bleeding and gingival abrasion: a randomized clinical trial. *Int J Dent Hyg.* 2017;16(3):380-388.

12. Johnson TM, Worthington HV, Clarkson JE, Pericic TP, Sambunjak D, Imai P. Mechanical interdental cleaning for preventing and controlling periodontal diseases and dental caries. *Cochrane Database Syst Rev.* 2015;(12):1-17. doi: 10.1002/14651858.CD012018.

13. Berchier CE, Slot DE, Haps S, Van der Weijden GA. The efficacy of dental floss in addition to a toothbrush on plaque and parameters of gingival inflammation: a systematic review. *Int J Dent Hyg.* 2008;6(4):265-279.

14. Poklepovic T, Worthington HV, Johnson TM, et al. Interdental brushing for the prevention and control of periodontal diseases and dental caries in adults. *Cochrane Database Syst Rev.* 2013;(12):CD009857.

15. Larsen HC, Slot DE, Van Zoelen C, Barendregt DS, Van der Weijden GA. The effectiveness of conically shaped compared with cylindrically shaped interdental brushes—a randomized controlled clinical trial. *Int J Dent Hyg.* 2017;15(3):211-218.

16. Ciancio SG, Shibly O, Farber GA. Clinical evaluation of the effect of two types of dental floss on plaque and gingival health. *Clin Prev Dent.* 1992;14(3):14-18.

17. Dörfer CE, Wündrich D, Staehle HJ, Pioch T. Gliding capacity of different dental flosses. *J Periodontol.* 2001;72(5):672-678.

18. Azcarate-Velazquez F, Garrido-Serrano R, Castillo-Dali G, Serrera-Figallo MA, Ganan-Calvo A, Torres-Lagares D. Effectiveness of flossing loops in the control of the gingival health. *J Clin Exp Dent.* 2017;9(6):e756-e761.

19. Hallmon WW, Waldrop TC, Houston GD, Hawkins BF. Flossing clefts. Clinical and histologic observations. *J Periodontol.* 1986;57(8):501-504.

20. Wolff A, Staehle HJ. Improving the mechanical properties of multiuse dental floss holders. *Int J Dent Hyg.* 2014;12(4):245-250.

21. Sharma NC, Lyle DM, Qaqish JG, Schuller R. Comparison of two power interdental cleaning devices on the reduction of gingivitis. *J Clin Dent.* 2012;23(1):22-26.

22. Lewis MW, Holder-Ballard C, Selders RJ Jr, Scarbecz M, Johnson HG, Turner EW. Comparison of the use of a toothpick holder to dental floss in improvement of gingival health in humans. *J Periodontol.* 2004;75(4):551-556.

23. Hoenderdos NL, Slot DE, Paraskevas S, Van der Weijden GA. The efficacy of woodsticks on plaque and gingival inflammation: a systematic review. *Int J Dent Hyg.* 2008;6(4):280-289.

24. Husseini A, Slot DE, Van der Weijden GA. The efficacy of oral irrigation in addition to a toothbrush on plaque and the clinical parameters of periodontal inflammation: a systematic review. *Int J Dent Hyg.* 2008;6(4):304-314.

25. Goyal CR, Lyle DM, Qaqish JG, Schuller R. Efficacy of two interdental cleaning devices on clinical signs of inflammation: a four-week randomized controlled trial. *J Clin Dent.* 2015;26(2):55-60.

26. Barnes CM, Russell CM, Reinhardt RA, Payne JB, Lyle DM. Comparison of irrigation to floss as an adjunct to tooth brushing: effect on bleeding, gingivitis, and supragingival plaque. *J Clin Dent.* 2005;16(3):71-77.

27. Goyal CR, Lyle DM, Qaqish JG, Schuller R. Evaluation of the plaque removal efficacy of a water flosser compared to string floss in adults after a single use. *J Clin Dent.* 2013;24(2):37-42.

28. Goyal CR, Lyle DM, Qaqish JG, Schuller R. Comparison of water flosser and interdental brush on reduction of gingival bleeding and plaque: a randomized controlled pilot study. *J Clin Dent.* 2016;27(2):61-65.

29. Goyal CR, Lyle DM, Qaqish JG, Schuller R. The addition of a water flosser to power tooth brushing: effect on bleeding, gingivitis, and plaque. *J Clin Dent.* 2012;23(2):57-63.

30. Lyle DM, Goyal CR, Qaqish JG, Schuller R. Comparison of water flosser and interdental brush on plaque removal: a single-use pilot study. *J Clin Dent.* 2016;27(1):23-26.

31. Nagarakanti S, Gunupati S, Chava VK, Reddy BVR. Effectiveness of subgingival irrigation as an adjunct to scaling and root planing in the treatment of chronic periodontitis: a systematic review. *J Clin Diagnostic Res.* 2015;9(7):ZE06-ZE09.

32. Pandya DJ, Manohar B, Mathur LK, Shankarapillai R. Comparative evaluation of two subgingival irrigating solutions in the management of periodontal disease: a clinicomicrobial study. *J Indian Soc Periodontol.* 2016;20(6):597-602.

28

Dentifrices and Mouthrinses

Kristeen Perry, RDH, MSDH

CHAPTER OUTLINE

CHEMOTHERAPEUTICS

DENTIFRICES

PREVENTIVE AND THERAPEUTIC BENEFITS OF DENTIFRICES
I. Prevention of Dental Caries
II. Remineralization of Early Noncavitated Dental Caries
III. Reduction of Biofilm Formation
IV. Reduction of Gingivitis/Inflammation
V. Reduction of Dentin Hypersensitivity
VI. Reduction of Supragingival Calculus Formation

COSMETIC EFFECTS OF DENTIFRICES
I. Removal of Extrinsic Stain
II. Reduction of Oral Malodor (Halitosis)

BASIC COMPONENTS OF DENTIFRICES: INACTIVES
I. Detergents (Foaming Agents or Surfactants)
II. Cleaning and Polishing Agents (Abrasives)
III. Binders (Thickeners)
IV. Humectants (Moisture Stabilizers)
V. Preservatives
VI. Flavoring Agents (Sweeteners)

ACTIVE COMPONENTS OF DENTIFRICES

SELECTION OF DENTIFRICES
I. Prevention or Reduction of Oral Disease
II. Considerations for the Pediatric Patient
III. Patient-Specific Dentifrice Recommendations

MOUTHRINSES

PURPOSES AND USES OF MOUTHRINSES
I. Before Professional Treatment
II. Self-Care

PREVENTIVE AND THERAPEUTIC AGENTS OF MOUTHRINSES
I. Fluoride
II. Chlorhexidine
III. Triclosan
IV. Phenolic-Related Essential Oils
V. Quaternary Ammonium Compounds
VI. Oxygenating Agents
VII. Oxidizing Agents

COMMERCIAL MOUTHRINSE INGREDIENTS
I. Active Ingredients
II. Inactive Ingredients
III. Patient-Specific Mouthrinse Recommendations
IV. Contraindications

PROCEDURE FOR RINSING

EMERGING ALTERNATIVE PRACTICES
I. Oil Pulling

UNITED STATES FOOD AND DRUG ADMINISTRATION
I. Brief History of the FDA
II. Purposes of the FDA
III. Dental Products Regulated
IV. Research Requirements and Documentation

AMERICAN DENTAL ASSOCIATION SEAL OF ACCEPTANCE PROGRAM
I. Purposes of the Seal Program
II. Product Submission and Acceptance Process
III. Acceptance and Use of the Seal

DOCUMENTATION

EVERYDAY ETHICS

FACTORS TO TEACH THE PATIENT

REFERENCES

LEARNING OBJECTIVES

After studying this chapter, the student will be able to:

1. Identify and define the active and inactive components in dentifrices and mouthrinses.

2. Explain the mechanism of action for preventive and therapeutic agents in dentifrices and mouthrinses.

3. Explain the purpose and use of dentifrices and mouthrinses.

4. Discuss Food and Drug Administration (FDA) and the purpose of FDA.

5. Explain the American Dental Association Seal of Acceptance program and its purpose.

CHEMOTHERAPEUTICS

Recent advances in understanding the pathogenesis of periodontitis have led to alternative therapies that focus on reduction of inflammation in the oral cavity using both mechanical devices and chemotherapeutics.

- Inflammation of periodontal tissues has an impact on the human body beyond the oral cavity, particularly in immunocompromised individuals.
- Oral inflammation has been linked to several conditions, including diabetes and heart disease.[1,2]
- Increased inflammation associated with diabetes can make a patient more susceptible to periodontal disease.[2,3]
- Oral pathogens can travel to the lungs, causing health-care-associated pneumonia.[4]
- Either the clinician or the patient can administer chemotherapeutics.

DENTIFRICES

The benefits of using dentifrices may be preventive, therapeutic, or cosmetic. A dentifrice is a substance applied with a toothbrush or other applicator for:

- Removal of biofilm, stain, and other soft deposits from the gingiva and tooth surfaces.
- Application of therapeutic agents.
- Superficial cosmetic effects.

PREVENTIVE AND THERAPEUTIC BENEFITS OF DENTIFRICES

I. Prevention of Dental Caries

- Although fluoride has long been recognized as an anti-cariogenic agent, the addition of stannous fluoride to a dentifrice was problematic because of lack of compatibility with abrasive agents.[5]
- The first caries-preventive dentifrice contained stannous fluoride (0.4%). It became available commercially in 1955.[6]
- Additional information about fluoride dentifrices is described in Chapter 34.
- Xylitol, a flavoring agent in some dentifrices, has been shown to provide anticaries benefits.[7]

II. Remineralization of Early Noncavitated Dental Caries

- Fluoride enhances remineralization as described in Chapters 25 and 34.

III. Reduction of Biofilm Formation

- Agents used:
  - Triclosan.
  - Zinc citrate.
  - Stannous fluoride.

IV. Reduction of Gingivitis/ Inflammation

- An antigingivitis dentifrice can contribute to the improved health of gingival tissue.
- Triclosan is the primary agent that has shown efficacy in reducing gingival inflammation.[8]
- Triclosan combined with a copolymer of polyvinyl methoxyethylene and maleic acid (PVM/MA) increases the substantivity after eating and drinking.[9]
- Use of a dentifrice-containing triclosan has demonstrated[8–11]:
  - Significantly reduced levels of *Aggregatibacter actinomycetemcomitans* and *Porphyromonas gingivalis* during induction of gingivitis.[11]
  - Research is inconsistent with regard to reduction in gingival inflammation and gingival bleeding, and a systematic review suggests that there is clinically no significant difference.[10,12]
  - There is weak evidence for a reduction of 15% in supragingival biofilm formation.[12]

V. Reduction of Dentin Hypersensitivity

- For in-home treatment of dentin hypersensitivity, chemical occlusion (potassium nitrate and sodium fluoride) of the dentinal tubules and nerve desensitization are most effective.[13]
- In-home treatment is the first intervention for dentin hypersensitivity, but if in-home treatments are not effective, then in-office treatments are recommended.[13]
- More information on reducing dentin hypersensitivity is discussed in Chapter 41.

VI. Reduction of Supragingival Calculus Formation

- "Tartar-control" dentifrices shown to help inhibit supragingival calculus may contain:
  - Pyrophosphate salts.[14]
  - Zinc salts (zinc chloride and zinc citrate).[14]
  - Sodium hexametaphosphate.[15]
  - Triclosan/copolymer.[10]

COSMETIC EFFECTS OF DENTIFRICES

I. Removal of Extrinsic Stain

- The pigments from foods, tobacco use, or chemical agents may become imbedded in the acquired pellicle and dental biofilm.
- Cosmetic results from dentifrice are based on:
  - Mechanical removal of the stained biofilm.
  - Delivery of a bleaching agent.
- Each commercially available product needs to be evaluated individually for efficacy and patient acceptance.
- More information on tooth stains is provided in Chapters 17 and 42.

II. Reduction of Oral Malodor (Halitosis)

◆ Certain ingredients added to a dentifrice can reduce oral malodor on a temporary basis by inhibiting the production of volatile sulfur compounds (VSCs).

◆ Chlorhexidine (CHX), cetylpyridinium chloride (CPC), and zinc formulations have a beneficial effect on reducing oral malodor via reduction of VSCs.[16,17]

◆ Triclosan/copolymer can control the bacteria associated with VSCs, thereby reducing oral malodor.[18]

◆ Stannous fluoride combined with sodium hexametaphosphate can reduce VSC production.[18]

BASIC COMPONENTS OF DENTIFRICES: INACTIVES

◆ Most dentifrices share a common composition of ingredients needed for a stable formulation.

◆ Dentifrices are sold primarily as pastes and gels. The common ingredients and their function are listed in Table 28-1.

◆ In addition to the inactive ingredients described in Table 28-1, a therapeutic dentifrice will have a drug or chemical agent stated as an active ingredient for a specific preventive or therapeutic action.

◆ The active ingredient represents approximately 1.5%–2% of the dentifrice's formulation.

◆ Therapeutic agents are described in Table 28-2.

TABLE 28-2 • Therapeutic Active Ingredients in Dentifrices

BENEFIT	ACTIVE INGREDIENTS
Antibiofilm/antigingivitis	Triclosan/copolymer, stannous fluoride, zinc citrate
Anticalculus	Tetrapotassium pyrophosphate, tetrasodium pyrophosphate, sodium hexametaphosphate, triclosan/copolymer, zinc compounds
Desensitizer	Potassium nitrate, potassium citrate, potassium chloride, stannous fluoride, strontium chloride
Oral malodor	Essential oils, chlorine dioxide, triclosan/copolymer, stannous fluoride/sodium hexametaphosphate

I. Detergents (Foaming Agents or Surfactants)

◆ *Purposes*
  • Lower surface tension.
  • Penetrate and loosen surface deposits.
  • Suspend debris for easy removal by toothbrush.
  • Emulsify/disperse the flavor oils.
  • Contribute to foaming action.

◆ *Substances used*
  • Sodium lauryl sulfate USP.
  • Sodium N-lauroyl sarcosinate.

II. Cleaning and Polishing Agents (Abrasives)

◆ *Purposes*
  • Cleans well with no damage to tooth surface.
  • A polishing agent is used to produce a smooth tooth surface.
  • A smooth surface can prevent or delay the reaccumulation of stains and deposits.

◆ *Primary abrasives used*[19]:
  • Silica, silicates, and hydrated silica gels.
  • Calcium carbonate.
  • Dicalcium phosphate.
  • Sodium bicarbonate.

III. Binders (Thickeners)

◆ *Purposes*
  • Stabilize the formulation.
  • Prevent separation of the solid and liquid ingredients during storage.

◆ *Types used*
  • Mineral colloids.
  • Natural gums.
  • Seaweed colloids.
  • Synthetic celluloses.

TABLE 28-1 • Ingredients and Function of Commercially Available Dentifrices

INGREDIENT	FUNCTION	AVERAGE FORMULATION PERCENTAGE (%)
Surfactant/detergent	Foaming and cleansing	1–2
Abrasive	Cleaning and polishing	20–40
Binder	Thickening agent and stabilizes formula	1–2
Humectant	Prevents water loss/hardening of dentifrice	20–40
Preservative	Prevents microorganisms from destroying the dentifrice in storage	2–3
Flavoring	Sweetener	1–1.5
Water	Maintains the ingredient in formulation	20–40

IV. Humectants (Moisture Stabilizers)

- *Purposes*
  - Retain moisture.
  - Prevent hardening on exposure to air.
- *Substances used*
  - Xylitol.
  - Glycerol.
  - Sorbitol.

V. Preservatives

- *Purposes*
  - Prevent bacterial growth.
  - Prolong shelf life.
- *Substances used*
  - Alcohol.
  - Benzoates.
  - Dichlorinated phenols.

VI. Flavoring Agents (Sweeteners)

- *Purposes*
  - Impart a pleasant flavor for patient acceptance.
  - Mask other ingredients that may have a less pleasant flavor.
- *Substances used*
  - Essential oils (peppermint, cinnamon, wintergreen, clove).
  - Artificial noncariogenic sweeteners (xylitol, glycerol, sorbitol).

ACTIVE COMPONENTS OF DENTIFRICES

Today's dentifrice selections offer a variety of active ingredients that may help prevent caries, dentin hypersensitivity, biofilm formation, gingivitis, calculus formation, and oral malodor.

- The first active ingredient introduced in a dentifrice was fluoride.
- Since then, there have been major developments in this area. These active ingredients provide benefits in the areas of:
  - Anticaries.
  - Antibiofilm/antigingivitis.
  - Anticalculus.
  - Antioral malodor (halitosis).
  - Antisensitivity.
  - Specific active ingredients are summarized in Table 28-2.

SELECTION OF DENTIFRICES

I. Prevention or Reduction of Oral Disease

- Dental caries.
- Fluoride-containing dentifrice during remineralization program (see Chapters 25 and 34).
- Dentin hypersensitivity.
- Gingivitis.
- Calculus formation.
- Oral malodor/reduction of VSCs.

II. Considerations for the Pediatric Patient

- *Birth to first tooth eruption*
  - Parents can clean the child's gingiva with a soft infant toothbrush or cloth and water.
- *Eruption of first tooth*
  - Parents can begin to start brushing twice daily using fluoridated toothpaste and a soft, age-appropriate sized toothbrush.
  - Use a very small "smear" or rice-sized amount of toothpaste to brush the teeth of a child less than 3 years of age.[20] The small smear of fluoride paste is shown in Chapter 47.
- *2–5 year old*
  - The parent can dispense a "pea-sized" amount of toothpaste for children over 3 years of age (Chapter 47) and perform or assist child's tooth brushing.[20]
  - Parents need to recognize that young children do not have the ability to brush their teeth effectively without help and supervision.
  - Parents can be role models for their child by brushing their teeth at the same time as the child.
  - Children should be supervised until they are able to adequate removal plaque biofilm, spit out toothpaste, and not swallow excess toothpaste during brushing.

III. Patient-Specific Dentifrice Recommendations

- Dentifrice recommendations are a key part of personal daily care planning and are patient-specific.
- Considerations include:
  - Patient's current oral condition.
  - Any patient complaint/concern.
  - Sensitivities or allergies to a specific ingredient.
  - Propensity of staining (stannous fluoride–containing dentifrice).
  - Patient's nontherapeutic/cosmetic choices.
  - Expectation of compliance. When a dentifrice does not appeal in either taste or texture, it will not be used no matter what its therapeutic benefits might be.
  - Personal trial is needed before a recommendation is made. Dental hygienists need firsthand experience with each product they recommend.

MOUTHRINSES

- Mechanical aids may not be sufficient to maintain optimum oral health for certain patients and may be supplemented with the use of a chemotherapeutic mouthrinse.
- The benefits of using a mouthrinse may be one or more of the following: preventive, cosmetic, and therapeutic.
- Chemotherapeutic rinses may have active ingredients to reduce inflammation.
- Cosmetic rinses can provide some extrinsic stain removal when it is superficial in unattached biofilm.
- Therapeutic rinses have healing properties that are delivered by rinsing or irrigation device.
- Delivery: Rinsing can deliver an agent less than 2 mm into the sulcus or pocket and is not a delivery of choice for patients with moderate or deep pockets.[21]
- Functions: A list of general functions of chemotherapeutic agents is provided in Box 28-1.

PURPOSES AND USES OF MOUTHRINSES

I. Before Professional Treatment

- To reduce the numbers of intraoral microorganisms available to aerosols.
- To reduce aerosol contamination during use of a handpiece or ultrasonic scaler.

II. Self-Care

- As part of personal oral self-care for specific needs.
- Biofilm control.
- Dental caries prevention through remineralization of noncavitated early dental caries.
- Prevention of gingivitis.
- Contribute to malodor control.

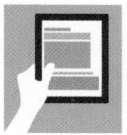

BOX 28-1
Functions of Chemotherapeutic Agents

- Remineralization: restore mineral elements.
- Antimicrobial: bactericidal or bacteriostatic.
  - Biofilm control.
  - Gingival health: reduction/prevention of gingivitis.
- **Astringent:** shrink tissues.
- Anodyne: alleviate pain.
- Buffering: reduce oral acidity.
- Deodorizing: neutralize odor.
- Oxygenating: cleansing.

- Posttreatment therapy following nonsurgical periodontal therapy:
  - Periodontal surgery.
  - Removal of teeth.

PREVENTIVE AND THERAPEUTIC AGENTS OF MOUTHRINSES

I. Fluoride

A. Mechanism of Action

- Stannous fluoride:
  - Deposit of fluoride ion on enamel.
  - Tin ion from stannous fluoride interferes with cell metabolism for antimicrobial effect.
- Sodium fluoride:
  - Deposit of fluoride ion on enamel.
  - Cariostatic: inhibits demineralization and enhances remineralization.

B. Availability and Use

- Available in varying concentrations.
- Uses:
  - Prevention of demineralization.
  - Reduction of hypersensitivity.
  - Reduction of gingivitis.

C. Efficacy

- Reduction in biofilm or dental caries when rinse is used topically by the patient.

D. Considerations

- Stannous: tooth staining; flavor.
- Instruct patient to expectorate/not to swallow.

II. Chlorhexidine

A. Mechanism of Action[22]

- A cationic bisbiguanide with broad antibacterial activity.
- Binds to oral hard and soft tissues.
- Attaches to bacterial cell membrane, thereby damaging the cytoplasm causing lysis.
- Binds to pellicle and salivary mucins to prevent biofilm accumulation.
- Bactericidal and bacteriostatic depending on concentration.
- Bactericidal concentrations cause cell lyses.
- Bacteriostatic concentrations interfere with cell wall transport system.
- The substantivity of CHX: 8–12 hours.
- Antimicrobial and antigingivitis agent.

B. Availability and Uses

- CHX is the most effective antimicrobial and antigingivitis agent available for clinical use.[22,23]

- Mouthrinse available by prescription in a 0.12% solution in the United States (higher concentrations are available in other countries); postsurgery for enhanced wound healing (Figure 28-1).
- ◆ Recommended uses:
  - Preprocedural rinse to reduce bacterial load before instrumentation-producing aerosols.
  - Before, during, and after periodontal debridement.
  - Patients who are at a high risk for dental caries.
  - Immunocompromised individuals who are more susceptible to infection.
  - Postsurgery for enhanced wound healing.

C. Efficacy

- ◆ CHX is safe and effective in:
  - Preventing and controlling biofilm formation.
  - Reducing viability of existing biofilm.
  - Inhibiting and reducing the development of gingivitis.[23]
  - Reducing *mutans streptococci*.[23]
- ◆ CHX varnish reduces dental caries in the following groups; however, evidence remains weak and more research is needed:
  - Children.[24]
  - People with xerostomia.[24]
  - During orthodontic treatment.[25]
  - Root caries.[26]

D. Considerations

- ◆ Low level of toxicity due to poor absorption through mucous membranes.
- ◆ Staining of teeth, including smooth surfaces, pits and fissures, restorations, and soft tissues (Figure 28-2).
- ◆ Increase in supragingival calculus formation.
- ◆ Altered taste perception.
- ◆ Minor irritation to soft tissues, lips, and tongue.

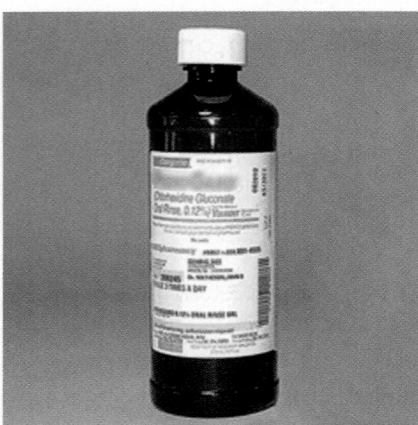

FIGURE 28-1 • Therapeutic Mouthrinse. Chlorhexidine gluconate mouthrinse aids in plaque biofilm control and requires a prescription for purchase. (Reprinted from Nield-Gehrig J, Willmann D. *Foundations of Periodontics for the Dental Hygienist*. Philadelphia, PA: Wolters Kluwer Health/Lippincott Williams & Wilkins; 2011.)

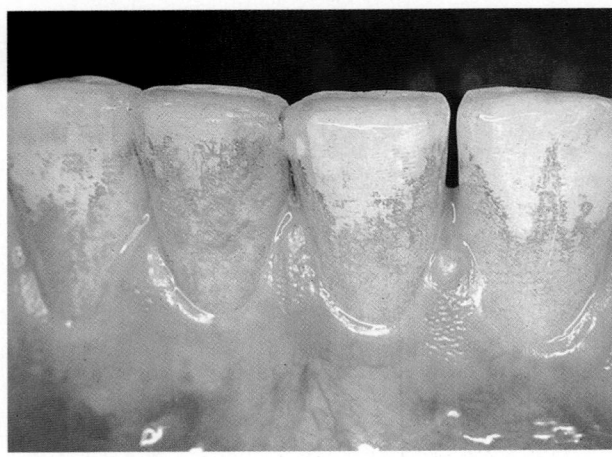

FIGURE 28-2 • Chlorhexidine Stain. (Reprinted from Nield-Gehrig J. *Fundamentals of Periodontal Instrumentation and Advanced Root Instrumentation*. Philadelphia, PA: Lippincott Williams & Wilkins; 2011.)

- ◆ Some research suggests CHX interacts with and is inactivated by sodium lauryl sulfate (a surfactant used in dentifrices) when rinsing is performed immediately after brushing. However, a recent systematic review and meta-analysis indicates that sodium lauryl sulfate does not interfere with the antiplaque effect of CHX.[27]

III. Triclosan

A. Mechanism of Action

- ◆ Bisphenol and nonionic antimicrobial agent.
- ◆ A broad-spectrum agent effective against both gram-negative and gram-positive bacteria.
- ◆ Acts on the microbial cytoplasmic membrane, causing leakage of the cell contents, or bacteriolysis.
- ◆ Antimicrobial and antigingivitis agent.
- ◆ Low toxicity.

B. Availability and Uses

- ◆ Triclosan-containing mouthrinses and dentifrices are available.
- ◆ Recommended uses:
  - Reduction of biofilm and gingivitis.
  - Reduced biofilm accumulation.
  - Reduced supragingival calculus formation.

C. Efficacy

- ◆ Reduction in biofilm and bleeding on probing (BOP).[28]

D. Considerations

- ◆ Easily released from oral tissue-binding sites such as tooth surface or soft tissue.
- ◆ Combining with PVM/MA increases substantivity and efficacy.[28]

IV. Phenolic-Related Essential Oils

A. Mechanism of Action

◆ Disrupt cell walls and inhibit bacterial enzymes.

◆ Decrease pathogenicity of biofilm.

◆ Antimicrobial and antigingivitis agent.

B. Availability and Uses

◆ A combination of thymol, eucalyptol, menthol, and methyl salicylate is available as a brand name product and generic product.

◆ Recommended uses:
  • Individuals unable to perform adequate brushing and flossing.
  • Initially or periodically to help improve oral hygiene.
  • Adjunct for mechanical self-care routines that are not sufficient in reducing biofilm, bleeding, and gingivitis.
  • Preprocedural rinse to reduce bacterial load before instrumentation-producing aerosols.

C. Efficacy

◆ Significant reduction in the levels of biofilm and gingivitis.[23,29]

D. Considerations

◆ Burning sensation.

◆ Bitter taste.

◆ Poor substantivity.

◆ Efficacy of individual rinses based on following the manufacturer's instructions and not casual use of the rinse.

◆ Contraindicated for current or recovering alcoholics due to alcohol content.

V. Quaternary Ammonium Compounds

A. Mechanism of Action[30]

◆ Cationic agents that bind to oral tissues.

◆ Rupture the cell wall and alter the cytoplasm.

◆ Initial attachment to oral tissue is very strong, but released rapidly.

◆ Decreases the ability of bacteria to attach to the pellicle.

◆ Low substantivity.

B. Availability and Uses

◆ The most commonly used agent is CPC, at 0.05%–0.07%.

◆ Recommended uses:
  • Reduction in biofilm accumulation.
  • Adjunct for mechanical self-care routines.

C. Efficacy

◆ Weak evidence for reductions in biofilm and gingivitis and more research is recommended.[31]

◆ Possible inhibition of calculus formation.[32]

D. Considerations

◆ Staining of teeth and tongue.[32]

◆ A burning sensation and occasional desquamation.[32]

VI. Oxygenating Agents

A. Mechanism of Action[33]

◆ Alters bacterial cell membrane, increasing permeability.

◆ Poor substantivity.

B. Availability and Uses

◆ The common agents available in commercial rinses are 10% carbamide peroxide and 1.5% hydrogen peroxide.

◆ Recommended for short-term use to reduce the symptoms of pericoronitis and necrotizing ulcerative gingivitis.[33]

C. Efficacy

◆ Negligible antimicrobial effect.

◆ Debriding agent.

D. Considerations

◆ Does not consistently prevent plaque biofilm accumulation short term, but when used long term, some reduction in gingival redness has been noted.[33]

◆ Occasional reports of erosive changes to oral mucosa.[33]

VII. Oxidizing Agents

A. Mechanism of Action

◆ Neutralization of VSCs that contribute to oral malodor.

B. Availability and Uses

◆ Common agents available in commercial rinses are chlorine dioxide (ClO_2) and chlorine dioxide/zinc combination.

C. Efficacy

◆ Mainly used for management of halitosis.[34]

D. Consideration

◆ Diluted 0.25%–0.5% sodium hypochlorite used as a mouthrinse twice per week showed significant reductions in BOP, dental biofilm, and gingival inflammation.[35,36]

COMMERCIAL MOUTHRINSE INGREDIENTS

Ingredients and their functions are listed in Table 28-3.

I. Active Ingredients

◆ Commercial mouthrinses generally contain more than one active ingredient and, therefore, may advertise multiple claims for use.

TABLE 28-3 • Typical Commercial Mouthrinse Formulation

INGREDIENT	FUNCTION
Alcohol	Enhances flavor impact and contributes to cleansing
Flavor	Adds pleasantness/freshness and makes breath temporarily fresh
Humectant	Adds "body" and inhibits crystallization around closure
Surfactant	Solubilizes the flavor and provides foaming action
Water	Major vehicle to carry other ingredients
Preservative	Preserves aqueous formulation
Dyes	Add color
Sweeteners	Contribute to overall flavor perception
Flavor	Makes mouthrinse pleasant to use
Active or functional ingredients	Provide therapeutic and/or benefits

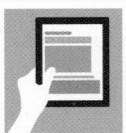

BOX 28-2
Characteristics of an Effective Chemotherapeutic Agent

- Nontoxic: The agent does not damage oral tissues or create systemic problems.
- No or limited absorption: The action is confined to the oral cavity.
- Substantivity: The ability of an agent to be bound to the pellicle and tooth surface and be released over a period of time with retention of potency.
- Bacterial specificity: May be broad-spectrum, but with an affinity for the pathogenic organisms of the oral cavity.
- Low-induced drug resistance: Low or no development of resistant organisms to agent.

- Factors that influence how effective an agent may be:
  - Dilution by the saliva.
  - Length of time the agent is in contact with the tissue or bacteria.
  - Evidence supporting the particular product.
- General characteristics of an effective chemotherapeutic agent are shown in Box 28-2.

II. Inactive Ingredients

A. Water
- Makes up the largest percentage by volume.

B. Alcohol[37]
- Increases the solubility of some active ingredients.
- Preservative.
- Percentage varies from 18% to 27%.
- Enhances flavor.
- No link to oral cancer has been found with regular use of an alcohol-containing mouthrinse.

C. Flavoring
- Essential oils and derivatives (eucalyptus oil, oil of wintergreen).
- Aromatic waters (peppermint, spearmint, wintergreen, or others).
- Artificial noncariogenic sweetener.

III. Patient-Specific Mouthrinse Recommendations

Mouthrinses are formulated for a variety of oral benefits, including mouth freshening, prevention of caries, biofilm control, and control of oral malodor. Several factors are considered when making a mouthrinse recommendation, including:
- Is the patient currently able to control biofilm through other methods?
- Does the patient consider rinsing a substitute for other mechanical procedures such as brushing and interproximal biofilm removal?
- Does the patient's substance abuse history contraindicate recommending an alcohol-containing mouthrinse?
- Could the patient's xerostomia be worsened by the drying effect of an alcohol-containing mouthrinse?

IV. Contraindications
- The use of a mouthrinse can enhance a patient's oral self-care regime. The patient needs to understand why rinsing is not a substitute for brushing or use of interproximal aids.
- Some agents are contraindicated for children less than 6 years of age who have a tendency to swallow instead of expectorate.
- Review manufacturer's instructions for age limits as they vary by product.
- Contraindicated in patients with physical or cognitive challenges who cannot follow rinsing instructions.

PROCEDURE FOR RINSING
- Many patients, particularly children, must be shown specifically how to rinse. The method can be practiced under supervision.
- Box 28-3 suggests steps for teaching a patient to rinse.

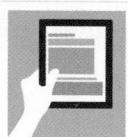

BOX 28-3
Steps: How to Rinse

1. Take a small amount of the fluid into the mouth.
2. Close lips; hold teeth slightly apart.
3. Force the fluid through the interdental areas with pressure.
4. Use the lips, cheeks, and tongue action to force the fluid back and forth between the teeth.
5. Balloon the cheeks, then suck them in, alternately several times.
6. Divide the mouth into three parts—front, right, and left.
7. Concentrate the rinsing first on the front, then on the right, and then on the left side.
8. Expectorate.
9. Follow manufacturer's directions on amount, length, and frequency of rinsing.

EMERGING ALTERNATIVE PRACTICES

I. Oil Pulling

- Ancient practice of swishing with 10 mL (one tablespoon) of sesame oil.[38,39]
- Reduction of biofilm.[38,39]
- Reduction of bacteria causing caries, gingivitis, halitosis, and oral thrush.[38,29]

UNITED STATES FOOD AND DRUG ADMINISTRATION

The purpose of the U.S. Food and Drug Administration (FDA) is to ensure the safety and efficacy of medical and dental drugs, equipment, and devices that affect living tissue. All drugs require FDA approval. Rinses and dentifrices are classified by the FDA as cosmetic, therapeutic, or a combination of cosmetic and therapeutic.[40]

I. Brief History of the FDA

- Oldest consumer protection agency in the U.S. federal government.
- Officially began in 1906 with the passage of the Pure Food and Drug Act.

II. Purposes of the FDA

- Regulate drugs, equipment, and devices.
- Some devices and equipment are exempt (dental water jets, power and manual toothbrushes, dental floss) if they have existing or reasonably similar characteristics as previously approved devices of the same type.

III. Dental Products Regulated

- Infection control products.
- Dental equipment such as ultrasonic instruments.
- Diagnostic test kits (i.e., dental caries detection devices).
- Prosthetic and restorative materials such as implants.
- Surgical and periodontal materials such as guided tissue regeneration membranes, bone-filling material, and growth factors.
- Prescription drugs, controlled and sustained-release devices, and chemotherapeutics.
- In the case of dentifrice and mouthrinses, FDA has reviewed active ingredients under over-the-counter (OTC) monographs, which are regulations that specify the active ingredients and permissible levels of those ingredients, as well as statements the product labels must bear.[41]
  - Recent removal of antiseptic products with triclosan has raised questions about the use in OTC antibacterial products because there is not testing to demonstrate benefit to human health.[42]
  - However, Colgate Total® toothpaste with triclosan underwent extensive testing to demonstrate effectiveness as a an antigingivitis agent as well as safety and was approved by the FDA in 1997.[42]

IV. Research Requirements and Documentation

- Table 28-4 outlines the documentation process for a product to receive FDA approval.[41]

AMERICAN DENTAL ASSOCIATION SEAL OF ACCEPTANCE PROGRAM

The American Dental Association (ADA) has promoted safety and effectiveness of dental products for over 100 years. The ADA Seal of Acceptance Program, which evaluates OTC products offered to consumers, has been in place since 1930, and is internationally recognized. The program is voluntary, and products are awarded the ADA Seal only after the ADA Council on Scientific Affairs has thoroughly evaluated clinical and laboratory studies on a product, and determined that it meets the ADA criteria for safety and effectiveness, when used as directed.[43]

For many years, the Seal Program website has provided a listing of all products that have the ADA Seal. Now there is a new Seal Program feature that provides detailed information on each of the accepted products to help consumers and dental professionals select OTC oral care products.[43]

- Unlike the FDA, the ADA Seal Program is voluntary, and a company must apply to obtain it by making a product submission.
- Each product has its ADA-approved Seal Statement that lists the indications for which the product is accepted.

TABLE 28-4 • Food and Drug Administration Clearance Documentation Process for Oral Care Products

PHASE	STUDY TYPE	PURPOSE
Preclinical	Animal studies	Safety/toxicity
I.	Clinical trial with small sample population (20–80)	Determine: dosing/safety how drug is metabolized and excreted identify side effects
II.	Clinical trial with a larger sample population (100–200) who have disease or condition that the product is designed to treat. The test drug is compared to a standard treatment or placebo known as a control	Provides further safety data and preliminary evidence of efficacy
III.	Clinical trial with a large sample population (1,000–3,000) who have a disease or condition to test efficacy, monitor side effects, and identify treatment parameters. The test drug is compared to a standard treatment or placebo known as a control	Identify possible less obvious side effects
IV.	Clinical trials on products that are already approved and on the market	Continue to measure long-term benefits, risks, and optimal protocol

◆ Information is included for each product on the basis for acceptance (i.e., the data on which acceptance is based), indications, directions for use, ingredients, label warnings, and company contact information.

◆ The Seal website also allows comparisons of the attributes of two to six products in a given product category.

◆ This information is printable and can be used to help consumers make informed decisions about the oral care products they use.

◆ It can also be useful to dental professionals in recommending OTC oral care products to their patients.

◆ Visit http://www.mouthhealthy.org for preventive oral health resources and ADA Seal product information for patients.

◆ Visit http://www.ada.org/seal for more information on the ADA Seal Program and for access to product information on ADA-accepted products.

I. Purposes of the Seal Program

The ADA Seal of Acceptance Program is designed to:
◆ Help the public and dental professionals make informed decisions about consumer dental products.

◆ Study and evaluate products for safety and efficacy, when used as directed.

◆ Inform members of the dental team and the public about the safety and efficacy of each product that is accepted.

◆ Maintain liaisons with regulatory agencies and research and professional organizations.

II. Product Submission and Acceptance Process

A. Information Required from the Company[43]:

◆ Complete ingredient listing.

◆ Objective data from clinical and laboratory studies that support the product's safety, and claimed effectiveness, when used as directed.

◆ Compliance with specific product category; acceptance guidelines if applicable (http://www.ada.org/3408.aspx).

◆ Evidence of good manufacturing processes.

B. Evaluation

◆ Involves more than 125 expert consultants, members of the ADA Council on Scientific Affairs, and Council staff scientists.

◆ Acceptance is for a 5-year period, after which the company can reapply for a new 5-year acceptance.

◆ When composition, manufacturer, or owner of an accepted product is changed, the company must resubmit for the Seal.

III. Acceptance and Use of the Seal[43]

◆ Claims of product effectiveness on labeling and in advertising and promotional materials must first be approved by the Council on Scientific Affairs.

◆ The use of the ADA Seal (Figure 28-3) on labeling and in promotional materials must be accompanied by an ADA-approved Seal Statement.

◆ The Seal Statement tells the consumer what specific claims have been reviewed and approved and indicates why the particular product was accepted.

DOCUMENTATION

◆ Information to be documented in the patient's permanent record will include a minimum of the following:
  • Recommended dentifrice and mouthrinse for personal oral care daily use: nonalcohol-containing mouthrinse and antibacterial dentifrice.

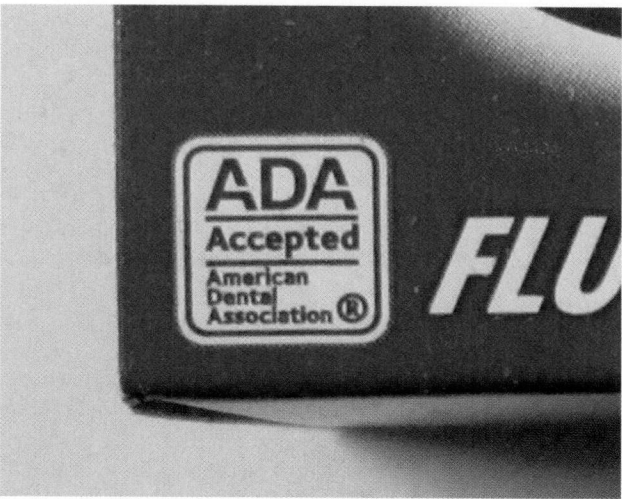

FIGURE 28-3 • ADA Seal of Acceptance, the American Dental Association, Council on Scientific Affairs. The Seal is awarded to consumer products that meet ADA guidelines for safety and effectiveness. (Reprinted with permission of the ADA Council on Scientific Affairs.)

- Patient instructed on proper usage, including amount and frequency of use.
- Summary of current oral findings indicating need for recommendations provided.
- Example documentation is provided in Box 28-4.

BOX 28-4

Example Documentation: Choosing a Mouthrinse for a Patient with Xerostomia

S—A 76-year-old male presented for a routine maintenance appointment. His chief complaint is a dry mouth. He reports no medication and although he has a history of smoking, he quit 40 years ago. Patient states he eats a lot of apples and other fruits. Patient stated he has been using a "great mouthwash" for the past 25 years. Patient believes it is helping "toughen up his gums" because his mouth is so dry.

O—Extraoral no significant findings. The intraoral examination reveals decreased salivary flow. The periodontal examination reveals generalized 3- to 4-mm pocket depths with no bleeding on probing present.

A—Patient presents with xerostomia and a history of smoking that increases his risk for caries, oral cancer, and periodontal disease.

P—Discussed xerostomia and probable causes and evaluated the amount of alcohol present in mouthwash currently being used. Discussed the effects of alcohol on the oral cavity and recommended mouthwash that does not contain alcohol to reduce the incidence of dry mouth.

Signed: _____, RDH

Date: _____

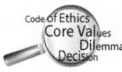

EVERYDAY ETHICS

Betty, a recent graduate, is just beginning her dental hygiene career in a private practice. Dr. Dadaman, the dentist she practices with, has no particular opinions regarding dentifrices and considers one as good as the other. He requests she hand out whatever sample-size products the office receives for free from visiting dental product reps. Betty has read up on the clinical support for many of the currently available products while in school and she is well versed on the differences. However, she is too shy and unsure of herself to challenge her employer and discuss the need to use an evidence-based approach to identifying the correct product for each patient.

When Betty gets home at the end of the day, she reflects that maybe something she learned in school might help her. She finds her *Wilkins* textbook and looks up the steps for ethical decision making.

Questions for Consideration

1. By answering some of the questions listed in Table VI-1 Decision Alternatives through Questioning (Section VI), identify and develop a rationale to support at least three different choices or alternative actions that Betty could take to resolve this issue.

2. Discuss this scenario in the context of the legal and ethical concepts. Which of these concepts might help support Betty's choice of actions as she reflects on her own professionalism and determines her responsibilities with regard to making product recommendations for her patients?

3. Whatever course of action Betty takes now will likely set the course for future discussions with her employer regarding patient recommendations or the way Betty practices her profession. Which dental hygienist roles (see Chapter 1) will Betty be filling when she determines the course of action she will take in this situation?

Factors to Teach the Patient

▶ Significance of American Dental Association product acceptance seal especially that it is a voluntary program and lack of a seal on a product does not signify it is unsafe or not effective.

▶ To ask the dental hygienist and dentist about new dentifrices and mouthrinses, best way to use, and appropriateness for personal needs.

▶ How to avoid impulse buying with regard to dentifrices, mouthrinses, and other chemical agents. To seek professional advice to avoid contraindications with oral condition and restorations.

▶ To understand compliance with recommended chemical agent is directly related to expected outcomes (results or improvements).

▶ Why the use of chemotherapeutics is not a substitute for proper and daily mechanical biofilm removal.

▶ To check the ingredients of mouthrinses to prevent the purchase of high-alcohol content if xerostomia is a problem.

ENHANCE YOUR UNDERSTANDING

ONLINE RESOURCES
(see the inside front cover for access information)
- Audio glossary
- Appendices

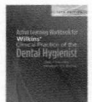

SUPPORT FOR LEARNING
(available separately)
- *Active Learning Workbook for Wilkins' Clinical Practice of the Dental Hygienist, 13th Edition*

INDIVIDUALIZED REVIEW
- Customized practice quizzing with Navigate 2 TestPrep for *Wilkins' Clinical Practice of the Dental Hygienist*

References

1. Holmlund A, Lampa E, Lind L. Poor response to periodontal treatment may predict future cardiovascular disease. *J Dent Res.* 2017;96(7):768-773.

2. Oberoi SS, Harish Y, Hiremath S, Puranik M. A cross-sectional survey to study the relationship of periodontal disease with cardiovascular disease, respiratory disease, and diabetes mellitus. *J Indian Soc Periodontol.* 2016;20(4):446-452.

3. D'Aiuto F, Gable D, Syed Z, et al. Evidence summary: the relationship between oral diseases and diabetes. *Br Dent J.* 2017;222(12):944-948.

4. Azarpazhooh A, Leake JL. Systematic review of the association between respiratory diseases and oral health. *J Periodontol.* 2006;77(9):1465-1482.

5. Mellburg JR. Fluoride dentifrices: current status and prospects. *Int Dent J.* 1991;41(1):9-16.

6. Fischman SL. The history of oral hygiene products: how far have we come in 6000 years? *Periodontol 2000.* 1997;15:7-14.

7. Janakiram C, Deepan Kumar CV, Joseph J. Xylitol in preventing dental caries: a systematic review and meta-analyses. *J Natural Sci Biol Med.* 2017;8(1):16-21.

8. Sälzer S, Slot D, Dörfer C, Van der Weijden GA. Comparison of triclosan and stannous fluoride dentifrices on parameters of gingival inflammation and plaque scores: a systematic review and meta-analysis. *Int J Dent Hyg.* 2015;13(1):1-17.

9. Loftsson T, Leeves N, Bjornsdottir B, Duffy L, Masson M. Effect of cyclodextrins and polymers on triclosan availability and substantivity in toothpastes in vivo. *J Pharm Sci.* 1999;88(12):1254-1258.

10. Riley P, Lamont T. Triclosan/copolymer containing toothpastes for oral health. *Cochrane Database Syst Rev.* 2013;(12):CD010514.

11. Pancer BA, Kott D, Sugai JV, et al. Effects of triclosan on host response and microbial biomarkers during experimental gingivitis. *J Clin Periodontol.* 2016;43:435-444.

12. Mankodi S, Bartizek RD, Winston JL, Biesbrock AR, McClanahan SF, He T. Anti-gingivitis efficacy of a stabilized 0.454% stannous fluoride/sodium hexametaphosphate dentifrice. *J Clin Periodontol.* 2005;32(1):75-80.

13. Moraschini V, da Costa LS, Dos Santos GO. Effectiveness for dentin hypersensitivity treatment of non-carious cervical lesions: a meta-analysis. *Clin Oral Investig.* 2018;22(2):617-631.

14. Netuveli GS, Sheiham A. A systematic review of the effectiveness of anticalculus dentifrices. *Oral Health Prev Dent.* 2004;2(1):49-58.

15. Winston JL, Fiedler SK, Schiff T, Baker R. An anticalculus dentifrice with sodium hexametaphosphate and stannous fluoride: a six-month study of efficacy. *J Contemp Dent Pract.* 2007;8(5):1-8.

16. Seemann R, Conceicao MD, Filippi A, et al. Halitosis management by the general dental practitioner—results of an international consensus workshop. *J Breath Res.* 2014;8(1):017101.

17. Mendes L, Coimbra J, Pereira A, Resende M, Pinto M. Comparative effect of a new mouthrinse containing chlorhexidine, triclosan and zinc on volatile sulphur compounds: a randomized, crossover, double-blind study. *Int J Dent Hyg.* 2016;14(3):202-208.

18. Farrell S, Barker ML, Gerlach RW. Overnight malodor effect with a 0.454% stabilized stannous fluoride sodium hexametaphosphate dentifrice. *Compend Contin Educ Dent.* 2007;28(12):658-661.

19. Schemehorn BR, Moore MH, Putt MS. Abrasion, polishing, and stain removal characteristics of various commercial dentifrices in vitro. *J Clin Dent.* 2011;22(1):11-18.

20. AAPD, Council on Clinical Affairs. Fluoride therapy. *Oral Health Policies & Recommendations (Reference Manual).* 2018;40(6):251-252. https://www.aapd.org/research/oral-health-policies--recommendations/fluoride-therapy/. Accessed July 8, 2019.

21. Wunderlich RC, Singelton M, O'Brien WJ, Caffesse RG. Subgingival penetration of an applied solution. *Int J Periodontics Restorative Dent.* 1984;4(5):64-71.

22. Van Strydonck DA, Slot DE, Van der Velden U, et al. Effect of a chlorhexidine mouthrinse on plaque, gingival inflammation and staining in gingivitis patients: a systematic review. *J Clin Periodontol.* 2012;39(11):1042-1055.

23. Neely AL. Essential oil mouthwash (EOMW) may be equivalent to chlorhexidine (CHX) for long-term control of gingival inflammation but CHX appears to perform better than EOMW in plaque control. *J Evid Based Dent Pract.* 2012;12(suppl 3):69-72.

24. James P, Parnell C, Whelton H. The caries-preventive effect of chlorhexidine varnish in children and adolescents: a systematic review. *Caries Res.* 2010;44(4):333-340.

25. Okada EM, Ribeiro LN, Stuani MB, et al. Effects of chlorhexidine varnish on caries during orthodontic treatment: a systematic review and meta-analysis. *Braz Oral Res.* 2016;30(1):e115.

26. Slot DE, Vaandrager NC, Van Loveren C, Van Palenstein Helderman WH, Van der Weijden GA. The effect of chlorhexidine varnish on root caries: a systematic review. *Caries Res.* 2011;45(2):162-173.

27. Elkerbout TA, Slot DE, Bakker EW, Van der Weijden GA. Chlorhexidine mouthwash and sodium lauryl sulphate dentifrice: do they mix effectively or interfere? *Int J Dent Hyg.* 2016;14(1):42-52.

28. Ciancio SG. Controlling biofilm with evidence-based dentifrices. *Compend Contin Educ Dent.* 2011;32(1):70-76.

29. Araujo MWB, Charles CA, Weinstein RB, et al. Meta-analysis of the effect of an essential oil-containing mouthrinse on gingivitis and plaque. *J Am Dent Assoc.* 2015;146(8):610-622.

30. Sanz M, Serrano J, Iniesta M, Santa Cruz I, Herrera D. Antiplaque and antigingivitis toothpastes. *Monogr Oral Sci.* 2013;23:27-44.

31. Gunsolley JC. Clinical efficacy of antimicrobial mouthrinses. *J Dent.* 2010;38(suppl 1):S6-S10.

32. Haps S, Slot DE, Berchier CE, Van der Weijden GA. The effect of cetylpyridinium chloride-containing mouth rinses as adjuncts to toothbrushing on plaque and parameters of gingival inflammation: a systematic review. *Int J Dent Hyg.* 2008;6(4):290-303.

33. Hossainian N, Slot DE, Afennich F, Van der Weijden GA. The effects of hydrogen peroxide mouthwashes on the prevention of plaque and gingival inflammation: a systematic review. *Int J Dent Hyg.* 2011;9(3):171-181.

34. Shinada K, Ueno M, Konishi C, et al. Effects of a mouthwash with chlorine dioxide on oral malodor and salivary bacteria: a randomized placebo-controlled 7-day trial. *Trials.* 2010; 11:14.

35. Gonzalez S, Cohen CL, Galván M, Alonaizan FA, Rich SK, Slots J. Gingival bleeding on probing: relationship to change in periodontal pocket depth and effect of sodium hypochlorite oral rinse. *J Periodontal Res.* 2015;50(3): 397-402.

36. De Nardo R, Chiappe V, Gómez M, Romanelli H, Slots J. Effects of 0.05% sodium hypochlorite oral rinse on supragingival biofilm and gingival inflammation. *Int Dent J.* 2012;62(4):208-212.

37. Gandini S, Negri E, Boffetta P, La Vecchia C, Boyle P. Mouthwash and oral cancer risk quantitative meta-analysis of epidemiologic studies. *Ann Agric Environ Med.* 2012;19(2): 173-180.

38. Naseem M, Khiyani M, Nauman H, Zafar M, Shah A, Khalil H. Oil pulling and importance of traditional medicine in oral health maintenance. *Int J Health Sci.* 2017;11(4): 65-70.

39. Shanbhag VK. Oil pulling for maintaining oral hygiene—a review. *J Tradit Complement Med.* 2017;7(1):106-109.

40. U.S. Food and Drug Administration, Division of Dermatology and Dental Products (DDDP). https://www.fda.gov/about-fda /center-drug-evaluation-and-research/division-dermatology -and-dental-products-dddp. Accessed July 8, 2019.

41. Food and Drug Administration. *Drug Applications for Over -the-Counter (OTC) Drugs.* Silver Springs, MD: FTC. https:// www.fda.gov/drugs/types-applications/drug-applications -over-counter-otc-drugs. Accessed July 8, 2019.

42. Food and Drug Administration, Federal Register. *21 CFR 310: Safety and Effectiveness of Consumer Antiseptics; Topical Antimicrobial Drug Products for Over-the-Counter Human Use.* April 2019:84:14847-14864. https://www.federalregister.gov /documents/2019/04/12/2019-06791/safety-and-effectiveness -of-consumer-antiseptic-rubs-topical-antimicrobial-drug -products-for#citation-2-p14851. Accessed July 8, 2019.

43. American Dental Association. *ADA Seal and Acceptance Program and Products.* Chicago, IL: American Dental Association. https://www.ada.org/en/science-research/ada-seal -of-acceptance. Accessed July 8, 2019.

29

The Patient with Orthodontic Appliances

Jessica August, RDH, MS

CHAPTER OUTLINE

CEMENTED BANDS AND BONDED BRACKETS
- I. Advantages of Bonded Brackets
- II. Disadvantages of Bonded Brackets
- III. Fixed Appliance System
- IV. Removable Aligner System

CLINICAL PROCEDURES FOR BONDING
- I. Assessment Examination
- II. Procedural Steps
- III. Characteristics of Bonding Relating to Debonding
- IV. Use of Fluoride-Releasing Bonding System

DENTAL HYGIENE CARE
- I. Complicating Factors: Risk Factors
- II. Disease Control

CLINICAL PROCEDURES FOR BAND REMOVAL AND DEBONDING
- I. Band Removal
- II. Clinical Procedures for Debonding

POSTDEBONDING EVALUATION
- I. Enamel Loss
- II. Demineralization (White Spots Lesions)
- III. Etched Enamel Not Covered by Adhesive

ORTHODONTIC RETENTION

POSTDEBONDING PREVENTIVE CARE
- I. Periodontal Evaluation
- II. Dental Examination
- III. Fluoride Therapy

DOCUMENTATION

EVERYDAY ETHICS

FACTORS TO TEACH THE PATIENT

REFERENCES

LEARNING OBJECTIVES

After studying this chapter, the student will be able to:

1. Recognize the key words and terminologies used in orthodontic therapy.

2. Explain the advantages and disadvantages of bonded brackets.

3. Summarize the clinical procedures for bonding and debonding.

4. Develop oral self-care recommendations for the orthodontic patient to address effective biofilm removal and reduce risk for dental caries and periodontal disease.

An individualized preventive program that includes a specific plan of instruction, motivation, and supervision is essential for the patient with orthodontic appliances.

CEMENTED BANDS AND BONDED BRACKETS

- Resin-bonded brackets have been used widely in orthodontic treatment.
  - Brackets are usually placed on the facial surfaces of the teeth; however, occasionally brackets are bonded to the lingual surfaces.
  - Brackets aid in the application and control of applied forces necessary to accomplish tooth movement and bone remodeling for orthodontic therapy.
  - Stainless steel or clear ceramic brackets may be used; their function is to retain the arch wire.
  - The two types of brackets are illustrated in Figures 29-1 and 29-2.
- In some cases, circumferential molar bands are used.
  - For example, for jaw stabilization following orthognathic surgery or when additional strength is needed to hold palatal bars, elastics, or other special devices.

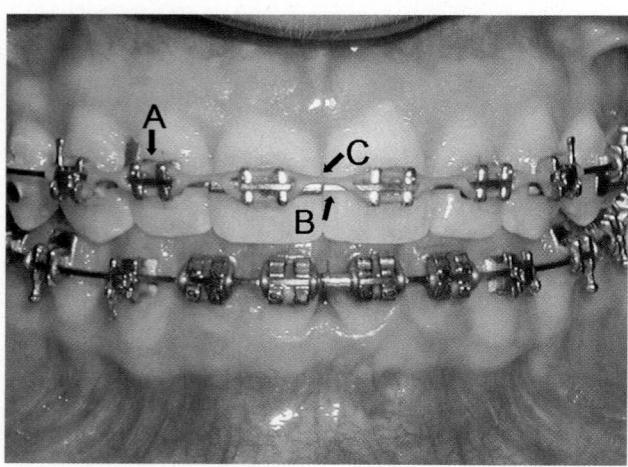

FIGURE 29-1 • Fixed Appliance System. A: Bonded brackets. **B:** With arch wire. **C:** Held in place by elastomers.

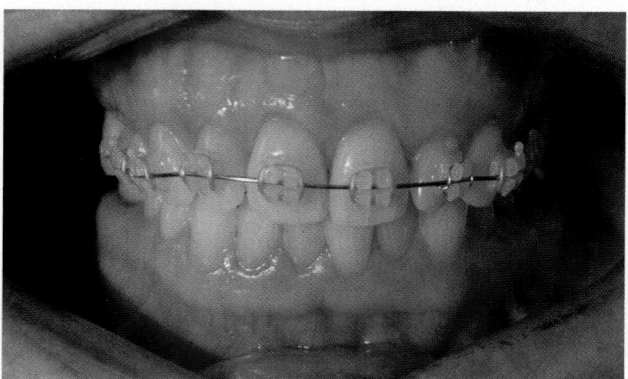

FIGURE 29-2 • Fixed Appliance System. Bonded clear brackets with arch wire.

I. Advantages of Bonded Brackets[1]

- Improved aesthetics.
- Improved gingival condition due to better access for control of dental biofilm at the cervical third of the teeth.
- Proximal surface dental caries can be detected and treated without bracket removal.
- Patient will immediately be aware when a bracket loosens, whereas an unsecured band may go undetected.
- Placement factors include:
  - No need for tooth separation (as required for band placement); results in less patient discomfort and no band spaces to close at the end of treatment.
  - Lingual brackets ("invisible braces") may be used for specially selected cases.
  - Placement of brackets is faster and easier than placement of bands.

II. Disadvantages of Bonded Brackets[1]

- Shear bond strength of the various materials differs, but all the generally available adhesives had higher than recommended bond strength.[2]
- Brackets may detach more readily than a band because attachment may be weaker with less surface area in contact with tooth.
- Rebonding a loose bracket is more time-consuming and requires more tooth preparation than recementing a loose band.
- Debonding at the end of treatment is more time-consuming than debanding, with more potential for damage to the tooth surface because of surface area covered by the adhesive.

III. Fixed Appliance System

- Figure 29-1 shows bonded metal brackets with arch wire held in place by elastomers.
- Figure 29-2 shows bonded clear brackets with arch wire.

A. Brackets

- *Materials*
  - Metal (stainless steel).
  - Plastic (polycarbonate).
  - Plastic with metal reinforcements.
  - Ceramic.
- *Forms:* Brackets are made in many styles, shapes, and sizes for different teeth, each designed to accomplish a specific objective of treatment. The basic forms are single or twin, as illustrated in Figure 29-3.
- *Base:* The base of the bracket is prepared with a mesh backing to assist in retaining the resin bonding agent.
  - The mesh backing, or bonding pad, is made to the exact size of the bracket to minimize the gaps between the composite–enamel junction, which can harbor bacteria that cause demineralization.

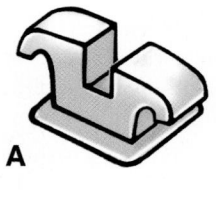
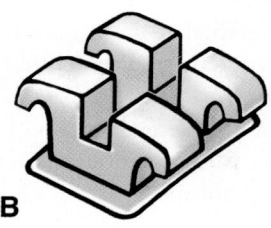

FIGURE 29-3 • Orthodontic Brackets. A: Single bracket with an incisal and a cervical wing. **B:** Twin, or Siamese, bracket with two wings on each side of the central groove where the arch wire is held. The shape and style of each bracket vary with the tooth on which the bracket will be located.

B. Arch Wire

◆ The arch wire attaches to the bracket to generate and distribute forces that guide orthodontic tooth movement.

◆ Arch wires are made of stainless steel or an alloy of chromium or titanium, and they may be round, rectangular, or multistranded. The arch wire is illustrated in Figures 29-1 and 29-2.

C. Elastomers

◆ Elastomers are available in latex and nonlatex materials and come in a wide variety of colors.

◆ Elastomers are used as chains and on individual teeth for the following purposes:
  • Hold wires in the brackets (Figure 29-1).
  • Apply light continuous force to close spaces between teeth.[3]

IV. Removable Aligner System

Clear aligner systems are an increasingly popular orthodontic technique for aligning teeth and correcting malocclusions.

A. Overview of Removable Aligner System[4]

◆ An individual treatment plan is developed and a series of custom, clear thermoplastic aligners are fabricated.

◆ With each set of aligners, the misaligned teeth are progressively moved.

B. Clinical Procedure

◆ A consultation with the orthodontist will determine the need for orthodontic treatment.
  • Fixed and removable orthodontic options are evaluated to meet the individual patient needs.
  • Not every patient is a candidate for removable aligner systems.

◆ Upper and lower impressions are taken and the aligners are fabricated.

◆ The study models are scanned into a computer to make a three-dimensional model of the step-by-step process for movement of the teeth.

◆ Retention attachments are bonded on the teeth so the aligner has a place to clip into place.

◆ A number of aligners are given to the patient to wear per instructions.
  • Each tray is worn for approximately 2 weeks.

◆ The patient will visit the orthodontist on a regular basis for adjustments and monitoring of progress.

◆ Impressions are taken to fabricate retainers to stabilize the tooth position after active treatment.

CLINICAL PROCEDURES FOR BONDING

I. Assessment Examination

Before bonding, documentation of any irregularities of the patient's teeth, such as white spots or cracks, is required to prevent misunderstanding by the patient after debonding.[5]

II. Procedural Steps

◆ The principles for pit and fissure sealants apply for bonding orthodontic brackets (see Chapter 35).
  • After bonding, the area around the bracket is carefully cleaned of excess material. Excess material around the bracket serves as a site for biofilm accumulation.[6]

III. Characteristics of Bonding Relating to Debonding

A. Nature of the Bond

◆ The acid etch exposes the prism structure of enamel and creates microclefts (see Chapter 35).

◆ On the bracket side, the resin becomes locked into the mesh base.

B. Effect of Filler Particles

◆ Adding fillers to the resin increases bond strength, hardness, and wear resistance.[7]
  • Heavily filled resins (composites) perform better for the posterior teeth because posterior attachments are subject to high forces of mastication.

◆ Ease of debonding is related to the type of resin and length of etching time.
  • Heavily filled composites are thicker and less viscous; they may be more difficult to remove.
  • Etching time of 30 seconds significantly improved bond strength for orthodontic brackets.[8]

◆ The bond is stronger when a thinner layer of resin is placed between the tooth surface and the bracket.

◆ Anterior brackets can be bonded with a lightly filled resin, whereas posterior teeth need a resin with more filler to prevent detachment.

IV. Use of Fluoride-Releasing Bonding System

- Demineralization around brackets can result in an increased risk of dental caries for even the most conscientious patient.[9]
- Use of fluoride-releasing bonding systems such as glass ionomers have been shown to have positive preventive results.[10]

DENTAL HYGIENE CARE

- The patient may be under orthodontic care with regular appointments for a long period, frequently years.
- Periodic communication between the orthodontist and the patient's referring dentist and dental hygienist is required to coordinate oral self-care instruction along with other essential dental and dental hygiene care.
- Regular dental hygiene preventive care and motivation for oral self-care are essential during orthodontic treatment.[11]

I. Complicating Factors: Risk Factors

A. Age Groups

- Many orthodontic patients are in the preteen and teenage years, periods when the incidence of gingivitis is high.
  - The incidence of periodontal infection increases from early childhood to late teenage years.
- There is a significant increase in the number of adult patients seeking orthodontic treatment.
  - As with younger patients, the risk factors for caries and periodontal diseases increase.
  - The adult orthodontic patient may be taking medications or have a systemic condition that can complicate therapy.
  - The adult patient may present with various classifications of periodontal disease, which can complicate orthodontic treatment as well as management of the periodontal status.[12,13]

B. Periodontal Health[14]

- Evidence suggests an increase in the quantity and quality of oral microorganisms with orthodonture, but this is short-term if the patient maintains good oral self-care.[6]
- It is essential for regular periodontal assessment including periodontal probing in adolescents and young adults during orthodontic treatment since this is an age group when periodontal disease may develop.
- Dental biofilm retention around orthodontic appliances may lead to gingivitis.
- The degree can vary from slight to severe with gingival enlargement, particularly of the interdental papillae.
- The tissue may greatly enlarge and cover the fixed appliance. In some cases, it may be necessary to remove the bracket until the patient can improve oral hygiene and resolve the inflammation.

C. Position of Teeth

- Teeth that are malpositioned are more susceptible to the retention of dental biofilm and are more difficult to clean.
- With the severe malocclusions presented by orthodontic patients at the outset, this factor becomes even more significant.

D. Problems with Appliances

- Orthodontic appliances retain biofilm and debris.
- Accidents may cause a bracket to become detached.

E. Self-Care Is Difficult

- The appliances interfere with the application of the toothbrush, interdental aids, and other devices used for dental biofilm control.
- Instruction needs to be very specific and reviewed at each appointment.

II. Disease Control

A meticulous program for dental caries and periodontal disease control is needed.

- The selection of biofilm control procedures for an individual patient is determined by the periodontal status, anatomic features of the gingiva, position of the teeth, and type and position of the orthodontic appliance.

A. General Oral Self-Care Instructions[11,14]

- Give oral self-care instructions before appliances are placed, with the goal of having the oral tissues healthy and the patient motivated to perform thorough daily biofilm removal.
- Encourage the patient to perform brushing and interdental care in front of a mirror so the technique is accurate and thorough.
  - Place emphasis on sulcular brushing and cleaning the area between the orthodontic bands and brackets and the gingiva.
- Disclosing solution is useful to help the patient self-evaluate biofilm removal; however, it may be difficult to remove from the bonding resin.
- *Interdental aids*
  - A floss threader may be helpful to provide access to interproximal areas around arch wires for biofilm removal.
  - Tufted dental floss used in the floss threader can remove the biofilm more efficiently than regular dental floss.
  - A single-tuft brush can be particularly beneficial around individual teeth that are hard to access with a regular toothbrush.
  - Travel interdental brushes can provide access to areas around and under the arch wires and come in a container that is easy for patients to use away from home.
  - Review Chapter 27 for interdental aids, such as tufted floss, interdental brushes, floss threaders, and irrigation options that may be effective for each patient.

◆ Caries prevention is a necessary part of minimizing and preventing white spot lesions.
  • Recommend an approved fluoride dentifrice, professionally applied fluoride varnish, and prescribe home fluoride gel or paste to aid in dental caries control (review Chapter 34 for recommendations for fluoride dentifrices, gels, and mouthrinses).[15]
  • Sugar-free mints or gum containing xylitol may be used between meals.
  • Dietary counseling is needed to ensure a patient understands the foods and beverages most likely to impact future dental caries.
  • For patients with xerostomia, saliva substitutes and dry mouth products may help reduce caries risk.
◆ Recommend an approved mouthrinse to aid in dental caries control and periodontal inflammation control.

B. Toothbrush Selection

Research found manual and power toothbrushes were not significantly different in terms of effectiveness.[16]
◆ *Power brush*
  • Sonic toothbrushes performed slightly better than other power or manual toothbrushes in reducing gingivitis, plaque, and interdental bleeding.[16]
  • See Chapter 26 for more information on power brushes.
◆ *Manual brush*
  • Soft brush: A soft brush with end-rounded filaments is recommended.
  • Bi-level: A special bi-level orthodontic brush designed with spaced rows of soft nylon filaments and a shorter middle row that can be applied directly over the appliance is shown in Figure 29-4. It is used with a short horizontal stroke.

C. Toothbrushing Procedure

◆ *Sulcular brushing*: A sulcular method is needed by most patients for cleaning the appliances and maintaining the gingiva.
◆ *Adapt toothbrush for appliance*
  • Place the brush with filament ends directed toward the occlusal surface (Charters' position, Figure 29-5D) to clean under the wire and bracket for mandibular arch, place in Stillman position for the opposite side (Figure 29-5C).
◆ *Clean all surfaces of biofilm and food debris*
  • Insert the brush from below, over, and above the arch wire; rotate and vibrate to remove biofilm and debris.
◆ *Lingual and palatal*: Approach to brushing is similar to the basic strokes used on the facial surfaces.

D. Additional Measures

◆ Keep the oral self-care routine as simple as possible; it can be a challenge to find the most effective therapeutic aids for the individual needs of the patient.
  • When suggesting a new aid, be sure to eliminate one that did not work well for the patient so the patient does not become overwhelmed.

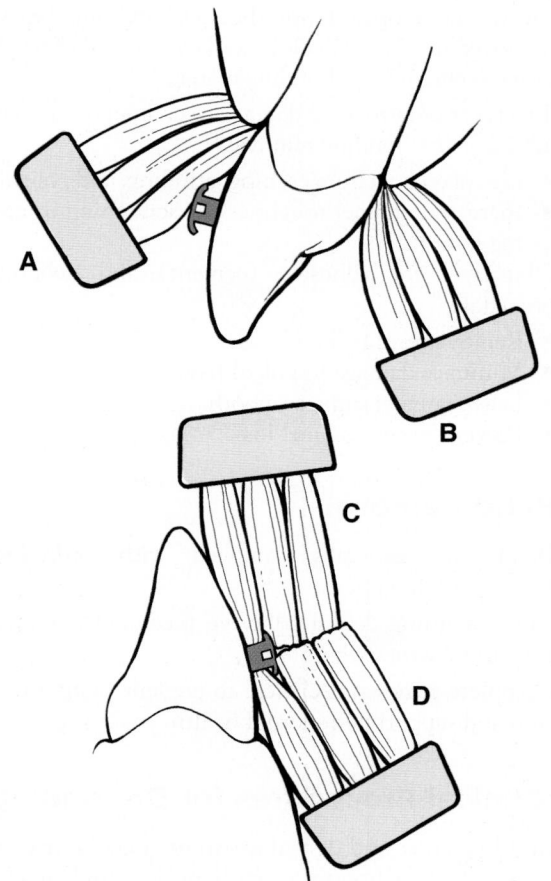

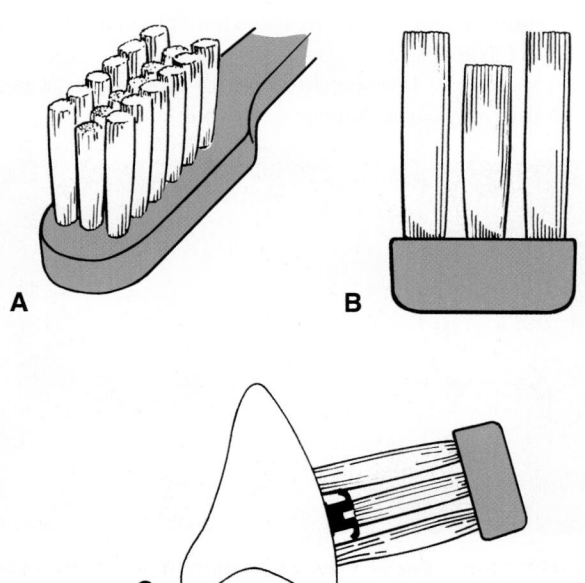

FIGURE 29-4 • Orthodontic Bi-level Toothbrush. A: Middle row of filaments trimmed shorter to fit over a fixed appliance. **B:** Cross section. **C:** Brush held over a bracket.

FIGURE 29-5 • Toothbrushing for Orthodontic Appliance. A and B: Sulcular brushing for periodontal tissues. **C:** Brush in Stillman position for occlusal side of bracket and arch wire. **D:** Cleaning the gingival side of bracket using brush in Charters' brushing position.

◆ Document changes to the oral care plan in the patient's chart.
◆ *Oral irrigation:*
  • Most patients who wear orthodontic appliances can benefit from the regular use of water irrigation for removal of loose dental biofilm and food debris.[17]
  • Oral irrigation, particularly with an orthodontic tip (see Chapter 27), before brushing is recommended so debris is removed to provide access to enamel surfaces for the fluoride dentifrice.

E. Dental Hygiene Instrumentation

◆ Manual instrumentation around orthodontic bands and brackets is challenging. The use of an ultrasonic or piezoelectric scaler may be helpful for debridement.
◆ The use of an air-powder polisher (Chapter 42) may be indicated to remove debris since the bands and brackets can tear polishing cups and the agent is less abrasive than polishing paste.[18,19]

CLINICAL PROCEDURES FOR BAND REMOVAL AND DEBONDING

Following active orthodontic therapy, bands and brackets are removed mechanically followed by removal of residual adhesive (cement) and bonding material.

◆ Two types of iatrogenic damage to enamel occur during adhesive and bonding removal[20]:
  • Loss of enamel from etching, grinding, and polishing.
  • Increased enamel roughness by scratching or creating wear facets.
◆ Objectives for adhesive (cement) and debonding procedure[20]:
  • Remove resin bulk.
  • Minimize damage to pulpal tissue.
  • Leave enamel surface smooth.
  • Prevent excess enamel loss.

I. Band Removal

◆ Bands are generally removed with orthodontic band-removing pliers.
◆ The remaining dental adhesive (cement) is removed primarily by rotary burs.
◆ Complete removal is critical to prevent biofilm retention and support periodontal health.

II. Clinical Procedures for Debonding

Dental hygienist and dental assistants may be involved in removal of orthodontic appliances, which may include use of slow- and/or high-speed handpieces depending on the scope of practice; so, it is important that clinicians know the scope of practice in their state, province, or county.

A. Method Types

◆ Mechanical, electrothermal, laser, and ultrasonic methods have been studied in an attempt to determine which debonding method is the most efficient and effective, provides the least discomfort for the patient, and causes the least damage to enamel.[20]
  • Tungsten-carbide burs are the fastest and most effective but require a multistep process to polish the enamel for finishing.
  • The most destructive tools for resin removal include Arkansas stones, green stones, diamond burs, steel burs, and lasers.[20]

B. Steps in Removal of Residual Resin Bonding

1. *Examination*
   • Varying amounts of resin remain after the bracket is removed, particularly in normal anatomic grooves, as shown in Figure 29-6.
   • During debonding, frequent examination is necessary using visual and tactile methods.
   • Box 29-1 contains a summary of the steps necessary for complete removal of the orthodontic adhesive resin.
2. *Identification of residual resin*
   • *Visual:* When dry, the resin appears dull and opaque compared to the shiny enamel.
   • *Tactile:* Application of an explorer reveals a rough surface, sometimes with catches along the margin of a resin tag. Filler particles from the resin may abrade the metal explorer tip, leaving a gray line on the resin surface.
   • Use of loupes for magnification to evaluate the tooth surface.
3. *Removal of resin from tooth surface*[20]
   • *Bur selection:* Use a tapered, plain-cut, tungsten-carbide finishing bur with a low-speed handpiece, as illustrated in Figure 29-7.
   • *Speed:* Use low speed to control production of heat that may cause damage to the pulp.

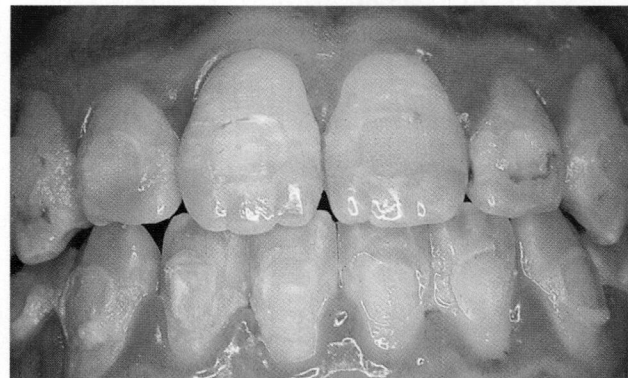

FIGURE 29-6 • Facial View of Anterior Teeth with Adhesive Resin Remaining Following Removal of Orthodontic Brackets. (Reprinted with permission from Gutmann ME. Composite adhesive resin removal following orthodontic treatment. *J Pract Hyg.* 1996;5:16.)

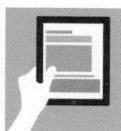

BOX 29-1

Steps for Orthodontic Adhesive Resin Removal Using Burs and Polishing Instruments

1. Identify the location and extent of the resin with an explorer, disclosing solution, and patient feedback.
2. Using a tapered, tungsten-carbide finishing bur in a low-speed handpiece, move the bur from the cervical to incisal/occlusal portion of the resin in a light, brush-like stroke.
3. Evaluate progress frequently by rinsing and drying the tooth surfaces.
4. Polish each surface with aluminum oxide polishing points, followed by aluminum oxide polishing cups.
5. Use a rubber cup in a slow-speed handpiece to polish each surface with a fine pumice slurry. Use intermittent strokes.
6. Use a brown polishing cup in a slow-speed handpiece to polish the enamel surfaces.
7. Use a green polishing cup in a slow-speed handpiece to provide the final finish to the enamel surfaces.

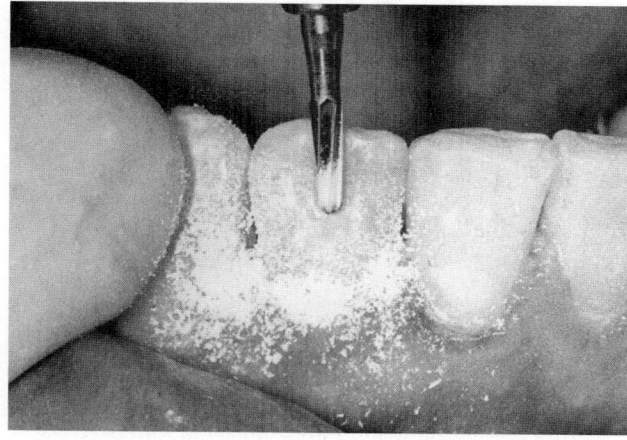

FIGURE 29-8 • **Adhesive Shavings Following Use of Bur.** (Reprinted with permission from Gutmann ME. Debonding orthodontic adhesives. *J Dent Hyg.* 1985;59:369.)

4. *Final finish*[20]
   * *Objective*: Restore pretreatment enamel surface finish.
   * *Examination*: Perform visual and tactile examination to distinguish areas of normal enamel from irregularities.
   * *Application of aluminum oxide finishing points and cups*
      * Use the finishing points first to remove any fine scarring resulting from the burs (Figure 29-9).
      * Use a low-speed handpiece.
      * Follow with aluminum oxide cups and move from area to area in a cervical to incisal/occlusal direction (Figure 29-10).
   * *Application of the rubber cup*
      * Use a fine pumice water slurry, as shown in Figure 29-11.
      * Polish in a wet field to prevent overheating.
      * Use intermittent strokes to avoid overheating and move from tooth to tooth.
   * *Final polish*: Use brown followed by green polishing cups to produce a natural-appearing, glossy enamel surface (Figures 29-12 and 29-13).
5. After debonding, topical fluoride varnish application is recommended for caries prevention and to reverse white spot lesions.[21]

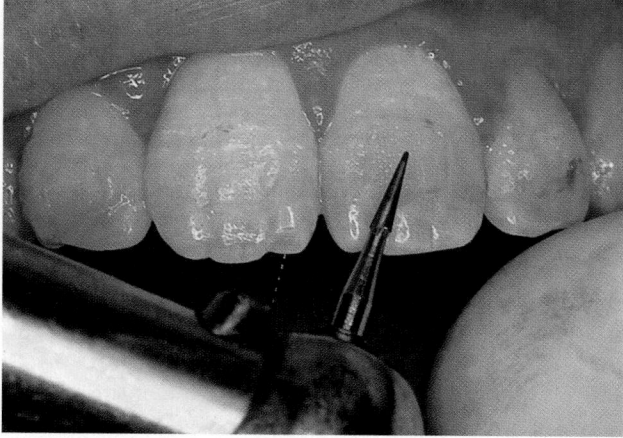

FIGURE 29-7 • **Use of Tapered, Tungsten-Carbide Finishing Bur on Low-Speed Handpiece to Remove Bulk of Adhesive Resin.** (Reprinted with permission from Gutmann ME. Composite adhesive resin removal following orthodontic treatment. *J Pract Hyg.* 1996;5:16.)

* *Stroke*: Use a smooth, evenly applied, light brush stroke in one direction to prevent faceting.
* *Direction*: Work systematically from cervical portion of the resin; move toward incisal or occlusal third. When removed, the resin resembles fine white shavings, as seen in Figure 29-8.
* *Evaluate frequently* to prevent excessive removal of enamel. Rinse frequently, dry, and evaluate the surface. The resin will appear opaque in contrast to the glossy enamel.

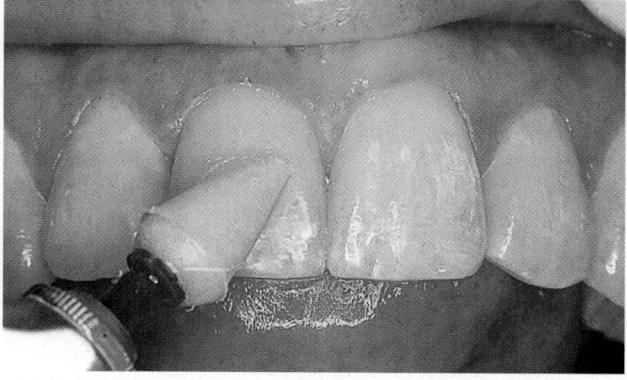

FIGURE 29-9 • **Aluminum Oxide Finishing Point to Remove Any Enamel Scarring Resulting from Bur.** (Reprinted with permission from Gutmann ME. Composite adhesive resin removal following orthodontic treatment. *J Pract Hyg.* 1996;5:16.)

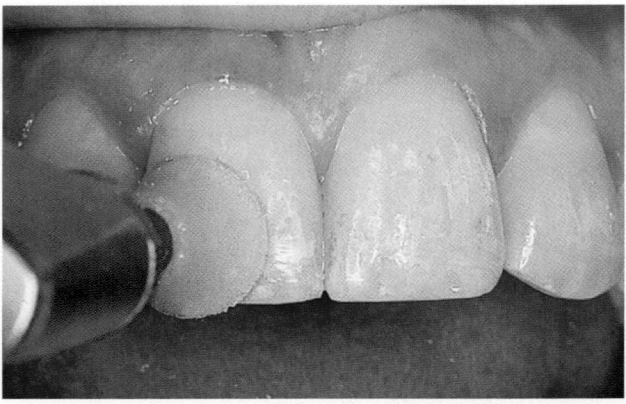

FIGURE 29-10 • Aluminum Oxide Finishing Cup to Remove Any Enamel Scarring Resulting from Bur. (Reprinted with permission from Gutmann ME. Composite adhesive resin removal following orthodontic treatment. *J Pract Hyg.* 1996;5:16.)

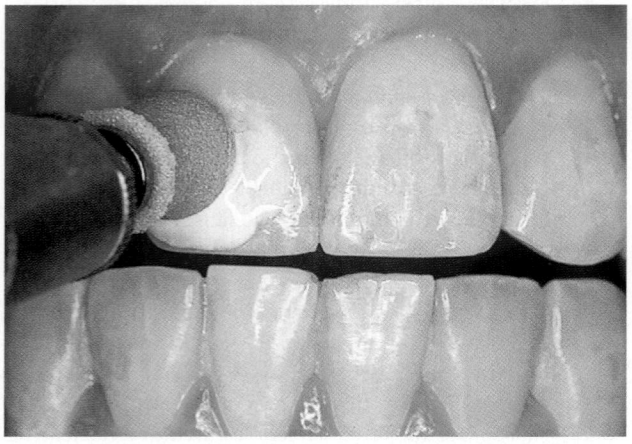

FIGURE 29-11 • Polishing with Fine Pumice Slurry and Rubber Cup. (Reprinted with permission from Gutmann ME. Composite adhesive resin removal following orthodontic treatment. *J Pract Hyg.* 1996;5:16.)

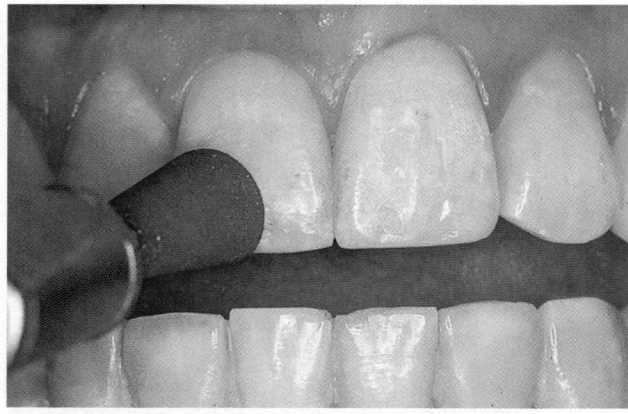

FIGURE 29-12 • Brown Polishing Cup Provides Maximum Gloss to Enamel Surface. (Reprinted with permission from Gutmann ME. Composite adhesive resin removal following orthodontic treatment. *J Pract Hyg.* 1996;5:16.)

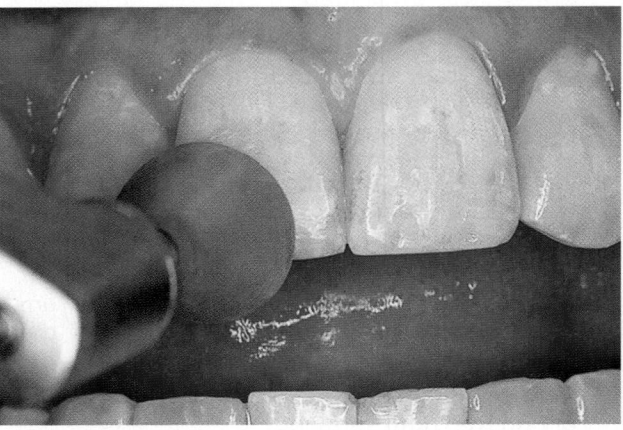

FIGURE 29-13 • Final Polishing with Green Polishing Cup. (Reprinted with permission from Gutmann ME. Composite adhesive resin removal following orthodontic treatment. *J Pract Hyg.* 1996;5:16.)

POSTDEBONDING EVALUATION

◆ Each step of bonding and debonding has a damaging effect on the enamel surface.
◆ The clinician must avoid unnecessary trauma during the various procedures.

I. Enamel Loss

◆ Total enamel loss from etching, bracket removal, residual resin removal, surface finishing, and application of pumice averages approximately 55 μm.[20]
  • Use of a tungsten-carbide finishing bur results in enamel loss from 22.8 to 50.5 μm.[20]
◆ Enamel loss is greater when filled resins (composites) are used for bonding than when unfilled resins are used.
◆ The loss is also greater when a rotating bristle brush rather than a rubber cup is used with the abrasive for finishing.
◆ The external layer of enamel is the most fluoride-rich enamel.[20]
  • Without care during debonding, the entire protective layer can be removed.
◆ When multiple bonding and debonding procedures are performed, such as when a bracket becomes detached, the enamel loss is compounded.
◆ Careful selection of instruments and abrasives, along with minimal instrumentation, is necessary to minimize enamel loss.

II. Demineralization (White Spot Lesions)

◆ White demineralization areas or dental caries are relatively common findings after orthodontic treatment.[22]
◆ Dental biofilm retention on appliances and the resin, along with the difficulty of biofilm removal by the patient, contribute to demineralization and dental caries.

III. Etched Enamel Not Covered by Adhesive

◆ Surface areas etched but not covered with adhesive resin may be remineralized when the fluoride contact is increased through regular patient and professional applications.

◆ Etched enamel has a high fluoride uptake.

ORTHODONTIC RETENTION

◆ After fixed appliances have been removed, a retainer is worn to prevent movement of the teeth while the bone and other supporting tissues are stabilizing.

    • One type of removable retainer is the Hawley retainer, as shown in Figure 29-14.

◆ The use of a fixed retainer appliance provides another source for retention of dental biofilm.

◆ General care and cleaning procedures for a removable retainers include:

    • Clean the appliance after each meal and before bedtime.

    • Instructions for cleaning procedures and agents for removable appliances are described with the care of the removable denture (Chapter 30).

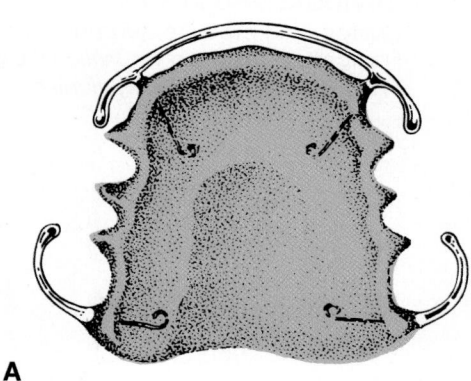

A

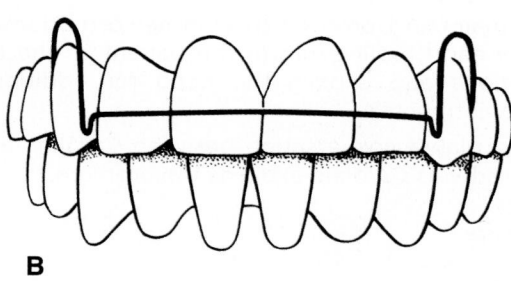

B

FIGURE 29-14 • Hawley Retainer. A: Removable acrylic retainer with facial retaining wire and clasps to be worn after removal of a fixed orthodontic appliance. **B:** Anterior view shows a Hawley appliance in position. The method for cleaning the appliance is similar to that for cleaning a removable denture.

    • Brush and rinse teeth and gingival tissue under the appliance each time the appliance is removed.

    • Keep appliance in a container with water when it is out of the mouth.

POSTDEBONDING PREVENTIVE CARE

I. Periodontal Evaluation

◆ A complete examination with a careful periodontal assessment is necessary because many changes take place during treatment.

◆ Thorough periodontal debridement.

◆ Intraoral images assist the patient in comparing gingival tissue changes and teeth before and after treatment.

◆ Apply disclosing agent for documentation of biofilm and patient instruction.

II. Dental Examination

◆ Examination for demineralization (white spots) and dental caries is essential.

◆ Dental biofilm retention by orthodontic appliances can be problematic for the patient.

    • The configurations of the appliances make biofilm control efforts by the patient extremely difficult.

    • Biofilm collects on brackets and some resins even when the patient's oral hygiene is generally good.[6]

◆ Composite resin may remain on the tooth surface where the bracket was removed leading to biofilm retention.

III. Fluoride Therapy

◆ A complete program of fluoride therapy, professionally applied at frequent maintenance appointments and used by the patient on a daily basis, is essential both during and following orthodontic therapy.[15]

◆ Application of a fluoride varnish immediately following bonding can help to reduce demineralization by up to 38%–44%.[21,23,24] Varnish applications need to become a part of every maintenance appointment.

DOCUMENTATION

◆ Document treatment goals and progress toward goals with any changes at each appointment.

◆ Assess the patient's oral health along with changes in risk for oral disease and record in the dental chart.

◆ Evaluation of effectiveness of the patient's oral self-care and adjustments needed for continued improvement.

◆ Monitoring of compliance with use of home fluorides.

◆ A sample progress note may be found in Box 29-2.

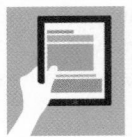

BOX 29-2

Example Documentation:
Patient Following Completion
of Orthodontic Treatment

S—A 16-year-old female patient presents for 6-month maintenance appointment. Patient has recently completed orthodontic treatment. Patient reports the soreness she had following band removal has subsided.

O—Assessment data collected include marginal redness with bleeding on probing on the mandibular anterior teeth. Hard-tissue examination findings include areas of demineralization on the maxillary anterior teeth. Calculus localized to the mandibular anterior teeth.

A—Patient is at a high caries risk level. Caries prevention and remineralization of enamel is essential.

P—Assessment data collected and documented. Health history update, intra- and extraoral examination, full-mouth periodontal assessment, and biofilm score using disclosing solution. Manually scaled to completion and applied fluoride varnish. Oral self-care instructions reviewed. Demonstrated flossing and positioning of her toothbrush for more effective biofilm removal. Patient observed while brushing and flossing mandibular anterior teeth. Recommended prescription fluoride toothpaste.

Next steps: Schedule continuing care appointment in 3 months to reevaluate demineralized areas.

Signed: _____, RDH

Date: _____

Factors to Teach the Patient

▶ The significance of dental biofilm around orthodontic appliances and the teeth.

▶ How to apply the toothbrush (power or manual) and adjunctive aids to remove dental biofilm from the bracket, the arch wire, and the teeth.

▶ How, when, and why to use fluoride rinses, toothpaste, and prescription gels/pastes.

▶ The frequency for professional follow-up during and after orthodontic therapy.

ENHANCE YOUR UNDERSTANDING

ONLINE RESOURCES
(see the inside front cover for access information)

• Audio glossary
• Appendices

SUPPORT FOR LEARNING
(available separately)

• *Active Learning Workbook for Wilkins' Clinical Practice of the Dental Hygienist, 13th Edition*

INDIVIDUALIZED REVIEW

• Customized practice quizzing with Navigate 2 TestPrep for *Wilkins' Clinical Practice of the Dental Hygienist*

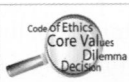

EVERYDAY ETHICS

Dorothy, a patient who had recently completed orthodontic therapy, presents for a maintenance appointment with Caroline, the dental hygienist in her general dentist's practice. The facial surfaces of tooth numbers 4–13 and 20–29 appear to have remnants of composite adhesive resin.

Caroline, the dental hygienist, feels an obligation to remove these adhesive remnants but does not want to make any disparaging comment about the orthodontist, whose responsibility was to remove the adhesive. There is not enough time to remove all the resin and complete the examination, radiographs, and dental hygiene therapy at the current appointment.

Questions for Consideration

1. Which of the dental hygiene core values have particular significance in this setting? How and why?

2. To maintain Dorothy's trust in her orthodontist, how can Caroline inform the patient of the accretions and explain the need for additional appointments?

3. Role play a conversation between Caroline and Dorothy as Caroline explains the problem.

References

1. Zachrisson BU. Bonding in orthodontics. In: Graber TM, Vanarsdall RL, eds. *Orthodontics: Current Principles and Techniques*. 3rd ed. St. Louis, MO: Mosby; 2000:557-639.

2. Sharma S, Tandon P, Nagar A, Singh GP, Singh A, Chugh VK. A comparison of shear bond strength of orthodontic brackets bonded with four different orthodontic adhesives. *J Orthod Sci.* 2014;3(2):29-33.

3. Baratieri C, Mattos CT, Alves M Jr, et al. In situ evaluation of orthodontic elastomeric chains. *Braz Dent J.* 2012;23(4):394-398.

4. Rossini G, Parrini S, Castroflorio T, Deregibus A, Debernardi CL. Efficacy of clear aligners in controlling orthodontic tooth movement: a systematic review. *Angle Orthod.* 2015;85(5):881-889.

5. Heravi F, Rashed R, Raziee L. The effects of bracket removal on enamel. *Aust Orthod J.* 2008;24(2):110-115.

6. Freitas AO, Marquezan M, Nojima Mda C, Alviano DS, Maia LC. The influence of orthodontic fixed appliances on the oral microbiota: a systematic review. *Dental Press J Orthod.* 2014;19(2):46-55.

7. Najafi-Abrandabadi A, Najafi-Abrandabadi S, Ghasemi A, Kotick PG. Microshear bond strength of composite resins to enamel and porcelain substrates utilizing unfilled versus filled resins. *Dent Res J.* 2014;11(6):636-644.

8. Firoozmand LM, Brandão JV, Fialho MP. Influence of microhybrid resin and etching times on bleached enamel for the bonding of ceramic brackets. *Braz Oral Res.* 2013;27(2):142-148.

9. Farronato G, Giannini L, Galbiati G, et al. Oral tissues and orthodontic treatment: common side effects. *Minerva Stomatol.* 2013;62(11-12):431-446.

10. Prabhakar AR, Dhanraj K, Sugandhan S. Comparative evaluation in vitro of caries inhibition potential and microtensile bond strength of two fluoride releasing adhesive systems. *Eur Arch Paediatr Dent.* 2014;15(6):385-391.

11. Migliorati M, Isaia L, Cassaro A, et al. Efficacy of professional hygiene and prophylaxis on preventing plaque increase in orthodontic patients with multibracket appliances: a systematic review. *Eur J Orthod.* 2015;37(3):297-307.

12. Gkantidis N, Christou P, Topouzelis N. The orthodontic-periodontic interrelationship in integrated treatment challenges: a systematic review. *J Oral Rehabil.* 2010;37(5):377-390.

13. Christensen L, Luther F. Adults seeking orthodontic treatment: expectations, periodontal and TMD issues. *Br Dent J.* 2015;218(3):111-117.

14. Levin L, Einy S, Zigdon H, Aizenbud D, Machtei EE. Guidelines for periodontal care and follow-up during orthodontic treatment in adolescents and young adults. *J Appl Oral Sci.* 2012;20(4):399-403.

15. Benson PE, Parkin N, Dyer F, Millett DT, Furness S, Germain P. Fluorides for the prevention of early tooth decay (demineralised white lesions) during fixed brace treatment. *Cochrane Database Syst Rev.* 2013;12:CD003809.

16. Sharma R, Trehan M, Sharma S, Jharwal V, Rathore N. Comparison of effectiveness of manual orthodontic, powered and sonic toothbrushes on oral hygiene of fixed orthodontic patients. *Int J Clin Pediatr Dent.* 2015;8(3):181-189.

17. Barnes CM, Russell CM, Reinhardt RA, Payne JB, Lyle DM. Comparison of irrigation to floss as an adjunct to tooth brushing: effect on bleeding, gingivitis, and supragingival plaque. *J Clin Dent.* 2005;16(3):71-77.

18. Leite Bdos S, Fagundes NC, Aragón ML, Dias CG, Normando D. Cleansing orthodontic brackets with air-powder polishing: effects on frictional force and degree of debris. *Dental Press J Orthod.* 2016;21(4):60-65.

19. Camboni S, Donnet M. Tooth surface comparison after air polishing and rubber cup: a scanning electron microscopy study. *J Clin Dent.* 2016;27(1):13-18.

20. Janiszewska-Olszowska J, Szatkiewicz T, Tomkowski R, Tandecka K, Grocholewicz K. Effect of orthodontic debonding and adhesive removal on the enamel—current knowledge and future perspectives—a systematic review. *Med Sci Monit.* 2014;20:1991-2001.

21. Vicente A, Ortiz Ruiz AJ, García López M, Martínez Beneyto Y, Bravo-González LA. Enamel resistance to demineralization after bracket debonding using fluoride varnish. *Sci Rep.* 2017;7(1):15183.

22. Heymann GC, Grauer D. A contemporary review of white spot lesions in orthodontics. *J Esthet Restor Dent.* 2013;25(2):85-95.

23. Vivaldi-Rodrigues G, Demito CF, Bowman SJ, Ramos AL. The effectiveness of a fluoride varnish in preventing the development of white spot lesions. *World J Orthod.* 2006;7(2):138-144.

24. Demito CF, Vivaldi-Rodrigues G, Ramos AL, Bowman SJ. The efficacy of a fluoride varnish in reducing enamel demineralization adjacent to orthodontic brackets: an in vitro study. *Orthod Craniofac Res.* 2004;7(4):205-210.

30

Care of Dental Prosthesis

Tammy K. Swecker, BSDH, MEd, and Linda D. Boyd, RDH, RD, EdD

CHAPTER OUTLINE

MISSING TEETH

THE EDENTULOUS MOUTH
I. Bone
II. Mucous Membranes

PURPOSE FOR WEARING A FIXED OR REMOVABLE PROSTHESIS
I. Replacement Options
II. Consequences of Not Replacing Missing Teeth

FIXED PARTIAL DENTURE PROSTHESES
I. Description
II. Types of Fixed Partial Dentures
III. Criteria for Fixed Partial Dentures

REMOVABLE PARTIAL DENTURE PROSTHESES
I. Description
II. Types of Removable Partial Dentures

COMPLETE DENTURE PROSTHESIS
I. Types of Complete Dentures
II. Components of a Complete Denture

COMPLETE OVERDENTURE PROSTHESES
I. Root-Supported Overdenture
II. Implant-Supported Overdenture

OBTURATOR
I. Description
II. Purposes and Uses
III. Clinical Applications
IV. Professional Continuing Care

DENTURE MARKING FOR IDENTIFICATION
I. Criteria for an Adequate Marking System
II. Inclusion Methods for Marking
III. Surface Markers
IV. Information to Include on a Marker

PROFESSIONAL CARE PROCEDURES FOR FIXED PROSTHESES

PATIENT SELF-CARE PROCEDURES FOR FIXED PROSTHESES
I. Debris Removal
II. Biofilm Removal from Abutment Teeth
III. Preventive Agents
IV. Care of the Fixed Prosthesis

PROFESSIONAL CARE PROCEDURES OF REMOVABLE PARTIAL PROSTHESIS

PATIENT SELF-CARE PROCEDURES FOR REMOVABLE PARTIAL PROSTHESES
I. Biofilm Removal for Abutment Teeth and Implants
II. Patient Education on Proper Use of Removable Prosthesis
III. Cleaning the Prosthesis

PROFESSIONAL CARE PROCEDURES FOR COMPLETE DENTURES
I. Denture Deposits
II. Removal of Denture
III. Care of Dentures during Intraoral Procedures

PATIENT SELF-CARE PROCEDURES FOR THE COMPLETE DENTURE
I. General Education Prior to Denture Placement
II. Education for the New Denture Wearer
III. Denture Cleaning

DENTURE-INDUCED ORAL MUCOSAL LESIONS (OML)
I. Contributing Factors for Denture-Induced OMLs
II. Types of Denture-Induced OMLs

DOCUMENTATION

EVERYDAY ETHICS

FACTORS TO TEACH THE PATIENT

REFERENCES

LEARNING OBJECTIVES

After studying this chapter, the student will be able to:

1. Identify the causes and prevention of tooth loss.

2. Describe the anatomic features of an edentulous oral cavity.

3. Describe the types and components of fixed and removable oral prostheses.

4. Describe the methods for marking a denture for permanent identification.

5. Develop an individualized patient oral self-care regimen for fixed and removal prostheses.

6. Provide a careful evaluation of an oral prosthesis to include clinical examination of the prosthesis, related soft tissue, and patient concerns.

7. Explain the causes and prevention of denture-induced oral lesions.

8. List the steps to provide professional cleaning of fixed and removable prostheses.

MISSING TEETH

◆ A patient may have one or more missing teeth or may have a treatment plan for tooth extractions.

◆ A patient should be informed of the various options to replace missing teeth as well as the risk factors associated with not replacing the missing teeth.

- Providing objective information on treatment alternatives and acting as a patient advocate allows the patient to make informed, autonomous decisions about personal oral health.

◆ A long history of poor oral self-care, carious lesions, and periodontal infections may have led to tooth loss; trauma is another common cause of tooth loss.

◆ A fully edentulous patient has no teeth.

- Absence of teeth may be congenital or due to loss from a variety of causes such as a traumatic accident or lack of knowledge about oral disease prevention.

- Inadequate oral self-care practices without professional dental and dental hygiene care may have resulted in progression of dental carious lesions and periodontal infections that result in removal of teeth.

- An edentulous patient may have dental implants to improve the function and stability of an overdenture dental prosthesis.[1]

◆ A partially edentulous patient may have a complete denture opposing an arch with all natural teeth or various kinds of fixed or removable partial prostheses.

THE EDENTULOUS MOUTH

I. Bone

◆ *Residual ridges*[2]

- After the teeth are removed, the residual ridges enter into a continuing bone remodeling process.

- The alveolar bone, which had supported the teeth, undergoes resorption. The rate and amount of bony resorption vary with each individual.

- Major bony changes occur during the first year after the teeth are removed, but changes continue throughout life.

- Mandibular bone loss is generally greater than maxillary bone loss.

- Bone remodeling and soft-tissue healing may make it necessary to have dentures rebased, relined, or remade at intervals.

◆ *Tori and exostoses*

- Benign bony outgrowths may interfere with the fabrication and wearing of dentures.

- Because of the size, shape, or location, excess bone often needs to be removed surgically before a denture can be constructed.

- *Torus palatinus*: bony enlargement located over the midline of the palate.

- *Torus mandibularis*: bony mass generally located on the lingual in the region of the premolars.

- *Exostosis*: a bony protuberance generally located on the buccal aspects of maxilla and/or mandible.

II. Mucous Membrane

◆ *Composition: mucosa*

- Oral mucosa is composed of masticatory, lining, and specialized mucosa.

- *Masticatory* mucosa covers the edentulous ridges and the hard palate. The mucous membrane covering the bony ridges is made up of two layers—the lamina propria and the surface-stratified squamous epithelium—which is keratinized in the healthy mouth.

- *Lining* mucosa covers the floor of the mouth, vestibules, and cheeks.

- *Specialized* mucosa covers the dorsal surface of the tongue and contains filiform, fungiform, and circumvallate papillae, as shown in Chapter 13.

◆ *Composition: submucosa*

- Underneath the mucous membrane is the submucosa, which is attached to the underlying bone.

- The submucosa is composed of connective tissue with vessels, nerves, adipose tissue, and glands.
- The support or cushioning effect for the denture depends on the makeup of the submucosa, which varies in different parts of the mouth.

◆ *Tension test*
- Examine the edentulous mouth by retracting the lips and cheeks using a tension test technique described in Chapter 20.
- A line of demarcation similar to the mucogingival junction is apparent, separating the attached tissue over the bony ridge and the loose lining mucosa of the vestibule.
- Frenal attachments can be observed.

PURPOSES FOR WEARING A FIXED OR REMOVABLE PROSTHESIS

The benefits of replacing missing teeth with dentures include the following[3]:
◆ Replace missing teeth and adjacent structures.
◆ Presence of teeth has an esthetic role.
◆ Restore facial contour, including lip support and temporomandibular joint position.
◆ Provide function.
◆ Enhance ability to eat a variety of healthy foods such as chewy meat and fresh vegetables/fruit.
◆ Promote proper speech and enunciation.

I. Replacement Options

◆ Replacement options include the following (see Box 30-1):
- Fixed prosthesis.
- Removable prosthesis.
- Dental implants (see Chapter 31).
◆ Dental hygienist's role.
- Explain each choice for the patient.
- Answer questions from the patient.
- Prepare notes from the patient's medical and dental histories, risk factors, intraoral/extraoral examination, and other pertinent observations to assist the dentist.

II. Consequences of Not Replacing Missing Teeth

◆ Replacement for a missing tooth may not be indicated for a patient who has sufficient remaining teeth for function, for example:
- Third molars are generally not replaced after extraction.

BOX 30-1
Types of Oral Prostheses and Appliances

Fixed
Fixed partial denture
Periodontal splint
Implant-supported complete denture
Orthodontic appliance
Space maintainer

Removable
Removable partial denture
Natural tooth supported
Implant supported
Complete denture
Overdenture
Obturator
Removable orthodontic appliance
Removable space maintainer
Hawley appliance

- Second molars that are extracted and have no opposing teeth.
- Teeth extracted for orthodontic purposes.
◆ Consequences of not replacing missing teeth include:
- *Migration of adjacent teeth*: Tilting and rotation of teeth may complicate future replacement options or lead to periodontal problems due to difficulty in biofilm control and misdirected occlusal forces when chewing.
- *Migration of opposing teeth*: An unopposed tooth may supererupt.
- *Remaining teeth may suffer from the added function and stress*: may lead to fractures and tooth loss.
- *Loss of occlusal vertical dimension*: Missing teeth may result in overclosure of the occlusion or bite and can lead to temporomandibular joint disorders.
- Loss of vertical dimension may promote angular cheilitis at the corners of the mouth from pooling of saliva.

FIXED PARTIAL DENTURE PROSTHESES

I. Description

◆ Fixed partial dentures, commonly called *bridges*, are composed of the following, as shown in Figure 30-1:
- Abutments.

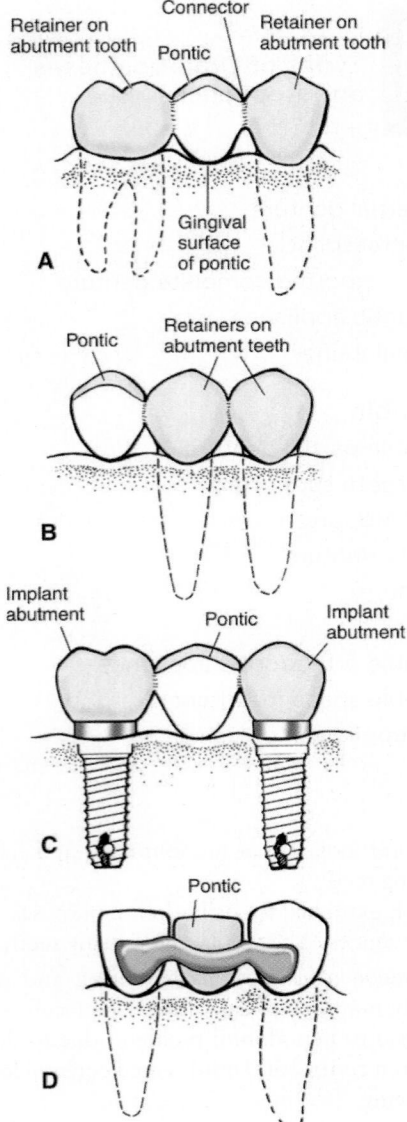

FIGURE 30-1 • Fixed Partial Dentures. A: Characteristic parts of a mandibular three-unit fixed partial denture. Cast gold crowns on the abutment teeth serve as the retainers for the bridge. **B:** Cantilever bridge supported by a double abutment. **C:** Fixed partial denture with implant abutments. **D:** Fixed resin–retained partial prosthesis.

- Connectors.
- Pontics.
◆ Bridges can be fabricated from various materials including:
  • Metals.
  • Ceramics.
  • Combination of both.
◆ A fixed partial denture is affixed to the teeth or implants with special cement and is not removable.

II. Types of Fixed Partial Dentures

◆ *Natural tooth supported*
  • *Traditional/bilateral*: supported by one or more natural teeth at each end, as shown in Figure 30-1A.
  • *Cantilever*: pontic supported by one or more teeth at one end only, as shown in Figure 30-1B.
  • *Resin retained*: Wing-like extensions are bonded with resin cement to etched enamel. Requires minimal or no preparation for tooth structure. Also called a Maryland Bridge and shown in Figure 30-1D.
◆ *Implant supported*
  • Most often the endosseous (endosteal) implant is used to support fixed partial dentures and overdentures and shown in Figure 30-1C.

III. Criteria for Fixed Partial Dentures

◆ Biologically and esthetically harmonious with the teeth and surrounding periodontium.
◆ All parts accessible for cleaning by the patient and the dental professional.
◆ Does not interfere with the cleaning regimen for the remaining natural dentition.
◆ Does not traumatize oral tissues.
◆ Restores function of the missing tooth or teeth.

REMOVABLE PARTIAL DENTURE PROSTHESES

I. Description

◆ A removable partial denture (RPD) replaces one or more, but less than all, of the natural teeth and associated structures.
◆ The partial denture can be removed from the mouth.
◆ The denture base rests on the oral mucosa and houses the artificial teeth.

II. Types of Removable Partial Dentures

◆ A typical partial denture consists of a stable metal framework made of chrome cobalt.
◆ The framework engages abutment teeth or an abutment implant with a wide variety of clasp assemblies and **rest** seats or **precision attachments**.
◆ Depending on the location and number of remaining natural teeth, a partial denture may receive all its support from the teeth or it may be partially tooth-borne, partially implant-borne, or partially tissue-borne.
◆ The base is made of plastic acrylic resin.
◆ The teeth are made of porcelain, plastic resin, or metal.
◆ The basic parts of an RPD are shown in Figure 30-2.

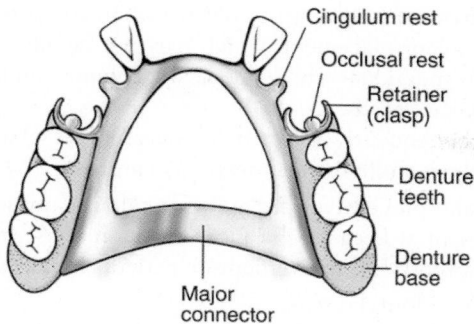

FIGURE 30-2 • Removable Partial Denture (RPD). Components of a RPD shown for a maxillary prosthesis.

COMPLETE DENTURE PROSTHESIS

◆ The initial adjustment to wearing a prosthesis is challenging for the patient.

◆ The entire dental team needs to work together to assist the patient through the process of losing teeth and adjusting to a new prosthesis.

◆ A new prosthesis requires several adjustment visits with the dentist.

◆ Components of a complete denture are shown in Figure 30-3.

I. Types of Complete Dentures[4]

◆ *Tissue-supported complete denture*: A removable dental prosthesis that replaces the entire dentition and associated structures of the maxilla or the mandible and rests on the denture foundation area, the mucosal-covered alveolar ridge.

◆ *Implant denture*: A complete dental prosthesis supported in part or whole by one or more dental implants. The denture itself is not an implantable device.

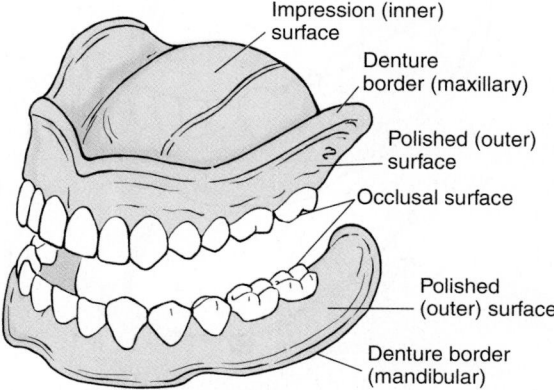

FIGURE 30-3 • Complete Denture. The surfaces and borders of maxillary and mandibular dentures.

◆ *Overdenture*: A removable prosthesis that rests on one or more remaining natural teeth and/or dental implants (Chapter 31). It is also called an overlay prosthesis.

◆ *Interim denture*: A removable dental prosthesis designed to enhance esthetics, stabilization, and/or function for a limited period, after which it is to be replaced by a definitive prosthesis.

 • Often such prostheses are used to assist in determining the therapeutic effectiveness of a specific treatment plan or the form and function of the planned definitive prosthesis.

 • Interim denture is also called a *provisional prosthesis*.

◆ *Immediate denture*: A denture fabricated for placement immediately following the removal of a natural tooth or teeth.

 • An immediate or interim denture tends to loosen after the significant remodeling of bone and soft tissue that follows surgery.

 • The denture may be relined temporarily with a soft liner or a tissue conditioning material.

 • The patient may use a denture adhesive until the majority of healing occurs.

 • After approximately 6 months, dentures are remade, relined, or rebased.

◆ *Denture for primary teeth*

 • Dentures occasionally must be constructed to replace primary teeth.

 • The teeth may be congenitally missing (anodontia) or may have been extracted due to rampant caries or trauma.

 • Early childhood dental caries can break down the teeth severely soon after eruption.

 • To provide esthetics and function, dentures can be constructed for the cooperative child.

 • As the permanent teeth begin to erupt, the denture is adjusted to allow for eruption.

 • A caries management program (see Chapter 25) based on caries risk is essential to prevent caries.

II. Components of a Complete Denture

◆ *Denture base*

 • The part of a denture that rests on the oral mucosa and to which the teeth are attached.

 • Most denture bases are made of plastic acrylic resin.

 • Others may be metal such as chrome cobalt or gold, in combination with a plastic resin.

◆ *Impression surface*[4]

 • The tissue or inner surface of the denture that is not polished.

 • Lies directly on the residual ridges and adjacent tissues.

 • The surface may be lined with a long-term material for removal to be removed by the patient, such as a temporary soft liner, a tissue conditioner, or a permanent soft silicone liner.

- A patient may place a denture-adhesive material on the impression surface of the denture before inserting the denture.
  - A denture adhesive is a commercially available paste or powder preparation.
  - The adhesive is used to improve denture retention, stabilization, and comfort, as recommended by the dentist.
  - The denture adhesive should be removed from the denture during daily cleaning and from soft tissues to enable visual examination.
  - The patient should be discouraged from using an adhesive indefinitely in the attempt to cope with ill-fitting dentures that need to be adjusted or remade.
- *Polished surface*: The external or outer surface is polished.
- *Occlusal surface*: The surface of a denture that makes contact or near-contact with the corresponding surface of the opposing denture or natural teeth.
- *Teeth*
  - The denture teeth may be made of plastic acrylic resin, composite resin, porcelain, or polymethyl methacrylate.
  - A patient may request to have decorative facings incorporated into certain teeth.
  - Metal occlusal surfaces may be present, for example, to maintain a stable vertical dimension of occlusion when opposing teeth may cause excessive wear.

COMPLETE OVERDENTURE PROSTHESES

An overdenture is a complete denture supported by both retained natural teeth and/or implants and the soft tissue of the residual alveolar ridge.

I. Root-Supported Overdenture

- An overdenture may be possible for any patient when the clinical crowns are not restorable and the root is caries-free and periodontally healthy.
  - Tooth crowns are reduced to short, rounded preparations or to the level and contour of the gingival margin and require endodontic therapy.
- The advantages of maintaining tooth roots as abutments to support an overdenture include[5,6]:
  - Significantly less alveolar bone resorption in the maxilla and mandible when compared with edentulous patients with complete dentures.
  - Better stability and retention of a mandibular prosthesis.
  - Improved masticatory (chewing) ability and efficiency.
  - Retain some tactile and proprioceptive senses for the patient because the periodontal ligament is present.
  - Increase the patient's psychological acceptance of the denture. The patient does not feel that all natural teeth have been lost.

- Invasive surgery is not needed when compared with implant placement, which may not be advisable in an individual who is medically complex and/or has special needs.
- Teeth frequently selected for overdenture abutments are the mandibular and maxillary canines.
- Regular preventive care and meticulous daily self-care is essential because the most common cause of abutment tooth loss in overdenture patients includes[7]:
  - Periodontal disease.
  - Caries.

II. Implant-Supported Overdenture

- Implants can be placed to help stabilize dentures and are becoming more widely used than root-supported overdentures.
  - Recent systematic review of the literature suggest a mandibular overdenture supported by two implants was cost-effective with good long-term survival.[8]
  - However, for maxillary overdentures, four or more implants are necessary for the best long-term success making them less cost-effective.[9]
- Mandibular implants are generally placed in the position of the mandibular canine as shown in Figure 30-4.
- The advantages of an implant-supported overdenture include[10]:
  - No risk for dental caries as seen with the abutment roots used in a root-supported overdenture.
  - Less alveolar bone loss when compared with complete dentures.
  - Improved stability and retention when compared with a complete denture.
  - Better chewing ability and quality of life.
- Peri-implant hygiene is described in Chapter 31.

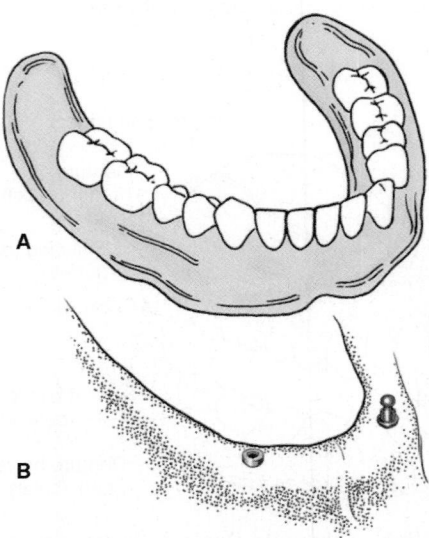

FIGURE 30-4 • Overdenture. A: Mandibular complete denture. **B:** Examples of two different types of implant abutments. Generally, the same type of abutments is used in a denture.

OBTURATOR

I. Description

◆ An obturator is a prosthesis designed to close a congenital or acquired opening, such as a cleft of the hard palate.

◆ Made with a resin base and retainer clasps that provide stability for the appliance.

◆ Depending on the exact location of the palatal defect, an obturator may extend to include anterior prosthetic teeth.

◆ See Figure 30-5A and B for an example of a palatal defect and corresponding obturator.

II. Purposes and Uses

◆ A variety of medical and physical conditions benefit from use of an obturator including:
  • Loss or perforation of the palate due to chronic cocaine abuse.[11]
  • Patient with a loss of the palate due to trauma.
  • Patients with previous cancers involving the maxilla.
  • Patients with cleft palate (see Chapter 49).

III. Clinical Applications

◆ Depending on the size of the palatal defect, the obturator may need to stay in place in the mouth during parts of the intraoral and extraoral examination and treatment procedures to prevent choking or aspiration of water or other materials used in the oral cavity.

◆ Obturators need to be removed during exposure of radiographic images. An appliance with metal clasps will interfere with the radiolucency of the teeth and surrounding tissues.

◆ Removal of an obturator during dental hygiene therapy may be necessary to ensure access for complete calculus and biofilm removal and treatment of natural tooth surfaces.

◆ Professional care of an obturator follows procedures for cleaning an RPD.

◆ Instruction for patient's daily cleaning and care of the obturator is the same as the care given to an RPD.

◆ Patients may need to sleep with the obturator in place when the defect is severe, which may cause the underlying mucosa to become desiccated and the tissue may spontaneously begin to bleed.

◆ Sleeping with an obturator in place increases the risk for demineralization and dental caries in the abutment teeth as well as the incidence of denture stomatitis.

◆ When the patient must sleep with the obturator in place, it is advisable the obturator be removed for short periods during the day to allow the tissue to rest.

IV. Professional Continuing Care

◆ A minimum of three visits each year to the dentist and dental hygienist is recommended for continuing care depending on patient compliance and risk factors.

◆ The palatal defect will change over time and the dentist will need to adjust the obturator along with providing routine preventive dental care.

DENTURE MARKING FOR IDENTIFICATION

Marking is required by law in some countries and in most states of the United States. However, there is not a universal denture marking system. The need for denture marking is apparent in a variety of situations as listed[11]:

◆ In forensic dentistry, or for identification of victims of war, such disasters as flood or fire, or transportation catastrophes, the dentition has been used increasingly as a means of identification.

◆ Prompt identification can be urgent when an individual is found unconscious from illness or injury or is suffering from amnesia as a result of psychiatric or traumatic causes, as well as suffering from Alzheimer disease.

◆ The dentures of people in long-term residence or care facilities must be marked.

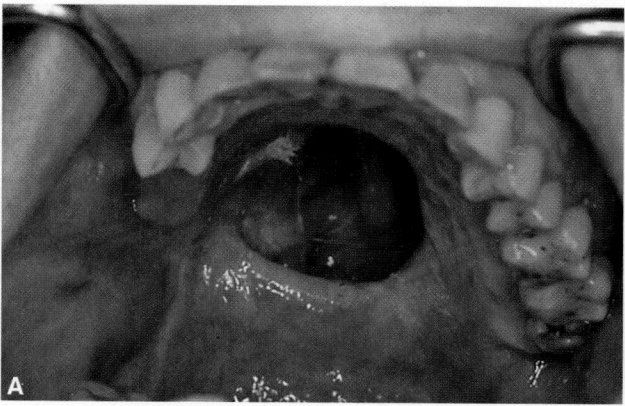
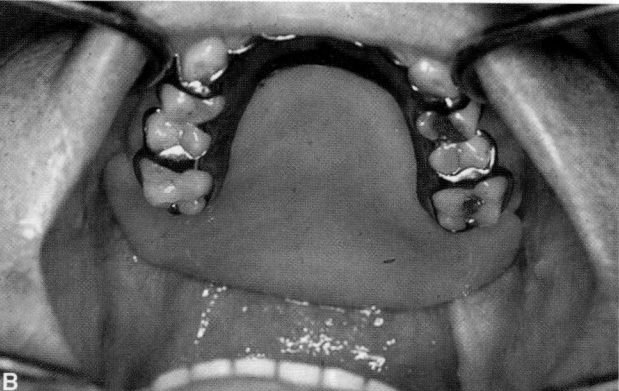

FIGURE 30-5 • **A:** Palatal defect. **B:** Corresponding obturator. (Picture Courtesy of Altug Kazanoglu DMD, MS, FAAMP, Virginia Commonwealth University.)

I. Criteria for an Adequate Marking System[12]

Information on the denture must be specific so that rapid identification is possible.

- *Relative to the denture*
  - Must have no adverse effects on denture material.
  - Must not change the strength, surface texture, or fit of the denture.
  - Must be cosmetically acceptable; the label must be placed in an unobtrusive position.
- *Relative to the procedure*
  - Marking system must be easy to learn and simple to carry out.
  - Inexpensive.
  - Durable result. When the information is incorporated during denture processing, it is permanent. A surface marker for a denture already in use needs to be able to withstand denture-cleaning methods for a reasonable period of time.
- *Characteristics of the material used*
  - *Fire and humidity resistant*: When the label is placed inside the posterior section of a denture, the surrounding tongue and maxillofacial parts offer protection.
  - *Radiopaque*: A metal marker can be of use as a means of identification by radiographic examination in the event the radiolucent acrylic denture is accidentally swallowed.

II. Inclusion Methods for Marking[12,13]

Inclusion methods are more permanent, but tend to be more expensive, require special equipment, and require trained personnel.

- *ID-Band*
  - A shallow indentation is made on the denture for a stainless steel metal band containing the patient identification and covered with clear acrylic resin.
  - The Swedish ID-Band is the international standard.
- *ID-Strip*
  - Identification information can be placed on the surface of the impression to be incorporated when the denture is fabricated.
- *Electronic microchip*
  - A microchip can be incorporated in the denture because of the small size and esthetic acceptability.
  - A disadvantage is higher cost.
- *Laser etching*
  - Copper vapor laser has been used to mark dentures with metal frameworks, removable partial dentures, and other metallic restorations.
  - This method is expensive and requires specialized equipment and personnel.
- *Radio-frequency identification (RFID) tags*
  - RFID tags are small and can be incorporated into the denture resin.

- They permit rapid identification and can store large amounts of data.
- Not widely used due to the high cost.
- *Bar codes*
  - Bar codes can be printed on silk and incorporated into a denture with clear acrylic resin.
  - A disadvantage is that it requires expensive special equipment.

III. Surface Markers

Surface markers are not as durable, but instruction can be provided for persons not trained in dental laboratory methods. In a skilled nursing facility or other long-term institution that has no resident dentist or dental hygienist, it may be possible to teach a nurse or other staff member to mark dentures of residents as they are admitted. The methods described as follows have been used for this purpose[12,13]:

- *Indelible pen or ballpoint*
  - After cleaning and drying the denture, a small area near the posterior of the outer or polished denture surface is rubbed with an emery board until it is rough.
  - Name, initials, or other identification is printed on the roughened area with an indelible pen and dried.
  - Two or three coats of a fingernail acrylic (heavy nail protector) are painted over the area; each layer is dried before applying the next.
  - Surface markings have been found to last up to 6 months.
  - Light-cured materials may also be used.
- *Engraving tool or dental bur*
  - An engraving tool or round dental bur may be used to enter the name on the denture.
  - The engraving should be covered with a denture acrylic and processed to provide a smooth surface that will not retain food debris.

IV. Information to Include on a Marker

- For residents of a home or institution, using only the person's name and initials can suffice for temporary surface marking.
- In a community, country, or international situation, the name alone would not provide enough identification, and the social security number, armed services serial number, or the equivalent in other countries have been included.
- Other identification, such as blood type and vital drug or disease condition, has been suggested.
- In certain countries, the dentist's registration or hospital number has been used. In Sweden, the patient's date of birth and national registration number have been marked on the dentures.
- Markings that can provide *immediate* identification are preferred.

PROFESSIONAL CARE PROCEDURES FOR FIXED PROSTHESES

Guidelines for professional care of fixed dental prostheses include the following[14]:

◆ Medical, dental, psychosocial history, and vital signs (see Chapters 11 and 12).

◆ Extraoral/intraoral examination (see Chapter 13).

◆ Risk assessments for oral disease.

◆ Radiographs according to recognized guidelines (see Chapter 15).

◆ Comprehensive dental and periodontal examination (see Chapters 16 and 20). The following should be carefully evaluated[15]:
  • Margins of fixed prostheses for possible dental caries and other irregularities.
  • Monitoring of periodontal health and changes in mobility or loss of attachment.
  • One or more bridge abutments can become lose or fracture.
  • Abutment teeth may also fracture.
  • Monitor for radiographic or clinical signs of loss of pulp vitality.

◆ Dental and dental hygiene diagnosis and care planning.

◆ Oral hygiene education for existing natural dentition along with fixed prostheses (see Chapters 26 and 27).

◆ Prophylaxis or periodontal treatment as indicated by the examination findings.
  • See Chapter 31 for care of implant-supported fixed prostheses.

◆ Preventive services to address modifiable risk factors such as fluoride varnish, prescription fluorides, chlorhexidine mouthrinse, tobacco intervention, and nutrition counseling (see Chapters 32, 33, and 34).

◆ Continuing care at a minimum of 6-month interval with more frequent intervals needed for those who are at higher risk or unable to perform adequate oral self-care.

PATIENT SELF-CARE PROCEDURES FOR FIXED PROSTHESES

I. Debris Removal

◆ Use an oral irrigator for loose debris removal throughout the dentition for a first step.
  • Facilitates next step: biofilm removal with a toothbrush and other aids.
  • Procedure for use of an oral irrigator is described in Chapter 27.

II. Biofilm Removal from Abutment Teeth

◆ Nearly all the methods proposed for dental biofilm control (see Chapters 26 and 27) are applicable to abutment teeth.

◆ The proximal surface of an abutment tooth and the gingiva adjacent to a pontic require special attention.

◆ *Toothbrushing*
  • Sulcular brushing is generally indicated.

◆ *Dentifrice selection*
  • A *nonabrasive* dentifrice is indicated to prevent the abrasion of the prosthesis surfaces and areas of exposed root on abutment teeth.
  • *Fluoride-containing* dentifrice is recommended for protection of remaining natural tooth surfaces, particularly exposed cementum.

◆ *Additional interdental care*
  • The method of interdental care is selected based on the manual dexterity of each patient and the type of prosthesis.
  • An interdental cleaning device is adapted specifically to the proximal surfaces of the abutments.

◆ Interdental cleaning methods and devices are described in Chapter 27.

III. Preventive Agents

◆ Those at risk for caries or periodontal disease may also benefit from prescription fluoride (5000 ppm fluoride).[14]

◆ Short-term chlorhexidine as needed.[14]

IV. Care of the Fixed Prosthesis

◆ *Areas requiring emphasis*
  • The pontics and beneath the connectors are particularly prone to biofilm retention.

◆ *Toothbrushing*
  • A toothbrush in the Charters' position (see Chapter 26) may be helpful for cleaning the gingival surface of the pontic from the facial aspect.
  • The filaments can be directed under the pontic to clean the gingival surface.

◆ *Dental floss for threader*
  • Tufted dental floss is most efficient for cleaning a fixed partial denture as it can be passed under the pontic(s) (see Chapter 27).
  • Thread a 12- to 15-inch length into a floss threader. Several types are available and are shown in Figure 30-6.
  • Apply threader between abutment, pontic, and gingiva (Figure 30-7).
  • Draw the floss through and use a single or double thickness for oral self-care.

◆ *Other interdental devices*
  • A single-tuft brush (see Chapter 26) can be recommended and demonstrated as needed for individual prosthesis.
  • Small interdental brushes (see Chapter 27) may be used mesial and distal to the pontic and natural teeth when space allows access.

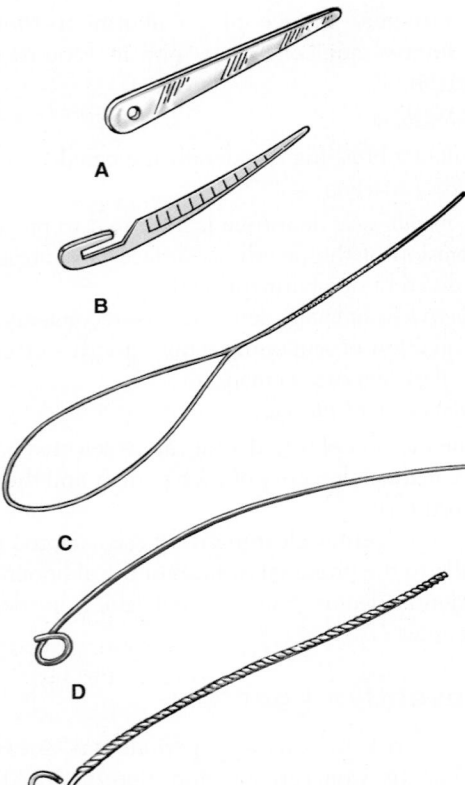

FIGURE 30-6 • Floss Threaders. A: Clear plastic with closed eye. **B:** Tinted plastic with open eye. **C:** Soft plastic loop. **D:** Flexible wire. **E:** Twisted wire.

◆ *Additional factors*
  • Instruct the patient to inform the dental team when any problem or change with the fixed prosthesis becomes apparent.

PROFESSIONAL CARE PROCEDURES FOR REMOVABLE PARTIAL PROSTHESIS

The guidelines for the care of removable partial prostheses are similar to the fixed prostheses in regard to the examination and care of the natural dentition present.[14]

◆ Medical, dental, psychosocial history, and vital signs (see Chapters 11 and 12).

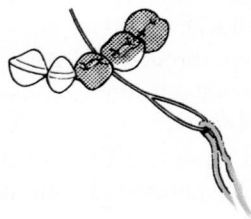

FIGURE 30-7 • Use of Floss Threader to Draw the Floss or Tufted Floss between Abutment and Pontic.

◆ Remove prosthesis for evaluation and cleaning (described in next section).
  • It is typically easiest to have the patient remove the prosthesis because the patient is familiar with the path of insertion and removal.
  • When a patient is unable to remove the appliance, the dental hygienist proceeds as follows:
    • Exert an even pressure on both sides of the denture simultaneously as the clasps slide up over their abutment teeth.
    • The line of insertion and removal of a partial denture is designed and constructed for an even, vertical movement.
    • Avoid grasping the clasp assemblies of the prostheses, which may damage or bend a clasp.
  • Prevent cross-contamination when receiving a removable prosthesis from a patient by wearing personal protective equipment and offering a disposable cup or re-sealable plastic bag to place the prosthesis in, rinse the prosthesis to remove any loose debris.
◆ Extraoral/intraoral examination (see Chapter 13).
  • Careful monitoring of the palatal tissue and edentulous ridges for signs of oral mucosal lesions (OMLs) is essential as about one-third of removable prosthesis wearers exhibit stomatitis.[16,17]
◆ Risk assessments for oral disease.
◆ Radiographs according to recognized guidelines (see Chapter 15).
◆ Comprehensive dental and periodontal examination (see Chapters 16 and 20). The following should be carefully evaluated[14]:
  • Check the condition of the removable prostheses by looking for fractures, cracks, chipped and worn teeth, and broken clasps.
  • Evaluate the fit and function of the prostheses.
◆ Dental and dental hygiene diagnosis and care planning.
◆ Oral hygiene education for existing natural dentition (see Chapters 26 and 27) along with prostheses.
  • Biofilm control is a major factor in maintaining the long-term health of abutment teeth for an RPD.[16]
  • The biofilm or oral microbiome is different in those who are dentate with partial dentures versus those who are edentulous with complete dentures.[17] When natural teeth are present, there are higher levels of *Actinomyces, Haemophilus, Corynebacterium,* and *Veillonella,* with fewer *Lactobacillus* and *Streptococcus.*[17]
◆ Prophylaxis or periodontal treatment as indicated by the examination findings.
  • See Chapter 31 for care of implant-supported fixed prostheses.
◆ Clean removable prosthesis.
  • Place in a cleaning solution in a resealable plastic bag in an ultrasonic cleaner as shown in Figure 30-8.
  • After removal from the cleaning solution, carefully brush the prosthesis with a denture brush and wrap

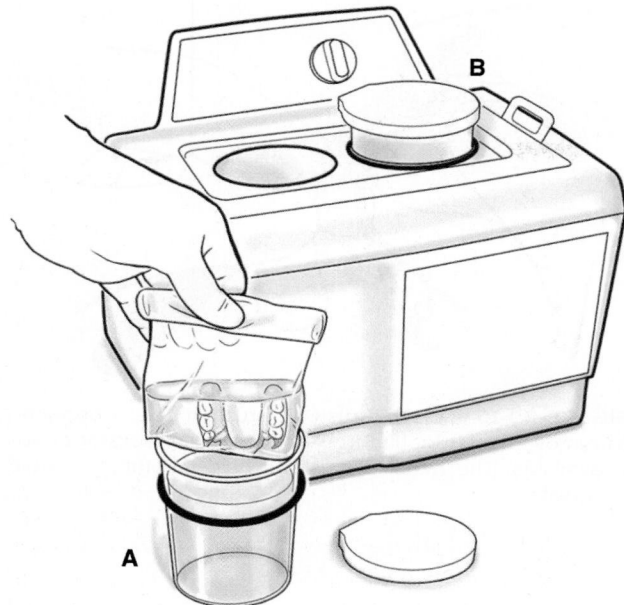

FIGURE 30-8 • Ultrasonic Denture Cleaner. A: First, the removable prosthesis is placed in a sealed bag with cleaning solution and placed in a beaker filled with water. **B:** Beaker is then placed in an ultrasonic unit and set according to manufacturer directions.

in a wet paper towel or put in a new resealable plastic bag with water to keep it moist until patient care is complete.

◆ Preventive services to address modifiable risk factors such as fluoride varnish, prescription fluorides, chlorhexidine mouthrinse, tobacco intervention, and nutrition counseling (see Chapters 28, 32 to 34).

◆ Continuing care at a minimum of 6-month interval with more frequent intervals needed for those who are at higher risk or unable to perform adequate oral self-care.

PATIENT SELF-CARE PROCEDURES FOR REMOVABLE PARTIAL PROSTHESES

Poor oral hygiene increases risk of OMLs like stomatitis in both partial and complete prosthesis wearers.[17,18]

I. Biofilm Removal for Abutment Teeth and Implants

See Chapters 26, 27, and 31 for oral self-care procedures for the abutment teeth and implants.

◆ *Biofilm control*
  • Prior to oral hygiene procedures, remove the RPD to access the natural teeth and/or implants.
  • Oral hygiene aids should be chosen according to patient's risk assessment, specific oral health needs, abilities, and preferences.

• Meticulous biofilm removal must be emphasized to prevent dental caries and/or periodontal infection involving abutment tooth, which can lead to additional tooth loss. Tooth loss impacts the longevity of the RPD and may impact options for replacement.

◆ *Dental caries and periodontal disease prevention*
  • Abutment teeth are at increased risk for dental caries and periodontal disease.[7,8]
  • Daily oral self-care, topical fluoride use (e.g., fluoridated toothpaste, 5000-ppm prescription fluoride paste or gel), and diet may be necessary to reduce caries risk (see Chapter 25).[14]

II. Patient Education on Proper Use of Removable Prosthesis

◆ Partial dentures should be removed at night or for a 6- to 8-hour-period daily.[14,16,18,19]
  • Not removing the RPD overnight may result in inflammation from exposure to microorganisms.
◆ Clean the prosthesis as recommended at least twice a day.[14,18,19]
◆ Proper storage at night in a recommended cleaning solution.[14]
◆ Regular dental examinations are needed to identify when the RPD needs to be replaced.[14]

III. Cleaning the Prosthesis

A. Rinsing

◆ Rinsing is used to remove food debris when complete cleaning of the prosthesis is not possible.
  • Remove the partial denture; rinse under running water.
  • Rinsing does not remove biofilm, which is attached firmly, so it is not a substitute for complete biofilm removal and disinfection.

B. Mechanical Denture Cleansing

◆ Guidelines recommend brushing the RPD twice a day.[14]
  • Brushing is primarily for biofilm removal but is considered the least effective method to disinfect a partial or complete prosthesis.[18]
◆ Precautions to take when brushing an RPD include:
  • Partially fill the sink with water and line the sink with a wash cloth or towel to prevent breakage if the prosthesis is dropped.
  • Carefully holding the RPD in the palm of the hand as described in Box 30-2.
◆ *Denture brush:* A good-quality soft denture brush with end-rounded filaments is recommended.[14,20] The styles of denture brushes vary.
  • One type shown in Figure 30-9 is designed with two arrangements of filaments:
  • Round arrangement to access the inner, curved impression surface.

BOX 30-2
Procedure for Cleaning Denture by Brushing

1. Spread a towel, wash cloth, or rubber mat over the bottom of the sink to serve as a cushion should the denture be dropped; partially fill the sink with water.

2. Grasp denture in palm of hand securely but without squeezing because dentures can be broken.

3. Apply warm water, nonabrasive cleanser, and brush to all areas of the denture. Pay particular attention to the impression surfaces where configurations of the surface correspond with those of the oral topography. The anterior areas of the inner surfaces of both the maxillary and mandibular dentures require special adaptations of the brush.

4. Rinse denture and brush under running water. Use the brush to remove denture cleanser that may be retained in the grooves.

5. Visually check each area carefully for biofilm.

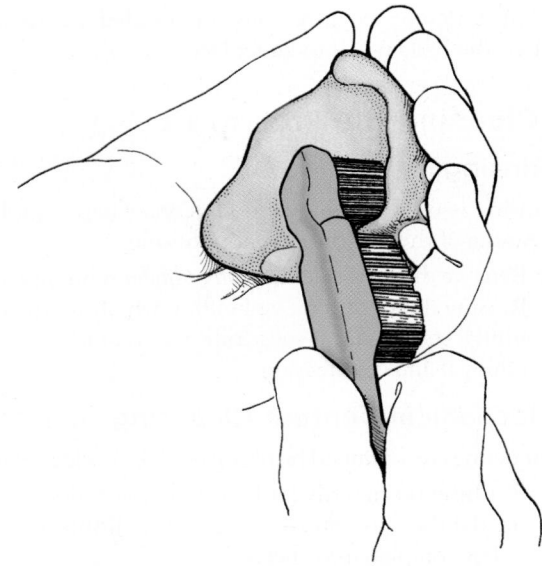

FIGURE 30-9 • Denture Brush. The denture is held securely, but without squeezing, in the palm of the nonworking hand. Place a face cloth in the bottom of the sink and partially fill with water. The specially designed brush is preferred because one group of tufts is arranged to provide access to the inner impression surface of the denture, as shown.

- Rectangular portion for convenient adaptation to the polished and occlusal denture surfaces.
- ◆ *Clasp brush*
  - A specially designed narrow, tapered brush about 2–3 inches long that can be adapted to the inner surfaces of clasps or **precision attachments** is recommended and shown in Figure 30-10.

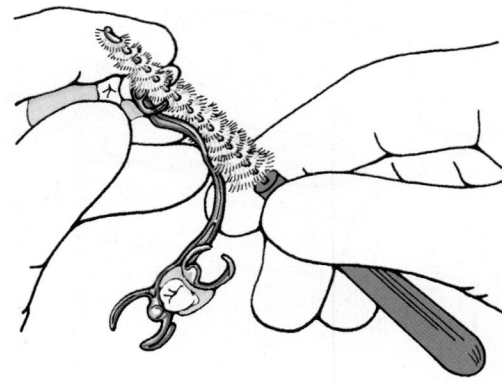

FIGURE 30-10 • Clasp Brush. A brush specially designed to remove dental biofilm from the inside surfaces of clasps is available. The denture must be held carefully to avoid accidents.

- Difficult-to-clean clasp assemblies have internal surfaces prone to biofilm accumulation that can be removed carefully with a clasp brush.
- ◆ *Brushing the RPD with denture-cleaning creams and pastes*
  - *Precaution:* All denture creams and pastes are to be used extraorally and may cause adverse effects such as damage to the esophagus, seizures, vomiting, and so on, if misused.[21]
  - The American College of Prosthodontists does not recommend use of traditional toothpastes on RPDs because they may be too abrasive for the acrylic resin and may scratch it leading to a nidus for biofilm attachment.[16,20,22]
  - Choose a cream or paste specifically designed for RPDs or dentures. Choices may also include a dishwashing liquid.[22] However, it should be noted that brushing alone has not been shown to eliminate *Candida*, so immersion in a denture cleanser is recommended in addition to brushing.[21]

C. Chemical Denture Cleansers
- ◆ Procedure
  - Denture cleansers should be used with the RPD outside the mouth to prevent adverse effects as previously noted.[21]
  - The procedure for soaking an RPD in a commercially available denture cleanser is discussed in Box 30-3.
  - The solution should be changed and the container should be cleaned daily to prevent contamination and growth of microorganisms.
- ◆ Types of denture cleansers
  - Generally available in powder or tablet form and include a variety of active agents such as hypochlorites, peroxides, and enzymes.[21]
    - Research has shown denture cleansers with sodium hypochlorite are most effective at killing pathogens such as *Candida* and methicillin-resistant *Staphylococcus aureus*.

BOX 30-3
Procedure for Cleaning a Denture by Immersion

- Place denture in a plastic container with a fitted cover specifically for this purpose.
- Use only warm water, which promotes the action of the cleanser, for rinsing and mixing the solution. Hot water is never used because it can distort plastic resin.
- Follow manufacturer's specifications to ensure correct dilution of cleanser and time length for immersion.
- Check that the denture is completely submerged in the solution; cover the container.
- When the denture is removed, rinse under running water and remove loosened debris and chemicals before proceeding to clean by brushing.
- Empty and clean container daily. Mix fresh solution to prevent contamination and growth of microorganisms.

- However, soaking for longer than 10 minutes in a sodium hypochlorite solution may damage the RPD.
- Manufacturer instructions vary and should be carefully followed.
    - The dental hygienist should ask the patient what kind of cleaning products are being used and review the instructions with them.
- Carefully rinse after using denture-cleaning solutions prior to reinserting them in the oral cavity.
- Immerse the RPD in water or cleansing solution when not in the mouth to avoid warping.

PROFESSIONAL CARE PROCEDURES FOR COMPLETE DENTURES

At the continuing care appointments, the dental hygienist and the dentist will evaluate the health of the oral mucosa, the prosthesis, the patient's compliance with personal care, prosthesis retention, and any issues the patient has with the appliance.
- A professional denture cleaning in a dental office or clinic needs is suggested annually to minimize calculus and biofilm accumulation over time.[21]
    - Ultrasonic cleaning can be done in the dental office with an approved denture-cleaning solution such as Biosonic Enzymatic and Ultra-Kleen (Sterilex) and has been shown to improve bacterial kill rates.[21]
    - An example of dentures placed in sealed bag filled with denture cleaner to be placed in an ultrasonic cleaner is shown in Figure 30-8.

- Avoid scaling the prosthesis with a sharp instrument to remove calculus deposits as it may scratch the resin or denture teeth resulting in a nidus for biofilm and calculus accumulation.

I. Denture Deposits

- Accumulation of stains and deposits on dentures varies between individuals in a manner similar to that on natural teeth. The phases of deposit formation may be divided as follows:
- *Mucin and food debris on the denture surfaces*
    - Readily removed by rinsing, brushing, and irrigation.
- *Denture pellicle and denture biofilm*
    - Denture pellicle forms readily after a denture is cleaned.
    - Denture biofilm or oral microbiome is different in those who are edentulous with complete dentures versus those who are dentate with partial dentures.[13]
    - For edentulous denture wearers, the biofilm is much less diverse and consists primarily of *Actinobacteria* and *Bacilli* with over 70% of dentures showing colonization by *Candida*.[17]
    - In stomatitis, denture biofilm contains *Candida albicans* along with higher levels of *Prevotella* and *Veillonella*.[17]
- *Denture calculus*
    - When biofilm is not thoroughly removed on a regular basis, calcification occurs within 3 days and is completely calcified by 2 weeks.[23]
- *Stains*
    - Dentures can become stained similarly to natural teeth.
    - Frequent causes of stain include tobacco, marijuana betel nut, red wine, coffee, and tea.

II. Removal of Denture

- It is usually most comfortable for the patient to remove the denture.
- The clinician may remove dentures for certain patients, particularly those with a physical limitation or in an emergency situation.
- Although denture removal may be complicated by anatomic features of an individual mouth, a general procedure is outlined in Box 30-4.

III. Care of Dentures during Intraoral Procedures

- Provide a disposable cup and tissue for the patient's use when requesting the patient to remove or insert the denture.
- Rinse in running water being careful to avoid splashing to remove any unattached debris.
- Professionally clean the denture in an ultrasonic denture cleaner, following manufacturer's instructions, with appropriate cleaning solution.

BOX 30-4
Method for Removal of a Complete Denture

The clinician follows standard procedures for infection control while removing and handling the denture from the patient's mouth.

The Complete Maxillary Denture

1. Clinician is positioned at 11–12 o'clock; left-handed clinician is at 12–1 o'clock.
2. Grasp the anterior portion of the denture firmly with the thumb on the facial surface at the height of the border of the denture under the lip and the index finger on the palatal surface.
3. With the other hand, elevate the lip to expose the border of the denture to break the seal.
4. Remove the denture gently in a downward and forward direction.
5. If the retention of the denture cannot be relieved by elevation of the lip, the patient may be able to blow into the mouth with the lips closed to break the suction seal.

The Complete Mandibular Denture

1. Clinician is positioned at 8–9 o'clock; left-handed clinician is at 3–4 o'clock.
2. Grasp the denture firmly on the facial surface with the thumb and on the lingual surface with the index finger.
3. With the other hand, retract the lower lip forward and remove the denture gently.

◆ Follow strict procedures to protect the denture from exposure to unclean areas during transportation and when in the ultrasonic cleaner.
◆ Provide a clean disposable cup or sterile container with a fitted cover to hold the prosthesis after rinsing.
◆ Immerse denture in water after cleaning to prevent drying, which can cause distortion of the denture.[21]
◆ Place container in a safe place away from treatment area to prevent spilling or inadvertently discarding it.
◆ At the end of the appointment, remember to rinse and return the moist denture before dismissing the patient from the dental chair.

PATIENT SELF-CARE PROCEDURES FOR THE COMPLETE DENTURE

I. General Education Prior to Denture Placement

◆ The preparation for denture insertion has to begin well in advance of delivery.

◆ Be sensitive to the patient's emotional state about becoming edentulous and be prepared to help them adapt to the new prosthesis.[24]
◆ Patient expectations about esthetics and function may impact satisfaction, so this must be carefully assessed prior to beginning treatment.[24]
◆ Develop an individualized plan appropriate for educating the patient on the self-care for the new prosthesis.

II. Education for the New Denture Wearer

The dental hygienist plays a valuable role in educating the new prosthesis wearer on its use, limitations, and functions. Education should include the following[25]:

◆ Each patient is different and progress in adjusting to new dentures cannot be compared with someone else.
◆ Patients may have to adapt to their appearance with new dentures. Many people may have had missing or broken teeth, so the change in vertical dimension and appearance require time for adjustment.
◆ Chewing or mastication with new dentures is a challenge for some and may take 6–8 weeks.
  • It may take time for the facial and masticatory muscles to learn to keep the denture in place and to go through the motion of chewing.
  • Hypersalivation may occur for the first few days; however, in individuals with xerostomia the lack of saliva can affect the comfort of the denture as well as swallowing ability.
  • Initially, the patient may want to eat a softer diet, eat more slowly, and cut fibrous foods into small pieces.
  • Avoid biting with the front teeth and bite into food such as a sandwich more toward the corners of the mouth, distributing food on both sides of the mouth to avoid dislodging the denture.
◆ Cover the mouth when coughing and sneezing as dentures may loosen and come out.
◆ An upper denture can affect taste and swallowing.
◆ New dentures can affect speech so they may need to practice.
◆ Choosing a high protein, healthy diet is important as those with dentures typically eat a less nutrient dense diet with higher levels of sucrose and refined carbohydrates.
  • Patients may choose to lightly steam fresh vegetables or cut them into small pieces to make them easier to chew.
  • Cooked whole-grain cereals and grains are also a good source of fiber and B vitamins.
  • Cutting fresh fruit will also make it easier for new denture wearers to eat a healthy diet.
  • Those who are edentulous tend to be at risk of malnutrition, so including good sources of protein (dairy, fish, meat, chicken, and eggs) will be important for new denture wearers.
◆ Denture care will be discussed in more detail in the next section.

III. Denture Cleaning

A. Purpose

◆ Prevent prosthesis-related OMLs such as traumatic ulcers, hyperplasia, angular cheilitis, and denture stomatitis.[18,21]

◆ Reduce levels of dental biofilm, bacteria, and fungi.[21]

◆ Prevent halitosis (oral malodor).

◆ Maintain appearance of the denture.

B. Denture Care Recommendations[21]

The recommendations for the patient self-care of the complete denture are essentially the same as for RPDs, so refer back to that section for additional detail.

◆ Thoroughly remove dental biofilm on the oral tissues with a soft toothbrush and complete denture with a denture brush daily.

  • Ideally the patient should clean (or at least rinse) the denture after meals to remove loose food debris.

  • At least once a day a soft toothbrush with end-rounded filaments should be applied lightly over the ridges and in the vestibules using long, straight strokes from posterior to anterior to remove debris and biofilm.

  • Clean the tongue daily.

◆ A nonabrasive denture cleanser is used only when the denture is not in the mouth.

◆ Thoroughly rinse to remove denture cleanser prior to reinsertion in the mouth.

  • Residual chemical agents, such as essential oils, may cause inflammatory or allergic reactions of the oral mucosa, and phenolic agents can have deleterious effects on plastic resin.

◆ Soaking the denture in a denture cleanser when not in the mouth may reduce bacterial levels and dental biofilm.

  • Denture cleansers have a variety of active ingredients, for example, peroxide, enzymes, and hypochlorite.

  • Recommend products shown to be safe and effective for denture use by looking for the American Dental Association Seal of Acceptance.

  • The patient should follow manufacturer's instructions.

◆ Recommend the patient remove the denture and leave it out overnight or for another extended period during the day as those who wear them continually have a greater risk of *Candida*-related denture stomatitis.[18,21]

◆ When the denture is not in the mouth, it should be stored in water.

◆ Those wearing upper and lower dentures need an annual dental examination to assess the oral tissues and the prosthesis.[21]

C. Denture Adhesives

◆ Benefits of denture adhesives[21]:

  • Patients may feel denture adhesives improve the stability, retention of a denture along with overall quality of life.

◆ An adhesive may be necessary for the new denture patient as the immediate, interim denture begins to loosen with healing of the underlying tissues.

◆ However, use of dental adhesives longer than 6 months have not been conducted so extended use is not recommended.[21]

  • The patient needs regular evaluation to determine the need for possible reline or rebase of the denture. In some cases, a new denture may be indicated.

◆ The practitioner needs to provide education on the use of a denture adhesive and include the following[21]:

  • Clean and dry the surface where the denture adhesive will be applied.

  • Use only three or four pea-sized dollops of denture-adhesive cream on each denture.

  • For power denture adhesives, dampen denture surface and apply a thin film to the entire surface and shake off the excess.

  • If using pad adhesives, adapt the size to the surface to be placed against the tissue.

  • Avoid zinc-containing adhesives due to adverse side effects.

  • Once the adhesive is applied, seat the denture and hold firmly in place for 5–10 seconds.

  • Bite firmly to spread the adhesive.

  • It is not recommended dentures be worn continuously (24 hours/day) because of risk for denture stomatitis.

  • Denture adhesives need to be thoroughly removed from the prosthesis and oral tissues daily.

D. Reline or Rebase of Denture[4]

◆ A reline of a denture is used to resurface the base material of the tissue side of the denture to provide an improve fit and retention.

◆ A rebase of the denture is done by a dental laboratory and is replacement of the entire denture resin base material and resetting of the denture teeth.

DENTURE-INDUCED ORAL MUCOSAL LESIONS (OMLs)

Regular intraoral examination of the oral cavity and evaluation of the denture will help to identify and manage denture-induced oral lesions.[26]

◆ Education of the patient is essential as a majority of those with dentures think they no longer need to have regular dental visits.

I. Contributing Factors for Denture-Induced OMLs

The factors causing OMLs under dentures are complex. The literature suggests the following:

◆ Ill-fitting dentures[26]

  • Food particles become lodged under an ill-fitting denture and may irritate the soft tissues and provide an environment for growth of microorganisms.

A—Ill-fitting, unstable RPD with retained calculus is contributing to gingival inflammation and increased risk for oral trauma.

P—RPD placed in sealed bag with cleaning solution and placed in a beaker filled in the ultrasonic unit to remove calculus; upon subsequent visual inspection, all calculus was removed and there were no fractures or roughness noted. Advised patient to clean RPD daily, and remove nightly to rest the underlying mucosa. Reminded her to keep the denture soaking in water when it is out of her mouth during the night. Proper technique for denture cleaning was demonstrated and practiced by the patient. Dispensed new denture toothbrush and clasp brush and advised patient to purchase American Dental Association–recommended denture cleanser.

Next steps: Schedule with dentist for RPD evaluation to determine possible reline or replacement.

Signed: _____, RDH

Date: _____

Factors to Teach the Patient

▶ How to perform self-examination of the oral tissues.

▶ Dentures may need to be replaced periodically as the bone and tissue under the denture change.

▶ The importance of careful removal of dental biofilm from the prosthesis on a regular basis to prevent tissue inflammation and possible *Candida* infection.

▶ The need for careful oral self-care of abutment teeth whether natural tooth or implant.

▶ How tongue cleaning contributes to complete oral health.

▶ The significance of regular maintenance appointments: intraoral/extraoral screening for pathology, especially oral cancer screening; professional cleaning of remaining teeth and prostheses; and prosthesis evaluation and adjustments as needed.

▶ The importance of seeking professional evaluation if any problems arise with existing prostheses; never attempt to repair or adjust a prosthesis.

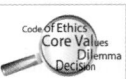

EVERYDAY ETHICS

Mr. Samuel wears an old maxillary complete denture that he has had for almost 30 years. He admits the denture moves around a bit and is sometimes difficult to chew with, but he refuses to have it remade because the removable lower partial denture he finally agreed to have remade last year was so expensive.

Bryce, a very caring dental hygienist who always tries to be sensitive to the financial concerns of his patients, decides to stop bothering Mr. Samuels about getting a new denture. He recommends an over-the-counter temporary soft reline material and the use of denture adhesive every day instead.

Questions for Consideration

1. What legal and ethical concepts are apparent in this scenario?

2. If he was asked, Bryce might say that his recommendations for this patient are supported by the core value of beneficence and that his personal values include helping Mr. Samuels keep the cost of his dental care low in any way he can. Do you agree or disagree? Explain why.

3. Explain how additional core values support a different approach to making recommendations.

ENHANCE YOUR UNDERSTANDING

ONLINE RESOURCES
(see the inside front cover for access information)

• Audio glossary

• Appendices

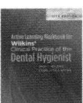

SUPPORT FOR LEARNING
(available separately)

• *Active Learning Workbook for Wilkins' Clinical Practice of the Dental Hygienist, 13th Edition*

INDIVIDUALIZED REVIEW

• Customized practice quizzing with Navigate 2 TestPrep for *Wilkins' Clinical Practice of the Dental Hygienist*

References

1. Tealdo T, Menini M, Bevilacqua M, et al. Immediate versus delayed loading of dental implants in edentulous patients' maxillae: a 6-year prospective study. *Int J Prosthodont.* 2014;27(3):207-214.

2. Mosnegutu A, Wismeijer D, Geraets W. Implant-supported mandibular overdentures can minimize mandibular bone resorption in edentulous patients: results of a long-term radiologic evaluation. *Int J Oral Maxillofac Implants.* 2015;30(6):1378-1386.

3. Yunus N, Masood M, Saub R, Al-Hashedi AA, Taiyeb Ali TB, Thomason JM. Impact of mandibular implant prostheses on the oral health-related quality of life in partially and completely edentulous patients. *Clin Oral Implants Res.* 2016;27(7):904-909.

4. Academy of Prosthodontics Foundation. The glossary of prosthodontic terms: ninth edition. *J Prosthet Dent.* 2017;117(5S):e1-e105.

5. Van Waas MA, Jonkman RE, Kalk W, Van 't Hof MA, Plooij J, Van Os JH. Differences two years after tooth extraction in mandibular bone reduction in patients treated with immediate overdentures or with immediate complete dentures. *J Dent Res.* 1993;72(6):1001-1004.

6. Ettinger RL, Qian F. Longitudinal assessment of denture maintenance needs in an overdenture population. *J Prosthodont.* 2019;28(1):22-29

7. Ettinger RL. Tooth loss in an overdenture population. *J Prosthet Dent.* 1988;60(4):459-62.

8. Zhang Q, Jin X, Yu M, et al. Economic evaluation of implant-supported overdentures in edentulous patients: a systematic review. *Int J Prosthodont.* 2017;30(4):321-326.

9. Raghoebar GM, Meijer HJ, Slot W, Slater JJ, Vissink A. A systematic review of implant-supported overdentures in the edentulous maxilla, compared to the mandible: how many implants? *Eur J Oral Implantol.* 2014;7(suppl 2): S191-S201.

10. Carlsson GE. Implant and root supported overdentures—a literature review and some data on bone loss in edentulous jaws. *J Adv Prosthodontics.* 2014;6(4):245-252.

11. Blanco GF, Madeo MC, Vázquez ME, Martínez M. Case for diagnosis. Palate perforation due to cocaine use. *An Bras Dermatol.* 2017;92(6):877-878.

12. Datta P, Sood S. The various methods and benefits of denture labeling. *J Forensic Dent Sci.* 2010;2(2):53-58.

13. Bathala LR, Rachuri NK, Rayapati SR, Kondaka S. Prosthodontics an "arsenal" in forensic dentistry. *J Forensic Dent Sci.* 2016;8(3):173.

14. Bidra AS, Daubert DM, Garcia LT, et al. Clinical practice guidelines for recall and maintenance of patients with tooth-borne and implant-borne dental restorations. *J Prosthodont.* 2016;25(suppl 1):S32-S40.

15. Tan K, Pjetursson BE, Lang NP, Chan ES. A systematic review of the survival and complication rates of fixed partial dentures (FPDs) after an observation period of at least 5 years. *Clin Oral Implants Res.* 2004;15(6):654-666.

16. Szalewski L, Pietryka-Michalowska E, Szymansky J. Oral hygiene in patients using removable dentures. *Polish J Public Health.* 2017;127(1):28-31.

17. O'Donnell LE, Robertson D, Nile CJ, et al. The oral microbiome of denture wearers is influenced by levels of natural dentition. *PLoS One.* 2015;10(9):e0137717.

18. Ercalik-Yalcinkaya S, Ozcan M. Association between oral mucosal lesions and hygiene habits in a population of removable prosthesis wearers. *J Prosthodont.* 2015;24(4):271-278.

19. Cakan U, Yuzbasioglu E, Kurt H, et al. Assessment of hygiene habits and attitudes among removable partial denture wearers in a university hospital. *Niger J Clin Pract.* 2015;18(4):511-515.

20. American Dental Association. Healthy Mouth: removable partial dentures. Available from https://www.mouthhealthy .org/en/az-topics/d/dentures-partial. Accessed June 3, 2018.

21. American College of Prosthodontists. Dentures FAQs. Available from https://www.gotoapro.org/dentures-faq/#445. Accessed June 2, 2018.

22. Felton D, Cooper L, Duqum I, et al. Evidence-based guidelines for the care and maintenance of complete dentures: a publication of the American College of Prosthodontists. *J Prosthodont.* 2011;20(suppl 1):S1-S12.

23. Matsumura K, Sato Y, Kitagawa N, Shichita T, Kawata D, Ishikawa M. Influence of denture surface roughness and host factors on dental calculi formation on dentures: a cross-sectional study. *BMC Oral Health.* 2018;18(1):78.

24. Roumanas ED. The social solution-denture esthetics, phonetics, and function. *J Prosthodont.* 2009;18(2):112-115.

25. Shigli K. Aftercare of the complete denture patient. *J Prosthodont.* 2009;18(8):688-693.

26. Mubarak S, Hmud A, Chandrasekharan S, Ali AA. Prevalence of denture-related oral lesions among patients attending College of Dentistry, University of Dammam: a clinico-pathological study. *J Int Soc Prev Community Dent.* 2015;5(6):506-512.

27. Gendreau L, Loewy ZG. Epidemiology and etiology of denture stomatitis. *J Prosthodont.* 2011;20(4):251-260.

28. Gleiznys A, Zdanavi ien E, Žilinskas J. *Candida albicans* importance to denture wearers. A literature review. *Stomatologija.* 2015;17(2):54-66.

The Patient with Dental Implants

Carol Tran, PhD, BOH, and Linda D. Boyd, RDH, RD, EdD

CHAPTER OUTLINE

BONE PHYSIOLOGY
I. Bone Classification
II. Biomechanical Force
III. Grafting and Regeneration

OSSEOINTEGRATION

IMPLANT INTERFACES
I. Implant–Bone Interface
II. Implant–Soft-Tissue Interface

TYPES OF DENTAL IMPLANTS
I. Subperiosteal
II. Transosseous (Transosteal)
III. Endosseous (Endosteal) Implant

PATIENT SELECTION
I. Systemic Health
II. Local Factors

EVALUATION FOR IMPLANT PLACEMENT

POST-RESTORATIVE EVALUATION

PERI-IMPLANT PREVENTIVE CARE
I. Care of the Natural Teeth
II. Implant Biofilm
III. Planning the Disease Control Program
IV. Maintenance of Implant-Supported Restorations
V. Antimicrobial Use
VI. Fluoride Measures for Dental Caries Control

CONTINUING CARE
I. Basic Criteria for Implant Success
II. Frequency of Appointments
III. The Continuing Care Appointment

CLASSIFICATION OF PERI-IMPLANT DISEASE
I. Peri-Implant Mucositis
II. Peri-Implantitis

DOCUMENTATION

EVERYDAY ETHICS

FACTORS TO TEACH THE PATIENT

REFERENCES

LEARNING OBJECTIVES

After studying this chapter, the student will be able to:

1. Describe the concepts, technology, and terminology relevant to implant dentistry.

2. Develop a knowledge base related to osseointegration and ancillary procedures in oral implantology.

3. Comprehend patient selection factors and education essentials.

4. Understand maintenance of dental implant in the clinical setting.

5. Recognize and manage dental implant problems, complications, and failures.

Dental implants offer a means of tooth replacement to preserve surrounding oral tissues normally compromised by a missing tooth.

◆ Dental implants simulate natural tooth roots.
  • Dental implants may replace one tooth or multiple teeth for a partially or completely edentulous patient.
◆ Knowledge of dental implants is essential for all dental hygienists who are responsible for professional maintenance and monitoring of peri-implant health.
◆ Patients often have questions and/or concerns for the dental hygienist regarding their treatment options, which presents an opportune time for education to dispel confusion, alleviate fears, or reinforce a decision to proceed with needed treatment.
◆ The success of a dental implant can depend on many factors, including patient understanding and skills for daily care of the prosthesis and the surrounding soft tissues.
◆ Frequent maintenance appointments for careful supervision and patient motivation are essential components of implant success.

BONE PHYSIOLOGY

Alveolar bone is of critical importance to the planning and execution of dental implants. A careful assessment of the quantity and quality of bone provides a foundation for proper treatment planning and a more predictable surgical outcome.
◆ Bone is a dynamic tissue that is cellular and vascular.
  • Osteocytes: mediate activity.
  • Osteoblasts: repair and regeneration.
  • Osteoclasts: remodeling and homeostasis.
◆ Key function: to provide structural support to various loads or stresses.

I. Bone Classification

◆ Bone is classified according to its density as follows[1]:
  • D1   dense cortical bone.
  • D2   thick dense to porous cortical bone on crest and coarse trabecular bone within.
  • D3   thin, porous cortical bone on crest and fine trabecular bone within.
  • D4   fine trabecular bone.
  • D5   immature, nonmineralized bone.
◆ The density of bone in a potential implant site determines factors such as:
  • Time frame for integration of the implant.
  • Window of time for prosthetic loading.

II. Biomechanical Force

◆ Wolff's law (1892) states bone is laid down in areas of greatest stress and is resorbed in areas where it is not stressed.[2]
◆ The patient needs to understand the implication of biomechanical force on the alveolar process.[2]
  • Bone will resorb when teeth are removed and mechanical stress is no longer applied to the bone.
  • Dental implants *preserve* surrounding bone through function, which supplies the needed load and stress.

III. Grafting and Regeneration

◆ Areas of insufficient bone due to previous resorption or tooth loss can be grafted to create a suitable recipient site for dental implant placement.
◆ Site preparation measures for implant therapy include:
  • Atraumatic extraction with ridge and/or socket preservation.
  • Ridge augmentation.[3]
  • Maxillary sinus augmentation is also called a "sinus lift."[4]
◆ Options for grafting and regeneration of recipient sites include[3]:
  • *Autograft*: bone obtained from the patient, harvested from a donor site.
  • *Allograft*: bone obtained from another human (cadaver bone).
  • *Xenograft*: bone obtained from another species (cow/bovine; horse/equine).
  • *Alloplast*: synthetic derivative of bone (e.g., beta-tricalcium phosphate).

OSSEOINTEGRATION

Successful tooth replacement is accomplished by osseointegration, which means direct bone anchorage to an implant body. When viewed at a light microscopic level, osseointegration reveals direct contact between bone and implant with no intervening connective tissue. The process of osseointegration is a dynamic process and includes the following stages[5]:
◆ Initial healing stage takes place up to 1 year.
◆ Second stage when bone actively remodels and may take up to 5 years.
◆ Third stage includes fewer osteocytes and less bone remodeling.

IMPLANT INTERFACES

An implant has an inner interface with the *bone* and a *soft-tissue* interface where the abutment, post, or other protruding portion of the implant is surrounded by the mucosal or gingival tissue.

I. Implant–Bone Interface

A. Osseointegration

◆ Refers to direct structural and functional union between the implant and healthy living bone.
◆ Indicates successful placement of the implant.
◆ No mobility evident.

B. Fibrous Encapsulation

◆ Fibrous encapsulation refers to the infusion of connective tissue cells between the implant body and surrounding bone.
◆ Indicates failure of osseointegration.
◆ Mobility of the implant is evident.

II. Implant–Soft-Tissue Interface

◆ The external environment of an implant is the oral cavity, with saliva, dental biofilm, and debris.

◆ Biologic seal (permucosal seal): Between the implant and the soft tissue, a biologic seal exists to prevent microorganisms and inflammation-producing agents from entering the tissues.

  • The peri-implant junction is similar to the junctional epithelium (JE) in a natural tooth.[6]

◆ The biologic width around an implant is 3–4 mm, which is slightly longer than in a natural tooth (~2 mm).[6]

◆ Soft-tissue connection: Peri-implant sulcular epithelium is in contact with the implant surface.[6]

  • The peri-implant epithelium (PIE) performs a similar function to the JE of a natural tooth.

  • Hemidesmosomes and basal lamina connect the PIE cells to the titanium of the implant much like JE cells connect to natural teeth.

  • The PIE attachment is weaker than the JE–tooth interface.

  • The long JE of an implant parallel to the implant, surrounding it, but with no attachment creating a cuff of tissue.

  • No connective tissue fibers (Sharpey's fibers) exist to hold the attachment as with a natural tooth.

  • Normal periodontal tissue has a blood supply from both alveolar bone and the periodontal ligament (PDL); however, the peri-implant tissue has no PDL, resulting a reduced blood supply.

  • The reduced blood supply and weaker PIE–titanium interface reduces resistance to bacterial invasion and to penetration of the periodontal probe during probing.[7,8]

  • Figure 31-1 illustrates the implant–soft tissue interface at the peri-implant epithelium.

TYPES OF DENTAL IMPLANTS

Over the years, a variety of dental implant systems have been tried clinically and studied with research.[9] They are subperiosteal, transosseous, and endosseous. Currently, endosseous or "root form" implants are the most widely used.

I. Subperiosteal

A. Definition

◆ Custom-fabricated framework of metal that rests over the bone of the mandible or maxilla, under the periosteum. Indicated under the following conditions[10]:

  • A removable denture cannot be retained because of lack of bone.

  • There is inadequate alveolar bone for endosseous implants.

B. Description[10]

◆ Material: titanium or Vitallium (cobalt–chromium–molybdenum).

◆ Two step: In the first step, a surgical flap is used to reflect mucosal tissues and to expose the underlying bone. An

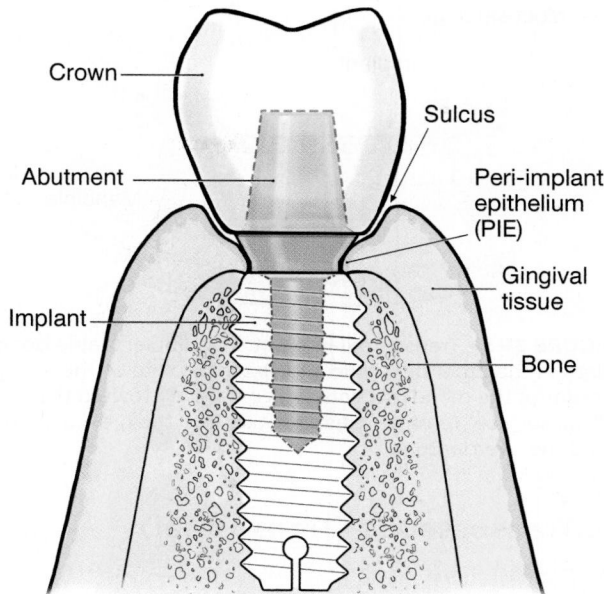

FIGURE 31-1 • The Implant–Soft-Tissue Interface. At the implant–soft-tissue interface, there can be no connective tissue fiber attachment as when bone is present. The peri-implant epithelium (PIE) attachment resembles a long junctional epithelial attachment.

impression is made of the bony ridge. The metallic unit is cast and then placed in a second surgical step. Usually, four posts protrude into the oral cavity to hold the complete denture.

◆ One step: Computer-assisted tomography design and manufacturing have been applied, using a reformatted computed tomography scan from which approximate casts of the maxilla or mandible can be made. The implant is designed on this replica and is placed in one surgical procedure (Figure 31-2).

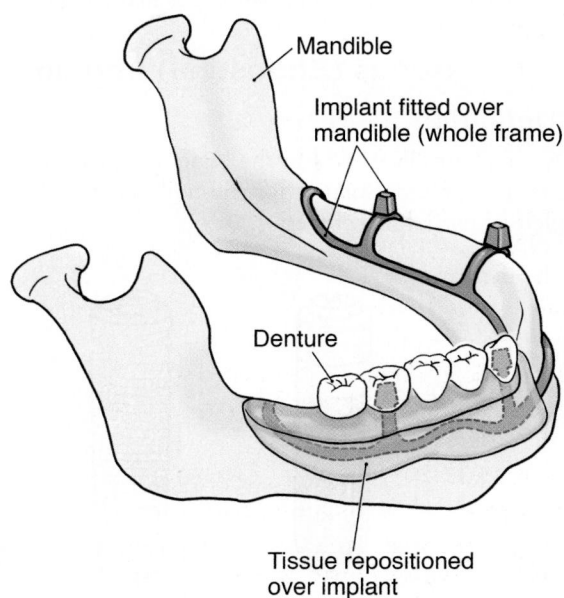

FIGURE 31-2 • Subperiosteal Implant. The custom-fabricated framework is shown on the left-hand side of the mandible; on the right-hand side, the framework is shown by dotted lines under the denture.

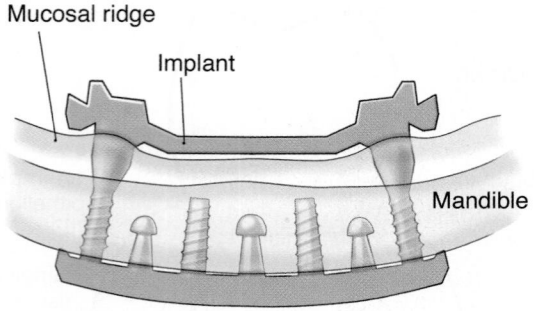

FIGURE 31-3 • Transosteal Implant. Mandibular staple bone plate in the anterior region shows metal plate at the lower border of the mandible, with pins extending toward the occlusal surface. Terminal pins protrude into the oral cavity to hold the overdenture.

II. Transosseous (Transosteal)

A. Definition

◆ A dental implant that penetrates both cortical plates and passes through the full thickness of the alveolar bone.

◆ Also known as a *mandibular staple implant* or *staple bone implant*.

B. Description[11]

◆ Materials: stainless steel, ceramic-coated materials, and titanium alloy.

◆ A metal plate, fitted to the inferior border of the mandible, has five to seven pins extending toward the occlusal surface.

◆ Usually, two terminal pins protrude into the oral cavity to hold the overdenture. The pins are connected by a crossbar (Figure 31-3).

◆ The transosteal implant can be used when the patient has an edentulous mandible with little mandibular bone.

III. Endosseous (Endosteal) Implant

A. Definition

◆ An implant placed within the bone to replace a single tooth or provide support for the replacement of complete or partial loss of teeth.

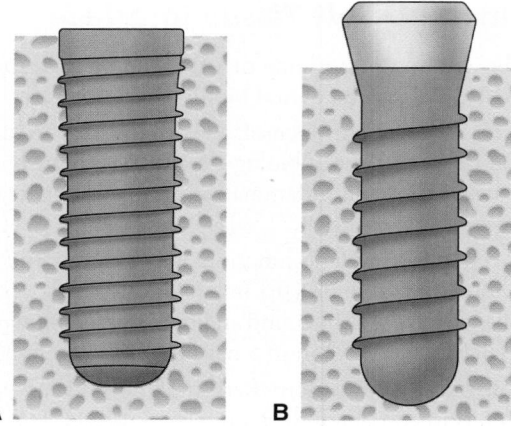

FIGURE 31-5 • Endosseous Implant Types. A: Bone level. **B:** Tissue level.

◆ Early forms (endosteal): blade or plate form.

◆ Current forms (endosseous): "root form" or cylindrical; can be threaded, smooth, perforated, or solid (Figure 31-4).[12]

◆ The endosseous implant may be placed so it emerges into the oral cavity at the bone level or tissue level (see Figure 31-5).

B. Description

◆ Material: primarily sandblasted and acid-etched titanium or titanium alloy (Ti-6Al-4V).

◆ May be placed in one or two phases[13]:
  • Immediate implant placement: The implant is placed immediately following extraction of the tooth. This approach has a lower survival rate versus a two-phase delayed implant approach.
  • Two-phase implant placement: after tooth extraction, the site is allowed to heal prior to placement of the implant fixture and left covered by a periodontal flap for several months while the implant integrates with the bone. In a second stage of the surgical procedure, the abutment post is exposed. Placement of the crown or prosthesis follows.

◆ Figure 31-6 illustrates the parts of an endosseous implant and the surrounding biologic tissues.

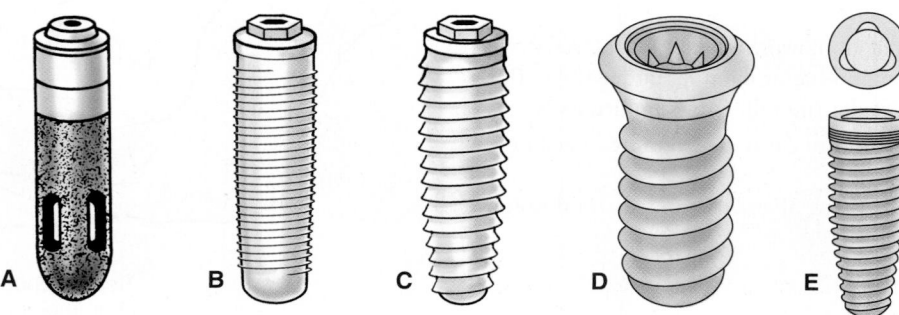

FIGURE 31-4 • Endosseous Root Form Implants. A: Cylinder type. **B and C:** Screw types (external hex). **D:** Screw type, tissue level, internal hex. **E:** Screw type, bone level, internal hex.

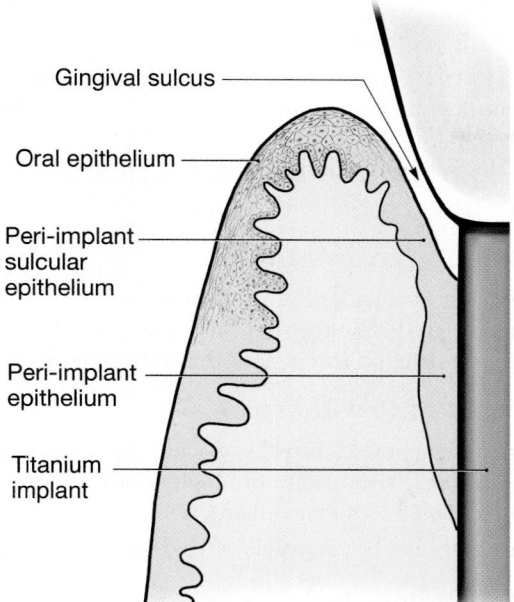

FIGURE 31-6 • Parts of an Endosseous Implant. The crown, abutment, and implant are shown in relation to the surrounding bone and soft tissues.

Labels in figure:
- Gingival sulcus
- Oral epithelium
- Peri-implant sulcular epithelium
- Peri-implant epithelium
- Titanium implant

PATIENT SELECTION

Patient selection depends on key factors that may impact osseointegration of the dental implant and success of treatment. These factors include primarily systemic health, condition of the jaws, and other local factors.[14]

I. Systemic Health

◆ *Medical history*: Careful review of the medical history and conditions is crucial to implant survival. Following are the conditions that most likely impact dental implant success[14]:
  • Tobacco may adversely affect wound healing, and jeopardize the success of dental implants and bone health.[15] Tobacco cessation should be addressed (see Chapter 32).
  • Alcohol abuse use may cause changes in alveolar bone healing impacting osseointegration and may result in implant failure.
  • Poorly controlled diabetes mellitus impacts osseointegration and increases risk for peri-implantitis and implant failure.[16]
  • Osteoporosis may have some impact on bone healing and osseointegration, but of greater concern is the bisphosphonate medication that patients may be taking to treat osteoporosis.
  • Patients using anticoagulant medications require consultation with the primary care provider to evaluate suitability for a dental implant.
  • Immunosuppressant therapy may also negatively impact healing.

◆ *Absolute contraindications*: There are a few conditions in which dental implants are not recommended which include[14]:
  • Liver disease.
  • Renal disease such as renal insufficiency and uremia.
  • Endocrine disorders such as hyperthyroidism and hypopituitarism.
  • Connective tissue disease and autoimmune diseases, such as lupus, that impact connective tissue.
  • Blood disorders.
  • High-dose radiotherapy.

II. Local Factors

Local factors include history and presence of oral disease along with status of oral soft and hard tissue in the area for the dental implant.[14]
◆ Periodontal disease
  • Presence of periodontal pathogens is a risk factor for development of peri-implantitis.
◆ Patient's dedication and ability to maintaining a high level of oral self-care.
◆ Soft-tissue architecture, that is, tissue height and adequate attached gingiva.
◆ Architecture of the implant site, including bone volume, soft tissue, and surrounding teeth, that is, root proximity.

EVALUATION FOR IMPLANT PLACEMENT

Implant therapy typically requires collaboration of a team, which may include the dentist or specialist placing the implant, general dentist or prosthodontist restoring the implant, dental hygienist, dental laboratory technician, and patient. Prior to placement, the following need to be evaluated[17]:
◆ Medical and psychological evaluation.
◆ Comprehensive dental examination.
  • Periodontal and restorative status of all teeth.
◆ Assessment of patient expectations of outcomes.
◆ Patient motivation and oral self-care abilities.
◆ Habits or conditions placing the patient at risk for implant failure, such as alcohol abuse, periodontal disease.
◆ Preparation of diagnostic aids:
  • Diagnostic models or casts.
  • Imaging.
  • Surgical template or computer-guided implant placement.

POST-RESTORATIVE EVALUATION

Once the implant is fully integrated in the bone and restorative work is complete, a post-restorative evaluation is made to establish a baseline for maintenance. Periodic evaluation of the implant includes the following[17]:

- *Radiographic* appearance of implant and surrounding alveolar bone.
- *Occlusal* evaluation including assessment of mobility.
- *Peri-implant tissue health*: no inflammation, no calculus or biofilm, and no suppuration or bleeding.
- *Peri-implant probing*: initial data serve as baseline for comparison during the maintenance phase.[18]
  - Although somewhat controversial, the seventh European Workshop of Periodontology consensus report and 2017 World Workshop on the Classification of Periodontal and Peri-Implant Diseases and Conditions indicates probing of implants is *necessary to detect peri-implant health*.[18,19]
  - Use very light pressure or force to gently probe (approximately 0.25 N) the implant. Remember the PIE–titanium interface is weaker and less resistant to bacterial invasion and penetration of the periodontal probe.[7]
  - Peri-implant pocket depths should be less than 5 mm and may not indicate pathology in the absence of bleeding or suppuration.[8,19]
  - Record presence of bleeding on probing and suppuration.
- *Sufficiency of patient's oral self-care.*
- *Patient comfort.*

PERI-IMPLANT PREVENTIVE CARE

A key requirement for implant success is the disease control program for the tissue surrounding the implant. Failure of dental implants is associated with increased plaque biofilm accumulation, so meticulous daily oral self-care is essential for implant success.[20,21]

I. Care of the Natural Teeth

- Periodontal disease is a risk factor for peri-implantitis and implant failure and must be controlled.[22,23]
- Before placement of the implants, the periodontal condition of surrounding natural teeth needs to be treated and maintained.
- After the placement of the implants, the maintenance program emphasizes care of the natural teeth and tissues as well as the peri-implant tissues.[21]

II. Implant Biofilm

- Although the biofilm formation process on implant surfaces is similar to that of teeth, the characteristics of the implant surface may also impact the amount and composition of the biofilm.[23]
- The oral microbiome of an implant may be more diverse when compared to natural teeth and continues to be studied.[24]

- The development of peri-implant disease is closely related to the host response to the microbiome composition.
  - Host response is impacted by diet, smoking, environmental factors, and the patient's general status.[23]

III. Planning the Disease Control Program

A. Relation to Treatment

Supervision of a patient's oral hygiene and oral self-care regimen begins before the surgical phase for implant placement and carries on throughout the treatment phases.

B. Types of Prostheses

- Implant-supported prostheses may be partial, complete, fixed, removable, or single-tooth replacements (see Chapter 30 for care instructions).
- Prostheses may be removable or fixed (cemented in place).

C. Monitoring Prostheses Fit

- Regular dental examinations are recommended to monitor implant-supported restorations and prostheses and adjust or repair as needed.[21]
- Instruct and demonstrate to the patient how to monitor the fit of the implant prosthesis.

IV. Maintenance of Implant-Supported Restorations

- Regular professional maintenance is required. Guidelines suggest at least a 6-month interval, but this may need to be more frequent dependent upon the patient's needs.[21]
- Each patient needs an individualized plan to effectively manage dental biofilm.
- Choose instruments and oral self-care aids compatible with the material and type of implant.
- *Toothbrushes*
  - Select either a manual or a powered toothbrush with smooth, soft, and end-rounded filaments to prevent damage to the titanium and peri-implant tissue.
- *Interdental care*
  - Interdental brushes with nylon-coated wires work well to clean embrasure spaces and areas around implant-supported restorations (see Chapter 27).
  - A floss threader can be used to position yarn or dental floss around an abutment and under a fixed prosthesis (see Chapter 30).
  - Clinical practice guidelines from the American College of Prosthodontists also suggest the option of a water flosser or air flosser.[20] However, the research on use of the water flosser is industry-supported, which introduces the chance of bias so further independent research is needed.[25]
  - The end tufted brush with soft filaments is used on distal surfaces of terminal teeth or in lingual and palatal embrasure spaces (see Chapter 27).

V. Antimicrobial Use

A. Toothpaste

◆ Research suggests a dentifrice with 0.3% triclosan was effective in improving microbial and periodontal parameters.[20,21]

B. Mouthwash

◆ Use of chlorhexidine gluconate is recommended as needed to manage inflammation of soft tissues around implants.[20,21]

◆ However, irrigation with chlorhexidine was more effective at reducing biofilm and reducing bleeding than use as a mouthwash.[26]

◆ Essential oil mouthrinse such as Listerine as an adjunct to mechanical biofilm removal resulted in reductions in plaque and marginal peri-implant bleeding.[26]

VI. Fluoride Measures for Dental Caries Control

◆ Patients with natural teeth and multiple or complex restorations should be advised to use a prescription fluoride such as a 5000-ppm sodium fluoride gel or toothpaste.[21]

◆ Avoid acidulated fluoride preparations due to possible effects on the implant surface.

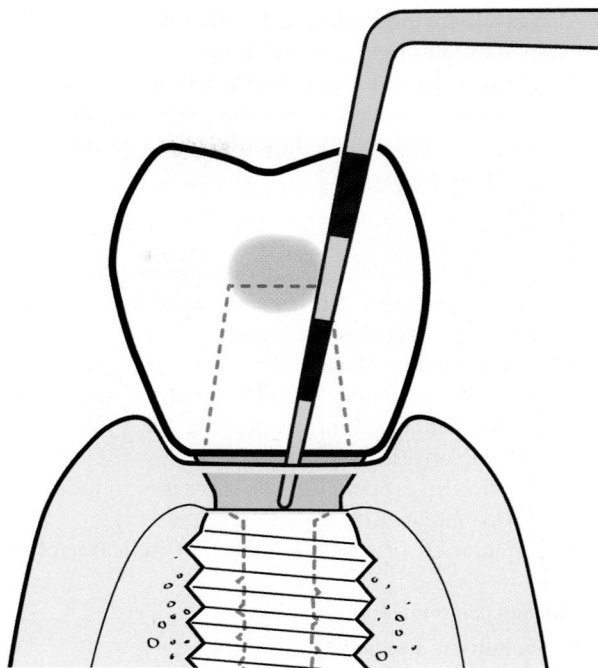

FIGURE 31-7 • Probing an Implant. Using a plastic probe, probe with gentle pressure to assess pocket depth and bleeding on probing.

CONTINUING CARE

Periodic care for professional maintenance and monitoring is scheduled according to the complexity of the restoration or prosthetic superstructure and the patient's ability to perform adequate oral self-care.[21]

I. Basic Criteria for Implant Success

◆ The long-term success of an implant is assessed during dental examinations at least every 6 months.[21]

◆ A successful implant meets the following criteria[27]:
  • No visible inflammation, pink as opposed to red, no tissue swelling, tissues appear to be firm compared to soft and loose.[19]
  • No pain or tenderness reported by the patient.
  • No mobility.
  • Radiograph: less than 2-mm radiographic bone loss from initial surgery.[19]
  • No bleeding, suppuration or increased depths beyond baseline on gentle probing with a plastic probe (Figure 31-7).
  • No movement or loose components in the prosthesis; check for cracks, fractures, missing, or unsecured screws by close visual inspection while applying coronally directed force to superstructure using a rigid single-ended instrument such as a mirror handle.

II. Frequency of Appointments

◆ When the original teeth were lost due to inadequate daily biofilm control by the patient, a more intense program of education and monitoring may be needed.

◆ Professional maintenance at least every 6 months based on individual needs is recommended.[21]

III. The Continuing Care Appointment

Once osseointegration has been achieved, maintenance of the soft tissues to prevent peri-implantitis is essential to minimize risk for implant failure.[17,20,21,26,28]

A. Health History Review, Vital Signs, and Intraoral/Extraoral Examination

◆ Basic review questions can reveal the present state of health, recent illnesses, changes in medications, and other current information.

◆ Comparisons with previous records permit assessment of vital signs and extraoral/intraoral observations.

B. Selective Radiographs

◆ A standardized procedure using a film placement device and a paralleling technique is recommended to allow comparison of marginal bone level changes from the original level.

◆ Remodeling of bone of 1.5 mm typically occurs in the first year and 0.2 mm annually thereafter.[8,27]

◆ Cone-beam computed tomography is gaining popularity to aid evaluation of the alveolar bone for implant placement.

C. Periodontal Assessment

◆ *Peri-implant tissue*: Visual examination to assess changes in color, size, shape, and consistency.

◆ *Dental biofilm*

- Use a disclosing solution to identify plaque biofilm and to aid in patient education.
- Utilize a plaque index to monitor biofilm to allow for comparison between maintenance appointments.[29]
- Assess biofilm accumulation patterns to aid in patient education.

◆ *Probing*
- A plastic probe is suggested.[29]
- Light pressure of 0.15–0.25 N is recommended.[7,18]
- Pressure-sensitive probes are available to guard against excess insertion pressure.
- Pocket depths should be compared with baseline measurements.[17] Probing depths more than 6 mm with bleeding on probing are indicators of peri-implantitis.[18-20,28]
- Bleeding on probing is recorded as it is an indication of peri-implantitis.[17-19,29]
- Suppuration or exudate is also an indicator of implant disease.[17-19,29]

◆ *Mobility determination*
- Mobility is assessed.[29]
- Inform the dentist and/or implant surgeon immediately of noticeable mobility.

◆ Recession
- Measure and document changes in location of the gingival margin in relation to the restoration margins.[29]

◆ *Calculus*
- Mineralized deposits usually are not extensive, hard, or firmly attached to implant abutments or other protruding parts.
- Semisoft, partially mineralized deposits can be effectively removed with floss or instruments designed for use on implants.

◆ *Residual cement*
- When the implant crown is permanently cemented to the abutment, residual cement is a significant risk factor for iatrogenic peri-implant disease.[28,30,31]
- Cement residue goes largely undetected on postrestorative radiographs.
- Be alert to clinical signs of inflammation, especially idiopathic change in an otherwise stable implant, since cement-associated peri-implantitis may not appear for many years following implant restoration.
- Typically cement cannot be removed with nonsurgical treatment, so these patients need to be referred back to the surgeon who placed the implant for further evaluation and treatment.[29]

D. Dental Biofilm Control

◆ Plaque biofilm control is essential for long-term implant success, so this must be continuously reinforced with the patient.[18,29]

◆ Review the patient's current oral self-care regimens and identify areas needing improvement based on plaque biofilm, pocket depth increases, and bleeding points.

◆ The patient should demonstrate oral self-care techniques and work with the clinician to refine techniques to improve effective biofilm removal.

E. Instrumentation

◆ *Biofilm removal*: Soft deposits are removed from the implant abutment with dental floss or implant instrument.
- Air polishing with glycine powder has been shown to be safe and effective in debriding the implant surface of plaque biofilm and is effective in treating sites of mucositis.[32]

◆ *Calculus removal*: Specialized implant-specific instruments typically made of plastic are indicated for hard deposits remaining after soft deposit removal.[29]
- Current implant-specific instruments mimic traditional universal curettes and sickle scalers in design.
- Implant-specific plastic-covered ultrasonic tips and inserts are available for peri-implant debridement. Use *low* power when instrumenting implant abutments with an ultrasonic device with tips designed to be safe around abutments.[29]

◆ *Stain removal*: Unless it is necessary for esthetics, stain removal is not included routinely.
- When selective stain removal with a rubber cup is indicated, only a nonabrasive agent is used and applied gently.
- Tin oxide or nonabrasive toothpaste may be suitable for polishing agents.

◆ *Professional subgingival irrigation*: The use of 0.12% chlorhexidine after professional instrumentation may be an alternative treatment when peri-implantitis has been identified. Irrigation with chlorhexidine gluconate has been shown to be a safe procedure around implants.[20,21,26]

CLASSIFICATION OF PERI-IMPLANT DISEASE

There are two basic peri-implant diseases: peri-implant mucositis and peri-implantitis.[19]

I. Peri-Implant Mucositis

Peri-implant mucositis is reversible. A recent meta-analysis found the prevalence of peri-implant mucositis to be approximately 30%.[34]

A. Diagnostic Criteria

The diagnostic criteria for peri-implant mucositis have not been universally agreed upon, but the most common signs include the following[18,33]:

◆ An inflammatory lesion in the mucosa similar to gingivitis.

◆ Bleeding and/or suppuration on gentle probing.

◆ An increase in probing depth (due to tissue inflammation and not bone loss).

◆ No bone loss has occurred.

B. Treatment

◆ Prevention and management of peri-implant mucositis includes patient compliance with meticulous plaque biofilm removal daily with either a manual toothbrush or a powered toothbrush and appropriate interdental aids. Regular reinforcement for oral self-care is an important part of managing peri-implant disease.

◆ Use of antimicrobial toothpaste.[21]

◆ Short-term daily 0.12% chlorhexidine gluconate mouthrinse for home use and chlorhexidine gel application in the dental office (if available in some countries).[21]

◆ Professional peri-implant debridement with appropriate hand instruments, that is, plastic scalers, and/or powered instruments such as a glycine polishing system.[20,32]

◆ Regular professional care may be required at short intervals such as 3–4 months to resolve the mucositis.[33]

II. Peri-Implantitis

The prevalence of peri-implantitis at the implant level varies in the literature from approximately 9%–13%.[35]

A. Diagnostic Criteria[18,19]

◆ Evidence of gingival inflammation in peri-implant tissues.

◆ Bleeding on gentle probing and exudate or suppuration is common.

◆ Increase in probing depths beyond baseline after implant healing, but probing depths more than 6 mm with bleeding on probing are at greater risk for progression of the peri-implantitis.

◆ Crestal bone loss on radiographs, and/or increasing probing depths compared to baseline.

◆ If no initial radiographs, or initial probing depths are available, greater than or equal to 6 mm and/or probing depths with bleeding.

B. Treatment

◆ Nonsurgical treatment[36]:
  • Plaque biofilm control daily by the patient is critical.
  • Professional debridement of plaque and calculus from the implant surface.
  • Adjunctive antimicrobials such as chlorhexidine may be used in conjunction with debridement.

◆ Surgical treatment[36]:
  • Guided bone regeneration.

◆ New treatment approaches include[36]:
  • Laser-assisted nonsurgical treatment using carbon dioxide and diode lasers to decontaminate the implant surface have shown some positive outcomes, but more research is recommended.
  • Photodynamic therapy has also shown positive results, but more research is needed.

DOCUMENTATION

The implant therapy team must collaborate when planning, treating, and maintaining an implant. For documenting appointments for a patient with a dental implant, the following factors are recorded in the progress note:

◆ Consultation before implant treatment plan:
  • Patient advised of all options to replace missing tooth/teeth.
  • Patient understands surgical, prosthetic, and maintenance phases of dental implant therapy.
  • Expected benefits, principal risks, and potential complications of dental implant therapy have been fully explained.
  • Alternatives to suggested dental implant treatment have been outlined.
  • The patient is ready to take responsibility for thorough daily oral self-care to manage plaque biofilm.

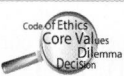

EVERYDAY ETHICS

Karen reviewed the permanent record progress notes before receiving Ms. Overly for her routine 4 months' continuing care. Dr. Richards had seen Ms. Overly within the week for an examination and radiograph of tooth #10 where a root canal had been placed 2 years ago and was giving her trouble. The endodontic therapy had failed and Dr. Richards had recorded that the tooth was now indicated for extraction.

While Karen was updating blood pressure and medical history, she noticed that her patient did not seem to be her usual talkative self. "I guess I have to have a bridge put in and *I am not happy* about it," Ms. Overly said.

Karen asked, "Have you discussed this with Dr. Richards?"

Ms. Overly replied, "To tell the truth I'm really confused. My brother asked me why I'm not getting an implant. Dr. Richards just said we need to do a bridge."

Questions for Consideration

1. What obligation does Karen have and what procedure does Karen need to follow in terms of assuring that Ms. Overly's treatment options have been fully presented and adequately explained and understood?

2. Is there an issue with societal trust in this incident? Which of the other dental hygiene core values are evident in this scenario?

3. With respect to core values and informed consent standards, role-play (1) additional conversation between Karen and Ms. Overly and (2) a dialogue that could ensue between Karen and Dr. Richards as Karen explains Ms. Overly's concerns about the treatment he has indicated for her.

- The need for ongoing professional maintenance appointments have been fully explained to patient.
- ◆ Examination as follows:
  - Verify dental implant locations with chart and current radiographs.
  - Peri-implant tissue tone, color, and texture.
  - Presence of inflammation: note erythema, edema, and/or exudate.
  - Probe implant with gentle pressure.
  - Assess implant mobility.
  - Take a radiograph if signs of peri-implant disease are present, and/or every 12 months to look for changes in bone level.
  - Prosthesis integrity and stability.
  - Note quantity and location of plaque biofilm and calculus accumulations.
- ◆ Carefully document continuing care procedures.
- ◆ An example of a progress note appears in Box 31-1.

Factors to Teach the Patient

- ▶ How dental implants preserve and maintain surrounding bone.
- ▶ How to care for implants; special needs related to the titanium surfaces.
- ▶ How the health of the periodontal tissues and the duration of the implants and prostheses depend on meticulous daily self-care by the patient.
- ▶ The role of biofilm in peri-implantitis.
- ▶ How a history of periodontitis may place a patient at increased risk for peri-implantitis.
- ▶ The complexity and dedication needed to maintain thorough daily oral self-care of complex restorations often associated with implant therapy.
- ▶ Why frequent, ongoing professional maintenance care and annual radiographs to document bone height around implants are necessary.
- ▶ When to call the office to address potential or suspected problems around an implant, for example, peri-implant bleeding, soreness, or pain.

ENHANCE YOUR UNDERSTANDING

ONLINE RESOURCES
(see the inside front cover for access information)

- Audio glossary
- Appendices

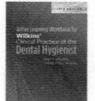

SUPPORT FOR LEARNING
(available separately)

- *Active Learning Workbook for Wilkins' Clinical Practice of the Dental Hygienist, 13th Edition*

INDIVIDUALIZED REVIEW

- Customized practice quizzing with Navigate 2 TestPrep for *Wilkins' Clinical Practice of the Dental Hygienist*

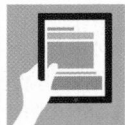

BOX 31-1
Example Documentation:
Patient with Implants

S—Patient presents for continuing care 3 months following final seating of implant prosthesis for tooth #3. No chief complaint or concerns.

O—Intraoral/extraoral examination within normal limits. Peri-implant soft tissue appears healthy with no bleeding. Biofilm score of less than 10%. One periapical radiograph within normal limits; no mobility evident of implant fixture or prosthesis; no biofilm or calculus accumulation on tooth #3.

A—Periapical implant appears healthy and well-integrated.

P—Treatment: Reinforce implant cleaning procedures with floss, periodontal debridement with implant safe instruments. Next: Three-month continuing care. Copy report to surgeon and general dentist.

Signed: _____, RDH

Date: _____

References

1. Misch DE. *Contemporary Implant Dentistry*. 3rd ed. St. Louis, MO: Mosby; 2008.
2. Huiskes R, Ruimerman R, Van Lenthe GH, Janssen JD. Effects of mechanical forces on maintenance and adaptation of form in trabecular bone. *Nature*. 2000;405(6787):704-706.
3. Milinkovic I, Cordaro L. Are there specific indications for the different alveolar bone augmentation procedures for implant placement? A systematic review. *Int J Oral Maxillofac Surg*. 2014;43(5):606-625.
4. Stern A, Green J. Sinus lift procedures: an overview of current techniques. *Dent Clin North Am*. 2012;56(1):219-233, x.
5. Insua A, Monje A, Wang HL, Miron RJ. Basis of bone metabolism around dental implants during osseointegration and peri-implant bone loss. *J Biomed Mater Res A*. 2017;105(7):2075-2089.
6. Atsuta I, Ayukawa Y, Kondo R, et al. Soft tissue sealing around dental implants based on histological interpretation. *J Prosthodont Res*. 2016;60(1):3-11.
7. Gerber JA, Tan WC, Balmer TE, Salvi GE, Lang NP. Bleeding on probing and pocket probing depth in relation to probing pressure and mucosal health around oral implants. *Clin Oral Implants Res*. 2009;20(1):75-78.
8. Coli P, Christiaens V, Sennerby L, Bruyn H. Reliability of periodontal diagnostic tools for monitoring peri-implant health and disease. *Periodontol 2000*. 2017;73(1):203-217.
9. Esposito M, Ardebili Y, Worthington HV. Interventions for replacing missing teeth: different types of dental implants. *Cochrane Database Syst Rev*. 2014(7):CD003815.
10. Homoly PA. The restorative and surgical technique for the full maxillary subperiosteal implant. *J Am Dent Assoc*. 1990;121(3):404-407.

11. Cranin AN, Sher J, Schilb TP. The transosteal implant: a 17-year review and report. *J Prosthet Dent.* 1986;55(6):709-718.

12. Niznick GA. Endosseous dental implant. Google Patents; 2006.

13. Mello CC, Lemos CAA, Verri FR, Dos Santos DM, Goiato MC, Pellizzer EP. Immediate implant placement into fresh extraction sockets versus delayed implants into healed sockets: a systematic review and meta-analysis. *Int J Oral Maxillofac Surg.* 2017;46(9):1162-1177.

14. Bryington M, De Kok IJ, Thalji G, Cooper LF. Patient selection and treatment planning for implant restorations. *Dent Clin North Am.* 2014;58(1):193-206.

15. Strietzel FP, Reichart PA, Kale A, Kulkarni M, Wegner B, Küchler I. Smoking interferes with the prognosis of dental implant treatment: a systematic review and meta-analysis. *J Clin Periodontol.* 2007;34(6):523-544.

16. Naujokat H, Kunzendorf B, Wiltfang J. Dental implants and diabetes mellitus: a systematic review. *Int J Implant Dent.* 2016;2(1):5.

17. Periodontology AAP. Parameter on placement and management of the dental implant. *J Periodontol.* 2000;71(5 suppl):870-872.

18. Lang NP, Berglundh T. Peri-implant diseases: where are we now?—Consensus of the Seventh European Workshop on Periodontology. *J Clin Periodontol.* 2011;38(suppl 11):178-181.

19. Renvert S, Persson GR, Pirih FQ, Camargo PM. Peri-implant health, peri-implant mucositis, and peri-implantitis: case definitions and diagnostic considerations. *J Periodontol.* 2018;89(suppl 1):S304-S312.

20. Bidra AS, Daubert DM, Garcia LT, et al. A systematic review of recall regimen and maintenance regimen of patients with dental restorations. Part 2: implant-borne restorations. *J Prosthodont.* 2016;25(suppl 1):S16-S31.

21. Bidra AS, Daubert DM, Garcia LT, et al. Clinical practice guidelines for recall and maintenance of patients with tooth-borne and implant-borne dental restorations. *J Am Dent Assoc.* 2016;147(1):67-74.

22. Sgolastra F, Petrucci A, Severino M, Gatto R, Monaco A. Periodontitis, implant loss and peri-implantitis. A meta-analysis. *Clin Oral Implants Res.* 2015;26(4):e8-16.

23. Stacchi C, Berton F, Perinetti G, et al. Risk factors for peri-implantitis: effect of history of periodontal disease and smoking habits. A systematic review and meta-analysis. *J Oral Maxillofac Res.* 2016;7(3):e3.

24. Pokrowiecki R, Mielczarek A, Zar ba T, Tyski S. Oral microbiome and peri-implant diseases: where are we now? *Ther Clin Risk Manag.* 2017;13:1529-1542.

25. Qaqish JG, Schuller R. Efficacy of two interdental cleaning devices on clinical signs of inflammation: a four-week randomized controlled trial. *J Clin Dent.* 2015;26:55-60.

26. Grusovin MG, Coulthard P, Worthington HV, George P, Esposito M. Interventions for replacing missing teeth: maintaining and recovering soft tissue health around dental implants. *Cochrane Database Syst Rev.* 2010(8):CD003069.

27. Misch CE, Perel ML, Wang HL, et al. Implant success, survival, and failure: the International Congress of Oral Implantologists (ICOI) Pisa Consensus Conference. *Implant Dent.* 2008;17(1):5-15.

28. Schwarz F, Derks J, Monje A, Wang HL. Peri-implantitis. *J Clin Periodontol.* 2018;45(suppl 20):S246-S266.

29. Todescan S, Lavigne S, Kelekis-Cholakis A. Guidance for the maintenance care of dental implants: clinical review. *J Can Dent Assoc.* 2012;78:c107.

30. Quaranta A, Lim ZW, Tang J, Perrotti V, Leichter J. The impact of residual subgingival cement on biological complications around dental implants: a systematic review. *Implant Dent.* 2017;26(3):465-474.

31. Staubli N, Walter C, Schmidt JC, Weiger R, Zitzmann NU. Excess cement and the risk of peri-implant disease—a systematic review. *Clin Oral Implants Res.* 2017;28(10):1278-1290.

32. Schwarz F, Becker K, Renvert S. Efficacy of air polishing for the non-surgical treatment of peri-implant diseases: a systematic review. *J Clin Periodontol.* 2015;42(10):951-959.

33. Jepsen S, Berglundh T, Genco R, et al. Primary prevention of peri-implantitis: managing peri-implant mucositis. *J Clin Periodontol.* 2015;42(suppl 16):S152-S157.

34. Lee C-T, Huang Y-W, Zhu L, Weltman R. Prevalences of peri-implantitis and peri-implant mucositis: systematic review and meta-analysis. *J Dent.* 2017;62:1-12.

35. Rakic M, Galindo-Moreno P, Monje A, et al. How frequent does peri-implantitis occur? A systematic review and meta-analysis. *Clin Oral Investig.* 2018;22(4):1805-1816.

36. Romanos GE, Javed F, Delgado-Ruiz RA, Calvo-Guirado JL. Peri-implant diseases: a review of treatment interventions. *Dent Clin North Am.* 2015;59(1):157-178.

32

The Patient with Nicotine Use Disorders

Lori Rainchuso, RDH, MS, DHSc

CHAPTER OUTLINE

HEALTH HAZARDS AND CURRENT TRENDS

COMPONENTS OF TOBACCO PRODUCTS AND TOBACCO SMOKE

METABOLISM OF NICOTINE
I. Nicotine from Smoking

ALTERNATIVE TOBACCO PRODUCTS
I. Smokeless Tobacco
II. Waterpipe Tobacco Smoking
III. Electronic Nicotine Delivery Systems

SYSTEMIC EFFECTS
I. Cardiovascular Diseases
II. Pulmonary Diseases
III. Cancer
IV. Tobacco and Use of Other Drugs

ENVIRONMENTAL TOBACCO SMOKE
I. Toxicity
II. Lung and Respiratory Effects
III. Cardiovascular Effects

PRENATAL AND CHILDREN
I. In Utero
II. Infancy
III. Young Children

ORAL MANIFESTATIONS OF TOBACCO AND NICOTINE USE

TOBACCO AND PERIODONTAL INFECTIONS
I. Effects on the Periodontal Tissues

II. Mechanisms of Periodontal Destruction
III. Response to Treatment

NICOTINE ADDICTION
I. Tolerance
II. Dependence
III. Addiction
IV. Withdrawal

TREATMENT
I. Reasons for Quitting
II. Self-help Interventions
III. Assisted Strategies

PHARMACOTHERAPIES USED FOR TREATMENT OF NICOTINE ADDICTION
I. Objectives and Rationale
II. Considerations
III. Contraindications
IV. Nicotine Replacement Therapy

NICOTINE-FREE THERAPY
I. Bupropion SR
II. Varenicline Tartrate
III. Combination Therapies
IV. Second-Line Medications
V. Alternative Cessation Therapies

DENTAL HYGIENE CARE FOR THE PATIENT WHO USES TOBACCO

ASSESSMENT
I. Patient History

II. Extraoral Examination
III. Intraoral Examination

CLINICAL TREATMENT PROCEDURES
I. Dental Biofilm Control
II. Nonsurgical Periodontal Therapy
III. Other Patient Instruction

TOBACCO CESSATION PROGRAM

MOTIVATIONAL INTERVIEWING

THE "5 A's"
I. Ask
II. Advise
III. Assess
IV. Assist
V. Arrange

THE TEAM APPROACH
I. Organize the Clinic Team
II. Organize a Tobacco-Free Environment
III. Organize a Tobacco User Tracking System

ADVOCACY
I. Public Health Policy
II. Community Oral Health Education Programs

DOCUMENTATION

EVERYDAY ETHICS

FACTORS TO TEACH THE PATIENT

REFERENCES

LEARNING OBJECTIVES

After studying this chapter, the student will be able to:

1. Recognize the health hazards associated with tobacco use.
2. Identify components of tobacco products.
3. Identify various alternative tobacco products.
4. Explain various mechanisms for nicotine delivery.
5. Describe the metabolism of nicotine.
6. Recognize the oral manifestations of tobacco use.
7. Recognize the effects of environmental tobacco smoke (ETS).
8. Assess and develop a dental hygiene care plan for the patient who uses tobacco.
9. Recognize protocols for developing a tobacco cessation program.
10. Identify the pharmacotherapies and behavioral therapies used for treatment of nicotine addiction.

In the 21st century, oral effects from tobacco use are well documented and show there is no safe form of tobacco.[1] Advice from health professionals has been shown to be a powerful influence on patients' decisions to stop or not begin using tobacco.[2] Dental and dental hygiene professionals are in an ideal position and have a responsibility to provide patients who use tobacco with the opportunity to enter a tobacco cessation program to assist in stopping tobacco use.[2]

HEALTH HAZARDS AND CURRENT TRENDS

- Tobacco is toxic to humans. Tobacco use is the single most preventable cause of disease and premature death in the world.[1]
- Approximately one in four adult Americans report using some type of tobacco product: any combustible tobacco product, cigars, cigarillos, regular pipe, waterpipe (hookah), electronic cigarettes, and smokeless tobacco.[3]
- Although cigarette smoking has declined in the past few years, it remains the most commonly used tobacco product.[3]
- An increased use of alternative tobacco products (ATPs), such as waterpipes, electronic nicotine delivery systems (ENDS), has emerged, especially among young adults.[3]
- The use of multiple forms of tobacco products is another growing trend, especially among noncigarette users, known as polytobacco use.[4]
- Offspring of smokers are more likely to become smokers.[1,5]
- As years of tobacco use accumulate, so do the systemic and oral health effects of all forms of tobacco.[1]
- Life expectancy is shortened.[1]
- Approximately 4.7 million middle- and high school–aged youth use tobacco products.[6]
- Approximately 16 million Americans suffer from a disease caused by smoking.[1]
- Eighty percent of deaths from lung cancer are attributed to smoking.[7]

COMPONENTS OF TOBACCO PRODUCTS AND TOBACCO SMOKE

- Nicotine is the chief psychoactive ingredient in tobacco that causes addiction.[8]
- Nicotine is considered toxic, and 60 mg can cause fatality.[9]
- Once tobacco is ignited, carcinogenic substances become part of mainstream smoke (smoke inhaled directly into the user's lungs) and are emitted in environmental tobacco smoke (ETS).[10]
- Cigarette smoke is a complex mixture containing an estimated 7,357 chemical compounds.[11]
- Over 90 of the chemical and chemical compounds in tobacco products and tobacco smoke are identified by the Food and Drug Administration (FDA) as being unsafe or having unsafe potential.[12]
- These chemicals or chemical compounds can be categorized as a carcinogen (cancer-causing), respiratory toxicant, cardiovascular toxicant, reproductive or developmental intoxicant, an addictive, or a combination of these agents.[12]
- The following chemical components in tobacco products have the greatest potential for harmful systemic effects: 1,3-butadiene (cancer), acrolein and acetaldehyde (respiratory), cyanide, arsenic, and cresols (cardiovascular).[1]
- Table 32-1 lists differences in the quantity of nicotine delivered by tobacco products: the amount and rate at which a nicotine-containing product delivers nicotine to the bloodstream is a determinant of its addiction potential.[12,13]

METABOLISM OF NICOTINE

- Absorption of nicotine occurs through most of the body's membranes: lungs, skin, and oral, buccal, nasal mucosa, and the gastrointestinal tract.[8,9]
- Delivery method affects the way nicotine is absorbed into the body. For example, inhaled tobacco is absorbed via the membranes in the lung.[9]

TABLE 32-1 • Nicotine Levels of Various Tobacco Products[13,93]

PRODUCTS	AMOUNT OF NICOTINE DELIVERY
Cigarette	0.7–2.0 mg
Bidi	1.5–4.1 mg
Kretek	1.9–2.6 mg
Moist snuff	0.01–7.8 mg/g
Hookah smoking (45 min–1 hr)	Equivalent to inhaling 100–200 times the volume of smoke from one cigarette

♦ Another factor affecting absorption is the pH level of the product. The more basic the medium, the easier the absorption.[11] For example, chewing tobacco has an alkaline pH to improve absorption.[8]

♦ Several factors influence absorption from smoked tobacco (cigarettes, pipes, and cigars), as identified in Figure 32-1. Regardless of the type of tobacco used, nicotine is primarily metabolized by the liver and excreted in the urine.[8,9]

I. Nicotine from Smoking

A. Absorption: Lungs

Nicotine enters the lungs and quickly passes into arterial circulation by way of blood vessels lining the sacs of the bronchi.[8]

B. Distribution

♦ *To the brain*: Nicotine is delivered efficiently to the brain by the bloodstream in 20 seconds or less.[8]

♦ *Peak plasma concentration*: Figure 32-2 illustrates the peak blood plasma concentrations from various tobacco products and nicotine replacement therapies (NRTs).

• Following the onset of cigarette smoking, peak plasma concentration of nicotine in the brain occurs in approximately 5 minutes.[9]

♦ *Dissemination*: Nicotine is spread to nearly all body tissues.[9]

♦ *Changes in the liver*: Nicotine is metabolized in the liver primarily as cotinine.[8]

• Cotinine concentrations in the blood, urine, hair, and saliva are used to assess[8]
  • Whether a person uses tobacco.
  • The extent of use.
  • The level of exposure of nonsmokers to passive or environmental smoke.

ALTERNATIVE TOBACCO PRODUCTS

ATPs are products that deliver nicotine via alternative methods other than cigarettes, such as smokeless tobacco,

ENDS (known as e-cigarettes or vape pens), waterpipes, cigars, and dissolvable and gel tobacco forms.

♦ ATPs contain nicotine and other harmful or potentially harmful constituents.[14]

♦ ATPs are not considered safe, nor a safe alternative to cigarette smoking.[14]

♦ Evidence shows individuals who use an ATP are at higher risk using of other forms of tobacco.[14,15]

♦ The FDA regulates the manufacturing, importing, packaging, labeling, advertising, and distribution of ATP-associated components, excluding accessories.[16]

♦ All ATP packages and advertisements require a warning statement, regarding nicotine and addiction.[16]

I. Smokeless Tobacco

Smokeless tobacco is the term applied to snuff (moist or dry), chewing tobacco products, and dissolvable products, which are not smoked but placed in the mouth.[17]

♦ Snuff is a fire-cured, finely ground, or powdered tobacco sold in both dry and moist forms or baglike pouches; not chewed but a small amount ("pinch" or "quid") is placed and held between cheek and gingiva or lower lip, gingiva, and mucosa.[17,18]

♦ Snuff can also be sniffed or inhaled into the nose.[17,18]

♦ Snus is moist snuff distributed in a prepackaged pouch and does not require spitting.

♦ Chewing (spit) tobacco is available in loose-leaf, twist/roll, and plug forms manufactured by air-drying tobacco leaves; it is held inside the cheek or lower lip and gingiva, and/or chewed.[17,18]

♦ Of the 28 carcinogens found in chewing tobacco and snuff, the most harmful are the tobacco-specific nitrosamines (TSNAs). These chemical compounds are usually formed during the growing, curing, fermenting, and aging of tobacco process.[18]

♦ Other cancer-causing substances found in smokeless tobacco include benzo(a)pyrene, formaldehyde, acetaldehyde, arsenic, nickel, cadmium, and polonium-210.[18]

A. Absorption: Oral Cavity

♦ Nicotine is directly absorbed through the oral mucous membranes.[8]

♦ Once smokeless tobacco is placed in the mouth, the amount of nicotine absorbed is three to four times the amount delivered by a cigarette.[11] Per day, a user may keep snuff in the mouth for approximately 11–14 hours.

♦ Nicotine concentration steadily increases with use and slowly declines over 2 hours and is at a negligible level within 24 hours.[8]

♦ Smokeless tobacco users experience nicotine blood plasma levels similar to the nicotine blood levels of smokers.[8]

CENTER FOR TOBACCO PRODUCTS

How a Cigarette Is Engineered

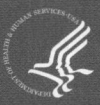

The design and content of cigarettes continue to make them attractive, addictive, and deadly.[1] Every day, more than 1,300 people in the United States die because of cigarette use.[2]

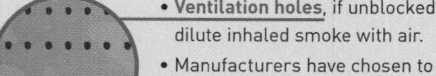

Filter [3,4,5]

- Typically made from bundles of thin, hair-like fibers.
- Designed to trap smoke, but only stops a small portion of the smoke from being inhaled.
- The filter (and ventilation holes) in most cigarettes may lead smokers to inhale more deeply, pulling dangerous chemicals farther into their lungs.

Cigarette paper [3]

- Holds the tobacco filler.
- Manufacturers add chemicals to the paper to control how fast the cigarette burns.
- Smokers inhale everything that is burned—the tobacco filler, the paper... everything.

Tobacco filler [7,8,9]

- Made up of chopped tobacco leaves, stems, reprocessed pieces, and scraps.
- Dangerous chemicals can form in and be deposited on tobacco during the processing of the tobacco leaves.
- Other dangerous chemicals are created when the tobacco filler is burned.

Tipping paper [6]

- Wraps around the filter, connecting it to the rest of the cigarette.

- **Ventilation holes**, if unblocked, dilute inhaled smoke with air.
- Manufacturers have chosen to place the ventilation holes where they are. The holes are largely ineffective. Because of their location, most smokers unknowingly block them with their fingers or lips.

Additives [10,11,12]

Manufacturers can **add hundreds of ingredients** to a cigarette to make smoking more appealing and to mask the harshness of smoke.

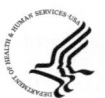 Certain **additives**, like sugars, can form cancer-causing chemicals when they are burned.

Sugar and **flavor*** additives can change the taste of smoke and make it easier to inhale, but no less harmful.

 Ammonia and other **chemicals** added to tobacco may increase the absorption of nicotine, which is addictive.

Some additives are **bronchodilators** that could increase the amount of dangerous chemicals absorbed by the lungs.

*In 2009, The Family Smoking Prevention and Tobacco Control Act banned characterizing flavors in cigarettes, except for tobacco and menthol flavors.

FDA'S REGULATORY AUTHORITY: The FDA Center for Tobacco Products (CTP) has broad authority, via the Tobacco Control Act, to regulate the manufacturing, distribution, and marketing of tobacco products. To protect public health, CTP has the authority to regulate what ingredients tobacco manufacturers can put into their products.

(1) U.S. Department of Health and Human Services. A Report of the Surgeon General: How Tobacco Smoke Causes Disease (Fact Sheet). Atlanta, GA: U.S. Department of Health and Human Services, Centers for Disease Control and Prevention, National Center for Chronic Disease Prevention and Health Promotion, Office on Smoking and Health; 2010. (2) U.S. Department of Health and Human Services. The Health Consequences of Smoking—50 Years of Progress: A Report of the Surgeon General. Atlanta, GA: U.S. Department of Health and Human Services, Centers for Disease Control and Prevention, National Center for Chronic Disease Prevention and Health Promotion, Office on Smoking and Health; 2014. (3) Taylor MJ. The role of filter technology in reduced yield cigarettes. Filtrona. World Tobacco Exhibition Kunming. (4) Kiefer JE, Mumpower RC II. Parameters That Affect the Pressure Drop and Efficiency of Cellulose Acetate Cigarette Filters. Research Laboratories, Tennessee Eastman Company; 2004; Bates number: 81052204/2269. (5) U.S. Department of Health and Human Services. Let's Make the Next Generation Tobacco-Free: Your Guide to the 50th Anniversary Surgeon General's Report on Smoking and Health (Consumer Booklet). Atlanta, GA: U.S. Department of Health and Human Services, Centers for Disease Control and Prevention, National Center for Chronic Disease Prevention and Health Promotion, Office on Smoking and Health; 2014. (6) Browne CL. The Design of Cigarettes. 3rd ed. Charlotte, NC: C Filter Products Division, Hoechst Celanese Corporation; 1990. (7) Spears AW. Effect of manufacturing variables on cigarette smoke composition. CORESTA Bulletin d'Information. 1974;665-78. (8) Geiss O, Kotzias D. Tobacco, Cigarettes, and Cigarette Smoke: An Overview. European Commission, Directorate-General, Joint Research Centre; 2007. (9) Baker R. A review of pyrolysis studies to unravel reaction steps in burning tobacco. Journal of Analytical and Applied Pyrolysis. 1987;11:555-573. (10) U.S. Department of Health and Human Services. How Tobacco Smoke Causes Disease: The Biology and Behavioral Basis for Smoking-Attributable Disease: A Report of the Surgeon General. Atlanta, GA: U.S. Department of Health and Human Services, Centers for Disease Control and Prevention, National Center for Chronic Disease Prevention and Health Promotion, Office on Smoking and Health; 2010. (11) Rabinoff M, Caskey N, Rissling A, Park, C. Pharmacological and chemical effects of cigarette additives. American Journal of Public Health. 2007;97(11):1981-1991. (12) Talhout R, Opperhuizen A, Amsterdam J. Sugars as tobacco ingredient: Effects on mainstream smoke composition. Food and Chemical Toxicology. 2006;44(11):1789-1798.

Last Updated October 2016
CTP-62-P

www.fda.gov/tobacco   @FDATobacco   facebook.com/fda

FIGURE 32-1 • Components of Mainstream Smoke and Factors Influencing Absorption by the Lungs.

Nicotine-Containing Products

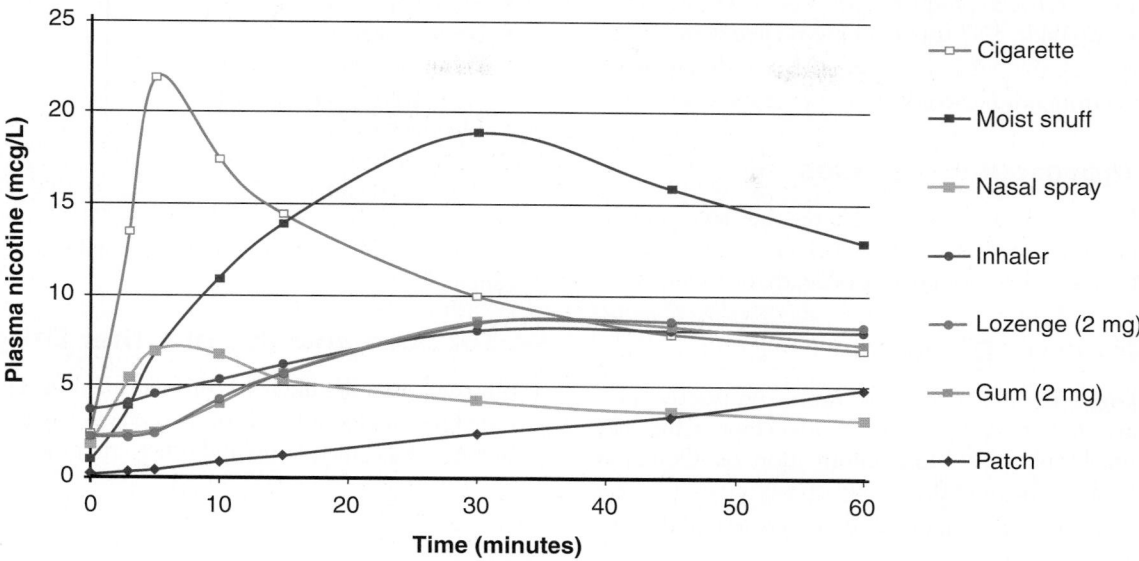

FIGURE 32-2 • Plasma Concentrations for Tobacco Products and Nicotine Pharmacotherapies. (From Choi JH, Dresler CM, Norton MR, et al. Pharmacokinetics of a nicotine polacrilex lozenge. *Nicotine Tob Res*. 2003;5:635-644; Fant RV, Henningfield JE, Nelson RA, et al. Pharmacokinetics and pharmacodynamics of moist snuff in humans. *Tob Control*. 1999;8:387-392; Schneider NG, Olmstead RE, Franzon MA, et al. The nicotine inhaler: clinical pharmacokinetics and comparison with other nicotine treatments. *Clin Pharmacokinet*. 2001;40:661-684.)

B. Absorption: Intestinal[18]

◆ Most tobacco juice produced by smokeless tobacco is spit out.

◆ Juice that is intentionally and/or accidentally swallowed by the user is absorbed through the blood vessels lining the small intestine.

II. Waterpipe Tobacco Smoking

A **waterpipe** is a device used to smoke tobacco, also known as hookah, shisha, and hubble-bubble.[19,20]

◆ Tobacco used in the waterpipe is available in a variety of flavors.[19]

◆ Waterpipe smoking can lead to nicotine dependence and has similar health risks as smoking of cigarettes.[20,21]

◆ A waterpipe commonly has a head, body, water bowl, and a hose with a mouthpiece and is indirectly heated by charcoal.[22]

◆ Significant association with respiratory diseases, oral cancer, cardiovascular disease, lung cancer, delivering a low birth weight child, metabolic syndrome, and mental health disorders.[22]

III. Electronic Nicotine Delivery Systems

◆ An **electronic cigarette** or e-cigarette does not contain tobacco but delivers vaporized nicotine through a device made to look similar to a regular cigarette, cigar, or pipe. Additionally, some e-cigarettes are manufactured to look different than a typical cigarette, and more like an everyday item such as a USB flash drive (or jump drive), to conceal its true identity.[23]

◆ The device consists of a battery, a heater, and a cartridge.[15]

◆ Puffing on the device activates the heating element, and the solution is then vaporized and inhaled through a mouthpiece.[15]

◆ Contains nicotine (typically derived from tobacco plant), water, propylene glycol, vegetable glycerin, additives, and flavorants.[15]

◆ Although found at lower levels than cigarette smoke, carcinogens such as carbonyl compounds, heavy metals, and nitrosamines have been detected in the liquid and vapor of ENDS.[15]

◆ Adverse health effects from components such as solvents, flavorants, and toxicants when heated and aerosolized are unknown.[15]

◆ To date, the FDA has not approved the safety of ENDS, its use in NRT, nor as an effective method of smoking cessation.[15,24]

◆ To understand health effects of the long-term use of ENDS, additional high-level research is necessary.[25,26]

◆ Using ENDS may lead youth/young adults to try conventional tobacco products, which are known to increase morbidity and mortality rates.[1,15]

SYSTEMIC EFFECTS

- The use of tobacco products influences every system of the body.[1] Table 32-2 lists smoking-related conditions.
- The diseases that affect each system have consequences ranging from mild to deadly.[1]

I. Cardiovascular Diseases

- Smoking aggravates and accelerates the development of atherosclerosis and is a major risk factor for coronary heart disease, the leading cause of death for Americans.[1]

II. Pulmonary Diseases

- Smoking is the major cause of chronic obstructive pulmonary disease (COPD), including emphysema and chronic bronchitis.[1] More information on COPD is provided in Chapter 60.
- Emphysema slowly diminishes a person's ability to breathe.[1]
- Chronic bronchitis is a condition in which the airways produce excess mucus, which forces the smoker to cough frequently.[1]

III. Cancer

- Smoking is responsible for 80% of lung cancers in the United States.[1]
- Lung cancer is currently the leading cause of death among cancers, for both men and womenv.[27]
- Smoking can cause many different types of cancers including[1]:
  - Lung cancer
  - Larynx/throat cancer
  - Oropharynx cancer
  - Esophagus cancer
  - Trachea cancer
  - Stomach cancer
  - Liver cancer
  - Pancreas cancer
  - Kidney and ureter cancers
  - Bladder cancer
  - Cervix cancer
  - Colorectal cancer
- Tobacco use causes most oral cancers. The increase use of tobacco products increases the risk of developing oral cancer.[28,29]

IV. Tobacco and Use of Other Drugs

- Smokers are more likely to consume alcohol. The combined use of alcohol and tobacco places the patient at higher risk for neoplasms and other oral problems.[1,7]

ENVIRONMENTAL TOBACCO SMOKE

- Also called passive, involuntary, or secondhand smoke when nonusers are exposed.[1]
- ETS is tobacco smoke present in room air resulting from ignited tobacco products.[10]
- A complex mixture of chemicals generated during the burning of tobacco products.
- The principal contributor is sidestream smoke, the material emitted from burning tobacco products between puffs.[10]
- Other components include exhaled mainstream smoke and vaporized compounds diffused through a cigarette wrapper.[10,30]
- In indoor areas, environmental smoke can last for many hours, depending on ventilation. Exposure for certain workers and family members can be extensive.[10]

TABLE 32-2 • Disease Consequences of Tobacco Use[1]

CANCER	RESPIRATORY DISEASES	CARDIOVASCULAR DISEASES	PREGNANCY INFANT HEALTH	OTHER CONDITIONS
Oral cavity	Chronic obstructive pulmonary disease	Atherosclerosis	Ectopic pregnancy	Immune function
Lung	Emphysema	Coronary heart disease	Fetal neonatal death/ stillbirth	Diabetes
Larynx	Asthma	Aortic aneurysm	Preterm delivery	Rheumatoid arthritis
Trachea	Pneumonia	Early abdominal aortic	Congenital defects	Male sex function (erectile dysfunction)
Oropharynx	Tuberculosis	Atherosclerosis in young adults	Orofacial clefts	Blindness
Esophagus	Pulmonary infections	Stroke	Reduced fertility	Cataracts
Stomach			Growth delay	Age-related macular degeneration
Bladder			Sudden infant death syndrome	
Cervix			Low birth weight	
Bronchus				
Kidney and ureter				
Pancreas				
Acute myeloid leukemia				
Liver				
Breast				
Colorectal				

- Secondhand smoke at any level is deemed unsafe.[1,31]
- Approximately 58 million Americans are exposed to passive smoke.[31]
- Exposure to secondhand smoke is most prevalent among children, African Americans, those living below the poverty level, and those living in multi-units rental housing.[31]
- Thirdhand smoke is defined as tobacco smoke residue absorbed by furnishings.[32,33]
  - Smoke reacts with a common pollutant on indoor surfaces, nitrous acid, which then forms TSNAs.
  - The TSNAs cling to the smoker's body, household dust, and every surface of the home, vehicle, or enclosed area where the smoking takes place. This process represents a health hazard.
- Although ENDS do not emit a sidestream, the aerosol emission from ENDS is potentially another toxicant secondhand and thirdhand exposure for nonusers.[15]

I. Toxicity

- Many chemicals are contained in passive smoke, including the same carcinogenic compounds, as those in mainstream smoke. Some toxic components are actually in higher concentrations in sidestream smoke than in mainstream smoke.[11]
- Chemicals present in ETS include irritants and systemic toxicants (hydrogen cyanide and sulfur dioxide), mutagens and carcinogens (benzo[a]pyrene and formaldehyde), and reproductive toxicants (nicotine, cadmium, and carbon monoxide).[30]
- Of the 250 toxic chemicals in ETS, there are at least 50 associated with cancer.[10]

II. Lung and Respiratory Effects

- Exposure to cigarette smoke, whether active or passive, is the primary cause of lung cancer.[7]
- Eye and nasal irritation are the most commonly reported symptoms among adult nonsmokers.[10]

III. Cardiovascular Effects

- Both active and passive exposure to smoke have similar effects on the cardiovascular system.[1,10]
- ETS is a major preventable cause of coronary heart disease and death.[10]
- A causal relationship exists between secondhand smoke exposure and increased risk of stroke.[1]

PRENATAL AND CHILDREN

The fetus, infant, and growing children are exposed to ETS through the following[1,10,31]:
- Homes and cars where smoking is permitted.
- Public environments in which smoking is permitted.

- Other enclosed environments that allow smoking, such as restaurants and sporting events.
- Nonsmoking mothers, who are exposed to ETS, expose their unborn child to tobacco smoke constituents, such as carbon monoxide, nicotine, and cotinine.
- Parental smoking is a strong determinant to smoking uptake among children and adolescents.[34]

I. In Utero

- Nicotine crosses the placenta and concentrates in the fetus at slightly higher levels than the mother.[1,5]
- Adverse pregnancy risks include miscarriage, low birth weight, placenta previa, preterm delivery, spontaneous abortion, and stillbirth.[1,5,35]
- Evidence shows maternal smoking in early pregnancy can cause orofacial clefts.[1]
- Evidence shows a causal relationship between maternal smoking and ectopic pregnancy.[1]

II. Infancy[1,10,36]

- Chemicals are passed to the baby in the breast milk of mothers who smoke.
- Acute effects include increased incidence of upper respiratory tract illness.
- ETS increases risk of an infant developing a lower respiratory illness.
- Nicotine can increase the risk of sudden infant death syndrome in infants of smokers.

III. Young Children[1,10,31,37,38]

- ETS affects lung development with symptoms of coughing, phlegm, and wheezing.
- Children who are exposed to passive smoking, particularly prenatal and postnatal maternal smoking, are at significant risk for onset of wheezing illness and asthma.
- Children have an increased incidence of middle ear infections.

ORAL MANIFESTATIONS OF TOBACCO AND NICOTINE USE

- The numerous oral conditions attributed to tobacco use vary with the type of tobacco used (smoking or smokeless) and the form in which it is used (cigarettes, pipes, cigars, chewing tobacco, moist, and dry snuff).[1]
- Pattern and severity of clinical presentation vary with frequency and duration of tobacco use.[29]
- Research indicates ENDS have shown oxidative stress and cell death to the epithelium tissue.[39]
- Table 32-3 lists examples of the wide variety of oral consequences of tobacco use; periodontal diseases and oral cancers provide the most serious destructive effects.

TABLE 32-3 • Oral Consequences of Tobacco Use

CANCER AND PRECANCER	PERIODONTAL FACTORS	SOFT-TISSUE PROBLEMS	HARD-TISSUE PROBLEMS	ESTHETIC FACTORS	EXCERBATION—ORAL SIGNS IN SYSTEMIC DISEASES
Squamous cell leukoplakia (ST)	Acute necrotizing ulcerative gingivitis (ANUG) and acute necrotizing ulcerative periodontitis (ANUP)	Nicotine stomatitis (P)	Occlusal or incisal abrasion (P, ST)	Halitosis	HIV/AIDS
Homogeneous		Smoker's melanosis		Dental stains	Type 1 and type 2 diabetes
Nonhomogeneous		Black hairy tongue	Cervical abrasion (ST)	Prosthesis stains	
Verrucous		Median rhomboid glossitis	Dehiscence of bone (ST)	Orthodontic appliance stains	
	Relapse during maintenance	Median rhomboid glossitis	Tooth loss	Discoloration of restorations	
	Increased risk for peri-implantitis and peri-implant bone loss	Median rhomboid glossitis		Impaired taste and smell	
		Leukodema (P)			
	Localized recession and clinical attachment loss	Hyperkeratosis (ST)			
		Dry socket			
		Delayed wound healing			

P, pipe; ST, smokeless tobacco; no notation, smoked tobacco.

◆ An extraoral/intraoral examination is the most efficient and effective method for detecting tobacco-related conditions in and around the mouth.
  • The extraoral/intraoral examination gives visual examples to use in encouraging the patient to begin a tobacco cessation program.

TOBACCO AND PERIODONTAL INFECTIONS

◆ Tobacco use is a major risk factor for the development and progression of periodontitis.[1,19,40,41]
◆ Users are at a high risk for developing more severe periodontitis than nonusers.[40]
◆ There is a positive association between periodontitis and nonsmokers exposed to ETS.[42]

I. Effects on the Periodontal Tissues

◆ *Gingivitis*[19,43]
  • The degree of inflammatory response to dental biofilm accumulation is reduced compared with nonsmokers.
  • Smoking may affect treatment and therapeutic outcomes for plaque-induced gingivitis.
◆ *Periodontitis in tobacco users*[22,44,45,46,47]
  • Increased rate and severity of periodontal destruction.
  • Increased bone loss, attachment loss, and pocket depths.
  • Diminished gingival blood flow and gingival crevicular flow.
  • Increased tooth loss from periodontal causes.[48]
  • Prevalence and severity may lessen with cessation.

II. Mechanisms of Periodontal Destruction

◆ Host response: lowered immune response.[49]
◆ Impaired neutrophils: decreased chemotaxis, phagocytosis, and adherence.[11]
◆ Altered antibody production; decreased serum immunoglobulin G.
◆ Impairment of revascularization; disruption of immune response; impact on healing; increased risk of periodontal disease.[1,50]
◆ Negative effect on bone metabolism; after menopause, women smokers have a deficit in bone density; smoking can also influence osteoporosis.[1]

III. Response to Treatment

◆ People who use tobacco products have a weakened response to conventional therapy.[51,52]
◆ Smoking has a negative impact on bone regeneration after periodontal therapy.[46]
◆ Implants have higher risk for failure due to implantitis.[53]
◆ Delayed healing after surgical and nonsurgical procedures.[52]
◆ Therapeutic effects of nonsurgical procedures may improve with cessation.[54,55]

NICOTINE ADDICTION

◆ Nicotine is tobacco's psychoactive agent (one that produces feelings of pleasure and well-being), and its use leads to tolerance, dependence, and addiction.[56]
◆ No one starts using tobacco to become addicted to it.

◆ Users seldom can explain why they use tobacco but often say it helps their physical performance, mood, or ability to think. In fact, physical performance does not improve, mood is not better, and intellectual stimulation is minor.[57]

I. Tolerance

◆ *Physiologic adaptation*
  • Tolerance refers to the user's need for more smoking or chewing the same amount of the same product over time as it becomes less and less effective in creating the desired feeling of well-being.[56]
◆ *Amount of use*
  • To sustain the positive feelings associated with tobacco use, more and more has to be used.[56]

II. Dependence

◆ *Characteristics*
  • As increased amounts are needed over time, the loss of control over the amount and frequency of tobacco use show evidence of dependence.[56]
  • Facts about nicotine dependency are included in Box 32-1, and criteria for nicotine dependency are outlined in Box 32-2.

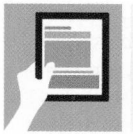

BOX 32-1
Facts about Nicotine Dependency

• Nicotine is the most addictive drug in the United States.
• Nicotine addiction is similar to that produced by other substances such as alcohol, cocaine, and heroin.
• Those who have a high tolerance to nicotine experience less nausea and dizziness following initial use.
• Tobacco abuse: Any use of tobacco products is considered a health hazard. Therefore, the use of any amount is considered abuse.
• Nicotine addiction may be the most challenging of all addictions for complete recovery.
• Many tobacco users make many unsuccessful quit attempts before stopping use for indefinite or extended periods of time.
• Successfully quitting smokeless tobacco use may be equally or more difficult than stopping smoking.

Source: National Institute on Drug Abuse. *Research Report Series: Is Nicotine Addictive?* Bethesda, MD: National Institutes of Health, National Institute on Drug Abuse; 2012; American Psychiatric Association. *Diagnostic and Statistical Manual of Mental Disorders (DSM-IV).* 5th ed. Washington, DC: American Psychiatric Association; 2013:571-589.

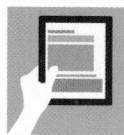

BOX 32-2
Criteria for Nicotine Dependency

• Tolerance:
  ◆ A need for markedly increased amounts of the substance to achieve intoxication or desired effect.
  ◆ Markedly diminished effect with continued use of the same amount.
• Withdrawal, as manifested by either:
  ◆ Daily use of nicotine for several weeks.
  ◆ Abrupt stopping or reducing nicotine may result in four or more of the signs of nicotine withdrawal found in Box 32-3 and they will occur within 24 hours.
• Used in greater amounts over longer period of time than intended.
• A persistent desire or unsuccessful efforts to cut down or quit.
• A great deal of time spent using the substance.
• Giving up important social, occupational, or recreational activities because of use of the substance.
• Continued use despite knowledge of medical problems related to use and/or social and legal problems resulting from use.

Source: American Psychiatric Association. *Diagnostic and Statistical Manual of Mental Disorders (DSM-IV).* 5th ed. Washington, DC: American Psychiatric Association; 2013:571-589.

◆ *Reinforcing effect*[56]
  • Nicotine intensifies the release of dopamine by the brain, thereby increasing a feeling of pleasure and the compulsion to use tobacco.
  • Positive reinforcement is produced with tobacco use, and abrupt stopping produces withdrawal symptoms.

III. Addiction

◆ Under Federal Law, tobacco companies are required to make the following statements regarding nicotine addiction and nicotine manipulation[58]:
  • Here is the truth: Smoking is highly addictive. Nicotine is the addictive drug in tobacco.
  • Cigarette companies intentionally designed cigarettes with enough nicotine to create and sustain addiction.
  • It's not easy to quit.
  • When you smoke, the nicotine actually changes the brain—that is why quitting is so hard.
  • Defendant tobacco companies intentionally designed cigarettes to make them more addictive.
  • Cigarette companies control the impact and delivery of nicotine in many ways, including designing

filters and selecting cigarette paper to maximize the ingestion of nicotine, adding ammonia to make the cigarette taste less harsh, and controlling the physical and chemical makeup of the tobacco blend.[58]

◆ Addiction is a chronic, progressive, relapsing disease characterized by compulsive use of a substance.[56]

◆ The effects result in physical, psychological, and/or social harm to the user, but use continues despite that harm.

◆ Smoking is more addictive than alcohol and other drugs of abuse in terms of the proportion of those who are exposed and subsequently become dependent.

◆ The pattern of relapse is identical for tobacco, alcohol, and heroin.

◆ Factors affecting the development of addiction include:
  • Properties of psychoactive drug (dose).
  • Family, peer influences, and social acceptance.
  • Existing psychiatric disorders.
  • Cost and availability of the drug.
  • Influence of advertising.

IV. Withdrawal

◆ Withdrawal refers to the effects of cessation of nicotine use by an individual in whom dependence is established.[56]

◆ When users of nicotine products stop abruptly, within 24 hours, they can experience maximal physical and/or psychological withdrawal symptoms.[56]

◆ Box 32-3 identifies typical nicotine withdrawal symptoms.

◆ Duration[2,56]
  • Patients experience withdrawal symptoms almost immediately, and relapse within a week is common.
  • Most symptoms diminish over a few weeks when relapse does not occur.

◆ Cravings for tobacco, increased appetite, and weight gain may persist for months or years.[56]

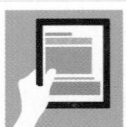

BOX 32-3
Criteria for Nicotine Withdrawal Syndrome

- Dysphoric or depressed mood
- Insomnia
- Irritability, frustration, and anger
- Anxiety
- Difficulty concentrating
- Restlessness
- Decreased heart rate
- Increased appetite or weight gain
- Cravings for tobacco

Source: American Psychiatric Association. *Diagnostic and Statistical Manual of Mental Disorders (DSM-IV).* 5th ed. Washington, DC: American Psychiatric Association; 2013:571-589.

TABLE 32-4 • Alleviating Nicotine Withdrawal Symptoms

SYMPTOMS	ACTIVITIES
Mood changes; anxiety, nervousness, feeling stressed	Breathe deeply; exhale through pursed lips. Take a walk or other relaxation exercise. Know your triggers, get more rest, and take multivitamin. Make a list of things to do instead of smoking. Avoid places where you most commonly used tobacco.
Sleep disturbances	Avoid caffeine, drink a glass of warm milk instead. Avoid alcohol. Take a long walk before bed. Avoid naps, take a warm bath or meditate. Read a book, listen to soothing music.
Appetite increase	Eat only when you are hungry. Eat low-fat, low-calorie snacks. Chew sugarless gum or eat sugarless hard flavorful candy. Drink additional glasses of water. Exercise.
Cravings	*Delay smoking or dipping.* Use tactics such as waiting 1 more minute; often cravings pass in 5 or 10 min. *Distract yourself.* Exercise; take a walk; call a friend. *Drink water.* to fight off cravings. *Deep breaths.* Relax! Close your eyes and take 10 deep breaths; exhale through pursed lips. *Discuss your feelings.* with someone close to you or a support group.[a]

[a]National Advisory Committee on Health and Disability. *Guidelines for Smoking Cessation, Revised 2002.* Wellington, New Zealand: National Advisory Committee on Health and Disability (National Health Committee); 2002.
Source: Adapted from Fiore MC, Jaén CR, Baker TB, et al. Treating tobacco use and dependence: 2008 update. In: *Quick Reference Guide for Clinicians.* Rockville, MD: U.S. Department of Health and Human Services. Public Health Service; 2009.

◆ *Alleviation of symptoms*
  • Table 32-4 lists activities to help overcome withdrawal symptoms.
  • The goal is to prevent relapse.[2]

TREATMENT

Cessation from cigarette smoking has increased over the past years, with two-thirds of smokers reporting an interest in quitting.[59] Tobacco cessation methods or treatment for nicotine addiction fall into two categories: *self-help* (unassisted) and *assisted strategies.*

I. Reasons for Quitting

Success cannot be expected unless the individual makes a concentrated effort and believes in the significance of the effort. Typical reasons include the following[2,60]:

◆ General health awareness.

◆ Specific health problem directly or indirectly related to tobacco use.

◆ Coughing and lack of breath while exercising.

◆ Halitosis and yellow-stained teeth.

◆ Effect on family
   • Need to act as a role model.
   • Awareness of effects of ETS.

◆ Effect of smoking and/or ETS on fetus during pregnancy.

◆ Cost.

◆ Social pressure and restrictions on smoking in many settings.

◆ Personal recognition of the dangers of nicotine addiction and the desire to regain control of one's life.

◆ Reported among young adults: Fear of becoming sick when older and not wanting to smoke as an older adult.[60]

II. Self-help Interventions

When attempting to quit, less than one-third of smokers currently use an evidence-based cessation treatment. As a result, fewer than one in ten reported success in cessation.[59]

◆ The following methods are used either singularly or, most commonly, in conjunction with one another[61]:
   • Go "cold turkey" all at once.
   • Reduce number of daily tobacco exposures.
   • Substitute cigarette smoking with ENDS.
   • Join a family member or friend in the tobacco cessation effort.
   • Select over-the-counter (OTC) nicotine replacement patches, gum, or lozenges.
   • Transitioned to a "light" version of cigarettes.

◆ Customized printed cessation material tailored for an individual can be helpful.[62]

◆ Recent evidence, although of low quality, indicates ENDS may reduce the frequency of smoking.[25] However, current clinical guidelines do not recommend ENDS for tobacco cessation.

◆ Recent evidence supports the reduction of smoking as a short-term harm reduction strategy and the cessation of smoking using NRTs as a long-term strategy.[63]

III. Assisted Strategies

◆ *Counseling*
   • Interventions provided by oral health professionals can help patients in tobacco cessation.[64]
   • Provide a brief intervention for cessation to all tobacco users at every appointment.[2,65,66]
   • Tailor cessation discussion to the individual[67] to-bacco users specific needs.[67]
   • Provision of practical counseling, including problem-solving and skills training.[2]
   • Provision of in-office social support: "Our office staff and I are willing to assist you."[2]
   • Customized Internet-based interventions with and without behavioral support can be an effective method for cessation.[68]

◆ *Pharmacotherapies*

◆ Table 32-5 provides an overview of FDA-approved first-line pharmacotherapies.

◆ *Combination*
   • Counseling combined with pharmacotherapy has been shown to be effective in helping patients to quit using tobacco.[69]

PHARMACOTHERAPIES USED FOR TREATMENT OF NICOTINE ADDICTION

I. Objectives and Rationale

◆ Make it easier to abstain from tobacco by partial replacement of nicotine or by counteracting nicotine's action.[70]

◆ Reduce withdrawal symptoms.[70]

◆ Fulfill, in part, the craving for tobacco by sustaining tolerance.[63]

◆ Provide some effects (mood, cognitive changes) previously delivered from nicotine.[63]

II. Considerations

◆ Discourage casual use of pharmacotherapies. Failure as a result of improper use can discourage future quit attempts.[2]

◆ Inform patient of potential adverse effects: nausea and vomiting.[63]

◆ Consult primary care provider before use if younger than 18 years, has a medical contraindication, or pregnant.[71]

III. Contraindications

◆ NRTs, bupropion and varenicline, have few associated risks.[72]

◆ Self-medication without professional examination and advice.

◆ Nicotine gum, lozenge, and inhaler: avoid eating or drinking acidic beverages for 15 minutes before and during use due to decreased nicotine absorption.[2]

◆ Pregnancy: nicotine in the bloodstream, even in small amounts, can reach the fetus.[1,73]

◆ Patients with history of seizures and history of eating disorders are cautioned in using bupropion SR.[2,72]

IV. Nicotine Replacement Therapy

◆ The objective of NRTs is to help prevent withdrawal symptoms and to promote tobacco cessation.[70]

◆ NRTs are less likely to cause dependence compared to tobacco products.[70]

◆ Dental hygienists are in an ideal position to discuss the immediate delivery of nicotine to the brain during smoking and to educate patients about the differences in nicotine delivery of various NRTs, particularly those that are available OTC.

TABLE 32-5 • Suggestions for the Clinical Use of Pharmacotherapies for Smoking Cessation

PHARMACOTHERAPY	PRECAUTIONS/ CONTRAINDICATIONS	SIDE EFFECTS	DOSAGE	DURATION	AVAILABILITY
Bupropion SR	History of seizure History of eating disorder Using monoamine oxidase inhibitor	Insomnia, dry mouth	Days 1–3: 150 mg each morning Day 4—end: twice daily; take evening dose 8 hr before sleep	Start 1–2 wk before quit date Use 2–6 mo	Zyban Wellbutrin SR Generic (prescription only)
Varenicline[a]	Kidney problems or on dialysis Has not been studied in pregnant or nursing women; FDA warning re: potential for agitation, depressed mood, atypical behavior, or suicidal thoughts	Nausea, insomnia, abnormal, vivid, or strange dreams Constipation, gas, and/or vomiting	Days 1–3: 0–5 mg once in morning Days 4–7: 0.5 mg twice daily Day 8 though end of treatment: 1 mg twice daily	Use 3–6 mo Start 1 wk before quit date	Chantix (prescription only)
Nicotine gum	Temporomandibular disorders disease Caution for denture wearers	Mouth soreness Dyspepsia Headaches	1–24 cigs/day 2 mg gum (up to 24 psc/day) 20+ cigs/day or smokeless tobacco—4 mg gum (up to 24 psc/day)[b]	Up to 12 wk or as needed	Nicorette gum (OTC only) Generic available
Nicotine inhaler	Asthma COPD	Local irritation of mouth and throat	6–16 cartridges/day[b]	Up to 6 mo; taper at end	Nicotrol inhaler (prescription only)
Nicotine nasal spray	Nasal polyps Rhinitis Sinusitis Asthma	Nasal and throat irritation Dependence potential	8–40 doses/day (no more than 48 sprays in 24 hr)	3–6 mo; taper at end	Nicotrol NS (prescription only)
Nicotine transdermal patch	Allergy to patch adhesive Do not use if have severe eczema or psoriasis Do not cut patches	Local skin reaction Insomnia Changes in dreams Headache	One patch per day If 10 cigs/day: 21 mg 4 wk 14 mg 2–4 wk 7 mg 2–4 wk If <10/day: 14 mg 4 wk, then 7 mg 4 wk One patch per day	8–12 wk	Nicoderm CQ (OTC only) Generic patches (prescription and OTC) Nicotrol (OTC only)
Nicotine lozenge	One lozenge at a time	Mouth soreness Dyspepsia Nausea Headache Cough Hiccups Heartburn Flatulence	2 mg if smoke/chew after 30 min of waking; 4 mg if smoke/chew within 30 min of waking Maximum 20 lozenges in 24 hr[b]	3–6 mo Wks 1–6:1 every 1–2 hr Wks 7–9:1 every 2–4 hr; Wks 10–12:1 every 4–8 hr	Commit • Mint • Cherry • Original (OTC only) Generic available
Nicotine mini lozenge	Same as above	Same as above	2 mg if smoke/chew after 30 min of waking; 4 mg if smoke/chew within 30 min of waking Maximum 24 mini lozenges/day[b]	Same as above	Nicorette mini • Mint (OTC only)

[a]Varenicline (Chantix) information. March 17, 2014. Available from https://www.chantix.com/index.aspx
[b]Nothing to eat or drink 15 min prior to or during use.
COPD, chronic obstructive pulmonary disease; FDA, Food and Drug Administration; OTC, over-the-counter.
Source: Adapted from Fiore MC, Jaén CR, Baker TB, et al. Treating tobacco use and dependence: 2008 update. In: *Quick Reference Guide for Clinicians.* Rockville, MD: U.S. Department of Health and Human Services. Public Health Service; 2009.

- NRTs have not been shown to be an effective cessation method for adolescents, 20 years and younger.[74]
- Nicotine gum[2]
  - *Transmucosal delivery*: Nicotine is released in the mouth during "chewing."
  - *Description*: Nicotine gum is sweetened with xylitol and has either a mild mint, cinnamon, or orange flavor.
  - *Directions*: Chew one piece slowly until tingling or peppery taste is achieved; "park" gum in buccal vestibule; resume chewing when peppery taste or tingle fades; and repeat chew/park activity.
- Nicotine patch[2]
  - *Transdermal delivery*: Nicotine is released through skin.
  - *Directions*: Place a new patch on a hairless location upon rising; if sleep disruption occurs, remove 24-hour patch before bedtime or use 16-hour patch.
- Nicotine inhaler[2]
  - *Transmucosal delivery*: Nicotine is released in mouth during inhalation or puffing; hold vapor in oral cavity for absorption, but do not inhale.
  - *Requirements*: Store inhaler and cartridges in a warm place when temperatures drop below 40°F to prevent a decline in delivery of nicotine from the inhaler to the oral cavity.
- Nicotine nasal spray[2]
  - *Nasal mucous membrane delivery*: Nicotine is released through lining of nose.
  - *Dose delivery*: Avoid sniffing, swallowing, or inhaling while administering doses, as these increase irritating effects.
  - *Directions*: Tilt head slightly back while delivering spray.
  - *Precaution for heavy smoker*: Increased dose.
- Nicotine lozenge[2]
  - *Transmucosal delivery*: Nicotine is released in mouth as lozenge dissolves.
  - *Description*: The lozenge is sweetened with mannitol and aspartame and flavored with a mild mint or cherry.
  - *Dose delivery*: see Table 32-5.
  - *Directions*: Do not bite or chew lozenge as it dissolves in the mouth; this can cause more nicotine to be swallowed quickly and may result in indigestion and/or heartburn.

NICOTINE-FREE THERAPY

I. Bupropion SR[2]

- The first non-nicotine medication shown to be effective for tobacco cessation and approved by the FDA for that use.
- *Mechanism of action*: blocks neural uptake of dopamine and/or norepinephrine.
- Additional dosing information is listed in Table 32-5.
- Take second dose 8 hours after first and with evening meal to reduce sleep disturbances.

- Bupropion SR can be used in combination with NRTs.
- Bupropion has not been shown to be an effective cessation method for adolescents, 20 years and younger.[74]

II. Varenicline Tartrate[2]

- The second non-nicotine medication shown to be effective for smoking cessation and approved by the FDA for that use.
- *Mechanism of action*: a partial nicotine agonist (blocks nicotine receptors in brain). It also causes reduction in dopamine release.
  - Always take after meals with full glass of water, to reduce nausea.
  - Take second dose 8 hours after first and with evening meal to reduce sleep disturbances.
  - Additional dosing information is listed in Table 32-5.
- Not currently recommended for use in combination with NTRs.

III. Combination Therapies[69]

- Certain combinations of first-line medications have been shown to be effective smoking cessation treatments.
- Effective combination medications are:
  - Long-term (>14 weeks) nicotine patch + nicotine gum or spray
  - Nicotine patch + nicotine inhaler
  - Nicotine patch + bupropion SR.

IV. Second-Line Medications

- Second-line medications are pharmacotherapies for which there is evidence of efficacy for treating tobacco dependence, but they have a more limited role because of the following reasons[2]:
  - The FDA has not approved them for a tobacco dependence treatment indication.
  - Second-line treatments, clonidine and nortriptyline, can be considered for use on a case-by-case basis after first-line treatments have been used or considered and while under a primary care provider's supervision.

V. Alternative Cessation Therapies

- Research suggests alternative aids such as acupuncture and hypnotherapy may help with smoking cessation.[75]
- It is unclear whether these alternative smoking aids are as effective as pharmocotherapies.[75]

DENTAL HYGIENE CARE FOR THE PATIENT WHO USES TOBACCO

- The majority of people who smoke state they would like to quit, and almost half say they have tried to quit in the past 12 months.[59]

- The tobacco-using patient presents a unique challenge to the oral health team. Specific treatment modifications are indicated.
- Helping the patient to quit using tobacco becomes an integral part of the dental hygiene care plan.

ASSESSMENT

I. Patient History

- Tobacco use status is assessed at each appointment.
- The basic history form in Chapter 11 used by all patients includes questions to determine whether the patient currently uses tobacco and, if so, the types of tobacco (cigarette, ATPs, and/or smokeless). A sample of a tobacco use assessment form is shown in Figure 32-3.
- Concomitant use of alcohol and other psychoactive drugs (substances that can alter mood, behavior, cognitive processes, or mention tension) with tobacco may necessitate modifications of clinical procedures.[56]
- Healthcare providers should consider tobacco use status as a *vital sign* along with temperature, pulse, respiratory rate, and blood pressure.[65,67]

II. Extraoral Examination

- *Breath and body odor*
  - Halitosis.[76]
  - Smoke from tobacco products clings to skin, hair, and clothes and results in body odor.[30]

- *Fingers*
- Smokers of nonfiltered cigarettes have a yellowish-brown discoloration of the fingers and fingernails.
- *Skin*
- Smokers experience premature and more extensive facial wrinkling.[1]
- *Lips*
  Cigar smokers are at risk for development of precancerous and cancerous lip lesions.[4]

III. Intraoral Examination

An excellent outline for conducting a thorough intraoral examination for the patient who uses tobacco is provided in Chapter 13. Oral consequences of tobacco use are listed in Table 32-3.

CLINICAL TREATMENT PROCEDURES

- Patients who use tobacco may require longer and more frequent appointments due to the presence of increased risk for the following[1,52,77,78]:
  - Dental stain
  - Calculus
  - Dental caries
  - Gingival inflammation
  - Periodontal problems

Tobacco Products			
Cigarettes	YES ( )	NO ( )	Number of cigarettes per day or week:
Cigars	YES ( )	NO ( )	Number of cigars per week:
E-cigarettes	YES ( )	NO ( )	Number of cartridge per day or week:
Waterpipe/hookah	YES ( )	NO ( )	Approximate amount of time per day or week:
Smokeless	YES ( )	NO ( )	Number of cans/pouches per day/week:
Dissolvable strips, sticks, orbs, etc.	YES ( )	NO ( )	Amount per day or week:
Other types of tobacco products?	YES ( )	NO ( )	Amount per day or week:
Have you tried quitting tobacco use in the past?	YES ( )	NO ( )	If you have tried to quit: How long did you quit last time? What did you use to help you quit? What was the longest time you have quit? What has caused you to relapse?

FIGURE 32-3 • Sample Tobacco Use Assessment Form.

I. Dental Biofilm Control

- Self-care for daily dental biofilm control is the first priority in the care plan.
- Meticulous oral self-care is required by this group of high-risk patients owing to their susceptibility to dental caries, periodontal infections, and other soft-tissue alterations.

II. Nonsurgical Periodontal Therapy

- Inform the patient healing will be jeopardized by continued tobacco use, and users cannot expect the same treatment results as nonusers.[52,54]
- Inform the patient tobacco cessation would improve the results of treatment.[79]
- When using power-driven instruments:
  - Take precautions to protect the patient from aerosols-containing bacteria and debris (smokers often have pulmonary and cardiovascular complications).[1]

III. Other Patient Instruction

- *Diet and nutrition*
  - Tobacco users may be poorly nourished because tobacco use suppresses appetite.[80]
  - Conversely, the desire to control body weight through tobacco use may impede a patient's willingness to quit.[2]
  - Suggestions about diet and exercise are included as a part of the cessation program.[2]

TOBACCO CESSATION PROGRAM

- A program for tobacco cessation is an essential component of the oral healthcare plan for all tobacco-using patients.[2,64,81]
- The treatment of tobacco use and dependence will often require multiple appointments, repeated interventions, and multiple attempts to quit.[2,81]
- The dental setting provides an excellent opportunity to assist tobacco users in tobacco cessation.[2,64,81]
- Interventions and their outcomes will vary depending on the motivation and experience of the clinician and the patient's acceptance of, and adherence to, the regimen.[2,81]
- Even a minimal intervention conducted by a clinician may help a patient become tobacco free.[67]

MOTIVATIONAL INTERVIEWING

The use of brief motivational interviewing is an effective method of tobacco cessation. Motivation and improving self-confidence increase likelihood of tobacco cessation.[78,79]

Motivational interviewing techniques are described in Chapter 24, which can be useful in conversing with patients concerning behavior change.

THE "5 A's"

The "5 A's"—ask, advise, assess, assist, arrange—provide the basis for a brief, simple, but effective tobacco dependence intervention for clinicians.[2,82,83] A cessation program flowchart is presented in Figure 32-4.

I. Ask

- *Health history*
  - Ask all patients about tobacco use.[2,81]
  - Include questions about tobacco use on the health history (Chapter 11) and document tobacco use at every appointment.
- *Present questions carefully*[2]
  - During review of the health history, present questions related to tobacco use nonjudgmentally.
  - Address tobacco use as a health issue, not as a moral and/or social issue.
  - Obtain facts without placing the patient on the defensive.
- *Obtain patient's confidence*[2]
  - Express empathy and support patient's decision to choose or reject change.
  - Social disapproval of tobacco use is increasing, and patients may hesitate to disclose their habit.
- *Children and adolescents*
  - E-cigarettes are the most common tobacco product used among adolescents.[84]
  - In the United States, 6.6% of adolescents reported smoking a whole cigarette before 13 years of age.[85]
  - The two greatest factors effecting a child or adolescent smoking are parents who smoke and parental nicotine dependence.[86]
  - Brief counseling, including risk assessment, needs to be implemented to prevent initiation of tobacco use. Assessment should include parent's history of smoking, product access, smoking among peers, and tobacco advertisement exposure.[86]
  - Most smokers try their first cigarette at approximately 11 years of age.[85]
  - Children need to hear negative impact messages to counter messages produced by the tobacco industry.[38]
  - Discuss with the parents about the effects of ETS on health, developmental risks, and how tobacco use sets a bad example for children.[1]
  - Group-based behavioral interventions may be helpful in adolescent tobacco cessation.[74]

II. Advise[2,81]

A. Never Users/Former Users

- Advise every patient about tobacco use.
- Praise "never users" and "former users" for their tobacco-free behavior.
- Reinforcement counters the tobacco industry's message and other enticements to begin tobacco use and can help prevent relapse.

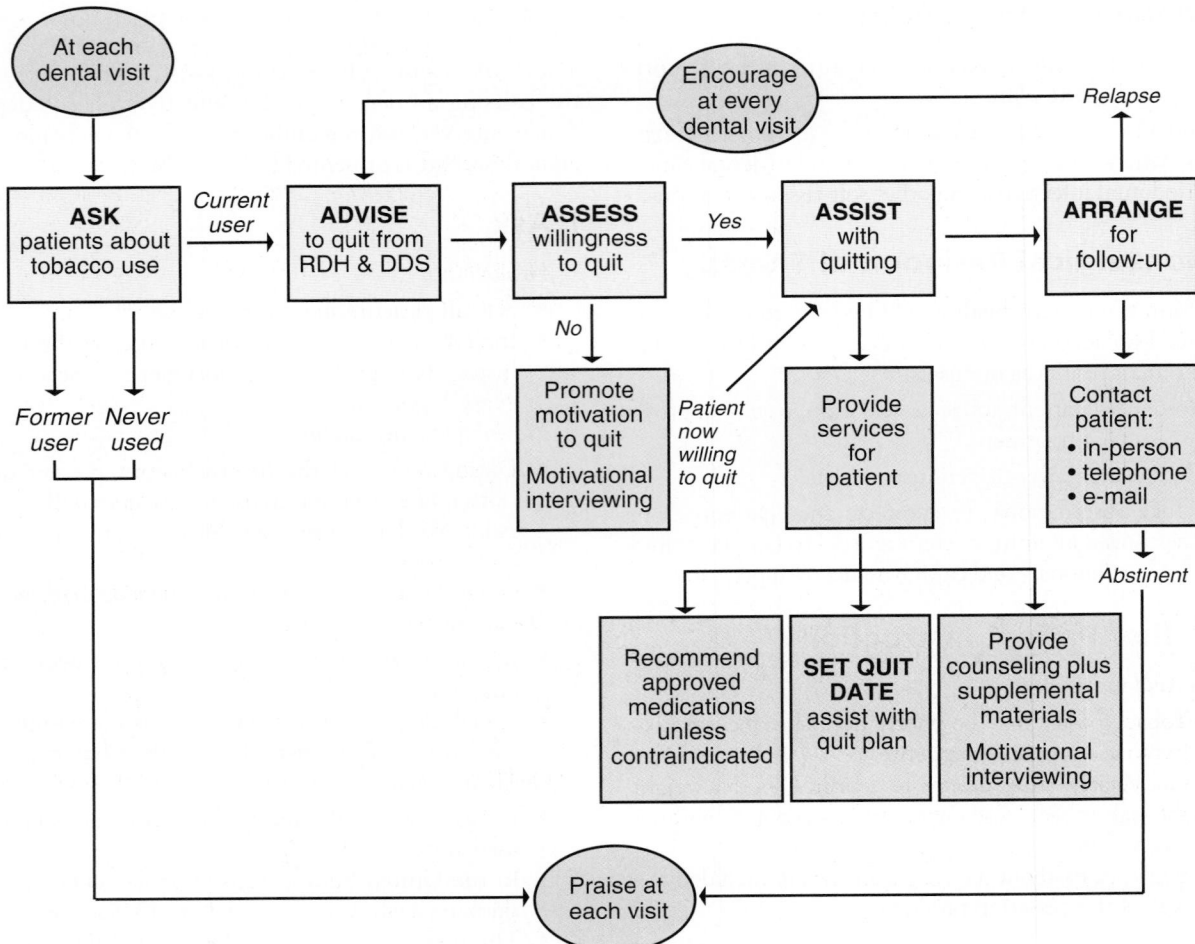

FIGURE 32-4 • Tobacco Cessation Flowchart. Flowchart to show how the 5 A's can be incorporated into the clinical setting. (Adapted from Fiore MC, Jaén CR, Baker TB, et al. Treating tobacco use and dependence: 2008 update. In: *Quick Reference Guide for Clinicians*. Rockville, MD: U.S. Department of Health and Human Services. Public Health Service; 2009.)

B. Current Users: Stop–Look–Listen Approach

1. *Stop now*: Clearly advise the patient about the importance of *stopping* now. Present the advice in a caring, compassionate manner so patients realize clinicians are interested in their health and well-being.

2. *Show*: Have patients *look* in their mouths during the initial oral examination to observe the clinical effects of tobacco use.
   - Patients may or may not be impressed by a discussion of possible future health problems or of the effect of tobacco use on others.
   - Advice needs to be relevant to existing conditions.
   - Existing oral conditions that may serve as strong motivators to quit.

3. *Listen*[2]:
   - Ask patients whether they want to quit and their reasons. Most users want to quit. Their reasons may have little to do with health, but verbalizing the reasons force patients to focus and strengthen their reasons.

- *Listening* to the patient allows the clinician to support the patient's thoughts and provide appropriate reinforcement.

III. Assess[2,81]

1. Ask the patient: "Are you ready to quit?"

2. If the patient is ready:
   - Determine whether the patient could best be treated in your practice. (A patient may have multiple problems necessitating referral.)
   - If treatment is provided in your office, go to the *assist* step.

3. If the patient is not ready to quit, use the "5 R's":
   - *Relevance*: Patient indicates personal importance of quitting.
   - *Risks*: Patient identifies negative consequences of continued use.
   - *Rewards*: Patient identifies personal benefits of quitting.

- *Roadblocks*: Patient identifies barriers to quitting, and clinician helps address barriers.
- *Repetition*: Reinforce the motivational message at every visit.

IV. Assist

A. Establish a Quit Plan

- Set a quit date, preferably within 2 weeks.[2,81]
- Have the patient tell family, friends, and coworkers about quitting and request their understanding and support.[2,81]
- Warn the patient to anticipate challenges to the planned quit attempt, particularly during the first few weeks. This includes nicotine withdrawal symptoms.
- Ask the patient to remove all tobacco-related products from home and work sites.[2]

B. Provide Practical Counseling

- Total abstinence is essential: "not even a single puff or dip after the quit date."
- Review past quit attempts and identify what helped and what factors contributed to relapse.
- Discuss challenges/triggers and how the patient will overcome them successfully.
- Because alcohol can cause relapse, the patient needs to limit/abstain from alcohol use.
- Quitting is more difficult when there is another smoker in the household. Tobacco-using housemates are encouraged to avoid use in the presence of the patient attempting to quit.
- Prolonged use of varenicline may assist in relapse prevention.[87]

C. Pharmacotherapy

- The combination of smoking cessation counseling and medication is more effective than either counseling or medication alone.[69]
- Suggest the use of approved OTC or prescription pharmacotherapy. Refer to Table 32-5.

D. Provide Educational Information

- Agencies publishing motivational materials are listed in Table 32-6.
- Web-based tobacco interventions have demonstrated promising evidence over the past few years. An e-referral program www.decide2quit.org is funded by the National Institutes of Health and is free service.[88,89]
- Specific educational materials are available for:
  - Various cultures and ethnic groups.
  - Different levels of education and literacy.
  - Readers of all ages.
    Keep a supply of these materials in the office for distribution to patients.
- Online communities can be supportive, providing motivation and reinforcing cessation.[90]

TABLE 32-6 • Sources for Tobacco Cessation Patient Educational Materials

NAME OF SOURCE	QUIT LINES	LINKS
American Cancer Society	1–877—yes quit 1–877—937–7848	www.yesquit.com https://www.cancer.org/treatment.html
American Lung Association	1-800-LUNGUSA	http://www.lung.org/support-and-community/
National Cancer Institute		www.cancer.gov
CDC Tobacco Information and Prevention Tips		www.cdc.gov/tobacco/
Nicotine Anonymous		www.nicotine-anonymous.org
QuitNet		www.quitnet.com
National Alliance for Tobacco Cessation		www.becomeanex.org
You Can Quit Smoking—Agency for Healthcare Research and Quality		www.ahrq.gov/consumer/tobacco
Smokefree.gov	National Quit Line 1–800—Quit-Now (1–800-784–8669)	www.smokefree.gov

V. Arrange

A. Follow-up

- Essential for successful quit rates.[2,81]
- Provide written documentation as a reminder, listing their quit date.
- Suggest posting quit-date reminders in visible locations, such as refrigerator door or bathroom mirror or placing index card, with the quit date between cellophane and paper of the cigarette package.[2,81]

B. Contact the Patient before the Quit Date

- Assure patient of care provider's sincere interest in their tobacco cessation attempt via telephone call, e-mail, or text message.[2]
- Inquire:
  - If information provided at initial contact has been helpful.
  - If the patient has any questions regarding the information received.
- *Follow-up contact*[2,81]
  - Follow-up, either in person or via telephone or e-mail.
  - Timely intervals would be once within the first week after the quit date when the patient's physical withdrawal symptoms are most intense, and again at the

end of the first, second, and third months of their tobacco cessation.

- More than four contacts with patient help to increase long-term abstinence.
- Follow-up at regularly scheduled continuing care appointments.

◆ *Actions during follow-up contact*[2,81]

- Congratulate and praise patients who have remained tobacco free.
- Provide the opportunity for patients to ask questions. If they have none, encourage the patient to contact you if questions arise.
- If relapse has occurred, ask the patient to recall and record the circumstances that led to reuse.[2,81]
- Encourage the patient to set another quit date, reminding the patient that a lapse can be a learning experience.[2,81]
- Review the use of pharmacotherapy.[2,81]
- Provide agencies and local contact numbers for the patient who requests a more intensive cessation program.

THE TEAM APPROACH

Evidence concludes that oral health professionals are more effective than other healthcare professionals in providing tobacco cessation interventions.[2,64]

I. Organize the Clinic Team[2]

◆ *Select a team coordinator*
◆ The coordinator does not do everything, but sees that everything is done.
◆ *Responsibilities*

- Identify tobacco use status at patient's first visit.
- Record appropriate documentation in patient's records.
- Ensure all tobacco-using patients are offered the opportunity to enter a cessation program.

- Contact patients for follow-up.
- Act as a coach for patients who relapse.
- Maintain a supply of literature for patients.

II. Organize a Tobacco-Free Environment[2]

◆ Display tobacco use prevention and cessation materials prominently.
◆ Eliminate magazines that contain tobacco advertising from reception area.

III. Organize a Tobacco User Tracking System

◆ *Tobacco use assessment form*: Figure 32-3.
◆ *Patient permanent progress report*: Records include dated case notes for all advice to quit, responses and interest in quitting, and progress.[2]
◆ *Tobacco status on records*: Clearly mark records (paper or electronic) so status can be immediately seen by any clinic staff.

ADVOCACY[1]

I. Public Health Policy

◆ The Surgeon General's Report on Oral Health was the first report of a Surgeon General focused on oral health, and the report specifically identified tobacco use as a risk factor for oral cavity and pharyngeal cancer.[91]
◆ Healthcare providers can help tobacco users quit and can become partners with one another and with community programs to prevent diseases and promote good health habits.
◆ The Centers for Disease Control and Prevention has been supporting state-based tobacco control coalitions in all 50 states. Many local communities

---

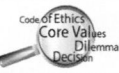

EVERYDAY ETHICS

Fifteen-year-old Jason comes with his mother for a regular maintenance appointment. During the oral examination, Edith, the dental hygienist who has been providing dental hygiene treatment for Jason and his family for many years, notices small red and white patches in the vestibular areas of the mandible adjacent to the molar teeth. She also records moderate brownish staining on the teeth and plans to use the air-powder polisher after scaling. She questions Jason about smoking and the use of smokeless tobacco, but he states he has tried cigarettes only once or twice.

Questions for Consideration

1. What approach can Edith use to further assess and enhance Jason's understanding of the oral effects of tobacco use if she suspects he is not telling the truth?

2. What alternatives does Edith have in reporting her assessment findings to maintain Jason's right to confidentiality but still inform his mother of the potentially serious oral tissue changes she has observed?

3. Which legal and ethical concepts apply to this situation?

and municipalities are considering or have adopted smoke-free workplace ordinances.[92]

◆ Oral health professionals can be valuable and collaborative partners in these programs.[64]

II. Community Oral Health Educational Programs

No community oral health program can be considered complete without inclusion of tobacco prevention, control, and cessation education. Excellent materials are available from many nonprofit and professional organizations.

DOCUMENTATION[2]

Careful and complete documentation of tobacco use is a component of each patient assessment. It is part of the health history for new patients and part of the clinical (progress) notes for maintenance patients.

◆ Include tobacco history and/or current use, type of tobacco, and amount typically used.

◆ Age, ethnicity, gender, periodontal, and overall dental status as well as oral cancer screening findings.

◆ Patient interest/confidence motivation/readiness to quit and previous quit attempts and techniques used.

◆ Options for cessation presented to patient and referrals to primary care provider for examination/treatment.

◆ Box 32-4 contains an example for tobacco use assessment and cessation treatment.

Factors to Teach the Patient

▶ The most effective method to stop using tobacco or nicotine use is never to start.

▶ How to perform a regular self-examination of the oral cavity.

▶ Pregnant women who use tobacco products can harm the developing fetus and the newborn infant.

▶ Young children may experiment with or use tobacco products. Parents can be educated so that they are prepared to provide guidance.

▶ All forms of social tobacco use can lead to addiction.

▶ Nonsmokers who breathe ETS can incur the same serious health problems as smokers; children are especially susceptible.

▶ Smokeless tobacco use is *not* a safe alternative to smoking.

▶ Oral health team members can help patients become tobacco free.

▶ Learn about local or state tobacco legislation and public health policy to make informed choices related to a tobacco smoke-free society.

BOX 32-4
Example Documentation:
Tobacco Use Assessment and Cessation Treatment

S—A 45-year-old African American male presents for second quadrant scaling, upper left (UL) with local anesthesia, and postscaling evaluation of first quadrant, upper right (UR). Cigarette smoker for 15 years; 1–2 packs a day. Patient states his oral self-care has improved since the initial quadrant scaling. Patient's chief complaint: Gums still sore from previous scaling appointment.

O—Intraoral assessment reveals slow healing for first quadrant scaling with localized inflammation and erythematous areas, evidence of nicotine stomatitis, other oral cancer finding negative, and no cavitated carious lesions. Periodontal examination findings: UL quadrant with generalized 5–6 mm pocket depths, and 7 mm pocket on #15 MB, bleeding on probing #14 and 15 buccal.

A—Patient presents with a high risk for oral and systemic disease due to tobacco dependence. Provided patient with smoking cessation basics, and explanation of oral and systemic effects of tobacco use. Brief discussion indicated patient is motivated to quit because he and his wife are expecting their first baby, but reports previous attempts to quit "Cold Turkey" were unsuccessful due to weight gain, mood swings, and increased stress.

P—Patient congratulated on wanting to quit and reminded previous attempts at quitting should not be looked upon as failures. Introduced various options for cessation support. Patient agreed to Internet option www.smokefree.gov, with quitting apps; walked patient through the website. Additionally, patient agreed to 21 mg nicotine transdermal patch, transitioning to 14 mg, then 7 mg patch over 8–10 weeks, combining patch therapy with nicotine gum to help prevent weight gain and provide relief for additional withdrawal symptoms and cravings. Follow-up by telephone in 1 week and re-evaluate at next visit scheduled in 2 weeks.

Next visit: Scale lower right quadrant with local anesthesia, reassess UL quadrant, and continue tobacco cessation counseling.

Signed: _____, RDH

Date: _____

ENHANCE YOUR UNDERSTANDING

ONLINE RESOURCES
(see the inside front cover for access information)
- Audio glossary
- Appendices

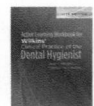

SUPPORT FOR LEARNING
(available separately)
- *Active Learning Workbook for Wilkins' Clinical Practice of the Dental Hygienist, 13th Edition*

INDIVIDUALIZED REVIEW
- Customized practice quizzing with Navigate 2 TestPrep for *Wilkins' Clinical Practice of the Dental Hygienist*

References

1. U.S. Department of Health and Human Services. *The Health Consequences of Smoking—50 Years of Progress: A Report of the Surgeon General*. Atlanta, GA: Centers for Disease Control and Prevention (US); 2014.

2. Fiore MC, Jaen CR, Baker TB, et al. *Treating Tobacco Use and Dependence: 2008 Update. Quick Reference Guide for Clinicians*. Rockville, MD: U.S. Department of Health and Human Services. Public Health Service; 2009.

3. Hu S, Neff L, Agaku I, et al. Tobacco product use among adults—United States, 2013-2014. *MMWR Morb Mortal Wkly Rep*. 2016;65:685-691. doi:10.15585/mmwr.mm6527a1.

4. Sung H, Wang Y, Yao T, Lightwood J, Max W. Polytobacco use of cigarettes, cigars, chewing tobacco, and snuff among U.S. adults. *Nicotine Tob Res*. 2016;18:817-826.

5. Ko T, Tsai L, Chu L, et al. Parental smoking during pregnancy and its association with low birth weight, small for gestational age, and preterm birth offspring: a birth cohort study. *Pediatr Neonatol*. 2014;55(1):20-27.

6. Singh T, Arrazola RA, Corey CG, et al. Tobacco use among middle and high school students—United States, 2011-2015. *MMWR Morb Mortal Wkly Rep*. 2016;65(14):361-367. doi:10.15585/mmwr.mm6514a1.

7. American Cancer Society. Cancer facts and figures 2017. 2017. https://www.cancer.org/content/dam/cancer-org/research/cancer-facts-and-statistics/annual-cancer-facts-and-figures/2017/cancer-facts-and-figures-2017.pdf. Accessed November 28, 2017.

8. Benowitz NL, Hukkanen J, Jacob P. Nicotine chemistry, metabolism, kinetics, and biomarkers. *Handb Exp Pharmacol*. 2009;192:29-60. doi:10.1007/978-3-540-69248-5_2.

9. Maisto SA, Galizio M, Connors GJ. *Drug Use and Abuse*. 8th ed. Boston, MA: Cengage Learning, Inc.; 2019.

10. Office on Smoking and Health. Centers for Disease Control and Prevention (CDC). *The Health Consequences of Involuntary Exposure to Tobacco Smoke: A Report of the Surgeon General*. Atlanta, GA: U.S. Department of Health and Human Services; 2006.

11. U.S. Department of Health and Human Services. *How Tobacco Smoke Causes Disease: The Biology and Behavioral Basis for Smoking-Attributable Disease: A Report of the Surgeon General*. 2010. http://www.cdc.gov/tobacco/data_statistics/sgr/2010/index.htm.

12. Food and Drug Administration. *Harmful and Potentially Harmful Constituents in Tobacco Products and Tobacco Smoke; Established List*. Atlanta, GA: U.S. Department of Health and Human Services; 2012.

13. Djordjevic MV, Doran KA. Nicotine content and delivery across tobacco products. *Handb Exp Pharmacol*. 2009;192:61-82. doi:10.1007/978-3-540-69248-5_3.

14. McMillen R, Maduka J, Winickoff J. Use of emerging tobacco products in the United States. *J Environ Public Health*. 2012;2012:989474. doi:10.1155/2012/989474.

15. U.S. Department of Health and Human Services. *E-Cigarette Use among Youth and Young Adults. A Report of the Surgeon General*. Atlanta, GA: U.S. Department of Health and Human Services, Centers for Disease Control and Prevention, National Center for Chronic Disease Prevention and Health Promotion, Office on Smoking and Health; 2016.

16. U.S. Food and Drug Administration. Deeming Tobacco Products to Be Subject to the Federal Food, Drug, and Cosmetic Act, as Amended by the Family Smoking Prevention and Tobacco Control Act; Restrictions on the Sale and Distribution of Tobacco Products and Required Warning Statements for Tobacco Products. Federal Register. https://www.federalregister.gov/documents/2016/05/10/2016-10685/deeming-tobacco-products-to-be-subject-to-the-federal-food-drug-and-cosmetic-act-as-amended-by-the. Published May 10, 2016. Accessed November 28, 2017.

17. Centers for Disease Control and Prevention, Office on Smoking and Health. Smokeless tobacco: products and marketing. https://www.cdc.gov/tobacco/data_statistics/fact_sheets/smokeless/products_marketing/index.htm. Accessed November 19, 2017.

18. World Health Organization. Smokeless tobacco and some tobacco-specific N-Nitrosamines. 2007. https://www.cabdirect.org/cabdirect/abstract/20083307001. Accessed January 20, 2018.

19. Munshi T, Heckman CJ, Darlow S. Association between tobacco waterpipe smoking and head and neck conditions: a systematic review. *J Am Dent Assoc 1939*. 2015;146(10):760-766. doi:10.1016/j.adaj.2015.04.014.

20. Maziak W, Ben Taleb Z, Jawad M, et al. Consensus statement on assessment of waterpipe smoking in epidemiological studies. *Tob Control*. 2017;26(3):338-343. doi:10.1136/tobaccocontrol-2016-052958.

21. U.S. Food and Drug Administration. Hookah Tobacco (Shisha or Waterpipe Tobacco). https://www.fda.gov/TobaccoProducts/Labeling/ProductsIngredientsComponents/ucm482575.htm#stats. Accessed November 28, 2017.

22. Waziry R, Jawad M, Ballout RA, Al Akel M, Akl EA. The effects of waterpipe tobacco smoking on health outcomes: an updated systematic review and meta-analysis. *Int J Epidemiol*. 2017;46(1):32-43. doi:10.1093/ije/dyw021.

23. U.S. Food and Drug Administration. Vapes, E-Cigs, Hookah Pens, and other Electronic Nicotine Delivery Systems (ENDS). https://www.fda.gov/TobaccoProducts/Labeling/Products IngredientsComponents/ucm456610.htm. Accessed November 28, 2017.

24. U.S. Food and Drug Administration. Electronic cigarettes (e-cigarettes). 2014. http://www.fda.gov/newsevents /publichealthfocus/ucm172906.htm.

25. Hartmann-Boyce J, McRobbie H, Bullen C, Begh R, Stead LF, Hajek P. Electronic cigarettes for smoking cessation. *Cochrane Database Syst Rev.* 2016;(9):CD010216. doi:10.1002/14651858.CD010216.pub3.

26. Glasser AM, Collins L, Pearson JL, et al. Overview of electronic nicotine delivery systems: a systematic review. *Am J Prev Med.* 2017;52(2):e33-e66. doi:10.1016 /j.amepre.2016.10.036.

27. U.S. Cancer Statistics. https://nccd.cdc.gov/uscs/. Accessed January 21, 2018.

28. National Institute of Dental and Craniofacial Research. Oral cancer. https://www.nidcr.nih.gov/oralhealth/Topics /OralCancer/. Accessed November 28, 2017.

29. National Cancer Institute at the National Institutes of Health. *What You Need to Know about Oral Cancer.* U.S. Department of Health and Human Service. NIH Publication No. 09-1574. http://www.nidcd.nih.gov.

30. National Cancer Institute at the National Institutes of Health. *Health Effects of Exposure to Environmental Tobacco Smoke: The Report of the California Environmental Protection Agency. Smoking and Tobacco Control Monograph no. 10..* Bethesda, MD. U.S. Department of Health and Human Services, National Institutes of Health, National Cancer Institute; 1999.

31. Centers for Disease Control and Prevention. Secondhand smoke: an unequal danger. *Vital Signs.* 2015. https://www .cdc.gov/vitalsigns/pdf/2015-02-vitalsigns.pdf.

32. Sleiman M, Gundel LA, Pankow JF, Jacob P, Singer BC, Destaillats H. Formation of carcinogens indoors by surface-mediated reactions of nicotine with nitrous acid, leading to potential thirdhand smoke hazards. *Proc Natl Acad Sci USA.* 2010;107(15):6576-6581. doi:10.1073 /pnas.0912820107.

33. Schick SF, Farraro KF, Perrino C, et al. Thirdhand cigarette smoke in an experimental chamber: evidence of surface deposition of nicotine, nitrosamines and polycyclic aromatic hydrocarbons and de novo formation of NNK. *Tob Control.* 2014;23(2):152-159. doi:10.1136 /tobaccocontrol-2012-050915.

34. Leonardi-Bee J, Jere ML, Britton J. Exposure to parental and sibling smoking and the risk of smoking uptake in childhood and adolescence: a systematic review and meta-analysis. *Thorax.* 2011;66(10):847-855. doi:10.1136/thx.2010.153379.

35. Hackshaw A, Rodeck C, Boniface S. Maternal smoking in pregnancy and birth defects: a systematic review based on 173 687 malformed cases and 11.7 million controls. *Hum Reprod Update.* 2011;17(5):589-604. doi:10.1093/humupd /dmr022.

36. Homa DM, Neff LJ, King BA, et al. Vital signs: disparities in nonsmokers' exposure to secondhand smoke—United States, 1999-2012. *MMWR Morb Mortal Wkly Rep.* 2015;64(4):103-108.

37. Burke H, Leonardi-Bee J, Hashim A, et al. Prenatal and passive smoke exposure and incidence of asthma and wheeze: systematic review and meta-analysis. *Pediatrics.* 2012;129(4):735-744. doi:10.1542/peds.2011-2196.

38. U.S. Department of Health and Human Services. *Preventing Tobacco Use among Youth and Young Adults: A Report of the Surgeon General.* Atlanta, GA: U.S. Department of Health and Human Services, Centers for Disease Control and Prevention, National Center for Chronic Disease Prevention and Health Promotion, Office on Smoking and Health; 2012. http://www.surgeongeneral.gov/library.

39. Ji EH, Sun B, Zhao T, et al. Correction: characterization of electronic cigarette aerosol and its induction of oxidative stress response in oral keratinocytes. *PLoS One.* 2016;11(12):e0169380. doi:10.1371/journal.pone.0169380.

40. Eke PI, Wei L, Thornton-Evans GO, et al. Risk indicators for periodontitis in U.S. adults: NHANES 2009 to 2012. *J Periodontol.* 2016;87(10):1174-1185. doi:10.1902/jop.2016.160013.

41. The American Academy of Periodontology. The parameters of care. *J Periodontol.* 2000;71(5 suppl):847-848.

42. Akinkugbe AA, Slade GD, Divaris K, Poole C. Systematic review and meta-analysis of the association between exposure to environmental tobacco smoke and periodontitis endpoints among nonsmokers. *Nicotine Tob Res Off J Soc Res Nicotine Tob.* 2016;18(11):2047-2056. doi:10.1093/ntr/ntw105.

43. Johannsen A, Susin C, Gustafsson A. Smoking and inflammation: evidence for a synergistic role in chronic disease. *Periodontol 2000.* 2014;64:111-126.

44. Mavropoulos A, Brodin P, Rosing KC, Aass AM, Aars H. Gingival blood flow in periodontitis patients before and after periodontal surgery assessed in smokers and non-smokers. *J Periodontol.* 2007;78(9):1774-1782.

45. Bahrami G, Vaeth M, Kirkevang L-L, Wenzel A, Isidor F. The impact of smoking on marginal bone loss in a 10-year prospective longitudinal study. *Community Dent Oral Epidemiol.* 2017;45(1):59-65. doi:10.1111/cdoe.12260.

46. Patel RA, Wilson RF, Palmer RM. The effect of smoking on periodontal bone regeneration: a systematic review and meta-analysis. *J Periodontol.* 2012;83(2):143-155.

47. Visvanathan R, Mahendra J, Ambalavanan N, Pandisuba, Chalini. Effect of smoking on periodontal health. *J Clin Diagn Res.* 2014;8(7):ZC46-ZC49. doi:10.7860 /JCDR/2014/8359.4597.

48. Hanioka T, Ojima M, Tanaka K, Matsuo K, Sato F, Tanaka H. Causal assessment of smoking and tooth loss: a systematic review of observational studies. *BMC Public Health.* 2011;11:221. doi:10.1186/1471-2458-11-221.

49. Karasneh JA, Al Habashneh RA, Marzouka NAS, Thornhill MH. Effect of cigarette smoking on subgingival bacteria in healthy subjects and patients with chronic periodontitis. *BMC Oral Health.* 2017;17(1):64. doi:10.1186 /s12903-017-0359-4.

50. Ramôa CP, Eissenberg T, Sahingur SE. Increasing popularity of waterpipe tobacco smoking and electronic cigarette use: implications for oral healthcare. *J Periodontal Res.* 2017;52(5):813-823. doi:10.1111/jre.12458.

51. Heasman L, Stacey F, Preshaw PM, McCracken GI, Hepburn S, Heasman PA. The effect of smoking on periodontal treatment response: a review of clinical evidence. *J Clin Periodontol.* 2006;33(4):241-253.

52. Research, Science and Therapy Committee of the American Academy of Periodontology. Position paper: tobacco use and the periodontal patient. *J Periodontol.* 1999;70(11):1419-1427. doi:10.1902/jop.1999.70.11.1419.

53. Chrcanovic BR, Albrektsson T, Wennerberg A. Smoking and dental implants: a systematic review and meta-analysis. *J Dent.* 2015;43(5):487-498. doi:10.1016/j.jdent.2015.03.003.

54. Chambrone L, Preshaw PM, Rosa EF, et al. Effects of smoking cessation on the outcomes of non-surgical periodontal therapy: a systematic review and individual patient data meta-analysis. *J Clin Periodontol.* 2013;40(6):607-615. doi:10.1111/jcpe.12106.

55. Rosa EF, Corraini P, de Carvalho VF, et al. A prospective 12-month study of the effect of smoking cessation on periodontal clinical parameters. *J Clin Periodontol.* 2011;38(6):562-571.

56. American Psychiatric Association. Tobacco-related disorders. In: *Diagnostic and Statistical Manual of Mental Disorders (DSM-5).* 5th ed. Arlington, VA: American Psychiatric Association; 2013:571-576.

57. Picciotto MR, Mineur YS. Molecules and circuits involved in nicotine addiction: the many faces of smoking. *Neuropharmacology.* 2014;76:545-553.

58. Tobacco Control Legal Consortium. Addiction. In: *The Verdict Is In: Findings From United States v. Philip Morris.* St. Paul, MN: Tobacco Control Legal Consortium; 2006.

59. Babb S, Malarcher A, Schauer G, Asman K, Jamal A. Quitting smoking among adults—United States, 2000-2015. *MMWR Morb Mortal Wkly Rep.* 2017;65(52):1457-1464. doi:10.15585/mmwr.mm6552a1.

60. Wellman RJ, O'Loughlin EK, Dugas EN, Montreuil A, Dutczak H, O'Loughlin J. Reasons for quitting smoking in young adult cigarette smokers. *Addict Behav.* 2018;77:28-33. doi:10.1016/j.addbeh.2017.09.010.

61. Rodu B, Plurphanswat N. Quit methods used by American smokers, 2013–2014. *Int J Environ Res Public Health.* 2017;14(11):1403. doi:10.3390/ijerph14111403.

62. Hartmann-Boyce J, Lancaster T, Stead LF. Print-based self-help interventions for smoking cessation. *Cochrane Database Syst Rev.* 2014;3(6):CD001118.

63. Lindson-Hawley N, Hartmann-Boyce J, Fanshawe TR, Begh R, Farley A, Lancaster T. Interventions to reduce harm from continued tobacco use. *Cochrane Database Syst Rev.* 2016;10:CD005231. doi:10.1002/14651858.CD005231.pub3.

64. Carr AB, Ebbert J. Interventions for tobacco cessation in the dental setting. *Cochrane Database Syst Rev.* 2012;13(6). doi:10.1002/14651858.CD005084.pub3.

65. Fiore MC. The new vital sign: assessing and documenting smoking status. *JAMA.* 1991;266(22):3183-3184.

66. Aveyard P, Begh R, Parsons A, West R. Brief opportunistic smoking cessation interventions: a systematic review and meta-analysis to compare advice to quit and offer of assistance. *Addiction.* 2010;107(6):1066-1073. doi:10.1111/j.1360-0443.2011.03770.x.

67. Van Schayck OCP, Williams S, Barchilon V, et al. Treating tobacco dependence: guidance for primary care on life-saving interventions. Position statement of the IPCRG.

NPJ Prim Care Respir Med. 2017;27(1):38. doi:10.1038/s41533-017-0039-5.

68. Taylor GMJ, Dalili MN, Semwal M, Civljak M, Sheikh A, Car J. Internet-based interventions for smoking cessation. *Cochrane Database Syst Rev.* 2017;(9):CD007078. doi:10.1002/14651858.CD007078.pub5.

69. Stead LF, Koilpillai P, Fanshawe TR, Lancaster T. Combined pharmacotherapy and behavioural interventions for smoking cessation. *Cochrane Database Syst Rev.* 2016;(3):CD008286. doi:10.1002/14651858.CD008286.pub3.

70. Stead LF, Perera R, Bullen C, et al. Nicotine replacement therapy for smoking cessation. *Cochrane Database Syst Rev.* 2012;(11). doi:10.1002/14651858.CD000146.pub4.

71. Agency for Healthcare Research and Quality. *Clinical Guidelines for Prescribing Pharmacotherapy for Smoking Cessation.* Rockville, MD: Agency for Healthcare Research and Quality; 2012. https://www.ahrq.gov/professionals/clinicians-providers/guidelines-recommendations/tobacco/prescrib.html. Accessed November 30, 2017.

72. Cahill K, Stevens S, Perera R, Lancaster T. Pharmacological interventions for smoking cessation: an overview and network meta-analysis. *Cochrane Database Syst Rev.* 2013;(5):CD009329. doi:10.1002/14651858.CD009329.pub2.

73. Chamberlain C, O'Mara-Eves A, Porter J, et al. Psychosocial interventions for supporting women to stop smoking in pregnancy. *Cochrane Database Syst Rev.* 2017;(2):CD001055. doi:10.1002/14651858.CD001055.pub5.

74. Fanshawe TR, Halliwell W, Lindson N, Aveyard P, Livingstone-Banks J, Hartmann-Boyce J. Tobacco cessation interventions for young people. *Cochrane Database Syst Rev.* 2017;(11):CD003289. doi:10.1002/14651858.CD003289.pub6.

75. Tahiri M, Mottillo S, Joseph L, Pilote L, Eisenberg MJ. Alternative smoking cessation aids: a meta-analysis of randomized controlled trials. *Am J Med.* 2012;125(6):576-584. doi:10.1016/j.amjmed.2011.09.028.

76. Mark AM. Knocking tobacco out. *J Am Dent Assoc 1939.* 2017;148(12):948. doi:10.1016/j.adaj.2017.09.028.

77. Kumar PS, Matthews CR, Joshi V, de Jager M, Aspiras M. Tobacco smoking affects bacterial acquisition and colonization in oral biofilms. *Infect Immun.* 2011;79(11):4730-4738. doi:10.1128/IAI.05371-11.

78. Shah SA, Ganesan SM, Varadharaj S, Dabdoub SM, Walters JD, Kumar PS. The making of a miscreant: tobacco smoke and the creation of pathogen-rich biofilms. *NPJ Biofilms Microbiomes.* 2017;3:26. doi:10.1038/s41522-017-0033-2.

79. Fiorini T, Musskopf ML, Oppermann RV, Susin C. Is there a positive effect of smoking cessation on periodontal health? A systematic review. *J Periodontol.* 2014;85(1):83-91. doi:10.1902/jop.2013.130047.

80. Audrain-McGovern J, Benowitz N. Cigarette smoking, nicotine, and body weight. *Clin Pharmacol Ther.* 2011;90(1):164-168. doi:10.1038/clpt.2011.105.

81. Ramseier CA, Warnakulasuriya S, Needleman IG, et al. Consensus report: 2nd European workshop on tobacco use prevention and cessation for oral health professionals. *Int Dent J.* 2010;60(1):3-6.

82. Siu AL, U.S. Preventive Services Task Force. Behavioral and pharmacotherapy interventions for tobacco smoking

cessation in adults, including pregnant women: U.S. Preventive Services Task Force recommendation statement. *Ann Intern Med.* 2015;163(8):622-634. doi:10.7326/M15-2023.

83. Agency for Healthcare Research and Quality, U.S. Department of Health and Human Services. *Five Major Steps to Intervention (The "5A's").* https://www.ahrq.gov/sites/default/files/wysiwyg/professionals/clinicians-providers/guidelines-recommendations/tobacco/5steps.pdf. Accessed January 27, 2018.

84. Jamal A, King BA, Neff LJ, Whitmill J, Babb SD, Graffunder CM. Current cigarette smoking among adults—United States, 2005-2015. *MMWR Morb Mortal Wkly Rep.* 2016;65(44):1205-1211. doi:10.15585/mmwr.mm6544a2.

85. Kann L, McManus T, Harris WA, et al. Youth risk behavior surveillance—United States, 2015. *Morb Mortal Wkly Rep Surveill Summ.* 2016;65(6):1-174. doi:10.15585/mmwr.ss6506a1.

86. Moyer VA, U.S. Preventive Services Task Force. Primary care interventions to prevent tobacco use in children and adolescents: U.S. preventive services taskforce recommendation statement. *Pediatrics.* 2013;132(3):560-565. doi:10.1542/peds.2013-2079.

87. Hajek P, Stead LF, West R, Jarvis M, Hartmann-Boyce J, Lancaster T. Relapse prevention interventions for smoking cessation. *Cochrane Database Syst Rev.* 2013;(8):CD003999. doi:10.1002/14651858.CD003999.pub4.

88. Ray MN, Funkhouser E, Williams JH, et al. Smoking-cessation e-referrals: a national dental practice-based research network randomized controlled trial. *Am J Prev Med.* 2014;46(2):158-165. doi:10.1016/j.amepre.2013.10.018.

89. Sadasivam RS, Kinney RL, Delaughter K, et al. Who participates in Web-assisted tobacco interventions? The QUIT-PRIMO and National Dental Practice-Based Research Network Hi-Quit studies. *J Med Internet Res.* 2013;15(5). doi:10.2196/jmir.2385.

90. Cutrona SL, Sadasivam RS, DeLaughter K, et al. Online tobacco websites and online communities-who uses them and do users quit smoking? The quit-primo and national dental practice-based research network Hi-Quit studies. *Transl Behav Med.* 2016;6(4):546-557. doi:10.1007/s13142-015-0373-5.

91. U.S. Department of Health and Human Services PHS National Institutes of Health, National Institute of Dental and Craniofacial Research. *National Call to Action to Promote Oral Health.* Rockville, MD: National Institute of Dental and Craniofacial Research (US); 2003.

92. Centers for Disease Control and Prevention, National Center for Chronic Disease Prevention and Health Promotion, Office on Smoking and Health. *Best Practices for Comprehensive Tobacco Control Programs-2014.* Atlanta, GA: Centers for Disease Control and Prevention. https://www.cdc.gov/tobacco/stateandcommunity/best_practices/pdfs/2014/comprehensive.pdf. Accessed January 28, 2018.

93. World Health Organization. *Waterpipe Tobacco Smoking: Health Effects, Research Needs, and Recommended Actions by Regulators.* 2005. http://www.who.int/tobacco/global_interaction/tobreg/Waterpipe%20recommendation_Final.pdf.

33

Diet and Dietary Analysis

Lisa F. Mallonee, RDH, RD, LD, MPH

CHAPTER OUTLINE

NUTRIENT STANDARDS FOR DIET ADEQUACY IN HEALTH PROMOTION
I. Government Standards
II. Dietary Standards
III. Dietary Guidelines for Americans
IV. MyPlate Food Guidelines
V. Recommended Food Intake Patterns

ORAL HEALTH RELATIONSHIPS
I. Skin and Mucous Membrane
II. Periodontal Tissues
III. Tooth Structure and Integrity
IV. Dental Caries

COUNSELING FOR DENTAL CARIES CONTROL

THE DIETARY ASSESSMENT
I. Purposes of a Dietary Assessment
II. Preliminary Preparation for Dietary Assessment
III. Forms Used for Assessment
IV. Presentation of the Food Diary to the Patient
V. Receiving the Completed Food Diary
VI. Analysis of Dietary Intake

PREPARATION FOR ADDITIONAL COUNSELING
I. Define Objectives
II. Planning Factors
III. Appropriate Teaching Materials

COUNSELING PROCEDURES
I. Setting

II. Setting the Stage for a Successful Counseling Session
III. Presentation of Findings
IV. Specific Dietary Recommendations

EVALUATION OF PROGRESS
I. Immediate Evaluation
II. Three-Month Follow-up
III. Six-Month Follow-up
IV. Overall Evaluation

DOCUMENTATION

EVERYDAY ETHICS

FACTORS TO TEACH THE PATIENT

REFERENCES

LEARNING OBJECTIVES

After studying this chapter, the student will be able to:

1. Recognize oral manifestations of vitamin and mineral deficiencies.

2. Explain the function of nutrients in maintaining oral and overall health.

3. Identify good food sources for each micronutrient relevant to oral health.

4. Determine the caries risk potential of a patient's food record.

5. Access and utilize the MyPlate website for diet analysis and as a tool for patient education.

Nutrition is an integral part of an individual's general health as well as the health status of the oral cavity. The health of oral tissues can be affected by nutrition, diet, and food habits.

- The interrelationship between nutritional status, systemic diseases, and oral conditions supports the need for timely and effective diet intervention.
- Within the scope of practice, the dental hygienist has a responsibility to assess, screen, and deliver nutritional information and instruction as part of comprehensive education in health promotion and disease prevention and intervention.
- Dietary and nutritional counseling, as part of a dental caries control program and periodontal maintenance, is an essential part of the dental hygiene care plan.

NUTRIENT STANDARDS FOR DIET ADEQUACY IN HEALTH PROMOTION

- Patient education centers on helping patients learn about selection of foods that make up a healthy diet.

I. Government Standards

A. Purposes of Standards

- Facilitate education for individuals about dietary needs and goals to achieve and maintain health.
- Prevent deficiency diseases and help achieve diet adequacy for the public.
- Make recommendations relative to poor food habits, such as missed meals, omission of essential foods and nutrients, and fad dieting.
- Make specific recommendations for oral health.
- Motivate for behavioral modification.

B. Guidelines

- Provide guidelines through printed and web-based educational materials.
- Guidelines reflect public health concerns as they relate to nutrition.

II. Dietary Standards

A. Dietary Reference Intakes (DRI)

- Dietary reference intakes (DRI) is a comprehensive term for categories of reference values to meet the general nutrient needs for the healthy population to prevent deficiencies, toxicities, and chronic disease.
- Encompasses the current nutrient recommendations made by the Institute of Medicine (IOM), National Academy of Sciences, and Food and Nutrition Board.[1]
- The categories include:
  - Recommended Dietary Allowance (RDA).
  - Adequate Intake (AI).
  - Estimated Average Requirement (EAR).
  - Tolerable Upper Intake Level (UL).
- Established for vitamins and minerals.

B. Estimated Average Requirements

- Estimates the nutritional requirements of the average individual.[1]
- Categorized by age and gender.
- Provide the foundation for the RDAs.

C. Recommended Dietary Allowances

- Recommended amounts of macronutrients and micronutrients needed to consume daily to maintain good health and prevent deficiency.[2]
- Categorized by age and gender; do not include special needs such as illness.
- Based on gender and age; do not include special needs such as in illness.

D. Adequate Intakes

- The AI is the recommended nutrient intake utilized when there is not enough information to establish an EAR.[2,3]
- AIs have been established for calcium, vitamin D, and fluoride for all age groups.

E. Tolerable Upper Intake Levels

- The UL is the maximum intake by an individual that is unlikely to create risks of adverse health effects in almost all healthy individuals.
- ULs were established to avoid toxicity due to excess intake of specific nutrients from food, fortified food, water, and nutrient supplements.[2,3]

III. Dietary Guidelines for Americans

- Established by U.S. Department of Agriculture (USDA) and U.S. Department of Health and Human Services as the basis for a federal nutrition policy based on the most recent scientific evidence review.
- Provides information and advice for choosing healthy eating patterns that focus on consuming nutrient-dense foods to promote a healthy weight and reduce risk of chronic disease.
- Includes food safety principles to avoid foodborne illness.
- Used as the basis for developing nutrition-related programs, educational materials, and consumer health messages to promote healthy eating patterns at home, school, work, community, and food retail.
- Box 33-1 lists key recommendations in the 2015–2020 Dietary Guidelines for Americans.

BOX 33-1

Key Recommendations: Dietary Guidelines for Americans, 2015–2020

- Follow a healthy eating pattern across the life span to maintain healthy weight and reduce risk of chronic disease.
- Choose a variety of nutrient-dense foods from each food group in recommended amounts.
- Consume an eating pattern low in added sugars, saturated fats, and sodium.
- Choose nutrient-dense food and beverages in place of less healthy choices.
- Support healthy eating patterns for all—locally and nationwide.

Source: U.S. Department of Health and Human Services and U.S. Department of Agriculture. *2015–2020 Dietary Guidelines for Americans.* 8th ed. December 2015. Available at http://health.gov/dietaryguidelines/2015/guidelines/. Accessed January 21, 2019.

IV. MyPlate Food Guidelines

- ◆ Originally developed as a "Food Pyramid" by the USDA in 1991.[4]
- ◆ Newest version established in June 2011 using the graphic representation of a "dinner-plate" icon as illustrated in Figure 33-1.
- ◆ Colorful graphic provides a visual reminder of the approximate proportions of five food groups necessary for a healthy diet.

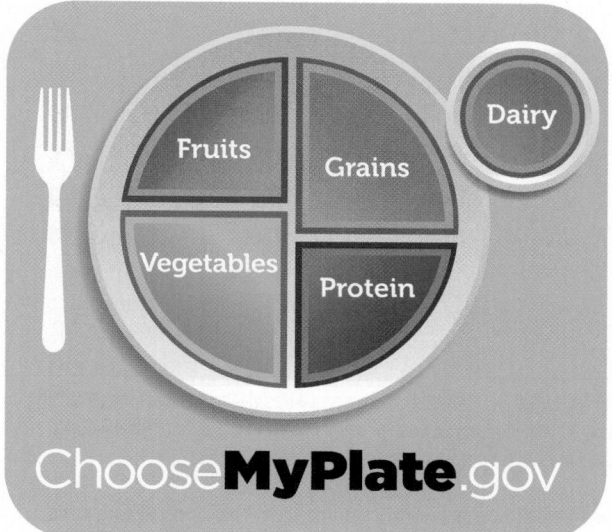

FIGURE 33-1 • ChooseMyPlate Guidelines Icon. (From U.S. Department of Agriculture, Center for Nutrition Policy and Promotion. ChooseMyPlate guidelines. 2011. http://www.choosemyplate.gov. Accessed January 18, 2019.)

- ◆ Educational materials accompanying the MyPlate food guidance system encourage consumers to build a healthy plate:
  - Make half the plate vegetables and fruits.
  - Switch to fat-free or low-fat milk.
  - Choose whole grains.
  - Vary protein choices to include seafood and legumes and keep meat portions small.
  - Cut back on foods high in solid fat, added sugars, and salt.
  - Eat the right amount of calories to maintain a healthy weight.
  - Enjoy food, but eat less and keep track of what is consumed.
  - Cook more often at home and choose lower calorie options when eating out.
  - Limit alcoholic beverages.
  - Be physically active.

V. Recommended Food Intake Patterns

- ◆ Including estimated calorie needs and recommended amounts of food from each food group accompany the MyPlate food guidelines.
- ◆ Individual plans based on age, gender, weight, height, and activity levels can be created.
- ◆ Provide option to create a plan to maintain current weight or achieve a healthy weight.
- ◆ Estimated calorie needs based on gender, age, and activity level are presented in Table 33-1.
- ◆ Twelve-calorie patterns ranging from 1,000 to 3,200 kilocalories provide specific amounts of food consumption from each of the food groups, subgroups, oils, and limits on calories from solid fats and added sugars, as presented in Table 33-2.

ORAL HEALTH RELATIONSHIPS

- ◆ Nutrition, diet, and oral health are closely interrelated.
- ◆ The oral cavity is the gateway to the body.
- ◆ Healthy masticatory function of the dentition contributes to proper dietary selection for maintenance of the nutritional status of the entire body.
- ◆ Healthy diet selection provides essential nutrients for optimum health of oral tissues and prevention of nutrient deficiency. Table 33-3 outlines micronutrients relevant to oral health, their function, associated deficiency state(s), and food sources.

I. Skin and Mucous Membrane

- ◆ Relevant vitamins: vitamin A, vitamin B complex, and ascorbic acid (vitamin C).
- ◆ Relevant minerals: zinc and iron.

TABLE 33-1 • Estimated Calorie Needs Per Day by Age, Gender, and Physical Activity Level

| | MALE | | | FEMALE[b] | | |
| | ACTIVITY LEVEL[a] | | | | | |
AGE (YEARS)	SEDENTARY	MODERATELY ACTIVE	ACTIVE	SEDENTARY	MODERATELY ACTIVE	ACTIVE

Estimated amounts of calories[c] needed to maintain calorie balance for various gender and age groups at three different levels of physical activity. The estimates are rounded to the nearest 200 calories for assignment to a USDA Food Pattern. An individual's calorie needs may be higher or lower than these average estimates.

AGE (YEARS)	SEDENTARY	MODERATELY ACTIVE	ACTIVE	SEDENTARY	MODERATELY ACTIVE	ACTIVE
2	1,000	1,000	1,000	1,000	1,000	1,000
3	1,200	1,400	1,400	1,000	1,200	1,400
4	1,200	1,400	1,600	1,200	1,400	1,400
5	1,200	1,400	1,600	1,200	1,400	1,600
6	1,400	1,600	1,800	1,200	1,400	1,600
7	1,400	1,600	1,800	1,200	1,600	1,800
8	1,400	1,600	2,000	1,400	1,600	1,800
9	1,600	1,800	2,000	1,400	1,600	1,800
10	1,600	1,800	2,200	1,400	1,800	2,000
11	1,800	2,000	2,200	1,600	1,800	2,000
12	1,800	2,200	2,400	1,600	2,000	2,200
13	2,000	2,200	2,600	1,600	2,000	2,200
14	2,000	2,400	2,800	1,800	2,000	2,400
15	2,200	2,600	3,000	1,800	2,000	2,400
16	2,400	2,800	3,200	1,800	2,000	2,400
17	2,400	2,800	3,200	1,800	2,000	2,400
18	2,400	2,800	3,200	1,800	2,000	2,400
19–20	2,600	2,800	3,000	2,000	2,200	2,400
21–25	2,400	2,800	3,000	2,000	2,200	2,400
26–30	2,400	2,600	3,000	1,800	2,000	2,400
31–35	2,400	2,600	3,000	1,800	2,000	2,200
36–40	2,400	2,600	2,800	1,800	2,000	2,200
41–45	2,200	2,600	2,800	1,800	2,000	2,200
46–50	2,200	2,400	2,800	1,800	2,000	2,200
51–55	2,200	2,400	2,800	1,600	1,800	2,200
56–60	2,200	2,400	2,600	1,600	1,800	2,200
61–65	2,000	2,400	2,600	1,600	1,800	2,000
66–70	2,000	2,200	2,600	1,600	1,800	2,000
71–75	2,000	2,200	2,600	1,600	1,800	2,000
76+	2,000	2,200	2,400	1,600	1,800	2,000

[a]Sedentary means a lifestyle that includes only the light physical activity associated with typical day-to-day life. Moderately active means a lifestyle that includes physical activity equivalent to walking about 1.5–3 miles/d at 3–4 miles/hr, in addition to the light physical activity associated with typical day-to-day life. Active means a lifestyle that includes physical activity equivalent to walking more than 3 miles/d at 3–4 miles/hr, in addition to the light physical activity associated with typical day-to-day life.

[b]Estimates for females do not include women who are pregnant or breastfeeding.

[c]Based on estimated energy requirements (EER) equations, using reference heights (average) and reference weights (healthy) for each age-gender group. For children and adolescents, reference height and weight vary. For adults, the reference man is 5 feet 10 inches tall and weighs 154 pounds. The reference woman is 5 feet 4 inches tall and weighs 126 pounds. EER equations are from the Institute of Medicine. *Dietary Reference Intakes for Energy, Carbohydrate, Fiber, Fat, Fatty Acids, Cholesterol, Protein, and Amino Acids.* Washington, DC: The National Academies Press; 2002.

USDA, U.S. Department of Agriculture.

Source: U.S. Department of Agriculture, Center for Nutrition Policy and Promotion. Mission. 2015. www.cnpp.usda.gov.

TABLE 33-2 • USDA Food Patterns-Healthy U.S.-Style Pattern

CALORIE LEVEL OF PATTERN[a] FOOD GROUP[b]	1,000	1,200	1,400	1,600	1,800	2,000	2,200	2,400	2,600	2,800	3,000	3,200
	DAILY AMOUNT[c] OF FOOD FROM EACH GROUP (VEGETABLES AND PROTEIN FOODS SUBGROUP AMOUNTS ARE PER WEEK)											
Fruits (c-eq)	1	1	1½	1½	1½	2	2	2	2	2½	2½	2½
Vegetables (c-eq)	1	1½	1½	2	2½	2½	3	3	3½	3½	4	4
Dark green vegetables (c-eq/wk)	½	1	1	1½	1½	1½	2	2	2½	2½	2½	2½
Red/orange vegetables (c-eq/wk)	2½	3	3	4	5½	5½	6	6	7	7	7½	7½
Beans and peas (c-eq/wk)	½	½	½	1	1½	1½	2	2	2½	2½	3	3
Starchy vegetables (c-eq/wk)	2	3½	3½	4	5	5	6	6	7	7	8	8
Other vegetables (c-eq/wk)	1½	2½	2½	3½	4	4	5	5	5½	5½	7	7
Grains (oz-eq)	**3**	**4**	**5**	**5**	**6**	**6**	**7**	**8**	**9**	**10**	**10**	**10**
Whole grains[d] (oz-eq/day)	1½	2	2½	3	3	3	3½	4	4½	5	5	5
Refined grains (oz-eq/day)	1½	2	2½	2	3	3	3½	4	4½	5	5	5
Protein foods (oz-eq)	**2**	**3**	**4**	**5**	**5**	**5½**	**6**	**6½**	**6½**	**7**	**7**	**7**
Meats, poultry, eggs (oz-eq/wk)	10	14	19	23	23	26	28	31	31	33	33	33
Seafood (oz-eq/wk)	3	4	6	8	8	8	9	10	10	10	10	10
Nuts, seeds, soy products (oz-eq/wk)	2	2	3	4	4	5	5	5	5	6	6	6
Dairy (c-eq)	**2**	**2½**	**2½**	**3**	**3**	**3**	**3**	**3**	**3**	**3**	**3**	**3**
Oils (g)	**15**	**17**	**17**	**22**	**24**	**27**	**29**	**31**	**34**	**36**	**44**	**51**
Limit on calories for other uses[e,f]												
Calories	150	100	110	130	170	270	280	350	380	400	470	610
Percent of calories	15	8	8	8	9	14	13	15	15	14	16	19

[a]Food intake patterns at 1,000, 1,200, and 1,400 calories are designed to meet the nutritional needs of 2- to 8-year-old children. Patterns from 1,600 to 3,200 calories are designed to meet the nutritional needs of children aged 9 years and older and adults. If a child aged 4 to 8 years needs more calories and, therefore, is following a pattern at 1,600 calories or more, his or her recommended amount from the dairy group should be 2.5 cups/d. Children aged 9 years and older and adults should not use the 1,000-, 1,200-, or 1,400-calorie patterns.
[b]Foods in each group and subgroup are:

Vegetables
- Dark green vegetables: All fresh, frozen, and canned dark green leafy vegetables and broccoli, cooked or raw: for example, broccoli, spinach, romaine, kale, and collard, turnip, and mustard greens.
- Red and orange vegetables: All fresh, frozen, and canned red and orange vegetables or juice, cooked or raw: for example, tomatoes, tomato juice, red peppers, carrots, sweet potatoes, winter squash, and pumpkin.
- Legumes (beans and peas): All cooked from dry or canned beans and peas: for example, kidney beans, white beans, black beans, lentils, chickpeas, pinto beans, split peas, and edamame (green soybeans). Does not include green beans or green peas.
- Starchy vegetables: All fresh, frozen, and canned starchy vegetables: for example, white potatoes, corn, green peas, green lima beans, plantains, and cassava.
- Other vegetables: All other fresh, frozen, and canned vegetables, cooked or raw: for example, iceberg lettuce, green beans, onions, cucumbers, cabbage, celery, zucchini, mushrooms, and green peppers.

Fruits
- All fresh, frozen, canned, and dried fruits and fruit juices: for example, oranges and orange juice, apples and apple juice, bananas, grapes, melons, berries, and raisins.

Grains
- Whole grains: All whole-grain products and whole grains used as ingredients: for example, whole-wheat bread, whole-grain cereals and crackers, oatmeal, quinoa, popcorn, and brown rice.
- Refined grains: All refined grain products and refined grains used as ingredients: for example, white breads, refined grain cereals and crackers, pasta, and white rice. Refined grain choices should be enriched.
- Protein foods.
- All seafood, meats, poultry, eggs, soy products, nuts, and seeds. Meats and poultry should be lean or low fat, and nuts should be unsalted. Legumes (beans and peas) can be considered part of this group as well as the vegetable group, but should be counted in one group only.

Dairy
◆ All milk, including lactose-free and lactose-reduced products and fortified soy beverages (soymilk), yogurt, frozen yogurt, dairy desserts, and cheeses. Most choices should be fat free or low fat. Cream, sour cream, and cream cheese are not included due to their low calcium content.

^cFood group amounts shown in cup-(c) or ounce-equivalents (oz-eq). Oils are shown in grams (g). Quantity equivalents for each food group are:
◆ Fruits and vegetables, 1 cup-equivalent is: 1 cup raw or cooked fruit or vegetable, 1 cup fruit or vegetable juice, 2 cups leafy salad greens, ½ cup dried fruit or vegetable.
◆ Grains, 1 ounce-equivalent is: ½ cup cooked rice, pasta, or cereal; 1 ounce dry pasta or rice; 1 medium (1 ounce) slice bread; 1 ounce of ready-to-eat cereal (about 1 cup of flaked cereal).
◆ Protein foods, 1 ounce-equivalent is: 1 ounce lean meat, poultry, or seafood; 1 egg; ¼ cup cooked beans or tofu; 1 tablespoon peanut butter; ½ ounce nuts or seeds.
◆ Dairy, 1 cup-equivalent is: 1 cup milk, yogurt, or fortified soymilk; 1½ ounces natural cheese such as cheddar cheese or 2 ounces of processed cheese.

^dAmounts of whole grains in the patterns for children are less than the minimum of 3 oz-eq in all patterns recommended for adults.

^eAll foods are assumed to be in nutrient-dense forms, lean, or low fat and prepared without added fats, sugars, refined starches, or salt. If all food choices to meet food group recommendations are in nutrient-dense forms, a small number of calories remain within the overall calorie limit of the pattern (i.e., limit on calories for other uses). The number of these calories depends on the overall calorie limit in the pattern and the amounts of food from each food group required to meet nutritional goals. Nutritional goals are higher for the 1,200- to 1,600-calorie patterns than for the 1,000-calorie pattern, so the limit on calories for other uses is lower in the 1,200- to 1,600-calorie patterns. Calories up to the specified limit can be used for added sugars, added refined starches, solid fats, alcohol, or to eat more than the recommended amount of food in a food group. The overall eating pattern also should not exceed the limits of less than 10% of calories from added sugars and less than 10% of calories from saturated fats. At most calorie levels, amounts that can be accommodated are less than these limits. For adults of legal drinking age who choose to drink alcohol, a limit of up to 1 drink/d for women and up to 2 drinks/d for men within limits on calories for other uses applies (see Appendix 9. Alcohol in the 2015–2020 Dietary Guidelines for Americans for additional guidance); and calories from protein, carbohydrate, and total fats should be within the acceptable macronutrient distribution ranges.

^fValues are rounded.
USDA, U.S. Department of Agriculture.
Source: www.cnpp.usda.gov/USDAFoodPatterns

TABLE 33-3 • Nutrients Relevant to Oral Health

NUTRIENT	FUNCTION	DEFICIENCY DISEASE	FOOD SOURCE
Vitamin A (retinol, provitamin A carotene)	• Fat soluble • Antioxidant • Bone and tooth development • Skin and mucous membrane integrity • Cell differentiation; essential for reproduction • Vision in dim light • Immune system integrity	• Night blindness • Xerophthalmia • Poor growth • Keratinization of epithelium • Dry, scaly skin • Toxic in large doses: double vision, hair loss, dry mucous membranes, joint pain, liver damage	Egg yolk, liver, fish liver oils, fortified milk, cream, cheeses; green leafy vegetables, orange, red, yellow pigmented fruits and vegetables
Vitamin D (calciferol)	• Fat soluble • Aids in the absorption of calcium and phosphorus • Mineralization of bone	• Rickets in children • Osteomalacia in adults • Osteoporosis • Toxic in large doses: calcification of soft tissues, growth retardation	Exposure to UV sunlight, fortified milk, fish oils
Vitamin E (tocopherol)	• Fat soluble • Antioxidant	• Low incidence of deficiency • Low toxicity	Whole grains, wheat germ, plant oils, margarines, legumes, seeds, nuts, greens
Vitamin K (quinone)	• Fat soluble • Synthesis of prothrombin in blood clotting and bone proteins	• Prolonged clotting time • Hemorrhage • Toxic in large doses: patients on blood thinners need to limit use in diet	Synthesized by intestinal bacterial flora; dark green leafy vegetables, liver
Thiamin (B₁)	• Acts as coenzyme in carbohydrate and amino acid metabolism	• Essential for synthesis of acetylcholine for healthy nerves • Beriberi: weight loss, fatigue, edema, depression • Toxicity: not seen	Enriched whole grains and cereals, pork, meats, poultry, nuts, seeds, legumes
Riboflavin (vitamin B₂)	• Coenzyme in energy metabolism of fat, carbohydrate, and protein	• Ariboflavinosis • Angular cheilosis • Growth failure • Eye disorders • Toxicity: not seen	Milk, cheese, enriched and whole grains and cereals, rice, mushrooms, liver

TABLE 33-3 • Nutrients Relevant to Oral Health (*Continued*)

NUTRIENT	FUNCTION	DEFICIENCY DISEASE	FOOD SOURCE
Niacin (vitamin B$_3$)	• Coenzyme in energy metabolism of fat, carbohydrate, and protein	• Pellagra: diarrhea, dermatitis, dementia, and death • Toxicity not seen in food sources • Toxicity with large doses of supplements for treatment of hypercholesterolemia: skin redness and flushing, gastric ulcers	Enriched whole grains and cereals, rice, meat, poultry, fish, green leafy vegetables
Pyridoxine (vitamin B$_6$)	• Coenzyme in amino acid and lipid metabolism • Hemoglobin synthesis • Homocysteine metabolism	• Dermatitis • Depression • Convulsions • Peripheral neuritis • Toxicity not seen in food sources • Toxicity from supplements: neuropathy, irreversible nerve damage	Widespread food sources with exception of fat and sugar
Cobalamin (vitamin B$_{12}$)	• Maturation of RBC • Requires intrinsic factor from parietal cells for absorption • Cofactor in folate and homocysteine metabolism	• Pernicious anemia secondary to lack of intrinsic factor and total vegan diet • Toxicity: not seen	All animal foods, fortified cereals
Folate (folic acid)	• Maturation of RBC • DNA synthesis • Homocysteine metabolism	• Megaloblastic anemia • Neural tube defects: spina bifida • Masks B$_{12}$ deficiency • Toxicity not seen	Green leafy vegetables, fruits, legumes, fortified grains
Ascorbic acid (vitamin C)	• Antioxidant • Collagen synthesis • Wound healing • Aids in absorption of iron	• Scurvy • Poor wound healing • Petechial hemorrhages • Increased periodontal symptoms • Toxicity: potential for rebound scurvy	Citrus fruits, broccoli, strawberries, peppers, tomatoes, cantaloupe
Calcium	• Muscle contraction • Blood clotting • Nerve impulse transmission • Calcification of bone and tooth structure	• Osteoporosis • Incomplete calcification of hard tissues • Toxicity: not seen	Dairy products, tofu, fortified orange juice, soy milk, green leafy vegetables, canned salmon, sardine bones
Phosphorus	• Required for bone and teeth strength • Acid–base balance • Muscle contraction	• Poor bone maintenance • Incomplete calcification of teeth • Compromised alveolar integrity • Toxicity: skeletal porosity	Dairy products, meat, poultry, processed foods, soft drinks, nuts, legumes, whole-grain cereals
Magnesium	• Bone strength and rigidity • Hydroxyapatite crystal formation • Nerve impulse • Muscle contraction	• Muscle weakness • Alveolar bone fragility • Toxicity seen in medications containing magnesium	Wheat bran, whole grains, green leafy vegetables, legumes, nuts, chocolate
Fluoride	• Prevention of dental caries • Remineralization	• Increased incidence of caries • Toxicity: tooth mottling, enamel hypoplasia	Fluoridated water, tea, seaweed, toothpaste
Iron	• Component of hemoglobin • Carries oxygen to cells • Immune function • Cognitive development	• Anemia: pallor of face, conjunctiva, lips, mucosa, and gingiva • Shortness of breath • Fatigue • Decreased immunity • Toxicity: gastrointestinal upset, pigmentation, seen in persons with hemochromatosis	Meat, poultry, fish, whole grains, dried fruit, enriched grains

(Continues)

TABLE 33-3 • Nutrients Relevant to Oral Health (*Continued*)

NUTRIENT	FUNCTION	DEFICIENCY DISEASE	FOOD SOURCE
Zinc	• Required for over 100 enzymes • Normal growth and development • Taste and smell sensitivity • Sexual development and reproduction • Immune integrity • Wound healing	• Altered taste • Growth retardation • Decreased wound healing • Impaired immunity • Toxicity: rare (stomach irritation, cramps, diarrhea, vomiting)	Seafood, meats, whole grains, greens
Copper	• Aids in iron metabolism • Collagen formation	• Anemia • Poor growth • Low white blood cells • Bone demineralization • Tissue fragility • Decreased trabeculae of alveolar bone • Toxicity: vomiting, diarrhea	Whole grains, nuts, dried fruits, meats legumes, shell fish, organ meats

RBC, red blood cell; UV, ultraviolet.

Source: Palmer CA, ed. *Diet and Nutrition in Oral Health.* 3rd ed. Upper Saddle River, NJ: Pearson Prentice Hall; 2017. Adapted from Palmer CA, Papas A. Chapter 8: The minerals and mineralization. In: *Diet and Nutrition in Oral Health.* Upper Saddle River, NJ: Pearson Prentice Hall; 2003; Palmer CA. Chapter 9: Vitamins today. In: *Diet and Nutrition in Oral Health.* Upper Saddle River, NJ: Pearson Prentice Hall; 2017.

II. Periodontal Tissues

Periodontal diseases are not caused by nutritional deficiencies, but malnutrition may contribute to the progression of periodontal disease symptoms and influence healing following treatment.

◆ *Nutritional deficiencies do not cause periodontal diseases.* Without local factors, including the periodontal pathogens in biofilm, biofilm-retentive factors (such as calculus and defective restorations), and lack of the oral self-care to remove biofilm, periodontal infections cannot occur.

◆ *Severe deficiencies are rare in developed countries.* Symptoms of deficiencies such as those listed in Table 33-4 may be seen in cases of severe deprivation, starvation, and patients with long-term alcoholism or other drug addictions.

◆ *RDAs are essential to the health of the periodontal tissues.* As part of total body health, the daily diet nourishes the oral tissues.

◆ *The physical characteristic of the diet contributes.* A soft, sticky diet that stays on the tooth surfaces, especially cervical third and proximal areas, encourages biofilm buildup and proliferation of bacteria, including the periodontal pathogens.

◆ *Malnutrition suppresses the immune system and impairs the host's reaction to infections.* Increased activity of pathogenic microorganisms may result in increased periodontal disease.

◆ *Nutrients contribute to healing and tissue repair.*[5] The elements strongly associated with wound healing include vitamin B complex, vitamin C (ascorbic acid), and dietary calcium.

• *B complex* refers to all the water-soluble vitamins, except vitamin C. They are thiamin (vitamin B_1), riboflavin (vitamin B_2), niacin (vitamin B_3), pyridoxine (vitamin B_6), cobalamin (vitamin B_{12}), biotin,

TABLE 33-4 • Oral Manifestations of Nutrient Deficiencies

ORAL SYMPTOMS ASSOCIATED WITH THE TONGUE	NUTRIENT DEFICIENCY
Altered taste sensations	Riboflavin, thiamin, zinc, vitamin A, vitamin B_{12}
Glossitis	Folate, niacin, riboflavin, vitamin B_6, vitamin B_{12}
Glossodynia	Niacin, vitamin B_6, vitamin B_{12}
Sore or burning tongue	Iron, niacin, riboflavin, thiamin, vitamin B_6, vitamin B_{12}
ORAL SYMPTOMS ASSOCIATED WITH MUCOSAL TISSUE	
Angular cheilosis	Folate, iron, riboflavin, vitamin B_6, vitamin B_{12}
Candidiasis	Folate, iron, zinc, vitamin A, vitamin C
Delayed wound healing	Riboflavin, zinc, vitamin A, vitamin C
Mucositis/stomatitis	Folate, niacin, thiamin, vitamin B_{12}

Source: Palmer CA, ed. *Diet and Nutrition in Oral Health.* 3rd ed. Upper Saddle River, NJ: Pearson Prentice Hall; 2017. Adapted from Palmer CA, Papas A. Chapter 8: The minerals and mineralization. In: *Diet and Nutrition in Oral Health.* Upper Saddle River, NJ: Pearson Prentice Hall; 2003; Palmer CA. Chapter 9: Vitamins today. In: *Diet and Nutrition in Oral Health.* Upper Saddle River, NJ: Pearson Prentice Hall; 2017.

folic acid, and pantothenic acid. Each member of the B complex has individual functions.

- *Vitamin C* is needed for collagen formation and intercellular material, and healing tissues after procedures including periodontal debridement.
- *Dietary calcium.* About 99% of the calcium in the body is in the bones and teeth; 1% is in the body tissues and fluids; essential for cell metabolism, muscle contraction, and nerve impulse transmission. Vitamin D is necessary for the continuous exchange of calcium between the blood, skeletal bones, and other cells.
- *Low dietary intake of calcium and vitamin D can impact alveolar bone integrity in periodontal disease.* Loss of alveolar bone and soft-tissue attachment are typical of periodontal disease progression.[6]
- *Current and former smokers with low dietary vitamin C intake are at risk for more severe periodontal disease.*[7] The IOM suggests smokers need 35 mg more vitamin C per day than nonsmokers.[8]

◆ *Obesity and periodontal disease*
- Obesity and periodontal disease have an association with each other, and inflammation is the proposed mechanism for this relationship.[9,10]
- Higher body mass index and waist circumference have been correlated with increased incidence of periodontal disease.[9,10]
- As with all chronic diseases, it is the dental professional's role to promote healthy lifestyle choices, including, but not limited to, oral self-care, tobacco cessation, healthy nutrition, adequate physical exercise, and weight control to manage and/or prevent progression of disease.

◆ *Dietary assessment for periodontal conditions*
- Following surgical intervention, patients may need to alter diet consistency during the healing period.
- A soft diet of high-quality protein is indicated for adequate wound healing. Puddings, scrambled eggs, milkshakes, yogurt, and cottage cheese have high-quality protein to promote healing.
- Chewing firm foods increases salivary flow. Saliva acts as a buffer, and increased saliva aids in oral clearance.

III. Tooth Structure and Integrity

◆ *Nutrients and health of tooth structure*
- Adequate nutrition during tooth development is essential for mineralization.
- Relevant minerals: calcium, phosphorus, magnesium, and fluoride.
- Relevant vitamin: vitamin A.

◆ *Dietary assessment*
- Diet assessment during early tooth development is essential to assist parents in caries prevention.

- Anticipatory guidance for the parents of infants, children, and adolescents can be found in Chapters 46 and 47.

IV. Dental Caries

◆ *Prevention*[11]
- Fluoride is an essential mineral for dental caries prevention.
- The complexity of dental caries formation is illustrated in Figure 33-2.

◆ *Role of cariogenic foods*[12]
- Dental caries is a result of biofilm and excess cariogenic foods, not a nutrient deficiency.
- *Streptococcus mutans*, *Lactobacilli*, and other acid-forming organisms use fermentable carbohydrate from the diet to produce acids.

◆ *Consistency of food*[12]
- Soft, sticky foods cling to the teeth and gingiva and encourage biofilm accumulation.
- Microorganisms are protected and nourished in dental biofilm on the tooth, leading to increased acid formation.

◆ *Dietary assessment and counseling*
- Use of dietary assessment and patient instruction relative to dental caries control.
- Personal recommendations foster behavioral modification in disease prevention.

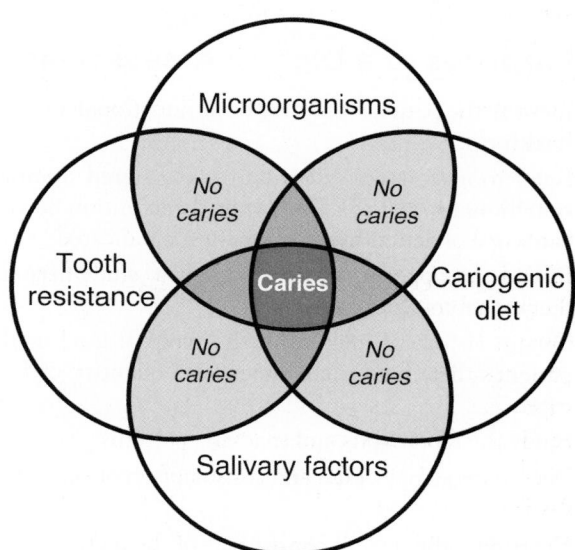

FIGURE 33-2 • Dental Caries Process. Four overlapping circles illustrate the factors involved in the development of dental caries. All four act together, and as shown by the center, dental caries results. (Adapted from U.S. Department of Health and Human Services, Public Health Service, National Institute of Dental Research. *Broadening the Scope. Long-Range Research Plan for the 1990s.* Washington, DC: U.S. Government Printing Office; 1990. NIH Publication No. 90-1188.)

COUNSELING FOR DENTAL CARIES CONTROL

◆ *Risk factors (see Chapter 25)*
  • Inadequate biofilm removal.
  • Inadequately mineralized tooth enamel, such as in enamel hypoplasia, or demineralization.
  • Frequent snacks with fermentable carbohydrates and acidic beverages between meals.
  • Altered salivary flow such as in drug-induced xerostomia.
  • Figure 33-2 illustrates the intricate relationship of all four factors in the development of dental caries.
◆ *Preventive measures that support dietary control*
  • Adequate plaque biofilm removal.
  • Modification of intake of cariogenic foods and beverages.
  • Strengthening the tooth surface to resist caries activity with appropriate office and home fluorides.
  • Pit-and-fissure sealants.
  • Restoration of existing carious lesions.

THE DIETARY ASSESSMENT

◆ The dietary assessment is an integral part of disease prevention and health promotion in the scope of dental hygiene care.[13]
◆ The patient and dental hygienist have the opportunity to collaborate in the evaluation of diet adequacy and in diet intervention.

I. Purposes of a Dietary Assessment

◆ Identify the patient who may be at nutritional and oral health risk.
◆ Refer to a registered dietitian or registered dietitian nutritionist (RD or RDN) when intervention beyond the scope of dental hygiene practice is indicated.
◆ Provide an opportunity for a patient to study personal dietary habits objectively.
◆ Obtain an overall picture of the types of food in the patient's diet, food preferences, and quantity of food eaten.
◆ Study the food habits and snacking patterns.
◆ Record frequency of use and consumption of cariogenic food.
◆ Determine the overall consistency of the diet.
  • Identify fibrous foods regularly consumed.
  • Identify soft, sticky foods regularly consumed.
◆ Identify the nutritional status of an individual with regard to overall requirements and then collaborate with the patient to make suggestions for modification in nutritional adequacy of the diet in health promotion.

◆ Plan with the patient for necessary changes to improve the health of the oral mucosa and periodontium and to prevent dental caries.

II. Preliminary Preparation for Dietary Assessment

A. Patient History

◆ Information obtained from medical, dental, and social histories is essential in assessing oral health and nutritional status:
  • Disease states
  • Medications
  • Disabilities
  • Learning limitations
  • Significant unintentional change in body weight
  • Factors influencing food use and food intake.
◆ Dietary influences can be identified by intraoral and extraoral examination, which may reveal oral tissue changes suggestive of nutritional deficiencies.

B. Clinical Evaluation

◆ High-risk patients can be identified by noting factors suggestive of a dietary problem.
◆ Clinical examination and charting of cavitated carious lesions and demineralizing areas.
◆ Identification of any abnormalities in the patient's overall appearance: weight, skin, nails, and hair.
◆ Table 33-4 lists oral manifestations of severe deficiencies.

III. Forms Used for Assessment

A. Twenty-Four Hour Recall

◆ A detailed account of the patient's dietary intake over the previous 24 hours (Table 33-5).
◆ Obtained during face-to-face interview with patient.
◆ Assesses nutrients, food groups, diet adequacy, form and frequency of the carbohydrate intake, and snacking patterns.
◆ Results are reviewed and appropriate instruction given at appointment or a follow-up appointment.
◆ It is quick and easy to administer and can be done chairside in one visit.
◆ Is limited to 1-day intake; therefore, it is not necessarily representative of a patient's normal diet.

B. Dietary Analysis Recording Form 3–7 Days

◆ A more accurate account of a patient's intake (Table 33-6).
◆ Patient completes food diary for 3, 5, or 7 days, inclusive of one-weekend day.

TABLE 33-5 • Dietary Intake Form

Type of Foods/ Beverages	Quantity Eaten (cup, oz, tbsp, tsp, etc.)	Preparation Method
BREAKFAST		
SNACK		
Lunch		
SNACK		
Dinner		
SNACK		

Sample of a form for patients to use to record the daily intake of foods. Can be used for the 24-hour recall or multiple forms used in the 3- to 7-day food diary.

NAME_____TEL_____

AGE_____SEX_____Height_____Weight_____BMI_____

7:30 AM		
Orange juice	½ cup	Bagel shop
Bagel	Whole	
Cream cheese	2 tablespoons	
Coffee	2 cups	
Milk	½ cup	
Sugar	2 packets	
10:00 AM		
Chocolate chip cookies	2	
Orange soda	12 oz can	
1:00 PM		
Mushroom pizza	2 slices	School cafeteria
Orange soda	12 oz can	
Cheese cake	1 slice	
4:00 PM		
Whole-wheat pretzels	1 bag	Vending machine
7:00 PM		
Turkey	6 oz	Roasted
Potato	1 medium	Baked
Sour cream	2 tablespoons	
Broccoli	1 cup	Sautéed
Oil	2 tablespoons	
Gravy	½ cup	Canned
9:30 PM		
Popcorn	3 cups	Microwave

◆ Affords the patient a more active role in the dietary assessment and a chance to observe areas that require modification.

◆ Provide patient with three to seven copies of the Dietary Intake Form (Table 33-6). Request patient to return the forms at follow-up visit.

◆ At follow-up visit, the patient's diary is evaluated for:
 • Eating patterns.
 • Consumption and frequency of fermentable carbohydrates.
 • Nutritional adequacy.

IV. Presentation of the Food Diary to the Patient

◆ *Explain the purpose*
 • Briefly describe how diet relates to oral health.
 • Provide a foundation for the education to follow.
 • Avoid mention of specific foods to prevent patient bias.

◆ *Explain the form*
 • Provide written and oral instructions for use of the food diary.
 • Provide suggestions for listing various foods and use of household measurements for indicating quantity (see examples in Box 33-2).
 • Instruction for completing the food diary encourages the patient to provide a more accurate portrayal of eating behaviors.

◆ *Complete the current day's food diary with the patient*
 • Helps to illustrate how to itemize and list foods eaten.
 • Provides an example while completing the patient's own daily diary.

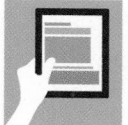

BOX 33-2
Food Diary Instructions

• Write down all foods consumed on the Dietary Intake Form (Table 33-5).

• Record each meal as soon after eating as possible to avoid forgetting.

• Record all fluids; include water and alcoholic beverages.

• Do not choose days when dieting, fasting, or ill.

• Be accurate in determining the amounts eaten, using household measurements (e.g., 1/2 cup cereal, 1 tsp margarine, 3 oz fish). A 3-oz serving size can be compared to the size of a deck of cards.

• Use brand names whenever possible.

• Record added sauces, gravies, condiments, and all extras (e.g., sugar or cream in coffee, mayonnaise, chewing gum, cough drops).

• Record food preparation methods (e.g., baked, fried, boiled, grilled).

TABLE 33-6 Dietary Analysis Recording Form

From the dietary intake form(s) completed by the patient (Table 33-5), each serving is entered as a check in the space beside the appropriate food group. Each category is totaled, averaged, and compared with the recommendation on the right.

Name _____

Date _____ Age _____

Dietary Analysis

FOOD GROUPS	DAY 1	2	3	4	5	6	7	DAILY AVERAGE	USDA FOOD PATTERNS FOR FIVE MOST USED CALORIC LEVELS (12 TOTAL LEVELS)					ADEQUATE	
									1,000 KCALS	1,600 KCALS	1,800 KCALS	2,200 KCALS	2,800 KCALS	YES	NO
Grains									3 oz-eq	5 oz-eq	6 oz-eq	7 oz-eq	10 oz-eq^a		
Vegetables									1 cup	2 cups	2.5 cup	3 cups	3.5 cups		
Fruits									1 cup	1.5 cups	1.5 cups	2 cups	2.5 cups		
Dairy									2 cups	3 cups	3 cups	3 cups	3 cups		
Protein Foods									2 oz-eq	5 oz-eq	5 oz-eq	6 oz-eq	7 oz-eq		
Oils^b									15g/4tsp	22g/tsp	24g/6tsp	29g/7tsp	36g/9tsp		

SWEETS

		TOTAL	
Liquid	With meal		Total all liquid exposures and multiply by 20 minutes and divide by total number of days to equal daily acid attack from liquid.
	End of meal		**Total Liquid Minutes** _____
	Between meal		
Soft/solid sticky/retentive	With meal		Total all soft and hard solid exposures and multiply by 40 minutes and divide by total number of days to equal daily acid attack from solids.
	End of meal		**Total Solid Minutes** _____
	Between meal		
Hard/solid slowly dissolving	With meal		Add both liquid and solid totals to determine the number of minutes per day teeth are under acid attack.
	End of meal		**Total Daily Minutes of Acid Attack** _____
	Between meal		

^{a}eq is the abbreviation for the word equivalents. See MyPyramid Food Intake Patterns (Figure 33-2) for more details on equivalents.

^{b}k 4.2 grams = 1 tsp.

◆ *General directions*

- Emphasize the importance of completing the diary for each meal as soon after eating as possible to avoid forgetting.
- Encourage use of typical days, uncomplicated by illness, dieting, holidays, or other unusual events.
- Review details of recording the component parts of a combination dish, such as a sandwich: 2 slices of whole-wheat bread, 4 oz of turkey, 1 teaspoon of mayonnaise, 2 slices tomato with lettuce, and 1 slice of cheddar cheese.
- Indicate need for recording nutritional supplements and all fluids consumed, including water and alcoholic beverages.
- The patient needs to indicate where the meal was eaten, such as at home, restaurant, or friend's house.
- Instruct patient to select consecutive days and at least one-weekend day for a realistic representation of diet pattern.
- Encourage patient to include oral hygiene methods performed before or after meals.

V. Receiving the Completed Food Diary

◆ *Obtain supplemental data*

- Receive the food diary soon after its completion.
- Question the patient to clarify presented information.
- Does food diary represent a typical day or week?
- Identify influences on appetite such as illness or stress.
- Identify food likes and dislikes, food preferences, intolerances, and food allergies.
- Frequency of dining out.
- Identify special diets being followed at home.
- Average alcohol intake.
- Which family member is doing the cooking and food shopping?
- Ask about common food habits, such as snacking at night.

◆ *Review patient's food diary*

◆ Common omissions include:

- Garnishes: frosting, whipped cream, butter or margarine on vegetables, salad dressings, and oil.
- Beverages: quantity and sweetened.
- Snacks: type, brand, and quantity.
- Chewing gum or mints: sugarless, noncariogenic sweetener such as xylitol, and quantity.
- Canned fruit: packed in water, heavy or light syrup, own juices, or sweetened with sugar substitute, and quantity.
- Fruit and vegetables: canned, fresh, or frozen.
- Cereal: sugar-coated or low sugar brand, type of milk and/or sugar added, and quantity.
- Potato: baked, mashed, or fried.
- Seasonings or sauces: quantity and type.

VI. Analysis of Dietary Intake

Three principal parts of the food diary to analyze are the number of servings in each food group, frequency of cariogenic foods, and consistency of the diet.

A. Nutritional Analysis for Adequacy of 24-Hour Recall Intake

- ◆ When time is a factor, a 24-hour analysis is appropriate.
- ◆ Compare intake of food groups recorded in the patient's 24-hour food diary with individual needs identified using MyPlate.
- ◆ Determine nutritional adequacy.
- ◆ Calculate the patient's "sweet score," as outlined in Table 33-7.
- ◆ Cariogenic foods are listed and categorized as solid, liquid, or slowly dissolving.
- ◆ Totals for the 1 day are multiplied by respective time factors and a score determines patient's caries risk.

B. Nutritional Analysis for Adequacy of Food Intake from the Food Diary

- ◆ Use the Dietary Analysis Recording Form to summarize adequacy of daily portions of each food group (Table 33-6).
- ◆ Each food eaten is entered into a food group with number of servings.
- ◆ Comparison of intake reported on patient's food diary with individual caloric needs for age, gender, height, weight, and activity level identified using MyPlate food guidance system (Figure 33-1; Tables 33-1 and 33-2).
- ◆ Totals for the week are added, and the average per day calculated.
- ◆ The average is compared to the recommended servings for each food group.
- ◆ Assist patient when inadequacies or deficiencies are identified.
- ◆ Analysis of cariogenic foods.
- ◆ Identify physical form of carbohydrate.
  - Liquids: sweetened or unsweetened soft drinks; fruit juice with added sugars.
  - Soft solid/sticky and retentive: retentive cakes, cookies, chips, pretzels, jellybeans, and chewy, sticky candies.
  - Hard solid/slowly dissolving: hard candies, mints, and cough drops.
- ◆ Identify frequency of meals and snacks.
  - When snacks are consumed.
  - Number of between-meal snacks consumed daily.
  - Circle in red and tally the number of cariogenic foods, both solid and liquids.
  - Frequency more relevant than quantity in caries incidence.
  - High frequency of eating events decreases the ability of calcium and phosphate to remineralize teeth between episodes.

TABLE 33-7 • Scoring the Sweets

SCORING THE SWEETS (CARIES-PROMOTING POTENTIAL)

FOOD ITEMS (from patients 24-hour recall)	REFERENCE FOODS CONSIDERED CAROGENIC	FREQUENCY (place a check for each exposure to cariogenic food)	WEIGHTED SCORE	TOTAL POINTS EACH CATEGORY
1. 2. 3. 4.	**Liquid** Soft drinks, fruit drinks, cocoa, sugar and honey in beverages, nondairy creamers, ice cream, sherbet, flavored or frozen yogurt, pudding, custard, jello	_____ _____ _____ _____	X 1	
1. 2. 3. 4. 5. 6.	**Solid and sticky** Cakes, cupcakes, doughnuts, sweet rolls, potato chips, pretzels, pastry, canned fruit in syrup, ba-nanas, cookies, chocolate candy, caramel, toffee, jelly beans, other chewy candy, chewing gum, dried fruit, marshmallows, jelly, jam	_____ _____ _____ _____ _____ _____	X 2	
1. 2. 3.	**Slowly dissolving** Hard candies, breath mints, antacid tablets, cough drops	_____ _____ _____	X 3	

Total Score _____

Using the 24-hour reall dietary intake form:
• Classify each sweet into liquid, solid and sticky, or slowly dissolving. (Use reference food list)
• For each time a sweet was eaten, either at a meal or between meals (at least 20 minutes apart), place a check in the frequency column
• In each category, tally the number of sweets eaten and multiply by the weighted score. Record the category points in the respective column
• Tally all the category points to determine the total score.

SWEET SCORE: (Risk for dental caries)	HOW TO LOWER YOUR RISK FOR CARIES:
0–1 low risk 2–4 5–7 moderate risk 8–9 >10 high risk	1. Cut down on the frequency of between-meal sweets 2. Don't sip constantly on sweetened beverage 3. Avoid using slowly dissolving items like hard candy, cough drops, and so on. 4. Eat more **cariostatic**: exerting an inhibitory action on the progress of dental caries by consuming foods such as low-fat cheese, protein-rich foods, raw vegetables, nuts, popcorn.

Form to be used to determine patient's caries risk when doing a 24-hour recall at chairside. (Adapted with permission from Carole A. Palmer EdD, RD. Division of Nutrition and Oral Health Promotion, Department of General Dentistry, Tufts University School of Dental Medicine.)

◆ During counseling appointment, show the patient how to:
  • Select and circle in red the cariogenic foods on the Scoring the Sweets form (Table 33-6).
  • Select liquid, soft solid, hard solid, and time of eating.
  • Total the number of sweets for both liquid and solids and multiply total by 20 minutes (liquids) and 40 minutes (solids).
  • Divide by number of days (3-, 5-, or 7-day diary).
  • Add both liquid and solid scores to determine total minutes teeth are exposed to sweets and acid attack (Table 33-6).

C. Analysis of Diet Consistency

◆ Help patient to identify the types of firm and fibrous foods from the food diary such as:
  • Uncooked fruits and vegetables.
  • Cooked; crisp–tender vegetables.

◆ Help patient to identify the frequency of cariogenic food patterns:
  • Daily or occasionally.
  • During meal, end of meal, or between meals.

D. Benefits of Food Diary Analysis

◆ Patient can identify appropriate and inappropriate practices for dental caries control.
◆ Corroborate findings with clinical findings and patient's oral health problems in preparation for counseling session.

PREPARATION FOR ADDITIONAL COUNSELING

I. Define Objectives

◆ To help patient understand the individual oral problems and appreciate the need for changing habits.

- To explain specific alterations in the diet necessary for improved general and oral health.
- For dental caries control.
  - Promote minimal consumption of cariogenic foods, particularly between meals.
  - Substitute noncariogenic foods or include anticariogenic foods, when possible, into the diet.

II. Planning Factors

A. Patient Attitude

- Consider patient's willingness and ability to cooperate as evidenced by keeping appointments and following personal oral care procedures.
- Consider patient's healthcare beliefs and nutrition and dental knowledge.

B. Possible Barriers

- Difficulty and resistance to change of normal habits.
- Patient dissatisfaction with loss of usual or customary foods.
- Patient may not attempt to make modifications if recommendations are numerous or overwhelming.
- Lack of appreciation of need for change due to limited knowledge of diet, nutrition, and oral health relationship.
- Common misconception about concentrated sugar as an indispensable energy source.
- Cultural and religious patterns significant to food selection and preparation.
- Financial considerations in food purchasing.
- Emotional eating patterns and cravings for sweets.
- Parental attitude toward sweets in the diet.
  - Elimination of all sugars would deprive a child of normal childhood pleasures.
  - All sugars may be viewed as "bad" foods for children. Foods are not "good" and "bad," rather it is the frequency and amount that may be a concern for oral and overall health.

III. Appropriate Teaching Materials

- Patient's radiographs, dental charting, and food diary.
- Diagrams, food models, food labels, or charts of dietary standards and requirements.
- Educational leaflets or pamphlets to illustrate patient's special dietary or oral health needs.
- An outline of a realistic diet plan with specific suggestions for food substitutes that is created based on patient preferences.
- A list of snack suggestions.

COUNSELING PROCEDURES

I. Setting

- An environment free from interruptions and distracting background sounds.
- Apart from the clinical treatment room.

- Patient comfort promotes environment conducive to learning.
- Provide limited but pertinent educational information.
  - Posters and pamphlets.
  - Food labels and food models of portion sizes.
  - Avoid overloading with too much new information to minimize confusion.
- Persons involved in promoting change:
  - For a younger patient, the primary caregiver is present since this individual supervises the child's eating and oral care.
  - Person preparing meals and grocery shopping needs to be present to learn about appropriate food choices.

II. Setting the Stage for a Successful Counseling Session

- Be prepared and on time.
- Plan for only a few simple visual aids.
- Concentrate on the factors related to the patient's diet-based dental problem.
- Encourage parents to exclude small children (other than the patient) from the conference; they may create distractions.
- Develop a friendly atmosphere; establish eye contact with a warm, nonthreatening environment.
- Adequately discuss all questions from patient or parent using a conversational tone without lecturing.
- Keep session brief, informative, and engaging for the patient without taking notes.

III. Presentation of Findings

A. Review Purpose of the Meeting

- Provide explanation of the relevance between diet and patient's oral disease.
- Emphasize health promotion and disease prevention.

B. Clarification of "Cariogenic" Foods

- Calculate the sugar score from the Scoring the Sweets or Dietary Analysis Recording Form to emphasize caries risk.
- Clarify confusion of hidden sugars, added sugars, and natural sugars.
- Clarify the moderation of sugar intake and help patient identify substitutions.

C. Review of Dental Caries Initiation

- The sucrose from cariogenic food on the tooth surface can be changed to acid in minutes.
- The pH drops to below 5.5, which is the critical level for demineralization of enamel.
- Acid left undisturbed will be cleared from the mouth from 20 minutes to up to 2 hours, depending primarily on salivary flow. For a patient with xerostomia, clearance takes much longer.

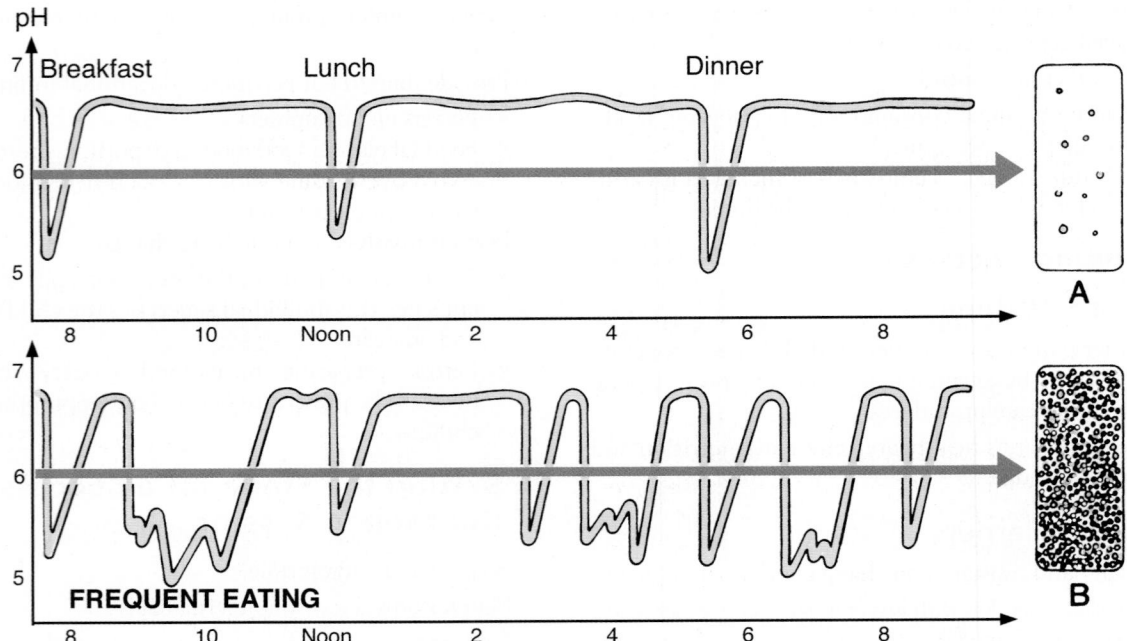

FIGURE 33-3 • Cariogenic Foods and Biofilm pH. The range of pH in dental biofilm from 5 to 7 is shown on the left. Time intervals are shown across the bottom of each graph. The double-line curve represents the variations in biofilm pH throughout a day. Each time sugar or a cariogenic food is taken in, the pH of the dental biofilm drops to or below the critical pH (5.2–5.5). As shown in the lower graph, frequent eating keeps the pH at the critical level below which enamel demineralization can occur. On the right, **(A)** shows that bacterial counts are lower, whereas in **(B)**, aciduric microorganisms are greatly increased in numbers. The critical pH for the root surfaces is 6.0–6.7. (Adapted with permission from Larmas M. Simple test for caries susceptibility. *Int Dent J.* 1985;35 (2):109–117.)

◆ Figure 33-3 illustrates how the frequent intake of sucrose lowers the pH for several hours in the course of the day.

D. Frequency and Time of Exposure

◆ Each exposure of the tooth surface to sucrose or other cariogenic food in a meal or snack increases the amount of acid on the tooth.

◆ The quantity of a cariogenic food is not as significant as when and how often the tooth is exposed to a cariogenic food.[14]

◆ Prolonged intake of a cariogenic liquid or solid, such as continuous sipping of a sucrose-containing beverage while working at a desk, does not allow for a remineralization period to occur in which the pH can rise above the critical level.

E. Retention

◆ Cariogenic foods consumed after brushing and flossing before bedtime are not cleared readily because salivary flow decreases during sleep.

◆ Cariogenic liquids are cleared from the mouth faster than solids.

◆ Oral retentiveness of cariogenic foods is related to length of time food debris with fermentable carbohydrate remains on the teeth and exposure to decreased biofilm pH.[15–17]

• Highly retentive fermentable carbohydrates have a delayed rate of oral clearance, increasing exposure of teeth to a decreased pH and higher potential for demineralization.[15,16,18]

◆ Sequence of food consumption within a meal pattern is related to caries incidence.[17–20]

• Eating fermentable carbohydrates at the beginning of a meal or between other noncariogenic foods (protein and fat) is less cumulative in cariogenic potential.

• Protein and fat are not metabolized by oral bacteria or broken down by salivary amylase and are recommended to be eaten at the end of a meal.

• Cheese eaten after sweets or at the end of a meal prevents the decrease in pH and production of acids in the oral cavity.[20]

◆ Noncariogenic sweeteners may be incorporated for caries prevention and management of a healthy weight in patients at risk for obesity.[11,21]

◆ Sugar-free gums decrease lactic acid production and increase salivary flow, potentially buffering acids.

• Chewing a gum with xylitol immediately after each meal reduces the levels of S. *mutans* and promotes remineralization.

• Xylitol is the sugar substitute of choice because it is not fermentable by caries-promoting bacteria. Sorbitol can be fermented by S. *mutans* at a very slow rate.[11,22]

IV. Specific Dietary Recommendations

A. Examination of the Patient's Food Diary

- After analyzing the diet, assist the patient in identifying the deficiencies and excesses in intake.
- Consult Chapter 24 for guidance on working collaboratively with the patient to develop a plan.
- Try to retain as many as possible of the patient's present food habits.
- Make recommendations that can be adapted to the patient's lifestyle.
- Discuss foods from each food group that the patient likes and can be added to the diet.
- Limit the use of cariogenic foods to mealtimes.
  - Evaluate the final food in a meal because it may remain on the teeth if rinsing is not possible.
  - Recommend chewing a gum containing xylitol at the end of each meal, especially for a caries-susceptible person.
  - Recommend specific stores in the area where patients can purchase gum containing xylitol.
- Assist patient in finding acceptable substitutions for the cariogenic food choices.
  - Unflavored milk.
  - Cheese.
  - Peanut butter (check the label of the peanut butter to choose one without added sugar) on sliced apples.
  - Sugar-free gelatin or pudding.
  - Crunchy vegetables.
- Explore ways to decrease sugar in food preparation and when purchasing ready-made food.
  - Decrease the amount of granulated or brown sugar by half when baking.
  - Consider substituting alternative sweeteners, such as xylitol.
  - Carefully read nutrition labels of prepared foods and choose foods with no added sugar when possible.
  - Natural sugars are just as detrimental as refined sugars (e.g., honey, maple syrup).
- To enhance compliance, help patients create their own meal plans for 1 day.
  - Incorporate the principles discussed during the counseling.
  - Collaborate on modifications the patient can achieve realistically and is willing to try.
  - Avoid too many changes that may be overwhelming.
  - Determine patient comprehension of information presented and patient's motivational level.
  - Include morning, afternoon, and evening snacks as well as breakfast, lunch, and dinner in a meal plan for a day.
- Encourage daily use of fluoride in water, foods, dentifrices, and rinses.
- When toothbrushing and flossing are not possible, encourage rinsing with water.

EVALUATION OF PROGRESS

I. Immediate Evaluation

- The patient's verbal and nonverbal interest, comprehension, and participation in the dietary analysis and counseling session.

II. Three-Month Follow-Up

- Request patient to keep a 3-, 5-, or 7-day food diary for assessment and evaluation.
- Review personal oral care procedures and provide suggestions as needed.
- Scaling as needed; fluoride varnish application.
- Collaborate on ideas for further modifications when indicated. Smaller goals may need to be established for greater compliance.
- Document progress, additional material reviewed, and plan for continued behavior modification.

III. Six-Month Follow-Up

- Perform examination and clinical procedures.
  - Charting of carious lesions and demineralized areas.
  - Disclose and evaluate biofilm score and reteach as needed with new biofilm removal brush, interdental, and tongue-cleaning devices.
  - Scaling as needed; fluoride varnish application.
- Compare dental caries incidence with previous chartings and completed restorative dentistry.
- Make collaborative dietary recommendations with patient in accord with new assessment.
- Document progress, education provided, and plan.

IV. Overall Evaluation

- Consistent reduction in dental caries rate in the years following the initial counseling shows sustained change in habits.
- Patient's and parents' attitudes toward maintaining adequate oral health habits.
- Attempts to maintain a diet containing minimum cariogenic foods.
- Compliance with keeping regular appointments for professional dental care.

DOCUMENTATION

The following factors are included when documenting patient care that includes diet analysis and patient counseling:
- Rationale for dietary analysis.
- The type of dietary intake utilized for dietary assessment.
- The results of the dietary analysis.
- The results of the sugar score and the level of caries risk.
- Instructions given on completing the food diary.
- Box 33-3 contains an example progress note for a patient receiving dietary analysis and counseling.

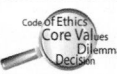

EVERYDAY ETHICS

Ms. Carlson presents with type 1 diabetes and several significant changes in her oral cavity since her last dental hygiene appointment, including angular cheilosis, glossitis, and several proximal carious lesions. The hygienist, Bettina, believes that Ms. Carlson has advanced dietary needs beyond the scope of practice of a dental hygienist and, therefore, avoids any chairside dietary assessment with the patient. Routine oral self-care instructions are given. On completion of the examination, Bettina mentions her concerns about Ms. Carlson's dietary status to the dentist but does not record any recommendations in the patient's permanent record.

Questions for Consideration

1. What professional protocol for referrals can be followed by the dental hygienist since she believes giving dietary advice to a patient with diabetes is beyond the scope of practice for a dental hygienist?

2. By eliminating the chairside dietary assessment for dental caries prevention, did Bettina act nonmaleficently toward the patient? Explain your response.

3. Which ethical principles would be ignored if Bettina does not educate the patient about the preventive measures for her dental caries or document this information in the patient's record?

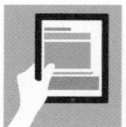

BOX 33-3

Example Documentation:
Patient Receiving a Dietary Analysis and Counseling

S— A 24-year-old, Hispanic female arrived for her annual examination and preventive care appointment. Her medical and dental history were unremarkable.

O—Caries, periodontal, and oral cancer risk assessments were performed. A comprehensive periodontal examination reveals biofilm-induced gingivitis with localized bleeding on probing. Dental examination reveals three new carious lesions.

A—Risk assessment indicates the patient is at high risk for dental caries because of the frequency of snacks. A 24-hour recall was performed chairside. Dietary analysis revealed a sweet score of 9, indicating a moderate caries risk. Evaluation of diet for nutritional adequacy revealed an inadequate representation of fruits and vegetables.

P—Preventive education included review of toothbrushing, flossing, and dietary changes to reduce the risk for caries. Reducing the frequency of snacks between meals was discussed. Recommendations include having desserts or sodas during meals. Rinsing with water or chewing xylitol gum were provided as options following desserts or sodas consumed between meals to reduce the caries risk. The patient was also provided with a prescription for a home fluoride for daily application prior to bedtime. A follow-up appointment was made in 2 weeks.

Signed: _____, RDH

Date: _____

Factors to Teach the Patient

Medications with Sucrose

▶ The need to avoid liquid or chewable forms containing sucrose.

▶ Reasons to avoid frequent daily use of medications with sucrose.

▶ Reasons for rinsing with water after a medication contained in a sucrose mixture.

Medications with Side Effect of Xerostomia

▶ Drugs the patient is using that cause xerostomia (dry mouth).

▶ How xerostomia increases the risk of dental caries development.

▶ Why it is necessary to use saliva substitutes, chew gum containing xylitol, and avoid slowly dissolving in the mouth candies containing sucrose.

▶ Effect of xerostomia on chewing and swallowing and how it compromises nutrient intake.

Facts about Dental Caries

▶ How dental caries on the tooth surface starts and progresses.

▶ How the interaction of cariogenic foods, tooth surface, saliva, and microorganisms act together, contributing as factors in the dental caries process (Figure 33-2).

▶ How repeated, frequent acid production and the pH in the dental biofilm adversely affect the teeth.

▶ Why there is a need to avoid frequent episodes of eating or drinking food or beverages that contain sucrose (Figure 33-3).

ENHANCE YOUR UNDERSTANDING

ONLINE RESOURCES
(see the inside front cover for access information)
- Audio glossary
- Appendices

SUPPORT FOR LEARNING
(available separately)
- *Active Learning Workbook for Wilkins' Clinical Practice of the Dental Hygienist, 13th Edition*

INDIVIDUALIZED REVIEW
- Customized practice quizzing with Navigate 2 TestPrep for *Wilkins' Clinical Practice of the Dental Hygienist*

References

1. National Research Council. *Dietary Reference Intakes: Applications in Dietary Planning*. Washington, DC: The National Academies Press; 2003.

2. National Research Council. *Dietary Reference Intakes: The Essential Guide to Nutrient Requirements*. Washington, DC: The National Academies Press; 2006.

3. Institute of Medicine. *Dietary Reference Intakes for Thiamin, Riboflavin, Niacin, Vitamin B6, Folate, Vitamin B12, Pantothenic Acid, Biotin, and Choline*. Washington, DC: The National Academies Press; 1998.

4. Department of Agriculture, Center for Nutrition Policy and Promotion. ChooseMyPlate guidelines. 2011. http://www.choosemyplate.gov. Accessed January 21, 2019.

5. Varela-López A, Navarro-Hortal MD, Giampieri F, Bullón P, Battino M, Quiles JL. Nutraceuticals in periodontal health: a systematic review on the role of vitamins in periodontal health maintenance. *Molecules*. 2018;23(5):pii: E1226. doi:10.3390/molecules23051226.

6. Miley DD, Garcia MN, Hildebolt CF, et al. Cross-sectional study of vitamin D and calcium supplementation effects on chronic periodontitis. *J Periodontol*. 2009;80(9):1433-1439.

7. Aziz AS, Kalekar MG, Suryakar AN et al. Assessment of some biochemical oxidative stress markers in male smokers with chronic periodontitis. *Indian J Clin Biochem*. 2013;28(4):374-380.

8. Institute of Medicine. Food and nutrition board. *Dietary Reference Intakes for Vitamin C, Vitamin E, Selenium, and Carotenoids*. Washington, DC: National Academy Press; 2000.

9. Martinez-Herrera M, Silvestre-Rangil J, Silvestre FJ. Association between obesity and periodontal disease. A systematic review of epidemiological studies and controlled clinical trials. *Med Oral Patol Oral Cir Bucal*. 2017;22(6):e708-e715. doi:10.4317/medoral.21786.

10. Keller A, Rohde Jf, Raymond K, Hetiman BL. Association between periodontal disease and overweight and obesity: a systematic review. *J Periodontol*. 2015;86(6):766-776.

11. Horst JA, Tanzer JM, Milgrom PM. Fluorides and other preventive strategies for tooth decay. *Dent Clin North Am*. 2018;62(2):207-234.

12. Sheiham A, James WP. Diet and dental caries: the pivotal role of free sugars reemphasized. *J Dent Res*. 2015;94(10):1341-1347.

13. Marshall TA. Chairside diet assessment of caries risk. *J Am Dent Assoc*. 2009;140(6):670-674.

14. Head D, A Devine D, Marsh PD. In silico modelling to differentiate the contribution of sugar frequency versus total amount in driving biofilm dysbiosis in dental caries. *Sci Rep*. 2017;7(1):17413. doi:10.1038/s41598-017-17660-z.

15. Bradshaw DJ, Lynch RJ. Diet and the microbial aetiology of dental caries: new paradigms. *Int Dent J*. 2013;63(suppl 2):64-72.

16. Chankanka O, Marshall TA, Levy SM, et al. Mixed dentition cavitated caries incidence and dietary intake frequencies. *Pediatr Dent*. 2011;33(3):233-240.

17. Botelho JN, Villegas-Salinas M, Troncoso-Gajardo P, Giacaman RA, Cury JA. Enamel and dentine demineralization by a combination of starch and sucrose in a biofilm—caries model. *Braz Oral Res*. 2016;30(1). doi:10.1590/1807-3107BOR-2016.vol30.0052.

18. Halvorsrud K, Lewney J, Craig D, Moynihan PJ. Effects of starch on oral health: systematic review to inform WHO guideline. *J Dent Res*. 2019;98(1):46-53. doi:10.1177/0022034518788283

19. Rugg-Gunn AJ, Edgar WM, Geddes DA, Jenkins GN. The effect of different meal patterns upon plaque pH in human subjects. *Br Dent J*. 1975;139(9):351-356.

20. Linke HA, Riba HK. Oral clearance and acid production of dairy products during interaction with sweet foods. *Ann Nutr Metab*. 2001;45(5):202-208.

21. Roberts MW, Wright JT. Nonnutritive, low caloric substitutes for food sugars: clinical implications for addressing the incidence of dental caries and overweight/obesity. *Int J Dent*. 2012;2012:625701. doi:10.1155/2012/625701.

22. Janakiram C, Deepan Kumar CV, Joseph J. 2017. Xylitol in preventing dental caries: a systematic review and meta-analyses. *J Nat Sci Biol Med*. 2017;8(1):16-21.

34

Fluorides

Erin E. Relich, RDH, BSDH, MSA

CHAPTER OUTLINE

FLUORIDE METABOLISM
I. Fluoride Intake
II. Absorption
III. Distribution and Retention
IV. Excretion

FLUORIDE AND TOOTH DEVELOPMENT
I. Pre-eruptive: Mineralization Stage
II. Pre-eruptive: Maturation Stage
III. Posteruptive

TOOTH SURFACE FLUORIDE
I. Fluoride in Enamel
II. Fluoride in Dentin
III. Fluoride in Cementum

DEMINERALIZATION–REMINERALIZATION
I. Fluoride in Biofilm and Saliva
II. Summary of Fluoride Action

FLUORIDATION
I. Historical Aspects
II. Water Supply Adjustment

EFFECTS AND BENEFITS OF FLUORIDATION
I. Appearance of Teeth
II. Dental Caries: Permanent Teeth
III. Root Caries
IV. Dental Caries: Primary Teeth
V. Tooth Loss
VI. Adults
VII. Periodontal Health

PARTIAL DEFLUORIDATION

SCHOOL FLUORIDATION

DISCONTINUED FLUORIDATION

FLUORIDES IN FOODS
I. Foods
II. Salt
III. Halo/Diffusion Effect
IV. Bottled Water
V. Water Filters
VI. Infant Formula

DIETARY FLUORIDE SUPPLEMENTS
I. Assess Possible Need
II. Available Forms of Supplements
III. Prescription Guidelines
IV. Benefits and Limitations

PROFESSIONAL TOPICAL FLUORIDE APPLICATIONS
I. Historical Perspective
II. Indications
III. Compounds

CLINICAL PROCEDURES: PROFESSIONAL TOPICAL FLUORIDE
I. Objectives
II. Preparation of the Teeth for Topical Application
III. Patient and/or Parent Counseling
IV. Tray Technique: Gel or Foam
V. Varnish Technique
VI. After Application
VII. Silver Diamine Fluoride

SELF-APPLIED FLUORIDES
I. Indications
II. Methods

TRAY TECHNIQUE: HOME APPLICATION
I. Indications for Use
II. Gels Used (Available by Prescription)

FLUORIDE MOUTHRINSES
I. Indications
II. Limitations
III. Preparations
IV. Benefits

BRUSH-ON GEL
I. Preparations
II. Procedure

FLUORIDE DENTIFRICES
I. Development
II. Indications
III. Preparations
IV. Patient Instruction: Recommended Procedures
V. Benefits

COMBINED FLUORIDE PROGRAM

FLUORIDE SAFETY
I. Summary of Fluoride Risk Management
II. Toxicity
III. Signs and Symptoms of Acute Toxic Dose
IV. Emergency Treatment
V. Chronic Toxicity
VI. How to Calculate Amounts of Fluoride

DOCUMENTATION

EVERYDAY ETHICS

FACTORS TO TEACH THE PATIENT

REFERENCES

LEARNING OBJECTIVES

After studying this chapter, the student will be able to:

1. Describe the mechanisms of action of fluoride in the prevention of dental caries.

2. Explain the role of community water fluoridation on the decline of dental caries incidence in a community.

3. Recommend appropriate over-the-counter (OTC) and professionally applied fluoride therapies based on each patient's caries risk assessment.

4. Compare use of fluoride home products (OTC and prescription).

5. Incorporate fluoride into individualized prevention plans for patients of various ages and risk levels.

The use of fluorides provides the most effective method for dental caries prevention and control. Fluoride is necessary for optimum oral health at all ages and is made available at the tooth surface by two general means:

◆ *Systemically*, by way of the circulation to developing teeth (pre-eruptive exposure).

◆ *Topically*, directly to the exposed surfaces of teeth erupted into the oral cavity[1] (posteruptive exposure).

◆ Maximum caries inhibiting effect occurs when there is systemic exposure before tooth eruption and frequent topical fluoride exposure throughout life.[2]

FLUORIDE METABOLISM[1,3]

I. Fluoride Intake

◆ Sources
   • Drinking water that contains fluoride naturally or has been fluoridated.
   • Prescribed dietary supplements.
   • Foods, in small amounts.
   • Foods and beverages prepared at home or processed commercially using water that contains fluoride.
   • Varying small amounts ingested from dentifrices, mouthrinses, supplements, and other fluoride products used by the individual.

II. Absorption

A. Gastrointestinal Tract

◆ Fluoride is rapidly absorbed as hydrogen fluoride through passive diffusion in the stomach:
   • Rate and amount of absorption depend on the solubility of the fluoride compound and gastric acidity.
   • Most is absorbed within 60 minutes.

◆ Fluoride that is not absorbed in the stomach will be absorbed by the small intestine.

◆ There is less absorption when the fluoride is taken with milk and other food.

B. Blood Stream

◆ Plasma carries the fluoride for its distribution throughout the body and to the kidneys for elimination.

◆ Maximum blood levels are reached within 30 minutes of intake.

◆ Normal plasma levels are low and rise and fall according to intake.

III. Distribution and Retention

◆ Fluoride is distributed by the plasma to *all* tissues and organs. There is a strong affinity for mineralized tissues.

◆ Approximately 99% of fluoride in the body is located in the mineralized tissues.

◆ Concentrations of fluoride are highest at the surfaces next to the tissue fluid supplying the fluoride.

◆ The fluoride ion (F) is stored as an integral part of the crystal lattice of teeth and bones.
   • Amount stored varies with the intake, the time of exposure, and the age and stage of the development of the individual.
   • The teeth store small amounts, with highest levels on the tooth surface.

◆ Fluoride that accumulates in bone can be mobilized slowly from the skeleton due to the constant resorption and remodeling of bone.

◆ Once tooth enamel is fully matured, the fluoride deposited during development can be altered by cavitated dental caries, erosion, or mechanical abrasion.[1]

IV. Excretion

◆ Most fluoride is excreted through the kidneys in the urine, with a small amount excreted by the sweat glands and the feces.

◆ There is limited transfer from plasma to breast milk for excretion by that route.[1]

FLUORIDE AND TOOTH DEVELOPMENT

◆ Fluoride is a nutrient essential to the formation of sound teeth and bones, as are calcium, phosphorus, and other elements obtained from food and water.

◆ A comprehensive review of the histology of tooth development and mineralization is recommended to supplement the information included here.[4,5]

I. Pre-eruptive: Mineralization Stage

◆ Fluoride is deposited during the formation of the enamel, starting at the dentinoenamel junction, after the enamel matrix has been laid down by the ameloblasts.

  • Figure 34-1A shows the distribution of fluoride in all parts of the teeth during mineralization.
  • The hydroxyapatite crystalline structure becomes fluorapatite, which is a less soluble apatite crystal.[2]
  • Pre-eruptive fluoride may contribute to shallower occlusal grooves and reduce the risk of fissure caries.[2]

◆ Chapter 47 lists the weeks in utero when the hard-tissue formation begins for the primary teeth.

◆ The first permanent molars begin to mineralize at birth as listed in Chapter 16.

◆ Effect of excess fluoride (fluorosis)[6,7]

  • Dental fluorosis is a form of hypomineralization that results from systemic ingestion of an excess amount of fluoride during tooth development.
  • During mineralization, the enamel is highly receptive to free fluoride ions.
  • The normal activity of the ameloblasts may be inhibited, and the defective enamel matrix that can form results in discontinuity of crystal growth.

◆ Dental fluorosis can appear clinically in varying degrees from white flecks or striations to cosmetically objectionable stained pitting, as listed in Chapter 21.

II. Pre-eruptive: Maturation Stage

◆ After mineralization is complete and before eruption, fluoride deposition continues in the surface of the enamel.

  • Figure 34-1B shows fluoride around the crown during maturation.
  • Fluoride is taken up from the nutrient tissue fluids surrounding the tooth crown.

III. Posteruptive

◆ After eruption and throughout the life span of the teeth, the concentration of fluoride on the outermost surface of the enamel is dependent on:

  • Daily topical sources of fluoride to prevent demineralization and encourage remineralization for prevention of dental caries.
  • Sources for daily topical fluoride include fluoridated drinking water, dentifrices, mouthrinses, and other fluoride preparations used by the patient.
  • The fluoride on the outermost surface is available to inhibit demineralization and enhance remineralization as needed.
  • Figure 34-2A depicts the areas on the tooth that acquire fluoride after eruption.

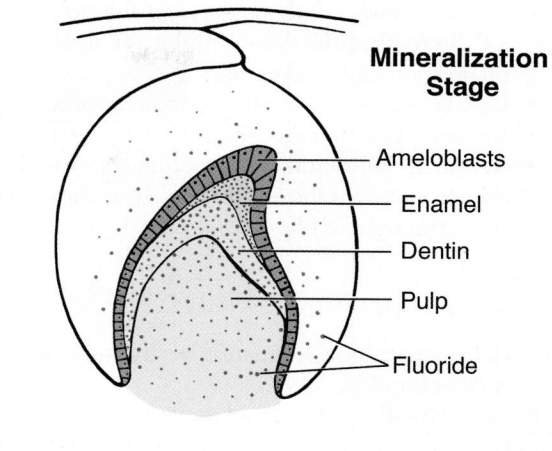

Mineralization Stage
— Ameloblasts
— Enamel
— Dentin
— Pulp
— Fluoride

A

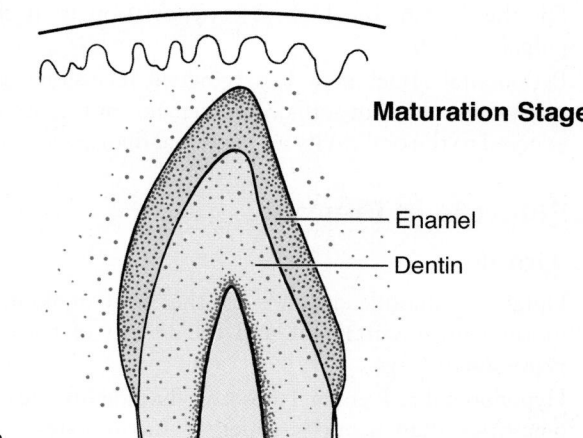

Maturation Stage
— Enamel
— Dentin

B

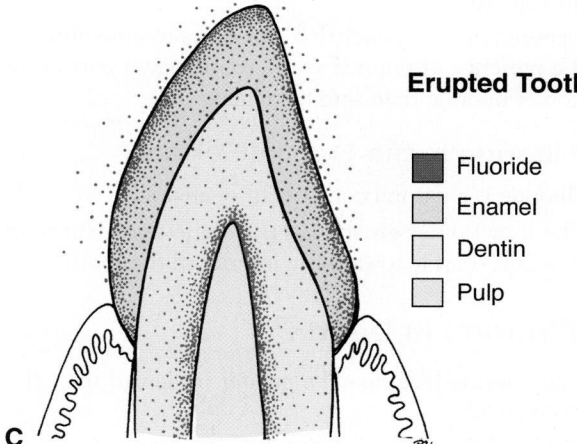

Erupted Tooth

▮ Fluoride
▯ Enamel
▯ Dentin
▯ Pulp

C

FIGURE 34-1 • Systemic Fluoride. Green dots represent fluoride ions in the tissues and distributed throughout the tooth. **A:** Developing tooth during mineralization shows fluoride from water and other systemic sources deposited in the enamel and dentin. **B:** Maturation stage before eruption, when fluoride is taken up from tissue fluids around the crown. **C:** Erupted tooth continues to take up fluoride on the surface from external sources. Note concentrated fluoride deposition on the enamel surface and on the pulpal surface of the dentin.

- The continuous daily presence of fluoride provided for the tooth surfaces can inhibit the initiation and progression of dental caries.
- Uptake is most rapid on the enamel surface during the first years after eruption.
- Repeated daily intake of drinking water with fluoride provides a topical source as it washes over the teeth throughout life.

TOOTH SURFACE FLUORIDE

Fluoride concentration is greatest on the surface next to the source of fluoride.

- For the enamel of the erupted tooth, highest concentration is at the outer surface exposed to the oral cavity.
- For the dentin, the highest concentration is at the pulpal surface.
- Periodontal attachment loss (gingival recession) can often cause the root surface and cementum to become exposed to the oral cavity and external fluoride sources.

I. Fluoride in Enamel

A. Uptake

- Uptake of fluoride depends on the level of fluoride in the oral environment and the length of time of exposure.
- Hypomineralized enamel absorbs fluoride in greater quantities than sound enamel; it incorporates into the hydroxyapatite crystalline structure to become fluorapatite.[6]
- Demineralized enamel that has been remineralized in the presence of fluoride will have a greater concentration of fluoride than sound enamel.

B. Fluoride in the Enamel Surface

- Fluoride is a natural constituent of enamel.
- The intact outer surface has the highest concentration that falls sharply toward the interior of the tooth.[8]

II. Fluoride in Dentin[9]

- The fluoride level may be greater in dentin than that in enamel.
- A higher concentration is at the pulpal or inner surface, where exchanges take place.
- Newly formed dentin absorbs fluoride rapidly.

III. Fluoride in Cementum[9]

- The level of fluoride in cementum is high and increases with exposure.
  - With recession of the clinical attachment level, the root surface is exposed to the fluids of the oral cavity.
  - Figure 34-2B shows fluoride acquisition to exposed cementum.

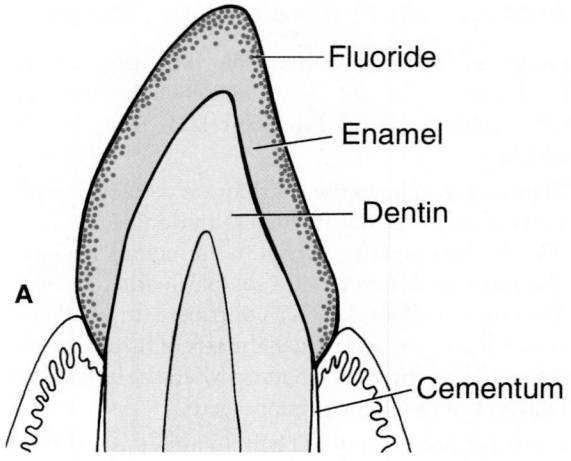

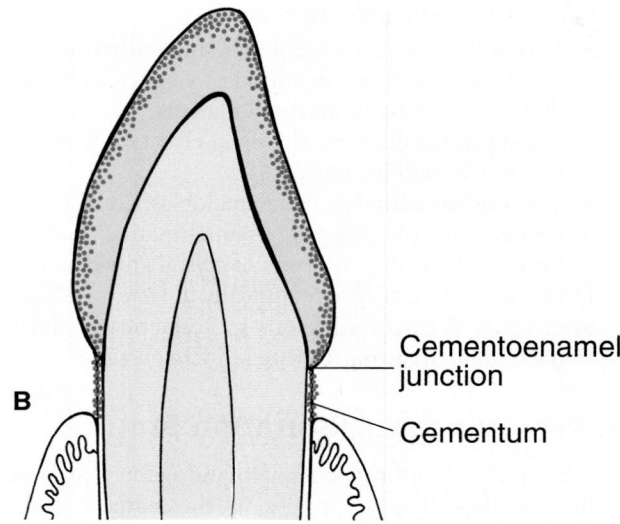

FIGURE 34-2 • Fluoride Acquisition after Eruption. A: Fluoride represented by green dots on the enamel surface is taken up from external sources, including dentifrice, rinse, topical application, and fluoridated drinking water passing over the teeth. B: Gingival recession exposes the cementum to external sources of fluoride for the prevention of root caries and the alleviation of sensitivity.

- Fluoride is then available to the cementum from the saliva and all the sources used by the patient, including drinking water, dentifrice, and mouthrinse.

DEMINERALIZATION-REMINERALIZATION[8]

Figure 34-3 illustrates the comparative levels of fluoride that may be found in the tooth surface and the sublevel lesion in early dental caries.

I. Fluoride in Biofilm and Saliva

- Saliva and biofilm are reservoirs for fluoride; saliva carries minerals available for remineralization when needed.

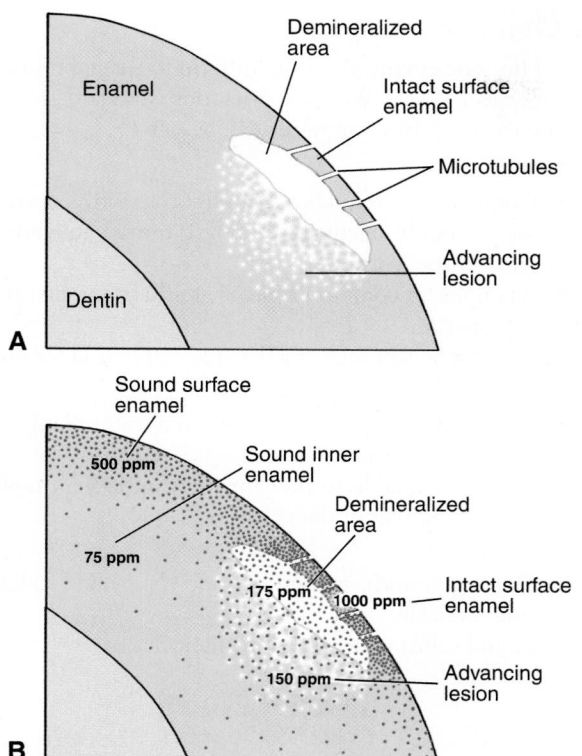

FIGURE 34-3 • Examples of Enamel Fluoride Content. A: Early stage of dental caries with an intact surface enamel and subsurface demineralized area. **B:** A demineralized area readily takes up available fluoride. As shown, the fluoride content (1,000 ppm) of the relatively intact surface over a subsurface demineralized white spot is higher than that of the sound surface enamel (500 ppm). The body of the advancing lesion has a higher fluoride content (150 ppm) than does the sound inner enamel (75 ppm). (From Melberg JR, Ripa LW, Leske GS. *Fluoride in Preventive Dentistry: Theory and Clinical Applications.* Chicago, IL: Quintessence; 1983:31.)

♦ Fluoride helps to inhibit demineralization when it is present at the crystal surface during an acid challenge.

♦ Fluoride enhances remineralization, forming a condensed layer on the crystal surface, which attracts calcium and phosphate ions.

♦ High concentrations of fluoride can interfere with the growth and metabolism of bacteria.

♦ Dental biofilm may contain 5–50 ppm fluoride. The content varies greatly and is constantly changing.

♦ Fluoride may be acquired directly from fluoridated water, dentifrice, and other topical sources and brought by the saliva or by an exchange of fluoride in the biofilm to the demineralizing tooth surface under the biofilm.

II. Summary of Fluoride Action

Having fluoride available topically to the tooth posteruptively is key to its effectiveness.

♦ Frequent exposure to fluoride, such as from fluoridated water, dentifrice, and mouthrinse, is recommended.

♦ There are three basic topical effects of fluoride to prevent dental caries:[8]

• Inhibit demineralization.

• Enhance remineralization of incipient lesions.

• Inhibit bacterial activity by inhibiting *enolase,* an enzyme needed by bacteria to metabolize carbohydrates.

FLUORIDATION

♦ *Fluoridation* is the adjustment of the natural fluoride ion content in a municipal water supply to the optimum physiologic concentration that will maximize caries prevention and limit enamel fluorosis.[10]

♦ Fluoridation has been established as the most efficient, effective, reliable, and inexpensive means for improving and maintaining oral health for all who use it.

♦ Fluoridation was named by the U.S. Centers for Disease Control and Prevention (CDC) as one of the 10 most significant public health measures of the 20th century.[10]

♦ The estimated annual cost per person per year is low, with lower cost per person for communities of more than 20,000 people.[11]

♦ In 2014, 66.3% of the total U.S. population received fluoridated water, whereas 74.4% of the population served by public (municipal) water systems received fluoridated water. These percentages vary greatly from state to state.[12]

I. Historical Aspects[13]

A. Mottled Enamel and Dental Caries

♦ Dr. Frederick S. McKay

• Early in the 20th century, Dr. McKay began his extensive studies to find the cause of "brown stain," which later was called mottled enamel and now is known as *dental fluorosis.*

• He observed that people in Colorado Springs, Colorado, with mottled enamel had significantly less dental caries.[14] He associated the condition with the drinking water, but tests were inconclusive.

♦ H.V. Churchill

• In 1931, H.V. Churchill, a chemist, pinpointed fluorine as the specific element related to the tooth changes that Dr. McKay had been observing clinically.[15]

B. Background for Fluoridation

♦ Dr. H. Trendley Dean

• Epidemiologic studies of the 1930s, sponsored by the U.S. Public Health Service (USPHS) and directed by Dr. Dean, led to the conclusion that the level of fluoride in the water optimum for dental caries prevention averages 1 ppm in moderate climates.

• Clinically objectionable dental fluorosis is associated with levels well over 2 ppm.[16]

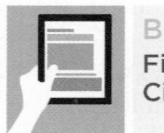

BOX 34-1

First Fluoridation Research Cities

RESEARCH CITY	CONTROL CITY
Grand Rapids, Michigan (January 1945)	Muskegon, Michigan
Newburgh, New York (May 1945)	Kingston, New York
Brantford, Ontario (June 1945)	Sarnia, Ontario
Evanston, Illinois (February 1947)	Oak Park, Illinois

- From this knowledge and the fact many healthy people had lived long lives in communities where the fluoride content of the water was much greater than 1 ppm, the concept of adding fluoride to the water developed.
- It was still necessary to show the benefits from controlled fluoridation could parallel those of natural fluoride.

C. Fluoridation—1945

- The first communities were fluoridated in 1945.
- Research in the communities began before fluoridation was started to obtain baseline information.

D. Control Cities

- Aurora, Illinois, where the natural fluoride level is optimum (1.2 ppm), was used to compare the benefits of natural fluoride in the water supply with those of fluoridation, as well as with a fluoride-free city, Rockford, Illinois.
- Original cities with fluoridation and their control cities in the research are shown in Box 34-1.
- The research conducted in those cities, as well as throughout the world, has documented the influence of fluoride on oral health.

II. Water Supply Adjustment

A. Fluoride Level

- In 2015, the U.S. Department of Health and Human Services updated the recommendation for the optimal concentration of water fluoridation to 0.7 ppm for all communities, regardless of climate.
  - The decision is based on the fact that Americans have access to many more sources of fluoride today than they did when water fluoridation was introduced in the United States.[17]
  - The change still provides an effective level of fluoride to reduce the incidence of dental caries while minimizing the rate of fluorosis.

B. Chemicals Used

- All fluoride chemicals must conform to the appropriate American Water Works Association standards to ensure that the drinking water will be safe.[18]
- Sources
  - Compounds from which the fluoride ion is derived are naturally occurring and are mined in various parts of the world.
  - Examples of common sources are fluorspar, cryolite, and apatite.
- Criteria for acceptance of a fluoride compound for fluoridation include:
  - Solubility to permit regular use in a water plant.
  - Relatively inexpensive.
  - Readily available to prevent interruptions in maintaining the proper fluoride level.
- Compounds used:
  - Dry compounds: sodium fluoride (NaF) and sodium silicofluoride.
  - Liquid solution: hydrofluorosilicic acid.

EFFECTS AND BENEFITS OF FLUORIDATION

Fluoridated water is a systemic source of fluoride for developing teeth and a topical source of fluoride on the surfaces of erupted teeth throughout life.[19]

I. Appearance of Teeth

- Teeth exposed to an optimum or slightly higher level of fluoride appear white, shining, opaque, and without blemishes.
  - When the level is slightly more than optimum, teeth may exhibit mild enamel fluorosis seen as white areas in bands or flecks. Without close scrutiny, such spots blend with the overall appearance.
- Today, the majority of fluorosis is mild and not considered an esthetic problem.[10,20]

II. Dental Caries: Permanent Teeth

A. Overall Benefits

- Maximum benefit is seen with continuous use of fluoridated water from birth.
- Estimates have shown the reduction in caries due to water fluoridation alone (factoring out other sources of topical fluoride) among adults of all ages is 27%.[19]
- The effects are similar to communities with optimum levels of natural fluoride in the water.
- Many more individuals are completely caries free when fluoride is in the water.

B. Distribution

- Anterior teeth, particularly maxillary, receive more protection from fluoride than do posterior teeth.[16]
  - Anterior teeth are contacted by the drinking water as it passes into the mouth.

C. Progression

- Not only are the numbers of carious lesions reduced, but the caries rate is slowed.
- Caries progression is also reduced in the surfaces that receive fluoride for the first time after eruption.[21]

III. Root Caries

- Root caries experience in lifelong residents of a naturally fluoridated community is in direct proportion to the fluoride concentration in the water compared with the experience of residents of a fluoride-free community.[22]
- The incidence of root caries is approximately 50% less for lifelong residents of a fluoridated community.[23]

IV. Dental Caries: Primary Teeth

- With fluoridation from birth, the caries incidence is reduced up to 40% in the primary teeth.[10]
- The introduction of fluoridation into a community significantly increases the proportion of caries-free children and reduces the decayed, missing, and filled teeth (dmft/DMFT) scores compared to areas that are non-fluoridated over the same time period.[20]

V. Tooth Loss

- Tooth loss due to dental caries is much greater in both primary and permanent teeth without fluoride[24] because of increased dental caries, which progresses more rapidly.

VI. Adults

- When a person resides in a community with fluoride in the drinking water throughout life, benefits continue.[25,26]

VII. Periodontal Health

- Indirect favorable effects of fluoride on periodontal health can be shown.
  - Fluoride works to decrease dental caries. The presence of carious lesions favors biofilm retention, which can lead to periodontal infection, particularly adjacent to the gingival margin.

PARTIAL DEFLUORIDATION

- Water with an excess of natural fluoride does not meet the requirements of the USPHS.
- Several hundred communities in the United States had water supplies that naturally contained more than twice the optimal level of fluoride.
- Defluoridation can be accomplished by one of several chemical systems.[27] The efficacy of the methods has been shown.

- Examples: The water supply in Britton, South Dakota, has been reduced from almost 7 to 1.5 ppm since 1948, and in Bartlett, Texas, from 8 to 1.8 ppm since 1952. Examinations have shown a significant reduction in the incidence of objectionable fluorosis in children born since defluoridation.[27,28]

SCHOOL FLUORIDATION

- To bring the benefits of fluoridation to children living in rural areas without the possibility for community fluoridation, adding fluoride to a school water supply has been an alternative.
- Because of the intermittent use of the school water (only 5 days each week during the 9-month school year), the amount of fluoride added was increased over the usual 1 ppm.
- Example: In the schools of Elk Lake, Pennsylvania, after 12 years with the fluoride level at 5 ppm in the school drinking water, the children experienced a 39% decrease in DMF surfaces compared with those in the control group.[29]
- Example: In the schools of Seagrove, North Carolina, after 12 years with the fluoride level at 6.3 ppm in the school drinking water, the children experienced a 47.5% decrease in DMF surfaces compared with those in the control group.[29]
- Such systems have significance in the long history of efforts for fluoridation for all people in the United States.
- School fluoridation has been phased out in several states, and the current extent of this practice is unknown. Operations and maintenance of small fluoridation systems are problematic.[10]

DISCONTINUED FLUORIDATION

- When fluoride is removed from a community water supply that had dental caries control by fluoridation, the effects can be clearly shown.
- Example: In Antigo, Wisconsin, the action of antifluoridationists in 1960 brought about the discontinuance of fluoridation, which had been installed in 1949.
  - Examinations in the years following 1960 revealed the marked drop in the number of children who were caries free and the steep increases in caries rates.
  - From 1960 to 1966, the number of caries-free children in the second grade decreased by 67%.[30]
  - Fluoridation was reinstated in 1966 by popular demand.

FLUORIDES IN FOODS

I. Foods[31]

- Certain foods contain fluoride, but not enough to constitute a significant part of the day's need for caries prevention.

◆ Examples: Meat, eggs, vegetables, cereals, and fruit have small but measurable amounts, whereas tea and fish have larger amounts.

◆ Foods cooked in fluoridated water retain fluoride from the cooking water.

II. Salt[32-34]

◆ Fluoridated salt has not been promoted in the United States, but is widely available and used in Germany, France, and Switzerland along with other European countries where 30%–80% of the domestic marketed salt is fluoridated.

◆ Another 30 countries or more use fluoridated salt worldwide for its effectiveness as a community health program.

◆ Fluoridated salt results in a reduced incidence of dental caries, but there is insufficient evidence for its overall effectiveness.

◆ Fluoridated salts currently available supply about one-third to one-half of the amount of fluoride ingested daily from 1 ppm fluoridated water.

◆ Fluoridated salt is recommended by the World Health Organization as an alternative to fluoridated water to target underprivileged groups.

III. Halo/Diffusion Effect

◆ Foods and beverages that are commercially processed (cooked or reconstituted) in optimally fluoridated cities can be distributed and consumed in nonfluoridated communities.

◆ The halo or diffusion effect can result in increased fluoride intake by individuals living in nonfluoridated communities, providing them some protection against dental caries.[31]

IV. Bottled Water

◆ Bottled water usually does not contain optimal fluoride unless it has a label indicating that it is fluoridated.

◆ Patients need to be advised to fill their drinking water bottles from a fluoridated water supply.

V. Water Filters[35]

◆ Reverse osmosis and water distillation systems remove fluoride from the water, but water softeners do not.

◆ Carbon filters (for the end of a faucet or in pitchers) vary in their removal of fluoride.

◆ Carbon filters with activated alumina remove fluoride.

◆ Patients need to be warned that water filters may remove fluoride from the drinking water and need to be checked with the manufacturer before purchase.

VI. Infant Formula[36-38]

◆ There has been an increase in breastfeeding in the United States, but infant formula remains a major source of nutrition for many infants.

◆ Ready-to-feed formulas do not need to be reconstituted, but water is added to powdered and liquid concentrate formulas.

◆ Breast milk may contain 0.02 ppm fluoride, and all types of infant formula themselves contain a low amount of fluoride (0.11–0.57 ppm).[37]

◆ The level of fluoride in the water supply used to reconstitute powdered or liquid concentrate formulas determines the total fluoride intake.

◆ The American Dental Association (ADA) recommends continuing to use optimally fluoridated water to reconstitute infant formula while being aware of the possible risk of mild enamel fluorosis in the primary teeth.[38]

DIETARY FLUORIDE SUPPLEMENTS[10,39,40]

◆ Prescribed dietary supplements were introduced in the late 1940s and are intended to compensate for fluoride-deficient drinking water.

◆ The current supplementation dosage schedule developed by the ADA and the American Association of Pediatric Dentistry (AAPD) and revised in 2010 includes children aged 6 months through 16 years.

  • Table 34-1 contains the daily dosage amounts based on the age of the child and the amount of fluoride in the primary water supply.

◆ Clinical recommendations from the ADA Council on Scientific Affairs include the use of fluoride supplements for children:

  • At high risk of developing dental caries
  • Those whose primary source of drinking water is deficient in fluoride.[41]

TABLE 34-1 • Fluoride Supplements Dose Schedule (MG NAF/D)[a]

AGE OF CHILD (Y)	WATER FLUORIDE ION CONCENTRATION (ppm)		
	LESS THAN 0.3	BETWEEN 0.3 AND 0.6	GREATER THAN 0.6
Birth–6 mo	0	0	0
6 mo–3 y	0.25 mg	0	0
3–6 y	0.50 mg	0.25 mg	0
6–16 y	1.0 mg	0.50 mg	0

[a]About 2.2 mg of sodium fluoride provides 1 mg of fluoride ion.
Source: Rozier, Adair S, Graham F, et al. Evidence-based clinical recommendations on the prescription of dietary fluoride supplements for caries prevention: a report of the ADA Council on Scientific Affairs. *J Am Dent Assoc.* 2010;141:1480-1489.
http://www.aapd.org/media/Policies_Guidelines/G_FluorideTherapy.pdf (2014)

I. Assess Possible Need

- Review the patient's history to be certain the child is not receiving other fluoride in such preparations as vitamin–fluoride supplements.
- Determine the fluoride level of all sources of drinking water is below 0.6 ppm.
- Refer to the list of fluoridated communities available from state or local health departments.
- Request water analysis when the fluoride level has not been determined, for example, in private well water.
- Determine the child's risk for dental caries is high or moderately high before considering the use of fluoride supplements.[39]
- Reassess the caries risk at frequent intervals as the status may be affected by the child's development, personal and family situations, and behavioral factors such as changes in oral hygiene practices.[33,41]

II. Available Forms of Supplements

- NaF supplements are available as tablets, lozenges, and drops in 0.25, 0.50, and 1.0 mg dosages.
- Prescribed on an individual patient basis for daily use at home.

A. Tablets and Lozenges

- Tablets are chewed thoroughly, swished/rinsed around in the oral cavity, and forced between the teeth before swallowing.
- Lozenges are dissolved for 1–2 minutes in the mouth to provide both pre-eruptive and posteruptive benefits.[41]
- Best taken at bedtime after teeth are brushed.
  - Avoid drinking, eating, or rinsing before going to sleep to gain maximum benefit.

B. Drops

- A liquid concentrate with directions that specify the number of drops for the prescription dose daily.
- Primary use for child aged 6 months to 3 years, and patient of any age unable to use other forms that require chewing and swallowing.

III. Prescription Guidelines

- No more than 264 mg NaF (120 mg fluoride ion) to be dispensed per household at one time.
- Take supplements with juice or water.
  - Avoid taking with dairy products because fluoride can combine with calcium and be poorly absorbed.
- Storage
  - Keep products out of reach of children.
  - Keep tablets in the original container, away from heat and direct light, and away from damp places such as a bathroom or kitchen sink area.

- Missed dose
  - Take as soon as remembered.
  - If near next dose time, skip that dose and go to the next regular time.

IV. Benefits and Limitations

- Prenatal use by pregnant women
  - Administration of prenatal dietary fluoride supplements is not recommended.
  - Some evidence has shown that fluoride crosses the placenta during the fifth and sixth months of pregnancy and may enter the prenatal deciduous enamel.[42]
  - Overall, there is weak evidence to support the use of fluoride supplements to prevent dental caries in primary teeth.
- Daily fluoride supplements offer caries preventive benefits in permanent teeth. School-aged children who chewed, swished, and swallowed 1 mg fluoride tablets daily on school days had significantly lower caries experience than those who did not use fluoride supplements.
- The use of fluoride supplements in children over 6 years of age shows a 24% decrease in DMF tooth surfaces in permanent teeth compared to no fluoride supplements.[43]
- Consider the child's age, caries risk, and all sources of fluoride exposure before recommending the use of fluoride supplements.[33,41]

PROFESSIONAL TOPICAL FLUORIDE APPLICATIONS

Topical fluorides are an essential part of a total preventive program for patients of all ages.

- Fluoridated water and fluoride toothpaste are the primary sources of topical fluoride for patients of all ages and levels of caries risk.
- Additional topical fluoride sources may be professionally applied and/or self-applied by the patient, primarily for those at an elevated caries risk.

I. Historical Perspectives

- Professionally applied fluoride has been instrumental in the reduction of dental caries in the United States and other industrialized countries since the early 1940s.
- Dr. Basil G. Bibby conducted the initial topical NaF study using Brockton, Massachusetts, schoolchildren.[44]
- More than one-third of the fewer new carious lesions resulted from a 0.1% aqueous solution applied at 4-month intervals for 2 years applied by a dental hygienist.
- The research led to extensive studies by Dr. John W. Knutson and others sponsored by the USPHS.
  - The aim was to determine the most effective concentration of NaF, the minimum time required for application, and procedural details.[45,46]

II. Indications

◆ The professional application of a high-concentration fluoride preventive agent is based on caries risk assessment for the individual patient.

◆ See Chapter 25 for the criteria to determine low, moderate, and high caries risk.

◆ Indications for a professional fluoride application are outlined in Box 34-2.[47]

III. Compounds

◆ Table 34-2 provides a summary of the available professional fluoride applications.

- 2.0% NaF as gel or foam delivered in trays.
- 1.23% acidulated phosphate fluoride (APF) as a gel or foam delivered in trays.
- 5% NaF as a varnish brushed on the teeth.

◆ *2.0% NaF gel*

- NaF, also called "neutral sodium fluoride" due to its neutral pH of 7.0, contains 9,050 ppm fluoride ion.
- Clinical trials demonstrating the efficacy of neutral NaF are based on a series of four or five applications on a weekly basis.[48]
- Quarterly or semiannual applications are most common in clinical practice.

◆ *2.0% NaF foam*

- There is limited clinical evidence to demonstrate foam's effectiveness in caries prevention.

◆ *1.23% APF gel*

- Contains 12,300 ppm fluoride ion.
- A 4-minute tray application is recommended at least every 3–6 months per year for individuals aged 6 years and older at an elevated risk for dental caries.[47]
- Widely used because of its storage stability, acceptable taste, and tissue compatibility.
- Low pH of 3.5 enhances fluoride uptake, which is greatest during the first 4 minutes.[49]

- APF may etch porcelain and composite restorative materials, so it is not indicated for patients with porcelain, composite restorations, and sealants.[50]
- The hydrofluoride component of APF can dissolve the filler particles of the composite resin restorations.
- Macroinorganic filler particles of composite materials demonstrate noticeable etched patterns generated by APF, whereas many of the more recently available microfilled composites/resins are not as sensitive to the APF.[50]
- The prevented fraction of dental caries ranged from 18% to 41% with the use of APF or NaF gels.[51]

◆ *1.23% APF foam*

- There is limited clinical evidence to show the effectiveness of foam in caries prevention.

◆ *5% NaF varnish*

- Fluoride varnishes (FVs) were developed during the late 1960s and early 1970s to prolong contact time of the fluoride with the tooth surface.[52]
- Varnishes are safe and effective, fast and easy to apply, and patient acceptance is good.
- The use of FV 2–4 times per year is associated with a 43% decrease in DMFT surfaces in permanent teeth and 37% in primary teeth.[53]
- Varnish has a higher concentration of fluoride than gel or foam (22,600 ppm fluoride ion), but an overall less amount of fluoride is used per application (<7 mg varnish vs. 30 mg of gel for a child).
- Varnish sets quickly and remains on the teeth for a number of hours, releasing fluoride into the pits and fissures, proximal surfaces, and cervical areas of the tooth where it is needed the most.[54]
- Application is recommended at least every 3–4 months per year for individuals at an elevated risk for dental caries.[47]
- Varnish is effective in reversing active pit and fissure enamel lesions in the primary dentition[55] and remineralizing enamel lesions, regardless of whether

TABLE 34-2 • Professionally Applied Topical Fluorides

AGENT	FORM	CONCENTRATION	APPLICATION MODE/FREQUENCY	NOTES
NaF neutral or 7 pH	2% Gel or foam[a]	9,050 ppm 0.90% F ion	Tray (4 min)/no currently recommended interval	Do not overfill: see Figure 34-5
Acidulated phosphate 3.5 pH	1.23% Gel or foam[a]	12,300 ppm 1.23% F ion	Tray (4 min)/at least every 3–6 mo[47]	Do not overfill: see Figure 34-5
NaF neutral or 7 pH	5% Varnish	22,600 ppm 2.26% F ion	Apply thin layer with a soft brush (1–2 min)/at least every 3–6 mo[47]	Sets up to a hard film
SDF pH 8–10	5.0–5.9% Fluoride	44,800 ppm 4.48% F ion	Apply a thin layer with a microbrush (1 min and let dry, then rinse with water)/at least every 6–12 mo[63]	Goes on clear, becomes black/gray upon application to cavitated areas

[a]There is limited published clinical evidence supporting the effectiveness of foam.[47]
NAF, sodium fluoride; SDF, silver diamine fluoride.

the varnish is applied over or around the demineralizing lesion.[56]

- Varnish is also effective in reducing demineralization (white areas) around orthodontic brackets.[57]
- Varnish received approval from the U.S Food and Drug Administration (FDA) for use as a cavity liner and for treatment of dentin hypersensitivity.[58] Varnish may be used for dentin hypersensitivity (Chapter 41).
- Varnish is the only professional topical fluoride to be used for children under the age of 6 years.
- Its use in the United States as a caries preventive agent is considered off-label, but has become a standard of care in practice.[54]
- Five percent NaF varnish is now offered with different formulations containing mineral enhancements:
  - Complex of casein phosphopeptide and amorphous calcium phosphate (ACP).
  - ACP.
  - Tri-calcium phosphate modified by fumaric acid.
  - Calcium and phosphate with xylitol.
  - Calcium sodium phosphosilicate.
  - Sodium trimetaphosphate.
- FV formulations have been adding both calcium and phosphate with the theory that making calcium ions bioavailable in the saliva will increase overall efficacy.[59]
- More in vivo research studies with human subjects are needed to determine the efficacy and benefits of mineral-enhanced FV formulations.[60]
- Only standard 5% NaF varnish formulations are recommended by the ADA for caries prevention.[47] There is no recommendation by the ADA at this time for FV with mineral enhancements.
- 38% silver diamine fluoride (SDF)[61-64]
  - No adverse issues have been reported in Japan since SDF was approved over 80 years ago.
  - 24.4%–28.8% silver (253,870 ppm Ag—antimicrobial effects)
  - 5.0%–5.9% fluoride (44,800 ppm F—promotes remineralization)
  - 8% ammonia (stabilizing agent/solvent)
  - pH 8–10, both colorless and tinted (blue) formulations available.
  - FDA cleared in 2015 as a Class II medical device for management of dentinal hypersensitivity.
  - Off-label use is caries arrest and prevention for high caries risk patients.
  - In 2017, the AAPD developed evidence-based guidelines for application of SDF on children, adolescents, and those with special needs.[64]
  - Individual state Dental Hygiene Practice Acts determine whether application is permitted for application by the RDH.

CLINICAL PROCEDURES: PROFESSIONAL TOPICAL FLUORIDE

I. Objectives

- *Prevention of dental caries*
  - Identify special problems, including areas adjacent to restorations, orthodontic appliances, xerostomia, and other risk factors.
  - Box 34-2 contains indications for the application of a professional fluoride.
  - Examples: Active or secondary caries, exposed root surfaces, current orthodontic treatment, low or no fluoride exposure, or xerostomia.
- *Remineralization of demineralized areas*
  - Demineralized white areas on the cervical third, especially under dental biofilm.
- *Desensitization*
  - Fluoride aids in blocking dentinal tubules, as explained in Chapter 41.
- Varnish covers and protects a sensitive area, and fluoride is slowly released for uptake.

II. Preparation of the Teeth for Topical Application

- *General preparation for tray and varnish applications*
  - Most patients will receive the professional topical application following their routine continuing care appointment with complete dental hygiene

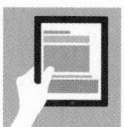

BOX 34-2

Indications for Professional Topical Fluoride Application[47]

- Patients at an elevated (moderate or high) risk of developing caries
- See Table 25-1 for the criteria to determine low, moderate, and high caries risk.
- **5% NaF varnish** at least every 3–6 months (for all ages and adult root caries)
  Or
- **1.23% APF gel** 4-minute trays at least every 3–6 months (for 6 years and older and adult root caries)
- Patients at a low risk of developing caries may not benefit from additional topical fluoride other than **OTC**-fluoridated toothpaste and fluoridated water daily.

Source: American Dental Association Council on Scientific Affairs. Topical fluoride for caries prevention: executive summary of updated clinical recommendations and supporting systematic review. *J Am Dent Assoc.* 2013;144(11):1279-1291.

procedures of personal oral hygiene care instruction, scaling, and stain removal.

- When the fluoride application is to be applied at a time other than following scaling and debridement, rubber cup polishing is not routinely necessary because fluoride will penetrate biofilm and provide the same benefits with or without prior polishing.[47,65]
- Calculus and stain removal are completed first.
- After calculus removal, apply principles of selective polishing for stain removal.
- Select an appropriate cleaning or polishing agent that will not harm the tooth surface or the restorative material present.
- A fluoride-containing polishing paste is not effective as a fluoride application.[66]
- Preparation and procedure for gel or foam tray application is included in Table 34-3; preparation and procedure for varnish application is described in Table 34-4.

III. Patient and/or Parent Counseling

- ◆ Help patients understand the purposes and benefits as well as the limitations of topical applications.
- ◆ Fluoride is one part of the total prevention program that includes daily biofilm control and limitation of cariogenic foods.

IV. Tray Technique: Gel or Foam

- ◆ *Tray application appointment preparation*
  - Schedule the appointment to end at least 30 minutes before the patient's eating time.
  - Prepare the patient for any discomfort, for example, the 4-minute timing when tray application is to be used.
  - Explain the need not to swallow but to expectorate immediately after the tray is removed.
- ◆ *Tray selection and preparation*
  - Figure 34-4 shows tray selection for coverage of all exposed root surfaces.
  - Design of trays: maxillary and mandibular trays may be hinged together or separated, are of a natural rounded arch shape to hold the gel and prevent ingestion, and are available in various sizes and brands.
  - Figure 34-5 shows the amount of gel to be placed in each tray.
  - Most gels are thixotropic to offer better physical and handling characteristics for use in trays.
  - Procedures for a professional gel or foam tray fluoride application are listed in Table 34-3.

V. Varnish Technique[54]

- ◆ *Varnish application appointment sequence:*
  - Dispense varnish: If dispensed from a tube (rather than a single-dose packet), discard any clear varnish

TABLE 34-3 • Procedure for Topical Gel or Foam Professional Tray	
Patient	• Determine need based on caries risk assessment (not to be used for children under 6 y of age) • Choose the type of fluoride (APF or NaF and gel or foam); data support use of APF Gel • Seat upright • Explain procedure including length: 4 min • Instruct not to swallow • Tilt head forward slightly
Tray coverage	• Choose appropriate size for full coverage • Complete dentition must be covered, including anterior and posterior vertical coverage, distal dam depth, and close fit to teeth • Check for coverage of areas of recession (if unable to cover exposed root surfaces, use varnish application) • Proper and improper tray coverage: see Figure 34-4
Place gel or foam	• Use minimum amount of gel or foam in the trays, as shown in Figure 34-5 • Fill tray one-third full with gel; completely fill, but do not overfill with foam
Dry the teeth	• Place a saliva ejector in the mouth during the drying procedure • Dry the teeth before insertion of trays starting with the maxillary teeth; facial, occlusal, and palatal surfaces and then the mandibular teeth; lingual, occlusal, and facial surfaces
Insert trays	• Place both filled trays in mouth • A two-step procedure (one tray at a time) may be required; if so, patient may not rinse but must expectorate after the removal of each tray to prevent swallowing
Isolation	• Use a saliva ejector with maximum efficiency suction
Attention	• Do not leave patient unattended
Timing	• Use a timer; do not estimate (4 min) • Procedure will take 8 min when a two-step procedure is used
Completion	• Tilt head forward for removal of tray • Request patient to expectorate for several minutes; do not allow swallowing • Wipe excess gel or foam from teeth with gauze sponge • Use high-power suction to draw out saliva and gel • Instruct patient that nothing is to be placed in the mouth for 30 min; do not rinse, eat, drink, or brush teeth

APF,   acidulated phosphate fluoride; NaF, sodium fluoride.

because the ingredients have separated and will contain only a fraction of the intended amount of fluoride.[67]

- Unit-dosed 5% NaF varnish is available in premeasured wells or individual packets of different dosages with an applicator brush to mix the varnish and then apply.

TABLE 34-4 • Procedure for Varnish Application (5% NaF)

Patient	• Determine need based on caries risk assessment (only professional fluoride recommended for children under 6 y of age) • Explain procedure • Seat supine • For the infant and toddler, the parent and clinician can sit knee to knee with the child held across the knees (Figure 46-4) • Instruct not to swallow during the procedure
Prepare product	• Dispense from a tube or open a single-dose packet • Have applicator brush available
Dry teeth	• Varnish sets up in the presence of saliva, but it is recommended to remove excess saliva by wiping the teeth with a gauze square
Apply varnish	• Dip applicator brush in varnish and mix well. Systematically brush a thin layer over all tooth surfaces. For prevention of early childhood caries in the infant, toddler, or very young child, apply to the maxillary anterior teeth first and then proceed to other areas of the dentition if patient is cooperative. For all other patients, use a systematic approach. Begin with mandibular teeth; facial, occlusal, and lingual surfaces and then the maxillary teeth; palatal, occlusal, and facial surfaces. Provide full coverage to all areas of the teeth including areas of recession and the cervical third of facial, lingual, and palatal surfaces and occlusal surfaces. Application time is approximately 1–3 min.
Completion	• Instruct patient that the teeth will feel like they have a coating or film, but this is not visible if clear product has been used. Ask the patient to avoid hard foods, drinking hot or alcoholic beverages, brushing, and flossing the teeth until the next day or at least 4–6 hr after application. It is advisable to drink through a straw for the first few hours after application

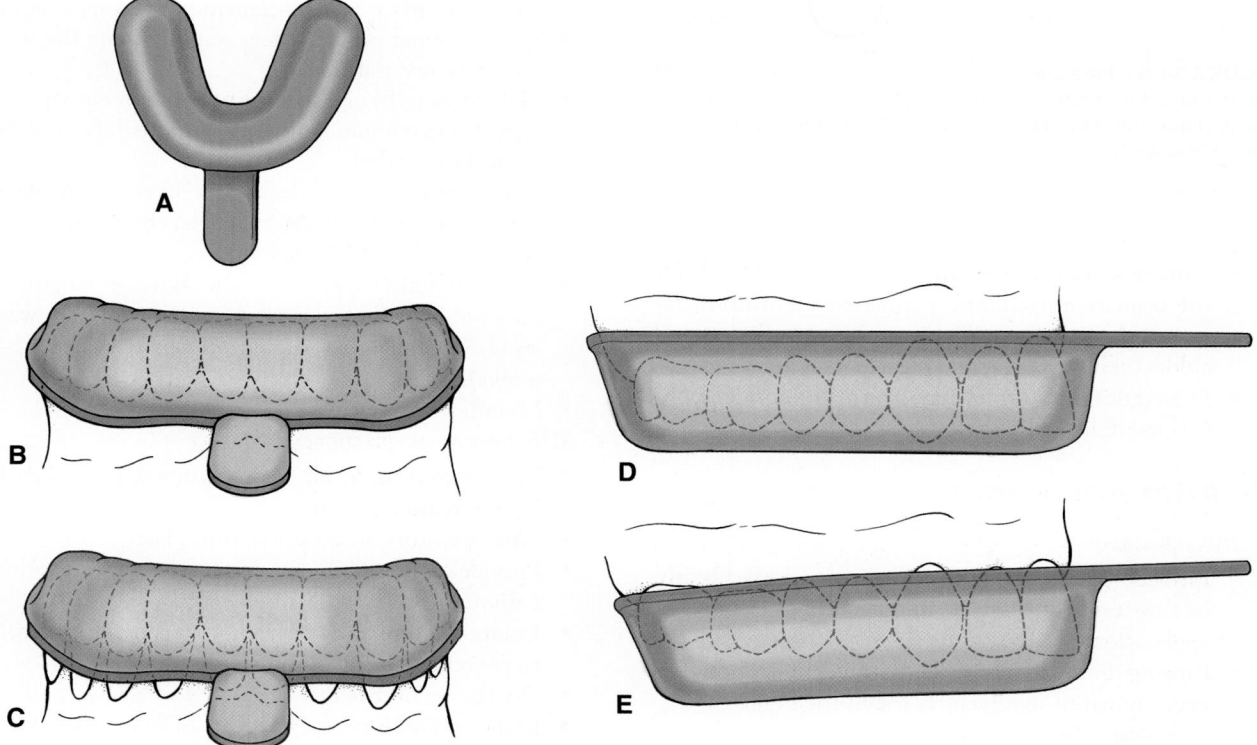

FIGURE 34-4 • Tray Selection. A: Mandibular tray held for try-in. **B:** Tray over teeth is deep enough to cover the entire exposed enamel above the gingiva. **C:** In the patient with recession and areas of root surfaces exposed, the tray may not be deep enough to cover the root surfaces where fluoride is needed for prevention of root caries or hypersensitivity. A custom-made tray is needed. **D:** Tray adequately covers the distal surface of the most posterior tooth. **E:** If the tray does not cover the distal surface of the most posterior tooth or the cervical third of canine and central incisor adequately, the tray may need to be repositioned to cover the distal surface, or a larger stock or custom-made tray is needed.

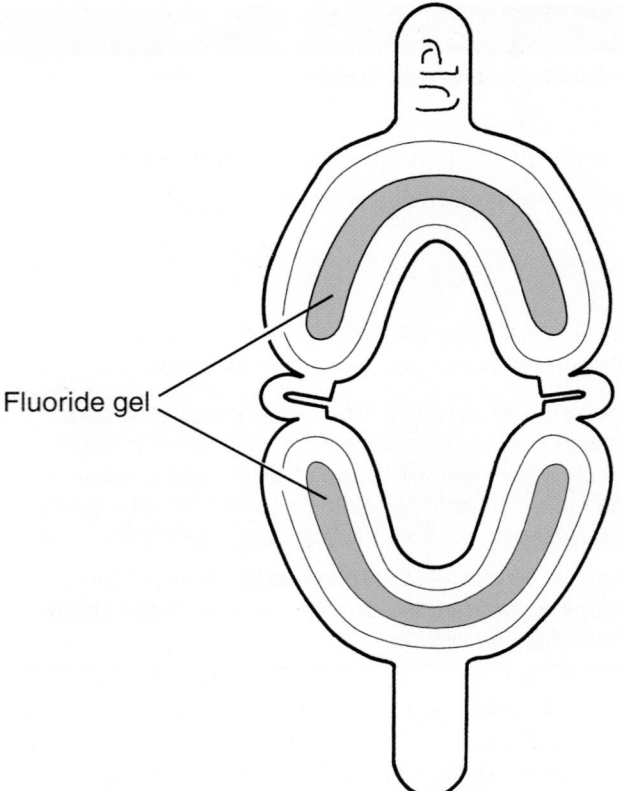

Fluoride gel

FIGURE 34-5 • Measured Gel in Tray. No more than 2 mL of gel is placed in each tray for children, and no more than 5 mL is placed in each tray for adults. This amount fills each tray size one-third full.

- Unit dosages are generally 0.25, 0.4, or 0.5 mL for the primary, mixed, and permanent dentitions, respectively, and are available in different flavors and colors (yellow, white, and clear).
- Procedures for a professional varnish fluoride application are listed in Table 34-4.

VI. After Application

- *Tray application*
  - Instruct patients not to rinse, eat, drink, brush, or floss until at least 30 minutes after gel or foam applications.
  - Rinsing immediately after a tray application has been shown to significantly lessen the benefits.[68]
- *Varnish application*
  - Instruct patients to avoid hot drinks and alcoholic beverages; eating hard, sticky, or crunchy foods; and brushing or flossing the teeth for 4–6 hours after application or until the next morning to allow fluoride uptake to continue undisturbed.
  - Varnish is removed by the patient using toothbrushing and flossing the next day.

VII. Silver Diamine Fluoride

- *Indications*[63]:
  - Extreme caries risk (xerostomia, severe early childhood caries, or cancer treatments—radiation/chemotherapy)
  - Treatment challenged by behavioral/medical management
  - Patients with carious lesions that may not all be treated in one visit (stabilize patient)
  - Difficult to treat dental carious lesions
  - Patients with no access to dental care (underserved populations)
- *Advantages*[69]:
  - Noninvasive (no needle or drill required)
  - Cariostatic agent
  - Reduces dentinal hypersensitivity
- *Contraindications/relative contraindications*[63]:
  - Allergy to silver
  - Pregnancy/breastfeeding
- Relative—Painful sores or raw areas on the gingiva or in the mouth (ulcerative gingivitis or stomatitis)
- *Potential limitations and risks*[63]:
  - Communicate effectively with the patient/parent/legal guardian/advocate and consider written informed consent form for SDF placement prior to application.
  - Sole placement of SDF does not eliminate the need for future restorations.
  - SDF needs to be applied one to two times at separate visits for maximum benefit (approximately once every 6–12 months).
  - The affected area of decay will likely stain black/gray permanently upon SDF placement; however, healthy enamel will not stain.
  - If accidentally applied to the skin or gingiva, a brownish stain may appear, which will not wash away immediately (should dissipate within 1–3 weeks).
  - Metallic/bitter taste.
- *SDF application appointment sequence*[63]:
  - Maximum dose 25 µL (1 drop) in a dappen dish/10 kg per treatment visit.
  - Line operatory and counter with plastic.
  - Provide a plastic bib and protective eyewear for the patient.
  - Isolate the tongue and cheek with gauze/cotton rolls to prevent staining of soft tissues.
  - Dry the lesion with air.
  - Immerse microsponge brush in SDF, remove excess on the side of the dappen dish.
  - Apply and allow the carious lesion to absorb for 1–3 minutes; may reapply.
- Rinse area thoroughly with water.
- Place gloves, cotton, and microsponge brush in a plastic bag for disposal.
  - Procedures for SDF application are listed in Table 34-5.

TABLE 34-5 • Procedure for SDF Application[63]

Patient	• Determine indications (e.g., extreme caries risk, xerostomia, severe childhood caries)
	• Review contraindications/relative contraindications
	• Communicate effectively regarding potential limitations and risks with the patient/parent/guardian and consider written informed consent prior to application
	• Inform the patient the affected area of decay will likely stain black/gray permanently upon placement of SDF
	• Provide protective eyewear and a plastic bib to the patient, and isolate both the tongue and cheek with gauze or cotton rolls to prevent staining
Prepare operatory & product	• Line counter and operatory with plastic. Dispense 1 drop in a dappen dish/10 kg per treatment visit
	• Have microsponge brush available
Dry the carious lesion and apply the SDF	• Dry the lesion with air. Immerse the microsponge in the SDF. Remove any excess product on the side of the dappen dish. Apply to the carious lesion and allow to absorb for 1–3 min; may reapply
Completion	• Rinse the area thoroughly with water. Place microsponge brush, cotton, and gloves into a plastic bag for disposal

SDF, silver diamine fluoride.

SELF-APPLIED FLUORIDES

◆ Self-applied fluorides (prescription [Rx] and OTC products) are available as dentifrices, mouthrinses, and gels.

◆ Concentrations of 1,500 ppm fluoride or less can be sold OTC.[39] Some products containing less than 1,500 ppm of fluoride are available only by Rx.

◆ May be applied by toothbrushing, rinsing, or trays that are custom-made or disposable.

I. Indications

◆ Patient needs are determined as part of total care planning.

◆ Indications for use of tray, rinsing, and/or toothbrushing depend on the individual patient prevention needs and caries risk assessment.

◆ Certain patients need multiple procedures combined with professional applications at the regular continuing care appointments. Special indications are suggested as each method is described in the following sections.

II. Methods

The three methods for self-application are by tray, rinsing, and toothbrushing.

◆ *Tray*
   • Custom-made or disposable tray: The tray is selected to fit the individual mouth and completely cover the teeth being treated.
   • Figure 34-4 shows adequate and inadequate tray coverage on the teeth.
   • Instruction is provided not to overfill the tray.

◆ *Rinsing*
   • The patient swishes for 1 minute with a measured amount of a fluoride rinse and expectorates.
   • Certain patients will need to learn how to rinse properly to force the solution between the teeth. Chapter 28 lists steps for teaching how to rinse.

◆ *Toothbrushing*
   • A fluoride-containing dentifrice is used for regular brushing after breakfast and before going to bed without further eating.
   • Brush-on gel is used after regular brushing to provide additional benefits.
   • Use an interdental brush to apply fluoride to proximal surfaces or open furcations.

TRAY TECHNIQUE: HOME APPLICATION

◆ The original gel tray studies using custom-fitted polyvinyl mouthpieces compared the use of 1.1% APF with plain NaF gel.

◆ The gel was applied daily over a 2-year period by schoolchildren aged 11–14 years during the school years. Dental caries incidence was reduced up to 80%.[70]

I. Indications for Use

◆ Rampant enamel or root caries in persons of any age to prevent additional new carious lesions and promote remineralization around existing lesions.

◆ Xerostomia from any cause, particularly loss of salivary gland function.

◆ Exposure to radiation therapy.

◆ Root surface hypersensitivity.

II. Gels Used (Available by Prescription)

◆ *Concentrations*[39]
   • 1.1% NaF; 5,000 ppm fluoride.
   • 1.1% APF; 5,000 ppm fluoride.

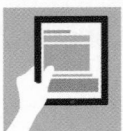

BOX 34-3
Instructions for Home Tray Application

1. One daily application just before bedtime; do not eat or drink until morning. If applied at other time of day, do not eat or drink for at least 30 minutes.
2. Brush and floss before applying tray to remove biofilm and food debris.
3. Use prepared custom-made polyvinyl trays. Disposable trays can be used if the appropriate fit can be obtained.
4. Distribute no more than 4–8 drops or a thin ribbon of the gel on the inner surface of each tray. Each drop is equivalent to 0.1 mL.
5. Expectorate to minimize saliva in the mouth.
6. Apply one tray at a time. Hold head upright.
7. Apply the mandibular tray first; close gently to hold the tray in place.
8. Time by a clock for 4 minutes. Do not swallow.
9. Expectorate several times when the tray is removed to prevent swallowing gel, and prepare the mouth for the other tray.
10. Apply the maxillary tray and follow steps 7–9 as for the mandibular tray.
11. After tray removal, do not eat, drink, or brush teeth for at least 30 minutes.
12. After both trays are removed, rinse the trays under running water and brush them clean.
13. Keep in open air for drying.

- *Precautions*[39]
  - Dispense small quantities.
  - Maximum adult dose is 16 drops per day (4–8 drops on the inner surface of each custom-made tray).
  - Use neutral sodium preparations on porcelain, composites, titanium, or sealants.
  - Patients with mucositis may experience irritation with the APF due to the high acidity.
- *Patient instructions*
  - Use the gel tray once each day, preferably just before going to bed without further eating and after tooth brushing and flossing.
  - Box 34-3 outlines the procedures for the patient to follow for a home tray application.
  - A printed copy of the instructions is given to the patient.

FLUORIDE MOUTHRINSES

- Mouthrinsing is a practical and effective means for self-application of fluoride for individuals at moderate or high caries risk.

- Do not use for patients aged 6 years or younger, or for those unable to rinse for a physical or other reason.[71]
- Rinsing can be part of an individual care plan or can be included in a group program conducted during school attendance.

I. Indications

- Mouthrinsing with a fluoride preparation may be an additional benefit for the following:
  - Young persons during the high-risk preteen and adolescent years.
  - Patients with areas of demineralization.
  - Patients with root exposure following recession and periodontal therapy.
  - Participants in a school health group program for children older than 6 years.
  - Patients with moderate-to-rampant caries risk who live in a fluoridated or nonfluoridated community.
  - Patients whose oral health care is complicated by biofilm-retentive appliances, including orthodontics, partial dentures, or space maintainers.
  - Patients with xerostomia from any cause, including head and neck radiation and saliva-depressing drug therapy.
  - Patients with hypersensitivity of exposed root surfaces.

II. Limitations

- Children under 6 years of age and those of any age who cannot rinse because of oral and/or facial musculature problems or other disability.
- Alcohol content:
  - Alcohol-based mouthrinses are not recommended; aqueous solutions are available.
  - Alcohol content of commercial preparations is not advisable for children, especially adolescents.
  - Alcohol-containing preparations are never to be recommended for a recovering alcoholic person; however, a history of former alcoholism would not necessarily be known to the clinician.
- Compliance is greater with a daily rinse than with a weekly rinse when practiced on an individual basis at home.

III. Preparations[39]

- Oral rinses are categorized as low-potency/high-frequency rinses or high-potency/low-frequency rinses.
- Most low-potency rinses may be purchased directly OTC, whereas most high-potency rinses are provided by Rx.
- Table 34-6 contains the compounds, concentration, and recommended frequency of use for currently available self-applied fluoride rinses.

TABLE 34-6 • Patient-Applied Fluoride Mouthrinses (Age 6 Years and Older)

TYPE/PERCENTAGE (RX OR OTC)	CONCENTRATION IN PPM	FREQUENCY OF USE (10 ML OR 2 TEASPOONS SWISHED FOR 1 MIN)
0.2% NaF (Rx)	905	Once daily or once weekly
0.044% NaF and APF (Rx and OTC)	200	Once daily
0.05% NaF (OTC)	230	Once daily
0.0221% NaF (OTC)	100	Twice daily

APF, acidulated phosphate fluoride; NaF, sodium fluoride; OTC, over-the-counter.

- *Low potency/high frequency (available OTC)*
  - *Preparations*
    - 0.05% NaF; 230 ppm.
    - 0.044% NaF or APF; 200 ppm (available by Rx or OTC depending on the brand).
    - 0.0221% NaF; 100 ppm.
  - *Specifications*
    - No more than 264 mg NaF (120 mg of fluoride) can be dispensed at one time.
    - A 500-mL bottle of 0.05% NaF rinse contains 100 mg of fluoride.
    - Bottle is required to have a child-proof cap.
    - Rinses are not to be used by children under 6 years of age or by children or adults with a disability involving oral and/or facial musculature.
    - Young children do not have sufficient control to expectorate, and they tend to swallow quickly.
    - The rinse is to be fully expectorated without swallowing.
  - *Procedure for use*
    - Low-potency rinses are used once or twice daily with 2 teaspoonfuls (10 mL) after brushing and before retiring. Follow manufacturer's ADA-approved specifications.
    - The adult and pediatric maximum dose is 10 mL of solution.
    - Swish between teeth with lips tightly closed for 60 seconds; spit out.
    - Have the patient practice rinsing at the dental chair.
    - Instruct patient: Do not eat or drink for 30 minutes after rinsing.
- *High potency/low frequency (available by Rx)*
  - *Preparation*
    - 0.20% NaF; 905 ppm.
    - Originally recommended as a weekly rinse, but can be used up to once per day.[47]
  - *Procedure for use*: the same as for high-frequency/low-potency rinses.

The prevented fraction of dental caries ranges from 30% to 59%, with the use of 0.2% fluoride rinse on various rinsing schedules.[51]

IV. Benefits

- Benefits from fluoride mouthrinsing have been documented many times since the original research using various percentages of various fluoride preparations.[72,73]
- Frequent rinsing with low concentrations of fluoride has the following effects:
  - A 26%–29% average reduction in dental caries incidence.[74]
  - Greater benefit for smooth surfaces, but some benefit to pits and fissures.
  - Greatest benefit to newly erupted teeth.
  - The program needs to be continued through the teenage years to benefit the second and third permanent molars.
  - Added benefits for a community with fluoridation.[74]
  - Effective in preventing and reversing root caries.[75]
  - Primary teeth present in school-aged children benefit by as much as a 42.5% average reduction in dental caries incidence.[76]

BRUSH-ON GEL

- Brush-on gel has been used as an adjunct to the daily application of fluoride in a dentifrice and as a supplement to periodic professional applications.
- Regular use has been shown to help control demineralization about orthodontic appliances.[77]
- Provides protection against postirradiation caries in conjunction with other fluoride applications.[78]

I. Preparations

Table 34-7 contains the type, concentration, and daily usage guidelines for currently available self-applied fluoride gels.

- *1.1% NaF (Neutral pH) or 1.1% APF (3.5 pH); 5,000 ppm*
  - Available as a gel to be used separate from toothbrushing.

TABLE 34-7 • Patient-Applied Fluoride Gels: Brush-On or Use in Custom-Made Trays (Age 6 Years or Older)

TYPE/PERCENTAGE (RX OR OTC)	CONCENTRATION IN PPM	DAILY USAGE GUIDELINES
1.1% NaF gel or paste (Rx)	5,000	Brush-on teeth, twice per day or 4–8 drops on inner surface of custom-made tray or brush-on teeth
1.1% APF (Rx)	5,000	Brush-on teeth, preferably at night or 4–8 drops on inner surface of custom-made tray
0.4% SnF (OTC)	1,000	Brush-on teeth, preferably at night

APF, acidulated phosphate fluoride; NaF, sodium fluoride; OTC, over-the-counter.

◆ 1.1% neutral NaF is also available as a dentifrice with an abrasive system added.

- The rationale for the dentifrice product is to increase compliance with one step (brushing only) rather than brushing, followed by application of the high-concentration gel with a toothbrush.
- Requires a prescription.

◆ *Stannous fluoride (SnF₂) 0.4% in glycerin base (1,000 ppm).*

◆ Available as a gel to be used separate from toothbrushing.

◆ Available OTC.

II. Procedure

◆ Teeth are cleaned first with thorough brushing and flossing before gel application with a separate toothbrush.

◆ Use once a day or more as recommended, preferably at night after toothbrushing and flossing.

◆ Place about 2 mg of the gel over the brush head and spread over all teeth.

◆ Brush 1 minute, then swish to force the fluid between the teeth several times before expectorating.

◆ Do not rinse.

FLUORIDE DENTIFRICES

I. Development

◆ Historically tried with various compounds, including stannous fluoride, NaF, sodium monofluorophosphate, and amine fluoride.

◆ Early research objectives: to find compatible fluoride, abrasive systems, and formulations containing available fluoride for uptake by the tooth surface.

◆ In 1960, the first fluoride dentifrice gained approval by the ADA, Council on Dental Therapeutics: 0.4% stannous fluoride.[79]

II. Indications

◆ *Dental caries prevention*

- Fluoride dentifrice approved by the ADA is an integral part of a complete preventive program and is a basic caries prevention intervention for all patients.[79]
- All patients regardless of their caries risk.
- Toothbrushing that covers all the teeth on all sides at least twice per day with fluoridated toothpaste is the foundation for all patients' fluoride regimen.
- Patients with moderate-to-rampant dental caries are advised to brush three or four times each day with a fluoride-containing dentifrice and to chew xylitol gum after a meal when they cannot brush.
- Expectorate, but do not rinse after toothbrushing, to give the fluoride a longer time to be effective.

III. Preparations

Fluoride dentifrices are available as gels or pastes. Amine fluorides are used in other countries, but not available in the United States.

◆ *Current fluoride constituents*[80]

- NaF 0.24% (1,100 ppm).
- Sodium monofluorophosphate (Na₂PO₃ F) 0.76% (1,000 ppm).
- Stannous fluoride (SnF₂) 0.45% (1,000 ppm).

◆ *Guidelines for acceptance*

The requirements for acceptance of fluoridated toothpaste by the ADA are described in Chapter 28. Look for ADA Seal of Acceptance.

IV. Patient Instruction: Recommended Procedures

Advise the patient in the selection of a fluoride dentifrice, the need for frequent use, the method for application to all the tooth surfaces, and the importance of using a fluoride dentifrice to promote oral health.

◆ Select an ADA accepted fluoride-containing dentifrice.

◆ Place recommended amount of dentifrice on the toothbrush.

◆ *Children (age less than 3 years)*: Twice-daily brushing (morning and night) with no more than a "smear" or the size of a grain of rice of fluoride dentifrice spread along the brushing plane.[81,82] Chapter 47 illustrates a small smear.

- Daily oral care begins with the eruption of the first primary tooth.
- The oral hygiene of parents and family with attention to daily biofilm removal by toothbrushing can make a significant impact on the small child's oral health.

◆ The paste is then spread over all the teeth before starting to brush so that all teeth benefit and large amounts of paste are not available for swallowing.

◆ *Older child (ages 3–6 years)*: Twice-daily brushing (morning and night) with fluoride toothpaste the size of a small pea.

- Demonstrate spreading this amount over the ends of the filaments, and explain that the child is not to swallow excess amounts of dentifrice.[81,82]

◆ *Adults*: Use 1/2 inch fluoride dentifrice twice daily.

◆ Spread dentifrice over the teeth with a light touch of the brush.

◆ Proceed with correct brushing positions for sulcular removal of dental biofilm (see Chapter 26).

◆ Do not rinse after brushing to keep fluoride in the oral fluids.[81,83]

◆ Keep dentifrice container out of reach of children.

V. Benefits

◆ Twice-daily use has greater benefits than once-daily use.[71]

◆ Moderate and high caries risk patients and those who live in a nonfluoridated community benefit from using a dentifrice several times per day to maintain salivary fluoride levels.

◆ The dentifrice is a continuing source of fluoride for the tooth surface in the control of demineralization and the promotion of remineralization.

◆ The use of a dentifrice with a fluoride concentration of 1,000 ppm and above compared to a dentifrice without fluoride can prevent dental caries up to an average of 23%.[84]

COMBINED FLUORIDE PROGRAM

◆ All patients, regardless of caries risk, benefit from at least twice-daily use of a fluoridated dentifrice and consumption of fluoridated water multiple times during each day.

◆ Patients at moderate-to-high caries risk benefit from additional methods of fluoride exposure.

◆ Additional caries reduction can be expected when another topical fluoride, such as a mouthrinse or gel tray, is combined with a fluoride dentifrice.[85]

◆ When self-administered methods are chosen, patient cooperation is a significant factor.

◆ Age and eruption pattern influence the method selected.

◆ Continuing care appointments are to be scheduled for frequent professional topical applications for those at moderate and high caries risk and for continuing instruction and motivation regarding daily fluoride use for all patients.

FLUORIDE SAFETY

◆ Fluoride preparations and fluoridated water have wide margins of safety.

◆ Fluoride is beneficial in small amounts, but it can be injurious if used without attention to correct dosage and frequency.

◆ All dental personnel need to be familiar with the following:
  • Recommended approved procedures for use of products containing fluoride.
  • Potential toxic effects of fluoride.
  • How to administer general emergency measures when accidental overdoses occur as listed in "Internal Poisoning" section of Chapter 9.

I. Summary of Fluoride Risk Management

◆ Use professionally and recommend only approved fluoride preparations for patient use.
  • Products may have approval from the FDA and the ADA in the United States.
  • Read about the programs of the ADA Council on Scientific Affairs and the Seal of Approval of Products in Chapter 28.

◆ Use only researched, recommended amounts and methods for delivery.

◆ Know potential toxicity of the various products, and be prepared to administer emergency measures for treating an accidental toxic response.

◆ Instruct patients in proper care of fluoride products.
  • Dentist prescribes no more than 120 mg of fluoride at one time (no more than 480 of the 0.25 mg tablets or 240 of the 0.5 mg tablets).[39] Do not store large quantities in the home.
  • Request parental supervision of a child's brushing or other fluoride administration. Rinses, for example, are not to be used by children under 6 years of age.
  • Fluoride products have child-proof caps and are to be kept out of reach of small children and other persons, such as the mentally challenged, who may not understand limitations.
  • In school health programs, dispensing of the fluoride product is to be supervised by responsible adults. Containers are to be stored under lock and key when not in active use.

II. Toxicity

◆ *Acute toxicity* refers to rapid intake of an excess dose over a short time.
  • Acute fluoride poisoning is extremely rare.[86]

◆ *Chronic toxicity* applies to long-term ingestion of fluoride in amounts that exceed the approved therapeutic levels.

◆ *Accidental ingestion* of a concentrated fluoride preparation can lead to a toxic reaction.

◆ *Certainly lethal dose (CLD)*[87]
  • A lethal dose is the amount of a drug likely to cause death if not intercepted by antidotal therapy.
  • *Adult CLD*: About 5–10 g of NaF taken at one time. The fluoride ion equivalent is 32–64 mg of fluoride per kilogram body weight (mg F/kg; Box 34-4A).
  • *Child*: Approximately 0.5–1.0 g, variable with size and weight of the child.

◆ *Safely tolerated dose (STD): one-fourth of the CLD*
  • *Adult STD*: About 1.25–2.5 g of NaF (8–16 mg F/kg).
  • *Child*: Box 34-4B shows STDs and CLDs for children.

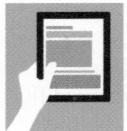

BOX 34-4
Lethal and Safe Doses of Fluoride

A. Lethal and Safe Doses of Fluoride for a 70-kg weight Adult CLD

5–10 g NaF

Or

32–64 mg F/kg

STD 5 1/4 CLD

1.25–2.5 g NaF

Or

8–16 mg F/kg

B. CLDs and STDs of Fluoride for Selected Ages

AGE (YEARS)	WEIGHT (LB/KG)	CLD (MG)	STD (MG)
2	22/10	320	80
4	29/13	422	106
6	37/17	538	135
8	45/20	655	164
10	53/24	771	193
12	64/29	931	233
14	83/38	1,206	301
16	92/42	1,338	334
18	95/43	1,382	346

Source: Reprinted with permission from Heifetz SB, Horowitz HS. The amounts of fluoride in current fluoride therapies: safety considerations for children. *ASDC J Dent Child.* 1984;51(4):257-269.

- Weights given for each selected age are minimal, and calculations for the doses are conservative.
- As can be noted in Box 34-4B, less than 1 g (1,000 mg) may be fatal for children aged 12 years and younger, and 0.5 g (500 mg) exceeds the STD for all ages shown.

For children under 6 years of age, however, 500 mg could be lethal.[87]

III. Signs and Symptoms of Acute Toxic Dose

Symptoms begin within 30 minutes of ingestion and may persist for as long as 24 hours.

- *Gastrointestinal tract*
- Fluoride in the stomach is acted on by the hydrochloric acid to form hydrofluoric acid, an irritant to the stomach lining. Symptoms include:
  - Nausea, vomiting, and diarrhea.
  - Abdominal pain.
  - Increased salivation and thirst.

- *Systemic involvements*
  - *Blood:* Calcium may be bound by the circulating fluoride, thus causing symptoms of hypocalcemia.
  - *Central nervous system:* Hyperreflexia, convulsions, and paresthesias.
  - *Cardiovascular and respiratory depression:* If not treated, may lead to death in a few hours from cardiac failure or respiratory paralysis.

IV. Emergency Treatment

- *Induce vomiting*
  - *Mechanical:* Digital stimulation at the back of tongue or in throat.
- *Second person*
  - Call emergency service; transport to hospital.
- *Administer fluoride-binding liquid when patient is not vomiting*
  - Milk.
  - Milk of magnesia.
  - Lime water (CaOH$_2$ solution 0.15%).
- *Support respiration and circulation*
- *Additional therapy indicated at emergency room*
  - Calcium gluconate for muscle tremors or tetany.
  - Gastric lavage.
  - Cardiac monitoring.
  - Endotracheal intubation.
  - Blood monitoring (calcium, magnesium, potassium, pH).
  - Intravenous feeding to restore blood volume, calcium.

V. Chronic Toxicity

- *Skeletal fluorosis*[86]
  - Isolated instances of osteosclerosis, an elevation in bone density, can result from chronic toxicity after long-term (10 years or more) ingestion of water with 8–10 ppm fluoride or from inhalation of industrial fumes or dust.
  - Skeletal fluorosis in its early stages is characterized by stiff and painful joints and becomes crippling in its later stages.
  - It has never been a public health concern in the United States, even in communities that naturally have had high levels of fluoride in the water for generations.
  - Is endemic in certain countries such as China and India with high levels of natural fluoride in the water.
  - Predisposing factors, dietary deficiencies, and population differences with regard to fluoride metabolism may play a role in its development in addition to exposure.
  - Methods for defluoridation have been developed, as described in this chapter.

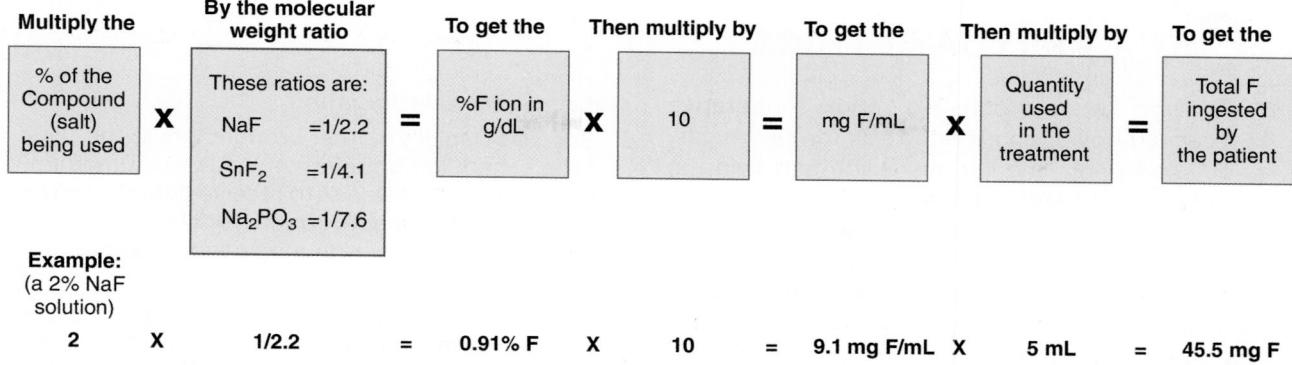

FIGURE 34-6 • Fluoride Calculation. Flowchart shows steps for the calculation of the amount of fluoride in a compound used in treatment. The example shows that 5 mL of a 2% solution of NaF contains 45.5 mg F, an amount slightly greater than half of the STD for a 2-year-old child (Box 34-4B). NaF, sodium fluoride; STD, safely tolerated dose. (From Heifetz SB, Horowitz HS. The amounts of fluoride in current fluoride therapies: safety considerations for children. *ASDC J Dent Child.* 1984;51(4):257-269.)

◆ *Dental fluorosis*
- Ingestion of naturally occurring excess fluoride in the drinking water and/or fluoride dental products can produce visible fluorosis only when used during the years of development of the crowns of the teeth, namely, from birth until age 16 or 18 years, or when the crowns of the third permanent molars are completed.
- No systemic symptoms result from the fluoride, and the individual has protection against dental caries.
- Scoring system used to describe dental fluorosis is found in Chapter 21.

◆ *Mild fluorosis*
1. *Clinical evaluation*
   - Mild and very mild forms, dental fluorosis appears as "white spots" or enamel opacities in the enamel surface.
   - No esthetic or health problem is involved. Many such white spots are not visible, except when scrutinized under a dental light and the surface is dried.
   - All white spots in the enamel are not related to fluoride intake; distinction can be made by reviewing the patient's dental and fluoride intake history, by noting the location and distribution of the white spots, and by considering the sequence of tooth development.
2. *Relation to fluoride sources*
   - Mild fluorosis may result from inadvertent ingestion of excess fluoride by young children during topical procedures, both self-applied and professional.
   - No problem exists when care is taken to follow basic steps, such as those listed in Tables 34-3 to 34-5, for professional applications.
   - Mouthrinses are not indicated for children less than 6 years of age.
   - Small amounts of dentifrice may be swallowed incidentally at each brushing. A child aged 4 years who lives in a nonfluoridated community uses a daily supplement (0.5 mg) and swallows two or three small amounts of dentifrice ingests far less than the STD of 106 mg, as shown in Box 34-4B.

VI. How to Calculate Amounts of Fluoride[87,88]

Figure 34-6 is a flowchart that shows the steps necessary to determine the amount of fluoride in a fluoride compound. By doing so, one can then calculate the amount ingested by the patient.

◆ Multiply the percentage of fluoride ion in the compound by the molecular weight conversion ratio, as shown in Figure 34-6.
◆ Obtain the ratio by dividing the molecular weight of the compound by the atomic weight of fluoride.
◆ Example: The molecular weight of NaF is 42 (Na = 23, F = 19). When divided by 19, a 1–2.2 ratio results, as shown in Figure 34-6.

DOCUMENTATION

A patient receiving a topical fluoride application and/or counseling regarding fluoride needs the following documented in the permanent record:
◆ Caries risk level (document as low, moderate, high, or extreme).
◆ Current use of fluoride toothpaste and exposure to fluoridated water.
◆ Type, concentration, mode of delivery, and postoperative instructions if a professional fluoride application is provided.
◆ Type, amount, and instructions for the use of any Rx or OTC patient-applied fluoride products recommended.
◆ A sample documentation using the SOAP format is provided in Box 34-5.

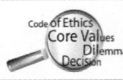

EVERYDAY ETHICS

Daniel was a well-behaved and cooperative 4.5-year-old boy at an elevated risk for dental caries due to having one carious lesion and living in a nonfluoridated area. At the time for the fluoride treatment, the dental hygienist, Nina, spent a few extra minutes explaining to Daniel how she will brush a coating on his teeth to make them stronger. Although Daniel's parents did not have insurance coverage, the hygienist decided it would be important for him to receive a fluoride application regardless of the fee. Daniel tolerated the procedure well. After the appointment, Nina explained to Daniel's mother the varnish postoperative instructions. Daniel's mother became upset and said, "Why did you give my son a fluoride treatment without my permission? My husband just lost his job, and I cannot afford this added cost."

Questions for Consideration

1. Because Daniel's mother brought him to the clinic for a scheduled appointment, Nina assumed *implied consent* for Daniel to receive dental hygiene treatment. Was it appropriate for Nina to assume consent for the fluoride application was also implied? Why or why not?

2. Discuss ways in which the legal/ethical concepts of professional liability, scope of practice, standard of care, and informed consent are related to this scenario.

3. Answer the questions in for resolving ethical issues or dilemmas found in "Ethical Applications" section of Chapter 1. Use the answers to determine at least one course of action Nina can take now to resolve the issue. Make sure to consider all individuals who might be affected by the decision.

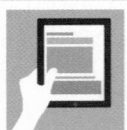

BOX 34-5

Example Documentation:
Professional Fluoride Application and Prescribing Home Fluoride

S— A 26-year-old male patient presents for a periodic oral examination, radiographs, and dental prophylaxis. Patient states that he drinks high-sucrose beverages on a frequent, daily basis. He also states that he uses toothpaste with fluoride twice daily and consumes fluoridated water.

O—Patient presents with medication induced xerostomia. Two proximal cavitated lesions were discovered on bitewing X-rays.

A—Patient was classified as being high risk for caries after conducting a caries risk assessment analysis.

P—Applied 5% NaF varnish to the entire dentition and provided postoperative instructions. Prescribed 1.1% NaF gel (two refills) to apply with a separate toothbrush at night. Discussed the need for an additional varnish application in 3 months to help prevent the future onset of dental caries.

Signed: _____, RDH

Date: _____

Factors to Teach the Patient

I. Personal Use of Fluorides
▶ Purposes, action, and expected benefits relative to the specific forms of fluoride treatment the patient will receive based upon individual caries risk.
▶ Specific instructions concerning self-applied techniques that will be performed at home.

II. Need for Parental Supervision
▶ Supervise daily care of child's teeth and mouth with the recommended amount of fluoridated toothpaste to prevent excess ingestion of fluoride.
▶ Keep fluoride products out of reach of small children.

III. Determine Need for Fluoride Supplements
▶ Must determine child is at high caries risk and consumes fluoride-deficient drinking water.
▶ Where to send private water source sample for fluoride analysis.

IV. Fluorides are Part of the Total Preventive Program
▶ Emphasize fluoride toothpaste and fluoridated water as the cornerstone for prevention of dental caries.
▶ Regular professional supervision and care.

V. Fluoridation
▶ How drinking fluoridated water helps people of all ages.
▶ How to access the CDC Community Water Fluoridation website to obtain reliable information about fluoridation in the United States.

VII. Bottled Drinking Water/Water Filters
▶ When bottled water does not have a label indicating that it is fluoridated, recommend filling a water bottle from a fluoridated water supply.
▶ Check with the water filter manufacturer to be certain the fluoride will not be removed through filtration.
▶ Distillation and reverse osmosis systems remove fluoride from drinking water, but water softeners do not.

VIII. Infant Formula
▶ Educate parents that powdered or liquid concentrate infant formula and the water used to reconstitute this formula may contain fluoride.

ENHANCE YOUR UNDERSTANDING

ONLINE RESOURCES
(see the inside front cover for access information)
- Audio glossary
- Appendices

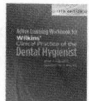

SUPPORT FOR LEARNING
(available separately)
- *Active Learning Workbook for Wilkins' Clinical Practice of the Dental Hygienist, 13th Edition*

INDIVIDUALIZED REVIEW
- Customized practice quizzing with Navigate 2 TestPrep for *Wilkins' Clinical Practice of the Dental Hygienist*

References

1. Ellwood R, Fejerskov O, Cury JA, Clarkson B. Chapter 18: Fluorides in caries control. In: Fejerskov O, Kidd E, eds. *Dental Caries: The Disease and Its Clinical Management.* 2nd ed. Oxford, England: Blackwell Munksgaard; 2008:293-294.

2. Newbrun E. Systemic benefits of fluoride and fluoridation. *J Public Health Dent.* 2004;64(suppl s1):35-39.

3. Ekstrand J. Chapter 4: Fluoride metabolism. In: Fejerskov O, Ekstrand J, Burt BA, eds. *Fluoride in Dentistry.* 2nd ed. Copenhagen, Denmark: Blackwell Munksgaard; 1996:55-67.

4. Bath-Balough M, Fehrenbach M. *Dental Embryology, Histology, and Anatomy.* 2nd ed. St. Louis, MO: Saunders; 2006:179-189.

5. Melfi RC, Alley KE. *Permar's Oral Embryology and Microscopic Anatomy.* 10th ed. Philadelphia, PA: Lippincott Williams & Wilkins; 2000:43-87.

6. Levy S. An update on fluorides and fluorosis. *J Can Dent Assoc.* 2003;69(5):286-291.

7. Aoba T, Fejerskov O. Dental fluorosis: chemistry and biology. *Crit Rev Oral Biol Med.* 2002;13(2):155-170.

8. Featherstone JD. The science and practice of caries prevention. *J Am Dent Assoc.* 2000;131(7):887-899.

9. Yoon SH, Brudevold F, Gardner DE, Smith FA. Distribution of fluoride in teeth from areas with different levels of fluoride in the water supply. *J Dent Res.* 1960;39:845-856.

10. Centers for Disease Control and Prevention. Recommendations for using fluoride to prevent and control dental caries in the United States. *MMWR Recomm Rep.* 2001;50(RR-14):1-42.

11. Centers for Disease Control and Prevention. Populations receiving optimally fluoridated public drinking water–United States, 1992–1996. *MWWR Morb Mortal Wkly Rep.* 2008;57(27):737-741.

12. Department of Health and Human Services, Centers for Disease Control and Prevention. *Community Water Fluoridation.* Atlanta, GA: Water Fluoridation Data and Statistics;

2014. [about 4 screens]. Updated July 11, 2017. Retrieved from https://www.cdc.gov/fluoridation/statistics/2014stats.htm. Accessed July 11, 2017.

13. Herschfeld JJ. Classics in dental history: Frederick S. McKay and the "Colorado brown stain." *Bull Hist Dent.* 1978;26(2):118-126.

14. McKay FS. The relation of mottled enamel to caries. *J Am Dent Assoc.* 1928;15:1429-1437.

15. Churchill HV. Occurrence of fluorides in some waters of United States. *J Ind Eng Chem.* 1931;23:996-998.

16. Dean HT, Arnold FA Jr, Elvove E. Domestic water and dental caries. V. Additional studies of the relation of fluoride domestic waters to dental caries experience in 4425 white children, aged 12 to 14 years, of 13 cities in 4 states. *Public Health Rep.* 1942;57:1155-1179.

17. Department of Health and Human Services (US). U.S. Public Health Service Recommendation for Fluoride Concentration in Drinking Water for the Prevention of Caries. *Public Health Rep.* 2015;130:1–14. Retrieved from http://www.cdc.gov/fluoridation/index.htm

18. Centers for Disease Control and Prevention. Engineering and administrative recommendations for water fluoridation, 1995. *MMWR Recomm Rep.* 1995;44(RR-13):1-40.

19. Griffin SO, Regnier E, Griffin PM, Huntley V. Effectiveness of fluoride in preventing caries in adults. *J Dent Res.* 2007;86(5):410-415.

20. Yeung CA. A systematic review of the efficacy and safety of fluoridation. *Evid Based Dent.* 2008;9(2):39-43.

21. Dirks OB, Houwink B, Kwant GW. Some special features of the caries preventive effect of water fluoridation. *Arch Oral Biol.* 1961;4:187-192.

22. Burt BA, Ismail AI, Eklund SA. Root caries in an optimally fluoridated and a high-fluoride community. *J Dent Res.* 1986;6(9):1154-1158.

23. Stamm JW, Banting DW, Imrey PB. Adult root caries survey of two similar communities with contrasting natural water fluoride levels. *J Am Dent Assoc.* 1990;120(2):143-149.

24. Ast DB, Fitzgerald B. Effectiveness of water fluoridation. *J Am Dent Assoc.* 1962;65:581-587.

25. Russell AL, Elvove E. Domestic water and dental caries. VII. A study of the fluoride-dental caries relationship in an adult population. *Public Health Rep.* 1951;66(43):1389-1401.

26. Englander HR, Wallace DA. Effects of naturally fluoridated water on dental caries in adults: Aurora-Rockford, Illinois, Study III. *Public Health Rep.* 1962;77(10):887-893.

27. Horowitz HS, Maier FJ, Law FE. Partial defluoridation of a community water supply and dental fluorosis. *Public Health Rep.* 1967;82(11):965-972.

28. Horowitz HS, Heifetz SB. The effect of partial defluoridation of a water supply on dental fluorosis—final results in Bartlett, Texas, after 17 Years. *Am J Public Health.* 1972;62(6):767-769.

29. Horowitz HS. Effectiveness of school water fluoridation and dietary fluoride supplements in school-aged children. *J Public Health Dent.* 1989;49(5 Spec No):290-296.

30. Lemke CW, Doherty JM, Arra MC. Controlled fluoridation: the dental effects of discontinuation in Antigo, Wisconsin. *J Am Dent Assoc.* 1979;80(4):782-786.

31. Jackson RD, Brizendine EJ, Kelly SA, Hinesley R, Stookey GK, Dunipace AJ. The fluoride content of foods and

beverages from negligibly and optimally fluoridated communities. *Community Dent Oral Epidemiol*. 2002;30(5):382-391.

32. Burt BA, Marthaler TM. Chapter 16: Fluoride tablets, salt fluoridation, and milk fluoridation. In: Fejerskov O, Ekstrand J, Burt BA, eds. *Fluoride in Dentistry*. 2nd ed. Copenhagen, Denmark: Blackwell Munksgaard; 1996:291-310.

33. Espelid I. Caries preventive effect of fluoride in milk, salt and tablets: a literature review. *Eur Arch Paediatr Dent*. 2009;10(3):149-156.

34. European Academy of Paediatric Dentistry. Guidelines on the use of fluoride in children: an EAPD policy document. *Eur Arch Paediatr Dent*. 2009;10(3):129-135.

35. American Dental Association. *Fluoridation Facts*. Chicago, IL: American Dental Association; 2005.

36. Hujoel PP, Zina LG, Moimaz SA, Cunha-Cruz J. Infant formula and enamel fluorosis: a systematic review. *J Am Dent Assoc*. 2009;140(7):841-854.

37. Siew C, Strock S, Ristic H, et al. Assessing the potential risk factor for enamel fluorosis: a preliminary evaluation of fluoride content in infant formulas. *J Am Dent Assoc*. 2009;140(10):1228-1236.

38. Berg J, Gerweck C, Hujoel P, et al. Evidence-based clinical recommendations regarding fluoride intake from reconstituted infant formula and enamel fluorosis. *J Am Dent Assoc*. 2011;142(1):79-87.

39. Burrell KH. Chapter 10: Fluorides. In: Mariotti AJ, Burrell KH, eds. *American Dental Association, Council on Scientific Affairs: ADA/PDR Guide to Dental Therapeutics*. 5th ed. Chicago, IL: American Dental Association and Thomson PDR; 2009:323-337.

40. Ismail AI, Hasson H. Fluoride supplements, dental caries, and fluorosis: a systematic review. *J Am Dent Assoc*. 2008;139(11):1457-1468.

41. Rozier RG, Adair S, Graham F, et al. Evidence-based clinical recommendations on the prescription of dietary fluoride supplements for caries prevention. *J Am Dent Assoc*. 2010;141(12):1480-1489.

42. Toyama Y, Nakagaki H, Kato S, et al. Fluoride concentrations at and near the neonatal line in human deciduous tooth enamel obtained from a naturally fluoridated and a non-fluoridated area. *Arch Oral Biol*. 2001;46(2):147-153.

43. Tubert-Jeannin S, Auclair C, Amsallem E, et al. Fluoride supplements (tablets, drops, lozenges or chewing gums) for preventing dental caries in children. *Cochrane Database Syst Rev*. 2011;(12):CD007592.

44. Bibby BG. Use of fluorine in the prevention of dental caries. II. The effects of sodium fluoride applications. *J Am Dent Assoc*. 1944;31:317.

45. Knutson JW. Sodium fluoride solutions: technique for application to the teeth. *J Am Dent Assoc*. 1948;36(1):37-39.

46. Galagan DJ, Knutson JW. The effect of topically applied fluorides on dental caries experience; experiments with sodium fluoride and calcium chloride; widely spaced applications; use of different solution concentrations. *Public Health Rep*. 1948;63(38):1215-1221.

47. Weyant RJ, Tracy SL, Anselmo T, et al. Topical fluoride for caries prevention: executive summary of the updated clinical recommendations and supporting systemic review. *J Am Dent Assoc*. 2013;144(11):1279-1291.

48. Warren DP, Chan JT. Topical fluorides: efficacy, administration, and safety. *Gen Dent*. 1997;45(2):134-140, 142.

49. Ripa LW. An evaluation of the use of professionally (operator applied) topical fluorides. *J Dent Res*. 1990;69(Spec No):786-796.

50. Soeno K, Matsumura H, Atsuta M, Kawasaki K. Influence of acidulated fluoride agents and effectiveness of subsequent polishing on composite material surfaces. *Oper Dent*. 2002;27(3):305-310.

51. Poulsen S. Fluoride-containing gels, mouth rinses and varnishes: an update of evidence of efficacy. *Eur Arch Paediatr Dent*. 2009;10(3):157-161.

52. Beltrán-Aguilar ED, Goldstein JW, Lockwood SA. Fluoride varnishes: a review of their clinical use, cariostatic mechanism, efficacy and safety. *J Am Dent Assoc*. 2000;131(5):589-596.

53. Marinho VC, Worthington HV, Walsh T, Clarkson JE. Fluoride varnishes for preventing dental caries in children and adolescents. *Cochrane Database Syst Rev*. 2013;(7):CD002279.

54. Bawden JW. Fluoride varnish: a useful new tool for public health dentistry. *J Public Health Dent*. 1998;58(4):266-269.

55. Autio-Gold JT, Courts F. Assessing the effect of fluoride varnish on early enamel carious lesions in the primary dentition. *J Am Dent Assoc*. 2001;132(9):1247-1253.

56. Castellano JB, Donly KJ. Potential remineralization of demineralized enamel after application of fluoride varnish. *Am J Dent*. 2004;17(6):462-464.

57. Demito CF, Vivaldi-Rodrigues G, Ramos AL, Bowman SJ. The efficacy of fluoride varnish in reducing enamel demineralization adjacent to orthodontic brackets: an in vitro study. *Orthod Craniofac Res*. 2004;7(4):205-210.

58. Association of State and Territorial Dental Directors Fluorides Committee. *Fluoride Varnish: An Evidence-Based Approach Research Brief*. Retrieved from https://astdd.org/docs/fl-varnish-brief-september-2014-amended-05-2016.docx. Accessed October 20, 2017.

59. Shen P, Bagheri R, Walker GD, et al. Effect of calcium phosphate addition to fluoride containing dental varnishes on enamel demineralization. *Aust Dent J*. 2016;61:357-365. doi:10.111/adj.12385.

60. Majithia U, Venkataraghavan K, Choudary P, Trivedi K, Shah S, Virda M. Comparative evaluation of application of different fluoride varnishes on artificial early enamel lesion: an in vitro study. *Indian J Dent Res*. 2016;27:521-527.

61. Chu CH, Lo ECM. Promoting caries arrest in children with silver diamine fluoride: a review. *Oral Health Prev Dent*. 2008;6(4):315-321.

62. Rosenblatt A, Stamford TC, Niederman R. Silver diamine fluoride: a caries "silver-fluoride bullet." *J Dent Res*. 2009;88(2):116-125.

63. Horst J, Ellenikiotis H, Milgrom P. UCSF protocol for caries arrest using silver diamine fluoride: rationale, indications and consent. *J Calif Dent Assoc*. 2016;44(1):16-28.

64. Crystal, YO, Marghalani AA, Ureles SD, et al. Use of silver diamine fluoride for dental caries management in children and adolescents, including those with special health care needs. *Pediatr Dent*. 2017;39(5):E135-E145.

65. Ripa LW. Need for prior toothcleaning when performing a professional topical fluoride application:

review and recommendations for change. *J Am Dent Assoc.* 1984;109(2):281-285.

66. Vrbic V, Brudevold F, McCann HG. Acquisition of fluoride by enamel from fluoride pumice pastes. *Helv Odontol Acta.* 1967;11(1):21-26.

67. Shen C, Autio-Gold J. Assessing fluoride concentration uniformity and fluoride release from three varnishes. *J Am Dent Assoc.* 2002;133(2):176-182.

68. Stookey GK, Schemehorn BR, Drook CA, Cheetham BL. The effect of rinsing with water immediately after a professional fluoride gel application on fluoride uptake in demineralized enamel: an in vivo study. *Pediatr Dent.* 1986;8(3):153-157.

69. Castillo J, Rivera S, Aparicio T, et al. The short-term effects of diammine silver fluoride on tooth sensitivity: a randomized controlled trial. *J Dent Res.* 2011;90(2):203-208.

70. Englander HR, Keyes PH, Gestwicki M, Sultz HA. Clinical anticaries effect of repeated topical sodium fluoride applications by mouthpieces. *J Am Dent Assoc.* 1967;75(3):638-644.

71. Adair SM. Evidence-based use of fluoride in contemporary pediatric dental practice. *Pediatr Dent.* 2006;28(2):133-142.

72. Torell P, Ericsson Y. The potential benefits derived from fluoride mouth rinses. In: Forrester DJ, Schulz EM, eds. *International Workshop on Fluorides and Dental Caries Reductions.* Baltimore, MD: University of Maryland School of Dentistry; 1974:114-176.

73. Birkeland JM, Torell P. Caries-preventive fluoride mouthrinses. *Caries Res.* 1978;12(suppl 1):38-51.

74. Driscoll WS, Swango PA, Horowitz AM, Kingman A. Caries-preventive effects of daily and weekly fluoride mouthrinsing in a fluoridated community: final results after 30 months. *J Am Dent Assoc.* 1982;105(6):1010-1013.

75. Heijnsbroek M, Paraskevas S, Vav der Weijden GA. Fluoride interventions for root caries: a review. *Oral Health Prev Dent.* 2007;5(2):145-152.

76. Ripa LW, Leske GS, Varma A. Effect of mouthrinsing with a 0.2 percent neutral NaF solution on the deciduous dentition of first to third grade school children. *Pediatr Dent.* 1984;6(2):93-97.

77. Stratemann MW, Shannon IL. Control of decalcification in orthodontic patients by daily self-administered application of a water-free 0.4 percent stannous fluoride gel. *Am J Orthod.* 1974;66(3):273-279.

78. Wescott WB, Starcke EN, Shannon IL. Chemical protection against postirradiation dental caries. *Oral Surg Oral Med Oral Pathol.* 1975;40(6):709-719.

79. American Dental Association, Council on Dental Therapeutics. Evaluation of Crest toothpaste. *J Am Dent Assoc.* 1960;61:272.

80. Mariotti MJ, Burrell K. Mouthrinses and dentifrices. In: *American Dental Association, Council on Scientific Affairs: ADA/PDR Guide to Dental Therapeutics.* 5th ed. Chicago, IL: American Dental Association and Thomson PDR; 2009:305-321.

81. American Academy of Pediatric Dentistry Liaison with Other Groups Committee; and American Academy on Pediatric Dentistry Council on Scientific Affairs. Guideline on fluoride therapy. *Pediatr Dent.* 2013;36:171-174.

82. American Dental Association Council on Scientific Affairs. Fluoride toothpaste use for young children. *JADA.* 2014;145(2):190-191.

83. Sjogren K, Melin NH. The influence of rinsing routines on fluoride retention after toothbrushing. *Gerodontology.* 2001;18(1):15-20.

84. Walsh T, Worthington HV, Glenny AM, Appelbe P, Marinho VC, Shi X. Fluoride toothpastes of different concentrations for preventing dental caries in children and adolescents. *Cochrane Database Syst Rev.* 2010;(1):CD007868.

85. Marinho VC. Cochrane reviews of randomized trials of fluoride therapies for preventing dental caries. *Eur Arch Paediatr Dent.* 2009;10(3):183-191.

86. Whitford GM. Acute and chronic fluoride toxicity. *J Dent Res.* 1992;71(5):1249-1254.

87. Heifetz SB, Horowitz HS. The amounts of fluoride in current fluoride therapies: safety considerations for children. *ASDC J Dent Child.* 1984;51(4):257-269.

88. Bayless JM, Tinanoff N. Diagnosis and treatment of acute fluoride toxicity. *J Am Dent Assoc.* 1985;110(2):209-211.

Sealants

Jill C. Moore, RDH, BSDH, MHA, EdD

CHAPTER OUTLINE

INTRODUCTION
I. Development of Sealants
II. Purposes of the Sealant
III. Purposes of the Acid Etch

SEALANT MATERIALS
I. Criteria for the Ideal Sealant
II. Classification of Sealant Materials

INDICATIONS FOR SEALANT PLACEMENT
I. Patients at Risk for Dental Caries (Any Age)
II. Selection of Teeth
III. Contraindications for Sealant Placement

PENETRATION OF SEALANT
I. Pit and Fissure Anatomy
II. Contents of a Pit or Fissure

III. Effect of Cleaning
IV. Amount of Penetration

CLINICAL PROCEDURES
I. Patient Preparation
II. Tooth Preparation
III. Tooth Isolation
IV. Acid Etch
V. Rinse and Air Dry Tooth
VI. Evaluate for Complete Etching
VII. Place Sealant Material
VIII. Cure Sealant
IX. Evaluate Cured Sealant
X. Check Occlusion
XI. Follow-Up

MAINTENANCE
I. Retention
II. Factors Affecting Retention
III. Replacement

SCHOOL-BASED DENTAL SEALANT PROGRAMS
DOCUMENTATION
EVERYDAY ETHICS
FACTORS TO TEACH THE PATIENT
REFERENCES

LEARNING OBJECTIVES

After studying this chapter, the student will be able to:

1. Describe the development and purposes of dental sealant materials.

2. Explain the types of sealant material and list the criteria of an ideal dental sealant material.

3. List indications and contraindications for placement of dental sealants.

4. Describe the clinical procedures for placement and maintenance of a dental sealant.

5. Explain the factors that affect sealant penetration.

6. Identify factors to document a dental sealant placement in the patient record.

INTRODUCTION

A pit and fissure sealant is an organic polymer (resin) that flows into the pit or fissure of a posterior tooth and bonds by mechanical retention to the tooth.

- Placement of dental sealants is an evidence-based preventive recommendation that can significantly reduce the incidence of dental caries.[1]
- As part of a complete preventive program, pit and fissure sealants are indicated for selected patients.
- Topically applied fluorides protect smooth tooth surfaces more than occlusal surfaces; dental sealants reduce the incidence of occlusal dental caries.
- The incidence of new pit and fissure caries can be lowered by 86% if the sealant is retained at 1 year, 78.6% at 2 years, and 58.6% at 4 years.[2]
- Sealant application is a part of a complete prevention program, not an isolated procedure.
- As an isolated procedure, the patient (and parent) may misunderstand the specific role of sealants in prevention.
- Other surfaces and other teeth still need other methods of preventive protection.

I. Development of Sealants

Sealants were developed by Dr. Michael Buonocore and a group of dental scientists at the Eastman Dental Center in Rochester, New York.

1. Early research focused on the need to prepare the enamel surface so a dental material would adhere.
2. They demonstrated that, by using an acid-etchant process, the enamel could be altered to increase retention.
3. The research proved to be a major breakthrough, particularly in esthetic and preventive dentistry.[3,4]

II. Purposes of the Sealant

- Provide a physical barrier to "seal off" the pit or fissure.
- Prevent oral bacteria and their nutrients from collecting within the pit or fissure to create the acid environment necessary for the initiation of dental caries.[5,6]
- Fill the pit or fissure as deep as possible and provide tight smooth margins at the junction with the enamel surface.[5,6]
- Provide continued protection in the depth of the micropore even when the sealant material is worn or cracked away on the surface around the pit or fissure, and new sealant material can be added for repair and to reseal the enamel/sealant junction.[5]

III. Purposes of the Acid Etch

- To produce irregularities or micropores in the enamel.
- To allow the liquid resin to penetrate into the micropores and create a bond or mechanical locking.
- Figure 35-1 illustrates the sealant placed on a smooth enamel surface in contrast with placement on an etched surface with retention.

SEALANT MATERIALS

The variety of available sealant materials provides options for both the patient and clinician. The clinician decides which material will be most beneficial depending on:

- An assessment of patient needs.
- Sealant placement environment.
- Available supplies.

I. Criteria for the Ideal Sealant[3]

- Achieve prolonged bonding to the enamel.
- Be biocompatible with oral tissues.
- Offer a simple application procedure.
- Be a free-flowing, low-viscosity material capable of entering narrow fissures.
- Have low solubility in the oral environment.

II. Classification of Sealant Materials

- A majority of sealants in clinical use are made of Bis-GMA (bisphenol A–glycidyl methylacrylate). The techniques of application vary slightly among available products; follow manufacturer's directions.

A. Classification by the Method of Polymerization

- *Self-cured* or *autopolymerized*
  - Preparation: material supplied in two parts. When the two are mixed, they quickly polymerize (harden).
  - Advantage: no curing light required.

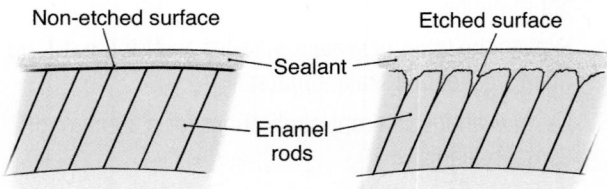

FIGURE 35-1 • Enamel–Sealant Interface. Diagram of enamel–sealant interface to compare nonetched with etched surface. Etching produces microscopic porosities in the enamel to increase the area of retention. The unpolymerized resin flows into the porosities and hardens in tag-like projections, as shown on the right. (From Buonocore MG, Matsui A, Gwinnett AJ. Penetration of resin dental materials into enamel surfaces with reference to bonding. *Arch Oral Biol.* 1968;13(1):61-70.)

- Disadvantages: mixing required; working time limited because polymerization begins when the material is mixed.
- *Visible light-cured or photopolymerized*
  - Preparation: material hardens when exposed to a special curing light.
  - Advantages: no mixing required; increased working time due to control over start of polymerization.
  - Disadvantages: extra costs and disinfection time required for curing light, protective shields, and/or glasses.

B. Classification by Filler Content

- *Filled*
  - Purpose of filler: to increase bond strength and resistance to abrasion and wear.
  - Fillers: glass and quartz particles give hardness and strength to resist occlusal forces.
  - Effect: viscosity of the sealant is increased. Flow into the depth of a fissure varies.
- *Unfilled*
  - Clear, does not contain particles.
  - Less resistant to abrasion and wear.
  - May not require occlusal adjustment after placement, so provides an advantage for school and community health programs where sealants are placed.
- *Fluoride releasing*
  - Purpose: to enhance caries resistance.
  - Action: remineralization of incipient caries at the base of the pit or fissure.

C. Classification by Color

- Available: clear, tinted, and opaque.
- Purpose: quick identification for evaluation during maintenance assessment.
- Effect: clear, tinted, or opaque sealants do not differ in retention.

INDICATIONS FOR SEALANT PLACEMENT

Individual patient benefit will depend on the following:
- Health, diet, and lifestyle.
- Age of tooth and past caries experience.
- Tooth anatomy.

I. Patients at Risk for Dental Caries (Any Age)

The following risk factors will lead to an increased risk of dental caries:
- Xerostomia: from medications or other reasons.
- Patient undergoing orthodontic treatment.
- Incipient pit and fissure caries (limited to the enamel) with no radiographic evidence of caries on an adjacent proximal surface.
- Low socioeconomic status.
- Diet high in sugars.
- Inadequate daily oral health care.

II. Selection of Teeth

- Newly erupted: place sealant as soon as the tooth is fully erupted.[7]
- Occlusal contour: when pit or fissure is deep and irregular, as illustrated in Figure 35-2.
- Caries history: other teeth restored or have carious lesions.
- Figure 35-3 is a flowchart to assist in decision making.

III. Contraindications for Sealant Placement

- Radiographic evidence of adjacent proximal dental caries.
- Pit and fissures are well coalesced and self-cleansing; low caries risk.
- Tooth not completely erupted.
- Primary tooth near exfoliation.

PENETRATION OF SEALANT

Penetration of sealant material to the depth of the fissure depends on the following:
- Configuration of the pit or fissure.
- Presence of deposits and debris within the pit or fissure.
- Properties of the sealant itself.

I. Pit and Fissure Anatomy

The shape and depth of pits and fissures vary considerably even within one tooth. Anatomic differences include:
- *Wide V-shaped* (Figure 35-4B) or *narrow V-shaped fissures*.

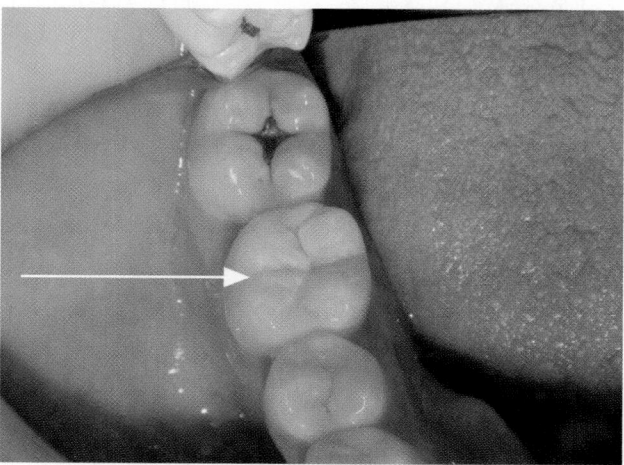

FIGURE 35-2 • Molar Tooth with Pits and Fissures. Tooth #30 with deep fissures is selected for placing a dental sealant. Note the amalgam filling on tooth #31, which is evidence of previous dental caries experience. (Photograph courtesy of Jill Moore, RDH, BSDH, MHA, EdD, School Oral Health Consultant, Michigan Department of Health and Human Services.)

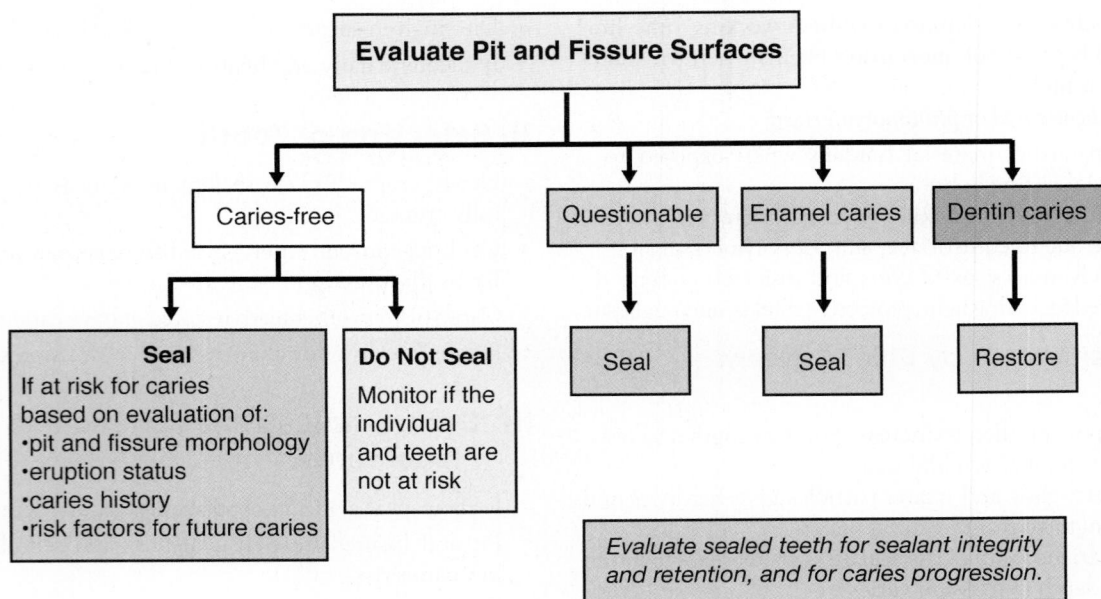

FIGURE 35-3 • **Tooth Selection for Sealant Placement.** Flowchart to assist in decision making for placement of sealants. (Adapted from Workshop on guidelines for sealant use: recommendations. The Association of State and Territorial Dental Directors, the New York State Health Department, the Ohio Department of Health and the School of Public Health, University of Albany, State University of New York. *J Public Health Dent.* 1995;55(5 Spec):263-273.)

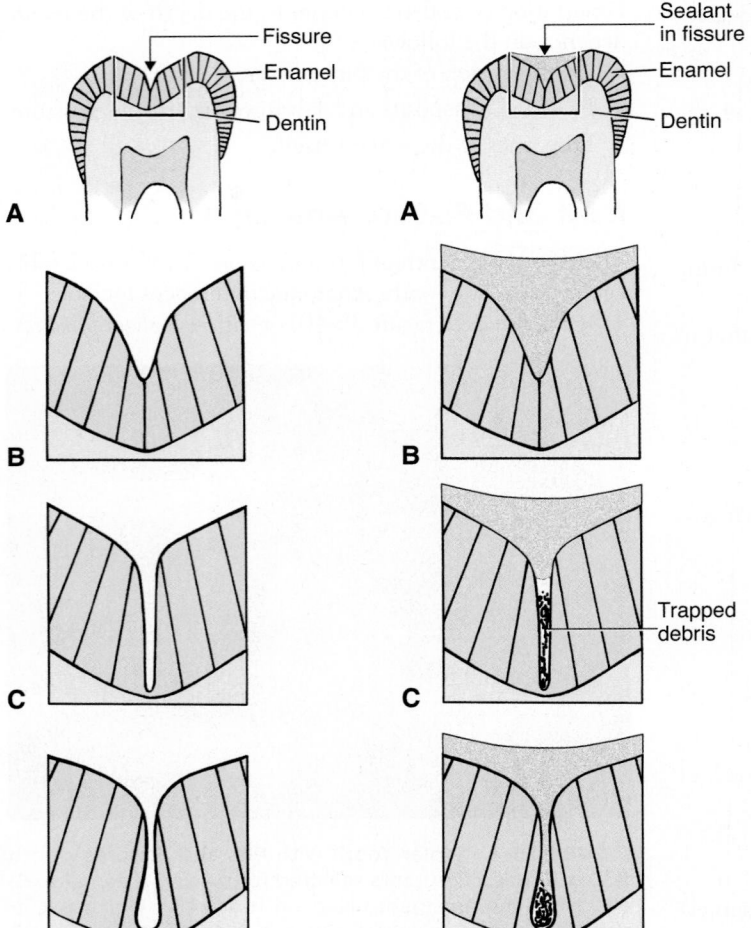

FIGURE 35-4 • **Occlusal Fissures.** Drawings made from microscopic slides show variations in the shape and depth of fissures both before and after sealant placement. **A:** Tooth with section enlarged for **(B-D)**. **B:** Wide V-shaped fissure shows full sealant penetration. **C:** Long narrow groove that nearly reaches the dentinoenamel junction. **D:** Long constricted form with a bulbous terminal portion.

- *Long narrow pits* and grooves reach, or nearly reach, the dentinoenamel junction (Figure 35-4C).
- *Long constricted fissures with a bulbous terminal portion* (Figure 35-4D) that may take a wavy course, which may not lead directly from the outer surface to the dentinoenamel junction.

II. Contents of a Pit or Fissure

A pit or fissure may contain the following:
- Dental biofilm, pellicle, debris.
- Rarely but possibly intact remnants of tooth development.

III. Effect of Cleaning

- Cleaning the tooth prior to acid etching can increase sealant retention.
- Use of an air polisher or laser prior to acid etching is not well supported by the literature, mainly because of added cost.[8]
- Cleaning the tooth with a toothbrush and water is ideal because the narrow, long fissures are difficult to clean completely.[9]
- Cleaning the tooth with pumice prior to dental sealant placement is avoided; if used, complete removal of pumice is necessary.
- Retained cleaning material can block the sealant from filling the fissure and can also get mixed with the sealant.
- Removal of pumice used for cleaning and thorough washing are necessary for retention of the sealant.

IV. Amount of Penetration

- Wide V-shaped and shallow fissures are more apt to be filled by sealants (Figure 35-4B).
- Although ideally the sealant penetrates to the bottom of a pit or fissure, such penetration is frequently impossible.
- Microscopic examination of pits and fissures after sealant application has shown the sealant material often does not penetrate to the bottom because residual debris, cleaning agents, and trapped air prevent passage of the material (Figure 35-4C and D).
- The bacteria in incipient dental caries at the base of a well-sealed pit or fissure have no access to nutrients required for survival.

CLINICAL PROCEDURES

To achieve high dental sealant retention rates:
- Treat each quadrant separately while placing sealants on all eligible teeth.
- Use the four-handed method with an assistant:
  - To ensure moisture control.
  - To work efficiently and save time.
- Follow manufacturer's directions for each product.
- Success of treatment (retention) depends on the precision in each step of the application.
- Retention of sealant depends on maintaining a dry field during etching and sealant placement.
- Step-by-step clinical procedures and equipment/supplies needed for the placement of a dental sealant are illustrated in Table 35-1. Additional details for each step are provided in Sections I through IX.

I. Patient Preparation (Step 1)

- Explain the procedure and steps to be performed.
- Provide patient with ultraviolet (UV) protective safety eyewear for protection from:
  - Chemicals used during etching and sealant placement.
  - The UV light from the curing lamp.

II. Tooth Preparation (Step 2)

A. Purposes

- Remove deposits and debris.
- Permit maximum contact of the etch and the sealant with the enamel surface.
- Encourage sealant penetration into the pit or fissure.

B. Methods

- Examine the tooth surfaces: remove calculus and stain.
- For a patient with no stain or calculus, apply toothbrush filaments straight into occlusal pits and fissures.
- Suction the pits and fissures with a high-velocity evacuator.
- Gently use the explorer tip to remove debris and bacteria from the pit or fissure and suction again to remove loosened material.
- Evaluate the need for additional cleaning; brushing may be sufficient.

III. Tooth Isolation (Step 3)

A. Purposes of Isolation

- Maintaining a dry tooth is the single most important factor in sealant retention.
- Keep the tooth clean and dry for optimal action and bonding of the sealant.
- Eliminate possible contamination by saliva and moisture from the breath.
- Keep the materials from contacting the oral tissues, being swallowed accidentally, or being unpleasant to the patient because of their flavor.

TABLE 35-1 • Steps for Placement of a Dental Sealant

STEP	ILLUSTRATION	DESCRIPTION	EQUIPMENT AND SUPPLIES
Step 1	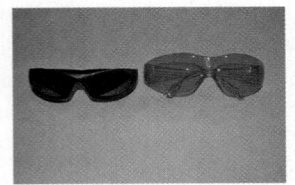	**Patient preparation** • Seat patient comfortably • Provide patient education materials and answer questions • Provide UV protective eyewear for protection from chemicals and curing light	• Patient education materials • Safety glasses for patient
Step 2	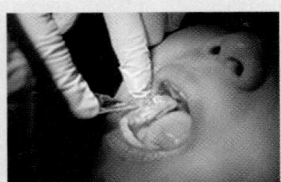	**Tooth preparation** • Clean the tooth with a toothbrush • Ensure the tooth is free from debris, external stain, and calculus prior to sealant placement	• Toothbrush • Examination instruments (mirror and explorer)

Step 3	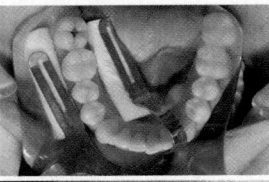	**Tooth isolation**
		• Maintain a working field that is not contaminated by saliva during all steps of sealant placement
		• Options include:
		  • rubber dam (not shown)
		  • cotton rolls on the mandibular arch (top left)
		  • triangular bibulous pad to cover the parotid duct for the maxillary arch (lower left)
		  • commercial isolation system with light and high speed suction (see Figure 35-5A)
		  • Note: Take care to moisten all cotton prior to removal to avoid sticking to dry mucosa
			• Rubber dam set up (optional)
			• Cotton rolls and holders Figure 35-5B
			• Bibulous pads (lower left)

Step 4	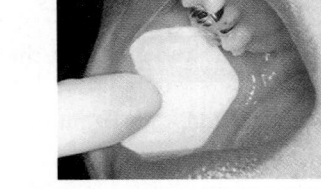	**Acid etch** • Dry entire area for 20–30 sec with air/water syringe • Maintain a dry field. Use a commercial etchant applicator (shown), brush, or cotton pellet to dispense etchant material • Place the acid etch only within the grooves and fissures where the sealant will be placed (shown at lower left) • Note: Follow manufacturer's directions for application time; usually between 15 and 60 sec	• Air/water syringe • Acid-etch material and applicator, brush, or cotton pellet
Step 5	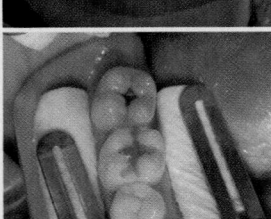	**Rinse and air dry tooth** • Place the high-velocity evacuation system over the tooth • Rinse the tooth with the air/water syringe • Spray water until the surface is free of etch (30–60 sec) • Spray air with an air/water syringe until dry • Re-isolate if necessary	• High-velocity evacuation system • Air/water syringe
Step 6	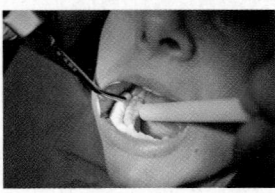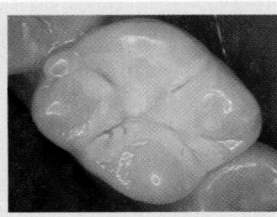	**Evaluate for complete etching** • A completely etched tooth will have a chalky-white appearance when dry • If the surface does not appear chalky, repeat the acid-etch step	• Air/water syringe • Mouth mirror for retraction and indirect vision

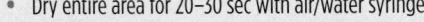

TABLE 35-1 • Steps for Placement of a Dental Sealant (*Continued*)

STEP	ILLUSTRATION	DESCRIPTION	EQUIPMENT AND SUPPLIES
Step 7	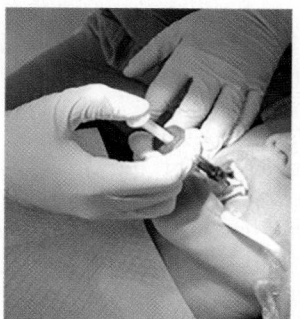	**Place sealant material** • Continue to maintain a dry field • Use external fulcrum (fingers resting lightly on patient's chin or cheek) • Place the wet sealant material in the prepared pits and fissures • Adjust flow so sealant material is deposited only within the grooves, pits, and fissures	• Sealant material and applicator • Slow-speed saliva ejector to help maintain dry field
Step 8	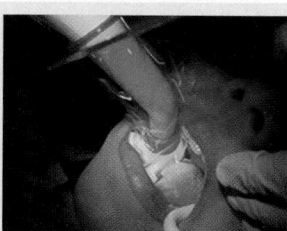	**Cure sealant** If using light-polymerized sealant material: • Ensure clinician and patient have UV protective eye protection • Cover entire tooth with light and cure for 20–30 sec in accordance with manufacturer's instructions If using self-curing sealant material: • Maintain dry field and allow drying time as indicated in manufacturer's instructions	• UV protective goggles/glasses for patient and clinicians • Curing light • Saliva ejector to help maintain dry field
Step 9	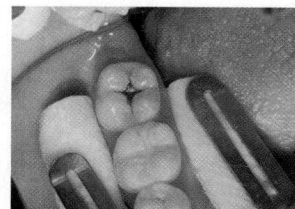	**Final/cured sealant** • Gently check for voids in the sealant material with explorer • Additional material can be added if the surface is not contaminated or wet	• Mirror and explorer • Saliva ejector to help maintain dry field • Additional sealant material, if needed, to fill voids
Step 10	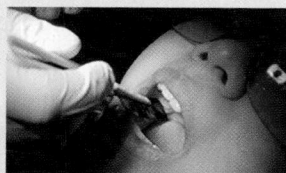	**Check occlusion** • Use articulating paper to locate high spots and adjust as needed • Unfilled sealant material will wear down via normal attrition • Filled sealant material will require occlusal adjustment	• Articulating paper • Holder
Step 11	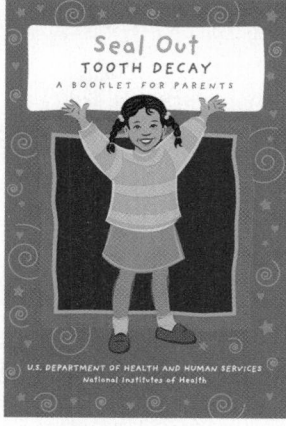	**Follow-up** • Provide patient education materials for the patient to take home • Answer patient's questions • Re-evaluate sealants at each subsequent maintenance appointment	• Excellent patient education materials are available for free from the National Institute of Dental and Craniofacial Research website. Available at: https://www.nidcr.nih.gov/orderpublications/

Source: Photographs in Steps 2, 4A, 7, 8, and 10 courtesy of Susan J. Jenkins, RDH, MS, CAGS, Forsyth School of Dental Hygiene, MCPHS University. Photograph in Step 11 courtesy of National Institute of Dental and Craniofacial Research. Available at: https://www.nidcr.nih.gov/sites/default/files/2017-11/seal-out-tooth-decay-parents.pdf. Additional photographs courtesy of Jill Moore, RDH, BSDH, MHA, EdD, School Oral Health Consultant, Michigan Department of Health and Human Services.

B. Rubber Dam Isolation

◆ Rubber dam application is the method of choice for complete isolation. This method is especially helpful when more than one tooth in the same quadrant is to be sealed.

◆ Rubber dam is essential when profuse saliva flow and overactive tongue and oral muscles make retraction and consistent maintenance of a dry, clean field impossible.

◆ When a quadrant has a rubber dam and anesthesia for restoration of other teeth, teeth indicated for sealant can be treated at the same time.

◆ Use local anesthesia when application of the clamp cannot be tolerated by the patient.

◆ Rubber dam may not be possible when a tooth needed to hold the clamp is not fully erupted.

C. Cotton-Roll Isolation

◆ Patient position: tilt the head to allow saliva to pool on the opposite side of the mouth.

◆ Position cotton-roll holder. Figure 35-5B shows the placement of two types of cotton-roll holders.

◆ Place a saliva ejector.

◆ Apply triangular saliva absorber (bibulous pad) over the opening of the parotid duct in the cheek.

◆ Take care to prevent saliva contamination from entering the area to be etched.

D. Additional Isolation Options

◆ Commercially available isolation systems (Figure 35-5A) that can be attached to the dental unit offer intraoral quadrant isolation, illumination, and suction.

IV. Acid Etch (Step 4)

A. Dry the Tooth

◆ Purposes
  • Prepare the tooth for acid etch.
  • Eliminate moisture and contamination.

◆ Use clean, dry air
  • Clear water from the air/water syringe by releasing the spray into a sink.
  • Test for absence of moisture by blowing on a mouth mirror or other dry surface.

◆ Air dry the tooth for at least 10 seconds.

B. Apply Etchant

◆ Action
  • Creates micropores to increase the surface area and provide retention for the sealant.
  • Removes contamination from the enamel surface.
  • Provides antibacterial action.

◆ Etchant solution forms
  • *Phosphoric acid:* 15%–50%, depends on the product and manufacturer.
  • *Liquid:* low viscosity allows good flow into the pit or fissure but may be difficult to control.
  • *Gel:* tinted gel with thick consistency allows increased visibility and control but may be difficult to rinse off the tooth surface.
  • *Semi-gel:* tinted, with enough viscosity to allow good visibility, control, and rinsing ease.

◆ Etchant timing varies from 15 to 60 seconds. Follow manufacturer's instructions for each product.

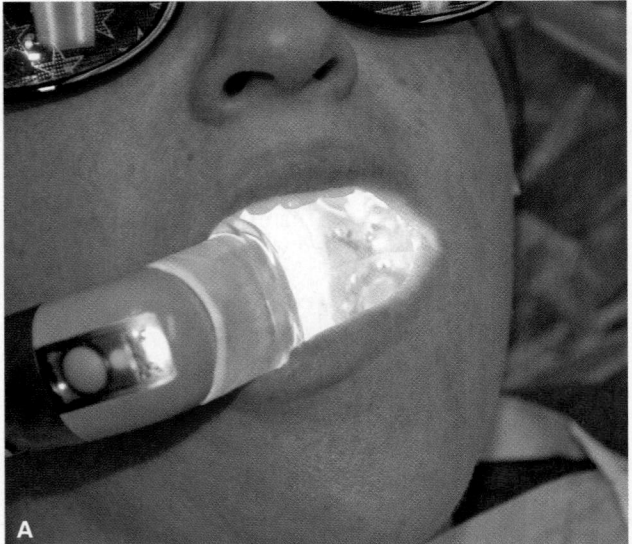
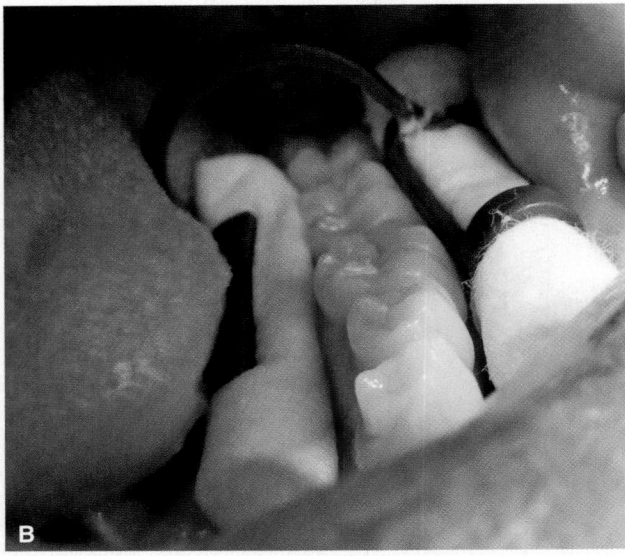

FIGURE 35-5 • Tooth Isolation. A: Demonstrates a commercial isolation system which has an internal light and high evacuation suction. This system will allow for two-handed sealant placement. **B:** Illustrates a disposable plastic cotton-roll holder used to isolate teeth in a mandibular quadrant. (Photographs courtesy of Jill Moore, RDH, BSDH, MHA, EdD, School Oral Health Consultant, Michigan Department of Health and Human Services.)

- ◆ Etchant delivery
  - *Liquid etch:* use a small brush, sponge, or cotton pellet; continuously pat rather than rub, when applying to keep the surface moist.
  - *Gel and semi-gel:* use a syringe, brush, or manufacturer-supplied single-use cannula.

V. Rinse and Air Dry Tooth (Step 5)

- ◆ Rinse thoroughly; apply continuous suction to prevent saliva from reaching the etched surface.
- ◆ Dry for 15–20 seconds and maintain a dry field through isolation.

VI. Evaluate for Complete Etching (Step 6)

- ◆ Dry, and examine the etched surface.
- ◆ Repeat etching process if the surface does not appear chalky white.

VII. Place Sealant Material (Step 7)

Follow manufacturer's instructions included in the sealant material package. General instructions include:

- ◆ Avoid over-manipulation of sealant materials to prevent producing air bubbles.
- ◆ Use the disposable implement supplied in the sealant material package for application.
- ◆ Flow minimal amount into all pits and fissures; do not overfill to a high, flat surface.
- ◆ Figure 35-6 illustrates a correctly filled dental sealant surface.

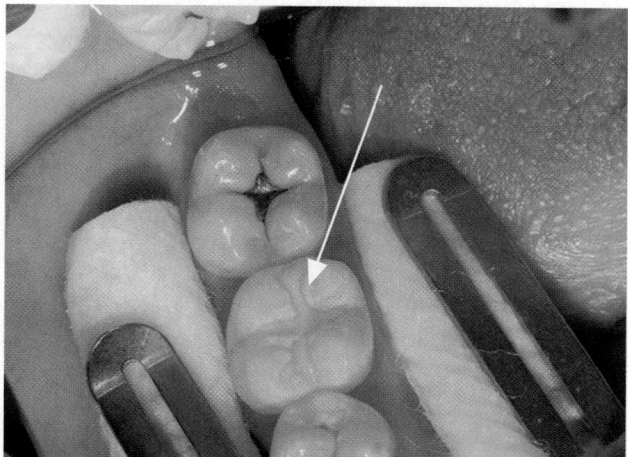

FIGURE 35-6 • Placement of Dental Sealant Material. Appropriate placement of a dental sealant will completely fill pits and fissures, but not compromise occlusion by overfilling to a high, flat surface. (Photograph courtesy of Jill Moore, RDH, BSDH, MHA, EdD, School Oral Health Consultant, Michigan Department of Health and Human Services.)

VIII. Cure Sealant (Step 8)

- ◆ If using a light-cured sealant material:
  - Leave the liquid sealant material in place for 10 seconds to allow for optimum penetration.
  - Use UV blocking eye protection for both the clinician and patient.
  - Apply the curing light for 20–30 seconds in accordance with the manufacturer's instructions. Cover the entire tooth surface with the light to ensure complete polymerization.
- ◆ If using an autopolymerized sealant material, consult the manufacturer's instructions for curing time.

IX. Evaluate Cured Sealant (Step 9)

- ◆ Check for voids gently with explorer: additional sealant material can be added if the surface is not contaminated or wet.

X. Check Occlusion (Step 10)

- ◆ Use articulating paper to locate high spots; adjust as required.
- ◆ Occlusal wear: unfilled sealants wear down via normal attrition to the correct height; filled sealants require occlusal adjustment.

XI. Follow-Up (Step 11)

- ◆ Educate the patient.
- ◆ Administer fluoride treatment.
- ◆ Re-evaluate at each subsequent appointment.

MAINTENANCE

Dental sealants need to be in place to prevent caries, and should be checked for the following:

- ◆ Retention.
- ◆ Need for replacement.

I. Retention

- ◆ At each continuing care appointment, or at least every 6 months, each sealant needs to be examined for retention and to identify deficiencies that may have developed.
- ◆ Properly placed dental sealants can be retained for many years.[1]

II. Factors Affecting Retention

- ◆ *During placement:* precision of technique with exclusion of moisture and contamination.
- ◆ *Patient self-care:* advise patient to avoid biting or chewing on hard surfaces such as a pencil or ice cubes.

◆ *Dental hygiene care:* avoid using an air-powder polisher on intact existing sealants during maintenance appointments.[10]

III. Replacement

◆ Consult the manufacturer's instructions.

◆ Tooth preparation: same as for original application.

◆ Removal of firmly attached sections of retained sealant is not usually necessary.

◆ Re-etching of the tooth surface prior to replacement of a dental sealant is always essential.

SCHOOL-BASED DENTAL SEALANT PROGRAMS

◆ Healthy People 2020 Objectives call of an increase in children and adolescents who have received dental sealants.

◆ Many states in the United States are not meeting national goals for delivering dental sealants to low-income children.[11]

◆ Delivery of dental sealants in school-based settings is a proven strategy[11,12] that can:
  ● Effectively increase the percentage of children in communities who receive dental sealants.
  ● Reduce the risk for decay for high-risk children.

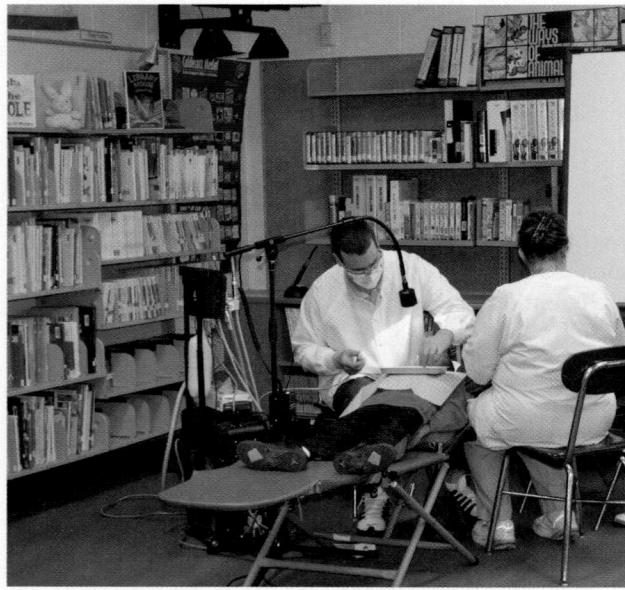

FIGURE 35-7 • Delivery of Dental Sealants in a School-Based Program Using Portable Dental Equipment Set Up in the School Library. (Photograph courtesy of Jill Moore, RDH, BSDH, MHA, EdD, School Oral Health Consultant, Michigan Department of Health and Human Services.)

◆ Many such school-based programs provide additional preventive services such as screening, prophylaxis, topical fluoride application, and oral health education.[11]

◆ Programs that provide sealants are an effective adjunct to preventive care provided in traditional dental care settings.[13]

◆ Figure 35-7 shows a portable dental unit set up in a school library.

DOCUMENTATION

Documentation in the record of a patient receiving a sealant contains a minimum of the following:

◆ Reason for selection of certain teeth for sealants; informed consent of patient, parent, or other caregiver.

◆ Type of sealant used, preparation of tooth, manner of isolation, patient cooperation during administration; post-insertion instructions given.

◆ Sample documentation for placement of dental sealants may be reviewed in Box 35-1.

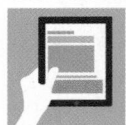

BOX 35-1

Example Documentation:
Placement of Dental Sealants

S—A 12-year-old male patient presents for dental sealant placement.

O—Occlusal contour and previous history of dental caries in primary dentition indicate need for sealant placement for second molars; X-rays indicate no dental caries on proximal surfaces of second molars. Tooth #30 partially erupted with operculum.

A—Need to wait until #30 is completely erupted to place sealant.

P—Reviewed sealant education materials with mother and patient. Mother provided consent for placement of the recommended sealants. Sealants placed on #3-O, 14-O, 14-L, 19-O, 19-B pit using right side, then left-side isolation. Autopolymerized opaque sealant material used with 15% acid etch, applied as per manufacturer's directions. Patient tolerated treatment well, no gagging, minimal saliva, easy isolation.

Next steps: Schedule in 1 month to re-examine for sealant placement on #30 and retention check on 3, 14, and 19.

Signed: _____, RDH

Date: _____

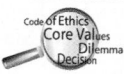

EVERYDAY ETHICS

Mackenzie is a prevention-driven hygienist who evaluates each patient closely to determine if he or she will benefit from dental sealants. One day, she had an 8-year-old boy in her chair, named Caden, who has significant past experience with caries in his primary teeth. Caden now has four permanent molars that she would like to protect with dental sealants. Mackenzie discussed the application with his mother and his mother wants him to receive dental sealants, but her insurance does not cover the cost of them. His mother mentioned the school dentist will be visiting Caden's classroom next month and knows that they can place dental sealants for free and asks Mackenzie if she thinks it is a good idea to have Caden get sealants at his school. Mackenzie knows the hygienist who provides care at the local schools and trusts her clinical skills, but she knows Dr. Carter, her employer, does not like the school dentist to see any of his patients. How should Mackenzie reply?

Questions for Consideration

1. Knowing that receiving the sealants at a reduced cost will be the only way that Caden will receive them, how might Mackenzie respond to Caden's mother's question?

2. What ethical issues may be involved here? How can they be resolved?

3. What practice-based discussions might Mackenzie and Dr. Carter have about how to make sure that children who are vulnerable to dental caries will have access to preventive treatments, such as dental sealants?

Factors to Teach the Patient

▶ Sealants are part of a total preventive program. They are not substitutes for other preventive measures. Limitations of dietary sucrose, use of fluorides, and dental biofilm control are major factors with sealants for prevention of dental caries.

▶ What a sealant is and why such a meticulous application procedure is required.

▶ What can be expected from a sealant; how long it lasts, and how it prevents dental caries.

▶ Need for examination of the sealant at frequent, scheduled maintenance appointments, and need for replacement when missing or chipped.

▶ Avoid biting hard items such as a pencil or ice cubes to increase sealant retention.

ENHANCE YOUR UNDERSTANDING

ONLINE RESOURCES
(see the inside front cover for access information)

• Audio glossary
• Appendices

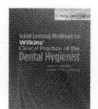

SUPPORT FOR LEARNING
(available separately)

• *Active Learning Workbook for Wilkins' Clinical Practice of the Dental Hygienist, 13th Edition*

INDIVIDUALIZED REVIEW

• Customized practice quizzing with Navigate 2 TestPrep for *Wilkins' Clinical Practice of the Dental Hygienist*

References

1. Ahovuo-Saloranta A, Forss H, Walsh T, et al. Sealants for preventing dental decay in the permanent teeth. *Cochrane Database Syst Rev.* 2013;(3):CD001830. doi:10.1002/14651858.CD001830.pub4.

2. Beauchamp J, Caufiel PW, Crall JJ, et al. Evidence-based clinical recommendations for the use of pit-and-fissure sealants: a report of the American Dental Association Council on Scientific Affairs. *J Am Dent Assoc.* 2008;139(3):257-268.

3. Handleman SL, Shey Z. Michael Buonocore and the Eastman Dental Center: a historic perspective on sealants. *J Dent Res.* 1996;75(1):529-534.

4. Cueto EI, Buonocore MG. Sealing of pits and fissures with an adhesive resin: its use in caries prevention. *J Am Dent Assoc.* 1967;75(1):121-128.

5. Wright JT, Tampi MP, Graham L, et al. Sealants for preventing and arresting pit-and-fissure occlusal caries in primary and permanent molars. *J Am Dent Assoc.* 2016;147(8):631-645.

6. Wright JT, Crall JJ, Fontana M, et al. Evidence-based clinical practice guideline for the use of pit-and-fissure sealants. A report of the American Dental Association and the American Academy of Pediatric Dentistry. *J Am Dent Assoc.* 2016;147(8):672-682.

7. Lindemeyer RG. The use of glass ionomer sealants on newly erupting permanent molars. *J Can Dent Assoc.* 2007;73(2):131-134.

8. Bagherian A, Sarraf Shirazi A. Preparation before acid etching in fissure sealant therapy: yes or no?: a systemic review and meta-analysis. *J Am Dent Assoc.* 2016;147(12):943-951.

9. Kolavic GS, Griffin SO, Malvitz DM, Gooch BF. A comparison of the effects of toothbrushing and handpiece prophylaxis on retention of sealants. *J Am Dent Assoc.* 2009;140(1):38-46.

10. Pelka MA, Altmaier K, Petschelt A, Lohbauer U. The effect of air-polishing abrasives on wear of direct restoration materials and sealants. *J Am Dent Assoc.* 2010;141(1):63-70.

11. PEW Center on the States. *States Stalled on Dental Seal-ant Programs: A 50-State Report.* Washington, DC: The PEW Charitable Trusts; 2015. http://www. pewtrusts.org /~/media/assets/2015/04/dental_sealantreport_final.pdf. Accessed March 8, 2018.

12. Children's Dental Health Project. *Dental Sealants: Proven to Prevent Decay.* Washington, DC: Children's Dental Health Project; 2014:21. https://www.cdhp.org/resources/314-dental -sealants-proven-to-prevent-tooth-decay. Accessed May 16, 2014.

13. Gooch BF, Griffin SO, Gray SK, et al. Preventing dental caries through school-based sealant programs: updated rec-ommendations and reviews of evidence. *J Am Dent Assoc.* 2009;140(11):1356-1365.

Implementation: Treatment

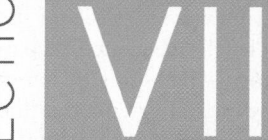

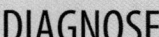

DIAGNOSE
Problem identification

PLAN
Selection of interventions

ASSESS
Data collection

IMPLEMENT
Provide preventive, clinical, educational, and motivational interventions

DOCUMENT
Comprehensive record-keeping

EVALUATE
Feedback on effectiveness

FIGURE VII-1 • The Dental Hygiene Process of Care.

INTRODUCTION FOR SECTION VII

The first objective of dental hygiene treatment is to create an environment in which the tissues can return to health.

In the sequence of patient care, introduction to preventive measures occurs first to help ensure the success of dental hygiene treatment. Professional treatment interventions make a limited contribution to arresting the progression of disease without daily biofilm control measures performed by the patient. Dental hygiene treatment interventions include:

◆ Anxiety and pain control.

◆ Instrumentation for scaling and root planing.

◆ Extrinsic stain removal.

◆ Care of dental restorations.

◆ Posttreatment care procedures.

◆ Placement and removal of dressings.

◆ Removal of sutures.

◆ Treatment of hypersensitive teeth.

◆ Immediate evaluation, short-term follow-up, and maintenance assessment of treatment outcomes.

THE DENTAL HYGIENE PROCESS OF CARE

◆ Dental hygiene treatment uses nonsurgical periodontal therapy combined with preventive care as a part of the dental hygiene process of care (Figure VII-1).

◆ Dental hygiene care can comprise the total treatment needed for certain patients with uncomplicated disease or the initial preparatory phase of treatment for others with more advanced disease.

◆ General objectives of dental hygiene instrumentation are as follows:

  • Create an environment in which the tissues can return to health and be maintained.

  • Aid in the prevention and control of gingival and periodontal infections by removal of periodontal pathogenic microorganisms and factors that predispose to the retention of dental biofilm.

  • Prepare the teeth and gingiva for dental procedures, including those performed by the restorative dentist, prosthodontist, orthodontist, pedodontist, and oral surgeon.

  • Improve oral esthetics and biofilm control of the oral cavity.

ETHICAL APPLICATIONS

◆ The professional dental hygienist acknowledges the ethical implications of all aspects of providing patient care.

◆ Many ethical facets of dental hygiene care can:

  • Relate directly to the provider–patient or intraprofessional relationships.

  • Affect the overall delivery of dental services.

◆ Practicing a consistent and professional demeanor with all patients and all members of the patient care team can be achieved and will uphold high standards and quality of care.

◆ The conduct of the professional dental hygienist prior to, during, and following the dental hygiene appointment is subject to moral assessment.

◆ Several ethical and professional issues to be considered are listed in Table VII-1.

TABLE VII-1 • Ethical and Professional Issues		
PROFESSIONAL ISSUES	EXPLANATION	APPLICATION EXAMPLES
Expressed or implied contracts	A written (third-party payment) or oral (between provider and patient) for specific services or a course of treatment.	Coding of dental hygiene services based on current edition of Current Dental Terminology guidelines.
Whistle-blowing	The disclosure of illegal or immoral wrongs committed by an individual practitioner. May involve negligent acts.	• Reporting the lack of infection control procedures. • Reporting the actions of an impaired colleague to a state dental board.
Privacy rights	Involves the handling of health information through protection of privacy, insurance access, preventing fraud and abuse, and standardization within the healthcare industry.	Health Insurance Portability and Accountability Act (HIPAA); seeks to protect the confidentiality of dental records, especially where computers are used to document patient data.
Supervision	The ethical and legal working relationship between the dentist, dental hygienist, and other healthcare providers.	A dental hygienist in a collaborative practice treating patients who reside in a nursing home.

36

Anxiety and Pain Control

Debra November-Rider, RDH, MSDH

CHAPTER OUTLINE

COMPONENTS OF PAIN
I. Pain Perception
II. Pain Reaction
III. Pain Threshold

PAIN CONTROL MECHANISMS
I. Remove the Painful Stimulus
II. Block the Pathway of the Pain Message
III. Prevent Pain Reaction by Raising Pain Reaction Threshold
IV. Depress Central Nervous System
V. Use Psychosedation Methods (Also Called Iatrosedation)

NONOPIOID ANALGESICS
I. Drugs
II. Indications for Use

NITROUS OXIDE–OXYGEN SEDATION

CHARACTERISTICS OF NITROUS OXIDE
I. Anesthetic, Analgesic, and Anxiolytic Properties
II. Chemical and Physical Properties
III. Blood Solubility
IV. Pharmacology of Nitrous Oxide

EQUIPMENT FOR NITROUS OXIDE–OXYGEN
I. Compressed Gas Cylinders
II. Gas Delivery System
III. Nasal Hood, Nose Piece, and Mask
IV. Scavenger System
V. Safety Features
VI. Equipment Maintenance

PATIENT SELECTION
I. Indications
II. Contraindications

CLINICAL PROCEDURES FOR NITROUS OXIDE–OXYGEN ADMINISTRATION
I. Patient Preparation
II. Equipment Preparation

III. Technique of Gas Delivery
IV. Completion of Sedation

POTENTIAL HAZARDS OF OCCUPATIONAL EXPOSURE
I. Issues of Occupational Exposure
II. Methods for Minimizing Occupational Exposure

ADVANTAGES AND DISADVANTAGES OF NITROUS OXIDE/OXYGEN SEDATION ANESTHESIA
I. Advantages
II. Disadvantages

LOCAL ANESTHESIA

PHARMACOLOGY OF LOCAL ANESTHETICS
I. Contents of a Local Anesthetic Cartridge
II. Ester and Amide Anesthetic Drugs
III. Specific Characteristics of Amide Drugs
IV. Vasoconstrictors
V. Criteria for Local Anesthetic Selection

INDICATIONS FOR LOCAL ANESTHESIA
I. Dental Hygiene Procedures
II. Patient Factors

PATIENT ASSESSMENT
I. Sources of Information for Complete Preanesthetic Assessment
II. Treatment Considerations Based on Assessment Findings
III. General Medical Considerations
IV. Specific Medical Considerations

ARMAMENTARIUM FOR LOCAL ANESTHESIA
I. Syringe
II. Needle
III. Cartridge or Carpule
IV. Additional Armamentarium
V. Sequence of Syringe Assembly
VI. C-CLAD System

CLINICAL PROCEDURES FOR LOCAL ANESTHETIC ADMINISTRATION
I. Injection(s) Selection
II. Aspiration
III. Sharps Management

POTENTIAL ADVERSE REACTIONS TO LOCAL ANESTHESIA
I. Adverse Drug Reactions
II. Psychogenic Reactions
III. Local Complications

ADVANTAGES AND DISADVANTAGES OF LOCAL ANESTHESIA
I. Advantages
II. Disadvantages

NONINJECTABLE ANESTHESIA
I. Armamentarium and Pharmacology
II. Technique

TOPICAL ANESTHESIA
I. Indications for Use
II. Action of a Topical Anesthetic
III. Agents Used in Surface Anesthetic Preparations
IV. Topical Drug Mixtures
V. Adverse Reactions to Topical Anesthetics

APPLICATION OF TOPICAL ANESTHETIC
I. Patient Preparation
II. Application Techniques
III. Completion of Topical Anesthetic Application

NEW DEVELOPMENTS IN PAIN CONTROL
I. Anesthesia Reversal Agent
II. Buffered Local Anesthetic
III. Intranasal Dental Anesthetic

DOCUMENTATION

EVERYDAY ETHICS

FACTORS TO TEACH THE PATIENT

REFERENCES

LEARNING OBJECTIVES

After studying this chapter, the student will be able to:

1. Describe the components of pain.

2. Summarize the advantages and disadvantages of nitrous oxide–oxygen administration.

3. Define titration and explain application during nitrous oxide–oxygen sedation.

4. List the local anesthetics of short, intermediate, and long duration and indications for use.

5. Give examples of absolute and relative contraindications for local anesthetic administration.

6. Identify items in local anesthesia armamentarium and describe the purpose of each.

7. Summarize the different local and systemic complications from the administration of local anesthesia and how to manage them.

8. List the components of a complete patient record entry following the administration of local anesthesia or nitrous oxide/oxygen sedation.

According to the 2000 U.S. Surgeon General's Report—Oral Health in America, 50% of Americans are afraid of visiting the dental office, with one-third so frightened that they avoid seeking any type of oral health services.[1,2]

◆ There are many contributing causes, one of which is the association of pain with dental procedures. Ranking of negative dental stimuli is presented in Box 36-1.

◆ Concern for patient anxiety and pain is an integral part of a dental hygiene appointment.

◆ Recognizing and managing a patient's anxiety and pain is an essential part of dental hygiene care planning.

◆ The decision to use a pharmacologic agent for management of anxiety and pain is dependent on a number of factors including the following:

  • Periodontal health status, the treatment being rendered.

  • Patient's pain threshold.

BOX 36-1
Ranking of Negative Dental Stimuli

1. Getting an injection (68.1%).
2. Dental radiographs (61.4%).
3. Use of curets and scalers (56%).
4. The sight of the dental needle (54.1%).
5. The sight of curets and scalers (49.4%).
6. The use and sound of power instruments (45.7%).
7. Use of air or water spray (36.4%).
8. Wearing of personal protective equipment (7.5%).

Source: Doebling S, Rowe MM. Negative perceptions of dental stimuli and their effects on dental fear. *J Dent Hyg.* 2000;74(2):110-116.

COMPONENTS OF PAIN

I. Pain Perception

◆ Relates to the physical process of receiving a painful stimulus and transmitting the information through the nervous system to the brain where it is interpreted as pain.

◆ Little variability in pain perception between individuals with intact nervous systems.

II. Pain Reaction

◆ Pain reaction is a combination of interpretation of and response to the pain message.

◆ It is highly variable between individuals and even in the same individual at different times.

◆ Accounts for much of the variability seen between patients in personal pain management needs.

◆ Many factors influence pain reaction, including age fatigue, emotional state, and both cultural and ethnic learned behaviors.

◆ Anxiety has special significance: The anxious patient is predisposed to feel pain. Research has shown an association between individuals with red hair and higher levels of dental fear and anxiety.[3]

III. Pain Threshold

◆ Varies between individuals with some having a low pain threshold and others having a high pain threshold.

◆ Highly reproducible.

◆ May be altered by drugs such as local anesthesia.

PAIN CONTROL MECHANISMS

◆ Match the pain control method to the patient's treatment needs and medical status.

◆ All pain management techniques are more effective if utilized before the patient experiences pain. The following five pain control mechanisms are often combined for optimum effect.

I. Remove the Painful Stimulus

◆ Affects pain perception.

◆ Example: clinician repositions fulcrum to avoid pinching the patient's lip during instrumentation.

II. Block the Pathway of the Pain Message

◆ Affects pain perception.

◆ Examples: use of local anesthetic, topical anesthetic.

III. Prevent Pain Reaction by Raising Pain Reaction Threshold

◆ Affects pain reaction.

◆ Examples: use of nitrous oxide–oxygen conscious sedation; nonopioid analgesics such as nonsteroidal anti-inflammatory drugs (NSAIDs).

IV. Depress Central Nervous System

◆ Affects pain reaction.

◆ Example: use of general anesthesia.

V. Use Psychosedation Methods (Iatrosedation)

◆ Iatrosedation or psychosedation helps reduce patient anxiety.

◆ Affects both pain perception and pain reaction.

◆ Includes any nonpharmacologic technique to reduce patient anxiety.
  • Builds a trust relationship.
  • Allows the patient to feel more in control.

◆ May be used alone or combined with pharmacologic pain management.

◆ Examples: Explain procedures carefully; allow patient to express concerns; use relaxation or distraction techniques.

NONOPIOID ANALGESICS

Over-the-counter (OTC) analgesics are an effective adjunct for preventing or reducing the mild-to-moderate discomfort patients experience during dental hygiene therapy or postoperatively.[4,5]

I. Drugs

◆ NSAIDs.

◆ Block prostaglandin synthesis at peripheral nerve endings to inhibit generation of pain message.

  • Suppress onset of pain.
  • Decrease pain severity.
  • Drugs of choice for dental pain.
  • If hemostasis is a consideration during treatment or postoperative bleeding is a concern, use caution when recommending NSAIDs.

◆ Acetaminophen (e.g., Tylenol).

II. Indications for Use

◆ Mild-to-moderate pain during treatment and postprocedure healing.

NITROUS OXIDE–OXYGEN SEDATION

◆ Nitrous oxide–oxygen sedation (N_2O-O_2) has been safely used in dental settings for pain control and anxiety management.[6]

◆ A state of conscious sedation is produced with the patient awake, relaxed, responsive to commands, able to cooperate with treatment, and having intact protective reflexes.

◆ The patient has some degree of analgesia and a higher pain reaction threshold.

CHARACTERISTICS OF NITROUS OXIDE

◆ Inhalation sedation with nitrous oxide provides a safe method of pain control, reduces patient anxiety, and produces few adverse reactions.[6,7]

◆ Gaseous agent (nitrous oxide) is absorbed from the lungs into the cardiovascular system.

◆ Is not biotransformed in the body; eliminated through the lungs.
  • Recommended to start with 10–15% N_2O (1–1.5 L) and add incrementally as needed to achieve desired result.[6]
  • Onset: rapid, less than 30 seconds; peak effect occurs less than 5 minutes.
  • Duration: terminated as soon as delivery of nitrous is stopped.
  • The clinician has the unique ability to control the amount of sedation based on the patient's psychological needs and level of pain control.
  • Food and Drug Administration (FDA) pregnancy category: C.

I. Anesthetic, Analgesic, and Anxiolytic Properties

◆ Produces analgesia.
  • Achieves optimum analgesia and patient cooperation at 20–40% nitrous oxide for most patients.[6]
  • The need for higher or lower concentrations depends on individual biologic variability.

- Reduces the intensity of pain but does not block it; only mildly potent as an anesthetic gas.
  - Use with local anesthetics when the patient experiences significant discomfort.
- Anxiolytic (sedative) effects.
  - Sedation reduces patient's level of fear and anxiety; has a positive effect on pain threshold.
- Possesses slight amnestic properties.

II. Chemical and Physical Properties

- Gas at room temperature and pressure.
- Heavier than air.
- Colorless; sweet smelling.
- Nonirritating and nonallergenic. No allergic reaction has ever been reported.
- Nonflammable but will support the combustion of flammable substances.

III. Blood Solubility

- Relatively insoluble in blood; primary saturation of blood occurs in 3–5 minutes.
- The gas molecules at the alveoli–blood interface and blood–brain interface pass readily to the tissue with the lowest concentration of nitrous oxide.
- Results in rapid onset and recovery.
- Diffusion hypoxia can occur at completion of sedation procedure if 100% oxygen is not administered.

IV. Pharmacology of Nitrous Oxide

- Is not metabolized in the body; remains unchanged in blood and tissues.
- Enters and exits almost entirely through the lungs.

EQUIPMENT FOR NITROUS OXIDE–OXYGEN

- Available as a portable unit or a central storage system with gas piped to individual treatment rooms.
- Units have several built-in safety features to ensure a minimal level of oxygen is delivered and the two gases cannot be reversed during delivery.
- The equipment can be divided into three basic parts:
  - Gas storage cylinders.
  - A gas delivery system.
  - A scavenger system with the nasal hood (mask) having components of both the gas delivery and scavenger portions.

I. Compressed Gas Cylinders

- *Nitrous oxide*
  - *Color code:* blue.
  - *Physical state:* gas and liquid.
  - *Tanks:* 95% liquid and 5% vapor; full tanks = 750 psi.

- *Oxygen*
  - *Color code:* green (International = white).
  - *Physical state:* gas.
- *Handle carefully*
  - Do not use grease, oil, lubricant, or hand cream around the cylinder valves or any fittings that come in contact with the gases.
  - Store vertically on a rack or in another stable and secure manner.
  - Open cylinder valves slowly in a counterclockwise direction.

II. Gas Delivery System

- *Regulator or reducing valve*
  - Converts high pressure of gas in the cylinders to a usable, lower level.
  - Subject to extreme high temperature if compressed gas cylinders are opened quickly.
- *Flow meter*
  - Visual indicator of liters per minute (L/min) flow of oxygen and nitrous oxide.
  - Gas flow rates of nitrous oxide and oxygen are adjusted independently and the sum of the two is the total gas flow rate.
  - A total combined gas flow rate is established and respective concentrations of the two gases are adjusted concurrently.
- *Reservoir bag*
  - Reservoir of gases to accommodate an exceptionally deep breath.
  - Allows for visualization of respirations for monitoring.
  - Degree of inflation can be used to help establish total flow rate of gas needed by the patient for comfortable respirations.
  - May be used to provide oxygen in assisted ventilation if attached to a full-face mask with relief valve.
- *Conducting or breathing tubes*

III. Nasal Hood, Nose Piece, and Mask

- Deliver gas for patient inhalation.
- Collect exhaled gas and direct it into scavenger system.
- Good fit and seal around patient's nose are essential in size selection.
- Ideally, use a disposable item or sterilize before each use.

IV. Scavenger System

- Removes exhaled gas to keep nitrous oxide levels low in the ambient air of the treatment room.
- Connects to the office central evacuation system.
- Vents to outside of building and away from windows and air intakes.

V. Safety Feature

◆ *Universal color coding* of cylinders, hoses, flow controls for each gas.

◆ *Pin index* and *diameter index* safety systems physically prevent gas cylinders or hoses from being interchanged by mistake between the gases due to incompatible placement of pins (projections) and diameter differences in the couplings.

◆ *Minimum oxygen flow*, 30% or 3 L/min.

◆ *Oxygen fail-safe system* automatically shuts off nitrous oxide if the oxygen falls below a minimum level.

◆ *Emergency air inlet* to provide room air if system shuts down.

◆ *Oxygen flush button* to supply 100% oxygen quickly.

VI. Equipment Maintenance

◆ *Function checks*
  • Maintain working order and safe practice by periodic checking of equipment.

◆ *Gas leaks*
  • All equipment connections and rubber goods are subject to leaking. Figure 36-1 shows the places that need to be examined for tight connections, defects, and wear. Apply soapy water to connections; bubbles will form if leaks are present.

PATIENT SELECTION

I. Indications

◆ Patient with mild-to-moderate anxiety.

◆ Medically compromised patient who would benefit from additional oxygen and/or anxiety reduction.
  • Examples: patient with cardiovascular or cerebrovascular disease, or stress-induced bronchial asthma.

◆ Procedures of short duration with low level of pain. The analgesic effect is most pronounced on soft tissues, making it especially useful during dental hygiene procedures.

◆ Patient with strong gag reflex.

II. Contraindications

◆ Absolute contraindications include:
  • significant respiratory compromise.[8]
  • ophthalmic surgery with intraocular gas.[9-11]

◆ Nitrous oxide–oxygen sedation may be contraindicated in the following conditions:
  • Upper respiratory tract infection or other acute respiratory conditions (cold, sinus problems, mouth breather, allergies, bronchitis, and cough)[8]: if nose breathing would be difficult or breathing apparatus cannot be sterilized or replaced.

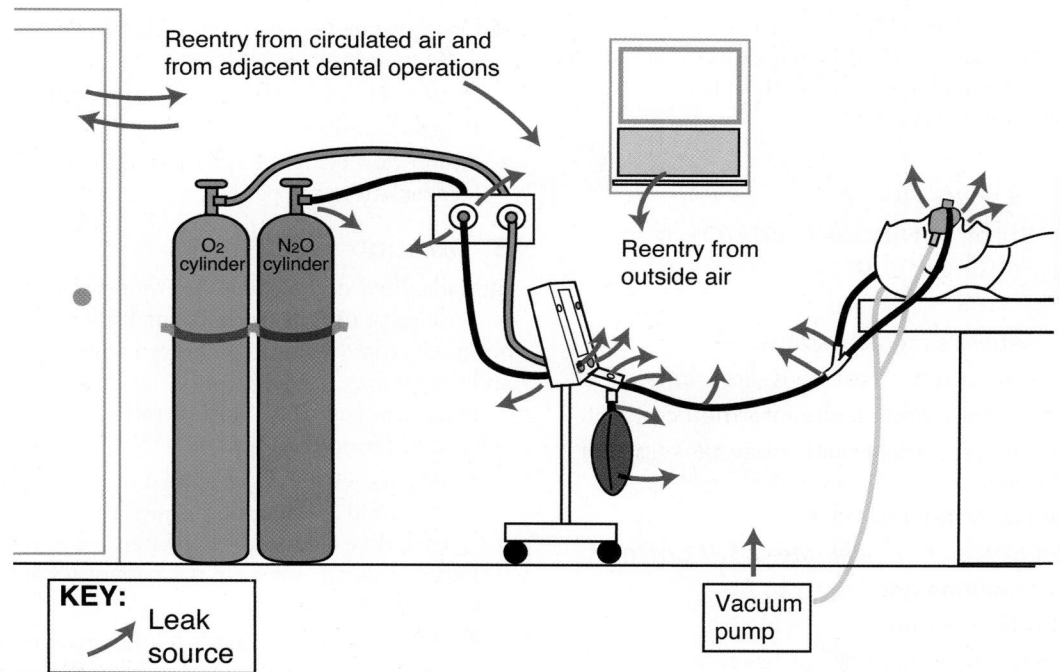

FIGURE 36-1 • Potential Sources of Leaks from Nitrous Oxide/Oxygen Delivery Systems. Arrows show locations where regular inspection and testing is necessary. The most common sites of leakage are: *high-pressure connections*: from the gas delivery cylinders, the wall connectors, the hoses connecting to the anesthetic machine, and the anesthesia machine itself (especially the on-demand valve). *Low-pressure connections*: from the anesthetic flow meter and the scavenging mask. Look for loose-fitting connections, loosely assembled or deformed slip joints and threaded connections, defective or worn seals, and gaskets. *Rubber goods*: hoses and reservoir bag. Look for cracks and tears. (Adapted from National Institute for Occupational Safety and Health (US). *Alert: Controlling Exposures to Nitrous Oxide during Anesthetic Administration* [Joint Publication of Public Health Service, Centers for Disease Control, National Institute for Occupational Safety and Health]. Cincinnati, OH: U.S. Department of Health, Education, and Welfare; 1994:5. Publication No. 94-100.)

- Chronic respiratory conditions: chronic obstructive pulmonary disease, emphysema, cystic fibrosis, chronic bronchitis, and tuberculosis.
- Recent ophthalmic surgery using intraocular gases: vision damage could result from increased pressure on the eye during healing.[9–11]
- Current or recovering drug addiction: may trigger an episode or promote addictive behavior.
- Pregnancy: first-trimester nitrous oxide crosses the placenta; effects on fetus are inconclusive; not metabolized in the body; however, safest of all anxiety-lowering techniques so a consult with physician may be required to determine whether it can be safely used.[12]

CLINICAL PROCEDURES FOR NITROUS OXIDE–OXYGEN ADMINISTRATION

Box 36-2 lists the sequence of steps for nitrous oxide–oxygen administration.

I. Patient Preparation

- *Inform before appointment*
  - No specific food limitations, but generally avoid fasting or heavy meals just before the appointment.
  - Wear comfortable clothing and loosen tight collars.
- *Inform at time of appointment*
  - Explain procedure in positive terms.
  - Stress the pleasant sense of relaxation; the patient will be aware and in control at all times.
  - Obtain informed consent.

BOX 36-2
Steps in Nitrous Oxide/Oxygen Administration

1. Assess patient's medical status.
2. Take and record pretreatment vital signs.
3. Educate patient and secure informed consent.
4. Prepare delivery equipment (open tanks, select nasal hood).
5. Activate scavenger system.
6. Turn on oxygen to a flow rate of 5-7 L/min.
7. Place nasal hood and adjust to fit.
8. Adjust gas flow rate.
9. Begin nitrous oxide at about 10-20%.
10. Titrate to optimum level.
11. Monitor throughout treatment.
12. Return to 100% oxygen.
13. Take and record posttreatment vital signs.
14. Remove nasal hood when patient feels fully recovered.
15. Record progress notes.

- *Assess and perform*
  - Evaluate patient's medical status; determine the American Society of Anesthesiologists' (ASA) classification (see Chapter 11).
  - Take and record vital signs.
  - Place patient in a supine position.

II. Equipment Preparation

- *Nasal hood*
  - Select the appropriate size for optimum comfort and minimum gas leakage.
  - Attach to tubing.
- *Scavenger system*
  - Connect, usually to high-speed volume evacuation, and activate system.
  - Adjust setting of scavenger system.
- *Turn on gas cylinders*
  - Open slowly, first oxygen, then nitrous oxide.
  - Confirm that all equipment are operating correctly.

III. Technique for Gas Delivery

A. Establish Volume of Gas Flow

- Based on patient's size and medical/psychological condition; determine the total liters flow per minute.[6]
- Begin with 6 L 100% oxygen/min for adults.
- Gas flow rate between 6 and 7 L/min for average adults, 4–5 L/min for most children.[6]
- Place nasal hood, adjust for comfort; patient may assist in positioning; establish good seal.
- Adjust flow using the inflation of the reservoir bag and feedback from the patient.

B. Titration

Individualized drug dose is determined by increasing the percentage of nitrous oxide in small increments until the optimum sedation level is achieved based on clinical signs and symptoms.

- *Initial concentration*: Start **titration** at about 10–15% concentration of nitrous oxide.[6]
  - Because of the rapid uptake of nitrous oxide in the lungs and distribution through the body, the effect of each dose can be assessed after 1–2 minutes.
- *Patient response*: Observe the patient for signs of relaxation or other changes.
  - Ask the patient what is felt. Use the patient's signs and symptoms to determine when the optimum level of sedation has been reached.
  - Table 36-1 lists signs and symptoms for various levels of nitrous oxide–oxygen sedation.
- *Adjust dose*: Increase or decrease the nitrous oxide by 5–10% when the optimum individual dose has not been achieved. Wait 1–2 minutes and reassess. Repeat as needed.
  - Distribution of optimum sedation dose for different individuals follows a bell curve. Generally 20–40%

TABLE 36-1 • Signs and Symptoms of Nitrous Oxide–Oxygen Sedation

LEVEL OF SEDATION	SIGNS AND SYMPTOMS
Minimal sedation (ideal)	Comfortable/relaxed; reduced fear and anxiety; tingling of extremities and/or near mouth; body warmth; glazed eyes; responds to directions; intact protective cough and gag reflex; light feeling; vasodilation of neck and face
Oversedation	Disassociation from surroundings; hallucinating; feeling of floating or flying. Inability to follow directions and keep mouth open; dizziness; drowsiness
Oversedation (serious)	Delayed responses; slurred words; agitated and/or combative behavior; vomiting; loss of consciousness

nitrous oxide results in adequate sedation for dental treatment.

- At high altitudes, greater nitrous oxide concentrations will be needed because of the change in the partial pressure of the gases.

◆ *Time*: Allow approximately 5 minutes for titration.

◆ *Monitor*: Continue to monitor and adjust the concentration throughout the appointment.

- As the appointment proceeds or during less anxiety-producing parts of the appointment, a lower dose may be more comfortable.
- Avoid excessive fluctuations.

◆ *Attend patient*: Never leave a sedated patient unattended; sedation can become deeper without some stimulation or interaction.

◆ *Outcome*: Titration increases clinical success rate of nitrous oxide–oxygen conscious sedation and decreases adverse responses.

◆ *Advantages*: Only the amount of drug required by the patient is given.

- Allows for individual biovariability.
- Uncovers idiosyncratic reactions early.
- Minimizes negative experiences with oversedation.

IV. Completion of Sedation

◆ *Recovery*

- *Procedure*: At the completion of sedation, return the patient to 100% oxygen for a minimum of 5 minutes, or longer if needed for full recovery.
- *Factors affecting recovery time*: Biologic variation, duration of sedation procedure, and concentration of nitrous oxide administration.
- *Signs of recovery*: Patient's report of feeling "back to normal" and is alert and able to respond appropriately to questions.
- Comparable presedation and postsedation vital signs are recorded.

- *Elimination*: Within 5–10 minutes, 99% removed completely from the body.

◆ *Diffusion hypoxia*

◆ If the patient is returned directly to room air rather than 100% oxygen, diffusion hypoxia can result.

- Nitrous oxide diffuses into an area of lower concentration more rapidly than oxygen, causing inadequate oxygen in the alveoli if the patient is not given supplemental oxygen at the completion of sedation.
- Hypoxia can result in patient discomfort or syncope.
- Inadequate postsedation oxygen may result in a feeling of lethargy, headache, or nausea.
- Prevention: Administer 100% oxygen for no less than 5 minutes.

◆ *Dismissal follows full recovery*

- Patients should be fully alert and show no signs of disorientation.
- Usually the patient is able to return to all normal activities, including driving.
- Vital signs should return to baseline readings.
- Recovery time varies for each patient.

◆ *Record keeping*

◆ As with every dental procedure, complete documentation is essential and good practice. The following items need to be included in the patient's record when administering nitrous oxide–oxygen analgesia (see Box 36-3):

- Medical and psychological history review, including determination of the ASA classification.
- Reason for nitrous oxide use.
- Presedation and postsedation vital signs.

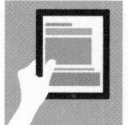

BOX 36-3

Example Documentation: Nitrous Oxide/Oxygen Conscious Sedation

S—Patient presents with gag reflex and anxiety about dental treatment.

O—Medical history nonsignificant. ASA I.

A—No contraindication for use of nitrous oxide/oxygen.

P—Total gas flow rate: 5 L/min; 35% (2 L/m) nitrous oxide and 65% (4 L/min) oxygen for 40 minutes. Patient reports tingling in extremities and relaxed feeling. 100% oxygen administered for 5 minutes following treatment; patient said he felt fully recovered.

Vital Signs	Pretreatment	Posttreatment
Blood pressure	124/84	120/82
Pulse	75	70
Respirations	12	12

Signed: _____, RDH

Date: _____

- Concentrations of both nitrous oxide and oxygen administered.
- Total gas flow rate (L/min).
- Length of time for sedation procedure.
- Length of time on recovery oxygen.
- Statement of patient's recovery status and any post-care instructions given.
- Any adverse reactions. Summary of patient's response to nitrous oxide can be helpful for subsequent appointments.
- Signature and date.

POTENTIAL HAZARDS OF OCCUPATIONAL EXPOSURE

Chronic occupational exposure to nitrous oxide may have deleterious effects on healthcare providers. Overexposure must be prevented.

I. Issues of Occupational Exposure

- *Potential health problems*[6,13,14–17]
  - Reduced fertility with unscavenged nitrous oxide exposure.
  - Spontaneous abortion.
  - Increased rate of neurologic, renal, and liver disease.
  - Decreased mental performance, audiovisual ability, and manual dexterity.
- *Recommended exposure levels*
  - Consensus has not been reached on occupational exposure limits; there is currently no exposure standard.
  - National Institute of Occupational Safety and Health recommends no more than 25 parts per million (ppm) during administration.

II. Methods for Minimizing Occupational Exposure

- Use an effective scavenging system that can move 45 L/min of air.
- Maintain equipment and inspect regularly for gas leaks, especially at the locations shown in Figure 36-1. Shut off and secure equipment at the end of each day's use.
- Improve general air quality:
  - Introduce fresh air.
  - Use a nonrecycling air-conditioning system, or open a window.
  - Vent the scavenger system gases outside the building and away from windows and air intakes.
- Use an air sweep fan to direct nitrous oxide away from the clinician's breathing zone; periodically monitor air quality in the clinicians' breathing zone.
- Minimize patient conversations and mouth breathing; fit the nasal hood carefully to avoid leaks.
- Set conservative limits on the duration and concentration of nitrous oxide use per patient.

ADVANTAGES AND DISADVANTAGES OF NITROUS OXIDE/OXYGEN SEDATION ANESTHESIA

I. Advantages

- Both a mild analgesic and sedative: reduces patient's reaction to pain by raising pain threshold.
- Increases relaxation and cooperation during treatment.
- Reduces the gag reflex.
- Very safe with few side effects and few medical contraindications. Excellent for management of many medically compromised patients:[6,8]
  - Respiratory disease: asthma–nitrous is nonirritating and will not precipitate an attack.
  - Cerebrovascular disease: elevated level of oxygen given, which is beneficial.
  - Hepatic disease: nitrous not metabolized in body like other drugs.
  - Epilepsy: does not increase risk of seizure development.
  - Diabetes: no contraindication.
- Allergy: no reported allergy to nitrous oxide.[6]
- Provides oxygen enrichment as well as stress reduction.
- Helps prevent emergencies because of anxiety and pain management.
- Readily absorbed and excreted from the body; rapid onset and recovery from drug effect.
- Able to titrate to optimum level.
- Recovery complete so patient can be dismissed to return to normal activities.
- Appointments less stressful for clinician because of relaxed, conscious, cooperative patient.

II. Disadvantages

- A low-potency analgesic drug.
  - Not effective with all patients because of low potency; does not block all perceptions.
  - Severely distressed or phobic patient may need a more potent drug or combination of drugs.
- Patient must be able and willing to breathe through the nose.
- Equipment and gases are expensive.
- Use of poor techniques such as failure to titrate or use a scavenger system results in undesirable patient experiences and potential staff health risks.[6,13,15–17]
- Potential for recreational abuse by health professionals.
- May stimulate sexual phenomena in some patients.[18]

LOCAL ANESTHESIA

- Local anesthesia is the main modality for the management of dental pain.
- It blocks sensations, especially of pain, from teeth, soft tissues, and bone in the anesthetized area.

- Root instrumentation without discomfort requires a profound pulpal and periodontal tissue anesthesia to increase patient comfort and compliance during the appointment.

PHARMACOLOGY OF LOCAL ANESTHETICS

- Local anesthetics are the most frequently used drugs for dental and dental hygiene treatment.
- When administered correctly, local anesthesia is a safe and effective method for pain control.

I. Contents of a Local Anesthetic Cartridge

A dental cartridge is prefilled by the manufacturer. Cartridges contain either 1.7 or 1.8 mL of solution.[19] Anesthetic cartridges include the following:

- *Amide anesthetic*: blocks the transfer of ions across the nerve membrane, which stops the transmission of pain messages.
- *Vasoconstrictor*: constricts local blood vessels to offset the vasodilation caused by the amide anesthetic. Provides greater duration, more profound anesthesia, and hemostasis to the immediate area.
- *Antioxidant*: preservative added to prevent the oxidation of the vasoconstrictor, usually sodium metabisulfite or sodium bisulfite.
- *Sterile water*: diluting agent.
- *Sodium chloride*: creates a biocompatible solution with the body.

II. Ester and Amide Anesthetic Drugs

Dental local anesthetic drugs can be divided chemically into two major groups: esters and amides. The first dental anesthetic was procaine (Novocain), an ester, which has not been available in dental cartridges in the United States since 1996.[20]

A. General Characteristics of Ester Anesthetics

- Widely used in topical anesthetic agents.
- Causes vasodilation of local blood vessels.
- High incidence of allergic reactions from by-product, para-aminobenzoic acid (PABA).[19]
- Hydrolyzed in plasma by the enzyme pseudocholinesterase.
- Elimination via the kidneys.
- Atypical plasma cholinesterase may result in slow removal of the drug from the blood resulting in toxicity (see "General Medical Considerations" section).[19]

B. General Characteristics of Amide Anesthetics

- Safe and effective with minimal side effects when administered correctly.[19-24]
- Cause vasodilation of local blood vessels.
- Extremely low incidence of allergic reactions.[19]
- Metabolized by the liver (all amides with the exception of articaine are primarily biotransformed in the liver)[19-24] (see "General Medical Considerations" section).
- Elimination via the kidneys.

C. Duration of Amide Drugs

- There are three categories of duration for dental local anesthetics:
  - Short acting (~30 minutes of pulpal anesthesia).
  - Intermediate acting (~60 minutes of pulpal anesthesia).
  - Long acting (~90 minutes of pulpal anesthesia).
- Factors influencing the duration include:
  - Individual response to the drug.
  - Type of injection administered (supraperiosteal/infiltration versus nerve block).
  - Accuracy of the injection.
  - Anatomical barriers (ligaments, tendons, fascial planes, density of bone).
  - Vascularity at site of injection.
  - Presence of inflammation and/or infection.
  - Injecting a plain local anesthetic versus a local anesthetic with a vasoconstrictor.

III. Specific Characteristics of Amide Drugs

A. Lidocaine Hydrochloride (HCl)

- *Properties*
  - Proprietary name: Xylocaine.
  - Duration: intermediate acting.
  - Considered the "gold standard" of all the local anesthetics.[19]
  - Metabolized in the liver and excreted by the kidneys.
- *Dosage*
  - Concentration: 2%.
  - Vasoconstrictor: epinephrine 1:50,000 (for hemostasis) or 1:100,000.
  - mg/cartridge: 36 mg (1.8 mL), 34 mg (1.7 mL).
- *Safety and precautions*
  - MRD (maximum recommended dose) = 500 mg; 3.2 mg/lb; 7.0 mg/kg.[19]
  - FDA pregnancy category: B (Box 36-4).
  - Calculate the MRD, confirm a negative aspiration prior to depositing, deposit a full cartridge no less than 1 minute.

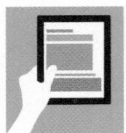

BOX 36-4
FDA Pregnancy Categories

Category A

Adequate and well-controlled studies have failed to demonstrate a risk to the fetus in the first trimester of pregnancy (and there is no evidence of risk in later trimesters).

Category B

Animal reproduction studies have failed to demonstrate a risk to the fetus and there are no adequate and well-controlled studies in pregnant women.

Category C

Animal reproduction studies have shown an adverse effect on the fetus and there are no adequate and well-controlled studies in humans, but potential benefits may warrant use of the drug in pregnant women despite potential risks.

Category D

There is positive evidence of human fetal risk based on adverse reaction data from investigational or marketing experience or studies in humans, but potential benefits may warrant use of the drug in pregnant women despite potential risks.

Category X

Studies in animals or humans have demonstrated fetal abnormalities and/or there is positive evidence of human fetal risk based on adverse reaction data from investigational or marketing experience, and the risks involved in use of the drug in pregnant women clearly outweigh potential benefits.

Source: U.S. Department of Health & Human Services; Chemical Hazards Emergency Medical Management. FDA pregnancy categories. April 2017. https://chemm.nlm.nih.gov/pregnancycategories.htm. Accessed July 18, 2019.

- *Absolute contraindication*: allergy to the local anesthetic or sodium bisulfite; cocaine or methamphetamine use in the previous 24 hours.
- *Relative contraindication*: cardiovascular disease, angina, cerebrovascular accident (CVA), hypertension, hyperthyroidism, significant liver or kidney disease, patients taking beta-blockers, cimetidine on a regular basis, steroid-dependent asthmatics, avoid 1:50,000 for ASA 3 cardiac, CVA, hyperthyroidism, and patients sensitive to epinephrine.
- *Recommended for*: pediatric patients, pregnant women, most procedures and treatment requiring intermediate duration; best choice for bleeding control (1:50,000).

B. Mepivacaine HCl

- *Properties*
  - Proprietary name: Carbocaine.
  - Duration: short acting (3% plain solution); intermediate acting (2% 1:20,000 levonordefrin).
  - Weak vasodilator.
  - Metabolized in the liver and excreted by the kidneys.
- *Dosage*
  - Concentration: 2% (with vasoconstrictor), 3% (plain).
  - Vasoconstrictor: levonordefrin 1:20,000.
  - mg/cartridge: 2% = 36 mg (1.8 mL); 34 mg (1.7 mL).
  - mg/cartridge: 3% = 54 mg (1.8 mL), 51 mg (1.7 mL).
- *Safety and/or precautions*
  - MRD = 400 mg; 3.0 mg/lb; 6.6 mg/kg.[19]
  - FDA pregnancy category: C.
  - Calculate the MRD, confirm a negative aspiration prior to depositing, deposit a full cartridge in no less than 1 minute.
  - *Absolute contraindication*: allergy to the local anesthetic or sodium bisulfite; cocaine or methamphetamine use in the previous 24 hours (2% 1:20,000).
  - *Relative contraindication*: patients taking tricyclic antidepressants (TCAs)—interacts with levonordefrin, significant liver or kidney disease.
  - *Recommended for*: short duration (3% plain solution), when a vasoconstrictor is contraindicated (3% plain solution), pediatric patients, patients who are epinephrine sensitive.

C. Prilocaine HCl

- *Properties*
  - Proprietary name: Citanest.
  - Duration: short acting administered as an infiltration; intermediate acting when administered as a nerve block.[19]
  - Weak vasodilator.
  - Metabolized: liver, small percentage by lungs as alternate site and excreted by the kidneys.
- *Dosage*
  - Concentration: 4%.
  - Vasoconstrictor: epinephrine 1:200,000.
  - mg/cartridge: 72 mg (1.8 mL); 68 mg (1.7 mL).
- *Safety and precautions*
  - MRD = 600 mg; 3.6 mg/lb; 8.0 mg/kg.[19]
  - FDA pregnancy category: B.
  - Calculate the MRD, confirm a negative aspiration prior to depositing, deposit a full cartridge in no less than 1 minute; may cause increased risk of paresthesia with an inferior alveolar (IA) nerve block.[24–27]
  - Metabolic by-products may cause acquired methemoglobinemia, a condition that reduces the blood's oxygen-carrying capacity (see "Specific Medical Considerations" section).
  - May cause increased risk of paresthesia with an IA nerve block.[25–27]

- *Absolute contraindication*: allergy to the local anesthetic or sodium bisulfite; cocaine or methamphetamine use in the previous 24 hours (1:200,000).
- *Relative contraindication*: significant liver or kidney disease, methemoglobinemia, sickle cell anemia, anemia, respiratory or cardiac failure, patients on acetaminophen long term.
- *Recommended for*: patients when a vasoconstrictor is contraindicated (4% plain solution); plain solution provides intermediate duration when administered as a nerve block.

D. Articaine HCl

◆ *Properties*
- Duration: intermediate acting.
- Shortest half-life of all the amide anesthetics; reported to diffuse through soft and hard tissues better than other amides.[19]

◆ *Dosage*
- Concentration: 4%.
- Vasoconstrictor: epinephrine 1:100,000 and 1:200,000.
- mg/cartridge: 72 mg (1.8 mL); 68 mg (1.7 mL).
- MRD = determined by weight; 3.2 mg/lb; 7.0 mg/kg.
- Metabolized: blood plasma (approx. 90–95%) and the liver (approx. 5–10%).
- Excreted: kidneys.
- Half-life: 30–45 minutes; shortest of all amide anesthetics.
- FDA pregnancy category: C.
- Calculate the MRD, confirm a negative aspiration prior to depositing, deposit a full cartridge in no less than 1 minute.
- May cause increased risk of paresthesia with an IA nerve block.[24–27]
- *Absolute contraindication*: allergy to the local anesthetic or sodium bisulfite; cocaine or methamphetamine use in the previous 24 hours.
- *Relative contraindication*: significant liver or kidney disease.
- *Recommended for*: patients with moderate systemic disease (liver, cardiac); lowest risk of systemic toxicity; shortest half-life allows for safer reinjections.[19]

E. Bupivacaine HCl

◆ *Properties*
- Proprietary name: Marcaine.
- Duration: long acting; longest onset of all the local anesthetics.
- Most potent of the local anesthetics.
- Metabolized by the liver and excreted by the kidneys.

◆ *Dosage*
- Concentration: 0.5%.
- Vasoconstrictor: Epinephrine 1:200,000.
- mg/cartridge: 9 mg (1.8 mL), 8.5 mg (1.7 mL).

◆ *Safety and precautions*
- MRD = 90 mg; 0.9 mg/lb; 2.0 mg/kg (no mg/lb recommended for the United States, only for Canada).[19]

- FDA pregnancy category: C.
- Safety and/or precautions: calculate the MRD, confirm a negative aspiration prior to depositing; deposit a full cartridge in no less than 1 minute; highly toxic, stay below the MRD, use caution with reinjection.
- *Absolute contraindication*: allergy to the local anesthetic or sodium bisulfite; cocaine or methamphetamine use in the previous 24 hours.
- *Relative contraindication*: children or adults who are prone to self-mutilation postinjection.
- *Recommended for*: posttreatment pain control; procedures requiring greater than 60 minutes of pulpal anesthesia.

IV. Vasoconstrictors

A. Reasons for Use

◆ *Safety*: Potential for toxic reaction (overdose) to the local anesthetic is reduced by slowing the rate at which it enters circulation.

◆ *Longevity*: Duration of anesthetic effect is increased.

◆ *Effectiveness*: Depth and profoundness of anesthetic is increased.

◆ *Hemostasis*: Only if drug is locally injected directly into the area; epinephrine 1:50,000 is most effective.[19,28]

B. Potential Risks with Use of Vasoconstrictors

◆ Hypersensitivity to the drugs.

◆ Medical problems (see "Specific Medical Considerations" section).

◆ Drug interactions (see "Potential Drug Interactions" section).

◆ Degree of risk to medically compromised patients, including those with heart disease varies. The use of vasoconstrictors in low doses is considered safe.[19,28]

C. Preservatives

◆ *Sodium bisulfite*
- Preservative added to local anesthetic cartridges that contain a vasoconstrictor.
- Prevents the oxidation of the vasoconstrictor.
- Provides a shelf-life of approximately 18 months.
- Most likely offending agent in a dental cartridge when an allergic reaction occurs.[19,28]
- Avoid administering any local anesthetic with a vasoconstrictor for patients that have a confirmed bisulfite allergy.
- Best alternative choice: 4% prilocaine plain as a nerve block or 3% mepivacaine.

D. Drugs

◆ *Epinephrine (Adrenalin)*
- Potent sympathomimetic amine.
- Rare occurrences to have an allergy since it is produced endogenously.[19]

- Concentrations: 1:50,000, 1:100,000, or 1:200,000.
- MRDs for healthy patients and for medically compromised, especially those with cardiac disease are listed in Table 36-2.
- *Absolute contraindication*: bisulfite allergy, myocardial infarction (MI; within 6 months), coronary bypass surgery (within 6 months), uncontrolled angina, arrhythmias, hypertension, hyperthyroidism or diabetes, pheochromocytoma (catecholamine producing tumors), cocaine, or methamphetamine use within 24 hours.
- *Relative contraindication*: cardiac conditions (ASA 3), taking nonselective beta-blockers or antidepressants, controlled hypertension, hyperthyroidism, or diabetes.

- *Levonordefrin (Neo-Cobefrin)*
  - About 15% as potent as equal doses of epinephrine and with less cardiac and central nervous system stimulation. Used at higher concentration (1:20,000) to accomplish adequate vasoconstriction.[19]
  - Not a good choice if hemostasis is required.
  - *Absolute contraindications*: bisulfite allergy, uncontrolled angina, arrhythmias, blood pressure, hyperthyroidism or diabetes; cocaine or methamphetamine within 24 hours.
  - *Relative contraindication*: patients taking TCAs.[19,28]
  - MRDs for healthy patients and for medically compromised, especially those with cardiac disease, are given in Table 36-2.

V. Criteria for Local Anesthetic Selection

- Length of time needed for pain control is a primary criterion for drug selection. Table 36-3 lists the typical duration of action for common local anesthetics.
- Need for hemostasis.

- Medical status of the patient.
- Potential for prolonged discomfort after treatment.
- Potential for self-inflicted injury before anesthetic wears off.

INDICATIONS FOR LOCAL ANESTHESIA

- Local anesthesia is indicated for treatment that has the potential to cause discomfort or pain.
- Anesthesia prevents both the patient and clinician from the anticipation of discomfort, reducing stress, and making treatment comfortable.

I. Dental Hygiene Procedures

- Scaling and root debridement in areas with probing depths of 4 mm or greater.
- Extensive instrumentation with either manual or power-driven instruments.
- Treatment in areas of challenging pocket topography, furcations, or other difficult root anatomy.
- Instrumentation of sensitive root surfaces.
- Instrumentation in areas of painful, inflamed soft tissue.
- Treatments involving soft-tissue manipulation.
  - Gingival curettage.
  - Suture removal.
  - Removal of subgingival overhanging restoration.
- Treatment in areas with excessive hemorrhage.

II. Patient Factors

- Extent of patient's oral status and periodontal condition directly influence the extent or rigor of the needed treatment.
- Patient's pain reaction or pain threshold.

TABLE 36-2 • Vasoconstrictors: Concentrations and Maximum Recommended Dose (MRD)				
VASOCONSTRICTORS AND CONCENTRATIONS	**MRD IN HEALTHY PATIENTS**		**MRD IN MEDICALLY COMPROMISED PATIENTS**	
	MG/APPT	CARTRIDGES/APPT	MG/APPT	CARTRIDGES/APPT
Epinephrine (based on 1.8 mL)				
1:50,000 (0.036 mg/cart.)	0.2	5.5	0.04	1.1
1:100,000 (0.018 mg/cart.)	0.2	11	0.04	2.2
1:200,000 (0.009 mg/cart.)	0.2	22[a]	0.04	4.4
Levonordefrin (based on 1.8 mL)				
1:20,000 (0.09 mg/cart.)	1.0	11.1	0.2	2.2

MG/APPT, milligram per appointment.
[a]Local anesthetic is the limiting drug.

TABLE 36-3 • Duration of Local Anesthetics (Currently Available in the United States)

LOCAL ANESTHETIC DRUGS	SOFT TISSUE (MINUTES)	PULPAL (MINUTES)	DURATION CATEGORY
4% Articaine 1:100,000 Epinephrine	180–360	60–75	Intermediate
4% Articaine 1:200,000 Epinephrine	120–300	45–60	Intermediate
0.5% Bupivacaine 1:200,000 Epinephrine	240–540	90–180	Long
2% Lidocaine 1:50,000 Epinephrine	180–300	60	Intermediate
2% Lidocaine 1:100,000 Epinephrine	180–300	60	Intermediate
3% Mepivacaine plain	120–180	20 (infiltration) 40 (nerve block)	Short Intermediate
2% Mepivacaine 1:20,000 Levonordefrin	180–300	60	Intermediate
4% Prilocaine plain	90–120 (infiltration) 120–240 (nerve block)	10–15 (infiltration) 40–60 (nerve block)	Short Intermediate
4% Prilocaine 1:200,000 Epinephrine	180–480	60–90	Intermediate

PATIENT ASSESSMENT

The goal of patient assessment is to ensure an effective and safe local anesthesia experience. Pretreatment evaluation is the first and most important step for avoiding a medical emergency.

I. Sources of Information for Complete Preanesthetic Assessment

◆ Chief complaint.
◆ Vital signs.
◆ Medical history; ASA status (see Chapter 11).
◆ Current medications.
◆ Emotional status/anxiety level.
◆ Dental history related to local anesthesia.
◆ Presence of infection or inflammation.

II. Treatment Considerations Based on Assessment Findings

Amide local anesthetics and the vasoconstrictor normally incorporated into the dental anesthetic cartridge can be administered safely to almost all patients. Options for treatment include:

◆ Use local anesthetic without special precautions.
◆ Avoid use of local anesthetic or of a specific local anesthetic because of high medical risk.
◆ Select an alternative drug to minimize or avoid risk.
◆ Limit the dose of drug given at any specific appointment.
◆ Use local anesthesia combined with stress reduction techniques; use in combination with nitrous oxide–oxygen conscious sedation.
◆ Seek medical intervention, consult, or additional testing before proceeding.
◆ Administer block (or regional) anesthesia rather than infiltration in inflamed tissue which has a low pH that inhibits drug distribution and effectiveness.

III. General Medical Considerations

◆ Regular utilization of safeguards such as medical history questionnaire, dialogue history, physical examination, and vital screenings (blood pressure, heart rate, and respiration) can help prevent most medical emergencies in the dental office or clinic.
◆ The ASA Classification System is a tool (see Chapter 11) to help assess medical risk of a patient receiving anesthesia and undergoing surgical procedures.
  • ASA 4 patients and some ASA 3 patients (especially those who are anxious about injections) may not have the functional reserve to tolerate the injection procedure and the subsequent treatment.
  • Elective treatment for patients who are too medically compromised for local anesthesia (ASA 4 and

some ASA 3) are not performed except in the case of emergency procedures until medical status improves; may not be appropriate for any elective dental therapy.

◆ When performing a risk–benefit analysis for use of local anesthesia, consider the potential for medical distress that can result from inadequate pain control.

◆ Seek a medical consult when there is doubt about the safety of a local anesthetic choice.

◆ Calculate the MRD for all patients, especially children or adults weighing less than 150 pounds. Every drug has an MRD in mg/lb and mg/kg that is used for the calculation (Table 36-2).

   • Determine and administer the smallest effective dose for each patient.

   • Always use the smallest effective dose.

◆ *Contraindications to local anesthesia administration*

   • The clinician may need to either limit (relative contraindication) or completely avoid use (absolute contraindication) of a local anesthetic drug or vasoconstrictor depending on specific medical or psychological considerations of the patient or medications.

IV. Specific Medical Considerations

A. Allergy

◆ *Amide anesthetics*: True allergy is rare. If confirmed, avoid offending drug, choose a different amide, a slight chance of cross-allergenicity may occur;[19,24] refer to allergist for testing.

◆ *Ester anesthetics*: Allergy is fairly common. If confirmed, avoid all ester anesthetics including topical anesthetics.

◆ *Bisulfites*: Sodium bisulfite and sodium metabisulfite are used as the preservatives for the vasoconstrictor. If allergy is known, avoid anesthetics containing vasoconstrictors.[19,24]

◆ Best choice: 3% mepivacaine or 4% prilocaine plain if sodium bisulfite is the allergen.

B. Hyperthyroidism

◆ *Uncontrolled*: avoid vasoconstrictor.

◆ *Controlled*: can choose local anesthetic with a vasoconstrictor, but stay below the MRD and use the weakest vasoconstrictor concentration.[29,30]

◆ Best choice: 4% prilocaine plain, 3% mepivacaine plain, 2% mepivacaine 1:20,000, or vasoconstrictor with 1:200,000 (articaine, prilocaine, or bupivacaine).

C. Impaired Liver or Kidney Function

◆ Only severe impairment is clinically relevant (ASA 3 or 4).

◆ Half-life of amide anesthetic could be prolonged, which could result in overdose.

◆ Best choice: 4% articaine (1:100,000 or 1:200,000) since very little is biotransformed through the liver.[19]

D. Malignant Hyperthermia (MH)

◆ Life-threatening complications associated with the administration of general anesthesia.

◆ Syndrome—transmitted genetically; defect in the distribution of myoplasmic calcium.

◆ MH most often occurs after first exposure to general anesthesia.

◆ Clinical signs: tachycardia, high fever, tachypnea, cardiac dysrhythmias, muscle rigidity, cyanosis, and death.

◆ Absolute contraindication for patients to receive general anesthesia (succinylcholine).

◆ Local anesthetics with or without vasoconstrictors can be used. No current evidence to support avoidance of local anesthetics or vasoconstrictors.[19,22,23]

◆ Medical consult is recommended prior to treatment.

E. Methemoglobinemia

◆ A congenital or acquired condition; hemoglobin molecule is converted to methemoglobin, which has less oxygen-carrying capacity. A cyanosis-like state may develop if a high percentage of molecules convert.

◆ Prilocaine, articaine, and topical benzocaine can cause a dose-related methemoglobinemia.[19,31] Avoid their use in patients with a pre-existing condition.

◆ Avoid prilocaine or benzocaine if on long-term acetaminophen use.

◆ Best choice: lidocaine, mepivacaine, or bupivacaine.

F. Heart Failure

◆ Reduced circulation resulting from heart failure slows elimination of amide anesthetic, which increases potential for anesthetic overdose.

◆ Patient is stress intolerant—pain and anxiety must be carefully managed. Consider use of nitrous oxide–oxygen sedation alone or in combination with local anesthesia.[6,30]

◆ Obtain medical consult and clearance before treating.

◆ Best choice: 2% lidocaine 1:100,000.

G. Coronary Heart Disease, MI, Recent Heart Surgery, and Stroke

◆ Do not treat within the first 6 months; higher risk of a subsequent event or complication.[19,30] Consult with the cardiologist.

◆ Concern is for the use and amount of vasoconstrictor. Epinephrine cardiac dose = 0.04 mg per appointment; levonordefrin cardiac dose = 0.2 mg per appointment; do not use 1:50,000 epinephrine concentration for these patients.[19]

◆ Decision based on patient ASA category, procedure to be performed, duration needed for pain control, medical consultation recommended.

◆ Best choice: plain anesthetic (if adequate depth and duration of pain control can be achieved); 1:200,000 epinephrine concentrations (if hemostasis is not a consideration); 2% mepivacaine 1:20,000.

H. Angina

◆ Uncontrolled—avoid all dental procedures; controlled—limit amount of vasoconstrictors.[19]

◆ Best choice: plain local anesthetic*; 2% mepivacaine 1:20,000 or 1:200,000 anesthetics.

I. Hypertension

◆ Uncontrolled—avoid all dental procedures; controlled—limit amount of vasoconstrictors.[19]

◆ Best choice: plain anesthetics*; 1:200,000 epinephrine concentrations (if hemostasis is not a consideration); 2% mepivacaine 1:20,000.

J. Hemophilia

◆ Excessive bleeding may result from needle contact with a blood vessel.

◆ Decision based on severity of condition can range from treatment in hospital to avoiding injections into highly vascularized areas (e.g., the posterior superior alveolar [PSA]).

◆ Best choice: local anesthetic that has a vasoconstrictor; avoid plain anesthetics.

K. Pregnancy and Lactation

◆ Local anesthetics and vasoconstrictors are not teratogens and may be safely administered.

◆ Select a drug in the FDA pregnancy risk category B (lidocaine or prilocaine). The FDA classifies drugs according to their safety for the fetus. Refer to Box 36-4 for FDA pregnancy categories.

◆ Elective dental treatment is recommended during the second trimester.[32]

◆ All local anesthetics are expressed in breast milk; use smallest effective dose.

◆ It is prudent practice to limit any elective drug administration, especially during the first trimester.

◆ There are no clinical trials showing the safety of local anesthetics and breast feeding.

◆ Best choice (pregnancy): 2% lidocaine 1:100,000; 4% prilocaine plain or 1:200,000 (FDA drug category B).

◆ Best choice (lactation): articaine 1:200,000 due to its half-life compared to the other anesthetics.

L. Diabetes

◆ Epinephrine opposes action of insulin and may raise blood glucose levels and should be used with caution.[33]

◆ Best choice: plain local anesthetic*; 1:200,000 concentrations; 2% mepivacaine 1:20,000.

M. Glaucoma

◆ Avoid or limit amount of vasoconstrictor, may increase ocular pressure due to vasoconstriction.

◆ Best choice: plain local anesthetic*; 1:200,000 concentrations; 2% mepivacaine 1:20,000.

N. Atypical Plasma Cholinesterase

◆ Uncommon, autosomal recessive trait; inability to metabolize ester drugs.

◆ Relative contraindication: ester drugs; avoid topical benzocaine.

◆ Best choice: amide topical and local anesthetics.[19]

O. Potential Drug Interactions

All medications reported in a patient's medical history need to be reviewed for potential drug interactions before selecting the local or topical anesthetic.

◆ Following are examples of frequently prescribed or OTC drugs that interact with an anesthetic or a vasoconstrictor.[34] Precaution is needed.

• Histamine (H_2) receptor blockers (e.g., Tagamet) and lidocaine: reduce liver ability to metabolize lidocaine; limit amount of lidocaine especially if have congested heart failure (ASA 3) and taking a histamine blocker.[34]

• Nonselective beta-blockers (e.g., Inderal, Corgard) and vasoconstrictors: increased risk of serious hypertension, cardiac dysrhythmias, and a potential cardiac event; use plain anesthetic unless hemostasis is needed.

• TCAs (Tricyclic Antidepressants) (e.g., Elavil, Norpramin) and vasoconstrictors: increased risk of hypertension and cardiac dysrhythmias; limit epinephrine and avoid levonordefrin.

• Phenothiazines (e.g., Thorazine) and vasoconstrictors: possible severe hypotension; be aware of potential postural hypotension; use cardiac dose and avoid 1:50,000 epinephrine.

• Cocaine, methamphetamine, and vasoconstrictors: increased risk of hypertensive crisis, MI or stroke; avoid all vasoconstrictors for 24 hours of using offending drug.[35]

*plain local anesthetics (if can achieve adequate depth and duration of pain control).

ARMAMENTARIUM FOR LOCAL ANESTHESIA

I. Syringe

◆ *Nondisposable types*

• Breech-loading, metallic, aspirating (most frequently used).

• Breech-loading, metallic, aspirating, petite (smaller thumb ring diameter makes handling easier for clinicians with small hands).

• Breech-loading, metallic, self-aspirating (easier aspiration for smaller hand clinicians).

• Breech-loading, plastic, aspirating.

• Pressure syringe for periodontal ligament (PDL) injection.

• Jet injector (needleless syringe); used for topical anesthesia of the palate.

◆ *Safety syringes* (single-use, self-sheathing to prevent needle stick injury) (Figure 36-2).
  ● Computer-controlled local anesthesia delivery (C-CLAD) system.
◆ *Design features of syringes*
  ● Durable metal or plastic can be sterilized and reused with the addition of a new needle and cartridge.
  ● Single-use, disposable safety syringes have features to prevent inadvertent needle stick after use.
  ● Provide good visibility of the cartridge to determine whether a positive aspiration has occurred.
◆ *Promote easy aspiration*
  ● Manual aspiration is the traditional design.
  ● Self-aspirating syringe works well for small hands.

II. Needle

◆ *Disposable*.
◆ Intended only for single-patient use.
◆ *Parts and lengths of the needle* (Figure 36-3).
◆ Needle lengths are not standardized and therefore can vary depending on the manufacturer.
  ● *Long needle*: approximately 30–35 mm (1½ inches).
  ● *Short needle*: approximately 20–25 mm (1 inch).
  ● *Extra-short needle*: approximately 10–12 mm (1/2 inch); used for palatal injections.

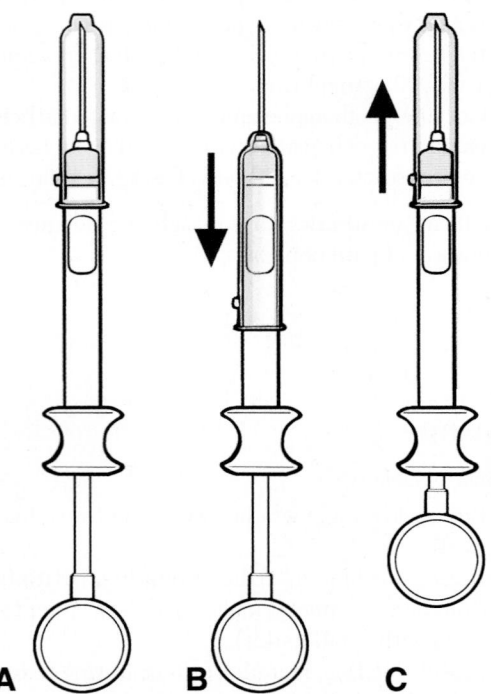

FIGURE 36-2 • Prevention of Percutaneous Injury: Self-sheathing Safety Needle. A: Syringe with protective sheath over the needle. **B:** As the injection is made, the sheath slides back. **C:** After injection, the sheath returns to cover the needle and protect the clinician during disposal.

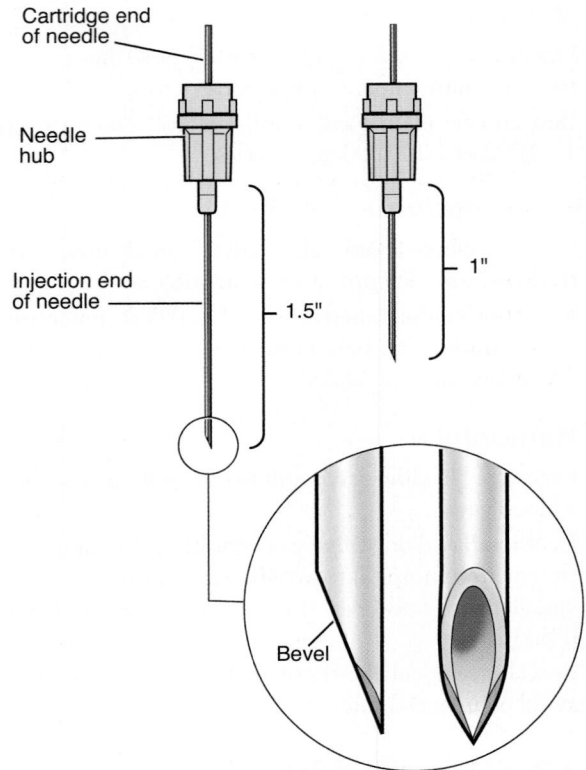

FIGURE 36-3 • The Dental Anesthetic Needle. Dental needles are available in three lengths, long, short, and extra-short. Lengths vary slightly between manufacturers. The components of the needle are cartridge end, which penetrates the rubber diaphragm of the dental cartridge; hub, which attaches the needle to the syringe (made of plastic or metal); injection end or shank or shaft, which penetrates the oral tissue so that anesthetic solution is deposited at the desired site. Inset: shows an enlargement of the tip of the needle with sharp terminus and bevel. When giving an injection, the needle is oriented so that the bevel is parallel to the bone to help prevent the needle from catching the periosteum, the sensitive covering over the bone. Needles should be changed after three to four uses to prevent unnecessary discomfort to the patient from a dull or barbed needle.

◆ *Gauge or needle diameter*
  ● *Size*: Ranked from largest to smallest, 25-, 27-, and 30-gauge needles are used in dentistry.
  ● *Rigidity*: 25-gauge needles are stiffer and have less needle deflection as it passes through tissue. Increased accuracy with deep tissue penetration (IA and Gow–Gates [GG] nerve blocks).
  ● *Aspiration*: Larger-gauge needles provide easier and more accurate aspiration.

III. Cartridge or Carpule

◆ Volume: 1.7 or 1.8 mL of solution.
◆ Storage:
  ● Store at cool room temperature and away from the light.
  ● Do not store in an alcohol or disinfectant solution.

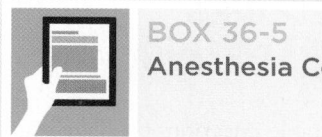

BOX 36-5
Anesthesia Color Code

Color Codes for Local Anesthetics Currently Available in the United States

A uniform system for easy recognition and safety

Lidocaine 2% with epinephrine 1:100,000

Lidocaine 2% with epinephrine 1:50,000

Mepivacaine 2% with levonordefrin 1:20,000

Mepivacaine 3% plain

Prilocaine 4% with epinephrine 1:200,000

Prilocaine 4% plain

Articaine 4% with epinephrine 1:100,000

Articaine 4% with epinephrine 1:200,000

Bupivacaine 0.5% with epinephrine 1:200,000

◆ Label on each cartridge: drugs, manufacturer, and expiration date.

◆ Color coding: local anesthetic drug is identified by color on cartridge. Color codes are standardized and shown in Box 36-5.

IV. Additional Armamentarium

◆ Topical antiseptic (e.g., povidone–iodine) to prevent postinjection infections.

◆ Topical anesthetic to increase patient comfort.

◆ Cotton gauze to wipe the injection site to clean, dry, and remove the topical anesthetic. May also be used to improve grasp for lip or cheek retraction.

◆ Needle recapping device, if self-sheathing needle is not used.

◆ Hemostat for broken needle removal from soft tissues if it occurs.

◆ Sharps disposal system to meet safe practice standards for used needle disposal.

V. Sequence of Syringe Assembly

◆ Figure 36-4A illustrates the assembly of the conventional, metallic, breech-loading anesthetic syringe; sequence makes the attachment between the harpoon and rubber stopper easier without applying excess force to the glass cartridge.

◆ Figure 36-4B demonstrates attachment of the dental needle to the needle adapter end of the syringe.

VI. C-CLAD System

◆ Pressure, volume, and rate of deposit of local anesthetic delivery are precisely regulated by a computer.

◆ Device includes a light, pen-like handpiece attached to a computer-controlled motor that is activated by a foot or finger control. Any gauge Luer Lock needle and standard anesthetic cartridge may be used.

◆ Slow, controlled delivery of anesthesia solution promotes more comfortable injections, especially palatal and PDL injections; allows unique injections, the anterior middle superior alveolar and the palatal anterior superior alveolar, as well as all traditional dental injections.

◆ Good option for needle phobic and pediatric patients.

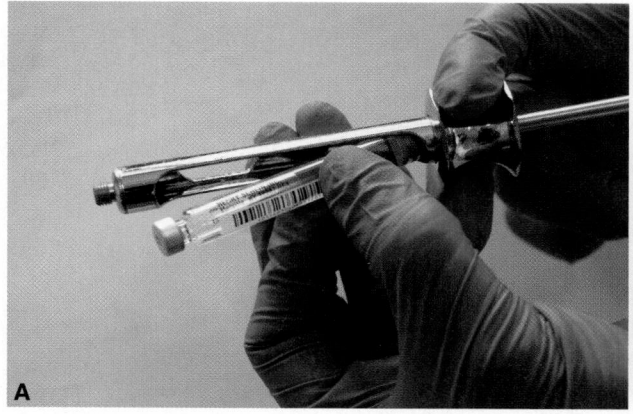
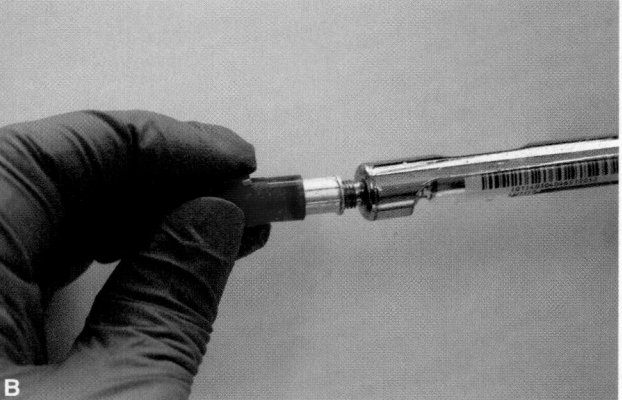

FIGURE 36-4 • Sequence for Assembling a Breech-Loading Aspirating Syringe. A: 1. Pull back on thumb ring. 2. Insert anesthetic cartridge, rubber stopper end first, toward the thumb ring, then the diaphragm end toward the needle opening. 3. Set harpoon and test for lock into rubber stopper. 4. Remove safety cap from needle. **B:** 5. Screw needle onto the syringe.

BOX 36-6
Example Documentation:
Local Anesthesia

S—Patient reported general root sensitivity and gum bleeding when brushing.

O—Reviewed medical history, no contraindications to treatment, ASA I; IOE—negative; BP = 115/75, HR = 65.

A—Moderate generalized chronic periodontitis. Plaque score: 50%.

P—NSPT on mandibular left quadrant; 20% benzocaine topical applied; 1:00 PM administered one cartridge of 2% Xylocaine 1:100,000 epinephrine using a 25-gauge long needle; 36 mg lidocaine and 0.018 mg epinephrine given for a left IA and buccal nerve blocks. Patient tolerated procedure well, no adverse reactions. Post-BP = 120/76; HR = 66; written posttreatment instructions given to the patient.

Signed: _____, RDH

Date: _____

CLINICAL PROCEDURES FOR LOCAL ANESTHETIC ADMINISTRATION

Administer the most comfortable injections possible by using gentle tissue manipulation, careful needle penetration, slow deposition of solution, and good patient communication. An example progress note for a patient receiving local anesthesia is found in Box 36-6.

I. Injection(s) Selection

◆ *Basic injections*

◆ Table 36-4 lists injections with hard and soft tissues anesthetized, and the branches of the trigeminal nerve involved.

◆ *Areas anesthetized*
  • Figure 36-5 shows the areas to be anesthetized.

◆ *Steps and procedures*
  • Box 36-7 outlines the sequence and procedures for the administration of local anesthesia.

TABLE 36-4 • Common Local Anesthetic Injections for Dental Hygiene Procedures

INJECTION	TISSUES ANESTHETIZED	BRANCH OF THE TRIGEMINAL NERVE
Maxillary Arch		**Maxillary Division**
Supraperiosteal	*Teeth:* individual teeth *Periodontium and soft tissues:* periodontium of teeth anesthetized including facial or buccal tissue overlying individual teeth	Individual terminal branches
PSA	*Teeth:* second and third molars; first molar including mesiobuccal root (72% completely anesthetized) *Periodontium and soft tissues:* periodontium of teeth anesthetized including overlying buccal tissues	PSA
MSA	*Teeth:* first and second premolars, mesiobuccal root of first molar (28%) *Periodontium and soft tissues:* periodontium of teeth anesthetized including overlying buccal tissues	MSA
ASA	*Teeth:* canine and incisors *Periodontium and soft tissues:* periodontium of teeth anesthetized and overlying facial tissues and lip	ASA
IO)	*Teeth:* incisors, canine, premolars, and MB root of first molar if MSA nerve is present (28%) *Periodontium and soft tissues:* periodontium of teeth including overlying facial tissues including the lower eye lid, side of nose cheek, and upper lip	IO (includes both anterior and middle superior alveolar)
GP	*Teeth:* none *Periodontium and soft tissues:* lingual gingiva and palatal tissue from distal of third molar to mesial of first premolar medial to midline of palate	GP
NP	*Teeth:* none *Periodontium and soft tissues:* palatal tissues from distal of right canine to distal of left canine	NP
Mandibular Arch		**Mandibular Division**
IA	*Teeth:* entire quadrant of teeth *Periodontium and soft tissues:* buccal periosteum and soft tissues from premolars to midline	IA (includes mental and incisive nerves)
L	*Teeth:* none *Periodontium and soft tissues:* lingual gingiva, floor of the mouth, anterior two-thirds of tongue	L

TABLE 36-4 • Common Local Anesthetic Injections for Dental Hygiene Procedures (*Continued*)

INJECTION	TISSUES ANESTHETIZED	BRANCH OF THE TRIGEMINAL NERVE
LB	Teeth: none *Periodontium and soft tissues:* buccal periosteum and soft tissues of molars	Long Buccal (LB)
Mental (M)	*Teeth:* none *Periodontium and soft tissues:* buccal gingival tissue and mucous membranes from mental foramen to mid-line, lower lip, skin of chin	Terminal branches of IA nerve
Incisive (I)	*Teeth:* premolars to central incisor in same quadrant *Periodontium and soft tissues:* buccal periosteum, gingival tissue, and mucous membranes from premolars to central incisor in same quadrant, lower lip, skin of chin	Terminal branches of IA nerve
Gow–Gates technique	*Teeth:* entire mandibular quadrant of teeth *Periodontium and soft tissues:* buccal and lingual tissues; anterior two-thirds of tongue and floor of mouth; lower lip; skin over the zygoma; posterior portion of the cheek and temporal regions	Mandibular nerve—V_3 nerve block (includes IA, mental, incisive, lingual, mylohyoid, auriculotemporal, and buccal nerves)
Either Arch		
Intraseptal	*Teeth:* unreliable; primarily soft-tissue anesthesia; good technique for hemostasis of moderate inflamed tissue (e.g., curettage) *Periodontium and soft tissues:* periosteum and gingiva of anesthetized area	Terminal nerve endings
PDL	*Teeth:* individual tooth *Periodontium and soft tissues:* periosteum, gingiva and mucous membrane associated with anesthetized tooth	Terminal nerve endings

ASA, American Society of Anesthesiologists; GP, greater palatine; IA, inferior alveolar; IO, infraorbital; L, lingual; LB, long buccal; MSA, middle superior alveolar; NP, nasopalatine; PDL, periodontal ligament; PSA, posterior superior alveolar.

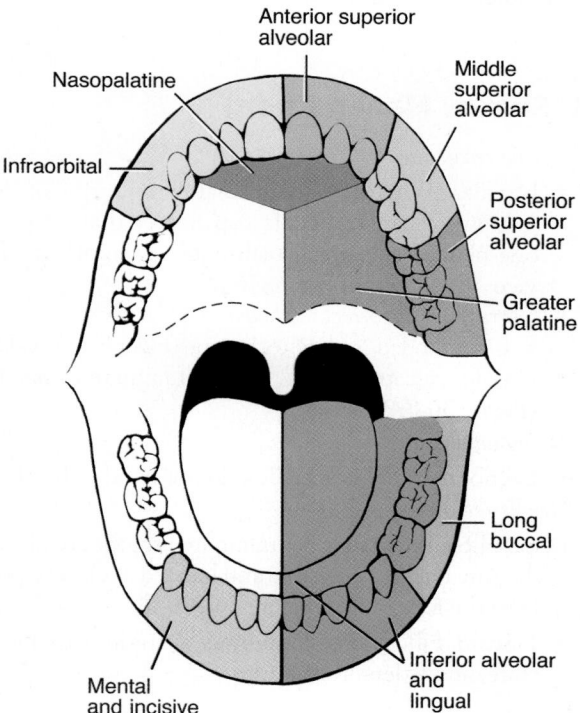

FIGURE 36-5 • Diagrammatic Representation of Teeth and Soft Tissues Anesthetized by Common Dental Injections.

Labels:
- Anterior superior alveolar
- Nasopalatine
- Middle superior alveolar
- Infraorbital
- Posterior superior alveolar
- Greater palatine
- Long buccal
- Inferior alveolar and lingual
- Mental and incisive

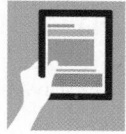

BOX 36-7
Steps in the Administration of Local Anesthesia

1. Assess patient medical status, treatment, and pain control needs in order to select injection(s) and anesthetic drug.
2. Assemble and test the syringe setup (Figures 36-3 and 36-4A and B).
   a. Orient the needle so the bevel will be toward the bone during the injection.
   b. Test the assembled syringe.
3. Position patient for good visibility and to prevent syncope with head level with or lower than heart.
4. Use topical anesthetic.
   a. Apply topical to dry tissue at the injection site for the appropriate time. For benzocaine, 1–2 minutes is optimal.
   b. Remove residual topical anesthetic.
5. Wipe injection site with gauze to dry and clean surface bacteria, saliva, and topical anesthetic from the area before injection.

6. Retract the lip or cheek for good visibility; gently stretch the tissue for easier needle penetration.

7. Keep the syringe out of the patient's sight.

8. Pick up the syringe so that the large window is facing the clinician.

9. Establish a fulcrum or hand rest for stability during the injection.

10. Insert the needle into the tissue and gently advance to desired site for administration of anesthetic.

11. Aspirate before depositing solution; reaspirate as needed throughout procedure.

12. Deposit the anesthetic solution slowly (1–2 minutes for full cartridge) to prevent patient discomfort and to reduce potential for a toxic reaction.

13. Withdraw the needle carefully at the completion of the injection, and recap the needle using a safe technique.

14. Remain with and observe the patient. Adverse drug reactions (ADRs) are most likely to occur during or shortly after the injection.

15. Record injection information in patient chart.

16. Use positive, supportive communication with the patient throughout the procedure.

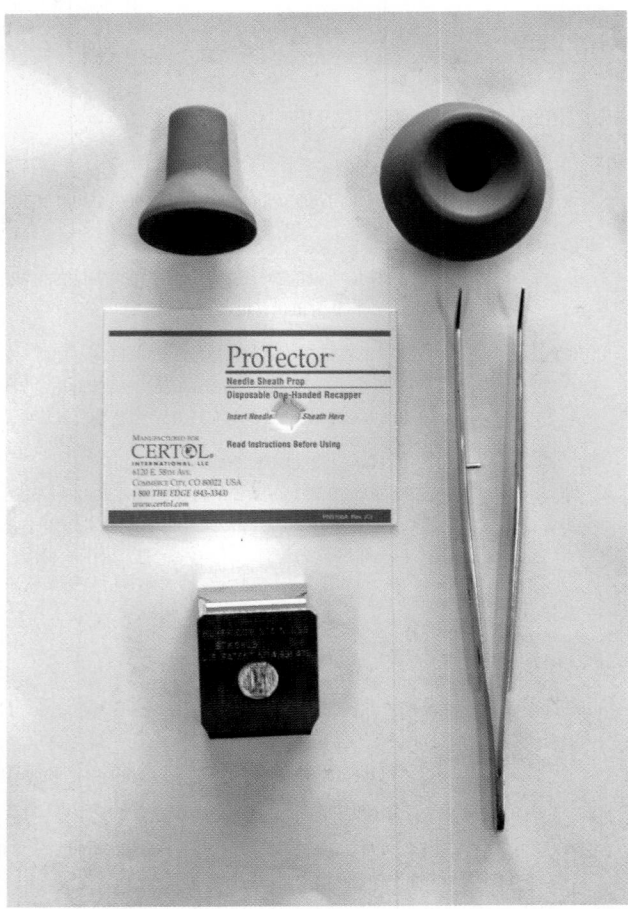

FIGURE 36-6 • Commercially Available Holders for Needle Caps. One-handed capping or recapping with a safety mechanical device to hold the needle sheath is acceptable.

II. Aspiration

◆ *Purpose*
  • To confirm the tip of the needle is not within a blood vessel prior to depositing the local anesthetic.
  • An anesthetic solution must be deposited extravascular to be effective and to prevent toxicity.

◆ *When to aspirate*
  • Before depositing anesthetic solution.
  • Periodically throughout injection to confirm that the needle has not moved and is now in a blood vessel; to slow the rate of deposit.

◆ *Interpretation*
  • Any fluid at the tip of the needle will be drawn into the cartridge. If the tip of the needle is in an artery or vein, blood will become visible; it may only be a small amount at the needle end of the cartridge.
  • *Negative aspiration:* No blood in cartridge; proceed with injection.
  • *Positive aspiration:* Blood in the cartridge.
    • A small amount of blood with most of the cartridge clear: move to a new location and reaspirate.
    • Cartridge generally bloody: withdraw needle, replace cartridge, and repeat injection.

III. Sharps Management

◆ *Needle recapping*
  • Needles are recapped immediately following an injection utilizing a needle cap holder that allows a one-handed recapping technique. Examples of devices are shown in Figure 36-6.
  • *Correct and incorrect methods:*
    • One-handed "scoop" technique (Figure 36-7 A–D).
    • Unsafe recapping of a contaminated needle (Figure 36-8A and B).
◆ *No manipulation*
  • Do not manipulate needles; do not bend or break.
◆ *Needle removal*
◆ Disposal containers for contaminated sharps are placed so they are readily accessible and located as close as possible to the area of use (Figure 36-9A–C).
  • Discard full sharps containers according to local, state, and federal regulations.

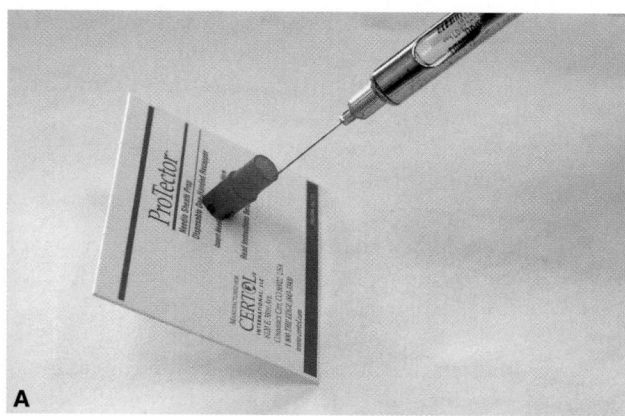

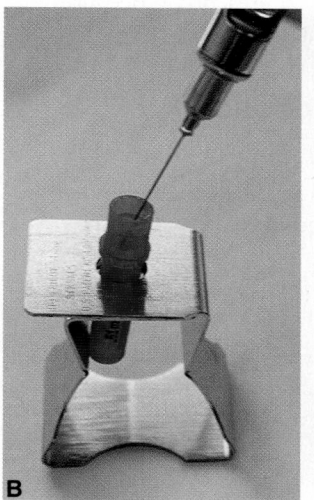

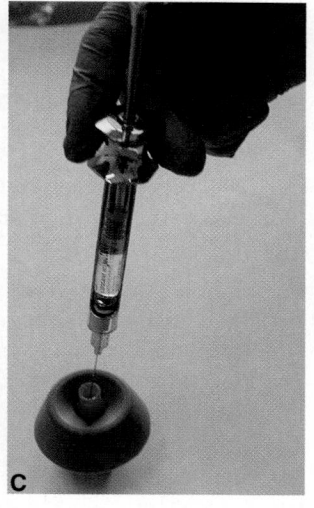

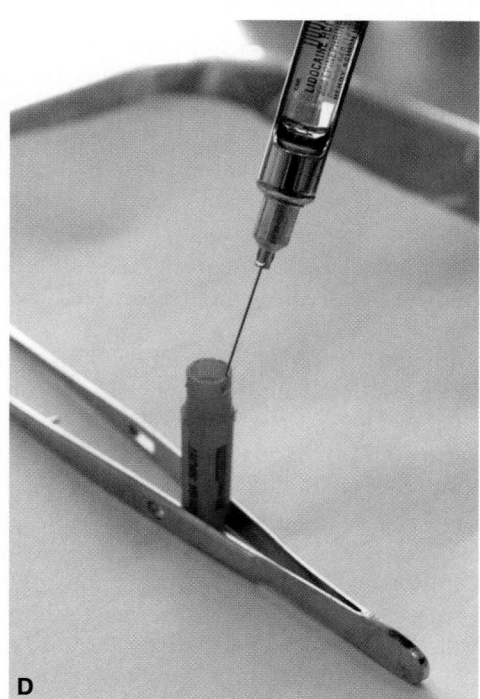

FIGURE 36-7 • Safe Needle Recapping Techniques. A to D:
Correct utilization of the various needle cap holders will allow for a safe one-handed needle recapping method.

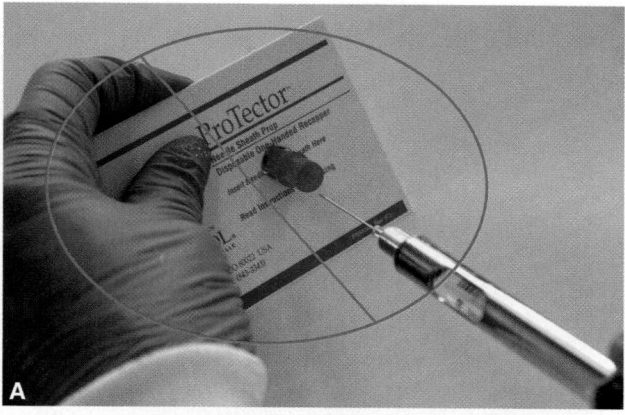

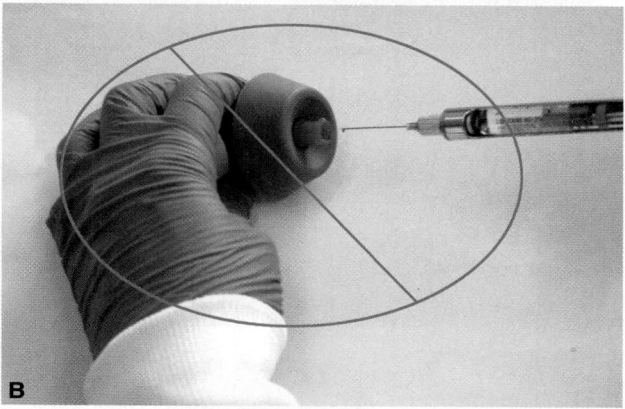

FIGURE 36-8 • Unsafe Needle Recapping Techniques.
A and B: Increases risk of needle exposure to the clinician.

POTENTIAL ADVERSE REACTIONS TO LOCAL ANESTHESIA

I. Adverse Drug Reactions

◆ *Overdose (toxicity)*
  • Overdose is the most common adverse drug reaction (ADR).[19]
  • Occurs when the circulating blood level of the drug becomes too high and reaches a toxic level for the individual.
  • Reaction continues as long as the local anesthetic plasma level remains above threshold for overdose.
◆ *Typical causes of overdose*
  • *Intravascular injection*: prevented by aspiration before deposition of the anesthetic drug.
  • *Excessive total drug dose*: affected by drug volumes, drug choice, patient's lean weight, age, and physical/medical status.
  • *Rapid absorption into the circulatory system*: affected by rate of injection, presence or absence of a vasoconstrictor, or vascularity of injection site.
  • *Reduced elimination and/or metabolism of drug*: reduced kidney or liver function or reduced circulation as a result of congestive heart failure may reduce the rate at which the drug is removed from circulation.

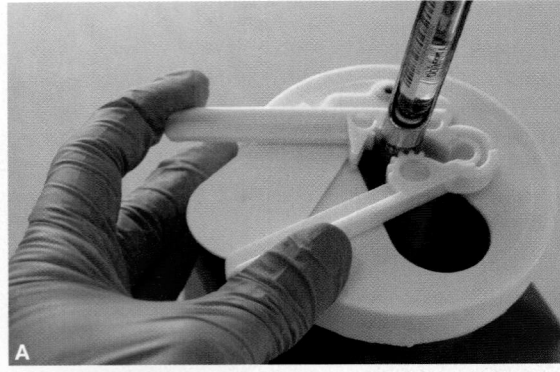

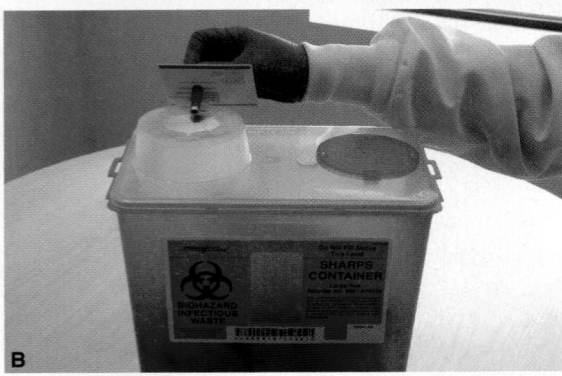

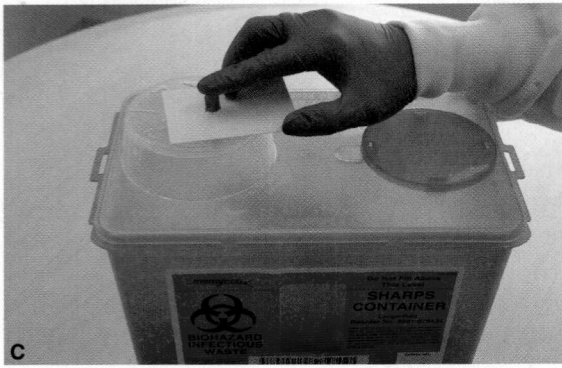

FIGURE 36-9 • Needle Disposal Technique. A to C: Dental needles must be disposed of in the appropriate sharps containers using a one-handed technique.

◆ *Reducing risk of overdose in the pediatric population*
- Treat only one quadrant at a time with local anesthesia.
- Do not administer full cartridges per injection.
- Avoid using local anesthetic solutions with no vasoconstrictor.
- Choose the lowest effective local anesthetic concentration.
- Stay below the MRD specific for that patient.

◆ *Primary prevention*
- Thorough review of medical history including any anxiety, fear, or phobias.
- Limit amount of topical anesthetic.
- Use vasoconstrictor when not contraindicated.
- Position patient in a supine or semi-supine position to prevent syncope.

- Administer lowest concentration and amount necessary to achieve adequate pain control.
- Aspirate and inject slowly (no less than 1 minute for a full cartridge).
- Continue to observe patient before, during, and after administration.

◆ *Allergy*
- *Incidence:* Although often reported, incidence is rare with amide drugs.[19,36] (Review allergy in "Specific Medical Considerations" section above.)
- *Symptoms:* Response may range from mild, such as localized erythema or itching, to life-threatening, such as generalized anaphylaxis or laryngeal edema.
- *Onset:* May range from a few seconds to hours.
- *Management:* Chapter 9 presents procedures for managing an allergic reaction.

II. Psychogenic Reactions

◆ *Cause.*
◆ A psychogenic reaction is an emotional or anxiety response to the injection procedure.
◆ *Symptoms:*
- Vasodepressor syncope (fainting) and hyperventilation are most common.[19,30]
- Symptoms can be highly varied and may mimic drug reactions or other medical conditions.
- Reactions reported by patients as allergies are often psychogenic in nature.

III. Local Complications

Local and topical anesthetics can cause a variety of local complications ranging from mild to severe; transient to permanent. The clinician is responsible to recognize, prevent, and manage any complications that may arise.

◆ *Trismus:* caused from trauma to muscles resulting in spasm of the jaw muscles that restricts opening or is painful; most often results from IA nerve block.
- Prevention: Use aseptic technique; do not contaminate the needle; avoid repeated insertions into muscle.
- Management: Apply warm, moist cloth to outside of face; warm saline rinses; analgesics for pain; light physiotherapy to exercise jaw.

◆ *Hematoma* (bruise): Blood from a nicked artery or vein leaks into the surrounding tissue.
- Prevention: Minimize number of needle penetrations; know the anatomy of the area; do not use needle as a probe.
- Management: Apply ice and pressure to the area immediately, continue over next 6 hours (20 minutes on/20 minutes off) for first day; avoid aspirin for pain.

◆ *Paresthesia:* caused from physical trauma to nerve or chemical insult; generally last for short period (hours–days), but can be long-term lasting months to years (permanent).[23–25]

- Prevention: proper infection control (needle sterility) and handling of dental cartridge (do not immerse in solutions, e.g., alcohol); thorough assessment whether to administer 4% solution for an IA nerve block.
- Evidence has shown an increased risk of paresthesia from injecting with a 4% anesthetic (articaine or prilocaine).[26,27] The risk and benefit of use of a 4% solution must be considered when choosing a local anesthetic.
- Management: reassure patient; determine extent of paresthesia and document; re-evaluate 1–2 months for any changes; refer to oral surgeon for consult if no improvement.
- *Facial paralysis*: from injecting anesthetic into parotid gland capsule.
  - Prevention: good IA injection technique; must touch periosteum prior to depositing; use alternative techniques: PDL, GG nerve block.
  - Management: discontinue treatment; manually close patient's eye (have patient remove contact lenses if wearing them) on affected side, place a gauze patch over eye and tape closed; paralysis lasts as long as the duration of soft-tissue anesthesia.
- *Broken needle*: caused from bending the needle, sudden movement by patient, using smaller gauge needles for deep insertions (e.g., 30 gauge); inserting needle to the hub.
  - Prevention: use larger-gauge needles (25 or 27); do not insert the needle to the hub; do not bend the needle; do not force against resistance.
  - Management: instruct patient to keep mouth open, do not allow the patient to close; if visible, use a hemostat or locking cotton pliers to remove needle from soft tissue; if unable to retrieve, refer to oral surgeon for consult.
- *Epithelial desquamation* (tissue sloughing): may follow prolonged application of topical anesthetic.
  - Prevention: Apply topical anesthetic correctly (follow manufacturer's instructions); avoid high concentrations of vasoconstrictor (1:50,000 on palatal injections).
  - Management: topical analgesics for pain.
- *Infection*: caused by nonsterile technique; injecting into an area of infection.
  - Prevention: use sterile armamentarium; change needle if injecting into area of infection.
  - Management: evaluate as soon as possible; antibiotics may need to be prescribed.
- *Pain on injection*: caused by careless injection technique; fast rate of deposit; using a dull or barbed needle.
  - Prevention: follow proper injection technique; use topical anesthetic prior to injection; use a sharp needle; slow rate of deposit; anesthetic solutions need to be kept at room temperature.
- *Burning on injection*: low pH of anesthetic solution containing a vasoconstrictor; contaminated solutions.
  - Prevention: use a higher pH solution; inject small amount of a plain local anesthetic solution prior to injecting local anesthetic with a vasoconstrictor (patient will then not feel burning from the low pH of anesthetic with a vasoconstrictor).

- Management: reassure patient; will subside by the time the injection is completed. May also consider using a buffered local anesthetic.
- *Self-inflicted soft-tissue injury*: occurs mainly in children.
  - Prevention: use shorter duration local anesthetics; inform parent/caregiver of duration of soft-tissue anesthesia; insert cotton roll to prevent biting of lip.
  - Management: analgesics for pain; lukewarm saline rinses; topical analgesics.

ADVANTAGES AND DISADVANTAGES OF LOCAL ANESTHESIA

I. Advantages

- Patient experiences no pain or discomfort during treatment procedure.
- Clinician has increased confidence to provide complete treatment when the patient is pain-free.
- Local effect results in loss of sensation in area of treatment without a change in level of consciousness or patient cooperation.
- Completely reversible without residual side effects.
- Rapid onset of action.
- Adequate duration of clinical action that is reasonably predictable and that can be varied by choice of commercially available drugs.
- Relatively free of allergic reactions.
- Achieves hemostasis if injected directly into area where bleeding is a factor.

II. Disadvantages

- Anticipating and receiving dental injections may cause high anxiety for patient. Effects may include:
  - Need for special anxiety reduction technique.
  - Undesirable psychogenic reactions.
  - Avoidance of needed care.
- Significant potential exists for toxicity (overdose).
- There are systemic side effects from both the local anesthetic drug and vasoconstrictor.
- Potential for soft-tissue injury postinjection, especially for the pediatric population and mentally challenged adolescents and adults.

NONINJECTABLE ANESTHESIA

The anesthetic drugs are applied to the surface of the pocket lining tissue making this a topical application. It provides adjacent soft-tissue anesthesia and in varying degrees of dental anesthesia.[38]
- Trade name: *Oraqix*®.
- Drugs: 2.5% lidocaine and 2.5% prilocaine; subgingival liquid-to-gel delivery thermosetting system.

◆ Indications: adults who require localized anesthesia during scaling and/or root planing; initial or maintenance treatment of periodontal pockets where profound pulpal anesthesia is not needed; needle phobic adults.

◆ Onset: ~1 minute; duration: ~20 minutes with a range of 14–31 minutes.

◆ MRD: 5 cartridges/appointment.

◆ Pregnancy category: B (see Box 36-4).

◆ Contraindicated: allergy to lidocaine or prilocaine; history of methemoglobinemia; children (not approved for use).[38]

◆ Precautions: do not inject.

I. Armamentarium and Pharmacology

A unique dispenser with a blunt-tipped applicator delivers a gel containing both lidocaine and prilocaine into the periodontal pocket. Both the dispenser and the anesthetic gel are contraindicated for injections.[38]

◆ *Dispenser cartridge and blunt-tipped applicator*
  ● Packaged together; for single-patient use.
  ● For use only with special dispenser and not for injection.
  ● Blunt-tipped applicator is individually bent by clinician with either a single or double bend.
  ● Cartridge contains 42.5 mg lidocaine and 42.5 mg prilocaine; 1.7 mL cartridge.
  ● Store at room temperature.

◆ *Anesthetic gel composition*
  ● *Anesthetics*: 2.5% lidocaine and 2.5% prilocaine amide anesthetics.
  ● *Poloxamers*: thermosetting agents.
  ● *pH adjuster*: hydrochloric acid.
  ● *Purified water*.

◆ *Anesthetic gel characteristics*
  ● Low-viscosity fluid at room temperature.
  ● Gel at oral temperature.

TOPICAL ANESTHESIA

◆ A topical anesthetic is a drug applied directly to the surface of the mucous membrane to produce a loss of sensation.

◆ A topical anesthetic is used with varying degrees of success for short-duration desensitization of the gingiva, but it does not affect pulpal anesthesia.

◆ Anesthetizes terminal nerve endings 2–3 mm beneath surface.[24]

◆ Topical anesthetic is not a substitute for local anesthetic administered by injection.

I. Indications for Use

A topical anesthetic can be used conservatively for selected dental hygiene and dental services, including the following:

◆ Reduce discomfort of an injection.

◆ Prevention of gagging in radiographic techniques and impression taking.

◆ Temporary relief of pain from localized diseased areas, such as oral ulcers, wounds, or inflammation.

◆ Suture removal.

II. Action of a Topical Anesthetic

◆ *Purpose*
  ● The purpose of a topical anesthetic is to desensitize the mucous membrane by anesthetizing the terminal nerve endings.
  ● The superficial anesthesia produced is related to the amount of absorption of the drug by the tissue.

◆ *Factors that affect efficacy*
  ● Type of drug.
  ● Duration of application.
  ● Site of application: thickness of stratified squamous epithelial covering; degree of keratinization.
    • Highly resistant: skin, lips, palatal mucosa.
    • Slow absorption: attached gingiva, palatal gingiva.
    • Fast absorption: tissue without keratinization, such as vestibular mucosa.

III. Agents Used in Surface Anesthetic Preparations

Table 36-5 provides onset and duration of topical anesthetics.

◆ *Benzocaine (ester)*
  ● Types and formulations: Used in 6–20% (20% most common in dentistry) formulations; available as liquid, gel, ointment, spray, and gel patch; most widely used topical agent.
  ● Onset: 30 seconds–2 minutes; duration: 5–15 minutes.
  ● Not readily absorbed into circulation; potential for toxicity is minimal.
  ● May cause allergic reaction at site of application after prolonged or repeated use.
  ● Precautions: fast absorption on nonkeratinized tissue—concern for toxicity; can cause methemoglobinemia (dose related); children.
  ● Pregnancy category: C (see Box 36-4).

◆ *Tetracaine HCl (ester)*
  ● Types and formulations: Used in 0.25–0.5% formulations; typically available as part of a combination of drugs in liquid, gel, and controlled-dose spray.
  ● Most potent; readily absorbed causing deeper penetration, longer effect, and more potential for toxicity. Not to be used over a large area.
  ● Onset: slow, within 20 minutes; duration: 20–60 minutes.
  ● Precautions: rapid absorption on mucous membranes, abraded tissues; children.
  ● Pregnancy category: C (see Box 36-4).

◆ *Lidocaine HCl (amide)*
  ● Types and formulations: Used in 2% or 5% formulations; available in ointment, metered spray, and in combination with prilocaine.
  ● The only amide used alone as a topical.

TABLE 36-5 • Topical and Noninjectable Anesthetic Characteristics

TYPES	DRUG	MRD	ONSET	DURATION
Noninjectable local anesthetic	Amide *2.5% Lidocaine and 2.5% prilocaine*	Five cartridges per appointment	~1 min	14–31 min 20 min average
Topical anesthetics	Ester *Benzocaine (6–20%)*	No established MRD; follow manufacturer's recommendations	30 sec–2 min	5–15 min
	Ester *Tetracaine (0.25–0.5%);* combined with other drugs	20 mg (1 mL of 2% solution)	Slow up to 20 min	20–60 min
	Amide *Lidocaine ointment (2% and 5%)*	2% and 5%—200 mg	1–2 min	15 min

MRD, maximum recommended dose.

- Toxicity unlikely from topical alone but would be additive with other amide anesthetics. Greatest risk from sprays.
- Onset: 1–2 minutes, peak between 5 and 10 minutes; duration: 15 minutes.
- Precautions: abraded tissues; large areas; children.
- Pregnancy category: B (see Box 36-4).

◆ *Dyclonine HCl (ketone)*
- Types and formulations: 0.5% or 1% formulation from a compounding pharmacy; available as a liquid, lozenges, and spray.
- As a gargle is good for gag reflex suppression.
- Onset: slow, up to 10 minutes; duration: 30 minutes (average), but up to 1 hour.
- Precautions: abraded tissues; reduce dosage in children and medically compromised adults.
- Pregnancy category: C (see Box 36-4).

IV. Topical Drug Mixtures

◆ *Eutectic mixture of local anesthetics (EMLA; amide)*
- EMLA is a combination of two or more drugs, provides more rapid onset on intact skin.
- Types and formulations: 2.5% lidocaine and 2.5% prilocaine; cream; lidocaine and prilocaine periodontal gel (Oraqix®).
- Pregnancy category: B (see Box 36-4).

◆ *Benzocaine, butamben, and tetracaine (ester)*
- Types and formulations: 14% benzocaine, 2% butamben, 2% tetracaine; by prescription only as a liquid, spray, and gel.
- Onset: rapid, less than 1 minute; duration: 30–60 minutes.
- Pregnancy category: C (see Box 36-4).
- Precautions: fast absorption into tissues—higher risk for toxicity; not to be injected.

V. Adverse Reactions of Topical Anesthetics

◆ Ester topical anesthetics have a higher incidence of allergic reactions from primary metabolite, PABA.

◆ Redness.
◆ Tissue sloughing.
◆ Edema.
◆ Pain and burning at site.
◆ Greater risk of toxicity compared to local anesthetics (higher drug concentrations).

APPLICATION OF TOPICAL ANESTHETIC

I. Patient Preparation

◆ Consult medical and dental history for pertinent information concerning patient's previous experiences with anesthetics. A patient with an allergy to a local anesthetic may also be allergic to a topical anesthetic.

◆ Determine the most appropriate anesthetic agent and method of application.

◆ Explain purpose and anticipated effect to the patient.

II. Application Techniques

Several application techniques are available. Not all methods are applicable to all products. Select the most appropriate method from the following:

◆ *Surface application*
- May be used with liquid, gel, or ointment formulations of any of the available topical agents.
- Topical is applied with a cotton-tipped swab or cotton roll.
- Time before becoming effective varies with the drug used.
- After application, excess topical is removed by rinsing or gentle wiping.

◆ *Aerosol spray*
- Prevent inhalation by avoiding spray preparations when another method would be as effective. A spray must never be directed toward the throat.
- Use metered- or controlled-dose spray dispensers to prevent overdose.

III. Completion of Topical Anesthetic Application

◆ Wait appropriate length of time for anesthetic to take effect before proceeding.

◆ Limit drug exposure.
- Apply only to the area of need.
- Use the smallest effective amount.
- Remove residual drug after application time.

◆ Apply to a limited area when using a drug with a short duration of action for a long procedure such as scaling.

◆ Record topical anesthetic drug information in the patient's record.

NEW DEVELOPMENTS IN PAIN CONTROL

I. Anesthesia Reversal Agent

A. Properties

◆ Drug: phentolamine mesylate (trade name: *OraVerse®*); nonselective alpha adrenergic blocking agent.

◆ Formulation: 0.4 mg/1.7 mL.

◆ Indications: reversal of soft-tissue anesthesia (~50% reduction time).[39–42] Recent research has shown that it will impact to a lesser degree reversal of pulpal anesthesia.[39]

◆ Metabolized by the liver and excreted by the kidneys.

◆ Onset: rapid; duration: 30–45 minutes.

◆ Dosage and MRD: 1:1 ratio (cartridge containing a vasoconstrictor).

◆ Contraindicated: children under 6 years of age and/or 33 pounds; postsurgical patients; post-PDL or intraosseous injections.

◆ Pregnancy category: C (see Box 36-4).

B. Advantages

◆ Patients can return to normal function faster.[39–42]

◆ Decrease risk of soft-tissue injury from prolonged anesthesia.

C. Technique

◆ Administered by injection in same location and with same technique as the local anesthesia being reversed approximately 20–30 minutes prior to the end of the procedure.

◆ Dosage:
- Adult: 1:1 ratio; one cartridge of phentolamine mesylate per cartridge of anesthetic containing a vasoconstrictor, not to exceed two cartridges.
- Children: (1/2 cartridge MRD).

◆ Candidates for use: adult patients with no contraindications to use; pediatric patients; geriatric patients; diabetic patients; special needs patient.

◆ Not candidates: sensitivity to phentolamine mesylate; children less than 6 years of age or weighing less than 33 pounds; postsurgical patients; (increased bleeding); history of MI, angina; coronary artery disease.

II. Buffered Local Anesthetic

A. Properties

◆ Buffered local anesthetic; sodium bicarbonate (8.4% neutralizing additive solution); Brands: *Onset®*, Anutra.

◆ Increases the pH of the local anesthetic solution with a vasopressor to a more physiologic range.

◆ Reduces stinging on injection and provides faster onset.[43–46]

◆ Higher nerve block injection success and the need for a smaller concentration claims needs further research.[43,45,46]

◆ Increased effectiveness in areas of inflammation.

B. Advantages

◆ Greater patient comfort.

◆ More rapid onset.

◆ Decreased postinjection tissue injury.

III. Intranasal Dental Anesthetic

A. Properties

◆ Drug: trade name: Kovonaze™.

◆ FDA approval June 2016.

◆ Intranasal anesthesia.

◆ 3% Tetracaine and 0.05% oxymetazoline (vasoconstrictor).

◆ Provides maxillary pulpal and soft-tissue anesthesia from first premolar to second premolar in the adjacent quadrant.

◆ Biotransformed: plasma.

◆ Excreted: kidneys.

◆ Half-life: 5.2 hours.

B. Advantages

◆ Anesthesia of maxillary teeth (#4–#13) with no needle.[47–50]

◆ Good for pediatric (88 pounds; 40 kg or more) and needle phobic patients.

C. Contraindications and ADRs

◆ *Absolute contraindication*: known hypersensitivity to tetracaine, benzyl alcohol, other ester drugs, PABA, oxymetazoline; uncontrolled hypertension or thyroid disease.

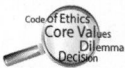

EVERYDAY ETHICS

Mr. Denver, in your office for a dental hygiene appointment, stated that he has not been to a dental office for the past 5 years because he is fearful of oral treatment because of painful experiences when he was young. Oral examination revealed bleeding on probing, generalized 5- to 6-mm pockets, and heavy biofilm, and calculus deposits. Proposed treatment is four appointments for nonsurgical periodontal therapy (NSPT) with anesthesia and patient instruction, followed by a re-evaluation. Mr. Denver does not want local anesthesia because he is fearful of the needle and wants to try the NSPT without it.

Questions for Consideration

1. What anxiety and pain management methods could be used for this patient? Refer to pain control mechanisms to make your list as complete as possible. Which of these methods are legal for a dental hygienist to utilize in your state or province?

2. In the past, this patient has had painful treatment, you plan to provide comfortable treatment, how do the core values of dental hygiene (Table II-I in Section II Introduction) relate to these two approaches for patient care?

3. Thinking of ethics as expressed by the core values is the patient's expectation for pain management different if a dentist or a dental hygienist provides the NSPT? Explain.

- *Relative contraindications*: monoamine oxidase inhibitors, nonselective beta-blockers, TCAs, drugs causing methemoglobinemia, history of frequent nose bleeds.

- *Adverse reactions*: rhinorrhea, nasal congestion, increased lacrimation, nasal discomfort, oropharyngeal pain; asymptomatic increase in blood pressure.

DOCUMENTATION

Documentation in the permanent record for each appointment when a pain control drug or technique is used includes a minimum of the following factors:

- Date.

- Medical status and vital signs (both pre and post treatment). Document any contraindications to the administration of either the local anesthetic or vasoconstrictor.

- Review of dental and psychological history as it pertains to the administration of local anesthesia.

- Informed consent was obtained (oral and/or written).

- Rational for pain control use.

- Location and type of injection.

- Time of administration.

- Number of cartridges; type and concentration of the local anesthetic including milligram of drugs administered.

- Type and concentration of vasoconstrictor including milligrams administered if applicable.

- Any adverse reactions that occurred.

- Posttreatment instructions given (specify written or oral).

- Full signature.

- Example documentation for a patient receiving nitrous oxide–oxygen conscious sedation is found in Box 36-4 and for a patient receiving local anesthesia in Box 36-7.

Factors to Teach the Patient

I. Nitrous Oxide–Oxygen Conscious Sedation

▶ Inform the clinician if the sedation becomes too strong or is too weak so that adjustments can be made. The level of sedation should be adjusted individually for optimum relaxation and comfort.

▶ The gas will not result in unusual or undesirable behavior; the patient will maintain control of all personal actions.

▶ Eat normally before treatment; avoid fasting or heavy meals.

II. Local and Topical Anesthesia

▶ Be careful not to bite lip, cheek, or tongue while tissues are without normal sensations. Warn and watch children to prevent injury. Do not test anesthesia by biting the lip.

▶ Avoid chewing hard foods and avoid hot food and drinks until normal sensation has returned.

ENHANCE YOUR UNDERSTANDING

ONLINE RESOURCES
(see the inside front cover for access information)
- Audio glossary
- Appendices

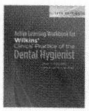

SUPPORT FOR LEARNING
(available separately)
- *Active Learning Workbook for Wilkins' Clinical Practice of the Dental Hygienist, 13th Edition*

INDIVIDUALIZED REVIEW
- Customized practice quizzing with Navigate 2 TestPrep for *Wilkins' Clinical Practice of the Dental Hygienist*

References

1. Department of Health and Human Services. *Oral Health in America: A Report of the Surgeon General*. Rockville MD: U.S. Department of Health and Human Services, National Institute of Dental and Craniofacial Research, National Institutes of Health; 2000.

2. Doebling S, Rowe M. Negative perceptions of dental stimuli and effects on dental fear. *J Dent Hyg*. 2000;74(2):110-116.

3. Binkley CJ, Beacham A, Neace W, Gregg RG, Liem EB, Sessler DI. Genetic variations associated with red hair color and fear of dental pain, anxiety regarding dental care and avoidance of dental care. *J Am Dent Assoc*. 2009;140(7):896-905.

4. Smith EA, Marshall G, Selph SS, Barker DR, Sedgley CM. Nonsteroidal anti-inflammatory drugs for managing postoperative endodontic pain in patients who present with preoperative pain: a systematic review. *J Endod*. 2017;43(1):7-15.

5. Jeske A, Zahrowski J. Good evidence supports ibuprofen as an effective and safe analgesic for postoperative pain. *J Am Dent Assoc*. 2010;141(5):567-568.

6. Clark MS, Brunick AL. *Handbook of Nitrous Oxide and Oxygen Sedation*. 3rd ed. St. Louis, MO: Mosby; 2008.

7. American Dental Association. Guidelines for the use of sedation and general anesthesia by dentists. October 2016. http://www.ada.org/~/media/ADA/Advocacy/Files/anesthesia_use_guidelines.pdf?la=en. Accessed February 3, 2018.

8. Sun R, Jia WQ, Zhang P, et al. Nitrous oxide-based techniques versus nitrous oxide-free techniques for general anesthesia. *Cochrane Data Base Syst Rev*. 2015;(11):CD008984.

9. Tanchyk A, Tanchyk A. The absolute contraindication for using nitrous oxide with intraocular gasses and other dental considerations associated with vitreoretinal surgery. *Gen Dent*. 2013;61(6):e6-e7.

10. American Dental Association. Nitrous oxide use dangerous after intraocular gas injection: FDA. *J Am Dent Assoc*. 2002;133(11):1476.

11. Lockwood AJ, Yang YF. Nitrous oxide inhalation anaesthesia in the presence of intraocular gas can cause irreversible blindness. *Br Dent J*. 2008;204(5):247-248.

12. Malamed SF. *Sedation: A Guide to Patient Management*. 4th ed. St. Louis, MO: Mosby; 2003.

13. National Institute for Occupational Safety and Health. *Control of Nitrous Oxide in Dental Operatories*. Washington, DC: National Institute for Occupational Safety and Health. https://www.cdc.gov/niosh/topics/nitrousoxide/. Accessed July 18, 2019.

14. Donaldson M, Donaldson D, Quarnstrom FC. Nitrous oxide-oxygen administration: when safety features no longer are safe. *J Am Dent Assoc*. 2012;143(2):134-143.

15. Rowland AS, Baird, DD, Weinberg CR, Shore DL, Shy CM, Wilcox AJ. Reduced fertility among women employed as dental assistants exposed to high levels of nitrous oxide. *N Engl J Med*. 1992;327(14):993-997.

16. Cohen EN, Gift HC, Brown BW, et al. Occupational disease in dentistry and chronic exposure to trace anesthetic gases. *J Am Dent Assoc*. 1980;101(1):21-31.

17. National Institute for Occupational Safety and Health (US). *Alert: Controlling Exposures to Nitrous Oxide During Anesthetic Administration* [Joint Publication of Public Health Service, Centers for Disease Control, National Institute for Occupational Safety

and Health]. Cincinnati, OH: U.S. Department of Health, Education, and Welfare; 1994:1. Publication No. 94-100.

18. Jastak T, Malamed SF. Nitrous oxide sedation and sexual phenomena. *J Am Dent Assoc*. 1980;101(1):38-40.

19. Malamed SF. *Handbook of Local Anesthesia*. 6th ed. St. Louis, MO: Mosby; 2013.

20. Moore PA, Hersh EV. Local anesthetics: pharmacology and toxicity. *Dent Clin North Am*. 2010;54:587-599.

21. Haas DA. An update on local anesthetics in dentistry. *J Can Dent Assoc*. 2002;68(9):46-51.

22. Becker DE, Reed KL. Essentials of local anesthetic pharmacology. *Anesth Prog*. 2006;53:98-109.

23. Becker DE, Reed KL. Local anesthetics: review of pharmacological considerations. *Anesth Prog*. 2012;59:90-102.

24. Ogle OE, Mahjoubi G. Local anesthesia: agents, techniques, and complications. *Dent Clin North Am*. 2012;56:133-148.

25. Haas DA, Lennon D. A 21 year retrospective study of reports of paresthesia following local anesthetic administration. *J Can Dent Assoc*. 1995;61(4):319-330.

26. Garisto GA, Gaffen AS, Lawrence HP, Tenenbaum HC, Haas DA. Occurrence of paresthesia after dental local anesthetic administration in the United States. *J Am Dent Assoc*. 2010;141(7):836-844.

27. Moore PA, Haas DA. Paresthesias in dentistry. *Dent Clin North Am*. 2010;54:715-730.

28. Hersh EV, Giannakopoulos H. Beta-adrenergic blocking agents and dental vasoconstrictors. *Dent Clin North Am*. 2010;54:687-696.

29. Becker DE. Preoperative medical evaluation, part 2: pulmonary, endocrine, renal and miscellaneous considerations. *Anesth Prog*. 2009;56:135-145.

30. Malamed SF. *Medical Emergencies in the Dental Office*. 7th ed. St. Louis, MO: Mosby; 2015.

31. Trapp L, Will J. Acquired methemoglobinemia revisited. *Dent Clin North Am*. 2010;54:665-675.

32. Fayans EP, Hunter SR, Carsten D, Ly Q, Kim H. Local anesthetic use in the pregnant and postpartum patient. *Dent Clin North Am*. 2010;54:697-713.

33. Kaur P, Bahl R, Kaura S, Bansal S. Comparing hemodynamic and glycemic response to local anesthesia with epinephrine and without epinephrine in patients undergoing tooth extractions. *Natl J Maxillofac Surg*. 2016;7(2):166-172.v

34. Moore PA. Adverse drug interactions in dental practice: Interactions associated with local anesthetics; sedatives and anxiolytics. *J Am Dent Assoc*. 1999;130(4):541-554.

35. Blanksma CJ, Brand HS. Cocaine abuse: orofacial manifestations and implications for dental treatment. *Int Dent J*. 2005;55(6):365-369.

36. Speca SJ, Boynes SG, Cuddy MA. Allergic reactions to local anesthetic formulations. *Dent Clin North Am*. 2010;54:655-664.

37. Piccinni C, Gissi DB, Gabusi A, Montebugnoli L, Poluzzi E. Paraesthesia after local anaesthetics: an analysis of reports to the FDA Adverse Event Reporting System. *Basic Clin Pharmacol Toxicol*. 2015;117(1):52-56.

38. Dentsply Pharmaceutical. Oraqix: the only FDA-approved needle-free anesthetic. York, PA: Dentsply Pharmaceutical; 2010. https://www.cdc.gov/niosh/docs/94-100/default.html. Accessed July 18, 2019.

39. Hersh EV, Lindemeyer RG. Phentolamine mesylate for accelerating recovery from lip and tongue anesthesia. *Dent Clin North Am.* 2010;54:631-642.

40. Daublander M, Liebaug F, Niedeggen G, Theobald K, Kürzinger ML. Effectiveness and safety of phentolamine mesylate in routine dental care. *J Am Dent Assoc.* 2017;148(3):149-156.

41. Prados-Frutos JC, Rojo R, Gonzalez-Serrano J, et al. Phentolamine mesylate to reverse oral soft-tissue local anesthesia: a systematic review and meta-analysis. *J Am Dent Assoc.* 2015;146(10):751-759.

42. Elmore S, Nusstein J, Drum M, Reader A, Beck M, Fowler S. Reversal of pulpal and soft tissue anesthesia by using phentolamine: a prospective randomized, single-blind study. *J Endod.* 2013;39(4):429–434.

43. Phero JA, Reside GJ, Turner BH, Philips C, White R Jr. A comparison of buffered and non-buffered 2% lidocaine with epinephrine, a pilot study. *J Oral Maxillofac Surg.* 2016;74(9):e41.

44. Malamed SF, Tavana S, Falkel M. Faster onset and more comfortable injection with alkalinized 2% lidocaine with epinephrine 1:100,000. *Compend Contin Educ Dent.* 2013;34 Spec No 1:10-20.

45. Saatchi M, Khademi A, Baghaei B, Noormohammadi H. Effect of sodium bicarbonate-buffered lidocaine on the success of inferior alveolar nerve block for teeth with symptomatic irreversible pulpitis: a prospective, randomized double-blind study. *J Endod.* 2015;41(1):33-35.

46. Hobeich P, Simon S, Schneiderman E, He J. A prospective, randomized, double-blind comparison of the injection pain and anesthetic onset with 2% lidocaine with 1:100,000 epinephrine buffered with 5% and 10% sodium bicarbonate in maxillary infiltrations. *J Endod.* 2013;39(5):597-599.

47. Ciancio SG, Hutcheson MC, Ayoub F, et al. Safety and efficacy of a novel nasal spray for maxillary dental anesthesia. *J Dent Res.* 2013;92(suppl 7):43S-48S.

48. Hersh EV, Pinto A, Saraghi M, et al. Double-masked, randomized, placebo-controlled study to evaluate the efficacy and tolerability of intranasal K305 (3% tetracaine plus 0.05%) in anesthetizing maxillary teeth. *J Am Dent Assoc.* 2016;147(4):278-287.

49. Ciancio SG, Marberger AD, Ayoub F, et al. Comparison of 3 intransal mists for anesthetizing maxillary teeth in adults—a randomized, double-masked, multicenter phase 3 clinical trial. *J Am Dent Assoc.* 2016;147(5):339-347.

50. Hersh EV, Saraghi M, Moore PA. Intranasal tetracaine and oxymetazoline: a newly approved drug formulation that provides maxillary dental anesthesia without needles. *Curr Med Res Opin.* 2016;32(11):1919-1925.

37

Instruments and Principles for Instrumentation

Uhlee (Yuri) Oh, RDH, BS, MSDH, Linda D. Boyd, RDH, RD, EdD, and Esther M. Wilkins, BS, RDH, DMD

CHAPTER OUTLINE

OVERVIEW OF PERIODONTAL INSTRUMENTS
I. Instrument Classification
II. Instrument Identification

INSTRUMENT DESIGN
I. Handle
II. Shank
III. Working End

GRASPS AND FULCRUM
I. Dominant Hand
II. Nondominant Hand
III. Palm Grasp
IV. Modified Pen Grasp
V. Neutral Wrist
VI. Fulcrum

INSTRUMENTATION BASICS
I. Adaptation
II. Angulation
III. Activation (Stroke)

SCALERS
I. Uses
II. Instrument Design
III. Types
IV. Scaler-Specific Instrumentation

CURETS
I. Uses
II. Instrument Design
III. Types
IV. Curet-Specific Instrumentation

PERIODONTAL FILES
I. Working Files
II. Finishing Files

POWERED INSTRUMENTS
I. Mode of Action
II. Indications for Use
III. Contraindications
IV. Risks and Considerations
V. Types

SONIC SCALERS
I. Mechanism of Action
II. Equipment

MAGNETOSTRICTIVE ULTRASONIC SCALERS
I. Mechanism of Action
II. Equipment

PIEZOELECTRIC ULTRASONIC SCALERS
I. Mechanism of Action
II. Equipment

POWERED INSTRUMENTATION TECHNIQUE
I. Insert/Tip Selection
II. Power Setting
III. Water Setting
IV. Grasp
V. Finger Rest
VI. Adaptation
VII. Activation (Stroke)

DEXTERITY DEVELOPMENT
I. Squeezing
II. Stretching
III. Pen/Pencil Exercises
IV. Refining Use of Mouth Mirror and Cotton Pliers
V. Increasing Tactile Sensitivity

CUMULATIVE TRAUMA
I. Risk Factors for Trauma
II. Preventing Trauma

DOCUMENTATION

EVERYDAY ETHICS

FACTORS TO TEACH THE PATIENT

REFERENCES

LEARNING OBJECTIVES

After studying this chapter, the student will be able to:

1. Identify the three main parts of a periodontal instrument.

2. Differentiate between various types of removal instruments based on their design.

3. State the indications and contraindications for the use of various removal instruments.

4. Describe and demonstrate fundamental techniques for manual and power instrumentation.

5. Practice exercises designed to develop hand dexterity and prevent trauma.

Instrumentation begins with the knowledge of instrument parts and identification of each instrument during dental hygiene assessment and treatment.

- ◆ The fundamentals of instrumentation technique include:
  - • *Stabilization* by means of a correct *grasp* and *fulcrum*.
  - • Instrument *adaptation*, *angulation*, and *activation*.
- ◆ A study of oral and dental anatomy and histology needs to accompany learning instrumentation procedures and skills.
- ◆ Development of a thorough, efficient, and safe procedure for treatment depends on an understanding of the normal, healthy, and disease characteristics of the dental and periodontal tissues being treated.
- ◆ A high degree of skill in the care and use of the instruments is required.
- ◆ Skill depends on knowledge and understanding of the goals of therapy and how the goals can be reached through application of the fundamental principles of instrumentation.

OVERVIEW OF PERIODONTAL INSTRUMENTS

Periodontal instruments refer to instruments that are utilized around ("perio") the teeth ("odont"). With the increasing number of periodontal instruments available on the market today, it is essential to understand the fundamentals of instrument design and the basic principles of periodontal instrumentation.

I. Instrument Classification

Periodontal instruments can be classified into two main categories: assessment and removal instruments. Each category serves a different purpose, which dictates the design of the instrument.

A. Assessment Instruments

- ◆ The instruments used for assessment include the mouth mirror, explorers, and periodontal probes. These instruments are described in Chapter 20.

- ◆ This chapter focuses on instruments used for scaling and related procedures.

B. Removal Instruments

- ◆ Consists of instruments used for scaling, or removal of hard and soft dental deposits.
- ◆ Includes manual scalers, manual curets, periodontal files, and powered scalers.

II. Instrument Identification

A. Instrument Design

- ◆ Each instrument can be distinguished at a glance by the design of the instrument.
- ◆ The ability to quickly identify instruments contributes to organization of instrument cassettes and efficiency of services rendered.
- ◆ In instances when an instrument cannot be quickly identified visually, the clinician can refer to the instrument design name and number labeled on the instrument handle.

B. Design Name

- ◆ Instruments are often named after the institution or individual responsible for their design or development.
- ◆ Popular instruments named after *institutions* include the UNC-15 probe (University of North Carolina at Chapel Hill), TU-17 explorer (Tufts University), and ODU-11/12 explorer (Old Dominion University).
- ◆ Popular instruments named after *individuals* include the Gracey curets (named after Dr. Clayton H. Gracey) and the Nevi scalers (named after craftsman Neville Hammond).

C. Design Number

- ◆ Instruments are also designated with a number following the design name.
- ◆ This number indicates the specific design of the working end and the area of the dentition indicated for use.
- ◆ The same instrument may be made by various manufacturers using the same design number.

INSTRUMENT DESIGN

The three major parts of a periodontal instrument include the *handle*, *shank*, and *working end*. The relationship of these parts is illustrated by the curet in Figure 37-1.

I. Handle

Depending on the instrument manufacturer, instrument handles come in various forms and designs. Figure 37-2 shows a few types of handles available. Selecting efficient and comfortable, or *ergonomic*, handles can reduce the risk of developing musculoskeletal disorders of the hand and wrist.

A. Weight

◆ Handles may be heavy and composed of solid metal, or they may be lightweight and hollow.
◆ Handles with lighter weight enhance tactile sensitivity and lessen fatigue related to a tighter grasp.
◆ Ergonomic handles ideally weigh less than 15.0 g.[1]

B. Diameter

◆ Diameters of instrument handles vary widely from standard handles that are 6.5 mm in diameter to larger handles that are 10 mm in diameter.
◆ Instruments with thin, small diameter handles increase muscle activity and pinch force, which over time can lead to musculoskeletal injuries.
◆ Ergonomic instruments have a 10-mm diameter handle.[1]

C. Texture

◆ Instrument handles may have either smooth or varying degrees of raised textures.
◆ A smooth handle may require a tighter grasp to prevent slipping in wet oral environments, which can lessen tactile sensitivity and increase clinician's fatigue.
◆ The textured handle created by ribbed or knurled patterns and serrations can provide better control with a firm, yet lighter grasp without lessening tactile sensitivity.[1]

II. Shank

◆ The shank connects the working end with the handle, as shown in Figure 37-1.

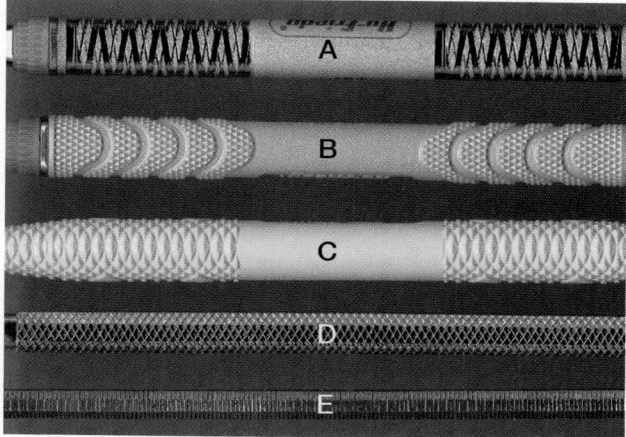

FIGURE 37-2 • **Handle Diameter and Texturing.** The diameter and texturing of a handle varies greatly from manufacturer to manufacturer. Shown here are examples of the variations in design characteristics of instrument handles. Instruments **(A, B, and C)** with large diameter handles and raised textures would be easy to hold and reduce muscle fatigue. Instruments **(A, B, and C)** have additional texturing on the tapered portion of the handle to reduce muscle strain for short-fingered clinicians who must grip the tapered portion of the handle. Instrument **(D)** has a smaller diameter handle and less pronounced texturing. Instrument **(E)** has a small diameter handle and very limited texturing.

◆ The section of the shank between the working end and the first bend in the instrument closest to the working end is called the terminal shank or *lower shank*, as labeled in Figure 37-1. With many instruments, the terminal shank can provide a cue for correct positioning for treatment.
◆ The shape, length, and rigidity of the shank govern the access of the working end to various teeth and tooth surfaces in the mouth.

A. Shape

◆ *Straight/simple:* The lack of bends and flat nature make it ideal for adaptation to tooth surfaces with unrestricted access, such as for anterior teeth.
◆ *Angled/complex:* Contains many bends, which makes it ideal for adaptation to tooth surfaces with restricted access, such as proximal surfaces of posterior teeth.

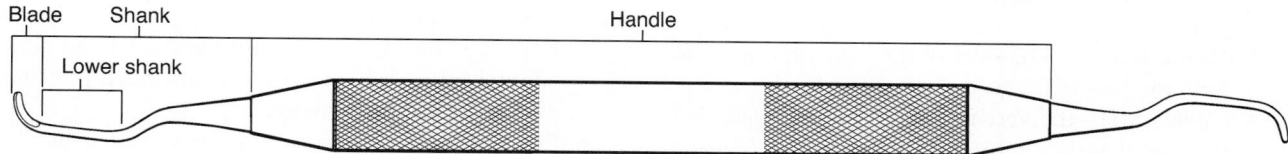

FIGURE 37-1 • **Parts of an Instrument.** Curet shows the relationship of the working end (blade), shank, and handle. The section of the shank next to the blade is referred to as the terminal or lower shank.

- In general, the more restricted the access, the more bends there are, and the deeper the bends in the instrument shank.
- Examples: Gracey curets 11/12, 13/14, and 15/16 are used on posterior teeth and have three bends.
- Because the *distal* surfaces of molars and premolars are much less accessible than are the *mesial* surfaces, the angles in the shank of the 13/14 are designed with deeper bends than the 11/12 to make access possible.

B. Length

- The distance from the working end to the junction between the shank and handle in most instruments is 35–40 mm (1.5 inches).
- Too short a distance limits action subgingivally.
- Extended lower shank length:
    - Adding on 3 mm permits the blade to access deep pockets along narrow roots, and into furcation areas.[2]
    - Examples: after five, mini-five, and micro-mini five curets (see Figure 37-15).

C. Rigidity

- Instruments are made with shanks of varying degrees of thickness and rigidity that relate to the purpose for which the instrument is used.
- *Rigid:* A thicker shank is stronger and is able to withstand greater pressure applied during instrumentation. Strong instruments are needed for removal of heavy calculus deposits that are firmly attached to the tooth surface.
- *Flexible:* A thinner shank may provide more tactile sensitivity and is used, for example, for removal of fine deposits of calculus and for maintenance root debridement.

III. Working End

- The **working end** refers to the part used to carry out the purpose and function of the instrument. Each working end is unique to the particular instrument.
- The working end of a scaler or curet is called a blade.
- The parts of a blade of a curet are illustrated in Figure 37-3. The blades of both a scaler and curet include the:
    - *Face*—the inner surface of the blade opposite to the back.
    - *Back*—the outer surface of the blade opposite to the face.
    - *Lateral surfaces*—the sides of the blade that meet to form the *back* of the instrument.
    - *Cutting edge*—the very fine line where the *face* and the *lateral surface* meet to form the sharp cutting edge of a scaler or curet.

A. Single-Ended

Handle has one working end (e.g., mouth mirror).

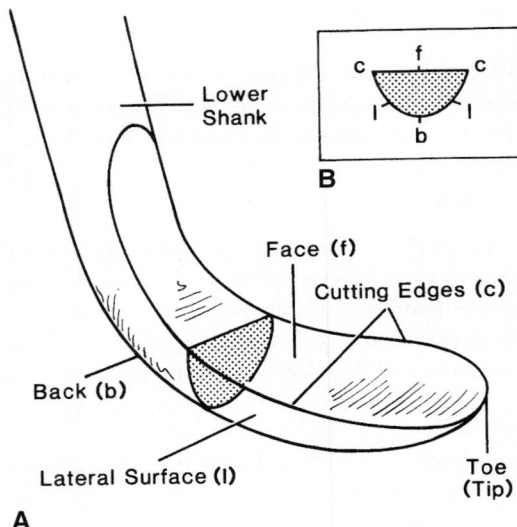

FIGURE 37-3 • Parts of a Curet Blade. A: Curet with parts labeled. The curet has a rounded toe, whereas the scaler has a pointed tip. **B:** Cross section of a curet labeled f (face), c (cutting edges), l (lateral surfaces), and b (back).

B. Double-Ended; Unpaired

Handle has two working ends, but working ends differ in design and function (e.g., probe on one end and an explorer on the other end).

C. Double-Ended; Paired

Handle has two working ends that are mirror images of each other. One end is used for access from the facial and the other end from the lingual or palatal of the same tooth (e.g., universal curet).

GRASPS AND FULCRUM

I. Dominant Hand

- During periodontal instrumentation, the dominant hand is used to hold and activate the treatment instrument.
- The manner in which the instrument is held influences the entire procedure.
- The appropriate grasp is controlled, displays the confidence of the clinician in the work being done, and provides the following effects:
    - Increased fingertip tactile sensitivity.
    - Positive control of the instrument with balance and flexibility during motion.
    - Decreased hazard of trauma to the dental and periodontal tissues, which in turn results in less postcare discomfort for the patient.
    - Prevention of fatigue to clinician's fingers, hands, and arms.
- A rigid grasp, in which the instrument is gripped tightly, lessens the tactile sensitivity and, hence, the effectiveness of instrumentation.

II. Nondominant Hand

- ◆ The nondominant hand is oftentimes used for essential supplementary functions to assist the dominant hand.
- ◆ With the appropriate grasp and finger rest, the following are functions of the nondominant hand:
  - Use of the mouth mirror for indirect vision, indirect lighting, and retraction.
  - Assistance in providing the dominant hand with an auxiliary finger rest.

III. Palm Grasp

- ◆ *Description*: The handle of the instrument is held in the palm by cupped index, middle, ring, and little fingers (Figure 37-4).
- ◆ *Used to grasp*:
  - Air/water syringe.
  - Periodontal instruments with nondominant hand when adjusting the light with dominant hand.
  - Periodontal instruments with nondominant hand when stabilizing the instrument for sharpening.

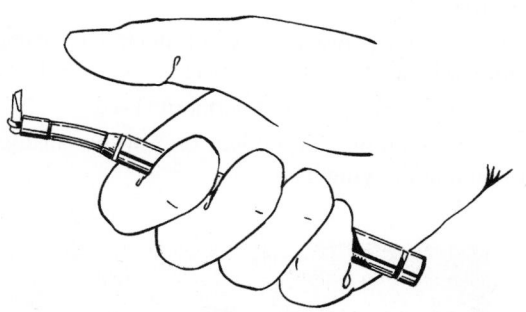

FIGURE 37-4 • Palm Grasp of Instrument. The instrument handle is held in the palm by cupped index, middle, ring, and little fingers. Thumb is free and serves as the finger rest.

IV. Modified Pen Grasp

- ◆ The modified pen grasp is a three-finger grasp with specific target points of the thumb, index finger, and middle finger all in contact with the instrument (Figure 37-5).
- ◆ The instrument is held by the pads of the thumb and index fingers, placed opposite of each other on the handle.
- ◆ The inner corner of the middle finger is placed on the upper portion of the shank to guide the movement of the instrument, to prevent the instrument from slipping during adaptation and activation, and to optimize application of lateral pressure.
- ◆ The ring finger is used to establish a finger rest/fulcrum.
- ◆ The side-to-side contact of the index, middle, and ring fingers allows for greater stability, strength, and control during instrumentation.

V. Neutral Wrist

- ◆ A neutral wrist is important to prevent *carpal tunnel syndrome*, a musculoskeletal disorder brought on by pressure on the median nerve in the carpal tunnel due to inappropriate work habits, such as working with a bent wrist.[3]
- ◆ During instrumentation, the wrist should be straight, and the forearm and hand are in the same horizontal plane when in the neutral position.
- ◆ Figure 37-6 illustrates the straight wrist versus a bent wrist.

VI. Fulcrum

A fulcrum is the support, or point of rest, on which a lever turns or pivots.

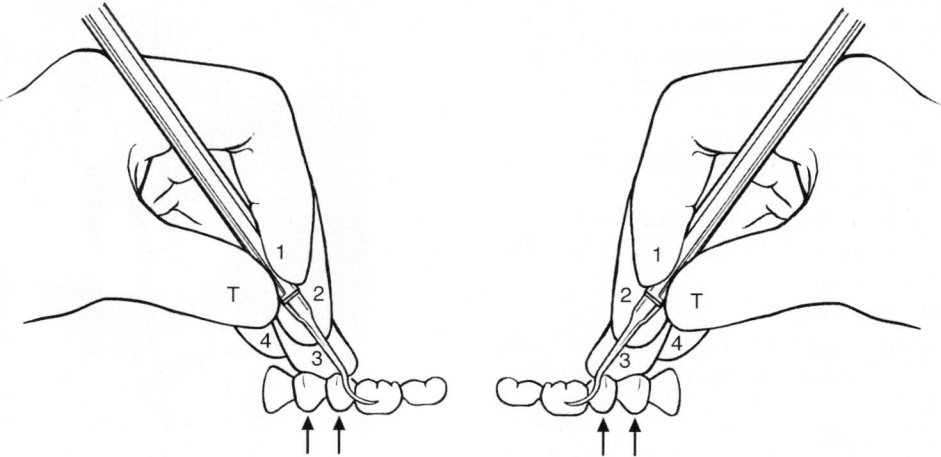

FIGURE 37-5 • Modified Pen Grasp for Left and Right Hands. An instrument is held by the thumb (T), index finger, and (1) the second, or "middle," finger (2), which also provides support. The third, or "ring," finger (3) serves as the finger rest, and the fourth, or "little," finger (4) is positioned beside the ring finger to supplement the finger rest.

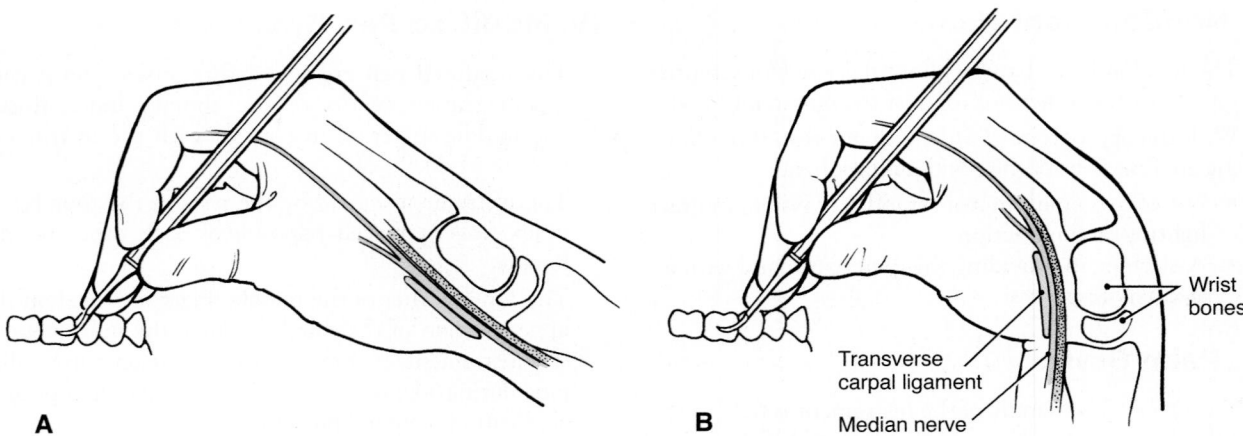

A

B

Wrist
bones

Transverse
carpal ligament

Median nerve

FIGURE 37-6 • **Effect of Wrist Position. A:** Wrist in neutral position in straight line with forearm. **B:** Bent wrist shows cramping of median nerve in the carpal tunnel of the wrist. Repeated pressure on the median nerve can cause carpal tunnel syndrome.

A. Purpose

- An effective, well-established fulcrum is essential for the following reasons:
- *Stability*—provides a focal point from which the whole hand can move as a unit.
- *Control of unit and stroke*—allows controlled action of the instrument and limits instrumentation to where it is needed.
- *Prevention of injury*—prevents irregular pressure and uncontrolled movement that can cause injury to the patient's oral tissues.
- *Patient comfort*—patients may sense a securely applied instrument, which may increase their confidence in the clinician's ability.

B. Intraoral Fulcrum

- The intraoral fulcrum is a finger rest inside the patient's mouth that serves to provide stabilization of the hand during instrumentation.
- Figure 37-7 shows the fingers grouped together with the fulcrum established where the ring finger maintains its position on a tooth adjacent to the tooth being treated.
- The ideal finger rest or fulcrum:
  - Is a tooth adjacent to the tooth being treated.
  - Allows ease in instrument adaptation.
  - Prevents accidental finger injury during instrumentation if the patient were to move suddenly or the instrument were to slip.
  - Is a firm and stable tooth.
  - Allows for stability and control of instrument during activation (strokes) compared to the patient's chin, lips, and cheeks, which are less reliable because they are mobile and flexible.
  - Is in the same arch and quadrant as the tooth being instrumented when possible.
  - Allows convenient access to the working area.
  - Promotes an effective grasp.

C. Extraoral Fulcrum

- An intraoral fulcrum cannot always be established in areas that are difficult to access, such as in maxillary posterior regions, and an extraoral fulcrum may be more effective.[4]
- Maximize the contact of the clinician's instrumentation hand with the patient's face.
- Cheek and chin are most commonly used.
- A secure fulcrum is dependent on pressure against the face and underlying bone.

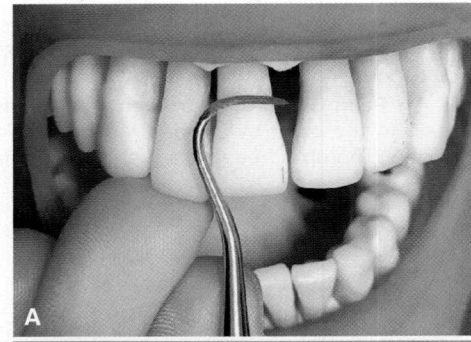

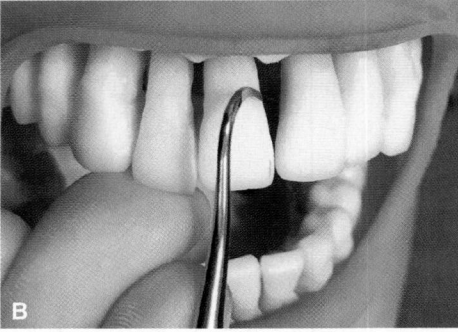

FIGURE 37-7 • **Instrument Adaptation.** Sickle scaler adaptation at the line angle of an anterior tooth. **A:** Incorrect adaptation can result in soft-tissue trauma and discomfort for the patient. **B:** Correct adaptation as a result of rolling the instrument handle.

◆ The grasp on the instrument will need to be modified so that it is farther from the working end than what is used with a traditional intraoral fulcrum.

D. Alternative Fulcrums

◆ In some instances, establishing an intraoral or extraoral fulcrum may not be possible or sufficient due to the following reasons:

- Limited access to posterior teeth.
- Limited access to tenacious calculus in difficult to reach areas (e.g., deep periodontal pockets) where greater support and pressure are required for instrumentation.[5]
- Patient's facial musculature.
- Small mouth opening (microstomia).
- Difficulty opening the mouth (trismus).
- Large tongue (macroglossia).
- Malocclusions of individual teeth.
- Physical disabilities interfering with the oral cavity.

◆ In such cases, a variation in finger fulcrum may be used; however, basic rules for stability and control are still applied, and fulcrums on movable tissues are avoided.

◆ Three types of variations are suggested here: *substitute*, *supplementary*, and *reinforced* finger rests.

- *Substitute finger rest:* used for missing or mobile teeth.
  - For an edentulous area, a cotton roll or gauze sponge may be packed into the area to provide a dry finger rest. Otherwise, a rest across the dental arch or in the opposite arch may be required to provide stability.
  - For mobile teeth with inadequate bony support, use only with minimal pressure for brief periods, or avoid altogether for finger rests since they are not only unstable, but undue stress on the tooth could also traumatize and tear the periodontal ligament fibers.
  - For areas with inadequate space or visibility, an index finger of the nondominant hand may be placed in the vestibule over a cotton roll or a dry gauze square, and the usual finger rest can be placed on the index finger to aid retraction and visibility, particularly in the mouth of a small child.
- *Supplementary finger rest:* also known as a "finger-on-finger" rest.
  - Place the index finger of the nondominant hand on the occlusal surfaces of teeth adjacent to the working area. The finger rest can then be applied to the nondominant index finger.
  - Such supplements are helpful for achieving a parallel orientation of the terminal shank to proximal surfaces.
  - Supplemental rests are not useful for certain distal surfaces where the mouth mirror is essential for vision.
- *Reinforced finger rest:* used to provide additional strength and force, particularly for hard, tenacious calculus in pockets.[4]

- Index finger of nondominant hand can be rested on the tooth adjacent to the one being scaled, while the thumb is placed on the instrument shank (or handle) for a reinforcement.
- When applied correctly, greater control of the instrument can result, and the danger of instrument breakage is reduced.
- A definite rest for both hands is needed to distribute the pressure.

INSTRUMENTATION BASICS

I. Adaptation

◆ With an appropriate grasp and fulcrum, the instrument is next ready for application. The working end of the instrument is **adapted** to the surface of the tooth where instrumentation is to take place.

◆ Select the correct end of a double-ended paired instrument.

◆ The blade of an instrument is divided into thirds, referred to as the heel-third, the middle-third, and the tip- or toe-third.

◆ The working end is applied to adapt to the contour of the tooth surface being examined or treated so that the side of the tip or toe is adapted for maximum usefulness.

◆ Example: About 2–3 mm of the toe third of a curet may be adaptable when on a "flat" surface of the tooth, whereas at a line angle or convex surface of a narrow root, less than 2 mm may be adaptable.

- As the instrument is activated, it is adjusted to changes required by variations in the tooth surface topography.

◆ All line angles require the instrument be rolled between the fingers as the instrument is activated to turn the working end to keep the toe or tip third adapted to the tooth surface.

◆ At each change of direction around a line angle, the instrument must be rolled.

◆ Figure 37-7 shows the adaptation of a sickle scaler tip to a line angle.

◆ Additional areas requiring more attention, time, and careful application of skill include convex/rounded surfaces and concave grooves.

- A properly adapted instrument harms neither the tooth surface being treated nor the surrounding or adjacent tissues.

II. Angulation

◆ **Angulation** refers to the angle formed between the working end of an instrument and the tooth surface.

◆ Each instrument is applied to a surface in a specific manner for optimum adaptation and angulation.

- *Probe:* The usual adaptation of a probe is to maintain the side of the tip on the tooth, with the long axis of the working end parallel to the root surface.

- *Explorer:* The side of the explorer tip is kept adapted to the tooth at all times (at an angle of approximately 5° or less) to feel for changes in the surface, such as roughness. Chapter 20 illustrates the use of the subgingival explorer.
- *Scalers and curets:* Angulation refers to the angle formed by the face of the blade with the tooth surface to which the instrument is applied.
  - At 0° ("closed") angulation, the face of a curet is flat against the tooth surface (Figure 37-8A). This is crucial to prevent soft tissue trauma when inserting the blade beneath the gingival margin.
  - For both curets and scalers, a 70° ("open") angulation between the face of the instrument and the tooth surface permits effective calculus removal (Figure 37-8B).
  - Attempting to remove calculus at a 0° closed angulation uses only the lateral surface of a sharp blade, which can result in the burnishing of calculus.
  - Burnishing produces a smooth veneer, making the calculus difficult or impossible to detect with an explorer.

III. Activation (Stroke)

- A stroke is an unbroken movement made by an instrument; it is the action of an instrument in the performance of the task for which it was designed.
- *Stability:* During a stroke, the whole hand pivots or rotates on the fulcrum.
- *Motion:* generated by a unified action of the shoulder, arm, wrist, and hand.
- *Length:* limited by the extent of calculus deposit and by the anatomic features of the area where the deposit is located.

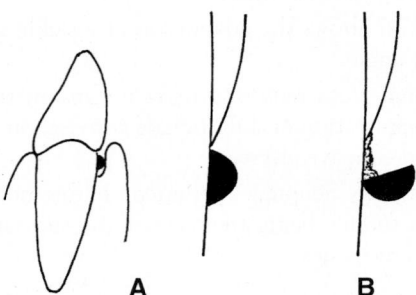

FIGURE 37-8 • Instrument Angulation. Enlargement of pocket area from the tooth on the left shows cross section of a curet blade in black. **A:** The face of the curet blade is closed, or angulated at 0° with the tooth surface during insertion into the pocket. At 0° the face of the blade is flat against the tooth surface. **B:** The face of the blade is opened or angulated at approximately 70° with the tooth surface for calculus removal.

- Strokes may be identified by the instrumentation being performed. Examples are the "probing or walking stroke," "exploratory or assessment stroke," "scaling or calculus removal stroke," or "root debridement stroke."

A. Lateral Pressure

- **Lateral pressure** refers to the pressure of the instrument against the tooth surface during activation.
- It is described as light, moderate, or heavy pressure.
- *Balance of pressure:* For control, a balance or an equalization of pressure is established between the instrument blade against the tooth surface and pressure on the fulcrum.
  - Keeping the two forces equal will facilitate a stable, intentional control of the instrument as it is activated.
- *Effects of Excessive Pressure:*
  - Excess removal of tooth structure; gouging of root surfaces.
  - Loss of instrument control.
  - Potential damage to soft tissue, pocket lining; bleeding.
  - Patient discomfort; discomfort during healing later.
  - Clinician fatigue.

B. Direction

- *Vertical:* Strokes are parallel to the long axis of the tooth being treated (Figure 37-9B).
- *Horizontal:* Strokes are parallel to the occlusal surface of the tooth being treated (Figure 37-9C).
- *Oblique:* Strokes are diagonal to the long axis of the tooth being treated (Figure 37-9A).
- Figure 37-9 shows direction of strokes for various instruments.

C. Walking Stroke

- Used with a probe to move up and down in small increments, gently touching the base of the sulcus or pocket with each down stroke (Chapter 20).
- Consists of a light grasp, light pressure, and vertical movement.

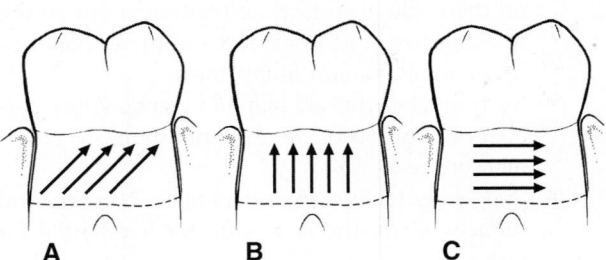

FIGURE 37-9 • Directions of Instrument Strokes. Arrows on root surface represent diagonal or oblique strokes **(A)**, vertical strokes **(B)**, and horizontal strokes **(C)**.

D. Exploratory/Assessment Stroke

- Used with assessment instruments to maximize tactile sensitivity when assessing tooth surfaces and detecting irregularities, such as the presence of:
  - Calculus.
  - Carious lesions.
  - Rough overhanging margins of crowns or restorations.
- Also used with manual/powered removal instruments to rehearse the movement of the instrument before activation to confirm correct adaptation.
- Consists of a light grasp, light pressure, and movement in vertical, horizontal, and oblique directions.

E. Scaling/Calculus Removal Stroke

- Used with manual removal instruments to remove calculus deposits.
- Defined as a short, well-controlled, and firm pull-stroke (emphasis on movement away from the base of the sulcus or pocket).
- Consists of a firm grasp, moderate-to-heavy pressure, and movement of the blade in vertical, horizontal, and oblique directions.
- The stroke is decisive and directed to protect the tissues from trauma.
- Avoid strokes long enough to pass over the whole crown when the calculus represents only a small area at the cervical third of the tooth.
- When transitioning from an assessment to removal stroke, the pressure on the tooth and fulcrum increases significantly to achieve stability and control of the instrument as it is activated.

F. Root Debridement Stroke

- Used when removing soft deposits from a tooth surface with minimal deposit.
- The grasp is consistent with the amount of lateral pressure placed on the blade to the tooth.
- Consists of light-to-moderate lateral pressure (depending on the texture and consistency of the deposits encountered) and movement in vertical, horizontal, and oblique directions.
  - When the texture of the deposits changes from grainy to heavy, the pressure on both the fulcrum and blade against the root surface will increase in order to remove the deposits.
  - Pressure is, therefore, responsive to the tactile information transmitted as the instrument progresses along the root surface.

SCALERS

I. Uses

- **Scalers** are used principally for removal of supragingival calculus.

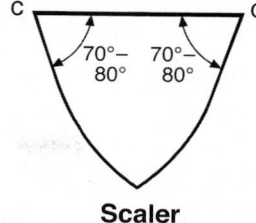

Scaler

FIGURE 37-10 • Internal Angles of a Scaler. Cross section of a scaler shows the 70°–80° internal angles. These angles are restored by sharpening techniques.

- May be useful for removal of gross calculus that is slightly below the gingival margin when it is continuous with the supragingival calculus, and when the gingival tissue is spongy and flexible to permit easy insertion of the instrument.[6]
- Extreme caution must be used since the pointed tip of the blade and back of the sickle scaler can traumatize the tissue.

II. Instrument Design

A. Blade

- Two cutting edges.
- The face converges with the two lateral surfaces to form the *tip* of the scaler, which is a sharp point.
- Has a triangular cross-section with a V-shaped back (Figure 37-10).
- Internal angles of 70°–80° are formed where the lateral surfaces meet the face at the cutting edges.

B. Shank

- *Straight*: unpaired instrument in which the relationships of the shank, blade, and handle are in a flat plane; adaptable primarily for anterior teeth, although may be used for scaling premolars when the lips and cheeks permit retraction for correct angulation.
- *Modified or contra-angle*: paired instruments that are mirror images of each other to provide access to posterior teeth; one end adapts from the buccal and the other from the lingual and palatal aspects.

III. Types

A. Sickles

- A scaler with a curved blade is referred to as a "sickle" (Figure 37-11).
- Face of the blade is curved from a lateral view.

B. Jacquettes

- A straight-bladed scaler is referred to as a "Jacquette" (Figure 37-12).
- Face of the blade is straight from a lateral view.

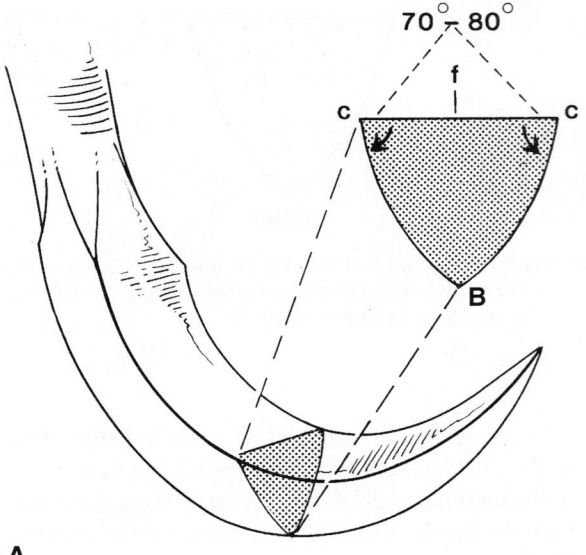

FIGURE 37-11 • Curved Scaler (Sickle Scaler). A: The curved blade terminates in a point. **B:** Cross section shows the face (f) and the two cutting edges (c) formed where the lateral surfaces meet the face at 70°–80° angles. This type of scaler is also called a sickle scaler.

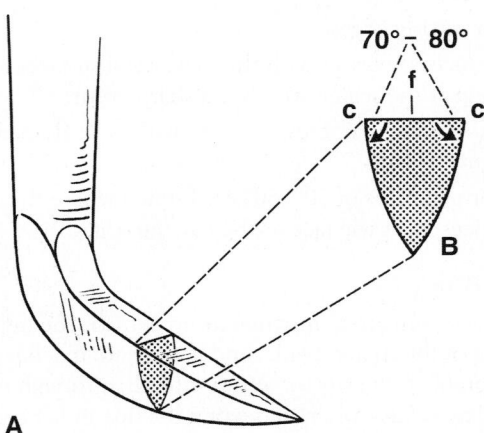

FIGURE 37-12 • Straight Scaler (Jacquette). A: The straight blade converges to a point where the two cutting edges meet at the tip. **B:** Cross section of the scaler shows the face (f), the two cutting edges (c), and the 70°–80° internal angles. This type of scaler is also known as the Jacquette scaler.

IV. Scaler-Specific Instrumentation

◆ *Adaptation:* Tip-third or terminal third of the cutting edge is maintained on the tooth surface at all times. On line angles, only the terminal 1–2 mm of the tip is used.

◆ *Angulation:* The face of the blade is adapted to the tooth surface at an angle of approximately 70°.

◆ *Activation:* Both light assessment strokes and heavy calculus removal strokes may be performed.

◆ Small scalers can be useful for removal of fine supragingival deposits directly under contact areas and between overlapping teeth.

◆ Tactile sensitivity is decreased with larger, heavier blades.

◆ The large size, thickness, and length of the blade may cause undue trauma to the gingival tissue.

◆ Pointed tip and straight cutting edges cannot be adapted to the curved root surfaces.

◆ There is increased risk of grooving or scratching the cemental surface.

CURETS

I. Uses

◆ **Curets** are used for removal of supra- and subgingival calculus and biofilm.

◆ Round back does not traumatize the gingival margin or base of sulcus or pocket when placed subgingivally.

◆ Necessary after powered scaling to remove residual deposits or "fine scale" for completion of periodontal debridement.

◆ Useful for obtaining a sample of subgingival biofilm to place on a glass slide for the phase microscope or for microbiologic tests.

II. Instrument Design

A. Blade

◆ Two cutting edges on a curved blade.

◆ The face converges with the two lateral surfaces to form a rounded *toe*.

◆ Has a semicircular cross-section with a rounded back (Figure 37-13).

◆ Internal angles of 70°–80° are formed where the lateral surfaces meet the face at the cutting edges.

◆ Figure 37-3 shows a curet blade with each part labeled.

B. Shank

◆ Angles or curves in the shank are specific to each of the many different curets available.

◆ Slender shanks allow entrance into the sulcus or pocket with minimal trauma to the gingival margin.

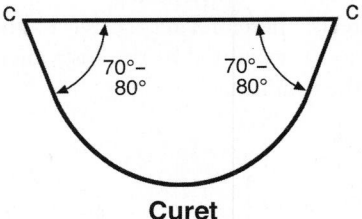

Curet

FIGURE 37-13 • Internal Angles of a Curet. Cross section of a curet shows the 70°–80° internal angles at the cutting edges. These angles are restored by sharpening techniques.

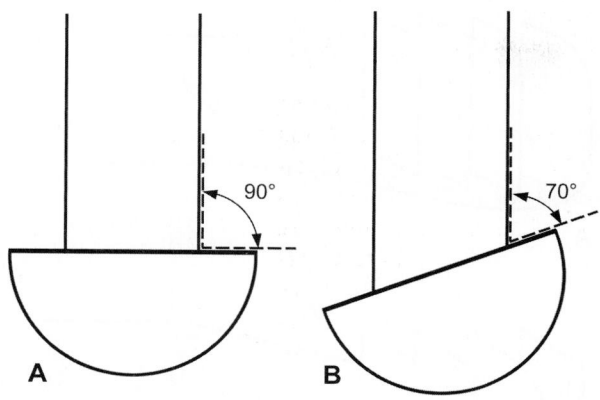

FIGURE 37-14 • Curet Design. A: A universal curet with the blade at a 90° angle to the lower shank. **B:** Offset blade of an area-specific curet at a 70° angle to the lower shank.

III. Types

A. Universal Curets

- Universal curets can be adapted for supra- and subgingival instrumentation on any tooth surface.
- Ideal for removing large deposits quickly and efficiently across multiple teeth.
- *Working ends:* Paired mirror images on a single handle.
- *Face:* Perpendicular (at a 90° angle) to the lower shank (Figure 37-14A).
- *Cutting edges:* Two per working end.
  - Cutting edges are parallel and level with each other.
  - Both cutting edges are used; therefore, blade is sharpened on both sides and around the toe.

B. Area-Specific Curets

- Area-specific curets are designed for adaptation to specific surfaces.
- Ideal for fine scaling and root planing.
- *Working ends:* Paired mirror image, usually placed on a single handle. The typical pairs are numbers 1/2, 3/4,

5/6. 7/8, 9/10, 11/12, 13/14, 15/16, and 17/18 (e.g., Gracey curet series).
- *Face:* Has an offset blade (at an approximate 70° angle) in relation to the lower shank (Figure 37-14B).
- *Cutting edge:* One per working-end ending with the curved toe.
  - The cutting edge is the lower edge of the blade when the handle is held vertically.
  - Only the lower cutting edge is used; therefore, the blade is sharpened on one side (lower edge) and around the toe.

C. Advanced Area-Specific Curets

- Variations of area-specific curets provide clinicians with greater opportunities to complete advanced instrumentation,[2] such as:
  - in deep pockets.
  - within curvatures of root surfaces with moderate-to-severe attachment loss.
  - on furcations on multirooted teeth.
- **Terminal (lower) shank** can vary in length and thickness, while the blade can vary in length and width. Some common variations are listed below.
- *After five curet* (Figure 37-15B)
  - Terminal shank is 3 mm longer than a standard curet.
  - Blade width is decreased by 10%.
  - Allows improved access to pocket depths beyond 5 mm.
- *Mini-five curet* (Figure 37-15C)
  - Terminal shank is 3 mm longer than a standard curet.
  - Blade width is decreased by 10%.
  - Blade length is 50% shorter.
  - Shorter blade length facilitates adaptation to the curved features of root morphology including concavities; longitudinal depressions on proximal surfaces; root surfaces within furcations; and interradicular convexities.
- *Micro-mini five curet* (Figure 37-15D)

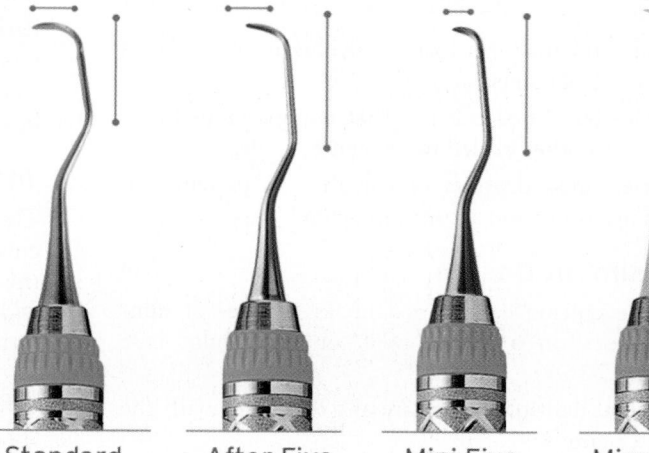

FIGURE 37-15 • Gracey Tip Comparison. A: A standard Gracey curet. **B:** The after five curet had a 3-mm longer shank than **(A)**. **C:** The minibladed curet has a 50% shorter blade and 3 mm longer shank than **(A)**. **D:** The micro-minibladed curet has a 50% shorter blade that is narrower and 20% thinner than **(A)**. (Courtesy of Hu-Friedy.)

A Standard Gracey Curet
B After Five Curet
C Mini-Five Curet
D Micro-Mini Five Curet

- Terminal shank is 3 mm longer and thicker than a standard curet.
- Blade width is decreased by 20% compared to a mini-five curet.
- Blade length is 50% shorter than a standard curet.
- The longer and more rigid shank, combined with its narrower and shorter blade, allows application of greater lateral pressure when scaling very deep and firmly attached calculus deposits.

IV. Curet-Specific Instrumentation

◆ *Adaptation:* Toe-third or lower third of the cutting edge is maintained on the tooth surface at all times. On line angles, the terminal 1–2 mm of the toe may be used only.
  - Either cutting edge of a universal curet may be adapted on a tooth surface.
  - Only the lower cutting edge of an area-specific curet may be adapted on a tooth surface.

◆ *Angulation:* The face of the blade is adapted to the tooth surface at various angles, depending on the action being performed (Figure 37-8).
  - When deposits are *removed supragingivally*, the blade face-to-tooth angulation is approximately 70°.
  - When the curet is *inserted subgingivally into the sulcus or pocket*, the blade is "closed" with the blade face-to-tooth angulation of approximately 0°.
  - When deposits are *removed subgingivally*, the blade is "opened" with the face-to-tooth angulation of approximately 70°.

◆ *Activation:* Light assessment strokes, moderate root debridement strokes, and heavy calculus removal strokes may be performed.

PERIODONTAL FILES

I. Working Files

Includes stainless steel Hirshfeld and Orban files.[7]

A. Uses

◆ Crushes and fractures heavy calculus into fragments prior to use of curets.
◆ Removes burnished calculus that is impervious to removal with other bladed instruments.
◆ Removes gross deposits of calculus on patients for whom ultrasonic use is contraindicated.

B. Instrument Design

◆ Multiple cutting edges lined up as a series of miniature hoes on a round, oval, or rectangular base (Figure 37-16A).
◆ The metal multiple blades are at a 90° angle with the shank (Figure 37-16B).
◆ Reduced tactile sensitivity because of the series of blades.

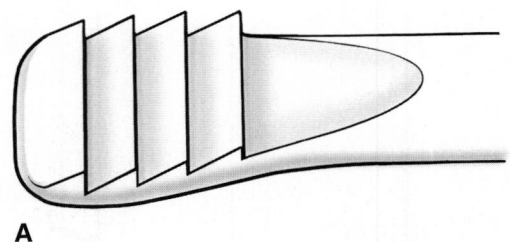

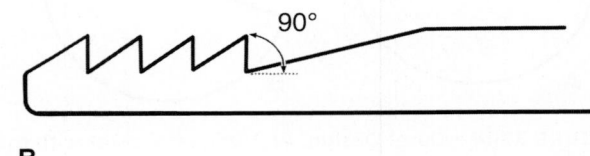

FIGURE 37-16 • Working File Scaler. A: A file has multiple cutting edges. **B:** Each blade is at a 90° angle with the shank.

◆ Shanks are variously angulated; most are paired instruments.

C. Instrumentation

◆ Can be used supra- and subgingivally.
◆ *Adaptation:* Entire working surface is placed flat against the area to be treated.
◆ Pressure applied permits the cutting edges to grasp the surface.
◆ *Activation:* pull-stroke only, using a linear motion.
◆ File use is always followed by curet instrumentation to leave a smooth surface on roots.

II. Finishing Files

These are not true files, scalers, or curets because there are no blades. These include Bedbug and diamond-coated files.[7]

A. Uses

◆ Used for finishing of root surfaces and accessing furcation areas.
◆ Early research suggests the use of diamond-coated curets after conventional curets may provide a tooth surface more compatible with attachment of periodontal ligament fibroblasts.[8]

B. Instrument Design

◆ The diamond coating, which is used to remove the calculus, is placed 180°–360° around the tip depending on the manufacturer (Figure 37-17).
◆ They have paired ends (buccal/lingual and mesial/distal) like other file scalers.

C. Instrumentation

◆ *Adaptation:* Working surface is placed flat against the root surface.

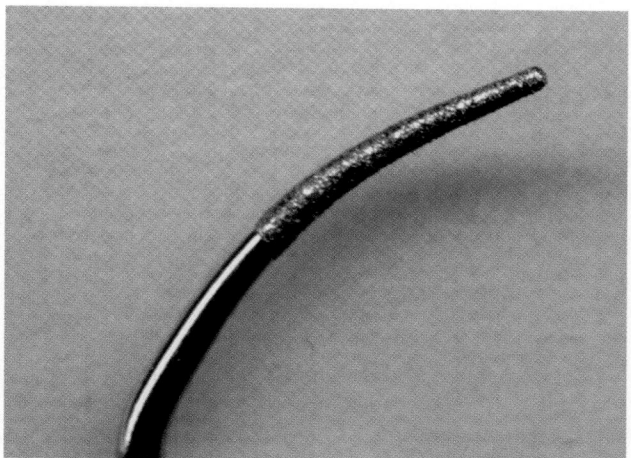

FIGURE 37-17 • Diamond-Coated Finishing File. A close-up view of a working end on a diamond-coated file. Note the textured coating on the working end.

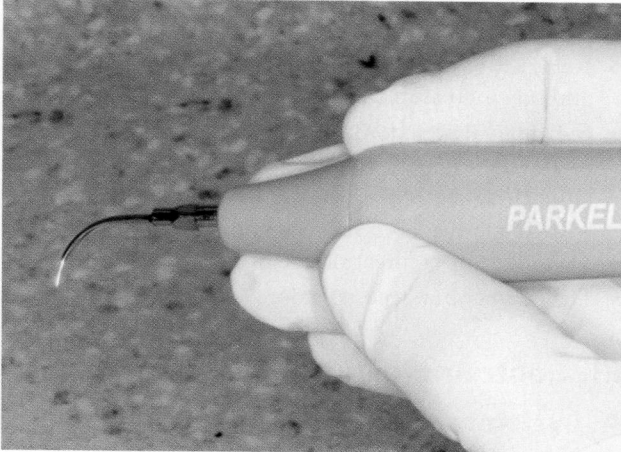

FIGURE 37-18 • Piezoelectric Handpiece and Universal Tip. An example of a piezoelectric ultrasonic handpiece and powered tip.

◆ Very light pressure is used to prevent damage to the root surface.

◆ *Activation:* Strokes are multidirectional (horizontal, vertical, and oblique) in a push–pull motion.

POWERED INSTRUMENTS

◆ Manual instrumentation was the only method of calculus removal until powered scalers were introduced in the 1950s.[9]

◆ The ultrasonic power-driven scaling device converted high-frequency electrical energy into mechanical energy in the form of rapid vibrations.

◆ Later, sonic scalers were developed that worked on the same principle but utilized an air turbine as an energy source.

◆ Technologic advances in powered scalers improved and allowed for rapid calculus removal that resulted in much less hand fatigue for the clinician.

◆ Powered instrumentation can produce equivalent results in calculus and dental biofilm removal as manual instrumentation when instruments are applied correctly and sensitive posttreatment evaluation is made.[10]

◆ Long-term goals of therapy are accomplished through a blended approach utilizing both powered and hand instrumentation.

I. Mode of Action

A. Mechanical Vibration

◆ Power-driven scaling devices convert electrical energy (ultrasonic) or air pressure (sonic) into high-frequency sound waves.

◆ Sound waves produce rapid mechanical vibrations in the specially designed scaling tips (Figure 37-18).

◆ Calculus is incrementally shattered from the tooth surface when the vibrations are applied to the deposit.

B. Cavitation

◆ When water meets the vibrating tip, cavitation, or the formation of microscopic bubbles, occurs.

◆ When the bubbles collapse, they release energy that creates adverse conditions of pressure and temperature that destroy bacterial cell walls.[10]

C. Irrigation

◆ Water is required to dissipate the heat produced by the vibrating tip.

◆ The water spray also creates a lavage that penetrates to the base of the pocket to provide a continuous flushing of blood, debris, microorganisms, and endotoxins.

◆ Oscillation of the ultrasonic tip causes acoustic turbulence, which has a disruptive effect on surface bacteria.[10]

◆ Ultrasonic debridement following manual instrumentation provides cleansing and rinsing of scaled tooth surfaces, which can promote healing of soft tissues.

D. Variable Elements

◆ Power-driven scaling devices feature variable elements, such as their amplitude and frequency output.

◆ Amplitude: distance of tip movement measured in micrometers.
  • Determines power output of the instrument.
  • Adjustable component on all ultrasonic devices.

◆ Frequency: speed of tip movement.
  • Number of cycles per second (cps) the tip moves.
  • Adjustable component available only on manually tuned ultrasonic devices.
  • Majority of available devices have tuning preset or "automatic."

II. Indications for Use

◆ Removal of dental biofilm, extrinsic stain, and supra- and subgingival calculus.
◆ Subgingival periodontal debridement, including:
  • Removal of calculus, attached biofilm, and endotoxins from the root surface.
  • Reduction of bacterial load in the periodontal pocket.
◆ Debridement of furcation areas.
◆ Debridement of deposits before oral surgery.

III. Contraindications

A. Systemic Health Conditions

◆ *Communicable disease*[11]
  • Patient with a communicable disease that can be transmitted by aerosols, such as tuberculosis.
◆ *Susceptibility to infection*[12]
  • Compromised patient with marked susceptibility to infection.
  • Examples: immunosuppression from disease or chemotherapy, uncontrolled diabetes, or kidney or other organ transplant.
◆ *Respiratory risk*[13]
  • Patient who may aspirate septic material and microorganisms from biofilm and periodontal pockets into the lungs.
  • Examples: history of chronic obstructive pulmonary disease, including asthma, emphysema, or cystic fibrosis.
◆ *Difficulty swallowing*[14]
  • Patient with a swallowing problem (dysphagia) or prone to gagging.
  • Dysphagia results in liquids being aspirated into the lungs along with oral bacteria and increases the risk of aspiration pneumonia. Consultation with the primary care provider is needed prior to dental treatment.
  • Examples: amyotrophic lateral sclerosis, muscular dystrophy, Parkinson's disease, paralysis, multiple sclerosis, and after stroke.
◆ *Cardiac pacemaker*[15]
  • Some studies have shown that ultrasonic devices may cause electromagnetic interference with implanted cardiac devices.[16,17]
  • Newer shielded cardiac devices may be less susceptible to interference.
  • Piezoelectric dental scalers may be safer than magnetostrictive scalers.[18,19]
  • Due to conflicting evidence, the clinician should consult with the patient's cardiologist to obtain medical clearance prior to use.

B. Oral Conditions

◆ *Demineralized areas*
  • Ultrasonic vibrations can remove the delicate remineralizing cover of a demineralized area.[20]

◆ *Exposed dentinal surfaces*
  • Tooth structure can be removed in excess and create sensitivity with too much lateral force and high-power settings.[20]
  • The smear layer can be removed and dentinal tubules uncovered, which can increase sensitivity or aggravate existing sensitivity.
◆ *Thermal injury*
  • Thermal damage to the pulp can occur if the ultrasonic tip overheats because of inadequate water cooling or excess pressure.[11]
  • Gingival tissues can experience thermal injury if water cooling is inadequate.
◆ *Children*
  • Young, growing, developing tissues are sensitive to ultrasonic vibrations.
  • Primary and newly erupted permanent teeth have large pulp chambers. Vibrations and heat from the ultrasonic scaler may damage pulp tissue.[11]
◆ *Restorations*[21]
  • Improper tip application may increase roughness, such as scratches, chips, or notches in restorative materials.
  • *Porcelain:* May remove the glaze of the porcelain and create pores on the surface where the tip was in contact with the porcelain.
  • *Amalgam:* Powered scaling may cause scratches, loss of material, and create pores in the restorative material.
  • *Composites:* May cause roughened surfaces.
◆ *Titanium implant abutments*
  • Ultrasonic instrumentation will damage titanium surfaces unless the insert is designed for use with implants and covered with a specially designed plastic tip.[22]

IV. Risks and Considerations

◆ *Hearing shifts*
  • Extended exposure to noises above a certain level, such as the noise of a high-speed handpiece or an ultrasonic scaler, may be damaging.
  • Temporary hearing shifts have been demonstrated for both clinicians and patients.[11]
◆ *Cumulative trauma*
  • Many dental hygienists suffer from musculoskeletal injuries related to cumulative trauma.
  • Scaling reduces the pinch force and finger–hand muscle activity needed to remove deposits, which can reduce operator fatigue.[9]
  • However, work with instruments that vibrate, such as the ultrasonic scaler, are associated with sensorineural dysfunction that include temporary loss of tactile sensitivity in the fingertips.[11]
◆ *Magnetic fields*
  • Ultrasonic scalers produce weak, time-varying magnetic fields similar to those produced by common household appliances.

- There is no scientific evidence that cumulative exposure to weak, time-varying magnetic fields has caused any biological harm to any dental personnel.[29]
- ◆ *Aerosols and spatter*[12]
  - *Aerosols:* Invisible airborne particles smaller than 50 μm that are dispersed into the surrounding environment by dental equipment.
  - Spatter: Droplets of airborne particulate matter larger than 50 μm that fall to the ground.
  - The use of powered scalers creates aerosols and spatter that contain patient's saliva, blood, microorganisms, debris, and other potentially infectious materials.
  - Aerosols can remain suspended in the air for up to hours following powered instrumentation.
  - It is important to follow the most current infection control guidelines to reduce the risk of contamination and infection from aerosols and spatter, including the use of more stringent personal protective equipment, a preprocedural mouth rinse, such as a chlorhexidine gluconate rinse (see Figure 37-19), and a high-volume evacuator.[11,12]

V. Types

- ◆ Sonic scalers.
- ◆ Ultrasonic scalers:
  - Magnetostrictive.
  - Piezoelectric.
- ◆ These various powered scalers are mainly distinguished by their frequency output and the direction and pattern of their tip motion, as shown in Figure 37-20.

SONIC SCALERS

I. Mechanism of Action

- ◆ Sonic scalers are driven by compressed air from the dental unit rather than electrical energy.

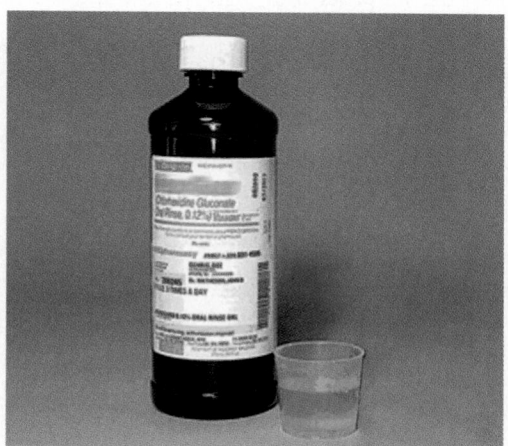

FIGURE 37-19 • Preprocedure Rinse. Administering a preprocedural rinse is recommended to reduce the numbers of bacteria and other oral pathogens in aerosols.

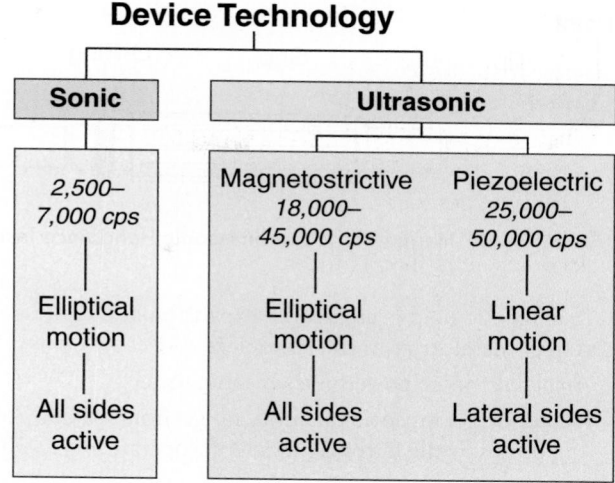

Device Technology

Sonic	Ultrasonic	
	Magnetostrictive	Piezoelectric
2,500–7,000 cps	18,000–45,000 cps	25,000–50,000 cps
Elliptical motion	Elliptical motion	Linear motion
All sides active	All sides active	Lateral sides active

FIGURE 37-20 • Power-Driven Scaling Devices Technology. For sonic and both magnetostrictive and piezoelectric ultrasonic scalers, the speed (cps), motion (linear or elliptical), and active part of the tip (lateral sides only or all sides) are identified.

- ◆ *Amplitude:* less powerful than ultrasonic scalers.
- ◆ *Frequency:* vibrates between 3,000 and 8,000 cps; fewer vibrations make calculus removal more difficult.
- ◆ *Tip movement:* elliptical pattern, but varies depending on tip and type of sonic scaler.
- ◆ *Active tip:* All surfaces of the tip are active.
  - Heat is not generated by the active tip.

II. Equipment

A. Unit Parts

- ◆ Handpiece.
- ◆ Interchangeable scaling tips.
- ◆ Handpiece attaches directly to the dental unit and is activated with the conventional handpiece foot control.

B. Unit Preparation

- ◆ Flush water lines in slow-speed-handpiece line for 2 minutes.
- ◆ Attach sonic handpiece to slow-speed handpiece line.
- ◆ Assemble the tip onto the handpiece.

MAGNETOSTRICTIVE ULTRASONIC SCALERS

I. Mechanism of Action

- ◆ Magnetostrictive ultrasonic devices are driven by electrical currents.
- ◆ *Conventional magnetostrictive units:* Utilize *inserts*, or longitudinal stack of metal strips, in the handpiece (Figure 37-21).
- ◆ *Ferromagnetic units:* Utilize a fragile ferric rod that generates less heat than the conventional metal stack.

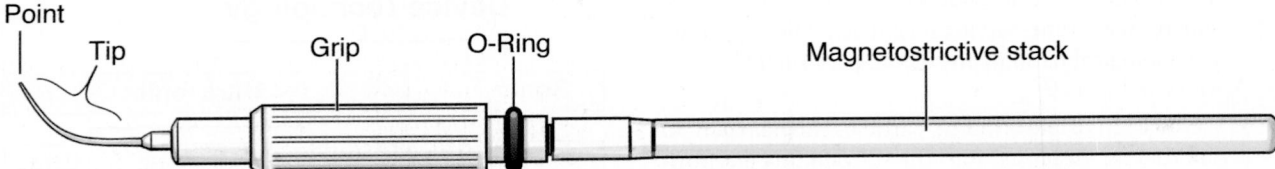

FIGURE 37-21 • Magnetostrictive Ultrasonic Handpiece Insert. With parts labeled.

- A magnetic field is created by expansion and contraction of metal strips in the handpiece.
- *Amplitude:* more powerful than sonic scalers.
- *Frequency:* Conventional units range from 18,000 to 45,000 cps, while ferromagnetic units operate at 42,000 cps.
  - Older conventional units are designed to operate at 25,000 cps and are called 25-kilohertz (kHz) machines.
  - Newer conventional units are designed to operate at 30,000 cps and are called 30-kHz machines.
- *Tip movement:* elliptical pattern.
- *Active tip:* All surfaces of the tip are active.
- Water cools the heat generated in the handpiece and tip.

II. Equipment

A. Unit Parts
- Electric generator.
- Handpiece assembly.
- Set of interchangeable scaling tip inserts.
- Foot control to activate the handpiece.

B. Unit Preparation
- Establish power and water connections.
- Flush lines for 2 minutes.
- Select the appropriate insert.
  - Insert needs to be compatible with ultrasonic unit available.
  - The metal stacks in the 30-kHz inserts are much shorter than the 25-kHz inserts.
- Hold handpiece upright as it is filled with water.
- Fill completely with water before seating the insert to eliminate trapped air bubbles and reduce heat.
- Select the appropriate power setting according to the task at hand.
- Adjust the water setting.

PIEZOELECTRIC ULTRASONIC SCALERS

I. Mechanism of Action
- Piezoelectric ultrasonic devices are driven by electrical currents.

- Uses a ceramic rod and crystal transducers housed in the handpiece to activate the tip.
- *Amplitude:* more powerful than sonic scalers.
- *Frequency:* ranges from 25,000 to 50,000 cps, varies according to manufacturer.
- *Tip movement:* linear pattern, forward and backward.
- *Active tip:* Only the lateral surfaces of the tip are active.
- Water cools the heat generated at the tip.

II. Equipment

A. Unit Parts
- Electric generator.
- Handpiece assembly.
- Set of interchangeable scaling tips.
- Foot control to activate the handpiece.
- Some piezoelectric ultrasonic units have reservoirs (see Figure 37-22) that hold antimicrobial solutions that can be used as irrigants for lavage.

B. Unit Preparation
- Establish power and water connections.
- Flush lines for 2 minutes.
- Select the appropriate tip.
- Securely screw the tip onto the handpiece using the tip wrench.
- Select the power setting according to the task at hand.
- Adjust the water setting.

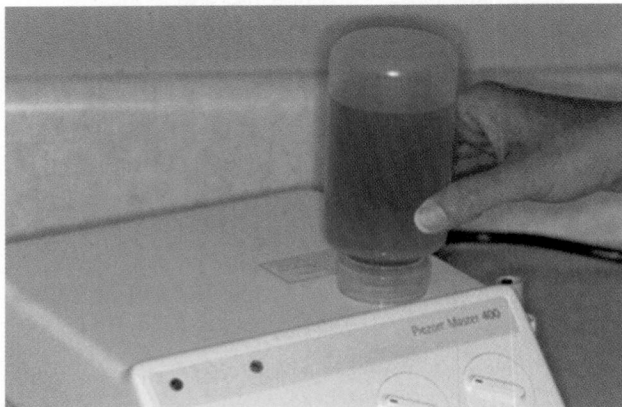

FIGURE 37-22 • Reservoir for Ultrasonic Unit. This ultrasonic device has an optional reservoir system for dispensing irrigant solutions—such as chlorhexidine gluconate—to an ultrasonic tip.

POWERED INSTRUMENTATION TECHNIQUE

I. Insert/Tip Selection

- Selecting the appropriate ultrasonic insert/tip is crucial for effectively and efficiently accomplishing the task at hand.
- Similarly to hand instruments, the inserts and tips of powered instruments can vary in design.

A. Size

- *Standard-diameter tips*: used for moderate-to-heavy calculus removal (Figure 37-23A).
- *Thin-diameter tips*: used for biofilm debridement and light calculus removal. Also ideal for accessing deep periodontal pockets (Figure 37-23C).

B. Shape

- *Straight design*: has a simple shank and is used universally on all tooth surfaces (Figure 37-23A).
- *Complex design*: has multiple bends in the shank to allow easy access to line angles and proximal surfaces (Figure 37-23B).
- *Left/right contra-angled inserts*: Complementary inserts have shanks that are curved to the left/right to better adapt to root concavities (i.e., furcations) and proximal surfaces of posterior teeth.
- *Beavertail design*: has a flat and wide working end; ideal for use on supragingival surfaces for the removal of heavy calculus, stain, and orthodontic cement (Figure 37-23D).

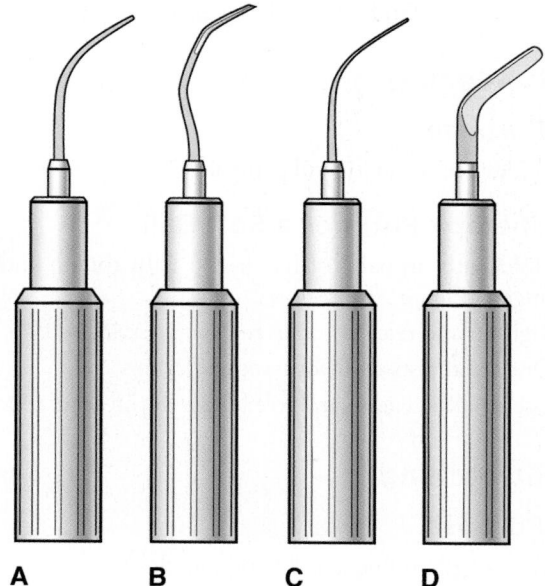

FIGURE 37-23 • Ultrasonic Tip Designs. A: Straight, standard-diameter tip. **B:** Triple-bend tip for access to line angles and proximal surfaces. **C:** Thin-diameter tip for access to deep pockets. **D:** Beavertail tip for supragingival surfaces needing removal of heavy calculus or cement.

II. Power Setting

- When selecting the appropriate power setting, it is important to consider the task at hand and the insert/tip selected.
- Consistent use of the unit on the lowest power setting for hard deposit removal will burnish the calculus present.
- Consistent use of the unit on the highest power setting for soft deposit removal will cause unnecessary discomfort to the patient.

A. Low-to-Medium Power

- Used with thin-diameter tips/inserts.
- Ideal for removal of biofilm, other soft deposits, and light-to-moderate calculus.

B. Medium-to-High Power

- Used with standard-diameter tips/inserts.
- Ideal for removal of moderate-to-heavy calculus.

III. Water Setting

- Proper water setting will create a halo of fine mist at the tip of the instrument with or without drips of water.
- If the tip becomes warm or hot, increase the water flow to prevent damage to hard and soft tissues.

IV. Grasp

- Balance the assembled instrument handle in the web between the thumb and index fingers.
  - This ensures a lighter grasp further away from the working end.
  - A light grasp will increase tactile sensitivity.
- Establish a modified pen grasp.
- The weight of the cord tends to pull on the handpiece and place additional strain on the wrist. Use the following strategies to manage cord drag:
  - Loop the cord and hold it between the ring finger and little finger.
  - Drape the cord over the clinician's shoulder.

V. Fulcrum/Rest

- A hard-tissue fulcrum is not required because force and pressure against the tooth surface are not indicated.
- A gentle finger rest is used to stabilize and guide the instrument tip in anterior segments.
- Extraoral and soft tissue rests allow for proper access and adaptation to deeper posterior segments.

VI. Adaptation

- Keep the side of the instrument tip closely adapted to the tooth surface.

◆ Do not hold the tip perpendicular to the tooth surface at any time because damage to the tooth surface can result.

◆ *Narrow periodontal pockets:*

- Narrow subgingival pockets interfere with proper adaptation and impede visibility.
- When instrumenting narrow pockets use an insert with appropriate length and limited width.
- Direct the tip apically and confirm access to the attachment prior to activating the tip.

◆ *Piezoelectric-specific technique:* placement and movement of the tip is specific.

- Position the lateral surface of the tip in contact with the tooth.
- Use the terminal 2–3 mm of the tip's *lateral surfaces* only (Figure 37-24).
- Keep terminal lateral surface adapted at all times around curvatures and line angles using wrist pivot.

VII. Activation (Stroke)

◆ Keep the instrument tip moving at a moderate-to-slow pace with a feather-light touch at all times to prevent the following:

- Scratches or gouging on the tooth surface.
- Excessive heat build-up.
- A galvanic shock-like effect to the patient.

◆ Use feather-light pressure to prevent tooth damage. Excessive lateral pressure can result in the following:

- Damage to the tooth surface.
- Dampening and deactivation of the tip vibrations.
- Burnishing of calculus.

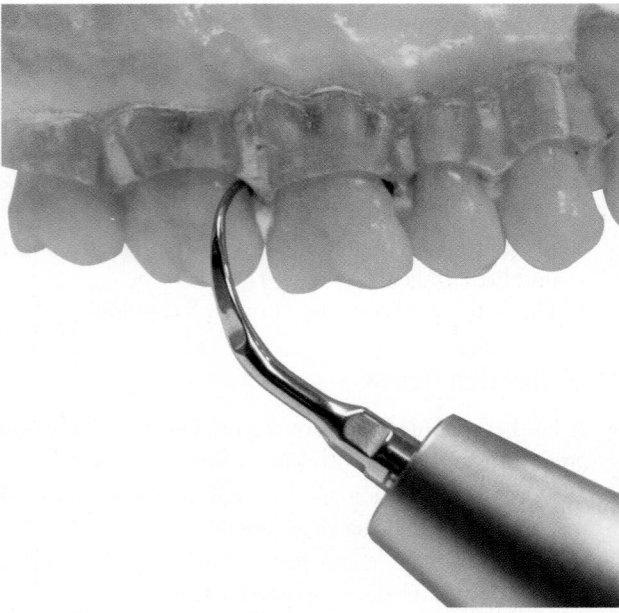

FIGURE 37-24 • Adaptation of Ultrasonic Tip. The side of the point of a tip is placed parallel to the tooth surface to prevent damage to the tooth structure. Damage occurs when the point is held perpendicular to the surface. (Courtesy of Hu-Friedy.)

◆ *Overlapping strokes*

- For comprehensive coverage of all surfaces.
- Strokes may be horizontal, vertical, oblique, or a combination.

◆ Procedure when the tip binds in an embrasure.

- Deactivate the power; remove the instrument tip from the embrasure.
- Reposition the instrument by lightly exploring with the tip to get in position and then reactivate the power.

DEXTERITY DEVELOPMENT

◆ The dental hygiene student or dental hygienist returning to practice after a temporary leave of absence can appreciate the need for exercises to develop dexterity and strength for the efficient and effective use of instruments.

◆ In addition, all students, returning retirees, and dental hygienists continuing in practice need an understanding of preventive measures to preserve the health of their hands, arms, shoulders, and all muscles and joints involved when undertaking patient care.

◆ The use of new or unusual instruments requires different procedures for coordination. Control is essential, and guided strength contributes to control.

◆ Proficiency during procedures comes from repeated correct use of the instruments.

- Exercises for the fingers, hands, and arms supplement experience.
- Directed exercises are needed for both hands, separately and together.
- During the training period, a regular period of time each day can be set aside for exercises.

I. Squeezing

A. Purpose

◆ To develop strength and control.

B. Therapy Putty or a Soft Ball

◆ Hold putty in palm of hand; grip with thumb and all fingers (Figure 37-25A).

◆ Tighten and release grip at regular intervals.

◆ One hand rests while other is exercising.

◆ Use a ball in each hand to exercise at the same time.

II. Stretching

A. Purpose

◆ To strengthen finger and hand muscles.

◆ To develop control of finger movements.

B. Rubber Band on Finger Joints

◆ Place band at joint between first phalanx and second phalanx.

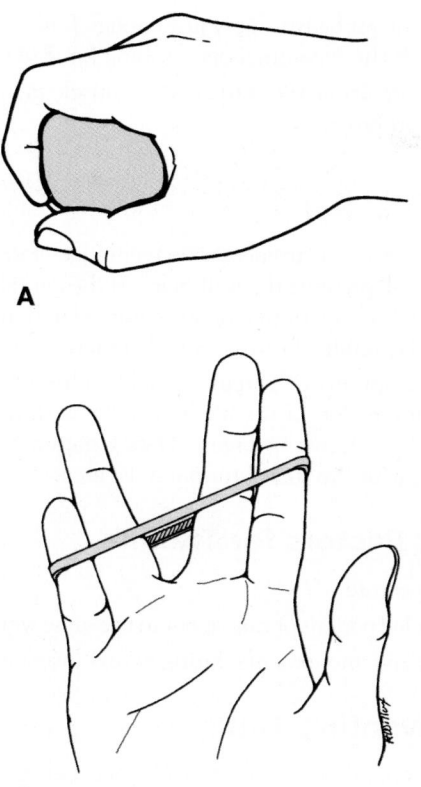

FIGURE 37-25 • Exercises for Dexterity Development. A: Squeezing therapy putty can aid in developing strength and control. **B:** A rubber band can be applied at each group of finger and thumb joints and stretched.

◆ Stretch band by separating middle and ring fingers (Figure 37-25B).

◆ Place band at joint between second phalanx and third phalanx and proceed as before.

◆ Place bands on both hands and do exercises together.

C. Rubber Band on Finger Joints with Use of Fulcrum

◆ Place band on joint between first phalanx and second phalanx.

◆ Establish fulcrum (ring finger) on tabletop with little finger closely adjacent to it; elbow and forearm are free, as they are during instrumentation. Keep wrist straight, in same horizontal line as the forearm, and hold elbow at 90°. Stretch band by separating middle and ring fingers.

◆ Touch thumb and index and middle fingers to simulate a modified pen grasp for holding an instrument. Stretch band by separating middle and ring fingers.

III. Pen/Pencil Exercises

A. Purpose

◆ To develop correct modified pen grasp.

◆ To propel instrument by activation from wrist and arm, without moving fingers.

◆ To practice instrument rolling.

◆ To develop control and precision.

◆ To practice use of instruments when indirect vision is required.

B. Everyday Penmanship

◆ Use modified pen grasp whenever possible for writing.

◆ Practice writing with the nondominant hand to increase dexterity for handling instruments.

◆ Practice rolling a pencil between the thumb and index fingers while keeping the two fingers opposite of each other and maintaining adequate space between them at all times.

C. Writing with Rubber Band around Grasp

◆ Hold a pencil with modified pen grasp.

◆ Place a rubber band around the grasp to keep the fingers together as one unit.

◆ Establish fulcrum (ring finger) on a piece of paper on tabletop.

◆ Keep wrist straight in line with forearm; elbow is at 90°, and shoulder is in neutral position. Forearm and elbow are free.

◆ Accomplish writing by activation of the wrist and upper arm only, without flexing or extending the thumb and fingers. This helps to prevent digital motions.

C. Using Mouth Mirror

◆ Hold mouth mirror with modified pen grasp in nondominant hand.

◆ Hold a pencil with modified pen grasp in the dominant hand.

◆ While looking only through the mouth mirror, practice writing exercises. Reverse hands.

◆ You may also practice tracing and outlining drawings or the small squares on a sheet of graph paper via indirect vision to develop precision and accuracy.

IV. Refining Use of Mouth Mirror and Cotton Pliers

A. Purpose

◆ To develop ability to turn mouth mirror at various angles.

◆ To develop dexterity in holding objects with cotton pliers.

B. Mouth Mirror

◆ Hold mouth mirror with modified pen grasp, ring finger on tabletop as fulcrum finger with little finger closely adjacent to it; elbow and forearm are free. The mirror is used most frequently in the nondominant hand.

◆ Practice turning mirror with fingers, adjusting as to the several surfaces of the tooth.

◆ Hold a small object in the dominant hand for viewing in mirror held in nondominant hand.

◆ Practice crossing the mirror over fulcrum finger as in position for retracting lower lip while viewing lingual surfaces of mandibular anterior teeth in mouth mirror.

C. Cotton Pliers

◆ Make small, tight cotton pellets with thumb and index and middle fingers of each hand; then make one in each hand simultaneously.

◆ Hold cotton pliers with modified pen grasp and establish fulcrum finger on tabletop; elbow and forearm are free.

◆ Practice picking up cotton pellets using mirror vision (right hand, then left).
  • Use in wiping motion on tabletop or other object.
  • Move to different area to release pellet as if to a waste-receiving cup.

V. Increasing Tactile Sensitivity

A. Purpose

◆ To establish desired grasp of the explorer and probe to ensure maximum tactile or touch sensitivity.

B. Explorer

◆ Mount small pieces of various grades of sandpaper on a card.

◆ Hold explorer with modified pen grasp, and establish fulcrum finger on tabletop, with upper arm and forearm free. With eyes closed, compare roughness of the various grades of sandpaper. Use a light, exploratory/assessment stroke.

◆ Various tools and educational aids (e.g., Calculus Detection PRO and Calculus Detection Calibrator) are available commercially to help develop tactile sensitivity required to detect cementum and varying degrees of calculus (see Figure 37-26).

C. Probe

◆ Hold a periodontal probe in the dominant hand using a modified pen grasp.

◆ Next to a precision scale (e.g., laboratory, kitchen, or food weighing scale), establish a level fulcrum, making sure not to fulcrum directly on the scale itself.

◆ With the probe tip, apply just enough force on the scale to reach the recommended probing force of 0.25 g.[23]

◆ Repeat multiple times to develop muscle memory of optimal probing force.

CUMULATIVE TRAUMA

Following proper instrumentation techniques and ergonomic practices will preserve the well-being of the dental hygienist.

◆ Primary occupational hazards are related to personal everyday habits during chairside practice.

◆ The symptoms of carpal tunnel syndrome are caused by compression of the median nerve within the carpal tunnel, as shown in Figure 37-6. Chapter 8 shows the anatomy of the carpel tunnel wrist area.

I. Risk Factors for Trauma

◆ Poor posture.

◆ Extended periods of time spent in the same work position.

◆ Repetitive movements during actual instrumentation.

II. Preventing Trauma

◆ Study and plan for action in advance, before serious disability can occur.

◆ Exercises performed chairside and between appointments can contribute greatly to long-range prevention.

◆ One easy and practical exercise that can be performed during patient treatment is stretching the fingers and wrists between returning an instrument to the cassette and picking up a new one (see Figure 37-27).

◆ Stretching exercises for stress release, improvement of posture, and counteracting repetitive movements used during instrumentation are suggested in Figure 37-28.

◆ Additional exercises are shown in Chapter 8.

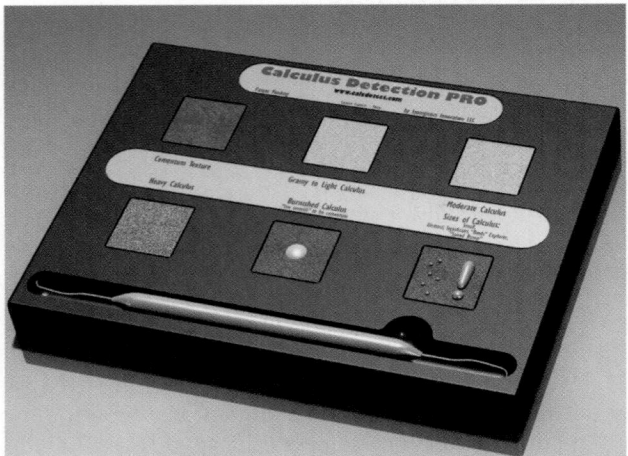

FIGURE 37-26 • Calculus Detection Tool. This tool consists of an explorer and mounted textured tiles that simulate different tooth structures and varying degrees of calculus. (Courtesy of Calculus Detection PRO.)

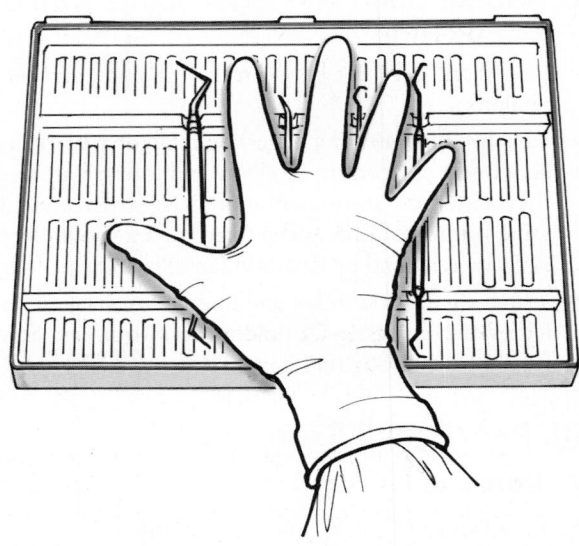

FIGURE 37-27 • Stretching Fingers Prior to Instrument Retrieval. One of the exercises that can be used during actual clinical practice.

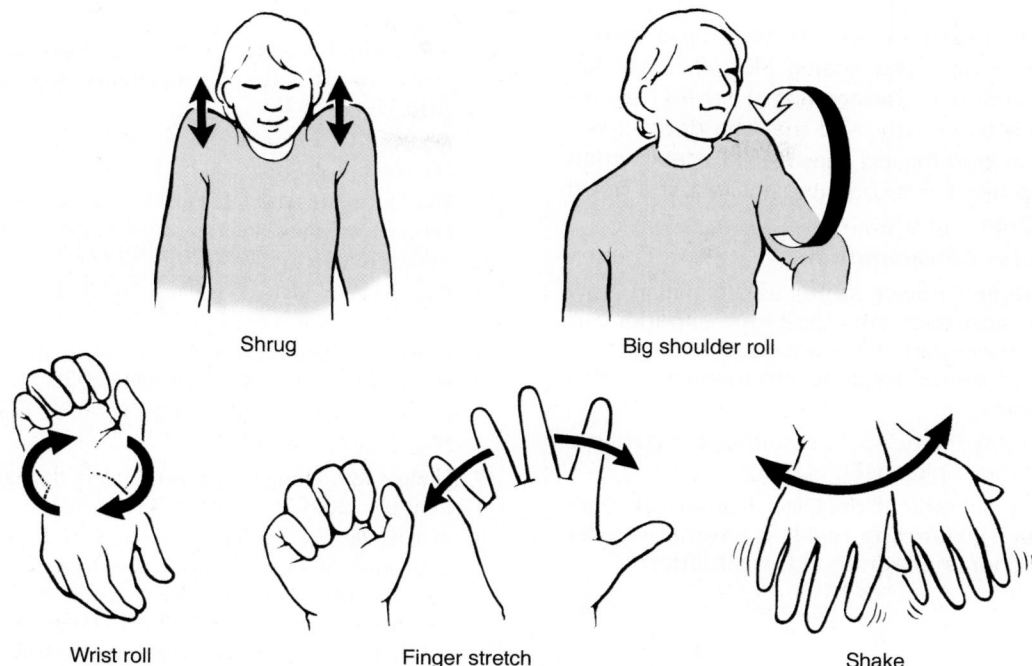

Shrug

Big shoulder roll

Wrist roll

Finger stretch

Shake

FIGURE 37-28 • Chairside Stretching Exercises. Stretching exercises to relax the back, shoulders, and neck are shown with the shrug and rolling the head around with the big shoulder roll. Hand and finger rolls, stretches, and shaking can be performed anytime, even while attending a patient.

DOCUMENTATION

Documentation of instrument selection and instrumentation techniques in a patient record can provide guidance during subsequent dental hygiene care. For example, notes made in the patient record may include the following:

◆ Areas in the patient's dentition that require more careful attention or careful application of skill.

◆ Specific instruments shown to be more effective in specific areas, such as minicurets in a particularly deep pocket.

◆ Instruments avoided due to patient contraindications or discomfort, such as an ultrasonic scaler due to dentinal hypersensitivity.

◆ An example progress note is found in Box 37-1.

BOX 37-1

Example Documentation:
Instrumentation

S— Female patient, 32 years old with cerebral palsy and dysphagia, presents to clinic with caregiver for first "long overdue" dental appointment in 5 years.

O— Generalized erythematous and inflamed gingiva with festooned margins and bulbous interdental papillae noted. Heavy, generalized calculus present on all teeth; bridge of calculus noted from #20 to #29 and occlusal calculus noted on all molars and premolars.

A— Unable to perform an accurate comprehensive periodontal examination today due to heavy supragingival calculus overlying soft tissues. Exposed six vertical bitewings using a NOMAD (mobile radiology unit) to assess for caries and bone loss.

P— Completed a full mouth debridement today for gross calculus removal. Did not use ultrasonic scaler due to patient's difficulty swallowing and risk for aspirating water into the lungs. Used the universal and rigid Gracey curets to remove heavy supragingival calculus.

Next steps: Patient to return with caregiver in 1 week for a full comprehensive periodontal examination.

Signed: _____, RDH

Date: _____

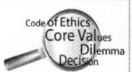

EVERYDAY ETHICS

Ryan, a recent dental hygiene graduate, joins his first small private practice office. There is a long-time hygienist, Margaret, at the practice who is in charge of making many important decisions, including which supplies, equipment, and instruments are ordered. During his first day of work, Ryan notices that all the hand instruments have been incorrectly or severely oversharpened and that there is not a single powered scaler in the entire office. When Ryan asks Margaret if the office could invest in several new hand instruments and a powered scaler, Margaret quickly denies his request, stating that ordering new instruments is too costly, and that she doesn't see the value of purchasing a powered scaler when extra sharp hand instruments can do just a good of a job of removing calculus.

Questions for Consideration

1. Given Ryan's novice status as a clinician, how will he approach Margaret—an experienced practitioner—with his concerns? Which core values of dental hygiene are involved in this scenario?

2. What harm, if any, could result for the patients and/or the clinicians?

3. Utilizing an ethical decision framework (see Chapter 1), describe realistic alternatives for Ryan's course of action in this situation.

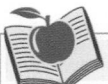

Factors to Teach the Patient

▶ The benefits and risks of using various types of instruments.

▶ Why it is necessary to use a variety of instruments for treatment.

▶ What sensations and experiences to expect during the use of certain instruments.

▶ How the patient can cooperate to help you instrument more effectively and efficiently.

ENHANCE YOUR UNDERSTANDING

ONLINE RESOURCES
(see the inside front cover for access information)

• Audio glossary
• Appendices

SUPPORT FOR LEARNING
(available separately)

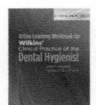

• *Active Learning Workbook for Wilkins' Clinical Practice of the Dental Hygienist, 13th Edition*

INDIVIDUALIZED REVIEW

• Customized practice quizzing with Navigate 2 TestPrep for *Wilkins' Clinical Practice of the Dental Hygienist*

References

1. Simmer-Beck M, Branson BG. An evidence-based review of ergonomic features of dental hygiene instruments. *Work.* 2010;35(4):477-485.

2. Hodges KO. Expanding your instrument armamentarium. *Dimensions Dent Hyg.* 2009;7(5):31-33.

3. You D, Smith AH, Rempel D. Meta-analysis: association between wrist posture and carpal tunnel syndrome among workers. *Saf Health Work.* 2014;5(1):27-31.

4. Pattison AM, Matsuda S, Pattison GL. Extraoral fulcrums. *Dimensions Dent Hyg.* 2004;2(10):20-23.

5. Nguyen M, Pattison AM. Activate alternative fulcrums. *Dimensions Dent Hyg.* 2014;12(5):24, 26, 28.

6. Pattison A. The secret use of sickle scalers. *Dimensions Dent Hyg.* 2008;6(9):46-47.

7. Hodges KO. Using files in periodontal therapy. *Dimensions Dent Hyg.* 2004;2(11):16, 18-20.

8. Eick S, Bender P, Flury S, Lussi A, Sculean A. In vitro evaluation of surface roughness, adhesion of periodontal ligament fibroblasts, and *Streptococcus gordonii* following root instrumentation with Gracey curettes and subsequent polishing with diamond-coated curettes. *Clin Oral Investig.* 2013;17(2):397-404.

9. Lea SC, Walmsley D. Mechano-physical and biophysical properties of power-driven scalers: driving the future of powered instrument design and evaluation. *Periodontol 2000.* 2009;51:63-78.

10. Krishna R, De Stefano JA. Ultrasonic vs. hand instrumentation in periodontal therapy: clinical outcomes. *Periodontol 2000.* 2016;71(1):113-127.

11. Trenter SC, Walmsley AD. Ultrasonic dental scaler: associated hazards. *J Clin Periodontol.* 2003;30(2):95-101.

12. Kohn WG, Collins AS, Cleveland JL, et al. Guidelines for infection control in dental health-care settings—2003. *MMWR Recomm Rep.* 2003;52(RR17):1-61.

13. Scannapieco FA, Bush RB, Paju S. Associations between periodontal disease and risk for nosocomial bacterial pneumonia and chronic obstructive pulmonary disease. A systematic review. *Ann Periodontol.* 2003;8(1):54-69.

14. Garcia JM, Chambers E IV. Managing dysphagia through diet modifications. *Am J Nurs.* 2010;110(11):26-33.

15. Elayi CS, Lusher S, Meeks Nyquist JL, Darrat Y, Morales GX, Miller CS. Interference between dental electrical devices and pacemakers or defibrillators: results from a prospective clinical study. *J Am Dent Assoc.* 2015;146(2):121-128.

16. Lahor-Soler E, Miranda-Rius J, Brunet-Llobet L, Sabate de la Cruz X. Capacity of dental equipment to interfere with cardiac implantable electrical devices. *Eur J Oral Sci.* 2015;123(3):194-201.

17. Roedig JJ, Shah J, Elayi CS, Miller CS. Interference of cardiac pacemaker and implantable cardioverter-defibrillator activity during electronic dental device use. *J Am Dent Assoc.* 2010;141:521-526.

18. Gomez G, Jara F, Sanchez B, Roig M, Duran-Sindreu F. Effects of piezoelectric units on pacemaker function: an in vitro study. *J Endod.* 2013;39(10):1296-1299.

19. Maiorana C, Grossi GB, Garramone RA, Manfredini R, Santoro F. Do ultrasonic dental scalers interfere with implantable cardioverter defibrillators? An in vivo investigation. *J Dent*. 2013;41(11):955-959.

20. Paramashivaiah R, Prabhuji ML. Mechanized scaling with ultrasonics: perils and proactive measures. *J Indian Soc Periodontol*. 2013;17(4):423-428.

21. Arabaci T, Ciçek Y, Ozgöz M, Canakçi V, Canakçi CF, Eltas A. The comparison of the effects of three types of piezoelectric ultrasonic tips and air polishing system on the filling materials: an in vitro study. *Int J Dent Hyg*. 2007;5(4):205-210.

22. Mann M, Parmar D, Walmsley AD, Lea SC. Effect of plastic-covered ultrasonic scalers on titanium implant surfaces. *Clin Oral Implants Res*. 2012;23(1):76-82.

23. Al Shayeb KN, Turner W, Gillam DG. Periodontal probing: a review. *Prim Dent J*. 2014;3(3):25-29.

Instrument Care and Sharpening

Esther M. Wilkins, BS, RDH, DMD, and Linda D. Boyd, RDH, RD, EdD

CHAPTER OUTLINE

INSTRUMENT SHARPENING
I. Benefits from Use of Sharp Manual Instruments
II. Consequences of Using Dull Manual Instruments
III. Dynamics of Sharpening
IV. Types of Sharpening Devices

BASIC SHARPENING PRINCIPLES
I. Sterilization of the Sharpening Stone
II. Instrument Handling
III. Preparation of Stone for Sharpening
IV. Sharpening Overview
V. Tests for Instrument Sharpness
VI. Evaluation of Technique
VII. After Sharpening
VIII. Instrument Wear

SHARPENING CURETS AND SCALERS
I. Technique Objectives
II. Selection of Cutting Edges to Sharpen

MOVING FLAT STONE: STATIONARY INSTRUMENT
I. Examine the Cutting Edge to Be Sharpened
II. Review the Angulation to Be Restored at the Dull Cutting Edge
III. Stabilize and Position the Instrument
IV. Apply the Sharpening Stone
V. Activate the Sharpening Stone
VI. Test for Sharpness

STATIONARY FLAT STONE: MOVING INSTRUMENT
I. Curet
II. Scaler: Sickle or Jacquette

SHARPENING THE FILE SCALER
I. Surface to Be Ground
II. Sharpening Procedure

CARE OF SHARPENING EQUIPMENT
I. Flat Sharpening Stone
II. Care of the Tanged File
III. Manufacturer's Directions

DOCUMENTATION

EVERYDAY ETHICS

FACTORS TO TEACH THE PATIENT

REFERENCES

LEARNING OBJECTIVES

After studying this chapter, the student will be able to:

1. Describe the benefits of using sharp instruments.

2. Describe the consequences of using dull instruments.

3. Demonstrate proper technique for sharpening procedures for a variety of periodontal instruments.

4. Explain how to preserve optimal instrument design when sharpening.

INSTRUMENT SHARPENING

*Objectives for techniques of sharpening emphasize the **preservation of the original shape of the blade** while restoring a sharp **cutting edge**.*

◆ Instruments designed for a particular purpose need to continue to be used in the manner for which they were designed.

- Inaccurate sharpening techniques can distort the blade and render the instrument useless for its intended purpose.

◆ Sharpening is an essential and integral part of instrumentation.

- Sharpening procedures are technique-sensitive and require skill and patience to become proficient.

- The clinician must test instrument sharpness at the beginning and during each appointment.

◆ Successful clinical outcomes with bladed instruments are dependent on correctly contoured and sharpened instruments.

◆ Maintaining instrument sharpness prevents loss of blade structure so recontouring to restore the original shape is not necessary.

I. Benefits from Use of Sharp Manual Instruments

Instruments must be sharp if scaling, root planing, or debridement is to be completed efficiently with minimal trauma to the tissues. When the instrument blade is maintained with its original contour and sharp cutting edges, the following may be expected[1]:

◆ Greater precision of treatment, improved quality of results, and less working time involved.

◆ Increased tactile sensitivity.

◆ Greater control with less blade slippage.

◆ Fewer strokes required.

◆ Less possibility of burnishing rather than removing the calculus.

◆ Prevention of trauma to gingival tissues and less discomfort and greater safety for the patient.

◆ Decreased possibility of nicking, grooving, or scratching the tooth surfaces.

◆ Less fatigue for the clinician.

II. Consequences of Using Dull Manual Instruments

◆ Stress and frustration of using ineffective instruments resulting in burnished or inadequate removal of calculus.

◆ Wasted time, effort, and energy.

◆ Loss of control and increased likelihood of slipping with instrument and lacerating the gingival tissue.

◆ Loss of patient confidence in clinician's ability.

◆ Increased likelihood of developing work-related musculoskeletal disorders from excessive muscle strain and increased number of stroke repetitions.

III. Dynamics of Sharpening

Instrument sharpening is accomplished by filing the surface or surfaces that form the cutting edge.

A. Cutting Edge

◆ The cutting edge is a very fine *line* formed where the face and lateral surface meet at an angle (see Figure 38-1).[2]

◆ The edge becomes dull when pressed against a hard surface (the tooth), or it may be nicked when drawn over a rough surface.

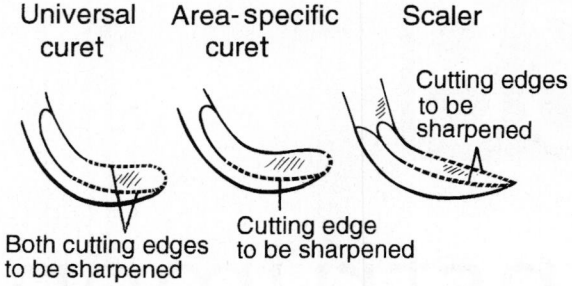

FIGURE 38-1 • Selection of Cutting Edge to Sharpen. Both cutting edges and the rounded toe are sharpened for a universal curet. An area-specific curet is sharpened on the longer cutting edge and the rounded toe. A scaler is sharpened on the two sides, and the tip is brought to a point.

◆ A dull edge (also called a *beveled* edge) is when the two planes of the blade no longer come to a fine edge and is flattened (Figure 38-2). *The object in sharpening is to reshape the cutting edge to a fine line while removing a minimal amount of material.*[2]

- Approximately 45 scaling strokes creates a very rounded cutting edge, even 15 strokes results in a slightly rounded cutting edge.[2]

B. Sharpening Stone Surface

◆ A sharpening stone acts as an abrasive to reshape a dulled blade by grinding the surface until the cutting edge is restored.

◆ The surface of the stone is made up of masses of minute crystals, which are the abrasive particles that accomplish the grinding of the instrument.

◆ A smaller particle size or a finer grit abrades or reduces more slowly and produces a finer cutting edge.[2]

IV. Types of Sharpening Devices

A. Stones

◆ *Natural abrasive stones:* Quarried from mineral deposits.

- Manual sharpening with an Arkansas stone (fine grit) produces a better cutting edge than synthetic stones or power-driven devices (Figure 38-3A).[2–5]

- India stones are also used for manual sharpening and come in a variety of grits[3] (Figure 38-3B).

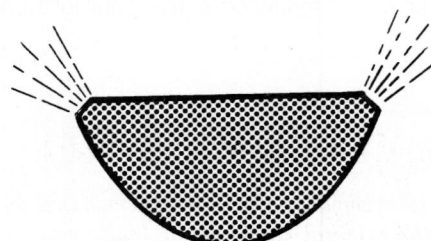

FIGURE 38-2 • Cross Section of a Dull Curet. A sharp curet has a fine line at the cutting edge that will not reflect light. A dull cutting edge is like a beveled or flattened surface and reflects light as shown.

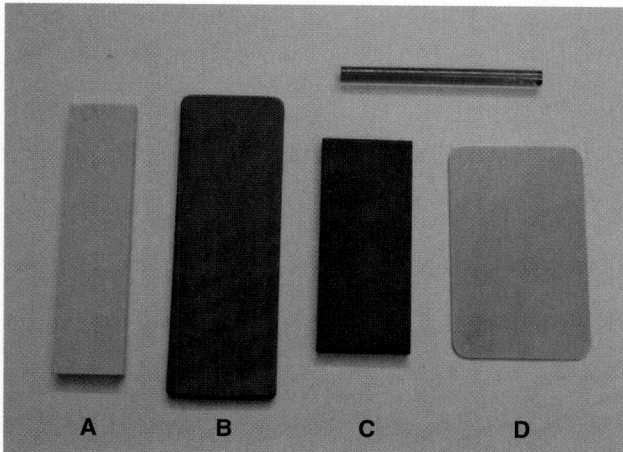

FIGURE 38-3 • Types of Sharpening Stones. A: Arkansas stone. **B:** India stone. **C:** Ceramic stone. **D:** Diamond-sharpening stone.

◆ *Artificial materials*
  • Hard, nonmetallic substances impregnated with aluminum oxide, silicon carbide, or diamond particles. Examples: ruby stone, carborundum stones, and the diamond stone.
  • Ceramic aluminum oxide (Figure 38-3C).
  • Steel alloys are metals that are harder than most dental instrument steel and, therefore, are capable of sharpening the instrument.
  • A diamond-coated stainless steel sharpening card is about the size of a credit card and used in the same way as other sharpening stones (Figure 38-3D). However, research suggests they remove significantly more metal than ceramic stones resulting in the need for more frequent replacement of scalers.[6]

B. Power-Driven or Mechanical Sharpening Devices

◆ A number of manufacturers offer power-driven sharpening devices.
◆ Research suggests a better cutting edge is created with manual sharpening.[2–4]

BASIC SHARPENING PRINCIPLES

I. Sterilization of the Sharpening Stone

◆ A sterile sharpening stone and testing stick are parts of a basic clinical setup for a scaling appointment.
◆ Sterilization of stones may be accomplished using any of the acceptable sterilization methods (Chapter 7) in accordance with specific manufacturer's recommendations.[1]
◆ Over time, the steam autoclave may dry out an Arkansas stone and lead to chipping or breakage.

II. Instrument Handling

All instruments must be handled with care to preserve sharpness and prevent accidental damage to the cutting edges.

III. Preparation of Stone for Sharpening

A. Dry Stone

◆ *Advantage:* The problems related to maintaining a sterile stone and preventing contamination when oil, tap water, or a lubricant is applied are eliminated.
◆ A dry stone contributes to the following effects:
  • Sharpens the cutting edge without nicks in the blade; nicks can be created from particles of metal suspended in a lubricant.
  • Allows the stone to be completely sterilized without the problem of interference by the oil left in and on the stone.

B. Water on Stone

◆ Water can be used for lubrication of ceramic stones, but they may also be used dry.

C. Lubricated Stone

◆ Oil lubrication is recommended with certain quarried stones such as the Arkansas stone to prevent drying out.
◆ Instruments are autoclaved before sharpening, and the stone and instruments are sterilized again after nonsterile lubricant is used.
◆ The lubricant can facilitate the movement of the instrument blade over the stone to prevent scratching of the stone.
  • Suspend the metallic particles removed during sharpening.
  • Help to prevent clogging of the pores of the stone (glazing).

IV. Sharpening Overview

A. Objectives

The objectives during sharpening are twofold:
◆ To produce a sharp cutting edge.
◆ To preserve the original shape of the instrument.
  • The contour of a curet toe is a smooth, continuous curvature with no points or flat edges.

B. When to Sharpen

◆ Sharpen at the first sign of dullness during an appointment.[1]
◆ Recontouring an overly dull instrument may result in more frequent instrument replacement.
  • Restoring original contour to a grossly dull instrument often leaves a blade that is not functional.
◆ Replace severely dulled instruments.

C. Angulation

- Before starting to sharpen, analyze the cutting edge and establish the proper angle between the stone and the blade surface.
- Maintain the angle through the firm grasp, secure hand rest, moderate pressure, short stroke, and other features of the technique appropriate to the individual instrument.

D. Maintain Control

- Maintain control so that the entire surface is reduced evenly.
- Care must be taken not to create a new bevel at the cutting edge.

E. Care of Sharpening Stone

- Prevent grooving of the sharpening stone by varying the areas for instrument placement.
- Cleaning and stain removal procedures are described in section "Care of Sharpening Equipment" in this chapter.

V. Tests for Instrument Sharpness

A. Visual or Glare Test

- Examine the cutting edge under adequate light using magnification.
- Because the sharp cutting edge is a fine *line*, it does not reflect light.
- The dull cutting edge presents a flat, shiny *surface*, which can reflect light.
  - Figure 38-2 shows the cross section of a dull universal curet.
  - The dull cutting edges are tiny surfaces that reflect light.

B. Plastic Testing Stick

- Use a sterile plastic or acrylic 1/4-inch rod, 3 inches long (see Figure 38-4).
- Place the fulcrum finger on the end of the stick.
- Apply the heel (shank end) of the cutting edge to the plastic stick, first at 90°, then closed to the correct angle for scaling (70°).
- Press lightly but firmly.
- Roll the cutting edge forward from the shank end to the toe by turning or rolling the instrument handle in the fingers to test the entire length of the blade.

C. Confirming Sharpness Using the Plastic Testing Stick

- The *sharp* cutting edge engages or grips the plastic as the length of the blade is tested. Each portion of the cutting edge will engage the plastic uniformly as the blade advances.
- The *dull* cutting edge does not catch without undue pressure and slides easily over the surface of the stick.

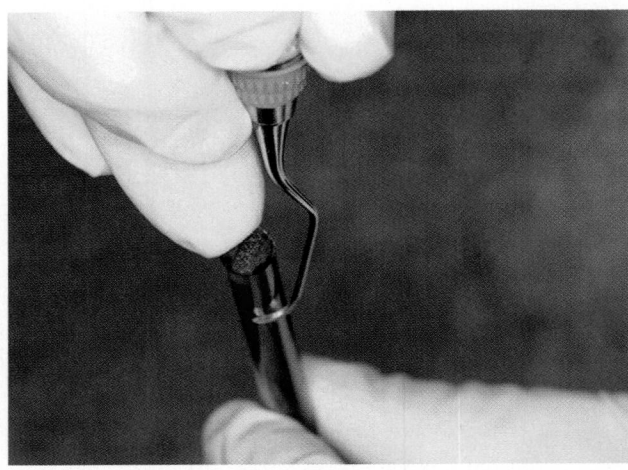

FIGURE 38-4 • Plastic Testing Stick. Sharpness can be evaluated using a test stick. A test stick is a cylindrical rod made of plastic or acrylic. (Reprinted from Nield-Gehrig J. *Fundamentals of Periodontal Instrumentation and Advanced Root Instrumentation.* Philadelphia, PA: Lippincott Williams & Wilkins; 2011.)

- Because the edge is not uniformly dulled during use, there will be portions of a blade that exhibit varying degrees of sharpness or dullness.
- As the instrument blade is rolled along the testing stick, the degree of slipping versus engagement will indicate the degree of sharpness or dullness. If only limited portions of the blade exhibit dullness, attempt to note the segments that slip as the blade is rolled along the testing stick.
  - The entire length of the cutting edge is always sharpened to maintain the original form.
  - Awareness of the portion(s) exhibiting dullness can guide pressure and the number of strokes.
  - This helps to minimize oversharpening.
  - Careful evaluation will increase efficiency and raise the likelihood that dull portions of the blade are restored to sharpness.

VI. Evaluation of Technique

- Observe closely the stabilization of both the instrument and stone, each kept aligned in a single plane, to evaluate sharpening technique.
  - *Self-check:* As the stone is activated for sharpening, observe the top of the instrument to ensure it is secure and not moving.
  - *Self-check:* Observe stone to ensure it remains in a single plane of movement back and forth as it is activated.
- Evaluate by turning the instrument over to examine the back of the lateral surfaces under well-lit magnification.
- A sharp cutting edge results from:
  - Instrument and stone positioned at the correct angle.
  - Movement occurring in a single plane.

- Irregular bevel is revealed by:
  - Breaks in the fine line of the blade edge.
  - Varying facets indicating the improper stone placement/movement.

VII. After Sharpening

A. Finishing the Instrument

Newly sharpened instruments are finished by carefully inspecting the edges for a clean consistent bevel with no particles or "wire edge" remaining.

B. How the Wire Edge Is Produced

- During sharpening, some of the metal particles removed during grinding remain attached to the edge of the instrument and create the wire edge (Figure 38-5).[2-4]
- If allowed to remain, the tiny particles may be removed when the instrument is applied to the tooth surface during treatment.

C. Removal of Wire Edge

- Wipe the instrument carefully with a dry gauze square or an alcohol wipe to remove particles.

VIII. Instrument Wear

- As curets are used, the cutting edge wears down, leaving a narrower face and shorter length over a period of time.
- Sharpening also contributes to the size reduction.
- After sufficient reduction, instruments must be retired and discarded.
  - Blades will no longer access or adapt to the tooth surface.
  - Thinner blades are more susceptible to breakage with lateral pressure.
- Used instruments that become narrow can be reserved for patients with minimal deposit and require biofilm debridement only.

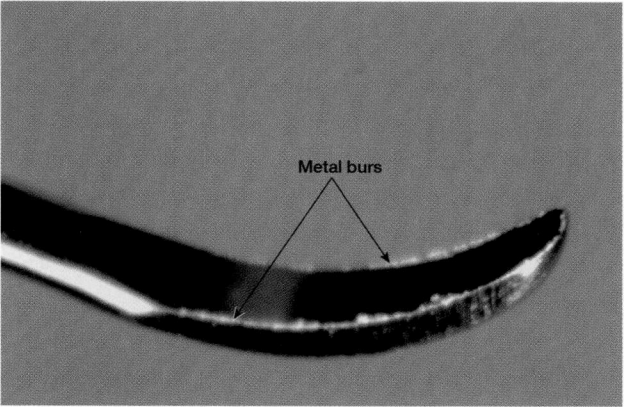

FIGURE 38-5 • Wire Edge After Sharpening. Sharpening can produce minute metal burs that project from the cutting edge. (Reprinted from Nield-Gehrig J. *Fundamentals of Periodontal Instrumentation and Advanced Root Instrumentation.* Philadelphia, PA: Lippincott Williams & Wilkins; 2011.)

- Exert care when using overly thinned curets. If strong lateral pressure is applied, they may break off at the tip, leaving the last few millimeters embedded in the sulcus or pocket.
- Evaluation during sharpening procedures provides the opportunity for proper attention to instrument maintenance.

SHARPENING CURETS AND SCALERS

In the following sections, procedures for a variety of sharpening techniques are outlined.

I. Technique Objectives

- Preserve the original contour of the blade.
- Sharpen frequently to maintain sharpness and prevent need for excessive recontouring of the blade.

II. Selection of Cutting Edges to Sharpen

A. Scalers/Sickles

- Most scalers are universal instruments.
- Cutting edges on both sides of the face are sharpened (Figure 38-1).
- A two-step sharpening procedure is used.

B. Curets: Universal

- Cutting edges on both sides of the face and the toe are sharpened (Figure 38-1).
- A three-step sharpening procedure is used.

C. Curets: Area Specific

- Cutting edges on one side of the face and the toe are sharpened.
- Sharpen the longer cutting edge; generally it will be the one farthest from the handle. In Figure 38-1, it is indicated by the dotted line.
- A two-step sharpening procedure is used: one side of the face and the toe.

MOVING FLAT STONE: STATIONARY INSTRUMENT

- Although widely used, research suggests this method is less effective in creating a fine cutting edge than a method where the stone is stationary and the instrument is moved across it.[4]
  - Greater irregularities in the cutting edge and wire edges (Figure 38-5) were created suggesting a loss of control during sharpening.[4]
- The side of the cutting edge formed by the lateral surface is reduced by this method.

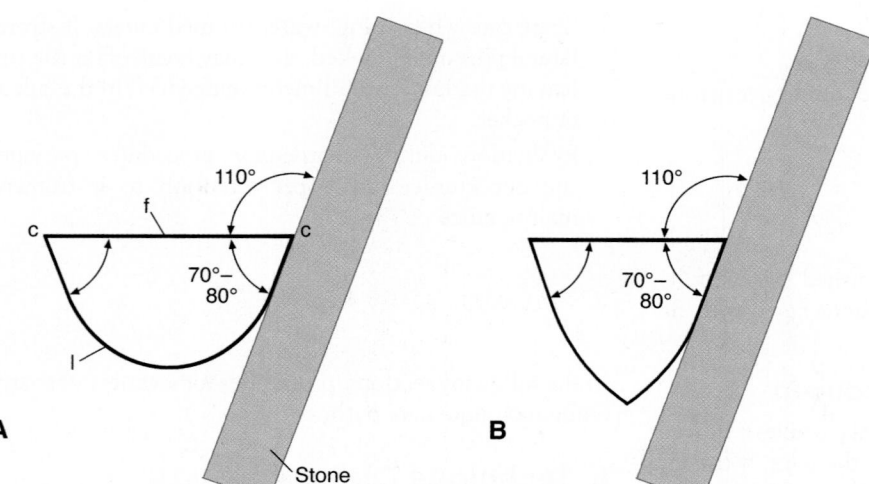

A

B

FIGURE 38-6 • Angulation for Sharpening. Cross sections of a curet **(A)** and a scaler **(B)** show correct angulation of the face (f) of the blade with the flat sharpening stone to reproduce the internal angle of the instrument at 70°. Note the cutting edges (c) and the lateral surfaces (l).

♦ The technique described applies to both curets and scalers.

♦ Because the scaler has a pointed tip and the curet has a round toe end, a variation is necessary in the adaptation of the sharpening stone to that portion of the blade (Figure 38-6).

I. Examine the Cutting Edge to Be Sharpened

Test for sharpness to determine specific areas that are dull, but plan to sharpen the whole cutting edge(s) to maintain original contour.

II. Review the Angulation to Be Restored at the Dull Cutting Edge

♦ Internal angle of the blade at the cutting edge(s) is 70° to 80° (see Chapter 37).

♦ Visible angle at which the stone will be placed will be 110°, as shown in Figure 38-6.

III. Stabilize and Position the Instrument

♦ Grasp the instrument in the nondominant hand in a palm grasp.

♦ Lean the hand against the edge of an immovable workbench or table under bright light (Figure 38-7A).

♦ The instrument is positioned low enough to allow the clinician to see the cutting edges clearly.

♦ Turn the face of the instrument up and parallel with the floor. Point the curet toe (or scaler tip) toward the clinician to provide better access for moving the stone (Figure 38-7B).

♦ The cutting edges begin at the lower shank.

♦ The cutting edges are parallel, until they converge.

♦ For the curet, the cutting edges curve to form the toe.

♦ For the scaler, the cutting edges taper to make the pointed tip.

IV. Apply the Sharpening Stone

♦ Hold the stone perpendicular to the floor, at the shank third of the cutting edge.

♦ From the 90° angle with the face of the instrument, open the stone to make an angle of 110° (Figures 38-7C, 38-8A and B).

V. Activate the Sharpening Stone

A. Steps One and Two

♦ Maintain the stone in contact with the blade and at the proper angle throughout the procedure.

♦ Tighten the grasp on the instrument (nondominant hand) while applying a smooth even pressure to the cutting edge to keep the instrument stable and motionless.

♦ Move the stone up and down with short rhythmical strokes about ½-inch high. Place more pressure on the down stroke. Maintain the 110° angle precisely. Finish each area with a down stroke.[4]

♦ *For the universal curet:*
  • Follow the cutting edge to where the curvature for the toe begins, applying three or four down strokes overlapping at each millimeter of the cutting edge.
  • Proceed to the opposite side to sharpen, repeating the steps just described (Figure 38-8).
  • Next, proceed to the third step to sharpen the toe.

♦ *For the area-specific curet:* Apply sharpening strokes **only** to the one selected side: proceed to the third step to sharpen all around the toe.

♦ *For the sickle scaler:* Follow the same procedure to where the cutting edge tapers to form the sharp tip and continue in that direction to finish that side of the blade. Proceed to the other side to sharpen the opposite cutting edge.

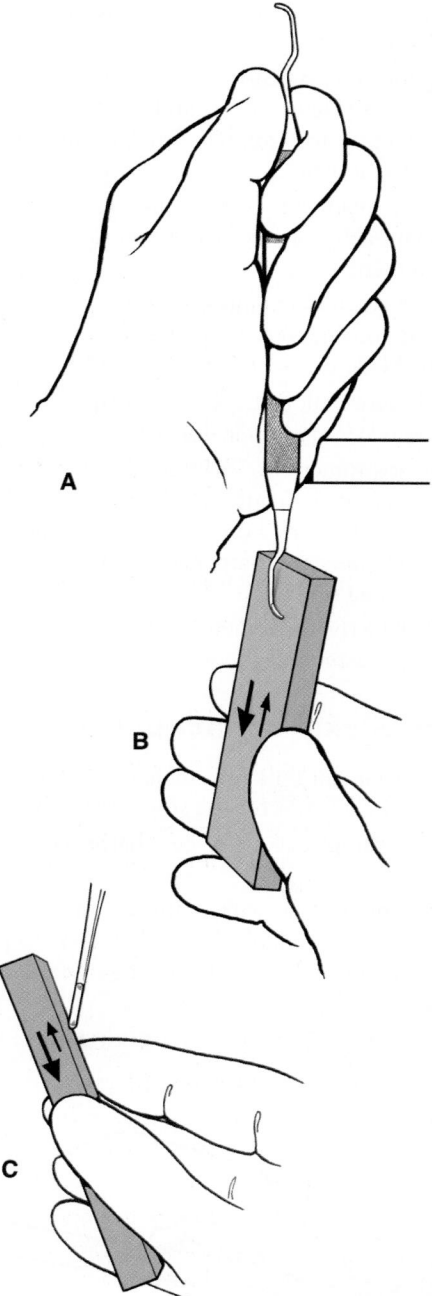

FIGURE 38-7 • Stationary Instrument—Moving Stone Technique. A: Grasp the instrument with the nondominant hand. Stabilize the hand on the edge of a stationary table or bench and provide good light on the instrument. **B:** The stone is angled with the face of the instrument at 110° to maintain the internal angle of the blade at 70° to 80°. **C:** Stone reversed to sharpen the opposite cutting edge of a universal curet.

B. Step Three: The Toe of a Curet

- Tip curet down to make the toe parallel with floor.
- Apply stone to make a 90° angle with the toe.
- Open the stone to make a 110° angle.
- Apply strokes for sharpening as described for the sides of the face of the blade.

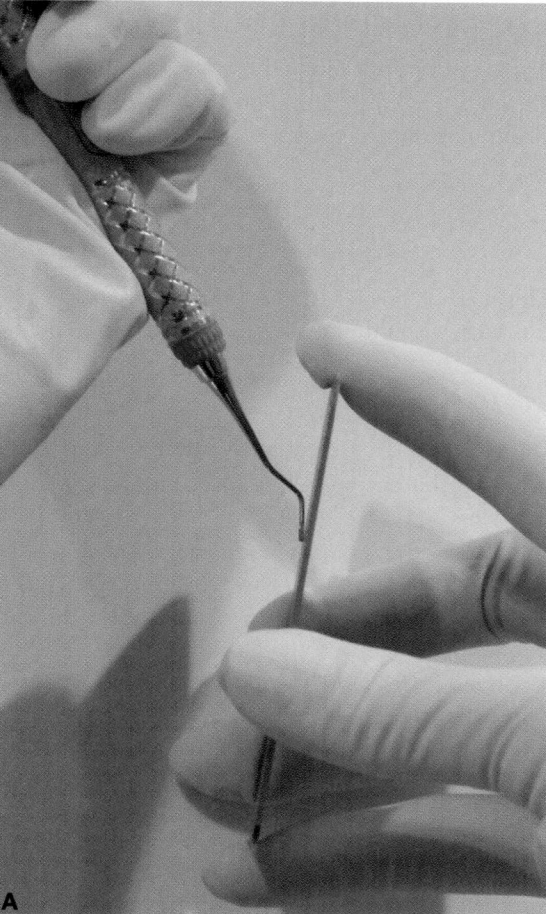

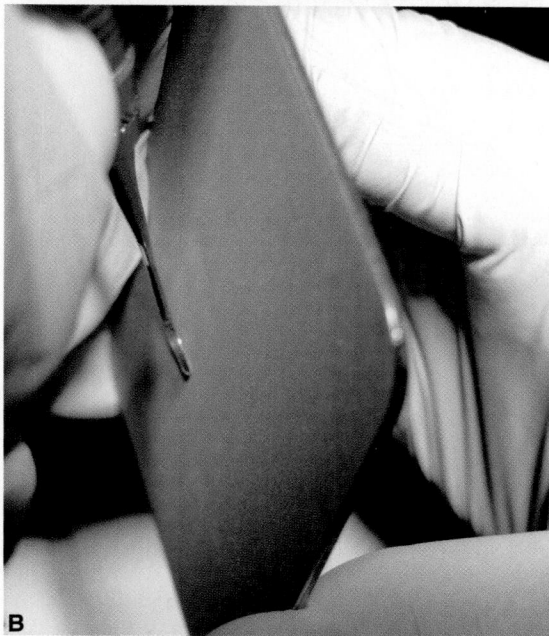

FIGURE 38-8 • Stationary Instrument—Moving Diamond-Sharpening Card. A and B: Grasp the instrument with the nondominant hand. Stabilize the hand. The card is angled with the face of the instrument at 110° to maintain the internal angle of the blade at 70° to 80°. Image **(B)** shows how the orientation of the diamond-sharpening card to the instrument face and blade look to the clinician during the sharpening process.

VI. Test for Sharpness

◆ Apply testing stick along the entire cutting edges.

◆ Repeat sharpening procedures as necessary to retain clean, sharp cutting edges.

STATIONARY FLAT STONE: MOVING INSTRUMENT

◆ This method creates the best result with a defined cutting edge with minimum irregularities or wire edges.[4]

I. Curet

◆ Place the stone flat on a steady surface.

◆ Examine the cutting edges to be sharpened. Test for sharpness.

◆ Hold the instrument in a modified pen grasp, and establish a secure finger rest (Figure 38-9A).

◆ Apply the cutting edge to the stone. An angle of 110° is formed by the stone and face.

  • Because the curet is curved, only a small section of the cutting edge can be applied at one time.

  • Sharpening is performed in a *series* of applications of the cutting edge to the stone, each overlapping

the previous, as the instrument is turned and drawn steadily along the stone.

  • The portion of the cutting edge nearest the shank is applied first (Figure 38-9A and B).

◆ Apply moderate to light but firm pressure while the instrument is activated.

◆ Use a slow, steady stroke to maintain control and to ensure that each portion of the cutting edge receives equal treatment.

◆ Move the blade forward into the cutting edge. Turn the instrument continuously until the center of the round end of the blade is reached (Figure 38-9).

◆ Test for sharpness along the entire cutting edge; reapply to stone as necessary for ideal sharpness.

◆ Turn the instrument to sharpen the second cutting edge. Overlap at the center of the round toe. Universal curets are sharpened on both sides and around the toe. Gracey curets are sharpened on one side only and around the toe (see Figure 38-1).

◆ Carefully wipe the instrument with a gauze square or an alcohol wipe to remove the wire edge.

II. Scaler: Sickle or Jacquette

◆ Place the stone flat on a firm table or bench top under adequate light. Do not tilt the stone while sharpening.

◆ Examine cutting edges to be sharpened. Test for sharpness.

◆ Hold the instrument with a firm pen grasp, using thumb, index, and middle (second) fingers to prevent the instrument from rotating or changing angles during sharpening (Figure 38-10A).

◆ Establish finger rest on side of stone using ring and little fingers.

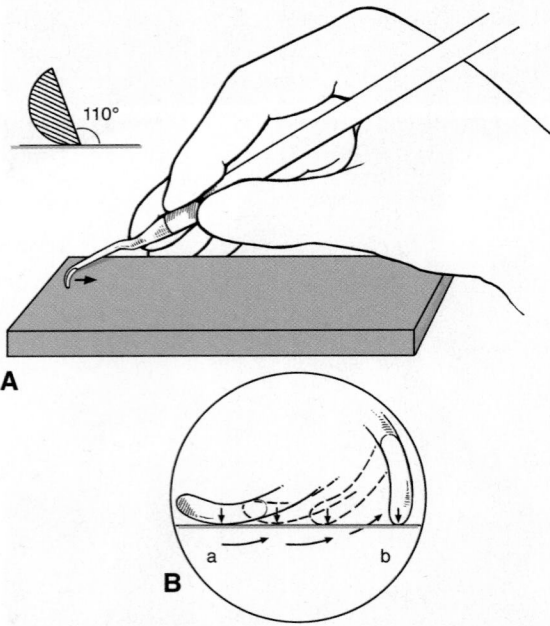

FIGURE 38-9 • Stationary Stone—Moving Instrument Technique for a Curet. A: Stone placed flat with blade in position at the beginning of the sharpening stroke. With the finger rest stabilized on the edge of the stone, the cutting edge is maintained at the proper angulation (110°) as the instrument is drawn along the stone with an even, moderate pressure. **B:** The movement of the blade is shown by the arrows, which indicate each portion of the cutting edge as the blade is turned on the stone from the beginning (a) to the completion (b) of the stroke at the center of the round toe of the curet. For a universal curet, the instrument is turned over and the opposite cutting edge is sharpened.

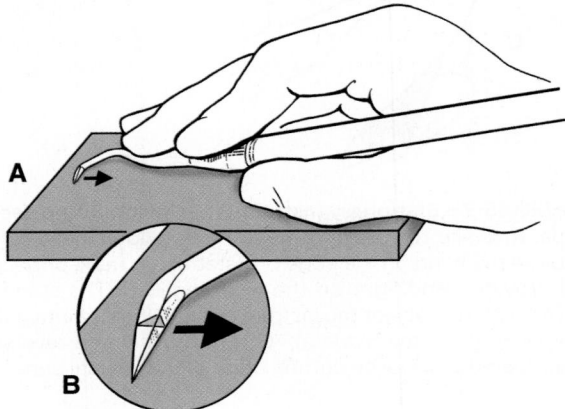

FIGURE 38-10 • Stationary Stone Technique for a Straight Scaler. A: With a modified pen grasp and a finger rest established on the side of the stone, the scaler is positioned for sharpening. **B:** The portion of the cutting edge nearest the lower shank is applied first with an angle of 110° between the face and the stone. The instrument is turned continuously to follow the arclike shape of the blade. The cutting edges are sharpened to the pointed tip.

◆ Stabilize stone with fingers of opposite hand.

◆ Apply cutting edge to be sharpened to the stone. Maintain 70° to 80° internal angle of the instrument (Figure 38-10B). The portion of the cutting edge nearest the shank is applied first.

◆ Apply moderate to light but firm pressure while instrument is in motion. Heavy pressure can reduce control of instrument, cause scratching of the stone, and produce an unfavorable bevel at the cutting edge.

◆ Use a short, slow stroke to maintain the exact relation of the cutting edge to the stone.
  • Pull blade forward, toward the cutting edge.
  • All fingers move with the arm as a unit.
  • Use a slow, steady stroke to maintain control and to ensure that each portion of the cutting edge receives equal treatment.
  • Turn the instrument continually to follow the shape of the blade to the pointed tip.

◆ Test for sharpness after one or two strokes. Repeat as needed for ideal sharpness.

◆ Turn instrument and proceed to sharpen other lateral surface. When instrument placement is awkward for a modified contra-angle scaler, use a narrow side of the stone.

SHARPENING THE FILE SCALER

◆ Files are sharpened with a flat sharpening instrument called a *tanged file*.
  • Diamond-coated files are *not* sharpened.

◆ Use of magnification and good illumination are necessary when sharpening files to ensure correct placement of the tanged file.

◆ Use a testing stick to check for the degree of sharpness to determine whether the file will need to be sharpened.

◆ If the file blades do not grasp the plastic testing stick when adapted lightly, they will need to be sharpened.

I. Surface to Be Ground

◆ Examine the file closely with the head of the working end positioned outward (Figure 38-11A).

◆ Note the two angular surfaces that meet to form a "V" shape (Figure 38-11B).

◆ The surface to be contacted with the tanged file and ground during sharpening is the surface of the "V" that is farthest away.

II. Sharpening Procedure

◆ Prepare a workplace with good illumination and some means of magnification such as loupes or a magnified light ring.

◆ Place the sterile file on a clean surface. Secure it with the series of teeth facing up.

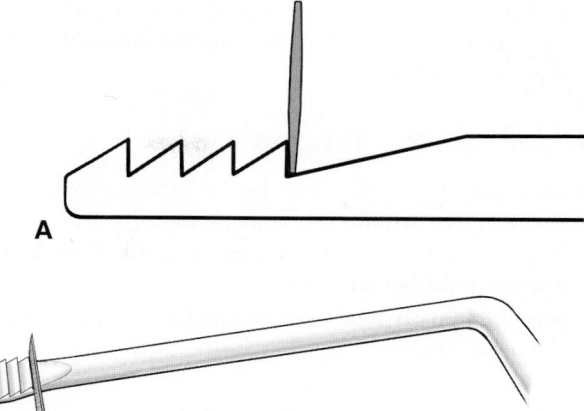

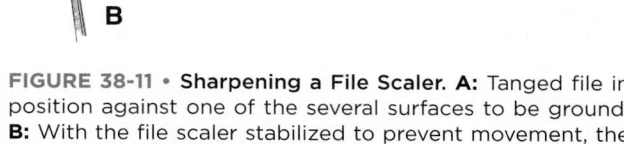

FIGURE 38-11 • Sharpening a File Scaler. A: Tanged file in position against one of the several surfaces to be ground. **B:** With the file scaler stabilized to prevent movement, the tanged file is pulled through the channel using a moderate, steady pressure against the surface to be ground.

◆ Position the right end of the tanged file in the channel as shown in the illustration (Figure 38-11A). (Left-handed clinicians reverse the process, positioning the left end of the tanged file in the channel.)

◆ With light-to-moderate steady pressure, pull the tanged file through the channel, moving in a straight line from one end to the other in one direction only.

◆ Release pressure and reposition the tanged file back at the starting point. Repeat the process. Two or three passes with the tanged file are usually sufficient to bring each edge back to sharpness.

◆ Sharpen the remaining blades using the same technique.

◆ Test for sharpness and repeat the sharpening stroke as needed for ideal edge sharpness.

CARE OF SHARPENING EQUIPMENT

I. Flat Sharpening Stone

A. Prepare for Sterilization

Submerge in ultrasonic cleaner or scrub with soap and water to remove metal particles left from sharpening.

B. Stain Removal

◆ Check manufacturer's recommendation.

◆ Alternate cleaning suggestions: Use powdered cleanser when stone becomes discolored. If the stone becomes "glazed" by metal particles ground into the surface, rub sandpaper over the stone placed on a flat, solid surface.

C. Storage

◆ Keep in sealed, sterilized packages for sharpening at instrument preparation area.

◆ A stone and testing stick should be stored with each instrument setup in the cassette for use during the treatment appointment.

II. Care of the Tanged File

Because the tanged file corrodes easily when exposed to moisture, it may require special handling.

◆ Wipe the tanged file with a sterile gauze soaked with isopropyl alcohol after use.

◆ Sterilize in a dry heat oven or chemical vapor sterilizer (Chapter 7).

III. Manufacturer's Directions

Follow manufacturer's directions for all artificial stones.

DOCUMENTATION

◆ See Box 38-1 for a sample documentation.

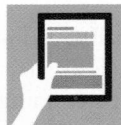

BOX 38-1

Example Documentation:
Monitoring of Sharpness of Instruments

S—Female patient, 48 years old and in good health, presents for the third in a series of scaling and root planing appointments (maxillary left quadrant).

O—Previously documented assessment findings for maxillary left quadrant include: heavy generalized calculus, generalized 4–5 mm probing depths, and 8 mm probing depth on the mesial of #12 and distal of #15 (furcation involvement).

A—Burnished calculus was noted on the quadrants completed.

P—Instrument sharpness carefully monitored. File scaler was used to break up burnished calculus and rigid Gracey curettes used for removal. Completed quadrant debridement with ultrasonic and manual instruments. Extended shank minicurets were used for root debridement in the mesial concavity of #12 and distal furcation of #15.

Next steps: Scheduled for scaling and root planing on mandibular left quadrant and re-evaluate completed quadrants, particularly pocket areas >4 mm.

Signed: _____, RDH

Date: _____

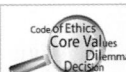
Code of Ethics
Core Values
Dilemma
Decision

EVERYDAY ETHICS

Leslie is eager to begin a new position in her first year of clinical practice as a dental hygienist. Dr. Shepherd has been in practice for 15 years and most staff members have been with him at least the past 10 years, including Ann, the dental hygienist with whom she will be practicing. Leslie is glad to have someone with experience take her under her wing. A dental assistant takes care of instrument sterilization and tray setups for the dental hygienists. As she sat down to her first patient, she noticed the instruments on her instrument cassette were all sickle scalers and she wanted curets. On closer inspection, however, she discovered that all but one instrument were indeed curets; they had just been sharpened incorrectly, leaving them with no contour (curvature) at the toe. She excused herself to go into the instrument supply room only to find that all of the curets had sharp, pointed toes. Going back to the clinical area, she peeked in to ask Ann if the assistant did the sharpening for her (as she glanced at Ann's tray she noted the curets were equally sharpened to a distinct point). Ann answered, "No, I do all the sharpening myself because I am very picky."

Leslie suddenly realizes nothing has ever been said in a work description about who orders new dental hygiene instruments. She had learned in school that dental hygiene practitioners took care of their own instruments. Leslie pondered what she would do to address this situation—especially how to approach it without alienating her new coworkers.

Questions for Consideration

1. Given Leslie's novice status as a clinician, how will she approach her new colleague—an experienced practitioner—with her concerns? Which core values of dental hygiene are involved in this scenario?

2. What harm, if any, is affecting Dr. Shepherd's patients? Discuss whether the dentist needs to be notified about the condition of the instruments.

3. Utilizing an ethical decision framework (see Chapter 1), describe realistic alternatives for Leslie's course of action in this situation.

Factors to Teach the Patient

▶ Benefits of using a finely sharpened instrument for calculus removal.

▶ Harmful effects of using dull instruments.

ENHANCE YOUR UNDERSTANDING

ONLINE RESOURCES
(see the inside front cover for access information)

- Audio glossary
- Appendices

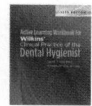

SUPPORT FOR LEARNING
(available separately)

- *Active Learning Workbook for Wilkins' Clinical Practice of the Dental Hygienist, 13th Edition*

INDIVIDUALIZED REVIEW

- Customized practice quizzing with Navigate 2 TestPrep for *Wilkins' Clinical Practice of the Dental Hygienist*

References

1. Wiebe CB, Hoath BJ, Owen G, Bi J, Giannelis G, Larjava HS. Sterilization of ceramic sharpening stones. *J Can Dent Assoc.* 2017 September;83:h11.

2. Balevi B. Engineering specifics of the periodontal curet's cutting edge. *J Periodontol.* 1996 Apr;67(4):374–378.

3. Nahass HE, Madkour GG. Evaluation of different re-sharpening techniques on the working edge of periodontal scalers: a scanning electron microscopic study. *Life Sci J.* 2013;10(1):589–593.

4. Andrade Acevedo RA, Cézar Sampaio JE, Shibli JA. Scanning electron microscope assessment of several resharpening techniques on the cutting edges of Gracey curettes. *J Contemp Dent Pract.* 2007 November 1;8(7):70–77.

5. Silva MV, Gomes DA, Leite FR, et al. Sharpening of periodontal instruments with different sharpening stones and its influence upon root debridement—scanning electronic microscopy assessment. *J Int Acad Periodontol.* 2006;8(1):17–22.

6. Hessheimer HM, Payne JB, Shaw LE, Spanyers EM, Beatty MW. A comparison of efficiency and material wear of diamond-plated versus ceramic sharpening stones. *J Dent Hyg.* 2017 October;91(5):64–67.

Nonsurgical Periodontal Therapy and Adjunctive Therapy

Linda D. Boyd, RDH, RD, EdD, Uhlee (Yuri) Oh, RDH, BS, MSDH, and
Esther M. Wilkins, BS, RDH, DMD

CHAPTER OUTLINE

NONSURGICAL PERIODONTAL THERAPY
I. Introduction to Components of Initial Periodontal Therapy
II. Overview of Nonsurgical Periodontal Therapy Outcomes

AIMS AND EXPECTED OUTCOMES
I. Interrupt or Arrest the Progress of Disease
II. Create an Environment to Encourage Healing and Resolution of Inflammation
III. Induce Positive Changes in the Quality and Quantity of Subgingival Bacterial Flora
IV. Provide Initial Preparation (Tissue Conditioning) for Surgical Periodontal Therapy in Advanced Disease
V. Educate and Motivate the Patient

NONSURGICAL PERIODONTAL THERAPY TREATMENT GOALS
I. Patient with Plaque (or Biofilm)-Induced Gingivitis
II. Patient with Mild-to-Moderate Periodontitis (Stage I or II)
III. Patients with Moderate-to-Severe Periodontitis (Stage III or IV), or Poor Response to Initial or Maintenance Therapy
IV. Patients Who Require Surgical or Other Advanced Periodontal Therapy

COMPONENTS OF NONSURGICAL PERIODONTAL THERAPY
I. Preventive Services
II. Dental Biofilm Removal
III. Calculus Removal
IV. Restorative Biofilm-Retentive Factors

DENTAL HYGIENE TREATMENT CARE PLAN FOR PERIODONTAL DEBRIDEMENT

APPOINTMENT PLANNING
I. Single Appointment
II. Multiple Appointments
III. Full-Mouth Disinfection
IV. Definitive Nonsurgical Periodontal Therapy

PREPARATION FOR PERIODONTAL DEBRIDEMENT
I. Review the Patient's Assessment Record
II. Review Radiographic Findings
III. Review Care Plan and Treatment Records
IV. Patient Preparation
V. Supragingival Examination
VI. Subgingival Examination
VII. Formulate Strategy for Instrumentation

ADVANCED INSTRUMENTATION
I. Definitions
II. Subgingival Anatomical Considerations
III. Instrumentation Technique

SPECIALIZED DEBRIDEMENT INSTRUMENTS
I. Furcation Debridement
II. Advanced Ultrasonic Tips
III. Microultrasonics
IV. Endoscope-Assisted Periodontal Debridement
V. Subgingival Air Polishing
VI. Laser Therapy

POST-OP INSTRUCTION FOR PERIODONTAL DEBRIDEMENT APPOINTMENTS
I. Management of Discomfort
II. Oral Self-Care

III. Diet
IV. Emergency Management
V. Instruction Format

RE-EVALUATION OF NONSURGICAL PERIODONTAL THERAPY
I. Clinical Endpoints
II. Re-evaluation Time Frame
III. Re-evaluation Procedure

ADJUNCTIVE THERAPY

ANTIMICROBIAL THERAPY
I. Systemic Delivery of Antibiotics
II. Systemic Subantimicrobial Dose Antibiotics
III. Local Delivery Antimicrobials Agents

INDICATIONS FOR USE OF LOCAL DELIVERY AGENTS
I. Nonsurgical Periodontal Therapy
II. Adjunctive Treatment: At Re-Evaluation
III. Recurrent Disease
IV. Peri-Implantitis

TYPES OF LOCAL DELIVERY AGENTS
I. Minocycline Hydrochloride
II. Doxycycline Hyclate
III. Chlorhexidine Gluconate

DOCUMENTATION

EVERYDAY ETHICS

FACTORS TO TEACH THE PATIENT

REFERENCES

LEARNING OBJECTIVES

After studying this chapter, the student will be able to:

1. Explain the goals and desirable clinical endpoints or outcomes for nonsurgical periodontal therapy.

2. Devise a care plan for a patient with slight-to-moderate chronic periodontitis.

3. Describe the changes in the subgingival bacteria after periodontal debridement.

4. Describe current evidence related to laser therapy for initial therapy.

5. Develop postoperative instructions for a patient following a nonsurgical periodontal therapy appointment.

6. List the steps in re-evaluation of nonsurgical periodontal therapy and the decisions that must be made based on the clinical outcomes.

7. Compare and contrast the risks and benefits of systemic antibiotics and local delivery antimicrobials.

8. Critically evaluate the benefit of local delivery antimicrobials on changes in pocket depth and clinical attachment level (CAL).

NONSURGICAL PERIODONTAL THERAPY

I. Introduction to Components of Initial Periodontal Therapy

◆ *Periodontal debridement* remains the "gold standard" for initial therapy in inflammatory gingival and periodontal infections and includes the following therapeutic interventions[1-4]:

• Management or elimination of modifiable risk factors for periodontal disease.

• Patient education for preventive strategies including control of biofilm, tobacco cessation, and nutritional counseling with ongoing evaluation and reinforcement.

• Nonsurgical periodontal therapy (NSPT) to remove dental biofilm, endotoxins, other bacterial products, and calculus.

• Administration of antimicrobial or antibiotic agents as appropriate to enhance periodontal treatment outcomes.

• Elimination of local factors contributing to periodontal disease, including:
  • Overhanging margins of restorations.
  • Unfinished, poorly contoured, or unpolished restorations.
  • Carious lesions.
  • Ill-fitting prosthetic devices.
  • Occlusal trauma.

• Re-evaluation of initial therapy to identify the need for surgical periodontal therapy or ongoing periodontal maintenance.

II. Overview of Nonsurgical Periodontal Therapy Outcomes

◆ The therapeutic goals of periodontal therapy are to manage or eliminate plaque biofilm and risk factors for periodontitis in order to stop progression of disease and maintain oral health.

◆ NSPT consisting of periodontal debridement can provide the definitive or complete treatment for many patients with mild-to-moderate periodontitis. Research shows the following outcomes[1-4]:

• Reduction in inflammation and infection.
• Reductions in pocket depth.
• Gains in clinical attachment.

◆ Research suggests NSPT plus certain adjunctive therapies may have an additive effect on improvements in clinical attachment level (CAL). The adjunctive therapies with moderate evidence of efficacy include[3]:

• Systemic subantimicrobial dose doxycycline (SSD).
• Systemic antimicrobials.
• Chlorhexidine gluconate (CHX) chips.
• Photodynamic therapy with a diode laser.

◆ The long-term success of treatment depends on the following[4]:

• *Control* of the dental biofilm by the patient on a daily basis.
• Management of modifiable periodontal risk factors.
• Regular periodontal maintenance based on risk factors and disease control.[5]
• A skilled clinician to provide definitive debridement initially and on an ongoing basis.

AIMS AND EXPECTED OUTCOMES

The effects and benefits of complete, carefully performed NSPT are summarized here.

I. Interrupt or Arrest the Progress of Disease

◆ Reduce formation of dental biofilm.

◆ Delay repopulation of pathogenic microorganisms.

◆ Change behavioral and lifestyle habits of the patient to reduce risk factors for periodontal infections.

II. Create an Environment to Encourage Healing and Resolution of Inflammation

- Facilitate resolution of disease to restore health.
- Reduce pocket depths.[1]
- Eliminate bleeding on probing (BOP).
- Restore the gingival tissues to normal texture, color, size, and contour.
- Increase attachment level.[1,3]
- Remove calculus and restorative dentistry irregularities to reduce biofilm retention.[4]

III. Induce Positive Changes in Quality and Quantity of Subgingival Bacterial Flora

- Before instrumentation, the predominant microorganisms are anaerobic, gram-negative, motile forms with many spirochetes and rods, high counts of all types of microorganisms, and many leukocytes.
- After instrumentation, the composition of the bacterial flora tends to shift to a predominance of aerobic, gram-positive, nonmotile, coccoid forms with lower bacterial load (Table 39-1).
  - However, in some individuals, periodontal pathogens may persist after NSPT, and further treatment may be necessary to manage periodontal disease progression.[6]

IV. Provide Initial Preparation (Tissue Conditioning) for Surgical Periodontal Therapy in Advanced Disease

- Reduce or eliminate etiologic and predisposing factors.[7]
- Re-evaluation following initial NSPT allows for identification of those areas requiring surgical intervention.[7]

TABLE 39-1 • Effect of Instrumentation on Pocket Microflora

PERIODONTAL INFECTION BEFORE TREATMENT	PERIODONTAL HEALTH AFTER TREATMENT
Predominant flora is: Anaerobic Gram negative Motile Spirochetes, motile rods; pathogenic	Predominant flora is: Aerobic Gram positive Nonmotile Coccoid forms; nonpathogenic
Total microbial count: Very high total count of all types of microorganisms	Total microbial count: Much lower total counts of all types of microorganisms
Leukocyte count: Many leukocytes	Leukocyte count: Lower leukocyte counts

V. Educate and Motivate the Patient

- To assume a co-therapist role in maintaining periodontal health following nonsurgical and/or surgical periodontal treatment.
- To make a commitment to perform daily personal biofilm control measures.
- To continue with periodontal maintenance appointments at intervals consistent with patient's individual risk factors to monitor and manage periodontal disease.[5,8]

NONSURGICAL PERIODONTAL THERAPY TREATMENT GOALS

I. Patient with Plaque (or Biofilm)-Induced Gingivitis

- Complete scaling.
- Patient compliance in personal daily biofilm removal.
- *Therapeutic goal*: Reversal of inflammation to establish gingival health through elimination of etiologic factors.[9]

II. Patient with Mild-to-Moderate Periodontitis (Stage I or II)

- Control of infection may be attained through NSPT.
- Maintaining the healthy state requires continuing routine appointments for professional scaling and supervision of the patient's biofilm removal methods.
- *Therapeutic goals*[4]:
  - Reduction in gingival inflammation and BOP.
  - Reduction in pocket depths.
  - CALs are stabilized or improved.
  - Decrease in detectable dental biofilm to a level consistent with health.

III. Patients with Moderate-to-Severe Periodontitis (Stage III or IV) or Patients with Poor Response to Initial or Maintenance Therapy

- Supplemental therapeutic measures, such as adjunctive chemotherapeutics, may be needed.
- Specialized instruments may be required for deep pockets, furcations, and complex anatomical features of involved diseased root surfaces.
- *Therapeutic goals*[7]:
  - Same goals as mild-to-moderate periodontal conditions.
  - Radiographic improvement in osseous lesions.
  - Occlusal stabilization.

IV. Patients Who Require Surgical or Other Advanced Periodontal Therapy

◆ Certain periodontal conditions will require surgical or other advanced therapeutic procedures. Examples of surgical periodontal procedures include[7]:

- *Gingival augmentation therapy:* periodontal plastic surgeries, gingival grafts.
- *Regenerative procedures:* bone grafting, guided tissue regeneration.
- *Resective therapy:* gingival flaps with or without osseous surgery, root resective therapy, gingivectomy.

◆ For these patients, thorough NSPT prepares the tissues for the surgical phase of treatment by reducing the bacterial load and reducing inflammation.

COMPONENTS OF NONSURGICAL PERIODONTAL THERAPY

I. Preventive Services

◆ Education for patients and collaboration with primary care providers for patients with systemic conditions for which periodontal infection is a risk factor (e.g., pregnancy, cardiovascular disease, diabetes).[4,7,9]

◆ Fluoride applications and other preventive measures, especially for root caries prevention in the patient with recession.

◆ At-home rinsing, irrigation, other selective use of antimicrobials, and fluorides (dentifrice, chlorhexidine, water fluoridation).

◆ Smoking cessation support and referral to services as appropriate.

◆ Dietary assessment and counseling.

◆ Desensitization of teeth.

◆ Care for dental implants and prostheses.

II. Dental Biofilm Removal

◆ Gingival inflammation and periodontal destruction result from the action of pathogenic microorganisms in dental biofilm and the host response.

◆ Endotoxin

- Lipopolysaccharides or endotoxins, derived from the cell walls of gram-negative pathogenic microorganisms, trigger an inflammatory host response, leading to periodontitis and destruction of the periodontal attachment.[8]
- Endotoxins exist in biofilm and can be removed with scaling.
- Calculus removal results in endotoxin levels consistent with health.[10,11]

◆ Cementum

- The cementum is thin at the cervical third of the root, and some removal of the cementum during

instrumentation for calculus removal is inevitable. However, the cementum should be preserved as much as possible as it serves as a source of growth factors for **new attachment**.[12]

III. Calculus Removal

◆ Calculus is not directly a cause of gingival inflammation, but it provides an environment for biofilm retention.[13]

◆ Although historically a smooth root surface was the endpoint for scaling, the current evidence suggests disruption of biofilm and removal of calculus along with preservation of the cementum is the ideal endpoint of root debridement.[12]

IV. Restorative Biofilm-Retentive Factors

◆ Overhanging margins and rough surfaces of restorations create a niche for biofilm development.

◆ Personal oral self-care efforts by the patient are impeded by overhanging margins, irregular margins that are breaking down, and poorly contoured restorations.

◆ Removal of an overhanging margin or replacement is a critical component of facilitating returning the periodontium to health.

DENTAL HYGIENE TREATMENT CARE PLAN FOR PERIODONTAL DEBRIDEMENT

◆ The needs of the individual patient are identified through patient assessment (refer to Chapter 20).

◆ The course of treatment is defined by the dental hygiene diagnosis and care plan (refer to Chapters 22 and 23). Included in the care plan are the following:

- Management of individual modifiable risk factors such as tobacco cessation.
- Periodontal diagnosis, including the distribution and severity of the periodontal infection.
- Treatment sequence needed for the individual.
- Length and number of appointments required to complete treatment.
- Plan for re-evaluation and continuing care (described in Chapters 44 and 45).

APPOINTMENT PLANNING

◆ Whether a single or multiple appointment plan is required, the initial step is patient education.

◆ The overall care plan should be reviewed and discussed to obtain informed consent of the patient, parent, or guardian obtained.

◆ Treatment begins with the patient taking responsibility for daily removal of biofilm.

I. Single Appointment

◆ The diagnosis may be gingivitis (Chapter 19) with minimal inflammation and small deposits near gingival margin; local anesthesia may not be needed.

◆ If only a few teeth are periodontally involved and require localized NSPT, limited areas of local anesthesia may be required.

◆ Patient presents with an acceptable biofilm score, and evidence of reasonable oral self-care without need for time to provide extended follow-up instruction.

◆ Patient acts responsibly in keeping appointments for periodontal maintenance and continued monitoring for disease control.

II. Multiple Appointments

Factors that determine the number of appointments needed include the extent of periodontal involvement as shown by probing measurements, distribution and extent of calculus deposits, and adequate biofilm removal.

A. Management of Modifiable Risk Factors

◆ At the initial appointment, education should begin to manage modifiable risk factors, such as tobacco cessation and biofilm removal. Chapter 24 provides guidance on motivational interviewing to assist with this component of treatment.

◆ Patient education to assess and refine daily oral self-care techniques for dental biofilm removal is initiated at the first NSPT appointment.

  • Interdental devices to complement the use of a toothbrush can be added as the patient demonstrates readiness. It is important not to overwhelm the patient at the first appointment.

◆ At each successive appointment, disclose the biofilm and review with the patient.

◆ Add new oral hygiene aids as needed based on patient's preferences and dexterity.

◆ Typically, inflammation and bleeding will gradually improve at each appointment as a result of improvement in biofilm removal and periodontal debridement.

B. Quadrant Scaling Appointments

◆ One system for appointment planning is by quadrants or sextants with local anesthesia for moderate-to-severe disease, such as stages III and IV periodontitis, at 1-week intervals.

  • This allows for review of oral self-care and healing of the area(s) previously treated.

◆ With less severe periodontitis, such as stage I or II, and a compliant patient, two quadrants on the same side (maxillary and mandibular arches) may be completed at an appointment.

◆ After periodontal debridement is completed, the need for re-evaluation should be reinforced to assess the need for additional care.

◆ The periodontal maintenance interval should be determined based on the patient risk for disease progression.

C. Evaluation

◆ At each appointment, the healing of the quadrants previously treated should be assessed.

◆ Any residual calculus remaining can be removed.

◆ Best done 4–8 weeks following completion of NSPT to allow for connective tissue healing.[14]

◆ Re-evaluation is important to determine the periodontal maintenance interval and the need for referral and/or surgical therapy.

III. Full-Mouth Disinfection

A. Definition

◆ System of performing NSPT in two long appointments completed within a 24-hour period with adjunctive chlorhexidine mouthrinse.[15]

◆ The procedures are best accomplished under local anesthesia with a chairside dental assistant.

◆ Systematic review of the research on full-mouth disinfection versus traditional NSPT found no clear evidence of a benefit for one approach over another.[15]

◆ The approach of NSPT selected needs to be based on patient preference and scheduling options.

B. Rationale

◆ The rationale is completing the procedure in one session or multiple sessions within 24 hours reduces likelihood of re-infection of previously treated sites.[15]

C. Limitations

◆ Case selection: Many patients would not be able to withstand such intense treatment.

◆ Patient instruction: Eliminates opportunities for review and repeated instruction at the patient's learning pace without a series of appointments with time in between for patient practice of oral self-care.

◆ The ability to re-evaluate immediate healing of each quadrant is also not possible.

IV. Definitive Nonsurgical Periodontal Therapy

A. Quadrant or Sextant Approach

◆ Quadrant or sextant treatment to completion is recommended.

◆ The decision between a quadrant and sextant approach is made according to what can reasonably be completed by the clinician and tolerated by the patient during an appointment.

◆ Treatment appointments are scheduled accordingly.

B. Factors to Consider in Care Planning

◆ *Access:* the relative ease of instrument insertion to the base of the soft-tissue pocket.
  • Tissue tone, such as fibrosity of the free gingiva.
  • Probing depths: attachment pattern around the full circumference of each tooth.
◆ *Deposit on tooth surfaces*
  • Extent and distribution of calculus.
  • Age of calculus/degree of mineralization.
  • Strength of attachment of calculus to the tooth.
◆ *Root anatomy*
  • Multirooted teeth with furcation involvement.
  • Deep concavities.
◆ *Patient factors*
  • Behavioral factors, such as apprehension.
  • Need for local anesthetic or nitrous oxide/oxygen sedation.
  • Limited capacity for opening mouth.

PREPARATION FOR PERIODONTAL THERAPY

I. Review the Patient's Assessment Record

◆ Document individual needs: from medical, dental, and psychosocial history along with previous appointment experiences.

◆ Identify systemic or physical problems with potential for emergency.

II. Review Radiographic Findings

A. Findings Applicable During Instrumentation

◆ Anatomic features of roots, furcations, and bone level, which may impact selection and adaptation of instruments.

◆ Overhanging restorations to be removed or scheduled for replacement.

B. Use Radiographs as Guide

◆ Keep radiographs on lighted viewbox or computer screen throughout the treatment for reference to observe bone level, root anatomy, and contour of restorations for each area.

III. Review Care Plan and Treatment Records

◆ Document flow and sequence of planned appointments.

◆ Document findings related to the instrumentation process.
  • Assess periodontal chart to review attachment topography and access limitations.
  • Assemble procedure tray setup or cassette to include appropriate instruments.
◆ Review previous appointment progress notes.
  • Read details of prior treatment, noting quadrants or sextants completed, which will be reassessed for healing.
  • Ascertain how previous treatment appointments have been tolerated by the patient.
  • Plan appropriate local anesthesia for pain management.
◆ Keep periodontal probing chart within view of the clinician throughout the treatment for reference.

IV. Patient Preparation

A. Premedication Requirements for High-Risk Patient

◆ Transient bacteremia can occur during and immediately after scaling procedures.
  • Flossing and a single quadrant of scaling and root debridement result in the same incidence and magnitude of bacteremia, so only high-risk patients are in need of antibiotic premedication.[16]
◆ Consult with the primary care provider to determine whether premedication is required (see Chapter 11 to identify patients who may be at risk for bacterial endocarditis and be in need of prophylactic premedication).

B. Provide Preprocedural Antimicrobial Rinse

◆ Preprocedural rinsing with chlorhexidine gluconate lowers bacterial aerosols and contamination produced by ultrasonic instrumentation.[17,18]

◆ Preprocedural rinsing with chlorhexidine rinse has not been shown to reduce bacteremia, or bacteria in the bloodstream following NSPT.[19]

C. Prepare for Local Anesthesia

◆ Adequate pain control tends to facilitate better patient outcomes and higher levels of patient satisfaction with treatment.

◆ Patients who refuse local anesthesia experience more discomfort, dental anxiety, longer treatment times, greater residual gingival inflammation, and more pocket depths greater than or equal to 5 mm.[20]
  • Rather than asking patients if they "want" local anesthesia, the clinician should state the best

treatment option and discuss the impact of pain control on improved outcomes to aid the patient in decision-making.

V. Supragingival Examination

A. Visual

◆ Gross deposits and tooth surface irregularities can be seen by direct vision. Fine, unstained, white, or yellowish calculus is frequently invisible when wet with saliva.

◆ Observe tooth surfaces closely while applying a gentle stream of compressed air. Dry calculus is more visible than wet calculus.

B. Tactile

◆ An enamel surface without deposits or anatomical irregularities is smooth.

◆ An explorer tip passed over the surface slides freely, smoothly, and quietly.

◆ When rough calculus deposits are present, the explorer tip does not slide freely, but meets with resistance over varying textures.

◆ Deposits can produce a surface that feels like sand paper or a click as the explorer passes over them.

VI. Subgingival Examination

A. Visual

◆ *Gingiva*: The clinical appearance suggestive of underlying calculus may be the following:
  • Soft, spongy, bluish-red gingiva, with enlargement of the interdental papillae over proximal surface calculus.
  • Dark-colored area beneath relatively translucent marginal gingiva.

◆ *Calculus*
  • A loose, edematous pocket wall can be deflected from the tooth surface with a gentle stream of compressed air.
  • Dark, subgingival calculus can be seen within the pocket on the root.

B. Tactile

◆ *Periodontal charting*
  • Use probing depth recordings as a basic guide for the depth of insertion of the curet.
  • Study the soft-tissue attachment pattern for instrument selection to provide access to the base of the pocket.

◆ *Identify shallow pockets (sulci)*
  • Scaling in shallow pockets of fewer than 3 mm can lead to loss of periodontal attachment due to detachment of periodontal ligament fibers, so it should be done with care.[1]
  • Root surfaces free of calculus require minimal lateral pressure for comprehensive biofilm removal.

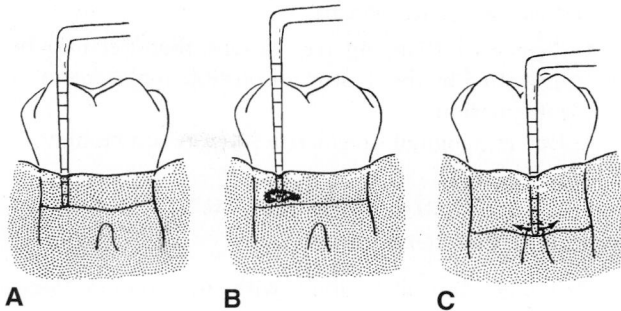

FIGURE 39-1 • **Subgingival Examination Using a Probe. A:** Probe inserted into the bottom of a pocket for complete examination prior to subgingival scaling. **B:** As the probe passes over the root surface, it may be intercepted by a hard mass of calculus. **C:** Using a horizontal probe stroke to examine the topography of a furcation area. Keep the side of the tip of the probe on the tooth surface and slide over one root, into the furcation, and across to the other root.

◆ *Determine distribution and extent of deposits*
  • Use an explorer, such as an ODU 11/12, for detection of calculus deposits.
  • The novice dental hygiene student will benefit from recording the location of calculus.
  • The periodontal probe may also detect the presence of calculus deposits, as shown in Figure 39-1.

◆ *Evaluate tooth topography*
  • Detect grooves and furcations using a horizontal stroke (Figure 39-1C).
  • Use a Nabers furcation probe to examine furcations (see Chapter 20).
  • Note anatomic root and furcation variations (Figure 39-2).

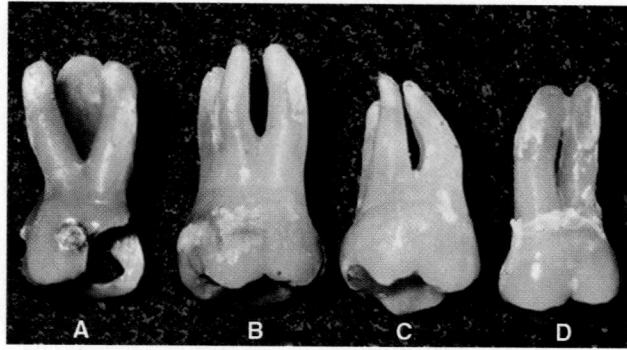

FIGURE 39-2 • **Anatomic Variations of Furcations. A:** Divergent roots with the furcation in the coronal one-third of the root with a short root trunk. **B:** Convergent roots with the furcation in the middle one half of the root with a longer root trunk. **C:** Very convergent roots. **D:** Fused roots with the furcation in the coronal one-third of the root. (Reprinted from Scheid R, Weiss G. *Woelfel's Dental Anatomy.* Philadelphia, PA: Lippincott Williams & Wilkins; 2016.)

◆ *Evaluate restorative margins*
  • Detect overhanging restorations that need to be evaluated by the dentist for possible replacement or margination.
  • Detect marginal irregularities that retain biofilm.

VII. Formulate Strategy for Instrumentation

◆ Combine clinical findings with information documented in the patient's record.
◆ Review overall treatment objectives for the patient.
◆ Determine a strategy for instrumentation.

ADVANCED INSTRUMENTATION

I. Definitions

◆ *Scaling and root planing (SRP)*: entails removal of calculus and "diseased" cementum. It was previously considered the desired endpoint necessary in order to achieve periodontal health.
  • Evidence now demonstrates removal of cementum is not necessary to reduce endotoxin levels and cementum needs to be preserved to facilitate new attachment.[10,11,21]
  • SRP is common terminology used in private practice and by insurance companies.
◆ *Periodontal debridement* or *root surface debridement*: involves disruption and removal of dental biofilm and associated endotoxins along with calculus from the root. Use of ultrasonic instrumentation, along with avoidance of excessive instrumentation time and pressure, helps to preserve cementum and dentin.[21]

II. Subgingival Anatomical Considerations

◆ *Tooth morphology*
  • Level of clinical attachment (normal or clinical attachment loss) varies; more attachment loss, resulting in deeper pocket depths exposing additional root concavities and possible furcations, complicates instrumentation.
  • The cementum is thin (0.03–0.06 mm), and care must be taken to minimize removal during instrumentation.[11]
◆ *Soft-tissue pocket wall*
  • The pocket is an extremely small area for manipulation of instruments.
  • The pocket narrows in the deeper area next to the clinical attachment.
  • Bleeding during instrumentation can impact visibility.
◆ *Variations in probing depths*
  • The periodontal charting is a guide to subgingival instrumentation and will serve as a road map to guide instrument depth of insertion.
◆ *Nature of subgingival calculus*
  • *Location*: Calculus may be located on the enamel or the root or both (Figure 39-3).
  • *Morphology of calculus*: Subgingival calculus is irregularly deposited. It can present as a spicule, ledge, smooth veneer, and other forms (Chapter 17).
  • Burnished calculus: Subgingival calculus that has been partially scaled and left after incomplete instrumentation may be smooth and may not be detected when an explorer is used to check the area.

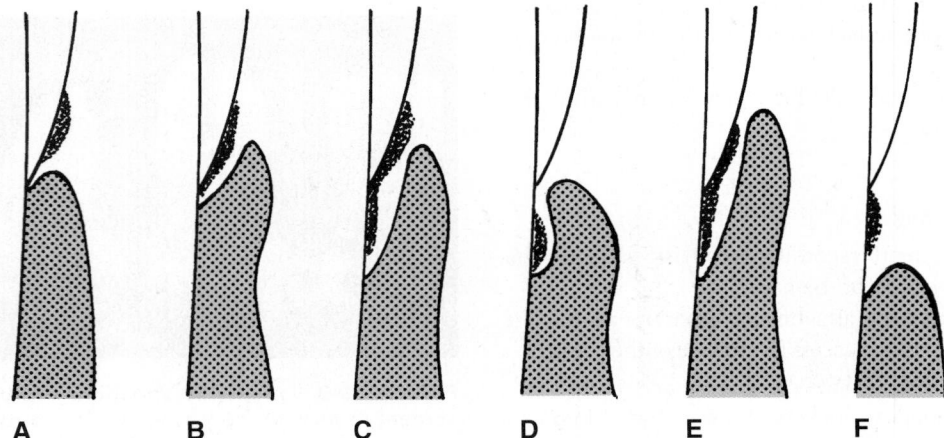

FIGURE 39-3 • Location of Instrumentation. The location of calculus deposits, level of periodontal attachment, depth of pocket, and position of the gingival margin determine the site of instrumentation. **A:** Supragingival calculus on the enamel. **B:** Gingival pocket with both supragingival and subgingival calculus on enamel. **C:** Periodontal pocket with both supragingival and subgingival calculus. **D:** Periodontal pocket with subgingival calculus only on the root surface. **E:** Periodontal pocket with subgingival calculus on both the enamel and the root surface. **F:** Calculus on the root surface exposed by gingival recession.

III. Instrumentation Technique

Types of instruments and the basic principles for their use are included in Chapter 37. This chapter focuses on the components of advanced instrumentation for deposit removal. Box 39-1 summarizes the steps.

BOX 39-1
Steps for Calculus Removal Using Manual Instruments

Assessment

- Probe to determine pocket/sulcus characteristics and confirm soft-tissue attachment topography.
- Explore to determine location and extent of deposits and tooth surface irregularities.
- Select correct instruments that will adapt and conform to concavities and other root morphology characteristics for areas being treated.

Preparation: Instrument Control

- Hold instrument with a modified pen grasp.
- Identify correct cutting edge of blade for surface being scaled.
  - For area-specific curets: terminal shank parallel with surface being scaled.
  - For universal curets: terminal shank *less* than parallel with surface being scaled (~20°).
- Establish a light finger rest for instrument placement to allow for adjustment and repositioning.
- Insert: use placement or exploratory stroke to locate apical edge of deposit.
- Adjust working angulation (average at 70°).

Action: Strokes

- Secure a stable, functional extraoral finger rest or intraoral fulcrum that can support instrument placement and activation at the correct working stroke angulation.
  - Pressure into the fulcrum equals the pressure against the tooth.
  - Balance fulcrum pressure with lateral pressure of the strokes.
- Activate for working stroke.
  - Apply firm lateral pressure for calculus removal.
  - Apply moderate lateral pressure to smooth the surface.
  - Apply light lateral pressure for biofilm debridement.
  - Control length and direction of stroke: respect to the **instrumentation zone**.
  - Maintain continuous adaptation throughout the stroke.

Channels: Overlap to Completion

- Continue channel scaling with overlapping multidirectional strokes.
  - Use an exploratory stroke to reposition blade for next stroke.
  - Activate instrument circumferentially around tooth.
  - Keep toe adapted around line angles by rolling handle.
  - Cover all surfaces comprehensively to remove all traces of calculus and biofilm.

Evaluation

- Use explorer to determine endpoint of treatment.

A. Instrument Selection and Sequence

- The order in which instruments are selected and used can impact the efficiency and quality of biofilm and calculus removal.
- Instrument selection sequence is recommended as follows (the order may vary depending on the depth of the periodontal pocket and tenacity of the calculus):
  - For stages I and II periodontitis, the following instruments are used in this order:
    1. Straight/*universal* and *triple bend-type* ultrasonic tips/inserts used on moderate-to-high power.
    2. Sickle scalers and/or periodontal files.
    3. Universal curets.
    4. Gracey curets.
    5. Precision-thin ultrasonic tips/inserts for final finishing.
  - For stages III and IV periodontitis where greater clinical attachment loss is involved, the following instruments may also be needed to access the base of pockets and furcation areas for debridement:
    1. Thin left/right ultrasonic tips/inserts used on low-to-moderate power.
    2. Mini-bladed area-specific Gracey curets.
    3. Micro-mini–bladed Gracey curets.
    4. Diamond files—used with light pressure only.
    5. Periodontal files.

B. Finger Rest

- Various factors such as tooth position and calculus tenacity may impact the fulcrum chosen.
- Review Chapter 37 for basics on fulcrums, which may include intraoral, extraoral, and alternative fulcrums such as supplementary, substitute, and reinforced.

C. Adaptation

- Keep working-end closely aligned with the surface of the tooth throughout the stroke.
- Convex surfaces, concavities, and furcations all require precise adaptation (Figure 39-4).

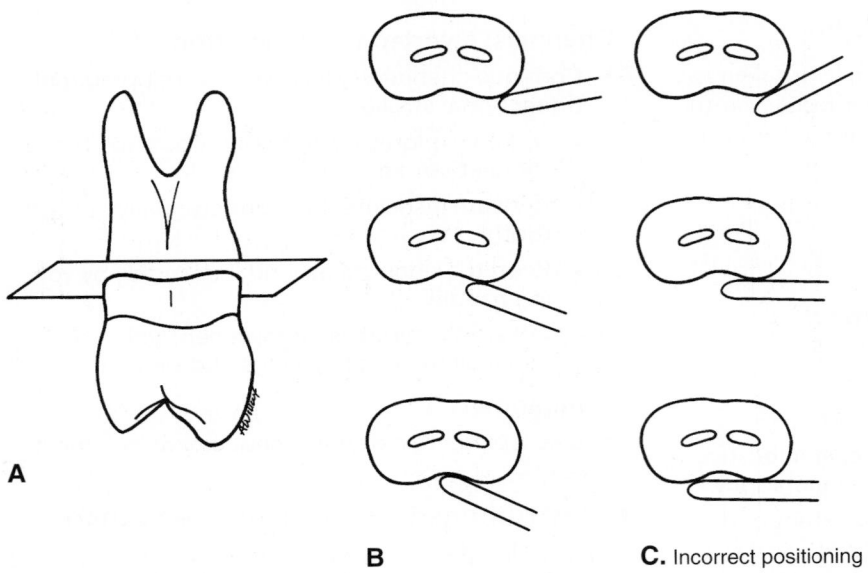

A

B

C. Incorrect positioning

FIGURE 39-4 • **Instrument Adaptation. A:** Maxillary first premolar shows cross section of root drawn for **(B)** and **(C)**. **B:** Diagram of three positions of a curet shows correct adaptation at a line angle and on the concave mesial surface with toe third of the instrument maintained on the tooth as the instrument is adapted. **C:** Diagram shows incorrect adaptation with toe of curet extended away from the tooth surface.

D. Lateral Pressure

◆ Light pressure is needed for exploration to position blade below the calculus deposit and to debride biofilm while preserving cementum.

◆ Moderate-to-heavy pressure is needed for manual working strokes depending on the degree of mineralization or tenacity of the calculus attachment.

◆ Factors affecting lateral pressure are as follows:

  • *Sharp instrument*
    • A minimum degree of pressure allows the cutting edge to "grab" the calculus.
    • Less time, with fewer strokes, is required.
    • Fatigue is kept to a minimum.

  • *Dull instrument*
    • When dull, the blade cannot engage the deposit and will slide over it, burnishing it on the surface, making it difficult to detect and remove.
    • Stroke control is reduced with the heavier pressure needed to activate a dull blade; this can lead to instrument slippage and trauma to the patient's gingival tissues.
    • Grasp and lateral pressures increase to compensate for the sliding effect.
    • More strokes are needed, causing increased fatigue.
    • Inefficiency increases treatment time.

E. Activation/Stroke

◆ Confine the strokes to the pocket to minimize the need for repeated reinsertion of the curet to prevent trauma to the gingival margin.

◆ Make strokes in channels (Figure 39-5).

  • At the completion of each stroke, move the instrument laterally a very short distance to assure overlap.

  • Maintain the same finger rest.

• Overlap strokes in channels to ensure complete coverage of subgingival surface for thorough removal of deposits.

• Repeat strokes until surface has been completely debrided.

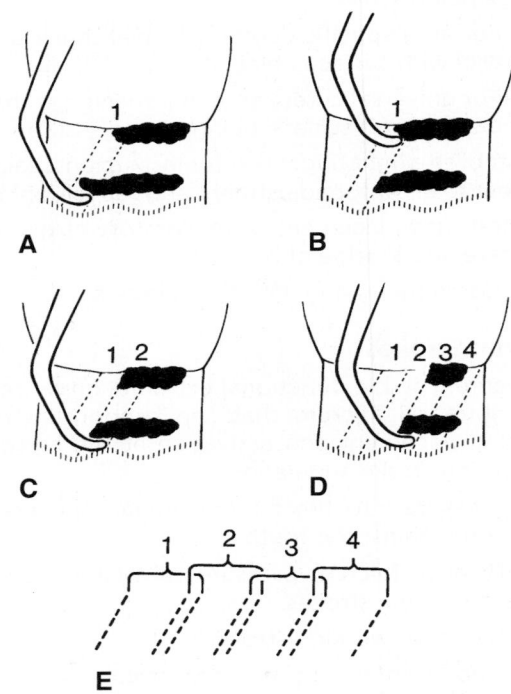

A

B

C

D

E

FIGURE 39-5 • **Channel Scaling. A:** Curet adapted in position for channel 1 stroke from the base of the pocket under the calculus deposit. **B:** Completion of stroke for channel 1. **C:** Using an exploratory stroke, the curet is lowered into the pocket and is positioned for calculus removal in channel 2. **D:** Curet positioned for channel 3. Several strokes in each channel may be needed to ensure complete calculus removal. **E:** Strokes of each channel overlap strokes of the previous channel. (Adapted from Parr RW, Green E, Madsen L, et al. *Subgingival Scaling and Root Planing.* Berkeley, CA: Praxis; 1976.)

F. Channeling

◆ Overlap strokes in channels to ensure complete coverage of subgingival surface for thorough removal of deposits (Figure 39-5).

◆ Maintain the same finger rest.

◆ At the completion of each stroke, move the instrument laterally a very short distance to assure overlap.

◆ Repeat strokes until surface has been completely debrided.

◆ As a surface area becomes smooth, a gradual change in the sound of the instrument stroke may occur as the calculus is removed.

SPECIALIZED DEBRIDEMENT INSTRUMENTS

I. Furcation Debridement

◆ Specialized instruments for furcation debridement include:
  • Precision-thin left/right ultrasonic tips/inserts *used at low power* may be used alone or in combination with hand instrumentation.
  • Mini-bladed Gracey numbers 5–6, 11–12, 13–14.
  • Micro-mini–bladed Gracey numbers 1–2, 11–12, 13–14.
  • Diamond files: *use only with light pressure.*

◆ Close adaptation of precision ultrasonic insert or blade to the contour of the furcation area.

◆ Use explorer such as regular or extended ODU 11/12 with light lateral pressure to assess root debridement.

II. Advanced Ultrasonic Tips

◆ Straight/*universal* and *triple bend-type tips* are used for moderate-to-heavy deposit removal on most surfaces; however, periodontal involvement may call for use of more specialized and area-specific tips, such as those listed in the subsequent section.

A. Thin/Periodontal Tip

◆ Thinner and longer tips provide better access to subgingival surfaces.

◆ Allow superior coverage of deep pockets and furcations.

◆ The limitation for magnetostrictive thin tips is they can only be used on low-to-medium power to prevent breakage and may burnish and/or not remove moderate-to-heavy calculus deposits. This limits their use to light calculus and biofilm debridement.[22]

◆ Piezoelectric thin tips may be used on high power.

B. Diamond-Coated Tip

◆ Limited evidence is available for diamond-coated tips.

◆ A small study suggests the diamond-coated tips appear to remove calculus efficiently.[23]

◆ It is not clear if cementum is preserved.[24]

C. Plastic, Silicone, or Carbon Composite Tip

◆ An insert with a plastic, silicone, or carbon composite tip may be used to protect vulnerable restorative surfaces, such as titanium abutments of implants or esthetic materials surfaces.[25,26]

◆ A low power, light pressure is all that is needed to remove biofilm and mineralizing deposits.

III. Microultrasonics

◆ Microultrasonics is a term used to describe the use of slimmer ultrasonic tips in conjunction with a dental endoscope to visualize subgingival calculus for debridement (Figure 39-6).[27]

◆ Advantages of microultrasonics include:
  • Reduce overinstrumentation.
  • Minimize excessive removal of cementum.

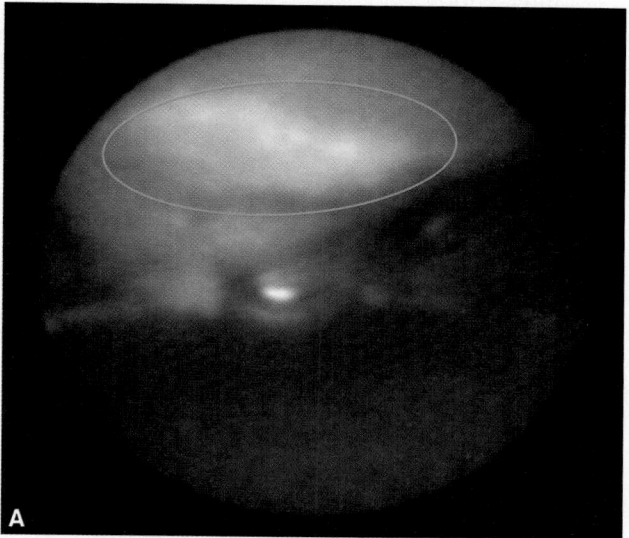

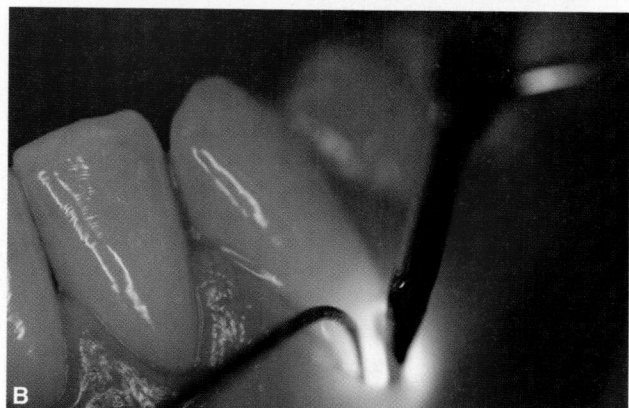

FIGURE 39-6 • Endoscope-Assisted Calculus Detection and Removal. A: The calculus is a cream white color because of the mineralization. The explorer for the endoscope is to at the bottom of the picture. **B:** In this image, the precision or slimline ultrasonic tip (left) is being used with the endoscope to the right. (Courtesy of Judy Carroll, RDH.)

- Improves outcomes and minimizes the need for periodontal surgery.
- *Quality of end product*: Enhance the quality of instrumentation by providing an objective means of evaluating root surface.
- *Patient education*: Create a new means of engaging, motivating, and educating the patient in the treatment.
- Provide opportunity for noninvasive, definitive root debridement:
  - When access is limited during routine instrumentation.
  - For sites unresponsive to traditional nonsurgical therapy.
  - In anterior regions where preservation of soft tissue is necessary for optimum esthetics.
  - When surgical therapy may be contraindicated for the patient.
- Provide confirmation of clinical findings that might otherwise go undiagnosed or require surgical intervention.
  - Root fractures.
  - Restorative following perforations.
  - Open margins.
  - Subgingival caries.
  - Residual cement.
  - Anatomical anomalies.
- Disadvantages
  - *Learning curve*: Using the endoscope to visualize root accretions is of significant benefit, but learning to utilize the endoscope is challenging and takes

regular use to become proficient. Some of the challenges include:
  - The clinician must work two-handed and hold the endoscope in the nondominant hand while adapting instruments and ultrasonic to the root surface with the dominant hand.
  - The clinician has to watch the monitor in order to assess the presence of calculus and adaptation for removal, which may impact ability to adapt to the root surface.
- The cost of the endoscope system and fiberoptic sheaths for each patient could be a disadvantage.

IV. Endoscope-Assisted Periodontal Debridement

The dental endoscope is a device developed to visualize below the gingival margin for use during diagnosis and instrumentation for treatment of periodontally diseased root surfaces.

- *Objectives*
  - Visualization of the root surface during instrumentation.
  - Explore, instrument, and evaluate the root surface using indirect visual observation on the device monitor.
  - Increase the effectiveness and thoroughness of root debridement.[28,29]
  - Augment subjective data collection with objective confirmation.
- *Dental Endoscope Components* (Figure 39-7A and B):

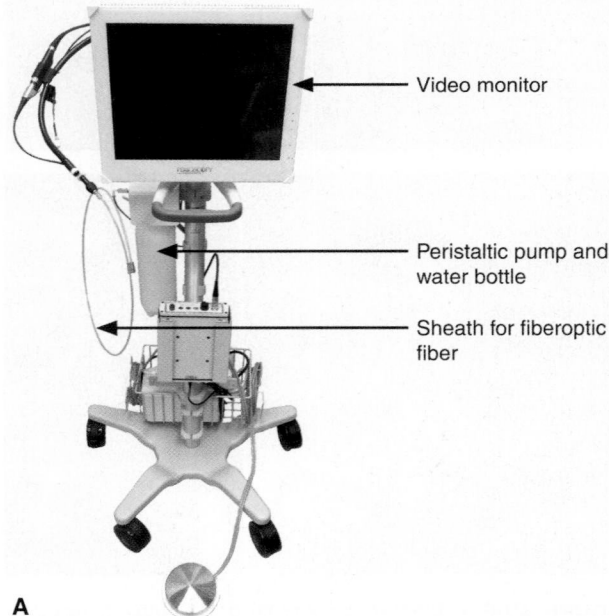

Video monitor

Peristaltic pump and water bottle

Sheath for fiberoptic fiber

A

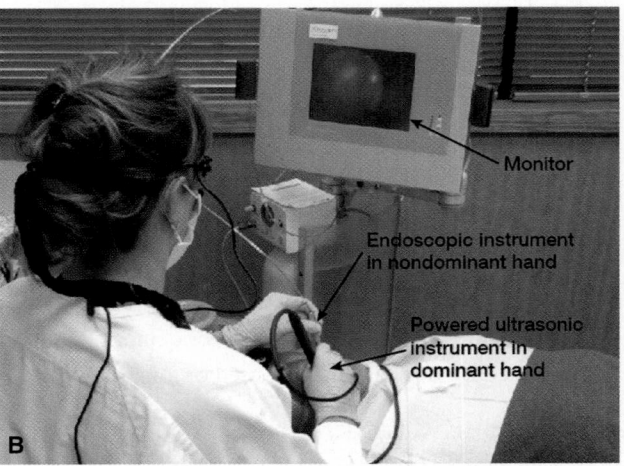

Monitor

Endoscopic instrument in nondominant hand

Powered ultrasonic instrument in dominant hand

B

FIGURE 39-7 • A: Dental endoscopic system. **B:** The clinician holds the endoscopic instrument in her nondominant hand. In this photo to visualize calculus and the root surface. The clinician uses microultrasonics in her dominant hand. (Courtesy of John Y. Kwan, DDS. Reprinted from Nield-Gehrig J. *Fundamentals of Periodontal Instrumentation and Advanced Root Instrumentation.* Philadelphia, PA: Lippincott Williams & Wilkins; 2011.)

- *Subgingival probe*: adapted to provide fiberoptic imaging with magnification.
- *Sheath* to provide a sterile barrier between the patient and the endoscope.
- *Peristaltic pump* to provide irrigation to the working field.
- *LED lamp* to provide illumination to the working field.
- *Video camera* to capture images of the working field for display.
- *Video monitor* for live viewing of the working field.
- *Specialized probes*, *curets*, and *retracting instruments* to maximize tissue visualization.

◆ *Indications for Use*
- During maintenance to detect and remove remaining deep burnished calculus deposits, which are the cause of continued BOP (Figure 39-6A and B).
- Advanced root debridement for patients unable or unwilling to have recommended surgical procedures.

V. Subgingival Air Polishing

◆ Over the years, subgingival air polishing has become a popular alternative to hand and ultrasonic instrumentation for subgingival biofilm management.[30]

◆ Subgingival air polishers deliver a stream of compressed air, water, and a nonabrasive powder (e.g., glycine or erythritol powder) through a nozzle to debride biofilm from shallow sulci, periodontal pockets, and around implants (Figure 39-8A).

◆ Subgingival air polishing has been shown to be equally effective as ultrasonic instrumentation in reducing BOP, periodontal probing depths, and attachment loss.[31]

◆ Advantages
- More effective than hand instrumentation at lowering bacterial counts in deep periodontal pockets.[32]
- Nonabrasive and safe to use on soft tissues, round restorations, and titanium implants.[33]
- Faster and more time-efficient than hand instrumentation.[34,35]
- Greater comfort for patients and less perceived pain than hand and ultrasonic instrumentation.[31,34,35]

A. Contraindications

Due to the production of water and aerosols, contraindications remain similar to those for the use of an ultrasonic scaler:

◆ Communicable diseases.

◆ Immunosuppression.

◆ Respiratory risk.

◆ Difficulty swallowing.

◆ Allergies to powder used.

B. Use

◆ Infection control protocol is also similar to that used for ultrasonic instrumentation, including the use of:
- Antimicrobial preprocedural mouth rinse.
- High-volume evacuator.
- Face mask with a high bacterial filtration efficiency (e.g., American Society for Testing and Materials level 3 mask).

◆ Technique for debriding shallow sulci:

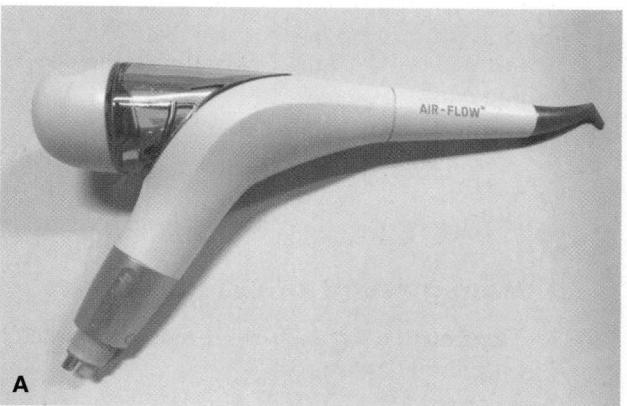

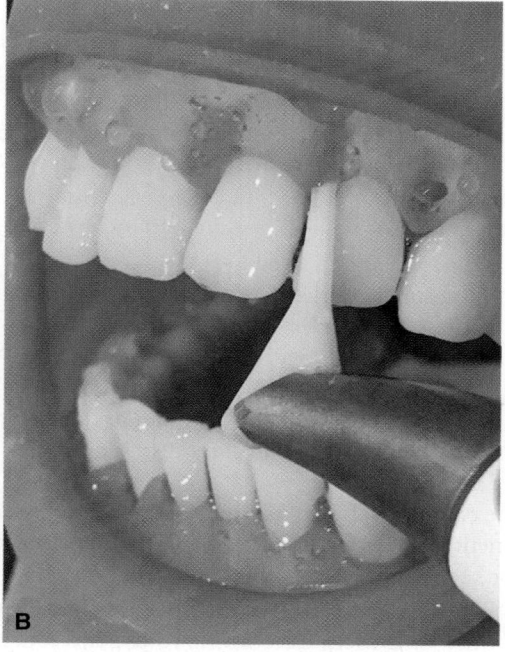

FIGURE 39-8 • Air Polisher. A: A handheld air polisher that connects to the dental until. Can be filled with appropriate powder and used supragingivally and subgingivally. **B:** Air polisher with a disposable periodontal nozzle that is inserted subgingivally into a deeper pocket to flush out biofilm.

- Keeping a distance of 3–5 mm away from the tooth surface, direct the nozzle toward the gingival margin anywhere from 30 to 60°.
- Press the device pedal for no longer than 5 seconds per site.
- Make small horizontal or circular strokes.
◆ Technique for debriding periodontal pockets up to 5 mm using a disposable periodontal nozzle (Figure 39-8B):
- Gently insert nozzle into the periodontal pocket.
- Once inserted, press the device pedal for 5 seconds per site.
- Use short vertical strokes.

VI. Laser Therapy

◆ Use of lasers in periodontal treatment is controversial, but continues to increase despite conflicting research findings.[36,37]
- The American Academy of Periodontology's best evidence consensus summary suggests the evidence to support use of lasers for treatment of chronic periodontitis is weak.[36,37]
- Evidence suggests that as an adjunct to conventional NSPT, laser therapy has modest additional benefit of less than 1 mm of improvement in pocket depth and CAL.[36,37]
◆ Significantly more well-designed research is needed to further explore the benefit of laser-assisted periodontal therapy.[37]

A. Types of Lasers

◆ Lasers emit light through a process called stimulated emission.
- When the light reaches the tissue, it is reflected, scattered, absorbed, or transmitted to surrounding tissues.
- The wavelength of the light influences how the light interacts with the tissue.
◆ The wavelength of lasers most often used in periodontal treatment is 635–10,600 nm and includes[36]:
- Semiconductor diode lasers.
- Solid-state lasers: neodymium-doped yttrium, aluminum, and garnet (Nd:YAG); neodymium-doped yttrium, aluminum, and perovskite (Nd:YAP); erbium-doped yttrium, aluminum, and garnet (Er:YAG); and erbium, chromium-doped yttrium scandium, gallium, and garnet (Er,Cr:YSGG).
- Gas lasers (CO_2).
◆ The equipment for laser therapy is expensive, and cost–benefit over traditional periodontal debridement has not been evaluated.
- Each manufacturer requires the purchaser to contract with them for training to use the equipment, which further impacts the cost and standardization of therapy.

B. Purported Benefits of Lasers in Nonsurgical Periodontal Therapy

◆ Enhances pocket disinfection by reduction of subgingival bacterial load.
◆ Promotes wound healing.
◆ Hemostasis.
◆ Root debridement.
- Erbium lasers (Er:YAG) show the most potential as an adjunct in root debridement of deep periodontal pockets (≥ 7 mm).[37]
- There is potential for damage to the root surface because the Er:YAG is a hard-tissue laser.

C. Technique

◆ For calculus removal:
- Insert laser fiber into the pocket parallel to the long axis of the tooth.
- Angulation is 45°.
- A horizontal and vertical stroke is used as the fiber is advanced around the root surface.
- Water spray along with high-volume evacuation is used to keep the area clear of debris.
◆ For reduction of bacterial load (a.k.a. pocket sterilization) and curettage of granulation tissue (a.k.a. laser curettage) as an adjunct to traditional root debridement[38,39]:
- Insert laser fiber into the pocket parallel to the long axis of the tooth.
- The fiber is directed toward the soft-tissue wall of the pocket.
- Move fiber in a horizontal and apical direction in a sweeping motion at a slow-to-moderate speed.
- Use moistened gauze to remove debris from the fiber periodically.
- Use high-volume evacuation for debris and to aspirate fumes.

POST-OP INSTRUCTION FOR PERIODONTAL DEBRIDEMENT APPOINTMENTS

◆ Instructions following NSPT should include information on:
- Management of discomfort.
- Oral self-care.
- Diet.
- Where to call in case of a problem or question.

I. Management of Discomfort

◆ There may be some soft-tissue discomfort when the local anesthesia wears off.
- Any discomfort can usually be managed with over-the-counter analgesics, including acetaminophen (Tylenol®), aspirin, or ibuprofen (Advil®).

- A nonsteroidal anti-inflammatory drug such as ibuprofen can also help reduce inflammation and swelling.
- On occasion, a cold compress or ice pack may help with discomfort.
- If the patient experiences dentin hypersensitivity, a toothpaste for sensitivity, such as a 5% potassium nitrate dentifrice, may be recommended.
  - The patient should understand that it may take several weeks of repeated used for the dentin hypersensitivity for improvement of sensitivity.

II. Oral Self-Care

A. Rinsing

- A warm solution may be soothing to the tissues helping healing.
- Possible solutions for rinsing may include:
  - *Hypertonic salt solution*: 1/2 teaspoonful of salt in 1/2 cup (4 oz) of warm water.
  - *Sodium bicarbonate solution*: 1/2 teaspoonful of baking soda in 1 cup (8 oz) of warm water.
  - *Rinsing directions*: Every 2 hours; after eating; after toothbrushing; before retiring.
- Chlorhexidine gluconate 0.12% has been shown to provide a small reduction in pocket depths when used in conjunction with periodontal debridement.[40] It may be especially helpful in the presence of significant gingival inflammation.
  - *Directions*: twice daily, after breakfast and before going to bed, without eating after rinsing to take advantage of the substantivity property of chlorhexidine.
  - Rinsing is not a substitute for personal biofilm removal with toothbrush and interdental aids.
  - Limit use to 2 weeks following the final periodontal debridement appointment to minimize tooth staining or other adverse effects of chlorhexidine.

B. Biofilm Management

- The patient needs to understand the significance of daily biofilm disruption/removal, particularly in the quadrant or sextant receiving treatment to support optimal healing.
- A soft toothbrush should be used. The patient may find that moistening the toothbrush with warm water and brushing without toothpaste initially may be more comfortable for the tissues. The fluoride toothpaste can then be added at the end of brushing.
- There may be slight bleeding during oral self-care, but this should stop as the tissues heal.
- The patient should continue to use the interdental cleaning aid recommended. If an interdental brush will fit interproximally, this can be very helpful for tissue healing.

III. Diet

- The patient should be instructed to avoid chewing solid food or drinking hot liquids until the anesthetic has worn off to avoid trauma to the tongue, cheek, and lips.
- If the tissues are tender during healing, consume bland foods without strong, spicy seasonings, as well as use of nutrient-dense, high-protein foods to promote healing.

IV. Emergency Management

- The patient should be given information about who to call in the following situations:
  - Bleeding that does not stop within a few hours.
  - Pain not stopped by use of ibuprofen or Tylenol, particularly pain that wakes the patient during the night.
  - Swelling that increases after the first 1-2 days.

V. Instruction Format

- The instructions may be handed out in paper form at the appointment with notes specific to the patient.
- Some offices may choose to provide instructions via email or may have general instructions on their office website.
- Patients particularly appreciate a call the evening or day after the appointment to check on how they are doing.

RE-EVALUATION OF NONSURGICAL PERIODONTAL THERAPY

I. Clinical Endpoints

- *BOP*: eliminated.
- *Probing depths*: reduced.
- *Attachment levels*: same or improved.
- *Inflammation*: resolved.
- *Gingival appearance*: size reduced, color normal.
- *Subgingival microflora*: lowered in numbers, delay in repopulation.
- *Dental biofilm control record*: improvement in scores approaching 100% biofilm free.
- *Tooth surfaces*: smooth; no biofilm-retentive irregularities.
- *Quality-of-life factors*: oral comfort with freedom from pain.

II. Re-evaluation Timeframe

- Recommendations are for the initial therapy re-evaluation to occur 4–8 weeks after NSPT.[14]
  - At least 2 weeks after instrumentation is complete for the re-establishment of the junctional epithelium.[14]
  - Four to 8 weeks are needed for the connective tissue to heal following NSPT.[14]

- Waiting longer than 2 months may allow the pathogenic bacteria to repopulate the periodontal pockets. In addition, it is necessary to identify and remediate any residual subgingival calculus at the re-evaluation appointment to facilitate continued healing.[14]

III. Re-evaluation Procedure

A. Periodontal Examination

- A comprehensive periodontal examination is performed and documented to compare pre- and post-treatment findings.[41]
  - Changes in BOP, CAL, biofilm, and inflammation in particular are evaluated and discussed with the patient.
  - Assessment for subgingival calculus is also needed. According to the literature, 17%–69% of surfaces may have residual calculus.[14] Re-instrument as needed.
- Review oral self-care techniques with the patient and offer assistance in continued refinement is essential to aid in continued healing and disease management.

B. Establish Continuing Care Interval

- The patient may have reached the point of being able to be managed under the care of the dental hygienist, and a maintenance interval should be determined based on the following:
  - Soft-tissue response to instrumentation and degree of healing.
  - Changes and/or stabilization in probing depth.
  - Patient factors: use of tobacco; systemic influences such as control of diabetes.
  - Currently demonstrated biofilm control efforts; level of skill.
  - Motivation and responsibility assumed for daily oral self-care.
  - Psychosocial factors; stress, mental health issues impacting oral self-care.
- There may be localized activity, and adjunctive therapy may be considered.
- In case of advanced disease that has not responded adequately to NSPT, a referral to a periodontist is necessary, as described in Chapter 45.

ADJUNCTIVE THERAPY

- Pharmacologic agents are used as adjuncts to mechanical therapy.

ANTIMICROBIAL TREATMENT

- Objectives of antimicrobial therapy include:
  - Arresting of infection using antimicrobial drugs to slow or arrest loss of periodontal attachment and other periodontal tissue destruction caused by microorganisms.
  - Suppression and elimination of pathogenic microorganisms to allow the recolonization of the microbiota compatible with health.

I. Systemic Delivery of Antibiotics

- Systemic administration of antibiotics is well known and highly successful in the world of medical care. Antibiotics have saved the lives of many people with generalized infectious diseases.
- A significant disadvantage to use of systemic antibiotics over the past 50 years is an increase in antibiotic resistance, so they need to be used with caution after a careful risk–benefit analysis.[39]

A. Action of Systemically Administered Antibiotic

- In contrast to locally applied agents placed directly into a pocket, antibiotics administered systemically reach the pathogenic organisms in the pocket through blood circulation via the cardiovascular system.
- The antibiotic is absorbed into the circulation from the intestine. From the bloodstream, the drug is passed into the body tissues.
- The antibiotic enters the periodontal tissues and passes into the pocket by way of the gingival crevicular fluid.

B. Selection of Antibiotic

- Systemic antibiotics may be prescribed as an adjunct to NSPT for a patient who does not respond to traditional periodontal therapy and experience continued loss of attachment; however, evidence is inconsistent on the benefit of their use.[40–44]
- Ideally, the specific microorganism causing a certain periodontal disease needs to be determined, and the antibiotic selected needs to be specific for the organism.[7,40]
  - Microbiologic testing is available and can be used to guide clinical decisions.
  - Periodontal diseases are caused by mixed infections of microorganisms. The pathogens tend to work in clusters, that is, in combination with other organisms so microbiological testing has limitations in mixed infections.
- Antibiotics regimens used with periodontal debridement include the following:
  - Metronidazole is effective against *Porphyromonas gingivalis* and *Prevotella intermedia* and a meta-analysis found reductions in pocket depths and clinical attachment gain.[45]
  - Tetracycline, specifically doxycycline or minocycline, to treat *Aggregatibacter actinomycetemcomitans* in more aggressive periodontitis.
  - Azithromycin with NSPT has shown reductions in pocket depths and gain in clinical attachment.[46]

C. Limitations

- The precautions and adverse effects, as well as the acquisition of antibiotic resistance by the organisms, preclude the widespread use of systemic antibiotics for periodontal problems.[40]

◆ Limitations include the following[40]:
  • Side effects of certain antibiotics.
  • Potential for the development of resistant strains.
  • Local concentration diluted by the time the drug reaches the pathogens; drug is "wasted" in that it covers a large area not needing the treatment.
  • Superimposed opportunistic infection can develop, such as candidiasis.
  • Low compliance of the patient in following the prescription for the required number of days.

D. Use of Systemic Therapy

◆ Most periodontal infection responds well to NSPT, meticulous biofilm control, and antimicrobial mouthrinses/dentifrices. However, there are groups of people who do not respond to initial therapy who would benefit from systemic antibiotics, including those with[40-44]:
  • Continued loss of attachment despite initial therapy and thorough biofilm control.
  • Recurrent or refractory periodontitis.
  • Acute periodontal infection, such as necrotizing ulcerative gingivitis or periodontitis, periodontal abscess.
  • Aggressive types of periodontitis.
  • Medical conditions predisposing to periodontal disease, such a poorly controlled diabetes.

II. Systemic Subantimicrobial Dose Antibiotics

◆ A subantimicrobial dose (SSD) does not have antimicrobial or antibiotic effects, and to date, antibiotic resistance has not been identified.[47]

◆ Doxycycline in a low dose modulates the host inflammatory response and inhibits the continued breakdown of collagen.[47,48]
  • The only approved systemic SDD is Periostat®.

◆ SDD (20 mg/twice a day) has been used for moderate-to-severe periodontitis as an adjunct to NSPT for 3–9 months.[47]

◆ Evidence shows small gains in clinical attachment and reductions in pocket depths.[48]

III. Local Delivery Antimicrobial Agents

◆ The concept of a controlled local delivery system for treatment of periodontal pathogens in a pocket infection was developed over many years by Goodson et al. with the introduction of a tetracycline fiber placed subgingivally.[49]
  • Improvements in probing depth, CAL, BOP, and reduction of sites with periodontal pathogenic microorganisms laid the groundwork for continuing research and development in local delivery agents.[49]

◆ Local delivery means the medication is concentrated at the site of the infection to reduce the bacterial load and inflammation to enhance healing.

◆ Local drug antimicrobial agents (LDAs) can be divided into two classes[50]:
  • Sustained-release formulations release a drug for a period less than 24 hours and are used in a variety of ways. The nicotine patch, used to assist a person trying to break a smoking addiction, is an example.
  • Controlled delivery refers to providing the medication over an extended period of time that exceeds 1 day.

A. Requirements

A local delivery method can place high concentrations of the antimicrobial in an infected pocket. To be successful, the medication must:

◆ Provide adequate bactericidal drug concentration.

◆ Reach site of disease activity, such as the bottom of the pocket and furcation.

◆ Stay in contact long enough in the effective concentration for the antimicrobial action to take place.

◆ Be easy to apply.

◆ Be biocompatible and biodegradable.

◆ Cost and the benefit for the patient must be carefully evaluated, given the average reduction in pocket depth ranges from 0.25 to 0.50 mm and the gains in clinical attachment of approximately 0.20 mm.[50,51]

B. Advantages of Local Delivery Agents

◆ Local delivery agents have the potential to enhance therapy at localized sites unresponsive to NSPT.

◆ Advantages include[51]:
  • Direct placement at site of infection.
  • Reliable drug delivery without reliance on patient compliance.
  • Safer with fewer side effects.
  • Noninvasive and typically painless.

C. Limitations to Local Delivery Agents

◆ Therapies other than LDAs should be considered in the following situations[52]:
  • Multiple sites with pocket depths greater than or equal to 5 mm in a quadrant.
  • LDAs have been attempted and did not control the localized infection.
  • Intrabony defects are present, which require surgical intervention.

INDICATIONS FOR USE OF LOCAL DELIVERY AGENTS

I. Nonsurgical Periodontal Therapy

◆ NSPT is considered the "gold" standard and results in reduction in inflammation and gain in clinical attachment gains of 0.49 mm.[44]

◆ The adjunctive use of local antimicrobials may enhance the effect of the mechanical instrumentation.

- Use of an LDA in addition to NSPT may result in an additional 0.24–0.64 mm gain in clinical attachment.[44]

II. Adjunctive Treatment: At Re-Evaluation

◆ At the completion of initial periodontal therapy, a re-evaluation is completed 4–6 weeks later.

- Residual calculus is removed.
- Control of dental biofilm is assessed, and reinforcement is provided for the patient.
- For areas of residual pocket depth and/or BOP, adjunctive therapy may be considered, such as systemic antibiotics or a local delivery antimicrobial agent.

III. Recurrent Disease

◆ Periodontal disease tends to be cyclical with periods of stability and progression.

◆ Recurrence or progression of periodontal disease may be due to:

- Noncompliance with periodontal maintenance schedule.
- Inadequate daily control of dental biofilm.
- Inadequate periodontal debridement.
- Continued tobacco use.
- Unknown.

◆ Recurrence of periodontal infection may be localized, particularly in pockets associated with root concavities, furcations, and areas of complex root morphology, where definitive debridement is most challenging.

- Burnished calculus is difficult to detect with an explorer and becomes recolonized with pathogenic microbes soon after debridement, which interferes with healing.
- Bleeding may indicate residual burnished calculus from insufficient instrumentation.

◆ Localized areas of recurrence of disease are candidates for application of an antimicrobial agent.

IV. Peri-Implantitis

Peri-implantitis may respond to a local delivery antimicrobial.[53]

TYPES OF LOCAL DELIVERY AGENTS

◆ Average improvement in clinical attachment with use of adjunctive agents versus periodontal debridement alone ranges from 0.18 to 0.64 mm (Table 39-2).[44]

I. Minocycline Hydrochloride

◆ Bioresorbable minocycline hydrochloride (HCl) is a sustained-release agent delivered in microsphere form and placed in periodontal pockets after periodontal debridement.

◆ Research indicates the following benefits to use of the minocycline HCl microspheres with NSPT:

- Overall pocket depth reduction was an additional 0.47 mm over SRP alone.[54]
- Gain in clinical attachment was an average of 0.24 mm.[44]

TABLE 39-2 Local Delivery Antimicrobials

	ARESTIN	ATRIDOX	PERIOCHIP
ACTIVE INGREDIENT	MINOCYCLINE HCL (1 mg)	DOXYCYCLINE HYCLATE (10%)	CHLORHEXIDINE GLUCONATE
Method of delivery	Unit-dose cartridge inserts into cartridge handle.	Doxycycline hyclate (10%); single use syringe suspended in 450 mg of ATRIGEL [poly(DL-lactide): NMP].	Chlorhexidine in a gelatin matrix is used for placement in the periodontal pocket.
Mechanism of action	Exerts antimicrobial activity by inhibiting protein synthesis in the bacterial cell wall that causes leakage and destroys the cell.	Subgingival controlled release; upon contact with crevicular fluid, the liquid product solidifies and then permits controlled release for a period of 7 days.	Controlled release over a 7–10 day period; bacteriostatic and bactericidal against gram-negative organisms.
Indications	As an adjunctive therapy to scaling and root debridement for reduction of pocket depth and BOP in patients with adult periodontitis.	For use in the treatment of chronic adult periodontitis for reduction in probing depth, reduction in BOP, and a gain in clinical attachment.	In conjunction with periodontal debridement.
Contraindications	Sensitivity to minocycline and/or tetracycline; children; pregnant or nursing women.	Sensitivity to doxycycline or any of the tetracycline class.	Hypersensitivity to chlorhexidine.

BOP, bleeding on probing.

A. Description

- Unit-dose cartridge contains 1 mg minocycline.
- Once the minocycline microspheres come in contact with gingival crevicular fluid, they hydrolyze allowing them to adhere to the surrounding surfaces.
- Sustained release for 14 days.
- Does not block the flow of subgingival fluid.
- Contraindications[54]:
  - Patients sensitive to tetracycline.
  - Women who are pregnant or breastfeeding.
  - Do not use in children less than 8 years of age due to possible enamel hypoplasia or permanent tooth discoloration.
  - Gastrointestinal issues.
  - Photosensitivity may occur, so protect the skin from prolonged sun exposure.
  - Prolonged use can result in fungal or bacterial superinfection.

B. Administration

- Site selection:
  - Use as an adjunct to periodontal debridement.
  - Probing depth of at least 5 mm.
- Cartridge loading:
  - Insert unit-dose cartridge into dispenser handle.
  - Exert slight pressure.
  - Twist cartridge until it locks securely into place.
- Tip preparation
  1. Cartridge tip can be manipulated to reposition the angle for difficult-to-reach areas.
  2. Leave cap covering the cartridge in place prior to manipulating the angle to prevent agent from being inadvertently expelled.
  3. Remove cap.
- Delivery of agent:
  1. Place cartridge tip into the site selected for treatment.[55]
  2. Keep tip parallel to the long axis of the tooth as it enters the periodontal pocket (Figure 39-9).
  3. Do not force the tip to the base of the pocket.
  4. Gently press thumb ring of handle to express the agent while withdrawing cartridge tip coronally from the base of the pocket.[54]
  5. With delivery complete, retract thumb ring and remove cartridge with free hand.
  6. Discard contaminated cartridge.
  7. Sterilize handle prior to reuse.[54]

C. Post-treatment Instructions

Instruct patient on proper care of treated areas. Give written guidelines to prevent misunderstanding.

- Avoid touching treated area(s).
- Do not use interdental cleaners or floss between teeth that have been treated for at least 10 days.

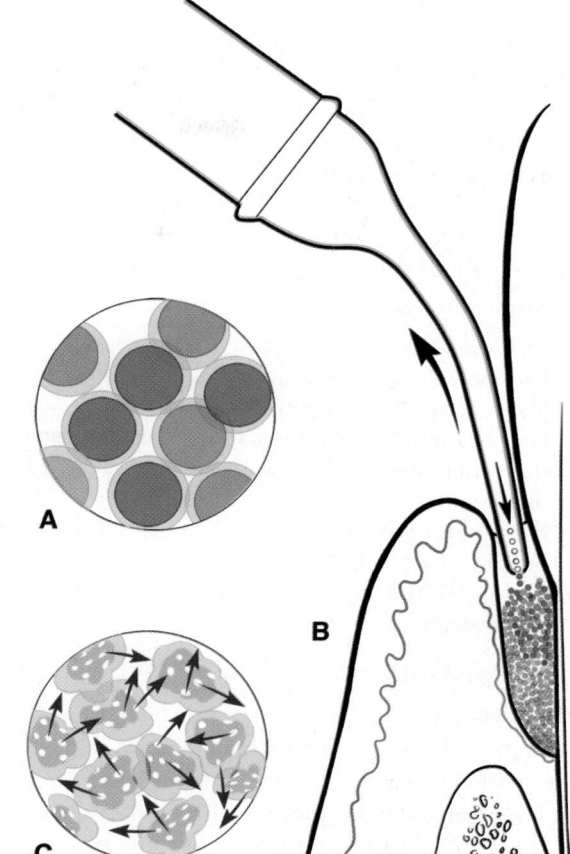

FIGURE 39-9 • **Minocycline HCl. A:** Minocycline microspheres intact within cannula, prior to application. **B:** Deposition: cannula is withdrawn from periodontal pocket as plunger is depressed. **C:** Once deposited, microspheres dissipate, releasing activated minocycline HCl into the subgingival space.

- Avoid eating hard, crunchy, or sticky foods that could disturb retention of the product for 1 week.
- Avoid brushing for 12 hours.
- Some mild-to-moderate sensitivity may be present the first week after scaling and root debridement and placement of minocycline HCl, but the patient needs to contact the dentist if pain or swelling occurs.
- Schedule a follow-up appointment for continuing maintenance care.

II. Doxycycline Hyclate

A. Description

- Biodegradable doxycycline polymer in liquid form is controlled-release agent delivered by cannula into a pocket and solidifies on contact with the sulcular fluid.
- Research indicates the following benefits to use of the minocycline doxycycline hyclate with NSPT:
  - Overall pocket depth reduction was an additional 0.57 mm over periodontal debridement alone.[55]
  - Gain in clinical attachment with periodontal debridement was an average of 0.64 mm.[44]

B. Equipment

◆ *Syringe*: Two syringe mixing system consisting of the following[55]:

• Syringe A contains 450 mg of the bioabsorbable polymeric formulation.

• Syringe B contains 50 mg of doxycycline hyclate.

• Once combined the solution contains 10% of doxycycline hyclate.

◆ *Cannula*: Blunt ended, 23-gauge, narrow diameter.

◆ Controlled release of drug for 7 days.[55]

◆ Contraindications[55]:

• Patients sensitive to tetracycline.

• Women who are pregnant or breastfeeding.

• Do not use in children less than 8 years of age due to possible enamel hypoplasia or permanent tooth discoloration.

• Photosensitivity may occur, so protect the skin from prolonged sun exposure.

• Prolonged use can result in fungal or bacterial superinfection.

C. Administration

◆ Site selection

• Probing depth of at least 5 mm.

◆ Preparation of agent

• If refrigerated, take pouches with product out of refrigerator at least 15 minutes before mixing.

• *Mixing*: Two syringes are coupled, and the substances are passed back and forth, which is one mixing cycle. Mixing continues for 100 mixing cycles (Figure 39-10A). Follow the manufacturer's instructions.[55]

• *Adapt cannula*: Attach 23-gauge blunt cannula to syringe. As the cap is removed, the cannula is held part way and bent against the wall of the cover to provide an angle appropriately similar to a periodontal probe for insertion into the periodontal pocket (Figure 39-10B).

◆ Delivery of agent[56]

1. Place cartridge tip into the site selected for treatment.

2. Keep tip parallel to the long axis of the tooth as it enters the periodontal pocket.

3. Do not force the tip to the base of the pocket.

4. Express the agent as the cannula is withdrawn to the gingival margin (Figure 39-10C).

5. Use a blunt instrument to pack the agent down.

6. Placing a periodontal dressing or adhesive over the area to aid retention.

D. Post-treatment Instructions

◆ Instruct patient on proper care of treated areas including the following:

• Prevent accidental removal.

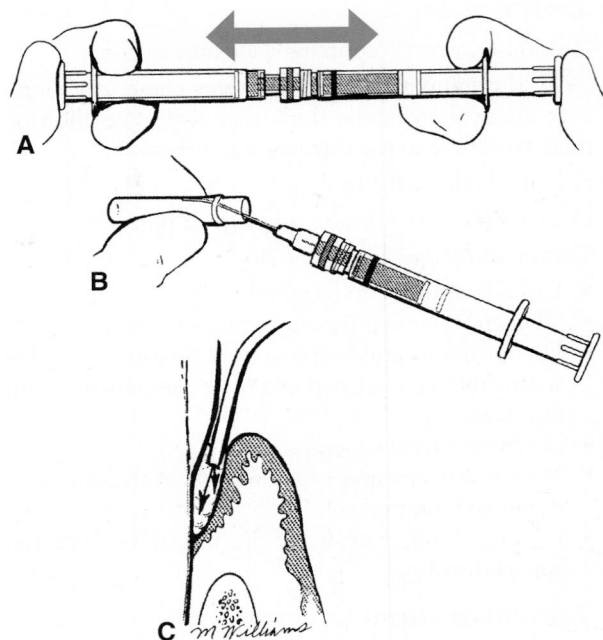

FIGURE 39-10 • Doxycycline Polymer Gel. A: Syringes are coupled, and the contents passed back and forth until mixed. **B:** The cannula is attached to the syringe with the agent; as the cap is removed, the cannula is pressed against the side to bend it to an angle appropriate for accessing the pocket to be treated. **C:** The cannula is inserted into the base of the pocket, and the agent is released to fill the pocket.

• Routine brushing and other oral self-care on all other areas, but avoid toothbrushing or flossing the treated areas for 7 days.[55]

• Schedule a follow-up appointment to remove periodontal dressing and evaluate tissue response.

◆ Schedule periodontal maintenance.

III. Chlorhexidine Gluconate

◆ The chlorhexidine gluconate chip is biodegradable and intended for use as an adjunctive therapy with periodontal debridement.[44,54,56]

◆ Research indicates the following benefits to use of the chlorhexidine chip with periodontal debridement:

• Overall pocket depth reduction was an additional 0.40 mm over periodontal debridement alone.[54]

• Gain in clinical attachment with periodontal debridement was an average of 0.40 mm.[44]

A. Description

◆ *Size*: 4 mm × 5 mm and 0.35-mm thick (Figure 39-11).

◆ *Shape*: orange-brown, rectangular, rounded at one end.

◆ *Contents*: matrix of hydrolyzed gelatin with 2.5 mg chlorhexidine gluconate.

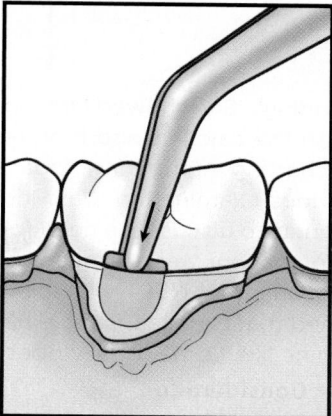

FIGURE 39-11 • Chlorhexidine Gluconate Chip. The gelatin chip is inserted into periodontal pockets greater than or equal to 5 mm. The gelatin chip adheres to the tooth surface and dissolves slowly—releasing the chlorhexidine antimicrobial agent trapped in the gelatin.

- Controlled delivery with 40% of dose in first 24 hours and remaining dose is delivered over a period up to 10 days.[56]
- Store product at controlled room temperature 15°C–25°C (59°F–77°F).
- Contraindications:
  - Do not use in acute periodontal abscess.
  - Exercise caution in pregnant or breastfeeding women.

B. Administration

- Site selection
  - *Pocket depth:* pockets greater than or equal to 5 mm.[56]
  - *Chips placed:* up to eight chips can be inserted at one appointment.
- Steps in placement[56]
  - Isolate with cotton rolls and dry area prior to chip placement. Chip may start to soften and become more difficult to place if it gets wet before placement in the pocket.
  - Insert by grasping the chip with cotton pliers position chip with round side away from the cotton pliers.
  - Insert the chip to the bottom of the pocket. The chip can be maneuvered with the tips of the cotton pliers or a flat instrument.

C. Post-treatment Instructions

- Instruct patient on proper care of treated areas, including the following:
  - Prevent accidental removal.
  - Avoid flossing the treated areas for 10 days.[56]
- Schedule periodontal maintenance.

DOCUMENTATION

Documentation for the second in a series of appointments for a quadrant of scaling and root debridement with local anesthesia:

- Complete health history and assessment examination findings.
- Record new blood pressure.
- Oral preliminary examination to evaluate progress of healing for the previously treated quadrant(s).
- Note patient's biofilm successes: provide instructions for care of newly treated area.
- Treatment completed during the appointment, including description of the amount of bleeding, necrotic tissue, and tenacity of subgingival calculus. Also note any areas that will need re-evaluation at the next appointment.
- A sample progress note may be reviewed in Box 39-2.

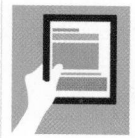

BOX 39-2

Example Documentation: Special Attention to Instrument Adaptation on a Compromised Tooth Surface

S—Female patient, 26 years old, presents for routine continuing care after being away for 2 years in the Peace Corps in Africa. Patient states she had tried hard to care for her teeth daily, but safe water was never assured, and she ran out of floss without a place to shop for more. She pointed to the upper left quadrant and said it was sore and bleeding up there. No basic changes in health history

O—Vital signs normal (BP 121/70). Generalized moderate calculus, with generalized 4 mm probing depths. Tooth #12 mesial has 6 mm pocket, BOP, and calculus (visible on the BW radiograph).

A—Tooth #13 may have a mesial concavity that requires careful adaptation of both hand and ultrasonic instrument tips.

P—Careful adaptation of the ultrasonic tip and a mini curet on the mesial surface of #13 to assure the base of a mesial concavity has been reached to remove calculus and root plane the root surface, followed by careful evaluation with an explorer.

Next Steps: Appointment made in 2 weeks for re-evaluation of #13 mesial.

Signed: _____, RDH

Date: _____

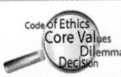

EVERYDAY ETHICS

Lorna and Caroline practice as dental hygienists in the same office approximately 2½ days per week. Lorna graduated from dental hygiene school about 15 years ago, while Caroline was licensed just 3 years ago. The front desk tries to schedule patients with the same hygienist. One day, Mrs. Border, a patient routinely scheduled with Lorna, showed up in Caroline's appointment book because she wanted to fit in her regular maintenance appointment before going to live with her daughter for several months. The receptionist scheduled her with the first available hygienist. Caroline reviewed the patient's medical history and recorded the blood pressure. During the periodontal examination, she found many areas of pocket depth increases with BOP in molar areas. Upon review of the radiograph taken that day, subgingival calculus was noted in many areas. Caroline raised Lorna's chair to an upright position to discuss the findings. She showed Mrs. Border the radiographs with the calculus and then reviewed the periodontal charting comparing today's numbers with her previous examination. Caroline then went to get Dr. Bennett to discuss the need for NSPT with Ms. Border. The patient was outraged at the recommendation for quadrant NSPT with local anesthesia and complained that Caroline "should have used the sprayer-machine like Lorna usually does."

Questions for Consideration

1. Is this an ethical dilemma or an issue for Caroline? For Lorna? For Dr. Bennett? Why?

2. Caroline realizes the deep calculus could not all have formed since the previous appointment. How should Caroline have addressed this problem with the patient? With Lorna? With Dr. Bennett?

3. Outline three or four possible avenues for Caroline to consider in resolving this difficult situation.

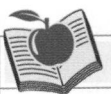

Factors to Teach the Patient

- The significance of dental biofilm in periodontal infection.
- The nature, occurrence, and etiology of calculus; its role as a biofilm reservoir.
- The importance and necessity for thorough daily removal of biofilm by the patient to prevent and manage periodontal infection. It is essential for the patient to understand their role in success of treatment.
- Reasons for multiple appointments to complete the scaling and root debridement or periodontal debridement.
- The rationale for re-evaluation following the completion of scaling and root debridement.
- The importance of the patient's role in maintenance of therapeutic gains.
- The limits of what can be accomplished nonsurgically and the rationale for referral to a periodontist so the patient understands all their treatment options.
- The rationale for adjunctive therapy to aid in healing following periodontal debridement.

ENHANCE YOUR UNDERSTANDING

ONLINE RESOURCES
(see the inside front cover for access information)

- Audio glossary
- Appendices

SUPPORT FOR LEARNING
(available separately)

- *Active Learning Workbook for Wilkins' Clinical Practice of the Dental Hygienist, 13th Edition*

INDIVIDUALIZED REVIEW

- Customized practice quizzing with Navigate 2 TestPrep for *Wilkins' Clinical Practice of the Dental Hygienist*

References

1. Drisko CL. Periodontal debridement: still the treatment of choice. *J Evid Based Dent Pract.* 2014;14(suppl):33.e1-41.e1.

2. Suvan JE. Effectiveness of mechanical nonsurgical pocket therapy. *Periodontol 2000.* 2005;37:48-71.

3. Smiley CJ, Tracy SL, Abt E, et al. Systematic review and meta-analysis on the nonsurgical treatment of chronic periodontitis by means of scaling and root planing with or without adjuncts. *J Am Dent Assoc.* 2015;146(7):508.e5-524.e5.

4. American Academy of Periodontology. Parameter on chronic periodontitis with slight to moderate loss of periodontal support. *J Periodontol.* 2000;71(suppl 5):853-855.

5. Farooqi OA, Wehler CJ, Gibson G, Jurasic MM, Jones JA. Appropriate recall interval for periodontal maintenance: a systematic review. *J Evid Based Dent Pract.* 2015;15(4):171-181.

6. Charalampakis G, Dahlén G, Carlén A, Leonhardt A. Bacterial markers vs. clinical markers to predict progression of chronic periodontitis: a 2-yr prospective observational study. *Eur J Oral Sci.* 2013;121(5):394-402.

7. American Academy of Periodontology. Parameter on chronic periodontitis with advanced loss of periodontal support. *J Periodontol.* 2000;71(suppl 5):856-858.

8. Lee CT, Huang HY, Sun TC, Karimbux N. Impact of patient compliance on tooth loss during supportive periodontal

therapy: a systematic review and meta-analysis. *J Dent Res.* 2015;94(6):777-786.

9. American Academy of Periodontology. Parameter on plaque-induced gingivitis. *J Periodontol.* 2000;71(suppl 5S):851-852.

10. Strachan A, Harrington Z, McIlwaine C, et al. Subgingival lipid A profile and endotoxin activity in periodontal health and disease. *Clin Oral Investig.* 2018; [Epub ahead of print].

11. Cadosch J, Zimmermann U, Ruppert M, Guindy J, Case D, Zappa U. Root surface debridement and endotoxin removal. *J Periodontal Res.* 2003;38(3):229-236.

12. Bozbay E, Dominici F, Gokbuget AY, et al. Preservation of root cementum: a comparative evaluation of power-driven versus hand instruments. *Int J Dent Hyg.* 2018;16(2):202-209.

13. Akcalı A, Lang NP. Dental calculus: the calcified biofilm and its role in disease development. *Periodontol 2000.* 2018;76(1):109-115.

14. Segelnick SL, Weinberg MA. Reevaluation of initial therapy: when is the appropriate time? *J Periodontol.* 2006;77(9):1598-1601.

15. Eberhard J, Jepsen S, Jervøe-Storm PM, Needleman I, Worthington HV. Full-mouth treatment modalities (within 24 hours) for chronic periodontitis in adults. *Cochrane Database Syst Rev.* 2015;(4):CD004622.

16. Zhang W, Daly CG, Mitchell D, et al. Incidence and magnitude of bacteraemia caused by flossing and by scaling and root planing. *J Clin Periodontol.* 2013;40(1):41-52.

17. Shetty SK, Sharath K, Shenoy S, et al. Compare the efficacy of two commercially available mouthrinses in reducing viable bacterial count in dental aerosol produced during ultrasonic scaling when used as a preprocedural rinse. *J Contemp Dent Pract.* 2013;14(5):848-851.

18. Gupta G, Mitra D, Ashok KP, et al. Efficacy of preprocedural mouth rinsing in reducing aerosol contamination produced by ultrasonic scaler: a pilot study. *J Periodontol.* 2014;85(4):562-568.

19. Balejo RDP, Cortelli JR, Costa FO, et al. Effects of chlorhexidine preprocedural rinse on bacteremia in periodontal patients: a randomized clinical trial. *J Appl Oral Sci.* 2017;25(6):586-595.

20. Leung WK, Duan YR, Dong XX, et al. Perception of non-surgical periodontal treatment in individuals receiving or not receiving local anaesthesia. *Oral Health Prev Dent.* 2016;14(2):165-175.

21. Ciantar M. Time to shift: from scaling and root planing to root surface debridement. *Prim Dent J.* 2014;3(3):38-42.

22. Walmsley AD, Lea SC, Landini G, Moses AJ. Advances in power driven pocket/root instrumentation. *J Clin Periodontol.* 2008;35(suppl 8):22-28.

23. Yukna RA, Vastardis S, Mayer ET. Calculus removal with diamond-coated ultrasonic inserts in vitro. *J Periodontol.* 2007;78(1):122-126.

24. Ioannou I, Dimitriadis N, Papadimitriou K, Sakellari D, Vouros I, Konstantinidis A. Hand instrumentation versus ultrasonic debridement in the treatment of chronic periodontitis: a randomized clinical and microbiological trial. *J Clin Periodontol.* 2009;36(2):132-141.

25. Park JB, Kim N, Ko Y. Effects of ultrasonic scaler tips and toothbrush on titanium disc surfaces evaluated with confocal microscopy. *J Craniofac Surg.* 2012;23(5):1552-1558.

26. Kawashima H, Sato S, Kishida M, Yagi H, Matsumoto K, Ito K. Treatment of titanium dental implants with three piezoelectric ultrasonic scalers: an in vivo study. *J Periodontol.* 2007;78(9):1689-1694.

27. Kwan JY. Enhanced periodontal debridement with the use of micro ultrasonic, periodontal endoscopy. *J Calif Dent Assoc.* 2005;33(3):241-248.

28. Geisinger ML, Mealey BL, Schoolfield J, Mellonig JT. The effectiveness of subgingival scaling and root planing: an evaluation of therapy with and without the use of the periodontal endoscope. *J Periodontol.* 2007;78(1):22-28.

29. Wilson TG Jr, Carnio J, Schenk R, Myers G. Absence of histologic signs of chronic inflammation following closed subgingival scaling and root planing using the dental endoscope: human biopsies—a pilot study. *J Periodontol.* 2008;79(11):2036-2041.

30. Bastendorf KD, Becker C, Bush B, et al. A paradigm shift in mechanical biofilm management? Subgingival air polishing: a new way to improve mechanical biofilm management in the dental practice. *Quintessence Int.* 2013:44(7):475-477.

31. Wennström JL, Dahlén G, Ramberg P. Subgingival debridement of periodontal pockets by air polishing in comparison with ultrasonic instrumentation during maintenance therapy. *J Clin Periodontol.* 2011;38(9):820-827.

32. Flemmig TF, Arushanov D, Daubert D, Rothen M, Mueller G, Leroux BG. Randomized controlled trial assessing efficacy and safety of glycine powder air polishing in moderate-to-deep periodontal pockets. *J Periodontol.* 2012;83(4):444-452.

33. Schwarz F, Ferrari D, Popovski K, Hartig B, Becker J. Influence of different air-abrasive powders on cell viability at biologically contaminated titanium dental implants surfaces. *J Biomed Mater Res B Appl Biomater.* 2009;88(1):83-91.

34. Moëne R, Décaillet F, Andersen E, Mombelli A. Subgingival plaque removal using a new air-polishing device. *J Periodontol.* 2010(1);81:79-88.

35. Crispino A, Figliuzzi MM, Iovane C, et al. Effectiveness of a diode laser in addition to non-surgical periodontal therapy: study of intervention. *Ann Stomatol.* 2015;6(1):15-20.

36. Mizutani K, Aoki A, Coluzzi D, et al. Lasers in minimally invasive periodontal and peri-implant therapy. *Periodontol 2000.* 2016;71(1):185-212.

37. da Costa LFNP, Amaral CDSF, Barbirato DDS, Leão ATT, Fogacci MF. Chlorhexidine mouthwash as an adjunct to mechanical therapy in chronic periodontitis: a meta-analysis. *J Am Dent Assoc.* 2017;148(5):308-318.

38. American Academy of Periodontology. Parameter on comprehensive periodontal examination. *J Periodontol.* 2000;71(suppl 5):847-848.

39. Frieri M, Kumar K, Boutin A. Antibiotic resistance. *J Infect Public Health.* 2017;10(4):369-378.

40. Slots J; Research, Science and Therapy Committee. Systemic antibiotics in periodontics. *J Periodontol.* 2004;75(11):1553-1565.

41. Santos RS, Macedo RF, Souza EA, Soares RS, Feitosa DS, Sarmento CF. The use of systemic antibiotics in the treatment of refractory periodontitis: a systematic review. *J Am Dent Assoc.* 2016;147(7):577-585.

42. Keestra JA, Grosjean I, Coucke W, Quirynen M, Teughels W. Non-surgical periodontal therapy with systemic antibiotics in patients with untreated chronic periodontitis:

a systematic review and meta-analysis. *J Periodontal Res.* 2015;50(3):294-314.

43. Garcia Canas P, Khouly I, Sanz J, Loomer PM. Effectiveness of systemic antimicrobial therapy in combination with scaling and root planing in the treatment of periodontitis: a systematic review. *J Am Dent Assoc.* 2015;146(3):150-163.

44. Smiley CJ, Tracy SL, Abt E, et al. Evidence-based clinical practice guideline on the nonsurgical treatment of chronic periodontitis by means of scaling and root planing with or without adjuncts. *J Am Dent Assoc.* 2015;146(7):525-535.

45. Sgolastra F, Severino M, Petrucci A, Gatto R, Monaco A. Effectiveness of metronidazole as an adjunct to scaling and root planing in the treatment of chronic periodontitis: a systematic review and meta-analysis. *J Periodontal Res.* 2014;49(1):10-19.

46. Zhang Z, Zheng Y, Bian X. Clinical effect of azithromycin as an adjunct to non-surgical treatment of chronic periodontitis: a meta-analysis of randomized controlled clinical trials. *J Periodontal Res.* 2016;51(3):275-283.

47. Preshaw PM. Host modulation therapy with anti-inflammatory agents. *Periodontol 2000.* 2018;76(1):131-149.

48. Sgolastra F, Petrucci A, Gatto R, Giannoni M, Monaco A. Long-term efficacy of subantimicrobial-dose doxycycline as an adjunctive treatment to scaling and root planing: a systematic review and meta-analysis. *J Periodontol.* 2011;82(11):1570-1581.

49. Goodson JM, Haffajee A, Socransky SS. Periodontal therapy by local delivery of tetracycline. *J Clin Periodontol.* 1979;6(2):83-92.

50. American Academy of Periodontology. Statement on local delivery of sustained or controlled release antimicrobials as adjunctive therapy in the treatment of periodontitis. *J Periodontol.* 2006;77(8):1457-1458.

51. Joshi D, Garg T, Goyal AK, Rath G. Advanced drug delivery approaches against periodontitis. *Drug Deliv.* 2016;23(2):363-377.

52. Jepsen K, Jepsen S. Antibiotics/antimicrobials: systemic and local administration in the therapy of mild to moderately advanced periodontitis. *Periodontol 2000.* 2016;71(1):82-112.

53. Esposito M, Grusovin MG, Worthington HV. Treatment of peri-implantitis: what interventions are effective? A Cochrane systematic review. *Eur J Oral Implantol.* 2012;5(suppl):S21-S41.

54. Lexicomp for Dentistry. *Minocycline Hydrochloride.* Updated December 14, 2018. Hudson, OH: Wolters Kluwer Clinical Drug Information.

55. Lexicomp for Dentistry. *Doxycycline Hyclate Periodontal Extended-Release Liquid.* Updated January 15, 2019. Hudson, OH: Wolters Kluwer Clinical Drug Information.

56. Lexicomp for Dentistry. *Chlorhexidine Gluconate (Oral).* Updated March 20, 2019. Hudson, OH: Wolters Kluwer Clinical Drug Information.

40

Sutures and Dressings

Susan J. Jenkins, RDH, PhD

CHAPTER OUTLINE

SUTURES
  I. The Ideal Suture Material
  II. Functions of Sutures
  III. Characteristics of Suture Materials
  IV. Classification of Suture Materials
  V. Selection of Suture Materials

NEEDLES
  I. Needle Components
  II. Needle Characteristics

KNOTS
  I. Knot Characteristics
  II. Knot Management

SUTURING PROCEDURES
  I. Blanket (Continuous Lock)
  II. Interrupted
  III. Continuous Uninterrupted

  IV. Circumferential
  V. Interdental
  VI. Sling or Suspension

PROCEDURE FOR SUTURE REMOVAL
  I. Review Previous Documentation
  II. Sterile Clinic Tray Setup
  III. Preparation of Patient
  IV. Steps for Removal
  V. Safety Measures

PERIODONTAL DRESSINGS
  I. Purposes and Uses
  II. Characteristics of Acceptable Dressing Material

TYPES OF DRESSINGS
  I. Zinc Oxide with Eugenol Dressing
  II. Chemical-Cured Dressing
  III. Visible Light–Cured Dressing
  IV. Collagen Dressing

CLINICAL APPLICATION
  I. Dressing Placement
  II. Characteristics of a Well-Placed Dressing
  III. Patient Dismissal and Instructions

DRESSING REMOVAL AND REPLACEMENT
  I. Patient Examination
  II. Procedure for Removal
  III. Dressing Replacement Procedure
  IV. Patient Oral Self-care Instruction
  V. Follow-up

DOCUMENTATION

EVERYDAY ETHICS

FACTORS TO TEACH THE PATIENT

REFERENCES

LEARNING OBJECTIVES

After studying this chapter, the student will be able to:

1. State the functions and purposes of sutures and periodontal dressings.

2. Describe the differences between absorbable and nonabsorbable sutures.

3. Describe the procedure for suture removal.

4. Describe the procedure for periodontal dressing placement and periodontal dressing removal.

5. Explain approaches for managing biofilm with the periodontal dressing in place and upon removal.

Many periodontal surgical procedures require sutures and dressings. The dental hygienist will often participate in the patient's oral self-care instruction at initial placement and during postoperative care.

SUTURES

I. The Ideal Suture Material

- A suture is a strand of material used to control bleeding, stabilize the wound edges in the proper position, protects the wound, and aids in patient comfort.[1]
  - Sutures are necessary in many oral surgical procedures when a surgical wound must be closed, a flap positioned, or tissue grafted.
- Historically a wide range of suture materials has been used including silk, cotton, linen, and animal tendons and intestines.
- The ideal suture material is nonallergic, easy to handle, has adequate tensile strength, sterile, does not interfere with healing, causes minimal inflammatory reaction, and has some capacity to stretch to allow for wound edema.[1,2]
  - Ultimately, the ideal suture does not exist and each surgeon must select the best suture material based on the surgical procedure to be performed, patient, and wound characteristics.[2]

II. Functions of Sutures

- Close periodontal wounds and secure grafts in position.
- Assist in maintaining hemostasis.
- Reduce posttreatment discomfort.
- Promote primary intention healing.
- Prevent underlying bone exposure.
- Protect a healing surgical wound from foreign debris and trauma.

III. Characteristics of Suture Materials

A. Biological Characteristics[1]

- Sterility.
- Reabsorption ability.
- Tolerability: creates minimal inflammatory reaction in the tissue.

B. Physical Characteristics[1]

- Tensile strength.
- Flexibility: ability to twist and tie know without breaking.
- Plasticity: ability to maintain new shape.
- Elasticity: ability of material to stretch and return to original shape.
- Maneuverability: easy to handle and able to create a small knot.

- Fluency: passes through tissue with minimal trauma.
- Length and diameter: various lengths and diameters are available.

IV. Classification of Suture Materials

A. Type of Material Used[1]

- *Natural*: classified into animal origin (i.e., catgut and silk) and vegetal origin (i.e., cotton and linen).
- *Synthetic*: developed to reduce tissue reactions and unpredictable rates of absorption commonly found in natural sutures.

B. Absorption Properties

- Absorbable sutures:
  - *Natural absorbable sutures*: digested by body enzymes.
    - *Plain gut*: monofilamentous, derived from purified collagen of sheep or cattle and lasts about 8 days before beginning to degrade.[1]
    - *Chromatic gut*: chromatic salts to delay enzyme resorption for 18 days.[1]
  - *Synthetic resorbable sutures*: broken down by hydrolysis, a process in which water slowly penetrates the suture filaments to cause a breakdown of the suture's polymer chain.
    - Example: polyglactin (Vicryl), poliglecaprone (Monocryl), and polydioxanone (PDS II).
- Nonabsorbable sutures: not digested by body enzymes or hydrolyzation; patient returns for removal usually after 1 week.
  - *Natural nonabsorbable*
    - Braided silk.
  - *Synthetic nonabsorbable*
    - Nylon (Ethilon).
    - Polyester (Ethibond).
    - Polypropylene (Prolene).
    - Polytetrafluoroethylene (PTFE) (Gore-Tex®).
    - *Coated sutures:* Suture material coated with the antibacterial agents triclosan and chlorhexidine may provide antibacterial efficacy and oral biofilm inhibition.[1,3]

C. Number of Strands

- *Monofilament suture*: single strand of material; typical of gut, nylon, PTFE, and other synthetic sutures.[1]
- *Multifilament suture*: several strands twisted or braided together: typical of silk, nylon, polyglycolic acid, polyester, and other synthetic sutures.[1]

D. Diameter of Suture Material

- Diameters range from 1–0 to 11–0.
- More zeros = smaller the diameter.
- Fewer zeros = larger the diameter.
- Example: 3–0 is larger than 5–0; size 4.0 and 3.0 are the most common intraoral sutures.

TABLE 40-1 • Selection of Suture Material	
SUTURE TYPES	SPECIFIC DENTAL PROCEDURES
Silk, nonresorbable, braided	Periodontal flaps and closure
Nylon, monofilament	Periodontal flaps and closure
Polyester, braided	Periodontal flaps and closure
Gut, resorbable	Extraction socket, bone grafting, free-gingival grafting
Resorbable preferred: nonresorbable used when pain and swelling may be anticipated	Implant flap closure

V. Selection of Suture Materials

Choosing the appropriate suture material for a specific procedure is critical both for patient comfort and tissue health. Suture selection is based on the following[2]:

◆ Preference and experience of the surgeon.

◆ Characteristics of the patient such as age.

◆ Characteristics of the wound such as length and tissue type (mucosa vs. attached gingiva).

◆ Cosmetic implications.

 • Examples of suture types surgeons may use for specific procedures are listed in Table 40-1.

NEEDLES

Many types of suturing needles are available. Their use and selection are primarily based on specific procedures, location for use, and clinician's preference.

I. Needle Components

◆ *Swaged end (eyeless)*

 • Swaged allows suture material and needle to act as one unit (Figure 40-1).

◆ *Body*

 • *Shape/curvature*

  • Straight.

  • Half-curved.

  • Curved 1/4, 3/8, 1/2, 5/8 (Figure 40-2).

 • *Diameter*

  • Gauge or size; finer for delicate surgeries.

  • Body is the strongest part of the needle that is grasped with the needleholder during the surgical procedure.

  • Swaged end is the weakest part of the body.

◆ *Point*

 • Point of the needle extends from the extreme tip of the needle to the widest part of the body.

 • Each needle point is designed and manufactured to penetrate tissue with the highest degree of sharpness.

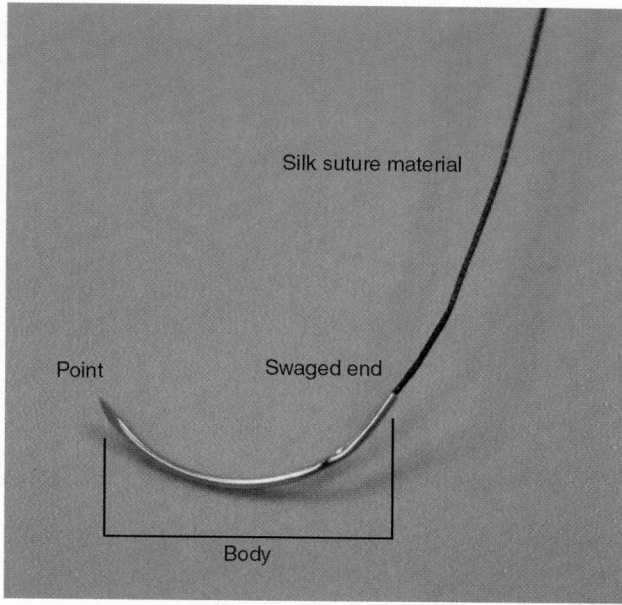

FIGURE 40-1 • **Suture Needle Components.** (Courtesy of Susan Jenkins, MCPHS University Forsyth School of Dental Hygiene.)

II. Needle Characteristics

◆ *Material*

 • Most needles are made of stainless steel formulated and sterilized for surgical use.

◆ *Attachment*

 • Majority of needles are permanently attached to suture material.

 • Eliminates need for threading and unnecessary handling.

◆ *Cutting edge* (Figure 40-3)

 • *Reverse cut*: the sharpest needle[3]; has two opposing cutting edges, with a third located on outer convex curve of needle.

 • *Conventional cut*: consists of two opposing cutting edges and a third within the concave curvature of the needle.

◆ *Requirements*

 • *Needle point*: designed to meet the needs of specific surgical procedures.

  • Sharp enough to penetrate tissues with minimal resistance.

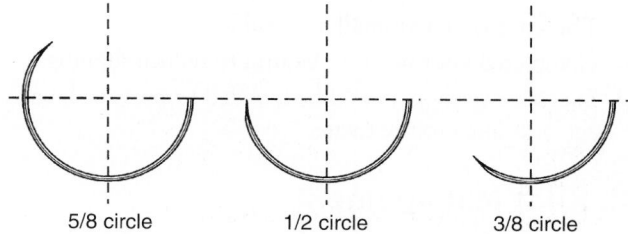

5/8 circle   1/2 circle   3/8 circle

FIGURE 40-2 • **Suture Needles.** A curved needle is manipulated with a needleholder. The 3/8 curve is most effective for closure of skin and mucous membranes and is a needle of choice in many dental and periodontal surgeries.

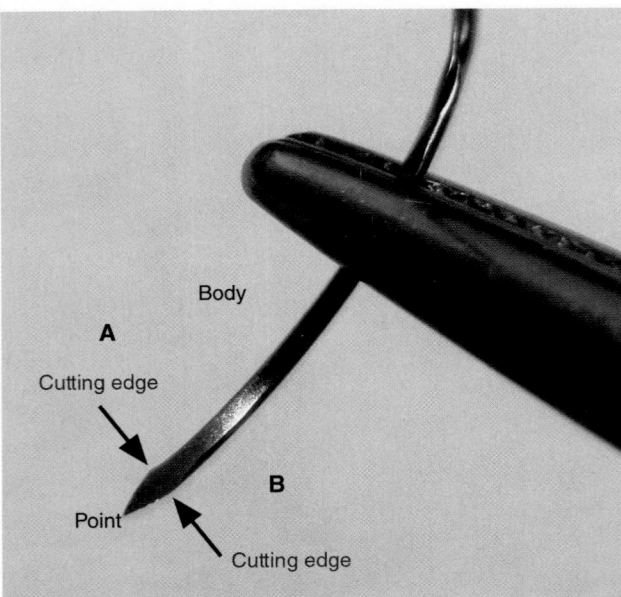

FIGURE 40-3 • Suture Needles. Shapes of Points. Triangle shows cross section of needle point. **A:** Conventional cutting with third cutting edge on the inside of the needle curvature. **B:** Reverse cutting with third cutting edge on the outer curvature of the needle, used for difficult-to-penetrate tissue, such as skin. (Courtesy of Susan Jenkins, MCPHS University Forsyth School of Dental Hygiene.)

- Rigid enough to resist bending, yet are flexible.
- Sterile and corrosion resistant.
- *Surgical needles*: intended to carry suture material through tissues with minimal trauma.

KNOTS

The book *Surgical Knots and Suturing Techniques*[4] describes a variety of surgical knots. Only a few are used in dentistry.
- Type of knot used will depend on the specific procedure.
- Location of the incision.
- Amount of stress the wound will endure.
- Square knots are most frequently used in dentistry because they are the easiest and most reliable.

I. Knot Characteristics

- The knot is tied as small as possible.
- Completed knot needs to be firm to reduce slipping.
- Excessive tension should be avoided to prevent breakage or trauma to the tissue.

II. Knot Management

- The knot is tied on the facial aspect for easier access for removal.
- A 2- to 3-mm suture "tail" is left to assist in locating the suture for removal.

SUTURING PROCEDURES

- Many different patterns of suturing are used. Assisting and observing during the surgical procedure can be an educational experience for the dental hygienist.
- General types of sutures used in the oral cavity are described in Figure 40-4.

I. Blanket (Continuous Lock)

- Each stitch is brought over a loop of the preceding one, thus forming a series of loops on one side of the incision and a series of stitches over the incision (Figure 40-4A).
- Uses: to approximate the gingival margins after alveolectomy.

II. Interrupted

- Figure 40-4B shows a series of interrupted sutures.

III. Continuous Uninterrupted

- A series of stitches tied at one or both ends.
- Examples of sutures that may be applied in a series are the sling or suspension and the blanket.

IV. Circumferential

- Suture that encircles a tooth for suspension and retention of a flap.

V. Interdental

- Flaps are on both the lingual and facial sides; interdental ligation joins the two by passing the suture through each interdental area (Figure 40-4C). Coverage for the interdental area can be accomplished by coapting the edges of the papillae.

VI. Sling or Suspension

- When a flap is only on one side, facial or lingual, the sutures are passed through the interdental papilla, around the tooth, and into the adjacent papilla (Figure 40-4D).
- The suture is adjusted so that the flap can be positioned for correct healing.

PROCEDURE FOR SUTURE REMOVAL

Removal schedule: 7 days after the surgery and no longer than 14 days to prevent tissue infection and promote healing.

I. Review Previous Documentation

- Medical history.
- Surgical procedures.

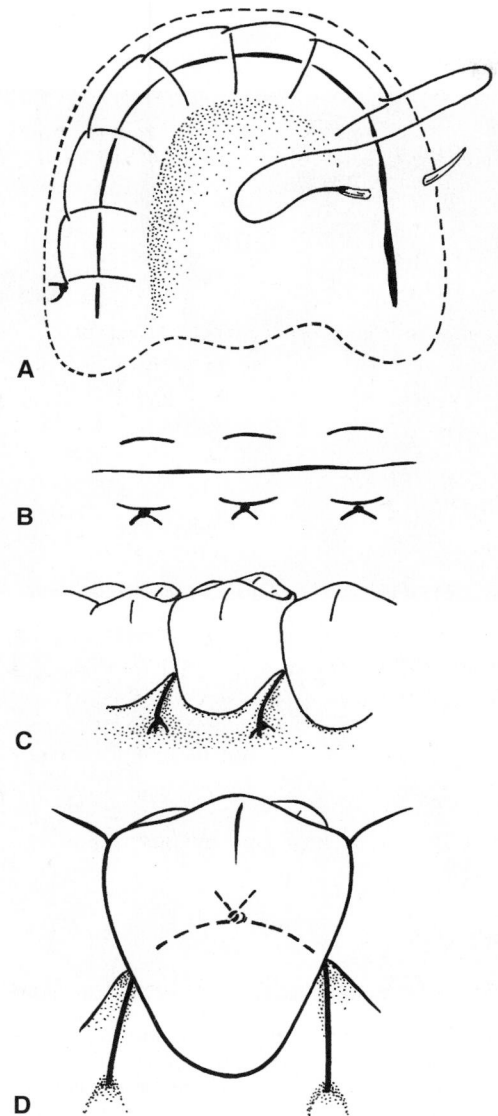

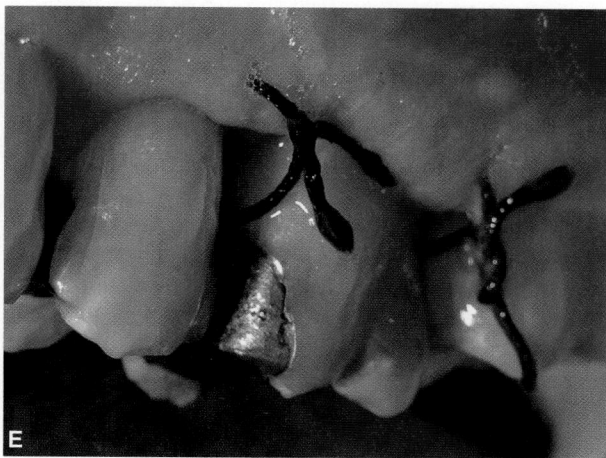

FIGURE 40-4 • **Types of Sutures. A:** Blanket stitch. **B:** Interrupted, individual sutures. **C:** Interdental individual sutures. **D:** Sling or suspension suture tied on the lingual (*dotted line*) **E:** Interrupted silk sutures in place 1-week postsurgery. (Courtesy of Dr. Robert Lewando, Boston, MA.)

◆ Patient reactions to healing.

◆ Current surgery: number and type of sutures placed.

II. Sterile Clinic Tray Setup

◆ Sterile mouth mirror.

◆ Sterile cotton pliers.

◆ Sterile curved sharp scissors with pointed tip (suture scissors).

◆ Gauze, that is, 2 × 2.

◆ Topical anesthetic: type that can be applied safely on an abraded or incompletely healed area.

◆ Cotton pellets.

◆ Saliva ejector tip.

III. Preparation of Patient

◆ *Patient history check*
  • Patients with valvular heart disease require consultation with the cardiologist.[5]
    • Sutures are colonized by bacteria and should be removed as soon as possible once adequate wound healing has occurred.[1,2,6]
    • Suture removal can cause bacteremia.[7–9]

◆ *Patient examination*
  • Observe healing tissue around the suture(s) (Figure 40-4E).
  • Record any deviations in color, size, shape of the tissue, adaptation of a flap, or coaptation of an incision healing by first intention.

◆ *Preparation of the sutured area*
  • Sutures placed without a dressing may have debris lodged in them at the time of removal.
  • Irrigate and/or swab with a cotton tip applicator or cotton pellet.
  • 0.12% chlorhexidine mouthrinse or 3% peroxide can be used to dip the cotton tip applicator to aid in debris removal.
  • Follow with another rinse or wipe gently with a gauze sponge.
  • Place and adjust saliva ejector.

IV. Steps for Removal

◆ The suture removal procedure described here and illustrated in Figure 40-5 is for a single interrupted suture.

◆ The same principles apply for the ends and each segment of a continuous suture, wherever suture material can pass through the soft tissue.

◆ *Steps*

1. Review the surgeon's chart notes to determine the number of sutures placed and visually locate them prior to beginning suture removal.

2. Use caution when removing a periodontal dressing to prevent tearing a suture that may have become embedded in the dressing causing the patient significant discomfort.

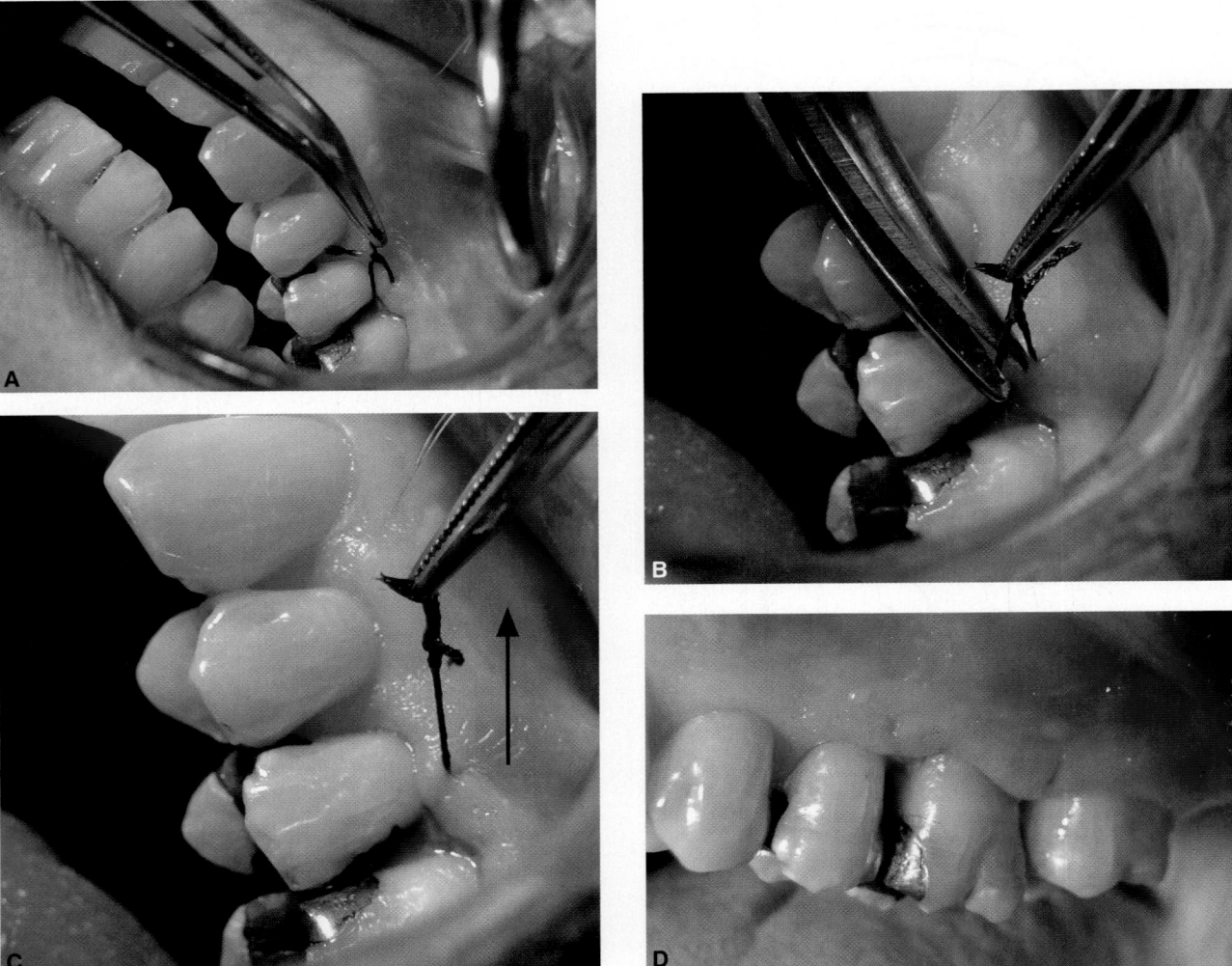

FIGURE 40-5 • Suture Removal. A: Suture grasped by pliers near the entrance into tissue. **B:** Suture pulled gently up while scissor is inserted close to the tissue. Suture is cut in the part previously buried in the tissue. **C:** Suture is held up for vertical removal. **D:** Suture is pulled gently to bring it out on the side opposite from where it was cut. The object is to prevent the external part of the suture from passing through the tissue and introducing infectious material. (Courtesy of Dr. Robert Lewando, Boston, MA.)

3. Once the sutures are exposed, carefully remove debris by irrigating with water and/or use antiseptic/antimicrobial like 0.12% chlorhexidine mouthrinse on a cotton tip applicator or cotton pellet.

4. Gently grasp the ends of the suture above the knot with the cotton plier held in the nondominant hand. Gently draw the suture up several millimeters if possible and hold with slight tension (Figure 40-5A). A finger rest is needed for control.

5. With the scissors in the dominant hand, insert one blade of the scissors just under the suture knot on one thread of the suture material (Figure 40-5B).

6. Hold knot end up with the cotton plier and pull gently to allow suture to exit through the side opposite where it was cut (Figure 40-5C).

7. Place each suture on a piece of gauze and proceed to remove the next suture.

8. Count the total number of sutures removed to ensure they were all removed.
   • During healing, sutures can become loosened, misplaced, or occasionally covered by tissue.
   • The effect of a remaining suture can lead to infection and possible abscess around the suture left behind.

9. Irrigate with water or antiseptic. Apply gauze with slight pressure on any bleeding spots.

10. Provide proper postsuture removal instructions both verbally and in writing.

11. Observe all tissue and record observations, noting any adverse reactions or bleeding.

PERIODONTAL DRESSINGS

Historically, periodontal dressing were thought to prevent wound infection and enhance healing; however, current evidence does not support this.[10,11] The use of a periodontal dressing is the personal preference and judgment of the clinician.

I. Purposes and Uses[10-12]

- Reduce pain following surgery.
- Provide a physical barrier to external irritation, trauma, and may reduce bacterial colonization of the suture material.
- Help prevent posttreatment bleeding by securing initial clot formation.
- Support mobile teeth during healing.
- Minimize tooth hypersensitivity.
- Assist in shaping or molding newly formed tissue, in securing a flap, or in immobilizing a graft.
- Possible use after nonsurgical periodontal therapy has also been proposed to enhance periodontal outcomes, but more research is needed.[13]

II. Characteristics of Acceptable Dressing Material

An acceptable dressing material has the following characteristics:
- Preparation, placement, and removal will take place with minimal discomfort to the patient.
- Material adheres to itself, teeth, and adjacent tissues and maintains retention within interdental areas.
- Provides stability and flexibility to withstand distortion and displacement without fracturing.
- Is nontoxic and nonirritating to oral tissues.
- Possesses a smooth surface that will resist accumulation of dental biofilm.
- Will not traumatize tissue or stain teeth and restorative materials.
- Possesses an aesthetically acceptable appearance.

TYPES OF DRESSINGS

Traditionally, dressings were classified into two groups: those that contained eugenol and those that did not. With the development of new products, "noneugenol-containing" dressings have been reclassified into *chemical-cure* and *visible light–cure* (VIC) materials. They are available as ready-mix, paste–paste, or paste–gel preparations.

I. Zinc Oxide with Eugenol Dressing

- Example: Kirkland periodontal pack.

B. Advantages

- *Consistency:* firm and heavy—provides support for tissues and flaps.
- *Slow setting:* extended working time.
- *Preparation and storage:* can be prepared in quantity and stored (frozen) in work-size pieces.

C. Disadvantages

- *Taste:* sharp, unpleasant taste.
- *Tissue reaction:* irritating; hypersensitivity reactions can occur.
- *Consistency:* the dressing is rough, hard and brittle, breaks easily, and encourages dental biofilm retention.

II. Chemical-Cured Dressing

- Two examples of chemical-cured dressings are PerioCare® and Coe-Pak™.

A. Basic Ingredients

- *Coe-Pak™:* Most commonly used two-paste system.[12]
  - Base paste: zinc oxide with added oils and gums.
  - Catalyst paste: resins, fatty acids, and chlorothymol as an antibacterial agent.
  - Coe-Pak™ is available in regular and fast set; hand mix or cartridge delivery.
- *PerioCare®:* two-paste system.[12]
  - One paste contains metal oxides and oil.
  - The other paste contains a gel rosin and fatty acids.

B. Advantages

- *Consistency:* pliable, easy to place with light pressure.
- *Smooth surface:* comfortable to patient; resists biofilm and debris deposits.
- *Taste:* acceptable.
- *Removal:* easy, often comes off in one piece.

III. VIC Dressing

- VIC dressing (*Barricaid®*) is available in a syringe for direct application.
- The same light-curing unit used for composite restorations and sealants is used.

A. Advantages

- *Color:* more like gingiva than other dressings and often preferred in anterior areas.
- *Setting:* cured in increments with a light-curing unit.
- *Removal:* easy, often comes off in one piece.

IV. Collagen Dressing

◆ Absorbable collagen dressings used to promote wound healing.[12]

◆ Special use in periodontal surgery for a collagen patch dressing: for protection of graft sites of the palate during healing.

◆ One form prepared in a bullet shape to use for deep biopsy sites.[12]

◆ Available in individual unit sterile packages.

◆ Collagen dressing may be placed on clean moist or bleeding wounds.

CLINICAL APPLICATION

I. Dressing Placement

◆ *General procedure*
  • For all types of dressing, follow the manufacturer's instructions. Each product has unique properties that require special handling.

◆ *Retention*
  • Mold the dressing by pressing at each interproximal site to cover interdental tissue (Figure 40-6A). Do not extend over the height of contour of each tooth.
  • Border mold to prevent displacement by the tongue, cheeks, lips, or frena (Figure 40-6 B and C).
  • Check the occlusion and remove areas of contact.

II. Characteristics of a Well-Placed Dressing

◆ Dressings placed in keeping with biologic principles contribute to healing and are tolerated more comfortably by the patient.

◆ A satisfactory dressing (Figure 40-6D) has the following characteristics:
  • Is secure and rigid. A movable dressing is an irritant and can promote bleeding.
  • Has as little bulk as possible, yet is bulky enough to give strength.
  • Locks mechanically interdentally and cannot be displaced by action of tongue, cheek, or lips.
  • Covers the entire surgical wound without unnecessary overextension.
  • Fills interdental area and adequately covers the treated area to discourage retention of debris and dental biofilm.
  • Possesses a smooth surface to prevent irritation to cheeks and lips while resisting debris and biofilm retention.

III. Patient Dismissal and Instructions

◆ Patient is not dismissed until bleeding or oozing from under a dressing has stopped.

◆ Written instructions are necessary to reinforce those that are provided verbally. Table 40-2 lists items to discuss with the patient before discharge.

DRESSING REMOVAL AND REPLACEMENT

During healing, epithelium begins to cover a wound in 5–6 days and complete epithelial healing in 7–14 days.[14] The dressing may be left in place for 7 to 10 days, as determined by the surgeon.

Keep the following factors relative to dressings in mind:

◆ If the dressing becomes dislodged before the removal appointment, the healing tissue needs to be evaluated.

◆ When the dressing remains intact for 4 or 5 days, replacement may not be necessary.

◆ When replacement is indicated, the dressing is replaced in its entirety rather than patched.

◆ Instruct the patient to proceed with daily biofilm removal and rinsing using an antimicrobial agent.

◆ Schedule patient's follow-up appointment.

I. Patient Examination

◆ Question patient about and record posttreatment effects or discomfort. Record length of time the dressing remained in place.

◆ Examine the mucosa around the dressing and record its appearance.

II. Procedure for Removal

◆ Insert a smooth instrument such as a plastic instrument under the border of the dressing and gently apply lateral pressure.

◆ Watch for sutures lodged in the dressing. If present, cut before removing the dressing.

◆ Remove fragments of dressing gently with cotton pliers to avoid scratching the thin epithelial covering of the healing tissue.

◆ Observe tissue and record its appearance. Note any deviations from normal healing that is expected within the number of days.

◆ Use a scaler for removal of fragments adhering to tooth surfaces and near the gingival margin.

◆ Use an air–water syringe with a gentle stream of *warm* water. Warm diluted mouthrinse may soothe the healing area.

III. Dressing Replacement Procedure

◆ Topical anesthetic may be necessary to prevent patient discomfort.

◆ Use a soft dressing with minimal pressure during application.

IV. Patient Oral Self-Care Instruction

Biofilm control follow-up is essential after final dressing removal.

◆ Use an extra soft or soft toothbrush on the treated area, paying careful attention to biofilm removal at the gingival margin.

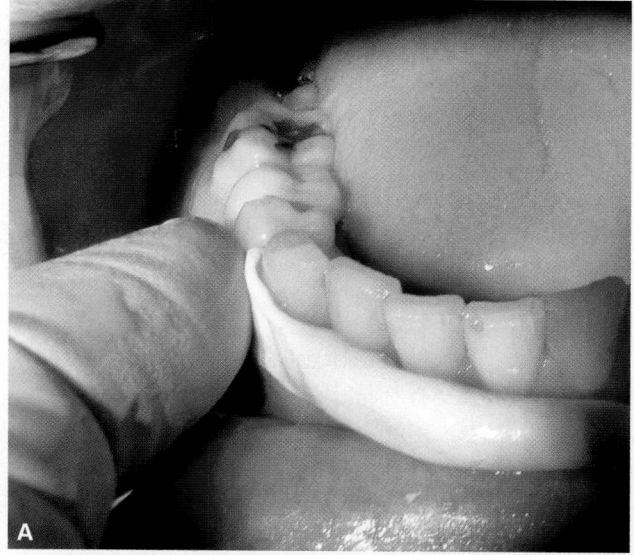

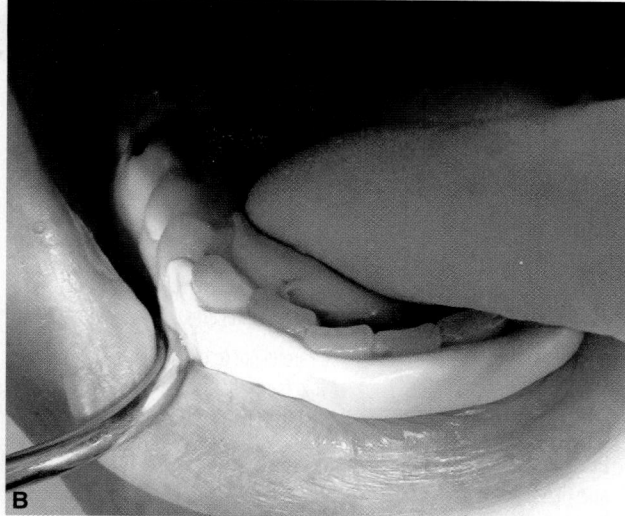

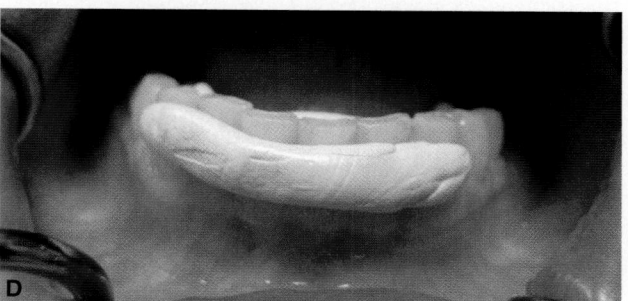

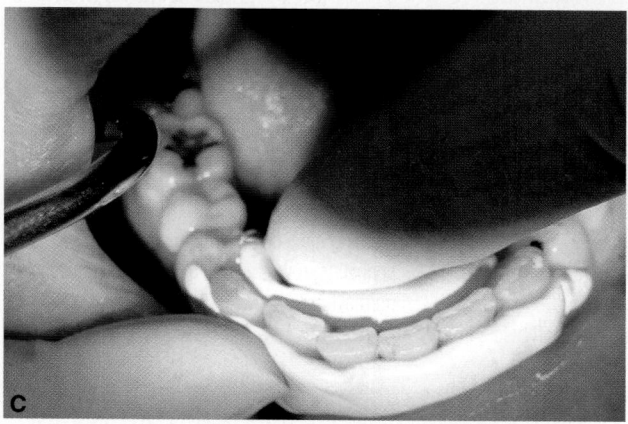

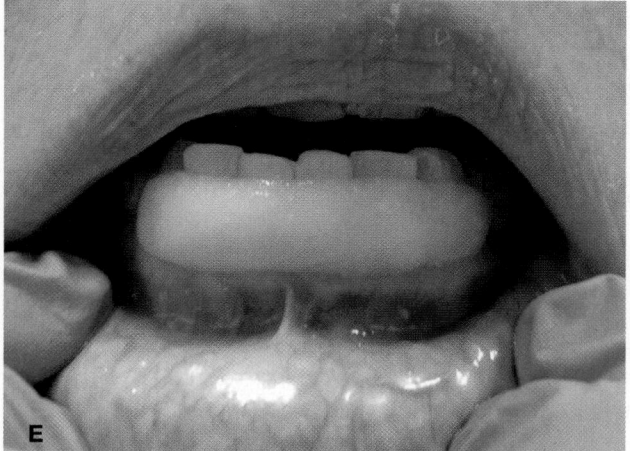

FIGURE 40-6 • Periodontal Dressing. A: Gently pressing the facial periodontal dressing into the interproximal space. **B:** Gently pushing the lingual periodontal dressing into the interproximal space. **C:** Gently pressing the dressing from the buccal and lingual to help "lock" the dressing in place. **D:** Correct placement of the periodontal dressing. A dressing must cover the surgical wound without unnecessary over-extension and fill interdental areas to lock the dressing between the teeth. It is molded in the vestibule and around frena to allow movement of the lips, cheeks, and tongue with no displacement of the dressing. **E:** Reso-Pac™-(Hager Worldwide), a hydrophilic, more esthetically pleasing periodontal dressing. (Courtesy of Susan Jenkins, MCPHS University Forsyth School of Dental Hygiene.)

◆ Increase intensity of care on the treated area each day, with a return to normal oral self-care procedures by day 3 or 4.

◆ Rinse with 0.12% chlorhexidine gluconate twice daily during the healing period. Gently force liquid between the teeth when swishing.

◆ Recommend a dentifrice with sodium fluoride for caries prevention and a prescription fluoride may be indicated depending on the patient's caries risk.

◆ If the patient experiences postsurgical sensitivity, recommend a dentifrice containing a desensitizing agent. Suggestions for coping with sensitivity are found in Chapter 41.

V. Follow-Up

The return for observation of the surgical areas can be scheduled in 1–2 weeks, depending on the patient's progress and treatment planning.

TABLE 40-2 • Instructions for Posttreatment Care

FACTOR	INSTRUCTIONS TO PATIENT	PURPOSE OF INSTRUCTION
Information for the patient about the dressing	• Dressing will protect the surgical wound. • Do not disturb the dressing. • Allow it to remain until the next appointment.	• An informed patient is more likely to be more compliant.
Care during the first few hours	• Do not eat anything that requires chewing. • Use only cool liquids. • Stay quiet and rest. • If a periodontal dressing was placed, it will not set for a few hours.	• Do not touch or disturb the surgical area. • Dressing will become set or become hard.
Local anesthesia	• Be careful not to bite lip, cheek, or tongue. • Avoid foods that require chewing, hot liquids, and spicy foods until anesthesia has worn off.	• Prevent trauma to lips, cheeks, and tongue. • Rest and be quiet.
Discomfort after local anesthesia wears off	• Fill any prescriptions provided by the dentist or periodontist and follow directions. • Do not take more than directed. • Avoid aspirin. • Call the dental office if pain persists.	• Pain control. • Aspirin can interfere with blood-clotting mechanism. • The patient will be more prepared to manage any postoperative discomfort when appropriately informed.
Ice pack or cold compress	• Apply every 30 min for 15 min; or 15 min on, then 15 min off. • Use as directed only.	• Prevent swelling from edema.
Bleeding	• Slight bleeding within the first few hours is not unusual. • Blood clot must not be disturbed. • Do not suck on the area or use straws.	• When bleeding seems persistent or excessive, please call the dental office immediately.
Dressing care and retention	• Avoid disturbing the dressing with the tongue or trying to clean under it. • Small particles may chip off, which is not a problem unless sharp edges irritate the tongue or the dressing becomes loose. • Call the dentist if the entire dressing or a large portion falls off before the fifth day. • Rinse with a saline solution; rinse with chlorhexidine 0.12% morning and evening after brushing teeth.	• Dressing is needed for wound protection. • Epithelium covers wound by fifth or sixth day in normal healing.
Use of tobacco and tobacco products	• Do not smoke; avoid all tobacco products. • A heavy smoker must make every effort to decrease quantity of tobacco used. The dental hygienist may suggest a nicotine patch to aid in preventing withdrawal symptoms and aid the patient in abstaining from tobacco use.	• Heat and smoke irritate the gingiva and delay healing.
Rinsing	• Do not rinse on the day of treatment. • Second day: Use saline solution made with 1/2 teaspoon (measured) in 1/2 cup of warm water every 2–3 hr. • Begin chlorhexidine 0.12% b.i.d. (twice a day).	• Might disturb blood clot. • Saline cleanses and aids healing.
FACTOR	INSTRUCTIONS TO PATIENT	PURPOSE OF INSTRUCTION
Toothbrushing and flossing	• Continue to maintain optimal personal oral self-care in untreated areas. • Lightly brush occlusal surface over dressing material. • Use extra soft or soft brush dampened with warm water, and carefully clean film from dressing. • Clean the tongue.	• Dental biofilm control essential to reduce the number of oral microorganisms. • Odor and taste control. • Oral sanitation.
Diet	• Use highly nutritious foods for healing. • Follow the MyPlate guide (Chapter 33). • Use soft-textured diet. • Avoid highly seasoned, spicy, hot, sticky, crunchy, and coarse foods.	• Healing tissue requires a healthy diet and specific comfort foods. • Use soft foods to protect the dressing from breakage or displacement.
Mastication	• Avoid foods that require excessive chewing such as hard, crunchy, or sticky foods. • Chew only on the untreated side. • Use ground meat or cut meat into small, bite-sized pieces.	• To protect the dressing while it protects the surgical site.

DOCUMENTATION

Detailed documentation is required at each patient visit. The appointment is dated and signed by the attending clinician.

◆ At the time of surgical treatment include in the patient's permanent record at least the following:
  • Vital signs.
  • Anesthesia: type, location, number and size of carpules, and patient response to anesthesia.
  • Sutures: type, location, and number placed.
  • Dressing: specific type and area placed.
  • Provide instructions to patient prior to dismissal.
  • Date and signature by attending dentist or periodontist and surgical assistant.
◆ Dressing and suture removal
  • Tissue examination: tissue response.
  • Patient comments of posttreatment effects, discomfort.
  • Number of sutures removed: compare with number placed.
  • Patient instruction for continued care.
  • Date and signature by attending dental hygienist.

Sample documentation may be reviewed in Box 40-1.

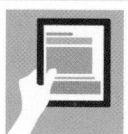

BOX 40-1
Example Documentation:
Sutures and Dressings

S—Patient presents for postsurgical dressing removal between teeth 11 and 15. Patient states no postsurgical problems.

O—Tissue bled slightly during dressing removal. Removed four sutures; confirmed four sutures were placed during surgery. Patient responded well.

A—Dr. examined area; no additional dressing needed; patient discharged with posttreatment instructions.

P—Patient instructed to call if any problems; patient to return for 3-month maintenance appointment.

Signed: _____, RDH

Date: _____

EVERYDAY ETHICS

Ms. Jean arrived for a suture removal appointment with Susan, the dental hygienist, and immediately explains the discomfort she is feeling. When asked why she didn't come in sooner to have the area observed, she said it was so close to the removal appointment she might as well wait. Susan notes from the chart notes that no dressing was placed. The area appeared inflamed, with a slight cyanotic appearance circumscribing the suture area. The patient prerinsed with a 0.12% chlorhexidine, and Susan began removing the sutures. Moderate bleeding and discomfort were present.

Upon removal, Susan noted that only three sutures could be found, but four silk sutures had been placed. When she conferred with Dr. Wynn, the periodontist, Susan was told to dismiss the patient and "prepare a prescription for an antibiotic to prevent an infection. Eventually the suture will be absorbed by body tissues."

Questions for Consideration

1. Given the sequence of events, what issues of ethical principles may be applied?

2. Does it seem clear that the patient understood the postoperative instructions? What suggestions do you have to improve communication?

3. Was the treatment provided within an acceptable standard of care for this patient? Which of the core values have application here?

4. You know the periodontist reviews all chart notes at the end of the day, prepare a progress note that you suggest Susan could write in the permanent record for Ms. Jean's appointment. Do you feel the note covers all the important information? Why or why not?

Factors to Teach the Patient

▶ Provide the posttreatment instructions as outlined in Table 40-2.

▶ Care of the mouth during the period after treatment while wearing a periodontal dressing.

▶ Reasons for not using aspirin for pain relief.

▶ Inform and explain why tobacco use is detrimental and delays healing. Encourage cessation of use of all forms of tobacco.

▶ Discuss the importance of regular periodontal maintenance after treatment is complete.

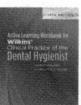

ENHANCE YOUR UNDERSTANDING

ONLINE RESOURCES
(see the inside front cover for access information)
• Audio glossary
• Appendices

SUPPORT FOR LEARNING
(available separately)
• *Active Learning Workbook for Wilkins' Clinical Practice of the Dental Hygienist, 13th Edition*

INDIVIDUALIZED REVIEW
• Customized practice quizzing with Navigate 2 TestPrep for *Wilkins' Clinical Practice of the Dental Hygienist*

References

1. Minozzi F, Bollero P, Unfer V, Dolci A, Galli M. The sutures in dentistry. *Eur Rev Med Pharmacol Sci.* 2009 May–June;13(3):217–226.

2. Selvi F, Cakarer S, Can T, et al. Effects of different suture materials on tissue healing. *J Istanb Univ Fac Dent.* 2016;50(1):35–42.

3. Burkhardt R, Lang NP. Influence of suturing on wound healing. *Periodontol 2000.* 2015 June;68(1):270–281.

4. Giddings FD. *Book of Surgical Knots and Suturing Techniques.* 3rd ed. Fort Collins, CO: Giddings Studio Publishing; 2009.

5. Nishimura RA, Otto CM, Bonow RO,et al. 2017 AHA/ACC focused update of the 2014 AHA/ACC guideline for the management of patients with valvular heart disease: A report of the American College of Cardiology/American Heart Association Task Force on clinical practice guidelines. *J Am Coll Cardiol.* 2017 July 11;70(2):252–289.

6. Giglio JA, Rowland RW, Dalton HP, et al. Suture removal-induced bacteremia: a possible endocarditis risk. *J Am Dent Assoc.* 1992;123(1):65–70.

7. Banche G, Roana J, Mandras N, et al. Microbial adherence on various intraoral suture materials in patients undergoing dental surgery. *J Oral Maxillofac Surg.* 2007 August;65(8):1503–1507.

8. Otten JE, Wiedmann-Al-Ahmad M, Jahnke H, Pelz K. Bacterial colonization on different suture materials: a potential risk for intraoral dentoalveolar surgery. *J Biomed Mater Res B Appl Biomater.* 2005 July;74(1):627–635.

9. King RC, Crawford JJ, Small EW. Bacteremia following intraoral suture removal. *Oral Surg Oral Med Oral Pathol.* 1988;65(1):23–27.

10. Soheilifar S, Bidgoli M, Faradmal J, Soheilifar S. Effect of periodontal dressing on wound healing and patient satisfaction following periodontal flap surgery. *J Dent.* 2015 February;12(2):151–156.

11. Dumville JC, Gray TA, Walter CJ, et al. Dressings for the prevention of surgical site infection. *Cochrane Database Syst Rev.* 2016 December 20;12:CD003091.

12. Kathariya R, Jain H, Jadhav T. To pack or not to pack: the current status of periodontal dressings. *J Appl Biomater Funct Mater.* 2015 July 4;13(2):e73–e86.

13. Monje A, Kramp AR, Criado E, et al. Effect of periodontal dressing on non-surgical periodontal treatment outcomes: a systematic review. *Int J Dent Hyg.* 2016 August;14(3):161–167.

14. Hämmerle CH, Giannobile WV; Working Group 1 of the European Workshop on Periodontology. Biology of soft tissue wound healing and regeneration: consensus report of Group 1 of the 10th European Workshop on Periodontology. *J Clin Periodontol.* 2014 April;41(suppl 15):S1–S5.

41

Dentinal Hypersensitivity

Amy N. Smith, RDH, MS, MPH

CHAPTER OUTLINE

HYPERSENSITIVITY DEFINED
I. Stimuli that Elicit Pain Reaction
II. Characteristics of Pain from Hypersensitivity

ETIOLOGY OF DENTINAL HYPERSENSITIVITY
I. Anatomy of Tooth Structures
II. Mechanisms of Dentin Exposure
III. Hydrodynamic Theory

NATURAL DESENSITIZATION
I. Sclerosis of Dentin
II. Secondary Dentin
III. Smear Layer
IV. Calculus

THE PAIN OF DENTINAL HYPERSENSITIVITY
I. Patient Profile
II. Pain Experience

DIFFERENTIAL DIAGNOSIS
I. Differentiation of Pain
II. Data Collection by Interview
III. Diagnostic Techniques and Tests

HYPERSENSITIVITY MANAGEMENT
I. Assessment Components
II. Educational Considerations
III. Treatment Hierarchy
IV. Reassessment

ORAL HYGIENE CARE AND TREATMENT INTERVENTIONS
I. Mechanisms of Desensitization
II. Behavioral Changes
III. Desensitizing Agents
IV. Self-Applied Measures
V. Professionally Applied Measures
VI. Additional Considerations

DOCUMENTATION

EVERYDAY ETHICS

FACTORS TO TEACH THE PATIENT

REFERENCES

LEARNING OBJECTIVES

After studying this chapter, the student will be able to:

1. Describe stimuli and pain characteristics specific to hypersensitivity and explain how this relates to differential diagnosis.

2. Describe the factors that contribute to dentin exposure and behavioral changes that could decrease hypersensitivity.

3. Explain the steps in the hydrodynamic theory.

4. Describe two mechanisms of desensitization and their associated treatment interventions for managing dentin hypersensitivity.

The dental hygienist is often the first oral health professional to become aware of the presence of hypersensitive teeth when a patient presents for care. Individuals who suffer from hypersensitivity may be uncomfortable during dental hygiene treatment, since exposure to stimuli such as a cold water spray or contact with metal instruments can elicit the pain of hypersensitive teeth.

◆ Patients often report activities of daily living such as eating or drinking cold foods or beverages cause pain and request information about causes and treatment for their discomfort.

◆ Hypersensitivity is often difficult to diagnose because the presenting symptoms can be confused with other types of dental pain with a different etiology.

◆ Management of hypersensitivity can be a challenge because there are numerous treatment approaches with varying degrees of efficacy.

◆ Knowledge of the predisposing factors that lead to gingival recession and loss of enamel or cementum and dentin can assist patients in preventing conditions that cause or exacerbate hypersensitivity.

HYPERSENSITIVITY DEFINED

A definitive characteristic associated with dentinal hypersensitivity is pain elicited by a stimulus and alleviated upon its removal. Numerous types of stimuli can lead to pain response in individuals with exposed dentin surfaces.

I. Stimuli That Elicit Pain Reaction

◆ *Tactile*: contact with toothbrush and other oral hygiene devices, eating utensils, dental instruments, and friction from prosthetic devices such as denture clasps.

◆ *Thermal*: temperature change caused by hot and/or cold foods and beverages, and cold air as it contacts the teeth. Cold is the most common stimulus for pain.

◆ *Evaporative*: dehydration of oral fluids as from high-volume evacuation or application of air to dry teeth during intraoral procedures.

◆ *Osmotic*: alteration of pressure in dentinal tubules through a selective membrane.

◆ *Chemical*: acids in foods and beverages such as citrus fruits, condiments, spices, wine, and carbonated beverages; acids produced by acidogenic bacteria following carbohydrate exposure; acids from gastric regurgitation; acidic formulation of whitening agents.

II. Characteristics of Pain from Hypersensitivity

◆ Sharp, short, or transient pain with rapid onset.

◆ Cessation of pain upon removal of stimulus.

◆ Presents as a chronic condition with acute episodes.

◆ Pain in response to a non-noxious stimulus, one that would not normally cause pain or discomfort.

◆ Discomfort that cannot be ascribed to any other dental defect or pathology.[1]

ETIOLOGY OF DENTINAL HYPERSENSITIVITY

A review of tooth anatomy facilitates an understanding of the mechanism of hypersensitivity.

I. Anatomy of Tooth Structures

A. Dentin

◆ The portion of the tooth covered by enamel on the crown and cementum on the root.

◆ Composed of fluid-filled dentinal tubules that narrow and branch as they extend from the pulp to the dentinoenamel junction or from the pulp to the dentinocementum junction (Figure 41-1).

◆ Only the portions of the dentinal tubules closest to the pulp are potentially innervated with nerve fiber endings from the pulp chamber.

◆ Tubules are wider and more numerous in sensitive areas.[2]

B. Pulp

◆ Highly innervated with nerve cell fiber endings that extend just beyond the dentinopulpal interface of the dentinal tubules.[3]

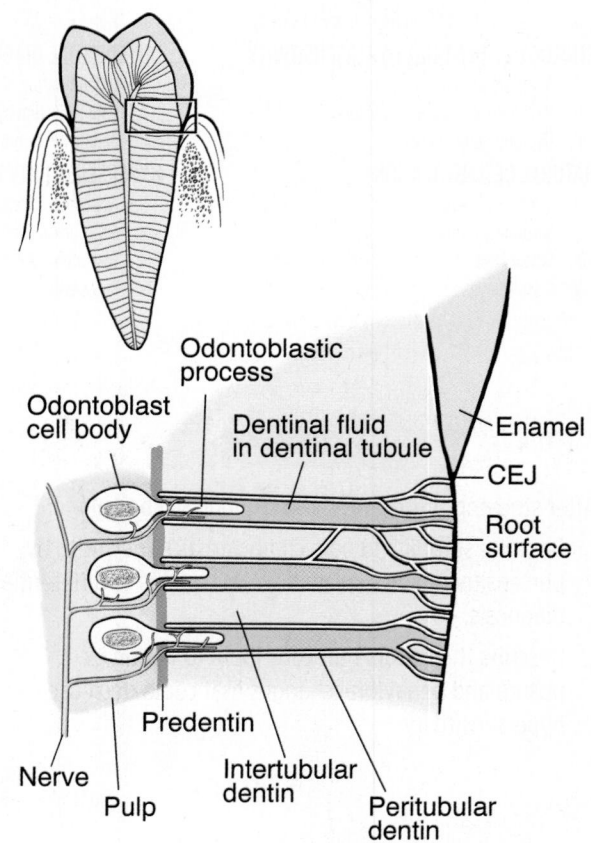

FIGURE 41-1 • Relationship of Dentinal Tubules and Pulpal Nerve Endings. Nerve endings from the pulp wrap themselves around the odontoblasts that extend only a short distance into the tubule. Fluid-filled dentinal tubules transmit fluid disturbances through the mechanism known as hydraulic conductance. CEJ, cementoenamel junction.

- Body portions of odontoblasts (dentin-producing cells) located adjacent to the pulp extend their processes from the dentinopulpal junction a short way into each dentinal tubule (Figure 41-1).

C. Nerves

- Nerve fiber endings extend just beyond the dentinopulpal junction[4] and wind around the odontoblastic processes as shown in Figure 41-1. However, not all dentinal tubules contain nerve fiber endings.
- Nerves react via the same neural depolarization mechanism (sodium–potassium pump), which characterizes the response of any nerve to a stimulus.

II. Mechanisms of Dentin Exposure

- The sequential events of gingival recession, loss of cementum or enamel, and subsequent dentin exposure, as seen in Figure 41-2, can result in hypersensitivity.
- Loss of enamel or cementum can expose dentin gradually or suddenly as in tooth fracture.
- As a result of the lower mineral content of cementum and dentin compared with enamel, demineralization occurs more rapidly and at a lower critical pH.
- Acute hypersensitivity may occur with sudden dentin exposure since gradual exposure allows for the development of natural desensitization mechanisms such as smear layer or sclerosis. After many years, secondary or tertiary/reparative dentin may form, which also protects the pulp.

A. Factors Contributing to Gingival Recession and Subsequent Root Exposure

The occurrence of gingival recession has a multifactorial etiology. Potential causes include:
- Effects of improper oral self-care:
  - Use of a medium- or hard-bristle toothbrush.
  - Frequent, long-term aggressive use of the toothbrush and/or other oral hygiene devices.

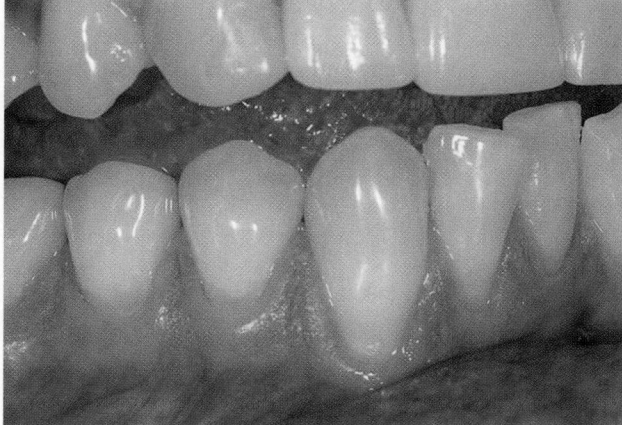

FIGURE 41-2 • Gingival Recession. Note recession from the mandibular right central incisor to the second premolar. If the thin cemental layer of the exposed root surface is lost, dentin hypersensitivity can develop.

- An anatomically narrow zone of attached gingiva is more susceptible to abrasion.
- Facial orientation of one or more teeth.
- A tight and short labial or buccal frenum attachment that pulls on gingival tissues during oral movement.
- Scaling and root debridement procedures that result in gingival tissue shrinkage.
- Subgingival instrumentation involving excessive scaling and debridement in shallow sulci.[5]
- Tissue alteration due to apical migration of junctional epithelium from periodontal diseases.
- Periodontal surgical procedures can alter the architecture of gingival tissues resulting in recession.
- Surgical procedures such as crown lengthening, repositioning of gingival tissues, or tooth extractions can affect gingival coverage of adjacent teeth.
- Orthodontic tooth movement may result in loss of periodontal attachment.
- Restorative procedures, such as crown preparation, that abrade marginal gingival tissues.
- Metal jewelry used in an oral piercing of the lip or tongue that repeatedly traumatizes the adjacent facial or lingual gingival tissue.

B. Factors Contributing to Loss of Enamel and Cementum

- Loss of tooth structure rarely develops from a single cause but rather from a combination of contributing factors.
- Cementum at the cervical area is thin and easily abrades when exposed.

Enamel and cementum do not meet at the cementoenamel junction in about 5–10% of teeth, leaving an area of exposed dentin.

C. Attrition, Abrasion, and Erosion

- Attrition can occur due to parafunctional habits such as bruxing.
- Effects of attrition and abrasion are exacerbated when acid erodes the tooth surface or when the tooth is brushed immediately after consumption of acidic foods and beverages.
- Hypersensitivity may be a clinical outcome of erosion.[6]
- Erosion can occur from dietary acids, such as citrus fruits/juices, wine, and carbonated drinks.[7]
- Dietary acid intake results in an immediate drop in oral pH; after normal salivary neutralization, a physiologic pH of 7 reestablishes within minutes.
- Frequent acid consumption is a critical factor; holding or "swilling" of acidic agents, holding low pH foods such as citrus fruits against teeth, or continual snacking increases erosion risk.
- Gastric acids from conditions such as gastric reflux, morning sickness, or self-induced vomiting (bulimia) repeatedly expose teeth to a highly acidic environment.

D. Abfraction

- Abfraction, a wedge-shaped cervical lesion, has a questionable etiology.[8–11]
- A cervical lesion caused by lateral/occlusal stresses or tooth flexure from bruxing.
- Microscopic portions of the enamel rods chip away from the cervical area of the tooth resulting in loss of tooth structure (Figure 41-3).
- Lesion appears as a wedge- or V-shaped cervical notch.
- A cofactor with abrasion for loss of tooth structure and potential sensitivity.

E. Other Factors

- Crown preparation procedures that remove enamel or cementum can expose dentin at the cervical area.

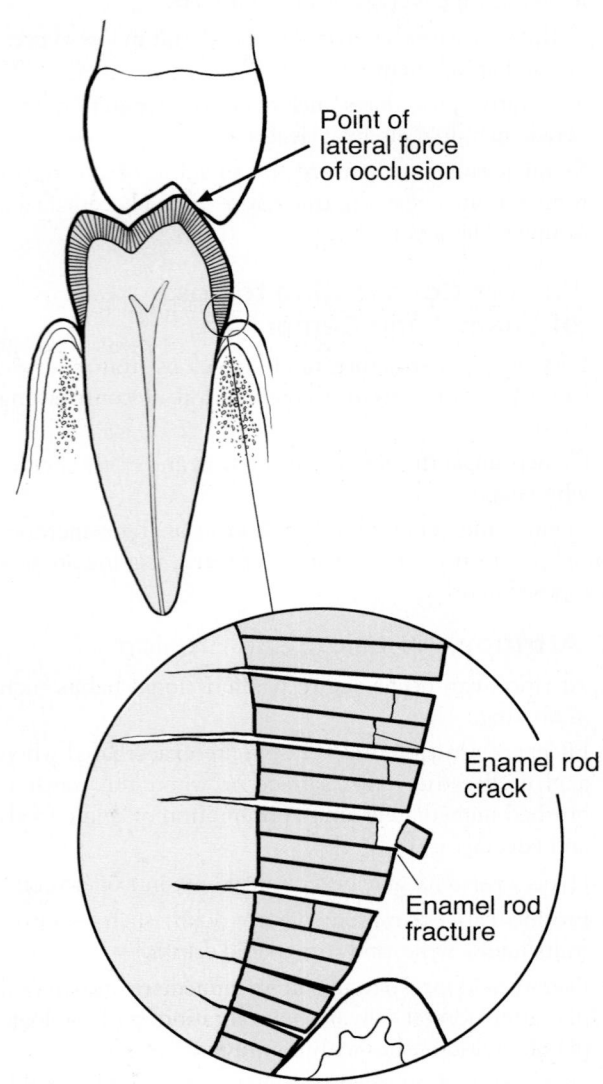

FIGURE 41-3 • Process of Abfraction. Lateral occlusal forces stress the enamel rods at the cervical area, resulting in enamel rod fracture over time. In an advanced stage, a wedge- or V-shaped cervical lesion is visible. Although minute cracks in the enamel rods may not be clinically evident, the tooth can exhibit hypersensitivity.

(Figure 41-3 labels: Point of lateral force of occlusion; Enamel rod crack; Enamel rod fracture)

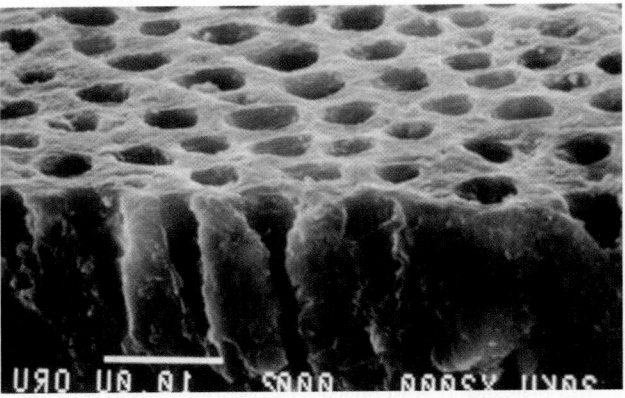

FIGURE 41-4 • Open Dentin Tubules. Note cross-section and transverse views of tubules. (Courtesy of Dr. Sheldon Newman.)

- Instrumentation during scaling or root debridement procedures on thinning cementum.
- Frequent or improper stain-removal techniques, in which abrasive particles wear away the cementum and dentin.
- Root surface carious lesions.
- Removal of proximal enamel using a sandpaper disk or strip to create additional space for orthodontic movement of crowded teeth, also known as "enamel stripping."

III. Hydrodynamic Theory

Hydrodynamic theory is a currently accepted explanation for transmission of stimuli from the outer surface of the dentin to the pulp.

- Described by Brännström in the 1960s,[12] who theorized that a stimulus at the outer aspect of dentin will cause fluid movement within the dentinal tubules.
- Fluid movement creates pressure on the nerve endings within the dentinal tubule, which transmits the pain impulse by stimulating the nerves in the pulp.
- Credibility for this theory is supported by the greater number of widened dentin tubules seen in hypersensitive teeth compared with nonsensitive teeth.[2] Figure 41-4 depicts open dentinal tubules at the microscopic level. Figure 41-5 depicts partially occluded dentinal tubules.

NATURAL DESENSITIZATION

- Hypersensitivity can decrease naturally over time, even without treatment interventions.
- These mechanisms include the following:

I. Sclerosis of Dentin

- Occurs by mineral deposition within tubules as a result of traumatic stimuli, such as attrition or dental caries.

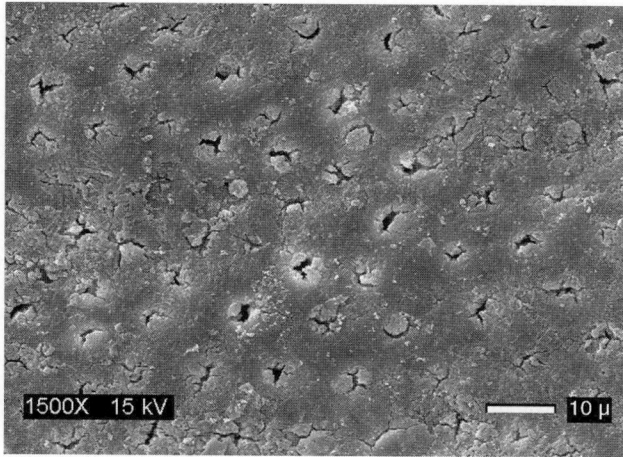

FIGURE 41-5 • Partially Occluded Dentin Tubules. These dentin tubules are nearly filled. (Courtesy of Anthony Giuseppetti.)

◆ Creates a thicker, highly mineralized layer of intratubular or peritubular dentin (deposited within the periphery of the tubules).

◆ Results in a smaller-diameter tubule that is less able to transmit stimuli through the dentinal fluid to the nerve fibers at the dentinopulpal interface.

II. Secondary Dentin

◆ Deposited gradually on the floor and roof of the pulp chamber after the apical foramen is completed.

◆ Formed more slowly than primary dentin; both types of dentin are created by odontoblasts.

◆ Creates a "walling off" effect between the dentinal tubules and the pulp to insulate the pulp from dentin fluid disturbances caused by a stimulus such as dental caries.

◆ With aging, secondary dentin accumulates, resulting in a smaller pulp chamber with fewer nerve endings and less sensitivity.

III. Smear Layer

◆ Consists of organic and inorganic debris that covers the dentinal surface and the tubules.[13]

◆ Accumulates following scaling and root instrumentation, use of toothpaste (abrasive particles), cutting with a bur, attrition, or abrasion.

◆ Occludes the dentinal tubule orifices, forming a "smear plug" or a natural "bandage" that blocks stimuli.

◆ The nature of the smear layer changes constantly since it is subject to effects such as mechanical disruption from ultrasonic debridement, or dissolution from acid exposure.

IV. Calculus

◆ Provides a protective coating to shield exposed dentin from stimuli.

◆ Postdebridement sensitivity can occur after removal of heavy calculus deposits; dentinal tubules may become exposed as calculus is removed.

THE PAIN OF DENTIN HYPERSENSITIVITY

Individuals react differently to pain based on factors such as age, gender, situation and context, previous experiences, pain expectations, and other psychological and physiological parameters.

I. Patient Profile

The prevalence of reported hypersensitivity varies due to differences in the stimulus, and whether data are gathered by patient report or standardized clinical examination. Patient accounts may not represent true hypersensitivity since the pain can be confused with other conditions.

A. Prevalence of Hypersensitivity

◆ Current systematic review articles reveal a global prevalence of dental hypersensitivity to be between 3% and 65% with most populations ranging from 10% to 30%.[14–16]

◆ Most commonly found among 30- to 40-year-olds.[14,15]

◆ Higher prevalence has been reported in periodontally involved populations.[14,16]

◆ Incidence and severity decline with advancing age due to the effects of sclerosis and secondary dentin.[14]

◆ Gingival recession is more prevalent with aging.[18] However, dentinal hypersensitivity is not more prevalent with aging.

◆ Hypersensitivity, when measured objectively, occurs more often in women.[14,17]

B. Teeth Affected

◆ Hypersensitivity has been reported to occur primarily at the cervical one-third of the facial surfaces of premolars and mandibular anterior teeth,[19] or on premolars and molars.[14]

◆ Can occur on any tooth exhibiting predisposing factors.

II. Pain Experience

A. Neural Activity

◆ Stimuli that affect the fluid flow within the dentinal tubules can activate the terminal nerve endings near to or surrounding the dentinal tubules; activation of these nerve fibers elicits the pain response.

◆ Occurs via the depolarization/neural discharge mechanism that characterizes all nerve activity.

◆ The sodium–potassium pump depolarizes the nerve as potassium leaves the nerve cell and sodium enters it.

B. Pain Perception

◆ The degree of pain is not always proportional to the amount of recession, the percentage of tooth structure loss, or to the quality or quantity of stimulus.

◆ Individuals experience the subjective phenomenon of pain differently. Many diverse variables such as stress, fatigue, and health beliefs can impact pain perception.

C. Impact of Pain

◆ Hypersensitivity can manifest as acute or chronic pain; acute pain may result in anxiety, whereas chronic pain may contribute to depression.

◆ Stress may exacerbate the pain response.

◆ Persistent discomfort from dentin hypersensitivity may affect quality of life.

DIFFERENTIAL DIAGNOSIS

◆ Etiology of pain can be systemic, pulpal, periapical, restorative, degenerative, or neoplastic.

◆ A differential diagnosis can rule out other causes of pain before treating for hypersensitivity.

◆ Skilled interviewing and diagnostics contribute to the differential diagnosis.

◆ Components to consider in the differential diagnosis of tooth pain are detailed in Table 41-1

TABLE 41-1 • Differential Diagnosis of Tooth Pain		
CONDITION	SIGNS AND SYMPTOMS	CLINICAL ASSESSMENT
Dentinal hypersensitivity	Thermal, mechanical, evaporative, osmotic, chemical sensitivity Sharp, sudden, transient pain	Clinical examination: gingival recession and loss of tooth structure
Caries extending into dentin	Thermal sensitivity Pain on pressure Pain with sweets	Clinical examination Radiographic examination
Pulpal caries	Thermal sensitivity Severe, intermittent, or throbbing pain Pain on chewing	Clinical examination Radiographic examination
Fractured restoration	Thermal sensitivity Pain on pressure	Clinical examination
Fractured tooth	Thermal sensitivity Pain on pressure	Occlusal examination Transillumination
Recently placed restoration	Thermal sensitivity Pain on pressure	Dental history Clinical examination Occlusal examination
Occlusal trauma	Chemical sensitivity Thermal sensitivity Pain on pressure Mobility	Occlusal examination
Pulpitis	Severe, intermittent, throbbing pain	Thermal and electric pulp tests Percussion
Sinus infection	"Nondescript" tooth pain Nasal congestion (drainage) Sinus pressure Headache	Clinical examination, including extraoral sinus palpation Radiographic examination
Galvanic pain	Sudden, sharp stabbing pain on tooth-to-tooth contact	Examination for contact between restoration of dissimilar nonprecious metals
Periodontal ligament inflammation	Pain on chewing Clinical examination, including palpation for apical tenderness	Percussion
Abfraction	"Cratered" areas of enamel or dentin at cementoenamel junction in the shape of a wedge- or V-shaped notch	Clinical examination Occlusal examination

I. Differentiation of Pain

- Hypersensitivity pain elicited by a non-noxious stimulus, such as cold water, can mimic pain elicited by a noxious agent, such as cavitated dental caries.

- The pain of hypersensitivity subsides when the stimulus is removed.

- It is difficult to distinguish between the pain of hypersensitivity and other causes of dental pain when both are in the mild-to-moderate range. Many types of dental pain can be intensified by thermal, sweet, and sour stimuli.

- Chewing pain (occlusal pressure) can be indicative of pulpal pathology.

- Pulpal pain is severe, intermittent, and throbbing. The pain results from deep dental caries, pulpal inflammation, vertical tooth fracture, or infection, and may occur without provocation and persist after stimulus is removed.

II. Data Collection by Interview

- Utilize direct, open-ended, and nonleading questions.
  - Establish the location, degree of pain, onset/duration, source of stimulus, intensity, and alleviating factors related to the painful response; patients may have difficulty characterizing the pain.
  - Ask trigger questions as suggested in Box 41-1 to elicit detailed information to characterize the pain and assist in the dental hygiene diagnosis.

BOX 41-1
Trigger Questions for Data Collection

- Which tooth or teeth surfaces is/are sensitive?
- On a scale from 1 to 10, with 10 being the most painful, what is your pain intensity?
- How long does the pain last?
- Which words best describe the pain: sharp, dull, shooting, throbbing, persistent, constant, pressure, burning, intermittent?
- Does it hurt when you bite down (pressure)?
- On a scale from 1 to 10, with 10 being a major impact, how much does the pain impact your daily life?
- Is the pain stimulated by certain foods? Sweet? Sour? Acidic?
- Does sensitivity occur with hot or cold food or beverages?
- Does discomfort stop immediately upon removal of the painful stimulus, such as cold food or beverage, or does it linger?
- Have you used whitening products lately?

- Establish rapport, combined with effective listening and counseling skills, to develop collaborative treatment/management strategies.

- Record a thorough dental history, including pain chronology, nature, location, aggravating and alleviating factors, and history of dental treatment/restorations.

III. Diagnostic Techniques and Tests

When patients have difficulty describing and localizing their pain, the following diagnostic techniques and tests can aid in differentiating among the numerous causes of tooth pain.

- Visual assessment of tooth integrity and surrounding tissues.
- Palpation of extra- and intraoral soft tissues.
- Evaluation of nasal congestion, drainage, or sinus expressed as tooth pain.
- Occlusal examination with use of marking paper to detect a premature contact or hyperfunction following placement of a new restoration.
- Radiographic assessment to determine signs of pulpal pathology, vertical tooth fracture, or other irregularities of the teeth or surrounding structures.
- Percussion with use of an instrument handle to lightly tap on each tooth. A pain response may indicate pulpitis.
- Mobility testing may detect trauma or periodontal pathology.
- Pain from biting pressure with use of a bite stick to assess pain indicative of tooth fracture.
- Transillumination with a high-intensity, focused light to enhance visualization of a cracked tooth; dye may also indicate a fracture line.
- Pulpal pathology assessment with thermal or electric pulp tests.

HYPERSENSITIVITY MANAGEMENT

When the differential diagnosis indicates dentinal hypersensitivity, the dental hygiene care plan includes further assessment and patient counseling combined with treatment interventions.

I. Assessment Components

- Determine extent and severity of pain.
  - Solicit a self-report of symptoms, including the eliciting stimuli.
  - Quantify and record the baseline pain intensity using objective measures such as the visual analog scale (VAS) and/or the verbal rating scale (VRS), as described in Box 41-2.
- Determine if oral self-care procedures contribute to loss of gingiva or tooth structure.

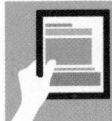

BOX 41-2

Subjective Pain Assessment Form

Name: _____

Date: _____

Teeth: _____

VAS—Visual Analog Scale

Please place an "X" on the line at a position between the two extremes to represent the level of pain that you experience.

| No Discomfort | | Severe Discomfort |

VRS—Verbal Rating Scale

0 = No discomfort/pain, but aware of stimulus

1 = Slight discomfort/pain

2 = Significant discomfort/pain

3 = Significant discomfort/pain that lasted more than 10 seconds

---

◆ Use a diet analysis to assess the frequency of acidic food and beverage intake; correlate intake with timing of toothbrushing.

◆ Explore parafunctional habits, such as bruxing, that may contribute to abfraction and attrition.

II. Educational Considerations

◆ Provide education regarding etiology and contributing factors. Explain the natural mechanisms for resolution of hypersensitivity over time.

◆ Discuss realistic oral self-care measures that the patient is likely to maintain and include technique demonstrations.

◆ Utilize effective communication and motivational interviewing skills to promote compliance and to decrease patient anxiety (see Chapter 24).

III. Treatment Hierarchy

◆ There are two basic treatment goals:
- Pain relief.
- Modification or elimination of contributing factors.

◆ Address mild-to-moderate pain with conservative approaches or agents; more severe pain may require an aggressive approach.

◆ Sequence treatment approaches from the most conservative and least invasive measures to more aggressive modalities.

◆ Prognosis of pain resolution is difficult to predict due to variable success with different treatment options among individuals.

BOX 41-3

The Ideal Desensitizing Agent

- Minimal application time.
- Easy application procedure.
- Does not endanger the soft tissues.
- Acceptable cost.
- Requires few dental appointments.
- Does not cause pulpal irritation or pain.
- Rapid and lasting effect.
- Causes no staining.
- Consistently effective.
- Acceptable taste.

- Historically, a vast array of treatment approaches have been utilized with varying degrees of success; no one best method has been identified due to lack of quality randomized controlled trial data, difficulties inherent in dentin hypersensitivity research design, and a significant placebo effect.
- A trial-and-error approach may be necessary to determine the most effective treatment option.
- Characteristics of an ideal desensitizing agent are listed in Box 41-3 and can be useful evaluation criteria when selecting a desensitizing agent.

◆ Treatment options that include both oral self-care measures and professional interventions with the same objective of reducing hypersensitivity have a synergistic effect.

IV. Reassessment

◆ Evaluate treatment interventions.
- Allow sufficient time to elapse (2–4 weeks) to evaluate effectiveness of treatment recommendations; assess and reinforce behavioral changes.
- Repeat the VAS and/or the VRS to compare changes in pain perceptions from baseline.

◆ If pain persists, a different option may provide relief.

ORAL HYGIENE CARE AND TREATMENT INTERVENTIONS

I. Mechanisms of Desensitization

Desensitization agents and oral self-care measures disrupt the pain transmission as described by the hydrodynamic theory in one of two ways[15]:

◆ Prevent nerve depolarization that interrupts the neural transmission to the pulp. This physiologic process is the mechanism of action for potassium-based products.[20]

◆ Prevent a stimulus from moving the tubule fluid by occlusion of dentin tubule orifices or reduction in tubule lumen diameter.

II. Behavioral Changes

◆ Encourage habits that allow tubules to remain occluded or that occlude patent tubules.

◆ Use a motivational interviewing approach (Chapter 24) to help the patient commit to appropriate oral hygiene self-care and dietary habits before or in conjunction with self-applied or professionally applied desensitizing agents.

◆ Educate the patient that some products may take 2–4 weeks to decrease sensitivity.

A. Dietary Modifications

◆ Have patient analyze acidic food and beverage habits that incite pain from dissolution of the smear layer, which covered open dentinal tubules.[21] Examples include citrus fruits and juices, acidic carbonated beverages, sharp flavors and spices, pickled foods, wines, and ciders.

◆ Counsel patient regarding change in dietary habits.

◆ Help patient determine if brushing is sequenced immediately after consuming acidic foods and beverages. Advise altering sequence to eliminate combined effects of erosion and abrasion, which can accelerate tooth structure loss.[22]

◆ Guide patient toward mouthrinses with a nonacidic formulation.

◆ Provide professional treatment referrals for patients with eating disorders such as bulimia or systemic conditions such as acid reflux that repeatedly create an acidic oral environment.

◆ The acidic environment created by bulimia and acid reflux can be neutralized by rinsing with water (particularly fluoridated water) or an alkaline rinse such as bicarbonate of soda in water.

◆ Counsel patient to eliminate or reduce extremes of hot and cold foods and beverages to avoid discomfort.

B. Dental Biofilm Control

◆ In the presence of dental biofilm, the dentinal tubule orifices increase to three times the original size; with reestablishment of biofilm control measures, there is a 20% decrease in size.[23]

◆ The presence/amount of dental biofilm on exposed root surfaces does not directly correlate with the degree of dentin sensitivity,[17] suggesting biofilm composition may be a factor.

C. Eliminate Parafunctional Habits

◆ Help patient assess bruxing and clenching behaviors and whether additional treatment is indicated.

◆ Determine need for occlusal adjustments to eliminate abfractive forces.

◆ Coach patient to monitor occurrence of subconscious parafunctional behaviors and levels of stress. Identify whether stress reduction protocols are needed.

◆ Introduce behavior modification techniques and refer when needed.

D. Toothbrush Type and Technique

◆ Brush one or two teeth at a time with a soft or ultrasoft toothbrush, rather than using long, horizontal strokes over several teeth to prevent further recession and loss of tooth structure.

◆ Identify brushing sequence and adjust by beginning in least sensitive areas and ending with more sensitive areas. In the initial phases of brushing, toothbrush filaments are stiffer and brushing is more aggressive.

◆ Explore option of brushing with the nondominant hand, if dexterity permits; nondominant hand exerts less pressure than the dominant hand.

◆ Help patient investigate current toothbrush grip. Adjust to a modified pen grasp rather than a traditional palm grasp to reduce the amount of pressure applied.

◆ Explore receptivity to use of a power toothbrush because it removes dental biofilm effectively with less than half the pressure of a manual toothbrush; an individual using a manual toothbrush typically exerts 200–400 g of pressure; 70–150 g of pressure is usually exerted with a power toothbrush.[24] Some power toothbrushes have a self-limiting mechanism to reduce filament action if too much pressure is applied.

◆ Recommend and demonstrate dental biofilm control measures that are meticulous, yet gentle, and do not contribute to abrasion of hard or soft tissues.

III. Desensitizing Agents

◆ There are study design challenges when researching desensitization due to subjectivity of the pain response, the strong placebo effect, and the process of natural desensitization.

◆ Despite widespread professional recommendation and use, there is little in vivo scientific evidence validating the efficacy and mechanisms of action of desensitizing agents.

◆ Randomized controlled trials (RCTs) are needed to support professional recommendation and treatment. The exception is fluoride, with a substantial body of knowledge validating its usefulness as a desensitizing agent.

◆ Desensitizing agents can be categorized according to their mechanisms of action, either depolarization of the nerve or occlusion of the dentinal tubule. Potassium salts are the only agents that are theorized to work by depolarization.

A. Potassium Salts

◆ Formulations containing potassium chloride, potassium nitrate, potassium citrate, or potassium oxalate reduce depolarization of the nerve cell membrane and transmission of the nerve impulse.[22]

◆ Potassium nitrate dentifrices containing fluoride are widely used[20] and readily available over the counter.

B. Fluorides

- Precipitate calcium fluoride (CaF_2) crystals within the dentinal tubule to decrease the lumen diameter.[22]
- Create a barrier by precipitating CaF_2 at the exposed dentin surface to block open dental tubules.[25]
  - Fluoride varnishes are Food and Drug Administration (FDA)-approved for tooth desensitization and a cavity liner, although they are frequently used "off-label" for dental caries prevention.
  - Fluoride gels and varnishes are most commonly used and are a successful treatment modalilty.[26,27]

C. Oxalates

- Block open dental tubules.[28]
- Oxalate salts such as potassium oxalate and ferric oxalate precipitate calcium oxalate crystals to decrease the lumen diameter.[28]

D. Glutaraldehyde

- Coagulates proteins and amino acids within the dentinal tubule to decrease the dentinal tubule lumen diameter.[28]
- Can be combined with hydroxyethylmethacrylate, a hydrophilic resin, which seals tubules.[28]
- Creates calcium crystals within the dentinal tubule to decrease the lumen diameter.[29]

E. Calcium Phosphate Technology

- Advocated for use as a caries control agent to reduce demineralization and increase remineralization by releasing calcium and phosphate ions into saliva for deposition of new tooth mineral (hydroxyapatite).[30]
  - Calcium phosphates can compromise the bioavailability of fluorides since calcium and fluoride react to form calcium fluoride.[31]
  - May be effective for patients with poor salivary flow and consequent deficient calcium phosphate levels.[32]
- Agents that support remineralization may lessen dentinal hypersensitivity by occluding dentinal tubule openings.
- Most studies in support of calcium phosphate technology are animal, in vitro, or in situ models designed to analyze remineralization rather than hypersensitivity.
  - One in vivo study found a reduction in bleaching-induced sensitivity at days 5 and 14 when amorphous calcium phosphate (ACP) was added to a bleaching gel.[33]
  - Additional research related to calcium phosphate technologies is needed.[34]
- ACP
  - Theorized to plug dentinal tubules with calcium and phosphate *precipitate*; promotes an ACP reservoir within the saliva.
  - Enhances fluoride delivery in calcium- and phosphate-deficient saliva.[32]
  - May remineralize areas of acid erosion and abrasion and reduce hypersensitivity.[32]

- Calcium sodium phosphosilicate (CSP)
  - Contains sodium and silica in addition to calcium and phosphorus.
  - Delivered in solid bioactive glass particles that react in the presence of saliva and water to release calcium and phosphate ions and create a calcium phosphate layer that crystallizes to hydroxyapatite.
  - Reacts with saliva; sodium buffers the acid, and calcium and phosphate saturate saliva to fill demineralized areas with new hydroxyapatite.
  - Claims include remineralizing enamel and dentin, positive impact on acid erosion and abrasion, a bactericidal effect, and reduction in hypersensitivity.
  - RCT comparing a CSP and a potassium nitrate toothpaste found, using a VAS, that CSP paste was significantly better at reducing dentin hypersensitivity.[35]
- Casein phosphopeptide (CPP)–ACP
  - CPP is a milk-derived protein that stabilizes ACP and allows it to be released during acidic challenges.
  - Researchers are exploring benefits such as remineralization of acid erosion, caries inhibition, and reduction of dentinal hypersensitivity.
- Tricalcium phosphate (TCP)
  - Developed in an effort to create a calcium material that can coexist with fluoride to provide greater efficacy than fluoride alone.[32] Additional components are added to β-TCP to "functionalize" it. Increased remineralization has been demonstrated in vitro[36]; in vivo evidence is needed.

IV. Self-Applied Measures

A. Dentifrices

- In many OTC sensitivity-reducing dentifrices, 5% potassium nitrate, sodium fluoride, or stannous fluoride separately or in combination are the active desensitizing agents. Studies have suggested that some of the desensitizing effects of dentifrices may be due to the blocking action of the abrasive particles.[22]
- Tartar control dentifrices may contribute to increased tooth sensitivity for some individuals, although the mechanism is unclear.
- Dentifrices containing highly concentrated fluoride (5,000 ppm fluoride) combined with an abrasive to facilitate extrinsic stain control are available by prescription. This formulation is also available with the addition of potassium nitrate.

B. Gels

- Gels containing 5,000 ppm fluoride are a prescription product brushed on for generalized hypersensitivity or burnished into localized areas of sensitivity.
- Contain no abrasive agents for biofilm and stain control.
- Can be self-applied with custom or commercially available fluoride or whitening trays.

C. Mouthrinses

◆ Mouthrinse containing 0.63% stannous fluoride mouthrinse can be prescribed for daily use to treat hypersensitivity.

◆ Short-term use (2–4 weeks) will limit staining concerns.

V. Professionally Applied Measures

A. Tray-Delivered Fluoride Agents

◆ A tray delivery system can be used to apply a 2% neutral sodium fluoride solution.

◆ Select trays of adequate height and fill with sufficient fluoride agent to cover the cervical areas of each tooth.

B. Fluoride Varnish

◆ A 5% sodium fluoride varnish maintains prolonged contact with the tooth surface by serving as a reservoir to release fluoride ions in response to pH changes in saliva and biofilm.[37]

◆ Does not require a dry tooth surface, which is advantageous since drying the tooth can be a painful procedure for a patient with dentin hypersensitivity.

◆ Use a microbrush to apply the varnish to the exposed dentin surface.

◆ Instruct the patient to avoid oral hygiene self-care for several hours to allow the fluoride to stay in contact with the tooth surface for as long as possible, preferably overnight.

C. 5% Glutaraldehyde

◆ Use a microbrush to apply to the affected tooth surface.

◆ Prevent excess flow into soft tissues with cotton roll isolation since contact with soft tissues may cause gingival irritation.

D. Oxalates

◆ Oxalate preparations are applied (burnished) to a dried tooth surface.

◆ May provide immediate and short-term relief, rather than long-term relief.

E. Unfilled or Partially Filled Resins

◆ Used to cover patent dentinal tubules.

◆ Resins are applied following an acid etch step that may remove the smear layer and cause discomfort.

◆ The tooth surface must be dehydrated before resin application, which can create discomfort.

◆ Use of local anesthetic may facilitate patient comfort during this procedure.

F. Dentin-Bonding Agents

◆ Obturates the tubule opening and does not require use of acid etch or dehydration; a single application may protect against further erosion for 3–6 months.

◆ Methylmethacrylate polymer is a common dentin sealer.

G. Glass Ionomer Sealants/Restorative materials

◆ Glass ionomer may be placed in the presence of moisture, which eliminates the need for drying the tooth.

◆ In addition to the glass ionomer restoration physically blocking the dentinal tubule, there is an added benefit of slow fluoride release.

H. Soft-Tissue Grafts

◆ Surgical placement of soft-tissue grafts to cover a sensitive dentinal surface.

I. Lasers

◆ Nd:YAG laser treatment can obliterate dentinal tubules through a process called "melting and resolidification." When used with an appropriate protocol, there is no resulting damage to the pulp or dentin surface cracking.[38,39]

◆ Low-level diode laser treatments have shown a reduction in dentinal hypersensitivity, but the exact mechanism of action is unclear.[40]

◆ Diode laser treatments combined with sodium fluoride varnish application have shown an immediate decrease in sensitivity.[41]

◆ Long-term, in vivo studies are needed to establish safety and efficacy of laser treatment for dentin hypersensitivity. The FDA has not approved these devices for this therapeutic modality.

VI. Additional Considerations

A. Periodontal Debridement Considerations

◆ *Preprocedure*

- Explain potential for sensitivity resulting from calculus removal and/or instrumentation of teeth with areas of exposed cementum or dentin.

- Patients are likely to respond more favorably to treatment when prepared for what might occur.

- When multiple teeth in the same treatment area are hypersensitive during scaling and root planing procedures, local anesthetics and/or nitrous oxide analgesia can be utilized.

- Desensitizing agents that are marketed for immediate relief from severe hypersensitivity can be used.

◆ *Postprocedure*

- Professionally applied desensitization agents can be used.

- Patient is instructed in daily oral health behavior changes and use of self-applied desensitizing agents.

B. Tooth Whitening–Induced Sensitivity

Tooth whitening agents, such as hydrogen peroxide and carbamide peroxide, may contribute to increased dentinal hypersensitivity.

◆ Thought to result from by-products of 10% carbamide peroxide (3% hydrogen peroxide and 7% urea) readily passing through the enamel and dentin into the pulp; the reversible pulpitis is caused from the dentin fluid flow and pulpal contact of the hydrogen peroxide without apparent harm to the pulp.[42]

◆ Hypersensitivity may dissipate over time, lasting from a few days to several months.

◆ Exposed dentin and preexisting dentin hypersensitivity increase hypersensitivity risk secondary to whitening.

◆ Some whitening products contain fluoride or potassium nitrate to eliminate or minimize the effects of sensitivity.

◆ Recommendations outlined in Chapter 43 to prevent or reduce tooth whitening–induced sensitivity include:

- Use of a potassium nitrate, fluoride, or other desensitization product before or concurrently with whitening.
- Some take home whitening gels incorporate, 5% potassium nitrate, fluoride, and ACP.
- Home-use whitening products are usually less concentrated than professionally applied in-office treatment options, with less hypersensitivity risk.
- Allow for a "recovery period" between whitening sessions during which desensitizing agents are used. Decrease frequency of use by whitening every second or third day.

C. Research Developments

◆ The search for the ideal desensitizing agent is ongoing.

◆ Evidence-based scientific research indicated as new products are developed; in vivo research protocols are needed to support clinical application.

DOCUMENTATION

The permanent record for a patient with a history of tooth sensitivity needs to include at least the following information:

◆ Medical and dental history, vital signs, extra- and intraoral examinations, consultations, and individual progress notes for each appointment and maintenance appointments.

◆ For dentin hypersensitivity: identify teeth involved (including measurements of recession, attached gingiva, abfractions, and attrition), differential diagnosis, and all treatments, along with patient instruction for ideal oral self-care, diet, and other for preventive recommendations.

◆ Outcomes and posttreatment directions.

◆ A progress note example for the patient with hypersensitive dentin may be reviewed in Box 41-4.

BOX 41-4

Example Documentation: Patient with Dentinal Hypersensitivity

S—Patient complains of pain when eating/drinking cold foods/beverages that disappears immediately after.

O—Generalized facial gingival recession of 1–2 mm on all teeth in the mandibular arch.

A—Based on patient symptoms, exposed roots, and no other evidence of dental disease, the working diagnosis is dentinal hypersensitivity.

P—Applied fluoride varnish and gave postoperative instructions; advised patient to avoid acidic beverages; or not to brush immediately after ingestion of citrus fruits or beverages; also advised to rinse with fluoridated water to buffer acidic conditions (to raise pH). Recommended purchase and use of an OTC potassium nitrate-containing dentifrice. Explained that relief from the dentifrice can take between 2 and 4 weeks. Advised to contact the office if pain persists or worsens.

Next Steps: Follow-up at next visit.

Signed: _____, RDH

Date: _____

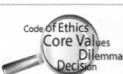

EVERYDAY ETHICS

Marcy, the dental hygienist, practices with Dr. Goldman, who only schedules time to examine a patient at alternate dental hygiene visits unless requested for special needs. Mrs. Stuart arrives for her dental hygiene appointment but is not scheduled to see Dr. Goldman until her next visit. She is complaining of discomfort "on the lower back teeth" when she chews and when she eats or drinks something cold. The pain may last up to an hour.

When she completes the scaling and debridement, Marcy determines that Dr. Goldman is running behind schedule. She knows it will be difficult to get him to come to her treatment room to examine her patient in a timely manner. Marcy gives Mrs. Stuart a sample of desensitizing toothpaste and suggests they will see how it is at the next appointment. Marcy then advises Mrs. Stuart to "Call if it gives you more trouble." The patient is not classified as having a periodontal condition, but is considered low-to-medium risk for dental caries. Her next visit will be in 4 months.

Questions for Consideration

1. How do each of the core values (Table II-1, Section II Introduction) apply in this event? Does the issue of informed consent enter this discussion? Explain why or why not.

2. What ethical issues can arise if Marcy and Dr. Goldman do not take time during this appointment to thoroughly assess Mrs. Stuart's situation to establish a differential diagnosis?

3. Answer the questions provided in the "Questions to Ask" column of Table VI-1 (Section VI Introduction) to determine at least two ethical alternative actions Marcy could have taken.

Factors to Teach the Patient

▶ Etiology and prevention of gingival recession.

▶ Factors contributing to dentin hypersensitivity.

▶ Mechanisms of dentin tubule exposure, which can allow various stimuli to trigger pain response.

▶ Natural desensitization mechanisms that may lessen sensitivity over time.

▶ Appropriate oral hygiene self-care techniques, such as using a soft toothbrush and avoiding a vigorous brushing technique that may contribute to gingival recession and subsequent abrasion of root surfaces.

▶ Connection between an acidic diet and dentin sensitivity; need to eliminate specific foods and beverages that can trigger sensitivity.

▶ Toothbrushing is not recommended immediately after consumption of acidic foods or beverages.

▶ Behavior modifications or treatments for eliminating parafunctional habits.

▶ The challenges of managing hypersensitivity, hierarchy of treatment measures, and variable effect of treatment options.

ENHANCE YOUR UNDERSTANDING

ONLINE RESOURCES
(see the inside front cover for access information)

- Audio glossary
- Appendices

SUPPORT FOR LEARNING
(available separately)

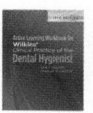

- *Active Learning Workbook for Wilkins' Clinical Practice of the Dental Hygienist, 13th Edition*

INDIVIDUALIZED REVIEW

- Customized practice quizzing with Navigate 2 TestPrep for *Wilkins' Clinical Practice of the Dental Hygienist*

References

1. Addy M. Etiology and clinical implications of dentine hypersensitivity. *Dent Clin North Am.* 1990;34(3):503-514.

2. Absi EG, Addy M, Adams D. Dentine hypersensitivity: the development and evaluation of a replica technique to study sensitive and non-sensitive cervical dentine. *J Clin Periodontol.* 1989;16(3):190-195.

3. Frank RM. Attachment sites between the odontoblast process and the intradental nerve fibre. *Arch Oral Biol.* 1968;13(7):833-834.

4. Thomas HF, Carella P. Correlation of scanning and transmission electron microscopy of human dentinal tubules. *Arch Oral Biol.* 1984;29(8):641-646.

5. Dufour LA, Bissell HS. Periodontal attachment loss induced by mechanical subgingival instrumentation in shallow sulci. *J Dent Hyg.* 2002;76(3):207-212.

6. Absi EG, Addy M, Adams D. Dentine hypersensitivity: the effect of toothbrushing and dietary compounds on dentine in vitro. *J Oral Rehabil.* 1992;19(2):101-110.

7. Prati C, Montebugnoli L, Supp P, et al. Permeability and morphology of dentin after erosion induced by acidic drinks. *J Periodontol.* 2002;74(4):428-436.

8. Staninec M, Nalla RK, Hilton JF, et al. Dentin erosion simulation by cantilever beam fatigue and pH change. *J Dent Res.* 2005;84(4):371-375.

9. Litonjua LA, Andreana S, Bush OJ, et al. Wedged cervical lesions produced by toothbrushing. *Am J Dent.* 2004;17(4):237-240.

10. Estafan A, Furnari PC, Goldstein G, et al. In vivo correlation of noncarious cervical lesions and occlusal wear. *J Prosthet Dent.* 2005;93(3):221-226.

11. Sarode GS, Sarode CS. Abfraction: a review. *J Oral Maxillofac Pathol.* 2013;17(2):222-227.

12. Brännström M, Linden LA, Astrom A. The hydrodynamics of the dental tubule and of pulp fluid: a discussion of its significance in relation to dentinal sensitivity. *Caries Res.* 1967;1(4):310-317.

13. Eldarrat AH, High AS, Kale GM. In vitro analysis of "smear layer" on human dentine using ac-impedance spectroscopy. *J Dent.* 2004;32(7):547-554.

14. Splieth CH, Tachou A. Epidemiology of dentin hypersensitivity. *Clin Oral Invest.* 2013;17(suppl 1):S3-S8.

15. Shiau HJ. Dentin hypersensitivity. *J Evid Base Pract.* 2012;12(suppl 1):220-228.

16. Kim JW, Park JC. Dentin hypersensitivity and emerging concepts for treatments. *J Oral Bio.* 2017;59(4):211-217.

17. Mantzourani M, Sharma D. Dentine sensitivity: Past, present, and future. *J Dent.* 2013;41(suppl 4):S3-S17.

18. Kassaba MM, Cohen RE. The etiology and prevalence of gingival recession. *J Am Dent Assoc.* 2003;134(2):220-225.

19. Gillam DG, Aris A, Bulman JS, et al. Dentine hypersensitivity in subjects recruited for clinical trials: clinical evaluation, prevalence and intraoral distribution. *J Oral Rehabil.* 2002;29(3):226-231.

20. Orchardson R, Gillam DG. The efficacy of potassium salts as agents for treating dentin hypersensitivity. *J Orofac Pain.* 2000;14(1):9-19.

21. Correa FO, Sampaio JE, Rossa C, et al. Influence of natural fruit juices in removing the smear layer from root surfaces—an in vitro study. *J Can Dent Assoc.* 2004;70(10):697-702.

22. Orchardson R, Gilla DC. Managing dentin hypersensitivity. *J Am Dent Assoc.* 2006;137(7):990-998.

23. Kawasaki A, Ishikawa K, Sug T, et al. Effects of plaque control on the patency and occlusion of dentine tubules in situ. *J Oral Rehabil.* 2001;28(5):439-449.

24. Van Der Weijden GA, Timmerman MF, Reijerse E, et al. Toothbrushing force in relation to plaque removal. *J Clin Periodontol.* 1996;23(8):724-729.

25. Suge T, Ishikowa K, Kawasaki A, et al. Effects of fluoride on the calcium phosphate precipitation method for dentinal tubule occlusion. *J Dent Res.* 1995;74(4):1079-1085.

26. Ritter AV, de L Dias W, Miguez P, et al. Treating cervical dentin hypersensitivity with fluoride varnish: a randomized clinical study. *J Am Dent Assoc.* 2006;137(7):1013-1020.

27. Cunha-Cruz J, Wataha JC, Zhou L, et al. Treating dentin hypersensitivity, therapeutic choices made by dentists of the Northwest PRECEDENT network. *J Am Dent Assoc.* 2010;141(9):1097-1105.

28. Haywood VB. Dentine hypersensitivity: bleaching and restorative considerations for successful management. *Int Dent J.* 2002;52(suppl 1):376.

29. Pashley DH, Kalathoor S, Burnham D. The effects of calcium hydroxide on dentin permeability. *J Dent Res.* 1986;65(3):417-420.

30. Featherstone JD. The continuum of dental caries-evidence for a dynamic disease process. *J Dent Res.* 2004;83(Spec No C):C39-C42.

31. Karlinsey RL, Mackey AC, Walker ER, et al. Surfactant-modified B-TCP: structure, properties, and in vitro remineralization of subsurface enamel lesions. *J Mater Sci Mater Med.* 2010;21(4):2009-2020.

32. Chow L, Wefel JS. The dynamics of de-and remineralization. *Dimensions Dent Hyg.* 2009;7(2):42-46.

33. Giniger M, MacDonald J, Ziemba S, et al. The clinical performance of professionally dispensed bleaching gel with added amorphous calcium phosphate. *J Am Dent Assoc.* 2005;136(3):383-392.

34. Yengopal V, Mickenautsch S. Caries-preventive effect of casein phosphopeptide-amorphous calcium phosphate (CPP-ACP): a meta-analysis. *Acta Odontol Scand.* 2009;21:1-12.

35. Pradeep AR, Sharma A. Comparison of clinical efficacy of a dentifrice containing calcium sodium phosphosilicate to a dentifrice containing potassium nitrate and to a placebo on dentinal hypersensitivity: a randomized clinical trial. *J Periodontol.* 2010;81(8):1167-1173.

36. Karlinsey RL, Mackey AC, Walker ER, et al. Preparation, characterization and in vitro efficacy of an acid-modified β-TCP material for dental hard-tissue remineralization. *Acta Biomater.* 2010;6(3):969-978.

37. Shen C, Autio-Gold J. Assessing fluoride concentration uniformity and fluoride release from 3 varnishes. *J Am Dent Assoc.* 2002;133(2):176-182.

38. Kara C, Orbak R. Comparative evaluation of Nd:YAG laser and fluoride varnish for the treatment of dentinal hypersensitivity. *J Endod.* 2009;35(7):971-974.

39. Lopes AO, Aranha ACC. Comparative evaluation of the effects of Nd:YAG laser and a desensitizer agent on the treatment of dentin hypersensitivity: a clinical study. *Photomed Laser Surg.* 2013;31(3):132-138.

40. Yilmaz H, Kurtulmus-Yilmaz S, Cengiz E. Long-term effect of diode laser irradiation compared to sodium fluoride varnish in the treatment of dentine hypersensitivity in periodontal maintenance patients: a randomized controlled clinical study. *Photomed Laser Surg.* 2011;29(11):721-725.

41. Corona S, Nascimento T, Catirse A, Lizarelli R, Dinelli W, Palma-Dibb R. Clinical evaluation of low-level laser therapy and fluoride varnish for treating cervical dentinal hypersensitivity. *J Oral Rehabil.* 2003;30(12):1183–1189.

42. Li Y, Greenwall L. Safety issues of tooth whitening using peroxide-based materials. *Br Dent J.* 2013;215(1):29-34.

42

Extrinsic Stain Removal

Heather Doucette, DipDH, BSC, Med

CHAPTER OUTLINE

INTRODUCTION

PURPOSES FOR STAIN REMOVAL

SCIENCE OF POLISHING

EFFECTS OF CLEANING AND POLISHING
  I. Precautions
  II. Environmental Factors
  III. Effect on Teeth
  IV. Effect on Gingiva

INDICATIONS FOR STAIN REMOVAL
  I. Removal of Extrinsic Stains
  II. To Prepare the Teeth for Caries-Preventive Procedures
  III. To Contribute to Patient Motivation

CLINICAL APPLICATION OF SELECTIVE STAIN REMOVAL
  I. Summary of Contraindications for Polishing
  II. Suggestions for Clinic Procedure

CLEANING AND POLISHING AGENTS
  I. Cleaning Agents
  II. Polishing Agents
  III. Factors Affecting Abrasive Action with Polishing Agents
  IV. Abrasive Agents
  V. Cleaning Ingredients

PROCEDURES FOR STAIN REMOVAL (CORONAL POLISHING)
  I. Patient Preparation for Stain Removal
  II. Environmental Preparation

THE POWER-DRIVEN INSTRUMENTS
  I. Handpiece
  II. Types of Prophylaxis Angles
  III. Prophylaxis Angle Attachments
  IV. Uses for Attachments

USE OF THE PROPHYLAXIS ANGLE
  I. Effects on Tissues: Clinical Considerations
  II. Prophylaxis Angle Procedure

AIR-POWDER POLISHING
  I. Principles of Application
  II. Specially Formulated Powders for Use in Air-Powder Polishing
  III. Uses and Advantages of Air-Powder Polishing
  IV. Technique
  V. Recommendations and Precautions
  VI. Risk Patients: Air-Powder Polishing Contraindicated

POLISHING PROXIMAL SURFACES
  I. Dental Tape and Floss
  II. Finishing Strips

THE PORTE POLISHER

DOCUMENTATION

EVERYDAY ETHICS

FACTORS TO TEACH THE PATIENT

REFERENCES

LEARNING OBJECTIVES

After studying this chapter, the student will be able to:

1. Describe the difference between a cleaning agent and a polishing agent.

2. Explain the basis for selection of the grit of polishing paste for each individual patient.

3. Discuss the rationale for avoiding polishing procedures on areas of demineralization.

4. Explain the effect abrasive particle shape, size, and hardness have on the abrasive qualities of a polishing paste.

5. Explain the types of powdered polishing agents available and their use in the removal of tooth stains.

6. Explain patient conditions that contraindicate the use of air-powder polishing.

INTRODUCTION

After treatment by scaling, root debridement, and other dental hygiene care, the teeth are assessed for the presence of remaining dental stains.

◆ The cleaning or polishing agents used must be *selected* based on the patient's individual needs such as the type, location, and amount of stain present.

◆ Preliminary examination of each tooth will reveal the surfaces to be treated may be tooth structure (enamel, or with recession, cementum or dentin) or when restored, a variety of dental materials (metal or esthetic, tooth-color restorations).

◆ *Preservation of the surfaces of both the teeth and the restorations is of primary importance during all cleaning and polishing procedures.*

◆ Stain removal requires the use of polishing agents with various abrasive grits. The smallest, least abrasive grit is used.

◆ Some patients will not consider their teeth "cleaned" unless they have been polished. This situation is ideal for a cleaning agent that will not abrade the dental hard tissues, but will remove dental biofilm and the patient's teeth will have the same clean feeling as they would if an abrasive prophylaxis paste were used.

◆ Incorrect selection of a prophylaxis paste can worsen hypersensitivity and cause significant damage to esthetic restorations.

◆ The longevity, esthetic appearance, and smooth surfaces of dental restorations depend on appropriate care by the dental hygienist and the daily personal care by the patient.

◆ It is the responsibility of the dental hygienist to be current in knowledge of the procedures to prevent damage to the restorations during professional healthcare appointments.

PURPOSES FOR STAIN REMOVAL

Stains on the teeth are not etiologic factors for oral disease.

◆ The removal of stains is for esthetic, not for therapeutic or health, reasons.

◆ The American Dental Hygienists' Association and the Academy of Periodontology include tooth polishing in their definitions of the term "oral prophylaxis."[1,2]

SCIENCE OF POLISHING

◆ Polishing is intended to produce intentional, selective and controlled wear. Within the science of tribiology, polishing is considered to be two-body abrasive polishing or three-body abrasive polishing.[3]

- Two-body abrasive polishing involves the abrasive particles attached to a medium, such as a rubber cup impregnated with abrasive particles that does not require a prophylaxis polishing paste.

- Three-body abrasive polishing is the type most commonly used by dental hygienists, in which loose abrasive particles (the abrasive particles in prophylaxis polishing paste) move in the interface space between the surface being polished and the polishing application device (rubber cup or brush).[4–6]

EFFECTS OF CLEANING AND POLISHING

Attention must be given to the positive and negative effects of polishing so evidence-based decisions can be made for the treatment of each patient.

I. Precautions

◆ As with all gingival manipulation with instruments, including a toothbrush,[7,8] bacteremia can be created during the use of power-driven stain removal instruments. Rotation of the rubber cup can force microorganisms into the tissues.

◆ An inflammatory response can be expected, and bacteria may gain access to the bloodstream to create a bacteremia.

◆ This is a concern for an immunocompromised patient and for a patient who requires prophylactic antibiotic coverage before dental treatment.

◆ A thorough medical history is essential before all treatments and must be reviewed and updated at each succeeding appointment.

◆ Patients at risk, particularly those with damaged or abnormal heart valves, prosthetic valves, and other conditions listed in Chapter 11, may require antibiotic prophylaxis as specified by the patient's cardiologist.

II. Environmental Factors

A. Aerosol Production

◆ Aerosols are created during the use of all rotary instruments, including a prophylaxis handpiece with a rubber cup to hold polishing paste, the air and water sprays used during rinsing, and air polishing.[9]

◆ The biologic contaminants of aerosols stay suspended for long periods and provide a means for disease transmission to dental personnel, as well as to other patients.

◆ Use of power-driven instruments is limited when a patient is known to have a communicable disease, a serious or chronic respiratory disease, or is immunocompromised.

◆ Standard personal protective procedures are used.

B. Spatter

◆ Protective eyewear is needed for all dental team members and for the patient.

◆ Serious eye damage has occurred because of spatter from polishing paste or from instruments.[10]

III. Effect on Teeth

A. Removal of Tooth Structure

◆ Polishing with coarse abrasive prophylaxis pastes may remove a few micrometer of the outer enamel. This is justification for using the least abrasive prophylaxis paste necessary to meet the patient's needs.

◆ The fluoride-rich outer surface of the enamel is necessary for protection against dental caries[11] and care must be taken to preserve it. The use of a cleaning agent in place of an abrasive prophylaxis polishing agent will not remove the outermost layer of enamel.

B. Areas of Demineralization

◆ *Demineralization:* Polishing demineralized white spots of enamel is contraindicated. More surface enamel is lost from abrasive polishing over demineralized white spots than over intact enamel.[12]

◆ *Remineralization:* Demineralized areas of enamel can remineralize as these areas are exposed to fluoride from saliva, water, dentifrices, and professional fluoride applications. Polishing procedures can interrupt enamel surface remineralization.

C. Areas of Thin Enamel, Cementum, or Dentin

◆ Areas of thin enamel are contraindicated for polishing.
  ● Amelogenesis imperfecta is an example of thin enamel resulting from imperfect tooth development (see Chapter 16).

◆ *Exposure of dentinal tubules:* Cementum and dentin are softer and more porous than enamel, so greater amounts of their surfaces can be removed during polishing than from enamel. Polishing of exposed cementum and dentin is contraindicated.

◆ Smear layer could be removed and dentinal tubules exposed[13] resulting in tooth sensitivity.[14]

D. Care of Restorations and Implants

◆ Use of coarse abrasives may create deep, irregular scratches in restorative materials. Figure 42-1 shows a scanning electron photomicrograph of the damaged

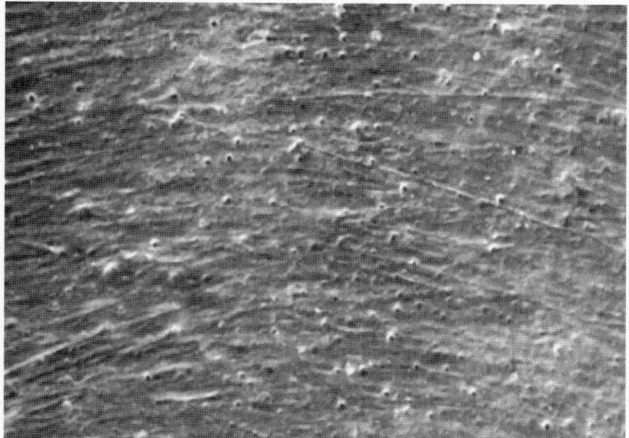

FIGURE 42-1 • Scanning Electron Photomicrograph of a Composite Restoration Polished with Coarse Prophylaxis Paste.

surface of a composite restoration polished with a rubber cup and coarse prophylaxis paste.

◆ It is imperative that prophylaxis polishing agents are not used on restorative materials. Polishing pastes not intended for use on restorative materials can destroy the surface integrity of the dental material.[15]
  ● Select a cleaning agent or a polishing agent recommended by the manufacturer of the restorative materials.[15,16]

E. Heat Production

◆ Steady pressure with a rapidly revolving rubber cup or bristle brush and a minimum of wet abrasive agent can create sufficient heat to cause pain and discomfort for the patient.

◆ The pulp chamber in the teeth of children are large and may be more susceptible to heat.

◆ The rules for the use of cleaning or polishing agents include:
  ● Use light pressure, slow speed of the rubber cup.
  ● Use a moist agent.
  ● Cleaning or polishing agents are never to be used as dry powders applied directly on teeth.

IV. Effect on Gingiva

◆ Trauma to the gingival tissue can result, especially when the prophylaxis angle is operated at a high speed with heavy pressure and the rubber cup is applied for an extended period of time adjacent to gingival tissues.

◆ It may be best to delay stain removal after nonsurgical periodontal treatments (NSPTs) to allow for healing of the sulcular tissue. If selective polishing is required, it can be done at the reevaluation appointment following initial NSPT therapy.

INDICATIONS FOR STAIN REMOVAL

I. Removal of Extrinsic Stains

A. Patient Instruction

◆ Discuss source of stain and how it can be prevented.

◆ Encourage patient to make necessary habit changes, especially to seek counseling for smoking cessation if that is the cause of the patient's stain. Tobacco cessation is described in Chapter 32.

◆ Practice toothbrushing to remove stains incorporated in dental biofilm.
  ● For example, educate the patient that careful dental biofilm removal when using chlorhexidine rinse can prevent and/or minimize stain accumulations. The less dental biofilm, the less chlorhexidine may stain the teeth.

B. Scaling and Root Debridement

◆ In addition to the use of cleaning or polishing agents during polishing procedures, stains can also be removed during scaling and root debridement instrumentation.

 • Example: Black line stain has been compared to calculus because it may be elevated from the tooth surface and may need to be removed by instrumentation. It is described in Chapter 17.[17]

II. To Prepare the Teeth for Caries-Preventive Procedures

A. Placement of Pit and Fissure Sealant

◆ Follow manufacturer's directions. Sealants vary in their requirements.

◆ Avoid commercial oral prophylaxis pastes containing glycerin, oils, flavoring substances, or other agents. Glycerin and oils can prevent an optimum acid-etch and interfere with the adherence of the sealant to the tooth surface, causing the sealant to fail.

 • Air-powder polishing is one method of choice for preparing tooth surfaces for sealants (see Chapter 35).[18,19]
 • An alternative is the use of a plain, fine pumice mixed with water when precleaning is necessary.

◆ After the use of pumice, the tooth surface(s) needs to be rinse thoroughly to remove the particles.

III. To Contribute to Patient Motivation

Removal of biofilm is a *daily* procedure to be carried out *by the patient*. When accomplished thoroughly at least twice daily and for some patients three times daily, infection can be controlled, the sanitation of the mouth maintained, and staining can be minimized or prevented.

◆ Motivation

Smooth, polished tooth surfaces may contribute in part to the following effects:

 • Help the patient to obtain more satisfactory results from oral self-care procedures. A smooth surface can be easier to achieve once the patient understands what a biofilm and debris-free mouth feels like after having the teeth professionally polished with a cleaning or polishing agent.
 • Show the patient the appearance and feeling of a clean mouth for motivational purposes. The change in behavior, or the true learning, can be obtained through patient participation in the use of a disclosing agent and personal visualization of the biofilm followed by removal of the biofilm with floss and toothbrush.

CLINICAL APPLICATION OF STAIN REMOVAL

The decision to polish teeth is based on the individual patient's needs.

I. Summary of Contraindications for Polishing

The following list suggests some of the specific instances in which polishing either can be performed with a cleaning agent or is contraindicated.

A. No Unsightly Stain

◆ If no stain is present, polishing with an abrasive polishing agent is not necessary; however, this is an ideal situation for using a cleaning agent.

B. Patients with Respiratory Problems

Polishing procedures typically require rinsing of the patient's mouth several times throughout the procedure.

◆ Care is taken to minimize the spray from the air–water syringe as much as possible as the aerosols are contraindicated for such conditions as asthma, emphysema, cystic fibrosis, lung cancer, patients requiring oxygen, or when breathing is a problem.

◆ This caution also applies to the use of air-powder polishers and spatter from prophylaxis polishing pastes.

C. Tooth Sensitivity

◆ Abrasive agents can uncover ends of dentinal tubules in areas of thin cementum or dentin.

◆ The polishing of dentin and cementum is contraindicated.

D. Restorations

◆ Restorations and titanium implants may be scratched by abrasive prophylaxis polishing pastes.

◆ Tooth-colored restorations need to be polished with a cleaning agent, a polishing paste specifically formulated for use on esthetic restorations, or the paste recommended by the manufacturer of the restorative material.[15]

E. Conditions That Require Postponement for Later Evaluation

◆ When instruction for personal biofilm removal (daily care) has not yet been given or when the patient has not demonstrated adequate biofilm control.

◆ Soft, spongy tissue that bleeds on brushing or gentle instrumentation.

◆ Communicable disease potentially disseminated by aerosol.

II. Suggestions for Clinic Procedure

A. Provide Initial Education

◆ Daily dental biofilm removal to assist in dental stain control.

◆ Explain to the patient that drinking coffee, tea, red wine, and color-added soft drinks and/or use of tobacco is responsible for most dental stains.

◆ Provide patients with information about the types of dentifrices that are safe for stain control and those contraindicated due to excessive abrasiveness or chemical harshness.

◆ Tobacco cessation introduction when stain is primarily from tobacco use (see Chapter 32).

B. Remove Stain by Scaling

◆ Whenever possible, stains can be removed during scaling and root debridement.

C. Stain Removal Techniques

◆ Cleaning agent or low-abrasion oral prophylaxis paste.

◆ Use the lightest pressure necessary for stain removal.

◆ Low-speed handpiece.

◆ Minimal heat production.

◆ Soft rubber cup at 90° to tooth surface with intermittent light applications.

CLEANING AND POLISHING AGENTS

There are two distinct types of agents used for "polishing" teeth: one is a cleaning agent and the other is a polishing agent.[20,21]

I. Cleaning Agents

◆ Unlike polishing agents, cleaning agents are round, flat, nonabrasive particles and do not scratch surface material but produce a higher luster than polishing agents.

◆ The most readily available cleaning agent (ProCare, Young Dental Mfg., Earth City, MO) is made of a combination of feldspar, alkali (sodium and potassium), and aluminum silicates.

  • This feldspar, sodium–aluminum silicate cleaning agent is formulated into a powder and can be mixed with water or sodium fluoride to make a paste for cleaning.[22,23]

◆ Because of the extremely low level of abrasion, cleaning agents can be used on any tooth surface, restorative surface, or implant surface without fear of creating deep scratches.

◆ Cleaning agents will not harm restorative surfaces, and any other polishing agent selected for restorative surfaces should be selected based on the formulation and appropriateness for the restorative material.[24]

II. Polishing Agents

◆ Traditionally, abrasive agents have been applied with polishing instruments to remove extrinsic dental stains and leave the enamel surface smooth and shiny.

◆ Polishing agents act by producing scratches in the surface of the tooth or restoration created by the friction between the abrasive particle and the softer tooth or restorative surface.

◆ The cleaning and polishing process progresses from coarse abrasion to fine abrasion until the scratches are smaller than the wavelength of visible light, which is 0.05 μm.[24]

◆ When scratches of this size are created, the surface appears smooth and shiny—the smaller the scratches, the shinier the surface.

◆ Unless the abrasive agent has been specially formulated for esthetic restorative surfaces, the use of prophylaxis polishing pastes is contraindicated for application to any esthetic restorative surfaces.[16,25]

III. Factors Affecting Abrasive Action with Polishing Agents

During polishing, sharp edges of abrasive particles are moved along the surface of a material, abrading it by producing microscopic scratches or grooves. The rate of abrasion, or speed with which structural material is removed from the surface being polished, is governed by hardness and shape of the abrasive particles, as well as by the manner in which they are applied.

A. Characteristics of Abrasive Particles

◆ *Shape:* Irregularly shaped particles with sharp edges produce deeper grooves and thus abrade faster than do rounded particles with dull edges.

◆ *Hardness:* Particles must be harder than the surface to be abraded; harder particles abrade faster.

  • Many of the abrasives used in prophylaxis polishing pastes are 10 times harder than the tooth structure to which they are applied.[24]

  • Table 42-1 provides a comparison of the Mohs hardness value of dental tissues compared to agents commonly used in prophylaxis polishing pastes and substances used in cleaning agents.

◆ *Body strength:* Particles that fracture into smaller sharp-edged particles during use are more abrasive than those that wear down during use and become dull.

◆ *Particle size (grit)*

  • The larger the particles, the more abrasive they are and the less polishing ability they have.

  • Finer abrasive particles achieve a glossier finish.

  • Abrasive and polishing agents are graded from coarse to fine based on the size of the holes in a standard sieve through which the particles will pass.

B. Principles for Application of Abrasives

◆ *Quantity applied:* The more particles applied per unit of time, the faster the rate of abrasion.

  • Particles are suspended in water or other vehicles for frictional heat reduction.

TABLE 42-1 • Mohs Hardness Value of Dental Tissues Compared to Commonly Used Polishing Abrasive Particles

	MOHS HARDNESS VALUE
Dental Tissues	
Enamel	5
Dentin	3.0–4.0
Cementum	2.5–3.0
Abrasive Agents in Polishing Pastes	
Zirconium silicate	7.5–8.0
Pumice	6.0–7.0
Silicone carbine	9.5
Boron	9.3
Aluminum oxide	9
Garnet	8.0–9.0
Emery	7.0–9.0
Zirconium oxide	7
Perlite	5.5
Calcium carbonate	3
Aluminum silicates	2
Sodium	0.5
Potassium	0.4

The Mohs hardness value of enamel, cementum, and dentin compared to the Mohs hardness value of abrasive materials commonly used in prophylaxis polishing pastes. The Mohs hardness value is indicative of a material's resistance to scratching. Diamonds have a maximum Mohs value of 10; talc has a minimum of Mohs hardness of 1.

- Frictional heat produced is proportional to the rate of abrasion; therefore, the use of *dry agents* is *contraindicated* for polishing natural teeth because of the potential danger of thermal injury to the dental pulp.
- *Speed of application:* The greater the speed of application, the faster the rate of abrasion.
  - With increased speed of application, pressure must be reduced.
  - *Rapid abrasion* is *contraindicated* because it increases frictional heat.
- *Pressure of application:* The heavier the pressure applied, the faster the rate of abrasion.
  - *Heavy pressure* is *contraindicated* because it increases frictional heat.
- *Summary:* When cleaning and polishing are indicated after patient evaluation, the following are observed:
  - Use wet agents.
  - Apply a rubber polishing cup, using low speed.
  - Use a light, intermittent touch.

IV. Abrasive Agents

The abrasives listed here are examples of commonly used agents. Some are available in several grades, and the specific use varies with the grade.

- For example, while a superfine grade might be used for polishing enamel surfaces and metallic restorations, a coarser grade would be used only for laboratory purposes.
- Abrasives for use daily in a dentifrice necessarily are of a finer grade than those used for professional polishing accomplished a few times each year.

A. Silex (Silicon Dioxide)

- *XXX Silex:* fairly abrasive.
- *Superfine Silex:* can be used for heavy stain removal from enamel.

B. Pumice

- Powdered pumice is of volcanic origin and consists chiefly of complex silicates of aluminum, potassium, and sodium.
- Pumice is the primary ingredient in commercially prepared prophylaxis pastes. The specifications for particle size are listed in the *National Formulary*[26] as follows:
  - *Pumice flour or superfine pumice:* least abrasive, and may be used to remove heavy stains from enamel.
  - *Fine pumice:* mildly abrasive.
  - *Coarse pumice:* not for use on natural teeth.

C. Calcium Carbonate (Whiting, Calcite, Chalk)

- Various grades are used for different polishing techniques.

D. Tin Oxide (Putty Powder, Stannic Oxide)

- Polishing agent for teeth and metallic restorations.

E. Emery (Corundum)

Not used directly on the enamel.

- *Aluminum oxide (alumina):* the pure form of emery. Used for composite restorations and margins of porcelain restorations.
- *Levigated alumina:* consists of extremely fine particles of aluminum oxide, which may be used for polishing metals but are destructive to tooth surfaces.

F. Rouge (Jeweler's Rouge)

- Iron oxide is a fine red powder sometimes impregnated on paper discs.
- It is useful for polishing gold and precious metal alloys in the laboratory.

G. Diamond Particles

- Constituent of diamond polishing paste for porcelain surfaces.

V. Cleaning Ingredients

◆ Particles for cleaning agents differ from abrasive agents in shape and hardness.

◆ Particles used for cleaning agents include feldspar, alkali, and aluminum silicate.

A. Clinical Applications

Numerous commercial preparations for dental prophylactic cleaning and polishing preparations are available. Clinicians need more than one type available to meet the requirements of individual restorative materials.

B. Packaging

◆ Commercial preparations are in the form of pastes or powders.

◆ Some are available in measured amounts contained in small plastic or other individual packets that contribute to the cleanliness and sterility of the procedure.

◆ Selection of a preparation is based on qualities of abrasiveness, consistency for convenient use, or flavor for patient pleasure.

C. Enhanced Prophylaxis Polishing Pastes

Additives are included in prophylaxis polishing pastes to provide a specific function, such as enhancing the mineral surface of enamel, diminishing dentin hypersensitivity, or tooth whitening.

◆ *Fluoride prophylaxis pastes*
  • Application of fluoride by use of fluoride-containing prophylaxis polishing pastes cannot be considered a substitute for or the equivalent of a conventional topical fluoride treatment.
  • *Enamel surface*: The greatest benefit of fluoride as a prophylaxis polishing paste additive occurs when the fluoride ions in the prophylaxis paste are released into the saliva.
    • The fluoride ions that become mixed in the saliva may become incorporated into the hydroxyapatite structure of the tooth, thus aiding in the remineralizing of the tooth and improving enamel hardness.
  • *Clinical application*: Use only an amount sufficient to accomplish stain removal to prevent a child patient from swallowing unnecessary fluoride. The paste may contain 4,000–20,000 ppm fluoride ion.[27]

◆ *Amorphous calcium phosphate and other forms of calcium and phosphate*
  • Amorphous calcium phosphate and other formulations of calcium and phosphate, as an additive to prophylaxis polishing pastes, have been shown to hydrolyze the tooth mineral to form apatite.
  • When prophylaxis polishing pastes containing calcium and phosphate become mixed with saliva, the mineral ions may become incorporated into the hydroxyapatite structure of the tooth, thus aiding in remineralizing the tooth and improving enamel hardness.
  • Polishing agents containing amorphous calcium phosphate have the potential to enhance tooth smoothness and the luster of the enamel surface.[28,29]

◆ *Fluoride, calcium, and phosphate*
  • Fluoride, calcium, and phosphate prophylaxis pastes have the potential to have all three minerals incorporated into the hydroxyapatite structure of the tooth, thus aiding in remineralization to improve enamel hardness.

◆ *Tooth whitening*
  • In addition to removing extrinsic stains, there are commercially available prophylaxis polishing pastes that contain 35% hydrogen peroxide to provide a whitening benefit.
  • A hydrogen peroxide gel is applied to the tooth and then "polished" into the tooth surface with a rubber cup and prophylaxis polishing paste.

◆ *Dentin hypersensitivity*
  • The purpose of prophylaxis polishing pastes containing arginine, calcium, and bicarbonate/carbonate is to minimize dentin hypersensitivity. Mixing these ingredients produces arginine bicarbonate and calcium carbonate. When applied with a rubber cup, these adjunctive ingredients can aid in temporarily occluding the dentinal tubules.[30]

PROCEDURES FOR STAIN REMOVAL (CORONAL POLISHING)

I. Patient Preparation for Stain Removal

A. Instruction and Clinical Procedures

◆ Review medical history to determine premedication requirements.

◆ Review intraoral charting and radiographs to locate all restorations.

◆ Provide education and hands-on practice with biofilm control techniques.

◆ Complete scaling, root debridement, and overhang removal.

◆ After scaling and other periodontal treatment, an evaluation is made to determine the need for coronal polishing for stain removal, polishing restorations, and dental prostheses.

◆ Inform the patient that polishing is a cosmetic procedure, not a therapeutic one.

◆ Explain the difference between cleaning and polishing agents.

◆ Check all restorations to ensure that the correct polishing agent has been selected.

B. Explain the Procedure

◆ Describe the noise, vibration, and grit of the polishing paste.

◆ Explain the frequent use of rinsing and evacuation with the saliva ejector.

C. Provide Protection for Patient

◆ Safety glasses worn for scaling should be kept in place to prevent eye injury or infection from the prophylaxis paste.

◆ Fluid-resistant drape over patient to keep moisture from skin and clothing.

D. Patient Position

◆ The patient is positioned for maximum visibility.

E. Patient Breathing

◆ Encourage the patient to breath only through the nose.

◆ Reduced potential for aspiration of oral pathogens into the lungs.

◆ Allows water to pool for evacuation with saliva ejector.

◆ Less fogging of mouth mirror.

◆ Enhanced patient comfort.

II. Environmental Preparation

Environmental factors are described in Chapter 7.

A. Procedures to Lessen the Extent of Contaminated Aerosols

◆ Flush water through the tubing for 2 minutes at the beginning of each work period and for 30 seconds after each appointment.

◆ Request the patient rinse with an antimicrobial mouthrinse to reduce the numbers of oral microorganisms before starting instrumentation.

◆ Use high-velocity evacuation.

B. Protective Barriers

◆ Protective eyewear and bib are necessary for the patient.

◆ The clinician should wear the standard barrier protection, namely, eyewear, mask, gloves, and clinic gown to cover clothing.

THE POWER-DRIVEN INSTRUMENTS

I. Handpiece

◆ A handpiece is used to hold rotary instruments.

◆ The three basic designs are straight, contra-angle, and right-angle.

◆ Instruments have been classified according to their rotational speeds, designated by revolutions per minute (rpm) as high speed and low (or slow) speed.

◆ Handpiece must be maintained and sterilized according to manufacturer's directions.

A. Low Speed

◆ Low-speed handpieces are used for cleaning or polishing the teeth with a prophylaxis angle and rubber cup.

◆ *Speed*: Typical range is up to 5,000 rpm for low-speed handpieces manufactured for dental hygienists. Other low-speed handpieces may have a higher range of rpms; air-driven.

II. Types of Prophylaxis Angles

◆ Types of prophylaxis angles are described in Table 42-2.

◆ Contra- or right-angle attachments to the handpiece for which polishing devices (rubber cup, bristle brush) are available.

◆ Contra-angle prophylaxis angles may have a longer shank and a wider angle between the rubber cup and shank to allow for greater reach when polishing posterior teeth and surfaces.

TABLE 42-2 • Types of Prophylaxis Polishing Angles

COMPARISON OF DISPOSABLE PROPHYLAXIS ANGLES AND STAINLESS STEEL PROPHYLAXIS ANGLES[a]

TYPE OF ANGLE	DISPOSABLE PROPHYLAXIS ANGLE	DISPOSABLE ANGLE WITH ABRASIVE-IMPREGNATED RUBBER CUP	STAINLESS STEEL PROPHYLAXIS ANGLE
Maintenance and care	One-time use, discard	One-time use, discard	Requires maintenance, sterilization
Attachments	Supplied with rubber cup from the manufacturer	Supplied with rubber cup from the manufacturer that is impregnated with one type of abrasive	Accepts variety of attachments: cups, brushes, and cone-shaped rubber points
Screw-in or snap-on rubber cups	Usually screw-in type cup		Will accept screw-in or snap-on cups and brushes
Advantages	Requires no maintenance or sterilization	Requires no additional prophylaxis paste	Can be used hundreds of times if maintained properly
Disadvantages	Not package with other attachments Creates refuse that is not biodegradable	Must have water and/or saliva as lubricant Creates refuse that is not biodegradable	Does require time to clean and maintain

[a]A comparison of the features of a disposable prophylaxis angle to a disposable prophylaxis angle with abrasive-impregnated rubber cup and a sterilizable stainless steel prophylaxis angle.

◆ Disposable with rubber cup impregnated with polishing agent (abrasive particles) embedded in the rubber cup.[20,21]

◆ Stainless steel with hard chrome, carbon, steel, or brass bearings.

◆ Figure 42-2 shows examples of disposable for one-time use[31] contra-angle and right-angle prophylaxis angles and a stainless steel prophylaxis angle.

◆ Stainless steel prophylaxis angles that are sealed will not allow saliva and debris into the head of the angle nor will they allow grease and debris to leak out of the head of the angle.[32,33]

◆ Stainless steel or any other type of metal autoclavable prophylaxis angle must be sterilized after every use and the manufacturer's instructions followed for the proper maintenance and care as well as the correct sterilization procedures.

◆ Unless they are disposable, only instruments that can be sterilized should be used.

III. Prophylaxis Angle Attachments

A. Rubber Polishing Cups

◆ *Types*: Figure 42-3 shows several types of rubber polishing cups from which to choose. The internal designs and sizes have the same purpose, which is to aid in holding the prophylaxis polishing paste in the rubber cup while polishing. The ideal rubber cup design retains the prophylaxis polishing paste in the cup and will release the paste at a steady rate.

- *Slip-on (snap-on)*: with ribbed cup to aid in holding polishing agent.
- *Threaded (screw type)*: with plain ribbed cup or flange (webbed) type.
- Mandrel mounted.

◆ *Materials*
- *Natural rubber*: more resilient; adapts readily to fit the contours of the teeth.
- *Synthetic*: stiffer than natural rubber.

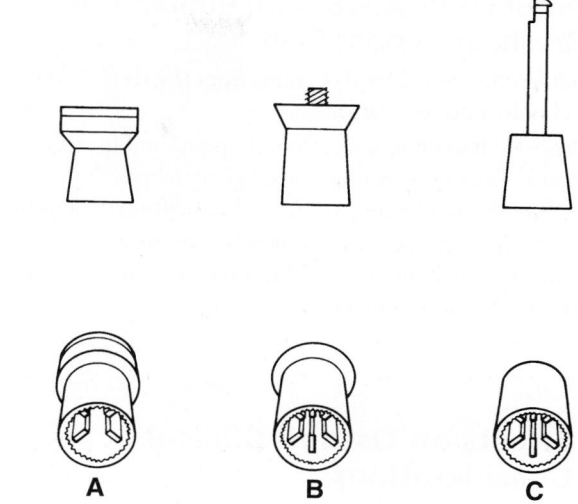

FIGURE 42-3 • **Rubber Cup Attachments. A:** Slip-on or snap-on for button-ended prophylaxis angle. **B:** Threaded for direct insertion in right-angle. **C:** Mandrel stem for latch-type prophylaxis angle.

B. Bristle Brushes

◆ *Types*
- *For prophylaxis angle*: slip-on or screw type.
- *For handpiece*: mandrel mounted.

◆ *Materials*: synthetic.

C. Rubber Polishing Points

◆ Figure 42-4 shows an example of a rubber point that screws into a prophylaxis angle.

◆ *Material*
- *Natural rubber*: flexible so that tip adapts to proximal surfaces, embrasures, and around orthodontic bands and brackets.

◆ *Use*: Because the ribs for holding the prophylaxis polishing paste onto the rubber polishing point are on the external surface, the polishing paste will have to be reapplied frequently.

IV. Uses for Attachments

A. Handpiece with Straight Mandrel

◆ Dixon bristle brush (type C, soft) for polishing removable dentures.

◆ Rubber cup on mandrel for polishing facial surfaces of anterior teeth.

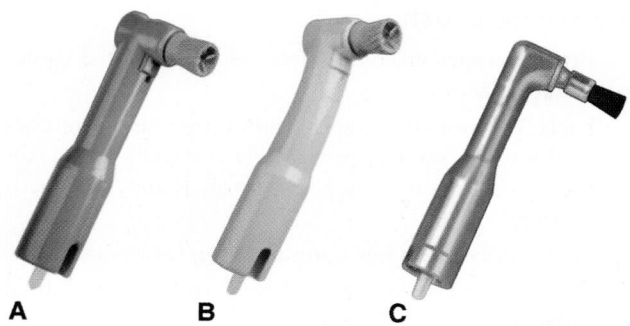

FIGURE 42-2 • **Prophylaxis Angles. A:** Disposable right-angled prophylaxis angle with rubber cup attached. **B:** Disposable contra-angled prophylaxis angle with an attached rubber cup impregnated with a polishing agent (abrasive particles). **C:** Sterilizable stainless steel prophylaxis angle holding a cleaning or polishing brush on a mandrel.

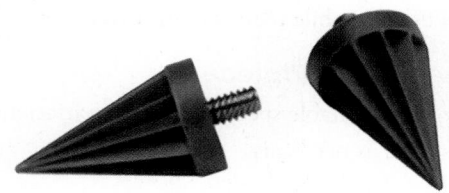

FIGURE 42-4 • **Flexible Rubber Point Has Screw Connection for a Prophylaxis Angle.** Made with ribs or grooves to carry cleaning or polishing agent to difficult-to-reach areas.

B. Prophylaxis Angle with Rubber Cup, Brush, or Rubber Point

- *Rubber cup*: for removal of stains from the tooth surfaces and polishing restorations.
- *Brush*: for removing stains from deep pits and fissures and enamel surfaces away from the gingival margin. A brush is contraindicated for use on exposed cementum or dentin.
- *Rubber polishing point*: for removing stains and biofilm from proximal surfaces, embrasures, and around orthodontic bands and brackets.

USE OF THE PROPHYLAXIS ANGLE

I. Effects on Tissues: Clinical Considerations

- Can cause discomfort for the patient if care and consideration for the oral tissues are not exercised to prevent unnecessary trauma.
- Tactile sensitivity of the clinician while using a thick, bulky handpiece is diminished and unnecessary pressure may be applied inadvertently.
- The greater the speed of application of a polishing agent, the faster the rate of abrasion. Therefore, the handpiece is applied at a low rpm.
- Trauma to the gingival tissue can result from too high a speed, extended application of the rubber cup, or use of an abrasive polishing agent.
- Tissue damage and the need for antibiotic premedication for risk patients are described in Chapter 11.

II. Prophylaxis Angle Procedure

- Apply the polishing agent only where it is needed. See section *Contraindications*.

A. Instrument Grasp

- Modified pen grasp (see Chapter 37).

B. Finger Rest

- Establish a fulcrum firmly on tooth structure or use an exterior rest.
- Use a wide rest area when practical to aid in the balance of the large instrument. For example, place cushion of rest finger across occlusal surfaces of premolars while polishing the molars.
- Avoid use of mobile teeth as finger rests.

C. Speed of Handpiece

- Use lowest available speed to minimize frictional heat.
- Adjust rpm as necessary.

D. Use of Rheostat

- Apply steady pressure with foot to produce an even, low speed.

E. Rubber Cup: Stroke and Procedure

- Observe where stain removal is needed to prevent unnecessary rubber cup application.
- Fill rubber cup with polishing agent, and distribute agent over tooth surfaces to be polished before activating the power.
- Establish finger rest and bring rubber cup almost in contact with tooth surface before activating power source.
- Using slowest rpm, apply revolving cup at a 90° angle lightly to tooth surfaces for 1 or 2 seconds. Use a light pressure so that the edges of the rubber cup flare slightly. The rubber cup needs to flare slightly underneath the gingival margin and onto the proximal surfaces.
- Move cup to adjacent area on tooth surface; use a patting or brushing motion.
- Replenish supply of polishing agent frequently.
- Turn handpiece to adapt rubber cup to fit each surface of the tooth, including proximal surfaces and gingival surfaces of fixed partial dentures.
- Start with the distal surface of the most posterior tooth of a quadrant and move forward toward the anterior; polish only the teeth that require stain removal. For each tooth, work from the gingival third toward the incisal third of the tooth.
- When two polishing agents of different abrasiveness are to be applied, use a separate rubber cup for each.
- Rubber cups, polishing points, and polishing brushes cannot be sterilized and are used only for one patient and then discarded.

F. Rubber Polishing Points

- Rubber polishing points can be used around orthodontic bands and brackets, on fixed bridges, and in wide interproximal spaces or embrasures.
- Rubber points are loaded with the cleaning or polishing agent in the grooves around the sides. The rubber points will need to be replenished frequently with paste after use on every 1–2 teeth.

G. Bristle Brush

- Bristle brushes are used selectively and limited to occlusal surfaces.
- Lacerations of the gingiva and grooves and scratches in the tooth surface, particularly the roots and restorations, can result when the brush is not used with caution.
- Soak stiff brush in hot water to soften bristles.
- Distribute mild abrasive polishing agent over occlusal surfaces of teeth to be polished.
- Place fingers of nondominant hand in a position to retract and protect cheek and tongue from the revolving brush.
- Establish a firm finger rest and bring brush almost in contact with the tooth before activating power source.

- Use slowest rpm as the revolving brush is applied lightly to the occlusal surfaces only. Avoid contact of the bristles with the soft tissues.
- Use a short stroke in a brushing motion; follow the inclined planes of the cusps.
- Move from tooth to tooth to prevent generation of excessive frictional heat. Avoid overuse of the brush. Replenish supply of polishing agent frequently.

H. Irrigation

- Irrigate teeth and interdental areas thoroughly several times with water from the syringe to remove abrasive particles. Avoid heavy water pressure to prevent forcing particles into the tissue.
- The rotary movement of the rubber cup or bristle brush tends to force the abrasive into the gingival sulci, thereby creating a potential source of irritation to the soft tissues.

AIR-POWDER POLISHING

- Principles of selective stain removal are applied to the use of the air-powder polishing system (Figure 42-5). After biofilm control instruction, instrumentation, and periodontal debridement are completed, follow with an evaluation of need for stain removal.

I. Principles of Application

- Air-powder systems manufactured by several companies are efficient and effective methods for mechanical removal of stain and biofilm.[34-36]
- Air-powder polishing systems use air, water, and specially formulated powders to deliver a controlled spray that propels the particles to the tooth surface.

- Only powders approved by each air-powder polishing manufacturer are used in each brand of air-powder polishing unit. The use of an unapproved powder in an air-powder polishing unit could void the warranty on the unit.[34,36]
- The handpiece nozzle is moved in a constant circular motion, with the nozzle tip 4–5 mm away from the enamel surface.
- The spray is angled away from the gingival margin.
- The periphery of the spray may be near the gingival margin, but the center is directed at an angle less than 90° away from the margin.
- Complete directions for care of equipment and preparation for use of the device are provided by the individual manufacturer.

II. Specially Formulated Powders for Use in Air-Powder Polishing

Several manufacturers make and sell air-powder polishing powders.

- The abrasiveness of one brand of powder may differ from another brand, even though it is the same type of powder.[37,38]

A. Sodium Bicarbonate[38]

- Sodium bicarbonate was the original powder used in air-powder polishing.
- It is specially formulated with scant amounts of calcium phosphate and silica to keep it free flowing.
- The Mohs hardness number for sodium bicarbonate is 2.5 and the particles average 74 μm in size.
- The *only* type of sodium bicarbonate that can be used in air-powder polishing units is the type specially formulated for air-powder polishing.

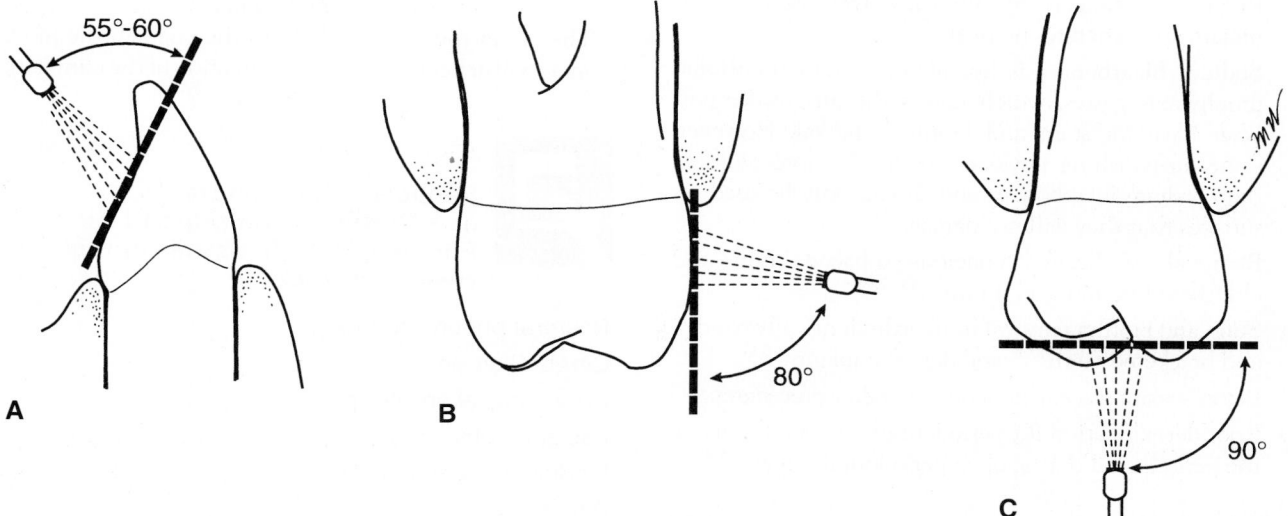

FIGURE 42-5 • Air-Powder Polishing. Direct the aerosolized spray for **(A)** the anterior teeth at a 60° angle. **B:** The posterior teeth facial and lingual or palatal at an 80° angle. **C:** The occlusal surfaces at a 90° angle to the occlusal plane.

- Sodium bicarbonate air-powder is available with flavorings. However, the patient will taste the salt and smell the flavor.

B. Aluminum Trihydroxide

- Aluminum trihydroxide was the first air-powder developed as an alternative to sodium bicarbonate for patients who are sodium bicarbonate intolerant.[37]
- Aluminum trihydroxide has a Mohs hardness value of 4 and the particles range in size from 80 to 325 μm.

C. Glycine

- Glycine is an amino acid. For use in powders, glycine crystals are grown using a solvent of water and sodium salt.
- Glycine particles for use in air polishing have a Mohs hardness number of 2 and are 20 μm in size.[38]
- Glycine has been shown to be safe and effective for subgingival plaque removal in pockets up to 5mm.[34]

D. Calcium Carbonate

- Calcium carbonate is a naturally occurring substance that can be found in rocks.
- It is a main ingredient in antacids, and is also used as filler for pharmaceutical drugs.
- Calcium carbonate has a Mohs number of 3.[38]

E. Calcium Sodium Phosphosilicate (Novamin)

- Calcium sodium phosphosilicate (Novamin) is a bioactive glass and has a Mohs hardness number of 6, making it the hardest air-polishing particle used in air-powder polishing powders.[38] The particles vary from 25 to 120 μm in size. This powder should not be used on any tooth structure or restorative material.[38]

III. Uses and Advantages of Air-Powder Polishing

- Requires less time, is ergonomically favorable to the clinician, and generates no heat.[35,37,39]
- Sodium bicarbonate is less abrasive than traditional prophylaxis pastes, which makes the air-powder polisher ideal for stain and biofilm removal. However, some air-polishing powders are much more abrasive than sodium bicarbonate and should only be used on surfaces that they will not damage.[38]
- Removal of heavy, tenacious tobacco stain and chlorhexidine-induced staining.[35,37,40]
- Stain and biofilm removal from orthodontically banded and bracketed teeth[40,41] and dental implants.[42,43]
- Before sealant placement or other bonding procedures.[18,19]
- Root detoxification for periodontally diseased roots by the periodontist during open periodontal surgery.[44,45]

IV. Technique

Proper angulation of the air-powder polishing handpiece is essential to reduce the amount of inherent aerosols created[46–48] and to remove stain and biofilm without iatrogenic soft-tissue trauma.

A. For Anterior Teeth

- Place the handpiece nozzle at a 60° angle to the facial and lingual surfaces of anterior teeth (Figure 42-5A).

B. For Posterior Teeth

- Place the handpiece nozzle at an 80° angle to the facial and lingual surfaces (Figure 42-5B).

C. For Occlusal Surfaces

- Place the handpiece nozzle at a 90° angle to the occlusal plane (Figure 42-5C).

D. Incorrect Angulation

- Incorrect angulation of the handpiece is probably the single most common cause of excess aerosol production.
- The handpiece nozzle is never directed into the gingival sulcus or into a periodontal pocket with little bony support remaining, as this could result in facial emphysema[36] (also known as a subcutaneous emphysema).
- Facial emphysemas occur due to the abnormal introduction of air into subcutaneous tissues or interstitial spaces.[36]
- Facial emphysemas can be prevented by avoiding the use of high-speed handpieces during third molar extractions,[49] air/water syringes near extraction or surgical sites or lacerations,[50–54] and airpolishing[55] spray in these areas.
- Facial emphysemas exhibit symptoms such as facial swelling, a "crackling" sensation of the face and neck area when touched, tenderness, and pain. If detected early, patients with facial emphysemas usually require observation, antibiotics, and analgesia.[36]
  - Box 42-1 contains a list of the sequelae that can develop as a result of compressed air forced into soft tissues of the head and neck.
  - Box 42-2 contains a list of sequelae that can develop as a result of a facial emphysema.
- The closer the nozzle is held to the enamel, the more spray will deflect back into the direction of the clinician.

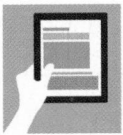

BOX 42-1

Sequelae That Can Develop as a Result of Compressed Air Forced into Soft Tissues of the Head and Neck

Bilateral pneumothorax

Cerebral air embolism

Cervicofacial emphysema

Facial emphysema

Mediastinal emphysema

Pneumediastinum

Pneumothorax

Retropharyngeal emphysema

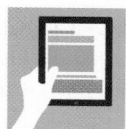

BOX 42-2
Sequelae That Can Develop as a Result of Facial Emphysema

Bilateral pneumothorax
Cerebral air embolism
Embolism
Pneumediastinum
Pneumothorax
Thrombosis

- When a clinician directs the handpiece at a 90° angle toward a facial, buccal, and some lingual surfaces, the result is an immediate reflux of the aerosolized spray back onto the clinician.
- Changing the angle of incidence to the proper angulations of 60° and 80° will result in a change in the angle of the reflection, thus reducing the amount of reflux of aerosolized spray.

V. Recommendations and Precautions

A. Aerosol Production

A copious spray containing oral debris and microorganisms is produced. As with all contaminated aerosols, a health hazard can exist. Suggestions for minimizing contamination and the effects of the aerosols include the following:

- Patient uses a preprocedural antibacterial mouthrinse.[56]
- High-volume evacuation is needed, using a wide tip held near the tooth where the spray is released from the nozzle or using a high-volume scavenger attachment for a high-volume evacuation suction tip or saliva ejector.[46–48]

B. Protective Patient and Clinician Procedures

- Use protective eyewear, protective gown, and hair cover.
- Lubricate patient's lips to prevent drying effect of the sodium bicarbonate using a nonpetroleum lip lubricant.
- Do not direct the spray on the gingiva, or other soft tissues, which can create patient discomfort, undue tissue trauma.
- Avoid directing the spray into periodontal pockets with bone loss or into extraction sites as a facial emphysema can be induced.

VI. Risk Patients: Air-Powder Polishing Contraindicated

The information from the patient's medical history is used and appropriate applications made. Antibiotic premedication is indicated for all the same patients who are at risk for any dental hygiene procedure (see Chapter 11).

A. Contraindications[36]

- Physician-directed sodium-restricted diet (only for sodium bicarbonate powder).
- Respiratory disease or other condition that limits swallowing or breathing, such as chronic obstructive pulmonary disease.
- Patients with end-stage renal disease, Addison's disease, or Cushing's disease.
- Communicable infection that can contaminate the aerosols produced.
- Immunocompromised patients.
- Patients taking potassium, antidiuretics, or steroid therapy.
- Patients who have open oral wounds, such as tooth sockets, from oral surgery procedures.

B. Other Contraindications

- *Root surfaces:* Avoid routine polishing of cementum and dentin.
  - There is some evidence they can be removed readily during air-powder polishing.[57]
  - However, research indicates that glycine powder is safe for use subgingivally.[57]
- *Soft, spongy gingiva:* The air-powder can irritate the free gingival tissue, especially if not used with the recommended technique.
  - When heavy stain calls for the use of an air-powder polisher, instruct the patient in daily bacterial biofilm removal.
  - Following scaling and periodontal debridement, postpone the stain removal until soft tissue has healed.
- *Restorative materials:* The use of air-powder polishing on composite resins, cements, and other nonmetallic materials can cause removal or pitting.[15,16,22]
  - Table 42-3 provides a guide as to which restorative materials can be safely treated with air-powder polishing agents, the sodium bicarbonate powder, and the aluminum trihydroxide powder.[33]
  - Significant damage to margins of dental castings has been shown.[32]

POLISHING PROXIMAL SURFACES

- Care must be exercised in the use of floss, tape, and finishing strips.
- Understanding the anatomy of the interdental papillae and relationship to the contact areas and proximal surfaces of the teeth is prerequisite to the prevention of tissue damage.
- As much polishing as possible of accessible proximal surfaces is accomplished during the use of the rubber cup in the prophylaxis angle.

TABLE 42-3 • Recommendations for Use of Air Polishing on Restorative Materials

	POLISHING POWDER CONTAINING	
RESTORATIVE MATERIAL	SODIUM BICARBONATE	ALUMINUM TRIHYDROXIDE
Amalgam	Yes	No
Gold	Yes[a]	No
Porcelain	Yes[a]	No
Hybrid composite	No	No
Microfilled composite	No	No
Glass ionomer	No	No
Compomer	No	No
Luting agents	No	No

[a]Only if margin is avoided.

- This can be followed by the use of dental tape with polishing agent when indicated.
- Finishing strips are used only in selected instances, when all other techniques fail to remove a stain.

I. Dental Tape and Floss

A. Uses During Cleaning and Polishing

- Techniques for tape and floss application are described in Chapter 27.
- The same principles apply whether the patient or the clinician is using the floss.
- Finger rests are used to prevent snapping through contact areas.
- *Stain removal with dental tape:* Polishing agent is applied to the tooth, and the tape is moved gently back and forth and up and down curved over the area where stain was observed.
- *Cleaning gingival surface of a fixed partial denture:* A floss threader is used to position the floss or tape over the gingival surface. Floss threaders are described and illustrated in Chapter 30. The agent is applied under the pontic, and the floss or tape is moved back and forth with contact on the bridge surface.
- *Flossing:* Particles of abrasive agent can be removed by rinsing and by using a clean length of floss applied in the usual manner.
- *Rinsing and irrigation:* Irrigate with water-spray syringe to clean out all abrasive agent.

II. Finishing Strips

A. Description

- Finishing strips are thin, flexible, and tape-shaped.
- Available in four widths: extra narrow, narrow, medium, and wide.

- Available in extra fine, fine, medium, and coarse grit. *Only extra narrow or narrow strips with extra fine or fine grit are suggested for stain removal, and then only with discretion.*
- Most finishing strips are now made of plastic; however, linen abrasive strips are available. Finishing strips have one side that is smooth and the other side serves as a carrier for abrasive agents bonded to that side.
- "Gapped" strips are available with an abrasive-free portion to permit sliding the strip through a contact area without abrading the enamel.
- Finishing strips are available with two different grits on one strip. One-half of the strip may have fine abrasives and the other one-half will have medium-grit abrasives. These strips are available in several different combinations.

B. Use

- *For stain removal on proximal surfaces of anterior teeth; when other techniques are unsuccessful.*
- *Precautions for use*
  - Edge of strip is sharp and may cut gingival tissue or the lip.
  - Use of a finishing strip is limited to enamel surfaces and some restorative materials, such as composite. It is of upmost importance to ensure the finishing strip selected has an appropriate grit abrasive for the surface to be polished. Manufacturers make finishing strips intended for use solely on composites or porcelain; other types of finishing strips are available for use on enamel.

C. Technique for Finishing Strip

- *Grasp and finger rest*
  - A strip no longer than 6 inches is most convenient to apply.
  - Grasp and finger rest must be well controlled.
  - Protection of the lip by retraction with the thumb and index finger holding the strip is a helpful safety measure.
- *Positioning*
  - Direct the abrasive side of the strip toward the proximal surface to be treated as the strip is worked slowly and gently between the teeth with a slight sawing motion.
  - Bring strip just through the contact area. If the strip breaks, immediately use floss to remove abrasive particles separated from the finishing strip.
  - When a space is clearly visible through an embrasure and the interdental papilla is missing, a narrow finishing strip may be threaded through. Prepare strip by cutting the end on a diagonal to facilitate threading.
- *Stain removal*
  - Press abrasive side of strip against tooth. Draw back and forth in a 1/8-inch arc two or three times, rocking on the established fulcrum.

- Remove strip. Do not attempt to turn the strip while it is in the interdental area.
- *Dental floss:* Follow each application of a finishing strip with dental floss to remove abrasive particles.

HISTORIAL PERSPECTIVE: THE PORTE POLISHER

- *Design*
  - The porte polisher is a manual instrument designed especially for extrinsic stain removal or application of treatment agents such as for hypersensitive areas.
  - It is constructed to hold a wood point at a contra-angle. The wood points may be cone or wedge-shaped and made of various kinds of wood, preferably orangewood. Figure 42-6 illustrates a typical porte polisher.
- *Grasp:* The instrument is held in a modified pen grasp or palm grasp.
- *Application:* The wood point is applied to the tooth surface using firm, carefully directed, massaging, circular or linear strokes to accommodate the anatomy of each tooth.
  - A firm finger rest and a moderate amount of pressure of the wood point provide protection for the gingival margin and efficiency in technique.
- *Features*
  - The porte polisher is useful for instrumentation of difficult-to-access surfaces of the teeth, especially malpositioned teeth.
  - No heat generation, no noise compared with powered handpieces, and minimal production of aerosols.
  - The porte polisher is readily portable and therefore is useful in any location, for example, for a bed bound patient.

DOCUMENTATION

Documentation for a patient receiving tooth stain removal as part of the dental hygiene care plan for a maintenance appointment would include a minimum of the following:

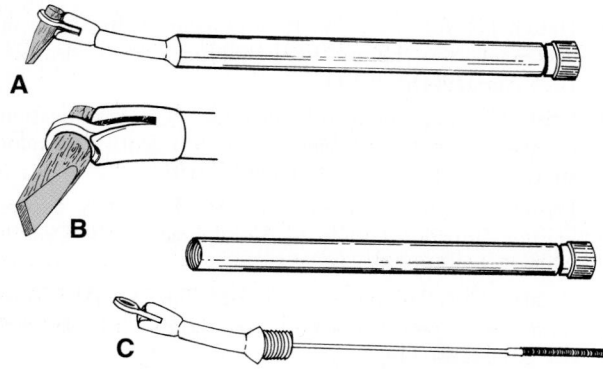

FIGURE 42-6 • Porte Polisher. A: Assembled instrument shows position of wood point ready for instrumentation. **B:** Working end shows wedge-shaped wood point inserted. **C:** Disassembled, ready for autoclave.

- Review patient medical history with questions to determine health problems, recent medical examinations and treatments, and changes in medications.
- *Current clinical examination findings:* intraoral, extraoral, periodontal, and dental.
- *With dental charting:* identification of dental materials used in restorations that can influence choice of polishing agents. Identification would require use of radiographs and the intraoral dental charting.
- Dental hygiene examination for state of patient's personal daily self-care, calculus and biofilm deposits, sources for dental stains, products used for oral care, and dietary factors influencing the dentition and all oral tissues: questions answered about best choices for various products.
- A sample progress note may be reviewed in Box 42-3.

BOX 42-3
Example Documentation: Selection of Polishing Agent for a Patient with Esthetic Restorations

S–A 36-year-old male patient presents for regular maintenance appointment, grinning to show that his new implant crown and other esthetic restorations are not distinguishable from the color of his teeth. Updated medical history, medications, no changes.

O–Blood pressure (115/75); extra-intraoral examinations: no findings; comprehensive periodontal examination: localized 3–4 mm, with bleeding on probing in 4 mm pockets in molar areas; supragingival calculus mand ant.; minimal biofilm with isolated areas of yellowish staining.

A–Checked his dental records for the material used for the various restorations and found that the patient has porcelain crowns on teeth numbers #2, 14, and anterior microhybrid composite restorations in teeth numbers #6, 7, 8, 10, and 11. Patient has an implant and porcelain crown on #9. Note: Microhybrid composite restorations and implant crown match the patient's natural teeth to the extent that it is difficult to identify the restorations.

P–Gave patient new toothbrush with tongue cleaner on back, and demonstrated the tongue cleaner. Went over places he had been missing on his teeth and gingiva. Calculus removal. Avoided use of air polishing with sodium bicarbonate (the only powder I have available) and also avoided prophy paste. Selected a cleaning agent to remove biofilm and isolated areas of yellowish staining.

Next regular appointment 4 months made at front desk.

Signed: _____, RDH

Date: _____

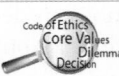

EVERYDAY ETHICS

Mr. Jackson, the 62-year-old chief executive officer of a major oil company, presents for his routine 3-month maintenance with Carol, his dental hygienist of several years. Mr. Jackson is meticulous about his appearance and is always handsomely dressed. He is well-known internationally and frequently seen in the news media being interviewed and having pictures taken for news articles.

Mr. Jackson had a complete cosmetic restoration of his teeth a year ago. Previously his teeth had been stained by the numerous cups of tea he drank every day. He has had porcelain veneers placed on his maxillary anterior teeth, and all restorations are now tooth-colored. Unfortunately, Mr. Jackson has not reduced intake of tea and during her assessment, Carol notes that generalized stain is starting to discolor most of the new restorations. Before the cosmetic restorations were placed, Carol used a coarse prophy paste to eliminate the tea stains and now Mr. Jackson asks her to "just use that gritty stuff again." He states that he absolutely does not want his teeth to appear stained.

Questions for Consideration

1. What role does each of the dental hygiene core values play as Carol contemplates a course of action to take in this situation?

2. What alternative actions are available that would respect Mr. Jackson's rights as well as allow Carol to provide treatment that meets standards of care?

3. What financial or legal considerations will Carol need to consider as she determines her course of action?

Factors to Teach the Patient

▶ How dental biofilm and stains form on the natural teeth and their replacements.

▶ The meaning of selective polishing and why it is not necessary to polish all teeth at every appointment when daily care is effective.

▶ Stains and biofilm removed by polishing can return promptly if biofilm is not removed faithfully on a schedule of two or three times each day.

▶ Polishing agents used during professional coronal polishing are too abrasive for daily home use.

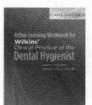

ENHANCE YOUR UNDERSTANDING

ONLINE RESOURCES
(see the inside front cover for access information)

• Audio glossary
• Appendices

SUPPORT FOR LEARNING
(available separately)

• *Active Learning Workbook for Wilkins' Clinical Practice of the Dental Hygienist, 13th Edition*

INDIVIDUALIZED REVIEW

• Customized practice quizzing with Navigate 2 TestPrep for *Wilkins' Clinical Practice of the Dental Hygienist*

References

1. American Academy of Periodontology. *Glossary of Periodontal Terms.* 4th ed. Chicago, IL: American Academy of Periodontology; 2001:42. https://members.perio.org/libraries/glossary.

2. American Dental Hygienists' Association. *Position Paper on the Oral Prophylaxis.* Chicago, IL: ADHA; 1998. www.adha.org/profissues/prophylaxis.htm.

3. Jeffries SR. Abrasive finishing and polishing in restorative dentistry: a state-of-the-art review. *Dent Clin North Am.* 2007;51(2):379-397.

4. Hutchings IM. Abrasion process in wear and manufacturing. *Proc Inst Mech Eng Part J: J Eng Tribol.* 2002;216(2):55-62.

5. Rémond G, Nockolds C, Phillips M, et al. Implications of polishing techniques in quantitative x-ray microanalysis. *J Res Natl Inst Stand Technol.* 2002;107(6):639-662.

6. Williams JA. Wear and wear particles: some fundamentals. *Tribol Int.* 2005;38(10):863-870.

7. Fine DH, Furgang D, McKiernan M, et al. An investigation of the effect of an essential oil mouthrinse on induced bacteraemia: a pilot study. *J Clin Periodontol.* 2010;37(9):840-847.

8. Hatzell JD, Torres D, Kim P, Wortmann G. Incidence of bacteremia after routine tooth brushing. *Am J Med Sci.* 2005,Apr;329(4):178-180.

9. Cristina ML, Spagnolo AM, Sartini M, et al. Investigation of organizational and hygiene features in dentistry: a pilot study. *J Prev Med Hyg.* 2009;50(3):175-180.

10. Farrier SL, Farrier JN, Gilmour AS. Eye safety in operative dentistry: a study in dental practice. *Br Dent J.* 2006;200(4):218-223.

11. Buzalaf MAR, Pessan JP, Honório HM, Ten Cate JM. Mechanisms of action of fluoride for caries control. *Monogr Oral Sci.* 2011;22:97-114.

12. Honório HM, Rios D, Abdo RC, et al. Effect of different prophylaxis methods on sound and demineralized enamel. *J Appl Oral Sci.* 2006;14(2):117-123.

13. Kubinek R, Zapletalova Z, Vujtek M, et al. Examination of dentin surface using AFM and SEM. In: Méndez-Vilas A, Díaz J, eds. *Modern Research and Educational Topics in Microscopy.* Vol 2. Zurbarán: Formatex; 2007:593-598.

14. Miglani S, Aggarwal V, Ahuja B. Dentin hypersensitivity: recent trends in management. *J Conserv Dent.* 2010;13(4):218-224.

15. Barnes CM. Polishing esthetic restorative materials. *Dimensions Dent Hyg.* 2010;8(1):24, 26-28.

16. Barnes CM. Care and maintenance of esthetic restorations. *J Prac Hyg.* 2004;14:19-22.

17. Zyla T, Kawala B, Antoszewska-Smith J, Kawala M. Black line stain and dental caries: a review of the literature. *Biomed Research International.* 2015. http://dx.doi.org/10.1155/2015/469392.

18. Botti RH, Bossu M, Zallocco N, Vestri A, Polimeni A. Effectiveness of plaque indicators and air polishing for the sealing of pits and fissures. *Eur J Paediatr Dent.* 2010;11(1):15-18.

19. Ahovuo-Saloranta A, Hiiri A, Nordblad A, et al. Pit and fissure sealants for preventing dental decay in the permanent teeth of children and adolescents. *Cochrane Database Syst Rev.* 2008;4:CD001830. Review.

20. Barnes CM. The science of polishing. *Dimensions Dent Hyg.* 2009;7(11):18-20, 22.

21. Covey D, Barnes C, Watanabe H, Johnson W. Effects of a paste-free prophylaxis polishing cup and various prophylaxis polishing pastes on tooth enamel and restorative materials. *G Dent.* November/December 2011:466-473. www.age.org.

22. Putt MS, Kleber CJ, Muhler JC. Enamel polish and abrasion by prophylaxis pastes. *J Dent Hyg.* 1982;56(9):38, 40-43.

23. Barnes CM. Adapting polishing procedures to maintain aesthetic restorations. *J Prac Hyg.* 2005;15:22.

24. Barnes CM, Covey DA, Walker MP, et al. Essential selective polishing: the maintenance of aesthetic restorations. *J Prac Hyg.* 2003;12(5):18-24.

25. Sawai MA, Bhardwaj A, Jafri Z, Sultan N, Daing A. Tooth polishing: the current status. *J Indian Soc Periodontal.* Jul-Aug 2015; 19(4):375-380.

26. Burrell KH, Chan JT. Fluorides. In: American Dental Association, ed. *Council on Scientific Affairs: ADA Guide to Dental Therapeutics.* 3rd ed. Chicago, IL: ADA; 2003:238.

27. Tung MS, Eichmiller FC. Amorphous calcium phosphates for tooth mineralization. *Compend Contin Educ Dent.* 2004;25 (9, suppl 1):9-13.

28. Tung M, Malerman R, Huang S, et al. Reactivity of prophylaxis paste containing calcium phosphate and fluoride salts. *J Dent Res.* 2005;84 (Special Issue A). Abstract #2156, IADR Abstracts, 2005.

29. Daniels A. Professionally applied enhanced polishing agents. *J Prac Hyg.* 2006;15:26.

30. Mattana D. Reducing dentin Hypersensitivity. *J Prac Hyg.* 2006;15:24.

31. Barnes CM, Fleming LS. An in vitro evaluation of commercially available disposable prophylaxis angles. *J Dent Hyg.* 1991;65(9):438-441.

32. Barnes CM, Anderson NA, Li Y, et al. Effectiveness of steam sterilization in killing spores of *Bacillus stearothermophilus* in prophylaxis angles. *Gen Dent.* 1994;42(5):456-458.

33. Barnes CM, Anderson NA, Michalek SM, et al. Effectiveness of sealed dental prophylaxis angles inoculated with *Bacillus stearothermophilus* in preventing leakage. *J Clin Dent.* 1994;5(2):35-37.

34. Graumann S, Sensat M, Stoltenberg J. Air polishing: a review of current literature. *J Dent Hygi.* August 2013; 87(4):173-180.

35. Weaks LM, Lescher NB, Barnes CM, et al. Clinical evaluation of the Prophy-Jet as an instrument for routine removal of tooth stain and plaque. *J Periodontol.* 1984;55(8): 486-488.

36. Barnes CM. An in-depth look at air polishing. *Dimensions Dent Hyg.* 2010;8(3):32, 34-36.

37. Barnes CM, Covey DA, Walker MP, et al. An in vitro evaluation of the effects of aluminum trihydroxide delivered via the Prophy Jet on dental restorative materials. *J Prosthet Dent.* 2004;13(3):166-172.

38. Barnes CM, Covey DA, Watanabe H, et al. An in vitro comparison of the effects of various airpolishing powders on enamel and selected esthetic restorative materials. *J Clin Dent.* 2014;25(4):76-87.

39. Kuar A, Gupta M, Das D, Sachdeva S, Jain S. Tooth polishing- a mouthful of history. *Int J Periodontol Implantol.* April-June 2018:3(2):63-67.

40. Barnes CM, Russell CM, Gerbo LR, et al. Effects of an air-powder polishing system on orthodontically bracketed and banded teeth. *Am J Orthod Dentofac Orthop.* 1990;97(1):74-81.

41. Shultz PH, Brockmann-Bell SL, Eick JD, et al. Effects of air-powder polishing on the bond strength of orthodontic bracket adhesive systems. *J Dent Hyg.* 1993;67(2):74-80.

42. Cochis A, Carassi F, Migilario M, Visai L, Rimondini L. Effect of air polishing with glycine powder on titanium abutment surfaces. *Clin Oral Implants Res.* 2013;24(8):904-9.

43. Barnes CM, Toothaker RW, Ross J. Polishing dental implants and dental implant restorations. *J Prac Hyg.* 2005; 14(8):6-8.

44. Berkstein S, Reiff RL, McKinney JF, et al. Supragingival root surface removal during maintenance procedures utilizing an air-powder abrasive system or hand scaling: an in vitro study. *J Periodontol.* 1987;58(5):327-330.

45. Agger MS, Hörsted-Bindslev P, Hovgaard O. Abrasiveness of an air-powder polishing system on root surfaces in vitro. *Quintessence Int.* 2001;32(5):407-411.

46. Barnes CM. The management of aerosols with airpolishing delivery systems. *J Dent Hyg.* 1991;65(6):280-282.

47. Harrel SK, Barnes JB, Rivera-Hidalgo F. Aerosol reduction during air polishing. *Quintessence Int.* 1999;30(9): 623-628.

48. Worrall SF, Knibbs PJ, Glenwright HD. Methods of reducing bacterial contamination of the atmosphere arising from use of an air-polisher. *Br Dent J.* 1987;163(4):118, 119.

49. Davies DE. Pneumomediastinum after dental surgery. *Anaesth Intensive Care.* 2001;29(6):638-641.

50. Tan WK. Sudden facial swelling: subcutaneous facial emphysema secondary to use of air/water syringe during dental extraction. *Singapore Dent J.* 2000;23 (1, suppl):42-44.

51. Josephson GD, Wambach BA, Noordzji JP. Subcutaneous cervicofacial and mediastinal emphysema after dental instrumentation. *Otolaryngol Head Neck Surg.* 2001;124(2):170, 171.

52. Yang SC, Chiu TH, Lin TJ, et al. Subcutaneous emphysema and pneumomediastinum secondary to dental extraction: a case report and literature review. *Kaohsiung J Med Sci.* 2006;22(12):641-645.

53. Heyman SN, Babayof I. Emphysematous complications in dentistry, 1960-1993: an illustrative case and review of the literature. *Quintessence Int.* 1995;26(8):535-543.

54. Arai I, Aoki T, Yamazaki H, et al. Pneumomediastinum and subcutaneous emphysema after dental extraction detected incidentally by regular medical checkup: a case report. *Oral Surg Oral Med Oral Pathol Oral Radiol Endod.* 2009;107(4):e33-e38.

55. Finlayson RS, Stevens FD. Subcutaneous facial emphysema secondary to use of the Cavi-Jet. *J Periodontol.* 1988;59(5):315-317.

56. Fine DH, Mendieta C, Barnett ML, et al. Efficacy of preprocedural rinsing with an antiseptic in reducing viable bacteria in dental aerosols. *J Periodontol.* 1992;63(10):821-824.

57. Buhler J, Schmidi F, Weiger R, Walter C. Analysis of the effects of air polishing powders containing sodium bicarbonate and glycine on human teeth. *Clin Oral Invest.* 2015;19(4):877-885.

43

Tooth Bleaching

Heather Hessheimer, RDH, MSDH

CHAPTER OUTLINE

OVERVIEW OF TOOTH BLEACHING
I. Bleaching versus Whitening
II. Vital Tooth Bleaching versus Nonvital Tooth Bleaching
III. History

VITAL TOOTH BLEACHING
I. Mechanism of Bleaching Vital Teeth
II. Tooth Color Change with Vital Tooth Bleaching
III. Materials Used for Vital Tooth Bleaching
IV. Vital Tooth Bleaching Safety
V. Factors Associated with Efficacy

VI. Reversible Side Effects of Vital Bleaching: Sensitivity
VII. Irreversible Tooth Damage
VIII. Modes of Vital Tooth Bleaching

NONVITAL TOOTH BLEACHING
I. Procedure for Bleaching Nonvital Teeth
II. Factors Associated with Efficacy

DENTAL HYGIENE PROCESS OF CARE
I. Patient Assessment
II. Dental Hygiene Diagnosis

III. Dental Hygiene Care Plan
IV. Implementation
V. Evaluation and Planning for Maintenance

DOCUMENTATION

EVERYDAY ETHICS

FACTORS TO TEACH THE PATIENT

REFERENCES

LEARNING OBJECTIVES

After studying this chapter, the student will be able to:

1. Discuss the mechanism, safety, and efficacy of tooth bleaching agents.

2. Identify specific tooth conditions and staining responses to tooth bleaching.

3. Differentiate reversible and irreversible side effects associated with the tooth bleaching process.

4. Assess appropriate interventions for tooth bleaching side effects.

OVERVIEW OF TOOTH BLEACHING

Patients of all ages have concerns about the appearance of their teeth and expect their dental hygienists to guide them in their esthetic choices with evidence-based information. Because there are many causes of tooth discoloration, a review of Chapter 17 is recommended.

◆ Tooth bleaching may result in significantly whiter teeth and contribute to an increase in patient's self-confidence.

◆ A whiter smile may motivate the patient to maintain improved oral health, which is a significant benefit.

I. Bleaching versus Whitening

The terms "bleaching" and "whitening" have been used interchangeably, but are not the same as described below[1]:

◆ Tooth whitening refers to use of abrasive agents and/or detergents contained in a dentifrice to remove extrinsic stain.

◆ Bleaching involves free radicals and the breakdown of pigment, which occurs in the tooth-bleaching procedures.

II. Vital Tooth Bleaching versus Nonvital Tooth Bleaching

◆ Teeth can be stained intrinsically and extrinsically.

◆ External tooth bleaching is used for both vital and nonvital teeth.

• Agents for bleaching are applied to the external surfaces of the teeth.

• Bleaching agent breaks down chemical bonds in chromogens making them refract light and appear lighter.[2]

◆ Color change can extend into the dentin to produce a whitened tooth.

◆ Nonvital teeth become intrinsically stained by blood breakdown products, or agents from root canal therapy.[1]

◆ Nonvital tooth bleaching is a procedure performed by a dentist after root canal therapy using a rubber dam or other type of isolation.

  • The bleaching agents are introduced into the pulp chamber.

  • The color of a single tooth is lightened to help it blend with the adjacent teeth.

III. History

A. Nonvital Tooth-Bleaching History

◆ Bleaching of discolored, nonvital teeth was first described as early as 1864.[3,4]

◆ In 1961, the *walking bleach method* was introduced. The *walking bleach method* sealed a mixture of sodium perborate and water into the pulp chamber and retained it there between the patient's visits.[5]

◆ By 1963, the *walking bleach method* was modified using water and 30%–35% hydrogen peroxide instead of the sodium perborate and water. Result: improved lighter color of nonvital teeth.[3]

B. Vital Tooth-Bleaching History

◆ In the 1960s, tooth lightening was observed after orthodontic patients used an antiseptic containing carbamide peroxide to promote tissue healing due to gingivitis.[3,6]

◆ In the 1980s, lighter tooth color was noted after advising patients to use carbamide peroxide in customized trays for antiseptic purposes following periodontal surgery.[6]

◆ In 1989, the use of carbamide peroxide for the primary purpose of tooth bleaching was introduced.[7]

  • A custom tray was used to maintain the bleaching gel on the tooth surface for an extended time.

  • The procedure was known as nightguard vital bleaching.

◆ No significant, long-term oral or systemic health risks have been associated with professional at-home tooth-bleaching materials containing 10% carbamide peroxide or 3.5% hydrogen peroxide when professionally supervised.[8,9]

VITAL TOOTH BLEACHING

The bleaching process is a subject of ongoing research and current theories about the mechanism of action involve a chemical change within the tooth structure.

I. Mechanism of Bleaching Vital Teeth

◆ Bleaching products penetrate enamel and dentin reaching the pulp[10] within 5–15 minutes.[8,11]

◆ Bleaching products break down larger pigmented organic molecules, called chromogens, into smaller, less

pigmented constituents that are locked in the enamel matrix and dentinal tubules.[2,12,13]

◆ The chemical reactions from bleaching products changes the optical qualities of the tooth color.[14]

II. Tooth Color Change with Vital Tooth Bleaching

◆ The color of the teeth is influenced by thickness of enamel and underlying color of dentin.

◆ Color of both dentin and enamel are changed; primarily the dentin color is changed.[15]

◆ Dentin color is either yellow or gray and can be seen through the enamel due to its translucency.

◆ Darker teeth take more time to lighten.

◆ Each tooth reaches a maximum color change. Additional bleaching product or contact time will not necessarily result in a lighter color.[15]

◆ Bleaching products cause teeth to become dehydrated during and after product administration. A lighter shade can result temporarily.

◆ Color will stabilize approximately 2 weeks after bleaching.[15,16]

III. Materials Used for Vital Tooth Bleaching

◆ Both hydrogen peroxide and carbamide peroxide are used to lighten vital teeth.

◆ Hydrogen peroxide is approximately three times stronger than carbamide peroxide.[6]

◆ Hydrogen peroxide has a short working time; carbamide peroxide has an extended working time.[11] Figure 43-1

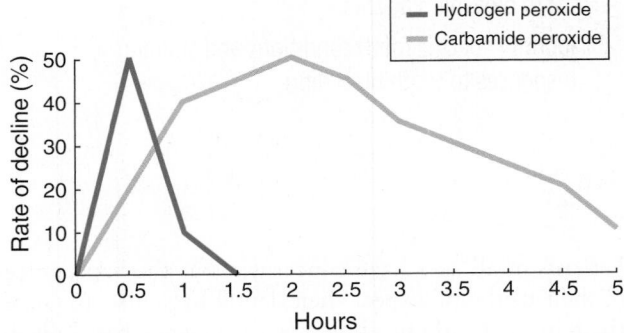

FIGURE 43-1 • Release Time of Carbamide Peroxide Compared to Hydrogen Peroxide. Hydrogen peroxide has a much shorter working time than carbamide peroxide and causes more sensitivity. Hydrogen peroxide releases all of the peroxide within 1.5 hours. Carbamide peroxide releases the peroxide over a much longer time. Hydrogen peroxide is approximately three times stronger than carbamide peroxide. (Figures courtesy of Dr. Van Haywood. Reprinted from Haywood VB. Treating sensitivity during tooth whitening. *Compend Contin Educ Dent.* 2005;28(9, suppl 3):11-20. © 2005, AEGIS Publications, LLC. Used with permission.)

compares the release or duration time of carbamide peroxide with hydrogen peroxide.

- The chemicals are used alone or in combination with each other.
- Bleaching materials need an appropriate viscosity to flow over the tooth surface but not so excessive as to spread onto gingival and other oral tissues.

A. Hydrogen Peroxide

- Used directly or produced through a chemical reaction when carbamide peroxide breaks down (see Figure 43-2).[15]
- Has a lower pH than carbamide peroxide, which may result in demineralization or erosion when used for longer treatment times than recommended.[2,17]
  - May result in dentin changes which never recover.[18]
- Takes less time per day, but more days to change tooth color effectively.[8]
- Higher concentrations of hydrogen peroxide may result in greater sensitivity and more color relapse after termination of bleaching.[18]

B. Carbamide Peroxide

- Active agent in most bleaching systems in a 10% concentration.
- Breaks down into hydrogen peroxide and urea. As shown in the flowchart (Figure 43-2), urea may further break down into ammonia with high pH to facilitate bleaching.
- Has slow release: 50% of peroxide released in 2–4 hours and remainder of peroxide in 2–6 hours resulting in less sensitivity.[11] In Figure 43-1, the release time is shown for carbamide peroxide compared with hydrogen peroxide.
- At neutral pH, 10% solution is both safe and effective as a bleaching agent.[8,19]
- Takes fewer days but more contact time to change tooth color effectively.[1]

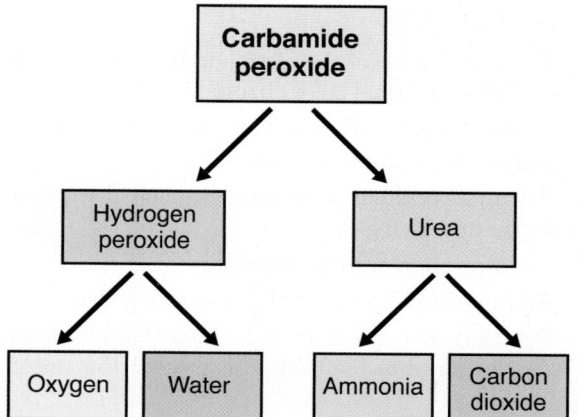

FIGURE 43-2 • Hydrogen Peroxide and Carbamide Peroxide Product Breakdown. Flowchart to show breakdown of bleaching products. Hydrogen peroxide breaks down into oxygen and water; carbamide peroxide breaks down into hydrogen peroxide and urea, which further break down as shown.

C. Desensitizers

- Materials to reduce the sensitivity side effect of bleaching may be added to bleaching systems.
- Materials can be:
  - Incorporated into the bleaching gel.
  - Applied to teeth before bleaching.
  - Given for use in trays before, during, and after treatment.
- Material used:
  - Potassium nitrate: creates a calming effect on pulp by affecting the transmission of nerve impulses.[20,11]
  - Sodium fluoride: aid in remineralization.[21]
  - Calcium phosphate and amorphous calcium phosphate: aid in remineralization.[20,11]

D. Other Ingredients

- Carbopol: a water-soluble resin used as a thickening agent, which:
  - Prolongs the release of hydrogen peroxide from carbamide peroxide.
  - Promotes quicker results.
- Glycerin: a gel to thicken and control the flow of bleaching agent to prevent overextending onto gingival tissues.
- Sodium hydroxide: a cleaning agent.
- Surfactants: help to lift and remove extrinsic stains.
- Flavoring: aids in patient satisfaction and compliance.

IV. Vital Tooth-Bleaching Safety

A. Tooth Structure

- Both hydrogen peroxide 3.5% and carbamide peroxide 10% are considered safe to lighten the color of teeth when professionally monitored.[8,9]
- Hydrogen peroxide at concentrations of 30% or higher may:
  - Remove the enamel matrix.
  - Create microscopic voids that scatter light.
  - Result in increased whiteness until remineralization occurs and color partly relapses.[1]
- Carbamide peroxide 10% will cause fewer changes in the enamel matrix.[1,13,22]
- Pulpal necrosis was noted when material combined with excessive heat or trauma.[23]

B. Soft Tissue

- Hydrogen peroxide is caustic and may cause burning and bleaching of the gingiva and any exposed oral tissue.[3]
- Hydrogen peroxide 10% concentration or higher has greater incidence of gingival irritation.[8]
- Ill-fitting or overfilled tray may cause product spillage onto soft tissues resulting in tissue burning.

C. Restorative Materials

- Restorative material color will not be lightened by bleaching.

◆ Complications with current restorations may include[13]:
  • Increased surface roughness.
  • Change in surface color.
  • Increased microleakage.
◆ After bleaching, new restorative procedures need to be delayed for 2 weeks to allow for color stabilization.[19]
◆ Bonding needs to be delayed for 2 weeks due to significantly reduced bonding strength associated with recently bleached tooth surface.[18]
◆ Bleaching chemicals containing hydrogen peroxide may:
  • Have a negative effect on restorations and restorative materials due to lower pH, although impact does not necessarily require the renewal of the restoration.[16]
  • Increase mercury release from amalgam restorations giving off a green hue.[16]
  • Increase solubility of some dental cements.[13]

D. Systemic Factors

◆ The use of tooth-bleaching products containing hydrogen peroxide or carbamide peroxide has not been shown to increase the risk of oral cancer in the general population, including those persons who are alcohol abusers and/or heavy cigarette smokers.[8]
◆ Accidental ingestion of small amounts of the product may cause sore throat, nausea, vomiting, abdominal distention, and ulcerations of the oral mucosa, esophagus, and stomach.[13]
◆ Medications that may be associated with photosensitivity and hyperpigmentation when light-activated bleaching agents are used are listed in Box 43-1.

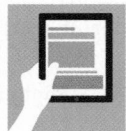

BOX 43-1

Medications Associated with Potential Photosensitivity and Hyperpigmentation

• Acne medications
• Antiarrhythmic drugs
• Antibiotics
• Anticancer drugs
• Antidepressants
• Antihistamines
• Antiparasitics
• Antipsychotics
• Antiseizure medications
• Arthritis medications
• Birth control medications
• Coal tar
• Diuretics
• Hypoglycemics
• Nonsteroidal anti-inflammatory drugs
• Steroids
• Tranquilizers
• Sulfur-containing drugs

E. Cautions and Contraindications Associated with Vital Tooth Bleaching

◆ Personal factors affecting acceptance for treatment may include:
  • Subjective determination when tooth shade is acceptable.
  • Patients with unrealistic personal expectations.
  • Poor patient compliance with treatment results in suboptimal results.
  • Patients with tooth conditions that do not respond favorably to vital tooth bleaching (see Table 43-1).
◆ Children and adolescents
  • The American Academy of Pediatric Dentistry discourages full-arch cosmetic bleaching for patients with a mixed dentition, but encourages judicious use of vital and nonvital bleaching due to the negative self-image that may arise from a discolored tooth or teeth.[24]
  • Current American Dental Association recommendations for children and adolescent use include[8]:
    • Delaying treatment until after permanent teeth have erupted.
    • Use of a custom-fabricated tray to limit amount of bleaching gel.
    • Close supervision.
◆ Tooth bleaching is contraindicated in the following patients:
  • Pregnant and lactating women.
  • Use of photosensitive medications (see Box 43-1).
  • Recent cosmetic procedures such as skin peels, facial waxing, or use of certain essential oils.
  • Laser light/power bleaching contraindicated for some patients as described in Box 43-2.

V. Factors Associated with Efficacy

◆ Some tooth conditions will not respond to tooth bleaching; other tooth conditions will respond slowly (Table 43-1).[1,9]
◆ The initial color of the teeth and type of stain present will affect the final color change.[1,9]
◆ Specific indications for bleaching and methods of treatments are listed in Table 43-2.
◆ Attrition: occlusal wear through enamel exposes the darker underlying dentin.
◆ Concentration of bleaching agent.
◆ Ability of agent to reach the stain molecules.
◆ Duration of contact of the active bleaching agent: the longer the duration, the greater the degree of bleaching.
◆ Number of times the agent is applied to obtain desired results: darker teeth tend to require more treatment applications.
◆ Temperature of agent: heat will result in faster oxygen release, but speed of color change may not be altered.

TABLE 43-1 • Decision Making for Tooth Bleaching

TOOTH CONDITION	RESPONSE TO TOOTH BLEACHING	SPECIAL CONSIDERATIONS
Yellow color	Normally excellent.	Resistant yellow may be tetracycline stain.
Enamel white spots	Do not bleach well or may get lighter during bleaching.	• Eventually background color lightens resulting in less noticeable white spots. • Goes through splotchy stage before background color whitens. • Microabrasion may lessen white spots if less than one-third through enamel.
Brown fluorosis stains	Respond 80% of the time.	Microabrasion techniques done after bleaching and color stabilization may improve final result.
Nicotine stains	Require longer treatment.	May take 2–3 mo of nightly application.
Tetracycline stains	Multicolored band may not respond well. • Gray most difficult. • Dark grays only get lighter. • Dark cervical has poorest prognosis.	Requires 2–12 mo of daily bleaching.
Minocycline stains	Will respond; will take longer than yellow stain.	• Type of tetracycline stain. • Gives gray hue.
Root exposure	Does not respond to bleaching.	Better treated with periodontal coverage.
Dentinogenesis imperfecta and amelogenesis imperfecta	No significant improvement with bleaching.	Inherited condition resulting in defective dentin and enamel, respectively.
Microcracks	Become whiter than rest of tooth.	Bright light or magnification required during assessment to view; may appear streaky during bleaching process.
Anterior lingual amalgams	Become more visible after bleaching.	Replacement with very light composite restoration before bleaching.
Dental caries	Not to be bleached.	• Decay removal. • Temporary restoration followed by bleaching and final restoration after color stabilization. Carbamide peroxide will increase sensitivity and is bactericidal.
Dark canines	Require longer bleaching.	Isolated canine treatment until color match.
Attrition	Incisal edges do not respond.	Composite restorations added to incisal edges after bleaching.
Aging	Excellent.	More youthful appearance; root surfaces exposure likely.
Translucent teeth	Bleaching will increase translucency at incisal.	Translucent areas will appear darker after bleaching due to contrast.

A. Intrinsic

◆ Tetracycline and minocycline staining
- Tetracycline particles incorporate into dentin calcium during mineralization of unerupted teeth. Result: discolored dentin resistant to bleaching.[25]
- Minocycline, a derivative of tetracycline, can discolor erupted teeth.[26]
- Tetracycline and minocycline staining severity varies. A comparison of before and after bleaching of brown tetracycline staining is shown in Figure 43-3.
  - *First-category staining*: light-yellow to light-gray responds to bleaching.
  - *Second-category staining*: darker and more extensive yellow-gray responds to extended bleaching time.
  - *Third-category staining*: intense dark gray-blue banding stains. Severe third-category staining may require porcelain veneers for satisfactory esthetic result.
  - Some tetracycline stains will require 1–12 months to achieve a satisfactory result.

◆ Fluorosis
- Fluorosis results from ingesting excessive fluoride during tooth development resulting in white or brown spots on teeth.

BOX 43-2
Issues Associated with Light-Activated Bleaching

Light-activated bleaching is contraindicated for patients who are:

- Light sensitive.
- Taking a photosensitive medication.
- Receiving photochemotherapeutic drugs or treatments such as psoralen and ultraviolet radiation.

Exposure to ultraviolet radiation produced by some lights is avoided by those at increased risk for or have a history of skin cancer, including melanoma.

TABLE 43-2 • Indications for Tooth Bleaching and Methods of Treatment

INDICATION	METHOD TO TREAT
Discolored, endodontically treated tooth	Internal bleaching; in-office or walking.
Single or multiple discolored teeth	External bleaching: in-office one to three visits or custom trays worn 2–6 wk.
Surface staining	Dental prophylaxis and brushing with whitening dentifrice.
Isolated brown or white discoloration, shallow depth in enamel	Microabrasion followed by neutral sodium fluoride applications.
White discoloration on yellowish teeth	Microabrasion followed by custom tray bleaching.

- Bleaching does not change white spots, but lightens the background color, making the contrast less noticeable.
- White spots go through a splotchy stage during bleaching but will return to baseline.
- Amorphous calcium phosphate may be effective in lessening the white spots if lesion is less than one-third through enamel.[27]
- Brown discoloration responsive to bleach 80% of the time.
- Resin infiltration or microabrasion may be recommended to decrease additional brown discoloration.[28,29]
◆ Nicotine
  - Nicotine stains: require 1–3 months of nightly treatment due to the tenacity of the stain.

B. Extrinsic
◆ Interactions with Bleaching Agents.
  - Staining agents may compromise treatment.[1] Advise patient to avoid:
    - Coffee and tea.
    - Dark sodas or soft drinks.
    - Red wine.
    - Soy sauce.
    - Tobacco.
◆ Chromogenic bacteria.
◆ Biofilm accumulation.
◆ Topical medications.

C. Longevity of Results
◆ Relapse of shade occurs almost immediately as newly bleached, dehydrated teeth rehydrate.
◆ As months and years pass, teeth may discolor and darken again, especially if stain-inducing activities continue.
◆ To maintain shade, periodic bleaching procedures are performed or repeated.

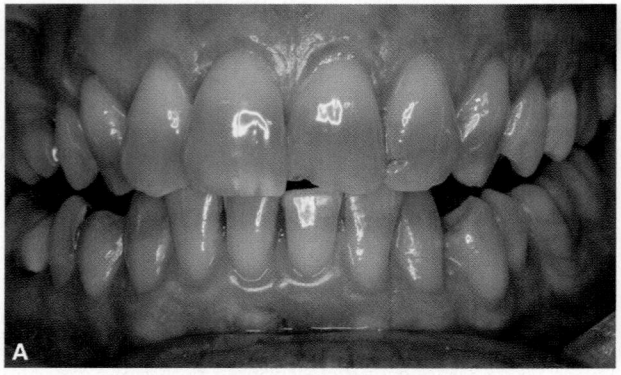
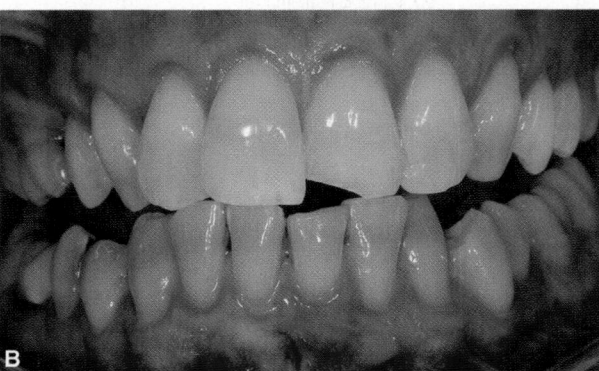

FIGURE 43-3 • Before and After Bleaching of Brown Tetracycline-Stained Teeth. A: Patient before treating. **B:** Patient treated with 10% carbamide peroxide for 2 months. Some tetracycline-stained teeth will require up to 12 months to achieve improved results. Those with severe gray stain or banded staining may require porcelain veneers to achieve an acceptable cosmetic result. (Images courtesy of Dr. Van Haywood. Reprinted from Haywood VB. The "bottom line" on bleaching 2008. *Inside Dent.* 2008;4(2):2-5. © 2008, AEGIS Publications, LLC. Used with permission.)

VI. Reversible Side Effects of Vital Bleaching: Sensitivity

The most common side effects of bleaching are tooth tingling and sensitivity. Aching sensation can occur because of insult of peroxide on nerves: a reversible pulpitis.[11,21]

◆ Up to two-thirds of patients will experience transitory mild-to-moderate tooth sensitivity.[8]

◆ Primarily occur in the first 2 weeks of treatment and may last days to months after cessation of bleaching.

◆ Side effects resolve completely as teeth become accustomed to bleaching.

◆ Not correlated with increased wear time.[20]

◆ Lower concentrations have been used for up to 12 months and do not exhibit greater sensitivity.[11]
  • Higher concentrations of hydrogen peroxide may result in greater sensitivity.[20]

◆ Patients with prior history of tooth sensitivity may be more at risk to develop sensitivity during bleaching.

◆ Vulnerable tooth surfaces include:
  • Exposed root surfaces and dentin appear to increase risk of developing sensitivity and need to be protected from bleaching material.
  • Teeth with unrestored abfraction lesions (see Chapter 41) tend to have more sensitivity.

◆ Addition of desensitizing materials decreases sensitivity.

◆ Treatments to reduce tooth sensitivity are listed in Table 43-3.

TABLE 43-3 • Desensitization Procedures for Bleaching	
Pretreatment	• Brush on or use with tray a desensitizing toothpaste containing potassium nitrate, without sodium lauryl sulfate, which removes smear layer from dentin, beginning 2 wk before bleaching.
	• Use toothpaste with prescription strength sodium fluoride.
	• Use toothpaste that includes calcium carbonate.
During treatment	• Continue to use desensitizing toothpaste, which includes sodium fluoride or potassium nitrate, daily between treatments. Amorphous calcium phosphate may be used as well.
	• Increase time intervals between treatments.
	• Reduce exposure time of bleaching materials.
	• Limit the amount in tray to prevent tissue contact.
Postbleaching	• Sensitivity diminishes with time.
	• Continue daily use of desensitizing dentifrice and amorphous calcium phosphate.
	• Have professional fluoride varnish application.
	• Avoid foods and beverages with temperature extremes or that contain acidic elements.

VII. Irreversible Tooth Damage

A. Root Resorption

◆ Can occur after bleaching, particularly after intracoronal, nonvital tooth bleaching when heat is applied during the technique.[1]

◆ Internal and external resorption may become apparent several years after bleaching.[1]

◆ Occurs usually in cervical third of the tooth.[1]

◆ Cause may be related to a history of trauma.[1]

◆ May lead to tooth loss.[1]

◆ Bleaching agents should not be placed on exposed cementum to avoid complications.[1]

B. Tooth Fracture

◆ May be related to removal of tooth structure or reduction of the microhardness of dentin and enamel.[30]

◆ More common with nonvital tooth bleaching.[31]

◆ May lead to tooth loss.[30]

C. Demineralization

◆ Demineralization with slight surface pitting can result from H_2O_2 concentration above 15%.[32]

◆ Patient with over-the-counter (OTC) product may not seek or follow professional advice and attempt to get the teeth whiter by using the product more often than recommended.

◆ Remineralization should be initiated early and fluoridated carbamide peroxide gels may be a good choice to aid remineralization.[33]

◆ Remineralization protocols are described in Chapter 25.

D. Erosion

◆ Products containing acidic pH may result in tooth erosion over time.[13]

◆ The higher the percentage of hydrogen peroxide, the lower the pH.

◆ More common with OTC bleaching products.

VIII. Modes of Vital Tooth Bleaching

◆ A comparison of the advantages and disadvantages of professionally applied and professionally dispensed/professionally monitored systems and the OTC systems is listed in Table 43-4.

◆ The different methods of tooth bleaching can achieve similar, effective results, although the mode of delivery, length of treatment, and ease of treatment vary.

A. Professionally Applied

◆ Professionally applied bleaching is performed with high concentrations of 30%–40% hydrogen peroxide or 35%–44% carbamide peroxide.

◆ Bleaching gels are administered by a dental professional and are not for at-home use.

TABLE 43-4 • Comparisons of Modes of Tooth-Bleaching Systems

METHODS	ADVANTAGES	DISADVANTAGES
Professionally applied utilizing laser/ultraviolet light system procedure	<ul><li>Performed as part of comprehensive care.</li><li>Treatment may be combined with trays and professional grade home bleaching materials.</li><li>Professional product selection.</li><li>Patient education.</li><li>Follow-up, evaluation of effectiveness.</li><li>Sensitivity treatment.</li><li>Compliance guaranteed.</li><li>Quickest result.</li></ul>	<ul><li>Higher cost.</li><li>Higher risk for sensitivity.</li></ul>
Professionally dispensed, includes professional grade product and trays	<ul><li>Performed as part of comprehensive care.</li><li>Appropriate patient selection.</li><li>Professional product selection.</li><li>Patient education.</li><li>Follow-up, evaluation of effectiveness.</li><li>Sensitivity treatment; patient can also use less often if sensitive.</li><li>Choice of comfortable time and place for application.</li><li>Potential for best result.</li></ul>	<ul><li>Cost.</li><li>Longer time to whiten than professionally applied.</li><li>Patient compliance.</li></ul>
Over-the-counter	<ul><li>Lowest cost.</li><li>Easier access to purchase.</li><li>Immediate start.</li><li>Results and tissue response not monitored.</li><li>Over-the-counter products have short exposure times, which limit effects.</li><li>Unsupervised.</li></ul>	<ul><li>No comprehensive exam.</li><li>Slowest and least effective results.</li><li>Noncustomized delivery.</li><li>Compliance issues.</li><li>Bulky fit for patient (see Figure 43-8).</li></ul>

◆ Some systems use activation or enhancement with a light or heat source.
  • Local anesthesia should not be used in order to monitor heat-provoked sensitivity.
  • Heat applied or produced by the use of light may cause an adverse effect such as necrosis of the pulp of the tooth.[34]
  • Additional issues associated with the use of a light-activated bleaching are listed in Box 43-2.
◆ Laser-safe/ultraviolet light protection of eyes for all in treatment room is required.
◆ Gingival sensitivity or irritation may occur.
  • Rubber dam or an equivalent technique, such as a liquid light-cured resin dam, should be used to isolate the caustic agents from contact with soft tissues.
  • Take care to assure the liquid light-cured resin dam is in the interproximal spaces to protect gingival tissue.
  • Improvements in paint-on rubber dams, cheek, lip retractors, and lower concentrations of peroxide have made in-office bleaching safer for patient and dentist.
◆ Treatment may take one to six applications for preferred results.
◆ Time for each application varies between different products; ranges from 30- to 60-minute treatment.
◆ Laser/power bleaching treatment plan may also involve use of bleaching trays for home use.

B. Professionally Dispensed/ Professionally Monitored

◆ Also called bleaching trays, external bleaching, at-home bleaching.
◆ Study model preparation:
  • An impression of the teeth is taken to prepare the cast for fabrication of the tray.
  • Inspect impression to ensure all anatomy is present without bubbles or voids.
  • Dental stone is poured into impression with little time delay to avoid distortion.
  • Place impression on vibration plate while slowly pouring stone mixture in impression to avoid bubbles on the cast surface.
  • After entire arch is filled with stone mixture, let solidify for one hour. Remove cast from impression and inspect for voids.
  • An ideal cast is trimmed into a horseshoe shape with the central incisors perpendicular to the base to allow proper suction during tray formation.
  • With a moderate grasp, place back of cast on model trimmer pushing lightly.
  • Hold the cast with the occlusal plane parallel to wheel until vestibule is removed.
  • Light-cured block-out resin can be placed on the surfaces of teeth to be bleached. A 1-mm border with no block-out should be maintained to allow proper fit of bleaching tray to the tooth.

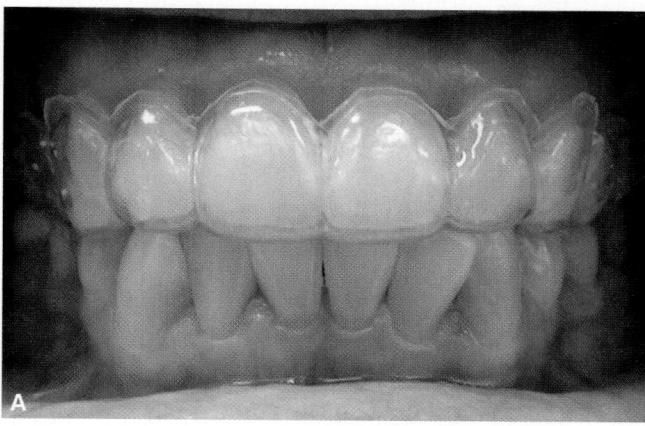
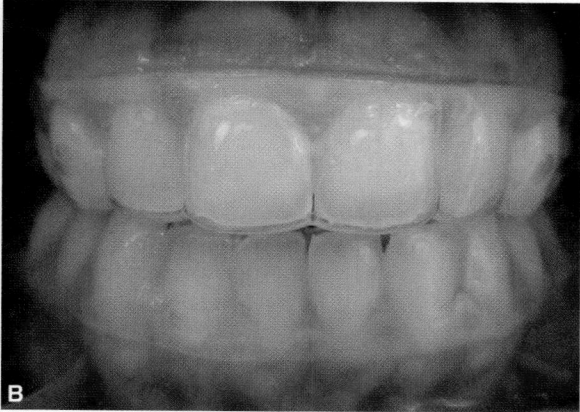

FIGURE 43-4 • Scalloped and Unscalloped Bleaching Tray Designs. Either scalloped or unscalloped trays may be used. **A:** Scalloped trays aim to protect the gingiva and exposed root surfaces. **B:** Unscalloped trays are more comfortable and take less preparation time. Patients need to be warned to avoid overfilling trays.

◆ Tray preparation:
- Thin, vacuum-formed custom trays are made for each dental arch to be bleached.
- Place prepared cast on base of vacuum former and place sheet of thin tray material in holder. Raise to heating element and heat tray material until sags one inch.
- Lower material to the vacuum base and allow machine to suction material around cast for one minute.
- Carefully remove from base since material may be hot. Cool completely before removing cast from material.
- Trays should be trimmed with small, sharp scissors in a smooth motion to produce uniform edges.
- As shown in Figure 43-4, trays are either scalloped at gingival margin or unscalloped and trimmed 1–2 mm from deepest portion of gingival margin, taking care to cut around the incisive papilla and frena.
- Nonscalloped trays seal better.
- Trays are fitted to the patient and adjusted to ensure bleaching material will not come into contact with soft tissues.

◆ Patient instruction:
- Instructions and bleaching materials for use in the trays at home should be provided.
- Patient should practice placing correct amount of bleaching gel to demonstrate understanding.
- Once or twice daily application for 1–2 weeks is usually recommended if lack of sensitivity and other side effects permit. Maximum color change obtained with consistent compliance (see Figure 43-5).
- The enamel may become more porous during treatment[13]; therefore, patient should be advised to avoid staining agents.

◆ Patient retains the trays after completion of bleaching to reuse for touch-ups as needed.

◆ Professionally dispensed bleaching products are commonly recommended after professionally applied bleaching procedures to maintain and promote results.

C. OTC Products

◆ Also called *at-home* or *self-directed* products.

◆ When asked about use of the self-directed product, a dental hygienist may stress the need for professional

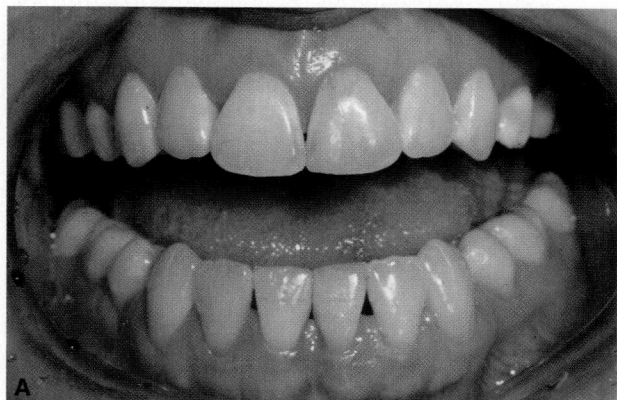
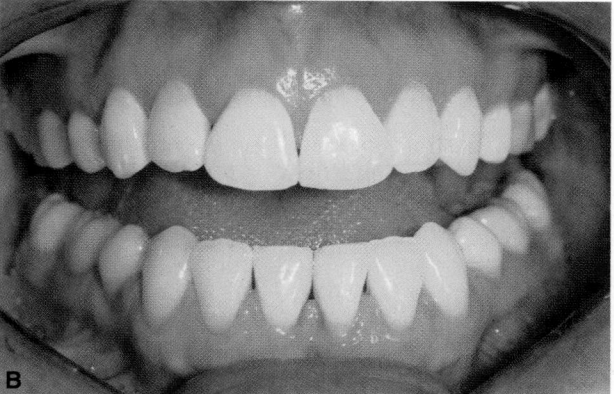

FIGURE 43-5 • Home Tray Bleaching Treatment. A: Before treatment. **B:** After treatment. (Photo courtesy of Gordon J. Christensen DDS MSD PhD. Used with permission.)

examination and supervision; the products can cause harm if misused, may irritate tissues, or cause systemic illness if ingested.

♦ May be recommended to help maintain results of professionally applied and professionally dispensed methods of bleaching.

♦ The dental professional must be informed of patient's proposed use of OTC products to discuss risks and possible interaction with any proposed dental treatment.

♦ An oral evaluation is recommended before use of the at-home or OTC products, as well as appropriate dental and periodontal treatment including calculus, stain, and biofilm removal.

♦ Delivered through various packaging, viscosities, and flavors (Box 43-3).

BOX 43-3
Over-the-Counter Bleaching Preparations

Strips
• Hydrogen peroxide is delivered on polyethylene film strips.
• Strips are placed on the teeth up to two times per day for 30 minutes for about 2 weeks.

Prefabricated Trays
• Thin-membrane tray loaded with bleaching agent is adapted to maxillary or mandibular arch.
• Usually worn 30–60 minutes daily for 5–10 days.

Paint-on
• Carbamide peroxide is incorporated into a thick gel that is painted on the teeth selected to be bleached.
• An advantage to this method is that individual teeth may be bleached.

Dentifrice
• Used to help keep teeth cleaner, and therefore look whiter.
• Some have more abrasive materials to remove extrinsic stains.
• Owing to short exposure time, the bleaching agent in the dentifrice has little effect on staining.
• Some contain hydrogen peroxide; others contain agents that may deter further attachment of stains to the teeth.

Mouthrinse
• Content of alcohol is avoided in selection of mouthrinse.

NONVITAL TOOTH BLEACHING

Also called *walking bleach method* and *internal bleaching*, nonvital tooth bleaching involves the bleaching of a single, endodontically treated tooth that is discolored.

♦ Alternative to more invasive correction, such as a post and core with crown.

♦ Performed by a dentist.

♦ Requirements for procedure:
  • Healthy periodontium.
  • Successfully obturated root canal filling.
  • Root canal filling is sealed off with a restorative material before treatment to prevent bleaching agent from reaching periapical tissue.

I. Procedure for Bleaching Nonvital Teeth

♦ Hydrogen peroxide and/or sodium perborate is placed in the pulp chamber, sealed, and left for 3–7 days, as outlined in Box 43-4.

♦ Hydrogen peroxide and sodium perborate may be synergistic and very effective in bleaching the tooth.

BOX 43-4
Procedure for Nonvital Tooth Bleaching

Periodontally healthy, endodontically treated tooth:
1. Photograph of the tooth to be bleached with shade guide.
2. Provide dental hygiene services to remove extrinsic stain and calculus.
3. Probe circumferentially to determine the outline of the cementoenamel junction.
4. Rubber dam isolation is applied to prevent contamination of root canal therapy.
5. Prepare access cavity. Remove all endodontic obturation material, sealer, cement, and necessary restorative material without removing more dentin than necessary.
6. Remove 2–3 mm of obturation material from the root canal to level below the crest of the gingival margin.
7. Irrigate access cavity with copious amount of water and dry well without desiccating.
8. Root canal therapy is sealed off, commonly with glass ionomer cement or other filling material.
9. Medicament is placed in pulp chamber.
10. Pulp chamber is sealed with a temporary restoration.
11. Patient returns in 3–7 days for evaluation.

Aforementioned procedure is repeated several times until desired result is obtained.

To finalize procedure:

1. Rubber dam isolation.
2. Temporary restoration on medicament is removed.
3. Pulp chamber is irrigated thoroughly with water.
4. Coronal restoration is placed; generally a composite material.
5. Photograph tooth with corresponding shade guide for records.

♦ The process is repeated until a satisfactory result is obtained.

♦ Once a satisfactory result is obtained, the pulp chamber is sealed with glass ionomer cement.

♦ Appoint patient 2 weeks later to place permanent, bonded, composite-resin restoration in access cavity to allow dissipation of residual oxygen that would interfere with efficacy of bonding agent.

♦ If unsuccessful after repeated attempts, techniques for vital tooth bleaching can be tried or an alternative restorative procedure can be tried, such as a post and core with crown.

II. Factors Associated with Efficacy

♦ Results usually last longer than external tooth bleaching.

♦ There is no universal standard for what is considered acceptable esthetics.

• Personal background, culture, and patient's image of esthetics are factors.

• The dentist initially may not identify a patient's esthetic issues in the same way that the patient identifies them.

♦ Careful communication and agreement about the course of treatment and the expected result of treatment before the start of bleaching by the patient is essential.

DENTAL HYGIENE PROCESS OF CARE

I. Patient Assessment

♦ Review of medical history; identify any contraindications for bleaching.

♦ Complete dental assessment include the following:

• Complete extraoral and intraoral examination including oral cancer screening.

• Updated radiographs.

• Comprehensive dental exam.

• The presence of cavitated dental caries is a contraindication for bleaching. A lesion is prepared and restored with a temporary restoration to be replaced with permanent matching restoration upon completion of bleaching.

• To identify abscesses or nonvital teeth, which would require endodontic therapy before bleaching.

♦ Comprehensive periodontal examination including areas of recession. Cementum needs to be protected from bleaching material to avoid potential internal and/or external resorption.

♦ Determine initial tooth shade either manually with a shade guide (Figure 43-6) or electronically with a spectrophotometer (Figure 43-7). Box 43-5 provides tips for manually selecting a tooth shade.

♦ Obtain photographic record of tooth shade without lipstick or strong clothing colors that may interfere with accurate assessment. Use the canine for base color. Color will be gray or yellow. Confirm with patient.

♦ Identify those factors that would lead to a guarded prognosis for bleaching such as:

• Unrealistic expectations of the patient.

• History of sensitive teeth.

• Extremely dark gingival third of tooth visible during a smile.

• Extensive white spots that are very visible.

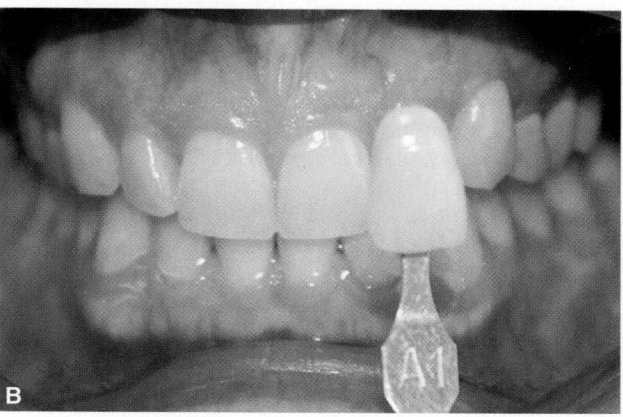

FIGURE 43-6 • Manual Selection of Tooth Shade. Patient's shade taken, recorded, and photographed in natural light or color-corrected lighting after extrinsic stain removal before bleaching. **A:** Several manufacturers provide color ranges with as many as 29 shades. **B:** Patient's shade and photograph are recorded at each visit while in bleaching treatment. (Photo courtesy Heather Hessheimer, RDH, MS.)

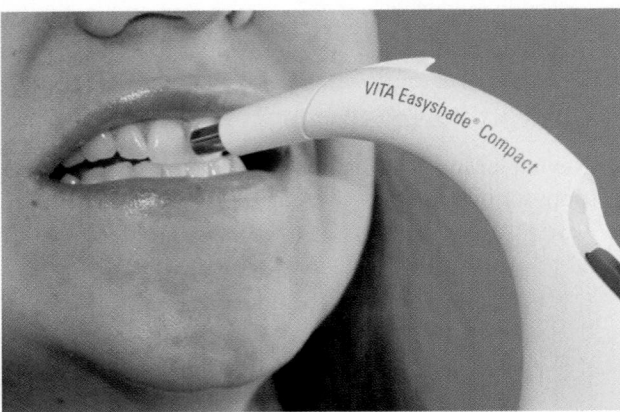

FIGURE 43-7. Digital Photographic Record of Tooth Shade. Electronic digital shade guides provide objective records. (Photo courtesy of Heather Hessheimer, RDH, MS.)

- Temporomandibular joint dysfunction or bruxism that would make wearing bleaching trays uncomfortable and potentially aggravate condition.
- Inability to tolerate the taste of the product.
- Identify contraindications for at-home bleaching including the following:
  - Presence of sensitive teeth.
  - Unwillingness or inability to comply with at-home treatment routines.

BOX 43-5
Tips for Manually Selecting Tooth Shade

Three concepts should be considered when determining tooth shade: hue, chroma, and value. *Hue* refers to the color of a tooth. Some teeth are more yellow while others are more red or gray. *Chroma* refers to the saturation, or intensity of the color. *Value* is the lightness or brightness of the color. When selecting tooth shade, it is best to start with selecting the proper *value*.

1. Arrange shade guide on the *value* scale with incisal edges oriented for maxilla.
2. Limit extra light sources in the room. Have patient face natural lighting if possible.
3. Remove any distracting colors from view, such as wiping off lipstick or covering brightly colored clothing.
4. Rest eyes by looking at light-gray color prior to shade matching.
5. Hold shade guide close to patient's teeth so shadow of the upper lip will be similar and select the *value* that best represents their tooth brightness. When debating between two shades, select the lighter of the two.
6. Next select the *chroma* that best correlates in that *value* range.
7. Finally, confirm the *hue* of the selected shade is appropriate for the tooth being matched.

- Excessive existing restorations not requiring replacement.
- Pregnancy or lactation.

II. Dental Hygiene Diagnosis

Deficit in wholesome body image as evidenced by patient statement related to dissatisfaction of tooth color.

III. Dental Hygiene Care Plan

- Plan dental hygiene therapy and preventive procedures.
- Choose appropriate bleaching method.
  - Discussion of procedure, risks, and realistic results.
  - Plan with patient for anticipated needs after bleaching, such as replacement of existing tooth-colored restorations that will not match after bleaching.
- List procedure and risks.
- Encourage questions.
- Obtain informed consent and patient's signature (see Chapter 23).

IV. Implementation

- *Dental hygiene therapy*: debridement of all soft and hard deposits along with extrinsic stains.
- Pretreatment desensitization when indicated. Recommended procedures for pretreatment, during treatment, and postbleaching are listed in Table 43-3.
- Premedication with anti-inflammatory pain medication when indicated for sensitivity.
- Preparation of trays: impression and construction.
- Provide patient education and instructions for use with an emphasis on the following:
  - Tooth sensitivity treatment and sensitivity prevention.
  - Effective daily biofilm removal before bleaching material use to prevent additional extrinsic stain accumulation.
  - Avoidance of foods that stain teeth such as coffee, red wine, and use of tobacco to maximize results.
  - Use of nonabrasive whitening dentifrice.
  - Avoidance of overfilling tray to protect soft tissue and exposed cementum.
  - Removal of excess bleaching material after use.
  - Avoidance of swallowing bleaching material due to irritation of materials to mucosa.

V. Evaluation and Planning for Maintenance

- Monitor appointments as needed to assess patient compliance, results, and sensitivity.
- At continuing care appointments, compare tooth color with tooth color guide. Take follow-up photos as appropriate for records.
- Tooth color from bleaching relapses with time.
- Plan for repeat of bleaching process at appropriate intervals.

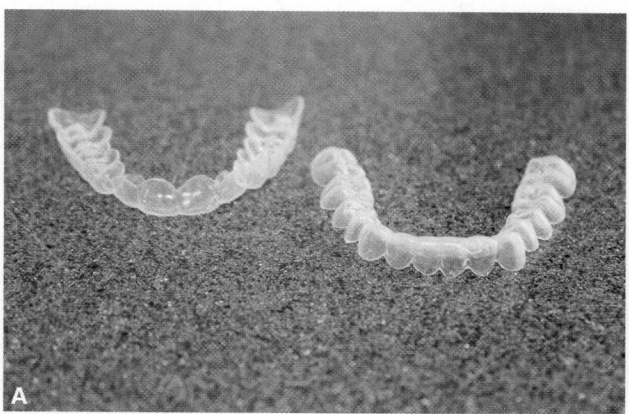
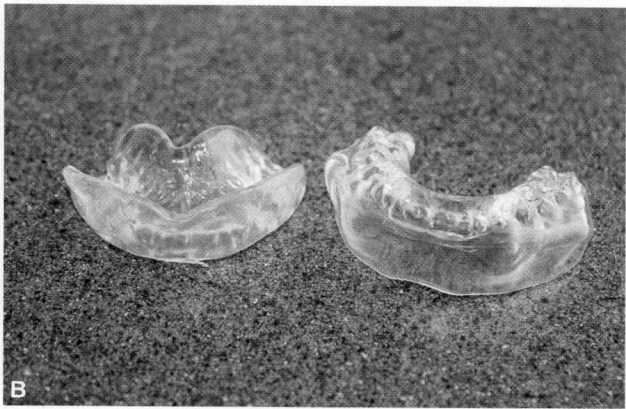

FIGURE 43-8 • Comparison of At-Home Bleaching Trays. A: Scalloped professionally dispensed bleaching trays. **B:** Over-the-counter (OTC) bleaching trays made by patient at home. Professionally dispensed trays are fitted to the patient using impressions, casts, and flexible plastic for custom fit. OTC trays are more bulky and prepared by patient at home. (Photo courtesy Heather Hessheimer, RDH, MS.)

DOCUMENTATION

Documentation in the patient's permanent record when planning tooth bleaching includes a minimum of the following:

- Current oral conditions.
- Consent to treat related to tooth bleaching.
- Services provided including necessary records for tooth shade.
- Impressions and preparation of the trays.
- Demonstration of tray filling, positioning, timing, and cleaning.
- Instructions given to patient.
- Planned follow-up care and appointments.
- Patient problems or complaints expressed.
- An example documentation is shown in Box 43-6.

obtained to document tooth color. Impressions and preparation of bleaching trays. Dispensed three syringes of carbamide peroxide 10%. Patient instructed to brush with potassium nitrate product for 2 weeks before beginning bleaching process; after beginning bleaching use of carbamide peroxide 10% every other day.

Patient demonstrated dispensing correct amount of bleaching gel into tray. Patient states: tray provides comfortable fit; understanding of sensitivity treatment; and willingness to return for follow-up appointment.

Next steps: Patient scheduled for follow-up appointment 2 weeks after bleaching process initiated.

Signed: _____, RDH

Date: _____

BOX 43-6

Example Documentation:
Patient Receiving Vital Tooth Bleaching

S–Patient states she is unhappy with the color of teeth. Patient states she has sensitive teeth.

O–Tooth shade: C-1; appears to have only yellow stain. Patient's medical and dental histories present no contraindications for tooth bleaching. Radiographs and dental examination reveal absence of cavitated caries.

A–Patient presents with a deficit in wholesome body image as evidenced by her statement she is self-conscious of tooth color.

P–Consent for treatment signed and copy given to patient. Completed prophylaxis with all extrinsic stain removed. Intraoral photographs

---

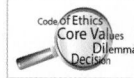

EVERYDAY ETHICS

Sarah is a 32-year-old female who presents as a new patient with the chief complaint of "wanting whiter teeth." Upon examination, multiple carious lesions and moderate periodontal disease is diagnosed. The dental hygienist, Sharron, educates Sarah about the need to control her diseases prior to proceeding with bleaching processes, but Sarah expresses her desire to start with bleaching and she will schedule for the other care after her results are achieved.

Questions for Consideration

1. Is it ethical to perform an elective bleaching procedure prior to treating the disease? Explain.

2. Consider the steps in resolving an issue or a dilemma (see Chapter 1). What are the rights of each of the individuals involved in this situation? Are there any conflicts of interest that Sharron must identify as she works through the steps in resolving this issue?

3. What financial, legal, or cultural factors need consideration if Sharron is to identify an alternative approach that will lead to a positive outcome? Describe her possible approaches.

Factors to Teach the Patient

▶ Why a complete oral cancer screening and dental examination, including radiographs and periodontal evaluation, is performed before any form of bleaching is initiated.

▶ During bleaching, teeth and gingival tissues may become sensitive for a period of time.

▶ If sensitivity is experienced, use a desensitizing product, discontinue bleaching, or delay next treatment.

▶ Regardless of method, color relapse occurs in a relatively short period of time.

▶ Excessive use of bleaching products may be harmful. Follow manufacturer's directions.

▶ Existing tooth-colored restorations will not change color, and therefore may not match and may need to be replaced after bleaching.

ENHANCE YOUR UNDERSTANDING

ONLINE RESOURCES
(see the inside front cover for access information)
- Audio glossary
- Appendices

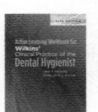

SUPPORT FOR LEARNING
(available separately)
- *Active Learning Workbook for Wilkins' Clinical Practice of the Dental Hygienist, 13th Edition*

INDIVIDUALIZED REVIEW
- Customized practice quizzing with Navigate 2 TestPrep for *Wilkins' Clinical Practice of the Dental Hygienist*

References

1. Byrne BE, McIntyre F. Chapter 12: Bleaching agents. In: *ADA/PDR Guide to Dental Therapeutics*. 5th ed. Chicago, IL: American Dental Association; 2009:351.

2. Carey CM. Tooth whitening: what we now know. *J Evid Based Dent Pract*. 2014;14:70-76.

3. Dahl JE, Pallesen U. Tooth bleaching—a critical review of the biological aspects. *Crit Rev Oral Biol Med*. 2003;14(4):292-304.

4. Truman J. Bleaching of non-vital discolored anterior teeth. *Dent Times*. 1864;1:69-72.

5. Spasser HF. A simple bleaching technique using sodium perborate. *NY State Dent J*. 1961;27:332.

6. Mokhlis GR, Matis BA, Cochran MA, et al. A clinical evaluation of carbamide peroxide and hydrogen peroxide whitening agents during daytime use. *J Am Dent Assoc*. 2000;131(9):1269-1277.

7. Haywood VB, Heymann HO. Nightguard vital bleaching. *Quintessence Int*. 1989;20(3):173-176.

8. ADA Council on Scientific Affairs. *Tooth Whitening/Bleaching Treatment Considerations for Dentists and Their Patients*. Chicago, IL: American Dental Association; 2009:12.

9. Albanai SR, Gillam DG, Taylor PD. An overview of the effects of 10% carbamide peroxide and its relationship to dentine sensitivity. *Eur J Prosthodont Restor Dent*. 2015;23(2):50-55.

10. Bharti R, Wadhwani KK. Spectrophotometric evaluation of peroxide penetration into the pulp chamber from whitening strips and gel: an *in vitro* study. *J Conserv Dent*. 2013;16(2):131-134.

11. Haywood VB. Treating sensitivity during tooth whitening. *Compend Contin Educ Dent*. 2005;26(9, suppl 3):11-20.

12. Ubaldini AL, Baesso ML, Medina Neto A, et al. Hydrogen peroxide diffusion dynamics in dental tissues. *J Dent Res*. 2013;92:661-665.

13. Alqahtani MQ. Tooth-bleaching procedures and their controversial effects: a literature review. *Saudi Dent J*. 2014;26:33-46.

14. Sanchez NP, Aleksic A, Dramicanin M, et al. Whitening-dependent changes of fluorescence of extracted human teeth. *J Esthet Restor Dent*. 2017;29(5):352-355.

15. Haywood VB. Chapter 1: Diagnosis and treatment planning for bleaching. In: *Tooth Whitening Indications and Outcomes of Nightguard Vital Bleaching*. Chicago, IL: Quintessence; 2007:1–26.

16. Sweeney MR. Tooth whitening. In: Gladwin M, Bagby M, eds. *Clinical Aspects of Dental Materials*. Philadelphia, PA: Lippincott, Williams & Wilkins; 2009:212-222.

17. Abou Neel EA, Aljabo A, Strange A, et al. Demineralization-remineralization dynamics in teeth and bone. *Int J Nano* 2016;11:4743-4763.

18. Haywood VB. The "bottom line" on bleaching 2008. *Inside Dent*. 2008;4(2):2-5.

19. Matis BA, Wang Y, Eckert GJ, et al. Extended bleaching of tetracycline stained teeth: a 5-year study. *Oper Dent*. 2006;31(6):643-651.

20. Pintado-Palomino K, Filno OP, Zanoito ED, et al. A clinical, randomized, controlled study on the use of desensitizing agents on bleaching. *J Dent*. 2015;43:1099-1105.

21. Wang Y, Gao J, Jiang T, et al. Evaluation of the efficacy of potassium nitrate and sodium fluoride as desensitizing agents during tooth bleaching treatment—a systematic review and meta-analysis. *J Dent*. 2015;43(8):913-923.

22. Zanolla J, Marques ABC, da Costa DC, et al. Influence of tooth bleaching on dental enamel microhardness: a systematic review and meta-analysis. *Aust Dent J*. 2017;62:276-282.

23. De Moor RJ, Verheyen J, Verheyen P, et al. Laser teeth bleaching: evaluation of eventual side effects on enamel and the pulp and the efficiency in vitro and in vivo. *Sci World J.* 2015;2015:835405.

24. American Academy of Pediatric Dentistry Council on Clinical Affairs. Policy on the use of dental bleaching for child and adolescent patients. *Oral Health Policies.* 2017-2018;39(6):90-92.

25. Mello HS. The mechanism of tetracycline staining in primary and permanent teeth. *J Dent Child.* 1967;34(6):478-487.

26. Basting RT, Rodrigues AL Jr, Serra MC. The effect of 10% carbamide peroxide, carbopol and/or glycerin on enamel and dentin microhardness. *Oper Dent.* 2005;30(5):608-616.

27. Reema SD, Lahiri PK, Roy SS. Review of casein phospho-peptides-amorphous calcium phosphate. *Chin J Dent Res.* 2014;17(1):7-14.

28. Gugnami N, Pandit IK, Gupta MG, et al. Comparative evaluation of esthetic changes in nonpitted fluorosis stains when treated with resin infiltration, in-office bleaching, and combination therapies. *J Esthet Restor Dent.* 2017;29:317-324.

29. Penumatsa NV, Sharanesha RB. Bleaching of fluorosis stains using sodium hypochlorite. *J Pharm Bioallied Sci.* 2015;7(suppl 2):5766-5768.

30. Elfallah HM, Bertassoni LE, Charadram N. Effect of tooth bleaching agents on protein content and mechanical properties of dental enamel. *Acta Biomater.* 2015;20:120-128.

31. Kazemipoor M, Shagheyegh A, Farnaz F. Concurrent effects of bleaching materials and the size of root canal preparation on cervical dentin microhardness. *Iran Endod J.* 2017;12(3):298-302.

32. Grazioli G, Valente LL, Isolan CP, Pinheiro HA, Duarte CG, Münchow EA. Bleaching and enamel surface interactions resulting from the use of highly-concentrated bleaching gels. *Arch Oral Biol.* 2018;87:157-162.

33. Bollineni S, Janga RK, Venugopal L, Reddy IR, Babu PR, Kumar SS. Role of fluoridated carbamide peroxide whitening gel in the remineralization of demineralized enamel: an in vitro study. *J Int Soc Prev Community Dent.* 2014 May;4(2):117-121.

34. Mondelli RF, Soares AF, Pangrazio EG, Wang L, Ishikiriama SK, Bombonatti JF. Evaluation of temperature increase during in-office bleaching. *J Appl Oral Sci.* 2016;24(2):136-141. doi:10.1590/1678-775720150154.

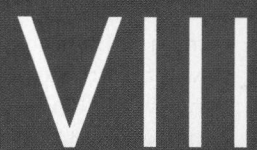

Evaluation

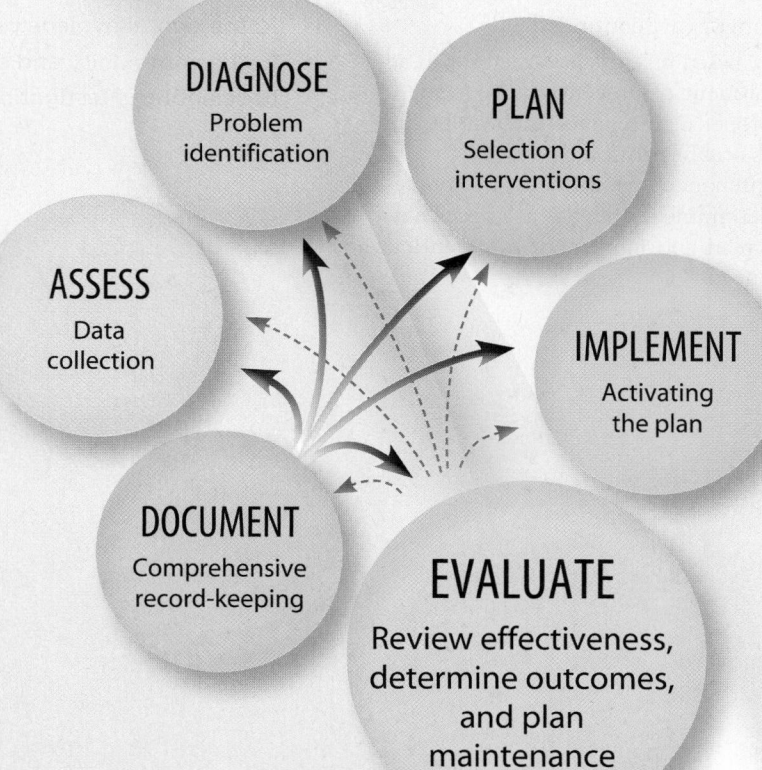

FIGURE VIII-1 • The Dental Hygiene Process of Care.

INTRODUCTION FOR SECTION VIII

Evaluation of dental hygiene care is a determination of whether the oral health goals identified in the patient's care plan have been met. The systematic evaluation of dental hygiene prevention and treatment interventions:

◆ Relies on the careful collection of data and comparison of posttreatment information with baseline data.

◆ Determines further treatment needs and appropriate periodontal maintenance interval.

◆ Allows comparison with both previous and future observations to determine changes in the patient's oral health status over time.

THE DENTAL HYGIENE PROCESS OF CARE

◆ Evaluation is an essential component of every step in the dental hygiene process of care, as illustrated by the arrows in Figure VIII-1.

◆ The dental hygienist who evaluates each step in the process during each patient appointment will assure that attention is paid to any changing circumstance that affects patient care or treatment outcomes.

◆ As the process of patient care continues:

• A new care plan, based on evaluation data, will address further treatment or preventive needs and/or determine the proper maintenance interval to support the patient's oral health status.

• During the maintenance appointment, the process will be used to determine if the patient's needs have changed and to plan and implement interventions that meet those needs.

ETHICAL APPLICATIONS

◆ It is beneficial to evaluate an ethical situation involving treatment outcomes or self-evaluation of professional skills and abilities based on the Standards of Professional Responsibility outlined in the ADHA Code of Ethics and listed in Box VIII-1.

◆ The ethical dental hygienist will:

• Assess how a particular decision could potentially affect each of the professional roles of a dental hygienist.

• Evaluate a choice of action that acknowledges each area of professional responsibility.

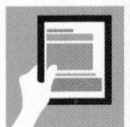

BOX VIII-1
Standards of Professional Responsibility

Professional dental hygienists acknowledge the following responsibilities:

• To ourselves as individuals and professionals.
• To family and friends.
• To patients.
• To employers and employees.
• To the dental hygiene profession.
• To the community and society.
• To scientific investigation.

44

Principles of Evaluation

Charlotte J. Wyche, BSDH, MS

CHAPTER OUTLINE

PRINCIPLES OF EVALUATION
I. Purposes of Evaluation
II. Evaluation Design
III. Evaluation Process

EVALUATION BASED ON GOALS AND OUTCOMES

EVALUATION OF CLINICAL (TREATMENT) OUTCOMES
I. Visual Examination
II. Periodontal Probing
III. Tactile Evaluation

EVALUATION OF HEALTH BEHAVIOR OUTCOMES
I. Visual Examination
II. Interview Evaluation

COMPARISON OF ASSESSMENT FINDINGS

STANDARD OF CARE

SELF-ASSESSMENT AND REFLECTIVE PRACTICE
I. Purpose
II. Skills and Methods
III. A "Critical Incident" Approach

DOCUMENTATION
I. Patient Care Outcomes
II. Self-assessment and Reflection

EVERYDAY ETHICS

FACTORS TO TEACH THE PATIENT

REFERENCES

LEARNING OBJECTIVES

After studying this chapter, the student will be able to:

1. Identify and define key terms and concepts related to the evaluation of dental hygiene interventions.

2. Discuss standards for dental hygiene practice.

3. Identify skills related to self-assessment and reflective dental hygiene practice.

PRINCIPLES OF EVALUATION

- Evaluation is a systematic determination of worth, value, or significance.[1]
- Ongoing evaluation is an important component of providing evidence-based dental hygiene care.
- Evaluation measures determine whether treatment and oral health education goals outlined in the dental hygiene care plan are achieved.[2-4]
- As illustrated in the dental hygiene process of care (Figure VIII-1), ongoing evaluation at each step provides feedback to determine success or indicate the need to modify procedures throughout the process.

I. Purposes of Evaluation

- Ongoing evaluation measures patient satisfaction with care provided.
- Assessing the outcome of both clinical and preventive interventions at the completion of a treatment cycle identifies need for further treatment and adapted self-care protocols.
- The evaluation process also helps to determine the appropriate continuing care interval to maintain an achieved increase in oral health status.

II. Evaluation Design

◆ The four most common types of evaluation design (listed with dental hygiene practice examples in Table 44-1) include[5]:
  - Formative evaluation
  - Process evaluation
  - Outcome evaluation
  - Impact evaluation.

◆ A plan for evaluation of patient care outcomes includes informal monitoring, feedback, and modifications in patient care provided during each patient appointment.

◆ Methods for evaluating the success of dental hygiene treatment have traditionally included collecting new clinical data, such as probing depths and areas of bleeding, to compare with the patient's health status at the beginning of treatment.

◆ The evaluation process includes measures to assess the extent to which disease prevention and health promotion interventions have been effective.

◆ A comparison of pre- and posttreatment outcomes indicates areas of success or areas of need for further intervention.

III. Evaluation Process

◆ When writing the dental hygiene care plan, indicators (evaluation measures) that will evaluate each oral health goal and outcome can be determined.

◆ Following treatment, new complete assessment data are documented.

◆ An evidence-based decision-making approach is used to determine any necessary modifications to the ongoing treatment sequence or to plan maintenance care.

TABLE 44-1 • Four Most Common Types of Evaluation

TYPES OF EVALUATION	DENTAL HYGIENE PRACTICE EXAMPLES
Formative evaluation	Information collected during dental hygiene assessment that will allow the dental hygienist to monitor patient needs (e.g., need for pain control) and adapt care to the patient's general health or oral health status
Process evaluation	**Immediate:** use of explorer to check for residual calculus **Ongoing:** monitoring of tissue trauma during instrumentation or evaluation of patient self-care during a multi-appointment treatment sequence
Outcome evaluation	Determination at end of treatment sequence to confirm whether oral health goals stated in the patient's treatment plan have been met
Impact evaluation	Assessment of the impact of oral health treatment on the patient's overall health status

◆ All assessment findings and any planned modifications for treatment or oral health education are documented in an evaluation summary.

EVALUATION BASED ON GOALS AND OUTCOMES

◆ The dental hygiene care plan establishes individualized short- and long-range patient goals for each dental hygiene intervention.

◆ The treatment, education, and self-care instruction goals listed in the patient's care plan provide the basis for evaluating whether the expected outcomes have been achieved at each level.

◆ Outcomes that can be evaluated following the completion of dental hygiene treatment and patient education in each area of a three-part plan for care are listed in Box 44-1.

◆ Selected outcomes are used to develop goals for patient care when writing a new dental hygiene care plan.

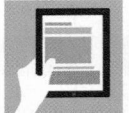

BOX 44-1
Expected Outcomes Following Dental Hygiene Interventions

Gingival/Periodontal Health Outcomes
- Reduced dental biofilm
- Smooth tooth surfaces with calculus removed
- Reduced probing depths
- No bleeding on probing, exudate, or suppuration
- Resolution of erythematous tissue
- Reduced swelling and edema
- No further loss in attachment level
- Decrease or no change in mobility

Dental Caries Risk Outcomes
- No new cavitated lesions
- Demineralized/non-cavitated areas resolved
- Reduced intake of cariogenic foods/beverages
- Dental sealants placed
- Increased fluoride use

Prevention Outcomes
- Elimination of iatrogenic factors (calculus, restoration overhangs)
- Increased percentage of biofilm-free areas
- Patient demonstration of recommended oral care procedures
- Patient report of compliance with daily care recommendations
- Compliance with recommended continuing care interval
- Tobacco-free status achieved
- Modification/stabilization of systemic risk factors

EVALUATION OF CLINICAL (TREATMENT) OUTCOMES

◆ Final evaluation of dental hygiene treatment outcomes is performed after initial therapy has been completed, when the response of the gingival tissue to therapy is apparent.

◆ When a treatment sequence consists of multiple appointments, evaluation of the previously treated areas at each subsequent appointment allows immediate intervention in an area that shows poor response to the previous treatment.

◆ The examinations used for initial assessment as well as evaluation assessment are described more completely in Chapters 13, 16, 17, and 20.

I. Visual Examination

◆ Obtain biofilm score after the soft tissue visual inspection has been completed so the use of disclosing solution does not interfere with soft tissue examination.

◆ Gingival examination looks for changes in tissue color, size, shape (contour), and consistency and compares them to examination findings documented prior to treatment.

◆ Visual examination can also determine whether a goal related to caries risk, such as restorative treatment or sealants, has been achieved.

II. Periodontal Examination

◆ A comprehensive periodontal examination is performed and documented using a form that allows comparison with pretreatment assessment data.

◆ Current pocket depths, bleeding points, exudate/suppuration, changes in attached gingiva or clinical attachment level noted during the comprehensive examination are documented in the periodontal record.

◆ See Chapter 31 for information about assessment of dental implants.

III. Tactile Evaluation

◆ All tooth surfaces, particularly in areas demonstrating bleeding points or exudate/suppuration, should be assessed for residual calculus deposits and other iatrogenic factors.

◆ Difficult-to-access areas require special attention during evaluation and include:
  • Concavities and depressions of the root anatomy.
  • Subgingival margins of crowns, fixed partial denture, or overhanging restoration.
  • Furcation involvement.

EVALUATION OF HEALTH BEHAVIOR OUTCOMES

◆ Evaluation of health behavior outcomes provides evidence of:
  • The patient's understanding and compliance with the clinician's counseling and education interventions.

  • Development of oral self-care skills.

◆ The dental hygiene care plan establishes self-care and health behavior goals developed in collaboration with the patient.

◆ If the evaluation process indicates goals have not been met, the data collected during evaluation can provide a baseline from which the dental hygienist can again collaborate with the patient to develop new or next step goals.

◆ Methods for evaluating self-care and health behavior outcomes are as follows.

I. Visual Examination

◆ Patient biofilm control is evaluated using the same dental indices used to determine original biofilm levels.

◆ Self-care skills are evaluated by observing a demonstration of each skill by the patient.

II. Interview Evaluation

◆ Patient interviewing techniques can be used to determine whether each goal established by the patient for health behavior change and daily self-care has been met.

◆ Patient interview and discussion can be used to evaluate:
  • Success of factors associated with patient comfort during treatment.
  • The patient's understanding of recommendations and self-care instructions.
  • Effectiveness of the clinician's communication approaches.

COMPARISON OF ASSESSMENT FINDINGS

◆ Analysis and comparison of pretreatment and outcome evaluation data determine the relative success of the therapy and can help determine whether the patient:
  • Is able to be managed under the care of the dental hygienist, requiring development of a new dental hygiene care plan.
  • Has not responded adequately to nonsurgical therapy and referral for specialized periodontal care may be necessary.

◆ On the basis of the findings, a recommended interval for continuing care appointments is determined.

◆ Additional factors taken into account when determining the next steps for patient care are listed in Box 44-2.

STANDARD OF CARE

◆ In addition to evaluating individual patient outcomes at all points in the dental hygiene process of care, the dental hygienist is responsible for evaluating personal adherence to a professional standard of care for practice.

BOX 44-2
Factors Considered When Determining the Need for

Retreatment, Referral, or Maintenance Interval

- Soft tissue response to instrumentation and degree of healing
- Changes and/or stabilization in probing depth and attachment loss
- Patient health behaviors, such as use of tobacco
- Systemic influences on oral health status, such as diabetes
- Level of skill and effectiveness in biofilm control
- Motivation and responsibility assumed for daily personal oral self-care
- Psychosocial factors that can affect oral status, such as stress

◆ Standards of care in dentistry evolved from early court cases that established a ruling of negligence when healthcare providers failed to possess a minimum standard of special knowledge and ability, or adhere to reasonable and recognized standards while providing patient care.[6]

◆ The *American Dental Hygienists' Association Standards for Clinical Dental Hygiene Practice*, based on the dental hygiene process of care, provides the standard of care for dental hygienists in the United States.[2]

◆ Canada also provides documents that outline standards for delivery of dental hygiene care.[3,4]

◆ Guidelines published by both dental and dental hygiene professional associations, such as the *American Academy of Pediatric Dentistry Guideline on Caries Risk-Assessment*,[7] are additional sources used for establishing a professional standard of care.

◆ Three sources for determining standard of care in a legal dispute are listed in Box 44-3.

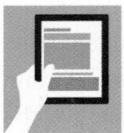

BOX 44-3
Three Sources for Determining Standard of Care in a Legal Dispute

- Opinion of **expert witnesses**
- Journals, guidelines, or other published documents from recognized professional associations or other authoritative sources
- Federal, state, or local statutes and/or regulations

Source: Curley AW. The legal standard of care. *J Am Coll Dent.* 2005;72(4):20-22.

◆ Failure to provide a minimally acceptable level of patient care is considered to be professional negligence.

◆ The professional dental hygienist recognizes that standards of care change over time as new knowledge is introduced and becomes commonly accepted by the profession and the public.

◆ Knowledge of and adherence to a professional dental hygiene standard of care are enhanced through continuous evidence-based inquiry and pursuit of life-long learning.

SELF-ASSESSMENT AND REFLECTIVE PRACTICE

◆ Dental hygiene education programs recognize ongoing self-assessment of skills as an essential component of evaluating clinical practice.[8,9]

◆ Although self-assessment and reflection in healthcare practice have been studied mainly in educational settings, there is evidence to suggest that development of these skills can:
  - Be successfully taught and developed, mainly through reflective writing.[9–11]
  - Be enhanced with practice.[10–12]
  - Help assure quality and positive outcomes in the delivery of patient care.[13]

I. Purpose

◆ Self-assessment of personal clinical and communication skills and knowledge can guide the dental hygiene practitioner toward an evidence-based approach to finding new information to support best-practice interventions for patient care.

◆ Reflecting on clinical experiences contributes to development of critical thinking skills that can help the practitioner determine and implement new and more successful approaches for patient care.[14]

◆ Self-assessment can assist the dental hygienist to determine a need to enhance specific clinical skills and abilities, or develop a plan for continuing education that supports personal professional goals.

II. Skills and Methods

◆ Key skills for reflective practice include:
  - Perceptive self-awareness.
  - Judgment and self-assessment.
  - Critical analysis and synthesis.
  - Access to and application of new knowledge.
  - Feedback and evaluation (continued reflection).
◆ Methods for informal assessment of professional practice include individual reflection (thinking about one's own practice habits) or discussing clinical issues with colleagues.

TABLE 44-2 • Components of a "Critical Incident" Approach to Reflection and Self-Assessment

STEP	SUMMARY/DEFINITION	SOME EXAMPLE QUESTIONS FOR GUIDING REFLECTION	CLINICAL PRACTICE EXAMPLE
Description "What?"	Brief description of what happened and what effect the situation had on those involved in the incident	What about the situation triggered a need to evaluate what happened? Who was involved? How did those involved feel about or react to the incident? What about this situation is interesting to explore further?	Patient presents for evaluation following scaling and root debridement. Residual calculus, resulting in areas of bleeding and need for patient to return for retreatment of those areas. Patient is not happy about the need for retreatment. Dental hygienist is concerned about her personal skill in calculus removal
Analysis "So What?"	Reflective phase that involves analysis and critical thinking to identify: potential causes and factors that influenced the outcome of the situation gaps related to standards of good practice changes that need to be made in current practice new knowledge required	Why did this happen? What gaps in knowledge or skill influenced the outcome? Does the knowledge base need to be updated? Were patient and/or clinician's goals met during this situation? How were values or ethical standards related to or applied during this situation?	The dental hygienist analyzes the situation using some of the questions in the previous column, and realizes that this is not the first time the personal patient care goal for complete calculus removal at each appointment has not been met. Recently, while participating in an advanced instrumentation continuing education course, it became clear that the problem is not deficient scaling and root debridement skills. Instrument-sharpening skills have not been updated (or applied) recently
Application "Now What?"	Summary of insights or learning from the situation and a plan for addressing need for new knowledge or alternative action	What was learned? What next steps can be taken to produce a different outcome in a future situation?	The dental hygienist learned that instrumentation skill alone might not be all that is necessary to meet the goal of complete calculus removal. Next steps: find an instrument-sharpening "how-to" booklet to begin practicing sharpening and attend a continuing education workshop related to instrument sharpening at the first opportunity

- Reflective practice can also take on a more formal aspect, as in developing a professional portfolio or maintaining a written "critical incident" journal.[10,15–17]

III. A "Critical Incident" Approach

A formal approach used to evaluate dental hygiene practice takes the form of answering questions about a specific situation, often called a critical incident, which prompts the practitioner to look for answers.[17]

- Three steps, sometimes referred to as the "What? So What? Now What" approach, can be used to structure written reflective journal entries or can also be used to guide a less formal means of thoughtful personal self-assessment.
- The approach to reflective self-assessment includes a basic progression of reflective actions with questions for each step to help guide thinking about the situation from a variety of perspectives.
- The steps and a brief clinical practice example are provided in Table 44-2. The same steps and similar questions can be used to guide self-assessment reflection

about situations involving communication skills, patient education approach, or adherence to ethical and legal standards of practice.

DOCUMENTATION

I. Patient Care Outcomes

- Evaluation of factors such as patient comfort, communication efforts, and treatment safety and efficacy is ongoing and occurs at each patient appointment. Documentation in the patient record provides guidance for future patient interactions.
- Documentation of outcomes evaluation following clinical dental hygiene treatment is similar to the documentation of clinical data during initial assessment.
- Evaluation data following treatment are recorded in an identical format to the pretreatment assessment data, which facilitates comparison and analysis of outcomes.
- Box 44-4 has an example progress note that documents evaluation of a patient care situation.

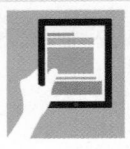

BOX 44-4

Example Documentation:
Evaluation of Patient Comfort During a Sequence of Treatment Appointments

S–A 79-year-old male patient presents for the third in a series of appointments scheduled for scaling and root debridement. Patient states: "Following both of the previous appointments, my back has significantly bothered me because of laying back so far in the dental chair for such a long time. Do we need to have such long appointments?"

O–Patient medical history form indicates history of osteoarthritis, but no previous problem with back pain.

A–Analyzed the problem through discussion with patient about how to balance his needs with the time necessary to complete planned care at each appointment. Decided together that placing a small cushion (or his jacket) beneath his knees as well as briefly bringing the chair to an upright position every 15 minutes could help to alleviate his discomfort.

P–Completed third quadrant scaling and provided flossing instruction as indicated in the patient's care plan for this appointment while using the new "comfort protocol." He indicated that he felt much better during this treatment session.

Next steps: Reevaluate at the next appointment, scheduled in 2 weeks.

Signed: _____, RDH

Date: _____

II. Self-assessment and Reflection

Self-assessment and reflective evaluation of personal professionalism and learning can be documented in several ways. Two suggestions are as follows:

◆ Regular written entries in a professional practice reflection journal that describe and critically analyze a variety of clinical, ethical, and professional situations the dental hygienist has found meaningful. Over time, this ongoing record will reflect how the practitioner's professional skills, actions, and knowledge have been enhanced through the process of reflective practice.

◆ A clinical practice portfolio can be developed to document a variety of factors related to professional development and self-evaluation of dental hygiene practice. A portfolio may contain artifacts such as:

  • Case presentations describing care provided for patients with special needs.

  • A personal practice philosophy describing ethical parameters that impact how the dental hygienist provides care.

  • Goals for future continuing education and courses taken or planned for reaching those goals.

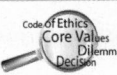

EVERYDAY ETHICS

Mrs. Midoun called in this morning and scheduled a visit during a cancelled appointment time in the afternoon. She states she is in a hurry and just wants her teeth "shined up" as her daughter is graduating this weekend. Salima, one of three dental hygienists in practice, has not provided care previously for Mrs. Midoun. She quickly scans the patient record, noticing that 3 months ago Mrs. Midoun received scaling and root debridement treatments in all four quadrants. Although she had signed a consent form outlining the entire sequence of appointments, including evaluation, Mrs. Midoun had cancelled the evaluation appointment at the last minute and never rescheduled it.

Salima explains that, before providing any further dental hygiene care, it would be necessary to complete the posttreatment evaluation. Mrs. Midoun objects strenuously to "wasting time" with evaluation of her previous treatment. She states that her oral health is much better now and she notices very little bleeding. She states emphatically that, unless Salima cleans her teeth today, she will "just leave now and find another office" where they will clean her teeth. Dr. Kim is out of the office and Salima hesitates, not knowing quite how to handle the situation without consulting him.

Questions for Consideration

1. Is this an ethical issue or a dilemma? Explain.

2. What are Mrs. Midoun's rights in this situation? What core values need to be considered during Salima's decision-making process?

3. What alternative decisions can Salima make about interventions she will provide at Mrs. Midoun's appointment today that will meet the standards of care for dental hygiene practice?

Factors to Teach the Patient

▶ The need for evaluation to establish the basis for "next step" treatment and maintenance decisions.

▶ Types of evaluation measures and indicators that measure outcomes for each goal.

▶ How outcomes from dental hygiene interventions are used to determine further treatment needs and maintenance interval.

ENHANCE YOUR UNDERSTANDING

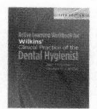

ONLINE RESOURCES
(see the inside front cover for access information)
- Audio glossary
- Appendices

SUPPORT FOR LEARNING
(available separately)
- *Active Learning Workbook for Wilkins' Clinical Practice of the Dental Hygienist, 13th Edition*

INDIVIDUALIZED REVIEW
- Customized practice quizzing with Navigate 2 TestPrep for *Wilkins' Clinical Practice of the Dental Hygienist*

References

1. Centers for Disease Control and Prevention. Program Performance and Evaluation Office (PPEO)—Program Evaluation. http://www.cdc.gov/eval/framework/. Accessed April 9, 2018.

2. American Dental Hygienists' Association (ADHA). Standards for Clinical Dental Hygiene Practice (Revised 2016). https://www.adha.org/resources-docs/2016-Revised-Standards-for-Clinical-Dental-Hygiene-Practice.pdf. Accessed April 9, 2018.

3. Canadian Dental Hygienists Association (CDHA). Dental Hygiene: Definition, Scope, and Practice Standards. https://www.cdha.ca/pdfs/Profession/Resources/DefinitionScope_public.pdf. Accessed April 9, 2018.

4. College of Dental Hygienists of Ontario. Standards of Practice. http://www.cdho.org/for-the-public/dental-hygienists/standards-of-practice. Accessed April 9, 2018.

5. Centers for Disease Control and Prevention (CDC). Types of Evaluation. https://www.cdc.gov/std/Program/pupestd/Types%20of%20Evaluation.pdf. Accessed April 9, 2018.

6. Graskemper JP. The standard of care in dentistry: where did it come from: how has it evolved? *J Am Dent Assoc.* 2004;135(10):1449-1455.

7. American Academy of Pediatric Dentistry (AAPD). Guideline on Caries Risk Assessment and Management for Infants, Children, and Adolescents. http://www.aapd.org/media/Policies_Guidelines/G_CariesRiskAssessment.pdf. Accessed April 9, 2018.

8. Commission on Dental Accreditation (CODA). Accreditation Standards for Dental Hygiene Education Programs. https://www.ada.org/~/media/CODA/Files/dental_hygiene_standards.pdf?la=en. Accessed April 9, 2018.

9. Mayes KA, Branch-Mays GL. A systematic review of the use of self-assessment in preclinical and clinical dental education. *J Dent Educ.* 2016; 80(8):902-913.

10. Mann K, Gordon J, MacLeod A. Reflection and reflective practice in health professions education: a systematic review. *Adv Health Sci Educ Theory Pract.* 2009; 14(4):595-621.

11. Tsang AK. Oral health students as reflective practitioners: changing patterns of student clinical reflections over a period of 12 months. *J Dent Hyg.* 2012;86(2):120-129.

12. Asadoorian J, Schönwetter DJ, Lavigne SE. Developing reflective health care practitioners: learning from experience in dental hygiene education. *J Dent Educ.* 2011;75(4):472-484.

13. Jackson SC, Murff EJ. Effectively teaching self-assessment: preparing the dental hygiene student to provide quality care. *J Dent Educ.* 2011;75(2):169-179.

14. Mould MR, Bray KK, Gadbury-Amyot CC. Student self-assessment in dental hygiene education: a cornerstone of critical thinking and problem-solving. *J Dent Educ.* 2011;75(8):1061-1072.

15. Gadbury-Amyot CC, Woldt JL, Siruta-Austin KJ. Self-assessment: a review of the literature and pedagogical strategies for its promotion in dental education. *J Dent Hyg.* 2015;89(6):357-364.

16. Gwozdek AE, Springfield EC, Kerschbaum WE. ePortfolio: developing a catalyst for critical self-assessment and evaluation of learning outcomes. *J Allied Health.* 2013;42(1):e11-e17.

17. Alpers RR, Jarrell K, Wotring R. Toward a reflective practice: using critical incidents. *Teach Learn Nursing.* 2013;8(1):33-35.

45

Continuing Care

Denise Zwicker, BDH, MEd, Linda D. Boyd, RDH, RD, EdD, and Esther M. Wilkins, BS, RDH, DMD

CHAPTER OUTLINE

GOALS OF THE CONTINUING CARE PROGRAM
  I. Periodontal Maintenance
CONTINUING CARE APPOINTMENT PROCEDURES
  I. Assessment
  II. Continuing Care Plan
  III. Criteria for Referral to a Periodontist

APPOINTMENT INTERVALS (FREQUENCY)
METHODS FOR CONTINUING CARE SYSTEMS
  I. Prebook or Preschedule Method
  II. Monthly Reminder Method

DOCUMENTATION
EVERYDAY ETHICS
FACTORS TO TEACH THE PATIENT
REFERENCES

LEARNING OBJECTIVES

After studying this chapter, the student will be able to:

1. Describe the goals of a continuing care program in dental hygiene practice.
2. Determine appointment intervals based on an individual patient's risk factors, compliance, and oral health history.
3. Name and discuss the contributing factors in recurrence of periodontal disease.
4. List steps in a continuing care appointment including assessment, care plan, and therapy.
5. Outline methods for continuing care systems in the dental office or clinic.

The overall therapeutic goals of treatment are to arrest disease and to provide optimal oral health, function, and comfort for the patient. Following active treatment, when reevaluation shows positive soft-tissue response and the function of the dentition has been restored, the patient enters a new phase of treatment for continuing care.

GOALS OF THE CONTINUING CARE PROGRAM

- Continue the healthy state attained during active therapy.
- Prevent recurrence of infection. The patient needs to understand that oral diseases recur, but *control* is possible through combined personal and professional effort.

- Prevent initiation of new disease.
- Monitor educational and behavioral changes.
- Monitor risk and clinical signs of health and disease including:
  - Periodontal infection.
  - Oral mucosal lesions.
  - Dental caries (noncavitated and continuum to cavitated lesions).
  - Eruption patterns and occlusion.
- Provide specialized instruction for implants, prostheses, orthodontic appliances, and restorations.
- Offer motivational encouragement for oral self-care. The success of the program depends on compliance by the patient with the daily oral self-care and regular professional maintenance.

I. Periodontal Maintenance

◆ Patients who comply with regular periodontal mainte-nance (PM) intervals have less attachment and tooth loss.[1,2]

◆ Evidence suggests it is optimal for patients with a his-tory of periodontal disease to be seen four times a year to decrease the risk for disease progression.[1]

◆ Therapeutic goals of PM are listed in Box 45-1 and in-clude the following[3]:

  • Prevent the recurrence of disease and maintain the state of periodontal health attained during surgical or nonsurgical periodontal therapy.

  • Prevent or reduce the incidence of tooth or implant loss with careful monitoring.

  • Increase timely identification of the need for treat-ment of other conditions or systemic disease mani-fested in the oral cavity such as poorly controlled diabetes mellitus.

CONTINUING CARE APPOINTMENT PROCEDURES

The dental hygiene process of care is described in Chapter 1. As with preparation of the diagnosis and initial dental hygiene care plan, discussed in Chapters 22 and 23, the steps in the process of care apply for the *dental hygiene continuing care plan*.

I. Assessment

◆ Preparation of assessment data follows the same proce-dure as that for a new patient.

◆ At every maintenance appointment, regardless of the interval, a patient of any age requires a complete reas-sessment, diagnosis, and care plan.

A. Review of Patient History

◆ Supplemental questions are asked to determine the present state of health with emphasis on changes since the previous appointment.

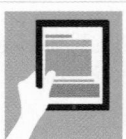

BOX 45-1
Purposes and Outcomes of Periodontal Maintenance

• Resolve inflammation
• Eliminate BOP
• Preserve clinical attachment levels
• Arrest disease progression
• Provide patient comfort
• Encourage patient oral self-care
• Control periodontal reinfection
• Patient motivation and reinstruction

◆ Recent illnesses, hospitalizations, current medications including prescription, over-the-counter and herbal/supplements, and other pertinent new data.

◆ Date of last physical examination with primary care provider.

B. Vital Signs

◆ Blood pressure and other vital signs are documented (see Chapter 12).

C. Extraoral and Intraoral Examination

◆ A thorough extraoral and intraoral examination is doc-umented, as described in Chapter 13.

D. Radiographs

◆ The frequency of radiographic surveys is in accord with the determination of an individual patient's need and recommendations for dental radiographs from the American Dental Association and Federal and Drug Administration (see Chapter 15).

E. Periodontal Examination

◆ Observe and record: gingival color, size, shape, and tex-ture; mucogingival changes.

◆ Complete periodontal examination: pocket depths, bleeding on probing (BOP), exudate or suppuration, attachment levels, furcation involvement, and gingival recession.[4]

  • Current findings are compared with previous peri-odontal assessments to assess changes since treat-ment was completed.

◆ Occlusion, fremitus, and mobility.

◆ Calculus: distribution and amount.

◆ Biofilm and soft deposits.

F. Examination of the Teeth

◆ Integrity of restorations and sealants.

◆ Dental caries: demineralization, white spot lesions, and cavitated lesions.

◆ Dentin hypersensitivity: location and severity.

G. Risk Assessment

◆ Evaluate the presence of systemic disease or other con-tributing factors such as smoking.

H. Evaluation of Oral Cleanliness and Self-Care Measures

◆ Apply a disclosing agent to evaluate the quantity of biofilm.

I. Examination of Specific Areas

◆ Areas of special interest include endodontically treated teeth, postsurgical areas, implants, occlusal factors, and prosthetic appliances.

II. Continuing Care Plan

A care plan is outlined on the basis of the new evaluation of the patient's oral condition and dental hygiene diagnosis.

A. Oral Hygiene Instruction/Motivation

- During continuing care, the patient is considered a co-therapist.
- To keep etiologic factors under control, compliance with daily oral self-care is a major feature in the total program (see Chapters 26 and 27).

B. Periodontal Instrumentation and Debridement

- The periodontal examination findings may indicate need for active disease requiring nonsurgical periodontal therapy.
- Plan appropriate pain control such as local anesthesia.
- Plan appropriate number of appointments.
- Local delivery of antimicrobials in isolated periodontal pockets with active disease that fail to respond to nonsurgical therapy (see Chapter 39).
- For areas of continued BOP, endoscopic examination or evaluation for surgical therapy by a periodontist may be indicated.

C. Dental Caries Control

- Prevention needs to address modifiable caries risk factors with attention to root caries, appropriate use of professional and home fluorides, and diet modifications.
- Implement or monitor previously introduced remineralization protocol (see Chapter 25).

D. Supplemental Care Procedures

- Smoking cessation assistance (see Chapter 32).
- Desensitization of dentin hypersensitivity (see Chapter 41).
- Special care for implants and fixed prostheses (see Chapters 30 and 31).
- Referral for retreatment evaluation.

III. Criteria for Referral to a Periodontist

A. Referral from General Practice

General practice dentists may include periodontal surgical therapy in their practice, but referral to a periodontist is recommended for care outside the scope of practice of a general dentist.

- Many general dentists refer severe or complicated periodontal cases to the periodontist.
- During patient care in a general practice, the dental hygienist should confer with the dentist to determine the need for referral to a periodontist in the following situations:

- *Initially* when a patient new to the practice is examined with the following findings:
  - Stage III or IV periodontitis with furcation involvement.
  - Periodontal disease classifications such as necrotizing ulcerative gingivitis or periodontitis.
  - Drug-induced gingival enlargement (such as in dilantin hyperplasia).
  - Areas of inadequate attached gingiva, especially when gingival margins are rolled, inflamed, and bleed easily.
- *During the reevaluation*, following nonsurgical periodontal therapy. Referral is required for any nonresponsive or refractory type of moderate or advanced periodontal condition (or any of the conditions mentioned earlier).
- *During PM*: If there are signs of recurrence of periodontal disease including, but not limited to bleeding or suppuration on probing, increasing pocket depths, increasing mobility or migration of teeth, or recurrent periodontal abscesses.

B. Recurrence of Periodontal Disease

- Recurrence of signs and symptoms of periodontal infection indicates recolonization of periodontal pathogens.
- Recolonization of a pocket can occur in an average of 42 days.[5]
  - Without daily personal dental biofilm control combined with regular professional maintenance procedures, infection can recur.
  - Colonization depends on the number, frequency of exposure, and virulence of the organisms.
  - Transmission of periodontal microorganisms has been shown between family members.[6–8]
  - Upon completion of treatment, the rate at which colonization may recur will vary with each patient depending on a number of contributing factors.
- *Contributing factors for recurrence:*
  - Inadequate biofilm control.
  - Lack of patient compliance with PM appointments.
  - Inadequate professional treatment.
    - *Inadequate or incomplete debridement*, particularly in areas of difficult access such as furcations and deep proximal pockets.
    - *Biofilm retention*: failure to remove or replace overhanging restorations and other biofilm niches that foster bacterial growth.
  - Failure of tobacco cessation including smoking tobacco, smokeless tobacco, or waterpipe tobacco smoking.[1,3,7,9–11]
  - Systemic diseases such as diabetes mellitus,[12] HIV/AIDS,[13] and certain other systemic diseases influence healing and may control factors related to bone loss and severity of infections.
  - Genetic factors: Future testing for genetic factors may be used as a component of risk assessment.[14,15]

C. Criteria for Referral during PM

During maintenance therapy, any of the aforementioned types of patients may still require referral. Other cases may include:

- Pocket depth that prohibits access for complete debridement during nonsurgical periodontal therapy.
- Furcation involvements and other complex anatomical areas that cannot be instrumented successfully by nonsurgical methods.
- Mucogingival problems; lack of attached gingiva.
- Periodontal disease that is refractory, or not responsive to usual treatment.[16]

APPOINTMENT INTERVALS (FREQUENCY)

- *Frequency planning*
  - The frequency of continuing care or maintenance depends on the needs of each individual patient.
  - Appointment intervals may vary from 2 to 6 months.
  - The time interval is reevaluated periodically and modified in accordance with changing needs of the patient.
- *Factors to consider in determining continuing care or maintenance frequency*
  - Risk for periodontal disease activity.
  - Risk for dental carious lesions.
  - Risk for oral cancer: frequent tobacco and alcohol users.
  - Predisposing diseases, conditions, and behaviors for periodontal diseases, including diabetes, HIV/AIDS, host genetic factors, smoking, and stress.
  - Compliance: keeping appointments and personal daily biofilm control.
  - Previous treatment: Patient who has a history of disease, either dental caries or periodontal infection, is at a greater risk for recurrence.
  - Local factors: rate of calculus formation.
  - Restorative complications: implants and prosthetic replacements.
- *Special appointment requirements*
  Intervals of 2 or 3 months are required for many patients. A few examples include:
  - *History of periodontal treatment:* Patients who have completed initial nonsurgical or surgical periodontal therapy. The first preventive maintenance appointment is scheduled based on the completion date of the initial nonsurgical periodontal therapy.
  - *Cognitive or physical disability:* Managing the toothbrush and other oral care devices may be difficult; when the disability involves the face, opening the mouth may be challenging.
  - *Diabetes:* Diabetes or other systemic disease can predispose patients to lowered resistance to infection.
  - *Cardiovascular disease or other condition:* Those who have been recently hospitalized may find oral self-care tiring and require some modifications to oral self-care routines. Appointments may need to be shorter due to patient fatigue.

- *Patient undergoing extensive dental care:* When extensive restorative, prosthetic, or other treatment is in progress, frequent tissue maintenance and reinstruction are essential.
- *Rampant dental caries:* Appointment for continuation of a caries control effort includes fluoride varnish applications, dietary supervision, and personal care factors for biofilm control.
- *Sealants:* need for regular examination for defects such as chipped or loss of a *sealant to repair, replace,* or *extend.*
- *Orthodontic therapy:* Appliances make cleaning and biofilm control difficult; frequent topical fluoride applications may be indicated; response of gingival tissue to biofilm accumulation to be monitored.

METHODS FOR CONTINUING CARE SYSTEMS

- The continuing care system is essential for managing the oral health of patients.
- Methods for administration of continuing care include prebooking or prescheduling an appointment or sending a reminder card to schedule an appointment.

I. Prebook or Preschedule Method

- Make each subsequent patient appointment prior to the patient leaving the office or clinic, either electronically or in a traditional appointment book.
- An appointment card is given to the patient with a reminder to enter it on their calendar.
  - If the patient uses a calendar application on their cell phone or tablet, encourage entering the new appointment before leaving the office or clinic.
- Appointment reminders can be done by:
  - Preparing a postcard for mailing a month or two before the scheduled appointment. The card can be prepared by the patient before leaving the office or postcards and labels can be printed from the patient management system.
  - Sending a reminder via e-mail, text, or other electronic media.
- The reminder requests the patient to confirm the appointment by calling or e-mailing. For unconfirmed appointments, a call to the patient the day before is made.

II. Monthly Reminder Method

- If an appointment is not prescheduled, a monthly list of all patients due for maintenance can be generated.
  - For a manual system, postcards can be filed alphabetically by the last name of the patient under the month when the patient is due.
  - Practice management systems can easily create patient-specific postcards or letters to be mailed to the patient. Many systems can be set up to automate the process.

DOCUMENTATION

For the patient's permanent record, the following information needs to be recorded for a patient who is scheduled for routine continuing care:

◆ Medical and dental histories updated with each continuing care appointment.

◆ Significant chief complaints and questions the patient may have concerning the treatment provided and of the personal self-care expected.

◆ Findings during routine examinations including vital signs, extraoral and intraoral, periodontal, dental, temporomandibular joint, occlusion, and all special examinations following individual treatments for other reasons.

◆ A sample progress note may be reviewed in Box 45-1.

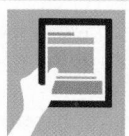

BOX 45-2
Example Documentation: Continuing Care Appointment

S— A patient presents for 3-month PM appointment and apologized for not being able to clean her teeth after lunch. She described her daily oral self-care regimen; a remarkable behavior change since her initial periodontal therapy and patient education 4 years ago.

O— Medical, dental, and medication reviews, no changes. BP 135/60, extra- and intraoral nothing remarkable. Vertical bitewings for molar areas were exposed based on patient risk factors. Periodontal examination with probing revealed numerous proximal areas of molars had 3–4 mm areas with BOP, subgingival calculus, and moderate-to-heavy biofilm suggesting lack of flossing.

A— Generalized Stage II, Grade B periodontitis. Interdental biofilm accumulation with need for more specific instruction to include interdental brushes.

P— Asked patient to demonstrate current brushing method and provided additional instruction to modify her technique with emphasis on Bass brushing for interdental cleaning. Advised brushing more than once a day with a focus on every tooth. Demonstrated use of interdental brush. Gave her sample interdental brushes and explained where to purchase them. Completed calculus removal for maxillary and mandibular right quadrant.

Next visit: two weeks to monitor healing and progress with improvement in oral self-care. Complete treatment for both left quadrants with local anesthesia due to extreme sensitivity in maxillary molars.

Signed: _____, RDH

Date: _____

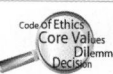

EVERYDAY ETHICS

There were two full-time dental hygienists in the practice. Susan had been working here for more than 15 years, and Jessica less than a year. Jessica had previously practiced with a periodontist in another city for 6 years, and she joined this practice shortly after moving here. Each hygienist had instruments of their own preference and cared for them relative to sharpening and preparation for the sterilizer. Patients usually had appointments with the same dental hygienist. Susan scheduled a maintenance appointment for 45 minutes, whereas Jessica felt she did not have enough time enough even with an hour.

Occasionally, certain long-standing patients who had been with Susan for many years would be scheduled with Jessica when Susan could not be in the office.

As Jessica saw more of Susan's regular patients, she began to see a pattern of residual subgingival calculus that could not have formed since the previous 3 or 4 months' maintenance appointment. She had decided to ask the receptionist to have Susan's patients wait for her return for their appointments.

Ms. Doubleday, a patient of Susan's, did not want to wait, and had come in for her appointment with Jessica. After reviewing the history and updating the periodontal charting, Jessica had to tell the patient that she needed two appointments and wanted to complete her scaling with local anesthesia. The patient was confused after having only short regular appointments and wanted to know whether to reschedule with Susan to finish once she was back from her vacation.

Questions for Consideration

1. Is this an ethical issue or a dilemma? Explain. How do the core values apply in this scenario?

2. Using the step procedure for solving an issue or a dilemma (see Chapter 1), suggest various possible actions for Jessica.

3. Prepare possible answers Jessica could use for her reply to Ms. Doubleday's immediate question.

Factors to Teach the Patient

▶ Purposes of follow-up and continuing care or maintenance appointments.

▶ The importance of the role of the patient and their personal oral care habits in relation to the overall maintenance provided through professional periodontal debridement.

▶ Importance of keeping all maintenance appointments.

ENHANCE YOUR UNDERSTANDING

ONLINE RESOURCES
(see the inside front cover for access information)
- Audio glossary
- Appendices

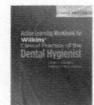

SUPPORT FOR LEARNING
(available separately)
- *Active Learning Workbook for Wilkins' Clinical Practice of the Dental Hygienist, 13th Edition*

INDIVIDUALIZED REVIEW
- Customized practice quizzing with Navigate 2 TestPrep for *Wilkins' Clinical Practice of the Dental Hygienist*

References

1. Lee CT, Huang HY, Sun TC, Karimbux N. Impact of patient compliance on tooth loss during supportive periodontal therapy: a systematic review and meta-analysis. *J Dent Res.* 2015;94(6):777-786.

2. Ng MC, Ong MM, Lim LP, Koh CG, Chan YH. Tooth loss in compliant and non-compliant periodontally treated patients: 7 years after active periodontal therapy. *J Clin Periodontol.* 2011;38(5):499-508.

3. Trombelli L, Franceschetti G, Farina R. Effect of professional mechanical plaque removal performed on a long-term, routine basis in the secondary prevention of periodontitis: a systematic review. *J Clin Periodontol.* 2015;42(suppl 16):S221-S236.

4. Preshaw PM. Detection and diagnosis of periodontal conditions amenable to prevention. *BMC Oral Health.* 2015;15(suppl 1):S1-S5.

5. Mousqués T, Listgarten MA, Phillips RW. Effects of scaling and root planing on the composition of the human subgingival microbial flora. *J Periodontal Res.* 1980;15:144–151.

6. Al Yahfoufi Z. Prevalence of periodontal destruction and putative periodontal pathogens in the same Lebanese family. *J Contemp Dent Pract.* 2017;18(10):970-976.

7. Do an B, Kipalev AS, Okte E, Sultan N, Asikainen SE. Consistent intrafamilial transmission of *Actinobacillus actinomycetemcomitans* despite clonal diversity. *J Periodontol.* 2008;79(2):307-315.

8. Monteiro MF, Casati MZ, Taiete T, et al. Salivary carriage of periodontal pathogens in generalized aggressive periodontitis families. *Int J Paediatr Dent.* 2014;24(2):113-121.

9. Chaffee BW, Couch ET, Ryder MI. The tobacco-using periodontal patient: role of the dental practitioner in tobacco cessation and periodontal disease management. *Periodontol 2000.* 2016;71(1):52-64.

10. American Academy of Periodontology, Research, Science and Therapy Committee. Position paper: tobacco use and the periodontal patient. *J Periodontol.* 1999;70(11):1419–1427.

11. Haddad L, Kelly DL, Weglicki LS, Barnett TE, Ferrell AV, Ghadban R. A systematic review of effects of waterpipe smoking on cardiovascular and respiratory health outcomes. *Tob Use Insights.* 2016;9:13-28.

12. Salvi GE, Carollo-Bittel B, Lang NP. Effects of diabetes mellitus on periodontal and peri-implant conditions: update on associations and risks. *J Clin Periodontol.* 2008;35(8 suppl):398-409.

13. John CN, Stephen LX, Joyce Africa CW. Is human immunodeficiency virus (HIV) stage an independent risk factor for altering the periodontal status of HIV-positive patients? A South African study. *BMC Oral Health.* 2013;13:69.

14. American Academy of Periodontology, Research, Science and Therapy Committee. Informational paper: implications of genetic technology for the management of periodontal diseases. *J Periodontol.* 2005;76(5):850-857.

15. Schaefer AS, Bochenek G, Manke T, et al. Validation of reported genetic risk factors for periodontitis in a large-scale replication study. *J Clin Periodontol.* 2013;40(6):563-572.

16. American Academy of Periodontology. Parameter on "refractory" periodontitis. *J Periodontol.* 2000;71(5 suppl):859-860.

Patients with Special Needs

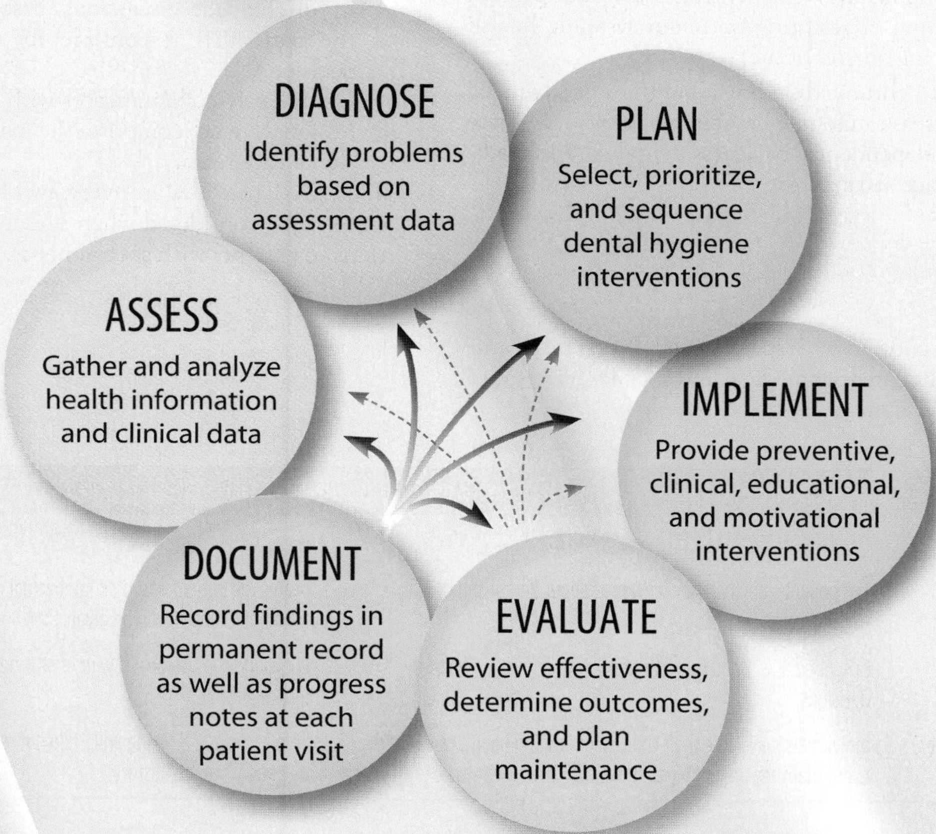

DIAGNOSE
Identify problems based on assessment data

PLAN
Select, prioritize, and sequence dental hygiene interventions

ASSESS
Gather and analyze health information and clinical data

IMPLEMENT
Provide preventive, clinical, educational, and motivational interventions

DOCUMENT
Record findings in permanent record as well as progress notes at each patient visit

EVALUATE
Review effectiveness, determine outcomes, and plan maintenance

FIGURE IX-1 • The Dental Hygiene Process of Care.

INTRODUCTION FOR SECTION IX

The dental hygienist's obligation is to see that no patient needs special rehabilitative dental or periodontal services because of any condition that could have been prevented by dental hygiene care.

◆ For every patient, dental hygiene interventions are selected and patient management strategies are considered according to individualized needs.

◆ Patients with special needs that may complicate the plan for dental hygiene care are those with significant concerns related to:
  ● Their age group.
  ● Specific oral and general systemic conditions.
  ● Degree of physical or cognitive disability.

◆ Dental hygiene care for patients with special needs may require:
  ● A more skillful application of dental hygiene knowledge and ability to accomplish a comparably favorable outcome.
  ● Pursuit of current evidence-based information about individuals with specific health concerns and successful patient management strategies.
  ● Collaboration with an interprofessional team of both healthcare and home care providers to assure the patient's needs are met.

◆ Optimum oral health is frequently a contributing factor in maintaining or restoring optimum systemic health and enhancing quality of life.

◆ Patients with chronic disabling conditions or advanced stages of disease may not be able to perform self-care regimens independently or access dental care in traditional practice settings.

THE DENTAL HYGIENE PROCESS OF CARE

◆ The care of patients with special needs integrates learning from other areas of medical and social sciences into the dental hygiene process of care.

◆ The importance of each step in the process (Figure IX-1) is enhanced when providing care for a patient with health concerns that affect patient management or increase risk for poor treatment outcomes.

ETHICAL APPLICATIONS

◆ The complex medical and dental conditions of certain patients may translate into a need to identify unique treatment approaches that consider:
  ● The quality of care provided.
  ● The patient's quality of life.

◆ Increasingly, medically compromised patients are ambulatory and appear in a dental practice or clinic for maintenance and preventive procedures.

◆ A dental hygienist may also provide care in alternative settings such as a long-term care facility or the patient's home.

◆ The ethical dental hygienist:
  ● Selects dental hygiene interventions consistent with the patient's physical, mental, and personal capabilities.
  ● Instructs patients and/or caregivers about oral hygiene problems and needs related to their systemic disorders and medications.
  ● Ensures that all appropriate persons are included in all chairside discussions, if someone other than the patient is responsible for making treatment decisions.
  ● Confidently communicates with all healthcare professionals who comprise the patient's interprofessional care team.

◆ Table IX-1 provides an overview of some ethical concerns to be considered when presenting treatment options to patients with special needs.

TABLE IX-1 • Ethical Concerns for Treatment Options		
QUALITY OF LIFE	DEFINITION	APPLICATION EXAMPLES
Competency	The patient's ability to make choices about dental and dental hygiene care.	Educates the patient based on intellectual capacity so autonomous consent can be given.
Surrogate	Described as a "substitute" or proxy with regard to healthcare decisions.	Acknowledges a "durable power of attorney" for a patient, where applicable.
Advanced directives	Individuals may write their choices for limiting health care in the event that they are unable to make choices in the future.	Examples include a "living will," "do not resuscitate" order, and "patient values" history.

46

The Pregnant Patient and Infant

Lori Rainchuso, DHSc, MS, RDH, and Esther M. Wilkins, BS, RDH, DMD

CHAPTER OUTLINE

INTRODUCTION

FETAL DEVELOPMENT
  I. First Trimester
  II. Second and Third Trimesters
  III. Factors That Can Harm the Fetus

ORAL FINDINGS DURING PREGNANCY
  I. Gingival Conditions
  II. Gingivitis
  III. Gingival Enlargement
  IV. Periodontal Infections
  V. Enamel Erosion

ASPECTS OF PATIENT CARE
  I. Assessment
  II. Radiography
  III. Overall Treatment Considerations
  IV. Dental Hygiene Care

PATIENT INSTRUCTION
  I. Dental Biofilm Control
  II. Diet
  III. Dental Caries Control
  IV. Fluoride Program

SPECIAL PROBLEMS REQUIRING REFERRAL
  I. Depression during Pregnancy
  II. Domestic Violence

TRANSITIONING FROM PREGNANCY TO INFANCY

INFANT ORAL HEALTH
  I. Anticipatory Guidance
  II. Infant Daily Oral Hygiene Care
  III. Feeding Patterns (Birth to 1 Year)
  IV. Nonnutritive Sucking
  V. Components of the First Dental Visit

DOCUMENTATION

EVERYDAY ETHICS

FACTORS TO TEACH THE PATIENT

REFERENCES

LEARNING OBJECTIVES

After studying this chapter, the student will be able to:

1. Describe the oral implications of fetal development in all stages of pregnancy.

2. Identify common oral findings during pregnancy.

3. Recognize the association between periodontal infection and pregnancy.

4. Assess and develop an appropriate care plan for the pregnant patient.

5. Identify considerations that may occur during pregnancy and need for referral.

6. Recognize the importance of infant oral health.

7. Describe anticipatory guidance considerations for the infant and caregiver education.

8. Define early childhood caries and recognize methods of bacterial transmission.

9. Describe the components and techniques for conducting an infant oral examination.

Pregnancy is a unique time during a woman's life. Attention is focused on healthy lifestyle practices for both the mother and *fetus*.[1]

◆ *Prenatal care* refers to supervised preparation for childbirth to help the mother enjoy optimum health during and after pregnancy and maximize chances for the baby to be born healthy.[2]

  • Prenatal care involves the combined efforts of the obstetrician and/or midwife, nurse practitioner, dentist, dental hygienist, dietitian, and expectant parents.

◆ There is no indication dental and dental hygiene treatment during any trimester of pregnancy can cause harm to the mother or developing fetus. However, most research indicates the second trimester is most ideal for dental treatment.[3]

INTRODUCTION

◆ Professional guidelines recommend medical providers (prenatal care specialists) refer patients for oral health examinations early in pregnancy.[4]

  • Referrals from medical providers may bring many women to the private dental practice or dental clinic who would not routinely access dental care. Many of these women may not have had education about the value of daily oral self-care and diet related to the health of the oral tissues.[5]

  • Numerous misconceptions can be addressed when providing information about the relationship of pregnancy and oral health.[5]

◆ Women who do not receive routine oral health care may appear for emergency dental services and once the emergency situation is resolved, they may be receptive to a preventive program of care and instruction.[5]

◆ The dental hygienist in public health, especially maternal and child health clinics, participates in community educational programs with public health nurses. In these programs, women not well informed about oral health may learn of the need for professional dental and dental hygiene care and education during pregnancy.

FETAL DEVELOPMENT

◆ Pregnancy is arbitrarily divided into three periods of 3 months each called the first, second, and third trimesters.[6]

◆ Physiologic changes in the mother occur in nearly every body system.

◆ Early development of the embryo is greatly influenced by heredity and the general health of the mother.[7]

◆ Normal pregnancy, or period of *gestation*, is approximately 40 weeks. Premature birth refers to a birth before 37 weeks of gestation.[7]

I. First Trimester

◆ During the early stages of pregnancy, the embryo is highly susceptible to injuries, malformations, and mortality.[8]

◆ Teratogenic effects can be produced by many sources, including maternal poor nutrition, infections, and drug intake.

◆ All organ systems are formed (organogenesis) during the first trimester. By 12 weeks, the fetus moves and swallows.[7]

A. Oral Cavity Development Includes the Teeth, Lips, and Palate

◆ Tooth buds develop between the 5th and 6th week. Initial mineralization occurs from the 4th to 5th month (see Table 47-4).[9]

◆ Lips form during the 4th–7th week and the palate forms between the 8th and the 12th week.[9]

◆ Cleft lip is apparent by the 8th week; cleft palate, by the 12th week (see Chapter 49).

II. Second and Third Trimesters

◆ The organs are completed, and growth and maturation continue.[7]

◆ Rapid fetal growth and weight changes occur during the second and third trimesters.

◆ The second trimester is the ideal time for dental treatment.[3]

III. Factors That Can Harm the Fetus

A. Infections

◆ Studies indicate a correlation between periodontitis and increased risk for adverse pregnancy outcomes.[10,11]

◆ The American Academy of Periodontology recommends women who are planning to become pregnant or currently are pregnant to have a periodontal examination and receive preventive or therapeutic treatment, when needed.[12]

◆ Protection from periodontal infection and infectious diseases is necessary to prevent potential damage to the developing fetus.[12,13]

◆ Women of childbearing age need to take advantage of all recommended immunizations prior to conception.[13]

◆ Defects, deformities, and life-threatening infections in the fetus can result from infection acquired during pregnancy or during delivery and after birth.[13]

◆ Rubella (German measles), rubeola, varicella, herpes viruses, hepatitis B, human immunodeficiency virus (HIV) infection, syphilis (congenital syphilis), and gonorrhea all can have serious effects on the fetus (see Chapter 5).

B. Pharmacokinetics

◆ During pregnancy, normal physiologic changes occur; as a result, drug movement within biologic systems is unique.[14]

◆ Nearly all drugs pass across the placenta to enter the circulation of the developing fetus and may have teratogenic effects based on factors such as gestational age, route of administration, absorption, dose, and maternal serum levels.[14]

◆ However, the majority of medications/drugs prescribed or used by an oral health professional and dispensed during pregnancy are not associated with teratogenic effects or adverse effects of fetal development.[1,15]

◆ Table 46-1 lists selected drugs with indications, contraindications, and special considerations for pregnant women.

◆ *Effect of tetracycline*
  • Tetracycline is well known for intrinsic staining of tooth structure.

TABLE 46-1 • Pharmacological Considerations for Pregnant Women[a]	
PHARMACEUTICAL AGENT	**INDICATIONS, CONTRAINDICATIONS, AND SPECIAL CONSIDERATIONS**
Analgesics	
Acetaminophen	May be used during pregnancy. Oral pain can often be managed with nonopioid medication. If opioids are used, prescribe the lowest dose for the shortest duration (usually <3 days), and avoid issuing refills to reduce risk for dependency.
Acetaminophen with codeine, hydrocodone, or oxycodone	
Codeine	
Meperidine	
Morphine	
Aspirin	May be used in short duration during pregnancy; 48–72 hr. Avoid in first and third trimesters.
Ibuprofen	
Naproxen	
Antibiotics	
Amoxicillin	May be used during pregnancy.
Cephalosporins	
Clindamycin	
Metronidazole	
Penicillin	
Ciprofloxacin	Avoid during pregnancy.
Clarithromycin	
Levofloxacin	
Moxifloxacin	
Tetracycline	Never use during pregnancy.
Anesthetics	Consult with a prenatal care health professional before using intravenous sedation or general anesthesia. Limit duration of exposure to <3 hr in pregnant women in the third trimester.
Local anesthetics with epinephrine (e.g., bupivacaine, lidocaine, mepivacaine)	May be used during pregnancy.
Nitrous oxide (30%)	May be used during pregnancy when topical or local anesthetics are inadequate. Pregnant women require lower levels of nitrous oxide to achieve sedation; consult with prenatal care health professional.
Antimicrobials	Use alcohol-free products during pregnancy.
Cetylpyridinium chloride mouth rinse	May be used during pregnancy.
Chlorhexidine mouth rinse	
Xylitol	

[a]The pharmacological agents listed are to be used only for indicated medical conditions and with appropriate supervision.
From *Oral Health Care During Pregnancy: A National Consensus Statement—Summary of an Expert Workgroup Meeting* ©2012 by the National Maternal and Child Oral Health Resource Center, Georgetown University. Table updated 2017. Permission is given to photocopy this publication or to forward it, in its entirety, to others.

- The effect occurs during mineralization of the primary teeth beginning at about 4 months of gestation and of the permanent teeth near and after birth (see Table 47-4).
- When an antibiotic is required during pregnancy, the prescribing of tetracycline must be avoided.[1]

- *Therapy for HIV infection*
  - Prevention of perinatal HIV transmission and health for the fetus and neonate are considered with the plan for optimal health care for the mother with HIV/acquired immune deficiency syndrome (AIDS) infection.[16]
  - There are high morbidity and mortality rates among pregnant and postpartum women with HIV infection who have suspended their antiretroviral therapy (ART).[16]
  - Among HIV-infected pregnant women who are eligible, ART is considered a safe and effective treatment in maternal viral suppression and in decreasing mother-to-child transmission and infant mortality.[16]

C. Drugs of Abuse and Dependence

- Use of tobacco, alcohol, and substances of abuse during pregnancy can have severe influences on the developing fetus, as well as on the child after birth.[17]
- Pregnancy is an ideal time to motivate a patient to quit smoking and avoid the use of other harmful substances.
- Explain increased risks for reduced birth weight, spontaneous abortions, perinatal deaths, and sudden infant death syndrome (SIDS).[18,19]
- The effects of tobacco use on pregnancy and assistance for smoking cessation are discussed in Chapter 32.
- Explain the effects of second-hand and third-hand smoke on the fetus and child after birth.[18,20,21]
- Present the steps in a cessation program, as described in Chapter 32.
- Information on the effects of alcohol use during pregnancy and fetal alcohol syndrome is included in Chapter 59.

D. Herbal Dietary Supplements

- Herbal supplements are not regulated by the Food and Drug Administration as a drug product, but as a dietary supplement. Dietary supplements are not reviewed for safety or effectiveness prior to being marketed to the public.[22]
- Questions about the use of herbal dietary supplements, their amount, and duration of use are documented when taking a routine medical history. Information about possible problems when taking the supplements can be presented to the patient.[23]
- Common uses are for colds, burns, headaches, allergies, rashes, depression, and insomnia.[23]
- Several of these supplements have treatment implications and may require physician consult:
  - Echinacea used for upper respiratory infections (colds) activates cell-mediated immunity: may cause allergic reactions, decreased effectiveness of immunosuppressants, and immunosuppression with long-term use.[21]
  - Valerian used for insomnia and stress has a sedative effect.[24] There are possible risks also associated when administering local anesthesia.

ORAL FINDINGS DURING PREGNANCY

I. Gingival Conditions

- Increased gingival inflammation is a well-documented phenomenon occurring during pregnancy[25] and may occur because of the following:
  - Increased circulating levels of estrogen and progesterone hormones in pregnancy.[26]
  - Immunologic alterations that are pregnancy induced cause a weakening of the mother's cell-mediated immune response.[26]
  - Exaggerated response of the tissues to dental biofilm and local irritants.
  - Trauma, poor oral self-care, and local irritation from calculus or prostheses may be contributory factors.
- Gingival changes in pregnancy usually appear in the first trimester and can continue throughout the pregnancy unless instruction is given and daily oral self-care is improved.[27]
- When the periodontal tissues are in good health and the patient uses adequate oral self-care measures for biofilm control, major adverse gingival changes are not expected.
- When left untreated, gingival inflammation continues as the hormones rise to a maximum level by the 8th month.[25]
- Symptoms abate after the birth of the child,[25] but a completely healthy condition may not result. For instance, gingival inflammation present during pregnancy my continue after birth, especially if the mother is breastfeeding.

II. Gingivitis

- Considered the most common oral condition associated with pregnancy.[4,28]
- Commonly referred to as pregnancy gingivitis.[4]

A. Clinical Appearance

- Shows characteristics of inflamed tissues, including enlargement, redness, smooth and shiny surface.
- Bleeding on probing (BOP).[25]

B. Predisposing Factors

- Maternal immunologic changes.[26]
- Local irritation and infection because of poor oral self-care, leaving dental biofilm on the teeth and gingiva.
- Hormonal (estrogen and progesterone) changes during pregnancy that may alter the tissue reaction.[29]

◆ Increased proportions of oral microbiota such as *Aggregatibacter actinomycetemcomitans*, *Porphyromonas gingivalis*, *Prevotella nigrescens*, and *Campylobacter rectus* have been found during pregnancy.[30]

III. Gingival Enlargement

A. Oral "Pyogenic" Granuloma[31]

◆ Also referred to as pregnancy epulis, granuloma gravidarum, pregnancy granuloma, or a pregnancy tumor.

◆ The use of the word *tumor* is misleading; the lesion is not a tumor, but a hyperplasia and may also occur in nonpregnant women.

◆ Benign, inflammatory lesion; rapid growing gingival mass that reacts to a variety of stimuli.

◆ When the lesion is removed during pregnancy, there is some tendency for recurrence.

B. Clinical Appearance[31]

◆ The lesion appears as an isolated, discrete, soft, round enlargement near the gingival margin usually associated with an interdental area, as shown in Figure 46-1.

◆ It forms in a mushroom-like shape with a smooth, glistening surface.

◆ The pressure of the lip or cheek tends to flatten it.

◆ The color depends on the age of the lesion, with newer lesions having increased vascularity and may be purplish-red, magenta, or deep blue, sometimes dotted with red; older lesions may have a more pink color.

C. Symptoms[31]

◆ Bleeds readily with slight trauma.

◆ Painless unless it becomes large enough to interfere with occlusion and mastication.

D. Significance[31]

◆ Interference during mastication: can contribute to inadequate nutritive intake for mother and baby because of discomfort when chewing.

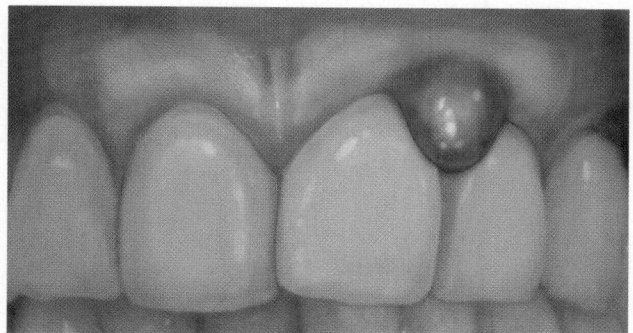

FIGURE 46-1 • "Pyogenic" Granuloma or "Pregnancy Tumor." Isolated, discrete, round, soft enlargement near the gingival margin; smooth, glistening surface, purplish-red in color.

◆ Provides a site for bacterial growth; potential development of periodontal attachment loss and eventual bone destruction.

◆ Results in bleeding and pain: may interfere with routine dental biofilm removal using toothbrush and interdental aids.

◆ Creates undesirable esthetic effects.

◆ Lesion must be ruled out for similar appearing malignancies and underlying systemic conditions. Referral for excision and biopsy may be indicated.

IV. Periodontal Infections

◆ Pregnancy-associated immunologic changes cause a suppression of the mother's cell-mediated immune response, particularly the neutrophil function.[26]

◆ Many epidemiologic studies suggest a causal relationship between periodontal infections and several adverse pregnancy outcomes, such as preeclampsia, preterm delivery, and low birth weight.[11,32]

◆ It is unclear if periodontal treatment during pregnancy can improve preterm delivery or low birth weight.[33]

◆ Evidence shows periodontal treatment is safe during pregnancy. The American Academy of Periodontology recommends that a pregnant woman undergo a routine periodontal examination.[12]

◆ Preventive services such as periodontal maintenance care can be rendered during pregnancy.[12]

◆ Periodontal therapeutic services can be rendered during pregnancy.[12]

V. Enamel Erosion

A. Development

◆ Morning sickness with vomiting over an extended period can lead to demineralization and acid erosion primarily on the maxillary palatal surfaces.[29]

B. Recommendations for the Patient[1,34]

◆ Eat small amounts of nutritious yet noncariogenic foods throughout the day.

◆ Use a sodium bicarbonate rinse after vomiting to neutralize acid on teeth: one cup of water to one teaspoon of sodium bicarbonate.

◆ Chew gum containing xylitol after eating.

◆ Use a soft toothbrush and low-abrasive fluoride toothpaste to prevent damage to demineralized tooth surfaces.

ASPECTS OF PATIENT CARE

I. Assessment

◆ Preventive oral health care needs to begin early and continue throughout the pregnancy, to keep the gingival tissues in optimum health and prevent oral infections.[1]

A. Medical History: Health Problems Need Identification during Examination

◆ Gestational diabetes: First recognition during pregnancy; needs insulin adjustment and careful supervision.[35] More information is included in Chapter 54.

◆ Women with hypertension are considered to be at high risk for complications during pregnancy. A consultation with the patient's physician and/or obstetrician is necessary.[4]

◆ Adolescent health: When the expectant mother is an adolescent, her own special needs differ from those of a mature woman.

◆ Complications such as delivery of a low-birth-weight baby and increased mortality for both mother and child occur more frequently in adolescent pregnant females.[36]

◆ Aspects of adolescent development are described in Chapters 47 and 53.

B. Consultations

◆ Treatment approval is not required when providing routine dental care. Consultation with the patient's physician and/or obstetrician may be indicated when underlying health conditions are present.[34]

◆ When a patient seeks dental and dental hygiene care and is not under the care of a physician, she is urged and assisted to obtain medical supervision for her health and the health of her baby.[28]

II. Radiography

A. Universal Safety Factors

◆ Guidelines for dental radiographs during pregnancy have been established.[37]

◆ ALARA (as low as reasonably achievable) principles to minimize the patient's exposure to radiation needs to be followed (see Chapter 15).

◆ Recommendations advise that dental radiographs are safe throughout pregnancy and X-ray exposure for a diagnostic procedure does not cause harmful effects to the developing embryo or fetus.[37]

◆ With safety factors of modern radiography, the patient can be assured essential radiographs can be taken safely during pregnancy.[38]

◆ When radiographs are required during pregnancy, the patient is covered with a lead apron and a thyroid collar.[38]

III. Overall Treatment Considerations

A. Dental Hygiene Care Goal

◆ The dental hygienist who is well informed about dental care can motivate the patient during her pregnancy and can alleviate fears related to certain services.

◆ When treating a pregnant patient, the dental hygienist's goal is to optimize the oral health of both the mother and child.

B. Dental Care

◆ Restorative: Complete restorative needs with permanent restorative materials, such as amalgam or composite materials. Recommended at any time during pregnancy.[4]

◆ Although silver diamine fluoride has not been specifically tested with pregnant women, protocol does not contraindicate its use. However, the use of potassium iodide to reduce staining from silver diamine fluoride is contraindicated during pregnancy and the first 6 months of breastfeeding.[39]

◆ Elective esthetic treatment: Postpone until postdelivery.[27]

C. Appointment Planning

◆ Appointment adaptations for the prenatal patient are listed in Table 46-2.

◆ Frequency depends on patient care plan.[1]
  • Monthly appointments or appointments three times during the 9-month period may be required.
  • Appointment frequency depends on the patient's needs as well as ability and motivation to maintain good oral self-care.

◆ Individual appointments
  • Patients are more comfortable with short appointments.[29]
  • A series of appointments is indicated when calculus deposits are heavy and/or periodontal infection is present.

◆ Postpartum continuing care appointments
  • Emphasis is placed on motivating the patient to continue regular appointments for dental hygiene and dental care after the baby is born.

D. Patient Positioning

◆ Effect of supine position[40]
  • The weight of the developing fetus in the uterus bears down directly on the major vessels, the aorta, and the inferior vena cava.
  • The vessels are pressed between the spinal column and the uterus.
  • Commonly occurs during the third trimester, symptoms of circulatory insufficiency can appear when venous return is decreased.

◆ Supine hypotensive syndrome: emergency[40]
  • Patient is lying in supine position.
  • Abrupt fall in blood pressure.
  • Bradycardia, sweating, nausea, weakness, air hunger.
  • Symptoms caused by impaired venous return resulting from pressure of the uterus with the developing baby on the inferior vena cava.
  • Leads to decrease in blood pressure, reduced cardiac output, and loss of consciousness.

TABLE 46-2 • Appointment Adaptations for the Prenatal Patient

CHARACTERISTIC	DENTAL HYGIENE IMPLICATION
Fatigues easily, may even fall asleep	Short appointments; several in series, as needed Work with an assistant to accomplish more at each appointment
General awkwardness because of new shape and weight gain	Attend to details, such as gently lowering and straightening chair for patient Make sure rinsing facilities are convenient; or preferably, an assistant attends to evacuation
Frequent urination	Allow sufficient appointment time for interruptions Suggest at beginning of appointment that patient indicate if a restroom break is needed
Discomfort of remaining in one position too long	Position the patient on her left side and not in supine or Trendelenburg position (Figure 46-2)
Backache	Encourage position changes throughout the appointment Assistance with evacuation during intraoral instrumentation can shorten appointment time
Faintness and dizziness	Be prepared for emergency (see Chapter 9)
Adverse reaction to strong smells and flavors	Recommend less strong-flavored dentifrice
Exaggerated reactions to odors and flavors of medicaments and other office materials	Determine particularly obnoxious odors for an individual patient and remove them; check office ventilation
Unpleasant taste in mouth	Advise: nonalcoholic mouth rinse; use a neutral sodium fluoride rinse Demonstrate tongue cleaning as in Chapter 26
Nausea and vomiting	To avoid tooth abrasion, do not brush immediately after vomiting. Rinse generously with fluoridated water or water and a teaspoon of sodium bicarbonate (baking soda) mixture after vomiting to neutralize the acid from the teeth
Gagging	Recommend a small toothbrush Turn head down over sink while brushing; helps to relax throat and allow saliva to flow out Take care in instrument and radiographic film placement
Physician's recommendation for alleviation of nausea symptoms: frequent eating of small amounts of foods	Encourage use of noncariogenic foods
Unusual food cravings	If cravings are for sweets, clearly define relationship of frequent snacking of cariogenic foods to dental caries Conduct a dietary analysis. Provide list of nutritious noncariogenic snacks

- *Emergency treatment*[29]
  - Roll the patient over to her left side to relieve pressure of the uterus on vena cava.
  - Blood pressure should return to normal promptly.
- *Alternate positions*[29] (Figure 46-2)
  - Elevate the right hip to displace the uterus to the left. Use a pillow or rolled-up blanket. (Figure 46-2A).
  - Patient lies on left side (Figure 46-2B).

IV. Dental Hygiene Care

A. Preventive Care and Measures

- Preventive oral health care needs priority attention, beginning with information and motivation.
- Areas of food impaction need to be corrected, and all overhanging restorations reshaped or replaced.

- All nonsurgical periodontal therapy procedures are thoroughly completed.
- When a patient has gingival enlargement and inflammation, instruction in biofilm control and other preventive measures including diet and eating patterns are needed.
- At the follow-up appointments, evaluation with disclosing agent is made and oral hygiene instruction is continued.

B. Instrumentation

- Careful instrumentation for complete calculus removal is indicated.[5]
- The use of ultrasonic scalers is not contraindicated for reasons related to pregnancy.[3]
- Nonsurgical periodontal therapy may be performed during pregnancy.[5]

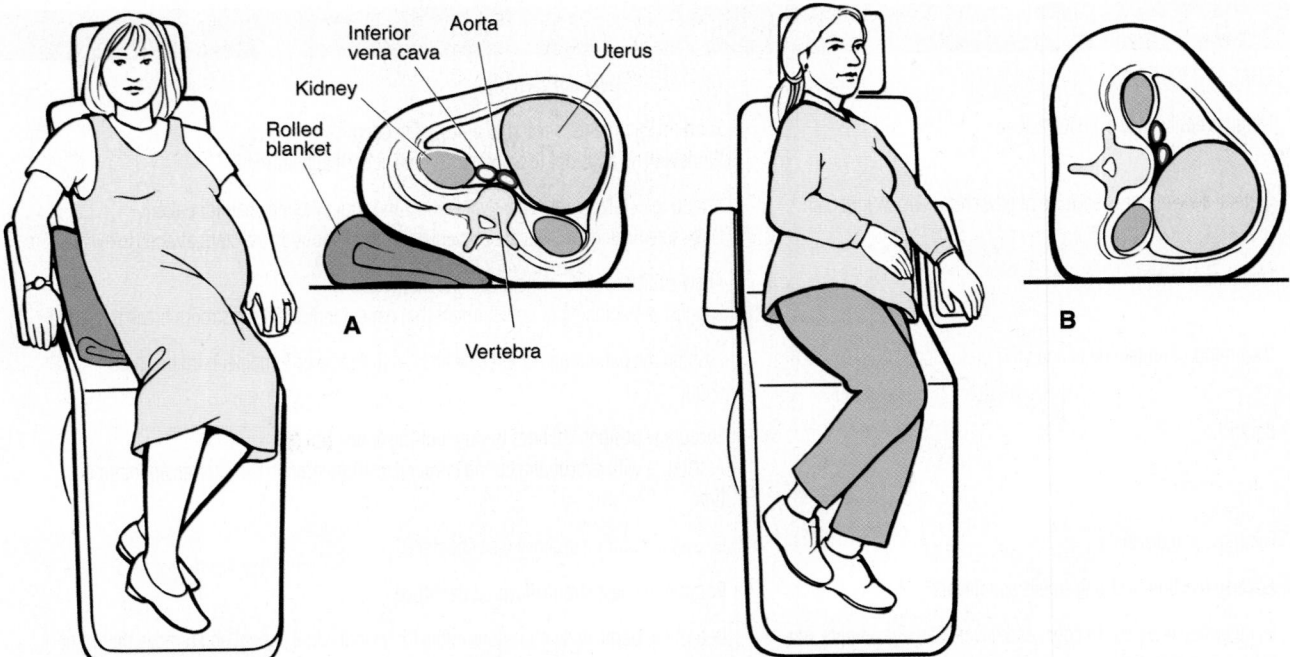

FIGURE 46-2 • Positions during Pregnancy. The supine position allows the weight of the developing fetus to bear down directly on the major vessels. **A:** Patient lies on left side with a pillow or blanket roll to elevate right hip. **B:** Patient turned farther to left. Note position of uterus in cross sections of the abdomen.

C. Anesthesia

◆ Local anesthetics containing epinephrine are allowed during pregnancy.[1,41]

◆ After consultation with the patient's physician, nitrous oxide/oxygen may be used in moderation.[1]

◆ If used in the second or third trimester, precaution is required, including minimizing the length to 30 minutes with oxygen percentage at 50%.[1]

PATIENT INSTRUCTION

◆ The emphasis on general health during pregnancy provides the ideal setting for instructions relative to many aspects of oral health for the mother, her expected child, and other family members.

◆ New developments in disease prevention and control need to be explained.

◆ Helping the mother learn what to expect before infant arrival is essential.[5]

I. Dental Biofilm Control[27]

◆ A schedule for oral self-care is established and specific methods are outlined and demonstrated. A series of instructional sessions is better for patient learning.

◆ Increased gingival inflammation is a common phenomenon during pregnancy.

◆ Gingival changes during pregnancy require daily self-care by the patient and periodic professional oral healthcare appointments.

II. Diet

◆ Instruction is provided in prevention of dental caries and maintenance of the health of the supporting structures of the teeth.[1]

◆ The use of a varied diet containing the essential protective food groups, with a minimum of cariogenic foods, is necessary.[34] The website www.choosemyplate.gov is a valuable resource with specifics for maternal nutrition. The ChooseMyPlate Food Guide is shown in Chapter 33.

A. Purposes of Adequate Diet during Pregnancy[42]

◆ Maintain daily strength and feeling of well-being.

◆ Provide the essential building materials for the developing fetus.

◆ Protect and promote the health of the oral tissues of the mother.[43]

◆ Minimize postpartum problems.

B. Dietary Needs during Pregnancy

◆ It is essential the mother's dietary needs are met to maintain her own nutritional status as well as the needs of the developing fetus. These particular needs are[42]:

• Proteins for general tissue construction.

• Minerals, especially calcium and phosphorus, for bone and tooth mineralization; iron for red blood cells.

• Vitamins, especially vitamin D, for calcium metabolism, folate to prevent neural tube defects and low birth weight.

- A prenatal vitamin supplement is commonly recommended during pregnancy.[44]

C. Dietary Assessment and Recommendations for Oral and General Health[45]

- Intake from food groups.
  - Consume a healthy diet from the fruit, vegetable, grain, meat/meat alternatives, and dairy food groups.
  - In addition to eating folate-rich foods, take a supplement containing folic acid.[44]
  - Low-fat/fat-free calcium-rich foods.
  - Recommended dietary allowance (RDA) of 1,300 mg of calcium per day is required for a pregnant adolescent (14–18 years) and 1,000 mg for those 19–50 years. The RDAs are the same for breastfeeding mothers.[46]
- Frequency and types of snacks per day.[42]
  - Limit cariogenic food occurrence.
  - Healthy snacks, such as carrots, fresh fruits, or almonds.
- Intake of sweetened and caffeinated beverages, such as ice tea or soda.
  - Limit or avoid drinking beverages sweetened with sugar and containing caffeine.[42]
  - Substitute with fluoridated water.[1]
- Avoiding sugar-containing chewing gum.[34]
  - Instead use a sugarless chewing gum containing xylitol.[1]

III. Dental Caries Control

A. Incidence during Pregnancy

- Complete a caries risk assessment survey to indicate patient's caries risk (see Chapter 25).[5]
- Some patients believe they have more dental caries during and because of pregnancy.
- Research has shown this is not true and any relationship is indirect.[5]
- Factors that result in dental caries formation are the same during pregnancy as at other times (Chapter 25).
- Mothers with poor oral health and high levels of cariogenic bacteria are at a greater risk for infecting their children with the bacteria and increasing their children's caries risk at infancy.[47]

B. Factors That May Contribute to an Increase in Dental Caries Rate

- *Previous neglect:* A patient may not have kept a regular dental appointment plan. The existing dental caries during pregnancy may represent years of accumulation.
- *Diet during pregnancy:* May increase the intake of cariogenic foods.
  - Unusual cravings may include sweet foods.
  - Frequency of eating: patient may be eating every few hours for prevention of nausea, and those foods may be cariogenic.[48]

- *Neglect of personal oral care procedures:* Patient may lack interest in daily dental biofilm removal or be lax about rinsing (with water) immediately following intake of a cariogenic food.
  - Vomiting associated with morning sickness may lead to tooth decalcification and erosion.[48]
  - The smell of toothpaste or the act of brushing may precipitate nausea and cause reduction in oral care.
- *Low socioeconomic status:* Women with lower income level and less education have been shown to have a higher rate of dental disease as well as untreated dental caries.[49]

C. Relationship of Fluoride

- There is no evidence prenatal fluoride supplementation intake by the mother influences the rate of dental caries in their newborn.[50]

IV. Fluoride Program

A. Professional Topical Application

- Professional fluoride varnish application for caries prevention.[51]
- Applications can be indicated, especially for patients with a tendency toward demineralization and those with numerous restorations. CAMBRA (Caries Risk Management by Risk Assessment) is described in Chapter 25.

B. Self-Applications

- A fluoride dentifrice.
- Drinking fluoridated water is recommended for all patients.[52]
- Other fluoride recommendations are individualized according to patient need.[1]
- A daily fluoride mouth rinse, gel tray, or other mode of application is essential for some patients; review how to rinse thoroughly.

SPECIAL PROBLEMS REQUIRING REFERRAL

I. Depression during Pregnancy

- Childbearing years place women at greatest risk for depression.[53] Oral healthcare professionals can learn to identify signs and symptoms of depression in pregnant patients. Treatment for depression and dental hygiene care for individuals with depression are described in Chapter 58.

A. Signs of Depression[54]

- Depressed mood; loss of interest or pleasure in ordinary activities.
- Fatigue and disturbed sleep.
- Loss of appetite.

- Difficulty making decisions.
- Feelings of worthlessness and suicidal thoughts.[42]

B. Impact on Health of the Fetus[55]

- Higher tendencies for preeclampsia.
- Fetal growth restriction.
- Low birth weight.
- Preterm delivery.

C. What to Do

- Explain that depression is a biologically based illness caused by a chemical imbalance in the brain.
- Indicate that depression is treatable and, when treated, can improve the quality of life.
- Refer patient to the physician of record or a community mental health resource center.

II. Domestic Violence

A. Identification

- Identification, assessment, and intervention with victims of domestic violence can be a significant part of a dental visit[56] (see Chapter 14).

B. Common Sites of Injury[57]

- Head.
- Soft tissue.
- Neck.

C. Obstetric and Other Manifestations

- Obstetric: miscarriages and spontaneous or multiple abortions.[57]
- Substance abuse.[58]
- Depression.[55]
- Suicide attempts.[58]

D. What to Do

- Address the issue with the patient.[34]
- Refer to a Domestic Violence Intervention Program in the community when domestic violence is suspected.

TRANSITIONING FROM PREGNANCY TO INFANCY

- Once the baby is born, the focus shifts to the oral health needs of both mother and child. The next section will address infant oral health and parental guidance through the first year of life.

INFANT ORAL HEALTH

- To optimize infant oral health, oral health counseling begins during prenatal dental visits.[59]

I. Anticipatory Guidance

- Dental care during pregnancy includes educating the mother about the importance of infant oral health, so she can be prepared (Table 46-3).[60]
- Anticipatory guidance helps a parent learn what to expect during the infant's early and future developmental stages.[60]
- Eruption patterns vary and are familial in nature; the primary maxillary and mandibular central and lateral incisors generally erupt prior to age 1.[9] This process is known as teething. See Chapter 47 for tooth eruption patterns.
- Teething[60] often causes the infant to experience mild irritability, increased salivation, and a low-grade fever.[59]
- To ease teething discomfort, a chilled teething ring or washcloth is recommended.
- Over-the-counter teething products containing anesthetics such as benzocaine are not recommended for children under 2 years.[59]
- Over-the-counter teething products containing benzocaine can cause a rare but potentially fatal condition, methemoglobinemia.[61]
- Homeopathic teething tablets and gels pose a risk for infants/children and should be avoided.[62]
- It is recommended an infant receive a dental examination at 12 months, or by the eruption of the first primary tooth.[60]
- Establishment of a dental home for infants by 12 months of age is recommended. Early establishment of a dental home is crucial in early childhood caries (ECC) prevention and intervention.[60]
- When discussing anticipatory guidance include the following: infant daily oral hygiene; fluoride exposure; nutrition and diet; nonnutritive oral habits such as pacifier use and thumb sucking; speech development; dental trauma and injury avoidance[60] (see Table 46-3).
- Developmental milestones to consider when providing patient education are outlined in Table 46-4.

II. Infant Daily Oral Hygiene Care

- Advise caregiver to brush the infant's teeth twice daily, with a child-size toothbrush.[60]
- A smear layer (approximately the size of a grain of rice) of fluoridated toothpaste is advised for an infant, up to the age of 3.[63]
- Brushing technique involves lifting of the lip to expose the cervical one-third portion of the erupted anterior teeth.[34]
- Advise caregiver to look frequently at the infant's teeth for demineralization (white chalky appearance) and early carious lesions[5] (Chapter 47).

A. Inquire about Fluoride Exposure

- History of exposure to fluoride.

TABLE 46-3 • Anticipatory Guidance: Birth to 12 Months

AREA OF CONCERN	BIRTH TO 6 MONTHS	6 TO 12 MONTHS
Developmental milestone	• Eruption of first tooth • Pattern of eruption	• Pattern of eruption • Expected new teeth
Nutrition and feeding	• Relation of improper bottle/breastfeeding to initiation of dental caries • No propping of bottles in bed • Avoid use of bottle as pacifier • Breastfeeding passage of alcohol and drugs to infant • Discuss weaning	• Begin weaning • Discontinue bottle feeding by age 1 y • Use small regular cup • Avoid at-will access to bottle or sippy cup • Discuss sugar use, sugar retention, and caries initiation • Discuss consumption of sugar-sweetened beverages • Snacking safety (aspiration) • Avoid use of food for behavior modification
Oral hygiene and caries prevention	• Oral health of parents; *Streptococcus mutans* transmission • Clean ridges after each feeding (soft, wet cloth or gauze) • Use of brush (water only) • Position of infant for brushing	• Use of brush • Review position of infant for brushing • Parents look for signs of disease • Importance of maintaining primary dentition
Fluoride information	• Explain the relation of fluoride to teeth • Anticipate need to supplement • Check water supply for fluoride content at home and daycare	• When water supply is deficient, prescribe supplement (see Table 34-1) • Discuss compliance • Review manner of storage: cool, dry, out of reach • Possible fluoride varnish application
Trauma prevention	• Car seat safety	• Discuss highest accident rate is 1–2 y • Car seat safety • Trauma proofing • Confirm emergency access to dental provider
Habits/function behaviors	• Discuss teething • Discuss nonnutritive sucking	• Discuss oral/head and neck signs of child abuse
Environmental (passive) smoke	• Detrimental at all ages; smoking parents encouraged to start tobacco cessation program	• Provide smoke-free environment
Dental/dental hygienist visit	• Provide rationale for timing of baby's first dental visit • Explain what happens at first dental visit • Encourage parents to make appointments for their own dental care to eliminate *S. mutans* and maintain oral health	• Schedule first dental visit within 6 mo of eruption of first tooth • Provide information about how to make the first dental/dental hygiene visit a happy experience • Review need for parents to complete their own dental care

TABLE 46-4 • Milestones in Child Development: Birth to Age 12 Months

AREAS	BIRTH TO 6 MONTHS	6 TO 12 MONTHS
Language	• 0–2 mo: quiets to sound • Reflects displeasure at noises • Coos and babbles	• Says dada or mama • Understands name • Pays attention to verbalization
Motor	• 2 mo: head control • 6 mo: transfer hand to hand • Grasps with forearm (ulnar grasp)	• 7–9 mo: sits • 9–10 mo: plays pat-a-cake • Waves bye, bye
Social/emotional	• 2 mo: gazes at human face • Alert to voices	• Inhibited by word "no" • Separation anxiety • Stranger awareness

◆ Fluoride level of current water supply, including childcare environments (check public health department records).

◆ Well water (have water tested for fluoride level).

◆ Use of fluoridated or unspecified bottled water.

◆ Use of fluoride supplementation can begin at 6 months of age (see Chapter 34).[64]

III. Feeding Patterns (Birth to 1 Year)

A. Frequency and Method of Feeding

◆ Explain the cariogenicity of certain foods and beverages, the consequence of frequent consumption of sugary beverages and foods, and the demineralization process (see Chapter 33).[65]

◆ Problems with feeding and sleeping.

• When the infant falls asleep after sucking, milk collects around teeth and causes demineralization.[65]

B. Breastfeeding

◆ The U.S. Surgeon General endorses exclusive breast-feeding for the first 6 months of life, and up to 12 months of age with additional nutritional supplementation after the first 6 months of life.[66]

◆ Evidence suggests breastfeeding can aid in dental caries prevention during early childhood.[67]

◆ Discourage prolonged, at-will breastfeeding after tooth eruption.[65]

◆ If the infant sleeps with the mother, discourage at-will breastfeeding, after the eruption of the first tooth.

C. Bottle Feeding

◆ The American Dental Association supports the use of fluoridated water with liquid or powdered concentrated infant formula.[68]

◆ Hold the child during feeding.

◆ Discourage putting the infant to bed with a bottle containing anything other than fluoridated water, after the first tooth eruption.[69]

◆ Do not put sweetened milk, juice, or other sweet liquids in a bottle or sippy cup.[69]

◆ Do not use the bottle as a pacifier.

◆ Inquire of the age other children in family were weaned.

◆ Encourage parents to have infant drink from a cup by age 1. The American Academy of Pediatrics recommends children be weaned from the bottle before 18 months of age.[70]

IV. Nonnutritive Sucking

◆ Suggestions for pacifier selection and use:
  • The use of pacifiers has been shown to decrease the incidence of SIDS.[19]
  • The American Academy of Pediatrics Task Force on SIDS recommends the use of a pacifier throughout the first year of life.[19]
  • Choose a pacifier with solid construction that cannot be pulled apart. Figure 46-3 shows two types of pacifiers: one has an orthodontic nipple and the other a nonorthodontic nipple. The orthodontic nipple is designed to be more like a mother's breast nipple during nursing.
  • The orthodontic nipple is reported to cause less severity of malocclusion when compared to the conventional nipple.[71]
  • Ventilated shield larger than the child's mouth, at least 1–1/2 inches (3.8 cm) wide, to prevent swallowing.[72]
  • Not tied to the crib, child's clothing, or around the neck or hand, which could lead to strangulation.[72]
  • Not cleaned in the parent's/caregiver's mouth since caries-producing bacteria could be transferred to the infant.[65]
  • Clean in warm, soapy water. Replace with a new pacifier regularly.[72]

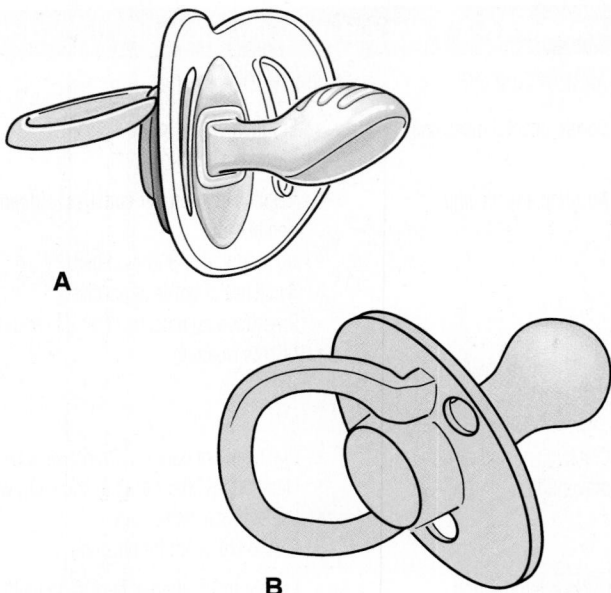

A

B

FIGURE 46-3 • Criteria for Selecting Pacifiers. Two styles of pacifier nipples: **(A)** orthodontic and **(B)** conventional. True orthodontic pacifiers expand to support the palate and maintain natural tongue posture. It is important to select the appropriate bulb size for each stage of development (0–2, 3–6, 6–18 months). Criteria for selection of a safe pacifier; size of shield is wider than child's mouth (at least 1.25 inches) in diameter; shield has air vents; plastic portion is of sturdy construction to prevent separation and possible choking; nipple is checked frequently for cracking and stickiness, at which time pacifier is replaced.

V. Components of the First Dental Visit

A first dental visit is recommended at the eruption of the first tooth, and no later than age 1.[60]

◆ One of the major reasons for this first visit is to establish a dental home (see Chapter 47).[60]

A. Components of Dental Visit

◆ To ensure patient cooperation, schedule the first visit at a time that is best for baby.

◆ A thorough medical history is necessary prior to beginning the infant oral examination.

◆ Explain to caregiver that crying is a normal reaction during the oral examination.

◆ Complete a caries risk assessment and discuss potential risk factors for ECC and Severe ECC.[73] Some of the risk factors include:
  • Diet and feeding patterns.[74]
  • Lack of daily oral hygiene care.[75]
  • Limited/no water fluoridation exposure.[52]
  • Poor maternal dental health. Research shows a strong association between maternal caries-producing bacterial loads and ECC development.[47]
  • The process known as vertical transmission occurs when mothers/primary caregivers exchange saliva with their infant. This can occur during kissing, sharing of food, drink, eating utensils, and the cleaning of pacifiers via the mother's mouth.[47]

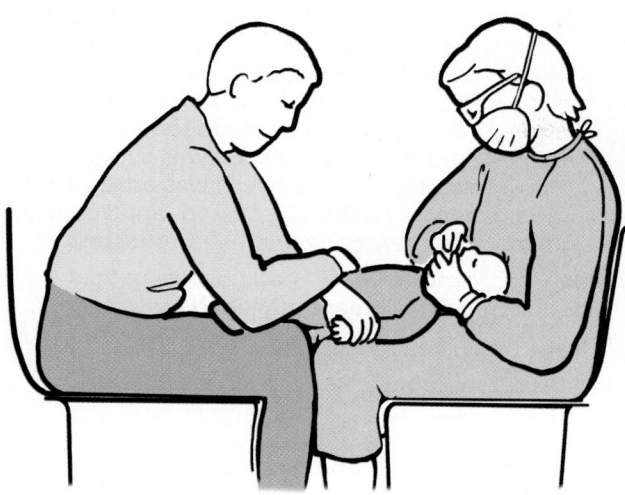

FIGURE 46-4 • Knee-to-Knee Infant Examination. The clinician makes the oral examination, discusses oral findings, and demonstrates proper oral care for the parent. The position of the infant then is reversed so that the parent has the opportunity to position the child and demonstrate proper oral care.

B. Oral Examination: Positioning to Access[3]

◆ Seat parent and clinician knee to knee.

◆ Place child's head on the lap of the examiner, as seen in Figure 46-4.

◆ Have caregiver crisscross arms gently across the infant's body, stabilizing the infant's hands and feet.

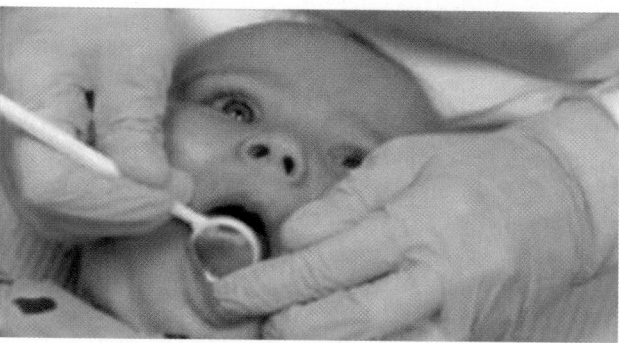

FIGURE 46-5 • Infant Oral Examination. Using a plastic mirror. Looking for presence of carious lesions on deciduous teeth.

C. Examination Sequence

◆ Examine the child's head and neck, legs, and arms for evidence of abuse. Signs of abuse are described in Chapter 14.

◆ When teeth are present, lift the lips away from the gingival margin to observe the condition of the anterior teeth (Figure 46-5).

◆ Examine all teeth for evidence of biofilm, discoloration.

◆ Look for malformations, dental caries, and white spot lesions (see Chapter 47).

◆ Assess for atypical frenum attachment that may potentially cause feeding issues.[59]

◆ Show parents the findings and inform them of the significance.

◆ Make referral to the dentist if evidence of pathology is noted (Tables 46-1 and 46-5).

TABLE 46-5 • Oral Soft and Hard Tissue Conditions/Pathology in Infants (1–6 Months)		
CONDITIONS	FINDINGS	SIGNIFICANCE
Soft Tissue		
Pseudomembranous candidiasis (thrush)	Mucosa or tongue; white, curdlike plaques; wipe-off leaving red and raw area	Discomfort; antifungal medication
Congenital epulis	Maxillary anterior ridge; pink, smooth, pedunculated mass; present at birth	Benign; spontaneous involution or surgical excision
Bohn's nodule	Buccal and lingual aspects of dental ridge; mucous gland remnant; smooth, translucent nodules	No treatment Shed spontaneously
Epstein's pearls	Palate near raphe; smooth, translucent nodules	No treatment
Dental lamina cysts	Crest of maxillary and mandibular ridges; dental lamina origin; smooth, translucent	No treatment
Bifid uvula	Cleft in uvula	Evaluate for possible submucous palatal cleft
Ankyloglossia	Short lingual frenum; may limit tongue mobility	Surgical reduction if interferes with nursing
Teeth		
Natal teeth	85% mandibular primary incisors; present at birth; commonly occur in pairs	Familial tendency; remove if mobile or have sharp edges causing injury
Neonatal teeth	Erupt within 30 d after birth	Same as above

Source: Dean JA. *Dentistry for the Child and Adolescent.* 10th ed. St. Louis, MO: Mosby; 2015.

D. Treatment

◆ Biofilm removal: use dampened cloth to clean gums[59] and a soft infant-size toothbrush when teeth are present.[76]

◆ Fluoride varnish application is recommended for children, beginning at age 1, who are moderate-to-high risk for ECC.[60]

DOCUMENTATION

◆ Documentation for the pregnant patient includes a minimum of the following:

◆ Thorough medical history, medications taken, use of tobacco, alcohol, or illicit drugs, history of gestational diabetes, miscarriage, hypertension, and morning sickness.

◆ Consultations with general physician and obstetrician along with their response.

◆ Oral examination findings with areas of concern that need treatment and follow-up.

◆ Changes from previous examinations with respect to oral self-care by the patient and record types of instruction provided.

◆ A sample progress note may be found in Box 46-1.

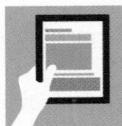

BOX 46-1
Example Documentation:
Pregnant Patient

S—A 32-year-old female presents for a 3-month recare appointment. Patient is in her second trimester, 15th week of pregnancy. Patient is currently taking folic acid (vitamin B9) supplement 600 mcg and prenatal vitamin daily. Patient reports mild nausea "morning sickness" during the morning hours. Patient's chief complaint: mild bleeding when brushing. States she hasn't been compliant with daily oral self-care, as her 1-year-old requires a lot of attention.

O—Intraoral assessment reveals generalized gingival inflammation, edematous and erythematous, with generalized light biofilm/plaque, new localized subgingival calculus deposits on mandibular posterior molars. Hard tissue examination: Cavitated carious lesion on #3. Periodontal examination findings: localized BOP #2, 3, 14, 18, 30, 31; localized 4 mm periodontal pocket depths on #2, 3, 14, 18, 31 were noted in periodontal chart.

A—Patient presents at a high caries risk. Periodontal condition: Gingivitis combination of plaque induced and pregnancy.

P—Patient congratulated on keeping the 3-month maintenance appointment, as last appointment was previously cancelled. Frequent bathroom breaks were offered. Dietary analysis completed and resources for improved nutritional intake were given. Relationship of nutritional intake for patient and baby was discussed, as well as dental caries relationship to carbohydrate foods. Patient demonstrated toothbrushing method, and better angulation was suggested. A powered electric toothbrush was advised for improved oral health. Discussed anticipatory guidance for new baby and 1-year-old son.

Next visit: Restorative #3. Additionally, patient scheduled son for 1-year oral health assessment.

Signed: _____, RDH

Date _____

EVERYDAY ETHICS

Anna, the dental hygienist, welcomed her patient Julie, a 20-year-old single woman. She is in the first trimester of pregnancy and was referred by a nurse from the Maternal and Child Health Clinic. Anna notices the way Julie holds a hand over her mouth when she talks. Julie's medical history appears negative except for smoking about a half pack of cigarettes daily. Examination reveals multiple carious lesions, heavy calculus, and 4–5 mm proximal probing depths in several molar areas. After making the radiographic survey and presenting initial patient instruction, there was time for one quadrant of scaling. Follow-up appointments were scheduled to complete treatment. The patient does not show up for any of the appointments.

Questions for Consideration

1. Which of the dental hygiene core values (Section II) apply to this situation? Explain.

2. What is the role of the dental hygienist, if any, to make further contact with this patient, and why? How will she go about it?

3. Describe two or three courses of action and the possible outcomes of the situation through a dental hygiene care plan.

Factors to Teach the Patient

► The relationship of oral health of the mother to the general health of the fetus and newborn.

► The serious effects of tobacco and other drugs on the health of the fetus, the infant, and the child.

► Reasons for dental hygiene appointments early during pregnancy, at regular intervals throughout pregnancy, and after birth of the baby.

► Rationale for receiving professional oral health care during pregnancy.

▶ The rationale for maintaining good personal oral hygiene care to control dental biofilm throughout the pregnancy and after the baby's birth.

▶ Self-examination of the oral cavity to evaluate the effectiveness of daily dental biofilm removal and the health of the soft tissues.

▶ Reasons for limiting fermentable carbohydrate intake, drinking fluoridated water, and maintaining a healthy diet from the fruit, vegetable, grain, meat and meat alternatives, and dairy food groups.

 ENHANCE YOUR UNDERSTANDING

ONLINE RESOURCES
(see the inside front cover for access information)

• Audio glossary

• Appendices

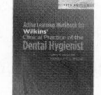 **SUPPORT FOR LEARNING**
(available separately)

• *Active Learning Workbook for Wilkins' Clinical Practice of the Dental Hygienist, 13th Edition*

INDIVIDUALIZED REVIEW

• Customized practice quizzing with Navigate 2 TestPrep for *Wilkins' Clinical Practice of the Dental Hygienist*

References

1. Oral Health Care during Pregnancy Expert Workgroup. *Oral Health Care during Pregnancy: A National Consensus Statement.* Washington, DC: National Maternal and Child Oral Health Resource Center; 2012. https://www.mchoralhealth.org/PDFs/OralHealthPregnancyConsensus.pdf. Accessed January 28, 2018.

2. U.S. Department of Health and Human Services, Office on Women's Health. Prenatal care. womenshealth.gov. https://www.womenshealth.gov/a-z-topics/prenatal-care. Published February 22, 2017. Accessed January 28, 2018.

3. New York State Department of Health. *Oral Health Care during Pregnancy and Early Childhood Practice Guidelines.* 2006. https://www.health.ny.gov/publications/0824.pdf. Accessed January 28, 2018.

4. American College of Obstetricians and Gynecologists Women's Health Care Physicians, Committee on Health Care for Underserved Women. Committee Opinion No. 569: oral health care during pregnancy and through the lifespan. *Obstet Gynecol.* 2013;122(2 pt 1):417-422. doi:10.1097/01.AOG.0000433007.16843.10.

5. California Dental Association Foundation, American College of Obstetricians and Gynecologists, District IX. Oral health during pregnancy and early childhood: evidence-based guidelines for health professionals. *J Calif Dent Assoc.* 2010;38(6):391-403, 405-440.

6. Barlow Pugh M. *Stedman's Medical Dictionary.* Vol. 2011. 28th ed. Baltimore, MD: Lippincott Williams & Wilkins; 2006.

7. Cunningham FG, Leveno KJ, Bloom SL, Hauth JC, Rouse DJ, Spong CY. Chapter 4: Fetal Growth and Development. In: Cunningham FG, Leveno KJ, Bloom SL, Hauth JC, Rouse DJ, Spong CY, eds. *Williams Obstetrics.* 23rd ed. New York, NY: McGraw-Hill; 2010.

8. Hardy K, Hardy PJ. 1(st) trimester miscarriage: four decades of study. *Transl Pediatr.* 2015;4(2):189-200. doi:10.3978/j.issn.2224-4336.2015.03.05.

9. Lunt RC, Law DB. A review of the chronology of calcification of deciduous teeth. *JADA.* 1974;89:599-606.

10. Boggess KA, Lieff S, Murtha AP, Moss K. Maternal periodontal disease is associated with an increased risk for preeclampsia. 2003;101(2):227.

11. Ide M, Papapanou PN. Epidemiology of association between maternal periodontal disease and adverse pregnancy outcomes—systematic review. *J Periodontol.* 2013;84(4 suppl):S181-S194. doi:10.1902/jop.2013.134009.

12. American Academy of Periodontology. American Academy of Periodontology statement regarding periodontal management of the pregnant patient. *J Periodontol.* 2004;75(3):495.

13. Advisory Committee on Immunization Practices (ACIP), Workgroup on the Use of Vaccines during Pregnancy and Breastfeeding. *Guiding Principles for Development of ACIP Recommendations for Vaccination during Pregnancy and Breastfeeding.* Centers for Disease Control and Prevention; 2008. https://www.cdc.gov/vaccines/acip/committee/guidance/rec-vac-preg.html. Accessed March 5, 2018.

14. Chisholm CA, Ferguson JE 2nd. Physiologic and pharmacologic factors related to the provision of dental care during pregnancy. *J Calif Dent Assoc.* 2010;38(9):663-671.

15. Hagai A, Diav-Citrin O, Shechtman S, Ornoy A. Pregnancy outcome after in utero exposure to local anesthetics as part of dental treatment: a prospective comparative cohort study. *J Am Dent Assoc.* 2015;146(8):572-580. doi:10.1016/j.adaj.2015.04.002.

16. Bernstein HB, Wegman AD. HIV infection: antepartum treatment and management. *Clin Obstet Gynecol.* 2018;61(1):122-136. doi:10.1097/GRF.0000000000000330.

17. Green PP, McKnight-Eily LR, Tan CH, Mejia R, Denny CH. Vital signs: alcohol-exposed pregnancies—United States, 2011-2013. *MMWR Morb Mortal Wkly Rep.* 2016;65(4):91-97. doi:10.15585/mmwr.mm6504a6.

18. U.S. Department of Health and Human Services. *The Health Consequences of Smoking—50 Years of Progress: A Report of the Surgeon General;* 2014.

19. Moon RY, Task Force on Sudden Infant Death Syndrome. SIDS and other sleep-related infant deaths: evidence base for 2016 updated recommendations for a safe infant sleeping environment. *Pediatrics.* 2016;138(5). doi:10.1542/peds.2016-2940.

20. Office on Smoking and Health. Centers for Disease Control and Prevention (CDC). *The Health Consequences of Involuntary Exposure to Tobacco Smoke: A Report of the Surgeon General.* Atlanta, GA: U.S. Department of Health and Human Services; 2006.

21. Centers for Disease Control and Prevention. Secondhand smoke: an unequal danger. *Vital Signs.* 2015. https://www.cdc.gov/vitalsigns/pdf/2015-02-vitalsigns.pdf. Accessed March 5, 2018.

22. Food and Drug Administration, Office of Dietary Supplement Programs. Dietary supplements. https://www.fda.gov/food/dietarysupplements/default.htm. Accessed January 30, 2018.

23. Ang-Lee MK, Moss J, Yuan C. Herbal medicines and perioperative care. *JAMA*. 2001;286(2):208-216.

24. National Institute of Health. Valerian. Valerian. https://ods.od.nih.gov/factsheets/Valerian-HealthProfessional/. Published 2013. Accessed February 1, 2018.

25. González-Jaranay M, Téllez L, Roa-López A, Gómez-Moreno G, Moreu G. Periodontal status during pregnancy and postpartum. *PLoS One*. 2017;12(5):e0178234. doi:10.1371/journal.pone.0178234.

26. Wu M, Chen S-W, Jiang S-Y. Relationship between gingival inflammation and pregnancy. *Mediators Inflamm*. 2015;2015:623427. doi:10.1155/2015/623427.

27. Hemalatha VT, Manigandan T, Sarumathi T, Aarthi Nisha V, Amudhan A. Dental considerations in pregnancy-a critical review on the oral care. *J Clin Diagn Res*. 2013;7(5):948-953. doi:10.7860/JCDR/2013/5405.2986.

28. Hartnett E, Haber J, Krainovich-Miller B, Bella A, Vasilyeva A, Lange Kessler J. Oral health in pregnancy. *J Obstet Gynecol Neonatal Nurs*. 2016;45(4):565-573. doi:10.1016/j.jogn.2016.04.005.

29. Amini H, Casimassimo PS. Prenatal dental care: a review. *Gen Dent*. 2010;58(3):176-180.

30. Borgo PV, Rodrigues VAA, Feitosa ACR, Xavier KCB, Avila-Campos MJ. Association between periodontal condition and subgingival microbiota in women during pregnancy: a longitudinal study. *J Appl Oral Sci*. 2014;22(6):528-533. doi:10.1590/1678-775720140164.

31. Jafarzadeh H, Sanatkhani M, Mohtasham N. Oral pyogenic granuloma: a review. *J Oral Sci*. 2006;48(4):167-175.

32. Corbella S, Taschieri S, Del Fabbro M, Francetti L, Weinstein R, Ferrazzi E. Adverse pregnancy outcomes and periodontitis: a systematic review and meta-analysis exploring potential association. *Quintessence Int*. 2016;47(3):193-204. doi:10.3290/j.qi.a34980.

33. Iheozor-Ejiofor Z, Middleton P, Esposito M, Glenny A-M. Treating periodontal disease for preventing adverse birth outcomes in pregnant women. *Cochrane Database Syst Rev*. 2017;6:CD005297. doi:10.1002/14651858.CD005297.pub3.

34. Massachusetts Department of Public Health. The Massachusetts oral health practice guidelines for pregnancy and early childhood. 2016. http://www.mass.gov/eohhs/docs/dph/com-health/data-translation/oral-health-guidelines.pdf. Accessed January 28, 2018.

35. Sanz M, Ceriello A, Buysschaert M, et al. Scientific evidence on the links between periodontal diseases and diabetes: consensus report and guidelines of the joint workshop on periodontal diseases and diabetes by the International Diabetes Federation and the European Federation of Periodontology. *J Clin Periodontol*. 2018;45(2):138-149. doi:10.1111/jcpe.12808.

36. The American Academy of Pediatric Dentistry. Guideline on oral health care for the pregnant adolescent. *Pediatr Dent*. 2016;38(5):59-66.

37. American College of Obstetricians and Gynecologists Committee. ACOG Committee Opinion Number 299: guidelines for diagnostic imaging during pregnancy. *Obstet Gynecol*. 2004;104(3):647.

38. American Dental Association and U.S. Department of Health and Human Services. Dental radiographic examinations: recommendations for patient selection and limiting radiographic exposure. 2012. www.ada.org/sections/professionalResources/pdfs/topics_radiography_examinations.pdf. Accessed March 6, 2018

39. Horst JA, Ellenikiotis H, Milgrom PM. UCSF protocol for caries arrest using silver diamine fluoride: rationale, indications, and consent. *J Calif Dent Assoc*. 2016;44(1):16-28.

40. Kinsella SM, Lohmann G. Supine hypotensive syndrome. *Obstet Gynecol*. 1994;83(5 pt 1):774-788.

41. Lee JM, Shin TJ. Use of local anesthetics for dental treatment during pregnancy; safety for parturient. *J Dent Anesth Pain Med*. 2017;17(2):81-90.

42. Kaiser L, Allen LH, American Dietetic Association. Position of the American Dietetic Association: nutrition and lifestyle for a healthy pregnancy outcome. *J Am Diet Assoc*. 2008;108(3):553-561.

43. Najeeb S, Zafar MS, Khurshid Z, Zohaib S, Almas K. The role of nutrition in periodontal health: an update. *Nutrients*. 2016;8(9). doi:10.3390/nu8090530.

44. United States Department of Agriculture. PregnancyFactSheet.pdf. https://wicworks.fns.usda.gov/wicworks//Topics/PregnancyFactSheet.pdf. Accessed February 1, 2018.

45. U.S. Department of Agriculture. Nutritional needs during pregnancy. Nutritional needs during pregnancy. https://www.choosemyplate.gov/moms/pregnancy-nutritional-needs. Accessed February 1, 2018.

46. National Institutes of Health, Office of Dietary Supplements (ODS). Calcium. https://ods.od.nih.gov/factsheets/Calcium-HealthProfessional/. Accessed February 1, 2018.

47. da Silva Bastos Vde A, Freitas-Fernandes LB, Fidalgo TK, et al. Mother-to-child transmission of Streptococcus mutans: a systematic review and meta-analysis. *J Dent*. 2015;43(2):181-191.

48. Jevtiá M, Pantelinaci J, Jovanović Ilić T, Petrović V, Grgić O, Blazić L. The role of nutrition in caries prevention and maintenance of oral health during pregnancy. *Med Pregl*. 2015;68(11-12):387-393.

49. Azofeifa A, Yeung LF, Alverson CJ, Beltrán-Aguilar E. Dental caries and periodontal disease among U.S. pregnant women and nonpregnant women of reproductive age, National Health and Nutrition Examination Survey, 1999-2004. *J Public Health Dent*. 2016;76(4):320-329.

50. Takahashi R, Ota E, Hoshi K, et al. Fluoride supplementation (with tablets, drops, lozenges or chewing gum) in pregnant women for preventing dental caries in the primary teeth of their children. *Cochrane Database Syst Rev*. 2017;10:CD011850.

51. Carey CM. Focus on fluorides: update on the use of fluoride for the prevention of dental caries. *J Evid-Based Dent Pract*. 2014;14(suppl):95-102.

52. Iheozor-Ejiofor Z, Worthington HV, Walsh T, et al. Water fluoridation for the prevention of dental caries. *Cochrane Database Syst Rev*. 2015;(6):CD010856.

53. Dennis C-L, Falah-Hassani K, Shiri R. Prevalence of antenatal and postnatal anxiety: systematic review and meta-analysis. *Br J Psychiatry*. 2017;210(5):315-323.

54. National Institute of Mental Health. Depression. https://www.nimh.nih.gov/health/topics/depression/index.shtml#part_145397. Accessed February 1, 2018.

55. Becker M, Weinberger T, Chandy A, Schmukler S. Depression during pregnancy and postpartum. *Curr Psychiatry Rep.* 2016;18(3):32.

56. O'Reilly R, Beale B, Gillies D. Screening and intervention for domestic violence during pregnancy care: a systematic review. *Trauma Violence Abuse.* 2010;11(4):190-201.

57. Petrone P, Jiménez-Morillas P, Axelrad A, Marini CP. Traumatic injuries to the pregnant patient: a critical literature review. *Eur J Trauma Emerg Surg.* 2019;45(3):383-392.

58. Sarkar NN. The impact of intimate partner violence on women's reproductive health and pregnancy outcome. *J Obstet Gynaecol.* 2008;28(3):266-271.

59. Guideline on perinatal and infant oral health care. *Pediatr Dent.* 2016;38(6):150-154.

60. Guideline on periodicity of examination, preventive dental services, anticipatory guidance/counseling, and oral treatment for infants, children, and adolescents. *Pediatr Dent.* 2016;38(6):133-141.

61. U.S. Food and Drug Administration. Drug Safety and Availability—FDA Drug Safety Communication: reports of a rare, but serious and potentially fatal adverse effect with the use of over-the-counter (OTC) benzocaine gels and liquids applied to the gums or mouth. https://www.fda.gov/drugs/drugsafety/ucm250024.htm#consumers. Accessed February 3, 2018.

62. U.S. Food and Drug Administration. Press Announcements—FDA warns against the use of homeopathic teething tablets and gels. https://www.fda.gov/NewsEvents/Newsroom/PressAnnouncements/ucm523468.htm. Accessed February 1, 2018.

63. American Dental Association Council on Scientific Affairs. Fluoride toothpaste use for young children. *J Am Dent Assoc.* 2014;145(2):190-191.

64. Rozier RG, Adair S, Graham F, et al. Evidence-based clinical recommendations on the prescription of dietary fluoride supplements for caries prevention: a report of the American Dental Association Council on Scientific Affairs. *J Am Dent Assoc.* 2010;141(12):1480-1489.

65. Anil S, Anand PS. Early childhood caries: prevalence, risk factors, and prevention. *Front Pediatr.* 2017;5:157.

66. U.S. Department of Health and Human Services. *The Surgeon General's Call to Action to Support Breastfeeding.* 2011 (Monograph).

67. Avila WM, Pordeus IA, Paiva SM, Martins CC. Breast and bottle feeding as risk factors for dental caries: a systematic review and meta-analysis. *PLoS One.* 2015;10(11):e0142922.

68. Berg J, Gerweck C, Hujoel PP, et al. Evidence-based clinical recommendations regarding fluoride intake from reconstituted infant formula and enamel fluorosis: a report of the American Dental Association Council on Scientific Affairs. *J Am Dent Assoc.* 2011;142(1):79-87.

69. Policy on early childhood caries (ECC): classifications, consequences, and preventive strategies. *Pediatr Dent.* 2017;39(6):59-61.

70. American Academy of Pediatrics. Weaning from the bottle. http://www.aap.org/en-us/about-the-aap/aap-press-room/aap-press-room-media-center/Pages/Weaning-from-the-Bottle.aspx

71. Lima AADSJ, Alves CMC, Ribeiro CCC, et al. Effects of conventional and orthodontic pacifiers on the dental occlusion of children aged 24-36 months old. *Int J Paediatr Dent.* 2017;27(2):108-119.

72. American Academy of Pediatrics. Caring for your baby and young child: birth to age 5. 2015. http://www.healthychildren.org/English/safety-prevention/at-home/Pages/Pacifier-Safety.aspx. Accessed March 5, 2018.

73. Guideline on caries-risk assessment and management for infants, children, and adolescents. *Pediatr Dent.* 2016;38(6):142-149.

74. Wong A, Subar PE, Young DA. Dental caries: an update on dental trends and therapy. *Adv Pediatr.* 2017;64(1):307-330.

75. Maheswari SU, Raja J, Kumar A, Seelan RG. Caries management by risk assessment: a review on current strategies for caries prevention and management. *J Pharm Bioallied Sci.* 2015;7(suppl 2):S320-S324.

76. American Academy of Pediatric Dentistry. Clinical Affairs Committee—Infant Oral Health Subcommittee. Guideline on infant oral health care. *Pediatr Dent.* 2012;34(5):e148-152.

47

The Pediatric Patient

Carolynn A. Zeitz, RDH, BS, RDA, MA

CHAPTER OUTLINE

PEDIATRIC DENTISTRY
  I.   The Specialty of Pediatric Dentistry
  II. American Academy of Pediatric Dentistry

THE CHILD AS A PATIENT
  I.   The Dental Home
  II. Barriers to Dental Care
  III. Child Dental Visits

PATIENT MANAGEMENT CONSIDERATIONS
  I.   Toddlers (1–3 Years of Age)
  II. Preschoolers (3–5 Years of Age)
  III. School-Age Children (6–12 Years of Age)
  IV. Adolescents (12–18 Years of Age)

COMPONENTS OF THE DENTAL HYGIENE VISIT
  I.   Initial Interview/New Patient Visit
  II. Child and Family Medical/Dental History
  III. Intraoral and Extraoral Examination
  IV. Developing Dentition, Occlusion, and TMJ

  V.   Radiographic Assessment
  VI.   Dietary Assessment
  VII. Dental Hygiene Treatment
  VIII. Prevention

PERIODONTAL RISK ASSESSMENT
  I.   Gingival and Periodontal Evaluation
  II. Periodontal Infections

CARIES RISK ASSESSMENT
  I.   Purpose
  II. Principles
  III. Steps
  IV. Classifications of Caries Risk
  V.   Early Childhood Caries

ANTICIPATORY GUIDANCE
  I.   Dietary and Feeding Pattern Recommendations
  II. Oral Health Considerations for Toddlers/
       Preschoolers

  III. Speech and Language Development
  IV.   Digit Habits
  V.   Accident and Injury Prevention
  VI.   Oral Malodor
  VII. Oral Health Considerations for Adolescents
  VIII. Tobacco/Piercings/Substance Abuse
  IX.   Referral

TREATMENT PLANNING AND CONSENT

DOCUMENTATION

EVERYDAY ETHICS

FACTORS TO TEACH THE PARENTS

REFERENCES

LEARNING OBJECTIVES

After studying this chapter, the reader will be able to:

1. Describe the specialty of pediatric dentistry.

2. Discuss the use of a caries risk assessment tool to identify an individual patient's risk and preventive factors.

3. Identify age-appropriate anticipatory guidance/counseling factors to educate parents/caregivers of toddlers, school-aged children, and adolescents.

4. Identify preventive and therapeutic oral healthcare interventions based on age and caries risk assessment.

5. Discuss oral health home care needs, adjunct aids, and continuing care recommendations for children.

Oral health for toddlers, preschoolers, school-aged children, and adolescents depends primarily on parental intervention for the young child, and gradually transitioning the child through parent involvement to independent management of daily oral self-care. Parents are:

- Provided with education through anticipatory guidance before a child's birth (see Chapter 46) and at regular intervals thereafter.
- Given the information needed to assess their child's oral health status.
- Taught how to intervene and to anticipate the child's oral health needs at various ages and stages of growth and development.

PEDIATRIC DENTISTRY

I. The Specialty of Pediatric Dentistry

- An age-defined specialty that provides both primary and comprehensive preventive and therapeutic oral health care for infants and children through adolescence, including those with special healthcare needs.[1]
- Requires 2 years of additional residency training (after the required 4 years of dental school) in dentistry for infants, children, teens, and children with special needs.[2]

II. The American Academy of Pediatric Dentistry

- The membership organization representing the specialty of pediatric dentistry and for general dentists who treat a significant number of children in their private practice.[3]
- Service as primary care and specialty providers for millions of children from infancy through adolescence.[3]
- The American Academy of Pediatric Dentistry's (AAPD) mission is to advance optimal oral health for all children by delivering outstanding service that meets and exceeds the needs and expectations of our members, partners, and stakeholders.[4]
- Professional and parental information is available at the AAPD website (www.aapd.org).[5]

THE CHILD AS A PATIENT

The age categories of pediatric patients are[6]:
- Infants: 0–1 year of age (see Chapter 46).
- Toddlers: 1–3 years of age.
- Preschoolers: 3–5 years of age.
- School-aged children (middle childhood): 6–11 years of age.
- Adolescents (young teens and teenagers): 12–17 years of age.

I. The Dental Home

- Dental home[7] is defined by the AAPD as, "An ongoing relationship between the dentist and the patient, inclusive of all aspects of oral health care delivered in a comprehensive, continuously accessible, coordinated, and family-centered way."
- The AAPD, the American Dental Association (ADA), and the American Academy of Pediatrics recommend a dental home should be established no later than 12 months of age and include referral to dental specialties when appropriate.
- Emphasis is placed on oral health counseling and prevention. One out of 10, 2-year-olds, toddlers already have one or more cavities.[8]

II. Barriers to Dental Care

- Availability of dental providers, which accept patient's insurance, in geographic area, office hours, and/or willing to see children.
- Financial (income/dental insurance).
- Lack of parental oral health literacy and the importance of oral health.
- Language.
- Transportation.

III. Child Dental Visits

A. Purposes

- The purposes of the dental hygiene visit are to:
  - Establish rapport, teach appropriate behaviors, and prevent management problems.
  - Develop and continue relationship with the child and the family.
  - Initiate and/or strengthen positive age-appropriate preventive measures, such as fluoride usage, appropriate nutritional practices, and daily dental biofilm removal.
  - Discover, intercept, and recommend changes in any parental practices that may be detrimental to the child's oral health.
- Appointments are planned for clinical oral examination, caries risk assessment, biofilm and calculus removal, professional fluoride application, radiographic assessment, treatment planning of dental disease, evaluation of developing dentition/malocclusion, anticipatory guidance/counseling, and introduction to dental hygiene.

B. Frequency of Continuing Care

- Visits to the dental hygienist and the dentist are scheduled according to the child's specific needs. A common appointment plan for children with little or no oral disease is every 4 or 6 months.
- Some patients may require more frequent intervals based upon the child's risk factors, historical, clinical, and radiographic findings.[9]
- Reevaluation and reinforcement of preventive activities contribute to improved instruction for the parent, child, and adolescent.[9]

C. Scheduling

The best time to schedule dental visits for toddlers and young school-aged children is:

◆ Early in the morning when the child is well rested and more cooperative.

◆ After naps when the child is not tired and is more apt to listen and cooperate.

PATIENT MANAGEMENT CONSIDERATIONS

Cooperation is usually gained with nonverbal communication such as smiling and talking with the child and the parent.

I. Toddlers (1–3 Years of Age)

◆ Primary teeth are vulnerable to tooth decay upon the eruption of the first tooth, usually between the ages of 6 and 12 months.

◆ Children who wait to have their first dental visit until 2 or 3 years of age are more likely to require restorative and emergency visits.

◆ Use of child-friendly terms instead of dental terms. See Box 47-1 for examples of child-friendly terms.

A. Oral Examination: Positioning for Access

◆ Utilize the knee-to-knee positioning for the oral examination and teach the parent to utilize this position at home to provide thorough biofilm removal with toothbrush and floss. Refer to Figures 46-4 and 46-5.

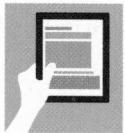

BOX 47-1
Child-Friendly Substitution Words for Dental Terminology

DENTAL TERM	CHILD-FRIENDLY TERM
Air/water syringe	Water squirter, wind
Amalgam restoration	Silver star
Dental light	Sunshine light
Explorer, scaler	Tooth counter
Fluoride varnish	Fluoride tooth vitamins
High-speed handpiece	Mr. Whistle
Low-speed handpiece	Tooth tickler, Mr. Bumpy
Mouth mirror	Tooth mirror
Mouth prop	Tooth pillow
Prophy paste	Special toothpaste
Dental hygiene treatment	Teeth cleaning
Saliva ejector	Mrs. Thirsty/special straw
Suction (high-speed)	Vacuum

◆ Prior to performing the examination, explain to the parent proper positioning—child's legs around parent's waist, parent's elbows restrain child's legs, and parent holds child's hands on his/her stomach.

◆ It is the clinician's responsibility to control the head during the examination.

◆ Crying during the examination is normal behavior and can provide better visibility of the child's mouth and throat.

B. Examination Sequence

◆ Examine the child's head and neck, legs, and arms for evidence of abuse. Abuse is described in Chapter 14.

◆ Oral soft tissues are assessed (see Table 47-1).[10]

◆ Lift the upper lip to observe the condition of the anterior teeth.

II. Preschoolers (3–5 Years of Age)

A. Prepare the Child for the Dental Visit

◆ Make the dental visit as pleasant as possible for the child.

◆ Children are told that the dental hygienist and dentist help them take good care of their teeth.

◆ Parents are instructed to avoid using negative words, such as "hurt, pain, and don't be scared."

◆ When the child is not present, parents are asked if the child has any fears or has had any prior negative experiences.

B. Positioning

◆ For young preschoolers (3-years-old) utilization of the knee-to-knee positioning may still be needed.

◆ May sit in the dental chair without any problems and can be encouraged with "being a big girl or boy."

◆ The dental chair possibly may be modified by removing the head rest or a portion of the backrest to better fit the child.

C. Parental Involvement

◆ Determine the expected developmental milestones of the child according to the chronological age, as outlined in Table 47-2.[11]

◆ Ask parents to identify actual developmental milestones so appropriate management can be initiated during the appointment.

◆ Ask parents to provide a general statement regarding the child's temperament and ability to cooperate.

◆ Evaluate whether the parent needs to accompany the child into the treatment room.

III. School-Age Children (6–11 Years of Age)

◆ Can be an active participant in the dental care visit.

◆ May still display signs of anxiety or uncooperativeness.

◆ Typically, once a child is in school full time having a parent present during their appointments is no longer necessary.

TABLE 47-1 • Oral Soft and Hard Tissue Conditions/Pathology in Children Approximately 6 Months to 5 Years

CONDITIONS	FINDINGS	SIGNIFICANCE
Soft Tissue		
Eruption cysts	Translucent, smooth; may appear blue to blue-black if bleeding in cystic space	Usually no treatment
Mucocele	Lower lip, floor of mouth, buccal mucosa most common in order of occurrence; fluid-filled vesicle or blister; trauma, tearing of minor salivary duct	May resolve or require surgical excision
Traumatic ulcer	Ulceration of the tongue, cheek, or lip after 24 hr of a dental appointment with local anesthesia	Due to patient chewing or biting soft tissue when area is numb; complications are rare, should be see within 24 hr; clean wound; warm saline mouthrinse; possible suture
Alveolar abscess	Smooth, red or yellowish nodule; tender; primary teeth—more diffuse infections; may be acute or chronic	Radiographic evaluation, drainage, and antibiotic may be required
Acute herpetic gingivostomatitis	Initially, yellow or white fluid-filled vesicles, which in a few days rupture and form painful ulcers; 1–3 mm diameter; whitish gray membrane cover; circumscribed area of inflammation; may have a fever; regional lymphadenopathy; diffuse, swollen erythematous gingiva; poor appetite; dehydration	Urgent care resolves in 10–14 d; antiviral medication; mild topical anesthetic; systemic analgesics; fluids; monitor for dehydration
Geographic tongue	Red, smooth areas devoid of filiform papillae on dorsum of tongue; margins well developed, slightly raised; pattern changes	No treatment; brush tongue to reduce bacteria
Verruca vulgaris	Multiple white sessile lesions; fingerlike projections, rough surface; human papilloma virus in origin	May resolve spontaneously or require excision
Teeth		
Enamel hypoplasia	Disturbance of enamel matrix during tooth development; irregular to round pits of varying size on enamel, usually in a row; multiple causes	Esthetics
Fluorosis	Infrequent in primary dentition; may be seen in cervical region of second primary molars; appearance ranging from fine white flecks to brown opaque lesions and/or pitting	Esthetics; daily biofilm removal
White-spot lesions	Opaque enamel, usually cervical and proximal areas of teeth at contacts; earliest clinical sign of the carious process; indicates that the surface and underlying enamel are demineralized	Twice daily biofilm removal with a fluoridate toothpaste; professional topical fluoride treatment every 3 mo; diet counseling; use of xylitol
Fused teeth	Usually limited to anterior teeth; union of two independently forming primary tooth buds; familial tendency	Possible caries at point of fusion; may be absence of one of corresponding permanent teeth
Gemination	More common in primary teeth; invagination of single tooth germ; bifid crown on single root; crown appears wide	None

Source: McDonald RE, Avery DR, Dean JA. *Dentistry for the Child and Adolescent.* 10th ed. Maryland Heights, MO: Mosby Elsevier; 2016:40, 41,49-53,71, 162-164, 245, 283, 603-604, 609.

◆ Child's dentition may be all primary or mixed dentition, or by 11 or 12 years of age all permanent dentition depending on individual development.

◆ Examine the need for pit and fissure sealants.

◆ A periodontal assessment needs to be completed even if there is no bone loss. Child may have pockets, bleeding, and subgingival calculus.

◆ Child is starting to develop independent skills and ability to perform their own oral care.

◆ Continue to avoid the use of negative words.

◆ Avoid lecturing or reprimanding with a negative tone. Suggest, advise, and highlight the positive.

◆ Use of pictures for explaining proper oral hygiene, calculus, and biofilm may help the child understand.

TABLE 47-2 • Milestones in Child Development: 12 Months to 5 Years

AREAS	12 MONTHS	18 MONTHS	2 YEARS	3 YEARS	4 YEARS	5 YEARS
Language/communication	• Responds to simple spoken requests • Uses simple gestures, like shaking head "no" or waving "bye-bye" • Makes sounds with changes in tone (sounds more like speech) • Says "mama" and "dad" and exclamations like "uh-oh!" • Tries to say words you say	• Says several single words • Says and shakes head "no" • Points to show someone what he wants	• Points to things or picture when they are named • Know names of familiar people and body parts • Says sentences with two to four words • Follows simple instructions • Repeats words overheard in conversation • Points to things in a book	• Follows instructions with two or three steps • Can name most familiar things • Understands words like "in," "on," and "under" • Says first name, age, and sex • Names a friend • Says words like "I," "me," "we," and "you," and some plurals (cats, dogs, cars) • Talks well enough for strangers to understand most of the time • Carries on a conversation using two to three sentences	• Knows some basic rules of grammar, such as correctly using "he" and "she" • Sings a song or says a poem from memory such as the "Itsy Bitsy Spider" or the "Wheels on the Bus" • Tells stories • Can say first and last name	• Speaks very clearly • Tells a simple story using full sentences • Uses future tense; for example, "Grandma will be here" • Says name and address
Movement/physical development	• Gets to a sitting position without help • Pulls up to stand, walks holding on to furniture. • May take a few steps without holding on • May stand alone	• Walks alone • May walk up steps and runs • Pulls toys while walking • Can help undress herself • Drinks from a cup • Eats with a spoon	• Stand on tiptoe • Kicks a ball • Begins to run	• Climbs well • Runs easily • Pedals a tricycle (three-wheel bike) • Walks up and down stairs, one foot on each step	• Hops and stands on one foot up to 2 sec • Catches a bounced ball most of the time • Pours, cuts with supervision, and mashes own food	• Stands on one foot for 10 sec or longer • Hops; may be able to skip • Can do a somersault • Uses a fork and spoon and sometimes a table knife • Can use the toilet on her own • Swings and climbs

(Continues)

803

TABLE 47-2 • Milestones in Child Development: 12 Months to 5 Years (Continued)

AREAS	12 MONTHS	18 MONTHS	2 YEARS	3 YEARS	4 YEARS	5 YEARS
Social/emotional	• Shy/nervous with strangers • Cries when mom or dad leaves • Has favorite things and people • Shows fear in some situations • Hands you a book when he wants to hear a story • Repeats sounds or actions to get attention • Puts out arm or leg to help with dressing • Plays "peak-a-boo" or "pat-a-cake"	• Likes to hand things to others as play • May have temper tantrum • May be afraid of strangers • Shows affection to familiar people • Plays simple pretend, such as feeding a doll • May cling to caregivers in new situations • Points to show others something interesting • Explores alone but with parent close by	• Copies others, especially adults and older children • Gets excited when with other children • Shows more and more independence • Show defiant behavior (doing what he has been told not to) • Plays mainly beside other children, but is beginning to include other children, such as chase games	• Copies adults and friends • Shows affection for friends without prompting • Takes turns in games • Shows concern for a crying friend • Understands the idea of "mine" and "his" or "hers" • Shows a wide range of emotions • Separates easily from mom and dad • May get upset with major changes in routine • Dresses and undresses self	• Enjoys doing new things • Play "Mom" or "Dad" • Is more creative with make-believe play • Would rather play with other children than by himself • Cooperates with other children • Often can't tell what's real and what's make-believe • Talks about what she likes and what she is interested in	• Wants to please friends • Wants to be like friends • More likely to agree with rules • Likes to sing, dance, and act • Is aware of gender • Can tell what's real and what's make-believe • Shows more independence (e.g., may visit a next-door neighbor by himself [adult supervision is still needed]) • Is sometimes demanding and sometimes very cooperative
Cognitive (learning, thinking, problem-solving)	• Explores things in different ways, like shaking, banging, throwing • Finds hidden things easily • Looks at the right picture or thing when it's named • Copies gestures • Starts to use things correctly: drinks from a cup, brushes hair • Bangs two things together • Puts things in a container; takes things out of a container • Let's things go without help • Pokes with index finger • Follows simple directions like "pick up the toy"	• Knows what ordinary things are for (telephone, brush, spoon) • Points to get the attention of others • Shows interest in a doll or stuffed animal by pretending to feed • Points one body part • Scribble on his own • Can follow one-step verbal commands without any gestures (sits when you say "sit down")	• Finds things even when hidden under two or three covers • Begins to sort shapes and colors • Completes sentences and rhymes in familiar books • Plays simple make-believe games • Builds towers of four or more blocks • Might use one hand more than the other • Follow two-step instructions such as "Pick up your shoes and put them in the closet" • Names items in a picture book such as a cat, bird, or dog	• Can work toys with buttons, levers, and moving parts • Plays make-believe with dolls, animals, and people • Does puzzles with three or four pieces • Understand what "two" means • Copies a circle with pencil or crayon • Turns book pages one at a time • Builds towers of more than six blocks • Screws and unscrews jar lids or turns door handle	• Names some colors and some numbers • Understands the idea of counting • Starts to understand time • Remembers parts of a story • Understands the idea of "same" and "differed" • Draws a person with two to four body parts • Uses scissors • Starts to copy some capital letters • Plays board or card games • Tells you what he thinks is going to happen next in a book	• Counts 10 or more things • Can draw a person with at least six body parts • Can print some letters or numbers • Copies a triangle and other geometric shapes • Knows about things used every day, like money and food

Source: Centers for Disease Control and Prevention. Learn the signs. Act early. https://www.cdc.gov/ncbddd/actearly/index.html. Published November 3, 2017. Accessed January 21, 2018.

♦ When teaching brushing and flossing techniques, demonstrate the techniques to the child and have the child demonstrate their ability to perform; modify as needed.

IV. Adolescents (11–18 Years of Age)

♦ Dental hygiene services provided during adolescence can impact oral health throughout the patient's lifetime.

♦ Adolescent's dentition is all permanent dentition.

♦ Need to assess for periodontal issues and diseases at each hygiene visit.

♦ May respond and wish to be treated as adults or as children at different times.

♦ Are learning to adapt to body changes, sexual impulses, secondary sex characteristics, and independence.

♦ May exhibit the different characteristics to one degree or another. Table 47-3 lists factors related to the psychological development of adolescents.

♦ May have anxiety due to family issues (i.e., divorce), school performance, sexual issues, peer pressures, violence, or substance abuse.

♦ Concern over physical characteristics and personal appearance. Want to dress/be like their peers.

♦ Teachers, coaches, and health professionals can have a powerful impact with this age group.

♦ Additional communication strategies for motivating adolescent patients are discussed in Chapter 3.

COMPONENTS OF THE DENTAL HYGIENE VISIT

Components of the dental visit are essentially the same for all pediatric patients. A clinical examination and diagnostic tools are utilized during a dental hygiene appointment to assess the child's overall oral health based on age and developmental milestones.

TABLE 47-3 • Psychosocial Development of Adolescents			
	EARLY ADOLESCENCE APPROXIMATELY 11–13 YEARS OF AGE	**MIDDLE ADOLESCENT APPROXIMATELY 14–17 YEARS OF AGE**	**LATE ADOLESCENT APPROXIMATELY 18–21 YEARS OF AGE**
Environment	• Home • Middle school • Extracurricular activities	• Home • High school • Extracurricular activities/employment	• Home/dorm • Secondary education • Employment
Identity/independence	• Struggles with identity • Increased need for privacy • Desire for independence	• Self-involvement increases; continual change between high expectations and poor self-concept • Tendency to distance selves from parents/parent conflicts peak • Continual drive for independence	• Firmer sense of identity • Increased independence or completely independent • Self-reliant
Physical	• Puberty is beginning • Physical growth: height and weight • Uncertain about changing appearance	• Puberty is complete • Physical growth continues for males, decreases for females as puberty progresses • Continued uncertainty regarding physical changes/appearance	• Females typically fully developed • Males continue to physically change (hair, muscle mass, height, weight) • Acceptance of pubertal changes
Cognitive	• Growing abstract thinking • Deeper moral thinking • Intellectual interests become more important and expand	• Continued growth of abstract thinking • Ability to set goals • Interest in moral reasoning	• Ability to think ideas through • Think or be interested about the future • Continued interest in moral reasoning
Peers	• Intense relationships with same sex friends • Increased influences of peer groups • Worried about being "normal"	• Need for friends, reliance of friends, and need to fit in/popularity • Increased sexual activity and experimentation • Risk-taking behaviors	• Peer relationships important • Development of intimate/serious relationships

Sources: AACAP. *Facts for Families.* Washington, DC: American Academy of Child & Adolescent Psychiatry; 1952–2013. AACAP Facts for Families: Normal Adolescent Development Part 1, No. 57; December 2015. https://www.aacap.org/AACAP/Families_and_Youth/Facts_for_Families/FFF-Guide/Normal-Adolescent-Development-Part-I-057.aspx and AACAP. *Facts for Families.* Washington, DC: American Academy of Child & Adolescent Psychiatry; 1952–2013. AACAP Facts for Families: Normal Adolescent Development Part II, No. 58; December 2015. https://www.aacap.org/AACAP/Families_and_Youth/Facts_for_Families/FFF-Guide/Normal-Adolescent-Development-Part-II-058.aspx.

I. Initial Interview/New Patient Visit

◆ Parents are seated in a quiet, private place so they can concentrate and feel comfortable while supplying the information requested.

◆ As rapport is established with the parent(s), an explanation is given as to why the information is needed.

◆ The initial medical and family history information is collected and reviewed.

II. Child and Family Medical/Dental History

A. Family Configuration

◆ Number of people in the household and their relationship to the child.

◆ Other caregivers, the time periods, and location.

◆ Socioeconomic status and educational level of parents/guardians.

B. Medical History of the Child

◆ An accurate, comprehensive, and up-to-date medical history is necessary for correct diagnosis and effective treatment planning.[8]

◆ Refer to Chapter 11 regarding the medical health history process.

◆ Other health problems: The child patient with diabetes; cardiovascular disease; a mental, physical, or sensory disability; or other systemic involvement requires special adaptations of procedures as described in the various chapters of Section IX of this book.

◆ Dental caries and periodontal disease infections of parents and children.

III. Intraoral and Extraoral Examination

◆ Table 47-1 lists child age-specific soft tissue and hard tissue conditions/pathology and identifies significance to dental hygiene care.[10]

◆ Evaluate head and extremities for any abnormalities or signs of child abuse.

◆ Refer to Chapter 13 for performing the intra- and extraoral examination.

IV. Developing Dentition, Occlusion, and Temporomandibular

A. Evaluation

◆ Retract the lips to expose facial aspect to evaluate cervical areas for demineralization.

◆ Assess and document amount of biofilm present and any discolorations.

◆ Document tooth eruption delays compared with normal averages (Table 47-4).

◆ Chapter 16 identifies general features to observe when examining the child's teeth.

◆ Adequate spacing for developing dentition.

◆ Classification of occlusion.

TABLE 47-4 • Tooth Development and Eruption: Primary Teeth

TOOTH	HARD TISSUE FORMATION BEGINS (WEEKS IN UTERO)	ENAMEL COMPLETED (MONTHS AFTER BIRTH)	ERUPTION (MONTHS)	ROOT COMPLETED (YEAR)
Maxillary				
Central incisor	14	1½	10 (8–12)	1½
Lateral incisor	16	2½	11 (9–13)	2
Canine	17	9	19 (16–22)	3¼
First molar	15½	6	16 (13–19 in boys; 14–18 in girls)	2½
Second molar	19	11	29 (25–33)	3
Mandibular				
Central incisor	14	2½	8 (6–10)	1½
Lateral incisor	16	3	13 (10–16)	1½
Canine	17	9	20 (17–23)	3¼
First molar	15½	5½	16 (14–18)	2¼
Second molar	18	10	27 (23–31 in boys; 24–30 in girls)	3

Source: Reprinted with permission from Lunt RC, Law DB. A review of the chronology of deciduous teeth. *J Am Dent Assoc.* 1974;89:372.

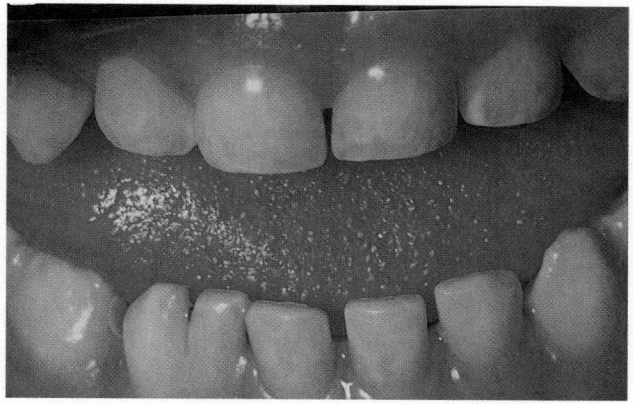

FIGURE 47-1 • Developmental Disturbance of Primary Teeth. Germination of mandibular right lateral incisor caused by invagination of a single tooth germ and resulting in a notched and grooved crown.

◆ Look for malformations (Table 47-1 and Figure 47-1) and dental caries (Figure 47-2).

◆ Loss of teeth and condition of present restorations.

◆ Evaluation of pits and fissures for indication for sealants or repair of previously placed sealants.

◆ Temporomandibular joint (TMJ) disorder for clicking, popping, grinding, or discomfort upon opening, closing, or mastication.

B. Indications for Referral

◆ Severely crowded, malposed, or congenitally missing teeth.

◆ Overbite, overjet, crossbites, or other malocclusions requiring intervention.

◆ Early loss of primary molars: This condition, if untreated, usually disrupts the eruption and alignment of permanent molars and premolars, as depicted in Figure 47-3.

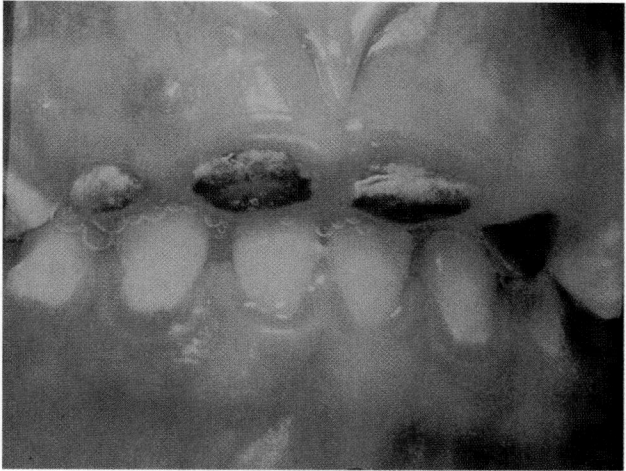

FIGURE 47-2 • Severe Early Childhood Caries. Nearly complete loss of tooth structure of maxillary incisors. Note the abscess on the gingival tissues between the maxillary right central and lateral incisor, and the cervical biofilm on the mandibular incisors.

V. Radiographic Assessment

Radiographs are a valuable diagnostic tool to aid in the overall oral health and developing an individualized treatment plan of the infant, child, or adolescent dental needs.

A. Radiographic Needs

◆ The dentist's professional judgment and ADA/Food and Drug Administration guidelines to prescribing needed dental radiographs for the child (see Chapter 15).

◆ A patient's age is not the indicator for initial radiographic needs.

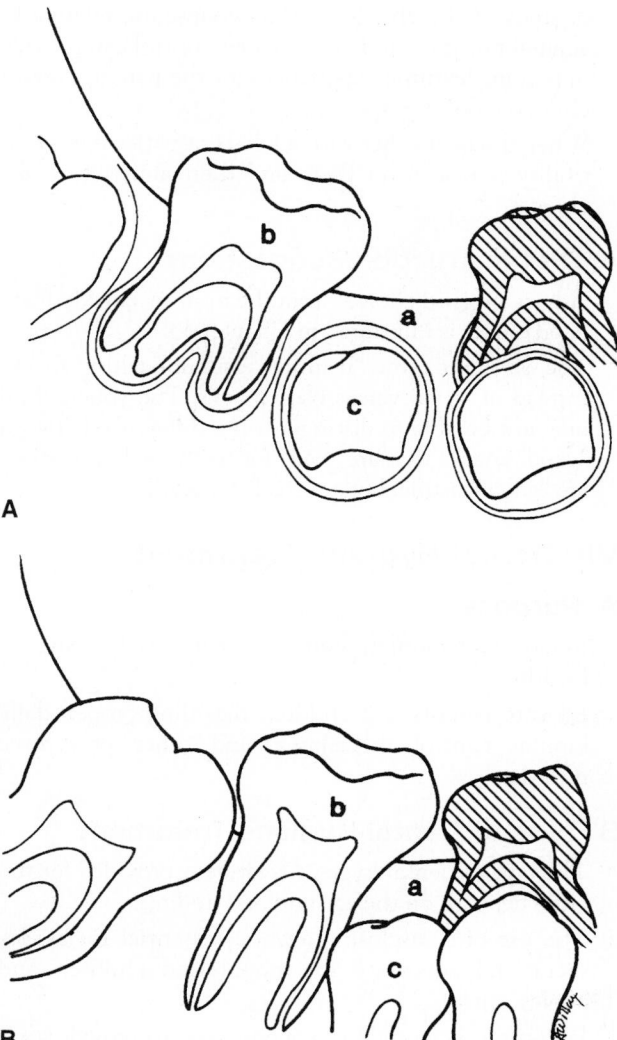

FIGURE 47-3 • Premature Loss of Second Primary Molar. A: Developing first permanent molar (*b*) inclines and drifts mesially into the space (*a*) from which the second primary molar was removed. Developing second permanent premolar (*c*) is crowded. **B:** Space from which molar was removed (*a*) is nearly closed by the mesial drift and eruption of the first permanent molar (*b*). Developing second premolar (*c*) is closed in and prevented from eruption. Note that the second permanent molar has impacted against the first molar.

◆ Each child is unique and the need can only be determined by the dentist after reviewing the patient's medical and dental histories, completing a clinical examination, and assessing the patient's vulnerability to environmental factors that affect oral health.

B. Cooperation

◆ Each child is different. Cooperation may depend on age and previous dental experiences.

◆ Use of tell–show–do, assistance of a parent, dental assistant or dentist, and/or using holding devices (see Chapter 15) will aid in taking radiographs.

VI. Dietary Assessment

◆ A study of the child's diet and counseling relative to general nutrition and dental caries control can provide important learning experiences for the parent, parent/child, or adolescent.

◆ When discussing diet with adolescent patients, responsibility is placed on them and their ability to make choices.

A. Diet Instruction Suggestions

◆ Advice on food choices from the most recent My Plate Food Guide is illustrated in Chapter 33.

◆ The use of the terms "healthy versus unhealthy" snacks instead of "good versus bad" snacks. The young child may not be able to distinguish the difference between "good" snacks that are "bad" for teeth, such as cookies are "good" tasting, but are "bad" for teeth.

VII. Dental Hygiene Treatment

A. Purpose

◆ Removal of biofilm, stain, and calculus for gingival health.

◆ Educate parents and children regarding proper, daily biofilm control procedures, and other preventive measures.

B. Type of Dental Hygiene Treatment

◆ The type of dental hygiene treatment provided for the child depends on the age and oral findings.

◆ The use of a disclosing agent is essential for assessment and education for school-aged children and adolescents.

◆ Perform at beginning of appointment to provide a visual tool for children to understand the presence of biofilm and removal with toothbrushing technique.

◆ Frequency of dental hygiene treatment is based on assessment of caries risk and periodontal health.

C. Instrumentation

◆ Presence of calculus is evaluated at each hygiene appointment for all ages.

◆ Removal of all local irregularities, including inadequate margins of restorations.

◆ When ultrasonic scaling is utilized for a pediatric patient with mixed dentition, it is only used on permanent teeth, never primary teeth.

◆ Ultrasonic scaling is effective for localized moderate-to-heavy calculus and orthodontic patients.

VIII. Prevention

A. Fluoride

Fluoride contributes to the prevention, inhibition, and reversal of caries.[12] Refer to Chapter 34 for additional fluoride information.

◆ *Professional application:*
  • Well water and nonfluoridated city water—have tested for fluoride level.
  • Use of nonfluoridated bottle water or water systems using reverse osmosis.
  • Application of professional fluoride treatment is based on the child's caries risk.
  • Children with moderate caries risk need to receive a professional fluoride application every 6 months; high caries risk receive at a greater frequency of 3–6 months.[9]

◆ *Supplementation:*
  • Fluoride supplementation may be considered if fluoride exposure is not optimal. The ADA and the AAPD guidelines are used for supplementation recommendations (see Chapter 34).
  • For children with moderate caries risk, over-the-counter fluoride rinses can be recommended as a supplement to daily brushing.

◆ Prescription fluoridated toothpaste is recommended for children with high risk or who have numerous carious lesions on proximal surfaces.

◆ A daily application of a fluoride gel in a custom-made tray may be necessary in select cases.

◆ *Fluorosis:*
  • Dental fluorosis occurs as a result of excess fluoride ingestion during tooth formation.[13]
  • Enamel fluorosis and primary teeth fluorosis can only occur when teeth are forming.[14]

B. Dental Sealants[15,16]

◆ As many as 90% of dental caries in school-aged children occurs in pits and fissures.

◆ Dentition is evaluated periodically for development defects and deep pits and fissures that may contribute to caries risk.

◆ Dental sealant is evaluated for repair or replacement as part of a periodic dental examination.

◆ Complete information about dental sealants can be found in Chapter 35.

C. Antibacterial Therapeutic Mouthrinses[17]

◆ Children younger than 6 years of age should not use mouthrinse, unless directed by a dentist, because they may swallow large amounts of the liquid inadvertently.

◆ Are available over-the-counter and by prescription, depending on the formulation.

◆ There are mouthrinses available that help reduce or control plaque, gingivitis, bad breath, and tooth decay.

◆ With over-the-counter products, look for mouthrinses that have the ADA Seal of Acceptance. The Seal shows that a product is safe and effective for the purpose claimed.

◆ Mouthrinses do not take the place of optimal brushing and flossing.

◆ Parent/main caregiver of the child may rinse at bedtime with a 0.12% chlorhexidine gluconate for 1 week per month to decrease risk of transferring cariogenic bacteria.[18]

PERIODONTAL RISK ASSESSMENT

I. Gingival and Periodontal Evaluation

Nondestructive gingival inflammation in childhood without appropriate intervention may progress to more significant periodontal diseases seen in adults.[19] The risk of periodontal disease is lowered by establishing excellent oral hygiene habits in children, which will carry over to adulthood.

◆ *Periodontal evaluation*
  • Significant changes occur in the periodontium as the dentition changes from primary to permanent teeth.[19]
  • Periodontal probing, periodontal charting, and radiographic periodontal diagnosis should be a consideration when caring for the adolescent.[20]
  • The extent and nature of the periodontal evaluation is determined professionally on an individual basis.[20]
  • Routine periodontal screening and probing is indicated following the eruption of permanent incisors and first molars.[21]
  • The use of the periodontal screening and recording (PSR) method can facilitate the early detection of periodontal diseases in children and the need for a comprehensive periodontal examination.[22] See Chapter 20 for more information about the PSR.

II. Periodontal Infections

◆ Significant changes occur in the periodontium as the dentition changes from primary to permanent teeth.[19]

◆ Adolescents are at risk for periodontal infections and gingival problems.

◆ Careful probing and study of radiographs are indicated for each patient.

◆ Emphasis is placed on preventive measures, early assessment, early treatment, and regular maintenance appointments.

◆ Development stages of gingivitis and periodontitis are discussed in Chapter 19.

A. Biofilm-Induced Gingivitis

◆ Most common periodontal disease among children.

◆ Incidence and severity may increase during puberty.

◆ Clinical changes and hormonal changes related to increased dental biofilm.

◆ Exaggerated response to dental biofilm.

B. Risk Factors for Periodontitis[23]

◆ Genetic factors.

◆ Host immune factors.

◆ Infrequent, inadequate dental and dental hygiene care.

◆ Local factors: supragingival and subgingival calculus; dental biofilm accumulations.

◆ Oral hygiene personal habits of care.

◆ Orthodontics—fixed or removable.

◆ Pathogenic microorganisms, viruses.

◆ Socioeconomic influences.

◆ Systemic diseases such as diabetes and hematological diseases.

◆ Untreated dental caries and defective restorations.

◆ Use of tobacco.

CARIES RISK ASSESSMENT

A caries management by risk assessment (CAMBRA) process uses a questionnaire to interview the parent and/or child in combination with other assessment data to determine caries risk level (see Table 47-5).

I. Purpose

◆ To identify and decrease contributing factors (biological and clinical findings).

◆ Identify current protective factors.

◆ Classifies the child's risk level (low, moderate, or high) of developing caries (see Box 47-2).

◆ A communication tool with the parent and/or age-appropriate child in discussing and eliminating risks.

◆ A balance of risk factors and protective factors is needed to prevent the progression of caries as visualized in Figure 47-4.

II. Principles

◆ Provide parent and/or patient education.

◆ Promote remineralization of noncavitated lesions by use of topical fluorides.

◆ Modify oral flora to favor oral health by use of topical antibacterial therapeutic agents.

TABLE 47-5 • Caries Risk and Protective Factors to Assess at Each Dental Visit

Assessment is based on provider's judgment of balance between risk factors/disease indicators and protective factors

CATEGORY	PATIENT AGE: 1–5 YEARS	PATIENT AGE: 6 YEARS AND ABOVE

Biological predisposing risk factors
Any one of these indicators signifies "high" overall caries risk
	• Mother/primary caregiver has active dental decay
	• Bottle with fluid other than water, plain milk, and/or plain formula
	• Continual bottle or sippy cup use
	• Child sleeps with a bottle or nurses on demand during night
	• Frequent (more than three times per day) intake of sugars, cooked starch, or sugared beverages
	• Saliva-reducing factors present, including:
	• Medications
	• Medical (cancer treatment or genetic factors)
	• Developmental delay or special healthcare needs
	• Low caregiver health literacy, Women, Infants, Children (WIC) program participant, and/or child participates in free lunch program and/or early head start
		• Visible, heavy dental biofilm
		• Frequent snacking (more than three times daily between meals)
		• Deep pits and fissures
		• Recreational drug use
		• Inadequate saliva flow by observation or measurement
		• Saliva-reducing factors:
		  • Medications
		  • Radiation
		  • Systemic/medical condition
		  • Exposed root surfaces
		  • Orthodontic appliances

Disease indicator/risk factors	• Obvious white spots, decalcification, enamel defects, or decay present • New remineralization since last examination • Past caries experience (restorations present) • Obvious biofilm or easily bleeding gingiva • Visually inadequate saliva flow	• Visible caries or radiographic penetration of the dentin • Radiographic proximal enamel lesions (not in dentin) • White spots on smooth surfaces • Caries experience (restorations) within last 3 y
Test results/saliva tests indicated for high risk	• Child: bacteria/saliva test • Caregiver: bacteria/saliva test	• MS and lactobacillus both medium or high (by culture) • Saliva flow rate
Protective factors Necessary protective factor(s) to be utilized to lower overall risk	• Lives in fluoridated community or takes fluoride supplements • Drinks fluoridated water (use of tap water instead of bottled water) • Use of fluoridated toothpaste at least once or twice daily • Fluoride varnish applied within last 6 mo • Xylitol chewing gum or application two to four times daily	• Lives in fluoridated community or takes fluoride supplements • Drinks fluoridated water (use of tap water instead of bottled water) • Use of fluoridated toothpaste at least once or twice daily • Use of 5,000 ppm fluoride toothpaste • Use of 0.05% NaF mouthrinse daily • Fluoride varnish or office topical fluoride treatment within last 6 mo • Chlorhexidine use at least 1 wk of last 6 mo • Xylitol chewing gum/lozenges four times daily during last 6 mo • Saliva flow >1 mL/min stimulated

Child's overall risk (circle): High Moderate Low
Assessed by: _____ Date: _____ Next assessment date: _____

MS, mutans streptococci; NaF, sodium fluoride.
Source: Ramos-Gomez FJ, Ng MW. CAMBRA—caries risk assessment form for age 0 to 5 years. *J Calif Dent Assoc.* 2011;3(10):723-733.

◆ Minimal restoration of cavitated lesions and defective restorations.

III. Steps

◆ Complete a caries risk assessment based on the child's specific age-related risk and preventive factors (Table 47-5).
◆ Determine level of caries risk (Box 47-2).
◆ Implement CAMBRA treatment guidelines for children aged 0–5 years, as listed in Table 47-6.
◆ CAMBRA treatment guidelines for individuals 6 years and older can be found in Chapter 25.

IV. Classification of Caries Risk

◆ Low: no or little history of carious lesions, restorations, or extractions due to caries; no risk factors indicated; adequate protective factors.
◆ Moderate: history of carious lesions, restorations, or extractions due to caries but none the last 2 years; some risk factors but show no signs of continuing caries; could easily move to high risk; some protective factors.
◆ High: one or more observable and/or radiographic carious lesions present; history of carious lesions, restorations, or extractions due to caries within last year; more

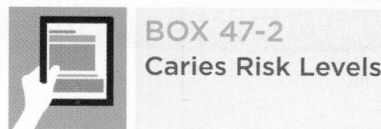

BOX 47-2
Caries Risk Levels

Low caries risk: no/little history of carious lesions, extractions, or restorations; no risk factors indicated; adequate protective factors.

Moderate caries risk: history of carious lesions, extractions, or restorations, some risk factors but show no signs of continuing caries; could easily move to high risk; some protective factors.

High caries risk: observable and/or radiographic carious lesions present; more than two risk factors; inadequate protective factors.

Extreme caries risk: high caries risk plus dry mouth or special needs.

than two risk factors; inadequate protective factors; special needs or medically compromised with parent intervention; continuous carious lesions; medications with diminished salivary function.

◆ Extreme: rampant decay; chronic medical condition or special needs; hyposalivary function; numerous risk factors, none or minimal protective factors.

V. Early Childhood Caries [24]

◆ The disease of early childhood caries (ECC) is the presence of one or more decayed (noncavitated or cavitated lesions), missing (due to caries), or filled tooth surfaces in any primary tooth in a child below the age of 6.

◆ A child below the age of 3 with any smooth-surface caries (white-spot lesion or cavitated lesion) is indicative of severe early childhood caries (S-ECC).

◆ This form of caries is usually seen in children who routinely have been given a bottle when going to sleep containing a cariogenic liquid (formula, milk, or juice) or have experienced prolong at-will breastfeeding.

◆ Nursing bottle caries, baby bottle tooth decay, and rampant caries are older terms. The AAPD adopted the term "ECC" to reflect the multifactorial etiology (frequency, tooth-adherent-specific bacteria, primarily mutans streptococci [MS] that metabolize sugars to produce acid that, over time, demineralizes tooth structure).

◆ Children experiencing caries as infants or toddlers are at higher risk for developing caries in primary and permanent teeth in the future.[25,26]

◆ ECC case definition criteria are found in Chapter 16.

A. Prevalence

◆ Tooth decay (dental caries) affects children in the United States more than any other chronic infectious disease.[27]

◆ Tooth decay affects one in four children aged 3–5 and 6–9 years who live in poverty.[28]

B. Microbiology

◆ Dental caries is a common chronic infectious transmissible disease resulting from tooth-adherent–specific bacteria, primarily MS.[27] *Lactobacilli* in large numbers are also in the dental biofilm.

◆ Transfer of MS from parent, caregiver, sibling, or other child by saliva sharing behaviors to the infant or young child.[29]

◆ Colonization of MS has been shown to occur before tooth eruption and as early as birth.[30]

◆ High levels of MS in saliva and dental biofilm are a strong risk indicator for ECC.[31]

◆ Avoid saliva sharing behaviors such as kissing on the mouth, tasting food before feeding, cleaning a dropped pacifier by mouth, and sharing of cups, toys, or utensils.[32]

C. Risk Factors

The areas of concern related to disease indicators/risk factors are listed in Table 47-5. Teaching parents about the cause and effects of ECC is a significant part of anticipatory guidance (Table 47-7).

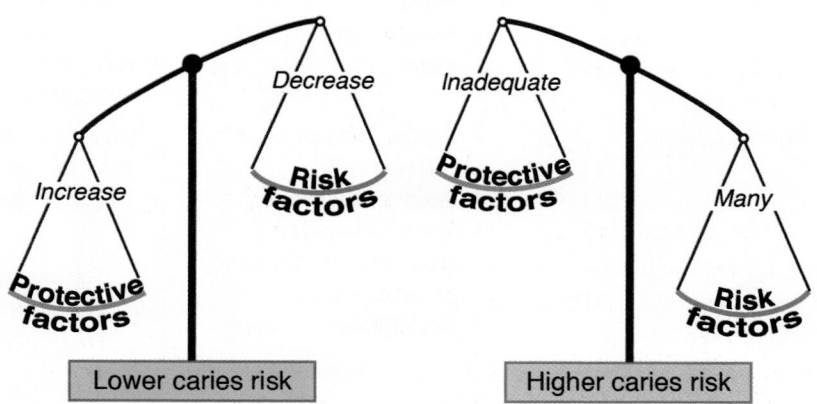

FIGURE 47-4 • Visualize the Caries Balance. Individualized assessment of risk factors can help determine the caries risk level of each patient. Providing interventions that increase protective factors such as adequate biofilm removal and fluoride exposure can change the balance and reduce caries risk.

TABLE 47-6 • Caries Management Based on Risk Level for Patients Up to Age 5 Years Old

RECOMMENDATIONS/ INTERVENTIONS	CARIES RISK LEVEL			
	LOW	MODERATE[a]	HIGH[a]	EXTREME[a]
Assessment				
Periodic oral examination	Annual	Every 6 mo	Every 3 mo	Every 1–3 mo
Radiographs—unless proximal surfaces can be visually examined	Posterior bitewings 12–24 mo interval	Posterior bitewings 12–24 mo interval	Anterior occlusal film and posterior bitewings 6–12 mo interval	
Saliva test	Optional for baseline	Suggested	Recommended	
Preventive interventions				
Fluoride: home	Fluoride toothpaste two times daily recommended: caregiver over-the-counter sodium fluoride rinses			
Fluoride: office	Not required	Varnish application at all preventive visits		
Xylitol[b] (wipes, syrup, lollipop, hard candy, mints, or chewing gum)	Not required	Recommended for both child and caregiver		
Sealants	n/a	In deep pits and fissures of fully erupted molars		
Antibacterials	n/a	n/a	Consider chlorhexidine rinse for caregiver	
Anticipatory guidance	Preventive oral health counseling and anticipatory guidance based on age-appropriate and caries risk–specific factors is recommended at all preventive visits			
Self-management goals (for parent)	Not required	Recommended		
White-spot lesions (noncavitated)	n/a	Fluoride application as indicated to promote remineralization		
Restorative interventions				
Existing lesions	n/a	**Interim therapeutic restoration** or conventional restorative treatment as patient cooperation and family circumstances allow		

[a]If the parent/guardian is noncompliant with recommended prevention protocols, assessment and radiographic intervals are decreased.
[b]Age-appropriate use of xylitol product recommendation.
Source: Ramos-Gomez F, Crall J, Gansky S, Slayton RL, Featherstone JD. Caries risk assessment appropriate for the age 1 visit (infants and toddlers). *J Calif Dent Assoc.* 2007;35(10):687-702.

TABLE 47-7 • Anticipatory Guidance: 12 Months to 6 Years of Age

AREA OF CONCERN	12–24 MONTHS	2–3 YEARS	4–6 YEARS
Developmental milestone	• Check tooth contacts • Close contacts: teach parents to floss • Normal/abnormal eruption pattern	• Primary dentition complete • Evaluate occlusion for crowding, overbite, overjet • Bruxing and occlusal wear • Evaluate for sealants on primary teeth based on caries risk	• Discuss exfoliation of primary teeth • Eruption patterns and expected new permanent teeth • Evaluate for sealants on first permanent molars
Nutrition and feeding	• Nutrition, snacking based on child's diet • Reduce snacking frequency • Review snacking safety • Avoid food as reward for behavior modification • Avoid dependence on sippy cup	• Suggest snacks from fruit, vegetable, dairy, and meat groups • Limit juice intake to 4 oz	• Snacking: suggest healthy snacks • Limit juice and soda

TABLE 47-7 • Anticipatory Guidance: 12 Months to 6 Years of Age (Continued)

AREA OF CONCERN	12–24 MONTHS	2–3 YEARS	4–6 YEARS
Oral hygiene and caries prevention	• Complete caries risk assessment • Oral hygiene index (OHI) with parent and daily oral hygiene completed by parent • Disclose for dental biofilm • Review brushing; continue with a "smear" of fluoridated toothpaste • Lift upper lip when brushing • Parents are the role models • Parents look for signs of disease • Review position of child for OH—knee-to-knee	• Complete caries risk assessment • OHI with parents and child. Parent continues with daily oral hygiene and child may "have a turn" • Ask about problems • Lift upper lip when brushing • Brush morning and night • Use a "pea"-sized amount of fluoridated toothpaste • Review signs of disease • Review position of child for OH—standing behind child	• Complete caries risk assessment • OHI including flossing with parents and child; parent continues with daily oral hygiene; child also performs brushing after parent • Review signs of disease
Fluoride information	• Update fluoride status • Store fluoride products out of reach of children • Use of small, thin smear of fluoride dentifrice on brush • Fluoride varnish application	• Parents control toothpaste • Evaluate changes in diet and water • Make appropriate fluoride recommendations • Fluoride varnish application	• Parents continue toothpaste control • Check fluoride status • Varnish applications
Trauma/injury prevention	• Car seat safety • Discuss oral electrical burns and child-proofing home • Care of avulsed tooth	• Provide trauma management plan at day care or preschool • Discuss head and neck, oral signs of child abuse • Review other safety measures (i.e., bike helmet, car seats)	• Trauma management plan at school • Review need for mouth guard • Discuss bike safety • Monitor for signs of child abuse • Review other safety measures
Habits/function behaviors	• Effects of continued thumb, finger, or pacifier sucking	• Nonnutritive sucking may still be present • Discuss elimination of thumb/finger sucking; possible early orthodontic referral	• Eliminate thumb/finger sucking; possible orthodontic referral needed
Environmental (passive) smoke	• Smoke-free environment required	• Smoke-free environment required	• Smoke-free environment required
Dental/dental hygiene visit	• Home preparation for dental visit • Frequency depends on caries risk and parent compliance with home preventive measures • Parents emphasize helping–caring nature of dentist/dental hygienist • Toothbrush dental biofilm removal • Discuss findings and recommendations with parents • Radiographic evaluation if indicated • Discuss findings and recommendations with parents	• Frequency of preventive care based on caries risk • Use disclosing solution to identify dental biofilm • Toothbrush or rubber cup dental biofilm removal • Radiographic evaluation if indicated • Discuss findings and recommendations with parents	• Frequency of preventive visits and radiographic evaluation based on risk factors • Emphasize helping–caring nature of providers • Use disclosing solution to identify dental biofilm • Assess for calculus requiring scaling • Rubber cup polishing • Discuss findings and recommendations with parents

Source: American Academy of Pediatric Dentistry. Guideline on periodicity of examination, preventive dental services, anticipatory guidance/counseling, and oral treatment for infants, children, and adolescents. [Revised 2018];40(6):104-203. http://www.aapd.org/media/Policies_Guidelines/G_Periodicity.pdf. Accessed January 27, 2018.

D. Predisposing Factors

◆ Placing bottle/sippy cup in bed.

◆ Bottle/sippy cup contain milk, formula, or sweetened fluid with sucrose.

◆ Prolonged at-will breast or bottle feeding as a sleep aid or behavioral control.

◆ Ineffective or no daily biofilm removal from the teeth.

E. Effects

◆ Maxillary anterior teeth and primary molars are the first to be affected, as noted in Figures 47-2 and 47-5.

◆ As the child falls asleep, pools of the sweet liquid can collect around the teeth.

◆ While the sucking is active, the liquid passes beyond the teeth.

◆ The nipple covers the mandibular anterior teeth; hence, they are rarely affected.

F. Recognition

◆ Demineralization or white-spot lesions may be noted along the cervical third of the maxillary anterior teeth and proximal surfaces when the upper lip is lifted (Figure 47-6).

◆ At a later stage, cavitation occurs and the lesions appear brown or dark brown (Figure 47-7). Eventually, the crowns may be destroyed to the gum line, abscesses may develop, and the child may suffer severe pain and discomfort. An advanced stage of dental caries is shown in Figure 47-2.

ANTICIPATORY GUIDANCE

◆ Anticipatory guidance is the process of providing practical, developmentally appropriate information about

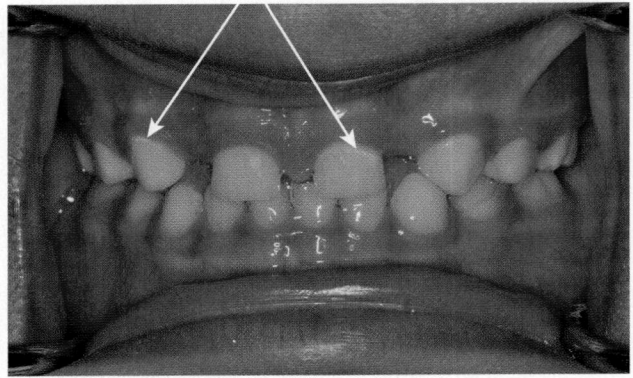

FIGURE 47-6 • **White-Spot Lesions.** Opaque, chalky enamel areas, usually on cervical or proximal areas of teeth at contacts, indicate that the surface and underlying enamel are demineralized. Subtle white lesions (indicated by the arrows) at the cervical margin of the maxillary canine and incisor provide the earliest clinical sign of the carious process. Note that the maxillary lateral incisors are missing. (Photograph courtesy of Dr. Samuel Blanchard, DDS, MS.)

children's health to prepare parents for the significant physical, emotional, and psychological milestones.[9]

◆ Involves both the parent and the child patient (when age-appropriate).

◆ Customized patient-centered recommendations presented orally, demonstration provided, and written documentation to be taken home for reference.

◆ Developmental milestones, nutrition and feeding, oral hygiene measures, dental caries prevention, health and safety precautions, and treatment measures are outlined in Tables 47-7 and 47-8.

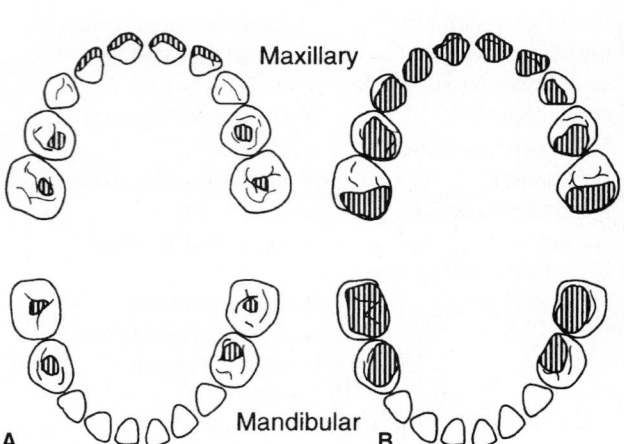

FIGURE 47-5 • **Progression of Early Childhood Caries. A:** Earliest caries affect the maxillary anterior teeth, followed by the molars as they erupt. **B:** Severe extensive lesions develop in all except the mandibular anterior teeth. Protection for the mandibular incisors and canines is provided by the tongue during the sucking process.

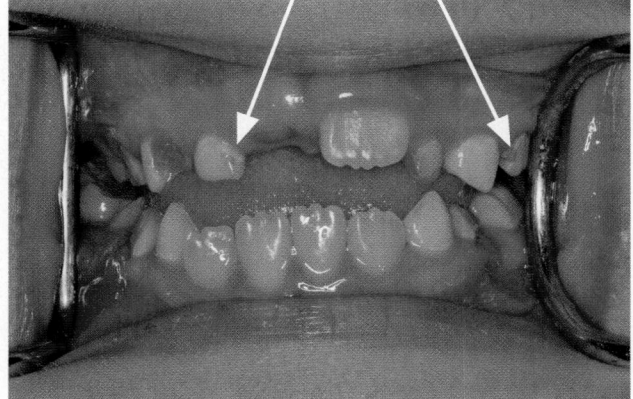

FIGURE 47-7 • **Cavitation of White Lesion Areas.** Small brownish-looking cavitated areas can be seen adjacent to white-spot lesions on the mesial–facial surface of the lateral incisor and the mesial–facial surface of the first primary molar. A large cavitated carious lesion can be seen on the maxillary right canine. Note additional white-spot lesions at the cervical margins of the maxillary left canine, the mandibular canines, and the left mandibular molar. (Photograph courtesy of Dr. Samuel Blanchard, DDS, MS.)

TABLE 47-8 • Anticipatory Guidance: 6 Years of Age to Adolescent

AREA OF CONCERN	6–12 YEARS	12 YEARS AND OLDER
Developmental milestone	• Eruption patterns; mixed dentition; missing teeth • Evaluate orthodontic needs • Evaluate for sealants on permanent molars	• Eruption patterns; permanent dentition; missing teeth • Evaluate orthodontic needs • Evaluate for sealants on second permanent molars
Nutrition and feeding	• Snacking: continue with healthy snack choices • Limit juice, soda, and sports drinks • Discussion with parent and child on hidden sugars, carbohydrate snacks, and frequency	• Snacking: continue with healthy snack choices • Limit juice, soda, and sports drinks • Discussion with parent and child on hidden sugars, carbohydrate snacks, and frequency
Oral hygiene and caries prevention	• Complete caries-risk assessment form • OHI with child; parent supervises daily oral hygiene; child performs daily oral hygiene • Reinforce daily brushing for 2 min, two times daily • Teach flossing and use of floss holders if needed; flossing daily • Review need for adjunct hygiene care products (disclosing tablets, fluoride rinses, floss threaders) • Review signs of disease	• Complete caries-risk assessment form • OHI with child; consult with parent as necessary • Reinforce daily brushing for 2 min, two times daily • Teach flossing and use of floss holders if needed; flossing daily • Review need for adjunct hygiene care products (disclosing tablets, fluoride rinses, floss threaders) • Review signs of disease
Fluoride information	• Check fluoride status • Varnish applications	• Check fluoride status • Varnish applications
Trauma/injury prevention	• Trauma management plan at school • Review need for mouth guard • Discuss bike safety • Monitor for signs of child abuse • Review other safety measures	• Trauma management plan at school • Review need for mouth guard • Discuss bike safety • Monitor for signs of child abuse • Review other safety measures
Habits/function behaviors	• Evaluation for orthodontic referral	• Evaluation for orthodontic referral
Environmental (passive) smoke	• Smoke-free environment required • Educate regarding tobacco use	• Smoke-free environment required • Educate regarding tobacco use
Dental/dental hygiene visit	• Frequency of preventive visits and radiographic evaluation based on risk factors • Emphasize helping–caring nature of providers • Use disclosing solution to identify dental biofilm • Evaluate periodontal status as permanent teeth erupt • Assess for calculus requiring scaling • Rubber cup polishing • Discuss findings and recommendations with parents • Age-appropriate counseling for substance abuse and/or smoking	• Frequency of preventive visits and radiographic evaluation based on risk factors • Emphasize helping–caring nature of providers • Use disclosing solution to identify dental biofilm • Evaluate periodontal status as permanent teeth erupt • Assess for calculus requiring scaling • Rubber cup polishing • Discuss findings and recommendations with parents • Assessment for removal of third molars • Age-appropriate counseling for: substance abuse, intraoral/perioral piercing, and/or smoking

Source: American Academy of Pediatric Dentistry. Guideline on periodicity of examination, preventive dental services, anticipatory guidance/counseling, and oral treatment for infants, children, and adolescents. [Revised 2018];40(6):104-203. http://www.aapd.org/media/Policies_Guidelines/G_Periodicity.pdf. Accessed January 27, 2018.

I. Dietary and Feeding Pattern Recommendations

A. Toddlers and Preschoolers

◆ Children need a series of small, healthy meals during the day.

◆ Healthy snacks include noncariogenic foods from the grain, vegetable, fruit, meat/meat alternatives, and dairy groups.

◆ Sweetened foods and drinks are limited to three or less per day and provided at mealtimes rather than between meals.

◆ Do not allow the child to sip or graze at will on a bottle or sippy cup containing milk or sweet liquids, which promotes demineralization and ECC.

◆ Milk and water should be the primary beverages with no more than 4-6 oz of juice per day with meals.

B. School-Aged

◆ Educate about healthy snacks and drinks; encourage tooth-healthy choices.

◆ School-aged children continue to have problems with likes and dislikes.

◆ Choices are strongly influenced by both their physical and social environments; easily accessible, parents' education, time constraints, ethnicity, eating together, TV viewing during meals, and the source of food (e.g., restaurants, schools), family, friends, and the media (especially TV) influence their food choices.[33]

◆ Parents have a direct role in children's eating patterns through their behaviors, attitudes, and feeding styles.[33]

C. Adolescent

◆ Adolescents' frequency of eating increases due to growth periods, emotional issues, or peer pressures.

◆ Cariogenic foods and drinks are often selected. Incidence of dental caries may increase during adolescence.

◆ Highest caries risk of any time in life for males; exceeded only during pregnancy for females.

◆ Inadequate nutrition is common.
  • Boys: due to over activity and poor food selection.
  • Girls: due to voluntary diet restrictions, with poor food selection and fad diets in the attempt to be trim.
  • Teens with a distorted body image may take concern to extremes.

◆ Eating disorders
  • Anorexia nervosa and/or bulimia can lead to severe health complications and even death.
  • Successful treatment usually requires an interdisciplinary team approach involving medical care, psychotherapy, and nutrition and family counseling (as described in Chapter 58).

◆ Iron-deficiency anemia
  • Common among teenage girls, particularly after the onset of menstruation.
  • Treated with iron supplements, changes in diet, or both.

II. Oral Health Considerations for Toddlers/Preschoolers

A. Gaining Cooperation

◆ At these ages, the child is becoming more independent.

◆ Parents can provide a fun activity by making up and singing a brushing song.

◆ For a 2- to 3-year-old, teach the child to take turns with the parent when brushing by using the phrase, "It's your turn to brush," followed by, "It's my turn to brush."

◆ To gain better cooperation, connect brushing with a fun activity such as first, we brush teeth and then, we read a story.

◆ Provide or recommend 2-minute timer to be used for motivation during brushing.

B. Brushing and Flossing

◆ Establish a routine: Make suggestions as to how to establish and maintain a brushing routine.

◆ Recommend brushing in the morning after breakfast and before bedtime.

◆ Specify that the most critical time for dental biofilm removal is before bedtime.

C. Parental Involvement and Supervision

◆ Parents keep fluoride toothpaste out of reach of the child and oversee/place the correct amount of toothpaste on the toothbrush.

◆ Until the child develops fine motor coordination, and can effectively remove biofilm, the parents/caregivers assist the child in cleaning the teeth by doing the brushing and flossing. The time to cease assistance depends on parental/caregiver assessment and varies markedly from child to child.

◆ Parents teach the child to brush and then evaluate to ensure effective and complete biofilm removal.

◆ Parents floss closely approximated primary teeth to remove biofilm from proximal surfaces.

D. Toothpaste

◆ Children's toothpastes manufactured in the United States contain the same amount of fluoride as adult toothpastes, whereas manufacturers in several countries around the world reduce the amount of fluoride in children's toothpastes.

◆ Parents/caregivers are informed that they need to prevent problems by controlling the amount of toothpaste used and placing it out of the child's reach.

◆ For children younger than 6 years, regularly ingesting pea-sized amounts or more can lead to mild fluorosis.[34]

◆ Appropriate amount of fluoridated toothpaste is to be used for children of all ages.[34]

◆ Children like the taste of toothpaste and may eat a large amount at one time resulting in acute fluoride toxicity.

E. Instructions for Parents

◆ An adult can brush the child's teeth with a tiny amount of fluoridated toothpaste as soon as the first tooth comes in.

◆ Children younger than 3 years old use a small "smear" of fluoride toothpaste (an amount about the size of a grain of rice), as illustrated in Figure 47-8.[34]

◆ Children who are 3 years of age and older use a "pea-size" amount of fluoride toothpaste.[34] See an illustration in Figure 47-8.

◆ Teach children to spit out toothpaste as soon as they are old enough to do so.[34]

◆ Continue to control the toothpaste and keep it out of reach.

◆ Teach parents how to examine the mouth for signs of gingival inflammation, dental caries, and injury.

◆ Evaluation of pits and fissure for caries-susceptible primary and permanent teeth (molars, premolars, and anterior teeth).

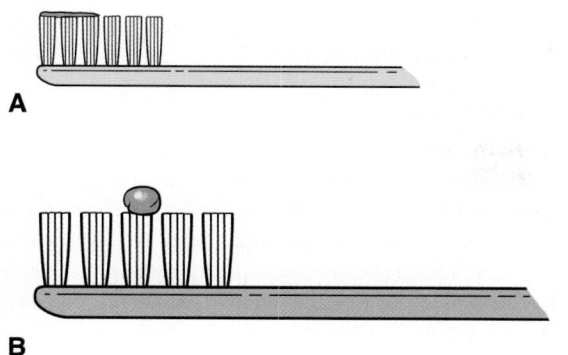

FIGURE 47-8 • Dentifrice for a Child. For children below 3 years of age, the parent is instructed to place a small smear of fluoridated toothpaste on a child-sized brush **(A)**. For all children aged 3–6 years, the appropriate size is that of a small pea **(B)**. The paste is spread in a thin layer over the brush surface and then spread over all of the teeth before brushing.

III. Speech and Language Development

◆ Premature loss of primary teeth, digit habits, and malocclusions can have direct implications on a child's development of speech and language.

◆ Early detection and referral can help correct speech or language development.

IV. Digit Habits

◆ Prolong thumb- and finger-sucking habits have been associated with narrow maxillary arch width, anterior open bite, posterior crossbite, increased overjet, and decreased overbite[35] (see Figure 47-9).

V. Accident and Injury Prevention

◆ Age-appropriate accident and injury prevention counseling for orofacial trauma is provided and/or evaluated at every hygiene visit.

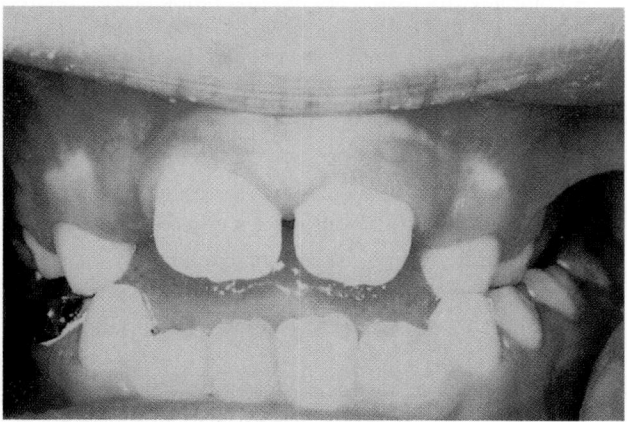

FIGURE 47-9 • Effects of Prolonged Thumb Sucking on Teeth. Anterior open bite with posterior crossbite.

◆ Written information regarding what to do in the event of a traumatic oral injury makes parents feel more prepared.

◆ Chapter 9 provides information on a dislocated jaw, facial fracture, and tooth forcibly displaced or avulsed.

A. Toddlers

◆ The greatest incidence of injury to the primary dentition occurs at 2–3 years of age. Toddlers have increased mobility and developing coordination and as a result are subject to injuries.

◆ Provide counseling regarding play objects, pacifiers, car seats, and electrical cords.

B. School-Aged Children

◆ House structures/furniture such as floors, steps, tables, and beds are most commonly associated with dental injuries in children below 7 years of age.

◆ Parents can be taught to protect the child by close supervision, anticipating problems, and making the environment safe by removing dangers.

C. Adolescents

◆ Common injuries to permanent teeth are related to car accidents, violence, and sports-related trauma.

◆ Counseling and providing athletic mouth guards for all contact sports and activities can enhance trauma prevention.

VI. Oral Malodor (Halitosis)

A. Causes[36]

◆ Biofilm build-up on the tongue and teeth.

◆ Diet.

◆ Dry mouth, low levels of saliva inhibit the ability to wash away food debris.

◆ Health conditions (e.g., infections in the nose, throat or lungs; chronic sinusitis; postnasal drip; chronic bronchitis; or disturbances in your digestive system).[37]

◆ Medications.

◆ Mouth breathing.

◆ Oral infections (e.g., dental caries, periodontal conditions, draining fistulas, oral surgery, oral sores).

◆ Smoking.

B. What to Teach Parents

◆ Explain bacterial causes.

◆ Emphasize thorough dental biofilm removal through daily brushing of the teeth.

◆ Teach how to floss their child's teeth.

◆ Show how to brush gently the dorsum of the tongue (refer to Chapter 26).

VII. Oral Health Considerations for Adolescents[20]

Increased risk for dental caries and periodontal infections during adolescence has already been described in this chapter. Some additional examples of oral problems related to adolescent development and behavior characteristics, including risky health behaviors, are listed here.

◆ Assess the presence, position, and development of third molars. Provide a referral if need of removal is indicated.

◆ Oral manifestations of sexually transmitted infections.

◆ Potential effects of hormonal fluctuations and use of oral contraceptives on periodontal tissues (see Chapter 53).

◆ Oral findings of anorexia nervosa or bulimia (see Chapter 58).

◆ Traumatic injury to teeth and oral structures.
  • Contact sports and skateboarding are risky behaviors.
  • Automobile and motorcycle accidents can also cause dental injuries.

◆ If pregnancy and parenting are issues for the adolescent patient, the dental hygienist can use anticipatory guidance to educate about important oral health issues for the mother and infant (see Chapter 46).

VIII. Tobacco/Obstructive Sleep Apnea/Piercings/Substance Abuse

◆ As the child approaches adolescence, the prevention discussion can be expanded to include the serious health consequences of tobacco use, intraoral/perioral piercings, obstructive sleep apnea (OSA), and substance abuse.

◆ Discussion of tobacco use (see Chapter 32) includes:
  • Smoking, smokeless tobacco, and exposure to second-hand smoke.
  • Current tobacco use trends (i.e., electric cigarettes, hookah).
  • Oral effects of tobacco, including leukoplakia, periodontal disease, and oral cancer.

◆ Discussion of identifiable signs, symptoms, and evaluation of OSA is a part of a child's regular clinical examination.
  • Pediatric OSA is a disorder of breathing characterized by prolonged, partial upper airway obstruction and or intermittent/complete obstruction (obstructive apnea) that disrupts normal ventilation during sleep and normal sleep patterns.[38]
  Signs and symptoms of OSA includes[38]:
    • Excessive daytime sleepiness.
    • Loud snoring three or more nights per week.
    • Episodes of breathing cessation witnessed by another person.
    • Abrupt awakenings accompanied by shortness of breath.
    • Awakening with dry mouth or sore throat.
    • Morning headache.

• Difficulty staying asleep.
• Attention problems.
• Mouth breathing.
• Sweating.
• Restlessness.
• Waking up a lot.
• Bed wetting (after at least 6 months of continence).
• Poor school performance due to misdiagnosed ADHD, aggressive behavior, or developmental delay.

◆ Referral to child's pediatrician if suspected of being at risk for OSA.

◆ Comorbidities with OSA can be cardiovascular problems, impaired growth, learning problems, and behavioral problems.

◆ Untreated OSA in combination with insulin resistance and obesity in a child sets the stage for heart disease and endocrinopathies.[39]

◆ Discussion of complications and nonreversible conditions that can result from intraoral/perioral piercings includes[40–47]:
  • Oral piercings, including the tongue, lips, cheeks, and uvula, have been associated with pathological conditions, including pain, infection, scar formation, tooth fractures, metal hypersensitivity reactions, localized periodontal disease, speech impediment, Ludwig angina, hepatitis, and nerve damages.
  • Increased plaque levels, gingival inflammation and/or recession, caries, diminished articulation, and metal allergy.
  • Life-threatening complications have been reported, including bleeding, edema, endocarditis, and airway obstructions.
  • Use of dental jewelry (e.g., grills) has been documented to cause dental caries and periodontal problems.[47]

◆ The patient who has or is considering an oral piercing is:
  • Educated regarding daily hygiene of the piercing site to avoid infection.
  • Counseled at every dental hygiene visit regarding possible complications.
  • Encouraged to remove the piercings.

◆ A complete discussion about oral complications related to the use of cocaine and other street drugs is found in Chapter 59.

IX. Referral

◆ Appropriate referrals are made when problems that require intervention by other health providers are identified.

◆ Conditions requiring referral include:
  • Evidence of systemic illness and pathology.
  • Child abuse or neglect and evidence of poor parenting skills.[48]
  • Failure to provide safety measures.
  • Substance abuse in the family.[48]

◆ Understand the reporting and licensing requirements for child abuse and neglect specific to the state.

TREATMENT PLANNING AND CONSENT

◆ The dental hygiene diagnosis is used to develop the dental hygiene care plan (see Chapters 22 and 23).

◆ Before treatment, the care plan is discussed with the dentist to integrate the dental hygiene plan into the comprehensive dental treatment plan.

◆ Inform parent/guardian of findings from the assessment and present the care plan both orally and in writing.

◆ Have parent/guardian sign an informed consent before treatment (see Chapter 23).

◆ *Medical clearance*: The parent/guardian will need to consent to medical clearance for conditions requiring antibiotic coverage, local anesthesia, or other medication for a patient under legal age.

◆ *Parental approval*: The dental hygienist care plan requires approval by the parent/guardian.

DOCUMENTATION

The following items are documented in the progress notes of pediatric patients:

◆ Overall appraisal of physical status and key health history findings.

◆ Existing pathology: soft tissue, gingiva, caries, occlusal status.

◆ Oral hygiene status and caries risk assessment.

◆ Anticipatory guidance provided, parent/patient recommendation, and any adjunct hygiene aids provided (disclosing tablets, prescriptions, proxy brush, and floss threader).

◆ Procedures completed: initial examination, recall examination, scaling and polishing, radiographs taken, type of fluoride provided.

◆ Child's behavior throughout the appointment and level of cooperation (e.g., patient's behavior quiet during appointment but cooperative with all aspects of the appointment).

◆ Treatment planned for next visit.

◆ Box 47-3 provides an example of documentation for a child's dental visit.

BOX 47-3
Example Documentation: Preventive Dental Hygiene Visit by Child Patient

S—An 8-year-old male presents for continuing care visit. Medical history reviewed w/mother. No health concerns, no medications, no chief complaint. Home care: brushing one time per day in the morning only and does not floss.

O—Intraoral/extraoral examination: within normal limits; buccal mucosa: bilateral linea alba; tongue: coated. Class II occlusion, 50% overbite, 3 mm overjet, lower anterior crowding. Clinical findings: sealants on #3, 14, 19, and 30 sound. Radiographic findings: no caries. Oral hygiene: generalized moderate biofilm, localized light calculus: supragingival mandibular anteriors—all surfaces, subgingival mandibular posterior linguals, and supra/subgingival facial of maxillary first molars. Periodontal evaluation of permanent teeth: 1–2 mm w/bleeding on probing.

A—Generalized gingivitis due to moderate biofilm, localized calculus, and generalized slight/moderate bleeding. OH is poor, "plaque-free score" = 20%, no improvement same as last visit, caries risk = low.

P—Scaled, polished, and flossed. Applied 5% sodium fluoride varnish. OHI and recommendations: using modified bass technique, two times per day brushing for 2 min w/fluoridated toothpaste, daily flossing using a floss holder, use of disclosing tablets every other day.

Goal for next appointment: "plaque-free score" improvement, and reduced areas of calculus present. Patient was well behaved and had genuine interest in improving his oral health care. Parent advised to supervise care at home.

Signed: _____, RDH

Date: _____

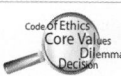

EVERYDAY ETHICS

Maria has practiced as a dental hygienist in the office of Dr. Reynolds for 3 years. She recently attended a continuing education course on dental caries risk assessment and prevention. At the course, recommendations from professionally applied topical fluoride, evidence-based clinical recommendations published by the ADA, were reviewed. She heard the results of systematic reviews on fluoride varnish, reviewed the ADA's recommendations of fluoride varnish as the only topical fluoride recommended for children below 6 years of age, and learned fluoride varnish can even be used on infants to prevent ECC.

Maria is convinced she needs to be using fluoride varnish on patients of all ages based upon caries risk. Dental hygienists at Dr. Reynolds' office are currently applying 2.0% sodium fluoride foam to patients below 18 years of age. At the weekly staff meeting, Maria presented an overview of fluoride varnish products, key research findings and a cost comparison of varnish versus fluoride tray and foam and distributed copies of the ADA fluoride recommendations. The following week, Dr. Reynolds told Maria that she had reviewed the fluoride varnish information and decided to continue using the fluoride foam and trays. When Maria asked why, Dr. Reynolds stated, "the increased costs of using fluoride varnish would really add up over a year and increasing patient fees is not an option. Anyway, patients expect to have smooth shiny teeth after dental hygiene treatment" Dr. Reynolds concluded.

Questions for Consideration

1. Because fluoride varnish is the safest professional fluoride application and recommended by the ADA for children below 6 years of age, how do the ethical principles of beneficence and nonmaleficence apply in this situation?

2. Do clinical recommendations or guidelines from professional associations, such as the ADA, constitute standards of care? Why or why not?

3. Maria has an ethical responsibility to her employer, who has expressed concerns about cost and patient acceptance of this "new" type of fluoride treatment, as well as to her patients. Which questions in the steps for resolving an ethical situation (see Chapter 1) might help Maria to balance those responsibilities as she makes a decision about an action to take in continuing this discussion with Dr. Reynolds?

Factors to Teach the Parents

▶ How the parents' own oral health affects their child's oral health.

▶ How the bacteria that cause dental caries can be transferred to the baby's mouth from parents or from other family members.

▶ How fluoride makes enamel stronger and more resistant to the bacteria that cause dental caries.

▶ Methods to prevent dental caries from developing in a young child's mouth.

▶ How feeding methods and snacking patterns can contribute to dental caries.

▶ How the parent can examine the infant's/child's mouth and what to look for during the examination.

▶ Reasons why the baby's mouth needs to be examined by an oral health professional at 6 months of age or as soon as the first tooth erupts.

▶ Reasons why maintenance of primary teeth is necessary for oral health, growth, and development.

▶ Ways parents can prepare their young children for visits to the dentist and dental hygienist.

▶ How parents can prevent accidents and injury in their infants and children.

ENHANCE YOUR UNDERSTANDING

ONLINE RESOURCES
(see the inside front cover for access information)
- Audio glossary
- Appendices

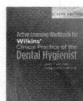

SUPPORT FOR LEARNING
(available separately)
- *Active Learning Workbook for Wilkins' Clinical Practice of the Dental Hygienist, 13th Edition*

INDIVIDUALIZED REVIEW
- Customized practice quizzing with Navigate 2 TestPrep for *Wilkins' Clinical Practice of the Dental Hygienist*

References

1. American Dental Association. Specialty definitions. In: ADA: America's Leading Advocate for Oral Health. Chicago, IL: American Dental Association; 1995–2013. http://www.ada.org/en/education-careers/careers-in-dentistry/dental-specialties/specialty-definitions. Accessed January 20, 2018.

2. HealthyChildren.org. What is a pediatric dentist? https://www.healthychildren.org/English/family-life/health-management/pediatric-specialists/Pages/What-is-a-Pediatric-Dentist.aspx. Published February 10, 2016. Accessed January 21, 2018.

3. Nickman J. An Overview of the Year Ahead for the American Academy of Pediatric Dentistry. 2018; LIII (4): 4. http://www.pediatricdentistrytoday.org/assets/3/7/2019JulyPDT.web.pdf. Accessed August 2, 2019.

4. American Academy of Pediatric Dentistry. Mission statement. https://www.aapd.org/about/about-aapd/who-is-aapd. Accessed January 21, 2018

5. American Academy of Pediatric Dentistry. Pediatrician Resources, Child Dental Health, AAPD I The American Academy of Pediatric Dentistry. https://www.aapd.org/about/about-aapd/. 2002–2018. Accessed January 21, 2018.

6. Centers for Disease Control and Prevention. Child development. https://www.cdc.gov/ncbddd/childdevelopment/positiveparenting/index.html. Published January 3, 2017. Accessed January 21, 2018.

7. American Academy of Pediatric Dentistry. Definition of a dental home. *Pediatr Dent.* 2015;39(6):12.

8. Shelov SP, Altmann TR, Hannermann RE. *Part 1.* In: *Caring for Your Baby and Young Child, Birth to Age 5.* 6th ed. Elk Grove Village, IL: American Academy of Pediatrics; 2014:395.

9. American Academy of Pediatric Dentistry. Guideline on periodicity of examination, preventive dental services, anticipatory guidance/counseling, and oral treatments for infant, children, and adolescents. *Pediatr Dent.* 2013;39(6):188-195.

10. McDonald RE, Avery DR, Dean JA. *Dentistry for the Child and Adolescent.* 10th ed. Maryland Heights, MO: Mosby Elsevier; 2016:40, 41, 49-53, 71, 162-164, 245, 283, 603-604, 609.

11. Centers for Disease Control and Prevention. Learn the signs. Act early. https://www.cdc.gov/ncbddd/actearly/index.html. Published November 3, 2017. Accessed January 21, 2018.

12. American Academy of Pediatric Dentistry. Guideline on fluoride therapy. *Pediatr Dent*. 2014;39(6):242-245.

13. Wong MC, Glenny AM, Tsang BW, Lo EC, Worthington HV, Marinho VC. Cochrane review: topical fluoride as a cause of dental fluorosis in children. *Evid Based Child Health*. 2011;6(2):388-439.

14. DenBesten P, Li W. Chronic fluoride toxicity: dental fluorosis. *Monogr Oral Sci*. 2011;22:81-96.

15. American Academy of Pediatric Dentistry. Policy on third-party reimbursement of fees related to dental sealants. *Pediatr Dent*. 2017;39(6):120-121.

16. Wright JT, Crall JJ, Fontana M, et al. Evidence-based clinical practice guideline for the use of pit-and-fissure sealants: A report of the American Dental Association and the American Academy of Pediatric Dentistry. *J Am Dent Assoc*. 2016 Aug;147(8):672-682.e12.

17. American Dental Association. Mouthwash (mouthrinse). http://www.ada.org/en/member-center/oral-health-topics /mouthrinse. Published September 13, 2017. Accessed January 22, 2018.

18. Ramos-Gomez FJ, Crall J, Gansky SA, Slayton RL, Featherstone JD. Caries risk assessment appropriate for the age 1 visit (infants and toddlers). *J Calif Dent Assoc*. 2007;35(10):687-702.

19. Carranza FA, Newman MG. *Carranzas Clinical Periodontology*. 11th ed. St. Louis, MO: Elsevier Saunders; 2012:104-110.

20. American Academy of Pediatric Dentistry. Guideline on adolescent oral health care. *Pediatr Dent*. 2013;35(6):142-149.

21. Clerehugh V, Tugnait A. Diagnosis and management of periodontal diseases in children and adolescents. *Periodontol 2000*. 2001;26(1):146-168.

22. Clerehugh V, Tugnait A. Periodontal diseases in children and adolescents: I. Aetiology and diagnosis. *Dent Update*. 2001;28(5):222-230, 232.

23. Albandar JM, Rams TE. Risk factors for periodontitis in children and young persons. *Periodontol 2000*. 2002;29(1):207-222.

24. American Academy of Pediatric Dentistry. Policy on early childhood caries (ECC): classifications, consequences, and preventive strategies. *Pediatr Dent*. 2016;39(6):59-61.

25. Peretz B, Ram D, Azo E, Efrat Y. Preschool caries as an indicator of future caries: a longitudinal study. *Pediatr Dent*. 2003;25(2):114-118.

26. Foster T, Perinpanayagam H, Pfaffenbach A, Certo M. Recurrence of early childhood caries after comprehensive treatment with general anesthesia and follow-up. *J Dent Child*. 2006;73(1):25-30.

27. Water, Sanitation & Environmentally-Related Hygiene. Centers for Disease Control and Prevention. Hygiene-related diseases. https://www.cdc.gov/healthywater/hygiene/disease /dental_caries.html. Published September 22, 2016. Accessed January 26, 2018

28. Dye BA, Li X, Thorton-Evans G. NCHS data briefs. National Center for Health Statistics. Centers for Disease Control and Prevention. https://www.cdc.gov/nchs/products/databriefs .htm. Published August 2012. Accessed January 26, 2018.

29. Berkowitz RJ. Mutans streptococci: acquisition and transmission. *Pediatr Dent*. 2006;28(2):106-109.

30. Wan AK, Seow WK, Purdie DM, Bird PS, Walsh LJ, Tudehope DI. Oral colonization of *Streptococcus mutans* in six-month-old predentate infants. *J Dent Res*. 2001;90(12):2060-2065.

31. Parisotto TM, Steiner-Oliveira C, Silva CM, Rodrigues LK, Nobre-dos-Santos M. Early childhood caries and mutans streptococci: a systematic review. *Oral Health Prev Dent*. 2010;8(1):59-70.

32. California Dental Association Foundation; American College of Obstetricians and Gynecologists, District IX. Oral health during pregnancy and early childhood: evidence-based guideline for health professional. *J Calif Dent Assoc*. 2010;38(6):391-426.

33. Patrick H, Nicklas TA. A review of family and social determinants of children's eating patterns and diet quality. *J Am Coll Nutr*. 2005;24(2):83-92. doi:10.1080/07315724.2005.1 0719448.

34. Wright JT, Hanson N, Ristic H, Whall CW, Estrich CG, Zentz RR. Fluoride toothpaste efficacy and safety in children younger than 6 years. *J Am Dent Assoc*. 2014; 145(2):182-189.

35. American Academy of Pediatric Dentistry. Management of the developing dentition and occlusion in pediatric dentistry. *Pediatr Dent*. 2014;39(6):334-347.

36. Bad breath: causes and tips for controlling it. *J Am Dent Assoc*. 2012;143(9):1053.

37. Kinberg S, Stein M, Zion N, Shaoul R. The gastrointestinal aspects of halitosis. *Can J Gastroenterol*. 2010;24(9):552-556.

38. Trosman I. Childhood obstructive sleep apnea syndrome: a review of the 2012 American Academy of Pediatrics guidelines. *Pediatr Ann*. 2013;42(10):195-199.

39. American Academy of Pediatric Dentistry. Policy on obstructive sleep apnea. *Pediatr Dent*. 2016;38(6):87-89.

40. Titus P, Titus S, Frances G, Alani MM, George AJ. Ornamental dentistry—an overview. *J Evol Med Dent Sci*. 2013;2(7):666-676. doi:10.14260/jemds/2015. Accessed January 27, 2018.

41. Durosaro O, El-Axhary R. A 10-year retrospective study on palladium sensitivity. *Dermatitis*. 2009;20(4):208-2013.

42. Ziebolz D. Hildebrand A, Proff P, Rinke S, Hornecker E, Mausberg R. Long-term effects of tongue piercing—a case-control study. *Clin Oral Investig*. 2012;16(1):231-237.

43. Plessa A, Pepelassi E. Dental and periodontal complications of lip and tongue piercing: prevalence and influencing factors. *Aust Dent J*. 2012;57(1):71-78.

44. Hennequin-Hoenderdos NL, Slot DE, Van der Weijden GA. The incidence of complications associated with lip and/or tongue piercings: a systematic review. *Int J Dent Hyg*. 2016;14(1):62-73.

45. Reyes P. Hole-y mouth jewelry! Piercings could lead to anterior tooth loss. *J Calif Dent Assoc*. 2008;36(9):651, 655.

46. Centers for Disease Control and Prevention, Division of Viral Hepatitis website. Hepatitis C FAQs for health professional. https://www.cdc.gov/Hepatitis/HCV/HCVfaq.htm. Accessed February 24, 2018.

47. Hollowell W, Childers N. A new threat to adolescent oral health: the grill. *Pediatr Dent*. 2007;29(4):320-322.

48. American Academy of Pediatric Dentistry. Guideline on oral and dental aspects of child abuse and neglect. *Pediatr Dent*. 2017;39(6):235-241.

48

The Older Adult Patient

Lisa M. LaSpina, RDH, MS, DHSc

CHAPTER OUTLINE

AGING
- I. Biological and Chronological Age
- II. Classification by Function
- III. Primary, Secondary, and Optimal Aging

NORMAL PHYSIOLOGIC AGING
- I. Musculoskeletal System
- II. Cardiovascular System
- III. Respiratory System
- IV. Gastrointestinal System
- V. Central Nervous System
- VI. Peripheral Nervous System
- VII. Sensory Systems
- VIII. Endocrine System
- IX. Immune System
- X. Cognitive Change

PATHOLOGY AND DISEASE
- I. Factors that Influence Disease
- II. Response to Disease

CHRONIC CONDITIONS ASSOCIATED WITH AGING
- I. Alzheimer Disease
- II. Osteoarthritis
- III. Alcoholism
- IV. Osteoporosis
- V. Sexually Transmitted Diseases
- VI. Respiratory Diseases
- VII. Cardiovascular Diseases

ORAL CHANGES ASSOCIATED WITH AGING
- I. Soft Tissues
- II. Teeth
- III. The Periodontium

DENTAL HYGIENE CARE FOR THE OLDER ADULT PATIENT
- I. Barriers to Care
- II. Assessment
- III. Preventive Care Plan
- IV. Dental Biofilm Control
- V. Relief for Xerostomia
- VI. Periodontal Care
- VII. Dental Caries Control
- VIII. Diet and Nutrition

DOCUMENTATION

EVERYDAY ETHICS

FACTORS TO TEACH THE PATIENT

REFERENCES

LEARNING OBJECTIVES

After studying the chapter, the student will be able to:

1. Describe physiologic and cognitive changes associated with aging.
2. Explain common chronic conditions associated with aging.
3. Identify common oral changes associated with aging.
4. Demonstrate best practices for communicating with the older adult patient.
5. Explain and document the dental hygiene process of care for the older adult patient.

The number of adults over 65 years of age continues to increase in the United States and is projected to grow to 98 million in 2060.[1] The first of the "baby boom" generation turned 65 in 2011. They are the first generation to benefit from systemic fluoride in community water supplies and topically in toothpastes.

- The older adult population is
  - retaining more natural teeth; many with full dentitions.
  - motivated to maintain and improve oral health.
  - seeking more preventive procedures for oral health than in previous years.[2]
- Dental hygienists will be challenged by the complex needs of the aging population.
- As the life span of individuals increases, so does the incidence of chronic diseases.
- Dental hygienists need to be competent in providing safe, preventive, and therapeutic services for the older adult patients in all types of dental settings.
- An increasing number of dental hygienists will specialize in the care of older adults and be employed in long-term care, home healthcare, and residential facilities.
- Tooth loss increases with age, but not because of the aging process.
- Dental caries and periodontal diseases are the major causes of tooth loss.
- Periodontal diseases in the older adult population represent the cumulative effects of long-standing, undiagnosed, untreated, or neglected chronic infection.
- Dental caries in the older adult population is associated with
  - Gingival recession.
  - Salivary hypofunction.
  - Use of xerostomic medications.
  - Diet in fermentable carbohydrates.
  - Poor oral hygiene.
- The use of fluoride can provide valuable protection to teeth and exposed root surfaces for all ages. It is unfortunate some older adults believe fluoride is only for children.

AGING

I. Biological and Chronological Age

- From a chronologic viewpoint, 65 years of age is the entry point for "old age." Gerontology has divided the period of 65 and older into subgroups:
  - Young-old, adults between the ages of 65 and 74.
  - Old-old, adults between the ages of 75 and 84.
  - Oldest-old, adults 85 and older.
  - Centenarians, adults over the age of 100.
  - Supercentenarians, adults over the age of 110.

- Biological age is not synonymous with chronological age:
  - Signs of aging appear at different chronologic ages in different individuals.
  - Aging is a process with many physiologic changes.
  - A person can be biologically old at age 65; others can be physically fit at age 75.

II. Classification by Function

- The degree of general health and physical activity provides a classification system, functional age, not based on chronologic age but on how the older adults actually performs various activities.
- Relative to the degree of impairment, older persons may be functionally independent, frail, or functionally dependent.
- Classification by function is more useful and is defined by activities of daily living and instrumental activities of daily living as described in Chapter 22.

III. Primary, Secondary, and Optimal Aging

- Primary aging (also referred to as normal aging): age-related changes that occur in the body's systems advancing at an individual rate. These age-related changes are universal, intrinsic, and progressive. Example: skin wrinkling.[3]
- Secondary aging (also referred to as impaired aging): age-related changes due to disease that leads to impairment. These age-related changes are associated to trauma and chronic diseases. Example: heart disease.[3]
- Optimal aging (also referred to as successful aging): aging is slowed or altered due to preventive measures to avoid negative changes. Example: eating a healthy diet and daily physical activity.[3]

NORMAL PHYSIOLOGIC AGING

- Primary normal changes with aging are physiologic.
- Secondary pathologic aging influences and accelerates the aging process.
  - Each age level brings changes in body metabolism, activity of the cells, endocrine balance, and mental processes.
  - In a healthy person, free of chronic diseases and medications with their potential side effects, the tissue changes of aging may be more subtle, appear at a later age, and be influenced by the person's lifestyle.
- Skin: thin, wrinkled, and dry, with pigmented spots, and loss of tone.
- Reduced tolerance to temperature extremes and solar exposure.

- Normal physiologic changes that occur as the individual ages are universal, progressive, intrinsic, and unavoidable. These changes vary between each individual and the body's systems.
- During aging, an overall gradual reduction in functional capacities occurs in most organs, with a decrease in cell metabolism and numbers of active cells.
- The following provides a summary of physiologic changes that occur due to the normal aging process.

I. Musculoskeletal System

- Bone volume (mass) decreases gradually after the age of 40.
- Loss of muscle function: diminished muscular strength and speed of response.
- Curvature of cervical vertebrae due to a decrease in bone density and atrophic changes to cartilage and muscle.
- Joints may stiffen because of loss of elasticity in the ligaments.

II. Cardiovascular System

- Decline in cardiac output; minimal increase in the size of the left ventricular wall.[4]
- Blood vessels become less elastic and flexible.[4]
  - Lumen of vessels decreases in size with resultant reduction of blood supply to organs, especially the liver and kidneys.
  - Increased peripheral resistance.
- Atherosclerosis (fatty deposits on inner walls of arteries) is associated with aging; diet, smoking, and lack of exercise can be an influence.
- Changes in cardiovasculature do not affect function under normal, non-stressful conditions.

III. Respiratory System

- Vital capacity is progressively diminished, leading to decreased efficiency of oxygen–carbon dioxide exchange.[5]
- Skeletal changes weaken respiratory muscles, which limit chest expansion and reduce effective ventilation.[5]
- Less effective cough reflex; increased risk for respiratory infections.[5]

IV. Gastrointestinal System

- Production of hydrochloric acid and other secretions gradually decrease.
- Peristalsis is slowed.
- Decreased absorptive functions can affect nutrition and medications.

V. Central Nervous System

- Intellectual or cognitive function is slowed, not lost.
- Complex tasks may be more difficult.
- Short-term memory declines; long-term memory remains constant.

VI. Peripheral Nervous System

- Decrease in tactile sensitivity.
- Decreased proprioception (sense of one's position in space); risk for falls.

VII. Sensory Systems

- Age-related vision changes include[6]:
  - Presbyopia.
  - Decreases in visual acuity (more light needed), peripheral vision, color clarity (problems with blues and greens).
  - Decreased dilation and constriction of pupils results in difficulty adjusting to changes in light and problems with glare.
- Age-related hearing changes include[7]:
  - Presbycusis.
  - Thicker and dryer cerumen (wax) contributes to hearing loss.
  - Decrease in the ability to hear high-frequency tones.
  - Tinnitus.
- Management of a dental hygiene patient with vision and hearing impairment is discussed in Chapter 51.

VIII. Endocrine System

- Decrease in thyroid efficiency; decreased basal metabolic rate.
- Altered thermoregulatory system; sensitive to cold; may not respond to infection with increased temperature.

IX. Immune System

- The immune system declines with age. Among individuals the degree of decline varies greatly.[8]
- Age-related changes in the skin and mucous membranes decrease effectiveness of the first line of defense against invading substances.
- Thymus gland decreases in size: decline in T-cell function.
- With age there may be an increase in autoimmune disorders.
- Changes in the immune system result in increased incidence of infections. Older adults need to seek immunizations for influenza, varicella–zoster virus, and pneumococcal pneumonia. Vaccinations for hepatitis A, hepatitis B, hepatitis C, varicella, and meningococcal infection are recommended.

X. Cognitive Change

◆ Cognitive change can distract the individual's attention away from their daily activities.[9]

◆ The older adult patient struggles with numerous demands, which can affect the ability to function, especially the ability to concentrate.

◆ Factors such as excess light and noise can distract the older adult from perceiving relevant information.

◆ Supportive interventions to aid an older adult with cognitive changes to maintain normal life activities are listed in Table 48-1.

◆ Tooth loss and gingival inflammation are associated with lower cognitive performance.[10]

PATHOLOGY AND DISEASE

I. Factors that Influence Disease

◆ An older person's health status is influenced by many factors. Biologic, environmental, psychosocial, psychologic, and lifestyle factors influence longevity.

◆ Genetically, a person may belong to a family that has exhibited resistance to disease factors.

◆ Healthy dietary habits and regular exercise can prevent or minimize disease.

◆ The following risk factors influence disease states:
  • Tobacco use: all forms.
  • Use of alcohol.
  • Obesity and overweight.

◆ Decreased immunologic functioning in aging is a factor for increased susceptibility of both men and women to human immunodeficiency virus (HIV) infection, acquired immune deficiency syndrome (AIDS), and other sexually transmitted diseases (STDs).

BOX 48-1

Characteristics of Altered Response to Disease in the Older Adult

• *Course and severity: disease may occur with greater severity and have a longer course, with slower recovery.*

• *Pain sensitivity: may be lessened.*

• *Body temperature response: may be altered so that a patient may be very ill without the expected increase in body temperature.*

• *Healing response:*
  ◆ Decreased healing capacity.
  ◆ More prone to secondary infection.

◆ Associations between periodontitis and specific systemic diseases include[11–14]:
  • Atherosclerotic diseases.[11,13,14]
  • Diabetes mellitus.[11,12,14]
  • Respiratory infections.[11,14]
  • Rheumatoid arthritis.[11,14]

◆ The incidence of disease is higher in individuals from lower educational and socioeconomic backgrounds.[15]

II. Response to Disease

◆ The diseases that affect the older adult age group also occur in younger people; however,
  • There are differences such as a lessened reserve capacity;
  • An older adult may not view the classic symptoms of disease as a younger person.

◆ Characteristics of the altered response of the older adult to disease are listed in Box 48-1.

CHRONIC CONDITIONS ASSOCIATED WITH AGING

◆ Although many older adults function well and live independently in the community, the incidence of chronic diseases increases with advancing age.

◆ Individuals may have more than one chronic illness.

◆ The most common chronic conditions are osteoarthritis, visual and hearing impairments, cardiovascular diseases, and diabetes.

◆ Because of the number of chronic conditions, patients may be taking a large number of medications (polypharmacy), which can exacerbate xerostomia and increase the possibility of drug interactions.

I. Alzheimer Disease

◆ Dementia is severe impairment of cognitive abilities, notably thinking, memory, and judgment. Alzheimer disease is a nonreversible type of dementia and the most common of all dementias.

TABLE 48-1 • Supportive Interventions to Aid an Older Adult with Cognitive Changes

SITUATION	SUPPORTIVE INTERVENTION
Physical surroundings—environmental	• Reduce clutter.
Informational	• Use 14-point font for paper and online reading materials. • Avoid unnecessary medical and legal jargon in patient reading materials. • Facilitate use of reminder devices and lists.
Behavioral	• When possible, alter situations that restrict behaviors, including transportation and mobility problems. • Provide assistive devices to promote independence and control.
Affective	• Assess for personal concerns and worries. • Manage to decrease anxiety.

A. Etiology

◆ Two types:
  • Early onset: rare, reported in individuals in their 30s and 40s.
  • Late onset: most common, in people over 65.
◆ Etiology unknown: theories include genetics, environment, nutrition, free radicals, and infectious agents.
◆ Average duration is 8–10 years from the onset of symptoms to death.

B. Symptoms and Stages

◆ The common impairments of Alzheimer disease may be divided into overlapping stages and may extend up to 20 years.
◆ Box 48-2 illustrates the progression of Alzheimer disease symptoms through stages that describes how a person's abilities change from normal function through advanced disability.

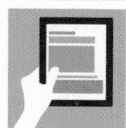

BOX 48-2
Stages of Alzheimer Disease

Stage 1: Normal Function
• No memory problems.

Stage 2: Very Mild
• Memory lapses; personal awareness of forgetting familiar words or the location of everyday objects.
• No medical diagnosis of dementia.

Stage 3: Mild
• Memory lapses; family members/friends begin to notice problems in memory or concentration.
• Observable difficulties include:
  ◆ Trouble remembering names or the right words.
  ◆ Performing tasks.
  ◆ Losing objects.
  ◆ Trouble organizing.

Stage 4: Moderate
• Able to clearly detect that there are problems.
• Observable difficulties include:
  ◆ Forgetting events and personal history.
  ◆ Increasing difficulty with complex tasks.
  ◆ Withdrawn.

Stage 5: Moderately Severe
• Noticeable lapses in memory and thinking.
• Does not remember own address/phone number.
• *Confused*; does not know what day it is.
• Still self-sufficient with eating or using the toilet.

Stage 6: Severe
• Memory worsens/personality changes.
• Observable difficulties include:
  ◆ Cannot recall recent experience.
  ◆ Trouble remembering the name of family members.
  ◆ Changes in sleep patterns.
  ◆ Needs assistance with toileting/unable to control bladder or bowels.
  ◆ Personality and behavior changes such as being more suspicious.
  ◆ Compulsive/repetitive behavior: example shredding tissue.
  ◆ Wanders easily/can become lost.

Stage 7: Very Severe
• Loss of ability to respond to environment.
• Cannot carry on a conversation or easily control movement.
• Observable difficulties include:
  ◆ Eating.
  ◆ Using the toilet.
  ◆ Smiling.
  ◆ Holding head upright.
  ◆ Swallowing.

Source: Stages of Alzheimer's Disease. Alzheimer's Association Web site. https://www.alz.org/alzheimers_disease_stages_of_alzheimers.asp#overview. Accessed January 15, 2018

◆ Keep in mind the stages are general guides; symptoms vary greatly. Not every individual with Alzheimer disease will experience the same symptoms or progress at the same rate.

C. Treatment

◆ There is no proven treatment to prevent or cure the disease.
◆ Treatment is designed to support the family as well as the patient.
◆ Requires a prolonged multidisciplinary effort.
◆ Medications are prescribed for patients with mild-to-moderate symptoms.
◆ Medications prescribed to address behavioral problems include:
  • Antidepressants.
  • Antianxiety medications.
  • Antipsychotics.
  • Anticonvulsants may be prescribed for the small percentage of individuals who have seizures.

D. Dental Hygiene Management Considerations

◆ Box 48-3 illustrates guidelines for caregivers of Alzheimer disease.

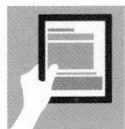

BOX 48-3
Alzheimer Disease: Guidelines for Caregivers

- Keep the same daily routine. Keep the environment calm.
- Promote the use of clocks, calendars, and newspapers to maintain the patient's orientation.
- Watch the patient's medical and oral health. Encourage exercise and regular dental visits.
- Keep communication open. Use laughter as a tool.
- Use positive reinforcement.

Source: Saxon S, Etten MJ, Perkins EA. *A Guide for the Helping Professions Physical Change & Aging.* 6th ed. New York, NY: Springer; 2014:98-99.

◆ Specific dental hygiene care considerations for the patient with early and later stages of Alzheimer disease are listed in Box 48-4.

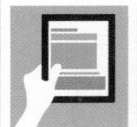

BOX 48-4
Dental Hygiene Care Considerations for a Patient with Alzheimer Disease

Early Stages
- Review of the patient's medical and dental history at each maintenance appointment may reveal lapses in memory and other signs of early disease.
- An early sign may be a slow decline of interest in oral hygiene and personal care.
- Provide routine care with initiation of aggressive preventive regimens.
- Three-month intervals for maintenance appointments are recommended.
- Topical fluoride applications; fluoride varnish.
- Oral hygiene instruction; involve caregivers early in the disease process.

Later Stages
- Routine intraoral examination to assess lesions due to cancer, medications, or injury.
- Sedation may be required.
- Possible need for mouth prop and physical restraint.
- Caregivers assume daily oral care. Power toothbrushes may improve dental biofilm removal for caregivers to use.
- Patient may reside in a long-term care facility. Dental hygienists who specialize in the treatment of this population may oversee care.

◆ Link between periodontal disease and Alzheimer disease; brain inflammation can result from periodontal bacteria and the entry of pathogen products into the brain.[16]
◆ Goals of dental hygiene care:
- Preserve oral health and function.
- Prevent future oral and systemic disease.
- Provide comfort.
◆ The dental hygiene care plan
- Considers the current stage of the patient's disease.
- Provides a plan for comprehensive care in anticipation of future decline in oral health.
◆ Undiagnosed patients: when patient's behavior is suspect, a referral to the patient's physician is made.

II. Osteoarthritis

◆ Osteoarthritis is the most common form of arthritis and involves a progressive loss of articular cartilage. Management of the patient with arthritis is discussed in more detail in Chapter 52.

A. Symptoms
◆ Intermittent joint pain.
◆ Stiffness upon arising.
◆ Crepitation (creaking joints).

B. Treatment
◆ Physical therapy.
◆ Exercise.
◆ Rest.
◆ Reduced stress on joints.
◆ Dietary modifications.
◆ Drug therapy.

C. Dental Hygiene Management Considerations
◆ Keep appointments short.
◆ Schedule afternoon appointments.
◆ Allow breaks to relax the jaw.

III. Alcoholism

A. Effects of Alcohol Use
◆ Owing to age-related primary physiologic changes, older drinkers may experience more detrimental health-related effects compared with younger drinkers.
◆ Older adults require less alcohol for adverse effects to occur.

◆ Excessive use of alcohol by older adults may[17]
  • Have more severe health-related consequences.
  • Exacerbate medical and emotional problems associated with aging.
  • Predispose to adverse drug reactions with prescription and over-the-counter medications.
  • Be associated with major depressive disorder.

B. Dental Hygiene Management Considerations

◆ Management of a dental hygiene patient with a substance-related disorder is discussed more completely in Chapter 59.

IV. Osteoporosis

◆ Osteoporosis is a bone disease involving loss of mineral content and bone mass.

◆ It is common in individuals older than age 60, and the incidence increases with age.

◆ Although most prominent in postmenopausal women, the condition may also occur at other ages and in men.

A. Causes

◆ Endocrine: hormonal disturbances; depletion of estrogen after menopause.

◆ Inadequate intake of calcium and/or vitamin D or defective absorption of calcium or vitamin D metabolism.

B. Prevention

◆ Prevention is the first line of defense against osteoporosis.

◆ Adequate calcium and vitamin D intake during adolescence and early adulthood is critical to forming peak bone mass.

◆ The minimum requirements for both calcium and vitamin D increase with age.

◆ Load-bearing exercise is necessary to maintain bone mass.

C. Risk Factors

A number of risk factors have been identified; some of which work together. From the risk factors, a list of methods for long-term prevention can be derived:

◆ Female gender; positive family history.

◆ Caucasian or Asian ethnicity (worldwide, Blacks are least affected).

◆ Low calcium and vitamin D intake (lifelong).

◆ Early menopause or early surgical removal of ovaries; use of corticosteroids; eating disorders.

◆ Sedentary lifestyle; lack of exercise.

◆ Alcohol abuse; tobacco use; high caffeine intake.

◆ High sodium intake.

◆ Low body mass index.

D. Relationship to Periodontal Disease[18,19]

◆ A relationship exists between the reduced bone mineral density of osteoporosis and oral bone loss in skeletal and mandibular bone; oral bone loss in the edentulous person pertains to[18]
  • Periodontal bone destruction.
  • Residual ridge loss.

◆ Mutual risk factors of osteoporosis and periodontal disease are
  • Smoking.
  • Nutritional deficiencies.
  • Alcohol use.
  • Hormonal status.

◆ Osteoporotic bone is
  • Less dense.
  • More readily absorbed.

E. Symptoms

Osteoporosis develops over many years; a long asymptomatic period of bone change can occur with no clinical symptoms.[19]

◆ Clinical symptoms may include
  • Backache: stooping posture. Figure 48-1 illustrates the posture of an older adult with osteoporosis.
  • Vertebral fractures or compression fractures that cause the spine to curve.
  • Fractures: hip, compression fractures of spine, ends of long bones.
  • Evidence of bone changes in the mandible: residual ridge resorption.

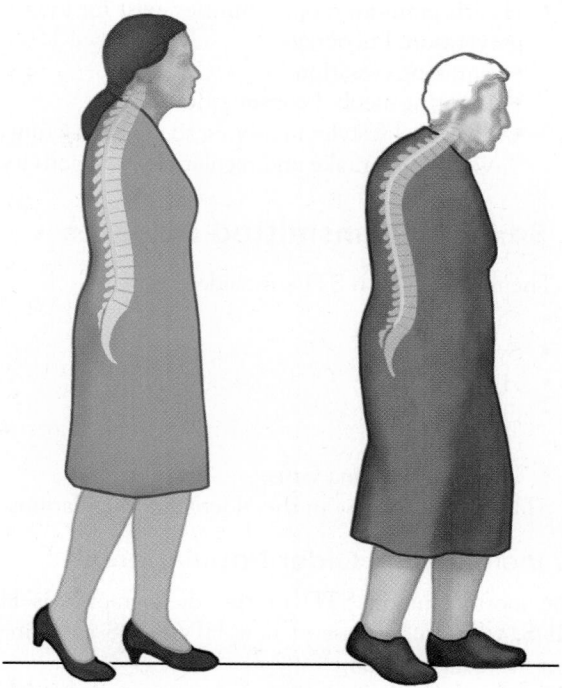

FIGURE 48-1 • Example of an Older Adult's Posture with Osteoporosis. Vertebral fractures or compression fractures cause the spine to curve.

F. Treatment/Medications

- A number of medications, with various mechanisms of action, decrease bone resorption, increase bone formation, or both.
- Whichever regimen of medications is prescribed, successful treatment and prevention requires simultaneous intake of calcium and vitamin D.
- Bisphosphonates: slows bone metabolism/increasing bone density.
- Selective estrogen receptor modulators: inhibits bone resorption.
- Calcitonin: inhibits bone resorption.
- Parathyroid hormone: stimulates bone formation.

G. Treatment and Prevention

- Weight-bearing physical activity, such as walking, has a beneficial effect on bone mass.
- Activities of daily living and physical activity require caution and preventive measures to avoid accidental falls.
- Avoid smoking and excessive alcoholic intake.
- Severe involvement of the spine may require orthopedic support and medication for pain.
- Dental hygiene management considerations:
  - Do not rush; try to prevent falls.
  - Provide extra time for positioning; provide cushioning.
  - Taking bisphosphonates is a contraindication for dental surgery due to increased risk for osteonecrosis (bone destruction) of the jaw.
  - Health promotion opportunities exist for long-term prevention. Encourage:
    - Smoking cessation.
    - Limiting alcohol consumption.
    - Healthy lifestyles involving adequate calcium and vitamin D intake and regular physical activity.

V. Sexually Transmitted Diseases

- The most common STDs include:
  - Chlamydia.
  - Syphilis.
  - HIV/AIDS.
  - Genital herpes.
  - Gonorrhea.
  - Human papilloma virus.
- STDs are on the rise in the older adult populations.

A. Incidence in Older Populations

The most common STD in this demographic is HIV/AIDS, with an increase of new HIV/AIDS cases in the over 50 years age group.[20]
- Factors that influence the increase in numbers include:
  - Increased use of medications to treat erectile dysfunction.
  - Increased divorce rate.
  - People living longer and generally in better health.

- Sexually active senior women more prone to acquiring STDs due to:
  - Thinning of the epithelium of the vaginal area.
  - Diminished immune system.
- Increased number of older adults living in assisted living centers or senior housing communities.
- Cultural and generational differences may explain why older adults are not as knowledgeable about the need for safe-sex practices.
- Older adults might not practice safe sex since the risk of pregnancy is eliminated.

B. Dental Hygiene Management Considerations

- Medical referral or consultation.
- An appointment with the patient's physician is necessary to determine what medication is needed to treat the STD.
- Goals of dental hygiene care include:
  - Open, nonjudgmental communication.[21]
  - Increased patient awareness of the transmission of STDs.
  - Importance of communication with the patient's physician.

VI. Respiratory Disease

- Older adults are at higher risk for respiratory disease.[22]
- Good oral hygiene practices can reduce the progression or occurrence of respiratory diseases among older adult patients.
- Chapter 60 provides more information regarding dental hygiene care for patients with respiratory disease.

A. Age-Related Disorders of the Respiratory System

- Pneumonia.
- Chronic obstructive pulmonary disease.
- Asthma.

B. Dental Hygiene Management Considerations

- Monitor vital signs.
- Adjust seating position as needed for comfortable breathing. Refer to Chapter 4 for information related to patient positioning.

VII. Cardiovascular Disease

- Heart disease is a common cause of death for the older adult patient over age 65.
- Health promotion and healthy behaviors initiated early can prevent heart disease.
- Chapter 61 provides more information regarding dental hygiene care for patients with cardiovascular disease.

- Age-related disorders of the cardiovascular system include:
  - Arteriosclerosis and atherosclerosis.
  - Hypertension and postural hypotension.
  - Angina pectoris.
  - Myocardial infarction.
  - Congestive heart failure.
  - Heart valve disease.
  - Transient ischemic attack (ministroke).
  - Cerebrovascular accident (stroke).
- Dental hygiene management considerations:
  - Monitor blood pressure.
  - Use of relaxation techniques.
  - Lifestyle changes.

ORAL CHANGES ASSOCIATED WITH AGING

- Healthy tissue features of primary aging need to be separated from the long-term effects of secondary aging due to chronic disease and medications.

I. Soft Tissues

A. Lips

- Tissue changes: dry, purse-string opening results from dehydration and loss of elasticity within the tissues.
- Angular cheilitis is not specifically an age-related lesion, but it is seen frequently among older adults.[23]
- Etiologic factors may be candidiasis and vitamin B deficiency.
- Appears as skin folds with fissuring at the angles of the mouth and can be related to reduced vertical dimension or inadequate support of the lips.
- Cheilitis in conjunction with dentures is described in Chapter 30.

B. Oral Mucosa

- Atrophic changes: The tissue may become thinner and less vascular, with a loss of elasticity; a smooth shiny appearance is related to thinning of the epithelium.
- Hyperkeratosis: White, patchy appearance of tissue may develop because of irritation from sharp edges of broken teeth, restorations, or dentures, and from use of tobacco.
- Capillary fragility: Facial bruises and petechiae of the mucosa are common.

C. Tongue

- Atrophic glossitis (burning tongue)
  - The tongue appears smooth, shiny, bald, and with atrophied papillae.
  - The condition is usually related to anemia that results from a deficiency of iron or combinations of deficiencies.
  - Deficiency anemia results from nutritional factors.

- Taste sensations
  - Taste buds are slower.[24]
  - The acuity of the perception for salt declines with age.
  - The perception of sweet and sour does not decline with age.
  - Olfactory acuity, which significantly affects taste, declines more than taste.
  - Flavoring agents and spices can be added to foods instead of salt and sugar to enhance taste.
  - Tongue cleaning increases taste perception.
- Sublingual varicosities
  - Clinical appearance: deep, red or bluish nodular dilated vessels on either side of the midline on the ventral surface of the tongue.
  - Significance: varicosities do not have a direct relation to systemic conditions.

D. Xerostomia

- Xerostomia, dryness of the mouth, is
  - Characterized by the absence or diminished quantity of saliva.[25]
  - Prevalent in the older adult.[26]
  - A symptom, not a disease entity.
- Lack of saliva and the effect of a dry mouth are significant contributing factors to oral discomfort and disease, particularly dental caries.
- Causes of xerostomia include:
  - Systemic medications, which provide the most common influence. Many drugs that are common prescription items produce dry mouth as a side effect.
  - Autoimmune diseases such as Sjogren's syndrome, rheumatoid arthritis, systemic lupus erythematosus.
  - Diabetes.
  - Radiation to head and neck for cancer therapy: permanent damage to the salivary glands can result.
- Clinical symptoms include:
  - Feeling of oral dryness; tongue sticks to the palate.
  - Difficulty with mastication, swallowing, and speech.
  - Impaired taste.
  - Burning, and soreness of mucosa and tongue.
- Oral effects of xerostomia
  - Heavy dental biofilm, material alba, and debris accumulation can lead to increased:
    - Severity of periodontal infection and demineralization of tooth surface.
    - Predisposition to dental caries, particularly root caries.
    - Problems of denture wearing.
    - Dietary changes during eating; may use increased quantities of liquid to soften food for swallowing.
- See Box 48-5 for a partial list of drug groups that may decrease salivary function.

E. Oral Candidiasis

- Oral candidiasis is an infection of the oral mucosal tissues.
- Denture stomatitis and angular cheilitis represent the two common forms, as described in Chapter 30.

BOX 48-5
Partial List of Classes of Drugs That Decrease Salivary Function

Anticholinergics
Antihistamines
Antihypertensives
Antianxiety
Anticonvulsants
Diuretics
Antidepressants (tricyclic)
Nonsteroidal anti-inflammatory

- Candidiasis is associated with the use of antibiotics, head and neck radiation therapy, chemotherapy, steroids, and other immunosuppressive drugs.
- Medical conditions that alter the immune system, including diabetes and HIV infection, permit overgrowth of the Candida organisms.
- Patients with xerostomia have an increased incidence of candidiasis.

II. Teeth

A. Color

- Darkening or yellowing is the result of changes in the underlying dentin.
- Color changes result from long use of tobacco and beverages such as tea and coffee.
- Dark intrinsic stains from dental restorations.

B. Dental Pulp

- Pulpal changes develop as reactions to wear, dental caries, restorations, bruxism, and other assaults during the elderly person's long life.[27]
- Narrowing of pulp chambers and root canals; increased deposition of secondary and tertiary dentin. Figure 48-2 provides examples of radiographs showing the narrowing of pulp canals with age.
- Progressive deposition of calcified masses (pulp stones or denticles).

C. Attrition

- Signs of wear, which may be long-term effects of diet, occupational factors, or bruxism.
- Attrition may be accompanied by chipping and teeth may seem more brittle.

D. Abrasion

- Abrasion at the cervical third of a tooth may result from extended use of a hard toothbrush in a horizontal direction with an abrasive dentifrice.

- With current preventive measures, use of soft-textured brushes, and attention to abrasiveness of dentifrices, future generations will be less likely to exhibit such tooth alterations.
- Figure 48-3 provides a photograph (A) and radiographic image (B) of abrasion.

E. Root Caries

- Prevalence: Older adults have more root caries than any other age group, except in communities with natural fluoride or community water fluoridation.[28]
  - A photograph in Figure 48-4 provides examples of root caries.
- Risk factors for root caries include:
  - Exposed root surfaces due to:
    - Periodontal infections that cause loss of attachment.
    - Horizontal toothbrushing technique results in abrasion.
  - Biofilm retention due to inadequate oral hygiene. Reasons include:
    - Cognitive and physical disabilities that hinder biofilm removal.
    - Inadequate oral care received.
    - Faulty restorations and partial dentures retain cariogenic food substances and biofilm.
    - Xerostomia and medications.
    - High carbohydrate diet; frequency of snacking on fermentable carbohydrates.
    - Combinations of these factors increase the risk.
  - Effect of fluoride:
    - Adults with longtime residence in a fluoridated community have substantially fewer root carious lesions than those in a non-fluoridated community.
    - The protective factor is especially true for lifelong residents of areas where there is natural fluoride in the water.[29]
  - Prevention:
    - Control of risk factors for dental caries is essential for older adults as it is for all age groups.
    - Emphasis is placed on periodontal health because attachment loss with resultant root exposure needs to be prevented.
    - Caries preventive agents need to be strongly recommended, including the professional application of fluoride varnish.

III. The Periodontium

- Bone
  - Osteoporosis may be present.
  - Depressed vascularity, a reduction in metabolism, and reduced healing ability affect bone.
- Cementum
  - The average overall thickness of the cementum at 20 years of age was 0.095 mm; cementum from 60-year-old persons measured 0.215 mm.[30]

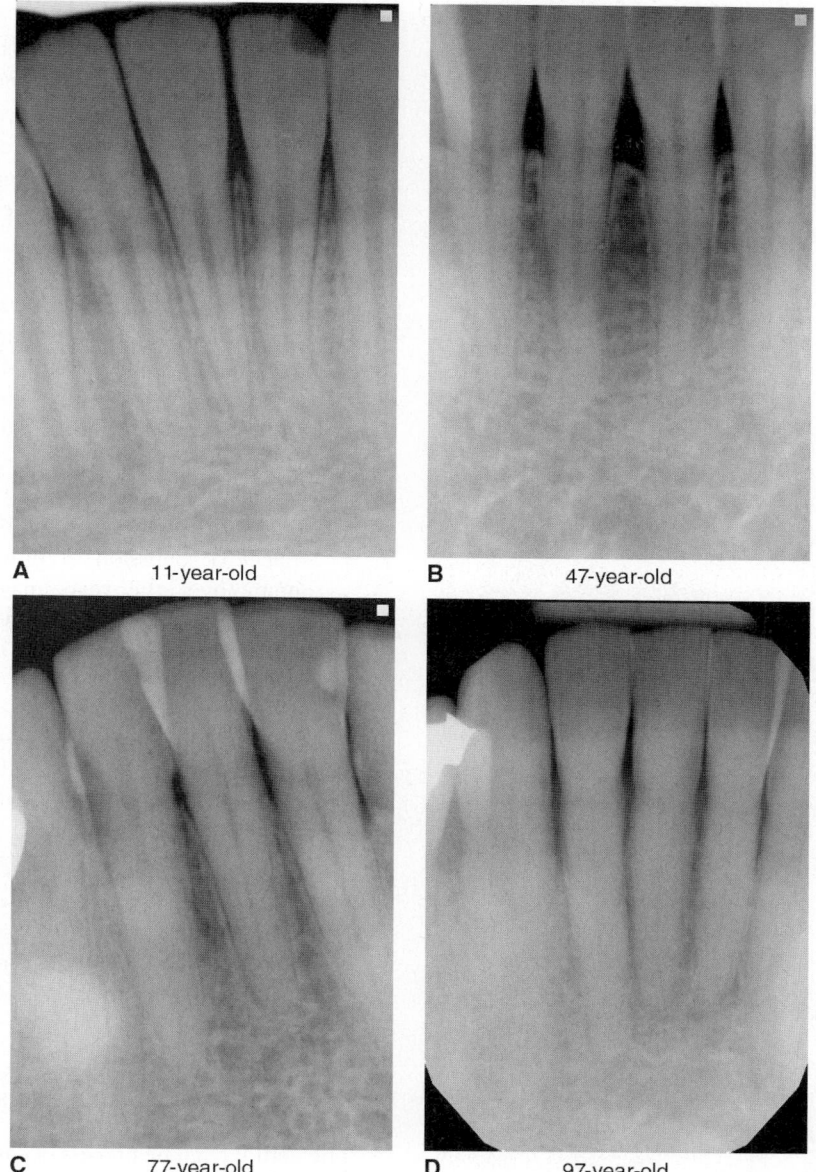

FIGURE 48-2 • Radiographs Provide an Example of Narrowing Pulp Canals with Age. The radiograph of an 11-year-old boy **(A)** illustrates pulp canals common in youth, radiographs **(B)** and **(C)** illustrate narrowing with advancing age, and the radiograph of a 97-year-old woman **(D)** shows pulp canals, which are significantly diminished.

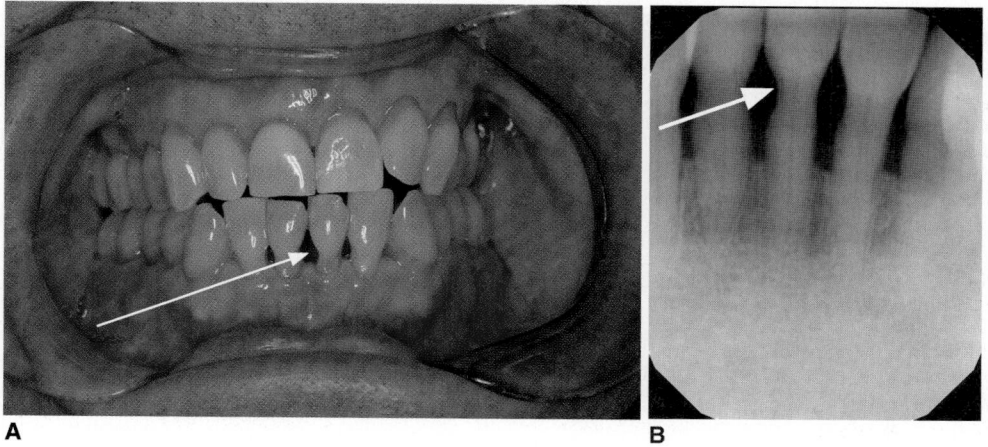

FIGURE 48-3 • In both the photograph **(A)** and the radiograph **(B)**, the arrow points to areas of abrasion present in the lower anterior teeth of a 66-year-old man. (Photograph courtesy of Dr. Paul Epstein, DMD.)

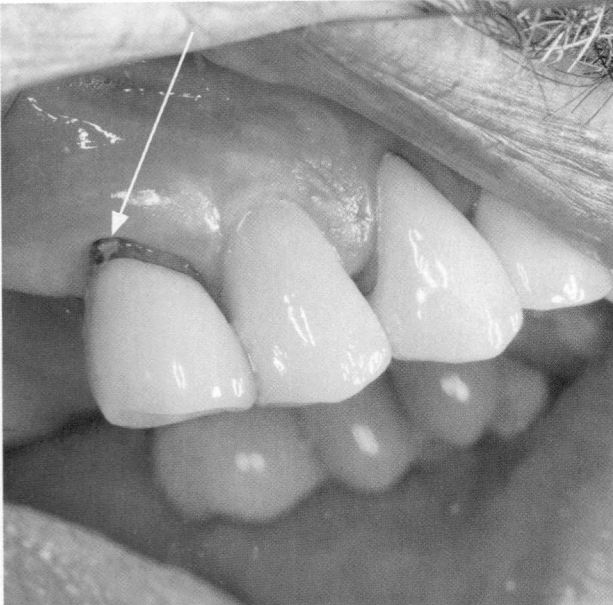

A

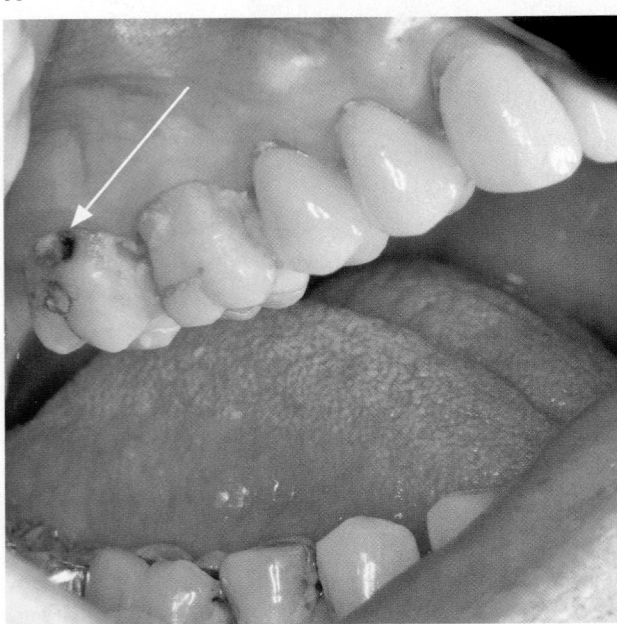

B

FIGURE 48-4 • Two Photographs Provide Examples of Root Caries in Older Adult Patients. A: Illustrates a cavitated lesion on the exposed root surface apical to the margin of a crown on tooth number 4. The arrow in photograph **(B)** points to dental caries apical to the cementoenamel junction on tooth number 3. Notice the previously restored areas on adjacent teeth. (Photographs courtesy of Dr. Paul Epstein, DMD.)

◆ Gingiva
  • Gingival changes can be traced to the effects of infection or to anatomic factors.
  • Gingival recession is common in older individuals.
  • Predisposing factors: lack of sufficient attached gingiva; malposition of the teeth.

◆ Risk factors for periodontal disease
  • Similar to younger individuals.
  • May be modified by chronic diseases and medications.
◆ Clinical findings
  • The periodontal tissues reflect the health and disease of the patient over the years.
  • Moderate periodontal disease may be more prevalent than advanced disease.
◆ The healthy periodontium
  • Healthy tissues that have been maintained over the years may have had a minimum of disease.
  • The radiographs show little, if any, attachment loss, the gingiva are firm, and the appearance is normal.
  • Probing reveals minimal sulcus depth with no bleeding.
  • The teeth are not mobile.
◆ The patient with periodontal infection
  • Neglect or omission of preventive measures and therapy over the years may have resulted in a chronic periodontal infection with extension of tissue destruction into the bone, periodontal ligament, and cementum.
  • Loss of attachment, deep periodontal pockets, tooth mobility, and radiographic signs of periodontitis may be present.
◆ The treated periodontal patient
  • The tissues may show effects of the disease, such as open interproximal embrasures.
  • Areas of recession with exposed cementum may also be evident.
  • The teeth are not mobile, especially when occlusal analysis and adjustment has been featured.

DENTAL HYGIENE CARE FOR THE OLDER ADULT PATIENT

◆ The dental hygiene process of care for the older adult is based on individual need as with all patients.
  • Many older adults value oral health as a component of overall health and wellness.
  • Care for the older adult patient needs to be planned in terms of comprehensive, not palliative treatment.
  • Increasing numbers of the older adult population avail themselves of esthetic dental services.
  • Adaptations need to be made to the process of care when cognitive, sensory, or physical conditions/limitations are present.
  • Long-term maintenance for the prevention of oral disease is the basic objective.

I. Barriers to Care

◆ Lack of perceived need is one of the most common reasons why older adults do not seek dental care.

◆ Older generations believed a decline in oral health was the result of the aging process.

◆ Economic and access barriers:
- Fixed income after retirement.
- Lack of dental insurance.

◆ Transportation problems.

◆ Functional disabilities affecting mobility limit access without assistance.

◆ Physical/architectural barriers:
- Accessibility to the dental office or clinic.
- Restrictions to access to care for institutional residents.
- Wheelchair access.
- Hazards, such as small rugs, which can slide on polished floors; loose corners of rugs, which can be tripped over; and irregularities in floor levels, need to be eliminated.
- Sitting for extended periods, keeping mouth open, and such might be difficult; provide frequent opportunities to change positions.
- Consider several short appointments as opposed to extended appointments.
- Raise the chair to a sitting position slowly due to the possibility of postural hypotension.

II. Assessment

◆ Patient history.

◆ Preparation of a careful and detailed medical and dental history takes on particular significance. Suggestions for good communication include the following:
- Allow sufficient time for reviewing complex histories.
- Eliminate distracting background music or sounds.
- Sit facing the patient and speak clearly with a low tone of voice.
- Speak directly to the patient even when a caregiver is present.
- Do not call the patient by his/her first name unless the patient suggests doing so.

◆ Medications.
- Because of the prevalence of chronic diseases, older patients are the largest consumers of both prescription and over-the-counter medications.
- Drug usage and the incidence of adverse drug reactions increase with age.
- Obtain a complete list. Include herbal and dietary supplements.
- Ask the patient to bring in either the bottles that contain the various medications (over-the-counter as well as prescription items) or a written copy of the labels so a list may be kept in the patient's record.

◆ References for checking drugs: Each practice center or clinic needs access to current references, such as the *Physician's Desk Reference*®, *Merck Manual*, or pharmacology reference websites (Lexi-Comp®) specifically directed to dental practice.

◆ Review the list of medications at each continuing care appointment.

◆ Review each medication to determine:
- Potential adverse side effects. Effects on the oral cavity such as xerostomia and gingival hyperplasia.
- Possible drug interactions with products recommended or used during the appointment.
- Certain medications may require frequent bathroom breaks.

◆ Vital signs.
- Blood pressure is determined and recorded at each visit.

◆ Intraoral and extraoral examination.
- The need for careful, periodic examination of the oral mucosa from the lips to the throat is especially crucial for the older adult patient because oral cancer occurs with increasing frequency with advancing years.
- Many oral lesions exist without the patient being aware of them.
- Document lesions with accurate descriptions and comparisons over time (see Chapter 13).
- When indicated, patient referral for biopsy is planned with the patient.

III. Preventive Care Plan

◆ Older adult patients may need frequent appointments to maintain a high level of oral health.

◆ The content of a care plan will address the control of dental biofilm and recommend fluoride use.

◆ Follow-up to assess healing of gingival tissues and daily biofilm removal.

◆ Give printed oral health instructions to the partner or caregiver to be posted in the bathroom or where the patient will be performing oral self-care.

IV. Dental Biofilm Control

◆ Implement the basic objectives of dental biofilm control.

◆ Infection needs to be eliminated and controlled.

◆ Factors affecting adequate biofilm control:
- Patients with cognitive, mental, and physical deficits can provide a challenge to the dental hygienist.
- Gingival recession with wide embrasures resulting from periodontal destruction provides a larger surface area for biofilm retention.
- Exposed cementum with areas of abrasion or dental caries at the cervical third of a tooth can create undercut areas where special adaptation of biofilm removal devices is needed.

- Decreased saliva production reduces or eliminates the cleansing and lubricating effects of saliva.
- Exposed untreated cementum may hold biofilm more readily than enamel. A smooth root surface is less likely to hold biofilm; therefore, biofilm removal efforts can be more successful.
- Restorations and prostheses provide more complex dentition and biofilm removal may require more time, patience, and motivation.
- Deficient restorations may have overhanging margins that provide areas for biofilm retention.
- Lack of dexterity related to disabling conditions resulting from chronic diseases, such as arthritis and Parkinson's disease, makes biofilm removal more difficult.

◆ Approach to instruction:

- Strategies to enhance communication with the older adult patient are listed in Table 48-2.
- Suggestions for providing oral health instruction for the older adult with specific characteristics are listed in Table 48-3.
- Motivation through expression of sincere interest on the part of dental personnel can be an influencing factor in helping the patient achieve better oral health.
- Allow sufficient time; do not leave instructions until the end of the appointment. Keep the session short and present small amounts of information at any one time.

TABLE 48-2 • Strategies for Enhancing Communication with the Older Adult Patient	
Before the appointment	• Schedule extra time for appointment • Ask patient to bring a list of medications
During the appointment	• Provide a friendly greeting • Eye contact • Be an active listener • Speak slowly • Present information one topic at a time • Use visual aids • Have the patient repeat instructions
After the appointment	• Provide written instructions

Source: Stein P, Aalboe J, Savage M, Scott AM. Strategies for communicating with older dental patients. *J Am Dental Assoc.* 2014;145(2):159-164.

- When appropriate, include the caregiver in instructions.
- Carefully assess the patient's ability to perform each technique. Avoid sudden changes or surprises.
- Base instruction on the patient's functional status.
- Determine what the patient already knows. Assist the older adult learner to relate new knowledge to past experiences.
- Make changes gradually over time.
- Repeated reinforcement and evaluation are critical.

TABLE 48-3 • Strategies for Providing Oral Health Instruction for Older Adult Patient	
CHARACTERISTIC OF THE OLDER ADULT PATIENT	**SUGGESTIONS FOR PATIENT INSTRUCTION**
Vision impaired	• Provide adequate lighting. • Provide instructional materials in large print on nonglare paper. • Avoid instructional materials in blue and green colors. • For the patient who wears prescription eyeglasses, make sure the glasses are worn while instruction is being given. • Recommend that eyeglasses be worn at home while performing biofilm control procedures.
Hearing impaired: loss of sensitivity to higher tones	• Speak distinctly in a normal voice. • Look directly at the patient while speaking; many are lip readers.
Hearing aid	• Reduce background noise; turn off music. • Ask patient if they prefer to turn down or turn off the hearing aid when the handpiece or ultrasonic is used.
Slowing of voluntary responses Slowing of speed of thought associations Rate of learning slowed, ability to learn not changed Changes in speed of vocalization	• Make suggestions gradually, over a series of appointments. • Be realistic and practical with expectations; go slowly, anticipate difficulties, give cues and clues. • Distinguish between slowness of learning and inability to learn. • Lower the pitch of your voice.
Memory difficulties	• Provide written instruction; spoken instructions may be forgotten or misunderstood. • Provide repeated reinforcement. • Give instructions to caregivers.
Apparent frustration with diminished functional abilities	• Acknowledge frustration; retain positive attitude; provide repeated reinforcement.
Symptoms of depression	• Acknowledge feelings; positive attitude but avoid overly cheerful demeanor; repeated reinforcement. • Appropriate use of affective ("caring") touch.

◆ Selection of dental biofilm removal devices:
  • Use of a power toothbrush may help patients with impaired hand function.
  • Power toothbrushes are often easier for caregivers to manage.
  • Adaptations to alter the handle of a manual brush are described in Chapter 51.
  • Interproximal brushes are recommended for open gingival embrasures. Methods for using interproximal brushes are described in Chapter 27.
◆ Dentifrice selection:
  • Fluoride ingredient mandatory for all surfaces including prevention for root caries.
  • Mild abrasive agent to prevent abrasion of root surfaces.
  • Desensitizing ingredient for exposed dentinal tubules.

V. Relief for Xerostomia

◆ Provide specific instructions for use of a saliva substitute.
◆ Instruction and motivation techniques are applied gradually and regularly at frequent intervals for best results.

VI. Periodontal Care

The incidence and severity of periodontal diseases tend to increase with age as an effect of disease accumulation. The extent of periodontal destruction reflects the length of time the tissues have been exposed to disease-producing factors, primarily biofilm microorganisms.
◆ Implementation of periodontal care includes complete debridement of calculus and biofilm.
◆ Follow-up evaluation to assess the need for additional therapy is essential.
◆ The patient's cognitive, mental, or physical condition may necessitate shorter appointments.
◆ Quadrant nonsurgical periodontal therapy with anesthesia may be appropriate.

VII. Dental Caries Control

◆ Assess diet; diet record covering several days.
◆ Diet adjustment to eliminate cariogenic foods and make appropriate substitutions.
◆ Emphasis on prevention of root caries.
◆ Professionally applied topical fluoride treatments: fluoride varnish.
◆ Daily self-applied fluoride therapy:
  • Fluoride dentifrice.
  • Fluoride rinses and gels; custom trays as applicable for a particular patient.
◆ Chlorhexidine rinses periodically for individuals with high bacterial counts; effective against *Streptococcus mutans* (Chapter 25).

◆ Xylitol chewing gum after meals and snacks for patients without chewing and swallowing difficulties.

VIII. Diet and Nutrition

◆ Dietary and resulting nutritional deficiencies are common in older people.
◆ Characteristic changes, such as burning tongue, angular cheilitis, and atrophic glossitis, may be related to vitamin B deficiencies.
◆ Factors contributing to dietary and nutritional deficiencies include:
  • Limited budget.
  • Not eating regular meals; frequently eating nonnutritious snacks.
  • Lack of interest in shopping for or preparing food.
  • Acuteness of senses (taste, smell) lowered; may seek highly seasoned or sweetened foods.
  • Inadequate masticatory efficiency because of tooth loss or dentures that no longer fit properly.
  • Adverse food selection may result from social embarrassment over inability to chew.
  • Following dietary fads that provide only a limited and unbalanced diet.
  • Difficulty in swallowing.
  • Alcoholism.
◆ Dietary/nutritional considerations for older adults include:
  • Reduced need for calorie intake as a result of decreased energy needs; to avoid overweight or obesity.
  • Protein, vitamins, minerals, and water are particularly important for body function, repair, and resistance to disease.
  • Increased need for calcium, vitamin D, and folate.
◆ A necessary objective in geriatric nutrition is to slow or prevent the progression of diet-induced chronic diseases. Examples are:
  • Atherosclerosis related to high dietary fat diets.
  • Anemias related to iron and folic acid deficiencies.
  • Osteoporosis resulting from inadequate intake of calcium and vitamin D.
◆ Fluoride intake over the years is beneficial in the prevention of osteoporosis and bone fractures, and water fluoridation is beneficial for direct application to the teeth.
◆ Instructions in diet and oral health:
  • Dietary analysis by means of a 4- or 5-day record of the patient's diet can provide information to guide recommended changes (see Chapter 33).
  • Patients with cognitive and/or memory deficits may be unable to provide an accurate food diary. When possible, enlist the help of family members or caretakers.
  • Minimally, an accurate 24-hour food diary needs to be obtained (see Chapter 33).

- Recommendations for older adult patients are based on establishing a well-balanced diet with limited amounts of cariogenic foods for dental caries prevention.
- Provide patient with dietary educational materials.
- Refer older adults with complex medical conditions to a registered dietitian nutritionist.
◆ Patient motivation may be enhanced by discussing the relationship of dietary deficiencies to:
  - Lowered resistance to disease.
  - Appearance (weight control).
  - Premature aging.

DOCUMENTATION

The permanent record for an older adult needs a complete personal health history followed from an initial appointment to include a minimum of the following:

◆ Detailed medical history.

◆ Current vital signs.

◆ History of medications.

◆ Current radiographs with exposure records.

◆ Extraoral and intraoral examination with particular emphasis on oral cancer and all pathologies.

◆ Dental history.

◆ Detailed dental charting and periodontal clinical examination including record of probing depths, clinical attachment level, furcations, mobility, occlusion, calculus classification, and biofilm control record.

◆ For each professional visit, a summary of current findings and planned treatment as well as outcomes from previous appointment treatments.

◆ A sample of documentation for an older adult dental visit may be reviewed in Box 48-6.

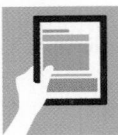

BOX 48-6

Example Documentation: Older Adult Patient with Xerostomia

S—A 78-year-old female presents for a 6-month continuing care appointment. Patient stated "I wake up in the middle of the night with my tongue sticking to the roof of my mouth. My tongue becomes sore."

O—Updating the medical health history, a new antihypertensive medication called hydrochlorothiazide is noted. During the intraoral examination, decreased salivary flow of saliva is observed.

A—Significant decrease in salivary flow is most likely due to the new antihypertensive medication. No previous clinical notes have documentation of complaints of xerostomia from the patient or noted findings of xerostomia from the intraoral examination. Patient is at high risk for caries based on the ADA caries risk assessment tool.

P—Patient is given instructions for the management of xerostomia such as the use of a saliva substitute and to drink plenty of water. Additional instructions were provided specifically for biofilm control and 5% sodium fluoride gel was prescribed with instructions for use to manage increased risk of dental caries. Fluoride varnish was applied due to high caries risk.

Next step: Reevaluate at the 3-month continuing care appointment.

Signed: _____, RDH

Date: _____

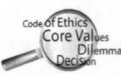

EVERYDAY ETHICS

Mr. and Mrs. Bracken were among Dr. Roberts' first patients when he began his practice almost 30 years ago. They keep a strict 4-month continuing care plan with the dental hygienist. Rosemary, the new hygienist, is looking forward to meeting and treating the Brackens for the first time as she has heard many wonderful things about this lovely older couple.

On completion of the oral examination with Mrs. Bracken, Rosemary recorded significant dental biofilm retention and evidence of xerostomia. She immediately begins to give the patient detailed home care instructions and asks for a complete listing of medications Mrs. Bracken is taking for her arthritis, angina, and diabetes. Mrs. Bracken left the appointment confused and upset.

Questions for Consideration

1. Which of the ethical core values (Table II-1 in the Section II Introduction) apply in this scenario? Considering that Mrs. Bracken seemed overwhelmed at the end of her appointment, how may Rosemary have erred in her judgment of the patient and the instruction she gave? Suggest alternative approaches.

2. To ensure the autonomy of Mr. and Mrs. Bracken while acknowledging their longevity in the practice, how can the medical status of these patients be clarified?

3. Using the questions in Table VI-1 in Section VI Introduction outline at least three alternative care plans that Rosemary could have used for her appointment with Mrs. Bracken.

Factors to Teach the Patient

▶ To remember to tell the dentist and dental hygienist all changes in personal health, medical care received since the last appointment, and all changes in prescriptions.

▶ The interrelationship of systemic and oral health.

▶ The dentition can last a lifetime. Daily preventive measures and a healthy lifestyle are essential.

▶ The value of a well-balanced diet with reduced calories and regular exercise for successful aging.

▶ Importance of drinking fluoridated water when it is available.

▶ Dental caries is a transmissible disease; therefore, it is urgent to have all cavitated lesions restored and dental biofilm removed from the teeth daily.

ENHANCE YOUR UNDERSTANDING

ONLINE RESOURCES
(see the inside front cover for access information)
- Audio glossary
- Appendices

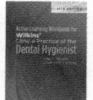

SUPPORT FOR LEARNING
(available separately)
- *Active Learning Workbook for Wilkins' Clinical Practice of the Dental Hygienist, 13th Edition*

INDIVIDUALIZED REVIEW
- Customized practice quizzing with Navigate 2 TestPrep for *Wilkins' Clinical Practice of the Dental Hygienist*

References

1. Population Reference Bureau. Fact sheet: aging in the Unites States. Retrieved from http://www.prb.org/Publications/Media-Guides/2016/aging-unitedstates-fact-sheet.aspx. Accessed February 25, 2018.

2. Manski RJ, Cohen LA, Brown E, Carper KV, Vargas C, Macek MD. Dental service mix among older adults aged 65 and over, United States, 1999 and 2009. *J Public Health Dent.* 2014; 74(3):219-226.

3. Whitbourne SK, Whitbourne SB. *Adult Development and Aging Biopsychosocial Perspectives.* 6th ed. Hoboken, NJ: John Wiley & Sons Inc; 2017:6-7.

4. Govindaraju DR, Pencina KM, Raj DS, Massaro JM, Carnes BA, D'Agostino RB. A systems analysis of age-related changes in some cardiac aging traits. *Biogerontology.* 2014; 15(2):139-152.

5. Lowery EM, Brubaker AL, Kuhlmann E, Kovacs EJ. The aging lung. *Clin Interv Aging.* 2013;8:1489-1496.

6. Chader GJ, Tayloe A. Preface: the aging eye: normal changes, age-related diseases, and sight-saving approaches. *Invest Opthalmol Vis Sci.* 2013;54(14):ORSF1-ORSF4.

7. Bainbridge KE, Wallhagen MI. Hearing loss in an aging American population: extent, impact, and management. *Annu Rev Public Health.* 2014;35:139-152.

8. Castelo-Branco C, Soveral I. The immune system and aging: a review. *Gynecol Endocrinol.* 2014;30(1):16-22.

9. Yam A, Marsiske M. Cognitive longitudinal predictors of older adults' self-reported IADL function. *J Aging Health.* 2013; 25(suppl 8):163S-185S.

10. Naorungroi S, Schoenbach VJ, Beck J, et al. Cross-sectional associations of oral health measures with cognitive function in late middle-aged adults: a community-based study. *J Am Dent Assoc.* 2013;144(112):1362-1371.

11. Linden GJ, Lyons A, Scannapieco FA. Periodontal systemic associations review of the evidence. *J Periodontol.* 2013;84(suppl 4):S8-S19.

12. Patel MH, Kumar JV, Moss ME. Diabetes and tooth loss: an analysis of data from the National Health and Nutrition Examination Survey, 2003–2004. *J Am Dent Assoc.* 2013;144(5):478-485.

13. Kelly JT, Avila-Ortiz G, Allareddy V, Johnson GK, Elangovan S. The association between periodontitis and coronary heart disease: a quality assessment of systematic reviews. *J Am Dent Assoc.* 2013;144(4):371-379.

14. Berkey D, Scannapieco F. Medical considerations relating to the oral health of older adults. *Spec Care Dentist.* 2013;33(4):164-178.

15. Griffin, SO, Jones JA, Brunson D, Griffin PM, Bailey WD. Burden of oral disease among older adults and implications for public health priorities. *Am J Public Health.* 2012;102(3):411-418.

16. Uppoor AS, Lhi HS, Nayak D. Periodontitis and Alzheimer's disease: oral systemic link still on the rise? *Gerodontology.* 2013;30:239-242.

17. Wang YP, Andrade LH. Epidemiology of alcohol and drug use in the elderly. *Curr Opin Psychiatry.* 2013;26(4):343-348.

18. Passos J, Gomes-Filho I, Vianna M, et al. Outcome measurements in studies on the association between osteoporosis and periodontal disease. *J Periodontol.* 2010;81(12):1773-1780.

19. Anil S, Preethanath RS, Almoharib HS, Kamath KP, Anand PS. Impact of osteoporosis and its treatment on oral health. *Am J Med Sci.* 2013;346(5):396-401.

20. Centers for Disease Control and Prevention. HIV among Older Americans. https://www.cdc.gov/hiv/group/age/olderamericans/index.html. Accessed January 15, 2018

21. Guneri P, Epstein J, Botto RW. Breaking bad medical news in a dental care setting. *J Am Dent Assoc.* 2013;144(4):381-386.

22. Vadiraj S, Nayak R, Choudhary GK, Kudyar N, Spoorthi BR. Periodontal pathogens and respiratory diseases—evaluating their potential association: a clinical and microbiological study. *J Contemp Dent Pract.* 2013;14(4):610-615.

23. Stoopler ET, Nadeau S, Sollecito TP. How do I manage a patient with angular cheilitis? *J Can Dent Assoc.* 2013;79:d68.

24. Toffanello ED, Inelmen EM, Imoscopi A, et al. Taste loss in hospitalized multimorbid elderly subjects. *Clin Interv Aging.* 2013;8:167-174.

25. Wiener C, Wu B, Crout R, et al. Hyposalivation and xerostomia in dentate older adults. *J Am Dent Assoc.* 2010;141(3):279-284.

26. Villa A, Polimeni A, Strohmenger L, Cicciù D, Gherlone E, Abati S. Dental patient's self-reports of xerostomia and associated risk factors. *J Am Dent Assoc.* 2011;142(7):811-816.

27. Tranasi M, Sberna MT, Zizzari V, et al. Microarray evaluation of age-related changes in human dental pulp. *J Endod.* 2009;35(9):1211-1217.

28. Sequeira-Byron P, Lussi A. Prevention of root caries. *Evid Based Dent.* 2011;12(3):70-71.

29. Ghezzi EM. Developing pathways for oral care in elders: evidence-based interventions for dental caries prevention in dentate elders. *Gerodontology.* 2014;31(suppl 1):31-36.

30. Zander HA, Hurzeler B. Continuous cementum apposition. *J Dent Res.* 1958;37(6):1035-1044.

The Patient with a Cleft Lip and/or Palate

Sara L. Beres, RDH, BA, MS

CHAPTER OUTLINE

CLASSIFICATION OF CLEFTS

ETIOLOGY
  I. Embryology
  II. Risk Factors

GENERAL PHYSICAL CHARACTERISTICS
  I. Other Congenital Anomalies
  II. Facial Deformities
  III. Infections
  IV. Airway and Breathing
  V. Speech
  VI. Hearing Loss

ORAL CHARACTERISTICS
  I. Tooth Development
  II. Malocclusion

  III. Open Palate
  IV. Muscle Coordination
  V. Periodontal Tissues
  VI. Dental Caries

TREATMENT
  I. Cleft Lip
  II. Cleft Palate
  III. Prosthodontics
  IV. Orthodontics
  V. Speech Therapy
  VI. Restorative Dentistry

DENTAL HYGIENE CARE
  I. Parental Counseling: Anticipatory Guidance
  II. Objectives for Appointment Planning

  III. Appointment Considerations
  IV. Patient Instruction
  V. Dental Hygiene Care Related to Oral Surgery

DOCUMENTATION

EVERYDAY ETHICS

FACTORS TO TEACH THE PATIENT

REFERENCES

LEARNING OBJECTIVES

After studying this chapter, the student will be able to:

1. Describe the types of cleft lip and palate that result from developmental disturbances.

2. Identify and describe the role of the professionals on the interdisciplinary team for the treatment of a patient with cleft lip and/or palate.

3. Recognize the oral characteristics a patient with cleft lip and/or palate may experience.

4. Explain how to adapt the dental hygiene appointment sequence for a patient with cleft lip and/or palate.

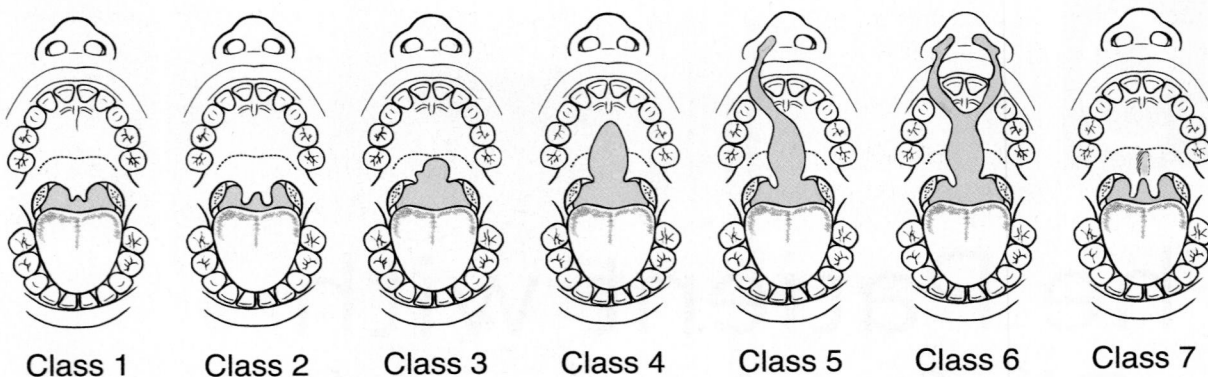

Class 1   Class 2   Class 3   Class 4   Class 5   Class 6   Class 7

FIGURE 49-1 • Classification of Cleft Lip and Cleft Palate. Class 1: cleft of the tip of the uvula; Class 2: cleft of the uvula (**bifid uvula**); Class 3: cleft of the soft palate; Class 4: cleft of the soft and hard palates; Class 5: cleft of the soft and hard palates that continues through the alveolar ridge on one side of the premaxilla, usually associated with cleft lip of the same side; Class 6: cleft of the soft and hard palates that continues through the alveolar ridge on both sides, leaving a free premaxilla, usually associated with bilateral cleft lip; and Class 7: submucous cleft in which the muscle union is imperfect across the soft palate. The palate is short, the uvula is often bifid, a groove is situated at the midline of the soft palate, and the closure to the pharynx is incompetent.

Cleft lip and palate are the most common of the many types of congenital craniofacial anomalies.[1] Cleft lip or palate may occur as isolated conditions, but frequently occur as part of a syndrome with other birth defects.

◆ The prevalence varies between 1 and 2 per 1,000 births, but this ratio varies based on geographic and ethnic distribution.[1]

◆ Cleft lip occurs more frequently in males, while cleft palate occurs more frequently in females.[1]

◆ The person with a cleft lip and/or palate can be dentally dysfunctional unless extensive habilitative care and supervision from birth is available.

◆ An interdisciplinary team of medical and dental specialists is required to provide adequate treatment and family counseling as needed.[1,2]

◆ The dental hygienist can be a member of the team with responsibilities to coordinate dental and periodontal care.

◆ Speaking ability and appearance are among the first factors considered when the long-range treatment program is planned because the objective is to help the patient lead a normal life.

◆ Dental personnel need to maintain a current list of the health agencies, clinics, and other community resources where the patient and family can obtain assistance for the various phases of treatment and rehabilitation.

CLASSIFICATION OF CLEFTS

◆ Classification is based on disturbances in the embryologic formation of the lip and palate as they develop from the premaxillary region toward the uvula in a definite pattern.

The seven classes are illustrated in Figure 49-1.[3]

ETIOLOGY

I. Embryology

◆ Cleft lip and palate represent a failure of normal fusion of embryonic processes during development in the first trimester of pregnancy.[4]

◆ Figure 49-2 shows the locations of the globular process and the right and left maxillary processes.

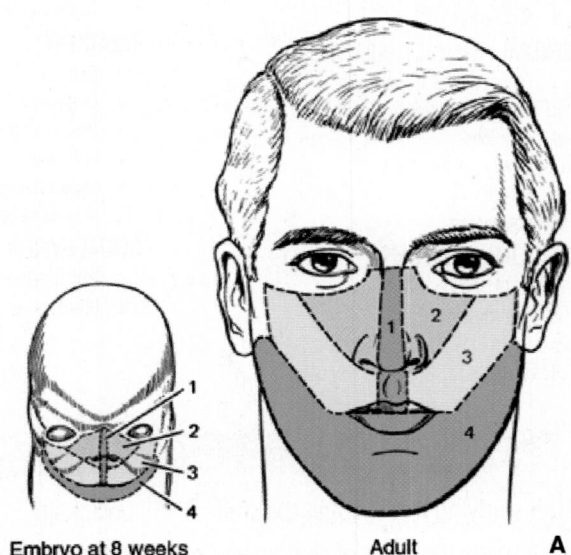

B Embryo at 8 weeks   Adult   **A**

FIGURE 49-2 • Developmental Processes of the Face. A: The nose, eyes, and mouth form between the fourth and sixth weeks of development. **B:** Development of the face illustrating derivatives of embryologic development. (1) Median nasal process; (2) lateral nasal process; (3) maxillary process; and (4) mandibular process. Clefts can occur at the midline of the maxillary and/or the mandibular process if fusion fails during development.

- With normal fusion, no cleft of the lip results.
- Fusion begins in the premaxillary region and continues backward toward the uvula.
- Formation of the lip.[4]
  - Occurs between the fourth and eight week in utero.
  - A cleft lip becomes apparent by the end of the second month in utero.
- Development of the palate.[4]
  - Takes place during the 6th–12th week.
  - A cleft palate is evident by the end of the third month.

II. Risk Factors

- Multifactorial genetic and environmental factors can be significant. Rarely, a single factor can be found as the specific cause of the cleft.[5]
  - Geographic: Cleft lip and palate are most common in Asian and American Indian children; African children are least likely to have clefts (1/2,500).[5,6]
  - Family history and genetics—Present or past members of a family increase the risk, as well as increased maternal age.[5]
  - Alcohol and tobacco.[5]
  - Diet: folic acid, vitamins, and zinc.[5]
  - Medication intake during pregnancy: teratogenic agents includes, phenytoin, vitamin A (isotretinoin), corticosteroids, and drugs of abuse.[5]
  - Occupational exposure: pesticides, lead, aliphatic acid, and organic solvents.[5]
  - Lack of adequate prenatal care and instruction is a risk factor that has influence on all the environmental factors.

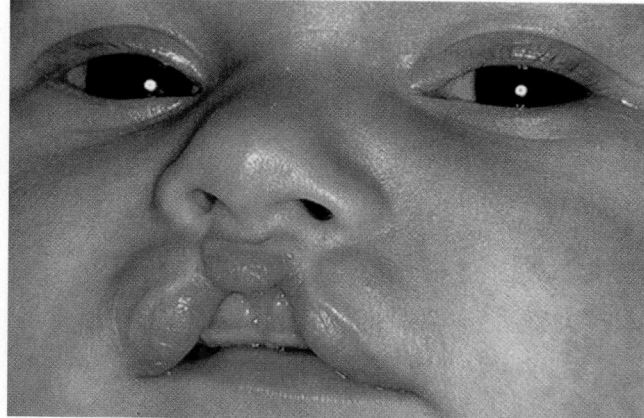

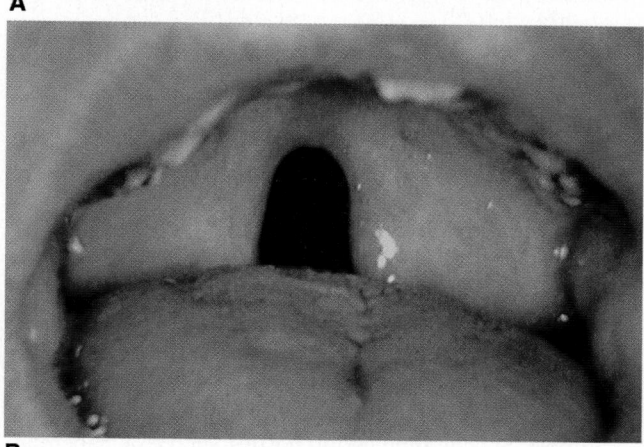

FIGURE 49-3 • **A:** Cleft lip. **B:** Cleft palate.

GENERAL PHYSICAL CHARACTERISTICS

I. Other Congenital Anomalies

- Incidence of multiple congenital anomalies is high with cleft lip and/or palate.
- At least 275 syndromes have been identified in which clefting is the primary feature.[6]

II. Facial Deformities

Facial deformities may include (see Figure 49-3):
- Depression of the nostril on the side with the cleft lip.
- Deficiency of upper lip, which may be short or displaced backward.
- Overprominent lower lip.

III. Infections

- Predisposition to upper respiratory and middle-ear infections is common.[7]

IV. Airway and Breathing

- Craniofacial anomalies of the nose and throat area predispose the child with a cleft palate to airway obstruction and breathing problems.[8]
- Early treatment intervention is necessary for the infant to cope with feeding problems.
- Speech involves breathing and swallowing.

V. Speech

- Patients with cleft lip and/or cleft palate have difficulty making certain sounds and may produce nasal tones.[1]
- Anatomic structure, airway and breathing problems, and hearing difficulties all contribute to speech problems.[1]

VI. Hearing Loss

- The incidence of hearing loss is significantly higher in individuals with cleft palate than in the noncleft population.[1]

ORAL CHARACTERISTICS

I. Tooth Development

◆ Disturbances in the normal development of the tooth buds occur more frequently in patients with clefts than in the general population.

◆ There is a higher incidence of missing and supernumerary teeth, as well as of abnormalities of tooth form.[9]

◆ Common missing teeth include:
  • Maxillary lateral incisors.
  • Maxillary premolar.
  • Mandibular second premolars.
  • Usually correspond to the side of the mouth that has the cleft.[9,10]

II. Malocclusion

◆ A high percentage of patients with cleft lip and palate require orthodontic care.[1]

◆ Orthodontic treatment may be required after each stage of surgical treatment for cleft palate.

III. Open Palate

◆ Before surgical correction, an open palate provides direct communication with the nasal cavity.

◆ A cleft lip makes it more difficult for a child to suck on a nipple. Special nipples and bottles, such as a Haberman feeder have been designed to make feeding easier.[11]

◆ A cleft palate may cause formula or breast milk to pass into the nasal cavity. A prosthetic palatal obturator may be constructed to aid during drinking and eating[11] (Figure 49-4).

IV. Muscle Coordination

◆ A lack of coordinated movements of lips, tongue, cheeks, floor of mouth, and throat may exist.

◆ Compensatory habits may be formed by the patient in the attempt to produce normal sounds while speaking.

V. Periodontal Tissues

◆ Dental biofilm accumulation is influenced by the irregularly positioned teeth, inability to keep lips closed,

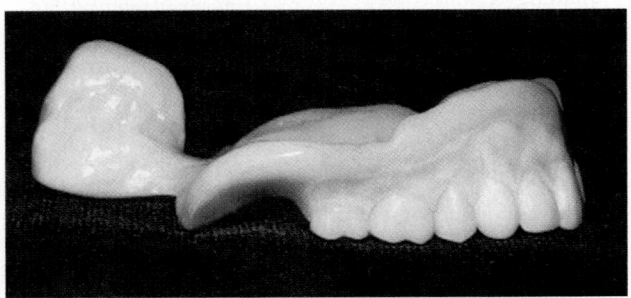

FIGURE 49-4 • Maxillary Obturator Prosthesis with Denture.

mouth breathing, and the difficulties in accomplishing adequate personal oral care, especially around the cleft areas.

◆ Patients with cleft palate and lip have increased levels of gingivitis and calculus accumulations.[12]

VI. Dental Caries

◆ Children with a cleft lip and/or palate are at higher risk for dental caries.[13]

◆ Risk factors relating to malpositioned teeth, problems of mastication, diet selection, and dental biofilm retention are intensified for the person with a cleft lip and/or palate.

◆ Feeding difficulties of infants and toddlers have contributed to early childhood caries also known as ECC (see Chapters 25 and 47).

TREATMENT

◆ Treatment is coordinated by a team of specialists and is based on the patient's progress at each age period.[1]

◆ Members of the interprofessional patient care team are listed in Box 49-1.

◆ The team is responsible for providing integrated case management. Quality and continuity of care are essential.[14]

◆ Need for attention to gingival health throughout the years of treatment cannot be overemphasized.

◆ Intraoral and/or extraoral appliances can be used in preparation for primary lip and palate surgery, including active and passive appliances, lip tapping/lip strapping, and the nasoalveolar molding technique technique.[2]

I. Cleft Lip

◆ Surgical union of the cleft lip is made at 2–3 months of age. A general well-known rule for scheduling surgery: when the child is approximately 10 weeks of age, weighs 10 pounds, and has achieved a serum hemoglobin of 10 mg/mL.[1]

◆ The infant's general health is a determining factor.

A. Purposes for Early Treatment

◆ Aid in feeding.

◆ Encourage development of the premaxilla.

◆ Help partial closure of the palatal cleft.

◆ Assist families in adjusting to the birth of a child with cleft lip and/or palate.

B. Orthodontics and Dentofacial Orthopedics

◆ In preparation for cleft closure, orthodontic and orthopedic treatment may be needed to reduce the protrusion and stabilize the premaxilla.[9]

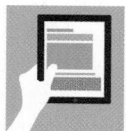

BOX 49-1
Interdisciplinary Team for Treatment of Patient with Cleft Lip and/or Palate[1,2,16]

Dental Profession
- Dental hygiene
- Oral and maxillofacial surgery
- Orthodontics
- Pediatric dentistry
- Prosthodontics
- Implantology
- Periodontics

Medical Profession
- Anesthesiology
- Genetics/dysmorphology
- Imaging/radiology
- Neurology
- Neurosurgery
- Ophthalmology
- Otolaryngology
- Pediatrics
- Physical anthropology
- Plastic surgery
- Psychiatry

Allied Medical
- Audiology
- Diet and nutrition
- Nursing
- Genetic counseling
- Psychology
- Social work
- Speech–language pathology
- Vocational counseling

II. Cleft Palate

- Primary surgery to close the palate is usually undertaken by age 18 months or earlier when possible.[14]
- The combined efforts of many specialists are required as listed in Box 49-2.

A. Goals for Treatment
- Produce anatomic closure.
- Maximize maxillary growth and development.
- Achieve normal function, particularly normal speech.
- Relieve problems of airway and breathing.
- Establish good dental esthetics and functional occlusion.

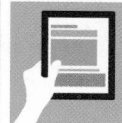

BOX 49-2
Types of Secondary Surgical Procedures

- **Rhinoplasty** and nasal septal surgery for an airway problem.[1]
- Velopharyngeal flap or other pharyngoplasty.[1]
- Closure of palatal fistulae.[1]
- Tonsillectomy and/or adenoidectomy.[1]

B. Types of Secondary Surgical Procedures
- Secondary surgical care (Box 49-2) refers to additional surgical procedures after primary closure of the clefts.
- Secondary surgery may involve the lips, nose, palate, and jaws.
  - Objectives are to improve function for coherent communication, improve appearance, or both.
- Treatment plans are individualized to fit the needs of the patient.
- Team evaluations on a periodic basis determine the effects of treatment and outline the next phase.

C. Use of Bone Grafting
- Bone grafting is used to repair residual alveolar and hard palate clefts.
  - *Alveolar graft*[15]
    - Placed before eruption of maxillary teeth at the cleft site.
    - Creates a normal architecture through which the teeth can erupt. A need for future prosthetic replacement of missing teeth is reduced.
    - Support is provided for teeth adjacent to the cleft areas.
  - *Hard palate graft*[15]
    - Provides closure of oronasal fistulae.
    - Helps to relieve a compromised airway.
  - *Sources for autogenous bone for graft*[15]
    - Rib, iliac crest, skull, mandible, or bone morphogenetic proteins.

D. Use of Osseointegrated Implant
After bone grafting, implants can be used to replace individual teeth.
- Implants also provide support for a complete prosthesis.

III. Prosthodontics

A. Types of Appliances
- *Obturator*: A removable prosthesis may be designed to provide closure of the palatal opening[16] (Figure 49-4).
- Speech aid prosthesis: A removable appliance to complete the palatopharyngeal valving required for speech.[16]

B. Purposes and Functions of a Prosthesis

The prosthesis may be designed to accomplish one or all of the following:

- Closure of the palate.
- Replacement of missing teeth.
- Scaffolding to fill out the upper lip.
- Masticatory function.
- Restoration of vertical dimension.
- Postorthodontic retainer.[16]

IV. Orthodontics

- Treatment may be initiated as early as 3 years of age, depending on dentofacial development.
- Each stage of surgery and treatment may require orthodontic intervention and follow-up.[1]
- Final formal orthodontic treatment for realigning the teeth and gaining a functional occlusion may start during the mixed dentition years or later.[1]
- During the orthodontic treatment period, an intensive program for dental caries prevention and gingival health is maintained.

V. Speech Therapy

- Training is started in very young children.[1]
- Therapy is essential following surgical or prosthodontic treatment.[1]

VI. Restorative Dentistry

- Dental hygienists practicing with a pediatric dentist or general dentist are involved in direct patient care.
- A major problem can be dental caries, leading to tooth loss. With missing teeth, major difficulties arise related to all phases of treatment.
- Preservation of primary teeth has special significance.

DENTAL HYGIENE CARE

- Preventive measures for the preservation of the teeth and their supporting structures are essential to the success of the special care needed for the habilitation of the patient with a cleft lip and/or palate.
- Teeth will often be poorly formed, lack enamel, and be at risk for loss due to decay.[1]
- Each phase of dental hygiene care and instruction takes on greater significance in light of the magnified problems of the patient with a cleft lip and/or palate.
- Every attempt is made to avoid the need to remove teeth, especially around the cleft area. In an area already weakened by lack of bone, removal of teeth creates further complications.
- The presence of teeth encourages optimum arch growth.

I. Parental Counseling: Anticipatory Guidance

- Understanding the value of preventive procedures by the patient and the parents is accomplished through explanation and instruction.
- When the patient has not had specialized care, the dental team has a responsibility to arrange referral to an available agency, clinic, or private practice specialist.
- Primary concerns are daily dental biofilm removal and prevention of early childhood dental caries.

II. Objectives for Appointment Planning

- Frequent appointments, scheduled every 3 or 4 months, are usually needed during the maintenance phase of the patient's care.
- *Objectives include* the following:
  - To review dental biofilm control measures.
  - To provide encouragement for the patient to maintain the health of the supporting structures and cleanliness of the removable prostheses (see Chapter 30).
  - To remove all calculus and biofilm as a supplement to the patient's personal daily care procedures.
  - To supervise a dental caries prevention program for both primary and permanent dentitions with fluorides (see Chapter 34) and sealants (see Chapter 35).

III. Appointment Considerations

A. Patient Apprehension and Self-Esteem

- A patient who has been seen often in hospital clinics may become apprehensive about dental and dental hygiene care.
- Lower self-esteem and difficulties in social interaction have also been noted with a patient with cleft lip and/or palate.[17]

B. Communication

- *Speech*: Speech may be difficult to understand. With repeated contact, understanding can be developed. Referral for speech assessment, if not already done, is recommended.
- *Hearing*: Depending on the severity of hearing loss, the approach is similar to that for speech difficulties. Suggestions for care of patients with hearing problems are described in Chapter 51.

C. Provide Motivation

- Use of a motivational interviewing approach can help patients gain a positive attitude toward oral health (see Chapter 24).

IV. Patient Instruction

A. Personal Oral Care Procedures

◆ For a small child, the caretakers may be afraid of damaging the deformed areas or hurting the child if cleaning methods are employed.

◆ An empathetic approach and plan for continued instruction over a long period is needed.

- *Personal daily care*: Select toothbrush, brushing method, and auxiliary aids according to the individual needs.
- *Fluoride*: Initiate daily self-application of fluoride by way of a fluoride dentifrice, and diet supplements for a young child in a nonfluoridated community (see Chapter 34).
- *Rinsing instruction*: Only older children (at least age 6 years, and evaluated for ability to rinse without swallowing) are given mouthrinse. Instruction on how to rinse is needed when this procedure is new to the patient (see Chapter 28).
- *Prosthesis or speech aid*: Halitosis may be a problem because mucous secreted in the nasal cavity, as well as biofilm, accumulates on the prosthesis and must be thoroughly cleaned on a regular basis (see Chapter 30).

B. Diet

◆ *Need for a varied diet*: Include adequate proportions of all essential food groups (see Chapter 33).

◆ *Need for prevention of dental caries*: Limit cariogenic foods, particularly for between-meal snacks.

C. Smoking Cessation

◆ The patient or family member who smokes or uses any form of smokeless tobacco should be informed about the effects of tobacco on all the oral tissues.

◆ Emphasis on the potential damage to the periodontal tissues can have special significance for the patient with a cleft palate.

◆ Offer assistance with a smoking cessation program.

V. Dental Hygiene Care Related to Oral Surgery

A. Presurgery (See Chapter 56)

◆ Treatment objectives have particular significance because the patient with a cleft palate is more susceptible to infections of the upper respiratory area and middle ear.

◆ Every precaution should be taken to prevent complications.

B. Postsurgery Personal Oral Care

◆ After each feeding (liquid diet for several days, soft diet for the next week), the mouth is rinsed carefully.

◆ Oral care is needed and accomplished with great care, usually by the parent or caregiver, to avoid damage to the healing suture lines.

◆ In selected cases, a toothbrush with suction attachment may be useful.

DOCUMENTATION

The documentation of care that the patient with cleft lip or palate receives over the individual's lifetime is imperative. Documentation includes the following:

◆ Description of location, classification, and extent of cleft.

◆ History and status of surgical interventions.

◆ Missing teeth and related recommendations for self-care regimens.

◆ Description of prosthetic appliances and recommendations for daily care regimens.

◆ A documentation example for a patient appointment is found in Box 49-3.

BOX 49-3
Example Documentation: Patient with Cleft Lip and/or Palate

S—A 12-year-old patient presented for routine maintenance appointment. Reviewed medical history: patient has recently started full mouth orthodontic treatment with local orthodontist. All vital signs are normal.

O—Extraoral examination: bilateral scarring on maxillary lip from cleft lip surgery at age 3 months. Intraoral examination: missing #D and G (permanent teeth are not present on recent pano). Dental biofilm free score: 50% primarily interproximally.

A—Bilateral cleft lip.

P—Disclosing solution used to show biofilm, demonstrated modified bass toothbrushing technique and "C" flossing. Showed patient and mother how to use floss threader to floss between wires and brackets. Showed patient and his mother how to use an interdental brush to clean between #E and #C and #F and #H. Hand scaled all four quads and applied 5% sodium fluoride varnish. Gave postoperative instructions. Patient tolerated appointment well. Three-month continuing care appointment scheduled.

Signed: _____, RDH

Date: _____

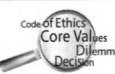

EVERYDAY ETHICS

Leona, a dental hygienist, has been working in her current position for 2 years. On most days she is scheduled for eight appointments, which are mostly maintenance appointments. Today she is scheduled for 12 appointments, which include Brian, a patient born with a bilateral clefting of the lip with partial involvement of the palate. He recently had another surgical procedure completed on his upper lip, and Brian's mother Joyce is concerned that several of his permanent teeth are not coming in. Joyce has depended on the guidance Leona has provided to help the family anticipate and meet Brian's oral health needs before, during, and after each of his multiple surgeries.

When Brian and Joyce arrive for their 4 PM appointment, Leona is 45 minutes behind schedule. Leona has dinner plans with friends at 5:30 PM and Leona is contemplating not taking the panoramic image and rescheduling the appointment.

Questions for Consideration

1. Consider the Basic Beliefs and Fundamental Principles identified in the ADHA Code of Ethics (see Chapter 1). Does Leona have an ethical responsibility to provide complete treatment during Brian's appointment? Why, or why not?

2. What strategies could Leona implement to allow for her to go to dinner with friends and provide complete treatment for Brain?

Factors to Teach the Patient

▶ Parental anticipatory guidance (see Chapters 47 and 48).

▶ Biofilm removal methods for cleft areas.

▶ Prevention of mouth odors by proper cleaning of tongue and removable appliances.

▶ Necessity for regular dental hygiene appointments to prevent oral infection and caries.

▶ Resources with addresses for team treatment clinics specializing in craniofacial developmental defects.

ENHANCE YOUR UNDERSTANDING

ONLINE RESOURCES
(see the inside front cover for access information)

· Audio glossary
· Appendices

SUPPORT FOR LEARNING
(available separately)

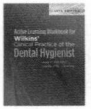

· *Active Learning Workbook for Wilkins' Clinical Practice of the Dental Hygienist, 13th Edition*

INDIVIDUALIZED REVIEW

· Customized practice quizzing with Navigate 2 TestPrep for *Wilkins' Clinical Practice of the Dental Hygienist*

References

1. Robin NH, Baty H, Franklin J, et al. The multidisciplinary evaluation and management of cleft lip and palate. *South Med J.* 2006;99(10):1111-1120.

2. Alzain I, Batwa W, Cash A, Murshid ZA. Presurgical cleft lip and palate orthopedics: an overview. *Clin Cosmet Investig Dent.* 2017;9:53-59.

3. Khan M, Ullah H, Naz S, et al. A revised classification of the cleft lip and palate. *Can J Plast Surg.* 2013;21(1):48-50.

4. Shkoukani MA, Chen M, Vong A. Cleft lip—a comprehensive review. *Front Pediatr.* 2013;1:53.

5. Kawalec A, Nelke K, Pawlas K, Gerber H. Risk factors involved in orofacial cleft predisposition—review. *Open Med.* 2015;10(1):163-175.

6. Leslie EJ, Marazita ML. Genetics of cleft lip and cleft palate. *Am J Med Genet C Semin Med Genet.* 2013;163(4):246-258.

7. Nagalo K, Ouédraogo I, Laberge J-M, Caouette-Laberge L, Turgeon J. Congenital malformations and medical conditions associated with orofacial clefts in children in Burkina Faso. *BMC Pediatr.* 2017;17:72.

8. Perkins JA, Sie KC, Milczuk H, Richardson MA. Airway management in children with craniofacial anomalies. *Cleft Palate Craniofac J.* 1997;34(2):135-140.

9. Menezes R, Vieira AR. Dental anomalies as part of the cleft spectrum. *Cleft Palate Craniofac J.* 2008;45(4):414-419.

10. Bartzela TN, Carels CE, Bronkhorst EM, Rønning E, Rizell S, Kuijpers-Jagtman AM. Tooth agenesis patterns in bilateral cleft lip and palate. *Eur J Oral Sci.* 2010;118(1):47-52.

11. Kumar Jindal M, Khan SY. How to feed cleft patient? *Int J Clin Pediatr Dent.* 2013;6(2):100-103.

12. Nagappan N, John J. Periodontal status among patients with cleft lip (CL), cleft palate (CP) and cleft lip, alveolus and palate (CLAP) in Chennai, India. A comparative study. *J Clin Diagn Res.* 2015;9(3):ZC53-ZC55.

13. Shashni R, Goyal A, Gauba K, Utreja AK, Ray P, Jena AK. Comparison of risk indicators of dental caries in children with and without cleft lip and palate deformities. *Contemp Clin Dent.* 2015;6(1):58-62.

14. American Cleft Palate-Craniofacial Association. *Parameters for Evaluation and Treatment of Patients with Cleft Lip/Palate or Other Craniofacial Differences.* Chapel Hill, NC: American Cleft-Palate-Craniofacial Association. 2009:1-34. https://acpa-cpf.org/team-care/standardscat/parameters-of-care/. Accessed August 7, 2019.

15. Guo J, Li C, Zhang Q, et al. Secondary bone grafting for alveolar cleft in children with cleft lip or cleft lip and palate. *Cochrane Database Syst Rev.* 2011;(6):CD008050.

16. Reisberg DJ. Dental and prosthodontic care for patients with cleft or craniofacial conditions. *Cleft Palate Craniofac J.* 2000;37(6):534-537.

17. Sousa AD, Devare S, Ghanshani J. Psychological issues in cleft lip and cleft palate. *J Indian Assoc Pediatr Surg.* 2009;14(2):55-58.

50

The Patient with a Neurodevelopmental Disorder

Lisa M. Byrne, RDH, BS, MHSc, Charlotte J. Wyche, BSDH, MS, and Linda D. Boyd, RDH, RD, EdD

CHAPTER OUTLINE

NEURODEVELOPMENTAL DISORDERS OVERVIEW

INTELLECTUAL DISORDERS
  I. Definition
  II. Model of Human Functioning and Disability
  III. Supportive Interventions
  IV. Classification of Intellectual Developmental Disabilities
  V. Etiology
  VI. Treatment
  VII. General Characteristics
  VIII. Factors Significant for Dental Hygiene Care

DOWN SYNDROME
  I. Physical Characteristics
  II. Cognitive and Behavioral Characteristics
  III. Comorbidity and Health Considerations

  IV. Oral Findings
  V. Factors Significant for Dental Hygiene Care

FRAGILE X SYNDROME
  I. Physical Characteristics
  II. Cognitive and Behavioral Characteristics
  III. Comorbidity and Health Considerations
  IV. Oral Findings
  V. Factors Significant for Dental Hygiene Care

AUTISM SPECTRUM DISORDER
  I. Prevalence
  II. Etiology
  III. Characteristics
  IV. Treatment Interventions

  V. Factors Significant for Dental Hygiene Care
  VI. Approaches to Dental Care for Patients with Autism

DENTAL HYGIENE CARE
  I. Oral Health Problems
  II. Dental Staff Preparation
  III. Dental Hygiene Care Plan
  IV. Appointment Considerations

DOCUMENTATION

EVERYDAY ETHICS

FACTORS TO TEACH THE PATIENT

FACTORS TO TEACH THE CAREGIVER

REFERENCES

LEARNING OBJECTIVES

After studying this chapter, the student will be able to:

1. Define and describe neurodevelopmental disorders.

2. Give examples of the characteristics, oral findings, and health problems significant for providing dental hygiene care for patients with:
   - Intellectual disability.
   - Down syndrome.
   - Autism spectrum disorder.

3. Recognize adaptations necessary for providing dental hygiene care for a patient with a neurodevelopmental disorder.

NEURODEVELOPMENTAL DISORDERS OVERVIEW

Neurodevelopmental disorders are a diverse group of chronic and potentially severe conditions that:

◆ Typically manifest in the early developmental period.

◆ Usually last throughout a person's lifetime.

◆ Lead to intellectual, social, and/or physical impairments.

◆ Create problems with major life activities such as language, mobility, learning, self-help, and independent living.

Many people with neurodevelopmental disabilities seek dental care in private and community settings, where opportunities are available to contribute to the health and well-being of these individuals. Down syndrome (DS) and autism spectrum disorder (ASD) are two major categories of patients with neurodevelopmental disabilities that dental professionals encounter in standard dental settings. Box 50-1 lists the major diagnostic categories of neurodevelopmental disorders.

INTELLECTUAL DISORDERS

I. Definition

Intellectual Disabilities (IDs) are characterized by[1]:

◆ Limitations in intellectual functioning.

◆ Limitations in adaptive functioning as expressed through conceptual, social, and practical skills.

◆ Origination and onset of symptoms during the developmental period, usually before the age of 18 years.

◆ Functional disability related to ID represents a more or less important symptom in well over 200 different conditions.

II. Models of Human Functioning and Disability

Several models of human functioning or disability have been proposed to better understand the interactions of disability with individual and environmental characteristics.[2] Based on these a model has been proposed to assess and support those with ID, which includes the following components[2]:

◆ Diagnosis: intelligence testing (problem solving, abstract thinking, judgment, academic learning abilities, ability to plan ahead, etc.) and assessment of adaptive functioning.[2,3] In individuals with ID, about one-third have comorbid psychiatric disorders and 10–20% have behavioral problems.[3,4]

◆ Assessment of functioning: establish baseline information for behavioral, social, and functional problems.

◆ Assessment of support needs.

◆ Planning and developing individual supports.

◆ Assessment of personal outcomes including quality of life.

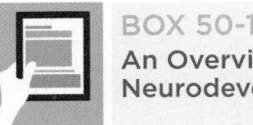

BOX 50-1
An Overview of Neurodevelopmental Disorders[1]

Intellectual Developmental Disorders Deficits in Intellectual and Adaptive Functioning

• **Global developmental delay**: Diagnosis used for individuals under 5 when assessment of reasons for not meeting developmental milestones is difficult.

• **Unspecified intellectual disability**: Used in exceptional circumstances for individuals over 5 years old when diagnosis is impossible because of the associated sensory deficits, physical impairments, severe behavioral problems, or mental disorders.

Communication Disorders

• **Language disorder**: Difficulty in acquisition and use of language, functional limitations in effective communication.

• **Speech sound disorder**: Persistent difficulty with sound production and speech intelligibility.

• **Childhood-onset fluency disorder (stuttering)**: Disturbances in fluency, timing, and repetition patterns of speech.

• **Social (pragmatic) communication disorder**: Difficulty using verbal and nonverbal communication in a manner that is appropriate for social context.

• **Autism spectrum disorder**: Severity of the condition is based on the level of social communication impairment and restrictive, repetitive behavior patterns.

• **Attention-deficit/hyperactivity disorder**: Persistent inattention, hyperactivity, and impulsivity.

• **Specific learning disorder**: Impairments in one or more academic domains (reading, writing, or mathematics).

• **Developmental coordination disorder**: Characterized by clumsiness, slowness, and inaccuracy of expected performance level of motor skills.

• **Stereotypic movement disorder**: Characterized by repetitive purposeless movements, with or without self-injurious behaviors.

• **Tic disorders**: Characterized by sudden rapid motor movement or vocalizations.

  • Tourette disorder: Both motor and vocal tics.

  • Persistent (chronic) motor or vocal tic disorder: Either motor or vocal tics, but not both, that have persisted for more than 1 year.

  • Provisional tic disorder: Motor and/or vocal tics present for less than 1 year since first onset.

III. Supportive Interventions

◆ Supportive interventions are strategies and resources selected after assessment of the individual level of ability and can help to improve the functioning of the individual with an ID. The rationale for supportive interventions includes:

- Promote development, education, interests, and personal well-being.
- Improve individual functioning and functional capabilities.
- Lessen the person's disorder by providing services and interventions that focus on prevention.
- Enhance personal outcomes related to independence, community participation, and personal well-being.

◆ Dental hygiene care is one of the supportive interventions needed to support the patient's:

- Freedom from oral discomfort and pain and maintain oral health.
- Learning self-care for daily oral biofilm removal.
- Improved quality of life.

IV. Classification of Intellectual Developmental Disabilities

◆ The traditional levels of intellectual functioning have included: *mild*, *moderate*, *severe*, and *profound*.[1] However, the International Classification of Disease 11 added the following classifications: *provisional* and *unspecified*.[5]

◆ Standardized intelligence tests are used to assess the overall intelligence quotient (IQ) as well as verbal comprehension, visual spatial skills, fluid reasoning, working memory, and processing speed.[3]

◆ Onset of the ID is before age 18.[1,3]

◆ A diagnostic category of "*unspecified*" is used when standardized tests cannot be performed because of lack of cooperation, severe impairment, or infancy.

A. Mild

◆ IQ approximate range 50–69 (in adults, mental age from 9 to under 12 years).

◆ Impairment of *adaptive behavior*[3,5]:

- Slower in acquisition and comprehension of complex language, academic, social, and daily living skills.
- Practical life skills such as basic personal self-care and domestic activities can be learned and these individuals can function with minimal support. They often can live semi-independently in group homes and maintain employment as adults with minimal support.

B. Moderate

◆ IQ approximate range 35–49 (adult mental age from 6 to under 9 years).

◆ Impairment of *adaptive behavior*[1,3,5]:

- A marked developmental delay occurs in the early years; child can be trained in personal care and hygiene with moderate support.
- Capacity for language and academic skills is limited to basic skills and they may not learn to read and write.
- Not completely capable of self-care and may require considerate, consistent support in order to be semi-independent and maintain employment as an adult.

C. Severe

◆ IQ approximate range 20–34 (adult mental age from 3 to under 6 years).

◆ Impairment of *adaptive behavior*[3,5]:

- Very limited language and communication skills. Limited capacity for academic skills.
- Motor impairments require daily support in a supervised setting; however, with extensive training they may be able to acquire basic self-care skills.

D. Profound

◆ IQ under 20 (adult mental age below 3 years).

◆ Impairment of *adaptive behavior*[3,5]:

- Severe limitation in self-care, continence, communication, and mobility.
- Close supervision and assistance with self-care and activities of daily living are necessary.
- These individuals are not able to live independently.

E. Provisional

◆ This diagnosis is assigned when there is evidence of an ID, but the individual is an infant or child under the age of 4 so it is not possible to conduct an assessment of intellectual functioning or adaptive behavior because of sensory or physical impairments, severe behavioral or mental disorders.[5]

V. Etiology

Anything that interferes with normal brain development can result in ID.

◆ Genetic[1,3]:

- DS is the most common cause of ID, 1 in every 700 live births.
- Fragile X syndrome (FXS) is the most common inherited cause of ID and occurs in 1 in 5,000 males.

◆ Nongenetic[1,3]:

- Exposure to toxic substances (e.g., prenatal alcohol exposure, prenatal/postnatal lead exposure).
- Nutritional deficiencies (e.g., iodine deficiency).
- Brain radiation.
- Childhood brain infections.
- Traumatic brain injury.
- Maternal infections (e.g., rubella, cytomegalovirus).
- Complications of prematurity (e.g., hypoxemia or periventricular hemorrhage).

◆ Etiology of some IDs is unknown.

VI. Treatment

Early diagnosis is essential to identify any comorbid medical, behavioral, or mental health disorders and determine services necessary to maximize their potential and quality of life. Treatment falls into three categories:

◆ Address or manage any underlying causes of ID such as the need to restrict phenylalanine in someone with phenylketonuria.

◆ Management of comorbid physical or mental health disorders to improve functioning and life skills.

◆ Early behavioral and cognitive interventions, special education, and psychosocial support to optimize functioning.

VII. General Characteristics

A. Physical Features

◆ Many individuals with ID may not have unusual physical characteristics.

◆ Delays in physical and motor functioning, such as walking, running, and jumping, is often associated with a lower IQ in this population.[6]

◆ Physical characteristics are most prominent in DS and FXS and may include:

• Facial or other characteristics may be pathognomonic for a particular condition or syndrome; for example, DS, described in this chapter.

• Skull anomalies include microcephalus (smaller), hydrocephalus (larger, contains fluid), spherical, conical, or otherwise asymmetrical shapes.

• Dysmorphic features, such as asymmetries of the face, malformations of the outer ear, anomalies of the eyes, or unusual shape of the nose, may become apparent as the child develops.

B. Oral Findings

◆ Higher levels of dental biofilm are present.[7]

◆ The gingival health of those with ID is worse than those without ID, but it remains unclear if the periodontal status is worse based on a systematic review and meta-analysis.[7]

◆ Dental caries

• Research on the caries rates of those with ID do not agree and at this time evidence suggests the risk for caries is similar to the general population.[7]

• However, the rate of untreated caries is higher with more missing permanent teeth due to caries.[7,8]

• Level of functioning, medication-induced xerostomia, and ability to perform oral self-care along with feeding issues (e.g., chewing and swallowing disorders, use of sugary foods as rewards, gastroesophageal reflux [GER]) are risk factors for dental caries.[9,10]

◆ Oral developmental malformations such as malocclusion, protruding tongue with macroglossia, narrow, short palate, microstomia, and delayed tooth development.[10]

◆ Oral habits: clenching, bruxing, mouth breathing, or tongue thrusting.

◆ Oral hypersensitivities, hyperactive bite or gag reflex.[10]

VIII. Factors Significant for Dental Hygiene Care

◆ Patients with ID often experience significant barriers to accessing dental care.[11]

◆ Individual factors include:

• Cognitive impairment may impact understanding of oral self-care procedures.

• Oral motor conditions may make oral self-care difficult (e.g., the individual may bite down on the toothbrush), or may make it difficult for a caregiver to assist with oral care.

• Oral tactile sensitivity such as gagging may make oral care difficult for those who support the individual.

• Challenging behaviors making it difficult to perform oral care at home and in a dental setting.

◆ Social factors include:

• Caregiver education and support for regular home and professional oral care.

◆ Environmental factors include:

• Transportation for professional care.

• Living in a residential setting may present a barrier to regular dental visits unless dental care is provided on-site.

DOWN SYNDROME

◆ Unique group of individuals with ID caused by a chromosomal abnormality; also referred to as trisomy 21 syndrome.

◆ Live birth prevalence is about 12.6 in 10,000 in the United States.[12]

◆ Life expectancy has increased dramatically from the 30s in 1980 to 55 years due to advancements in medical treatment and social support.[13]

◆ Most live with family in private homes or settings such as group residential homes and access healthcare as well as dental care services within their communities.

I. Physical Characteristics

◆ Poor muscle tone and altered gait (e.g., decreased walking speed, reduced step length, wider base of support to compensate for differences in muscle tone).[14]

◆ Short neck.

◆ Flattened facial profile with a flat nasal bridge.[13]

◆ Slanted eyes with the epicanthic fold of skin continuing from the upper eyelid over the inner angle of the eye (Figure 50-1).

◆ Small mouth and large tongue (hyperglossia).[13]

◆ Small hands with short fingers and the palm has a single, transverse palmar crease (Figure 50-2).[13]

◆ Gastrointestinal problems may include intestinal obstructions.[13]

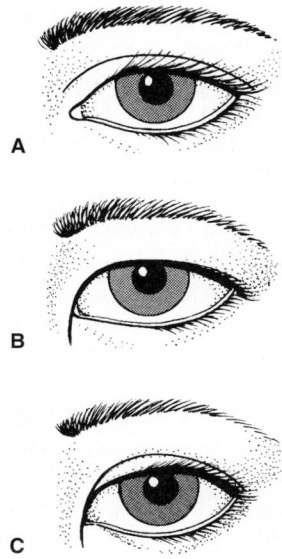

FIGURE 50-1 • Down Syndrome: Eye Characteristics. A: Absence of an epicanthic fold. **B:** Epicanthic fold in oriental populations. **C:** Epicanthic fold of a person with Down syndrome. (From Smith GF, Berg JM. *Down's Anomaly*. 2nd ed. Edinburgh: Churchill Livingstone; 1976.)

II. Cognitive and Behavioral Characteristics

Typical characteristics listed here may impact management approaches for dental and dental hygiene appointments.

◆ Many individuals with DS have mild to moderate ID.[15]

◆ Common cognitive functioning characteristics include[15,16]:

- Short attention span.
- Impulsive behavior.
- Slow learning.
- Delayed developmental milestones such as language and speech development.

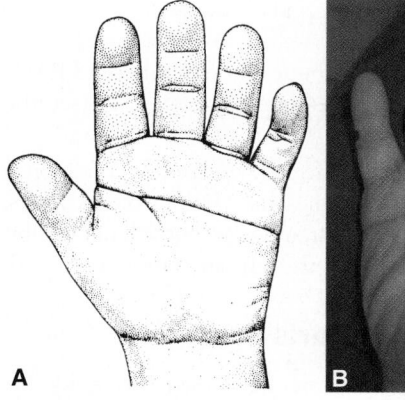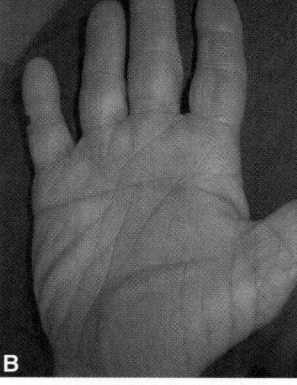

FIGURE 50-2 • Down Syndrome: Hand. (A) The artist's drawing and **(B)** the photograph both illustrate characteristic short, stubby fingers with the little finger curved inward and the single transverse palmar crease. (A: From Smith GF, Berg JM. *Down's Anomaly*. 2nd ed. Edinburgh: Churchill Livingstone; 1976.)

- Reduced working memory capacity (temporary memory) and long-term memory for explicit (factual) memory.
- Poorer ability to process information delivered verbally.
- Slower to gain new skills with more difficulty with stability of these new skills meaning they may not be able to repeat a skill at a later time.
- Nonverbal reasoning (ability to understand, interpret, and analyze visual information) and solve problems using visual reasoning.
- The DS individual may have difficulty with complex sentences.

III. Comorbidity and Health Considerations

Although improvements in health care and immunizations have resulted in a longer life expectancy, many patients with DS also present with additional special needs and comorbid health concerns. Common medical problems include[13]:

◆ Cardiac problems.
- 50% of DS babies have congenital heart disease.
- Ventricular septum defects affect 35%.

◆ Neurologic conditions.
- Seizures.
- Those with DS are at a greatly increased risk of early onset Alzheimer disease.[13]

◆ Hematologic problems.
- DS individuals have a 10–20 fold increased risk for leukemia.[13]

◆ Gastrointestinal problems.[15,17]
- 12% experience intestinal obstruction.
- GER is also common because of reduced muscle tone.
- Dysphagia is also common and may result in aspiration pneumonia.

◆ Vision problems.[15]
- Nearsightedness, eyes crossing inward, and congenital cataracts are common.
- White spots (Brushfield spots) on the colored part of the eye.

◆ Abnormalities of the immune system resulting in increased risk of infection and severity of disease, particularly respiratory tract infections.[17,18]

◆ Ear infections due to congenital ear abnormalities which may result in hearing loss.[18]

◆ Obstructive sleep apnea and airway obstruction is extremely common in DS due to airway abnormalities.[17]

IV. Oral Findings

◆ Anatomic anomalies[19]:
- Macroglossia with protruding tongue as illustrated in Figure 50-3.
- Macrosomia.
- Narrow, vaulted palate.

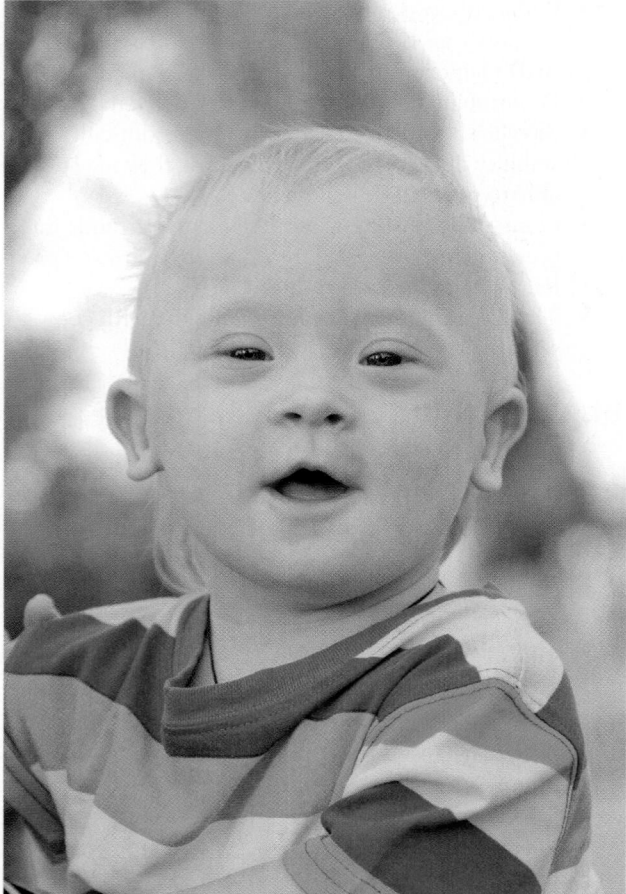

FIGURE 50-3 • Child with Down Syndrome. Common features in children with Down syndrome. Note the child's small rounded skull, small open mouth with protruding tongue, slanting almond-shaped eyes, flattened nose bridge, small lower set ears, and short neck. (Image from Shutterstock.)

◆ Dental anomalies[19]:
  • Delayed or irregular sequence of eruption.
  • Congenitally missing teeth.
  • Irregularities in tooth formation (hypoplastic enamel): microdontia fused teeth.
  • Class III malocclusion and posterior crossbite are common and relate to the flat face and underdevelopment of the midfacial region (prognathic appearance).
  • Teeth may be spaced because certain anomalous teeth take less space.
◆ Mouth breathing is common.
◆ Periodontal infections are more prevalent and often more severe in people with DS.[19]
◆ Poor oral hygiene.[19]
◆ Bruxism.[19]
◆ Xerostomia.[19]
◆ Children and young adults with DS have a lower prevalence of dental caries.[20] Factors that may contribute include:
  • Delayed eruption.

• Congenitally missing teeth and microdontia (small teeth) may result in wider interdental spaces reducing food accumulation.[20]

V. Factors Significant for Dental Hygiene Care

◆ Individual factors may include:
  • Review the medical and medication history with the caregiver and carefully investigate any medical conditions in order to plan safe dental/dental hygiene treatment. Consultation with a medical provider may be necessary.
  • Careful attention by the dental hygienist to effective communication by using simple, clear language along with visual aids to help educate the patient. In addition, repetition will be necessary due to memory issues.
  • Cognitive limitations along with impaired vision or hearing may impact understanding of oral self-care instructions.
  • Typically behavior is not an issue, but talk to the caregiver to determine the most effective way to manage any negative behaviors.
  • Minimize stimuli, that is, noise.
  • Positioning of the chair may need to be adjusted if the patient has respiratory problems.
  • More frequent periodontal maintenance may be necessary.
◆ Social factors include:
  • Children with DS may have access to occupational therapy (OT). OT assists people with self-care tasks and may be a resource to assist with oral hygiene skills.
  • Caregiver education and support for routine oral care will be important to prevent and manage oral disease.
◆ Environmental factors include:
  • Determine living arrangement as those living in a residential center may have more difficulty finding transportation for routine dental care.

FRAGILE X SYNDROME

FXS is the most common genetic cause of inherited ID.[21]
◆ The most common single-gene cause of ASD (see the following section).
◆ Boys are mostly severely affected because this condition is associated with the X chromosome. Girls are often carriers, carry the gene on one X chromosome, but will not exhibit the characteristics unless both X chromosomes are affected.

I. Physical Characteristics

In addition to ID, the following are often present (Figure 50-4)[21]:
◆ Prominent forehead.
◆ Narrow, long face.
◆ Protruding ears.
◆ Connective tissue dysplasia results in hyperflexibility of joints.

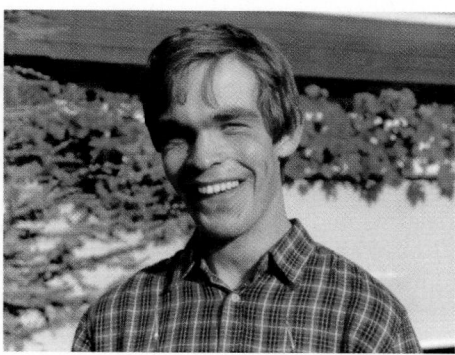

FIGURE 50-4 • Fragile X Syndrome. Fragile X syndrome in a 28-year-old man: broad nose, prognathism, and large ears.

II. Cognitive and Behavioral Characteristics

Common cognitive and behavioral considerations[22]:

◆ IDs.

◆ Hyperactivity disorder.

◆ ASD.

◆ Weaknesses in short-term and working memory limit the ability to retain and process new information.[23]

◆ Limitations in executive function which controls aspects of behavior such as attention.[23]

◆ Difficulty with visual-motor coordination which means they may have trouble with motor skills like toothbrushing.[23]

◆ Relative strengths include verbal reasoning (ability to understand and logically work through problems) and simultaneous processing (ability to see the big picture and understand relationships).[23]

III. Comorbidity and Health Considerations

◆ Recurrent otitis media because of collapsible eustachian tubes.

◆ Neurologic conditions may include[21]:
  • Seizures.
  • Movement disorders such as hand flapping is common in FXS.

◆ Gastrointestinal issues[21]:
  • GER.
  • Diarrhea.

◆ Ocular disorders are common and many individuals with FXS require glasses for correction.[21]

◆ Sleep problems occur in 10–25% of children and teens with FXS.[21]
  • Obstructive sleep apnea occurs in about one-third of individuals with FXS.
  • Airway obstruction is also common.

IV. Oral Findings

Common oral findings include[22]:

◆ High arched palate.

◆ Mandibular prognathism.

◆ Macroglossia.

◆ Enamel hypoplasia.

◆ Malocclusion.

◆ Dental caries.

◆ Gingivitis.

◆ Poor oral hygiene.

◆ Medication induced xerostomia with saliva with a low buffering capacity.

V. Factors Significant for Dental Hygiene Care

◆ Individuals factors may include:
  • The dental hygienist needs to carefully investigate the medical history and medications along with questioning the caregiver on behavioral considerations.
  • Explore cognitive and behavioral limitations as well as any vision or hearing issues prior to the first visit.
  • Behavior may result in lack of cooperation with caregivers for oral care.
  • Understand issues with short-term and working memory and adjust oral hygiene education accordingly.
  • Visual-motor coordination may make it more difficult for the patient to learn oral self-care techniques.
  • If GER is present along with medication-induced xerostomia, additional strategies may be needed to prevent caries such as prescription fluoride.

◆ Social factors include:
  • Caregiver education and support for routine oral care will be an important part of preventing and managing oral disease in the FXS patient.

AUTISM SPECTRUM DISORDER

Autism, first described by Dr. Leo Kanner in 1944, is a complex spectrum of developmental disorders marked by limitations in the ability to understand and communicate.[1]

◆ Usually appears during early childhood and persists throughout life, although many individuals with ASD can learn coping behaviors to enhance daily functioning.

◆ Manifests as a range of disorders, as listed in Box 50-2, rather than by the presence or absence of a single behavior or symptom.

◆ Comorbidity with other disabling and medical conditions is common.[1]

I. Prevalence

◆ Prevalence has increased in the past two decades; the prevalence of ASD according to the National Health Center for Health Statistics in 2016 was estimated to be 1 in 36 children.[24,25]

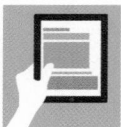

BOX 50-2
Autism Spectrum Disorders

Autistic Disorder

- Impairments in verbal and nonverbal communication and social (aka: classic autism) interaction, and restrictive or repetitive patterns of behavior, interests, and activities.
- Symptoms are usually measurable by 18 months of age; formal diagnosis is usually made between ages 2 and 3, when delays in language development are apparent.

Asperger Disorder

- Three to four times more likely in males.
- Characterized by impairments in social interactions and restricted interests and activities, without clinically significant delays in language, cognitive ability, or developmental age-appropriate skills.

Pervasive Developmental Disorder, not Otherwise Specified (PDD-NOS)

- Severe and **pervasive** impairment in specified behaviors, without meeting all of the criteria for a specific diagnosis (aka: atypical autism).

Rett Disorder

- An autism-like genetic disorder, which occurs only in girls, causing the development of autism-like symptoms after a period of seemingly normal development.
- Purposeful use of hands is lost and replaced by repetitive hand movements beginning between ages 1 and 4 years.

Childhood Disintegrative Disorder

- Rare autism-like disorder characterized by normal development for at least the first 2 years, followed by a significant loss of previously acquired skills.

- Some increase in prevalence may be attributable to better diagnostic criteria and more frequent screening.[24,25]
- Occurs in all racial, ethnic, and social groups worldwide.
- Frequency of occurrence is almost five times greater in males than in females.[24]

II. Etiology

- The etiology is multifactorial with genetic and environmental factors playing a role.[24,25]
  - Genetic factors are estimated to be between 30 and 35% of risk for autism.[26]

- There are about 40 prenatal, perinatal, and postnatal risk factors that may increase the risk for autism, but more research needs to be done to understand how the risk factors work in combination in the development of autism.[26]
- Prenatal risk factors include[26]:
  - Advanced maternal or paternal age greater than or equal to 35 years.
  - Mother or father's race: white or Asian.
  - Maternal and paternal education level beyond college graduate.
  - Gestational diabetes.
  - Gestational hypertension.
  - Antepartum hemorrhage (vaginal bleeding between the 20th and 24th week of pregnancy and birth of the baby).
  - Threatened miscarriage (bleeding and abdominal cramping).
- Perinatal risk factors include[26]:
  - Cesarean delivery.
  - Gestational age less than or equal to 36 weeks.
  - Breech birth.
  - Preeclampsia.
  - Fetal distress.
  - Induced labor.
- Postnatal risk factors include[26]:
  - Low birth weight.
  - Postpartum hemorrhage.
  - Male gender.
  - Brain anomaly.

III. Characteristics

- The onset of autism is typically before age 3 and some parents may notice signs in the first year of life. Signs may include delays or abnormal response in the following:
  - Social interaction.
  - Language.
  - Symbolic or imaginative play.
- Persistent deficits in social communication and interaction across multiple contexts such as the following[1]:
  - Impairment in nonverbal communication for social interaction (e.g., eye-to-eye gaze, facial expression, gestures).
  - Deficit in developing, maintaining, and understanding peer relationships appropriate for the developmental level.
  - Lack of social or emotional reciprocity or inability to initiate and respond to social interaction.
- Restricted interests and repetitive behaviors manifested by at least two of the following[1]:
  - Highly restricted patterns of interest that are abnormal in intensity or focus.
  - Insistence on sameness or inflexible adherence to routines or rituals (e.g., extreme stress with small changes).

- Repetitive body movements, use of objects, or speech.
- Hyper- or hyporeactivity to sensory input (e.g., adverse response to specific sounds or textures).

◆ Severity designation is based on the level of communication impairments and behavior patterns (see Box 50-3).

◆ Comorbidity: ASD is commonly associated with other intellectual impairments, structural language disorder, attention deficit and hyperactivity disorders, learning disabilities, and seizure disorders.[1]

IV. Treatment Interventions

◆ There is no "cure," in the medical sense, for autism.

◆ Interventions usually target behavioral issues and support behavioral adaptations.

A. Early Intervention Services

◆ Early intervention targets children from birth to 3 years old to provide services to improve development in the following areas:
- Physical, such as walking, crawling, etc.
- Cognitive, such as learning, problem solving, etc.

BOX 50-3
Autism Spectrum Disorders:
Levels of Severity[1]

Level 3: Requires Very Substantial Support
- Severe verbal and nonverbal communication deficits.
- Initiates social interactions only to meet immediate needs.
- Limited intelligible speech.
- Inflexible behavior, extreme difficulty in coping with change or changing focus.
- Repetitive behavior markedly interferes with functioning.

Level 2: Requires Substantial Support
- Limited initiation of social interactions; reduced response to overtures from others.
- Deficits in nonverbal communication/behavior.
- Inflexible, difficulty in switching between activities.
- Difficulty in changing focus or action.

Level 1
- Some difficulty in initiating social interactions; atypical response to social overtures from others.
- Inflexible behavior; difficulty switching between activities.
- Problems with organization and planning.

- Communication, such as speech.
- Social/emotional, such as play.
- Self-help, such as eating and dressing.

B. Pharmacologic

◆ Treatment is complex due to the heterogeneity or variation in the behaviors and severity of behaviors in an individual with ASD.

◆ Purpose: relief of negative behavioral symptoms (such as severely disruptive behaviors and hyperactivity).[27]

◆ The two medications with Food and Drug Administration approval for treatment of severely disruptive behaviors (also referred to as irritability) are *risperidone* and *aripiprazole*.[27]

◆ Treatment of repetitive or compulsive behaviors with serotonin reuptake inhibitors such as fluoxetine has shown promise in adults with ASD, but research in children has been inconsistent.[27]

◆ Medication for the management of hyperactivity has been mixed with some studies reporting psychostimulants like Ritalin (methylphenidate), but other studies show an increase in irritability.[27]

◆ Identification and medical management of comorbid, potentially treatable conditions (e.g., epilepsy seizures, allergies, gastrointestinal problems, or sleep disorders), can lead to quality-of-life improvements.

C. Cognitive-Behavioral Therapy

◆ A form of treatment that focuses on relationships between thoughts, feelings, and behaviors.

◆ Purpose: help people with autism lead more normal lives by decreasing anxiety and increasing their ability to respond to everyday stimuli with appropriate coping mechanisms.

◆ No one behavior-based or educational approach is effective in alleviating symptoms in all cases of autism because of the spectrum nature of the condition and the many behavior combinations that can occur.

◆ Examples: special teachers in intensive structured programs directed toward individual instruction, applied behavior analysis (ABA), sensory integration, music therapy, OT, speech and language therapy, and auditory integration training.
- ABA has been widely used and encourages positive behavior while discouraging negative behavior.

D. Controversial Treatment

◆ Dietary approaches for the treatment of ASD are not evidence-based; however, those with ASD often have a restricted diet which may impact overall health.
- In particular, evidence is emerging for lower protein, calcium, and phosphorus intake resulting in lower bone mass.[28]
- Caregivers should be discouraged from restricting diet choices without oversight by a medical provider.

◆ Complementary and alternative treatment currently have no conclusive evidence to support efficacy.[29]

- However, music therapy as a component of behavioral therapy may impact several aspects of ASD including communication, emotion, and social reciprocity (or response to social interaction).

V. Factors Significant for Dental Hygiene Care

◆ Poor oral hygiene and gingivitis are common.

◆ Impairment in social interaction and difficulty in shifting focus of attention make traditional oral health education approaches difficult.

◆ Repetitive body movements and mannerisms may compromise patient safety and impact infection control protocols.

◆ The dental hygienist needs to carefully investigate the medical history and medication along with questioning the caregiver on behavioral considerations.

◆ Patience and a consistent approach and patient preparation prior to the appointment can enhance the probability of a successful dental visit.

VI. Approaches to Dental Care for Patients with Autism

A. D-Termined Program (DTP) of Familiarization and Repetitive Tasking

◆ DTP is a behavior guidance approach based on ABA for dental professionals developed for use specifically for patients with ASD.[30,31]

- Pretreatment assessment form to gather information about behavior challenges and what motivates the child.
- Familiarization visits.
- Practicing and learning cooperation skills.

◆ Benefits of DTP include[30]:

- Improvement in behavior.
- Fewer referrals for dental treatment under general anesthesia resulting in lower costs for dental care.

◆ Cooperation skills to be learned include:

- Positioning oneself in the dental chair.
- Sitting with legs straight and hands at side or on the tummy.
- Making eye contact as instructions are given.
- Opening the mouth and remaining consistently open.
- Allowing instrumentation, and responding appropriately to instructions.

◆ The five "D" steps for learning cooperation skills[31]:

1. *Divide the skill into smaller parts*: the key for people with autism is to take each small step of a dental appointment one at a time, and master it before moving ahead.

2. *Demonstrate the skill*: use the tell–show–do technique.

3. *Drill the skill*: repeat/practice the skill many times until it becomes second nature.

4. *Delight the learner*: reward successful attainment of any small portion of the task with reinforcers.

5. *Delegate the repetition*: involve other members of the dental staff in reinforcing the skills, and have parents and caregivers rehearse/practice at home.

B. Autism Speaks Dental Tool Kit

◆ The tool kit is designed to[32]:

- Provide tips to dental professionals for patient care.
- Teach families how to prepare for the visit to the dentist.
- Decrease anxiety about the dental visit.
- Provide information for good oral health for a lifetime.

◆ Resources include a pre-visit assessment form, a dental professionals tool kit, video, information for caregivers to prepare the child for the dental visit, and instructions for brushing their child's teeth.

- The pre-visit assessment and interview is particularly important to learn what behaviors might be encountered and what reinforcement for positive behavior might be effective.
- Home-based preparation may include familiarization with procedures the child will encounter such as "open your mouth" and "counting teeth."

C. Additional Strategies for Dental Care

◆ In addition to the previously mentioned program, there are a variety of strategies for preparing to have a positive experience at the dental visit.[33]

- Desensitization with familiarization visits may also be planned.
- Visual pedagogy is a way to educate the child with ASD through pictures.
- Create a personalized picture book of the steps in the dental visit to be reviewed at home in preparation for the visit.
- Social stories are a widely used strategy for ASD and focus on a short story to provide an understanding of the social information for a setting and the behavioral expectations.
- Video modeling to teach behaviors related to the dental visit as well as to oral care at home.

DENTAL HYGIENE CARE

◆ Appointments for medical or dental health care may be overwhelming because of all the unfamiliar stimuli for many patients with neurodevelopmental disorders, especially for patients with an ASD.

◆ Dental care may have been neglected due to problems with social interactions, language and communication problems, or difficult behaviors.

- Severity of symptoms dictates the appropriate setting for the delivery of dental care services for these patients.
- With some modifications to the treatment plan and implementation of appropriate behavior guidance techniques, patients with mild-to-moderate manifestations of the condition may be treated successfully in the general dental setting.
- Patients with more severe symptoms may require sedation, general anesthesia, or immobilization in a hospital or specialized setting.

I. Oral Health Problems

Several factors can contribute to poor oral health for individuals with a neurodevelopmental disorder.

A. Previous Dental Care

- Dental care may have been a low priority due to challenges the caregiver encounters in completing the activities of daily living.
- Reasons for unmet dental needs:
  - The child's behavior and parent's embarrassment about the behavior are major barriers to dental care.[32,33]
  - Cost of treatment, particularly if general anesthesia was recommended.[33]
  - Parents may be resistant to the use of protective stabilization in children unable to follow direction or with behaviors that may cause them harm in the dental chair.[33]
  - Unpleasant experiences from previous dental visits.

B. Dental Caries

- Feeding problems can lead to offering foods that will be accepted, without regard for nutrient content or caries prevention.
- Dietary selection may have been limited by needs for sameness, with the possibility of serving an excess of cariogenic foods.
- Sweet food rewards for behavior modification/guidance, repeated frequently over time, promote dental caries development.
- Aversion to certain food textures can lead to extreme diets that result in either entirely soft food selections or entirely hard crunchy/crispy food selections with low nutritional value.
- Foods used in therapy sessions to stimulate speech or help develop the muscles necessary for improved language are frequently cariogenic (i.e., chewy or sticky candy).

C. Oral Hygiene

- Daily oral care procedures may be inadequate for the uncooperative individual, even when delivered by an informed caregiver.

- Strategies suggested in the resources for the child with autism such as those provided by Autism Speaks can be useful for most children with neurodevelopmental disorders.[32]
- OT may be able to assist with the sensory issues some individuals may experience to familiarize them with the sensations associated with routine oral home care.

II. Dental Staff Preparation

- Be familiar with the various neurodevelopmental disorders and prepare for the visit by doing the following:
  - Review medical, dental, and personal histories with the caregiver by telephone interview in advance of the first office appointment. Both the DTP and Autism Speaks resources previously discussed have a form that could be used to gather specific information about behavior, sensitivities, etc.
  - Discuss information with the parent/caregiver, primary care provider, or other healthcare provider associated with the patient.
  - Gather specific information about appropriate motivators and rewards that are safe and effective reinforcers for the individual.
- Consider some of the strategies previously mentioned for those with ASD for pre-appointment familiarization the parents/caregiver can do at home such as:
  - Place a plastic mirror and flashlight in and out of the mouth.
  - Follow commands such as "Hands on your tummy."… "Feet out straight."
- Plan several short orientation and familiarization appointments initially with not more than a week between visits.
- Involve the same members of the dental team at each appointment to avoid distressing the patient and losing time for reorientation.

III. Dental Hygiene Care Plan

- Plan four-handed dental hygiene for the resistant patient.
- Frequent appointments to prevent oral disease are recommended. As the patient becomes more cooperative, increase the preventive services they will tolerate which may include:
  - Dental biofilm control for the patient and the caregiver.
  - Debridement as needed.
  - Fluoride varnish therapy: simple easy to do procedure that can be especially helpful for patients unable to cooperate with biofilm control (see Chapter 34).
  - Dental sealants (see Chapter 35).

IV. Appointment Considerations

- Provide a predictable and consistent experience.

◆ Create a quiet environment free from sensory stimuli; patients with autism may have sensitivity to light, sounds, touch, and smell.

- Avoid loud, inconsistent background music, noisy dental equipment, and irrelevant conversations.
- Avoid unnecessary touching during treatment.
- Provide sunglasses for patients with light sensitivity.
- Placing the lead apron on the patient to induce deep pressure touch stimulation may help the patient feel more secure and stay calm.

◆ Desensitization/practice

- Begin with orientation to the setting and each part of the equipment.
- If the patient is not ready, instrumentation may not be included at the first appointment.
- Instruction takes the form of "tell–show–do" repeated many times. Patience and firmness are necessary elements.
- Have the caregiver help condition the patient by giving a plastic mouth mirror and a few dental films to take home for practice in the mouth each day.

◆ Use behavior guidance procedures when the patient condition is appropriate.

- Involve caregiver(s) while presenting preventive measures in a simple step-by-step manner.
- Ask the caregiver or parent if the ABA therapist could attend the first dental visit to provide guidance.
- Provide reinforcing rewards immediately following each success.
- Use inedible rewards (stickers, picture cards, child-safe tokens, or toys) and explain the rationale against cariogenic food rewards.

◆ Protective stabilization[34]

- Protective stabilization is considered an advanced behavior guidance technique in dental settings and the clinician must have adequate training in appropriate, safe, and effective use for a patient who is unable to cooperate.
- Other less restrictive approaches to behavior management should be attempted prior to using protective stabilization.
- Written informed parental/guardian consent is required from the parent or guardian pre-procedure.
- The risks and benefits must be explained prior to asking for informed consent.
- Parental presence in the operatory may be helpful for both the parent and child.

DOCUMENTATION

Factors to document include:

◆ Chronologic age versus developmental age.

◆ Communication strengths and weaknesses with patient and caregiver.

◆ Helpful behavioral supports and guidance techniques.

◆ Treatment that was accomplished and modifications to treatment that were helpful.

◆ Recommended home care oral hygiene and behavior practice skills.

◆ Box 50-4 provides an example documentation for a patient with an ID.

BOX 50-4
Example Documentation:
Patient with an ID

S—Patient presented as a 10-year-old boy with a developmental age of approximately 4 years. Used three-to-four word simple sentences and caregivers presented a picture board that showed the steps of the appointment. This helped the patient recognize how many more steps were needed until the end of the appointment. Patient needs to have his hands held to remind him not to touch and finds comfort in holding his favorite rubber tube toy that he brought from home. He also loves to hear quiet singing and counting throughout the appointment.

O—Mirror only examination performed. Biofilm score noted as roughly 50%. No visual decay found.

A—Dental hygiene diagnosis: biofilm-induced gingivitis.

P—Oral hygiene instruction with patient and caregiver. Rubber cup prophy completed. Flossing of entire mouth. Fluoride varnish applied to entire dentition. Caregivers congratulated on preparing the patient for the visit; patient congratulated on a successful visit.

Next steps: 3 months recall-examination with explorer and biofilm removal with toothbrush.

Signed: _____, RDH

Date: _____

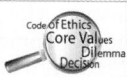

EVERYDAY ETHICS

At the Caring Community Dental Health Clinic, the first and third Mondays of each month are reserved for special needs patients referred by health professionals in the local area. Adults and children with Down syndrome, autism spectrum disorder, and other intellectual disabilities frequently are scheduled for dental hygiene appointments. With only one full-time and one part-time dental hygienist, more hygiene appointment time is needed. Dental hygiene students from a nearby dental hygiene program have been invited to rotate through the clinic as a community practicum experience.

Questions for Consideration

1. Two days before a scheduled assignment, Ellie, a student, confides to her classmate, Julie, that

she cannot participate in this field experience because she is too afraid of people with intellectual disabilities. Which core values are evident in this situation?

2. When arriving at the assignment, the students are greeted and oriented by the part-time hygienist, Ms. Gray. She advises the students, "Just get 'em in and get 'em out. They don't understand anything anyway and it's a waste of your time to try to talk to them for patient instruction." What are the ethical principles applicable to this situation?

3. How might the students handle these ethical issues using the steps in the resolution of an ethical issue or dilemma listed in Chapter 1 (Box 1-7) to determine an acceptable course of action?

Factors to Teach the Patient

When the patient is able to perform self-care skills independently and can expectorate, then proceed with instruction using language and methods appropriate to the intellectual level and abilities of each patient.

▶ Use a disclosing agent to show the biofilm to the patient and have the patient use the toothbrush or other appropriate oral hygiene aid to remove the biofilm. For someone who is visual, seeing the biofilm may be a helpful educational tool.

▶ Help the patient to refine their oral hygiene technique and identify which oral hygiene aids may be most appropriate based on the patient's dexterity.

▶ If the patient is unable to adequately remove dental biofilm, encourage the patient to accept assistance from the parents or caregiver.

▶ When needed, include the parent or caregiver in the oral self-care instruction.

▶ Identify ways to support the patient at home with the parent or caregiver.

▶ Identify ways to support the patient at home with the parent or caregiver. Provide a reminder or pictures of the technique that can be attached to the bathroom mirror.

▶ Identify what reinforcers work best for the patient, such as putting a sticker on the calendar each time they perform their oral self care.

ENHANCE YOUR UNDERSTANDING

ONLINE RESOURCES
(see the inside front cover for access information)
· Audio glossary
· Appendices

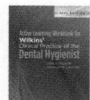

SUPPORT FOR LEARNING
(available separately)
· *Active Learning Workbook for Wilkins' Clinical Practice of the Dental Hygienist, 13th Edition*

INDIVIDUALIZED REVIEW
· Customized practice quizzing with Navigate 2 TestPrep for *Wilkins' Clinical Practice of the Dental Hygienist*

Factors to Teach the Caregiver

▶ Benefit of frequent intervals for oral health services to prevent disease and make the visits shorter and easier.

▶ Educate the parent or caregiver about the specific oral hygiene aids and techniques appropriate for the individual patient.

- ▶ Provide guidance on assistance of patients with limited abilities, such as:
  - ▶ Approach to stabilize the patient's head.
  - ▶ Effective retraction of the patient's lips to insert and adapt the toothbrush.
- ▶ How to incorporate behavior modification into oral care procedures.
- ▶ Emphasize the necessity of repeating tell-show-do instructions often.
- ▶ Discuss the need for coordination of the patient's medical and dental team to provide appropriate care.

References

1. American Psychiatric Association. Section II: diagnostic criteria and codes: neurodevelopmental disorders. In: *Diagnostic and Statistical Manual of Mental Disorders*. 5th ed. Arlington, VA: American Psychiatric Association; 2013:31-86.

2. Buntinx WHE, Schalock RL. Models of disability, quality of life, and individualized supports: implications for professional practice in intellectual disability. *J Policy Pract Intellect Disabil*. 2010;7(4);283-294.

3. Committee to Evaluate the Supplemental Security Income Disability Program for Children with Mental Disorders; Board on the Health of Select Populations; Board on Children, Youth, and Families; Institute of Medicine; Division of Behavioral and Social Sciences and Education; The National Academies of Sciences, Engineering, and Medicine; Boat TF, Wu JT, eds. *Mental Disorders and Disabilities Among Low-Income Children*. Washington, DC: National Academies Press (US); 2015.

4. Salvador-Carulla L, Bertelli M. "Mental retardation" or "intellectual disability": time for a conceptual change. *Psychopathology*. 2008;41(1):10-16.

5. World Health Organization. *ICD-11: Mental, Behavioural or Neurodevelopmental Disorders*. 06a Disorders of intellectual development. June 2018. https://icd.who.int/browse11/l-m/en#/http%3a%2f%2fid.who.int%2ficd%2fentity%2f334423054. Accessed August 5, 2019.

6. Almuhtaseb S, Oppewal A, Hilgenkamp TI. Gait characteristics in individuals with intellectual disabilities: a literature review. *Res Dev Disabil*. 2014;35(11):2858-2883.

7. Zhou N, Wong HM, Wen YF, Mcgrath C. Oral health status of children and adolescents with intellectual disabilities: a systematic review and meta-analysis. *Dev Med Child Neurol*. 2017;59(10):1019-1026.

8. Morgan JP, Minihan PM, Stark PC, et al. The oral health status of 4,732 adults with intellectual and developmental disabilities. *J Am Dent Assoc*. 2012;143(8):838-846.

9. Bakry NS, Alaki SM. Risk factors associated with caries experience in children and adolescents with intellectual disabilities. *J Clin Pediatr Dent*. 2012;36(3):319-323.

10. Ziegler J, Spivack E. Nutritional and dental issues in patients with intellectual and developmental disabilities. *J Am Dent Assoc*. 2018;149(4):317-321.

11. Chadwick D, Chapman M, Davies G. Factors affecting access to daily oral and dental care among adults with intellectual disabilities. *J Appl Res Intellect Disabil*. 2018;31(3):379-394.

12. de Graaf G, Buckley F, Dever J, Skotko BG. Estimation of live birth and population prevalence of Down syndrome in nine U.S. states. *Am J Med Genet A*. 2017;173(10):2710-2719.

13. Asim A, Kumar A, Muthuswamy S, Jain S, Agarwal S. Down syndrome: an insight of the disease. *J Biomed Sci*. 2015;22(1):41.

14. Almuhtaseb S, Oppewal A, Hilgenkamp TI. Gait characteristics in individuals with intellectual disabilities: a literature review. *Res Dev Disabil*. 2014;35(11):2858-2883.

15. Eunice Kennedy Shriver National Institute of Child Health and Human Development. What are the common symptoms of Down syndrome? https://www.nichd.nih.gov/health/topics/down/conditioninfo/symptoms. Updated January 31, 2017. Accessed September 22. 2108.

16. Patterson T, Rapsey CM, Glue P. Systematic review of cognitive development across childhood in Down syndrome: implications for treatment interventions. *J Intellect Disabil Res*. 2013;57(4):306-318.

17. Alsubie HS, Rosen D. The evaluation and management of respiratory disease in children with Down syndrome (DS). *Paediatr Respir Rev*. 2018;26:49-54.

18. Ram G, Chinen J. Infections and immunodeficiency in Down syndrome. *Clin Exp Immunol*. 2011;164(1):9-16.

19. Ziegler J, Spivack E. Nutritional and dental issues in patients with intellectual and developmental disabilities. *J Am Dent Assoc*. 2018;149(4):317-321.

20. Deps TD, Angelo GL, Martins CC, Paiva SM, Pordeus IA, Borges-Oliveira AC. Association between dental caries and Down syndrome: a systematic review and meta-analysis. *PLoS One*. 2015;10(6):e0127484.

21. Kidd SA, Lachiewicz A, Barbouth D, et al. Fragile X syndrome: a review of associated medical problems. *Pediatrics*. 2014;134(5):995-1005.

22. Amaral COFD, Straioto FG, Napimoga MH, Martinez EF. Caries experience and salivary aspects in individuals with fragile X syndrome. *Braz Oral Res*. 2017;31:e79.

23. Huddleston LB, Visootsak J, Sherman SL. Cognitive aspects of Fragile X syndrome. *Wiley Interdiscip Rev Cogn Sci*. 2014;5(4):501-508.

24. Sharma SR, Gonda X, Tarazi FI. Autism spectrum disorder: classification, diagnosis and therapy. *Pharmacol Ther*. 2018;190:91-104.

25. Zablotsky B, Black LI, Blumberg SJ. Estimated prevalence of children with diagnosed developmental disabilities in the United States, 2014–2016. NCHS Data Brief, no. 291. Hyattsville, MD: National Center for Health Statistics. 2017.

26. Wang C, Geng H, Liu W, Zhang G. Prenatal, perinatal, and postnatal factors associated with autism: a meta-analysis. *Medicine*. 2017;96(18):e6696.

27. Accordino RE, Kidd C, Politte LC, Henry CA, McDougle CJ. Psychopharmacological interventions in autism spectrum disorder. *Expert Opin Pharmacother*. 2016;17(7):937-952.

28. Ekhlaspour L, Baskaran C, Campoverde KJ, Sokoloff NC, Neumeyer AM, Misra M. Bone density in adolescents and young adults with autism spectrum disorders. *J Autism Dev Disord*. 2016;46(11):3387-3391.

29. Brondino N, Fusar-Poli L, Rocchetti M, Provenzani U, Barale F, Politi P. Complementary and alternative therapies for autism spectrum disorder. *Evid Based Complement Alternat Med*. 2015;2015:258589.

30. AlHumaid J, Tesini D, Finkelman M, Loo CY. Effectiveness of the D-TERMINED program of repetitive tasking for children with autism spectrum disorder. *J Dent Child.* 2016;83(1):16-21.

31. The Nancy Lurie Marks Family Foundation. D-Termined program of repetitive tasking and familiarization in dentistry. http://www.nlmfoundation.org/media/dental_clips.htm. Accessed October 6, 2018.

32. Autism Speaks. Dental tool kit. https://www.autismspeaks .org/tool-kit/dental-tool-kit. Accessed October 6, 2018.

33. Gandhi RP, Klein U. Autism spectrum disorders: an update on oral health management. *J Evid Based Dent Pract.* 2014;14(suppl):115-126.

34. Academy of Pediatric Dentistry, Council on Clinical Affairs. Protective stabilization for pediatric dental patients. 2017;40(6):18/19   :268-273.   https://www.aapd.org/research /oral-health-policies--recommendations/protective-stabilization -for-the-pediatric-dental-patients/. Accessed August 5, 2019.

DISABILITIES OVERVIEW

This chapter provides general guidelines for modifying dental hygiene care for a patient with a disability. People with disabilities may require a modified approach to oral health care in order to achieve and maintain oral health and prevent rampant dental disease.[1]

- An estimated 10.5% of individuals aged 17–64 years, 5.4% of children aged 5–17 years, and 35.4% of people aged above 65 years are affected by a disability and the number is increasing.[1]
- The Americans with Disability Act (ADA) defines 54 million individuals as disabled, including 1 million children below 6 years of age and 4.5 million between 6 and 16 years of age.[2]
- Progress in medical care has increased initial survival of those born with a disability and increased the survival rate of those experiencing a disabling condition.[3]
- Advances in medicine have increased the life span of people with comorbidities that would have shortened their life spans.[4]
- As life expectancy increases, so does the likelihood of acquiring a disability.[3]
- Individuals with disabilities often have less access to oral health services due to challenges for the patient, caregiver, and the dental personnel.[4,5]
- The patient may need to overcome numerous obstacles in daily living before the additional issues of oral self-care and access to dental care are addressed.
- Imagination, ingenuity, flexibility, persistence, and patience are necessary in order to individualize and modify dental hygiene interventions when caring for people with disabilities.[4]
- Successful management and treatment of patients depends largely on the interpersonal communication between the patient and the clinician.
- Services are provided in a manner that makes people less different and focuses on the needs of individuals and not their differences.

I. Americans with Disability Act

- *Purpose*
  - The ADA is civil rights legislation enacted into law on July 26, 1990 "that prohibits discrimination and guarantee that people with disabilities have the same opportunities as everyone else to participate in the mainstream of American life—to enjoy including employment opportunities, to purchase goods and services, and to participate in State and local government programs and services."[2]
- *Definition*
  - ADA defines an individual with a disability as a person who:
    - Has a physical or mental impairment that substantially limits one or more major life activities.

- Has a record of such impairment.
- Is regarded as having such an impairment.[2]
- "Major life activities include, but are not limited to, caring for oneself, performing manual tasks, seeing, hearing, eating, sleeping, walking, standing, lifting, bending, speaking, breathing, learning, reading, concentrating, thinking, communicating, and working."[2]

II. Definitions and Classifications

- Disability is an umbrella term for impairment, activity limitations, and participation restrictions.[3]
  - Impairment refers to a problem with body structure or function.[3]
  - Disabling condition can be developmental, communicative, medical, musculoskeletal, neurologic, or sensory.[6]
  - Activity limitations is when an individual has difficulty in executing a task associated with daily living.[3,6]
  - Participation restrictions is when an individual has a problem involving a life situation.
- The term "handicap," is no longer used, as it implies an individual with impairment is disadvantaged.
- *Person first language* is important to emphasize the person and not the disability. The disability is not a defining characteristic of an individual, but rather part of the whole person. For example, avoid saying "disabled child" and instead use "child with a disability."
- Table 51-1 outlines a classification system for disability and health that provides a standard language and framework for the description of health and health-related states.[7]

III. Types of Conditions

- Types of disabilities include:
  - Developmental: hereditary conditions that manifest symptoms before age 21.
  - Acquired: caused by chronic disease, acute medical conditions, or trauma.
  - Age-associated: usually occur after 65 years of age and often related to a chronic health condition.
- Some types of impairment can manifest as a stable condition; others may cause progressive disability.
- A temporary disability can result from a physical impairment such as a broken leg or because of a physiologic condition such as limitations that may occur during pregnancy.
- A variety of impairments are found among persons with disabilities, and an individual may have more than one type of disability.
- Many diseases and syndromes with associated symptoms of disability or impairment are described in various chapters throughout Section IX of this book.

TABLE 51-1 • International Classification of Functioning, Disability, and Health

PART 1: FUNCTIONING AND DISABILITY

Body Functions

Mental functions	The brain: both global mental functions, such as consciousness, energy and drive, and specific mental functions, such as memory, language, and calculation mental functions.
Sensory functions	Seeing, hearing, tasting, and touch, as well as the sensation of pain.
Voice and speech functions	Producing sounds and speech.
Functions of the cardiovascular, hematologic, immunologic, and respiratory systems	The heart and blood vessels, blood production, immunity, respiration, and exercise tolerance.
Functions of the digestive, metabolic, and endocrine systems	Ingestion, digestion, and elimination, as well as metabolism and the endocrine glands.
Genitourinary and reproductive functions	Urination and the reproduction, including sexual and procreative functions.
Neuromusculoskeletal and movement-related functions	Movement and mobility, including functions of joints, bones, reflexes, and muscles.
Functions of the skin and related structures	Skin, skin glands, nails, hair, and related structures.

Body Structures

Structures of the nervous system	Brain, spinal cord, meninges, and nervous system, including sympathetic and parasympathetic nervous systems.
The eye, ear, and related structures	Eye socket, eyeball, external ear, middle ear, inner ear, and related structures.
Structures involved in voice and speech	Nose, mouth, pharynx, larynx, and related structures.
Structures of the cardiovascular, immunologic, and respiratory systems	Heart, arteries, veins, and capillaries; central lymphoid tissue (bone marrow, thymus) and peripheral lymphoid tissue (lymph nodes, spleen, mucosa-associated lymphoid tissue); and pharynx, trachea, bronchi, and lungs.
Structures related to the digestive, metabolic, and endocrine systems	Salivary glands, esophagus, stomach, intestines, pancreas, liver, gall bladder and ducts, endocrine glands, and related structures.
Structures related to the genitourinary and reproductive systems	Kidneys, ureter, bladder, pelvic floor, and male and female reproductive structures.
Structures related to movement	Head, neck, shoulder, upper and lower extremities, pelvic regions, trunk, musculoskeletal system, and other structures related to movement.
Skin and related structures	Skin, skin glands, nails, hair, and related structures.

PART 2: CONTEXTUAL FACTORS

Activities and Participation

Learning and applying knowledge	Learning, applying the knowledge that is learned, thinking, solving problems, and making decisions.
General tasks and demands	Carrying out specific single or multiple tasks, organizing routines and handling stress; identifying the underlying features of the execution of tasks under different circumstances.
Communication	General and specific features of communicating by language, signs and symbols, including receiving and producing messages, carrying on conversations, and using communication devices and techniques.
Mobility	Moving by changing body position or location or by transferring from one place to another by carrying, moving, or manipulating objects; by walking, running, or climbing; and by using various forms of transportation.
Self-care	Caring for oneself and washing and drying oneself; caring for one's body and body parts; dressing, eating, and drinking; and looking after one's health.
Domestic life	Carrying out domestic and everyday actions and tasks; acquiring a place to live, food, clothing, and other necessities; household cleaning and repairing; caring for personal and other household objects; and assisting others.

(continues)

TABLE 51-1 • International Classification of Functioning, Disability, and Health (*Continued*)

Interpersonal interactions and relationships	Carrying out the actions and tasks required for basic and complex interactions with people (strangers, friends, relatives, family members, and lovers) in a contextually and socially appropriate manner.
Major life areas	Carrying out the tasks and actions required to engage in education, work, and employment and to conduct economic transactions.
Community, social, and civic life	Actions and tasks required to engage in organized social life outside the family in community, social, and civic areas of life.
Environmental Factors That Influence Functioning	
Products and technology	Natural or human-made products or systems of products, equipment, and technology in an individual's immediate environment that are gathered, created, produced, or manufactured.
Natural and human-made changes to environment	Animate and inanimate elements of the natural or physical environment, and components of that environment that have been modified by people, as well as characteristics of human populations within that environment.
Support and relationships	People or animals that provide practical physical or emotional support, nurturing, protection, assistance, and relationships to other persons in their home, place of work, school, at play, or in other aspects of their daily activities.
Attitudes	The observable consequences of customs, practices, ideologies, values, norms, factual beliefs, and religious beliefs that influence individual behavior and social life; individual or societal attitudes about a person's value as a human being that may motivate positive, honorific practices, or negative and discriminatory practices.
Services, systems, and policies	Governmental and private programs, infrastructure, regulations, and standards designed to meet the needs of individuals.

IV. Physical and Intellectual Disabilities

- Specific physical disabilities are described more completely in Chapter 52.
- Neurodevelopmental disorders are described in Chapter 50.

V. Sensory Disabilities

- Sensory disabilities are impairments of one of the senses: vision, hearing, touch, smell, and spatial awareness.[8]
- When a patient has either a vision or hearing impairment, modifications to the dental hygiene process of care, especially communication, is essential.

A. Visual Impairment

- There are an estimated 285 million individuals worldwide who have a visual impairment with 39 million blind and 246 million with low vision.[9,10]
- 23.7 Americans adults report have vision loss.[9,10]
- Limitations of sight cover a broad spectrum from the slightly affected to completely blind with no perception of light.
- Blindness may be secondary to another primary condition or chronic disease.
- "Legal blindness" is defined as having central vision (or acuity) of not more than 20/200 in the better eye with correction (glasses) or having peripheral fields (side vision) of no more than 20° diameter.[11]
- Individuals with visual impairment may use a white cane to aid them while walking and for identification purposes.[11]
- Technology and assistive devices available for the visual impaired include:
  - Computer screen readers that allow the individual to read displayed data with a speech synthesizer.
  - Screen magnifiers are available to help the low-vision user by enlarging the text and graphics on the screen.
  - Braille wristwatches and printers.[10,11]

B. Causes of Visual Impairment

- The leading age-related causes of blindness are diabetic retinopathy, macular degeneration, cataracts, glaucoma, trauma, and infections.[12]
- In individuals above the age of 60 years, the leading cause of blindness is macular degeneration, which affects the viewing of fine details, and can interfere with reading, driving, and performing daily tasks.[12]
- Blindness in children is of prenatal origin, resulting from maternal infections such as rubella, syphilis, and toxoplasmosis.[13]
- Other causes in childhood are neoplasms and retinopathy of prematurity.

- The incidence of retinopathy of prematurity has increased as more premature babies survive.[13]
- Major cause of unilateral blindness in North America is ocular trauma related to sport, work, assaults, traffic, and contact lens–induced keratitis.[13]
- Sport-related eye injuries are the leading cause of blindness in school-age children in the United States.[14–16]
- Current preventable strategies need to be implemented,[15] including wearing safety glasses during dental hygiene care.

C. Hearing Impairment

- 360 million people worldwide have disabling hearing loss and 32 million of those are children.[17]
- 2 to 3 out of 1,000 children in the United States are born with a detectable level of hearing loss.[18]
- 27.7 million American adults, aged 20–69 years, have hearing loss.[18]
- When hearing is impaired to the extent that it has no practical value for the purpose of spoken communication, a person is considered *deaf*.[17]
- A person who cannot hear as well as someone with normal hearing is referred to as having *hearing loss*.[17]
- "Hard of hearing" refers to people with mild to severe hearing loss, who communicate through spoken langange.[17]
- The hearing loss can be mild to severe or profound and can affect one or both ears.
- Hearing aids benefit people who have sensory cell damage in the inner ear.
- Assistive measures and devices for those who are deaf or have hearing loss include qualified interpreters, assistive listening headsets, text telephone devices readers, videotext displays, hearing aids, and closed caption.[17]
- People with significant hearing loss may benefit from cochlear implants.[17]

D. Causes of Hearing Impairment

- The cause of hearing loss may be associated with the outer-, middle-, or inner-ear mechanisms, singly or in combinations. Many factors may contribute to deafness.
  - Congenital: prenatal infection in the mother, especially rubella, low birth weight and birth asphyxia (lack of oxygen at birth), inappropriate use of medications during pregnancy, and severe jaundice in the neonatal period.[17]
  - Acquired: chronic inner-ear infections, infectious diseases (meningitis), injury to the head or ear, excessive noise (workplace and recreation), ageing, and toxic effects of drugs have all been implicated.[17]
- *Newborn screening*: The spread of these universal programs prevents future psychosocial, education, and linguistic implications related to hearing loss.[19]

- Partial deafness may not be diagnosed, or certain patients, particularly elderly ones, may not admit hearing limitation. Clues to the identification of a hearing problem are:
  - Lack of attention—fails to respond to conversation.
  - Focused, strained facial expression or stares when others are talking.
  - Turns head to one side—hearing may be good on one side only.
  - Answers are unrelated to the question.
  - Does one thing when told to do another.
  - Frequently asks others to repeat what was said.
  - Unusual speech quality.[18]

VI. Access to Oral Health Services

- People with disabilities "are the most underserved groups in receiving dental care and have the most significant oral health disparities of any group."[20]
- Progress is being made to ensure adequate access to dental care, but barriers exist related to the patient, family, caregivers, guardians, and dental professional (Table 51-2).
- Having adequate access to dental and dental hygiene services can make a significant contribution to the oral health, well-being, independence, and sense of personal esteem of a patient with a disability.
- Although providing care for patients with disabilities is challenging, training, experience, empathy, patience, and a desire to be successful can help.[21]

VII. Trends in Community-Based Delivery of Services

A. Overview

- Individuals with physical and intellectual impairments may be self-sufficient or may have community-based living, educational, and work arrangements.
- Barrier-free or assisted-living housing for individuals and staffed community-based residential facilities for group living are available for those who need daily assistance.
- Many home-care and community-based services are available for individuals with disabilities; however, access to dental services is often limited by traditional office-based dental care delivery systems.
- New healthcare delivery system models are being proposed to provide access to dental services where people live, work, play, go to school, or receive other social services.[20–22]
- Expansion of "direct access" regulations increase the ability of dental hygienists to provide preventive services in alternative settings and function as members of interprofessional patient care teams.[20,21]
- See Chapter 4 for information about providing dental hygiene care in alternative settings.

TABLE 51-2 • Examples of Barriers to Access for Dental Care

	PATIENT	FAMILY, CAREGIVER, AND GUARDIAN	DENTAL PROFESSIONAL
Attitude barriers	• May not comprehend importance of oral health. • May not be aware of needing oral care. • May not want to or be able to cooperate.	• May not care for own oral health. • May be overstressed with other patient health issues that seem more important than oral needs.	• May not feel adequately trained to or want to or be able to treat safely a physically, cognitively, or medically compromised patient.
Health literacy barriers	• May not understand the relationship of oral health to systemic health. • May have difficulty understanding insurance coverage, locating a provider, making appointments, or completing paperwork.	• May not understand the relationship of oral health to systemic health. • May have difficulty understanding insurance coverage, locating a provider, making appointments, or completing paperwork.	• May not understand that the patient has many barriers to accessing oral care. • May not have adequately assessed the patient's health literacy when providing previous care.
Physical barriers	• Fear of not being able to cope with architectural barriers. • Fear of falling. • Fear of attracting attention in an embarrassing way.	• May not be able to transport patient with wheelchair. • May not be able to lift or support patient in car or dental chair.	• Office facility or treatment rooms may not provide a barrier-free environment.
Financial barriers	• May have limited income. • May not have adequate dental insurance coverage or cannot find a provider who accepts specific insurance.	• May not be able to take time from employment to accompany patient to appointments.	• Cost of building accessible features or buying specialized equipment. • Lack of reimbursement for the additional cost of longer appointment times needed for care.

BARRIER-FREE ENVIRONMENT

◆ Healthcare facilities are required to follow guidelines and specifications for a barrier-free physical environment based on the ADA: Standards for Accessible Design.[23]

◆ A barrier-free facility for a patient in a wheelchair, who requires more space for turning and positioning, is deemed accessible to all individuals.

◆ Additional features for other specific disabilities are braille floor indicators on elevators; doorways, steps, and stairways can be outlined with bright colors to contrast with the background for people with limited vision.

I. External Features

A. Parking

◆ A reserved area, clearly marked, near the building entrance and 13-feet wide (8-foot car space with 5-foot access aisle permits opening car doors for exiting and reboarding).

◆ Curb ramps (cuts) from the street and from the parking area.

B. Walkways

◆ A 3-foot-wide walkway is needed for wheelchair accommodation.

◆ The surface is solid and nonslip, without irregularities.

C. Entrance

◆ At least one entrance to the building on ground level accessible by a gently sloping ramp (rise of 1 inch for every 12 inches).

◆ An easily grasped handrail (height 30–34 inches) is needed on both sides to accommodate left- and right-handed cane and one-crutch users.

D. Door

◆ The lightweight door with a lever type of handle opens at least 32 inches to accommodate a wheelchair.

II. Internal Features

Official regulations specify dimensions for accessibility of all aspects, including passageways, floors, drinking fountains, and restrooms. A few are described here.

A. Passageways

◆ Passageways must be at least 3 feet wide.

◆ Passageways must be free from obstructions, such as hanging signs, chairs, and large plants.

B. Floors

◆ Level floors with nonslip surfaces.

◆ Movable rugs or mats are obstacles or hazards for patients who use wheelchairs, walkers or canes, or are blind.

C. Reception Area

◆ Chairs should permit easy access during seating and rising.

  • Eighteen-inch-high, flat, firm seats, and arms to provide support when pushing oneself up by the arms.

  • Should not slide or tip as the person rises.

III. The Treatment Room

◆ Doorways are at least 32 inches wide.

◆ Enough room beside the dental chair to allow for turning the wheelchair.

◆ The dental chair is able to lower to 19 inches from the floor and accessible from both sides for wheelchair transfer.

◆ An x-ray machine in the same treatment room or a portable or handheld x-ray machine[24] can simplify the problems of moving the patient into a separate radiography room.

◆ For the patient with visual impairment, move equipment, such as the bracket tray and clinician's stool, from the pathway to the operatory chair and lower the chair before seating the patient.

RISK ASSESSMENT

Patients with disabilities may be at higher risk for oral disease due to characteristics related to the specific disability or disease.

◆ Risk factors associated with specific disabilities and medical conditions are described in the chapters in Section IX of this book devoted to the particular condition.

◆ Assessment of oral disease risk factors for a patient with a disability includes assessment of oral conditions, functional ability, and medical status.[25]

I. Oral Manifestations

People with disabilities have an increased risk for oral problems.

◆ Dental caries is common, often associated with diet and poor oral hygiene.

◆ Periodontal disease can occur more often and develop at an earlier age.

◆ Malocclusion is associated with muscular abnormalities, developmental delays, delayed tooth eruption, and oral habits such as bruxism or tongue thrusting.[6,25]

◆ Oral and craniofacial anomalies may be present, particularly in individuals with developmental disabilities. Examples include:
  • Enamel defects.
  • High lip lines and dry gingiva due to air exposure.
  • Variations in number, size, or shape of teeth.
  • Facial asymmetry and hypoplasia of the midfacial region.[25]
  • Cleft lip or palate (see Chapter 49).

◆ Damaging oral habits can affect both soft and hard oral tissues. Examples include:
  • Bruxism.
  • Food pouching.
  • Mouth breathing.
  • Tongue thrusting.

  • Self-injurious behavior.
  • Rumination (regurgitation of chewed food).
  • Pica (eating unusual objects and substances such as cigarette butts or gravel).[25]

◆ Evidence of trauma or injury may be present, especially in individuals with a seizure disorder or physical disability.

◆ Weakness or paralysis of facial muscles can compromise mastication and self-cleaning motion of the tongue. Food pouching is common.

◆ Drooling or impaired swallowing of saliva is a common feature of some disabling conditions involving head and neck musculature.[27]

◆ Potential oral side effects of medications include:
  • Increased dental caries risk due to sweetened elixirs or medication-induced xerostomia.
  • Drug-induced gingival enlargement, a potential side-effect of treatment with phenytoin or other antiepileptic medication (see Chapter 57).
  • Oral ulcerations, mucositis, and susceptibility to infection and frequent manifestations following chemotherapy cancer treatment or radiation to head and neck area are discussed in Chapter 55.

II. Functional Ability

◆ Functional ability refers to the ability of an individual to accomplish daily living skills (bathing, toothbrushing, dressing, answering the phone, etc.).[7,28,29]

◆ In children, functional ability may also include activities such as coloring a picture or catching a ball.[29]

◆ Assessment of functional ability determines what oral self-care tasks an individual can do alone, what range or degree of assistance is needed, or whether the person depends on others for complete care.

◆ An individual patient's functional level may be affected by:
  • Decrease in cognitive capability.
  • Behavioral problems.
  • Mobility problems.
  • Uncontrolled body movements.[28–30]

◆ Sensory impairments may mask a child's functional and intellectual capacity because responses may differ from other children.[31–33]
  • Children with blindness are limited in terms of learning by imitation.[31–33]
  • A child with blindness may learn to speak later than a child with average vision and may start school later.[31–33]
  • The earlier the hearing loss in a child, the more serious impact on the child's development.[33]
  • Communication delays may impact on social interactions and vocational choices.[33]

◆ Functioning levels and implications for oral self-care are described in Box 51-1 and in Chapter 22.

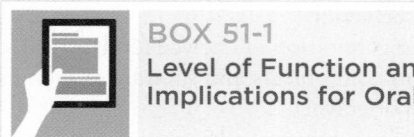

BOX 51-1
Level of Function and Implications for Oral Self-Care

ADL/IADL (based on ADL/IADL measures of patient functioning in Table 22-3) Level 0

- Individuals who are capable of flossing and brushing their own teeth.
- Children and those of all ages need varying degrees of encouragement, motivation, and supervision.

ADL/IADL Levels 1 and 2

- Includes those individuals capable of carrying out at least part of their oral hygiene needs but who require considerable training, assistance, and direct supervision.
- The assistance may be verbal, gestural, or hand-over-hand.

ADL/IADL Level 3

- Includes individuals who are unable to attend to their own care and are therefore dependent.
- Patients in this group may be confined to bed and nonambulatory, although others may be confined to wheelchairs. With training, some may be able to attempt a part of their own care.

III. Medical Status

- Assistance in completing the health history questionnaire may be needed, especially for the individual with visual impairment.[32]
- Specific details of the patient's limitations are recorded so that adaptations can be made during the current and future appointments.
- Having extensive knowledge of every health conditions patients have is impossible; however, having the knowledge about when to gather and apply additional information is essential.[4]
- Assessment and monitoring of the patient's medical status during treatment can reduce the risk of a medical emergency.
- Individuals with a disability may also experience additional medical comorbidities and health challenges such as:
  - Cardiac disorders.
  - Gastroesophageal reflux.
  - Seizures.
  - Visual and hearing impairments.
  - Latex allergies (due to spina bifida or frequent surgeries).[34]
- Medications the patient takes may enhance risk for oral disease.
  - Medications with a side effect of xerostomia contribute to dental caries.

- Medications that diminish appetite as a side effect influence eating an adequate diet.
- Sucrose-based liquid medications contribute to dental caries incidence.[35]

ORAL DISEASE PREVENTION AND CONTROL

I. Objectives

Whether care is being delivered in a traditional or an alternative practice, the dental hygienist's objectives are to:

- Provide regular professional examinations and treatment at appropriate intervals to maintain patient's oral health.
- Determine patients' ability for oral self-care and need for caregiver intervention.[4]
- Motivate the patient and caregiver to establish and maintain healthy oral tissue.
- Contribute to the patient's general health through preventing tooth loss, thus maintaining ability to masticate food, preventing malnutrition, and increasing resistance to infection.
- Prevent extensive dental and periodontal treatment the patient may not tolerate because of lowered physical stamina or the inability to cooperate.
- Prevent the need for dentures or other removable prostheses, which can be hazardous, difficult, or impossible for certain patients to tolerate.

II. Preventive Care Introduction

- Preventive interventions are selected based on individualized risk factors and level of assistance needed for daily oral care.[25]
- Depending on the disability and level of function, the patient may need:
  - Complete assistance.
  - Partial assistance.
  - No assistance with daily biofilm removal.
- Daily personal oral hygiene care can be compromised due to patient or caregiver:
  - Lack of knowledge and understanding about oral disease prevention and how it is accomplished.
  - Lack of motivation to carry out the necessary daily routines.
  - Lack of the necessary cognitive and/or physical coordination to carry out oral hygiene measures.

III. Dental Biofilm Removal

A. Provide Basic Information

- Individualized instruction is provided for each patient according to the patient's unique needs and functional ability.
- Determine the current daily care routine to identify if modifications are required.

◆ Biofilm formation and disease development are described on a level at which the patient and caregiver can learn and be motivated.

◆ Approaches for motivating the patient or caregiver's health behavior change are described in Chapter 24.

B. Toothbrushing

◆ Basic information about toothbrushes and methods is found in Chapter 26.

◆ Provide clear and concise instructions.

◆ Biofilm removal is more important than the specific technique used, as long as damage is not done to the gingiva or teeth.

◆ Use of a soft toothbrush and a scrub-brush or circular Fones method may be appropriate and within the capability of certain patients.

◆ Alternative positions for a parent or caregiver providing toothbrushing assistance are discussed more completely later in this chapter.

◆ Encourage independence in daily oral care.[25]

◆ Although a caregiver may be willing to brush the patient's teeth, as much as possible should be carried out by the patient.

◆ Adaptations for brush handles and other oral self-care aids can promote or make possible a patient's independent biofilm removal.

◆ Demonstrate toothbrushing in the patient's mouth and describe the feeling of the filament tips on and under the gingival margin and the feeling of clean teeth.

◆ Guide patient with hand-over-hand toothbrush technique to help with placement of the toothbrush in the mouth.

C. Adaptive Aids

◆ For patients whose main deterrent to oral self-care is related to grasp, manipulation, or control of a toothbrush, adaptations and self-care aids can help accommodate specific needs.

◆ Benefits to the patient may include feelings of self-esteem and accomplishment when able to manage the important task of brushing, particularly for patients who have physical but no cognitive disability.

◆ General prerequisites for a self-care aid include:
  • Disinfectable.
  • Durable: can withstand exposure to water and saliva.
  • Resistant to absorption of oral fluids.
  • Replaceable.
  • Inexpensive.

D. Adapted Manual Toothbrush

◆ Figure 51-1 illustrates attachments to insert and hold the brush handle against the patient's hand. This attachment is useful for a patient.
  • With fingers permanently fixed in a fist.
  • Who cannot grasp and hold.

◆ Aids to enlarge the diameter of the handle of an oral care implement, useful for a patient with limited hand closure, are illustrated in Figures 51-2 and 51-3.

◆ For patient with limited shoulder or elbow movement, lengthen handle of the brush using a material strong or rigid enough to provide sufficient lateral pressure to remove biofilm from the tooth surfaces. Examples include:
  • Attach a handle of a kitchen utensil, such as wooden spoon, to the brush handle with glue or tape (see Figure 51-4).
  • Tongue depressors taped to the brush handle, then one or two other tongue depressors taped to overlap and provide an extension.
  • Use other means by wrapping the object securely to the brush handle for elongation.[25,30]

◆ A specially designed toothbrush curved outer filaments and a short stiff center row of filaments that brush exposed tooth surfaces simultaneously is shown in Figure 51-5.

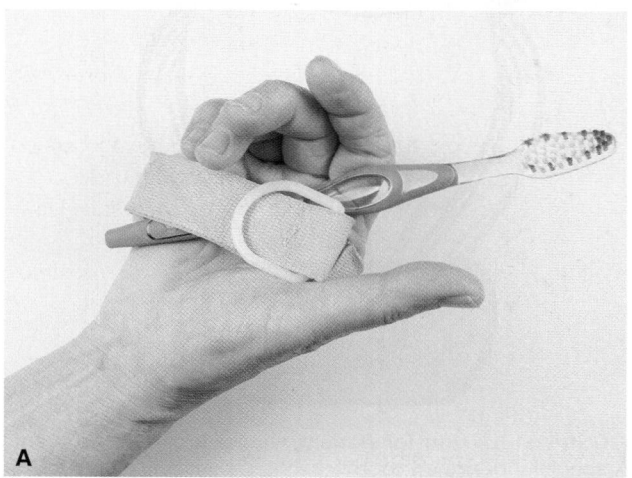

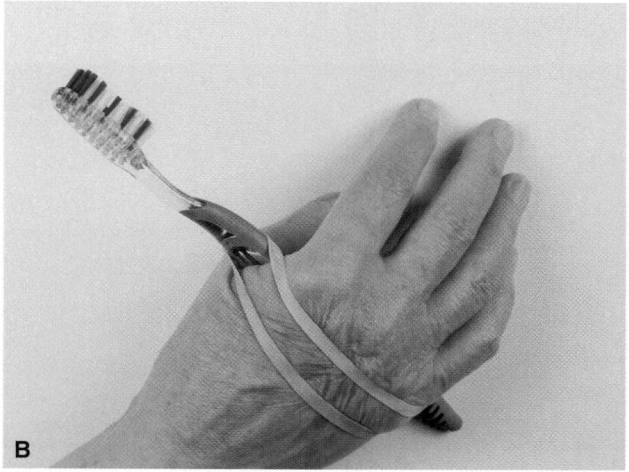

FIGURE 51-1 • Aids for Patient Who Cannot Grasp and Hold. Adjustable Velcro strap **(A)** or simple rubber band **(B)** around toothbrush handle enables patient to secure brush firmly across the palm of the hand. A floss holder also may be held by these methods.

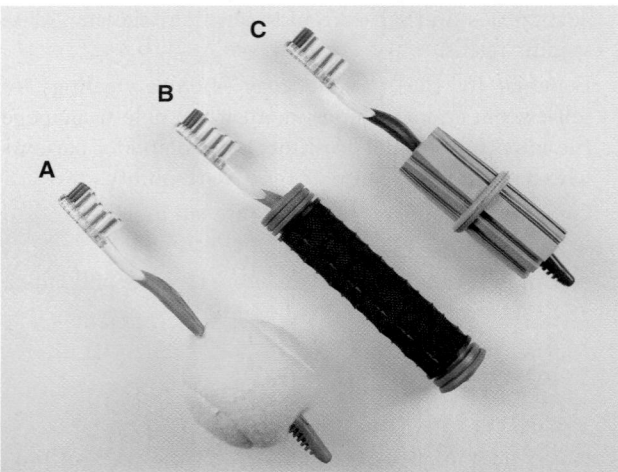

FIGURE 51-2 • Aids for Patient with Limited Grasp. A: Toothbrush inserted into tennis ball or other soft rubber ball. **B:** Toothbrush inserted into a bicycle handle grip. **C:** Toothbrush inserted into a clean, unused rubber pet toy.

◆ For a patient who can hold and position the toothbrush, but cannot make strokes for biofilm removal.

◆ For a patient with hand tremors, such as with Parkinson's disease.

◆ Can be used with patient moving their head side-to-side and up-and-down instead of moving their hand.

◆ Can be used by a caregiver who provides toothbrushing assistance.

◆ Provides similar reduction in biofilm compared with use of a conventional brush.[36]

E. Power-Aided Devices

◆ Use of a power toothbrush can provide independence and more effective biofilm removal for many patients and can motivate patients who have difficulty with a manual toothbrush.[37]

  • Can cause trauma if used incorrectly by, for example, a patient unable to hold the heavier weight of the power toothbrush or one lacking the comprehension for proper use.

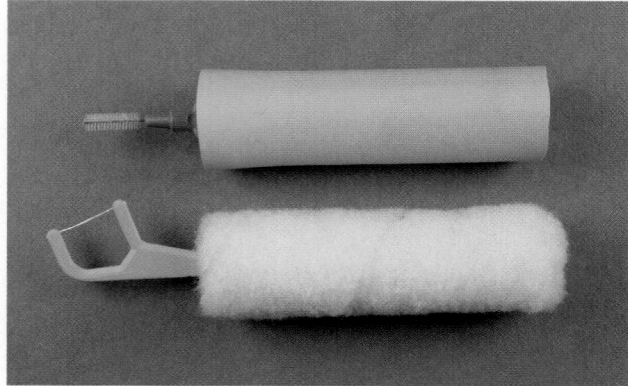

FIGURE 51-3 • Interdental Cleaning Aids for Patient with Limited Grasp. Floss aids and interdental cleaners can be inserted into commercially available foam tubing or the open end of a clean mini-sized paint roller cover.

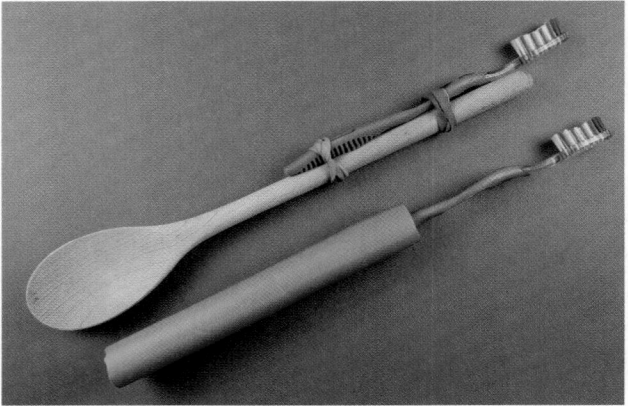

FIGURE 51-4 • Aid for Patient with Limited Shoulder or Elbow Movement. Toothbrush with added handle extension can be created using commercially available foam tubing or by securing a toothbrush to a long-handled wooden spoon with tape or an elastic band.

  • The extra size and weight of the handle may be advantageous for some patients or difficult for others with limited strength.

  • The on/off mechanism may be difficult to use for those lacking finger strength and coordination.

  • The larger handle can aid those who have difficulty grasping objects.

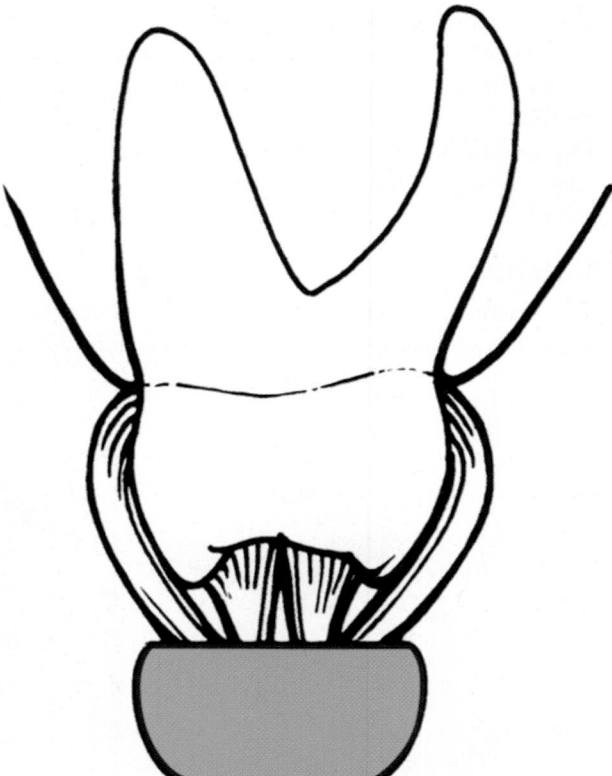

FIGURE 51-5 • Aid for Patient with a Brushing Problem. A specially designed toothbrush is shown on the mesial of a maxillary second primary molar. Used with a back-and-forth motion, the filaments remove debris and dental biofilm simultaneously from the facial, lingual (palatal), and occlusal tooth surfaces.

- The vibrations created during use cannot be tolerated by certain patients.
- Additional cost of the brush may be a consideration for some patients.

◆ Additional power-aided devices, such as flossers, are available and are recommended based on assessment of an individual patient's need and abilities.

◆ Patients are instructed to follow manufacturers' instructions for proper use as indicated on each package.

◆ A patient with limited grasp can adapt a cuff around the handle to aid in holding the power-aided brush, similar to those shown in Figure 51-1.

◆ Cross-contamination can be a problem, particularly in group-living situations. Ensure each patient has a separate marked toothbrush and is kept apart from others.

F. Dentifrice

◆ A dentifrice containing fluoride is recommended for patients who can use a dentifrice.

◆ When a patient cannot control saliva, rinse, or expectorate, use of a dentifrice may be contraindicated.

◆ A dentifrice may increase a gag reflex for certain patients.

◆ When a parent or other caregiver is assisting, the paste may limit visibility for thorough biofilm removal.

◆ When a paste is used, only a small, pea-sized amount is placed on the brush.
  - Dentifrice is not essential for biofilm removal, and another method of daily fluoride application may be more appropriate.

◆ The person who is severely disabled may be treated with a suction brush, as described in Chapter 4 to help prevent aspiration.

G. Interdental Cleaning

◆ If standard use of dental floss is not possible, due to limited dexterity or use of only one hand, the use of a floss holder or other interdental aid can make interdental cleaning possible.

◆ Certain aids may be useful for the caregiver.

◆ Methods for increasing the size of a toothbrush handle may be adapted for the handle of a floss holder.

◆ Some patients will need to use other interdental aids, as described in Chapter 27.

◆ Careful instruction for use and supervision are provided to prevent tissue damage.

H. Cleaning Removable Dental Prostheses

◆ The details for cleaning removable prostheses are described in Chapter 30.

◆ For the patient with difficulty grasping or holding the brush, a denture brush handle may be adapted by any of the methods described for the regular toothbrush.

◆ A fingernail brush may be used instead of a standard denture brush provided all denture surfaces can be reached for biofilm removal.

◆ For the patient with use of only one hand or who needs to grasp the denture with two hands to prevent accidents, the following are recommended:
  - Fingernail brush with suction cups.
  - Denture brush, as shown in Figure 51-6A.
  - Denture brush with suction cups, as shown in Figure 51-6B, can attach low inside the sink bowl.

IV. Fluorides

◆ Selection of a fluoride program for any patient depends on the assessment of the individual's caries risk status (see Chapter 25).

◆ The patient with a disability may be at increased risk for caries due to barriers that limit access to preventive services, decreased ability to provide or cooperate with assistance for self-care, and side effects of medications.

◆ Risk-based fluoride recommendations are described more completely in Chapter 34 and include:
  - Encouragement to drink fluoridated tap water where available.
  - Use of dentifrice with fluoride.
  - Dietary supplements for young children, when fluoride is below optimum level in the community water supply (see Chapter 34 for guidelines).
  - Some patients with disabilities cannot tolerate fluoride trays.
  - Fluoride varnishes are tolerated better than fluoride trays for many people with disabilities.[37]
  - Fluoride varnish treatment is quick, teeth do not need to be isolated, and the varnish is not sensitive to moisture.[37]
  - Self-applied home fluoride.

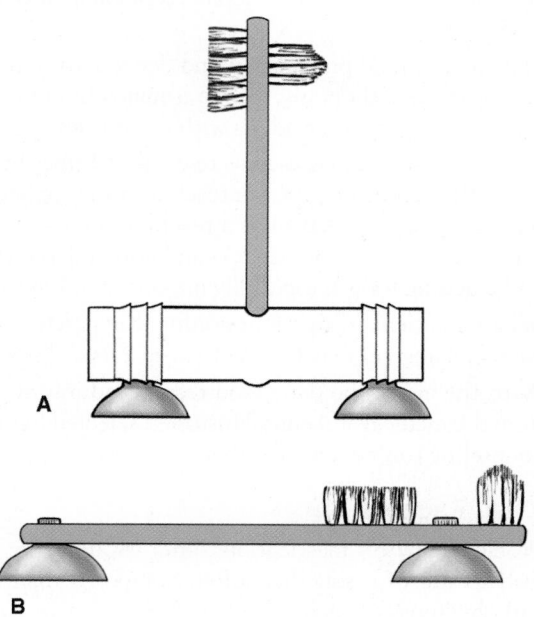

FIGURE 51-6 • Denture Brushes with Suction Cups. A: Denture brush in a commercially available mounting. **B:** Suction cups attached directly to a denture brush. Either brush may be positioned in a sink to aid the person who has one hand or who needs to grasp the denture with two hands to prevent accidental dropping and breakage.

◆ For a dependent, low-functioning person, brushing with a fluoride gel rather than a toothpaste can be recommended or the toothbrush could be soaked in a fluoridated mouth rinse before brushing.[37]

◆ Silver diamine fluoride is beneficial for people with disabilities, as it is noninvasive and could reduce the need for surgical-restorative work.[38,39]

V. Pit and Fissure Sealants

◆ Pit and fissure sealants can be provided for cooperative patients with developmental disabilities with satisfactory results.

◆ The principles for application are the same as those for all patients, as described in Chapter 35.

◆ Use of a dental assistant is imperative to help with patient management and to maintain a dry field to assure sealant retention.

◆ Use of a rubber dam is helpful for patients with excess saliva, hyperactivity of the tongue, or other management difficulties.

◆ When a patient who is severely disabled receive general anesthesia for restorative procedures, pit and fissure sealants are placed in all noncarious occlusal pits and fissures at that time.

VI. Diet Instruction

A. Eating Habits

◆ Current eating and snack habits, extent of oral health knowledge, family customs, and economic status are considered before specific dietary recommendations are made.

◆ Difficulty of food preparation and dependence on others for grocery shopping can be a major limitation to diet selection for some adults with disabilities.

◆ Sweets are sometimes used as rewards or bribes by unsuspecting family members or teachers using applied behavioral analysis (ABA) as a teaching tool,[40] and the introduction of sugarless snacks and nonfood as rewards and teaching tools is especially important.

◆ When a patient is high functioning, the parent, advocate, or caregiver may be able to keep a food diary.

◆ With the aid of the daily food record and information from the medical and dental histories, selected items for counseling can be selected, that is, caries.

B. Oral Factors

◆ Problems with mastication and swallowing can lead to use of a soft diet, often composed mainly of carbohydrates.

◆ Conditions affecting the integrity of facial musculature can compromise self-cleansing of oral structures and contribute to food pouching in the buccal vestibule.

C. Recommendations

◆ General procedures for dietary assessment and counseling are described in Chapter 33.

◆ Adaptations involve long-range planning for gradual modification of the patient's diet.

◆ The person who selects and prepares the food for the patient is involved in the planning.

◆ In an institutional setting, the dental hygienist can work as a member of the interprofessional patient care team with the administrative and medical personnel, teachers, dietitians, and aides to introduce dietary modifications.

PATIENT MANAGEMENT

◆ With a few modifications and attention to managing specific factors related to each individual's situation, most patients with disabilities can be treated in a clinical setting.

◆ Only a relatively small number of patients need hospitalization due to difficulties in management or a systemic condition that requires special medical supervision.

I. Objectives

◆ Increase the efficacy, efficiency, and safety of dental and dental hygiene treatment.

◆ Make patient appointments pleasant and comfortable.

II. Modes of Communication

◆ Basic behavioral support strategies, such as tell–show–do, modeling, positive reinforcement, and desensitization, can be adapted to address the unique needs of the patient with a disability.[32]

◆ Unless the patient has an extreme cognitive impairment, the patient is always addressed first and the caregiver second.

◆ Address the patient in *person first language*, describing them by their abilities rather than labeling them by their disabilities.[4]

◆ Parents and/or caregivers can explain how best to communicate with the patient, help interpret the changing moods of the patient, identify problems, and note changes in behavior that may indicate a dental problem.

◆ Using nonverbal communication, facial expressions, pointing, body language, and demonstration helps certain patients to respond.

◆ Kindness, patience, and empathy will help the clinician build trust.

◆ A person who is totally blind is more likely to accept a new experience if told about it in detail beforehand.

◆ A person with hearing loss may prefer a particular way of communication.

- Choices include speaking, speechreading, writing, manual, or a combination.
- Manual communication includes using sign language or "signing" and fingerspelling.
- *Always ask the patient which means of communication is preferred and how communication can be improved.*

A. American Sign Language

- American Sign Language (ASL) is a visual/gestural language with a unique grammar and syntax.
- Many people with deafness who prefer this mode of communication grew up using ASL and consider themselves part of a cultural group.
- Individuals who have become deaf in later years may learn sign language and use the signs in English word order, meaning the subject comes before the verb and the verb comes before the object in a sentence structure.
- Some people with deafness prefer to communicate using ASL in medical or dental situations. They can request the services of an ASL interpreter.
- A universal sign language has not been recognized, and many countries have their own.

B. American Manual Alphabet

- Fingerspelling "in the air" is often combined with sign language.
- When making an introduction, for example, the name may be fingerspelled.
- New words often do not have signs and are fingerspelled.

C. Oral Communication

Oral communication by a person with deafness or severe hearing impairment may require a combination of speech, residual hearing, and speechreading.

D. Speechreading

- Speechreading consists of recognizing spoken words by watching the lips, face, and gestures.
- Many of the mouth movements for spoken words have the same appearance as one or more other words, so speechreading may need to be combined with another method of communication.
- Speechreading is not a reliable means of communication for extended, complex discussions for most people with hearing loss.
- Speechreading is not a choice when the clinician must wear a mask.

E. Writing

- Writing may be an alternative when the patient is hard of hearing or when other methods are not satisfactory.
- Have a writing pad available with pen or pencil for communication purposes.

III. Pretreatment Planning

A. Preliminary Contact

- Information may be obtained from the patient, or with legal authority from the guardian, parent, relative, advocate, or other person responsible for the patient.
- The essential information can be obtained in advance by telephone interview, or medical forms can be mailed to the home for completion.
- Advanced information permits the dental team to be prepared to make the appointment a successful and positive experience for the patient and clinician.

B. Legal Guardianship

- When a person is declared incapacitated by a legal process, a guardian is appointed.
- Documented proof of legal guardianship is kept in the patient record.
- When the patient is unable to sign informed consent for treatment, the legal guardian provides this service.[41]

C. Information to Obtain

- In addition to the usual topics covered by the medical, personal, and dental histories, additional information is requested, using questions listed in Box 51-2.
- To avoid unpleasant situations and misunderstanding, ask direct questions about a patient's disability, rather than making assumptions.

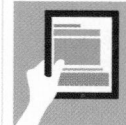

BOX 51-2

Patient with a Disability:
Additional Information to Obtain Before the Appointment

Basic Information

- Has a guardian been legally appointed? Obtain written documentation.
- Is there a caregiver, case worker, or counselor who works with the patient?
- Will someone accompany the patient to appointments?
- Does the patient give consent to discuss care with other individuals?
- Degree of independence, self-care, and communication preferences of the patient.

Medical History

- Specific list of disabilities or disabling conditions.
- When diagnosed.
- History of treatments, hospitalizations, or institutionalization.
- Current medications and other therapy.
- Names and addresses of specialists.
- Any restrictions, such as dietary or for safety (leg braces, helmet).

Dental History

- Previous dental experiences and patient's attitude.
- Barriers to previous dental care.
- Most recent care: procedures, setting, success.
- History of oral infections and oral habits.
- Fluoride history, including fluoridation levels in drinking water and self- or professionally applied topical methods.
- Current home-care methods: aids and special devices, frequency, degree of self-care.
- Concepts of perceived needs, attitudes, and apparent emphasis on oral care.
- Modifications and successful techniques used before and during appointments.

Supplemental Information

Are any of the following affected by disability?

- Muscular coordination, mobility, walking.
- Sitting tolerance.
- Sitting position.
- Ability to cooperate/involuntary movements.
- Communication: speech, hearing, vision.
- Breathing, including when reclined.
- Swallowing, control of saliva.
- Bowel or bladder control.
- Mental capacities.
- Dexterity, ability to brush and floss teeth.
- Ability to chew or eat.

Open-Ended Other Information

- Does patient require any additional assistance or have any other issues of concern?

D. Consultation with Interprofessional Care Team

- Management of a patient with disabilities can be very complex due to medical complications.
- Need to prevent aggravating a medical condition while rendering care.[41]
- Consultation with physicians, social worker, and other medical providers who form the patient's inter-professional care team may be required to help determine an oral health plan.[6]
- Extra time may be required to access information about the conditions and medications before an appointment.

E. Interaction with Caregiver

- A patient with a disability may depend on a caregiver for daily life activities.

- Caregivers may or may not be the legal guardian of the patient or the contact person to plan appointments.
- If the caregiver is not the legal guardian, the adult patient or guardian must be consulted to determine the limits of the caregiver's role.
- Caregivers can be an excellent source of information, help prepare the patient for the appointment, and offer suggestions for gaining cooperation from the patient.
- Invite the caregiver to the office before the appointment to see the facility and become familiar with the surroundings and staff.

IV. Appointment Scheduling

A. Special Requirements

- Allow time in the schedule for preparation needed before appointment, for example, to move furniture, retrieve and set up special equipment such as paper to write on for a patient with a hearing impairment, or to premedicate the patient.
- Identify special aids the patient is asked to bring to the appointment, such as a transfer board for transfer into the dental chair, hearing aid, dental prostheses, and biofilm control devices currently in use.
- Individuals who are deaf may require an ASL interpreter.
- Some individuals with disabilities are accompanied by service dogs, such as guide dogs for the visual, hearing, and other disabilities, which are allowed by law into all public buildings and on public transportation.
- When a patient brings a guide dog to the appointment:
  - Do not distract a dog on duty by touching, speaking, or making eye contact.
  - Do not walk on the dog's left side, which can distract the dog.
  - Do not offer the dog food.
  - Do not lead or grab the patient while the dog is guiding.
  - Ask the patient where the best place would be for the dog to stay during the appointment.[42]
- Service dogs are well-trained animals and will lie quietly as directed by the patient.
  - If you want to pet the dog, ask the guide dog-user first. Often the user will remove the harness before allowing someone to pet the dog.[42]

B. Transportation

- A patient may rely on the caregiver or another source for transport to appointment.
- A patient using a wheelchair may need to reserve wheelchair accessible transportation and be limited by the availability of transportation.
- The transportation service may need to be contacted when the patient has completed the appointment; forms may need to be completed.

C. Time Considerations

◆ Determine how the patient's daily schedule influences time selection for scheduling appointments.

◆ Inquire about the schedule of the caregiver who accompanies the patient.

◆ The cooperation of the patient may be decreased if basic routines are disturbed, for example:

- The appointment for the patient with diabetes cannot interfere with medication, meal, or between-meal eating schedules.
- The elderly person who rises early may want a morning appointment.
- Patients with arthritis may have greater mobility later in the day.
- Child's nap schedule should not be disrupted.
- Early morning appointment may be difficult for a patient who requires a long time for morning preparation, such as a patient with a spinal cord injury or colostomy.

◆ Arrange a time when the patient will not have a long wait.

◆ Allow sufficient time so the patient is not rushed; many persons with disabilities require more time.

◆ Consider incontinence issues, including time needed for restroom visits.

D. Patient Reception: The Initial Appointment

◆ The orientation of a patient with a disability paves the way for long-term success of dental and dental hygiene supervision and care.

◆ The first appointment includes and, when necessary, may be devoted entirely to a basic orientation to the facilities, the dental chair, and the personnel.

◆ Several orientation visits may be necessary to acclimate the patient to surroundings and to desensitize.

◆ Desensitization techniques and a "show–tell–do" approach can help reduce anxiety, particularly for a patient with cognitive impairment or one who is fearful.

◆ Assessment procedures and preventive personal care instructions are initiated, and participation of the caregiver is solicited as indicated.

V. Introduction of Clinical Settings

◆ Create a casual and relaxed environment.

◆ Create unique ways to communicate during treatment explaining the procedure step-by-step, always face the person when explaining the clinical procedures.[41,43]

◆ Describe each step in detail before proceeding.

◆ Introduce the patient to the dental office by utilizing their senses.[41,43]

◆ Start the oral examination slowly, use fingers first before introducing instruments.[6]

◆ Explain instruments, materials, and how each will be applied using the "show–tell–do" approach.[6]

◆ Prepare patient for power-driven instruments; avoid surprise applications of compressed air, water from syringe, or power-driven instruments.

◆ Explain to patient the sound of the suction before turning it on for the procedure.

◆ For a patient who is not familiar with dental procedures, permit patient to handle dull or blunted instruments if able to do so safely.

◆ Allow the patient to hear the equipment, such as the saliva ejector, that will be used during the appointment.[41,43]

◆ Introduce unusual smells or taste utilized during the different treatment.[41,43]

◆ Apply rubber cup to person's finger so they can experience how polishing feels.

A. Patient with a Visual Impairment

◆ Because of the visual impairment, the patient may tend to rely more on other senses such as touch and hearing.

◆ A person with total blindness tries to be neat and orderly. Avoid moving items belonging to a visually impaired person without alerting them.

◆ A person with total blindness learns to interpret and rely on tone of voice more than persons with sight, who can watch facial expressions.

◆ *Protective eyewear*: The patient may prefer to wear the personal glasses regularly worn.

◆ *Light*: Avoid directing the dental light in the patient's eyes.

- Sensitivity to light is characteristic of many eye conditions.[41,43]

◆ Position the patient for best vision. For example, a patient with glaucoma has no peripheral vision; thus, instruction must be given directly from in front of the patient.[44]

◆ Do not expect a patient to see fine detail, such as that in a radiograph without enlargement.

◆ When the dental hygienist leaves the treatment room during the appointment, explain absence to prevent embarrassment of the patient speaking to someone who is not present.

◆ For the patient with a visual impairment, ask their preference for how to guide them to the dental chair. Many prefer to hold the clinician's arm and follow them (Figure 51-7).

◆ Provide forewarning of potential hazards in the way.

B. Patient with a Hearing Impairment

◆ Full visibility is essential for communicating with a hearing impaired or deaf patient.

- Remove mask when talking.
- Wear a clear face shield.
- Do not demonstrate out of the patient's field of view.[6]

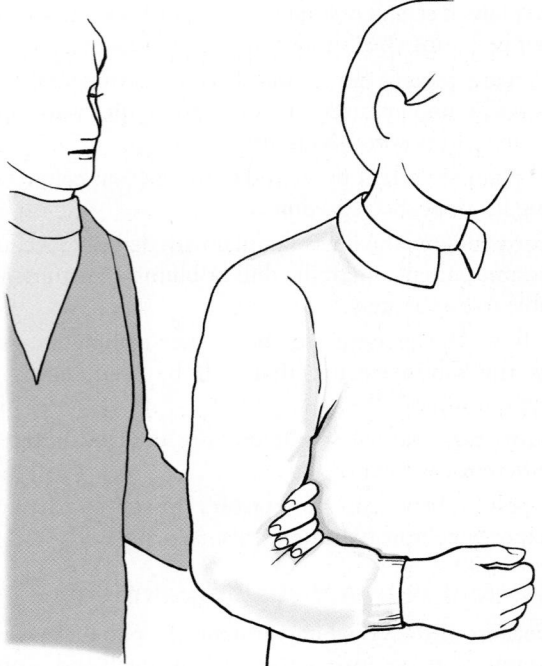

FIGURE 51-7 • Escorting a Visually Impaired Individual. A visually impaired person holds the arm of the guide just above the elbow and walks beside and slightly behind. The guide verbally gives advance notice of approaching changes. The blind person can sense the body movement of the guide and anticipate changes.

- Be careful not to touch a hearing aid when it is turned on.
- Adjust patient's head so ears are not compressed against the headrest or pillow, which can cause discomfort.
- Eliminate or minimize background noise.[45]
- Use visual tools, posters, brochures, and so on, to help explain procedures.[6]

VI. Continuing Care Appointments

The frequency of continuing care appointments for all patients is individualized, but frequent appointments are encouraged for some persons with a disability for the following reasons:

- To decrease the length of single appointment.
- To assist the patient who has limited ability to perform personal oral self-care adequately.
- To provide motivation through monitoring biofilm and review of procedures for the patient and the caregiver involved.
- To provide preventive procedures such as fluoride.

VII. Assistance for the Patient Who Is Ambulatory

- A patient may walk with one or more assistive aids such as braces, a cane, crutches, or a walker.

- Certain patients do better without assistance because they have developed their own method of balancing; many patients gain balance by holding both hands on the partially flexed forearm of a person walking beside them.

A. Seating the Patient

- Ask patient how much and what kind of assistance is needed.
- Raise chair slightly above the patient's knee level and adjust chair arm out of the way.
- Stand aside or assist while patient moves until back of legs touch chair and then bends knees to lower into dental chair.
- If assistance is needed, grasp ankles, lift legs, and turn patient into dental chair.
- Remove assistive aides and store out of the way.
- For patients who are blind, have the patient feel the chair, especially the seat and the back.

B. The Seated Patient

- After telling the patient, tilt chair back slowly.
- While tipping the chair back, place one hand on the patient's shoulder to offer assurance and support.
- Bring the feet up first to provide balance so that the patient cannot fall.
- If necessary, position supportive padding to maintain patient comfort.

C. Rising from the Chair

- After telling the patient, slowly raise the chair to upright position, with the seat slightly higher than the patient's knee level to minimize need to bend their knees when rising.
- Allow time for adjustment to upright position in order to avoid the effects of postural hypertension.
- Ask or assist patient with moving their feet to the floor.
- Retrieve assistive aids and hold them for patient to grasp with the dominant hand.
- Ask patient if assistance is needed to rise from the chair, and offer support if needed by placing the clinician's arm under the patient's arm on the nondominant side until balance is obtained for walking.

VIII. Patient Positioning

- The objectives for patient positioning during treatment are to let the patient feel comfortable while the clinician provides care in a position that provides adequate illumination, visibility, and accessibility.
- Extreme care should be given to slightly raising the head of any patient with a swallowing defect or respiratory compromise; the patient may be unable to prevent aspiration of fluids or object placed in the mouth during treatment.

A. Adapt Chair Position

◆ A patient with a respiratory or cardiac complication is positioned with the chair back raised to a level that is comfortable for the patient.

◆ The patient can be asked, "How many pillows do you use at night?" and the chair can be adjusted accordingly.

B. Body Adjustments

◆ Patients with a spinal cord injury do a "push up" and patients with quadriplegia shift their weight every 20 minutes for 10–15 seconds to maintain good circulation in the tissues that do not have sensation, such as the buttocks.

◆ Allowing movement prevents decubitus ulcers—this is a particular consideration during long procedures.

◆ Place patient in center of chair.

◆ Do not move limbs into unnatural positions.

◆ Allow patient to settle into a comfortable position.

◆ Place patient's chin in a neutral or downward position to prevent the gag reflex.[34]

IX. Supportive and Protective Stabilization

◆ Always obtain a signed informed consent from patient, guardian, or parent before any form of stabilization is performed.[46]

◆ Protective stabilization or medical immobilization techniques described below can help prevent injury to the patient, the caregiver, and the dental practitioner; however, the use of restraint is controversial and has the risk of causing injury or resulting in legal actions.[46]

◆ The method of stabilization is decided after communication-based or desensitizing techniques are tried and is individualized for each patient.

◆ When the patient is a child, the parent should be present to recognize immobilization protects their child from harm.[46]

◆ With basic knowledge of methods for maintaining patient stability, adequate visibility of working area, secure instrument grasps and finger rests, and well-controlled strokes, instrumentation can be effectively accomplished.

◆ Supportive stabilization, such as padding under flexed knees or bite block positioned to rest jaw muscles, can be used to facilitate patient comfort.

◆ Protective stabilization is never used as a form of punishment.

A. Extremity Movement

◆ A team member, parent, or caregiver employs a hand guarding or hold the patient's hands.

◆ If hand guarding is unsuccessful, wrist restraints may be used (seat belts, Velcro® straps).[46]

B. Body Enclosure

◆ Although a small patient may be held by a parent, such positioning can be tiring for the parent, insecure, and may not provide good body mechanics for the clinician.

◆ Pediwrap™ or Papoose Board™: Adjustable arm or leg immobilizer wraps with Velcro closures or a padded board with wide fabric wraps around upper body, middle body, and legs are available in adult and pediatric sizes, but not recommended unless the clinician has specialized training and informed consent has been obtained.[46]

C. Head Stabilization

◆ Arm of clinician: From a working position at 12 o'clock (top of the patient's head), the nondominant arm is placed around the patient's head to stabilize it in position.

◆ Head positioner or another person may also stabilize the head.[46]

D. Oral Stabilization

A mouth prop can be used to assist the patient who has difficulty maintaining an open mouth. Patience, a gentle but firm touch are essential. Training on the technique for safe use of mouth props is required. Verbal encouragement of the patient should continue throughout the appointment.

◆ The most stable mouth prop is a sterilized ratchet type (Molt mouth prop) that can be nearly closed for insertion between the teeth.

  • It can be opened gradually to hold the jaws to the necessary position.

  • The tips are covered with rubber tubing and are positioned over the maxillary and mandibular teeth on one side while the clinician treats the opposite side.

◆ Different types of rubber bite blocks are available; for example, Figure 51-8 shows one that allows for placement of a suction tip.

◆ A long piece of dental floss can be tied through the holes in a commercially available rubber mouth prop so, in case of a sudden respiratory change, the prop can be quickly pulled out and breathing normalized.

E. Precautions for Stabilization

◆ Patient and caregivers are informed of the risks and reassured all stabilization devices are for comfort and to make the work easier and they are in no way meant to hurt or punish.

◆ Ongoing monitoring of patient's physical and psychological well-being is necessary during stabilization.[46]

◆ Mobile teeth could be knocked out and aspirated.

  • Loose primary teeth in young patient.

  • Mobile teeth in advanced periodontal infection.

◆ Fatigue of the patient's facial and masticatory muscles and temporomandibular joint.

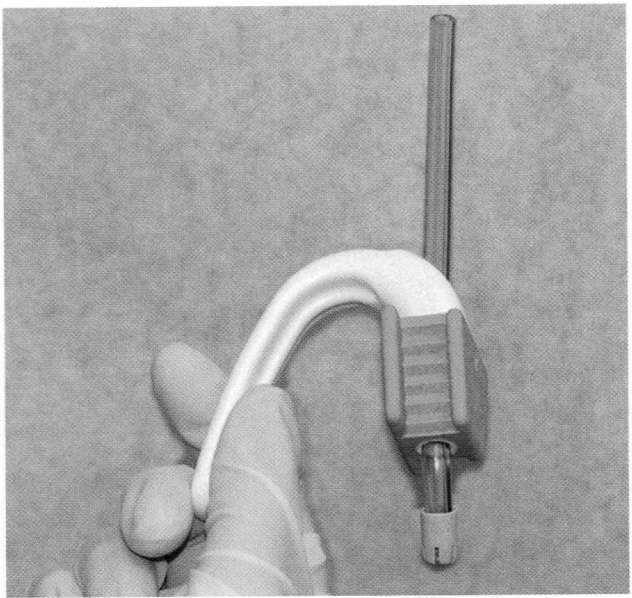

FIGURE 51-8 • Rubber Bite Block Mouth Prop with Saliva Ejector.

X. Four-Handed Dental Hygiene

◆ The use of a dental hygiene assistant during the appointment can enhance:
  • Efficiency.
  • Patient management.
  • Patient safety and comfort.
  • Safety and comfort for clinician.
  • Visibility during intraoral procedures.
◆ Excess drooling, common with some disabilities, requires continuous suction to maintain a clear visual field for instrumentation and to decrease the risk of aspiration.
◆ A patient with impaired respiratory function, swallowing, or gag reflex is at risk for aspiration; attention to patient position and continuous suction to keep passageways clear are vital.
◆ When the patient's disorder involves orofacial muscles and nerves, the risk for splashing of aerosols into the eye is increased during dental hygiene care.

XI. Instrumentation

◆ Biofilm control instruction should precede scaling to reduce the bacterial load during instrumentation.
◆ Unbreakable mirrors are recommended for use with a patient subject to spasm or sudden closure.
◆ Use single-end sharp instruments to prevent accidents. When an unrestrained patient moves involuntarily, the nonworking end of an instrument can be a hazard.
◆ Use of power instruments is contraindicated for a patient at risk for aspiration and for patients who overreact to sensory stimuli, such as a patient with autism.

◆ Introduce each procedure and sound to prevent startling a patient: Follow the basic instruction rule to "show, tell, then do."
◆ Finger rests: Firm, dependable finger rests are needed. Supplemental or reinforced rests can contribute to instrument stability. An external finger rest and handrest may be safer for the clinician.
◆ The occurrence of generalized heavy calculus deposits in patients with disabilities is not unusual due to factors related to the disabling condition.

XII. Pain and Anxiety Control

◆ For many patients with a disability, treatment can be easily accomplished in a dental clinic.
◆ Some patients with behavioral or cognitive dysfunction may need intervention beyond standard communication techniques and local anesthesia in order to receive dental care.
◆ Alternative methods of pain and anxiety control for patients who are unable to cooperate during dental treatment include[34]:
  • Pharmacologically induced sedation: minimal, moderate, or deep sedation; provided by trained dentist or anesthesiologist.
  • General anesthesia: delivered in hospital, surgery centers, or dental offices; provided by trained anesthesiologists.

WHEELCHAIR TRANSFER

Always inform the patient of intended actions before starting.[26] Ask patient, parent, or caregiver the preferred transfer method, and ability to help with the transfer.[26]

◆ Selection of a transfer technique is influenced by the size, weight, and mobility of the patient, along with any special physical conditions and patient's preferences.
◆ The patient may prefer to transfer from the left or the right side of the dental chair, depending on which side of the body is stronger.
◆ Transfer from the wheelchair can be a frightening experience to the patient owing to fear of falling and injury.

I. Preparation for Wheelchair Transfer

A. Clear the Area

◆ Before starting a transfer, clear the area: move the clinician's stool, bracket tray, foot controls, and operatory light.
◆ Remove or move the operatory chair armrest out of the transfer area.

B. Special Needs of Patient

◆ *Chair padding*: Special padding is used in a wheelchair as protection from pressure sores. Depending on the length of the appointment, the patient will decide whether the padding is moved to the dental chair. Pressure sores (decubitus ulcers) are described in Chapter 52.

◆ *Bags and catheters*: For patients wearing a urinary or colostomy bag, care must be taken during transfer and after transfer to ensure tubing is not bent or twisted.

◆ *Spasms*: Ask the patient about susceptibility to spasms and about procedures to follow for prevention.

◆ *Advice concerning transfer*: Ask the patient, family member, or caregiver how best the clinician can help during the transfer. The patient is allowed to do as much as possible.

II. Transfer of Patient Who Can Assist

When a patient can support his or her own weight, the "stand and pivot" technique can be used, as shown in Figure 51-9.

A. Position the Wheelchair

◆ Face the wheelchair in the same direction as the dental chair at approximately an angle of 30°, set brakes, and remove footrests and wheelchair armrests.

B. Prepare Dental Chair

◆ Adjust the chair to the same height as or lower than the wheelchair; clear a path for transfer by lifting or removing the chair arm.

◆ Always have a second person in the treatment room to help if required.

C. Approach to Patient

◆ Support the person while detaching safety belt if present.

◆ Face the patient and place feet outside the patient's feet for pivoting.

◆ Clinician's knees are placed close to or against the patient's knees to prevent buckling.

◆ Place hands under the patient's arms and grasp the waist belt in back. Patient places arms around clinician's neck or places hands on wheelchair to push up.

◆ Clinician lifts patient to standing position, as in Figure 51-9B.

D. Pivot to Dental Chair

◆ Pivot together slowly until the patient is backed up to the side of the chair, with the backs of the legs touching.

◆ The patient is gently lowered to a sitting position.

◆ Reposition the arm of the chair.

◆ Grasp the patient's legs together between the ankles and knees, and lift them onto the chair, as shown in Figure 51-9C.

E. After the Wheelchair Transfer

◆ Release the wheelchair brake to move it aside.

◆ In a small treatment room, the wheelchair may be folded and set aside.

◆ After the appointment, return the patient to the wheelchair in the reverse order of procedure.

III. Transfer of Patient Who Is Immobile

When the patient is unable to support his or her own weight, two aides are required. The parent or other caregiver may serve as the second person. Never attempt to do this alone.

A. Position the Wheelchair

◆ Position the wheelchair in the same direction and parallel with the dental chair, set brakes, and remove footrests.

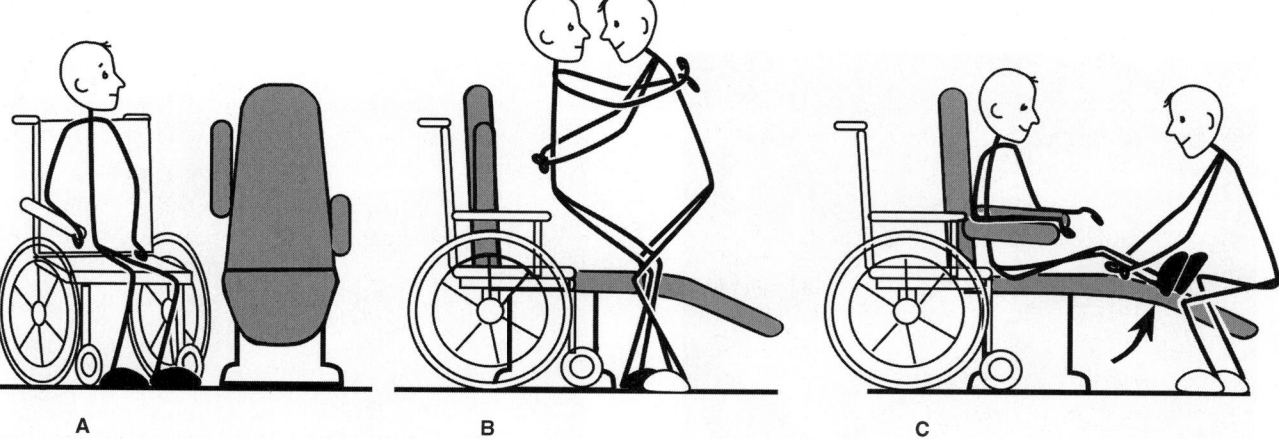

A   **B**   **C**

FIGURE 51-9 • **Wheelchair Transfer for a Mobile Patient. A:** Position the wheelchair at level of or lower than the dental chair; set wheel locks, remove footrests and armrests, and raise the dental chair arm. **B:** Clinician places feet outside of the patient's feet, grasps the patient around the waist under the arms, locks hands, or grasps belt in back; patient holds clinician around shoulders or neck; and patient is lifted up and pivoted to dental chair side. **C:** Patient is gently lowered to sitting position; dental chair arm is lowered; and clinician grasps legs together to lift onto dental chair.

♦ Adjust the dental chair to the same height as or lower than the seat of the wheelchair.

♦ Move the arm of the dental chair out of the transfer area and remove the arm of the wheelchair.

B. Clinician 1

♦ Is positioned behind the wheelchair.

♦ Help patient cross arms across chest.

♦ Will place arms under the patient's upper arm and grasp the patient's wrists.

C. Clinician 2

♦ Face patient and place both hands under patient's lower thighs.

D. Transfer

♦ On a prearranged signal and a steady motion, clinician 2 will initiate and lead the lift.

♦ Both clinicians should use their leg and arm muscles to lift the patient's torso and legs at the same time.

♦ Gently transfer the patient to the dental chair.

♦ Secure patient in chair and replace armrest.

E. Repeat in Reverse

After the appointment, the patient is returned to the wheelchair in the reverse order of procedure.

IV. Sliding Board Transfer

♦ A patient may bring a sliding board or one may be kept in the office or clinic. A transfer board is shown in Figure 51-10. Two persons are recommended during transfer and are required when the patient is heavy or less mobile.

A. Position the Wheelchair

♦ Position the wheelchair in the same direction as and parallel with the dental chair; set the brakes; remove the footrests.

♦ Adjust the seat of the dental chair to slightly lower than the wheelchair seat.

♦ Move the arm of the dental chair out of the transfer area and remove the arm of the wheelchair.

B. Adjust the Sliding Board

♦ Patient or clinician places the sliding board under the hip of the patient.

♦ The board is extended across the dental chair.

C. Transfer

♦ Patient shifts weight, balances on hands, and walks the buttocks across the board. The clinician can assist or do the transfer by holding the patient under the axillae (armpit).

♦ Board is removed and replaced after the appointment.

D. Repeat in Reverse

Dental chair is positioned slightly higher than the wheelchair seat for the return transfer.

V. Wheelchair Used During Treatment

When the patient is in a total support wheelchair, transfer to the dental chair may not be advisable. The wheelchair can be positioned for direct utilization.

♦ Some wheelchairs are self-reclining and have headrests (see Chapter 4).

♦ A portable headrest may be attached to the wheelchair handles, as shown in Figure 51-11.

♦ The dental chair can be swiveled to permit the wheelchair to be placed so the dental light can be directed into the patient's oral cavity.

♦ An automatic wheelchair lift that tilts the chair back can be obtained for a clinical facility where patients in wheelchairs are treated frequently.

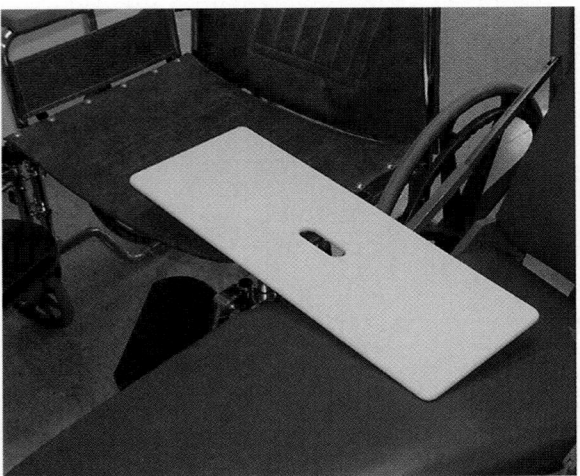

FIGURE 51-10 • Transfer Board. Transfer board placement between wheelchair and dental chair.

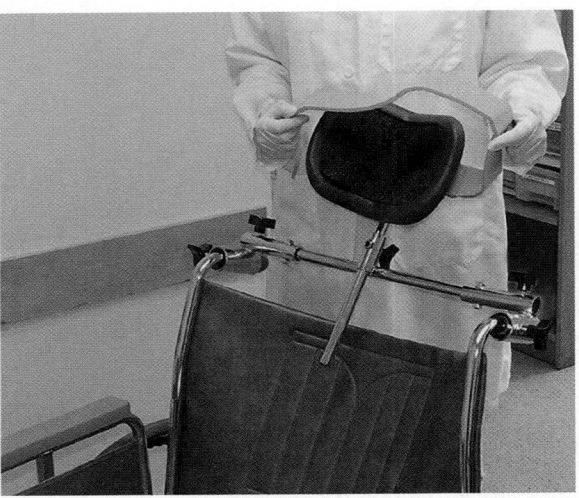

FIGURE 51-11 • Portable Headrest Attached to Wheelchair.

INSTRUCTION FOR CAREGIVERS

◆ Individuals who need partial or total care present with varying degrees of ability to cooperate, depending on the type of disability.

◆ The size of the patient and whether the patient is ambulatory, bedridden, or in a wheelchair are among the factors that influence the technique for management.

◆ The instructions for the caregiver are given where the specific techniques can actually be demonstrated as they will be done at home.

◆ Time and repeated practice sessions may be needed for successful biofilm removal.

I. Self-Care and Attitude

◆ Whenever possible, instruction for the parents, family members, or other caregivers begins with their own personal oral care.

◆ Success comes when those who care for the patient have knowledge and understanding of the purposes and techniques.

II. General Suggestions

A. Place

◆ The biofilm removal procedures are accomplished best when both the patient and the caregiver are comfortable and relaxed.

◆ A small bathroom may be the least desirable place because positioning the patient may be awkward, except when a standing position can be used.

◆ Good light, easy visibility of the teeth, and control of the head of the person with the disability are prerequisites.

B. Teaching Techniques for Biofilm Removal

◆ *Use of finger rest and handrest:* The person performing the biofilm removal balances the toothbrush, dental floss, floss aid, or any other implement with a finger or handrest on the side of the patient's face or chin. Such contact contributes to total patient control and to effective use of the biofilm-removal device.

◆ *Use of a mouth prop:* For certain patients, biofilm removal is impossible without a mouth prop, and demonstration for insertion on both sides is needed. For home use, a rolled and moist washcloth may be appropriate.

III. Positions

A. Caregiver Standing

◆ With the caregiver standing from behind, the arm is brought around the patient's head and the chin is cupped while using the thumb and index finger to retract the lips and cheeks.

◆ The other hand applies the toothbrush, floss aid, or other device.

◆ This technique requires the patient be able to bend the head back far enough for the parent to see the maxillary teeth.

◆ The procedure may be applicable for the following:
  • Short patient standing in front of and backed up to the caregiver.
  • Tall patient seated in a chair with the head tipped back to lean against the caregiver, or seated in a large chair or sofa with the head stabilized against the top of chair back.
  • Patient in a wheelchair leaning back against the caregiver. Wheelchair brakes are set.

B. Caregiver Seated

◆ Patient seated on pillow on floor in front of caregiver, with back close to the chair and head turned back into caregiver's lap, as shown in Figure 51-12A. The caregiver may place his/her legs over the shoulders of the patient to restrain arms and body movements, as shown in Figure 51-12B.

◆ Caregiver is seated at the end of a sofa or couch, and patient is lying down with the head in caregiver's lap, as shown in Figure 51-12C.

◆ For a patient who is confined to bed, the caregiver may sit at the patient's head and place the head in the lap. When body and arm movements need to be controlled, the caregiver can sit beside the patient, lean across the patient's chest, and hold the patient's arm against the body with the elbow. The hand of the clinician's restraining arm can hold the mouth prop, retract, or do whatever is necessary.

C. Two People

◆ In any of the positions previously mentioned, the parent may need the assistance of a second person to hold the hands and arms or otherwise restrain the patient.

◆ A small child may be placed across the laps of two persons seated facing each other. One stabilizes the head and brushes and flosses, while the other person holds hands, arms, and legs as needed, as shown in Figure 51-12D.

GROUP IN-SERVICE EDUCATION

◆ In-service programs are provided for teachers, registered nurses, other health professionals, parents, and volunteers in school and community preventive programs.

◆ In extended care institutions, many patients are unable to care for their own needs and may require total care, partial assistance, supervision, or regular reminders.

◆ Dental hygienists can provide in-service education sessions on oral health measures for those who provide daily personal care for others.

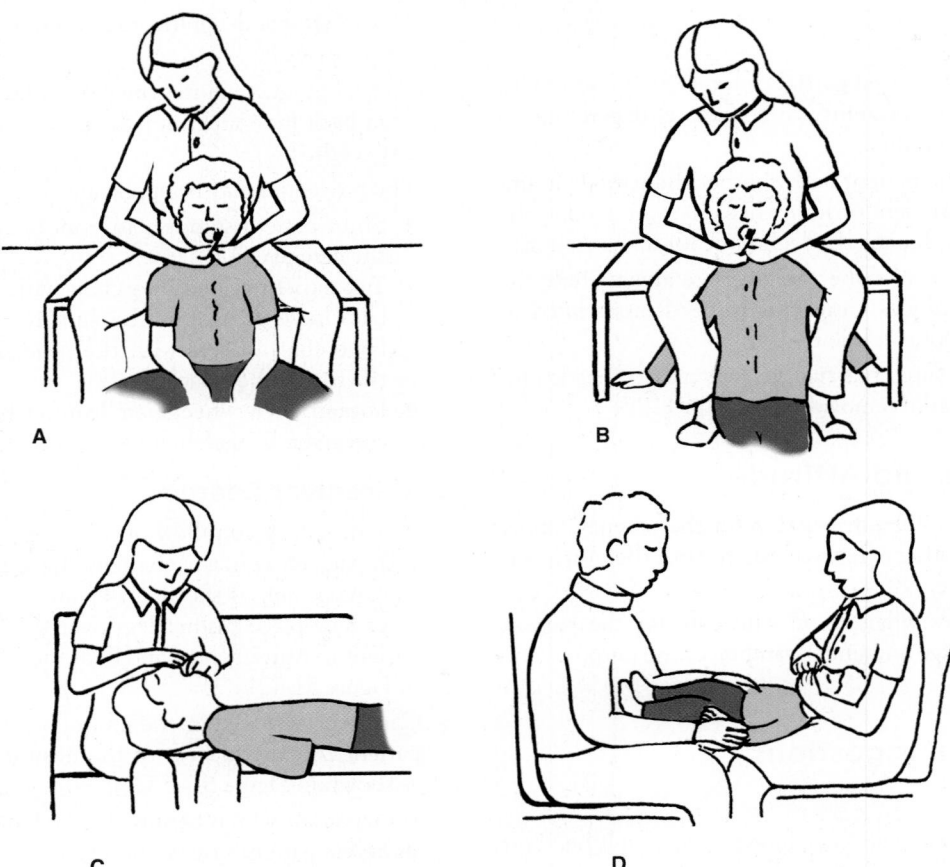

FIGURE 51-12 • Positions for Child or Disabled Patient During Biofilm Removal. A: Patient seated on floor with head turned back into the lap of the caregiver. **B:** Patient's arms restrained by legs of caregiver. **C:** Patient reclining on couch with head in lap of caregiver. **D:** Two people participating with small child between. One holds patient for stabilization while the other holds the head for toothbrushing and flossing.

I. Preparation for an In-Service Program

A. Planning

- An in-service program needs careful planning.
- Objectives are defined in writing and serve as a guide to preparation and evaluation.
- Effective learning materials are clear and to the point, interestingly presented with appropriate visual aids, and stimulating for learning.
- Staff concerns are recognized and addressed during the program.
- Initially, basic preparation includes learning about the functioning levels of the patient and assessing the procedures used for oral care.
- A survey of the biofilm control materials and devices available and in current use, methods for labeling or storing individual brushes, and the frequency of use are important.

- The dental hygienist invited to the institution for the specific purpose of presenting the workshop can arrange a preworkshop visit to observe and get to know the caregivers and the patient's needs.

B. Use of Patient Records

Health Insurance Probability and Accountability Act regulations may restrict access to individual patient records.

C. Gingival/Biofilm Index

- When the dental hygienist is providing hands-on instruction for oral care, use of a gingival or biofilm index can provide a baseline of information from which progress can be evaluated.
- The caregivers could carry out the daily biofilm program and see the changes that take place by comparing the before and after results.
- Continuing participation and receiving feedback of successful biofilm removal can provide real motivation to caregivers.

II. Program Content

- An oral health in-service program will be more successful if the content presented is based on an assessment of specific needs identified by the institution, patients, and caregivers.
- Content could include oral self-care, as motivation of self-care may contribute to caregivers prioritizing the oral needs of their patients.

A. Facts About Cause and Prevention of Oral Disease

- Basic information about biofilm, its formation, and how gingivitis and dental caries development are important to most groups.
- The progress of disease from reversible gingivitis to severe periodontitis can be explained, as can the process of dental caries.
- The concept of prevention through biofilm control, fluoride, dietary controls, sealants, and early treatment for restorations is carefully presented.
- Handout materials and colorful visual aids promote learning.

B. Oral Inspection

Caregivers can be trained to notice changes to the oral mucosa during daily cleaning and to report to the appropriate person.

C. Techniques of Mouth Care and Disease Control

- Caregivers working in pairs can be more efficient, particularly in the care of challenging patients.
- Individualized plans can be developed and training provided for caregivers to address specific problems relative to each patient's needs.
- *Information to teach caregivers about biofilm control* is discussed in Chapters 26 and 27.
- The use of a portable or bedside suction unit for removing debris from a patient's mouth is mentioned in Chapter 4.
- *Fluoride application* techniques are outlined in Chapter 34.
- *Denture care:* Procedures for care of dentures and of the mucosa under the denture are shown in Chapter 30.
- *Xerostomia relief:* Instruction for caregivers includes how to use a swab with saliva substitute to provide relief for certain patients.

D. Denture Marking Procedure

- All dentures are marked for patient identification.
- The techniques for denture marking are outlined in Chapter 30.

III. Records

- Oral care documentation for each patient is essential to evaluate the success of the in-service presentation.
- During instruction, the staff can learn appropriate information to include in each patient's record.
- Documentation for oral care provided by a caregiver may include implements and materials used, self-care instruction provided, successful techniques, and suggestions for future instruction.

IV. Follow-up

- After caregivers have tried their newly learned procedures, an opportunity to have questions answered is provided.
- Direct observation of techniques performed with and for the patients, advice concerning oral problems of particular patients, and corrections when necessary can motivate and encourage both patient and caregiver.
- The hygienist disclosing and recording the biofilm for comparison of scores before and after the program can show the progress being made.

V. Continuing Education

- In residential care facilities, individual instruction is provided for each new employee during the orientation period.
- Periodic in-service presentations for updating all employees can be provided. Questions and problems can be discussed, and plans can be introduced for changing a certain procedure based on new research evidence.

THE DENTAL HYGIENIST WITH A DISABILITY

- Disability is not necessarily an obstacle to dental hygiene licensure and provision of clinical care.[47]
- Adaptive technology, tax incentives for accessibility construction, and creative thinking can facilitate necessary workplace modifications.
- Additional dental hygiene roles, such as manager, advocate, or educator may provide employment opportunities for the dental hygienist with a disability.

DOCUMENTATION

In addition to the standard information recorded for a patient visit, documentation of care provided for a patient who has a disability includes:

- Individualized information about the patient's condition or level of functioning that will affect modifications needed during dental hygiene care. Some suggestions for information needed are listed in Box 51-3.

BOX 51-3
Basic Planning Questions for a Patient with Disability

- What is the patient's functioning level?
- Is the patient capable of all or part of the daily biofilm removal independently or will the patient require partial or total care?
- Is the patient involved in any community oral health programs (home, school, or day activity), and can the oral care provider in such a program be contacted to coordinate the instruction given?
- Which disabilities have the greatest influence on oral self-care abilities? What is the anticipated success of the overall preventive program?
- Which techniques and procedures will best fit the situation of the particular patient and the caregiver?
- How can the patient be helped to be as independent as possible?

◆ Specific details related to patient management or communication strategies used during the dental hygiene appointment, and an indication of whether those strategies were successful.

◆ Identification of self-care aids, modifications to standard oral hygiene instructions and aids, and details of any recommendations or instructions provided for caregivers.

◆ Box 51-4 provides an example of documentation for an appointment with a patient with a disability.

BOX 51-4
Example Documentation:
Self-Care Management for Patient with a Disability

S—A 25-year-old male patient with Down syndrome, who lives in an assisted-living group home, presents for routine 3-month continuing care appointment. Both the patient and his caregiver state the curved bristle toothbrush, introduced at the last appointment, is working quite well for him and his caregiver has affixed a rubber band to the handle in order to help stabilize the toothbrush in his hand.

O—No changes in medical history. His biofilm index is now below 20%.

A—Next step in patient's care plan is to help develop a system that will help patient take more personal responsibility for his own oral self-care with less need for caregiver assistance.

P—Congratulated patient and caregiver on their successful reduction in biofilm. Worked with caregiver to develop a personal "Daily Oral Care" list to identify all the steps and materials necessary for his daily oral care regimen. Caregiver will make up a large poster of the steps using pictures and will laminate and hang the poster by the bathroom sink in order to help the patient be more independent with his daily oral care regimen. Maintenance scaling and root planing completed. Used a "tell-show-do" approach to provide basic instructions for using a floss holder. First time efforts were clumsy, but patient is motivated to practice.

Next steps: Evaluate success at next visit scheduled in 3 months.

Signed: _____, RDH

Date: _____

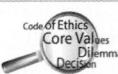

EVERYDAY ETHICS

When Mrs. Becker, who uses a wheelchair, arrives for her usual 6-month continuous care appointment, Chris, the dental hygienist, needs to rush to make time to go to the storage closet in the basement and get the transfer board. When Chris has to raise her voice and take extra time to ask questions more than once during a health history update, she suspects Mrs. Becker may have some hearing loss. After completing her assessment, Mrs. Becker's current oral health status indicates she needs to be placed on more frequent 2- to 3-month continuing care appointments. When Chris explains the new treatment plan, Mrs. Becker does not respond. The patient signs the electronic signature pad, but Chris is not sure she understands what was proposed. Chris feels stressed preparing for and treating Mrs. Becker in the time allowed for the appointment.

Chris is considering ignoring the plan for more frequent continuing care visits and just letting the front desk schedule Mrs. Becker in 6 months to avoid another unpleasant experience for both of them.

Questions for Consideration

1. Which core values of dental hygiene ethics apply to the way Chris handled treatment consent in this situation?

2. What are the legal implications related to standard of care if Chris follows through with the plan to reduce the frequency of Mrs. Becker's maintenance visits?

3. How can virtue ethics apply to a patient with special needs such as a hearing impairment or other loss of sensory functions? Go to Appendix II (The Canadian Dental Hygienists' Code of Ethics) to read about "virtue ethics."

Factors to Teach the Patient and Caregiver

▶ Seek regular dental and medical examinations.

▶ Have knowledge of current status, names and doses of medications including over-the-counter medications, and other changes in medical history.

▶ Recognize the early warnings of complications of disease.

▶ Recognize the side effects of treatments and medications.

▶ Seek immediate medical attention for any complications.

▶ Practice a healthy lifestyle, including healthy diet, daily exercise, no tobacco products, alcohol avoidance, attainment and maintenance of ideal weight, and stress reduction. Accept assistance for smoking cessation.

▶ Practice meticulous oral hygiene to prevent dental and periodontal diseases and adapt techniques as needed.

▶ Ways to overcome barriers to dental care.

ENHANCE YOUR UNDERSTANDING

ONLINE RESOURCES
(see the inside front cover for access information)
- Audio glossary
- Appendices

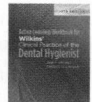

SUPPORT FOR LEARNING
(available separately)
- *Active Learning Workbook for Wilkins' Clinical Practice of the Dental Hygienist, 13th Edition*

INDIVIDUALIZED REVIEW
- Customized practice quizzing with Navigate 2 TestPrep for *Wilkins' Clinical Practice of the Dental Hygienist*

References

1. Kraus L, Lauer E, Coleman R, Houtenville A. 2017 Disability Statistics Annual Report. Durham, NH: University of New Hampshire. 2018. https://files.eric.ed.gov/fulltext/ED583258.pdf. Accessed July 9, 2019.

2. United States Department of Justice. Americans with Disabilities Act of 1990 as amended. https://www.ada.gov/pubs/adastatute08.htm. Accessed December 1, 2018.

3. World Health Organization. Disability and health. January 16, 2018. http://www.who.int/mediacentre/factsheets/fs352/en/. Accessed December 1, 2018.

4. Glassman P, Harrington M, Namakian M, Subar P. Interprofessional collaboration in improving oral health for special populations. *Dent Clin North Am.* 2016;60(4):843-855.

5. Naseem M, Shah AH, Khiyani MF, et al. Access to oral health care services among adults with learning disabilities: a scoping review. *Ann Stomatol (Roma).* 2017;7(3):52-59.

6. NYS Oral Health Center of Excellence. Oral health for children with special health care needs: tool box. https://www.mchoralhealth.org/PDFs/CSHCNExpertMeeting.pdf. Accessed July 9, 2019.

7. World Health Organization. International classification of functioning, disability and health (ICF). January 27, 2017. http://www.who.int/classifications/icf/en/. Accessed December 1, 2018.

8. National Library Services (NLS). Information resources for people with sensory disabilities. http://www.naric.com/sites/default/files/Sensory%20Disabilities.pdf. Accessed December 1, 2018.

9. World Health Organization. Vision impairment and blindness. http://www.who.int/mediacentre/factsheets/fs282/en/. Updated October 11, 2018. Accessed December 1, 2018.

10. National Federation of the Blind. Statistical facts about blindness in the United States. June 2018. https://nfb.org/blindness-statistics. Accessed December 1, 2018.

11. American Foundation for the Blind. Key definitions of statistical terms. August 2017. https://www.afb.org/research-and-initiatives/statistics/key-definitions-statistical-terms. Accessed July 9 2019.

12. National Institute of Health, Medline Plus. Leading causes of blindness. *NIH Medline Plus* 2012. https://medlineplus.gov/magazine/issues/winter12/articles/winter12pg12-13.html. Accessed September 25, 2017.

13. Gilbert C, Foster A. Childhood blindness in the context of VISION 2020—the right to sight. *Bull World Health Organ.* 2001;79:227-232. https://www.scielosp.org/pdf/bwho/v79n3/v79n3a11.pdf. Accessed September 25, 2017.

14. Haring RS, Sheffield ID, Canner JK, Schneider EB. Epidemiology of sports-related eye injuries in the United States. *JAMA Ophthalmol.* 2016;134(12):1382-1390.

15. Aghadoost D. Ocular trauma: an overview. *Arch Trauma Res.* 2014;3(2):e21639.

16. National Eye Institute. About sport eye injury and protective eyewear. June, 2017. https://nei.nih.gov/sports/. Accessed July 9, 2019.

17. World Health Organization. Deafness and hearing loss. February 2017. http://www.who.int/mediacentre/factsheets/fs300/en/. Accessed September 25, 2017.

18. U.S. Department of Health & Human Services. National Institute of Deafness and Other Communication Disorders (NIDCD). Quick statistics about hearing. https://www.nidcd.nih.gov/health/statistics/quick-statistics-hearing. Updated December 2015. Accessed September 25, 2017.

19. Delaney AM. Newborn hearing screening. Medscape. https://emedicine.medscape.com/article/836646-overview. Updated June 28, 2018. Accessed December 1, 2018.

20. American Dental Hygienists' Association. Direct access. http://www.adha.org/direct-access. Accessed December 1, 2018.

21. National Governors Report. The role of dental hygienists in providing access to oral health care. Washington, DC: National Governors Association. January 2014. https://

classic.nga.org/cms/home/nga-center-for-best-practices/center-publications/page-health-publications/col2-content/main-content-list/the-role-of-dental-hygienists-in.html. Accessed December 1, 2018.

22. Rodriguez TE, Galka AL, Lacy ES, Pellegrini AD, Sweier DG, Romito LM. Can midlevel dental providers be a benefit to the American public? *J Health Care Poor Underserved.* 2013;24(2):892-906.

23. United States Department of Justice. ADA standards for accessible design. https://www.ada.gov/2010ADAstandards_index.htm. Accessed December 1, 2018.

24. Jogezai U, Riches T, Townsend D, Abercrombie C. Introduction of a Nomad Pro hand held x-ray unit for radiography in a special care setting. *J Disability and Oral Health.* 2016;17(2):78-91.

25. Dental Care Every Day: A Caregiver's Guide. Dental Care Every Day: A Caregiver's Guide. https://www.nidcr.nih.gov/sites/default/files/2018-10/dental-care-everyday.pdf. Accessed July 9, 2019.

26. National Institute of Dental and Craniofacial Research. Wheelchair transfer: a health care provider's guide. July 2009. https://www.nidcr.nih.gov/sites/default/files/2017-09/wheelchair-transfer-provider-guide.pdf. Accessed December 1, 2018.

27. Meningaud JP, Pitak-Arnnop P, Chikhani L, Bertrand JC. Drooling of saliva: a review of the etiology and management options. *Oral Surg Oral Med Oral Pathol Oral Radiol Endod* 2006;101(1):48-57.

28. Millan-Calenti JC, Tubio J, Pita-Fernandez S, et al. Prevalence of functional disability in activities of daily living (ADL), instrumental activities of daily living (IADL) and associated factors, as predictors of morbidity and mortality. *Arch Gerontol Geriatr.* 2010;50(3):306-310.

29. Van der Linde BW, van Netten JJ, Otten B, Postema K, Geuze RH, Schoemaker MM. Activities of daily living in children with developmental coordination disorder: Performance, learning, and participation. *Phys Ther.* 2015;95(11):1496-1506.

30. Osakwe ZT, Larson E, Agrawal M, Shang J. Assessment of activity of daily living among older adult patients in home healthcare and skilled nursing facilities: an integrative review. *Home Health Now.* 2017;35(5):258-267.

31. Willings C. Impact on development & learning. Teaching students with visual impairment. August 27, 2017. https://www.teachingvisuallyimpaired.com/impact-on-development-learning.html. Accessed December 1, 2018.

32. Strickling C. Impact on visual impairment on development. Texas School for the Blind and Visually Impaired. http://www.tsbvi.edu/infants/3293-the-impact-of-visual-impairment-on-develop. Accessed December 1, 2018.

33. American Speech-Language-Hearing Association. Effects of hearing loss on development. https://www.asha.org/public/hearing/Effects-of-Hearing-Loss-on-Development/. Accessed December 1, 2018.

34. National Institute of Dental and Craniofacial Research. Practical care for people with developmental disabilities. https://www.nidcr.nih.gov/OralHealth/Topics/Developmental Disabilities/ContinuingEducation.htm. Accessed December 1, 2018.

35. Valinoti AC, da Costa LC, Farah A, Pereira de Sousa V, Fonseca-Goncalves A, Maia LC. Are pediatric antibiotic formulations potentials risk factors for dental caries and dental erosion? *Open Dent J.* 2016;10:420-430.

36. Vajawat M, Deepika PC, Kumar V, Rajeshwari P. A clinico-microbiological study to evaluate the efficacy of manual and powered toothbrushes among autistic patients. *Contemp Clin Dent.* 2015;6(4):500-504.

37. Baygin O, Tuzuner T, Kusgoz A, Senel AC, Tanriver M, Arslan I. Antibacterial effects of fluoride varnish compared with chlorhexidine plus fluoride in disabled children. Oral Health Prev Dent. 2014;12(4):373-382.

38. Crystal YO, Marghalani AA, Ureles SD, et al. Use of silver diamine fluoride for dental caries management in children and adolescents, including those with special health care needs. *Pediatr Dent.* 2017;39(5):135-145.

39. Hendre AD, Taylor GW, Chavez EM, Hyde S. A systematic review of silver diamine fluoride: effectiveness and application in older adults. *Gerontology.* 2017;34(4):411-419.

40. Autism Canada. See the Spectrum Differently. ABA. https://autismcanada.org/living-with-autism/treatments/non-medical/behavioural/aba/. Updated December 11, 2017. Accessed December 1, 2018.

41. American Academy of Pediatric Dentistry. Guideline on management of dental patients with special health care needs. *Pediatr Dent.* 2016;38(6):171-176.

42. CNIB. Seeing beyond vision loss. Guide dog etiquette. https://cnib.ca/en/programs-and-services/live/cnib-guide-dogs/guide-dog-education/guide-dog-etiquette?region=gta. Accessed July 9, 2019.

43. Association of State and Territorial Dental Directors, and The Oklahoma Association of Community Action Agencies. Oral health care for children with special health care needs: a guide for family members/caregivers and dental providers. http://studylib.net/doc/8524313/oral-health-care-Oklahoma-association-of-community-action. Accessed December 1, 2018.

44. Glaucoma Research Foundation. Symptoms of open-angle glaucoma. October 29, 2017. https://www.glaucoma.org/glaucoma/symptoms-of-primary-open-angle-glaucoma.php. Accessed December 1, 2018.

45. University of Washington, School of Dentistry. Oral health fact sheet for dental professionals: adults with hearing impairment. http://dental.washington.edu/wp-content/media/sp_need_pdfs/Hearing-Adult.pdf. Accessed December 1, 2018.

46. American Academy of Pediatric Dentistry. Protective stabilization for pediatric dental patients. *Pediatr Dent.* 2017;39(6):260-265.

47. Smith DS. Challenges in dental hygiene employment for dental hygienists with disabilities. *Access.* 2010;24(8):35-37.

52

Neurologic Disorders and Stroke

Betty Ann Pryzdial BSc, RDH, PID, and Lisa F. Mallonee, RDH, RD, LD, MPH

CHAPTER OUTLINE

NEUROLOGIC DISORDERS ASSOCIATED WITH PHYSICAL DISABILITY
I. Acute Disorders
II. Degenerative Disorders
III. Developmental Disorders

OTHER CONDITIONS THAT LIMIT PHYSICAL ABILITY

SPINAL CORD INJURY
I. Occurrence
II. Characteristics/Effects of SCI
III. Potential Secondary Complications
IV. Mouth-Held Implements
V. Dental Hygiene Care

CEREBROVASCULAR ACCIDENT (STROKE)
I. Etiologic Factors
II. Signs and Symptoms
III. Medical Treatment
IV. Dental Hygiene Care

BELL'S PALSY (IDIOPATHIC TEMPORARY FACIAL PARALYSIS)
I. Occurrence
II. Characteristics
III. Medical Treatment
IV. Dental Hygiene Care

AMYOTROPHIC LATERAL SCLEROSIS
I. Occurrence
II. Diagnosis

III. Etiology and Pathogenesis
IV. Two Forms of ALS
V. Symptoms
VI. Treatment
VII. Dental Hygiene Care

PARKINSON'S DISEASE
I. Occurrence
II. Characteristics
III. Treatment
IV. Dental Hygiene Care

POSTPOLIO SYNDROME
I. Description
II. Dental Hygiene Care

CEREBRAL PALSY
I. Description
II. Classifications
III. Accompanying Conditions
IV. Medical Treatment
V. Oral Characteristics
VI. Dental Hygiene Care

MUSCULAR DYSTROPHIES
I. Duchenne Muscular Dystrophy (Pseudohypertrophic)
II. Facioscapulohumeral Muscular Dystrophy
III. Myotonic Muscular Dystrophy (Steinert Disease)
IV. Other Types of Muscular Dystrophy
V. Medical Treatment

VI. Dental Hygiene Care

MYELOMENINGOCELE
I. Description
II. Types of Deformities
III. Physical Characteristics
IV. Medical Treatment
V. Dental Hygiene Care

ARTHRITIS
I. Degenerative Joint Disease (Osteoarthritis)
II. Dental Hygiene Care

SUMMARY OF CONSIDERATIONS FOR DENTAL HYGIENE CARE
I. Preparation for Appointments
II. Additional Considerations during Clinical Care
III. Assistance for the Ambulatory Patient
IV. Wheelchair Transfer
V. Patient Positioning and Body Stabilization
VI. Four-Handed Dental Hygiene
VII. Personal Factors that Affect Self-Care
VIII. Residence-Based Delivery of Care

DOCUMENTATION

EVERYDAY ETHICS

FACTORS TO TEACH THE PATIENT

REFERENCES

LEARNING OBJECTIVES

After studying this chapter, the student will be able to:

1. Identify and define key terms and concepts related to physical impairment.

2. Describe the characteristics, complications, occurrence, and medical treatment of a variety of physical impairments.

3. Identify oral factors and findings related to physical impairments.

4. Describe modifications for dental hygiene care based on assessment of needs specific to a patient's physical impairment.

INTRODUCTION

◆ Many conditions related to the neuromuscular system, joints, or connective tissue have as a symptom, or leave as a chronic after-effect, loss of function in the form of a physical impairment.

◆ Dental hygiene treatment modalities and oral care recommendations are adapted to the unique situations created by each disorder.

◆ General suggestions that may be adapted to a variety of patients with disabilities are described in Chapter 51.

◆ This chapter contains descriptions of selected diseases or conditions and describes modifications and adaptations needed by the patient during oral self-care, as well as by the dental hygienist during treatment appointments.

NEUROLOGIC DISORDERS ASSOCIATED WITH PHYSICAL DISABILITY

Most of the disabling conditions described in this chapter are considered neurologic disorders.

◆ A characteristic of many neurologic disorders is apoptosis, the death of cells, specifically the nerve cells in the central nervous system.[1]

◆ Disruption of sensory or motor neuron signals is the cause of partial or complete paralysis associated with neurologic disorders.

◆ Acute ischemia or traumatic injury to the brain or spinal cord causes necrotic (immediate) death of nerve cells in the most severely affected areas and immediate/complete destruction of transmission of neurologic signals.

◆ Apoptotic cell death, a slower, biochemical, or metabolic destruction of the nerve cell, occurs in chronic or degenerative neurologic conditions.

I. Acute Disorders

◆ Acute neurologic disorders can be caused when one or more neurons are injured by trauma or biologic assault or when there is disruption of blood flow to an area of the brain.

◆ Complete or partial loss of motor ability, sensory perception, or cognitive function can result.

◆ Acute neurologic disorders discussed in more detail in this chapter include spinal cord injury (SCI), stroke, and Bell's palsy.

II. Degenerative Disorders

◆ Degenerative neural disorders are a result of progressive destruction of nerve cells.

◆ Patients with these disorders typically become increasingly disabled and dependent on caregivers to help them with everyday activities and personal care as their disease progresses over time.

◆ Degenerative neural disorders discussed in this chapter include amyotrophic lateral sclerosis (ALS), Parkinson's disease, and postpolio syndrome.

III. Developmental Disorders

◆ Developmental impairments have their onset early in life, around the time of birth or before a child is 18 years old.

◆ Depending on the disorder, either a stable or a progressive impairment can result.

◆ Developmental disorders highlighted in this chapter include cerebral palsy, muscular dystrophies, and myelomeningocele.

OTHER CONDITIONS THAT LIMIT PHYSICAL ABILITY

◆ Joint and connective tissue diseases, such as arthritis, can affect a patient's ability to provide oral self-care and require adaptations during delivery of dental hygiene care.

◆ Autoimmune diseases, such as myasthenia gravis, scleroderma, and rheumatoid arthritis, which can limit physical ability, are discussed in Chapter 63.

SPINAL CORD INJURY

◆ The spinal cord extends down the middle of the back and carries both motor and sensory nerves that branch to send messages between the brain and specific areas of the body.

◆ External traumatic force can cause partial or complete loss of sensory and/or motor function related to the spinal cord level and the extent of the injury.

I. Occurrence

◆ There are more than 288,000 people in the United States living with SCI; approximately 17,700 new cases each year.[2]

◆ More than one-third of trauma cases result from motor vehicle accidents; other causes are falls, diving accidents, violence, and combat injuries.

◆ Nearly half of all injuries involve males aged between 16 and 30 years, but as the population ages, there has been an increase in average age of injury.

II. Characteristics/Effects of SCI

◆ The signs and symptoms of paralysis depend on the nature and level of injury to the spinal cord.

◆ There are 7 cervical (C), 12 thoracic (T), 5 lumbar (L), and 5 sacral (S) vertebrae, with paired spinal nerves extending from each; the areas of the body affected by injury at the different levels are illustrated in Figure 52-1.

   • *Complete lesion*: A complete transection or compression of the spinal cord leaves no sensation or motor function below the level of the lesion.

   • *Incomplete lesion*: Partial transection or injury of the spinal cord leaves some evidence of sensation or motor function below the level of the lesion. Some sensation and motor function may return within a few hours after injury, and maximum return may occur in 6–18 months.

◆ *Other possible effects*: Impairment of bladder and bowel control and sexual function; impairment of vasomotor and body temperature regulatory mechanisms.

III. Potential Secondary Complications

Patients with lesions at or above the T6 level are at greater risk for the complications described here.

A. Impaired Respiratory Function

◆ Pneumonia can significantly reduce life expectancy for a person with SCI.[2]

◆ Some quadriplegic patients are unable to elicit a functional cough and need assistance.

◆ By placing manual pressure over the abdomen, below the diaphragm, after the patient has inhaled, the patient may be assisted while an attempt to cough is made.[3]

B. Tendency for Decubitus Ulcers

◆ A pressure sore (*decubitus ulcer*) results from tissue anoxia or ischemia caused by pressure exerted on the skin and subcutaneous tissues by bony prominences and the object on which they rest, such as a mattress.[4]

◆ The cutaneous tissue becomes broken or destroyed, leading to destruction in the subcutaneous tissue.

◆ The ulcer that forms may become infected by secondary bacterial invasion and be slow to heal; anemia and poor nutrition may also contribute.[4]

C. Spasticity

◆ As spinal shock subsides following a traumatic injury, muscle-reflex spasticity develops from a slight to a severe degree.

◆ Stimuli, such as decubitus ulcers, infections, and sensory irritation, may bring on a spasm.

D. Body Temperature

High-level quadriplegic patients are unable to regulate body temperature, requiring careful monitoring and intervention to warm or cool the patient as necessary.

E. Vulnerability to Infection

Complications related to elimination, urinary tract infections, renal stones, secondary infection of decubitus ulcers, and respiratory infections occur more commonly in this population.

F. Cardiovascular Instability

◆ Bradycardia and hypotension are common because of the loss of the sympathetic autonomic nervous system.

◆ Deep vein thrombosis is another potentially serious complication.

G. Neurogenic Bladder and Bowel

Complications related to dysfunctions in emptying bladder and bowels require planning to avoid the complications of autonomic dysreflexia.

H. Autonomic Dysreflexia

◆ *Definition*

   • Autonomic dysreflexia, or hyperreflexia, is a life-threatening *emergency* condition in which the blood pressure increases sharply.[5]

   • It may occur in patients with lesions at T6 or above.

   • A variety of stimuli may precipitate dysreflexia, including irritation to the bowel or bladder distension.

   • Patients who require manual bowel or bladder management techniques are more susceptible.[6]

◆ *Symptoms*

   • Increased blood pressure with slowed pulse rate. The blood pressure may rise to 300/160 mm Hg.

   • Pounding headache.

   • Flushing, chills, perspiration, and stuffy nose.

   • Restlessness; increased spasticity.

◆ *Prevention*

   • Consult with physician when the patient has history of recurrent difficulties.

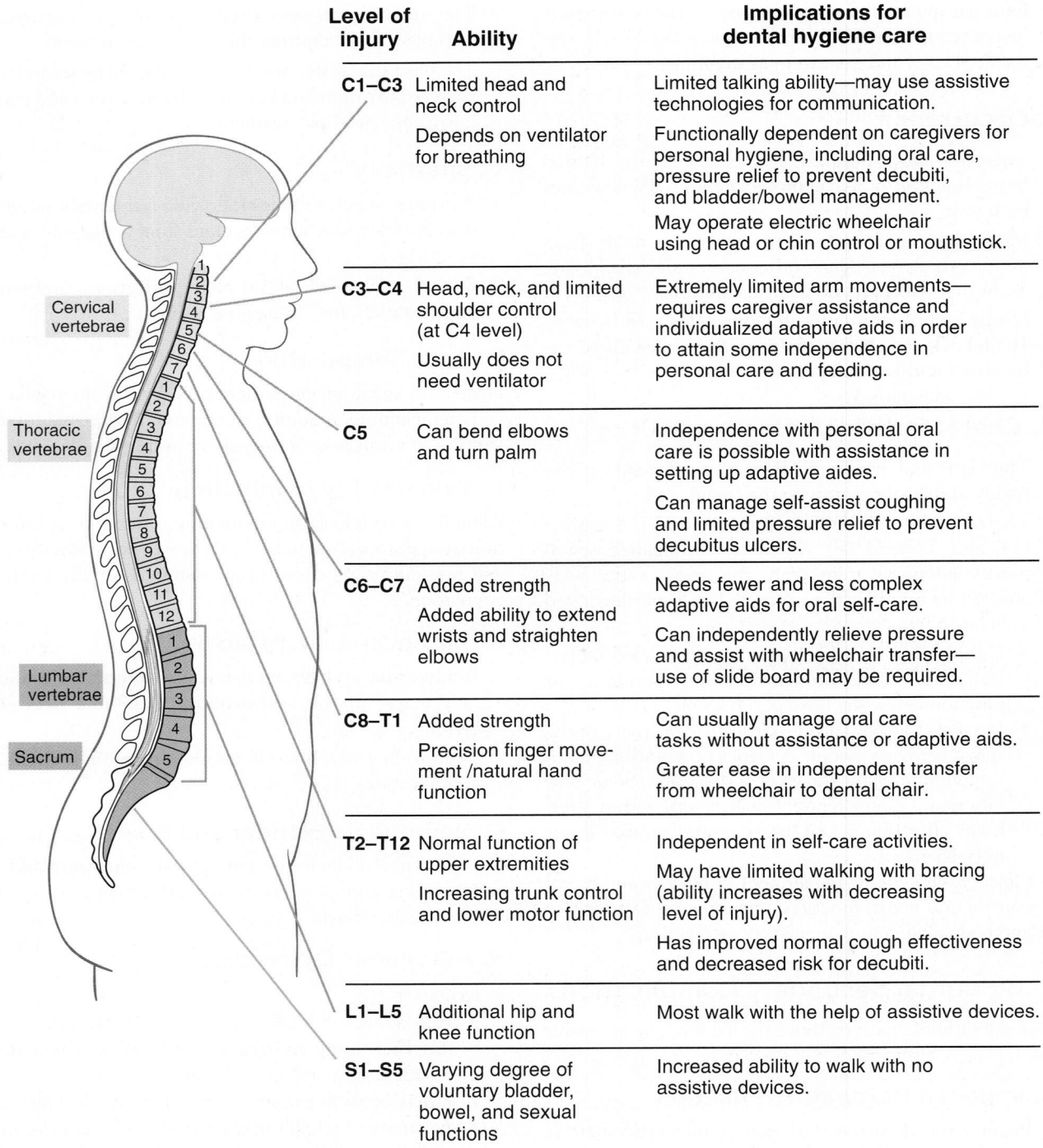

Level of injury	Ability	Implications for dental hygiene care
C1–C3	Limited head and neck control	Limited talking ability—may use assistive technologies for communication.
	Depends on ventilator for breathing	Functionally dependent on caregivers for personal hygiene, including oral care, pressure relief to prevent decubiti, and bladder/bowel management.
		May operate electric wheelchair using head or chin control or mouthstick.
C3–C4	Head, neck, and limited shoulder control (at C4 level)	Extremely limited arm movements—requires caregiver assistance and individualized adaptive aids in order to attain some independence in personal care and feeding.
	Usually does not need ventilator	
C5	Can bend elbows and turn palm	Independence with personal oral care is possible with assistance in setting up adaptive aides.
		Can manage self-assist coughing and limited pressure relief to prevent decubitus ulcers.
C6–C7	Added strength	Needs fewer and less complex adaptive aids for oral self-care.
	Added ability to extend wrists and straighten elbows	Can independently relieve pressure and assist with wheelchair transfer—use of slide board may be required.
C8–T1	Added strength	Can usually manage oral care tasks without assistance or adaptive aids.
	Precision finger movement /natural hand function	Greater ease in independent transfer from wheelchair to dental chair.
T2–T12	Normal function of upper extremities	Independent in self-care activities.
	Increasing trunk control and lower motor function	May have limited walking with bracing (ability increases with decreasing level of injury).
		Has improved normal cough effectiveness and decreased risk for decubiti.
L1–L5	Additional hip and knee function	Most walk with the help of assistive devices.
S1–S5	Varying degree of voluntary bladder, bowel, and sexual functions	Increased ability to walk with no assistive devices.

FIGURE 52-1 • Levels of Spinal Cord Injury (SCI). On the left, the vertebrae are designated as C (cervical), T (thoracic), L (lumbar), and S (sacral). The effects of SCI depend on the level of injury. (From The Spinal Cord Injury Information Network. *SCI Functional Goals for Specific Levels of Complete Injury.* Birmingham: University of Alabama at Birmingham—Spinal Cord Injury Model System (UAB-SCIMS); 2008. http://www.spinalcord.uab.edu/show.asp?durki=30166. Accessed August 6, 2010.)

- Avoid abrupt changes in body position and maintain a semi-upright chair position.
- Monitor bladder outflow catheter tubing, outflow of urine into catheter bag, and bladder distention.
- Schedule appointments that allow the patient to maintain the regular schedule for the bowel elimination program at home.

◆ *Emergency care*
- Position chair upright gradually.
- Do *not* recline the chair because increased blood pressure in the brain could result.
- Check bladder distention and straighten catheter if clamped.
- Manually relieve bowel impaction if necessary.
- Monitor the blood pressure and vital signs using a medical emergency report form (see Chapter 9).
- Call for medical aid if blood pressure does not begin to drop within 2–3 minutes.

IV. Mouth-Held Implements

The patient with a high-level SCI who does not have strong function of hands and arms may use mouth-held appliances to perform many tasks and the teeth for holding objects. Optimum oral health and effective biofilm control has special significance because many functions cannot be accomplished by an edentulous mouth.

A. Uses

Fabrication of mouth-held appliances contributes to increased independence and makes possible such activities as operating an electric wheelchair, typing on a computer, or turning the pages of a book.

B. Criteria

◆ Does not harm the oral tissues.[7,8]
- Stabilization of occlusion with contact for all fully erupted teeth and the biting forces distributed to as many teeth as possible.
- Is not traumatic to the periodontal supporting structures.
- Does not prevent eruption of teeth.
◆ Is comfortable and does not cause fatigue.[7,8]
- Patient can talk, swallow, and moisten the lips.
- Orthosis can be inserted and removed by the patient.
- Orthosis is adaptable for the various needs of the quadriplegic patient.
◆ Can be cleaned and cared for easily.
◆ Is relatively easy to construct; inexpensive.

V. Dental Hygiene Care

Factors to consider when planning dental hygiene care for the patient with an SCI include:
◆ Impaired motor and sensory ability.
◆ Risk for secondary complications during treatment; autonomic dysreflexia and aspiration due to decreased respiratory function.

◆ Risk for pressure sores, potential for spasticity, poor control of body temperature.
◆ Use of mouth-held implements.

CEREBROVASCULAR ACCIDENT (STROKE)

◆ Cerebrovascular accident (CVA) is sudden loss of brain function resulting from interference of the blood supply to a part of the brain.
◆ The clinical manifestation of cerebrovascular disease.
◆ Frequent disability caused by changes in motor function, communication, and perception or hemiparesis is common.
◆ The third leading cause of death, following heart disease and cancer, in the United States.
◆ The stroke may be severe and death can occur within minutes; a less severe attack leaves the patient with residual and chronic effects.

I. Etiologic Factors

◆ The blood flow decreases to an area of the brain and shuts off the oxygen supply to the portion of the brain supplied by that vessel, resulting in cerebral infarction.
◆ The two main causes or types of stroke are[9]:

A. Ischemic Stroke

◆ Occurs when a blood vessel to the brain is blocked.
◆ Can be caused by atherosclerotic plaque build-up in a blood vessel.
◆ A *thrombotic stroke* is caused when a clot within a blood vessel of the brain or neck closes or occludes an already narrowed vessel.
◆ An *embolic stroke* happens when a blood vessel is blocked by a clot or other material carried through the circulation from another part of the body.

B. Hemorrhagic Stroke

◆ Occurs when a cerebral blood vessel ruptures and bleeds into the brain tissues.
◆ Common causes include:
- Defects in blood vessels, such as aneurysm or malformation.
- Very high blood pressure.
- Use of blood thinner medication.
- An ischemic stroke that develops a burst blood vessel and causes bleeding.

C. Predisposing Factors

Early diagnosis and treatment for control of the following predisposing factors are necessary in the prevention of stroke and its devastating effects.
◆ Atherosclerosis (see Chapter 61).
◆ Hypertension, the greatest risk factor that leads to stroke (see Chapter 61).

◆ Hypercholesterolemia, hypertriglyceridemia.

◆ Tobacco use, smoking.

◆ Cardiovascular disease (rheumatic heart disease, congestive heart failure, history of transient ischemic attacks).

◆ Diabetes mellitus.

◆ Use of oral contraceptives (enhanced by hypertension, tobacco use, age over 35).

◆ Drug abuse (especially in adolescents and young adults).

II. Signs and Symptoms

The effects of a stroke depend on the location of the damage to the brain, as well as on the degree or extent of involvement.

A. Transient Ischemic Attack

◆ A brief event where the blood supply to a localized area of the brain is interrupted and the patient may have transient signs or symptoms of a stroke.

◆ These "little strokes" may last a few minutes to an hour and may leave no permanent damage.

◆ A history of transient attacks is a possible risk factor or warning for a stroke.

B. Acute Symptoms of a Stroke

Acute symptoms and emergency procedures are included in Chapter 9.

C. Residual or Chronic Effects

◆ Approximately two-thirds of those who survive have some degree of permanent disability.

◆ Temporary or permanent loss of thought, memory, speech, sensation, or motion results.

◆ The side of the face and body affected is opposite that of the brain injury (Figure 52-2).

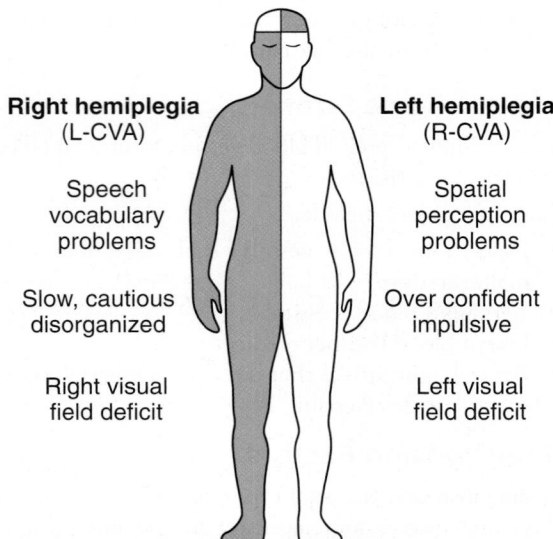

Right hemiplegia
(L-CVA)

Speech
vocabulary
problems

Slow, cautious
disorganized

Right visual
field deficit

Left hemiplegia
(R-CVA)

Spatial
perception
problems

Over confident
impulsive

Left visual
field deficit

FIGURE 52-2 • Cerebrovascular Accident (CVA) (Stroke). Right hemiplegia is the result of left-sided brain damage, and left hemiplegia results from right-sided brain damage.

◆ Persons with right hemiplegia have more difficulty with verbal communication and are more apt to be cautious, anxious, and disorganized.

◆ Patients with left hemiplegia have difficulty with action requiring physical coordination and may respond impulsively with overconfidence.

◆ Common signs and symptoms observed following a stroke are described in Box 52-1.

D. Disease Risk Detection

◆ Calcifications in the carotid artery are observable on a panoramic radiograph.[10,11] If present, the patient is referred for medical evaluation.

◆ Radiation therapy is associated with an accelerated form of atherosclerosis formation and risk of stroke.[12]

III. Medical Treatment

◆ Surgical correction of aneurysms, clots, or malformations may include removal of microscopic clots in the intracranial arteries or minute grafting to bypass blocked vessels and provide collateral circulation.

◆ Physical and occupational therapy and rehabilitation techniques are vital to the patient's recovery and functioning.

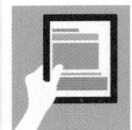

BOX 52-1
Description of Signs and Symptoms Following Stroke

• **Paralysis:** hemiplegia (one side of the body) or portions, such as an arm, leg, or the face.

• **Articulation:** difficulty of speech, which may be caused by involvement of the tongue, mouth, or throat, as well as aphasia by brain damage related to the speech centers, and the patient may have difficulty finding the right word.

• **Salivation:** difficulty in control of saliva complicated by difficulty in swallowing; aspiration.

• **Sensory:** loss in affected parts may result in superficial anesthesia, or the opposite may occur with resultant increased sensitivity to pain and touch.

• **Visual impairment:** blurred vision or diminished visual acuity.

• **Mental function:** may be unaffected, but slowness, poor memory, and loss of initiative are common. Brain deterioration may occur over a period of time.

• **Personal factors:** personality changes relate to emotional trauma, fear, discouragement, and dependency. Anxiety neuroses and periods of depression, which are common, may require assistance from a psychiatrist, psychologist, or social worker.

◆ Careful recording of the medical history includes the listing of medications. The patient who has experienced a stroke may be taking a variety of drugs for some or all of the purposes found in Box 52-2.

IV. Dental Hygiene Care

Particular factors to consider when planning dental hygiene care for the patient with a stroke-related disability:
◆ Impaired motor and/or cognitive ability.
◆ Hemiplegia; particularly if the dominant hand is affected. For example, the patient who wears dentures requires a suction cup brush, as illustrated in Chapter 51, to clean the dentures with one hand.
◆ Facial paralysis; decreased self-cleansing action of the tongue and lips; decreased control of saliva; risk for aerosol in eye during treatment.
◆ Medication for treatment of the condition: anticoagulant use is common following a stroke.

BELL'S PALSY (IDIOPATHIC TEMPORARY FACIAL PARALYSIS)

◆ Bell's palsy is paralysis of the facial muscles innervated by the facial or seventh cranial nerve.
◆ Although the cause is not known, various possible agents have been implicated, including:
  • Bacterial and viral infections; particularly herpes simplex.
  • Injury, trauma from tooth removal or oral surgery such as the removal of a tumor in the parotid gland area.

I. Occurrence

◆ Although relatively rare, the incidence increases with each decade of life.
◆ In younger age groups, women are more frequently affected than are men.
◆ After 50 years of age, the disorder is more common in men.

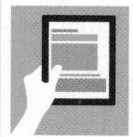

BOX 52-2
Categories and Purposes of Medications Used to Treat Strokes

• **Anticoagulant:** to thin the blood.
• **Antihypertensive:** to lower the blood pressure.
• **Thrombolytic:** to dissolve clots.
• **Vasodilator:** to relax the blood vessels of the brain.
• **Steroid:** to control brain swelling.
• **Antiepileptic:** to help to control seizures.

II. Characteristics[13]

A. Signs and Symptoms

Abrupt weakness or paralysis of facial muscles, usually without preceding pain, occurs on one side of the face.
◆ *Mouth*: The corner of the mouth droops, and salivation with drooling is uncontrollable.
◆ *Eye*: Eyelid on the affected side may not close; watering and drooping of the lower lid invites infection.
◆ When only the seventh nerve is affected, sensory responses are still intact.

B. Functional Problems

Speech and mastication may be impaired.

C. Prognosis

◆ A majority of patients experience a return to normal within a month with a spontaneous recovery.
◆ Others may have lasting residual effects or permanent paralysis.

III. Medical Treatment

A. Palliative

◆ Eye protection such as an eye patch during sleep and eye lubrication drops during waking hours.
◆ Hot compresses and massaging the involved muscles provides some relief.
◆ Analgesics may relieve pain.

B. Drugs

◆ Corticosteroids, administered within the first 72 hours, have been used to improve the prognosis.
◆ Antiviral drugs are prescribed sometimes, but the efficacy of such drugs is unclear.[14]
◆ Recent treatment protocols indicate combining corticosteroid, and antiviral treatment may have added benefits for satisfactory recovery.[15]

C. Surgical

◆ Surgical procedures to relieve pressure on the nerve or reduce deformities have been used but are controversial and seldom recommended.[16]

IV. Dental Hygiene Care

Particular factors to consider when planning dental hygiene care for the patient with Bell's palsy:
◆ Facial paralysis; decreased self-cleansing action of the tongue and lips; decreased control of saliva; risk for aerosol in eye during treatment.
◆ Medications used for treatment of the condition.

AMYOTROPHIC LATERAL SCLEROSIS

ALS (often referred to as Lou Gehrig's disease) is a progressive neurodegenerative disorder characterized by a progressive loss of motor neurons.

I. Occurrence

◆ Prevalence is approximately 5 per 100,000 population; more than 12,000 people in the United States.[17]

◆ Men are more often affected than women; Caucasians more frequently than other ethnic groups.

◆ Onset usually occurs at middle age or later; prevalence highest in those aged 70–79 years and lowest in those aged 18–39 years.[17]

II. Diagnosis

◆ There are no diagnostic tests for ALS.

◆ Diagnosis is usually made after ruling out other disorders with similar symptoms.

◆ Clinically diagnosed with both upper and lower neuron dysfunction, although variants include a pure upper motor and pure lower motor syndrome.[18]

III. Etiology and Pathogenesis

◆ Unknown cause.

◆ About 90% of cases are sporadic.

◆ About 5–10% are familial (predominantly autosomal dominant).

◆ Average life expectancy is 3–5 years; but the range is broad and some live much longer.

◆ Typically progressive degeneration of both upper and lower motor neurons with no periods of remission.

◆ More areas of the body are affected over time; nearly all systems eventually become involved.

◆ Respiratory failure is the usual cause of death.

IV. Two Forms of ALS

◆ *Spinal form*[19]
  • About two-thirds of patients.
  • Early symptoms include muscle weakness in upper and lower limbs and muscle wasting.
◆ *Bulbar onset form*[19]
  • Initially presents with dysarthria.
  • Sometimes dysphasia for solids or liquids is initial symptom.
  • Facial weakness and wasting/spasticity of the tongue are common.
  • Limb symptoms may develop simultaneously; or can happen later as the disease progresses.
  • Sialorrhea (excessive secretion of saliva; drooling) develops in almost all who have the bulbar-onset form of the disease.

V. Symptoms

◆ Symptoms include[20]:
  • Cramps and spasticity.
  • Muscle weakness, particularly in extremities.
  • Increasing respiratory difficulty.
  • Difficulty swallowing and chewing.
  • Excessive saliva.[21,22]
  • Depression and anxiety.
  • Cognitive[23] and behavioral disorders that can affect compliance with recommendations.

VI. Treatment

◆ There is Only one Food and Drug Administration-approved treatment (riluzole); treatment only extends survival about 2 months.[18]

◆ Palliative treatment is provided by interprofessional teams.[24]

◆ Treatment focused on progressive management of symptoms.

◆ Sialorrhea managed with medications, but in later stages treatment can include radiation or Botox injection into salivary glands.[18]

VII. Dental Hygiene Care

Factors to consider when planning dental hygiene care for the patient with ALS:

◆ Increased motor impairment over time.

◆ Need for body stabilization and support.

◆ Risk for respiratory difficulties.

◆ Effects of facial paralysis.

◆ Effects of treatment for sialorrhea.

PARKINSON'S DISEASE

◆ Progressive disorder of the central nervous system characterized by four primary symptoms[25]:
  • Tremor in hands, arms, legs, jaw, and face.
  • Rigidity of limbs and trunk.
  • Bradykinesia or slowness of movement.
  • Postural instability.

◆ It is also known as paralysis agitans and Parkinson's syndrome.

◆ Although the cause is not known, the basis for the specific group of symptoms is degeneration of certain neurons in the substantia nigra of the basal ganglia, where posture, support, and voluntary motion are controlled.

◆ In addition, a severe deficiency of dopamine, one of the substances that participates in nerve transmission, occurs.

I. Occurrence[26]

◆ Parkinson's disease affects as many as a million middle-aged and older persons in the United States; more than 10 million people worldwide.

◆ Incidence increases with age; only about 4% are diagnosed before age 50.

◆ Approximately 60,000 new cases are diagnosed each year.

◆ One and half times higher incidence in men than in women.

II. Characteristics

◆ The signs and symptoms center around tremor, rigidity, and loss or impairment of motor function (akinesia).

◆ These factors also occur in other conditions, which are differentiated by a physician when a diagnosis is made.

◆ The disease progresses through stages; from mild/early to severe/advanced with increasing impairment of motor function.

A. General Manifestations

◆ Body posture bent, with bent head and general stiffness.

◆ Motion and responses slowed; difficulty in keeping balance and turning.

◆ Gait slow and shuffling.

◆ Speech monotonous and slow.

◆ Resting tremor of one or both hands is common; the tremor can be reduced or stopped when the person engages in a purposeful action such as toothbrushing.

◆ The fingers may be involved in a "pill-rolling" motion in which the thumb and index finger are rubbed together in a circular movement.

◆ Nonmotor symptoms include variations in blood pressure, cardiac dysrhythmias, excessive sweating, bowel and bladder dysfunction, and sleep disorders.

◆ Cognitive ability is seldom affected, except in the advanced stages.

◆ Eventually, after 10–20 years, the person may become incapacitated and may require complete care.

B. Face and Oral Cavity

◆ Expression is fixed and mask-like, with diminished eye blinking.

◆ Tremor or exaggerated movement in lips, tongue, and neck, and difficulty in swallowing.

◆ Excess salivation and drooling.

III. Treatment

◆ Although no known cure exists for Parkinson's disease, symptomatic control can be accomplished, in part, by replenishing the dopamine shortage with levodopa in combination with other medications; side effects can include dizziness and confusion.

◆ Maintenance of good general health is encouraged, including plenty of rest and nutritious meals.

◆ Professional physical therapy and occupational therapy have particular significance for a patient's well-being.

◆ Surgical relief for symptoms is sometimes accomplished by deep brain stimulation or pallidotomy.

IV. Dental Hygiene Care

Particular factors to consider when planning dental hygiene care for the patient with Parkinson's disease include[27]:

◆ Increased motor impairment, tremor, and rigidity over time, which interferes with daily activities.

◆ Rigid, uncontrolled facial muscles; poor control of eyes, lips, tongue, and swallowing muscles.

◆ Increased drooling of saliva.

◆ Need for short appointments.

◆ Potential for cognitive deficits over time.

◆ Adverse drug interactions and reactions.

◆ Need for caregiver education.

POSTPOLIO SYNDROME

I. Description

◆ Condition that affects adults, years after recovery from an initial attack of the poliomyelitis virus when they were children.[28]

◆ Cause is unknown.

◆ Prevalence is currently unknown, but appears to be growing.

◆ Treatment focus is mainly palliative, with exercise often prescribed to strengthen specific muscle groups.

◆ Characterized by progressive muscle weakness, fatigue, muscle and joint pain, and potential muscle atrophy in muscles originally affected by the poliomyelitis as well as other muscles, including orofacial muscles.

II. Dental Hygiene Care

Particular factors to consider when planning dental hygiene care for the patient with multiple sclerosis:

◆ Impaired motor ability.

◆ Weakness in respiratory and swallowing muscles.

CEREBRAL PALSY

I. Description

◆ A group of disorders that involve the cerebral cortex, the part of the brain that directs motor function.[29]

◆ Damage to the developing brain can occur such as:
  • During fetal development, usually (congenital).
  • Natally, or postnatally (acquired).

◆ In many cases the cause is unknown, but can be related to:
  • Abnormal development of the brain.
  • Bleeding in the brain.
  • Severe lack of oxygen.

◆ Risk factors include[29]:

- Maternal infections, thyroid abnormalities, or seizures during pregnancy.
- Maternal exposure to toxic substances during pregnancy.
- Blood type incompatibility between mother and child.
- Complicated labor and delivery, breech position of baby during birth, or multiple births.
- Infant jaundice, infection, or seizures after birth.
- Severe head injury after birth.

◆ Symptoms usually can be observed during the first year after birth, but if symptoms are mild, it may not be noticed for several years.

◆ Cerebral palsy is not progressive.

II. Classifications

Cerebral palsy is classified into four types according to associated motor impairment.[29]

A. Spastic Palsy

◆ Muscles have increased tone, tension; can be in one limb or all four; sometimes includes oral structures.

◆ Condition characterized by spasms (sudden, involuntary contractions of single muscles or groups of muscles) and stiff, rigid muscles resistant to movement.

◆ Complete or partial loss of ability to control muscular movement; therefore, movements are awkward and stiff with resistance to movement. Lack of control causes patient to fall easily.

B. Dyskinetic or Athetoid Palsy

◆ Characterized by constant, slow, involuntary writhing movements with frequent changes of muscle tone.

◆ Lack of ability to direct muscles in the motions desired.

◆ Grimacing, drooling, and speech defects are common.

◆ Factors influencing movements:

- Effort by patient to control muscle activity results in exaggerated muscle movement.
- May be initiated and aggravated by stimuli outside body, such as sudden noises, bright lights, or quick movements by people or things in the area.
- Intensity influenced by emotional factors. Patient is least in control in an emotionally charged environment, such as the dental office or clinic.

C. Ataxic Palsy

◆ Loss of equilibrium, balance, and depth perception; walk uncertain; has difficulty in sitting straight.

◆ Lack of coordination; needs time to execute changes.

◆ Involuntary muscle quivering may affect part or all of the body; placing gentle firm pressure on the affected muscles will help calm the tremor.

D. Combined Palsy

A combination of the three named types.

III. Accompanying Conditions

A. Primitive Reflexes and Abnormal Response to Stimuli

◆ *Asymmetric tonic neck reflex*: When head is turned, same side extremities extend and stiffen, while opposite side extremities flex.

◆ *Tonic labyrinthine reflex*: If neck is extended back, extremities also extend and back is arched.

◆ *Startle reflex*: Any surprising stimuli can trigger uncontrolled body movement.

B. Contractures

◆ Muscles fixed in abnormal positions.

◆ Increase in muscle spasticity and joint deformities.

C. Seizures

◆ As many as half have seizures and those with seizure disorder are more likely to have an intellectual disability.[29]

D. Sensory Disorders

◆ Visual impairments and hearing loss are common.

E. Speech and Language Disorders

◆ Speech may be slow and difficult to understand due to lack of control of mouth and throat muscles (dysarthria).

◆ Difficulty processing auditory information.

F. Cognitive Impairment

◆ Some individuals with cerebral palsy also have significant cognitive impairment.

◆ More than 50% *do not* have intellectual or cognitive disabilities; therefore, an inability to communicate does not necessarily mean lack of comprehension.

◆ Of the 50% who are not significantly intellectually impaired, some may learn more slowly because of sensory impairments, perceptive-cognitive deficiencies, and speech difficulties.

IV. Medical Treatment

◆ Interprofessional teams of healthcare providers caring for the individual with cerebral palsy can include medical, surgical, orthopedic, and dental providers, as well as speech, physical, recreational, and occupational therapists.

◆ Orthotic devices to support the lower limbs and the use of cane, crutches, walker, or wheelchair may help to increase function.

◆ Surgery may be needed for addressing orthopedic deformities, correcting eye or ear difficulties, or severing nerves to relax muscles and reduce chronic pain.

◆ Oral medications may be used to reduce tension in affected muscles, aid in pain management, or control seizures.

V. Oral Characteristics

A. Disturbances of Musculature

◆ Facial grimacing, facial asymmetry, and abnormal function of muscles of mastication, swallowing, and speech are common.

◆ Spasticity of orofacial muscles can interfere with daily oral care.

◆ Inability to close lips contributes to increased drooling.

◆ Hyperactive bite and gag reflexes can present difficulties during dental and dental hygiene therapy, as well as during biofilm control at home.

B. Malocclusion

◆ The incidence of malocclusion is high; often a musculoskeletal abnormality rather than only misaligned teeth.[30]

◆ Oral habits of mouth breathing, tongue thrusting, and faulty swallowing contribute to open bite with protruding anterior teeth.[31]

C. Attrition and Erosion

◆ Severe, constant, involuntary bruxism is common and can severely wear down tooth structure and restorations.

◆ Gastroesophageal reflux can cause erosion of oral tissues.

D. Oral Injury

◆ Patients may fall frequently, which can damage and fracture teeth and jaws.

E. Dental Caries

◆ The rate of dental caries may be higher, but the risk factors for the patient with cerebral palsy are the same as the general population.

◆ Difficulties in maintaining biofilm control and problems of mastication can lead to the use of a soft diet, which increases risk for dental caries.

F. Periodontal Infections

◆ Periodontal or gingival infections are found in a high percentage of patients with cerebral palsy.[31]

◆ *Phenytoin-induced gingival overgrowth*: When phenytoin is used for the prevention of seizures, the patient is susceptible to gingival enlargement.

◆ *Risk factors for periodontal involvement*: Mechanical difficulties related to biofilm control, mouth breathing, and increased food retention because of ineffective self-cleansing all lead to increased periodontal involvement and biofilm collection.

◆ Many patients with cerebral palsy have heavy calculus deposits.

VI. Dental Hygiene Care

Particular factors to consider when planning dental hygiene care for the patient with cerebral palsy:

◆ Numerous associated oral characteristics and predisposing factors for oral disease.

◆ Impaired motor ability; uncontrolled movements, reflexive reactions.

◆ Compromised ventilatory capacity.[32]

◆ Involvement of muscles in head and neck.

◆ Need for body stabilization and support due to joint contractures.

◆ Potential cognitive impairment and compromised communication.[32]

◆ Increased risk for seizure.

MUSCULAR DYSTROPHIES

◆ The muscular dystrophies are a group of more than 30 genetic myopathies characterized by progressive severe weakness and loss of use of groups of muscles.[33]

◆ The term *dystrophy* means degeneration and is associated with atrophy and dysfunction.

◆ The syndromes of muscular dystrophy have been separated by clinical and genetic means and range from mild (Becker type) with a later onset to more severe types (Duchenne, facioscapulohumeral).

◆ All types of muscular dystrophy are genetically inherited and the underlying pathologic processes do not differ.

◆ Generally, the diseases are limited to skeletal muscles, with cardiac muscle only rarely involved.

◆ In the United States, more than 50,000 children and adults are affected with some form of muscular dystrophy.[33]

I. Duchenne Muscular Dystrophy (Pseudohypertrophic)

A. Occurrence

◆ The Duchenne muscular dystrophy (DMD) type is primarily limited to males and transmitted by female carriers.

◆ Prevalence of approximately 1:7,250 males 5–24 years of age.[34]

B. Age of Onset

The condition is present at birth and becomes apparent during early childhood, usually diagnosed at an average age of 4.9 years.[34]

C. Characteristics

◆ *Musculature*: Enlargement (pseudohypertrophy) of certain muscles, particularly the calves, is present in early years.

◆ *Weakness of hips*: Child falls frequently, has increasing difficulty in standing erect.

◆ *Lordosis*: With an abdominal protuberance.

◆ *Waddling*: Either walks on toes or flat foot because of muscle contracture.

◆ *Precarious balance:* Patient arches back in attempt to find center of gravity; gait is slow because balance needs to be sustained during each step.

◆ *Progressive muscular wasting:*
  • Eventual involvement of thighs, shoulders, trunk; weakness of respiratory muscles.
  • Inactivity is detrimental and increases the individual's helplessness and dependency.

◆ *Intellectual impairment:* A mild degree of mental impairment is noted in some persons with DMD.

◆ *Cardiac abnormalities:* Arrhythmia and cardiomyopathy are common.

D. Prognosis

◆ Disablement severe by puberty; child is confined to a wheelchair.

◆ Patients rarely live to reach their third decade.

II. Facioscapulohumeral Muscular Dystrophy

A. Occurrence

◆ Males and females are equally affected.

◆ Incidence is approximately 1 in 20,000.[35]

B. Age of Onset

◆ Between 6 and 20 years, with an average at 13 years, after puberty.

◆ Mild symptoms may appear at later ages; with rare cases occurring during infancy.[35]

C. Characteristics

◆ Facial muscles involved, particularly the orbicularis oris. The effect of gaping lips on oral tissues is similar to mouth breathing.

◆ Malocclusion and temporomandibular disorder problems have been noted.

◆ Scapulae prominent; shoulder muscles weak; difficulty in raising the arms.

◆ Difficulty in closing eyes completely.

◆ Cardiac involvement is rare.

D. Prognosis

◆ Progression is slower than that of the Duchenne type and progress may become arrested.

◆ Most patients live a normal life span and become incapacitated late in life.

III. Myotonic Muscular Dystrophy (Steinert Disease)

◆ Most common form in adults; can appear any time from early childhood to adulthood.[36]

◆ Affects both men and women.

◆ Prolonged spasm of muscles after use; usually worse in cold temperatures.

◆ Also affects central nervous system, heart, gastrointestinal tract, eyes, and hormone-producing glands.

IV. Other Types of Muscular Dystrophy

Other less common types of muscular dystrophy include[37]:

◆ *Becker:* Similar to Duchenne type, but more benign with a later onset (5–15 years).

◆ *Emery–Dreifuss:* Onset between 5 and 30 years; generally benign, but severe cardiomyopathy and risk for sudden death is a feature.

◆ *Limb-girdle:* Most severely affects muscles of the hips and shoulders; manifests in late childhood/early adolescence and ranges from rapidly to slowly progressive.

◆ *Oculopharyngeal and myotonic dystrophies:* Each is relatively rare, has onset between 20 and 50 years of age, is slowly progressive, and features extensive involvement of orofacial muscles.

V. Medical Treatment

◆ Supportive treatments consist of:
  • Physical, occupational, and speech therapy.
  • Respiratory therapy.

◆ Drug therapy includes[38]:
  • Corticosteroids.
  • Anticonvulsants.
  • Immunosuppressants.
  • Antibiotics (for treating respiratory infections).

◆ Preventive treatment consists of prenatal diagnosis, carrier detection, and genetic counseling.

VI. Dental Hygiene Care

Particular factors to consider when planning dental hygiene care for the patient with muscular dystrophy[37]:

◆ Impaired motor ability.

◆ Potential need for body stabilization and support.

◆ Some types involve orofacial muscles.

MYELOMENINGOCELE

◆ Spina bifida is a congenital defect or opening in the spinal column. A portion of the spinal membranes may protrude through the opening with or without spinal cord tissue.

◆ When the spinal cord protrudes through the spina bifida, the condition is called myelomeningocele.

◆ Anticipatory guidance prior to conception includes the use of multivitamins containing recommended levels of folic acid. A reduced risk of offspring with spina bifida and other neural tube defects has been shown when mothers received folic acid.[39]

◆ Patients with spina bifida appear to be specifically at risk for latex hypersensitivity.[40] Precautions and management of latex hypersensitivity are discussed in Chapter 6.

I. Description

◆ Embryologically, a neural tube forms during the first month of pregnancy.

◆ From the neural tube, the brain, brain stem, and spinal cord arise, and, eventually, the vertebrae form and enclose the spinal cord.

◆ When a place in the spinal column fails to close, the result is an open defect in the spinal canal, which is called a spina bifida.

II. Types of Deformities[41]

A. Myelomeningocele

◆ A myelomeningocele is a protrusion or outpouching of the spinal cord and its covering (meninges) through an opening in the bony spinal column.

◆ Because part of the spinal cord and nerve roots protrude, flaccid paralysis of the legs and part of the trunk results, depending on the level of the protrusion (herniation).

B. Meningocele

◆ A meningocele is a protrusion of the meninges through a defect in the skull or spinal column.

◆ No neural elements are contained in the protrusion, but can cause minor disabilities.

C. Closed Neural Tube Defect

◆ Malformations in fat, bone, or meninges of spinal cord.

◆ Few or no symptom in most instances, sometimes causes incomplete paralysis with urinary and bowel dysfunction.

D. Spina Bifida Occulta

◆ Spina bifida occulta is a congenital cleft in the bony encasement of the spinal cord in which no outpouching of the meninges or spinal cord exists.

◆ Usually, spina bifida occulta has no symptoms.

III. Physical Characteristics

Depending on the level of the myelomeningocele, some or all of the following signs and physical characteristics may be found.[42]

A. Bony Deformities

Muscle imbalance from paralysis can cause dislocation of the hip, club foot, and spinal curvatures, such as humpback (kyphosis), curvature (scoliosis), or swayback (lordosis).

B. Loss of Sensation

Lack of skin sensitivity to pain, temperature, and other sensations can lead to problems of inadvertent burn or trauma unrecognized by the patient or caregiver or to pressure sores. Frequent position changes are necessary during dental hygiene care.

C. Bladder and Bowel Paralysis

The nerve supplies to the bladder and bowel are usually affected. Lack of bowel and bladder control requires continual attention. Kidney infection with loss of kidney function is one cause of shorter life expectancy.

D. Hydrocephalus

◆ A high percentage of children with myelomeningocele have hydrocephalus. Hydrocephalus is a condition characterized by an excessive accumulation of fluid in the brain. The fluid dilates the cerebral ventricles, causes compression of brain tissues, and separates the cranial bones as the head enlarges (Figure 52-3).

◆ Development is slowed, and intellectual disability may be present.

◆ Many of these patients have seizures.

IV. Medical Treatment

Surgical, orthopedic, and urologic treatment as well as physical and occupational therapy may constitute a minimum of specialties involved in the care of a patient with myelomeningocele.

A. Neurosurgery

◆ *Closure of the myelomeningocele:* Surgical closure helps to prevent infections that may otherwise enter into the spinal cord. Paralysis is not lessened by surgery.

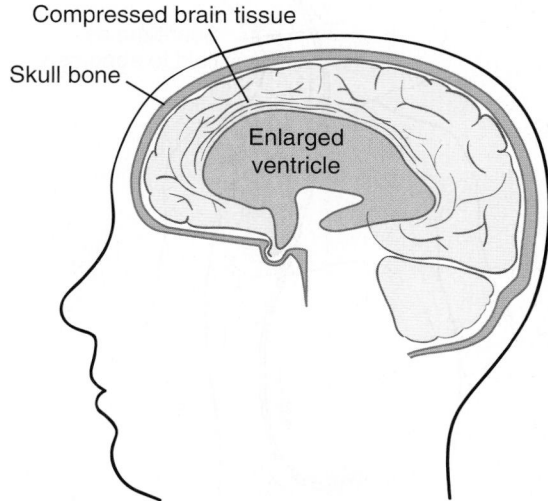

FIGURE 52-3 • Hydrocephalus. The ventricle is enlarged because of the accumulation of fluid. Brain tissues are compressed.

- *Treatment of the hydrocephalus*: Permanent drainage systems may be accomplished in the form of a ventriculoatrial shunt between the cerebral ventricle and the atrium of the heart. Sometimes, drainage by way of the abdomen in the form of a ventriculoperitoneal shunt is used (Figure 52-4).
- Individuals who have a cerebrospinal fluid shunt are at increased risk for transient infections. Need for premedication during dental treatment is established by medical consultation.[43]

B. Orthopedic Surgery

- Orthopedic surgical procedures can assist by reducing or correcting deformities.
- Bracing to support the trunk and lower limbs is used in accord with the extent of the individual's paralysis.
- Ambulation varies from dependency on a wheelchair, walker, crutches, or cane to near normal with only foot problems.

V. Dental Hygiene Care

Particular factors to consider when planning dental hygiene care for the patient with myelomeningocele:
- Impaired motor ability.
- Potential need for body stabilization and support.
- Increased risk for latex allergy and transient infections related to a cerebrospinal fluid shunt.

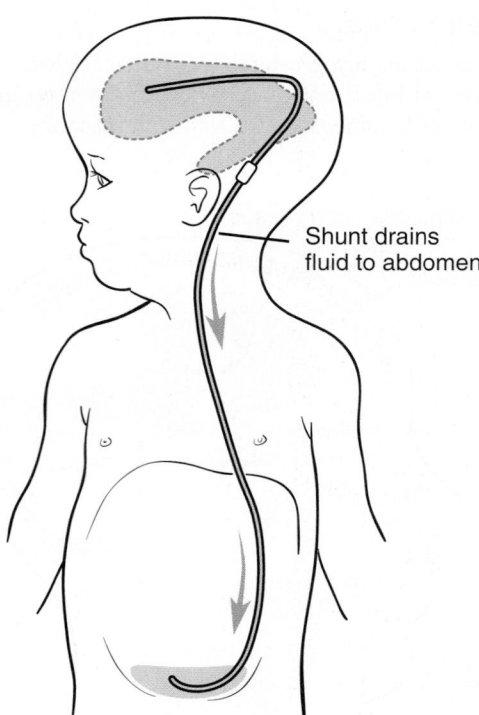

Shunt drains fluid to abdomen

FIGURE 52-4 • Shunt for Hydrocephalus Treatment. Fluid is drained by way of a ventriculoatrial or ventriculoperitoneal shunt.

ARTHRITIS

Diseases of the joints, including arthritis, are among the most common causes of chronic illness in the United States. In addition to arthritis as a disease entity, arthritic manifestations may occur as a symptom of various other chronic diseases. A person may suffer from more than one type at a time.
- Arthritis means inflammation in a joint. It may occur in an acute or chronic form and may be localized or generalized. When many joints are involved, the term *polyarthritis* may be applied.
- The resulting disability may be temporary or permanent, partial or complete.
- Factors implicated in the cause of rheumatic and arthritic diseases include infectious agents, traumatic disorders, endocrine abnormalities, tumors, allergy and drug reactions, and inherited or congenital conditions. When the cause is known, specific medical, physical, and surgical therapies may be available to alleviate pain and disability.

I. Degenerative Joint Disease (Osteoarthritis)

- Chronic condition related to breakdown and progressive loss of the hyaline cartilage cushion in the joints.[44]
- Eventually changes in underlying bone are noted.
- Inflammation is not a key symptom.
- Particularly affects the weight-bearing joints.
- No specific cause known, but predisposing risk factors may include:
  - Repeated trauma and mechanical stresses to the weight-bearing joints.
  - Obesity.
  - Age-related changes in the joint tissues.
  - Genetic predisposition.
  - Estrogen deficiency and high bone density may be factors.

A. Occurrence

- Affects approximately 14% of adults above 25 years of age and more than one-third of those above 65 years of age.
- Incidence increases with age and levels off around age 80.
- Women, particularly those above 50 years, have higher rates than men.

B. Symptoms

- At first insidious, the condition leads to pain, deformity, and limitation of movement.
- Hips, knees, fingers, and vertebrae affected most frequently.
- Swelling and inflammation rare; ankylosis does not occur.

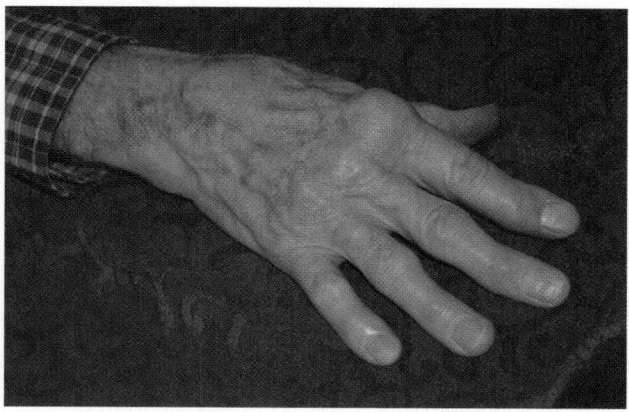

FIGURE 52-5 • Adult Hand Compromised by Degenerative Joint Disease. Pain and lack of ability to grasp the small handle of a toothbrush affect ability to hold and maneuver oral self-care implements.

◆ Stiffness in the morning on rising and after periods of inactivity; diminishes with exercise.

◆ Pain aggravated by temperature changes, bearing body weight, and strenuous activity.

◆ Temporomandibular joint usually without pain or other clinical symptoms, although crepitation, clicking, or snapping may occur when the joints are exercised.

C. Medical Treatment

◆ Treatments to reduce symptoms include:
  • Physical therapy and regular, moderate exercise.
  • Pain-relieving drug therapy.
  • Weight reduction for obese patients.

◆ Total joint replacement has proved satisfactory for many patients.

II. Dental Hygiene Care

Particular factors to consider when planning dental hygiene care for the patient with arthritis include:

◆ Joint pain contributes to impaired motor function and difficulty performing everyday activities of living (see Chapter 51).

◆ Affected areas, degree of impairment, and adaptations to provide for patient comfort are considered when planning care and providing instructions for oral self-care.

◆ The effect of osteoarthritis on the hands of an older patient is considered when planning for self-care procedures (see Figure 52-5).

SUMMARY OF CONSIDERATIONS FOR DENTAL HYGIENE CARE

◆ High cost, dental anxiety, and physical barriers are three main reasons individuals with physical disabilities experience difficulty accessing dental care in traditional settings.[45]

◆ Not being aware of oral health needs is another important barrier to oral care.[46]

◆ Dental professionals are essential members of the interprofessional patient care team for a patient with a physical impairment.[47,48]

◆ Early dental hygiene intervention and regular preventive care will aid in optimizing oral health status and minimizing oral problems.

◆ Knowledge and understanding of the specifics of a patient's particular condition will help the clinician become confident in managing adaptations needed during the dental hygiene appointment.

◆ Communication to determine and support the patient's wishes in adapting patient care procedures is essential, particularly when the patient is unable to perform daily life activities independently and is dependent on others.

◆ Most patients with a physical impairment do not have an intellectual impairment.

◆ Information provided in Chapter 51 is useful for planning dental hygiene care for a patient with a physical impairment, either in a dental clinic or in an alternative practice setting.

◆ General suggestions for the older adult patient in Chapter 48 may also prove useful.

I. Preparation for Appointments

◆ Information for appointment scheduling and providing a barrier-free environment is found in Chapter 51.

◆ Communication with the patient or caregiver prior to appointment to assess specific needs will help the clinician to identify and prepare for modifications necessary to provide care based on the individual patient's needs.

◆ Essential information, such as a completed health history and description of the patient's physical abilities and limitations, can be obtained by telephone.

◆ Ask specific questions about abilities and limitations in performing activities of everyday living.
  • Information about assistance needed from caregivers.
  • Adaptive aids the patient is currently using for oral self-care or other personal hygiene tasks.

◆ Determine factors related to the best time of day for dental appointments, for example:
  • Schedule of urinary/bowel management program for a patient with SCI.
  • The time of day when symptoms associated with the particular condition are most likely to be relieved or diminished.

◆ Assess methods preferred by the patient to communicate with healthcare providers or caregiver.

◆ Determine adaptations needed for the patient's comfort or safety during the appointment.
  • Blankets or increased air circulation if body temperature control is compromised.
  • Positioning and padding needed for stabilization.
  • Procedures for stress reduction.

◆ Identify medications that may put the patient at risk for:
- Xerostomia.
- Increased bleeding.
- Potential interactions with local anesthesia.

II. Additional Considerations during Clinical Care

◆ Frequent, short appointments in a warm, quiet, comfortable atmosphere lessen patient fatigue and emotional stress.

◆ Emergency care may be needed during the period of recovery, such as immediately following a stroke or traumatic spinal injury; nonemergency care is delayed until the patient is stabilized.

◆ When the patient's condition involves partial or complete paralysis of facial muscles:
- Decreased self-cleaning action of the tongue increases potential for collecting dental biofilm on oral surfaces.
- Rinsing may be difficult or impossible.
- When anesthesia is used, the affected cheek and lip may be at higher risk for biting injury until the anesthesia has worn off.
- If the eyelid lacks natural ability to close for protection, care is taken to ensure that calculus, polishing agent, or other foreign material does not splash into the eye by assuring that protective eyewear and suction are used during treatment.

◆ Potential effects from interactions with medications taken for many disorders and conditions require particular care when administering anesthetics.
- For example, epinephrine interaction with levodopa, often prescribed for Parkinson's disease, may cause the patient to experience an exaggerated effect on blood pressure and heart rate.

◆ Dental hygiene care is complicated if the patient has a disorder that involves involuntary movement; for example, athetoid movements in a patient with cerebral palsy.
- Involuntary movement is not interpreted as lack of cooperation.
- Ask the patient or caregiver for suggestions about assistance or management.
- Sedation through premedication may be possible.

III. Assistance for the Ambulatory Patient

Suggestions for how to aid patients who walk with one or more assistive aides such as braces, a cane, crutches, or a walker are found in Chapter 51.

IV. Wheelchair Transfer

◆ Most patients who use wheelchairs can be treated in a traditional clinical setting.

◆ Detailed information about wheelchair to dental chair transfer is available in Chapter 51.

V. Patient Positioning and Body Stabilization

◆ Danger for the patient and dental personnel can result from the uncontrolled movement of the patient.

◆ Communication with patient or caregiver prior to appointment to assess specific needs related to body positioning and use of specific measures such as padding, warm coverings, or other supportive devices will help enhance safety, patient comfort, and clinician efficiency.

◆ The patient is asked to provide direction for correct, individualized procedures.

◆ Slow and incremental adjustments of the patient chair during treatment will help maintain comfort and patient stability.

◆ Prevention of decubitus ulcers can be accomplished by:
- Appropriate positioning of the dental chair.
- Use of padding.
- Periodic repositioning to prevent or reduce pressure.

◆ Before dental hygiene treatment, the patient is asked about susceptibility to spasms and to describe the procedure to follow should one occur.

◆ Suggestions for body stabilization and use of mouth props are found in Chapter 51.

◆ Chapter 4 provides ideas for treatment adaptations when the patient is bed-bound or if care is provided in a nonclinical setting.

VI. Four-Handed Dental Hygiene

◆ Continuous assistance when providing dental hygiene care for patients with a physical impairment is essential.

◆ Use of a dental hygiene assistant will:
- Enhance the clinician's efficiency.
- Ensure the patient's comfort and safety.

VII. Personal Factors that Affect Self-Care

◆ Depression from limitations or discouragement from the pain and pressure of treatment and rehabilitation can affect attitude toward oral self-care practices for the patient who has a physical impairment.

◆ Daily oral care can become a part of the personal hygiene routine accomplished as independently as the patient's ability allows. Physical and occupational therapists provide self-care training to enable as much independence as possible for personal care.

◆ Paralysis or muscle contractions may make grasping and manipulating a toothbrush difficult or impossible.

◆ Adaptations that may assist in maintaining daily oral care include:
- Toothbrush handle modifications (see Chapter 51).
- A specially designed toothbrush (see Chapter 51).[49]
- A lightweight power-driven toothbrush.

- Instruction for the caregiver assistance, provided on the basis of patient ability and limitations.
- Hemiplegia, common after a stroke, can require the challenge of helping the patient develop dexterity in the nondominant hand in order to manipulate biofilm removal implements.

VIII. Residence-Based Delivery of Care

- People with physical disabilities may benefit from oral health service delivery models that provide care in their place of residence.
- Delivery of dental hygiene care in alternative settings is discussed in Chapter 4.

DOCUMENTATION

Documentation in the permanent record for each appointment with a physically impaired patient includes a minimum of the following factors:

- Description of the patient's impairment level and ability to provide oral self-care, with changes/updates noted for each dental hygiene visit, particularly if the patient has a degenerative condition.
- Recommendations for adaptive aids and modifications to daily oral care regimens.
- Description of oral hygiene care instructions provided to the caregiver.
- Description of patient position modifications and other adaptations during patient care.
- An example of documentation for an appointment with a patient with a physical disability is in Box 52-3.

BOX 52-3

Example Documentation: Maintenance Appointment for Patient with a Physical Impairment

S—A 32-year-old female patient presents for routine 3 months maintenance appointment. Patient is ambulatory with a walker and prefers no assistance at this time, but padding under knees helps her relax and enhances her comfort during treatment.

O—Medical history includes diagnosis of MS 2 years ago. Update today indicates no changes in health history or medications. Decreased ability to grasp a regular toothbrush was noted during oral hygiene instruction. No changes in oral status. Biofilm scores less than 20%.

A—Routine 3 months maintenance care today with the use of padding for patient comfort and reassessment of daily oral self-care procedures are indicated.

P—Full-mouth scaling/root debridement, polish, fluoride varnish application. Several options for modifying/enlarging a toothbrush handle to facilitate better grasp during oral care were discussed with patient. At patient request, instruction for using a power toothbrush was provided. The use of a floss holder was demonstrated and ideas for enlarging the handle were given to the patient.

Signed: _____, RDH

Date: _____

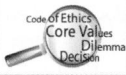

EVERYDAY ETHICS

John had an accident when diving into the surf at the beach 2 years ago at age 18. He has a complete transection lesion at the C5 level. John came today for his biannual dental visit with his mother, who is his primary caregiver. Amy, the dental hygienist, was assisting in the wheelchair transfer into the dental chair. During the transfer, John's t-shirt was inadvertently lifted slightly, and Amy noticed obvious decubitus ulcers that showed signs of secondary infection. Amy continues to transfer him safely into the dental chair and then stops to consider what to do next. Dramatic images from a lecture in dental hygiene school flash through her mind. She will never forget those photographs of patients suffering from neglect.

Questions for Consideration

1. It is possible, although not clearly established in this scenario, that John is the victim of neglect.

Is this an ethical issue or an ethical dilemma for Amy? What issues does Amy need to consider and what questions does she need to ask before she can proceed through the framework for making decisions about:

- Continuing today's appointment when she thinks that John's decubitus ulcers may be infected?
- Addressing the issue of potential neglect?

2. What does the core value of autonomy have to do with this scenario as Amy considers John's competency to make his own choices and treatment decisions versus his dependence on his mother for care?

3. What additional core values (Section II, Introduction) come into play as Amy contemplates how she can best advocate for her patient's safety and well-being?

Factors to Teach the Patient

▶ The need to communicate is key to successful dental treatment and oral health and is achieved by speaking openly about medical history, patient limitations, and adaptations needed for safe dental treatment and effective oral care.

▶ Daily thorough biofilm removal is necessary to reduce the occurrence of oral disease.

▶ Regular maintenance appointments are needed to promote oral health.

▶ Why maintaining periodontal health can help maintain teeth that are necessary as abutments in order to tolerate a mouth-held adaptive aid.

▶ How to clean and maintain a mouth-held aid.

ENHANCE YOUR UNDERSTANDING

ONLINE RESOURCES
(see the inside front cover for access information)
• Audio glossary
• Appendices

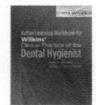

SUPPORT FOR LEARNING
(available separately)
• *Active Learning Workbook for Wilkins' Clinical Practice of the Dental Hygienist, 13th Edition*

INDIVIDUALIZED REVIEW
• Customized practice quizzing with Navigate 2 TestPrep for *Wilkins' Clinical Practice of the Dental Hygienist*

References

1. Wu HJ, Pu JL, Krafft PR, Zhang JM, Chen S. The molecular mechanisms between autophagy and apoptosis: potential role in central nervous system disorders. *Cell Mol Neurobiol.* 2015;35(1):85-99.

2. National Spinal Cord Injury Statistical Center. *Spinal Cord Injury: Facts and Figures at a Glance.* Birmingham, AL: University of Alabama at Birmingham. 2018. https://www.nscisc.uab.edu/Public/Facts%20and%20Figures%20-%202018.pdf. Accessed March 25, 2018.

3. Berlowitz DJ, Wadsworth B, Ross J. Respiratory problems and management in people with spinal cord injury. *Breathe (Sheff).* 2016;12(4):328-340.

4. Remaley DT, Jaeblon T. Pressure ulcers in orthopaedics. *J Am Acad Orthop Surg.* 2010;18(9):568-575.

5. Stephenson RO, Berliner J. Autonomic dysreflexia in spinal cord injury. Medscape Website. http://emedicine.medscape.com/article/322809-overview. Accessed March 25, 2018.

6. Furusawa K, Tokuhiro A, Sugiyama H, et al. Incidence of symptomatic autonomic dysreflexia varies according to the bowel and bladder management techniques in patients with spinal cord injury. *Spinal Cord.* 2011;49(1):49-54.

7. Berger VM, Pölzer S, Nussbaum G, Ernst W, Major Z. Process development for the design and manufacturing of personalizable mouth sticks. *Stud Health Technol Inform.* 2017;242:437-444.

8. Ruff JC. Selection criteria for static and dynamic mouth-sticks. *Gen Dent.* 1990;38(6):414-416.

9. U.S. National Library of Medicine, National Institutes of Health, Medline Plus. Stroke. http://www.nlm.nih.gov/medlineplus/ency/article/000726.htm. Accessed March 25, 2018.

10. Moshfeghi M, Taheri JB, Bahemmat N, Evazzadeh ME, Hadian H. Relationship between carotid artery calcification detected in dental panoramic images and hypertension and myocardial infarction. *Iran J Radiol.* 2014;11(3):e8714.

11. Alves N, Deana NF, Garay I. Detection of common carotid artery calcifications on panoramic radiographs: prevalence and reliability. *Int J Clin Exp Med.* 2014;7(8):1931-1939.

12. Friedlander AH, Freymiller EG. Detection of radiation-accelerated atherosclerosis of the carotid artery by panoramic radiography. A new opportunity for dentists. *J Am Dent Assoc.* 2003;134(10):1361-1365.

13. Warner MJ, Dulebohn SC. Bell Palsy. StatPearls [Internet]. Treasure Island, FL: StatPearls Publishing; 2018.

14. Hazin R, Azizzadeh B, Bhatti MT. Medical and surgical management of facial nerve palsy. *Curr Opin Ophthalmol.* 2009;20(6):440-450.

15. de Almeida JR, Al Khabori M, Guyatt GH, et al. Combined corticosteroid and antiviral treatment for bell palsy: a systematic review and meta-analysis. *JAMA.* 2009;302(9):985-993.

16. National Institute of Neurological Disorders and Stroke. Bell's palsy fact sheet. https://www.ninds.nih.gov/Disorders/Patient-Caregiver-Education/Fact-Sheets/Bells-Palsy-Fact-Sheet. National Institute of Health: Bethesda, MD. Accessed March 25, 2018.

17. Mehta P, Kaye W, Raymond J, et al. Prevalence of amyotrophic lateral sclerosis—United States, 2014. *MMWR Morb Mortal Wkly Rep.* 2018;67:216-218.

18. Holecek V, Rokyta R. Possible etiology and treatment of amyotrophic lateral sclerosis. *Neuro Endocrinol Lett.* 2018;38(8):528-531.

19. Wijesekera LC, Leigh PN. Amyotrophic lateral sclerosis. *Orphanet J Rare Dis.* 2009;4:3.

20. National Institute of Neurological Disorders and Stroke. Amyotrophic lateral sclerosis (ALS) fact sheets. NINDS/NIH Website. https://www.ninds.nih.gov/Disorders/Patient-Caregiver-Education/Fact-Sheets/Amyotrophic-Lateral-Sclerosis-ALS-Fact-Sheet. Accessed March 25, 2018.

21. Nakayama R, Nishiyama A, Matsuda C, Nakayama Y, Hakuta C, Shimada M. Oral health status of hospitalized amyotrophic lateral sclerosis patients: a single-centre observational study. *Acta Odontol Scand.* 2017;26:1-5.

22. Scott K, Shannon R, Roche-Green A. Management of sialorrhea in amyotrophic lateral sclerosis. *J Palliat Med.* 2016;19(1):110-111.

23. Cheng HWB, Chen WTT, Chu CKA, et al. The development of neurology palliative care service for motor neuron disease (MND) patients: Hong Kong experience. *Ann Palliat Med.* 2017 [Epub]. doi: 10.21037/apm.2017.08.17

24. Rooney J, Byrne S, Heverin M, et al. A multidisciplinary clinic approach improves survival in ALS: a comparative

study of ALS in Ireland and Northern Ireland. *J Neurol Neurosurg Psychiatry*. 2015;86(5):496-501.

25. National Institute of Neurological Disorders and Stroke. NINDS Parkinson's disease information page. NINDS/NIH Website. https://www.ninds.nih.gov/Disorders/All-Disorders/Parkinsons-Disease-Information-Page. Accessed March 25, 2018.

26. Parkinson's Disease Foundation. Understanding Parkinson's: Statistics. https://www.parkinson.org/Understanding-Parkinsons/Statistics. Accessed July 9, 2019.

27. Cicciù M, Risitano G, Lo Giudice G, Bramanti E. Periodontal health and caries prevalence evaluation in patients affected by Parkinson's disease. *Parkinsons Dis*. 2012;2012:541908.

28. National Institute of Neurological Disorders and Strokes. Post-polio syndrome fact sheet. NINDS/NIH Website. https://www.ninds.nih.gov/Disorders/Patient-Caregiver-Education/Fact-Sheets/Post-Polio-Syndrome-Fact-Sheet. Accessed March 25, 2018.

29. National Institute of Neurological Disorders and Stroke. Cerebral palsy: hope through research. NINDS/NIH Website: https://www.ninds.nih.gov/Disorders/Patient-Caregiver-Education/Hope-Through-Research/Cerebral-Palsy-Hope-Through-Research. Accessed March 25, 2018.

30. National Institutes of Health, National Institute of Dental and Craniofacial Research. Practical oral care for people with cerebral palsy. NIH Publication No. 09–519. https://www.nidcr.nih.gov/sites/default/files/2017-09/practical-oral-care-cerebral-palsy.pdf?_ga=2.207835090.1185165932.1522030188-79043338.1522030188. Accessed March 25, 2018.

31. Al-Allaq T, Debord TK, Liu H, Wang Y, Messadi DV. Oral health status of individuals with cerebral palsy at a nationally recognized rehabilitation center. *Spec Care Dentist*. 2015;35(1):15-21.

32. Dougherty NJ. A review of cerebral palsy for the oral health professional. *Dent Clin North Am*. 2009;53(2):329-338.

33. National Institute of Neurological Disorders and Stroke. NINDS muscular dystrophy information page. https://www.ninds.nih.gov/Disorders/All-Disorders/Muscular-Dystrophy-Information-Page. Accessed March 25, 2018.

34. Centers for Disease Control and Prevention. Muscular dystrophy: data and statistics. MD STARnet data and statistics. https://www.cdc.gov/ncbddd/musculardystrophy/data.html. Accessed March 25, 2018.

35. U.S. National Library of Medicine, National Institutes of Health, Department of Health and Human Services: Genetics Home Reference Website. Facioscapulohumeral muscular dystrophy. https://ghr.nlm.nih.gov/condition/facioscapulohumeral-muscular-dystrophy. Accessed March 25, 2018.

36. Muscular Dystrophy Association. Muscular dystrophy (DM). https://www.mda.org/disease/myotonic-dystrophy. Accessed June 6, 2018.

37. Balasubramaniam R, Sollecito TP, Stoopler ET. Oral health considerations in muscular dystrophies. *Spec Care Dentist*. 2008;28(6):243-253.

38. National Institutes for Health, Eunice Kennedy Shriver National Institute of Child Health and Human Development. What are the treatments for muscular dystrophy? https://www.nichd.nih.gov/health/topics/musculardys/conditioninfo/treatment. Accessed March 25, 2018.

39. Deavenport-Saman A, Britt A, Smith K, Jacobs RA. Milestones and controversies in maternal and child health: examining a brief history of micronutrient fortification in the US. *J Perinatol*. 2017;3(11):1180-1184.

40. Garg A, Utreja A, Singh SP, Angurana SK. Neural tube defects and their significance in clinical dentistry: a mini review. *J Investig Clin Dent*. 2013;4(1):3-8.

41. National Institute of Neurological Disorders and Stroke. Spina bifida fact sheet. NINDS/NIH Website. https://www.ninds.nih.gov/Disorders/Patient-Caregiver-Education/Fact-Sheets/Spina-Bifida-Fact-Sheet. Accessed March 25, 2018.

42. U.S. National Library of Medicine, National Institutes of Health, MedlinePlus. Myelomeningocele. http://www.nlm.nih.gov/medlineplus/ency/article/001558.htm. Accessed March 25, 2018.

43. American Academy of Pediatric Dentistry, Clinical Affairs Committee. Guideline on antibiotic prophylaxis for dental patients at risk for infection. Reference Manual, Revised. 2014. http://www.aapd.org/media/Policies_Guidelines/G_AntibioticProphylaxis.pdf. Accessed March 25, 2018.

44. Centers for Disease Control and Prevention. Osteoarthritis. http://www.cdc.gov/arthritis/basics/osteoarthritis.htm. Accessed March 25, 2018.

45. Yuen HK, Wolf BJ, Bandyopadhyay D, Magruder KM, Selassie AW, Salinas CF. Factors that limit access to dental care for adults with spinal cord injury. *Spec Care Dentist*. 2010;30(4):151-156.

46. Sullivan AL. Perception of oral status as a barrier to oral care for people with spinal cord injuries. *J Dent Hyg*. 2012;86(2):111-119.

47. Greig V, Sweeney P. Special care dentistry for general dental practice. *Dent Update*. 2013;40(6):452-454, 456-458, 460.

48. American Academy on Pediatric Dentistry; Council on Clinical Affairs. Guideline on management of dental patients with special health care needs. *Pediatr Dent*. 2016;38(6):171-176.

49. Yitzhak M, Sarnat H, Rakocz M, Yaish Y, Ashkenazi M. The effect of toothbrush design on the ability of nurses to brush the teeth of institutionalized cerebral palsy patients. *Spec Care Dentist*. 2013;33(1):20-27.

53

The Patient with an Endocrine Condition

Shannon K. Waldron, RDH, BSc(DH), MSc, and Katherine A. Yee, RDH, BSDH, MPH

CHAPTER OUTLINE

OVERVIEW OF THE ENDOCRINE SYSTEM
  I. Glands of the Endocrine System
  II. Hormones and Their Functions
  III. Regulation of Hormones

ENDOCRINE GLAND DISORDERS

PITUITARY GLAND
  I. Pituitary Tumors
  II. Common Symptoms of Pituitary Disorders
  III. Oral Health Risk Assessment
  IV. Patient Management Considerations

THYROID GLAND
  I. Hypothyroidism
  II. Hyperthyroidism

PARATHYROID GLANDS
  I. Hyperparathyroidism
  II. Hypoparathyroidism

ADRENAL GLANDS
  I. Hyperadrenalism/Cushing Syndrome
  II. Hypoadrenalism/Addison Disease/Adrenal Insufficiency

PANCREAS

PUBERTY
  I. Stages of Adolescence
  II. Pubertal Changes
  III. Patient Management Considerations

WOMEN'S HEALTH
  I. Menstrual Cycle
  II. Hormonal Contraceptives
  III. Menopause
  IV. Patient Management Considerations

DOCUMENTATION

EVERYDAY ETHICS

FACTORS TO TEACH THE PATIENT

REFERENCES

LEARNING OBJECTIVES

After studying this chapter, the student will be able to:

1. Identify the major endocrine glands and describe the functions of each.

2. Explain signs, symptoms, and potential oral manifestations of each endocrine gland disorder.

3. Describe hormonal effects and oral health risk factors commonly associated with puberty, menses, contraceptives, and menopause.

OVERVIEW OF THE ENDOCRINE SYSTEM

Endocrine glands secrete substances directly into the blood or lymph system. They secrete highly specialized substances (hormones) that, with the nervous system, maintain body homeostasis. Influences of the endocrine system on oral health and patient care are discussed in this chapter.

I. Glands of the Endocrine System

◆ The major endocrine glands, shown in Figure 53-1, are the pineal, hypothalamus, pituitary, thyroid, parathyroid, thymus, pancreas, adrenals, and gonads (ovaries and testes).

◆ The anterior pituitary is called the master gland because it regulates the output of hormones by other glands.

◆ In turn, the pituitary itself is regulated by the hormones produced by the other endocrine glands.

◆ The endocrine glands and the hormones produced by each are listed in Table 53-1.

II. Hormones and Their Functions

◆ Hormones affect a number of major functions and are transported by the blood or lymph.

◆ Hormones may act directly on body cells or indirectly to control the hormones of other glands.

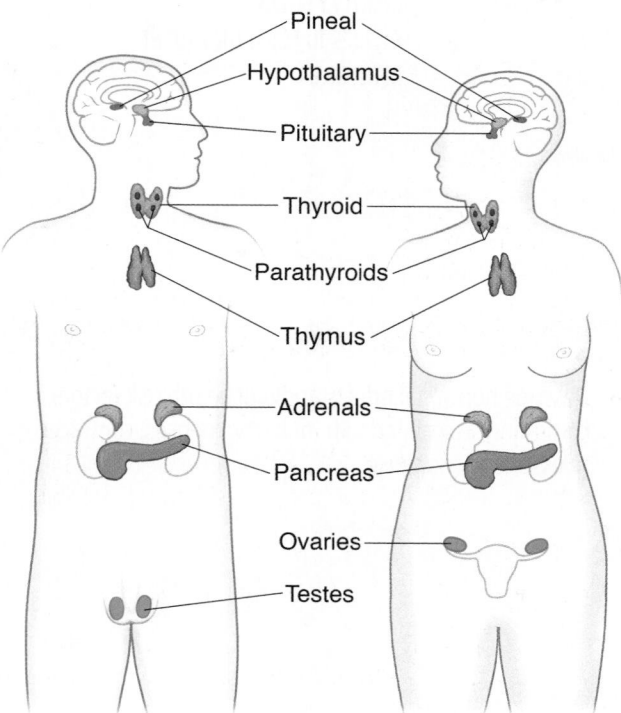

FIGURE 53-1 • The Major Endocrine Glands. Illustrated here for both male and female, these glands produce hormones that regulate body systems.

TABLE 53-1 • Endocrine Glands and the Hormones	
ENDOCRINE GLAND	**HORMONE(S) PRODUCED**
Pineal	Melatonin
Hypothalamus	Controls hormone production in the pituitary gland
Pituitary	
Anterior	Prolactin Growth hormone Adrenocorticotropin Thyroid-stimulating hormone Luteinizing hormone Follicle-stimulating hormone
Posterior	Oxytocin Antidiuretic hormone also called vasopressin
Thyroid	Triiodothyronine (T3) Thyroxin (T4)
Parathyroid	Parathyroid hormone
Thymus	Humoral factor hormones
Adrenals	
Adrenal cortex (outer portion)	Glucocorticoids (such as cortisol) Mineral corticoids (such as aldosterone)
Adrenal medulla (inner portion)	**Epinephrine** (adrenaline) **Norepinephrine**
Pancreas	Insulin
Gonads	
Testes (males)	Testosterone
Ovaries (females)	Estrogen Progesterone Inhibin

◆ Complex and unified actions of hormones produced by endocrine glands augment and regulate many vital functions, including[1]:
  • Growth and development.
  • Energy production.
  • Food metabolism.
  • Reproductive processes.
  • Responses of the body to stress and temperature.

III. Regulation of Hormones

◆ Regulation of hormonal secretion is complex, and the mechanisms are not fully understood. Normally, hormones are secreted when needed.

◆ The stimulus for hormone secretion is often a chemical signal in the blood.
  • When the hormone is released the signal disappears.
  • As more hormone is required, the signal reappears.

◆ This system of "negative feedback" works to provide hormones in optimal amounts and only in response to a need.

◆ Both hyposecretion and hypersecretion of a hormone can cause physical and mental disturbances.

ENDOCRINE GLAND DISORDERS

◆ When diseases affect the glands, hormones may be underproduced or overproduced, causing physical and biochemical changes that may have profound effects on the body, including the oral cavity.

◆ Presence or absence of a particular hormone may affect oral structures and may cause the host response to infection, healing, or stress to vary.[2]

◆ Many systemic diseases and disorders are risk indicators or risk factors for periodontal disease.

◆ Hormonal fluctuations associated with puberty, pregnancy, and menopause can affect the periodontium and directly modify the tissue's response to local factors.

PITUITARY GLAND

◆ The pituitary gland is composed of two functionally distinct portions:
  • Anterior pituitary.
  • Posterior pituitary.

◆ Each portion of the pituitary secretes different hormones.

◆ Excess or inadequate secretion of any of these hormones can cause severe problems for bodily functions.

◆ The anterior pituitary is called the "master gland" because of its great influence on body organs, other endocrine glands, and overall well-being.

I. Pituitary Tumors

◆ Adenomas are the most common pituitary tumors.

◆ These benign tumors:
  • Usually secrete too much of one hormone.
  • Can develop at any age.

◆ Types of pituitary adenomas include[3]:
  • Functioning tumor: causes the other endocrine glands to secrete excess hormones.
  • Nonfunctioning tumor: secretes excess hormones that are inactive due to cell development process and may not be detectible in blood tests.

◆ Other types of pituitary disorders include:
  • Craniopharyngiomas: benign tumors that grow near the pituitary gland; most common in children, teenagers, and adults older than 50.
  • Rathke cleft cysts: benign cysts in the pituitary gland.

II. Common Symptoms of Pituitary Disorders

◆ Headaches.
◆ Vision problems.
◆ Mood swings or behavioral changes.
◆ Weight change.
◆ Reproductive problems.
◆ Hypertension.

III. Oral Health Risk Assessment

During oral health assessment, the dental hygienist recognizes that the patient with a pituitary gland disorder is at increased risk for:

◆ Macrocephaly.
◆ Macrognathia.
◆ Disproportionate mandibular growth: mandibular prognathism.
◆ Open anterior bite.
◆ Large pulp chambers.
◆ Delayed eruption of primary and secondary teeth.[2]
◆ Increased risk for periodontal disease due to growth factors and hormone imbalances.[4]

IV. Patient Management Considerations

◆ Orthodontic evaluation.
◆ Increased risk of hypertension.
◆ Increased risk of developing insulin resistance or type 2 diabetes.
◆ General anesthesia may be contraindicated due to electrolyte imbalance.

THYROID GLAND

◆ Thyroid hormone receptors are present in almost every tissue in the body.

◆ This hormone plays a big role in normal physiologic function in the body including growth and development and energy metabolism.[5]

◆ Levothyroxine (Synthroid), used to treat thyroid gland disorders, is the third most common drug prescribed in the United States.[6]

I. Hypothyroidism

◆ Hypothyroidism, the most common thyroid disorder, occurs when the thyroid does not produce enough thyroid hormone.[7]

◆ It is more common in women than in men. Hypothyroidism develops slowly and is more common in people over the age of 60.

- Untreated or inadequately controlled hypothyroidism may cause an increased susceptibility to infections.
- The most common cause is an autoimmune disorder called Hashimoto disease.
- Characteristics and oral manifestations of hypothyroidism[8] are listed in Table 53-2.
- Oral health risk assessment: because of the autoimmune response, patients with hypothyroidism are at an increased risk for:
  - Periodontitis.[8]
  - Oral candidiasis.
  - Easily bleeding gingiva.
  - Poor wound healing.
- Medical management: treatment is levothyroxine, lifelong monitoring.
- Patient management considerations:
  - Monitor vitals: blood pressure and pulse.
  - Avoid aspirin due to increased gingival bleeding and poor wound healing.
  - Increased risk for myxedema coma due to long-standing low levels of thyroid hormone in the blood.
  - Myxedema coma is a life-threatening emergency. Triggers for myxedema coma are listed in Box 53-1.

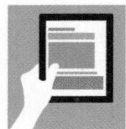

BOX 53-1

Triggers for Myxedema Coma in a Patient with Hypothyroidism

- Drugs (especially sedatives, narcotics, anesthesia).
- Infections.
- Stroke.
- Trauma.
- Heart failure.
- Gastrointestinal bleeding.
- Hypothermia.
- Failure to take thyroid medications.

II. Hyperthyroidism

- When the thyroid gland produces too much thyroid hormone, also referred to as overactive thyroid, it is called hyperthyroidism.[7,8]
- This can occur over a short or long period of time.
- Causes include:
  - Excess of iodine in the diet.
  - Graves disease (autoimmune disorder that affects the thyroid).
  - Viral infection.
  - Taking too much thyroid hormone medication.
- Characteristics and oral manifestations of hyperthyroidism are listed in Table 53-2.
- Oral health risk assessment:
  - Accelerated tooth development, potential for malocclusion.
  - Analgesics can increase the amount of thyroid hormones, making it more difficult to control hyperthyroidism.
  - Vasoconstrictors are used with caution in patients with uncontrolled hyperthyroidism, as these may increase symptoms of tachycardia.[7]
- Patient management considerations:
  - Check vitals: blood pressure and pulse.
  - Thyroid crisis (thyroid storm) is a sudden worsening of hyperthyroidism symptoms, which can be caused by an infection or stress. Immediate hospitalization is necessary.

PARATHYROID GLANDS

As the parathyroid glands develop, they become embedded in the thyroid gland. Secretion of the parathyroid hormone (PTH) is in response to the serum-ionized calcium.[9,10]

- The hormone controls calcium, phosphorus, and vitamin D levels in the blood and bone.
- All parathyroid gland disorders are rare. The most common cause of hypoparathyroidism is when the glands are accidently removed during a thyroidectomy.

TABLE 53-2 • Characteristics of Thyroid Disorders

HYPOTHYROIDISM

Hashimoto **thyroiditis**
Congenital hypothyroidism

GENERAL CHARACTERISTICS	ORAL MANIFESTATIONS
• Fatigue	• Macroglossia
• Intolerant to cold	• Salivary gland enlargement
• Weight gain—decreased metabolic rate	• Facial myxedema
• Constipation	• Increased dental caries
• Decreased concentration	• Compromised periodontal health
• Bradycardia	• Delayed tooth eruption
• Muscle cramps and pain	• Delayed wound healing
• **Myxedema**	• Hoarse voice
	• Burning mouth syndrome
	• Xerostomia
	• Lichen planus

HYPERTHYROIDISM

Graves disease—autoimmune
Thyroid storm (**thyrotoxic crisis**)

GENERAL CHARACTERISTICS	ORAL MANIFESTATIONS
• Fatigue	• Difficulty swallowing
• Intolerant to heat	• Increased dental caries
• Increased appetite	• Increased periodontal disease
• Weight loss	• Macroglossia
• Tremor	• Accelerated development of teeth and jaws
• Protrusion of the eyes	
• Excess sweating	
• Enlargement of thyroid gland	

I. Hyperparathyroidism

- Occurs when the parathyroid glands produce too much PTH.
- Can cause long-standing hypercalcemia, which may result in osteoporosis.
- Symptoms of hyperparathyroidism:
  - Bone pain.
  - Depression.
  - Fatigue.
  - Frequent broken bones.
  - Kidney stones.
  - Nausea.
  - Loss of appetite.
- Oral health risk assessment:
  - Loss of alveolar bone evident in dental images.
  - Spontaneous mandibular fracture.
  - Widened pulp chambers.
  - Demineralized teeth.
- Patient management considerations:
  - Home fluoride therapy.
  - Increased risk of osteoporosis.

II. Hypoparathyroidism

- Hypoparathyroidism occurs when the glands produce insufficient PTH.
  - Causes the blood calcium levels to decrease and phosphorus levels to increase.
  - Most common cause is injury to the parathyroid glands during thyroid and neck surgery.
- Symptoms[11]:
  - Abdominal pain.
  - Brittle nails.
  - Dry hair.
  - Muscle cramps.
  - Muscle spasms (tetany).
  - Increased muscular and peripheral nerve irritability.
- Oral care risk assessment[8]
  - Delayed teeth eruption.
  - Congenitally missing teeth.
  - Shortened roots.
  - Delay or cessation of dental development.
  - Enamel hypoplasia.
  - Poorly calcified dentin.
  - Widened pulp chambers.
  - Mandibular tori.
  - Chronic candidiasis.
  - Paresthesia of the tongue or lips.
  - Twitching or spasm of the facial muscles.
- Medical management: calcium supplements needed.
- Patient management considerations:
  - Home fluoride therapy.
  - Antifungal medication to treat chronic candidiasis.

ADRENAL GLANDS

- The adrenal glands consist of a pair of glands that sit at the top of each kidney.
- The glands are composed of an outer cortex and an inner medulla.
- The adrenal glands work with the hypothalamus and the pituitary gland to produce adrenaline, noradrenaline, dopamine, progesterone, and glucocorticoids.
- Treatment for adrenal gland disorders is corticosteroids.

I. Hyperadrenalism/Cushing Syndrome

Cushing syndrome is caused by too much cortisol production. Increased production of cortisol can be caused by a tumor in the anterior pituitary, a tumor in the adrenal gland, or exogenous administration of steroids.

- Symptoms[11]:
  - Weight gain.
  - Broad, round face.
  - "Buffalo hump."
  - Hypertension.
  - Impaired healing.
  - Hypokalemia.
  - Hyperglycemia, glycosuria, polydipsia (mimics diabetes mellitus).
  - Increased bone fractures.
  - Mood swings and depression.
- Oral health risk assessment:
  - Increased melanic pigmentation may develop black-bluish areas affecting the buccal mucosa, palate, tongue, and lips.
  - Delayed wound healing.
  - Loss of collagen.
  - Skin and oral tissues are fragile.
  - Oral candidiasis.
- Medical management: surgery or radiation.
- Patient management considerations:
  - Antifungal treatment.
  - Antiviral medication.

II. Hypoadrenalism/Addison Disease/ Adrenal Insufficiency

- Hypoadrenalism is divided into three categories:
  - Primary acute (adrenal crisis) failure of the gland to produce cortisol and aldosterone.
  - Primary chronic adrenocortical insufficiency: Addison disease (an autoimmune disease).
  - Secondary adrenocortical insufficiency: rapid withdrawal of steroids or insufficient steroid supplements combined with acute stress (infections, trauma, or surgical procedures) may precipitate an adrenal crisis.
- Symptoms of adrenal crisis, a life-threatening emergency, are listed in Box 53-2.

Dental professionals have a significant responsibility to:

◆ Recognize signs and symptoms of diabetes to promote early diagnosis in order to significantly reduce life-threatening complications of the disease and improve quality of life.

◆ Assess the management and control of diabetes to determine the impact on dental treatment and oral health of the patient.

◆ Work with the patient and other healthcare professionals to provide preventive oral care aimed at maintaining health and preventing infections and emergencies.

◆ Understand the presence of infection, including periodontitis, may make it more difficult to control the blood glucose levels in diabetes.

◆ Identify and treat acute emergencies.

DIABETES MELLITUS

I. Definition

◆ Diabetes mellitus is a group of metabolic diseases associated with hyperglycemia (high blood glucose).[1]

◆ Hyperglycemia results from an insulin deficiency, resistance to insulin action, or both.

◆ People with poorly controlled diabetes mellitus are at risk of complications including:
  • Retinopathy (loss of vision).
  • Kidney failure.
  • Atherosclerotic cardiovascular disease, that is, coronary heart disease, cerebrovascular disease (stroke), and peripheral arterial disease.
  • Peripheral neuropathy (nerve damage of extremities) with increased risk for amputation of toes, feet, and legs.

II. Diabetes Impact

A. Prediabetes Prevalence

◆ In the United States, 84.1 million adults, more than 1 in 3, have prediabetes.[2]
  • Nearly half (48.3%) of those aged 65 years and older have prediabetes.
  • Prediabetes prevalence is similar among racial and ethnic groups.

B. Diabetes Mellitus Prevalence

◆ In the United States, 30.3 million adults (9.4% of the population) have diabetes.[2]
  • Approximately 23 million people (7.2% of the population), or 1 in 4, with diabetes are undiagnosed.
  • American Indian/Alaska Natives (15%), non-Hispanic blacks (12.7%), and Hispanics (12.1%) have the highest prevalence of diabetes.
  • The southern states and the Appalachian regions have the highest prevalence of diagnosed diabetes.
  • 132,000 children and adolescents younger than age 18 (0.18%) had been diagnosed with diabetes.[2]

◆ As the population ages and with increases in obesity, diabetes has become more prevalent.

◆ Medical costs and lost work and wages for those with diabetes are 245 billion dollars annually in the United States.[2]

◆ The risk of death is 50% higher for individuals with diabetes compared to those without diabetes.

◆ Globally, 415 million adults (8.8% of men and 9.2% of women) have diabetes.[3]
  • Health expenditures due to diabetes globally are estimated to be 673 billion dollars.

ORAL HEALTH IMPLICATIONS OF DIABETES MELLITUS

◆ Infection that does not respond to treatment and/or tissues that do not heal may be a sign of undiagnosed diabetes.

◆ Oral findings associated with diabetes can be found in Table 54-1.

◆ Conducting a Diabetes Risk Test (www.diabetes.org) may help to identify those patients needing referral to a primary care provider for evaluation and diagnosis.

TABLE 54-1 • Extraoral/Intraoral Findings Associated with Diabetes

LOCATION	FINDINGS
Gingiva	Increased gingival inflammation
Periodontium	Periodontitis: more frequent, severe, longer duration Attachment loss: more frequent, more extensive Probing depths: more teeth with deep pockets Alveolar bone loss: more Tooth mobility and migration: increased Healing: delayed, increased infection after surgery
Teeth	Poorly controlled diabetes: increased risk of caries related to decreased saliva, diet, and less successful resolution of endodontic therapy related to decreased resistance to infection Well-controlled diabetes: decreased caries related to low sugar, regular eating habits, dental maintenance appointments
Saliva	Glucose in sulcular fluid Xerostomia: contributes to opportunistic infection such as oral candidiasis
Mucosa	Edematous and red color Oral candidiasis Burning mouth and/or tongue, burning mouth syndrome Poor tolerance for removable prostheses Delayed healing May have increased prevalence of lichen planus and aphthous stomatitis
Taste	Hypogeusia, diminished taste perception
Neck	Acanthosis nigricans is a skin condition with a light brown to black appearance in the creases on the neck and in other areas

I. Relationship between Diabetes and Periodontal Disease

◆ The association of diabetes mellitus with periodontal disease is hypothesized to be related to the inflammatory process involved in the pathogenesis of both diseases.[4]

A. Diabetes as a Risk Factor for Periodontitis

◆ Systematic reviews suggest patients with diabetes are at a two to four times greater risk for more severe periodontal disease than individuals without diabetes.[4]

B. Effect of Periodontitis on Glycemic Control

◆ Evidence indicates individuals with diabetes had more severe periodontal disease and a higher A1c than healthy individuals.[4]

C. Effect of Periodontal Treatment on Diabetes

◆ Nonsurgical periodontal therapy and management of periodontal disease have resulted in an average decrease in A1c of 0.36%–0.46%.[5,6]
  • This is roughly equivalent to decreases seen in physical activity and weight loss intervention studies.
  • Management of periodontitis along with lifestyle changes may have an additive effect in lowering A1c.

II. Dental Caries

◆ There is conflicting evidence for a direct relationship between diabetes and risk for coronal or root caries, but there is a reduction in salivary flow and higher levels of dental biofilm, which puts the patient at risk for dental caries.[7]

III. Endodontic Infections

◆ Patients with diabetes have increased periodontal disease in teeth involved endodontically and have a reduced likelihood of success of root canal treatment.[8]

IV. Dental Implants

◆ A meta-analysis found the failure rate for dental implants was similar between individuals with and without diabetes.[9]

BASICS ABOUT INSULIN

I. Definition

◆ **Insulin** is a hormone produced by beta cells in the pancreas.
◆ Insulin directly or indirectly affects every organ in the body.

II. Description

◆ The beta cells of the pancreas are responsible for releasing insulin when stimulated by nutrients, primarily glucose.[10]
◆ Insulin acts like a key to unlock the cell to allow uptake of glucose to use as energy.
◆ Figure 54-1A shows the healthy pancreas and the action of insulin as it is taken up by the body cells.

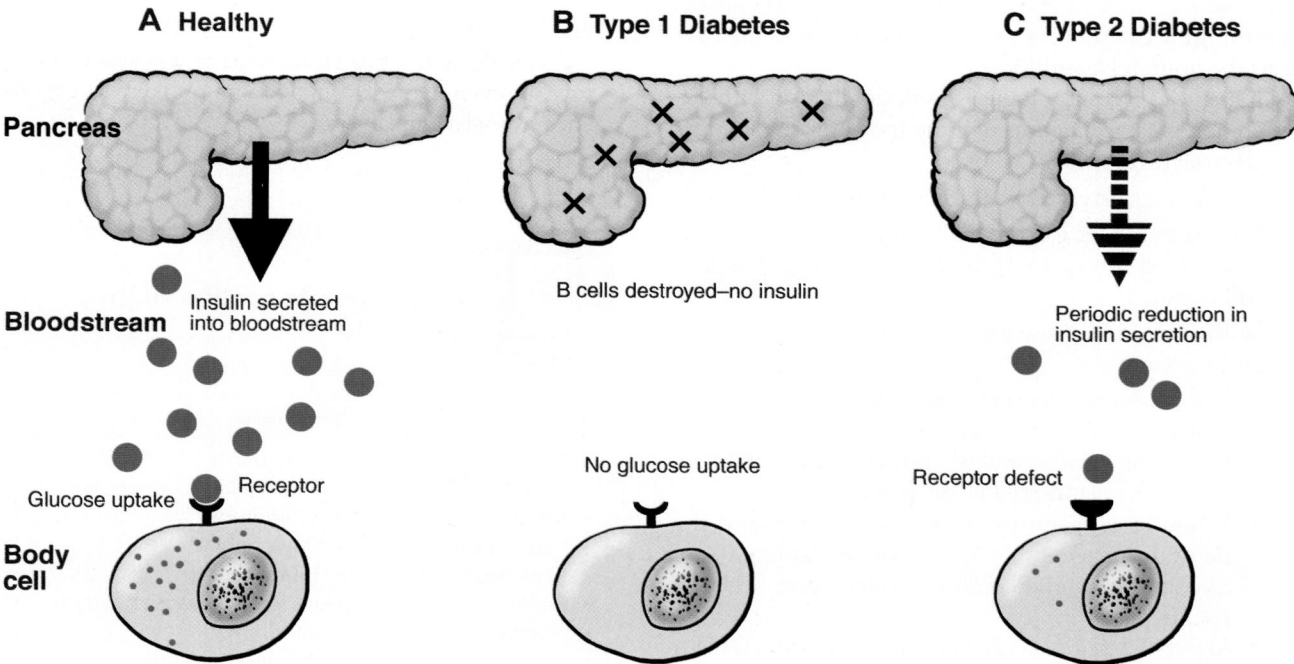

FIGURE 54-1 • Pancreas and Action of Insulin on Body Cell in Health, and Type 1 and Type 2 Diabetes. A: Healthy pancreas excretes insulin into bloodstream that enables glucose uptake by body cell. **B:** Type 1 diabetes shows no insulin produced by pancreas and no glucose uptake by cell. **C:** Type 2 diabetes shows normal, increased, or decreased insulin production by pancreas and the defective receptor on cell that hampers insulin uptake.

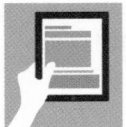

BOX 54-1
Functions of Insulin

1. Facilitates glucose uptake from blood into tissues, which lowers blood glucose level.
2. Speeds the oxidation of glucose within the cells to use for energy.
3. Speeds the conversion of glucose to glycogen to store in the liver and skeletal muscles and to prevent the conversion of glycogen back to glucose.
4. Facilitates the conversion of glucose to fat in adipose tissue.

III. Functions

The functions of insulin are listed in Box 54-1. Without insulin, glucose accumulates in the blood, resulting in hyperglycemia, which in the long-term results in damage to the cells and tissues throughout the body.

- Normal blood glucose levels in healthy individuals range from 60 to 99 mg/dL, and the hemoglobin A1c is less than 5.6%.[1]

IV. Effects of Absolute Insulin Deficiency (Type 1 Diabetes)

Glucose increases in the circulating blood (hyperglycemia) until a threshold is reached and glucose spills over into the urine (glycosuria).[1]

- Increased glycosuria induces osmotic diuresis with excretion of large amounts of urine (polyuria). Water and electrolytes are lost.
- Fluid loss signals excessive thirst to the brain (polydipsia).
- Cells starving for glucose may cause the patient to increase food intake (polyphagia), but weight loss may still occur.
- Without glucose to use for energy, the body metabolizes fat for energy.
  - End products of fat metabolism are harmful ketones that accumulate in the blood.
  - Ketones are acidic, and when they accumulate, they are usually neutralized in the blood.
  - When large quantities of ketones are present, the neutralizing effect of the blood is depleted rapidly and an acidic condition (metabolic acidosis) results.
  - Metabolic acidosis (diabetic ketoacidosis [DKA]) leads to a diabetic coma if not treated promptly.
- Figure 54-1B shows changes in pancreas function that occur in type 1 diabetes.

V. Effects of Impaired Secretion or Action of Insulin (Type 2 Diabetes)

- Deficient insulin action results from inadequate insulin secretion and/or diminished tissue responses to insulin.[1]
  - Cell surface insulin receptors develop defects, and glucose cannot be transmitted into the cells.
  - Blood glucose level increases as the insulin resistance of the cells increases. This stimulates more insulin to be released.
- Over time, insulin secretion may also decline and lead to both decrease of insulin in the blood and increased insulin resistance of the cells.
- Figure 54-1C shows the effects of decreased insulin and action of insulin that can occur in type 2 diabetes. Note the defective receptor on the body cell.

VI. Insulin Complications

- Earlier diagnosis, improved treatment, and better informed patient, family, and friends have reduced the occurrence of emergency insulin complications.
- Constant verbal and visual contact needs to be maintained with a patient during treatment to identify early behavioral and physical changes indicative of a developing medical emergency.

A. Hypoglycemia/Insulin Shock

- Too much insulin (hyperinsulinemia), which lowers the level of blood glucose (hypoglycemia).
- Hypoglycemia (low blood glucose) is an emergency more likely to occur in the dental setting. See Box 54-2 for symptoms of hypoglycemia.
- Individuals with a longer duration of diabetes and history of severe hypoglycemia are more likely to experience hypoglycemic events.[11]

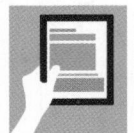

BOX 54-2
Symptoms of Low and High Blood Glucose

HYPOGLYCEMIA	HYPERGLYCEMIA
• Mental confusion	• Polyuria
• Sweating	• Polydipsia
• Irritability	• Weight loss
• Palpitations	• Polyphagia
• Shakiness	• Blurred vision
• Pallor	• Increased susceptibility to infections
• Headache	• Impaired growth
• Seizure	• Ketoacidosis
• Coma and death (if untreated)	

B. Hyperglycemic Reaction/Diabetic Coma (Ketoacidosis)

◆ Too little insulin (hypoinsulinemia) with increased levels of blood glucose (hyperglycemia).

◆ Table 54-2 compares the characteristics of hyperglycemic and hypoglycemic reactions, along with the respective treatment procedures.

IDENTIFICATION OF INDIVIDUALS AT RISK FOR DEVELOPMENT OF DIABETES

I. Diabetes Risk Factors

◆ Adults at risk for diabetes include those who are overweight with a body mass index (BMI) greater than 25 kg/m² and have other risk factors such as[1]:

TABLE 54-2 • Comparison of Hypoglycemia (Insulin Shock) and Hyperglycemia (Diabetic Coma)

	HYPOGLYCEMIA/INSULIN SHOCK	DIABETIC COMA/KETOACIDOSIS
History/predisposing factors	Too much insulin Too little food: omitted or delayed Excessive exercise Stress	Too little insulin: omission of dose or failure to increase dose when requirements increased Too much food Less exercise than planned Infection, illness of any sort Trauma, drugs, alcohol abuse Stress
Occurrence	More common complication than ketoacidosis, especially with less stable type 1 diabetes	Type 1 diabetes especially if poorly controlled, unstable
Onset	Sudden	Develops slowly over hours/days
Behavioral changes	Confusion, stupor Drowsy, restless Anxious, irritable, agitated Incoordination, weakness	Any hypoglycemia behavioral change
Physical findings	Skin: moist, sweaty, perspiration Hunger Headache Tremor, shakiness, weakness Pallor Dilated pupils, blurry vision Dizziness, staggering gait	Skin: flushed, dry Abdominal pain Nausea, vomiting Lack of appetite Dry mouth, thirst Fruity smelling breath Increased urination
Vital signs	Temperature: normal or below Respiration: normal Pulse: fast, irregular Blood pressure: normal or slightly elevated	Temperature: elevated when infection Respiration: hyperpnea, rapid and labored with acetone or fruity smelling breath Pulse: rapid, weak Blood pressure: lowered, person may go into shock
If left untreated	Possible convulsions, eventual coma, and death	Eventual coma and death
Treatment	Glucose gel (15–20 g) is the preferred treatment for the conscious individual with hypoglycemia After 15 min of treatment, if SMBG shows continued hypoglycemia, the treatment should be repeated. Once SMBG returns to normal, the individual should consume a meal or snack to prevent recurrence of hypoglycemia If unconscious/unresponsive: injection of glucagon or intravenous glucose	Immediate professional care Activate emergency medical system, hospitalize Monitor vital signs Keep patient warm Fluids for conscious patient Insulin injection after medical assessment
Prevention	Monitoring and regulation of blood sugar and frequent blood glucose monitoring	Monitoring and regulation of blood sugar and frequent blood glucose monitoring

SMBG: self-monitoring of blood glucose.

- Physical inactivity.
- First-degree relative with diabetes.
- High-risk race/ethnicity such as African American, Hispanic, Native American, Asian, and Pacific Islander.
- Women who have delivered a baby that weighs over 9 pounds or had gestational diabetes during pregnancy.
- Hypertension (>140/90 mm Hg) or taking antihypertensive medications.
- Women with polycystic ovarian syndrome.
- History of cardiovascular disease.
- A1c greater than 5.7%, impaired glucose tolerance, or impaired fasting glucose.

II. Prediabetes

- Individuals who have blood glucose levels above normal but do not meet the criteria for diagnosis of diabetes are considered to have prediabetes. (Diagnostic criteria are provided later in this chapter.)

- Prediabetes means the individual is at high risk for developing diabetes and cardiovascular disease.[1]
- The Diabetes Prevention Program (DPP) showed a 58% reduction in progression to diabetes in those with prediabetes with lifestyle changes including modest weight loss of 7% and a minimum of 150 minutes/week of physical activity.[12]
- The most frequent medication used to manage blood glucose level is metformin.

CLASSIFICATION OF DIABETES MELLITUS

- Classification is based on the etiology of the disease.
- The type of diabetes is based on the circumstances at the time of diagnosis, such as gestational diabetes during pregnancy.[1]
- A comparison of type 1 and 2 diabetes is found in Table 54-3.

TABLE 54-3 • Comparison of Type 1 and Type 2 Diabetes Mellitus

CHARACTERISTIC	TYPE 1	TYPE 2
Age of onset	Young, usually before or during puberty, but may appear later	Adult, usually after 30 years, but occurring with increasing frequency in children and adolescents
Body weight	Normal or thin	Most are obese, body fat particularly in abdominal area
Ethnicity	More common in Caucasians	More common in African Americans, Asian Americans, Hispanics, Native Americans, Pacific Islanders
Hereditary	Yes, but less frequent occurrence than in type 2	Much more frequent occurrence in families
Lifestyle	Restrictions very difficult for young patients	More frequent in sedentary individuals with high-fat diets
Onset of symptoms	Rapid, abrupt symptoms of hyperglycemia	Slow, insidious progression over years, frequently goes undiagnosed for years
Symptoms	Weight loss, weakness Polyuria Frequent/recurrent infections Polydipsia, slow healing Polyphagia Tingling/numb extremities Blurred vision Fatigue Mimic flu Eye/kidney/cardiovascular problems	Any type 1 symptom
Severity	Severe, life threatening	Early mild, but progressively serious
Complications	Acute hypoglycemic/hyperglycemic emergencies and chronic long-term complications common	Acute complications rare, chronic long-term complications common
Ketoacidosis	Common	Rare
Stability	Unstable, difficult, and much effort to control	More stable, easier to manage
Insulin	No insulin production, exogenous insulin required	Insulin levels normal, elevated, or low; exogenous insulin needed by some
Prevention	None, due to multiple genetic predispositions and unclear environmental factors	May be possible to prevent or delay with lifestyle changes, increased activity, and weight loss

I. Type 1 Diabetes Mellitus

A. Description

◆ Accounts for 5%–10% of those with diabetes.

◆ Results from the destruction of insulin-producing beta cells in the pancreas for one of the following reasons[1]:
  • Autoantibodies.
  • No known etiology.

◆ Results in an absolute insulin deficiency requiring exogenous insulin to sustain life.
  • Figure 54-1B illustrates the changes in pancreas function in type 1 diabetes.

◆ Patients are prone to ketoacidosis.[1]

◆ Typically arises in childhood or adolescence, but may appear in adulthood depending on the rate of beta-cell destruction.[1]

◆ Individuals with type 1 diabetes are also prone to other autoimmune disorders such as Graves disease or Hashimoto thyroiditis.[1]

B. Former Names

Insulin-dependent diabetes mellitus, juvenile diabetes, or juvenile-onset diabetes.

II. Type 2 Diabetes Mellitus

A. Description

◆ Most prevalent type of diabetes, accounts for 90%–95% of all patients with diabetes.[1]

◆ Pancreatic insulin secretion may be low, normal, or even higher than normal, but the patient exhibits an insulin resistance that impairs the use of insulin.[1]
  • Figure 54-1C shows changes that occur in type 2 diabetes.

◆ Onset typically occurs in adulthood, and the risk increases with age, obesity, and lack of physical activity.[1]

◆ Although traditionally thought of as occurring in adults, the incidence has increased in children and adolescents due to increases in lack of physical activity, overabundance of fast food, and obesity.[13]
  • In children, the average age of onset is 13 years.

B. Screening

◆ Type 2 diabetes is usually identified after acute symptoms of hyperglycemia prompt evaluation.

◆ Screening in asymptomatic adults is recommended for prediabetes and type 2 diabetes. Basic criteria for testing in healthcare setting are the following[1]:
  • Age 45 and above, repeated a minimum of every 3 years.
  • Screening begins earlier and more frequently if the patient is overweight or obese (BMI > 25 kg/m^2) and has one or more additional risk factors.
  • When tests are normal, they are repeated at least every 3 years.

◆ Screening should be done in children and adolescents who are overweight or obese (BMI >85th percentile for age and sex) and have other risk factors for diabetes.[1]

C. Former Names

◆ Noninsulin-dependent diabetes mellitus or adult-onset diabetes.

III. Gestational Diabetes Mellitus

◆ The prevalence of gestational diabetes mellitus (GDM) is as high as 9.2% of pregnancies in the United States and as high as 15% worldwide.[14,15]

◆ Defined as any degree of glucose intolerance first recognized during pregnancy.[1]

◆ Onset is related to genetics, obesity, and hormones causing insulin resistance.

◆ Insulin adjustment, carefully supervised prenatal care, and improved obstetric practices have lessened much of the potential danger for the mother.

◆ Infants are larger; premature births are more frequent; incidence of congenital malformations and perinatal death is high; and rates lower with improved prenatal care.

◆ More than 50% of women with GDM go on to develop type 2 diabetes within 5–10 years.[1]

A. Screening

◆ Pregnant women with risk factors for diabetes should be screened at the initial prenatal visit.[1]

◆ Women with no history of diabetes prior to pregnancy should be screened at 24–28 weeks of gestation.[1]

◆ Women with gestational diabetes should have lifelong screening for diabetes or prediabetes.[1]

IV. Other Specific Types of Diabetes Mellitus

A. Monogenic Diabetes Syndromes

◆ Neonatal diabetes occurs before the age of 6 months and is typically of genetic origin.[1]

◆ Maturity-onset diabetes of the young typically occurs before the age of 25 years and is also related to genetic abnormalities in at least 13 genes.[1]

B. Cystic Fibrosis–Related Diabetes

◆ Occurs in 20% of adolescents and 40%–50% of adults with cystic fibrosis.[1]

◆ Insufficient production of insulin from the pancreas is the primary cause and is related to poor nutritional status, more severe inflammatory lung disease, and greater mortality.[1]

C. Posttransplantation Diabetes Mellitus (PTDM)

♦ Also called "new-onset diabetes after transplantation."

♦ Immunosuppressants and glucocorticoid steroid use posttransplant are the major causes of PTDM.[1]

DIAGNOSIS OF DIABETES

I. Diabetes Symptoms

Careful review of the medical history with follow-up questions is used to identify risk factors and symptoms (Table 54-3) of diabetes.

♦ The classic symptoms of diabetes include the 3 Ps[1]:

  • Polyphagia (excessive hunger).
  • Polydipsia (excessive thirst).
  • Polyuria (excessive urination).

II. Diagnostic Tests

A. Glycated Hemoglobin Assay (HbA1c or A1c)

♦ A1c measures the quantity of the end product of high glucose bound to a hemoglobin molecule (glycated or glycosylated hemoglobin).

  • An easy way to remember this is to think of the red blood cell as your "donut" and the product of high glucose as the "glaze" on your "donut." The higher the level of end products of high glucose in the blood, the more "glazed" the "donut" (red blood cell).

♦ A1c value provides an average of glycemia (blood glucose levels) over a 3-month period.

♦ The HbA1c test is used to *diagnose* prediabetes and diabetes.[1]

  • Prediabetes is diagnosed with an A1c value of 5.7%–6.4%.
  • A1c greater than or equal to 6.5% is used to diagnose diabetes.

♦ The A1c is also used to *monitor* diabetes control[11]:

  • Testing is recommended twice a year for individuals with good glycemic control.
  • Patients with unstable glycemic control may require testing every 3 months.

♦ A1c goal may vary slightly for an individual based on risk for hypoglycemia, but the goal for most nonpregnant adults is less than 7%.[11]

  • Individuals with a history of severe hypoglycemia may have a less stringent goal such as less than 8%.

B. Fasting Plasma Glucose

♦ Measurement for fasting plasma glucose (FPG) is taken after fasting at least 8 hours and used for diagnosis in the following ways[1]:

  • FPG of 100–125 mg/dL is used to diagnose prediabetes.
  • FPG greater than 126 mg/dL is the criterion used for diagnosis of diabetes.
  • Repeat testing is recommended to confirm a diagnosis.

C. 2-Hour Plasma Glucose

Typically measured during an oral glucose tolerance test[1]:

♦ A 2-hour plasma glucose (PG) of 140–199 mg/dL is also used to diagnose prediabetes.

♦ A 2-hour PG greater than 200 mg/dL is used as a criterion for the diagnosis of diabetes.

♦ Repeat testing is recommended to confirm a diagnosis.

III. Diabetes Screening in the Dental Setting

♦ Dental visits provide an opportunity to screen patients for undiagnosed diabetes (see Figure 54-2).[16,17]

  • A type 2 diabetes risk test is available on the American Diabetes Association website and could be used chairside in the dental office for screening.[18]
  • Screening may also include point-of-care (POC) A1c testing using fingersticks or gingival crevicular bleeding.[16,17,19]

STANDARDS OF MEDICAL CARE FOR DIABETES MELLITUS

♦ Medical management depends on the severity of the disease and on individual characteristics.

  • Consideration is given to individualized needs related to age, activities, vocation, lifestyle, knowledge, attitudes, personality, culture, emotional and psychological needs, as well as the health and nutritional status and weight issues of the patient.

I. Early Diagnosis

♦ Identify individuals with prediabetes and undiagnosed diabetes through regular screening and/or monitoring.[1,18,20]

♦ Assess risk factors and refer for evaluation.

II. Management of Prediabetes

♦ The DPP that demonstrated lifestyle changes including physical activity, attaining and maintaining a healthy weight, and making wise food choices is effective in preventing or delaying the onset of diabetes.[20,21]

III. Diabetes Self-Management Education

♦ The National Standards for Diabetes Education and Support guidelines indicate diabetes self-management education is essential for those at risk for developing diabetes as well as for those individuals who are newly diagnosed.[22]

  • Diabetes self-management education and support has been shown to reduce HbA1c by 0.6%, which is equivalent to some medications.[22]

ARE YOU AT RISK FOR
TYPE 2 DIABETES? American Diabetes Association.

Diabetes Risk Test

1 How old are you?

   Less than 40 years (0 points)
   40–49 years (1 point)
   50–59 years (2 points)
   60 years or older (3 points)

Write your score in the box.

2 Are you a man or a woman?

   Man (1 point)   Woman (0 points)

3 If you are a woman, have you ever been diagnosed with gestational diabetes?

   Yes (1 point)   No (0 points)

4 Do you have a mother, father, sister, or brother with diabetes?

   Yes (1 point)   No (0 points)

5 Have you ever been diagnosed with high blood pressure?

   Yes (1 point)   No (0 points)

6 Are you physically active?

   Yes (0 points)   No (1 point)

7 What is your weight status?
   (see chart at right)

Height	Weight (lbs.)		
4' 10"	119–142	143–190	191+
4' 11"	124–147	148–197	198+
5' 0"	128–152	153–203	204+
5' 1"	132–157	158–210	211+
5' 2"	136–163	164–217	218+
5' 3"	141–168	169–224	225+
5' 4"	145–173	174–231	232+
5' 5"	150–179	180–239	240+
5' 6"	155–185	186–246	247+
5' 7"	159–190	191–254	255+
5' 8"	164–196	197–261	262+
5' 9"	169–202	203–269	270+
5' 10"	174–208	209–277	278+
5' 11"	179–214	215–285	286+
6' 0"	184–220	221–293	294+
6' 1"	189–226	227–301	302+
6' 2"	194–232	233–310	311+
6' 3"	200–239	240–318	319+
6' 4"	205–245	246–327	328+
	(1 Point)	(2 Points)	(3 Points)

You weigh less than the amount in the left column (0 points)

Adapted from Bang et al., Ann Intern Med 151:775-783, 2009.
Original algorithm was validated without gestational diabetes as part of the model.

If you scored 5 or higher:
You are at increased risk for having type 2 diabetes. However, only your doctor can tell for sure if you do have type 2 diabetes or prediabetes (a condition that precedes type 2 diabetes in which blood glucose levels are higher than normal). Talk to your doctor to see if additional testing is needed.

Add up your score.

Type 2 diabetes is more common in African Americans, Hispanics/Latinos, American Indians, and Asian Americans and Pacific Islanders.

Higher body weights increase diabetes risk for everyone. Asian Americans are at increased diabetes risk at lower body weights than the rest of the general public (about 15 pounds lower).

For more information, visit us at diabetes.org/alert or call 1-800-DIABETES (1-800-342-2383)

Lower Your Risk
The good news is that you can manage your risk for type 2 diabetes. Small steps make a big difference and can help you live a longer, healthier life.

If you are at high risk, your first step is to see your doctor to see if additional testing is needed.

Visit diabetes.org or call 1-800-DIABETES (1-800-342-2383) for information, tips on getting started, and ideas for simple, small steps you can take to help lower your risk.

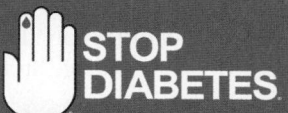 STOP DIABETES.

Special Thanks to our National Sponsor

Walgreens

FIGURE 54-2 • Diabetes Risk Test. "Are You at Risk for Type 2 Diabetes?" screening tool. (Copyright 2009 American Diabetes Association. From http://www.diabetes.org. Reprinted by permission of The American Diabetes Association.)

◆ Maintain tight glycemic control to reduce the complications of diabetes through regular self-monitoring of blood glucose (SMBG) at home.[11]

- Frequency and timing are individualized to patient needs, but are often recommended before breakfast, prior to meals, and prior to bedtime.
- More frequent monitoring is associated with better glycemic control and a lower A1c.
- Hypoglycemia is a limiting factor in setting a glycemic target.

◆ Monitoring devices for home may include the following:

- *Glucose meter (or glucometer)* is a device that requires a fingerstick to obtain a drop of blood for measurement of blood glucose.
- *Continuous glucose monitoring* (CGM) is done automatically with a device such as FreeStyle Libre throughout the day and night and may have an alarm for hypoglycemia and hyperglycemia.
  - Depending on the device, a sensor is placed on the abdomen or back of the upper arm, and a thin filament is inserted under the skin to measure the interstitial fluid glucose level.
  - A handheld reader is then used to scan the sensor and provide the current blood glucose, an 8-hour history, and an arrow to show the trends in the blood glucose to help the individual understand and manage his or her blood glucose.
  - Some devices may send the information to a cell phone, and the information can be downloaded to a computer.
  - CGM is most commonly used with an insulin pump (Figure 54-3).

A. Interprofessional Healthcare Team

◆ Initial and ongoing individualized education is provided by the interprofessional team.

- Members include physicians, registered nurses, nurse practitioners, physician assistant, registered dietitian, nutritionists, pharmacists, mental health professionals, dental professionals, and other specialists, such as endocrinologist, cardiologist, ophthalmologist, and podiatrist.

B. Educational Resources

◆ *Books and journals*: A number of excellent books, professional journals, and other printed materials have been prepared for the patients and for health professionals.

- Annually, the American Diabetes Association publishes evidence-based Clinical Practice Recommendations in the *Diabetes Care* journal. These can be accessed free of charge on www.diabetes.org.

◆ *Internet*: Access to diabetes education and support resources continues to expand rapidly (review strategies to determine the validity of information on websites in Chapter 2). In addition to static websites, the

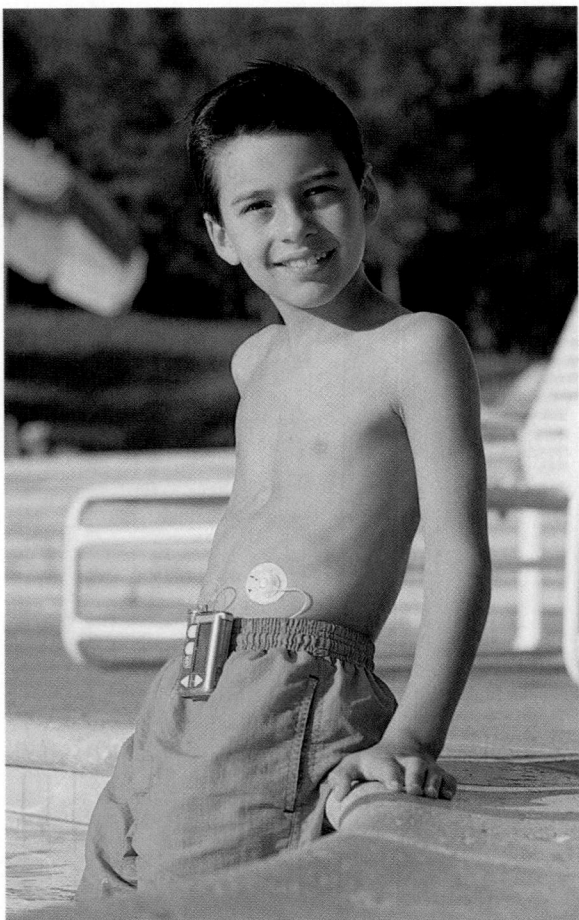

FIGURE 54-3 • Patient Wearing Insulin Pump. Young boy with active lifestyle wearing an insulin pump. (Photo courtesy of Minimed.)

Internet provides interactive resources that include the following:

- Interactive behavior change programs.
- Peer support through social media networks such as Facebook, blogs, and chat rooms.[23]

◆ *Technology*: Cell phone applications for tracking food intake, physical activity, weight, blood glucose, and blood pressure can be used to assist the individual with self-monitoring and can be shared with the healthcare team.[24]

IV. Medical Nutrition Therapy

◆ Medical nutrition therapy (MNT) is individualized to meet the needs of the patients to manage and control diabetes.[25]

◆ The American Diabetes Association recommends nutrition therapy be provided by a registered dietitian/nutritionist.[25]

◆ Goals for MNT include the following[25]:

- A variety of eating patterns are acceptable and should be individualized to meet overall health goals. The Mediterranean diet and Dietary Approaches to Stop Hypertension are examples of healthy eating patterns.

- Energy balance for modest weight loss (5–10 pounds) and weight maintenance.
- Carbohydrate intake needs to be balanced throughout the day, with focus on vegetables, fruits, whole grains, beans, and low-fat dairy products and an emphasis on higher fiber and lower glycemic loads over foods with added sugars.
- Similar to the Dietary Guidelines for Americans, individuals with diabetes need to limit or avoid added sugar and refined carbohydrates.
- Limit intake of saturated fat, trans fat, and cholesterol. Include foods rich in omega-3 fatty acids such as fatty fish, nuts, and seeds.
- Recommendations for sodium intake of less than 2,300 mg/day are the same as for the general population (see Chapter 33).
- Alcohol should be in moderation with an understanding about how it may increase the risk for hypoglycemia.

V. Physical Activity

- Adults are encouraged to engage in 150 minutes/week of moderate-intensity physical activity spread over at least 3 days/week.[25]
- Children and adolescents are encouraged to engage in 60 minutes/day of moderate- or vigorous-intensity physical activity at least 3 days/week.[25]
- Contributes to lowering insulin requirements by increasing the muscle sensitivity to insulin.

VI. Habits

A. Tobacco

- Patients must avoid all types of tobacco (see Chapter 32).
  - Tobacco use increases the risk of heart disease, stroke, myocardial infarction, limb amputations, periodontal disease, and numerous other health problems.[25]

B. Alcohol

- Avoid excessive alcohol; alcohol can raise blood pressure and contribute to other health problems as well as difficulty with diabetes management.[25]

VII. Psychosocial Issues

- Screening for diabetes distress (DD) should be done routinely by the primary care provider and requires interprofessional collaboration to manage.
  - DD refers to the psychological challenges of managing a chronic disease like diabetes.

PHARMACOLOGIC THERAPY

I. Insulin Therapy

All patients with type 1 diabetes require exogenous insulin for survival. Type 2 diabetic patients may need to use insulin in combination with other medications for glycemic control.[26]

A. Types of Insulin

Insulin is classified as rapid acting, regular or short acting, intermediate acting, or long acting based on the onset, peak, and duration of action. The types of insulin and range of peak action are found in Table 54-4.

B. Dosage

- *Objective*: Attain optimum utilization of glucose throughout each 24 hours.
- *Factors affecting the need for insulin*: Food intake, illness, stress, variations in exercise, or infections.
- *"Sick Day Rules"*: Insulin dose is adjusted if there are any factors that affect the need for insulin.

C. Methods for Insulin Administration

- *Subcutaneous injection with syringe*: A syringe is filled from vial of insulin. Injection sites are rotated usually on the abdomen, thigh, or upper arm.
- *Insulin pen*: Prefilled cartridge of single type of insulin injected with attached needle. May be disposable or a reusable type.
- *Continuous subcutaneous insulin infusion with a battery-operated insulin pump*:
  - The insulin pump delivers a preprogrammed continuous basal rate of insulin and bolus doses when needed.
  - Offers greater flexibility and smoother control of glycemia, but may increase the risk of hypoglycemia.

TABLE 54-4 • Types and Action of Insulin			
CLASS OF INSULIN	TYPE/NAME	PEAK ACTION	DURATION
Rapid acting	Lispro (Humalog), Aspart (NovoLog)	30 min to 3 hr	3–5 hr
Regular or short acting	Humulin R, Novolin R	2–5 hr	Up to 12 hr
Intermediate acting	NPH (Humulin N, Novolin N)	4–12 hr	Up to 24 hr
Long acting	Detemir (Levemir), Glargine (Lantus)	Minimal peak	Up to 24 hr
Inhaled, rapid acting	Afrezza®	15 min	

- The small cell phone–sized pump can be worn in a pocket or on a belt or a waistband, as shown in Figure 54-3.
- *Inhalable insulin*[27]:
  - Contraindicated for those who have long-term (chronic) lung problems such as asthma or chronic obstructive pulmonary disease (COPD)
  - Rapid-acting, "mealtime" insulin is taken through an inhaler.
  - Side effects include lower lung function, cough, dry mouth, bronchospasm, or chest discomfort.
  - Brand name: Afrezza®.
- Future modes for insulin administration include an insulin patch and implantable insulin pumps.

II. Antihyperglycemic Therapy

- The medications listed in Table 54-5 may be used individually or in combinations.[26]
- The most common medication used in prediabetes is metformin.
- Monotherapy: lifestyle management + metformin.[26]
  - A1c less than 9%.
- Dual therapy: lifestyle management + metformin + additional agent.[26]
  - A1c greater than or equal to 9%.
- Triple therapy: lifestyle management + metformin + two additional agents.[26]
  - A1c greater than or equal to 10%.

- The takeaway message for dental professionals is that when a patient is on multiple medications, it means the diabetes is not well controlled.

COMPLICATIONS OF DIABETES

Patients with well-controlled blood glucose levels tend to develop fewer complications later in life than those whose diabetes is less well controlled.[28]

I. Infection

- Individuals with poorly controlled diabetes are more susceptible to infections and impaired healing, which can worsen prognosis.[26,29,30]
- The presence of stress, trauma, and infection affects blood glucose levels.
- Failure to treat an infection intensifies the symptoms and increases the severity of diabetes, which can progress to life-threatening infections or precipitate DKA.[1,26,29]
- Insulin requirements may increase with fever, infection, inflammation, trauma, bleeding, pain, or stress. When the condition is eliminated, prescribed insulin may be reduced.
- Numerous factors are involved including impaired immune response, alterations in metabolism of carbohydrate and protein, vascular changes and impaired circulation, and altered nutritional state.[29]

TABLE 54-5 • Antihyperglycemic Agents Used for Treatment of Type 2 Diabetes

AGENT	EXAMPLE	ACTION/FUNCTION
Biguanides	Metformin (Glucophage)	• Prevent liver glycogen breakdown to glucose • Increase tissue sensitivity to insulin
Sulfonylureas	Glyburide (Diabeta, Micronase) Glipizide (Glucotrol)	• Stimulate pancreas to release more insulin after a meal • May cause hypoglycemia
Meglitinides	Repaglinide (Prandin) Nateglinide (Starlix)	• Stimulate pancreas to release more insulin after a meal • May cause hypoglycemia
Thiazolidinediones	Pioglitazone (Actos)	• Increase tissue sensitivity to insulin
Dipeptidyl peptidase-4 inhibitors	Sitagliptin (Januvia)	• Improve insulin level after meals and lowers glucose production
Alpha-glucosidase inhibitors	Acarbose (Precose)	• Slow digestion and absorption of glucose into bloodstream after eating
Bile acid sequestrants	Colesevelam (Welchol)	• Bind bile acids in intestinal tract, increasing hepatic bile production
SGLT2 inhibitors	Canagliflozin (Invokana®) Dapagliflozin (Farxiga®)	• Block glucose reabsorption in kidney
GLP-1 receptor agonists	Exenatide (Byetta®) Liraglutide (Victoza®)	• Increase insulin secretion • Decrease glucagon secretion • Slow gastric emptying • Increase satiety
Dopamine-2 agonists	Bromocriptine (Cycloset®)	• Increase insulin secretion

GLP: glucagon-like peptide; SGLT: sodium–glucose cotransporter.

Source: Adapted from American Diabetes Association. 8. Pharmacologic approaches to glycemic treatment: standards of medical care in diabetes—2018. *Diabetes Care*. 2018; 41(suppl 1):S73-S85.

II. Neuropathy

◆ Neuropathy can cause pain, numbness, or tingling of mouth, face, and extremities.

A. Peripheral Neuropathy

◆ Symptoms vary based on the sensory nerve fibers affected and may result in loss of sensation in the feet, hands, and fingers.[31]

◆ Numbness in the hands and fingers may make effective oral self-care difficult.

◆ As many as 50% of people with peripheral neuropathy may be asymptomatic and not recognize the loss of sensation, which can put them at risk for injury and resulting infection.[31]

◆ Leads to increased incidence of amputations and Charcot joints.[31]

B. Autonomic Neuropathy

◆ Manifestations include tachycardia, orthostatic hypotension, gastroparesis, and hypoglycemic unawareness.[31]

• Cardiovascular autonomic neuropathy can be symptomatic other than changes in the heart rate.

• Gastroparesis is a slowing of digestion and motility of the gastrointestinal tract.

• Hypoglycemic unawareness can quickly become an emergency situation because the patient is not able to recognize the usual symptoms of low blood glucose.

◆ Early management to maintain glycemic levels near normal can be effective in preventing or delaying neuropathy.[31]

III. Nephropathy

◆ Diabetes is a leading cause of renal disease and the most common cause of end-stage renal disease in the United States and Europe. Dialysis or kidney transplant is needed.[31]

◆ Patients diagnosed with diabetes are screened at least annually for microalbuminuria (protein in the urine).[31]

IV. Retinopathy

◆ Diabetes is a leading cause of new cases of blindness through the progression of diabetic retinopathy.[31]

◆ Patients are more likely to have glaucoma and cataracts.[31]

V. Cardiovascular Disease

◆ Individuals with diabetes are at high risk for cardiovascular disease, a major cause of morbidity and mortality. Conditions common in people with diabetes include the following[32]:

• Hypertension.

• Dyslipidemia (high total cholesterol and low-density lipoproteins [LDL]).

• Hypertriglyceridemia (high triglycerides).

◆ May lead to myocardial infarction and stroke.

◆ Owing to the excessive risk of coronary heart disease, aggressive treatment for dyslipidemia and hypertriglyceridemia is recommended.[32]

◆ Low-dose aspirin therapy may be recommended for the prevention of cardiovascular disease in patients with diabetes. Daily aspirin intake may increase bleeding time.[32]

VI. Amputation

Diabetes is a major cause of limb amputation (usually foot) from possible complications of neuropathy and vascular disease.[31]

VII. Pregnancy Complications

Patients with diabetes are at higher risk for spontaneous miscarriages, having babies with birth defects and increased weight.[33]

VIII. Mental Health

◆ Due to complications of diabetes, the daily life of the patient as well as those close to the patient are significantly affected. Diabetes distress (DD) was discussed in the previous section regarding psychosocial issues. However, mental health issues common in those with diabetes include the following[29]:

• Anxiety disorders.

• Depression.

• Disordered eating behavior characterized by omission of insulin to lose weight.

• Serious mental illness such as schizophrenia.

◆ Treatment regimens may be challenging to cope with and lead to emotional and social problems, including depression.

◆ A suggestion for the patient to discuss psychosocial issues with the physician may improve patient's compliance with treatment and daily oral personal care.

DENTAL HYGIENE CARE PLAN

◆ The control of oral infection is vital. Infections can progress more quickly and can alter the management of diabetes.

◆ Frequent, thorough oral care requires the patient's cooperation along with regular professional care.

◆ The patient with diabetes is prone to life-threatening emergencies.

◆ Emergency practice drills can help the dental team prevent an emergency, identify early indications of a developing emergency, and act swiftly and appropriately.

I. Appointment Planning

Stress, including stress created during a dental or dental hygiene appointment, can affect blood sugar levels. Appointment planning needs to center around many factors, including stress prevention.

A. Time

- Treat patient after a meal, preferably containint protein and fat to slow carbohydrate absorption.
- Avoid peak insulin level noted in Table 54-4.
- Ideal time of appointment varies with individual patient's lifestyle and method of insulin intake.
- Preferred time of appointment may be morning, soon after the patient's normal breakfast and medication, during the ascending portion of the blood glucose level curve.[34]

B. Precautions: Prevent/Prepare for Emergency

- Do not keep the patient waiting.
- Do not interfere with the patient's regular meal and between-meal eating schedule.
- Avoid long, stressful procedures; dental and dental hygiene care can be divided into short appointments appropriate to the individual's needs.

- Take additional precautions indicated for the patient with long-term diabetes with complications related to atherosclerosis and other cardiovascular diseases.
- Prevent and treat all infections promptly.
- Monitor for symptoms of hypoglycemia including dizziness, sweating (diaphoresis), mental confusion, shakiness, pallor, palpitations, and irritability. The symptoms of hypoglycemia and hyperglycemia are listed in Box 54-2.
- Prepare for hypoglycemic emergency.
  - Keep glucose gel as part of the office emergency kit for the conscious patient.
  - A glucometer should also be part of the emergency supplies to allow testing to identify hypoglycemia and monitor the effect of the glucose gel.

D. Emergency Management

- Recognize any change in patient behavior that signals a diabetes emergency.
  - If in doubt, it is safer to treat for hypoglycemia since it will only cause a brief increase in blood glucose.
  - Follow the *Rule of 15s* (see the flowchart in Figure 54-4 for the management of hypoglycemia).[11]

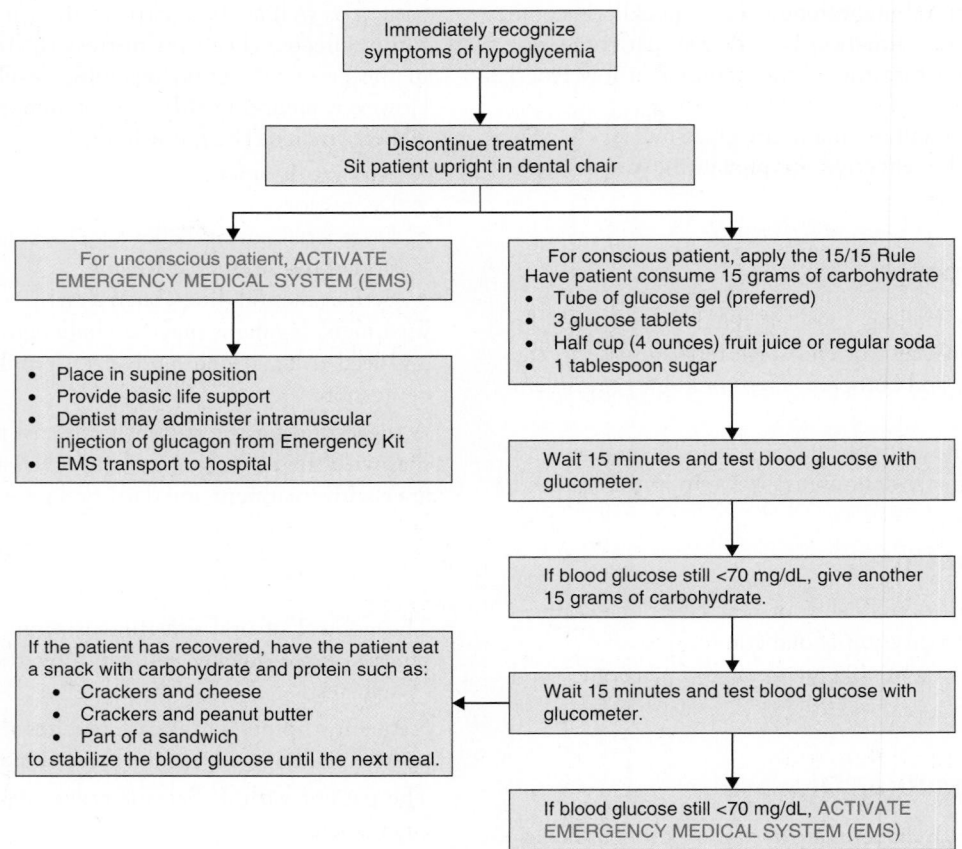

FIGURE 54-4 • Managing Hypoglycemia (Rule of 15s). Flowchart to show steps to take when the patient exhibits symptoms of hypoglycemia (insulin shock). (Reprinted from DeLong L, Burkhart N General and Oral Pathology for the Dental Hygienist. Philadelphia: Lippincott Williams & Wilkins; 2015.)

II. Patient History

A. Medical History

◆ Questions regarding signs and symptoms of diabetes are included in a standard medical history questionnaire. Appropriate questions to ask are listed in Box 54-3.

- Supplement the basic medical history with additional questions to obtain information about diabetes (suggested questions along with answers can be found in Box 54-4).
- If an unexplained positive response is present suggesting symptoms of diabetes, the patient is referred to a primary care provider for evaluation.

◆ Ask about physical activity and tobacco use; review effect on health.

◆ Update medical history at each appointment.

◆ Identify health problems or complications of diabetes that may influence dental treatment.

B. Screening for Diabetes

◆ The American Diabetes Association's diabetes risk test (Figure 54-2) can also be used to identify those at risk for diabetes.

◆ Using POC devices to test HbA1c and blood glucose has been shown to be a cost-effective approach to identifying undiagnosed and at-risk patients needing referral for further evaluation.[16]

- Note: Using these devices is not similar to laboratory tests, and verification is needed by a blood sample evaluated by a certified laboratory.

III. Consultation with Primary Care Provider

◆ Consultation with the primary care provider to obtain A1c values can be initiated either prior to or at the first visit.

- Table 54-6 provides a conversion for the A1c values to average blood glucose levels.

◆ Further consultation may be necessary in more advanced periodontal disease to obtain clearance for treatment.

IV. Dental Hygiene Assessment and Treatment

A. Extraoral/Intraoral Examination

◆ Acanthosis nigricans appears as a light brown to black discoloration of the skin in the creases of the neck and can indicate risk for diabetes (Figure 54-5).[35]

B. Dental Biofilm Control Instruction

◆ Because of the impact of diabetes on periodontal health and the effect of oral infection on diabetes status, daily meticulous oral self-care is crucial.

◆ Disclosing the biofilm and individualized self-care measures for biofilm control should be conducted at each visit.

C. Tobacco Cessation

◆ Refer to the information on Tobacco Cessation Programs in Chapter 32.

D. Instrumentation

◆ *Nonsurgical periodontal therapy*: Definitive nonsurgical periodontal therapy reduces the possibility of periodontal abscess formation. Allow several short appointments if needed for stress management.

◆ *Healing*: Avoid undue trauma to tissues to minimize the risk for complications associated with healing.

E. Fluoride

◆ Fluoride treatments, varnishes, and home use of fluoride should be recommended based on caries risk.

◆ Methods for daily self-fluoride application are described in Chapter 34.

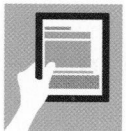

BOX 54-3
Common Medical History Questions to Screen for Diabetes

• Have you ever been diagnosed with prediabetes, borderline diabetes, or diabetes?	Yes	No
• Have any members of your family ever been diagnosed with diabetes?	Yes	No
• Do you urinate frequently? How many times per day?	Yes	No
• Are you frequently thirsty?	Yes	No
• Does your mouth feel dry?	Yes	No
• Have you had any unexplained weight loss?	Yes	No
• Do you experience excessive hunger?	Yes	No
• Did you have recent blurred vision?	Yes	No

Gather detailed information on all current prescribed and over-the-counter medications, including recommended dose.

Gather information on vitamins and homeopathic or herbal supplements.

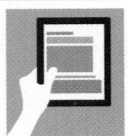

BOX 54-4
Questions to Ask a Patient with Diabetes to Gather Additional Information

- When was your last visit to your diabetes care healthcare provider?

    Answer: It is recommended individuals with stable glycemic control be seen twice/year and those with poor glycemic control at least quarterly.

- What medications and dose have you taken today?

    Answer: Medications need to be taken prior to the appointment, and patient knowledge about medications suggests personal responsibility for diabetes self-care.

- When did you eat last? What did you eat?

    Answer: Foods containing complex carbohydrates and protein and/or fat 1–2 hours before the appointment to prevent hypoglycemia is ideal.

- Do you monitor your blood sugar at home?

    Answer: Yes, self-monitoring of blood glucose is critical for diabetes self-care.

- How often do you monitor your blood glucose?

    Answer: Those taking multiple doses of insulin need to check the blood glucose levels three or more times daily. Once or twice daily is typical for those using oral medications.

- What is your usual fasting blood sugar in the morning?

    Answer: Glucose levels between 90 and 130 mg/dL premeal and below 180 mg/dL 2 hours postmeal (**postprandial**).

- What is your hemoglobin A1c? How often does your primary care provider check the A1c?

    Answer: About less than 7% and preferably less than 6.5%; A1c testing recommended twice/year in those with good glycemic control and quarterly in those with poor control.

- (If the patient reports poorly controlled diabetes) Are you experiencing frequent urination?

    Answer: Response of "yes" may indicate hyperglycemia and poor diabetes control and requires referral. The patient will not heal, and it is best to postpone treatment as healing will be suboptimal.

- Do you have frequent episodes of hypoglycemia (low blood sugar)? Can you tell when your blood sugar is getting low?

    Answer: Response of "yes" to the first question and "no" to the second identifies a patient at risk for a medical emergency. Hypoglycemic unawareness occurs as a result of neuropathy, and the patient is no longer able to identify when the blood sugar has dropped to dangerously low levels.

- (For those with a history of hypoglycemia, ask this question) What time of day does it usually happen and how do you treat it?

    Answer: If the appointment is during a critical time of day for hypoglycemia, precautions need to be taken to prevent and treat it or the appointment can be rescheduled. Mid-afternoon is typically when some types of insulin and oral medications reach their peak action and glucose from the midday meal reaches a low, resulting in a dangerous combination putting the patient at risk for hypoglycemia.

- Have you been hospitalized for hypoglycemia?

    Answer: Response of "yes" indicates extreme risk, and preparation needs to be made to rapidly treat hypoglycemia. Place a glucometer and glucose source near the treatment area for quick access.

- Are you having problems with your eyes, feet, hands, or legs? If so, what kind of problems are you experiencing?

    Answer: A patient experiencing complications may be poorly controlled, and a medical consult is advised.

Adapted from Boyd LD. Commentary on survey of diabetes knowledge and practices of dental hygienists. *Access.* 2008;22(8):40-43.

V. Continuing Care

- Appointment for supervision and examination on a regular 3- to 6-month basis as needed. Effectiveness of daily oral self-care is evaluated.
- Probe carefully to detect early bleeding on probing and evidence of pocket formation.
- Assess soft tissue with attention to areas of irritation related to fixed and removable prostheses.
- Identify any changes requiring consultation or referral to the patient's primary care provider, dietitian, mental health professional, or other specialist.
- Check for dental biofilm control and review control with the patient at each appointment. Gingival health is of major importance. Keep the patient motivated.

TABLE 54-6 • Comparison of Average Blood Glucose and A1$_c$

| A1$_c$ (%) | MEAN PLASMA GLUCOSE | |
	mg/dL	mmol/L
6	126	7.0
7	154	8.6
8	183	10.1
9	212	11.8
10	240	13.4
11	269	14.0

Source: Adapted from American Diabetes Association. 6. Glycemic targets: standards of medical care in diabetes—2018. *Diabetes Care.* 2018;41(suppl 1): S55-S64.

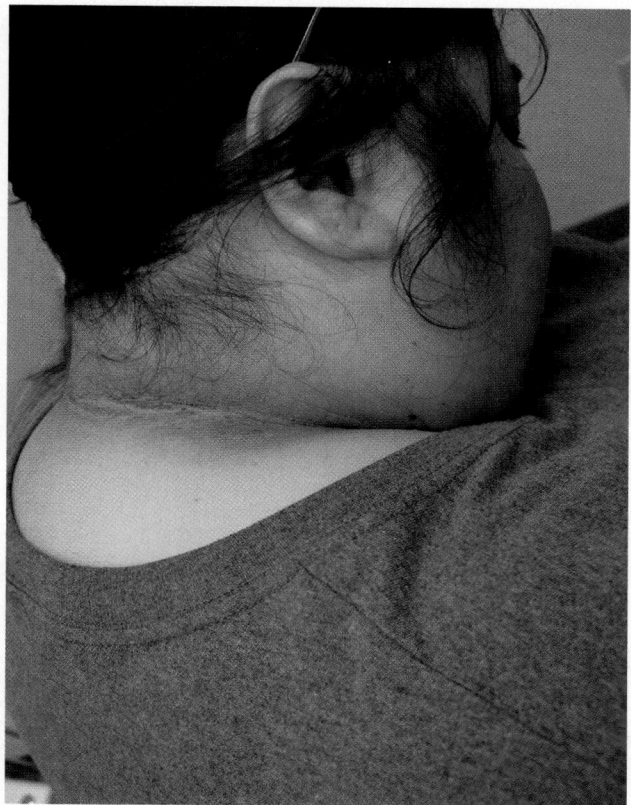

FIGURE 54-5 • Acanthosis Nigricans. This skin condition is seen in patients at risk for diabetes and typically appears on the creases in the neck as a light brown to black discoloration. (Reprinted from DeLong L, Burkhart N. *General and Oral Pathology for the Dental Hygienist.* Philadelphia, PA: Lippincott Williams & Wilkins; 2015.)

DOCUMENTATION

◆ Record status of blood glucose control, including most recent HbA1c and other daily monitoring such as fasting blood glucose levels the patient has performed.

◆ Update current medications and doses.

◆ Confirm compliance with medication intake and food consumption.

◆ Record discussion about relationship between oral health status, oral hygiene status, risk factors, and diabetes.

◆ Box 54-5 contains an example progress note for a patient with diabetes.

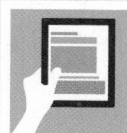

BOX 54-5

Example Documentation:
Patient with Diabetes Mellitus

S—A 66-year-old Hispanic female who presents for a periodontal maintenance. She reports bleeding when she flosses for the last couple of weeks. She was recently diagnosed with type 2 diabetes and is taking Metformin and Glipizide. Her initial HbA1c was 8.5, and she will have a follow-up test next month. She reports checking her blood glucose when she gets up in the morning and before dinner. Her fasting blood glucose this morning was 120. Patient reports taking her medications this morning.

O—Blood pressure: 131/79. Pulse: 88. Respirations: 24. Risk assessment for caries was moderate, periodontal disease was high, and oral cancer was moderate. Periodontal examination reveals localized bleeding on probing, and 1–2 mm pocket depth increases primarily in maxillary molar areas. Radiographic bone loss is 1–2 mm in maxillary posterior areas. Biofilm score: 30%. No new dental caries.

A—Localized periodontitis Stage 1, Grade 3 due to poorly controlled diabetes mellitus.

P—Discussed the association of periodontal infection with diabetes and need for meticulous oral self-care and regular professional periodontal maintenance appointments. Reviewed use of interdental brushes for molar areas where biofilm was located. The patient had difficulty removing biofilm on the lingual line angles of the molars, so careful wrapping of the floss was also reviewed. Complete periodontal debridement was performed. Applied 5% sodium fluoride varnish and provided a prescription for 0.12% chlorhexidine gluconate mouthrinse to use twice a day for 2 weeks to assist with healing.

Signed: _____, RDH

Date: _____

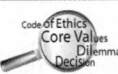

EVERYDAY ETHICS

Ed, a 45-year-old restaurant owner, presents for an appointment with Susan, the dental hygienist. She has treated this patient before, but he has not had an appointment for more than 2 years. The review of his medical history determines he is obese, complains of a dry mouth, has excessive thirst, gets up at night multiple times to urinate, and has not seen his primary care provider in several years. An intraoral examination reveals candidiasis on his hard palate. Susan suggests that he sees his physician, but he refuses to even talk about it. He insists that he just wants "clean teeth" for his daughter's upcoming wedding.

Questions for Consideration

1. Describe how each of the dental hygiene ethical core values apply to this scenario.

2. In what ways will Susan be violating the patient's rights if she agrees to Ed's request that she focus only on "cleaning" his teeth at this appointment? How may she be violating his rights if she refuses to clean his teeth unless he first has an examination with his primary care provider?

3. Explain choices or alternative actions Susan can consider as she decides how to continue treatment during Ed's appointment.

Factors to Teach the Patient

Factors to Teach Patients with Diabetes

▶ Importance of regular medical and dental care; eye examinations; blood pressure checks; blood tests for cholesterol, lipids, and kidney readings; and practicing self-examination, particularly of feet, for nerve involvement or delayed healing visits to prevent complications.

▶ Connection between oral health and diabetes and need for meticulous oral self-care.

▶ The patient's role in self-management of diabetes with an emphasis on the need to be compliant with lifestyle modifications including healthy eating, physical activity, weight management, glucose monitoring, tobacco cessation, good oral self-care, limiting or avoiding alcohol, stress management, and use of prescribed medications.

▶ The value of seeking immediate medical attention for any signs of complications from diabetes.

Factors to Teach Patients at Risk for Diabetes

▶ Need for regular medical examinations and screening for diabetes.

▶ How to recognize the early warning signs of diabetes and seek medical consult.

▶ Factors that affect a healthy lifestyle, including healthy diet, daily exercise, no tobacco products, avoiding alcohol, and maintaining ideal weight.

▶ How to practice meticulous oral hygiene to prevent dental caries and periodontal disease.

▶ Stress reduction techniques.

ENHANCE YOUR UNDERSTANDING

ONLINE RESOURCES
(see the inside front cover for access information)

· Audio glossary
· Appendices

SUPPORT FOR LEARNING
(available separately)

· *Active Learning Workbook for Wilkins' Clinical Practice of the Dental Hygienist, 13th Edition*

INDIVIDUALIZED REVIEW

· Customized practice quizzing with Navigate 2 TestPrep for *Wilkins' Clinical Practice of the Dental Hygienist*

References

1. American Diabetes Association. Classification and diagnosis of diabetes mellitus: standards of medical care in diabetes—2018. *Diabetes Care.* 2018;41(suppl 1):S13-S27.

2. Centers for Disease Control and Prevention. *National Diabetes Statistics Report, 2017.* Atlanta, GA: Centers for Disease Control and Prevention, U.S. Department of Health and Human Services; 2017. https://www.cdc.gov/diabetes/data/statistics/statistics-report.html. Accessed November 18, 2018.

3. Ogurtsova K, da Rocha Fernandes JD, Huang Y, et al. IDF Diabetes Atlas: global estimates for the prevalence of diabetes for 2015 and 2040. *Diabetes Res Clin Pract.* 2017;128:40-50.

4. Sanz M, Ceriello A, Buysschaert M, et al. Scientific evidence on the links between periodontal diseases and diabetes: consensus report and guidelines of the joint workshop on periodontal diseases and diabetes by the International diabetes Federation and the European Federation of Periodontology. *Diabetes Res Clin Pract.* 2018;137:231-241.

5. Botero JE, Rodríguez C, Agudelo-Suarez AA. Periodontal treatment and glycaemic control in patients with diabetes and periodontitis: an umbrella review. *Aust Dent J.* 2016;61(2):134-148.

6. Engebretson S, Kocher T. Evidence that periodontal treatment improves diabetes outcomes: a systematic review and meta-analysis. *J Clin Periodontol.* 2013; 40(suppl 14):S153-S163.

7. D'Aiuto F, Gable D, Syed Z, et al. Evidence summary: the relationship between oral diseases and diabetes. *Br Dent J.* 2017;222(12):944-948.

8. Segura-Egea JJ, Martín-González J, Cabanillas-Balsera D, Fouad AF, Velasco-Ortega E, López-López J. Association between diabetes and the prevalence of radiolucent periapical lesions in root-filled teeth: systematic review and meta-analysis. *Clin Oral Investig.* 2016; 20(6):1133-1141.

9. Moraschini V, Barboza ES, Peixoto GA. The impact of diabetes on dental implant failure: a systematic review and meta-analysis. *Int J Oral Maxillofac Surg.* 2016;45(10):1237-1245.

10. Newsholme P, Cruzat V, Arfuso F, et al. Nutrient regulation of insulin secretion and action. *J Endocrinol.* 2014;221(3):R105-R120.

11. American Diabetes Association. 6. Glycemic targets: standards of medical care in diabetes—2018. *Diabetes Care.* 2018;41(suppl 1):S55-S64.

12. Diabetes Prevention Program (DPP) Research Group. The Diabetes Prevention Program (DPP): description of lifestyle intervention. *Diabetes Care.* 2002;25(12):2165-2171.

13. Pulgaron ER, Delamater AM. Obesity and type 2 diabetes in children: epidemiology and treatment. *Curr Diab Rep.* 2014;14(8):508.

14. DeSisto CL, Kim SY, Sharma AJ. Prevalence estimates of gestational diabetes mellitus in the United States, pregnancy risk assessment monitoring system (PRAMS), 2007–2010. *Prev Chronic Dis.* 2014;11:E104.

15. Linnenkamp U. IDF diabetes atlas reveals high burden of hyperglycaemia in pregnancy. *Diabetes Voice.* 2014; 59:55-56.

16. Glurich I, Bartkowiak B, Berg RL, Acharya A. Screening for dysglycaemia in dental primary care practice settings: systematic review of the evidence. *Int Dent J.* 2018; 68(6):369-377.

17. Strauss SM, Russell S, Wheeler A, et al. The dental office visit as a potential opportunity for diabetes screening: an analysis using NHANES 2003–2004 data. *J Public Health Dent.* 2010;70(2):156-162.

18. American Diabetes Association. Type 2 diabetes risk test. http://www.diabetes.org/are-you-at-risk/diabetes-risk-test/. Accessed November 23, 2018.

19. Strauss SM, Tuthill J, Singh G, et al. A novel intraoral diabetes screening approach in periodontal patients: results of a pilot study. *J Periodontol.* 2012;83(6):699-706.

20. American Diabetes Association. 5. Prevention or delay of type 2 diabetes: standards of medical care in diabetes—2018. *Diabetes Care.* 2018; 41(suppl 1):S51-S54.

21. The Diabetes Prevention Program Research Group. The 10-year cost-effectiveness of lifestyle intervention or metformin for diabetes prevention: an intent-to-treat analysis of the DPP/DPPOS. *Diabetes Care.* 2012;35(4):723-730.

22. Beck J, Greenwood DA, Blanton L, et al. 2017 national standards for diabetes self-management education and support. *Diabetes Educ.* 2018;44(1):35-50.

23. Maher CA, Lewis LK, Ferrar K, Marshall S, De Bourdeaudhuij I, Vandelanotte C. Are health behavior change interventions that use online social networks effective? A systematic review. *J Med Internet Res.* 2014;16(2):e40. doi:10.2196/jmir.2952.

24. Fu H, McMahon SK, Gross CR, Adam TJ, Wyman JF. Usability and clinical efficacy of diabetes mobile applications for adults with type 2 diabetes: a systematic review. *Diabetes Res Clin Pract.* 2017;131:70-81.

25. American Diabetes Association. 4. Lifestyle management: standards of medical care in diabetes—2018. *Diabetes Care.* 2018;41(suppl 1):S38-S50.

26. American Diabetes Association. 8. Pharmacologic approaches to glycemic treatment: standards of medical care in diabetes—2018. *Diabetes Care.* 2018;41(suppl 1):S73-S85.

27. Mohanty RR, Das S. Inhaled insulin—current direction of insulin research. *J Clin Diagn Res.* 2017;11(4):OE01-OE02.

28. Nathan DM; DCCT/EDIC Research Group. The diabetes control and complications trial/epidemiology of diabetes interventions and complications study at 30 years: overview. *Diabetes Care.* 2014;37(1):9-16.

29. American Diabetes Association. 3. Comprehensive medical evaluation and assessment of comorbidities: standards of medical care in diabetes—2018. *Diabetes Care.* 2018;41(suppl 1):S28-S37.

30. Baltzis D, Eleftheriadou I, Veves A. Pathogenesis and treatment of impaired wound healing in diabetes mellitus: new insights. *Adv Ther.* 2014;31(8):817-836.

31. American Diabetes Association. 10. Microvascular complications and foot care: standards of medical care in diabetes—2018. *Diabetes Care.* 2018;41(suppl 1):S105-S118.

32. American Diabetes Association. 9. Cardiovascular disease and risk management: standards of medical care in diabetes—2018. *Diabetes Care.* 2018;41(suppl 1):S86-S104.

33. American Diabetes Association. 13. Management of diabetes in pregnancy: standards of medical care in diabetes—2018. *Diabetes Care.* 2018;41(suppl 1):S137-S143.

34. American Dental Association. Oral health topics: diabetes key points. https://www.ada.org/en/member-center/oral-health-topics/diabetes. Updated June 6, 2018. Accessed November 25, 2018.

35. Bustan RS, Wasim D, Yderstraede KB, Bygum A. Specific skin signs as a cutaneous marker of diabetes mellitus and the prediabetic state—a systematic review. *Dan Med J.* 2017;64(1):pii: A5316.

55

The Patient with Cancer

Dianna S. Weikel, RDH, MS, and Deborah S. Manne, RDH, RN, MSN, OCN

CHAPTER OUTLINE

DESCRIPTION
- I. Incidence and Survival
- II. Risk Factors
- III. Types of Cancer
- IV. How Cancer Is Treated

SURGERY
- I. Indications for Surgery

CHEMOTHERAPY
- I. Objectives
- II. Indications
- III. Types of Chemotherapy
- IV. Systemic Side Effects of Chemotherapy
- V. Oral Complications of Chemotherapy

RADIATION THERAPY
- I. Indications
- II. Types
- III. Doses
- IV. Systemic Effects
- V. Oral Complications

HEMATOPOIETIC STEM CELL TRANSPLANTATION
- I. Types
- II. Stages of Transplantation Process
- III. Acute Complications
- IV. Chronic Complications

MUCOSITIS MANAGEMENT
- I. Prevention/Oral Health Maintenance
- II. Treatment of Established Mucositis

DENTAL HYGIENE CARE PLAN
- I. Objectives
- II. Personal Factors
- III. Oral Care Protocol

DOCUMENTATION

EVERYDAY ETHICS

FACTORS TO TEACH THE PATIENT

FACTORS TO TEACH THE CAREGIVER

REFERENCES

LEARNING OBJECTIVES

After studying this chapter, the student will be able to:

1. Identify healthcare professionals involved in the multi-disciplinary oncology team.

2. Explain several systemic medical treatment options utilized in cancer management.

3. Describe common oral complications secondary to cancer treatment.

4. Provide examples of evidence-based dental hygiene care strategies for mucositis management.

Dental hygiene care of the patient with cancer before, during, and after therapy strives to not only attain but also maintain a patient's oral health at the highest possible level. This contributes to the patient's general health and overall quality of life.

◆ Cancer treatment modalities (radiation therapy, chemotherapy, surgery, and hematopoietic cell transplantation) have the potential to affect the oral cavity significantly.

◆ The patient will be under the care of a team of multidisciplinary specialists. Box 55-1 lists the members of the multidisciplinary team.

DESCRIPTION

◆ Cancer refers to:
- A group of neoplastic diseases in which there is transformation of normal cells into malignant ones.

BOX 55-1
Multidisciplinary Team for the Care of the Patient with Cancer

Cancer Specialists
- Medical oncologist: provides cancer management utilizing chemotherapeutic modalities.
- Radiation oncologist: responsible for the planning, delivery, and follow-up of radiation therapy.
- Surgeon (all subspecialties): biopsy and/or excision of cancer.
- Oncology nurse: provides clinical support in the medical, surgical, and/or radiation management of the cancer patient.
- Oncology dietitian: provides symptom management.
- Oncology social worker: provides psychosocial support and is often a liaison between clinical staff and patient/family.
- Oral care specialists: play a role in initial diagnosis and management of oral complications during cancer therapy.
- Dental hygienist.
- Dentist.
- Oral maxillofacial surgeon.
- Periodontist.
- Endodontist.
- Oral maxillofacial prosthodontist.
- Oral pathologist.

Other Health Specialists
- Speech pathologist.
- Physical therapist.
- Occupational therapist.
- Psychologist/psychiatrist.

- As cancer cells proliferate, the mass of abnormal tissue formed enlarges until it takes over the host site. It then sheds cells that spread to distant sites (metastasis).

◆ The characteristics of benign and malignant neoplasms are compared in Table 55-1.

◆ Cancers are classified on the basis of the following:
- Origin of the tissue involved: carcinomas from epithelial tissue and sarcomas from connective tissue.
- Type of cell from which they arise, namely, an epithelial or connective tissue cell.[1]

◆ Staging is:
- A succinct, standardized description of a tumor based on origin and extent.
- Made up of three components: T (tumor size), N (presence or absence of lymph nodes), and M (presence or absence of distant metastases).

◆ Common signs and symptoms of cancer are listed in Box 55-2.

I. Incidence and Survival

Cancer is the second leading cause of death in the United States for adults under the age of 85 years.[2] Survival depends on the following:

◆ Type of cancer.

◆ Location and size of the tumor.

◆ Presence of distant metastases.

◆ Tumor sensitivity to treatment.

◆ Physical condition: comorbidities and age.

II. Risk Factors

Numerous factors increase a person's risk for developing cancer, including the following[3]:

◆ *Tobacco*: both cigarette smoking and use of smokeless tobacco products are implicated in head and neck cancer, lung cancer, and bladder cancer.

◆ *Alcohol*: chronic, long-term use especially in combination with tobacco use implicated in head and neck cancer, bladder cancer, and liver cancer.

◆ *Sunlight*: especially occupations requiring work under the sun such as construction workers, farmers, as well as sunbathers.

◆ *Environmental/occupational*: exposure to asbestos, radon, coal dust, and chemicals, to name a few.

◆ *Viruses*:
- Epstein–Barr virus implicated in Burkett's lymphoma.
- Hepatitis C implicated in liver cancer.
- Human papillomavirus (16 and 18) implicated in cervical cancer and cancer of the oropharynx (tonsil and base of tongue).

◆ *Socioeconomic*: late diagnosis with poorer prognosis seen in lower socioeconomic populations (inner city, rural, and working poor).

TABLE 55-1 • Characteristics of Benign and Malignant Neoplasms

CHARACTERISTIC	BENIGN	MALIGNANT
Cell characteristics	Well-differentiated cells of the tissue from which the tumor originated	Cells are undifferentiated. **Anaplastic** features (lack of differentiation)
Mode of growth	Tumor grows by expansion and does not infiltrate the surrounding tissues; encapsulated	Tumor grows at the periphery and sends out processes that infiltrate and destroy the surrounding tissues
Rate of growth	Rate of growth is usually slow	Rate of growth is usually relatively rapid and is dependent on the level of differentiation; the more anaplastic the tumor, the more rapid the rate of growth
Metastasis	Does not spread by metastasis	Gains access to the blood and lymph systems to metastasize to other organs
Destruction of tissue	Does not usually cause tissue damage unless location interferes with blood flow	Often causes extensive tissue damage as the tumor outgrows its blood supply or encroaches on blood flow to the area; may also produce substances that cause cell damage

Source: Adapted from Grossman SC, Porth CM. *Pathophysiology: Concepts of Altered Health States.* 9th ed. Philadelphia, PA: Lippincott, William & Wilkins; 2014.

III. Types of Cancer

The most common types of cancer are as follows[2]:
- Men:
  - Prostate.
  - Lung and bronchus.
  - Colon and rectum.
- Women:
  - Breast.
  - Lung and bronchus.
  - Colon and rectum.

IV. How Cancer Is Treated

Cancer is treated using a variety of different approaches based on the following[3,4]:
- The location and size of the tumor.
- Treatment objectives (cure, control, or palliation).
- The different approaches including:

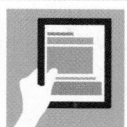

BOX 55-2
Common Signs and Symptoms of Cancer

C: A change in bowel or bladder habits (colon)

A: A sore that doesn't heal on skin or inside mouth (skin or oral)

U: Unusual bleeding or discharge (uterine, lung, and colon)

T: Thickening or lump in breast tissue or anywhere on the body (breast and testicle)

I: Indigestion/difficulty swallowing

O: Obvious change in wart or mole (skin)

N: Nagging cough or hoarseness (lung or throat)

Source: American Cancer Society. Signs and symptoms of cancer. http://www.cancer.org/cancer/cancerbasics/signs-and-symptoms-of-cancer. Accessed February 20, 2018.

- Surgery.
- Chemotherapy.
- Radiation therapy.
- Hematopoietic cell transplantation.
- Hormone therapy.
- Vaccine therapy.
- Biotherapy.
- Targeted therapies.
- A combination of two or more of the above.

SURGERY

Surgery is the most common form of treatment for solid tumors, both malignant and nonmalignant.

I. Indications for Surgery

- Tumors that are small in size, localized, and easy to remove.[5]
- Debulk or remove portions of large tumors before treatment (chemotherapy or radiation therapy).[5]
- Provide pain relief or prolong life when no chance of cure is possible (palliative/palliation).[5]

CHEMOTHERAPY

Chemotherapy involves the use of drugs that affect the rapidly dividing cancer cells at different points in the cell cycle. The drugs are used as a single agent or in combination. Side effects can be severe and frequently involve the oral cavity.

I. Objectives

- To destroy cancer cells and keep them from metastasizing.
- To prevent cancer from recurring.
- To provide an improved quality of life.

II. Indications

- Eliminate a localized tumor too large for surgical removal.
- Treat cancer that has metastasized to other parts of the body.
- Prevent cancer recurrence with maintenance therapy.
- Use before surgery to make a tumor easier to remove completely.
- Palliative.
- Treatment of "liquid tumors" such as leukemia.

III. Types of Chemotherapy

Box 55-3 lists the types of agents used for chemotherapy.

IV. Systemic Side Effects of Chemotherapy

Chemotherapy affects both rapidly dividing cancer cells and rapidly dividing normal cells (hair, oral/gastrointestinal mucosa, and bone marrow). Halting cell division of normal cells may cause side effects that range from mild to life threatening. The most common include the following:

- Alopecia (hair loss).
- Myelosuppression (bone marrow suppression causing a reduction in blood counts leading to anemia, leukopenia, and thrombocytopenia).
- Immunosuppression (inhibition of antibody responses resulting from leukopenia).
- Nausea, vomiting, and diarrhea.
- Loss of appetite.
- Gastrointestinal mucositis.

V. Oral Complications of Chemotherapy

The following are oral complications resulting from chemotherapy[4,6]:
- *Oral mucositis/stomatitis*: an inflammation of the oral mucosa characterized by erythema, ulceration, and pain.

BOX 55-3
Types of Agents Used for Chemotherapy

Alkylating agents

Antibiotics

Antimetabolites

Plant alkaloids

Steroids/hormones

Proteasome inhibitors, mammalian target of rapamycin inhibitors

Targeted therapies

- *Xerostomia*: subjective report of oral dryness.
- *Salivary gland hypofunction*: objective reduction in saliva production.
- *Infections*:
  - Bacterial.
  - *Viral*: herpes simplex, varicella zoster, and cytomegalovirus.
  - *Fungal*: *Candida albicans*.
- *Bleeding*: anywhere in the mouth; spontaneous or induced.
- *Neurotoxicity*: mimics toothache; usually bilateral.
- *Osteonecrosis of the jaw* exposed bone of at least 8 weeks duration in either the maxilla or mandible secondary to use of systemic bisphosphonates and/or other antiresorptive medication/therapies.[7]
- Also referenced as *medication-related osteonecrosis of the jaw* and *antiresorptive drug-related osteonecrosis of the jaw*.

RADIATION THERAPY

Radiation therapy uses ionizing radiation to treat cancer.
- Radiation impacts the cancer cell's ability to replicate and survive.
- Not all tumors are radiosensitive (ability of the radiation therapy to kill the tumor).
- Head and neck radiation therapy produces acute short-term and chronic long-term effects in the oral cavity.

I. Indications

- Treat a small localized tumor that is radiosensitive.
- Shrink a large tumor before surgery.
- Increase the effectiveness of chemotherapy when used concurrently.
- Prevent the spread of cancer or control residual tumor.
- Prevent a recurrence of the cancer.
- Provide symptom/pain relief for bone metastases or palliative therapy.

II. Types

A. External Beam

Conventional use of ionizing radiation applied outside the body.
- Intensity-modulated radiation therapy (IMRT)
  - Developed in the late 1990s.
  - Considered a high-precision delivery of radiation.
  - Accomplished via computer-guided images of target anatomy with radiation produced by a linear accelerator.
  - Used in treatment of head and neck cancer.
  - Radiation dose is elevated at the site of the gross tumor while simultaneously sparing the surrounding normal tissue.

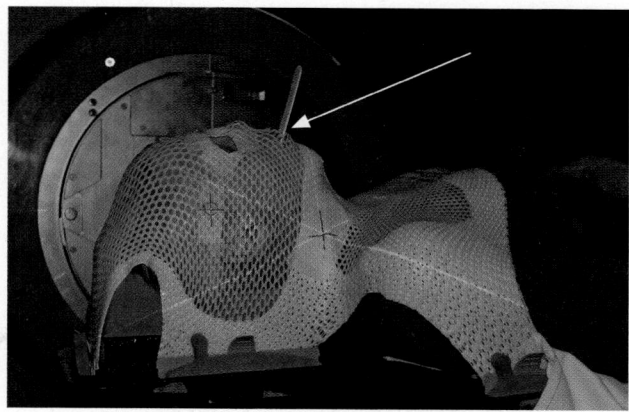

FIGURE 55-1 • Custom Patient Mask. This is worn by the patient at each radiation appointment. The mask, made out of firm mesh, snaps into the treatment table to assist immobilizing the patient for precise radiation delivery throughout the course of radiation therapy. A bite block is placed intraorally (arrow) to maintain the mouth in a static position. The linear accelerator (source of radiation) is seen in the background. (Used with permission from Dianna S. Wiekel.)

- Results in decreased side effects, better tumor targeting as compared to conventional external beam radiation.
- Figure 55-1 illustrates the patient preparation prior to IMRT.
- Proton therapy.[8]
- New method of radiation delivery, used in some head and neck cancer patients.
- Technique is considered more precise than IMRT with less damage to the surrounding oral structures, thus producing less acute and chronic oral complications.
- Not widely available, more expensive to deliver care.
- Presently lack of clinical trials comparing to photon (IMRT) delivery method.

B. Internal Source

- Radiation source (such as radium implants or seeds) is placed within the body.
- Less radiation is delivered to the surrounding tissues than when an external source is utilized.

III. Doses

- Total dose given depends on the type of tumor, treatment goals, and patient's ability to tolerate treatment.
- Total radiation dose is approximately 30–70 Gy.
- It is divided into equal doses (conventional) or modulated fractions (IMRT) per day.
- It is given once a day, 5 days a week, for 5–8 weeks.

IV. Systemic Effects

- *Skin reactions*: looks like a bad sunburn.
- Fatigue.
- Nausea, vomiting, diarrhea, and constipation.

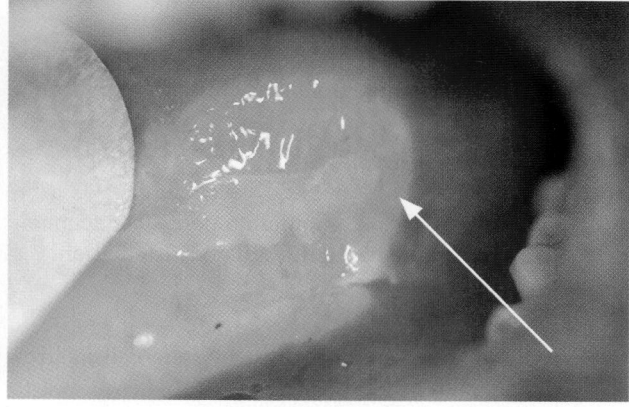

FIGURE 55-2 • Mucositis Left Lateral Border of Tongue, Secondary to Radiation to the Head and Neck Tissue. Note erythema distal to the ulcerated area (arrow). This lesion is characterized by pain, complicating the patient's ability to eat, speak, or swallow. (Used with permission from Dianna S. Wiekel.)

V. Oral Complications

- Oral mucositis[6] (see Figure 55-2).
- Xerostomia/salivary gland hypofunction.[4,6,8]
- Radiation caries.[6]
- Dysgeusia.[4]
- Infection[6]:
  - Bacterial.
  - *Viral*: herpes simplex and varicella zoster.
  - Fungal: *C. albicans*.
- Trismus.[6,8]
- Osteoradionecrosis.[6]

HEMATOPOIETIC STEM CELL TRANSPLANTATION

Hematopoietic stem cell transplantation is used to treat cancers involving the bone marrow, including leukemia. The purpose is to substitute peripheral blood stem cells from the patient or a healthy, compatible donor.[9,10]

I. Types

- Autologous: self.
- Allogeneic: human leukocyte antigen–matched donor, either related or unrelated.
- Syngeneic: identical twin.

II. Stages of Transplantation Process

A. Patient Selection

- *Indications*: patient not responsive to chemotherapy alone; relapse occurs after one or more remissions.
- *Evaluation*: medical and dental assessments completed to ensure the patient is free of infection and physically able to undergo the preparative regimen.

B. Donor Regimen

◆ Histocompatibility matching.

◆ Bone marrow aspirated from iliac crest, ribs, or sternum.

C. Conditioning of Patient to Receive Bone Marrow Graft

◆ Preparative high-dose immunosuppressive regimen: chemotherapy alone or with total body irradiation.

◆ Purposes:
  • Kill malignant cells.
  • Suppress immune system so new stem cells/marrow will engraft.

D. Transplantation

◆ Intravenous infusion of donor's marrow/stem cells.

E. Pancytopenia

◆ Pancytopenia is a reduction in all cellular elements of the blood, which includes white blood cells, red blood cells, and platelets.

◆ Protective isolation for the patient is required; the patient is highly susceptible to infection.

◆ Function of new marrow (to produce peripheral blood elements) begins after 10–20 days.

F. Recovery

◆ Immune recovery: 3–12 months; long-term recovery: 1–3 years.

III. Acute Complications

◆ Acute graft-versus-host disease (GVHD):[6,11]
  • Description: The donor's T-lymphocytes see the host cell antigens as foreign and react against the host tissue.
◆ Symptoms:
  • Present during the first 100 days posttransplant.
  • Painful red skin rash starting on the palms of hands and soles of feet and progressing to the upper trunk.
  • Severe, persistent diarrhea.
  • Jaundice, elevated liver enzymes, liver tenderness.
◆ Infection:
  • Bacterial.
  • *Viral:* herpes simplex, varicella zoster, and cytomegalovirus.
  • *Fungal: C. albicans.*
◆ Gastrointestinal, hepatic, cardiac, pulmonary, hematologic, and neurologic complications.
◆ Oral complications:
  • Oral mucositis: appears 10–14 days posttransplant.
  • Xerostomia.
  • Viral and fungal infections: herpes simplex virus and *C. albicans.*

IV. Chronic Complications

◆ Chronic GVHD[11]:
  • May affect all organs of the body.
  • Can appear up to 2 years posttransplant.
◆ Oral complications:
  • Oral mucositis.
  • Oral infection/periodontal infection.
  • Xerostomia/dental caries.
  • Poor oral hygiene.
  • Difficulty eating/chewing.

MUCOSITIS MANAGEMENT

I. Prevention/Oral Health Maintenance[12–14]

◆ Basic oral care using a soft toothbrush.

◆ As dental flossing is technique sensitive, use may be precluded during cytotoxic treatment.

◆ Use of a bland mouthrinse such as normal saline, three to four times/day.

◆ Cryotherapy (ice chips):
  • Recommended for selected patient populations such as multiple myeloma patients receiving high-dose Melphalan and head and neck cancer patients receiving bolus dosing of 5-fluorouracil.
  • Instruct patient to hold ice chips in mouth immediately prior to and during the administration of chemotherapy agent.
◆ Palifermin (a human recombinant keratinocyte growth factor):
  • Intravenous infusion in selected populations prior to peripheral blood stem cell transplant.
  • Given for three consecutive days before and after myelotoxic therapy for a total of six doses.
◆ Benzydamine mouthrinse (nonsteroidal anti-inflammatory agent) in patients receiving moderate dose radiation therapy (up to 50 Gy). Note: This drug is not available in the United States.

II. Treatment of Established Mucositis[15,16]

◆ Mouthrinse containing diphenhydramine hydrochloric acid in combination with other agents (usually coating agent and topical anesthetic).
  • Evidence does not support a direct effect of this antihistamine on the prevention or treatment of mucositis lesions.
  • This type of rinse is often used to palliate pain topically.
◆ *Systemic pain medication:* Patient-controlled analgesia with morphine for the management of pain due to oral mucositis in patients undergoing hematopoietic stem cell transplant.

◆ Transdermal fentanyl patch may be effective in the management of mucositis pain due to conventional and high-dose chemotherapy with or without total body irradiation.

◆ Morphine mouthrinse may reduce the severity and duration of mucositis pain in patients undergoing head and neck area radiation therapy.

◆ Doxepin mouthrinse (0.5%) may be effective for the management of pain due to oral mucositis.

DENTAL HYGIENE CARE PLAN

I. Objectives

◆ It is recommended patients be in optimal oral health before starting any type of cancer therapy. Overall objectives include the following[6]:

◆ Assess the oral cavity for any signs of hard or soft tissue infection.

◆ Eliminate or minimize sources of dental/periodontal or soft tissue infection.

◆ Eliminate or minimize any areas of chronic trauma or tissue irritation.

◆ Provide preventive oral care education to the patient and/or the caregiver.

II. Personal Factors

The very word *cancer* brings fear and anxiety to the patient, and many times it is viewed by the patient as *cancer equals death*. This will impact anything taught to the patient. Suggestions include the following:

◆ Encourage the patient to bring a friend or a family member along to take notes during teaching visits.

◆ Provide written instructions appropriate to the reading level of the patient. Make sure they are written in the patient's native language.

◆ Provide positive reinforcement and be creative in helping the patient maintain optimal oral health.

◆ Show acceptance and empathy. Acknowledge the appropriateness of the patient's concerns.

◆ Practice active listening skills.

III. Oral Care Protocol

The following sections are adapted from the *Oral Complications of Cancer Treatment: What the Oral Health Team Can Do* from the National Institute of Dental and Craniofacial Research (National Institutes of Health publication no. 09-4372).

◆ Similarities exist between the three forms of treatment (radiation therapy, chemotherapy, and hematopoietic stem cell transplantation).

◆ There are differences that dental hygienists need to know to provide appropriate oral care.

TABLE 55-2 • World Health Organization's Oral Mucositis Scale

GRADE	CLINICAL FEATURES
0	No oral mucositis
1	Soreness, erythema
2	Oral ulcers, solid foods tolerated
3	Oral ulcers, liquid diet only (due to mucositis)
4	Oral ulcers, alimentation impossible (due to mucositis)

Source: Lalla R, Sonis S, Peterson D. Management of oral mucositis in patients with cancer. *Dent Clin North Am.* 2008;52(1):61-68.

◆ Numerous grading scales have been developed to assess the severity of oral mucositis, but none for the other oral complications.

◆ Table 55-2 lists an example of one mucositis scale. Scales are useful to:
  • Measure mucositis in the nursing/medical setting.
  • Document treatment toxicity in the clinical and/or research setting.
  • Communicate intraprofessionally.

A. Pretreatment Therapy

◆ Patients who do intensive personal oral care in preparation for and during their cancer therapy have a reduced risk for the development of oral complications.

◆ Box 55-4 provides examples of dental hygiene/dental treatment options that may be beneficial before the start of cancer therapy.

B. Head and Neck Radiation Therapy[17–19]

◆ Patients receiving radiation therapy to the head and neck are at high risk for developing severe oral complications that will affect the patient in the short and long term.

◆ Box 55-5 lists an example oral care protocol to be followed during treatment.

◆ *During radiation therapy:*
  • Encourage daily oral care including biofilm removal at least twice daily.
  • Encourage daily fluoride use (in any form, i.e., tray, brush-on, rinse).
  • Monitor the patient for trismus; check for pain or weakness in masticating muscles in the radiation field.
  • Instruct the patient to exercise three times a day, opening and closing the mouth as far as possible without pain; repeat 20 times.

◆ *After radiation therapy:*
  • For the first 6 months after cancer treatment, recall the patient every 4–8 weeks as needed for nonsurgical periodontal therapy.
  • Review instructions for daily oral self-care.

BOX 55-4
Dental Hygiene/Dental Pretreatment Guidelines for Patients Planning to Undergo Cancer Therapy

Dental

- Conduct a pretreatment oral health examination.
- Schedule dental treatment in consultation with the oncologist (medical or radiation).
- Extract teeth with a poor or questionable prognosis at least 2 weeks before the start of cancer therapy.
- Restore or repair indicated teeth before the start of cancer therapy.
- Perform other necessary oral surgery procedures at least 2 weeks before the start of cancer therapy.

Dental Hygiene

- Conduct a pretreatment oral health assessment.
- Schedule dental hygiene treatment in consultation with the oncologist (medical or radiation).
- Perform dental hygiene treatment (periodontal scaling and root planing, polishing, and fluoride applications) before the start of cancer treatment.
- Evaluate the patient's oral health knowledge and provide an appropriate oral hygiene regimen based on the cancer management.
- Prevent tooth demineralization and dental caries:
  - Instruct the patient in the daily application of fluoride gel at home.
  - If receiving head and neck radiation therapy, fabricate custom gel-applicator trays for the patient.
  - Demonstrate application of a 1.1% neutral pH sodium fluoride gel or a 0.4% stannous, unflavored gel for use in the trays or brush-on when tray insertion may not be tolerated.
  - Use only a neutral pH sodium fluoride gel for porcelain crowns or glass or resin ionomer restorations.
  - The trays cover all tooth surfaces and are left in the mouth for 5 minutes. Instruct the patient to have nothing to eat or drink for 30 minutes after using the fluoride. Specific technique is located in Chapter 34.

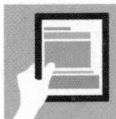

BOX 55-5
Oral Care Protocol during Treatment

Daily Biofilm Removal

- Gently brush teeth with a soft toothbrush and fluoride toothpaste after every meal and at bedtime. The tongue may be brushed with a soft toothbrush and water.
- Use interdental aids gently, but thoroughly clean between teeth before brushing at least once a day.

Mouthrinsing

- Every 2–3 hours while awake, rinse the mouth with a baking soda, salt, and water solution, followed by a plain water rinse. (Use one-fourth teaspoon baking soda and one-eighth teaspoon salt in a cup of lukewarm water.)
- Use of fluoridated water when available.

Xerostomia

- Sip water frequently.
- Suck on ice chips or use sugar-free gum or candy.
- Use saliva substitute spray or gel or a prescribed saliva stimulant.
- Avoid lemon glycerin swabs.
- Avoid hot, spicy, salty, sharp, or high-sucrose foods.
- Moisten foods with gravy or liquids before eating.

Dental Caries Prevention

- Use fluoride toothpaste every day.
- If prescribed, brush teeth with 1.1% neutral sodium fluoride gel for 60 seconds after usual tooth cleaning, just before going to bed. Do not eat, drink, or rinse for a minimum of 30 minutes afterward.
- If using custom-made polyvinyl trays, place gel in trays, apply to teeth, close mouth, and hold in place for 4 minutes. Set timer. Remove trays, expectorate several times, and do not eat or drink for at least 30 minutes afterward.

Oral Pain Management

- Swish and spit a prescribed mouthrinse containing topical anesthetic solution 30 minutes before eating.

- Reinforce the importance of daily oral self-care.
- After mucositis subsides, consult with the radiation/medical oncologist regarding timing of denture/appliance fabrication.
- Observe for trismus, demineralization, and caries.
- Lifelong, daily applications of prescription fluoride (in any form) are recommended for patients with chronic salivary gland hypofunction.
- Advise against oral surgery on irradiated bone, because of the risk of osteoradionecrosis.
- Tooth extraction, if unavoidable, is conservative.
- Prophylaxis against possible osteoradionecrosis is accomplished with Pentoxifylline 400 mg pre- and postextraction.

C. Chemotherapy

- ◆ The extent of oral complications of chemotherapy depends on the following[6,20,21]:
  - The degree of preexistent dental and oral disease.
  - The chemotherapy drugs used and their dosages.
  - The use of concurrent or adjuvant radiation therapy to the head/neck.
  - The patient's personal daily oral hygiene.
- ◆ Before any dental or dental hygiene clinical procedures during chemotherapy:
  - Consult the medical oncologist before any dental or dental hygiene clinical procedures.
  - Ask the medical oncologist to order blood work 24 hours before oral surgery or other invasive procedures (such as periodontal scaling/root planing). Postpone when the platelet count is less than $50,000/mm^3$ or abnormal clotting factors are present and/or neutrophil count is less than $1,000/mm^3$.
  - In patients with fever of unknown origin as determined by the medical oncologist, check for oral source of viral, bacterial, or fungal infection.
  - Encourage thorough oral self-care.
  - Review indications for use of antibiotic premedication for patients with central venous catheters or peripherally inserted catheters (also known as central lines). There is no evidence suggesting this is beneficial and as such varies from practitioner to practitioner.
  - Consult the medical oncologist for preference on using the American Heart Association's prophylactic antibiotic regimen or another antibiotic regimen.
- ◆ Refer to Box 55-5 for a suggested oral care protocol during treatment.
- ◆ *After chemotherapy:* Place the patient on a dental hygiene continuing care schedule when chemotherapy is completed and all side effects, including immunosuppression, have resolved.

D. Hematopoietic Stem Cell Transplantation

Some hematopoietic stem cell transplant patients develop acute oral complications, especially patients who had an allogeneic stem cell transplant and develop GVHD.

- ◆ *After transplantation*[22,23]
  - Monitor for oral infections of the soft tissues. Herpes simplex and *C. albicans* are common oral infections.
  - Delay elective dental procedures (such as implants) for 1 year.
  - Follow patients for long-term oral complications (changes in taste, xerostomia, and dental caries). Such problems are strong indicators of chronic GVHD.
  - Continue to monitor the patient's oral health for biofilm control, tooth demineralization, dental caries, and oral infection.
  - Follow transplant patients carefully for second malignancies in the oral region.

E. Special Care for Children

Children receiving chemotherapy and/or radiation therapy are at risk for the same oral complications as adults. Other actions to consider in managing pediatric patients include the following[24,25]:

- ◆ Extract loose primary teeth and teeth expected to exfoliate during cancer treatment.
- ◆ Remove orthodontic bands and brackets if myelosuppressive chemotherapy is planned or if the appliances will be in the radiation field.
- ◆ Continually monitor craniofacial and dental structures for abnormal growth and development.
- ◆ Encourage routine daily personal oral care including biofilm removal and fluoride application.
- ◆ Avoid cariogenic foods and drinks. If these are necessary to improve a child's weight, then have the child rinse with fluoridated water after eating or drinking.

DOCUMENTATION

Each patient appointment is carefully documented to include at least the following:

- ◆ Cancer diagnosis, type of treatment, treatment start and completion dates.
- ◆ Oncologists' names and contact information; note any consults done with the oncologists.
- ◆ Oral assessment, clinical care provided, patient teaching on each visit.
- ◆ Any oral complications present, grade of oral mucositis indicating severity and type of symptom management prescribed.
- ◆ Planned follow-up visit and plan of care with proposed symptom management treatment outcomes.
- ◆ Box 55-6 shows an example of a documentation for a patient with oral lesions related to cancer therapy.

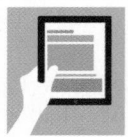

BOX 55-6

Example Documentation:
Patient with Oral Lesions Related to Cancer Treatment

S—The patient presents for 3-month periodontal maintenance appointment; medical history changes include diagnosis of stage IV floor of mouth (FOM) cancer; lesion found at previous periodontal maintenance visit and the patient evaluated by otolaryngology 3 months ago, surgery completed 10 weeks ago followed by 6 weeks of radiation therapy (total of 62 Gy) ending last week.

O—Complete oral examination performed; unable to perform periodontal maintenance due to severe oral ulcerations and inflammation involving the tongue bilaterally as well as the mandibular labial mucosa and vestibule; saliva appears thick and ropey; reviewed oral hygiene; the patient is not currently using fluoride.

A—Oral mucositis grade 4 and severe xerostomia following radiation to the oral cavity for squamous cell carcinoma of the FOM. Current health status precludes dental hygiene instrumentation today.

P—Recommend:

1. Discuss the above findings and today's recommendations with oncology team (primary oncologist and oncology nurse).

2. Use of extra soft toothbrush after meals and at bedtime.

3. Interproximal cleansing with appropriate aid.

4. Neutral sodium fluoride gel applied with brush 1× day following dental biofilm removal.

5. Baking soda mouthrinse—mix one-fourth teaspoon baking soda and one-eighth teaspoon salt in 8 oz of warm water; rinse with 20 mL 3× day.

6. Avoid mouthrinses containing alcohol.

Will follow 1× week until oral mucositis resolves; on next visit, assess xerostomia and make treatment recommendations as needed.

Signed: _____, RDH

Date: _____

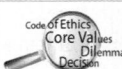

EVERYDAY ETHICS

It is the end of the day, and all of the patients, staff, and the dentist had left the office. Ashley, the dental hygienist, was reviewing the next day's patient records at the front desk.

The telephone rang, and Ashley answered it. It was Gina, the daughter of a longtime patient, Mr. Prisby. Gina, a pediatric registered nurse, lives out of state, but is visiting her 70-year-old father who is undergoing head and neck radiation therapy and chemotherapy treatments for tongue cancer. When she arrived, she was shocked to find her father having difficulty opening his mouth completely and a white coating on the inside of his cheeks. Gina also noticed multiple sores in his mouth. Her father has been unable to eat anything but the softest of foods due to the severe discomfort and dryness. Gina is concerned that her father cannot maintain a healthy weight during treatment. She asks Ashley what the white coating and the sores are in her father's mouth and what can be done for him.

Ashley puts Gina on hold and pulls Mr. Prisby's record. She sees that he had a complete examination and all treatment performed that left him in good dental health 3 months ago, just before he started his cancer treatment. The white coating that Ashley described may be candidiasis and require medication. But she is not sure how to treat the sores Gina sees. Ashley considers whether to refer Gina back to the oncologists treating her father or phoning in the prescription in the dentist's name to save time.

Questions for Consideration

1. What advice can Ashley give to Gina, considering the stipulations of patient confidentiality?

2. Describe the ethical and legal consequences of Ashley phoning in a prescription for Mr. Prisby.

3. What decisions and/or actions are appropriate for Ashley to pursue within the scope of her legal duties at this time?

Factors to Teach the Patient

- ▶ How to exercise the jaw muscles three times a day to prevent and treat jaw stiffness from head and neck radiation therapy.
- ▶ Why to avoid candy, gum, and soda unless they are sugar free.
- ▶ Why to avoid spicy or acidic foods and the use of toothpicks.
- ▶ Why to avoid the use of tobacco products and alcohol.
- ▶ Why the dental hygienist needs to conduct an oral soft tissue screening and complete oral examination at regular frequent intervals.
- ▶ How and when to use dental biofilm control methods, gel-tray application, use of saliva substitute, and all other details of personal oral care to reduce oral side effects caused by the disease and/or cancer treatment.
- ▶ Ideas for remembering to follow the instructions to keep the mouth healthier and more comfortable during cancer treatment.
- ▶ The reasons why a routine schedule of preventive periodontal scaling, fluoride application, and oral hygiene assessment by a dental hygienist contributes to the success of the cancer treatment.

Factors to Teach the Caregiver

- ▶ How maintaining optimal oral health throughout the treatment will contribute to the successful outcome of cancer therapy.
- ▶ The need to report any changes in the oral cavity to the oncologist and/or dentist/dental hygienist.
- ▶ Why it is necessary for the patient to receive preventive periodontal scaling, polishing if indicated, fluoride application, and oral hygiene assessment by a dental hygienist on a regular frequent basis.
- ▶ Why it is important to support the patient in stopping tobacco and alcohol use.

References

1. Hanahan D, Weinberg RA. Hallmarks of cancer. *Cell.* 2011;144(5):646-674.
2. Siegel R, Miller K, Jemal A. Cancer statistics, 2017. *CA Cancer J Clin.* 2017;67(1):7-30.
3. American Cancer Society. *CA Facts and Figures.* Atlanta, GA: American Cancer Society; 2018.
4. American Cancer Society. Find support and treatment. http://www.cancer.org/treatment/index. Accessed February 20, 2018.
5. Scarpa R. Surgical management of head and neck carcinoma. *Semin Oncol Nurs.* 2009;25(3):172-182.
6. National Institutes of Health Consensus. Development Conference on oral complications of cancer therapies: diagnosis,

ENHANCE YOUR UNDERSTANDING

ONLINE RESOURCES
(see the inside front cover for access information)
- Audio glossary
- Appendices

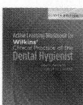

SUPPORT FOR LEARNING
(available separately)
- *Active Learning Workbook for Wilkins' Clinical Practice of the Dental Hygienist, 13th Edition*

INDIVIDUALIZED REVIEW
- Customized practice quizzing with Navigate 2 TestPrep for *Wilkins' Clinical Practice of the Dental Hygienist*

prevention, and treatment. Bethesda, Maryland, April 17-19, 1989. *NCI Monogr.* 1990;9:1-184.

7. Ruggiero S, Dodson T, Fantasia J, et al. American Association of Oral and Maxillofacial Surgeons position paper on medication-related osteonecrosis of the jaw—2014 update. *J Oral Maxillofac Surg.* 2014;72(10):1938-1956.
8. Leeman J, Romesser P, Ying Z, et al. Proton therapy for head and neck cancer patients expanding the therapeutic window. *Lancet Oncol.* 2017;18(5):e254-e265.
9. Gooley TA, Chien JW, Pergam SA, et al. Reduced mortality after allogeneic hematopoietic-cell transplantation. *N Engl J Med.* 2010;363(22):2091-2101.
10. Sheppard D, Bredeson C, Allan D, Tay J. Systematic review of randomized controlled trials of hematopoietic stem cell mobilization strategies for autologous transplantation for hematologic malignancies. *Biol Blood Marrow Transplant.* 2012;18(8):1191-1203.
11. Elad S, Jensen S, Raber-Durlacher J, et al. Clinical approach in the management of oral chronic graft-versus-host disease (cGVHD) in a series of specialized medical centers. *Support Care Cancer.* 2015;23(6):1615-1622.
12. McGuire DB, Fulton JS, Park J, et al.; Study Group of the Multinational Association of Supportive Care in Cancer/International Society of Oral Oncology (MASCC/ISOO). Systematic review of basic oral care for the management of oral mucositis in cancer patients. *Support Care Cancer.* 2013;21(11):3165-3177.
13. Peterson DE, Ohrn K, Bowen J, et al.; Mucositis Study Group of the Multinational Association of Supportive Care in Cancer/International Society of Oral Oncology (MASCC/ISOO). Systematic review of oral cryotherapy for management of oral mucositis caused by cancer therapy. *Support Care Cancer.* 2013;21(1):327-332.
14. Raber-Durlacher JE, von Bultzingslowen I, Logan RM, et al.; Mucositis Study Group of the Multinational Association of Supportive Care in Cancer/International Society of Oral Oncology (MASCC/ISOO). Systematic review of cytokines and growth factors for the management of oral mucositis in cancer patients. *Support Care Cancer.* 2013;21(1):343-355.

15. Nicolatou-Galitis O, Sarri T, Bowen J, et al; Mucositis Study Group of the Multinational Association of Supportive Care in Cancer/International Society of Oral Oncology (MASCC/ISOO). Systematic review of anti-inflammatory agents for the management of oral mucositis in cancer patients. *Support Care Cancer.* 2013;21(11):3179-3189.

16. Saunders DP, Epstein JB, Elad S, et al.; Mucositis Study Group of the Multinational Association of Supportive Care in Cancer/International Society of Oral Oncology (MASCC/ISOO). Systematic Review of antimicrobials, mucosal coating agents, anesthetics and analgesics for the management of oral mucositis in cancer patients. *Support Care Cancer.* 2013;21(11):3191-3207.

17. Buglione M, Cavagnini R, Di Rosario F, et al. Oral toxicity management in head and neck cancer patients treated with chemotherapy and radiation: Xerostomia and trismus (Part 2). Literature review and consensus statement. *Crit Rev Oncol Hematol.* 2016;102:47-54.

18. Hong CHL, Napenas JL, Hodgson BD, et al; Dental Disease Section, Oral Care Study Group, Multi-national Association of Supportive Care in Cancer (MASCC)/International Society of Oral Oncology (ISOO). A systematic review of dental disease in patients undergoing cancer therapy. *Support Care Cancer.* 2010;18(8):1007-1021.

19. Bueno A, Ferreira R, Barbosa F, et al. Periodontal care in patients undergoing radiotherapy for head and neck cancer. *Support Care Cancer.* 2013;21(11):969-975.

20. Rubenstein E, Peterson D, Schubert M, et al.; the Mucositis Study Section of the Multinational Association of Supportive Care in Cancer; and the International Society for Oral Oncology. Clinical practice guidelines for the prevention and treatment of cancer therapy-induced oral and gastrointestinal mucositis. *Cancer.* 2004;100(suppl 9):2026-2046.

21. Jensen S, Pedersen A, Vissink A, et al. A systematic review of salivary gland hypofunction and xerostomia induced by cancer therapies: prevalence, severity and impact on quality of life. *Support Care Cancer.* 2010;18(8):1039-1060.

22. Bos-den Braber J, Potting C, Bronkhorst E, Huysmans MC, Blijlevens NM. Oral complaints and dental care of haematopoietic stem cell transplant patients and their dentists. *Support Care Cancer.* 2015;23(1):13-19.

23. Meier J, Wolff D, Pavletic S, et al. Oral chronic graft-versus-host disease: report from the International Consensus Conference on clinical practice in cGVHD. *Clin Oral Investig.* 2011;15(2):127-139.

24. Effinger K, Migliorati C, Hudson M, et al. Oral and dental late effects in survivors of childhood cancer: a Children's Oncology Group report. *Support Care Cancer.* 2014;22(7):2009-2019.

25. Cheng K, Lee V, Li C, et al. Impact of oral mucositis on short-term clinical outcomes in paediatric and adolescent patients undergoing chemotherapy. *Support Care Cancer.* 2013;21(8):2145-2152.

56

The Oral and Maxillofacial Surgery Patient

Evie F. Jesin, RDH, BSc, Lisa F. Mallonee, RDH, RD, LD, MPH, and
Esther M. Wilkins, BS, RDH, DMD

CHAPTER OUTLINE

PATIENT PREPARATION
I. Objectives
II. Personal Factors

DENTAL HYGIENE CARE
I. Presurgery Treatment Planning
II. Patient Instruction: Diet Selection
III. Presurgical Instructions
IV. Postsurgical Care

PATIENT WITH INTERMAXILLARY FIXATION

FRACTURED JAW
I. Causes of Fractured Jaws
II. Emergency Care
III. Recognition
IV. Types of Fractures
V. Treatment of Fractures

MANDIBULAR FRACTURES
I. Closed Reduction
II. Intermaxillary Fixation
III. External Skeletal Fixation (External Pin Fixation)
IV. Open Reduction

MIDFACIAL FRACTURES
I. Principles
II. Description

ALVEOLAR PROCESS FRACTURE
I. Clinical Findings
II. Treatment

DENTAL HYGIENE CARE
I. Problems
II. Instrumentation

III. Diet
IV. Personal Oral Care Procedures

DENTAL HYGIENE CARE BEFORE GENERAL SURGERY
I. Patients in Whom Surgical Procedures Affect Their Risk Status
II. Preparation of the Mouth before General Inhalation Anesthesia
III. Patient with a Long Convalescence

DOCUMENTATION

EVERYDAY ETHICS

FACTORS TO TEACH THE PATIENT

REFERENCES

LEARNING OBJECTIVES

After studying this chapter, the student will be able to:

1. Discuss the role of the dental hygienist in the pre- and postsurgery care of the oral and maxillofacial surgery patient.

2. Discuss the pre- and postsurgical care planning for the maxillofacial surgery patient.

3. Identify the types of maxillary and mandibular fractures and discuss treatment options.

4. Describe the modifications for dental hygiene treatment, diet, and personal oral care procedures needed after maxillofacial surgery.

5. Explain the dental hygiene care needed before and after general surgery.

Oral and maxillofacial surgery is the specialty of dentistry that includes diagnostic, surgical, and adjunctive treatment of diseases, injuries, and defects involving both functional and aesthetic aspects of the hard and soft tissues in the oral and maxillofacial regions.[1] Box 56-1 lists the types of treatment included in this specialty.

◆ The oral surgeon may be based in a group clinical setting, in a hospital, or in a private practice with outpatient hospital facilities available.

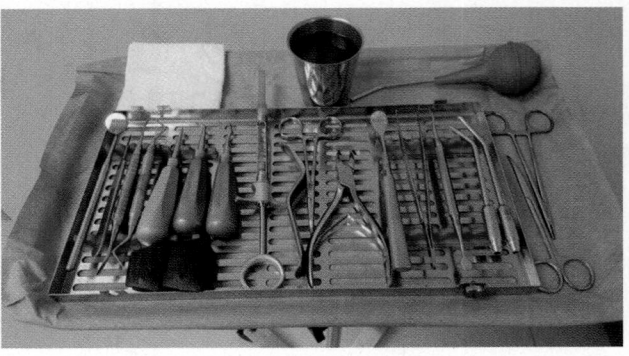

FIGURE 56-1 • **Tray Setup for Routine Extraction of Teeth.** Instrument identification from left to right: dental mirror, surgical scalpel, periosteal elevator, surgical curette, elevators (three), bite-blocks, syringe with needle, Minnesota retractor, hemostat, rongeurs, retractor, forceps, bone file, surgical aspirating tip, scissors, needle holder, cups with saline solution, and bulb syringe. (Evie F. Jesin, RRDH, BSc, Professor, Toronto, ON, Canada: George Brown College.)

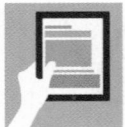

BOX 56-1
Categories of Oral and Maxillofacial Treatments

Dentoalveolar Surgery

Exodontics

Impacted tooth removal

Alveolar bone surgery: alveoloplasty, bone grafting, ridge augmentation

Infection

Abscesses

Osteomyelitis

Traumatic Injury Treatment

Fractures of jaws, zygoma

Fracture of teeth, alveolar bone

Neoplasm and Oral Pathology

Cysts

Tumors

Biopsy

Incisional biopsy

Excisional biopsy

Exfoliative biopsy

Dental Implant Placement

Preprosthetic Reconstruction

Maxillofacial prosthetics

Immediate denture

Orthognathic Surgery

Prognathism correction

Facial aesthetics

Cleft Lip/Palate

Temporomandibular Disorders

Salivary Gland Obstruction

◆ The oral surgeon is part of a team of specially trained individuals that includes surgical assistants, anesthetists, registered nurses, and dental hygienists.

◆ The oral surgeon may coordinate the surgical procedures with various dental practitioners, including general dentists, laboratory technicians, prosthodontists, orthodontists, dental implant specialists, and other specialists caring for the patient.

◆ Surgery for treatment of diseases and correction of defects of the periodontal tissues is categorized specifically as *periodontal surgery.*

• Within the scope of periodontal surgery are procedures for pocket elimination, gingivoplasty, treatment of furcation involvements, correction of mucogingival defects, treatment for bony defects about the teeth, and placing implants.

• Preparation for periodontal surgery is not specifically described in this chapter. Many of the surgical instruments are used by both a periodontist and an oral surgeon (Figure 56-1).

PATIENT PREPARATION

I. Objectives

Dental hygiene care and instruction before oral and maxillofacial surgery may improve a patient's health and well-being by one or more of the following.

A. Reduce Oral Bacterial Count

◆ Aid in the preparation of an aseptic field for the surgery.

◆ The human oral cavity harbors a variety of microbes. Recent investigative data indicate more than 400 species of microorganisms exist in the microflora of the human oropharynx.[2]

◆ Make postsurgical infection less likely or less severe.

B. Reduce Inflammation of the Gingiva and Improve Tissue Tone

- Lessen local bleeding at the time of the surgery.
- Promote postsurgical healing.

C. Remove Calculus Deposits

- Remove a source of dental biofilm retention and thus improve gingival tissue tone.
- Prevent interference with placement of surgical instruments.
- Prevent pieces of calculus from breaking away.
  - Danger of inhalation, particularly when a general anesthetic is used.
  - Possibility of calculus falling into a tooth socket or other surgical area and acting as a foreign body to inhibit healing.

D. Instruct in Presurgical Personal Oral Care Procedures

- Reduce inflammation and thus improve tissue tone.
- Help to prepare the patient for postsurgical care.

E. Instruct in the Use of Foods

- Foods that provide the elements essential to tissue building and repair during pre- and postsurgical periods.
- For the patient who will have teeth removed and immediate complete or partial dentures inserted, the importance of a diet containing all essential food groups is emphasized.

F. Interpret the Dentist's Directions

- Explanation is needed for the immediate presurgical preparation with respect to rest and dietary limitations, particularly when a general anesthetic is to be administered.

G. Motivate the Patient Who Will Have Teeth Remaining

- Motivation to prevent further tooth loss through routine dental and dental hygiene professional care and personal oral care procedures.

II. Personal Factors

- Extent of the surgery to be performed and previous experiences affect patient attitude.
- Many patients in greatest need of presurgical dental hygiene care and instruction may have neglected their mouths for many years. They may have been indifferent to or unaware of the importance of obtaining adequate oral care.
- Visits to a dentist may have been to have a toothache relieved. Patient knowledge of preventive measures may be limited.
- A few possible patient traits are suggested here:

A. Apprehensive and Fearful

- Apprehensive and indifferent toward need for personal care of teeth.
- Fearful of all dental procedures, particularly oral surgery and anesthesia.
- Fearful of personal appearance after surgery.

B. Resigned

- Feeling the situation is unavoidable.
- Lack of appreciation for preserving natural teeth.

C. Discouraged

- Over tooth loss or development of soft-tissue lesions.
- Toward time lost from work.
- By the financial aspects of dental care.
- About inconvenience and discomfort.

DENTAL HYGIENE CARE

I. Presurgery Treatment Planning

A. Initial Oral Preparation

- The pending date for the surgery and the patient's attitude may limit the time spent.
- Complete medical and dental history, extra- and intraoral examination, vital signs, and photographs are essential.
- Complete radiographs including the use of cone beam computed tomography (CBCT) are essential.[3]
- CBCT is more accurate in predicting implant length and width and the need for bone grafting procedures.
- For routine unguided implant placement in sites where anatomic structures and bone grafting are not a concern, the use of a panoramic radiograph could be adequate for determining the length and width of the implant.[4]
- Determine the need for prophylactic premedication (see Chapter 11).
- Antibiotics are not required as prophylaxis for third molar surgery. The standard of care after extraction of mandibular third molar surgery for all healthy patients should be a good anti-inflammatory regimen rather than an antibiotic prophylaxis.[5] Proper aseptic precautions and good anti-inflammatory regimen are more important than the prophylactic antibiotics. Antibiotics use increases the risk of bacterial resistance.[6]
- Develop rapport; explain purposes of presurgical appointments.
- Explain and demonstrate dental biofilm control principles. Demonstrate appropriate technique using new soft toothbrush and appropriate adjunctive interdental aids.
- Perform debridement to prepare for tissue healing; local anesthesia is used as needed.

◆ Provide postsurgical instruction for rinsing with basic saline or with chlorhexidine 0.12% for tissue conditioning.

◆ Encourage participation in a tobacco cessation program if patient is currently using tobacco products.

B. Follow-up Evaluation

◆ Complete or continue the debridement.

◆ More appointments may be needed for patients who will have surgery for oral cancer or who have a cardiovascular or other condition for which all periodontal and dental treatment is completed before surgery.

◆ When radiation or chemotherapy will be used following surgery for oral cancer, or when a prosthetic heart valve or total joint replacement will be involved, complete oral care is needed before surgery.

◆ Debridement is planned for a few weeks after oral surgery. Emphasis is placed on review and demonstration of personal daily oral self-care. The patient's oral self-care plan may require modification based on the oral surgery performed.

◆ Continue to provide support for tobacco cessation program if client uses tobacco products.

II. Patient Instruction: Diet Selection

◆ The nutritional status can influence the resistance to infection and wound healing, as well as general recovery powers.

◆ Nutritional deficiencies can occur because of the inability to ingest adequate nutrients orally.

◆ Specific recommendations of what to include and not to include in the diet are provided.

◆ Postsurgical suggestions may differ from presurgical suggestions; for example, when difficulty in chewing is a postsurgical problem, a liquid or soft diet may be required.

◆ When major oral surgery requires hospitalization, nasogastric tube feeding may be used during the initial healing period.

A. Nutritional and Dietary Needs

Diets outlined are designed to include the essential nutrients from key food groups from the current food guidance system MyPlate (see Chapter 33).

◆ *Essential for promotion of healing*: proteins and vitamins, particularly vitamin A, vitamin C, and riboflavin.

◆ *Essential for building gingival tissue resistance*: a varied diet that includes adequate portions of all essential food groups.

◆ *Essential for dental caries prevention*: noncariogenic foods. When a patient has not been able to masticate properly, the diet employed frequently may have included intake of the following:
  - Soft and cariogenic foods.
  - Frequent sugary snacks.
  - Intake of high-sucrose calorie-dense beverages.

B. Suggestions for Instruction

◆ Provide take-home instruction sheets that recommend specific pre- and postsurgery food options. Foods for liquid and soft diets are listed in the "Dental Hygiene Care" section of this chapter.

◆ Express nutritional needs in terms of quantity or servings of foods so that the patient clearly understands.

◆ For the patient who will receive dentures, careful instruction is provided over a period of time. Information for the patient with new dentures is described in Chapter 30.

◆ When the patient loses the teeth because of dental caries, the diet may have been highly cariogenic. Emphasis needs to be placed on helping the patient include nutritious foods for the general health of the body and, more specifically, the health of the alveolar processes, which will support the dentures.

III. Presurgical Instructions

◆ The objective of presurgical instruction is to educate the patient on what to expect during the oral surgery appointment and immediately afterward.[7]

◆ The patient may have concerns about the anesthesia, the surgical procedure, and the outcome.

◆ For surgery in a hospital setting, the presurgical instructions are often mailed to the patient.

◆ When surgery is done in the dental office, the dental hygienist may be responsible to deliver the instructions.

◆ Verbal instructions are supplemented with printed information.

◆ Instructions may include explanation of:
  - *Food and liquid restrictions before surgery*: Specify the number of hours before the time of the surgery when the patient stops further intake of food and fluids.
  - *Alcohol and medication restrictions*: The patient may be instructed to discontinue use of certain medications (prescribed and over-the-counter), supplements, herbal remedies, and alcohol, which are not compatible with the anesthetic and drugs to be used during and following the surgical procedure.
  - *Smoking*: The patient may be instructed to stop smoking or limit smoking well in advance of the surgery date.
  - *Clothing*: The patient may be instructed to wear loose fitting clothing around the neck and upper arms for intravenous delivery and assessment of vitals throughout the surgical procedure.
  - *Makeup*: The patient should not wear lipstick or excessive makeup, and nail polish color should be removed.
  - *Transport to and from the appointment*: When general anesthetic or light sedation is used, the patient is instructed not to drive. Plans for someone to accompany and assist the patient are made.

- *Ice packs*: The patient may be instructed to prepare ice packs well in advance of surgery. Ice cubes may be placed in a plastic bag. Alternatively, a disposable plastic glove may be filled with cold water and the end of the glove tied in a knot and then placed in a freezer. Ice packs are beneficial for the first 36 hours following the surgical procedure.

IV. Postsurgical Care

A. Immediate Instructions

Printed postsurgical instructions are provided following all oral surgery procedures. The prepared material is reviewed with the patient and/or caregiver or family member after surgery. Specific details vary, but basic information for postsurgical instruction sheets includes the following:

- *Control bleeding*:
  - Keep the gauze square in the mouth over the surgical area for half an hour and then discard it.
  - When bleeding persists at home, place a gauze square or cold wet tea bag over the area and bite firmly for 30 minutes.
- *Rinsing*:
  - Do not rinse for 24 hours after the surgical appointment.
  - Then use warm saltwater (1/2 teaspoonful salt in 1/2 cup [4 ounces] of warm water) after toothbrushing and every 2 hours.
- *Dental biofilm control*: Brush the teeth and use interdental aids more carefully than usual. Avoid the surgery site.
- *Rest*: Get plenty of rest; at least 8–10 hours of sleep each night. Avoid strenuous exercise during the first 24 hours, and keep the mouth from excessive movement. Avoid sleeping on the surgical site.
- *Diet*: Use a liquid or soft diet high in protein. Drink water, warm soups (not hot), and fruit juices freely. Avoid spicy, hard, hot, or chewy foods.
- *Smoking*: The patient should avoid smoking for at least 2 weeks postsurgery to allow for initial healing of the surgical site.
- *Pain*: If needed, use a pain-relieving preparation prescribed by the oral surgeon or general dentist. Prescribed medication will vary from nonsteroidal anti-inflammatory drugs to opioid-containing compounds depending on the procedure. Adhere to directions.
  - Pain relief medication may include ibuprofen and/or acetaminophen for atraumatic removal of teeth; acetaminophen with 30 mg of codeine or a compound using oxycodone may be prescribed for more invasive procedures.[8]
- *Limited opening*: Limited mouth opening will be present—two-finger opening is expected on the third day following surgery.
- *Exercise*: Limit strenuous exercises for the first few days after surgery.

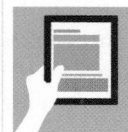

BOX 56-2
Five Ss for Patients to Avoid

No vigorous swishing.
No vigorous spitting.
No smoking.
No drinking from a straw.
No eating of solid food for first 24 hours.

- *Ice pack*:
  - When swelling is possible, apply ice pack (ice cubes in a plastic bag or water frozen in a disposable glove) for 15 minutes, followed by 15 minutes off, or as directed by the oral surgeon for the first 36 hours after surgery.
  - Heat is not used for swelling.
- *Complications*: Include the telephone number to call after office hours, should complications arise. Complications may include:
  - Uncontrolled pain, uncontrolled bleeding.
  - Temperature of 101°F or higher.
  - Difficulty in opening the mouth (trismus).
  - Unusual or excessive swelling after the surgery.
  - Nerve damage.
  - Infection in the surgical site or area.
  - Possible alveolitis or dry socket, especially in lower posterior molars. Alveolitis is extremely painful and usually occurs 2–4 days after tooth extraction whereby the blood clot is dislodged from the tooth socket. The surgical site is irrigated with warm saline solution followed by the placement of iodoform gauze, which is packed into the socket. The patient returns in 1–2 days to have the iodoform gauze changed and a new one placed, and the site is re-evaluated for healing.
- Box 56-2 identifies important habits for patients to avoid following surgery.

B. Follow-up Care

- The dental hygienist may participate in suture removal, irrigation of sockets, and other postsurgical procedures when the patient returns.
- Instruction concerning biofilm control, rinsing, oral irrigation, and other personal care, as well as diet supervision, can be continued as appropriate.

PATIENT WITH INTERMAXILLARY FIXATION

- Limited access for personal oral care procedures and the effect of the liquid diet required for most cases define the need for special dental hygiene care for the patient with intermaxillary fixation (IMF).

◆ Attention to rehabilitation of oral tissues during the period following removal of fixation appliances takes on particular significance to prevent permanent tissue damage and inadequate oral care habits from being continued indefinitely.

◆ Descriptions in this section are related to a fractured jaw, but IMF may be required for a variety of corrective surgeries and other conditions, including temporomandibular joint treatment and reconstructive and orthognathic surgeries.

◆ Regardless of the reason for IMF, instructions for dental hygiene care are similar, and the patient's problems are much the same.

FRACTURED JAW

◆ The patient with a fractured jaw may be hospitalized.

◆ A dental hygienist employed in a hospital would be called upon to assume part of the responsibility for patient care or to give oral hygiene instruction to direct care personnel.

◆ After dismissal from the hospital, the patient may require special attention in the private dental office for a long period.

◆ Treatment of a fractured jaw can be complex, and the patient may suffer considerably, both physically and mentally.

◆ Basic knowledge of the nature of fractures and treatment is helpful in understanding the patient's needs.

I. Causes of Fractured Jaws

A. Traumatic

Domestic violence, gunshots, sporting injuries, falls, road traffic accidents (including motorcycles and bicycles), and industrial accidents.

B. Predisposing

Pathologic conditions, such as tumors, cysts, osteoporosis, or osteomyelitis, weaken the bone; thus, slight trauma or even tooth removal can cause fracture.

II. Emergency Care

◆ Immediate attention is paid to measures for care of the patient's general condition.

◆ Monitor breathing, airway, and circulation, and prepare for possible basic life support measures (see Chapter 9).

◆ Hemorrhage, shock, and skull or internal head injuries are next in the sequence of concern.

◆ Almost any category of emergency care may be required (see Chapter 9).

◆ Although treatment for the fractured jaw cannot be postponed for any great length of time, its immediate care takes second place to the vital aspects of patient care.

III. Recognition

A. History

Except for a pathologic fracture, a history of trauma is usually described by the patient.

B. Clinical Signs

◆ Pain, especially on movement, and tenderness on slight pressure over the area of the fracture.

◆ Teeth may be displaced, fractured, or mobile. Because of muscle pull or contraction, segments of the bones may be displaced and the occlusion of the teeth may be irregular.

◆ Muscle spasm is a common finding, particularly when the fracture is at the angle or ramus of the mandible.

◆ Crepitation can be heard if the parts of bone are moved.

◆ Soft tissue in the area of the fracture may show laceration and bleeding, discoloration (ecchymosis), and enlargement.

IV. Types of Fractures

A fracture is classified by using a combination of descriptive words for its *location*, *direction*, *nature* (Figure 56-2), and *severity*. Fractures may be single or multiple, bilateral or unilateral, and complete or incomplete.

A. Classification by Nature of the Fracture

◆ *Simple*: has no communication with outside.

◆ *Compound*: has communication with outside.

◆ *Comminuted*: shattered.

◆ *Incomplete*: "Greenstick" fracture has one side of a bone broken and the other side bent.
  • It occurs in incompletely calcified bones (young children, usually).
  • The fibers tend to bend rather than break.

B. Mandibular (Described by Location)

◆ Alveolar process.

◆ Condyle.

◆ Angle.

◆ Body.

◆ Symphysis.

C. Midfacial

◆ *Alveolar process*: The alveolar process fracture does not extend to the midline of the palate.

◆ *Le Fort*[9]: The Le Fort classification is used widely to identify the three general levels of maxillary fractures, as shown in Figure 56-3.

◆ *Le Fort I*: A horizontal fracture line extends above the roots of the teeth, above the palate, across the maxillary sinus, below the zygomatic process, and across the pterygoid plates.

◆ *Le Fort II*: The midface fracture extends over the middle of the nose, down the medial wall of the orbits, across

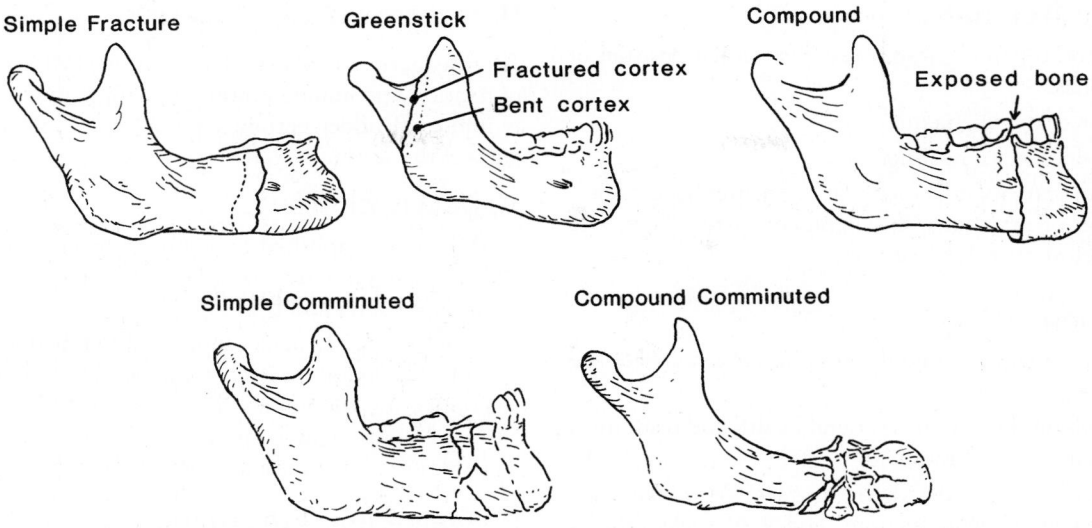

FIGURE 56-2 • Types of Fractures. (Reprinted with permission from Kruger GO. *Textbook of Oral and Maxillofacial Surgery.* 6th ed. St. Louis, MO: Mosby; 1984.)

the infraorbital rims, and posteriorly across the pterygoid plates.

- *Le Fort III*: The high-level craniofacial fracture extends transversely across the bridge of the nose, across the orbits and the zygomatic arches, and across the pterygoid plates.
- *Le Fort combination*: A combination of two levels is also possible such as a right Le Fort I and a left Le Fort II.

V. Treatment of Fractures

Each fracture differs from the next, and the methods used in treatment vary with the individual case.[10,11]

A. Treatment Planning

- Many factors are involved when the oral surgeon selects the methods to be used, particularly the location of the fracture or fractures, the presence or absence of teeth, existing injuries to the teeth, other head injuries, and the general health and condition of the patient.
- All fractures do not require active intervention. Examples are fractures of the condylar and coronoid processes, nondisplaced fractures of an edentulous mandible, and greenstick fractures of children.

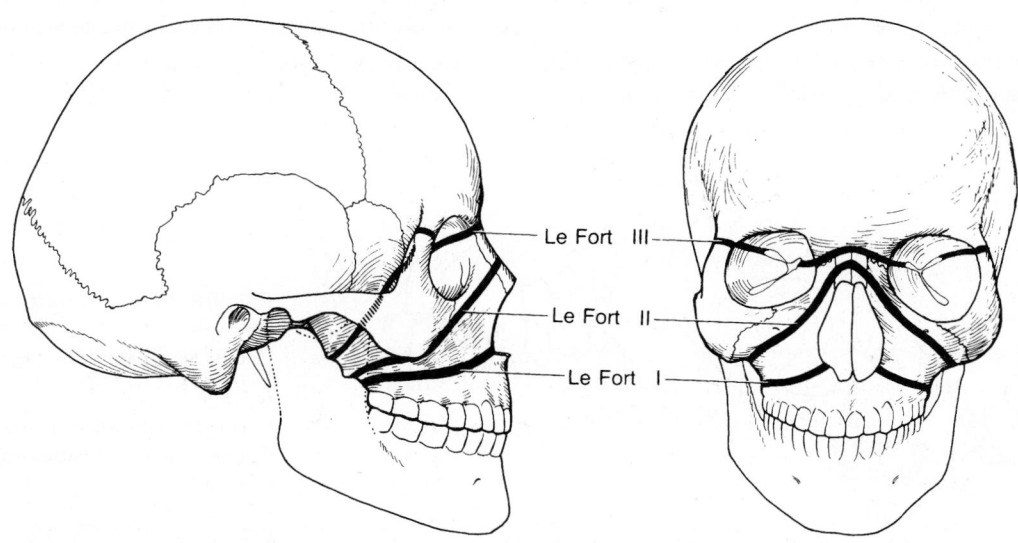

FIGURE 56-3 • Le Fort Classification of Facial Fractures. Le Fort I, horizontal fracture above the roots of the teeth, below the zygomatic process, and across the pterygoid plates. Le Fort II, midface fracture over the middle of the nose and across the intraorbital rims. Le Fort III, transversely across the bridge of the nose and across the orbits and the zygomatic bone. (Adapted with permission from Archer WH. *Oral and Maxillofacial Surgery.* 5th ed. Philadelphia, PA: Saunders; 1975. From American College of Surgeons, Committee on Trauma. *Early Care of the Injured Patient.* Philadelphia, PA: Saunders; 1972.)

B. Basic Treatment

◆ *Reduction* (open or closed) restores normal position of the bones.
◆ *Fixation* of the fragments.
◆ *Immobilization* for healing.
◆ Control of treatment complications centers around prevention of infections, misalignment of the parts, and malocclusion of the dentition.

C. Healing

◆ Union is affected by the location and character of the fracture.
◆ Depends on the patient's general health and resistance, as well as on cooperation.
◆ Six weeks is considered the average for the uncomplicated mandibular fracture, and 4–6 weeks for the maxillary.
◆ Major cause of complication is infection.

MANDIBULAR FRACTURES

Reduction means the positioning of the parts on either side of the fracture so they are in apposition for healing and restoration of function.

◆ *Open reduction* refers to the use of a surgical flap procedure to expose the fracture ends and bring them together for healing.
◆ *Closed reduction* is accomplished by manipulation of the parts without surgery.

I. Closed Reduction

◆ The closure of the teeth in normal occlusion for the individual is the usual guide for position of the fracture parts in the dentulous patient.
◆ To identify the customary relation of the teeth can be difficult, especially in the partially edentulous mouth.

II. Intermaxillary Fixation

After reduction, intermaxillary fixation (IMF) is a method of fixation and immobilization used for many years. It still is indicated under certain circumstances and in certain parts of the world.

A. Description

◆ IMF is accomplished by applying wires and/or elastic bands between the maxillary and mandibular arches (Figure 56-4A and B).
◆ *Arch bars*: Ready-made, contoured arch bars are adapted to fit accurately to each tooth and provide hooks for connecting the arches (Figure 56-4C). A small horizontal elastic may be positioned across the fracture to reduce the lateral displacement (Figure 56-4D).

B. Evaluation: Advantages

◆ Relative simplicity without surgical requirement: noninvasive.
◆ Lower cost; shorter hospital stay (depending on other injuries).
◆ Resources and trained surgeons may be limited in less developed countries.
◆ Patient can return to activity and work sooner; can use outpatient facility for follow-up.

C. Evaluation: Contraindications and Disadvantages

◆ Patients with chronic airway diseases who cough and expectorate: asthma and chronic obstructive pulmonary diseases.
◆ Patients who vomit regularly; notably, during pregnancy.
◆ Patients with a mental illness.
◆ Dietary problems: Patients lose weight with the liquid, monotonous diet, often with cariogenic content.
◆ Oral hygiene and dietary limitations lead to increased dental caries and periodontal infection.

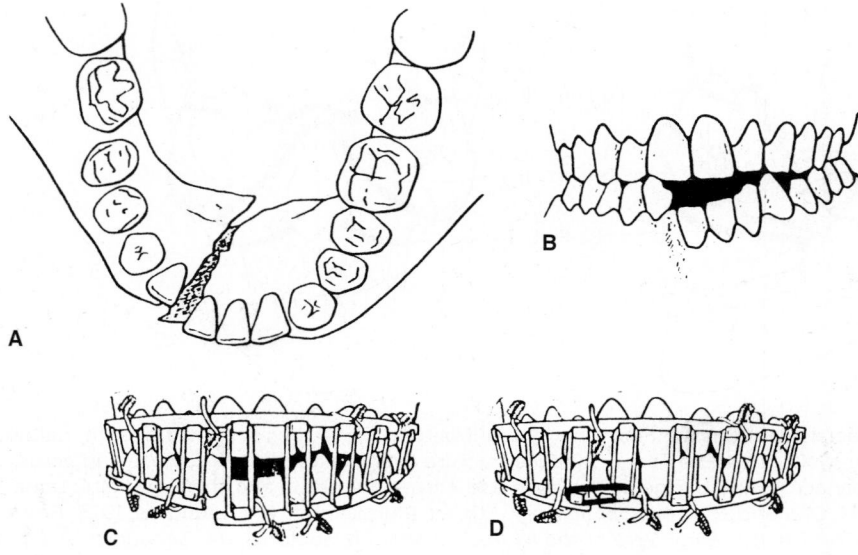

FIGURE 56-4 • Intermaxillary Fracture. A: Location of fracture of the mandible. **B:** Segments of bone on either side of the fracture are displaced by muscle pull or contraction. **C:** Arch bars with hooks for metal wires or rubber bands positioned to provide a steady pull for fracture reduction. **D:** Note small horizontal rubber band extending from the hook at the mandibular right central incisor to the mandibular right canine to reduce the lateral displacement. (Adapted with permission from Archer WH. *Oral and Maxillofacial Surgery*. 5th ed. Philadelphia, PA: Saunders; 1975.)

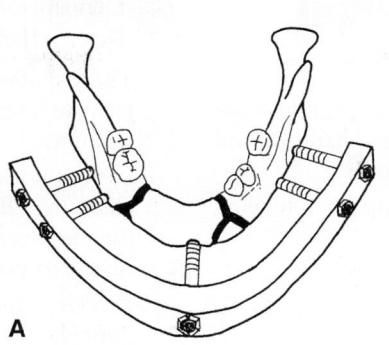
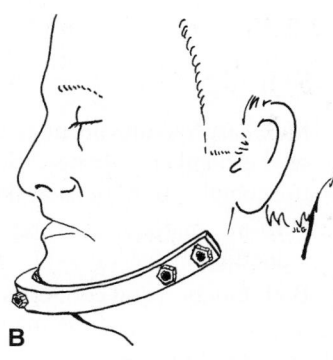

FIGURE 56-5 • External Skeletal Fixation. A: Precision bone screws placed on either side of the fractures shown by heavy black lines. **B:** Molded acrylic bar positioned over the bone screws and locked into position with nuts.

III. External Skeletal Fixation (External Pin Fixation)

A. Description

Precision bone screws are placed via skin incisions on either side of the fracture (Figure 56-5A). An acrylic bar is molded and, while still pliable, is pressed over the threads of the bone screws and locked into position with the screw nuts (Figure 56-5B).

B. Indications

Management of a fracture cannot always be accomplished satisfactorily by intermaxillary wiring alone. The following are indications for external fixation:

◆ Insufficient number of teeth in good condition for IMF.

◆ As a supplement to IMF when no teeth are present in the fractured portion of the mandible.

◆ Loss of bone substance.

• When bone substance is lost because of an accident, a gunshot wound, or a pathologic condition, a bone graft may be indicated.[12]

• The extraoral fixation is used first to hold the fractured parts in a normal relationship and then to immobilize the area during healing following the bone graft surgery.

◆ Some patients may be unable to have the jaws closed for a long period. Examples of these are:

• Patient with a vomiting problem, such as during pregnancy.

• Patient with a mental or physical disability, such as cerebral palsy, epilepsy, or mental retardation.

◆ Edentulous mandible when the fracture fragments are greatly displaced, when the fracture is at the angle of the mandible, or when the mandible is atrophic or thinned.

IV. Open Reduction

A. Principles for Treating Skeletal Fractures

◆ Anatomic reduction.

◆ Functionally stable fixation.

◆ Atraumatic surgical technique.

◆ Active function.

◆ Prevention of infection.

B. Description

◆ Surgical approach to bring the fracture parts together.

◆ *Anesthesia*: anesthesia selected in accord with patient history.

◆ Types of systems used for immobilization include:

• Transosseous wiring (osteosynthesis).

• Plates of various sizes.

• Titanium mesh.

• Bone clamps, staples, and screws.

• *Materials*: miniplates, screws, and other parts made of biodegradable or resorbable synthetic materials.

C. Clinical Example

◆ Figure 56-6 illustrates various positions for miniplate osteosynthesis to provide stability for the reduced fracture parts.

◆ Care is needed so the screws are not placed over a fracture line or over the roots of teeth and do not infringe on the mandibular canal.

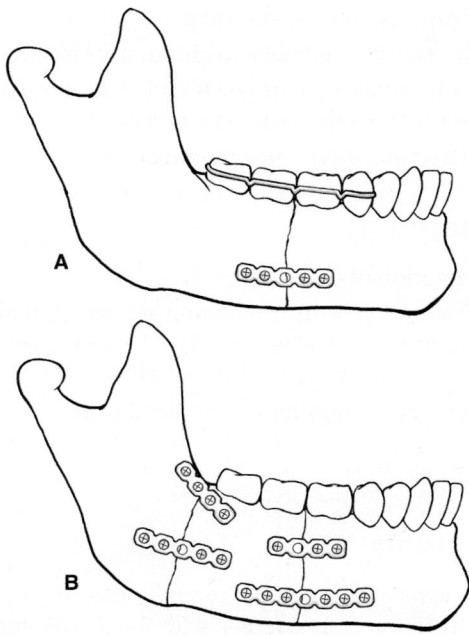

FIGURE 56-6 • Miniplates for Immobilization of Fracture. A: Tension band on the teeth to aid in maintaining correct occlusion, while miniplate holds fracture ends in apposition. **B:** Examples of possible positions for miniplates.

MIDFACIAL FRACTURES

I. Principles

- Maxillary fractures are more difficult to manage because of the number of bones, the associated anatomy, and the complications of basal skull fractures.
- Not all midface fractures need fixation following reduction.
- Both function and cosmetics are involved.

II. Description

A. Older Methods

- Internal wire suspension.
- External cranial suspension to a stable bone, such as uninvolved zygoma.
- Head caps.

B. Current Therapeutic Interventions

- Open reduction with internal fixation.
- Use of bone plates of various sizes.
- Grafts for reconstruction of midface defects.
- Early reconstruction before scarring and soft-tissue contracture deform the surrounding area.

ALVEOLAR PROCESS FRACTURE

The most common fracture is of the alveolar process, maxillary or mandibular.

I. Clinical Findings

- Face: bruising, areas of swelling.
- Teeth: fractures, mobility, avulsion, displacement.
- Lips and gingiva: bruising, bleeding lacerations from contact with teeth at the time of impact.
- Bone fracture: most frequently in anterior.

II. Treatment

- Replantation of displaced teeth.
- Immobilization with interdental wiring. A temporary fixed splint of acrylic may be placed over the wires. The teeth are tested periodically for vitality.
- Endodontic therapy may be required later.

DENTAL HYGIENE CARE

I. Problems

Fixation apparatus, however carefully placed to prevent tissue irritation, interferes with normal function. Identification of possible effects of treatment provides the basis for planning dental hygiene care.

A. Development of Gingivitis or Periodontal Complications

- Thick biofilm formation and food debris accumulation provide sources of irritation to the gingiva, resulting in gingivitis.
- Lack of normal stimulation of the periodontium and of cleansing effects usually provided by the action of the tongue, lips, and facial muscles contributes to stagnation of saliva and accumulation of debris and bacteria.
- Tender, sensitive gingiva makes biofilm control more difficult, even on available surfaces.

B. Initiation of Demineralization

- An appetizing soft or liquid diet is difficult to plan using limited cariogenic foods for dental caries prevention.

C. Loss of Appetite

- Loss of appetite related to monotonous liquid or soft diet may lead to weight loss and lowered physical resistance.
- Secondary infections, including those of the oral tissues, may result.

D. Difficulty in Opening the Mouth

- When there has been trauma to bony and/or soft tissues of the jaw that require fixation, there is going to be a degree of trismus following release of fixation.
- After removal of appliances, all patients have a degree of muscular trismus that limits personal oral self-care and mastication.

II. Instrumentation

A. Presurgical

Gross calculus is removed, as much possible, before open reduction procedures. Trauma to surrounding soft tissues of lip, tongue, and cheeks limits accessibility.

B. During Treatment

Periodic debridement contributes to oral health. Although access is only from the facial aspect for a patient with intermaxillary wiring, some benefit can be obtained. An assistant provides continual suction during treatment.

C. After Removal of Appliances

A few weeks after removal of appliances, when the patient can open the mouth normally and personal daily oral care has been initiated, complete debridement can be provided.

III. Diet

Many patients with fractured jaws tend to lose weight, which is generally related to an inadequate nutrient and caloric intake. Objectives in planning the diet are to:

- Prevent new carious lesions.
- Help the patient maintain an adequate nutritional state.

◆ Promote healing.

◆ Increase resistance to infection.

Attention is given to the patient's willingness and ability to follow the recommendations made. The patient may be in the hospital for a few days to a few weeks, depending on the severity of other injuries. A greater length of time is spent as an outpatient, when the diet is much more difficult to supervise. The patient's understanding of dietary instructions and what is expected may appear more significant than the specific components of the diet recommended.

A. Nutritional Needs

After a surgical fixation procedure, the diet is planned to promote tissue building and repair.

◆ All essential food elements.

◆ Emphasis on protein; vitamins, particularly A, C, and D; and minerals particularly calcium and phosphorus.

◆ Usual caloric requirements for patient's age, taking into consideration lack of physical exercise and loss of appetite when ill.

B. Methods of Feeding

◆ *Plastic straw*: Liquid is sucked through the teeth or through an edentulous area. Straw can be bent to accommodate a patient who cannot sit up.

◆ *Spoon feeding*: When a patient's arms are not functional, direct assistance is needed. The mouth may have injuries that prevent sucking food through a straw.

◆ *Tube feeding*: Tube feeding may be indicated following various types of extensive oral surgery, facial trauma, burns, immobilized fractured jaw, and other conditions that prevent ingesting sufficient calories and nutritional foods by way of the mouth.

  • A nasogastric tube is used. Blenderized food can be prepared, or special tube formulas are available commercially.

  • When commercial preparations are used, contents can be selected to meet the specific nutritional and caloric requirements of an individual patient.

C. Liquid Diet

A *clear liquid* diet to help prevent dehydration may be prescribed initially, but it can be nutritionally inadequate. A *full liquid* diet to provide high protein and other healing elements is of a consistency to be taken by a cup. A *blenderized liquid* diet can be passed through a straw.

◆ Indications

  • All patients with jaws wired together.

  • Patients with no appliance or single-jaw appliance who have difficulty opening the mouth because of a condition, such as temporomandibular joint involvement or tongue or lip injury, that hinders insertion of food or manipulation of food in the mouth.

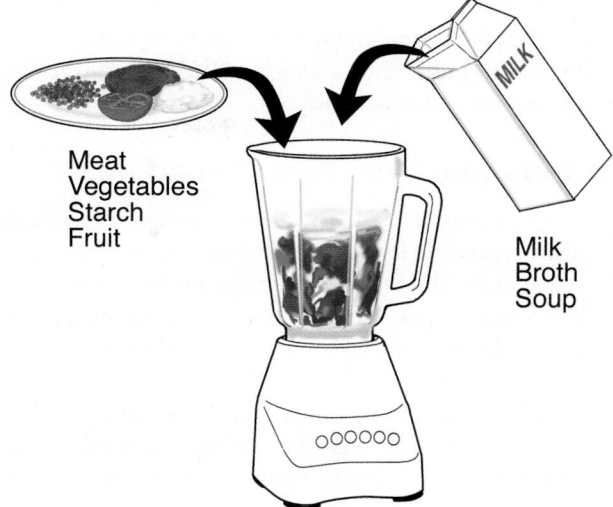

FIGURE 56-7 • Preparation of a Liquid or Soft Diet. Regular table foods can be blended with milk or other nutritious liquid.

◆ *Examples of foods*: fruit juices, milk, eggnog, smoothies, meat juices and soups, cooked thin cereals, and canned baby foods. Strained vegetables and meats (baby foods) may be added to meat juices and soups.

◆ *Use of a blender*: Regular table foods can be mixed in a food blender. With liquid, such as clear soup or milk, added, a fluid consistency can be obtained that will pass through a straw (Figure 56-7).

D. Soft Diet

◆ *Indications*

  • Patient with no appliance or with single-jaw appliance without complications in opening the mouth or in movement of the lips and tongue.

  • Patient who has been maintained on liquid diet throughout treatment period.

    • After appliances are removed, the soft diet is recommended for several days to 1 week to provide the stomach with foods that are readily digestible rather than making a drastic change to a regular diet.

    • A soft diet can also aid by protecting tender oral tissues from the rough textures of a regular diet until the tissues have had a chance to respond to softer foods.

◆ *Examples of foods*

  • Soft-poached, scrambled, or boiled eggs; fruit and yogurt smoothies, cooked cereals; mashed soft-cooked vegetables, including potato; mashed fresh or canned fruits; soft, finely divided meats; custards; plain ice cream.

E. Suggestions for Diet Planning with the Nonhospitalized Patient

◆ Provide instruction sheets that show specific food suggestions.

◆ Express nutritional needs in quantities or servings of foods.

- Show methods of varying the diet. A liquid or soft diet is at best monotonous due to similarity in texture.
- Encourage limitation of cariogenic foods as an aid to prevention of dental caries.

IV. Personal Oral Care Procedures

- Every attempt is made to keep the patient's mouth as clean as possible for comfort and sanitation, and as free of dental biofilm as possible for disease prevention.
- The extent of possible care depends on the appliances; the condition of the lips, tongue, and other oral tissues; and the cooperation of the patient.
- The patient is encouraged to begin toothbrushing as soon as possible after the surgical procedure, but until the patient is able, a plan for care is outlined for a caregiver.

A. Irrigation

- *Indications*: During the first few days after the surgical procedure, while the mouth may be too tender for brushing, frequent irrigations are required; irrigation also serves as an adjunct to toothbrushing.
- *Method*: In a hospital, irrigations with suction are possible. At home, the patient irrigates with the head lowered over a sink (see Chapter 27).
- *Mouthrinse selection*: The oral surgeon is consulted for specific instructions. Suggestions include:
  - Physiologic saline (1 tsp [5 g] of salt to 1 cup [250 mL] of warm water).
  - Chlorhexidine gluconate.
  - Fluoride rinse.

B. Early Mouth Cleansing

While the patient is in the hospital, a soft toothbrush with suction can be used. The toothbrush with suction is described in Chapter 4.

C. Personal Care by the Patient

- As soon as possible, the patient is instructed in personal care.
- A toothbrushing method and other aids, such as those used for orthodontic appliances, are recommended and demonstrated, as discussed in Chapter 29.
- Interdental and proximal tooth surface care is restricted to access only from the facial approach, making the choice of oral care devices limited.[13]
- Some spaces permit insertion of an interdental brush. With instruction, most patients can use a toothpick in a holder (Perio Aid®) to disturb biofilm around just under the free gingival margin, as shown in Chapter 27.
- When the tongue is not injured, the patient can be instructed to use the tongue as an aid in cleaning the lingual surfaces of the teeth and massaging the gingiva.
- The ambulatory patient can use a water irrigator. A low-pressure setting is used, and the spray is directed carefully to prevent tissue injury, as illustrated in Chapter 27.

D. After Appliances Are Removed

- Demineralization and dental caries can result from biofilm retention around the appliances.
- Except for the patient who had practiced good personal oral care before the accident, a step-by-step series of lessons is necessary.
- A method for daily self-applied fluoride, such as a mouthrinse or brush-on gel, can be introduced along with the use of a fluoride dentifrice.

DENTAL HYGIENE CARE BEFORE GENERAL SURGERY

- When emergency surgery is performed, preparation of the mouth is not possible, and postsurgical examination and care may be complicated by various limitations.
- When surgery is elective, or planned in advance, the patient can be encouraged to have a complete dental and periodontal treatment.
- Types of patients are described briefly here. Other examples are found in the various special patient chapters throughout this section of the book.

I. Patients in Whom Surgical Procedures Affect Their Risk Status

- Patients who receive chemotherapeutic agents following surgery for various types of cancer, and others who use immunosuppressant drugs, require special management to prevent complications during dental and dental hygiene appointments.
- Antibiotic premedication to prevent infective endocarditis and other infections is mandatory for certain patients, as described in Chapter 11.
- Before surgery for prostheses, transplants, cancer, and other serious conditions, patients are informed of the need for completing oral care treatments and practicing preventive daily personal care.

II. Preparation of the Mouth before General Inhalation Anesthesia

- Because the mouth is an entryway to the respiratory system, the possibility always exists that bacteria, debris, and fluids from the mouth may be inhaled.
- Inhalation could occur during the administration of an anesthetic or when the patient coughs.

III. Patient with a Long Convalescence

- Patients whose surgery requires a long convalescence may be unable to keep a regular continuing care appointment.
- When the patient has a healthy mouth before hospitalization and convalescence, the problems of postsurgical oral care are lessened, but not eliminated.

◆ Instruction for the caregiver may be needed. A home visit by the dental hygienist may be possible depending on the state or province practice act (see Chapter 4).

DOCUMENTATION

The permanent oral care record for most maxillofacial patients needs to include a summary of the hospital care when available, but may start when the patient returns to the general practice. At that time, the initial recording documentation needs a minimum of the following:

◆ Health history, radiographs interpretation, extra- and intraoral findings, and vital signs.

◆ Comprehensive periodontal examination and summary of current needs.

◆ Risk factors and dental caries review; complete examination for demineralization.

◆ Care planning for maintenance.

◆ A sample progress note is available for review in Box 56-3.

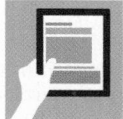

BOX 56-3

Example Documentation:
Postsurgical Dental Hygiene Appointment

S—A 20-year-old college student presents for first dental hygiene appointment following a mandibular fracture due to a motorcycle accident. Stabilizing interdental wiring and fixed splint were removed yesterday. Patient's chief complaint is "My mouth feels dirty and it smells bad." Past medical history: Patient admits to smoking a pack of cigarettes a day and an occasional beer on the weekends; otherwise unremarkable.

O—Healthy looking young male in no obvious distress. Oral cavity is remarkable for heavy dental biofilm and calculus buildup; tissues are inflamed, bleeding, and edematous. No pocket depths greater than 4 mm were charted. Mandibular fracture appeared completely healed.

A—A 20-year-old male status postwire removal from motorcycle accident with poor oral hygiene.

P—Complete periodontal debridement × 4 quadrants, and polishing; detailed oral hygiene instructions; tobacco cessation education; 4-week follow-up to assess healing and patient compliance to oral care instructions and success with tobacco cessation.

Signed: _____, RDH

Date: _____

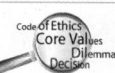

EVERYDAY ETHICS

Ms. Squires (age 79 years) was involved in a serious automobile accident that fractured her mandible and required fixation with intermaxillary wiring, which was recently removed. Apparently she is here because of pressure from her adult children who have been taking turns tending to her needs. The daughter who accompanied her to this appointment said her bad breath was bothering them even more than her complaining all the time.

This is her first appointment with William, the dental hygienist, since the accident 10 months ago. He documented the moderate amounts of calculus and heavy dental biofilm throughout the mouth. Mrs. Squires demonstrates difficulty opening her mouth and seems fussy and apprehensive when William attempts to go over a toothbrushing procedure and continually asks her to "open wider, please."

Questions for Consideration

1. Which of the dental hygiene core values (Section II) become involved with a patient with such complications? Explain each one.

2. Review the steps for decision making in Chapter 1 to help plan and present optimal oral health services to benefit this patient.

3. Describe the role of the dental hygienist in coordinating preventive care with the posttreatment examinations Mrs. Squires has with the oral maxillofacial surgeon.

Factors to Teach the Patient

Accident Prevention

▶ Always use seat belts in automobiles and other vehicles.

▶ Use mouthguards and all safety devices during contact sports.

▶ Wear motorcycle and bicycle helmets.

▶ Helmets protect against facial injuries in totality and appear to be more effective at preventing midfacial fractures when compared with mandible fractures.[14]

For the Patient Who Will Have General Surgery

▶ Significance of a clean mouth during general anesthesia.

▶ Postsurgery oral problems related to specific diseases.

ENHANCE YOUR UNDERSTANDING

ONLINE RESOURCES
(see the inside front cover for access information)
- Audio glossary
- Appendices

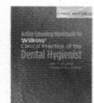

SUPPORT FOR LEARNING
(available separately)
- *Active Learning Workbook for Wilkins' Clinical Practice of the Dental Hygienist, 13th Edition*

INDIVIDUALIZED REVIEW
- Customized practice quizzing with Navigate 2 TestPrep for *Wilkins' Clinical Practice of the Dental Hygienist*

References

1. American Dental Association. Specialty definitions. http://www.ada.org/en/education-careers/careers-in-dentistry/dental-specialties/specialty-definitions. Accessed April 20, 2018.

2. Ferneini EM, Goldberg MH. Management of oral and maxillofacial infections. *J Oral Maxillofac Surg.* 2018;76(3):469-473.

3. Carter JB, Stone JD, Clark RS, Mercer JE. Applications of cone-beam computed tomography in oral and maxillofacial surgery: an overview of published indications and clinical usage in United States Academic Centers and Oral and Maxillofacial Surgery Practices. *J Oral Maxillofac Surg.* 2016;74(4):668-679.

4. Deeb G, Antonos L, Tack S, Carolein C, Laskin D, Deeb JG. Is cone-beam computed tomography always necessary for dental implant placement? *J Oral Maxillofac Surg.* 2017;75(2):285-289.

5. Prajapati A, Prajapati A, Sathaye S. Benefits of not prescribing prophylactic antibiotics after third molar surgery. *J Oral Maxillofac Oral Surg.* 2016;15(2):217-220.

6. Pasupathy S, Alexander M. Antibiotic prophylaxis in third molar surgery. *J Craniofac Surg.* 2011;22(2):551-553.

7. Chuong R. Perioperative management of the surgical patient. In: Peterson LJ, ed. *Oral and Maxillofacial Surgery.* Philadelphia, PA: Lippincott; 1992:63-85.

8. Dowell D, Haegerich TM, Chou R. CDC guideline for prescribing opioids for chronic pain—United States, 2016. *JAMA.* 2016; 315(15):1624-1645.

9. Haskell R. Applied surgical anatomy. In: Rowe NL, Williams JL, eds. *Maxillofacial Injuries.* London: Churchill Livingstone; 1985:21-24.

10. Bell RB. Contemporary management of mandibular fractures. In: *Peterson's Principals of Oral and Maxillofacial Surgery.* Philadelphia, PA: Lippincott; 2011:407-439

11. Banks P, Brown A. Treatment of fractures of the mandible. In: *Fractures of the Facial Skeleton.* Oxford: Wright; 2001:81-106.

12. Boyne PJ. Bone grafts. In: *Boyne and Peetz's Osseous Reconstruction of the Maxilla and the Mandible.* Chicago, IL: Quintessence; 1997:64-74.

13. Phelps-Sandall BA, Oxford SJ. Effectiveness of oral hygiene techniques on plaque and gingivitis in patients placed in intermaxillary fixation. *Oral Surg Oral Med Oral Pathol.* 1983; 56(5):487-490.

14. Christian JM, Thomas RF, Scarbecz M. The incidence and pattern of maxillofacial injuries in helmeted versus non helmeted motorcycle accident patients. *J Oral Maxillofac Surg.* 2014;72(12):2503-2506.

57

The Patient with a Seizure Disorder

Sharon M. Grisanti, RDH, BA, MCOH

CHAPTER OUTLINE

SEIZURES
I. Seizure Definition
II. Classification of Seizures
III. Diagnosis of a Seizure
IV. Types of Seizures
V. Etiology
VI. Prognosis
VII. Implications

CLINICAL MANIFESTATIONS
I. Precipitating Factors and Trigger Signs
II. Aura
III. Prevention of Seizure Injuries

TREATMENT
I. Medications
II. Surgery
III. Ketogenic Diet

ORAL FINDINGS
I. Effects of Accidents with Seizures
II. Gingival Overgrowth/Gingival Hyperplasia

DENTAL HYGIENE CARE PLAN
I. Patient History
II. Information to Obtain
III. Patient Approach
IV. Care Plan: Instrumentation
V. Care Plan: Prevention

EMERGENCY CARE
I. Objectives
II. Differential Diagnosis of Seizure
III. Preparation for Appointment
IV. Emergency Procedure
V. Postictal Phase
VI. Status Epilepticus

DOCUMENTATION

EVERYDAY ETHICS

FACTORS TO TEACH THE PATIENT

REFERENCES

LEARNING OBJECTIVES

After studying this chapter, the student will be able to:

1. Define each term associated with the type of seizure disorder.

2. Describe the etiology of seizure disorders.

3. Discuss clinical manifestations of seizure disorders.

4. Develop a dental hygiene care plan, including patient education prevention strategies, for working with patients with seizure disorders.

5. Prepare an emergency care protocol for a patient having a seizure.

INTRODUCTION

A seizure is a paroxysmal event resulting from abnormal brain activity. A seizure may involve loss of consciousness or awareness or impaired awareness with or without convulsive movements or spasms. Epilepsy is a term to describe a group of functional disorders of the brain characterized by recurrent seizures. Seizures are a symptom of epilepsy.

- The patient's medical history may reveal susceptibility to seizures. A complete evaluation is required prior to treatment.
- Treatment modalities of epilepsy and a seizure itself may affect the oral tissues as well as dental and dental hygiene treatment.
- Dental personnel need to be aware of the issues associated with seizures, know how to evaluate the patient, and how to apply emergency measures in and out of the dental office or clinic.
- Care of the oral cavity is necessary due to its relationship to overall health and to oral accidents that may occur during a seizure.
- All patients should consult their physicians regarding exercise and lifestyle.
- Occupation and lifestyle may be limited for patients who have recurrent seizures. A person susceptible to seizures cannot participate in activities that may precipitate a seizure such as driving or operating machinery. Such limitations may lead to depression.
- According to the Center for Disease Control, there are approximately 3.4 million adults and 470,000 children in the United States who have recurrent seizures associated with epilepsy. The World Health Organization estimates more than 50 million people worldwide have epilepsy.[1-4]
- New cases are most commonly found in children and in older adults.

SEIZURES

I. Seizure Definition

- An epileptic seizure is a transient occurrence of signs and symptoms due to abnormal neuronal activity in the brain.
- Epilepsy is a disease of the brain and a seizure is a symptom of the disease.
- Onset defines where the seizure begins in the brain.
- Unknown onset seizures mean the beginning of the seizure was unknown or was not witnessed by another person.
- Patient may have impaired awareness or be fully aware of their surroundings. Special care must be taken with impaired awareness seizures relating to the safety of the patient.
- Seizures are generally unprovoked and involuntary, but triggers may precipitate an epileptic seizure.
- A seizure begins with an abrupt onset of symptoms that may be of a motor, sensory, cognitive, or emotional nature, depending on which cells or part of the brain is involved.

- Non-movement during a seizure is considered nonmotor.
- As a seizure progresses, it may or may not cause loss of consciousness or awareness, tonic and/or clonic movements, incontinence, saliva foaming, or tongue biting.
- Length of a seizure is uncontrollable.
- Other terms: convulsion, fit, spell, ictus.

II. Classification of Seizures

The syndromes associated with seizures are complex. A summary of the classification of seizures is outlined in Table 57-1.[5,6]

TABLE 57-1 • Classifications of Seizure Types

CLASSIFICATIONS	DEFINITION	SEIZURE TYPES

Focal Onset
• Aware
• Impaired awareness
	Involving one side of the brain
	• Aware
	  • patient aware of surroundings and self
	  • able to recall events of seizure
	• Impaired awareness
	  • Patient is confused of surroundings
		Motor Onset
		• Spasms
		• Epileptic
		• **Automatisms**
		• Atonic
		• Clonic
		• Hyperkinetic
		• **Myoclonic**
		• Tonic
		Nonmotor Onset
		• Sensory
		• Emotional
		• **Autonomic**
		• **Behavior arrest**
		• Cognitive
		Focal to bilateral
		• Tonic-clonic

Generalized Onset • Impaired awareness	Affecting both sides of the brain • Impaired awareness • Patient is confused of surroundings	Motor • **Epileptic spasms** • Clonic • Tonic • Tonic-clonic • Myoclonic • Myoclonic-tonic-clonic • Myoclonic-atonic • Atonic Nonmotor (absence) • Eyelid myoclonic • Typical • **Atypical** • Myoclonic
Unknown Onset	Start of seizure is unknown • Seizure not witnessed	Motor Tonic-clonic Epileptic spasms Nonmotor Behavior arrest Unclassified

Source: Adapted from Epilepsy Foundation. Types of seizures. March 20, 2017. Available from https://www.epilepsy.com/learn/types-seizures

III. Diagnosis of a Seizure

◆ Clinical signs and symptoms:
  • A patient with a complex seizure disorder may exhibit a trance-like state with confusion that can last for a few minutes to hours.
  • Consciousness is impaired to varying degrees.
  • Patient may manifest purposeless movements or actions followed by confusion, incoherent speech, ill humor, unpleasant temper; does not remember what happened during the attack.
◆ History:
  • Medical history is the first step in the diagnosis of epilepsy seizures.
  • Documentation of initial onset and preliminary factors that led up to the seizure should be noted.
◆ Electroencephalography (EEG):
  • EEG shows patterns of normal and abnormal brain activity. This test can reveal slowing in rhythm due to trauma, stroke, brain tumor, or seizures.
◆ Type and symptoms:
  • Severity.
  • Age-related onset.
  • Cause.
  • Inherited and genetic.
  • EEG patterns and part of brain involved.

IV. Types of Seizures

◆ Seizures have three basic types, generalized, focal, and those of unknown onset.[5] The type depends on where and how the seizure begins in the brain.
  • Generalized onset affects both sides of the brain. Examples are tonic-clonic, absence or atonic seizures.
  • Focal onset begins in one area or group of cells of the brain. Examples are focal onset aware and focal onset impaired awareness.[5]

A. Generalized Onset Seizures

◆ Motor Category[5,6]:
  • Affecting both sides of the brain at the same time.
  • Tonic-clonic known as convulsive or grand mal seizures.
  • Muscles of the chest and pharynx may contract at the same time, forcing air out and a sound known as the "epileptic cry."
  • Loss of consciousness or awareness is sudden and complete; the patient becomes stiff and falls or may slide out of the dental chair.
  • Musculature contraction: with tonic phase body becomes rigid, with clonic phase there is intermittent muscular contraction and relaxation.
  • Atonic refers to weakened muscles.
  • Skin color turns pale to bluish, breathing is shallow or stops briefly.
  • Possible loss of bladder, and rarely, bowel control.
  • Tongue may be bitten.

  • Incident usually lasts 1–3 minutes.
  • Respiration returns.
  • Saliva, which previously could not be swallowed, may mix with air and appears foamy.
  • Patient begins to recover, may be confused, tired, complain of muscle soreness or injury; falls into a deep sleep.
  • Phases of seizures are aura, ictus, and postictal.
  • Seizure may continue without recovery and progress to *status epilepticus*, meaning lasting more than 5 minutes or experiencing two more seizures within a 5-minute period.
◆ Nonmotor or Absence Seizure[5,6]:
  • Previously known as petit mal.
  • Loss of consciousness or awareness begins and ends abruptly in about 5–30 seconds.
  • Most common in children, and may lead to learning difficulties if not identified.
  • Patient has a blank stare, usually does not fall, posture becomes fixed, may drop whatever is being held.
  • May become pale.
  • Myoclonus may occur: patient may have rhythmic twitching of the eyelids, eyebrows, head, or chewing movements.
  • Attack ends as abruptly as it begins. Patient quickly returns to full awareness, resumes activities, unaware of what occurred.

B. Focal Onset Seizures

◆ Focal seizures start with one group of cells in one part of the brain. Focal onset aware means patient is aware during the seizure.
◆ Focal onset impaired awareness means the patient is confused.

C. Unknown Onset Seizures

◆ Start of seizures is unknown.
◆ Seizure has not been witnessed.[5]
  Unclassified seizures may be classified once additional information has been brought to the neurologist's attention.

V. Etiology

In addition to epilepsy, seizures can be a symptom of many different conditions. The causes can be genetic, structural/metabolic, or unknown.[7]

A. Genetic

Genetic predisposition to seizures or to other neurologic abnormalities for which the seizure may be a symptom.

B. Structural/Metabolic

Seizures can arise during many neurologic and non-neurologic medical conditions, for example:
◆ Congenital conditions, such as maternal infection (rubella); toxemia of pregnancy.
◆ Maternal drug use.
◆ Perinatal injuries.

◆ Brain tumor.

◆ Cerebrovascular disease (stroke).

◆ Trauma (head injury).

◆ Infection (meningitis, encephalitis, opportunistic infections of human immunodeficiency virus).

◆ Degenerative brain disease.

◆ Metabolic and toxic disorders, including lead exposure, alcoholism, and other drug addictions; seizures are common during alcohol and/or drug withdrawal.

◆ Complication of cancer.

C. Unknown Cause

◆ The onset and cause of the epileptic seizure are unknown.

◆ A neurologic examination may diagnose the reason.

VI. Prognosis

◆ Prognosis for seizure control is favorable.

◆ Epilepsy Foundation reports that 56% of adults with epilepsy have uncontrolled seizures.

◆ Of the 90% of patients taking antiepileptic (antiseizure) drug (AED), only 44% have controlled seizures.

◆ The prevalence of seizures and seizure control increases with low family income.[8]

VII. Implications

Due to the possibility of severe injury, accidents, or embarrassment, patients who experience recurrent seizures may avoid or be legally restricted from certain activities: These may include:

◆ *Vocation*: occupations that involve use of machinery or require physical activity.

◆ *Licenses*: certain licenses, such as driver's license, may be restricted until the patient is seizure free.

◆ *Independent living*: assisted living may be advised.

CLINICAL MANIFESTATIONS

I. Precipitating Factors and Trigger Signs

The patient or caregiver can provide helpful information to prepare dental personnel in the management of an emergency. Triggers may occur frequently and are in response to specific stimuli. The dental hygienist should be prepared to eliminate or minimize these stimuli. Factors that may precipitate a seizure include[9–11]:

◆ Flashing/bright lights or noises.

◆ Stressor apprehension.

◆ Fatigue; sleep deprivation.

◆ A specific time of the day.

◆ Alcohol or drug use.

◆ Fever.

◆ Not eating resulting in low blood sugar.

◆ Noncompliance with antiseizure medications.

◆ Menstruation.

◆ Physical exercise/physical trauma.

II. Aura

◆ An aura can be described as a sensory stimulus, a visual disturbance, numbness, tingling, twitching, or stiffness of muscles.

◆ Not all patients have warning signs, or auras, before a seizure.

◆ A patient experiencing a warning may seek a safe place to sit or lie down.

◆ In the dental environment, the patient may inform the personnel so dental procedures can be terminated and preparations made.

III. Prevention of Seizure Injuries

A patient may experience more than one type of seizure. The primary method to control and prevent seizures is through antiepileptic drugs (AEDs). The injuries associated with seizures may be prevented through modification of behaviors[12]:

◆ Primary prevention of seizure injuries focuses on medication compliance, avoiding brain injury through the use of protective measures such as helmets, and mouth guards.

◆ Secondary prevention includes early detection, recognition, and preparation of the seizure.

◆ Tertiary prevention comprises training and education strategies for patients, teachers, caregivers, and health care practitioners.

TREATMENT

I. Medications

AEDs are the primary method used to prevent and control seizures.[13–15]

A. Choices

◆ Patients may be placed on one or a combination of AEDs.

◆ Choice of therapy is aligned to the type of seizure and desired side effect or the elimination of an undesirable side effect.

◆ Frequently prescribed medications are listed in Table 57-2.

B. Side Effects

◆ *Each* medication has side effects a patient may experience to varying degrees. It is imperative for patients to follow directions for the use of antiseizure medications from their primary care provider.

TABLE 57-2 • Antiepileptic Medications

GENERIC NAME	BRAND NAME
Carbamazepine	Tegretol, Carbatrol
Clonapam	Klonopin
Clorazepate	Tranxene
Ethosuximide	Zarontin
Felbamate	Felbatol
Gabapentin	Neurontin
Lamotrigine	Lamictal
Levetiracetam	Keppra
Oxcarbazepine	Trileptal
Phenobarbital	Luminal
Phenytoin	Dilantin
Primidone	Mysoline
Tiagabine	Gabitril
Topiramate	Topamax
Valproic acid/Valproate	Depakote
Zonisamide	Zonegran

◆ Side effects may include the following:
  • Allergic reaction, rash.
  • Fatigue, dizziness, drowsiness, weakness, ataxia, headache, slurred speech, blurred vision.
  • Nausea, vomiting.
  • Memory loss; behavioral and cognitive deficits.
  • Damage to the pancreas, liver, interactions of medications processed in the liver.
  • Leukopenia: delayed healing and infection.
  • Thrombocytopenia or decreased platelet aggregation: increased bleeding, petechiae.
  • Osteoporosis.
  • Increased or unknown risk of birth defects.
  • Hirsutism; hypertrichosis or excessive hair growth.
  • Gingival hyperplasia, gingival enlargement, is most common with phenytoin.
  • Numerous drug interactions, including other AEDs, acetaminophen, nonsteroidal anti-inflammatory drugs, erythromycins, and reduction in the efficacy of *oral contraceptives*.
◆ *Elderly and children*
  • Both age groups are more sensitive to side effects such as weakness, unsteadiness, and cognitive alterations.
  • Elderly are more likely to be on other medications with possible drug interactions and may forget to take medications.

C. Precaution: Herbal Supplements

◆ Certain over-the-counter herbal supplements are used as self-medications to help prevent seizures. These supplements may interfere with the prescribed AED.
◆ Herbal supplements have not been shown to effectively treat epileptic seizures and may make seizures worse.[16,17]
◆ Patients are asked to inform their primary care provider and dental team when using alternate forms of medication.
◆ Herbal supplements such as ginkgo biloba, St. John's wart, and some essential oils may also affect dental treatment, for example, causing increased bleeding.

II. Surgery

A variety of surgical interventions are available and indicated when epilepsy is refractory to traditional AED therapy. Surgical intervention has become more precise through advances in identifying the epileptogenic area with magnetic resonance imaging, tomography, electroencephalographic studies, neuropsychological testing, and other analyses. Surgical options include:
◆ *Lobe resection* of the epileptogenic area in the brain.[18,19]
◆ If total resection leads to unacceptable deficits, *multiple subpial transections*, which are a series of small parallel slices, are removed. *Gamma-knife radiosurgery* involves delivery of a focused dose of radiation to the epileptogenic area in the brain. This technique reduces the risk of infection, bleeding, and hospitalization.[20]
◆ Vagus nerve stimulation utilizes a pacemaker-like device to deliver signals to the vagus nerve known to reduce seizure activity without adverse effects to the patient.[21]

III. Ketogenic Diet

The goal of the ketogenic diet is to induce fat metabolism through ketosis by maintaining a diet high in fat and low in carbohydrates.
◆ The diet has been shown to be an effective treatment for patients with epilepsy, particularly children.[22,23]

ORAL FINDINGS

Epilepsy in itself produces no oral changes.
◆ Specific oral changes are related to:
  • Side effects of AEDs.
  • Oral accidents during a seizure.
  • Side effects of the epilepsy, such as depression leading to poor oral hygiene and neglect.[24]

I. Effects of Accidents with Seizures

A. Scars of Lips and Tongue

◆ Oral tissues, particularly tongue, cheek, or lip, may be bitten.

◆ Scars may be observed during the extraoral/intraoral examination; cause may be differentiated from other types of healed wounds.

B. Fractured Teeth

◆ Clenching and bruxing may be forceful enough to fracture teeth.

◆ Fractured teeth may be sharp, lacerate tissue and need to be smoothed or restored.

◆ Fractures may extend into the pulp of the tooth, allowing bacterial infection; requiring root canal therapy or extraction.

II. Gingival Overgrowth/Gingival Hyperplasia

◆ Gingival overgrowth occurs in 25–50% of persons using phenytoin for treatment.

◆ Phenytoin and other antiseizure drugs have been used in the treatment of other conditions besides epilepsy, including stuttering, headaches, neuromuscular disturbances, and cardiac conditions; therefore, their use should not lead to the assumption that the patient has epilepsy.

◆ Other antiseizure drugs can induce gingival overgrowth but less frequently.

◆ Other terms for gingival enlargement in the use of phenytoin may be referred to as Dilantin hyperplasia, diphenylhydantoin-induced hyperplasia, diphenylhydantoin gingival hyperplasia, Dilantin-induced gingival fibrosis, or phenytoin-induced hyperplasia.[25–27]

A. Mechanism

◆ Phenytoin may cause fibroblasts and osteoblasts to deposit excessive extracellular matrix, causing gingival overgrowth.

◆ Tissue color and texture are generally within normal limits with interdental papilla taking on a lobular shape.

◆ Local irritants such as biofilm, faulty restorations, or ill-fitting appliances cause a more exaggerated tissue response.

◆ Meticulous oral hygiene has been found to reduce the occurrence and severity of gingival overgrowth.

B. Occurrence

◆ Incidence is greater in younger patients just beginning drug therapy.

◆ The gingiva may start to enlarge within a few weeks or even after a few years following initial administration of drug therapy.

◆ The size of the dose and length of treatment are not necessarily factors in the incidence or nature of the gingival enlargement.

◆ The anterior gingivae are more likely affected than posterior, and the maxillary more than the mandibular arch.

◆ Facial and proximal areas are more affected than lingual or palatal areas.

◆ Although rare, an overgrowth of tissue may occur in an edentulous area. This is usually associated with trauma, irritation from a denture, the presence of retained roots, or unerupted teeth.[28,29]

◆ Overgrowth of tissue surrounding dental implants may occur.[30]

C. Effects

◆ Control of dental biofilm may be a problem.

◆ May affect mastication.

◆ May alter tooth eruption.

◆ May interfere with speech.

◆ May cause serious esthetic concerns.[31]

D. Tissue Characteristics

◆ *Early clinical features*:
  • Overgrowth appears as a painless enlargement of interdental papillae with signs of inflammation (Figure 57-1A).

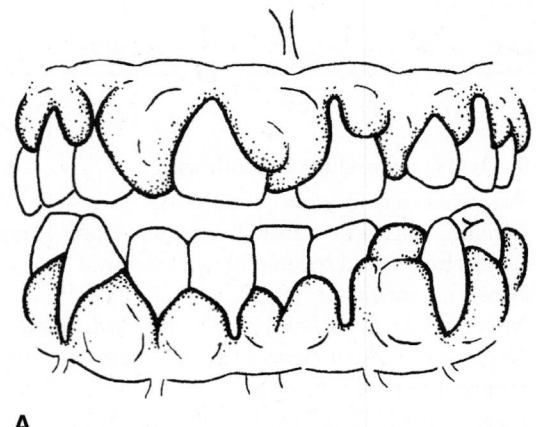

A

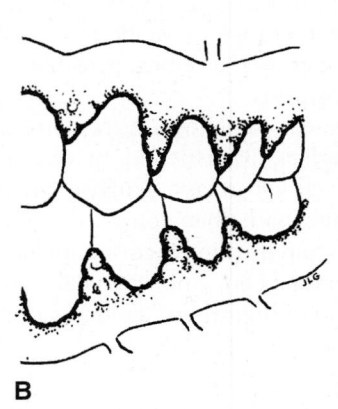

B

FIGURE 57-1 • Phenytoin-Induced Gingival Enlargement. A: Papillary enlargement with cleft-like grooves. Note the effect of the pressure of the fibrotic tissue on the position of teeth. Maxillary incisors and the mandibular left canine have been wedged away from normal positions. **B:** Mulberry-like shape of interdental papillae.

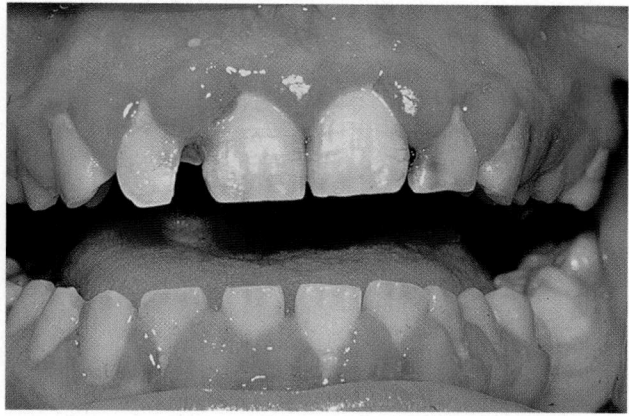

FIGURE 57-2 • Phenytoin-Induced Gingival Overgrowth. (Dr. James Cottone.)

- Eventually, the tissue becomes fibrotic, pink, and stippled, with a mulberry or cauliflower-like appearance, as in Figure 57-1B.
- *Advanced lesion*:
  - Tissue increases in size, extends to include the marginal gingiva, and covers a large portion of the anatomic crown.
  - Cleft-like grooves may occur between the lobules.
- *Severe lesion*:
  - Large, bulbous gingiva may cover the enamel, tend to wedge the teeth apart, and interfere with mastication and oral self-care (Figure 57-2).
- *Microscopic appearance*:
  - During therapy, phenytoin is present in the saliva, blood, gingival sulcus fluid, and dental biofilm.
  - Number of fibroblasts and the amount of collagen in connective tissue increase.
  - Stratified squamous epithelium is thick, with long rete ridges.
  - Inflammatory cells are in greatest abundance near the base of pockets.

E. Complicating Factors

- Dental biofilm:
  - Biofilm appears to be the most significant determinant in the severity of phenytoin-induced gingival enlargement.[32]
  - Adequate biofilm control, particularly if started prior to the administration of phenytoin, helps control the extent of gingival overgrowth.
- Contributing factors:
  - Mouth breathing.
  - Overhanging and defective restorations.
  - Malocclusion.
  - Large carious lesions.
  - Calculus and biofilm retention encourages gingival overgrowth.
  - Treatment should include removal of contributing factors by recontouring overhangs, placing or replacing restorations, effective biofilm and calculus removal.

F. Treatment

There are varying ways to treat gingival enlargement based on the medication used and clinical presentation of lesions.

- Change in seizure medication:
  - Collaboration with the primary care physician should be integrated into the treatment plan.
  - Change to a different drug with a lower chance of causing gingival enlargement.
- Medication change should be just prior to a surgical removal procedure.[33]
- Nonsurgical treatment:
  - Periodontal debridement along with strict biofilm control may help early lesions regress.
  - Where the tissue has become fibrotic, shrinkage cannot be expected.
  - Initiate prevention of biofilm control prior to, or simultaneously with, initial administration of the antiepileptic medication.
  - The use of 0.12% chlorhexidine gluconate rinses is linked to positive outcomes to prevent return of gingival enlargement caused by antiseizure medication.[34,35]
- Surgical removal:
  - *Gingivectomy*: A surgical procedure used for tissue removal when a sufficient band of attached gingiva exists.
  - A *periodontal flap procedure*: may be the choice for healing and esthetics.
  - Prior to surgery, a regulated program of biofilm control is introduced and continued after surgical dressings have been removed.
  - General health has special significance, and oral health contributes to general health.
  - Meticulous oral hygiene is required to minimize gingival overgrowth.

G. Differential Diagnosis of Medications Causing Gingival Enlargement

Numerous medications may cause gingival enlargement, including:

- Antiseizure medications, especially phenytoin and to a lesser extent ethosuximide, valproic acid, and primidone.[36,37]
- Calcium channel blockers used for the treatment of hypertension such as nifedipine, verapamil, and diltiazem.
- Immunosuppressant cyclosporine used frequently with organ transplant patients. Tacrolimus may be a substitute with less occurrence of gingival overgrowth.

DENTAL HYGIENE CARE PLAN

- The majority of patients with epilepsy or a history of seizures can and need to receive the same level of dental care as the general population.[38]

- Interprofessional collaboration plays an important role in the development of the dental hygiene care plan.
  - The patient with a seizure disorder may be under the care of other specialists including a neurologist, social worker, and primary care physician.

I. Patient History

- Most patients with epilepsy have regular, thorough medical examinations.
- Contact the primary care provider when the patient or caregiver is unable to provide needed information, is noncompliant, if seizure activity has increased or changed, or if treatment for epilepsy is impacting the patient's oral health.
- Patients with autism may present with social, communication, and/or behavioral problems, in addition to seizure disturbances.[39,40]
- A well-controlled patient with epilepsy may still be at risk to have a seizure.
- For seizure-prone patients: advise wearing medical alert jewelry.

II. Information to Obtain

Information to obtain from a patient with a history of seizures is listed in Box 57-1.

III. Patient Approach

- Provide a calm, reassuring atmosphere and treat with patience and empathy.
- Use a motivational interviewing approach to patient education, enabling patients to be partners in the decision-making process (see Chapter 24).
- Encourage self-expression, particularly if the patient tends to be quiet and withdrawn or has a narrow range of interests.
- Recognize possible impairment of memory when reviewing personal oral care procedures.
- Help the patient develop an interest in caring for the mouth, providing positive reinforcement for patient successes.
- Medications used for treatment of seizures may make the patient drowsy, and chronic illness sufferers tend to have more frequent health issues that interfere with appointments.
- Be understanding when the patient is late or misses an appointment; confirm with telephone reminders at opportune time; do not mistake drowsiness (effect of drugs) for inattentiveness.

IV. Care Plan: Instrumentation

- Patients should be considered an integral part in their daily oral health maintenance.
- All patients need to be instructed and motivated to comply with an effective biofilm control program.

BOX 57-1

Risk Assessment for Dental Hygiene Treatment:
Information to Obtain from Patient with a History of a Seizure Disorder

Basic Information:
- Thorough medical history review, including date of last physical examination, other medical conditions or risk factors present.
- Physician: name and phone number.
- Emergency contact person with phone number.

Additional Factors:
- Inquire about recent illness, stress, alcohol use, menstrual cycle, fatigue, or pain as factors that may provoke a seizure.
- General well-being; refer for evaluation if patient presents with signs or symptoms of other conditions such as depression.
- Ask if the patient has changed any aspect of their activities of daily living.

Treatment:
- Medication list, surgery, or diet.
- Effectiveness of seizure control treatment.
- Investigate each medication for possible interaction with the proposed dental treatment and side effects.
- Nonprescription, herbal supplement use.
- Medication compliance.

About the Seizures:
- Type of seizure(s) experienced, frequency, severity, and duration of episodes.
- Age at onset.
- The precipitating/trigger factors or cause of seizure if known.
- Description of prodrome, aura if known.
- Experience alteration or loss of consciousness.
- Characteristic motor movements.
- Urinary/fecal incontinence.
- History of injuries, including oral injuries, broken teeth, tongue lacerations.
- Postictal symptoms such as confusion.

Suggestions:
- Any other helpful information that the patient can provide for prevention, comfort, and management.

- Complete removal of all deposits on teeth, and thorough nonsurgical periodontal therapy is essential for patients who plan to or are taking an antiseizure medication such as phenytoin, which may cause gingival overgrowth.

A. Prior to and at the Start of Phenytoin Therapy

◆ A rigorous biofilm control program and complete periodontal debridement are needed in preparation for phenytoin therapy.

◆ The patient (and caregivers) should be guided in oral hygiene maintenance, emphasizing preventing or minimizing gingival overgrowth with effective biofilm management.

B. Initial Appointment Series for the Patient Treated with Phenytoin

Weekly appointments for complete biofilm control instruction and debridement are planned with the following objectives:

1. *Slight or mild gingival overgrowth.*
   - Nonsurgical treatment, including frequent thorough debridement, may lead to tissue reduction, provided the patient maintains daily biofilm control.
   - Frequent continuing care appointments can contribute to more appealing esthetics, function, and comfort with minimum periodontal involvement.
2. *Moderate gingival overgrowth.*
   - After the initial series of biofilm instruction and debridement, reevaluation of the gingival tissues will determine whether further treatment is needed.
   - An optimal level of oral health may be attained by changing the medication to another antiseizure drug, surgical removal of excess tissue, and more frequent continuing care appointments.
3. *Severe fibrotic overgrowth.*
   - Initial nonsurgical periodontal therapy and biofilm control should be provided in preparation for surgical gingival tissue removal.
   - Consultation with the primary care provider may be indicated for modifying a drug or altering the dose to limit gingival overgrowth.

C. Continuing Care Intervals

◆ Frequent appointments on 1-, 2-, or 3-month intervals may be indicated, depending on the severity of gingival enlargement as well as the ability and motivation of the patient in maintaining their oral health.

◆ Most patients need ongoing assistance and supervision.

V. Care Plan: Prevention

◆ Daily biofilm removal and fluoride therapy, the use of pit and fissure sealants, and dietary control.

◆ Initiation of preventive measures as soon as possible after epilepsy has been diagnosed contributes to the overall health and well-being.

EMERGENCY CARE

I. Objectives

1. Prevent body injury and accidents related to the oral structures, such as:
   - Tongue bite.
   - Broken or dislocated teeth.
   - Dislocated or fractured jaw.
   - Broken fixed or removable dentures.[41–43]
2. Ensure adequate ventilation.

II. Differential Diagnosis of Seizure

Other diseases or conditions with similar signs or symptoms include[44]:

◆ Syncope.

◆ Migraine headache.

◆ Transient ischemic attack.

◆ Cerebrovascular accident, stroke.

◆ Sleep disorder such as narcolepsy.

◆ Movement disorders such as dyskinesia, common, for example, in patients with cerebral palsy or multiple sclerosis.

◆ Overdose of local anesthetic.

◆ Hypoglycemia or insulin overdose in a patient with diabetes.

◆ Hyperventilation.

III. Preparation for Appointment

When the patient's medical history indicates susceptibility to seizures, advance preparation may prevent complications should a seizure occur.

◆ Place emergency materials in a convenient location.

◆ Have the patient remove dentures for the duration of the appointment.

◆ Provide a calm and reassuring atmosphere.

◆ Have other dental personnel available in case of an emergency.

IV. Emergency Procedure

Seizures are short lived. The dental clinic team should assign responsibilities during an emergency. Initiation of procedures for seizure emergency follows preplanned routines.

◆ Make no attempt to stop the convulsion or restrain patient.

◆ Terminate the clinical procedure; call for assistance.

◆ Protect patient from injury.
   - Position patient: lower chair and tilt to supine; raise feet.
   - Keep patient from falling out of the dental chair.
   - Push aside sharp objects, movable equipment, and instrument trays.
   - Loosen tight belt, collar, and necktie.
   - Do *not* place (or force) anything between the teeth.
   - Establish airway; check for breathing obstruction; provide basic life support when indicated. Place on side recovery position. Use high-speed suction with wide tip to remove vomit.
   - Monitor vital signs.
   - Stay beside the patient to prevent personal injury and reassure.

- Check for the level of consciousness and determine if emergency medical assistance is required.
- When a seizure is still occurring or has recurred within 5 minutes, activate emergency medical system.

V. Postictal Phase

◆ Document the emergency situation as described in Chapter 9.

◆ Allow the patient to rest.

◆ Talk to the patient in a quiet, reassuring tone.

◆ Check oral cavity for trauma to teeth or tissues. Palliative care can be administered. When a tooth is broken, the piece must be located so aspiration can be prevented.

◆ With patient's consent, contact the patient's family/friend to accompany the patient.

VI. Status Epilepticus

◆ Status epilepticus is when a seizure lasts longer than 5 minutes or when seizures occur close together without recovery.

◆ There are two types, convulsive and nonconvulsive.

◆ Prolonged seizure may result in brain injury and long-term morbidity or death.

◆ Emergency medical assistance is notified immediately, and the patient is transported to an emergency department.

◆ Basic life support is provided if necessary (see Chapter 9).

DOCUMENTATION

The patient who is subject to seizures will need complete permanent records indicating the following:

◆ Complete health history, vital signs, radiographs, findings of extra- and intraoral examination; periodontal history, charting, and tissue description; dental caries history, charting, and current demineralization and carious lesions.

◆ Progress notes for each appointment with abbreviated history and current clinical findings.

◆ Information about the type of seizure; the treatment patient is receiving; and what steps to take in the event of an emergency.

◆ A sample progress note may be reviewed in Box 57-2.

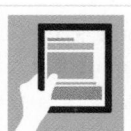

BOX 57-2

Example Documentation:
Patient with a Seizure Disorder

S—Steve, a healthy appearing 55-year-old man, presents for the first of four scheduled periodontal scaling appointments. He stated he recently had a seizure at work when his arms and legs stiffen and he felt confused.

When pressed for more information, he stated that he had seen a physician for the seizure. He also states he will be losing his job in 1 month and has started looking for another.

O—Vitals normal (see medical profile). No chief complaint, other than being upset due to impending job loss. Reassessed medical profile—added Tegretol; no other medications are taken. Noticed rash on the left side of the patient's neck. Patient stated the rash began when antiseizure medication was added. Contacted physician for advice on patient care post-seizure; physician recommended longer appointments to account for frequent breaks during treatment and for patient to call concerning rash. Intraoral assessment reveals generalized 4–5 mm pocketing on posterior teeth. No gingival enlargement found.

A—Increased risk for potential emergency situation during appointment until seizure disorder is stabilized. Need for use of stress-reduction protocols and extension of treatment time during patient visit. Potential for side effects of new medication, including current skin rash.

P—Patient Education—Discussed potential side effects of medications for the treatment of seizures. Recommended patient check with the medical provider about skin rash on the neck. Provided patient with information from the Epilepsy Foundation, also on local stress-reduction and exercise classes.

Oral self-care—Discussed need for meticulous oral hygiene to avoid gingival enlargement. Showed patient how to perform an intraoral examination to check for gingival enlargement and possible areas of trauma should he experience another seizure.

Treatment provided—Asked patient to verbalize any discomfort or uneasiness he may have during treatment. Completed debridement with hand and ultrasonic instruments using high-speed evacuation on quadrant one with no adverse reaction to additional sounds or light. Patient tolerated treatment well but required frequent breaks to relax and reduce stress.

Next visit: Assess tissue response to quadrant one debridement; reassess plaque score and home care technique, modify as needed. Assess skin condition and determine whether the patient contacted his physician. Monitor stress-reduction progress.

Signed: _____, RDH

Date: _____

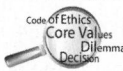

EVERYDAY ETHICS

Lillian, the dental hygienist, just finished treating her last patient of the day. Diana, the patient, is a very pleasant woman with excellent oral health and a history of a car accident with concussion over a month ago. She has no other medical findings. While passing the window, Lillian notices that Diana has collapsed in the parking lot and is convulsing. She calls for assistance from the dentist and dental assistant, and they rush out to the parking lot. By the time they reach Diana, she is getting to her feet and says she just tripped and fell.

Individuals with seizures may have their driver's license revoked because of the potential for serious automobile accidents that may occur during a seizure. Diana is about to get into her car to drive home.

Questions for Consideration

1. Which dental hygiene ethical core values have application in this scenario?

2. Given the patient's medical history, will this information be documented in Diana's dental record, remain confidential, or be otherwise handled? To evaluate one's responsibilities toward self, one's patients, and others, read over the Codes of Ethics professional responsibilities to help Lillian decide the correct procedure.

3. Describe the rights of the patient and professional duties of the dental hygienist who witnessed the incident.

Factors to Teach the Patient

► Relationship of systemic health to oral health.

► Significance of daily biofilm removal.

► Importance of antiepileptic drug compliance.

► Need for providing complete medical history information for dental appointments.

► Antiseizure medication side effects, including gingival enlargement and how to minimize its growth.

► Seek immediate care if any oral change or injury is suspected.

References

1. Azanzini G, Beghi E, de Boer H, Engel J, Sander JW, Wolf P. Epilepsy. In: *Neurological Disorders: Public Health Challenges*. Geneva: World Health Organization; 2006:14. http://www.who.int/mental_health/neurology/chapter_3_a_neuro_disorders_public_h_challenges.pdf. Accessed June 13, 2018.

ENHANCE YOUR UNDERSTANDING

ONLINE RESOURCES
(see the inside front cover for access information)

· Audio glossary

· Appendices

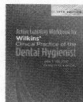

SUPPORT FOR LEARNING
(available separately)

· *Active Learning Workbook for Wilkins' Clinical Practice of the Dental Hygienist, 13th Edition*

INDIVIDUALIZED REVIEW

· Customized practice quizzing with Navigate 2 TestPrep for *Wilkins' Clinical Practice of the Dental Hygienist*

2. Centers for Disease Control and Prevention. National and state estimates or the number of adults and children with active epilepsy—United States, 2015. *MMWR Morb Mortal Wkly Rep.* 2017;66(31);821-825.

3. World Health Organization. *Epilepsy: key facts.* Geneva: World Health Organization; 2018. https://www.who.int/news-room/fact-sheets/detail/epilepsy. Accessed June 13, 2018

4. Centers for Disease Control and Prevention. Epilepsy in adults and access to care—United States, 2010. *MMWR Morb Mortal Wkly Rep.* 2012;61(45):909-913.

5. Fisher RS, Cross JH, French JA, et al. Operational classification of seizure types by the International League Against Epilepsy: Position Paper of the ILAE Commission for Classification and Terminology. *Epilepsia.* 2017;58:522-530.

6. Scheffer IE, Berkovic S, Capovilla G, et al. ILAE classification of epilepsies: Position paper of the ILAE Commission for Classification and Terminology. *Epilepsia.* 2017;58:512-521.

7. Brodie M, de Boer HM, Johannessen SI. Epidemiology. *Epilepsia.* 2003;44(6 suppl):17.

8. Centers for Disease Control and Prevention. Active epilepsy and seizure control in adults—United States, 2013 and 2015. *MMWR Morb Mortal Wkly Rep.* 2018;67(15):437-442.

9. Fattal-Valevski A, Nissan N, Kramer U, Constantini S. Seizures as the clinical presenting symptom in children with brain tumors. *J Child Neurol.* 2012;28(3):292-296.

10. Nakken KO, Solaas MH, Kjeldsen MJ, Friis ML, Pellock JM, Corey LA. Which seizure-precipitating factors do patients with epilepsy most frequently report? *Epilepsy Behav.* 2006;6(1):85-89.

11. Balamurugan E, Aggarwal M, Lamba A, Dang N, Tripathi M. Perceived trigger factors of seizures in persons with epilepsy. *Seizure.* 2013;22(9):743-747.

12. Dua T, Janca A, Kale R, Montero F, Muscetta A, Peden M. Public health principles and neurological disorders. In: *Neurological Disorders: Public Health Challenges*. Geneva: World

Health Organization; 2006:20. http://www.who.int/mental
_health/neurology/chapter1_neuro_disorders_public_h
_challenges.pdf. Accessed June 13, 2018.

13. Schoenberg MR, Frontera AT, Bozorg A, Hernandez-Frau P, Vale F, Benbadis SR. An update on epilepsy. *Expert Rev Neurother.* 2011;11(5):639-645.

14. Guncu G, Caglayan F, Dincel A, Bozkurt A, Saygi S, Karabulut E. Plasma and gingival crevicular fluid phenytoin concentrations as risk factors for gingival overgrowth. *J Periodontol.* 2006;77(12):2005-2010.

15. Burneo JG, McLachlan RS. When should surgery be considered for the treatment of epilepsy? *Can Med Assoc J.* 2005;172(9):1175-1177.

16. Schachter SC. Botanicals and herbs: a traditional approach to treating epilepsy. *Neurotherapeutics.* 2009;6(2):415-420. doi:10.1016/j.nurt.2008.12.004.

17. Li Q, Chen X, He L, Zhou D. Traditional Chinese medicine for epilepsy. *Cochrane Database Syst Rev.* 2009;(3):CD006454.

18. Schmeiser B, Daniel M, Kogias E, et al. Visual field defects following different respective procedures for mesiotemporal lobe epilepsy. *Epilepsy Behav.* 2017;76:39-45.

19. Mohan M, Keller S, Nicolson A, et al. The long-term outcomes of epilepsy surgery. *PLoS One.* 2018;13(5):e0196274.

20. Bates K. Epilepsy: current evidence-based paradigms for diagnosis and treatment. *Prim Care.* 2015;42(2):217-232.

21. Roberts HW. The effect of electrical dental equipment on a vagus nerve stimulator's function. *J Am Dent Assoc.* 2002;133(12):1657-1664.

22. Guerrini R. Epilepsy in children. *Lancet.* 2006;367(9509):499-524.

23. Martin K, Jackson CF, Levy RG, Cooper PN. Ketogenic diet and other dietary treatments for epilepsy. *Cochrane Database Syst Rev.* 2016;2:CD001903.

24. Pette GA, Siegel MA, Parker WB. Gingival enlargement. *J Am Dent Assoc.* 2011;142(11):1265-1268.

25. Thomason JM, Seymour RA, Rawlins MD. Incidence and severity of phenytoin-induced gingival overgrowth in epileptic patients in general medical practice. *Community Dent Oral Epidemiol.* 1992;20(5):288-291.

26. Rees TD, Levine RA. Systematic drugs as a risk factor for periodontal disease initiation and progression. *Compendium.* 1995;16(1):20, 22, 26, 42.

27. Hassell TM. Epilepsy and the oral manifestations of phenytoin therapy. *Monogr Oral Sci.* 1981;9:1-205.

28. Bredfeldt GW. Phenytoin-induced hyperplasia found in edentulous patients. *J Am Dent Assoc.* 1992;123(6):61-64.

29. McCord JF, Sloan P, Hussey DJ. Phenytoin hyperplasia occurring under complete dentures: a clinical report. *J Prosthet Dent.* 1992;68(4):569-572.

30. Chee WW, Jansen CE. Phenytoin hyperplasia occurring in relation to titanium implants: a clinical report. *Int J Oral Maxillofac Implants.* 1994;9(1):107-109.

31. Camargo PM, Melnick PR, Pirih FQ, Lagos R, Takei HH. Treatment of drug-induced gingival enlargement: aesthetic and functional considerations. *Periodontol 2000.* 2001;27:131-138.

32. Majola MP, McFadyen ML, Connolly C, Nair YP, Govender M, Laher MH. Factors influencing phenytoin-induced gingival enlargement. *J Clin Periodontol.* 2000;27(7):506-512.

33. Mavrogiannis M, Ellis JS, Thomason JM, Seymour RA. The management of drug-induced gingival overgrowth. *J Clin Periodontol.* 2006;33(6):434-439.

34. Saravia ME, Svirsky JA, Friedman R. Chlorhexidine as an oral hygiene adjunct for cyclosporine-induced gingival hyperplasia. *ASDC J Dent Child.* 1990;57(5):366-370.

35. Pilatti GL, Sampaio JE. The influence of chlorhexidine on the severity of cyclosporin A—induced gingival overgrowth. *J Periodontol.* 1997;68(9):900-904.

36. Jaiarj N. Drug-induced gingival overgrowth. *J Mass Dent Soc.* 2003;52(3):16-20.

37. Suneja B, Chopra S, Thomas AM, Pandian J. A clinical evaluation of gingival overgrowth in children on antiepileptic drug therapy. *J Clin Diagn Res.* 2016;10(1):ZC32-ZC36.

38. Mehmet Y, Senem Ö, Sülün T, Hümeyra K. Management of epileptic patients in dentistry. *Surg Sci.* 2012;3:47-52.

39. Friedlander AH, Yagiela JA, Paterno VI, Mahler ME. The neuropathology, medical management and dental implications of autism. *J Am Dent Assoc.* 2006;137(11):1517-1527.

40. Rada RE. Controversial issues in treating the dental patient with autism. *J Am Dent Assoc.* 2010;141(8):947-953.

41. Malamed SF. Knowing your patients. *J Am Dent Assoc.* 2010;141(suppl 1):3S–7S.

42. Reed KL. Basic management of medical emergencies: recognizing a patient's distress. *J Am Dent Assoc.* 2010;141(suppl 1):20S–24S.

43. Panayiotis PN, Spanaki MV, Mirski MA. Status epilepticus: an update. *Curr Neurol Neurosci Rep.* 2013;13(7):1-9.

44. Shneker BF, Fountain NB. Epilepsy. *Dis Mon.* 2003;49(7):426-478.

58

The Patient with a Mental Health Disorder

Linda D. Boyd, RDH, RD, EdD, and Esther M. Wilkins, BS, RDH, DMD

CHAPTER OUTLINE

OVERVIEW OF MENTAL DISORDERS
  I. Prevalence of Mental Disorders

ANXIETY DISORDERS
  I. Types and Symptoms of Anxiety Disorders
  II. Treatment
  III. Dental Hygiene Care

DEPRESSIVE DISORDERS
  I. Types of Depressive Disorders
  II. Signs and Symptoms
  III. Treatment
  IV. Dental Hygiene Care

BIPOLAR DISORDER
  I. Signs and Symptoms
  II. Treatment
  III. Dental Hygiene Care

FEEDING AND EATING DISORDERS
  I. Types and Symptoms of Feeding and Eating Disorders
  II. Medical Complications
  III. Treatment
  IV. Dental Hygiene Care

SCHIZOPHRENIA
  I. Signs and Symptoms
  II. Treatment
  III. Dental Hygiene Care

MENTAL HEALTH EMERGENCY
  I. Psychiatric Emergency
  II. Patients at Risk for Emergencies
  III. Prevention of Emergencies
  IV. Preparation for an Emergency
  V. Intervention

DOCUMENTATION

EVERYDAY ETHICS

FACTORS TO TEACH THE PATIENT

REFERENCES

LEARNING OBJECTIVES

After studying this chapter, the student will be able to:

1. Describe the various types of mental health disorders and major symptoms.

2. Summarize the side effects of treatment for mental health disorders that may have oral health implications.

3. Explain dental hygiene treatment considerations for each major category of mental health disorder.

OVERVIEW OF MENTAL DISORDERS

A psychiatric or mental health disorder is a complex, clinically significant behavioral or psychological syndrome that may impact the individual's ability to engage in daily activities of living. The causes may be related to behavioral, psychologic, or biologic dysfunction in the individual.[1]

◆ The American Psychiatric Association has classified more than 200 types of mental disorders in the document *Diagnostic and Statistical Manual of Mental Disorders* (DSM-5).[1]

◆ Each disorder has characteristic signs and symptoms.

◆ This chapter provides descriptions of common mental disorders including anxiety, mood, and eating disorders along with schizophrenia.

  ● Additional disorders are described in other chapters, for example, alcoholism (see Chapter 59), Alzheimer disease (see Chapter 48), autism spectrum disorder, and attention-deficit disorder (see Chapter 50).

◆ With the current policies of deinstitutionalization, more individuals with mental disorders are seeking dental and dental hygiene care in dental offices and clinics.

◆ *Person-first language* is used to refer to someone with a mental disorder, chronic disease, or disability.[2] The person is emphasized first and not the disorder, disease, or disability.

  ● For example, refer to the patient as "an individual with schizophrenia," not as "a schizophrenic."

I. Prevalence of Mental Disorders

◆ In a meta-analysis of 175 studies in 63 countries, 1 in 5 respondents met the criteria for a common mental disorder in the previous year.[3]

  ● About 29% of respondents had experienced a mental disorder during their lifetime.

  ● Women had higher rates of mood and anxiety disorders, while men had higher rates of substance abuse disorders.

  ● English-speaking countries had the highest lifetime prevalence of mental disorders with North and Southeast Asia among the lowest reported prevalence.

ANXIETY DISORDERS

◆ Anxiety disorders are the most common class of mental disorders in the general population.

  ● Anxiety disorders are common with a global prevalence of around 7%.

  ● Euro/Anglo countries having prevalence over 10%, suggesting 1 in 10 people have an anxiety disorder.[4]

◆ Anxiety is a normal reaction to stress.

  ● In anxiety disorders, the anxiety is exaggerated resulting in excess worry and avoidance behavior that can impact day-to-day functioning.

◆ For formal diagnosis, the symptoms must be present for at least 6 months.[1]

◆ Some individuals may have secondary problems of alcohol and other substance abuse.

  ● The abuse may be the result of an attempt at self-medication.

◆ Individuals with anxiety disorders often have comorbid conditions, including other mental health disorders, hypertension, gastrointestinal issues, thyroid disease, cardiovascular conditions, migraine headaches, allergies, and/or a respiratory disease.[5]

I. Types and Symptoms of Anxiety Disorders

A. Generalized Anxiety Disorder

◆ Persistent, pervasive anxiety and excessive worry, but are not associated with life-threatening fears or "attacks."[6,7]

◆ May be complicated by depression, alcohol abuse, or anxiety related to a general medical condition.

◆ Symptoms include[6,7]:

  ● Feeling restless, on-edge, irritable.

  ● Difficulty falling and staying asleep.

  ● Difficulty concentrating.

  ● Muscle tension.

B. Obsessive-Compulsive Disorder

◆ Frequent upsetting thoughts (obsessions), and when the individual tries to control them, there is an overwhelming urge (compulsion) to repeat routines or rituals over and over.[8]

◆ Symptoms include[8]:

  ● Spend at least 1 hour a day with obsessive thoughts and rituals that cause distress and interfere with normal daily functioning.

  ● Thoughts or obsessions might include fear of germs, dirt, or intruders.

  ● Rituals might include washing hands, locking and unlocking doors, or keeping unneeded items (hoarding).

C. Panic Disorder

◆ Panic disorder is characterized by sudden and repeated episodes of extreme fear (panic attacks).[9]

◆ Symptoms center on panic attacks[9]:

  ● A panic attack may be unexpected (uncued) or "situationally bound" (cued). A situationally bound panic attack invariably results from exposure to a specific trigger, such as the dental office.

  ● Fear of being out of control during a panic attack.

  ● Physical symptoms during an attack may include pounding or racing heart, sweating, difficulty breathing, chest pain, or dizziness (Box 58-1).

D. Posttraumatic Stress Disorder

◆ All individuals experience stressful or traumatic events, yet not everyone responds in the same way.

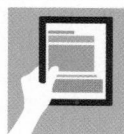

BOX 58-1
Symptoms of Panic Attack

1. Shortness of breath
2. Dizziness, unsteady feelings, or faintness
3. Palpitations or accelerated heart rate
4. Trembling or shaking
5. Sweating (clammy hands)
6. Choking
7. Nausea or abdominal stress
8. Paresthesia (numbness or tingling sensation)
9. Flushes (hot flashes) or chills
10. Chest pain or discomfort
11. Fear of dying
12. Fear of losing control

Source: American Psychiatric Association. *Diagnostic and Statistical Manual of Mental Disorders (DSM-5)*. Washington, DC: American Psychiatric Association; 2013:214.

Some people will develop posttraumatic stress disorder (PTSD) and others are resilient and manage the adversity and adapt.

- PTSD develops after a terrifying ordeal involving physical harm or threat of physical harm.[10]
- Onset may be triggered by destruction to the home or family or may result from a manmade disaster, such as war, imprisonment, torture, rape, physical or sexual abuse, or other exposure associated with intense fear or serious threat to life.
- Signs and symptoms include:
  - Flashbacks of the traumatic experience and terror may be triggered by a stimulus that can be readily associated with the original event.
  - Dreams or recollections may cause the individual to feel they are reliving the event.
  - Avoidance of places, events, or objects that are reminders of the triggering event.
  - Loss of interest in activities that were enjoyable in the past.
  - Hyperarousal symptoms including feeling tense, difficulty sleeping, angry outbursts, and may be easily startled.
  - In children, symptoms may be slightly different and include bedwetting, acting out the scary event during playtime, or being unusually clingy to a parent or other adult.
- Risk factors for PTSD may include[10]:
  - Living through a dangerous or traumatic event.
  - A history of mental illness or substance abuse.
- Resilience factors for PTSD include[10]:
  - Seeking out support either formal or informal from family and friends.

- A positive coping strategy.
- Ability to function despite feelings of fear.

II. Treatment

A. Basic Therapeutic Approach

- Lifestyle modifications include regular physical activity, adequate sleep, and avoidance of drugs and alcohol.[5,7]
- Diagnose and treat other medical and psychiatric problems.

B. Pharmacologic Treatment

- *Antidepressants*: antidepressants preferred as an initial treatment of anxiety disorders.[7,10,11]
  - Examples include fluoxetine (Prozac), paroxetine (Paxel), and sertraline (Zoloft).
  - Side effects: headache, weight gain, tremor, irritability, and xerostomia.
- *Anxiolytics*: These are used only short term because of the risk of dependency.[7]
  - Examples include benzodiazepines (Valium, lorazepam). These are highly addictive and must be carefully monitored.
  - Side effects: confusion, dizziness, muscle memory impairment, weakness, difficulty in speaking, skin rash, and xerostomia.
- *Beta-blockers*: taken on a short-term basis for anxiety, these medication help to relieve the physical symptoms of anxiety such as trembling, shaking, and rapid heartbeat.[7]

B. Psychotherapy

- Cognitive behavioral therapy (CBT)[5,7,11,12]
  - CBT is a combination of strategies to address the cognitive, behavioral, and emotional components of the anxiety disorder.
  - May be conducted in individual or group sessions.
  - Support groups are also helpful.
- Prolonged exposure (PE) therapy[7,12]
  - PE therapy is used in treatment of PTSD and gradually exposes an individual to the traumatic event in a safe way and helps them to cope with their feelings.
- Cognitive processing therapy (CPT)[7,12]
  - CPT is also used to treat PTSD and helps people to make sense of the traumatic event they experienced.

III. Dental Hygiene Care

A. Personal Factors

- Each anxiety disorder has its own characteristics.
- Relationships with other people can be strained.
- Physical complaints, such as rapid heartbeat, hyperventilation, tightness in the throat, and constant fatigue, are common.

B. Oral Implications

- Xerostomia related to medications put the patient at high risk for dental caries.[13]

◆ Individuals with a diagnosis of an anxiety disorders are at higher risk of tooth loss.[13]

◆ Individuals with mental health disorders have a 25% higher caries risk.[13]

◆ The odds for periodontal disease in a patient with panic disorder is three times that of someone without the disorder, but it was not higher in other mental health disorders.[14]

◆ A patient with obsessive-compulsive disorder may perform such excessive, vigorous toothbrushing that gingival and dental abrasion may result.

C. Appointment Interventions

◆ Review medical history and medications carefully.

◆ Enhance the patient's sense of control.[15]

  • One technique is to establish a "stop signal," which may consist of the patient raising the left hand when they are uncomfortable or need to stop treatment.

  • Explain each step to the patient and keep communication as open as possible.

◆ Cognitive distraction involves encouraging the patient to think about something besides the dental treatment.

  • Headphones for music and relaxation can help to reduce stress.

◆ Environmental changes can help reduce anxiety.

  • An example would be the smell of lavender in the waiting room to relax the patient, but this needs to be used in addition to the previously mentioned techniques.

◆ Nitrous oxide sedation may be helpful to relax the patient (see Chapter 36).

◆ Effective pain control is needed.

  • Use local anesthesia for nonsurgical periodontal therapy (NSPT).

  • Attention to technique to minimize discomfort is essential.

◆ Appointments are best scheduled in the morning; eliminate unnecessary waiting in the reception area; length of appointment can be minimized and planned to prevent stress.

◆ Be alert to symptoms of a panic attack (Box 58-1), such as sweating or hyperventilation. Allow the patient to sit up and take short breaks.

DEPRESSIVE DISORDERS

Mood disorders that include depressive disorders are another common classification of mental disorder.

◆ The prevalence of mood disorders for adults is 7.1% in the previous 12 months with a lifetime prevalence of nearly 31% in the United States.[16]

  • Women are more likely to experience mood disorders.

  • Onset is usually in the mid-20s, but it can occur at any age.

  • Depression is the leading cause of disability worldwide.[17]

I. Types of Depressive Disorders

A. Major Depressive Disorder

◆ Transient depressed moods occur in the lives of most people.

  • Sadness over unforeseen tragic events, illnesses, death, or disappointments in career or other life plans can cause depressed feelings.[18,19]

◆ Major depressive disorder interferes with daily life.

◆ Some individuals experience only one episode of major depression in their lifetime, but it is more common to have multiple episodes.

B. Postpartum Depression

During the postpartum period, many physiologic and psychologic stresses are related to the changes taking place in the mother's life.

◆ A moderate-to-severe depression within the first month postpartum, but postpartum depression (PPD) tends to peak at 2–6 months after delivery.[20]

  • The prevalence of PPD is estimated to be 10%–20%.[20]

  • Recent research suggests that fathers can also experience paternal PPD in the first 6 months after birth of the baby with prevalence rates of about 10%.[21]

◆ It is critical to identify women with PPD because it can lead to negative mother–infant bonding and interactions that include maternal withdrawal, disengagement, and abuse.[20]

  • The mother may be less likely to engage in preventive care and is less responsive to providing care to the infant; this may include engaging in appropriate feeding practices and oral health care for the infant/children.[20,21]

  • PPD may impact developmental milestones such as cognitive scores and nonverbal communication of the infant/toddler.[21]

  • Infants may also exhibit increased dysregulation of sleep and feeding.[21]

  • Negative infant behaviors are also typical including excessive infant crying and fussiness.[21]

II. Signs and Symptoms

◆ Symptoms vary between individuals, but common symptoms include[18,20]:

  • Depressed mood or loss of interest or pleasure in activities present for at least 2 weeks.

  • Feelings of hopelessness, worthlessness, or guilt.

  • Fatigue and lack of energy.

  • Difficulty with memory and concentration.

  • Appetite disturbance.

  • Insomnia, early-morning wakefulness.

  • Thoughts of suicide.

III. Treatment

In the case of depression, one of the first things assessed is suicide risk. Hospitalization may be indicated when potential danger of suicide or harm to others exists.[22]

A. Basic Therapeutic Approach

◆ Lifestyle modifications include regular physical activity, adequate sleep, and avoidance of drugs and alcohol.

◆ Diagnose and treat other medical and psychiatric problems.

B. Pharmacotherapy

Antidepressants are preferred as an initial treatment of depressive disorders.[22] However, they take 2–4 weeks to reach therapeutic levels.[22]

◆ *Selective serotonin reuptake inhibitors*

- Advantages: tolerability better than earlier drugs; better compliance; safety in overdose.
- Examples: fluoxetine (Prozac), paroxetine (Paxel), and sertraline (Zoloft).

◆ *Serotonin and noradrenergic reuptake inhibitors*

- Examples: duloxetine (Cymbalta) and venlafaxine (Effexor).

◆ *Dopamine norepinephrine reuptake inhibitor*

- Example: bupropion (Wellbutrin).

◆ *Monoamine oxidase inhibitors*

- Use is restricted to patients who do not respond to other medications due to drug–drug and drug–food interactions.[22]
- Example: phenelzine and tranylcypromine.

◆ *Alternative therapies*

- St. John's Wart may be used by some patients, but the evidence is not strong for its effectiveness and there are potential drug interactions, so patients should be encouraged to consult with their mental health provider.[22]

C. Psychotherapy

Psychotherapy combined with pharmacotherapy is more effective than either one alone for treating depressive disorders.[19,23]

◆ CBT.

◆ Problem-solving therapy.

◆ Psychodynamic therapy.

◆ Interpersonal psychotherapy.

D. Electroconvulsive Therapy

◆ Electroconvulsive therapy is used in severe major depression disorder when pharmacologic therapy and psychotherapy have not been effective. It is also indicated in situations where an immediate response is needed, such as for someone who is suicidal.[22]

◆ Patient may experience confusion and short-term memory loss.[22]

◆ May have cardiovascular side effect and is contraindicated in patients with a history of cardiac arrhythmia or recent myocardial infarction.

IV. Dental Hygiene Care

A. Personal Factors

◆ Self-care impairment and lack of motivation negatively impact oral health.[24]

◆ Symptoms not controlled by medication, such as difficulties with memory, may need to be considered when planning dental hygiene care.

◆ Individuals with depression may have poor diet quality such as higher intakes of energy-dense foods that tend to be higher in sugar, which may increase the risk of dental caries and impact healing after periodontal therapy.[24,25]

B. Oral Health Implications

◆ *Side effects of medications:* xerostomia along with poor dietary choices encourages growth of dental biofilm and increases the risk for dental caries.[13,25]

◆ Omission of general health habits and neglect of oral care make the person susceptible to oral diseases.

- Adults with a diagnosis of depression were at a 64% higher risk for having six or more teeth extracted.[26]
- Those with depression are at 37% greater risk of being edentulous.[26]

◆ Taste perception changes may contribute to a diet high in cariogenic foods with high levels of sucrose.[27]

C. Appointment Interventions

◆ *Assessment*

- Monitor the medical and medications histories closely; note side effects and contraindications related to new drug therapies.
- Review consultations with medical/psychiatric specialists caring for the patient.
- *Intraoral/extraoral examination:* check for signs of xerostomia.

◆ *Approach*

- Provide positive reinforcement and reassurance. Avoid negative guilt-inducing words. Depressed patients may needlessly blame themselves.
- Show genuine interest in the patient to build rapport.

◆ *Preventive instruction*

- *Dental biofilm control:* Teach patient and caregivers the need for daily measures to preserve the teeth and periodontal tissues.
- *Xerostomia:* Manage caries risk with dietary counseling, office and home fluorides, saliva substitutes, and xylitol gum between meals.

◆ *Implementation of care plan*

- Adjust dental light carefully and provide tinted protective eyewear for the patient with photosensitivity, a side effect of certain medications.
- Profound local anesthesia when needed for pain control.
- Provide in-office fluoride treatment after instrumentation.
- Use care to prevent postural hypotension. Sit the patient up slowly from a reclined position and have the patient remain seated a few moments before standing.

BIPOLAR DISORDER

- Bipolar disorder (BD) was formerly known as manic-depressive disorder and involves mood changes from extreme highs (mania) to extreme lows (depression).[28]
  - The lifetime prevalence in the United States is approximately 4%.[29]
  - It is more prevalent in women and the average age of onset is mid-20s.
  - In those with BD, suicide is a leading cause of death, so they need frequent monitoring by a mental health professional.[30]
- BD is the most costly behavioral health issue in part because of high rates of comorbidities such as anxiety disorder, metabolic syndrome, substance abuse, and attention-deficit disorder.[30,31]

I. Signs and Symptoms

- Manic episode symptoms include behaviors that are not consistent with the patient's usual behavior including the following[28]:
  - Inflated self-esteem.
  - Decreased need for sleep.
  - Irritable.
  - Attention gets focused on unimportant activities.
  - Excessive involvement in risky activities.
  - Extreme changes in energy, activity, sleep, and behavior based on the large swings in mood.
- Major depressive episode symptoms are the same as those described for depressive disorders.

II. Treatment

Both pharmacotherapy and psychotherapy are used during all phases of the disorder. Initially, hospitalization may be needed to protect the individual from harm to self or others.

A. Pharmacotherapy

- *Mood stabilizers*[29]
  - Example: lithium.
  - Side effects: xerostomia, restlessness, joint and muscle pain, salivary gland swelling, indigestion, and bloating.
- *Atypical antipsychotics* are sometimes used in conjunction with antidepressants.[29]
  - Examples: quetiapine (Seroquel), risperidone (Risperdal), olanzapine (Zyprexa), and aripiprazole (Abilify).
  - Side effects: dizziness, blurred vision, rapid heartbeat, skin rashes, and drowsiness.
- *Antidepressants* are usually taken with a mood stabilizer.[29]
  - Example: fluoxetine (Prozac), paroxetine (Paxil), sertraline (Zoloft), and bupropion (Wellbutrin).

B. Psychotherapy

- Cognitive behavioral therapy helps patients to learn to change harmful or negative thought patterns and behaviors.
- Family-focused therapy improves communication and coping strategies to aid in early recognition of manic or depressive episodes.

- Interpersonal and social rhythm therapy (IPSRT) is typically used in conjunction with other psychotherapies and is helpful in the maintenance phase of BD. IPSRT focuses on helping individuals to maintain consistent daily routines to promote stability in mood.[30,32]
  - If a patient was undergoing IPSRT, inclusion of oral hygiene procedures in the daily routines may be helpful in encouraging regular oral self-care.
- Psychoeducation educates the patient and family about BD and coping strategies.[30]

III. Dental Hygiene Care

A. Personal Factors

- In a manic episode:
  - Many patients talk quickly, jump from thought to thought, and have a short attention span.
  - A tendency to argue and become irritable may be apparent.
- In a depressive episode:
  - The patient may not be interested in oral self-care and be unmotivated.

B. Oral Health Implications

- Oral hygiene needs are often not a priority to the patient.
- Gingival tissues may appear abraded and lacerated because of overzealous toothbrushing with excessive pressure.
- Side effects of medications with implications for oral health and dental care include[33]:
  - Xerostomia.
  - Dysgeusia and impart a metallic taste in the mouth (lithium).
  - Stomatitis and glossitis.
  - Loss of taste acuity.
  - Dizziness.

C. Appointment Interventions

- Carefully review medical and medication history; consult with patient's physician/psychiatrist as needed.
- Simplify the surroundings; provide a comfortable, calm, and uncluttered environment.
- Patient instruction may be difficult due to a short attention span. Use direct, simple instructions.
  - When applicable, help the patient's caregiver to learn procedures for dental caries prevention and periodontal health.
- Manage caries and periodontal risk with saliva substitutes, office and home fluoride application, dietary counseling, and sugar-free xylitol gum or mints between meals.[33]
  - Chlorhexidine gluconate mouthrinse may be prescribed for short intervals to reduce caries risk and aid healing after NSPT.
- Three- to four-month continuing care appointments may be needed.

FEEDING AND EATING DISORDERS

Feeding and eating disorders are serious disturbances in the amounts and types of foods consumed.

◆ The lifetime prevalence ranges from 0.9% for women and 0.3% for men for anorexia nervosa to 1% for bulimia to 2.8% for binge-eating disorder.[34]

◆ Prevalence of other feeding disorders such as pica and rumination disorder is unclear.

◆ Identification and referral of a patient suspected of having an eating disorder for medical evaluation may be lifesaving because serious medical problems may exist and psychiatric therapy is indicated.

◆ An interdisciplinary team approach for successful rehabilitation of an individual with an eating disorder involves, at the least, medical, psychiatric, nutritional, dental, and dental hygiene professionals.

I. Types and Symptoms of Feeding and Eating Disorders

A. Pica

◆ Consumption of nonfood items typically occurs in children, but it also common in adults, particularly those with mental disorders and/or intellectual disabilities.[35]

◆ Diagnostic criteria include[35]:

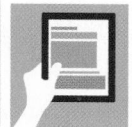

> **BOX 58-2**
> **Characteristics of Anorexia Nervosa**
>
> 1. Refusal to maintain body weight over a minimally normal weight for age and height.
> 2. Intense fear of gaining weight or becoming fat, even though underweight.
> 3. Disturbance in the way in which one's body weight or shape is experienced.
> 4. Denies the seriousness of the current low body weight.
> 5. In females, absence of menstrual cycles when otherwise expected to occur.
>
> **Types**
>
> **Restricting type:** does not regularly engage in binge-eating or purging behavior (i.e., self-induced vomiting or misuse of laxatives, diuretics, or enemas).
>
> **Binge-eating/purging type:** regularly engages in binge-eating or purging behavior (i.e., self-induced vomiting or the misuse of laxatives, diuretics, or enemas).

Source: American Psychiatric Association. Feeding and eating disorders. In: *Diagnostic and Statistical Manual of Mental Disorders (DSM-5)*. 5th ed. Washington, DC: American Psychiatric Association; 2013:329-354.

• Persistent eating of nonfood substances such as dirt, clay, starch, gum, or ice for at least 1 month.

• Consumption of nonfood items may replace healthy foods and lead to nutrient deficiencies that can impact immune response and healing.

B. Anorexia Nervosa

Anorexia nervosa is characterized by a refusal of the individual to maintain body weight over the minimal normal weight for age and height. The aversion to eating results in life-threatening weight loss.[35]

◆ Anorexia nervosa has the highest mortality rate of any mental disorder.[36]

◆ Commonly begins in adolescence or young adulthood.

◆ Signs and symptoms (Box 58-2) include[35,36]:

• Restriction of energy intake resulting in severe weight loss with emaciation; "waiflike" appearance.

• Intense fear of weight gain or becoming fat.

• Body image distortion (Figure 58-1).

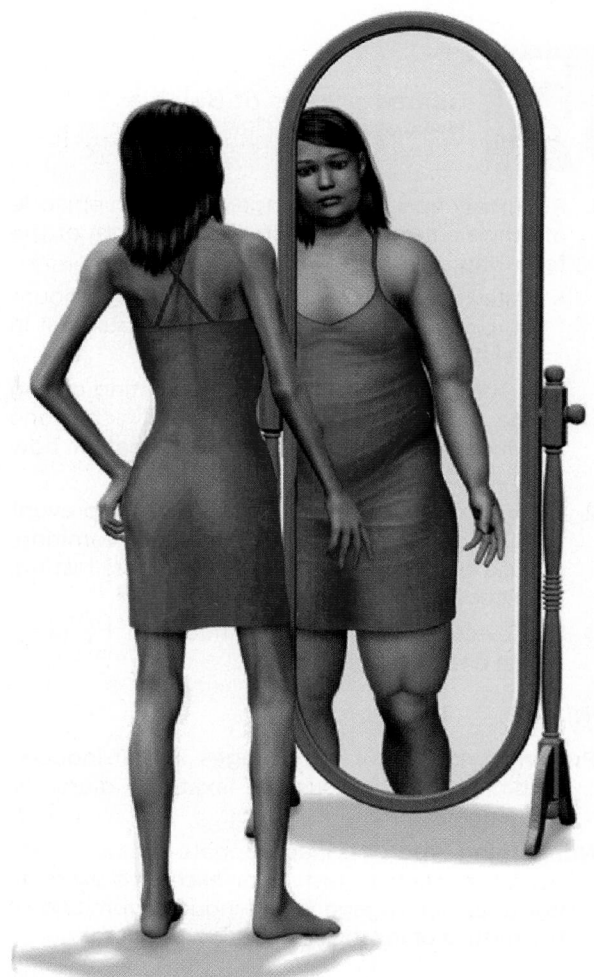

FIGURE 58-1 • Anorexia Nervosa. The person with anorexia typically has a distorted body self-image. Although small and waiflike in real life, the mirror image appears as an overweight individual. (Reprinted from Werner R. *Massage Therapist's Guide to Pathology*. Philadelphia, PA: Lippincott Williams & Wilkins; 2012.)

- Purging by vomiting, laxatives, and excessive exercise.
- Malnutrition can have long-term impact on bone mineral density (osteopenia or osteoporosis).
- *Vital signs*: low pulse rate, hypotension, decreased respiratory rate, and low body temperature.
- *Metabolic changes*: gastrointestinal, cardiovascular, hematologic, and renal system disturbances.
- Amenorrhea (missed menstrual periods).

C. Bulimia Nervosa

◆ Bulimia nervosa is a mental disorder marked by recurrent episodes of uncontrollable binge eating that occurs an average of once a week for 3 months.[35]

◆ Two types of compensatory behaviors are seen in individuals with bulimia nervosa known as the purging type and the nonpurging type (Box 58-3).

- Because of the fear of becoming overweight, self-induced vomiting after eating or the use of laxatives or diuretics is characteristic of the purging type (Figure 58-2).

BOX 58-3
Characteristics of Bulimia Nervosa

1. Recurrent episodes of binge eating. An episode of binge eating is characterized by both of the following:

   - Eating, within any 2-hour period, an amount of food larger than most people would eat in a similar period of time.

   - A sense of lack of control over eating during the episode, for example, a feeling that one cannot stop eating or control what or how much one is eating.

2. Recurrent inappropriate behavior to prevent weight gain, such as self-induced vomiting; misuse of laxatives, diuretics, enemas; fasting; or excessive exercise.

3. Self-evaluation is unduly influenced by body shape and weight.

Types

Purging type: regularly engages in self-induced vomiting or the misuse of laxatives, diuretics, or enemas.

Nonpurging type: uses inappropriate compensatory behaviors such as fasting or excessive exercise, but does not engage in self-induced vomiting or the misuse of laxatives, diuretics, or enemas.

Source: American Psychiatric Association. Feeding and eating disorders. In: *Diagnostic and Statistical Manual of Mental Disorders (DSM-5)*. 5th ed. Washington, DC: American Psychiatric Association; 2013:329-354.

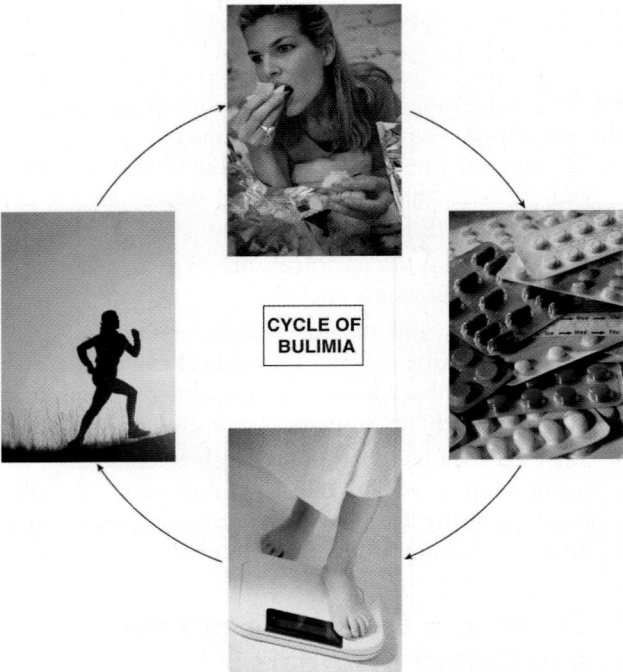

FIGURE 58-2 • Bulimia Nervosa. The person with bulimia becomes trapped in recurring behaviors involving food and weight management. They ingest a vast number of calories at once and then take measures to purge themselves of their binge (e.g., abuse of laxatives, diet pills, and diuretics). They monitor their weight several times a day; some exercise obsessively to burn off the calories. (Reprinted from Mohr W. *Psychiatric-Mental Health Nursing*. Philadelphia, PA: Lippincott Williams & Wilkins; 2012.)

- The nonpurging type uses strict dieting, fasting, and/or vigorous exercise.

◆ Signs and symptoms include[34–36]:
  - Normal body weight or slightly overweight is typical, in contrast to the thin anorectic person.
  - Comorbidity with other mental disorders is common, especially depression and BDs.
  - Lifetime prevalence of alcohol or substance abuse is 30% for people.
  - Chronically inflamed and sore throat.
  - Swollen salivary glands.
  - Enamel erosion and dentin hypersensitivity due to frequent exposure to acid gastric fluids.
  - Severe dehydration may result from purging.
  - Food consumed during a binge include 65% breads/pasta, 56% sweets, and 40% salty snacks, which may be more cariogenic.[37]

D. Binge-Eating Disorder

◆ Recurrent episodes of binge eating without compensatory behaviors seen in bulimia nervosa at least once a week for 3 months.[35,36]

◆ Signs and symptoms include[35,36]:

- Occurs in normal weight, overweight, and obese individuals.
- Binge eating is associated with feeling embarrassed or guilty about how much one is eating.
- Comorbid disorders include mental health disorders such as bipolar, depressive, and anxiety disorders.
- Eating large amounts of food quickly in a short time.
- Eating alone or in secret.
- Frequent dieting.

E. Diabulimia

◆ Diabulimia is defined as the restriction or omission of insulin in an individual with type 1 diabetes mellitus (T1DM) in order to lose or prevent weight gain.[38,39]

- This condition has been documented since the 1970s, but there are no recognized diagnostic criteria in the *DSM-5*.
- Diabulimia is most often seen in adolescent and young women.
- These individuals are at increased risk of microvascular complications such as renal failure, neuropathy, heart attack, stroke, and death.

◆ Signs and symptoms include[38]:

- Rapid weight loss.
- Obsession with body size and shape and dissatisfaction with body image.
- Ketone or "fruity" smell.
- Persistent high hemoglobin A1c.
- Eating behaviors similar to bulimia nervosa.
- Frequent emergency rooms visits or admission for diabetic ketoacidosis.

F. Orthorexia Nervosa

◆ Characterized by pathologic or disordered healthy eating with a focus on the quality of food choices resulting in negative effects on health.[40]

◆ This condition is not recognized by the American Psychiatric Association in the *DSM-5* and did not appear in the peer-reviewed literature until 2004.

◆ Proposed diagnostic criteria include[40]:

- Compulsive behavior or preoccupation with restrictive dietary practices believed to promote health.
- Dietary restriction tends to escalate over time with elimination of entire food groups and may engage in "cleanses" (partial fasts) to detoxify.
- Violation of dietary restriction causes anxiety and shame.
- Malnutrition or medical complications from the restricted diet.
- Impairment of social, academic, and/or vocational functioning.

II. Medical Complications

Medical complications are primarily associated with anorexia nervosa and people with bulimia who engage in purging behaviors.[35]

◆ Problems include dehydration, electrolyte imbalance, protein malnutrition, and cardiac arrhythmia.

◆ Self-medications include abuse of laxatives and diuretics, which contribute to gastrointestinal disturbances.

◆ Esophageal tears.

◆ Amenorrhea or menstrual irregularities.

III. Treatment

Multidisciplinary team treatment for eating disorders is considered best practice. The primary objectives are to promote weight gain and restore the nutritional status. Treatment may require months or even years.

◆ Typically outpatient treatment is recommended, so if someone has been hospitalized for treatment, it suggests they are at high risk for medical complications and a medical consult is needed.[41]

A. Pharmacotherapy

◆ *Antidepressants (primarily in bulimia nervosa)*[38,41]

- Example: fluoxetine (Prozac).
- Side effects: headache, weight gain, tremor, irritability, and xerostomia.

B. Psychotherapy

◆ The goal of therapy is to help the individual discover the underlying causes of the problems and source of the disordered eating behavior.[41]

- Cognitive behavioral therapy is the first line of treatment in bulimia nervosa and diabulimia.[38,41]
- Interpersonal therapy.
- Family-based therapy is recommended for younger patients.

C. Nutrition Therapy

◆ Registered dietitian nutritionists with advanced training in eating disorders work as part of the interprofessional team to conduct a full nutrition assessment, diagnosis, and individualize a plan for medical nutrition therapy in collaboration with the team.[42]

◆ This in-depth type of nutrition counseling is beyond the scope of practice for dental professionals.

IV. Dental Hygiene Care

A. Personal Factors

◆ Anorexia nervosa

- Individuals with anorexia are frequently engaged in excessive exercise and preoccupied with food and weight loss.

- Frequently the person is a high achiever and highly motivated scholastically, but may be socially isolated and withdrawn.
- Suicide risk is elevated in anorexia.[35,36]

◆ Bulimia nervosa and binge-eating disorder
- The patient is well aware that the eating habits are abnormal, and as a result may suffer low self-esteem and guilt feelings.

B. Oral Implications

◆ *Dental erosion (perimolysis):* This is the chemical erosion of the tooth surfaces by acid from the regurgitation of stomach contents.[43,44] After vomiting, acid is retained by the tongue papillae and provides longer contact with the palatal surfaces of maxillary teeth.
- Individuals who engage in self-induced vomiting have five times greater risk of dental erosion.[44]
- Because of perimolysis, the earliest evidence of bulimia or binge-eating/purging type of anorexia may be on the smooth palatal surfaces of the teeth.
- The lingual surfaces of the maxillary anterior teeth appear translucent and glasslike (Figure 58-3B).
- With time, the erosion extends over the occlusal and incisal surfaces and chipping may occur.
- Restorations in posterior teeth may appear raised because of erosion of the enamel around the margins.

◆ *Dental caries:* an increase in caries incidence is found,[44] particularly in cervical caries. Demineralization results from pH changes in the saliva, from xerostomia, and from the large quantities of cariogenic foods ingested during binges.

◆ *Mucosal lesions:* Nutrient deficiencies, especially in the B vitamins, may result in angular cheilitis (Figure 58-4), glossitis, inflammation of pharynx (Figure 58-3A), and a burning sensation.[43]

◆ *Periodontal manifestations:* Nutritional deficiencies with inadequate control of dental biofilm due to depression may predispose the patient to gingivitis.

◆ *Saliva:* The decrease in quantity, quality, and pH of the saliva limits its buffering and lubricating properties.[44] Dehydration of the oral soft tissues occurs.
- Body fluid is lost from vomiting and the use of diuretics may result in xerostomia.
- Xerostomia is also a side effect of antidepressant medication prescribed for patients with bulimia and anorexia.

◆ *Hypersensitive teeth:* The loss of enamel and the exposure of dentin results in sensitivity, which can be especially noticeable for the maxillary anterior teeth.

◆ *Trauma:*
- The soft palate can be traumatized by fingers, comb, pencils, or toothbrush used to induce vomiting. The same implement may injure the mouth at the commissures.
- Pharyngeal trauma is caused by a large food bolus that is swallowed or regurgitated.
- Callous formation or scars on fingers or knuckles used for self-induced vomiting may be observed.

◆ *Parotid gland:* Enlargement may occur for 2–6 days after a binge.[43] The cause of enlargement is not known.
- The degree of enlargement increases with the frequency of vomiting. The gland functions normally and is not sensitive to palpation.

◆ *Bruxism:* Tooth wear is related to stress and tension.[43]

◆ *Taste:* Taste perception may be impaired.

◆ *Temporomandibular joint disorders (TMD):* Self-induced vomiting may cause dislocation or subluxation of the mandibular condyle due to excessive opening and result in symptoms of TMD, including headaches, facial pain, and sensitivity to palpation.[43]

C. Appointment Interventions

◆ Present a nonthreatening, nonjudgmental demeanor. Develop rapport through mutual respect and a trusting relationship.

◆ Recognize that denial of an eating disorder is common.

◆ Be aware answers to medical and personal history questions concerning diet, medications, use of laxatives

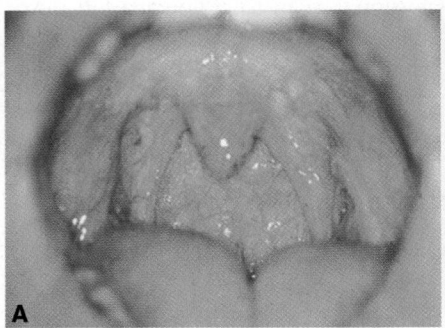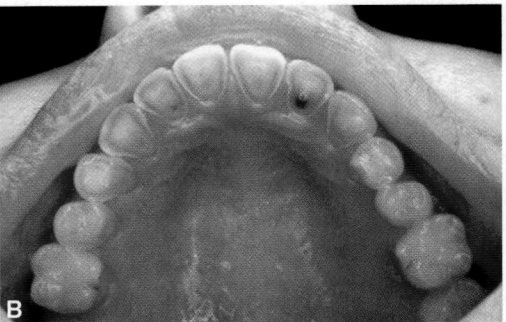

FIGURE 58-3 • Oral Manifestations of Purging-Type Eating Disorders. Signs of purging include **(A)** irritation and inflammation of the pharynx as well as the esophagus from chronic vomiting and **(B)** erosion of the lingual surface of the teeth, loss of dental enamel, periodontal disease, and extensive dental caries. (Reprinted from Timby B, Smith N. *Introductory Medical-Surgical Nursing.* Philadelphia, PA: Lippincott Williams & Wilkins; 2013.)

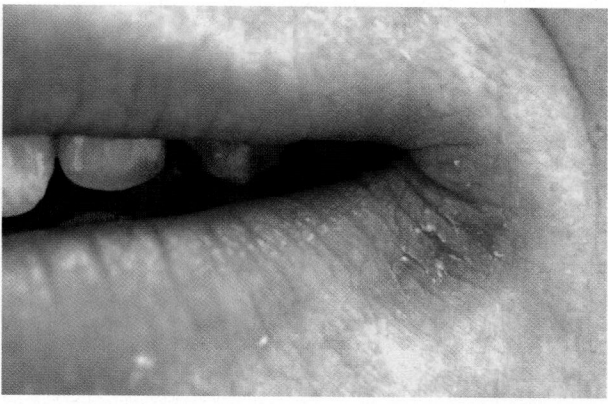

FIGURE 58-4 • Angular Cheilitis. Angular cheilitis may occur in vitamin B deficiencies, which can occur in patients with eating disorders. (Reprinted from Schalock P, Hsu J, Arndt K. *Lippincott's Primary Care Dermatology.* Philadelphia, PA: Lippincott Williams & Wilkins; 2010.)

and diuretics, and weight and weight loss may provide strong suspicions of a feeding or eating disorder.

◆ Assess the nutritional status through use of a dietary assessment.

◆ Record vital signs.

◆ *Perimolysis* and *dental caries* prevention strategies include:

  • Reduction in consumption of cariogenic foods; provide list of suggestions for substitutions.

  • Improvement in oral self-care. Show use of appropriate brushing and flossing with additional interdental aids if required for biofilm removal. Clean the tongue (see Chapter 26).

  • Avoidance of brushing after vomiting. Demineralization of the tooth surface by the acid from the stomach starts immediately on contact. Brushing may remove additional enamel/dentin.

  • Remineralization after vomiting with an alkaline rinse of sodium bicarbonate solution to neutralize the acid.[43]

◆ *Dental hypersensitivity* is managed as follows:

  • Office application of fluoride varnish.

  • Use fluoride dentifrice at least twice daily.

  • Daily application of 1.1% neutral sodium fluoride toothpaste or gel.

  • Avoid acidic foods and beverages.

◆ *Xerostomia* management includes:

  • Advise sugar-free mints or chewing gum containing xylitol to stimulate saliva flow.

  • Recommend saliva substitutes.

  • To reduce problems caused by hypersensitive teeth: choose sugar substitute and acid-free foods and beverages.

SCHIZOPHRENIA

◆ Schizophrenia is a complex, chronic mental disorder. Disturbances in feeling, thinking, and behavior significantly impair function to a level below normal for the individual.[35,45]

• Prevalence of schizophrenia is 0.3%–0.7%.

• The onset is usually between the age of 16 and 30 years.

• Men tend to develop symptoms at an earlier age than women.

◆ Genetic factors are strong contributors to risk for schizophrenia.[35,45]

◆ Associated medical issues such as cardiovascular disease, obesity, diabetes, and metabolic syndrome reduce life expectancy.[35]

◆ About 10%–13% of people with schizophrenia attempt suicide and 4%–6% die as a result of suicide.[46] However, research conducted with a large Canadian community–based sample found 39% of those with schizophrenia had a lifetime prevalence of attempted suicide and were 15 times more likely to attempt suicide than someone without schizophrenia.[47]

I. Signs and Symptoms

Symptoms fall into three categories: *positive symptoms*, *negative symptoms*, and *cognitive symptoms*.[35,45]

◆ *Positive symptoms* are those that reflect unusual, exaggerated behavior and include:

  • Hallucinations that may include hearing voices.

  • Delusions.

  • Disorganized thinking characterized by the person having difficulty organizing thoughts or connecting them logically.

  • Movement disorders such as agitated body movements.

  • People with positive symptoms may "lose touch" with reality and the symptoms may come and go.

◆ *Negative symptoms* are associated with disruptions in normal emotions or behaviors and may be mistaken for depression. Symptoms include:

  • The individual may have a "flat affect" meaning the person shows no emotion.

  • Lack of pleasure in activities once enjoyed.

  • Inability to start and carry out tasks.

  • Little communication even when forced to interact.

  • These individuals have difficulty with everyday tasks such as oral self-care.

◆ *Cognitive symptoms* are less obvious and may be difficult to recognize. Symptoms include:

  • Poor executive functioning, meaning difficulty with understanding information and using it to make decisions.

  • Difficulty paying attention.

  • Challenges with working memory or the ability to use information immediately after it is learned.

◆ Prevalence of substance-use disorder (SUD) is high among patients with schizophrenia.[48]

  • Prevalence of any SUD was approximately 42% with over 27% using illicit drugs, 26% using cannabis, 24% using alcohol, and 7% using stimulants.[48]

  • Over 60% of patients with schizophrenia use tobacco.[49]

II. Treatment

The response to initial treatment can be a predictor of the long-term prognosis. The prognosis has generally been considered guarded to poor. Evidence shows that although deterioration may occur during the early years, the condition may stabilize with treatment during middle age.[45–48]

A. Pharmacotherapy

◆ The objectives of treatment are to reduce or alleviate the delusions, hallucinations, and other symptoms and to enable the patient to function in daily living.[45]

◆ The use of antipsychotic medications has improved the outcomes of treatment.

◆ *Typical antipsychotics* are used to block dopamine receptors and are effective against positive symptoms with less effect on negative symptoms.[45]

  • Examples: chlorpromazine (Thorazine), haloperidol (Haldol), and perphenazine (Etrafon, Trilafon).
  • Side effects: xerostomia, persistent muscle spasms, tremors, and restlessness, and long-term use can lead to tardive dyskinesia (uncontrolled muscle movements), which commonly happens around the mouth.

◆ *Atypical antipsychotics* were developed in the 1990s and are second-generation antipsychotics:

  • Examples: clozapine (Clozaril), quetiapine (Seroquel), risperidone (Risperdal), olanzapine (Zyprexa), and aripiprazole (Abilify).
  • Side effects: xerostomia, dizziness, blurred vision, rapid heartbeat, skin rashes, and drowsiness.

◆ Table 58-1 lists a few of the many side effects of antipsychotic medications, with suggestions for appointment adaptations.

B. Psychosocial Therapy

◆ Psychosocial therapy is utilized once the patient is stabilized on antipsychotic medication.[45]

  • Treatment is to help give general support in dealing with the challenges of the illness such as self-care, work, interpersonal relationships, and communication.
  • Rehabilitation once stabilized includes social and vocational training, so a person with schizophrenia can function in the community.
  • Family education is also essential to help them learn coping strategies and problem-solving skills to support their loved one.

◆ CBT focuses on thinking and behavior and helps the person with schizophrenia manage symptoms that remain despite medication.

III. Dental Hygiene Care

A. Oral Implications

◆ Overall degeneration of health factors may have occurred because of neglect of diet, exercise, sleep, general cleanliness, personal grooming, and oral care.

TABLE 58-1 • Effects of Antipsychotic Medication

SIDE EFFECTS	IMPLICATIONS FOR DENTAL HYGIENE CARE
Dystonia	
Muscle contractions	Laryngeal spasm; coughing Unable to turn head
Dysarthria	
Difficult speech	Communication difficulty
Parkinson-like syndrome	
Shuffling gait Muscular rigidity Resting tremor (pill rolling) Facial grimacing **Bradykinesia**	Cooperation may be difficult Patient positioning Instrument positioning; retraction
Akathisia	
Restlessness, pacing	Plan short appointments
Akinesia	
Loss of voluntary movement Lethargy, fatigue feelings	Adjust patient position
Tardive dyskinesia	
Involuntary mouth and jaw movements	Difficulty in instrumentation Wearing dentures difficult or impossible Muscle fatigue; may need mouth prop
Anticholinergic effects	
Xerostomia Blurred vision	Dental caries prevention Fluoride dentifrice; saliva substitute Difficulty seeing visual aids
Cardiovascular	
Postural hypotension Tachycardia, palpitations	Have patient sit up slowly and wait before standing Monitor vital signs
Sedation	
Drowsiness	Interfere with patient's daily routine Patient may be late; needs reminders
Blood	
Reduced leukocytes Agranulocytosis	Increased susceptibility to infection Oral candidiasis may be present

- ◆ Concurrent alcohol and/or other drug abuse, as well as smoking, can influence dental and periodontal health.
- ◆ Individuals with schizophrenia have higher rates of dental caries, more missing teeth, and fewer filled teeth, suggesting either a lack of access to dental care or a failure to seek dental care.[50]
- ◆ Xerostomia coupled with lack of attention to self-care may lead to an increase in rampant dental caries.[51]
- ◆ Those with schizophrenia also have higher rates of periodontal disease, which may be a result of lack of self-care coupled with lack of dental care and tobacco use.[51]

B. Appointment Planning

- ◆ Elective dental and dental hygiene treatment cannot be carried out until the schizophrenia is stabilized.
- ◆ If the patient decompensates, such as hallucinations or exhibits bizarre behavior, during a dental or dental hygiene appointment, immediate referral is needed.
- ◆ Telephone numbers of the patient's mental healthcare provider should be kept in an easily accessible location for quick referrals.

C. Appointment Interventions

- ◆ Because schizophrenia is often a lifelong disorder, planning for future oral health is essential.
- ◆ Review medical and medication history; analyze drugs for possible side effects that require appointment modifications (Table 58-1).
- ◆ Consult with the mental health provider relative to medications, alcohol or other substance use, and medico-legal competence for informed consent.
- ◆ Negative symptoms are associated with poor oral health and a greater need for periodontal treatment.[51]
- ◆ Plan a simple routine. For a series of appointments and maintenance, use a familiar, organized routine that is comfortable for the patient.
- ◆ Decrease stimulation; create a restful atmosphere; if background music is present, keep it low and soft.
- ◆ Management of the risk for caries, periodontal, and oral cancer includes the following:
  - Oral self-care instruction to improve biofilm removal on a daily basis.
  - When applicable, evaluate the patient's personal caregiver for attitude and knowledge and provide information and instruction.
  - Diet assessment and counseling to assist patient in making noncariogenic food choices (see Chapter 33).
  - Encourage use of xylitol-containing gum or mints when cariogenic snacks or beverages are consumed between meals.
  - Office and home fluorides (see Chapter 34).
  - Saliva substitutes may be helpful in patients with severe medication-induced xerostomia.
  - Tobacco cessation (see Chapter 32) may be more difficult for people with schizophrenia because

nicotine withdrawal may cause psychotic symptoms to worsen, so the dental professional must collaborate with the medical treatment team to closely monitor the patient.[35]
- ◆ Use a mouth prop to assist the patient with tardive dyskinesia. The patient who does not have control of mouth movements might appreciate the stability.

MENTAL HEALTH EMERGENCY

I. Psychiatric Emergency

A psychiatric emergency in a dental clinic or private dental practice would be rare. The most common causes of emergency include panic attack, atypical drug reaction, and schizophrenic or manic decompensation.

II. Patients at Risk for Emergencies

- ◆ Patient with a significant psychiatric history.
- ◆ Patient with a known substance abuse history.
- ◆ Patient new to the clinic or office; not known by the practitioners.

III. Prevention of Emergencies

- ◆ Prepare a complete history; collect as much information as possible; consult with the patient's physician and psychiatrist.
- ◆ Be alert to risks and characteristic symptoms of each disorder.
- ◆ Apply all the principles of stress management.
- ◆ Know the patient's medications and when they are taken.
  - Request that patient (or caregiver if accompanied) have readily available any necessary medication that may be effective during an emergency.
- ◆ Develop rapport with each patient; avoid confronting the patient and present a nonthreatening demeanor.

IV. Preparation for an Emergency

- ◆ Attend to surroundings, such as door access, objects in the room.
- ◆ Arrange for colleagues to be aware of the possible needs of a special patient appointment; when possible plan for an assistant to participate in clinical procedures.
- ◆ Review characteristics of possible emergencies; have necessary equipment ready.
- ◆ Keep names and contact information of the patient's case manager, psychiatrist, and responsible family member in the record in a prominent position for ready reference.

V. Intervention

- ◆ Stay with the patient; request colleague to contact patient's case manager, psychiatrist, or other responsible person.

- Maintain a calm, serene manner; talk quietly but firmly.
- Move the patient to a quiet, less stimulating environment. The dental equipment and environment may have contributed to the patient's disturbance.
- If you think the patient might be suicidal because the individual mentions wanting to die or kill themselves, try to remain calm and implement the five action steps of #BeThe1To[52]:
  1. **#BeThe1To** *ASK:* Directly ask the patient "Are you thinking about suicide?" Asking in a direct manner can open the door for the individual to share their feelings.
  2. **#BeThe1To** *KEEP THEM SAFE:* Showing support for someone can put time and distance between the person and their chosen suicide method.
  3. **#BeThe1To** *BE THERE:* Being present shows support for the person at risk, this can be lifesaving.
  4. **#BeThe1To** *HELP THEM CONNECT:* Call the Suicide Prevention Lifeline 1-800-273-TALK (8255). Your call will be routed to a local call center and they will walk you through resources available to assist and if the patient is willing have them talk to a mental health professional.
  5. **#BeThe1To** *FOLLOW-UP:* Following up to see how the individual is doing has been shown to reduce the number of suicide deaths.

DOCUMENTATION

- The patient with a mental health disorder must complete a health history with details of the medical problem and medication history at the initial appointment.
- Follow-up with progress notes at each succeeding appointment to review all procedures and medications for changes.
- The following list suggests the minimum information to include in the permanent record:
  - Resources for assistance in a convenient place in the event of need to contact: telephones; e-mails; and working addresses for physicians, psychiatrist, family, and emergency sources.
  - Progress notes for each appointment and other contacts to update all personal data and treatment.
  - Contacts and correspondence with specialists and others.
  - A sample progress note may be reviewed in Box 58-4.

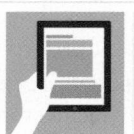

BOX 58-4
Example Documentation:
Patient with a Mental Disorder

S—Mary is a 23-year-old. Sporadic dental care mainly for emergency root canals and extractions. She presents for an examination and "cleaning" because her physician recommended she seek dental care for obvious dental caries.

O—Medical history: She reports trouble sleeping and waking at 2 or 3 every morning and not being able to get back to sleep. Mary reports hallucination of neon people walking down the hallway. She said when she was at work she experienced high levels of anxiety. Her psychiatrist has diagnosed Mary as suffering from panic attacks. She also reported a previous history of being hospitalized for schizophrenia. She has smoked 1 pack of cigarettes/day since she was 13 years old. Medications: Risperidone (Risperdal). Dental examination: Caries noted MOD-#2, 14, 15, 18, 30; M & D #7–10 and #22–27. Leukoplakia noted in vestibule buccal to #28–29. Generalized pocket depths 4–5 mm with bleeding on probing, indicating generalized Stage II, Grade B periodontitis. Biofilm score: 95%. Generalized moderate supra- and subgingival calculus.

A—Patient education to include oral self-care along with strategies to manage risk factors for caries and periodontal disease. Consult with primary care provider to coordinate tobacco cessation based on her history of schizophrenia. Disease control treatment phase to include restoration of carious lesions and NSPT.

P—Disclosed biofilm and patient demonstrated oral self-care techniques. Mary seems to have good toothbrushing and flossing technique, but motivation seems to be her main problem. Suggested putting a sticky note on her bathroom mirror to remind her to perform oral self-care. Another suggestion was to make it a family affair and brush and floss with her children to be a role model to them. Mary was anxious at the beginning of the appointment, but seem calmer toward the end. Nutrition counseling focused on reducing the frequency of sugar-sweetened snacks and beverages with recommendations to use xylitol gum or mints when she snacks between meals and cannot brush. She was given a prescription for 1.1% sodium fluoride paste to begin using at home. There was not adequate time to begin NSPT at today's appointment.

Next visit: Review oral self-care. Follow-up on diet and tobacco cessation. NSPT maxillary and mandibular right quadrants with two carpules, 2% lidocaine with 1:100,000 epinephrine for an inferior alveolar (IA), posterior superior alveolar (PSA), middle superior alveolar (MSA), and greater palatine (GP) injections.

Signed: _____, RDH

Date: _____

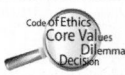

EVERYDAY ETHICS

Samuel, age 28, suffers from panic disorder and generally requests short appointments because he becomes very anxious while receiving dental care. Even with a moderate amount of generalized deposits, Ginny, the dental hygienist, usually schedules two visits to complete the treatment.

During his visit today, Samuel appears in an almost dream-like state. He was asked by the receptionist at the check-in about any new medications, but he stated that only a sleep aid was added to his pills, which he takes at night. Ginny suspects the patient may have taken his medication incorrectly and is concerned that Samuel is driving himself home after the appointment.

Questions for Consideration

1. Without breaching confidentiality, what ethical or other responsibility does Ginny have in verifying the type and amount of medication Samuel took and how does that influence the current day's dental hygiene appointment procedures?

2. Which of the dental hygiene core values are evidenced in this scenario? Describe each in terms of the concern Ginny shows relative to Samuel's "competency" at driving himself home after the appointment as well as management during the appointment.

3. Is this an ethical dilemma or issue for Ginny? Suggest several alternative procedures that Ginny can follow during this appointment.

Factors to Teach the Patient

► The significance of daily oral self-care of the oral cavity.

► How medications cause dry mouth and how it increases the risk for caries.

► The importance of minimizing sweets such as cake, candy, and sugar-sweetened drinks to prevent dental caries.

► The use of saliva substitutes to make a dry mouth more comfortable.

► For the patient with bulimia or the binge-eating/purging type of anorexia:

  • The causes and effects of enamel erosion; the high acidity of the vomitus from the stomach.

  • The importance of rinsing after vomiting but not brush immediately; demineralization begins promptly after the acid from the stomach reaches the teeth. Brushing can cause abrasion of the demineralizing enamel.

  • The need for multiple fluoride applications through office and home fluoride containing dentifrice, rinse, and brush-on gel, as well as professional application of varnish at regular dental hygiene appointments.

ENHANCE YOUR UNDERSTANDING

ONLINE RESOURCES
(see the inside front cover for access information)

• Audio glossary

• Appendices

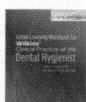

SUPPORT FOR LEARNING
(available separately)

• *Active Learning Workbook for Wilkins' Clinical Practice of the Dental Hygienist, 13th Edition*

INDIVIDUALIZED REVIEW

• Customized practice quizzing with Navigate 2 TestPrep for *Wilkins' Clinical Practice of the Dental Hygienist*

References

1. American Psychiatric Association. *Diagnostic and Statistical Manual of Mental Disorders (DSM-5)*. 5th ed., text revision. Washington, DC: American Psychiatric Association; 2013:19.

2. Centers for Disease Control and Prevention. Communicating with and about people with disabilities. 2014. http://www.cdc.gov/ncbddd/disabilityandhealth/pdf/disabilityposter_photos.pdf. Accessed September 10, 2018.

3. Steel Z, Marnane C, Iranpour C, et al. The global prevalence of common mental disorders: a systematic review and meta-analysis 1980–2013. *Int J Epidemiol*. 2014;43(2): 476-493.

4. Baxter AJ, Scott KM, Vos T, Whiteford HA. Global prevalence of anxiety disorders: a systematic review and meta-regression. *Psychol Med*. 2013;43(5):897-910.

5. Katzman MA, Bleau P, Blier P, et al. Canadian clinical practice guidelines for the management of anxiety, posttraumatic stress and obsessive-compulsive disorders. *BMC Psychiatry*. 2014;14(suppl 1):S1.

6. National Institute of Mental Health. Generalized anxiety disorder. Revised July 2018. http://www.nimh.nih.gov/health/topics/generalized-anxiety-disorder-gad/index.shtml. Accessed September 7, 2018.

7. American Psychiatric Association. Anxiety disorders. In: *Diagnostic and Statistical Manual of Mental Disorders*. 5th ed. Washington, DC: American Psychiatric Association; 2013:189-223.

8. National Institute of Mental Health. Obsessive-compulsive disorder. Revised January 2016. http://www.nimh.nih.gov/health/topics/obsessive-compulsive-disorder-ocd/index.shtml. Accessed September 7, 2018.

9. National Institute of Mental Health. Panic disorder. http://www.nimh.nih.gov/health/topics/panic-disorder/index.shtml. Accessed September 7, 2018.

10. National Institute of Mental Health. Post-traumatic stress disorder. http://www.nimh.nih.gov/health/topics/post-traumatic-stress-disorder-ptsd/index.shtml. Accessed September 10, 2018.

11. National Institute of Mental Health. Anxiety disorders. http://www.nimh.nih.gov/health/topics/anxiety-disorders/index.shtml. Accessed September 10, 2018.

12. American Psychological Association. *Clinical Practice Guideline for the Treatment of Posttraumatic Stress Disorder (PTSD) in Adults.* February 24, 2017. Washington, DC. http://www.apa.org/ptsd-guideline/ptsd.pdf. Accessed September 10, 2018.

13. Kisely S, Sawyer E, Siskind D, Lalloo R. The oral health of people with anxiety and depressive disorders—a systematic review and meta-analysis. *J Affect Disord.* 2016;200:119-32.

14. Khambaty T, Stewart JC. Associations of depressive and anxiety disorders with periodontal disease prevalence in young adults: analysis of 1999–2004 National Health and Nutrition Examination Survey (NHANES) data. *Ann Behav Med.* 2013;45(3):393-397.

15. Newton T, Asimakopoulou K, Daly B, Scambler S, Scott S. The management of dental anxiety: time for a sense of proportion? *Br Dent J.* 2012;213(6):271-274.

16. Kessler RC, Petukhova M, Sampson NA, Zaslavsky AM, Wittchen H-U. Twelve-month and lifetime prevalence and lifetime morbid risk of anxiety and mood disorders in the United States. *Int J Methods Psychiatr Res.* 2012;21(3):169-184.

17. World Health Organization. Depression. March 22, 2018. http://www.who.int/mediacentre/factsheets/fs369/en/. Accessed September 7, 2018.

18. American Psychiatric Association. Depressive disorders. In: *Diagnostic and Statistical Manual of Mental Disorders (DSM-5).* 5th ed. Washington, DC: American Psychiatric Association; 2013:155-188.

19. National Institute of Mental Health. Depression. February 2018. http://www.nimh.nih.gov/health/topics/depression/index.shtml. Accessed September 7, 2018.

20. Bobo WV, Yawn BP. Concise review for physicians and other clinicians: postpartum depression. *Mayo Clin Proc.* 2014;89(6):835-844.

21. Hoffman C, Dunn DM, Njoroge WFM. Impact of postpartum mental illness upon infant development. *Curr Psychiatry Rep.* 2017;19(12):100.

22. American Psychiatric Association. *Practice Guideline for the Treatment of Patients with Major Depressive Disorder.* 3rd ed. Reaffirmed October 31, 2015. Washington, DC: American Psychiatric Association; 2010:1-152.

23. Cuijpers P, Sijbrandij M, Koole SL, Andersson G, Beekman AT, Reynolds CF 3rd. Adding psychotherapy to antidepressant medication in depression and anxiety disorders: a meta-analysis. *World Psychiatry.* 2014;13(1):56-67.

24. Barbosa ACDS, Pinho RCM, Vasconcelos MMVB, Magalhães BG, Dos Santos MTBR, de França Caldas Júnior A. Association between symptoms of depression and oral health conditions. *Spec Care Dentist.* 2018;38(2):65-72.

25. Camilleri GM, Méjean C, Kesse-Guyot E, et al. The associations between emotional eating and consumption of energy-dense snack foods are modified by sex and depressive symptomatology. *J Nutr.* 2014;144(8):1264-1273.

26. Wiener R, Wiener M, McNeil D. Comorbid depression/anxiety and teeth removed: Behavioral Risk Factor Surveillance System 2010. *Community Dent Oral Epidemiol.* 2015;43(5):433-443.

27. Platte P, Herbert C, Pauli P, Breslin PAS. Oral perceptions of fat and taste stimuli are modulated by affect and mood induction. *PLoS One.* 2013;8(6):e65006.

28. American Psychiatric Association. Bipolar and related disorders. In: *Diagnostic and Statistical Manual of Mental Disorders (DSM-5).* 5th ed. Washington, DC: American Psychiatric Association; 2013:123-154.

29. National Institute of Health, National Institute of Mental Health. Bipolar Disorder. November 2017. https://www.nimh.nih.gov/health/statistics/bipolar-disorder.shtml. Accessed September 7, 2018.

30. Yatham LN, Kennedy SH, Parikh SV, et al. Canadian Network for Mood and Anxiety Treatments (CANMAT) and International Society for Bipolar Disorders (ISBD) 2018 guidelines for the management of patients with bipolar disorder. *Bipolar Disord.* 2018;20(2):97-170.

31. Jin H, McCrone P. Cost-of-illness studies for bipolar disorder: systematic review of international studies. *Pharmacoeconomics.* 2015;33(4):341-353.

32. Haynes PL, Gengler D, Kelly M. Social rhythm therapies for mood disorders: an update. *Curr Psychiatry Rep.* 2016;18:75. doi:10.1007/s11920-016-0712-3.

33. Clark DB. Dental care for the patient with bipolar disorder. *J Can Dent Assoc.* 2003;69(1):20-24.

34. National Institute of Health, National Institute of Mental Health. Eating Disorders. November 2017. https://www.nimh.nih.gov/health/statistics/eating-disorders.shtml. Accessed September 8, 2018.

35. American Psychiatric Association. Feeding and eating disorders. In: *Diagnostic and Statistical Manual of Mental Disorders (DSM-5).* 5th ed. Washington, DC.

36. National Institute of Health, National Institute of Mental Health. Eating Disorders. https://www.nimh.nih.gov/health/topics/eating-disorders/index.shtml. Accessed September 8, 2018.

37. Allison S, Timmerman GM. Anatomy of a binge: food environment and characteristics of nonpurge binge episodes. *Eat Behav.* 2007;8(1):31-38.

38. Callum AM, Lewis LM. Diabulimia among adolescents and young adults with type 1 diabetes. *Clin Nurs Stud.* 2014;2(4):12.

39. De Paoli T, Rogers PJ. Disordered eating and insulin restriction in type 1 diabetes: a systematic review and testable model. *Eat Disord.* 2018;26(4):343-360.

40. Dunn TM, Bratman S. On orthorexia nervosa: a review of the literature and proposed diagnostic criteria. *Eat Behav.* 2016;21:11-17.

41. Hilbert A, Hoek HW, Schmidt R. Evidence-based clinical guidelines for eating disorders: international comparison. *Curr Opin Psychiatry.* 2017;30(6):423-437.

42. Tholking MM, Mellowspring AC, Eberle SG, et al. American Dietetic Association: standards of practice and standards of professional performance for registered dietitians (competent, proficient, and expert) in disordered eating and eating disorders (DE and ED). *J Am Diet Assoc.* 2011;111(8):1242-1249.

43. Romanos GE, Javed F, Romanos EB, Williams RC. Oro-facial manifestations in patients with eating disorders. *Appetite*. 2012;59(2):499-504.

44. Kisely S, Baghaie H, Lalloo R, Johnson N. Association between poor oral health and eating disorders: systematic review and meta-analysis. *Br J Psychiatry*. 2015;207(4):299-305.

45. National Institute of Health, National Institute of Mental Health. Schizophrenia. February 2016. https://www.nimh.nih.gov/health/topics/schizophrenia/index.shtml. Accessed September 8, 2018.

46. Popovic D, Benabarre A, Crespo JM, et al. Risk factors for suicide in schizophrenia: systematic review and clinical recommendations. *Acta Psychiatr Scand*. 2014;130(6):418-426.

47. Fuller-Thomson E, Hollister B. Schizophrenia and suicide attempts: findings from a representative community-based Canadian sample. *Schizophr Res Treatment*. 2016;2016:3165243.

48. Hunt GE, Large MM, Cleary M, Lai HMX, Saunders JB. Prevalence of comorbid substance use in schizophrenia spectrum disorders in community and clinical settings, 1990-2017: systematic review and meta-analysis. *Drug Alcohol Depend*. 2018;191:234-258.

49. Dickerson F, Schroeder J, Katsafanas E, et al. Cigarette smoking by patients with serious mental illness, 1999-2016: an increasing disparity. *Psychiatr Serv*. 2018;69(2):147-153.

50. Yang M, Chen P, He MX, et al. Poor oral health in patients with schizophrenia: a systematic review and meta-analysis. *Schizophr Res*. 2018;201:3-9.

51. Arnaiz A, Zumβrraga M, Díez-Altuna I, Uriarte JJ, Moro J, Pérez-Ansorena MA. Oral health and the symptoms of schizophrenia. *Psychiatry Res*. 2011;188(1):24-28.

52. National Suicide Prevention Lifeline. *#BeThe1To: Join the Movement*. Rockville, MD. http://www.bethe1to.com/join/. Accessed September 9, 2018.

59

The Patient with a Substance-Related Disorder

Karen M. Portillo, RDH, MS, and Ernestine R. Daniels, RDH, BS

CHAPTER OUTLINE

INTRODUCTION

ALCOHOL CONSUMPTION
I. Clinical Pattern of Alcohol Use
II. Etiology

METABOLISM OF ALCOHOL
I. Ingestion and Absorption
II. Liver Metabolism
III. Diffusion
IV. BAC

HEALTH HAZARDS OF ALCOHOL
I. Brain
II. Heart
III. Liver Disease
IV. Digestive System
V. Nutritional Deficiencies
VI. Cancer Risk
VII. Immunity and Infection
VIII. Nervous System
IX. Reproductive System

FETAL ALCOHOL SPECTRUM DISORDERS
I. Alcohol Use during Pregnancy

ALCOHOL WITHDRAWAL SYNDROME
I. Predisposing Factors
II. Signs and Symptoms
III. Complications

TREATMENT FOR AUD
I. Types of Treatment
II. Treatment Settings

ABUSE OF PRESCRIPTION AND STREET DRUGS

RISK MANAGEMENT FOR PRESCRIPTION DRUGS OF ABUSE
I. Prevention of Opioid Addiction in the Dental Office

MOST COMMON DRUGS OF ABUSE
I. Cannabinoids (Marijuana)
II. Depressants
III. Dissociative Anesthetics
IV. Hallucinogens
V. Opioids and Morphine Derivatives
VI. Stimulants
VII. Other Compounds
VIII. Emerging Drugs

MEDICAL EFFECTS OF DRUG ABUSE
I. Cardiovascular Effects
II. Neurologic Effects
III. Gastrointestinal Effects
IV. Kidney Damage
V. Liver Damage
VI. Musculoskeletal Effects
VII. Respiratory Effects
VIII. Prenatal Effects
IX. Infections

TREATMENT METHODS
I. Behavioral Therapies
II. Drug Withdrawal Medications

DENTAL HYGIENE PROCESS OF CARE
I. Assessment
II. Intraoral Examination
III. Dental Hygiene Diagnosis
IV. Care Planning
V. Implementation
VI. Evaluation

DOCUMENTATION

EVERYDAY ETHICS

FACTORS TO TEACH THE PATIENT

REFERENCES

LEARNING OBJECTIVES

After studying this chapter, the student will be able to:

1. Explain key terms and concepts related to the metabolism, intoxication effects, and use patterns of alcohol.

2. Identify physical health hazards, medical effects, and oral manifestations associated with alcohol and substances of abuse.

3. Interpret names of the most commonly abused drugs and describe their intoxication effects and methods of use.

4. Discuss modifications for the dental hygiene process of care for patients who are chemically dependent. Recognize patients who are cognitively impaired and cannot be treated in a safe manner.

5. Employ the National Institute on Drug Abuse Quick Screen to assess patients who are at risk for alcohol or substance abuse and provide resources for the patient to seek help.

INTRODUCTION

◆ When an individual consumes a substance such as drugs or alcohol, their brain produces large amounts of dopamine. Dopamine is a neurotransmitter which triggers the brain's reward system. After repeated drug or alcohol use, the brain is unable to produce normal amounts of dopamine on its own, resulting in the individual to increase their usage of the substance leading to an addiction.[1]

◆ Patients who develop a drug or alcohol dependence may "premedicate" themselves when a stressful situation such as a dental appointment is anticipated; therefore, direct questions and observation of symptoms at each appointment are required to determine if a patient is cognitively impaired to prevent complications.

◆ There is no classic cultural, socioeconomic, or educational profile for one who has a substance abuse disorder.

◆ A patient's medical and dental history does not always provide the information necessary to determine whether the patient uses substances at all, or the level of dependency.

◆ It is a professional responsibility of the dental hygienist to:

• View substance dependency as an illness and to be aware of the characteristics that suggest a possible condition.

• Address the issues of an appropriate dental hygiene care plan for the patient who has become dependent on a substance.

ALCOHOL CONSUMPTION

I. Clinical Pattern of Alcohol Use

◆ Abstinence and low-risk use. For women, low-risk drinking is defined as no more than three drinks on any single day and no more than seven drinks per week. For men, it is defined as no more than four drinks on any single day and no more than 14 drinks per week.[2] Figure 59-1 shows what constitutes a standard drink.

◆ Moderate alcohol use is defined as up to one drink/day for women and two drinks per day for men.[2] The individual can function appropriately in work, family, and social situations.

◆ Unhealthy alcohol use increases an individual's risk for neuropsychiatric conditions, gastrointestinal diseases, cancers including oropharyngeal, intentional injuries such as suicide, unintentional injuries, and cardiovascular disease.

◆ Binge drinking occurs when an individual excessively drinks in a short period, typically four drinks for women and five drinks for men in about a 2-hour period, increasing blood alcohol concentration (BAC) levels to 0.08 g/dL.[2]

◆ Heavy alcohol use increases a patient's risk for infectious diseases such as pneumonia or tuberculosis (TB) as the immune system becomes more compromised. The Substance Abuse and Mental Health Services Administration defines heavy alcohol use as binge drinking on 5 or more days in the past month.[2]

◆ Alcohol Use Disorder (AUD), also known as alcoholism, is a pattern of alcohol use in which one has difficulty controlling his/her drinking, being preoccupied with alcohol, continuing to use alcohol even when it causes problems, having to drink more to get the same effect, or having withdrawal symptoms when blood alcohol levels decrease or if one ceases to drink.[3]

A. Effects of Alcohol Intoxication

The following are the effects of alcohol intoxication[4]:

◆ Behavioral changes: aggressiveness, mood instability, impaired judgment; impaired social or occupational functioning; impaired attention and memory; stupor or coma.

◆ Physical characteristics: slurred speech, lack of coordination, unsteady gait, and nystagmus.

◆ Complications: irresponsible actions in work and family settings.

◆ Accidents with resultant bruises, fractures, or brain trauma.

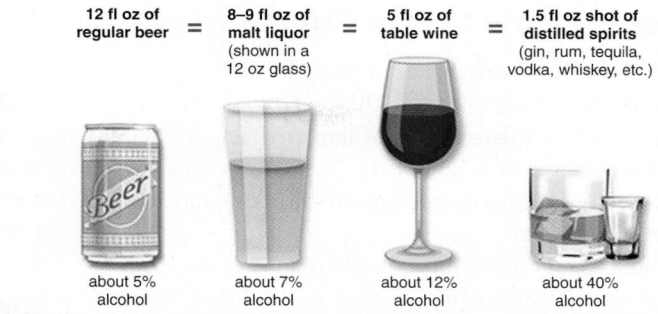

FIGURE 59-1 • What Is a Standard Drink? In the United States, one "standard" drink contains roughly 14 g of pure alcohol, which is found in: 12 ounces of regular beer, which is usually about 5% alcohol; 5 ounces of wine, which is typically about 12% alcohol; and 1.5 ounces of distilled spirits, which is about 40% alcohol. Graphic was designed by Anthony Portillo, adapted from the National Institute on Alcohol Abuse and Alcoholism. (From National Institute on Alcohol Abuse and Alcoholism. Retrieved from https://www.niaaa.nih.gov /alcohol-health/overview-alcohol-consumption /what-standard-drink.)

- Vehicular accidents.
- Suicide.

B. Consequences of Underage Drinking[5]

- Binge drinking.
- Drinking and driving.
- Suicide.
- Sexual assault.
- High-risk sex.
- Alcohol-induced mental impairment.

C. Signs of AUD

AUD, also known as alcoholism or alcohol dependence, is a disease which includes four main symptoms:

- *Craving*: A strong need or compulsion to drink.
- *Loss of control*: The inability to limit one's drinking to a safe level despite the negative impact it may be having on one's responsibilities to work, school, or family/ relationships.
- *Physical dependence*: Withdrawal symptoms, such as nausea, sweating, shakiness, and anxiousness, when alcohol use is stopped after a period of heavy drinking.
- *Tolerance*: The need to drink greater amounts of alcohol to reach a level of desired intoxication. Other signs include amnesia and binge drinking.[6]

II. Etiology

A. Genetics

- Although there is no single gene directly linked to alcoholism, a combination of genes related to alcoholism and mental illness can increase the risk of developing alcoholism by 20%.[7]

B. Biopsychosocial

- Alcohol-specific parenting is a distinct and influential predictor of adolescent alcohol use partially shaped by parents' own drinking experiences.
- Children of alcohol-dependent parents are two to six times more likely than the general population to develop AUDs. Additionally, children raised by alcohol-dependent parents are exposed to a higher level of multiple risk factors leading to alcohol-related problems[8]:
  - Mental and behavioral disorders and adverse family environments.
  - Decreased sensitivity to intoxication effects of alcohol.

C. Environmental

- Psychological stress, family, peers, and social forces.
- Current lifestyle, culture, advertisements, and economics.
- Motivational factors: both emotional (stress reduction, mood enhancement, social rewards) and cognitive (conscious and unconscious beliefs about alcohol) may play a role in an individual's decision to drink.

METABOLISM OF ALCOHOL

I. Ingestion and Absorption

- Upon intake, alcohol is absorbed promptly from the stomach and small intestine into the bloodstream.
- Transported to the liver for metabolism.[9]

II. Liver Metabolism

- More than 90% of ingested alcohol is converted into acetaldehyde, then acetone, and finally into carbon dioxide and water by the action of various liver enzymes.
- High acetaldehyde levels and chronic alcohol consumption impair liver function and lead to liver damage.[9]

III. Diffusion

- Within 5 minutes after ingestion, alcohol can be detected in the blood.
- Alcohol is quickly diffused into all cells and intercellular fluid of the body.
- Less than 10% is excreted directly through the lungs, skin, and kidney (breath, sweat, and urine).
- A person's alcohol level can be determined by several tests of the blood, urine, saliva, or water vapor in the breath.[9]

IV. Blood Alcohol Level (BAC)

◆ Alcohol-impaired driving accounted for 31% of the traffic-related fatalities in 2014 in the United States.

◆ Drivers are considered alcohol-impaired when their BACs are 0.08 g/dL or higher.

◆ BAC measurement reflects a person's drinking rate and rate of metabolism.

◆ Alcohol is metabolized more slowly than it is absorbed. The BAC increases when alcohol is consumed faster than previous drinks are metabolized.

◆ The rate at which the body will absorb and metabolize alcohol is based on factors such as age, gender, percentage of fatty tissue in the body, and whether food is also being metabolized.[10]

◆ The characteristic effects exhibited at various levels of blood alcohol can be seen in Figure 59-2.

HEALTH HAZARDS OF ALCOHOL

Prolonged alcohol use causes many serious medical disorders. Alcohol consumption has been identified as a cause for more than 200 diseases, health conditions, or injuries that can affect various organs or body systems. A few are mentioned here.

I. Brain

◆ Alcohol interferes with the brain's communication pathways, slowing down the transfer of neurotransmitters.

◆ These neurotransmitter disruptions can change mood and behavior, and make it harder for a person to think clearly or move with adequate coordination.[11]

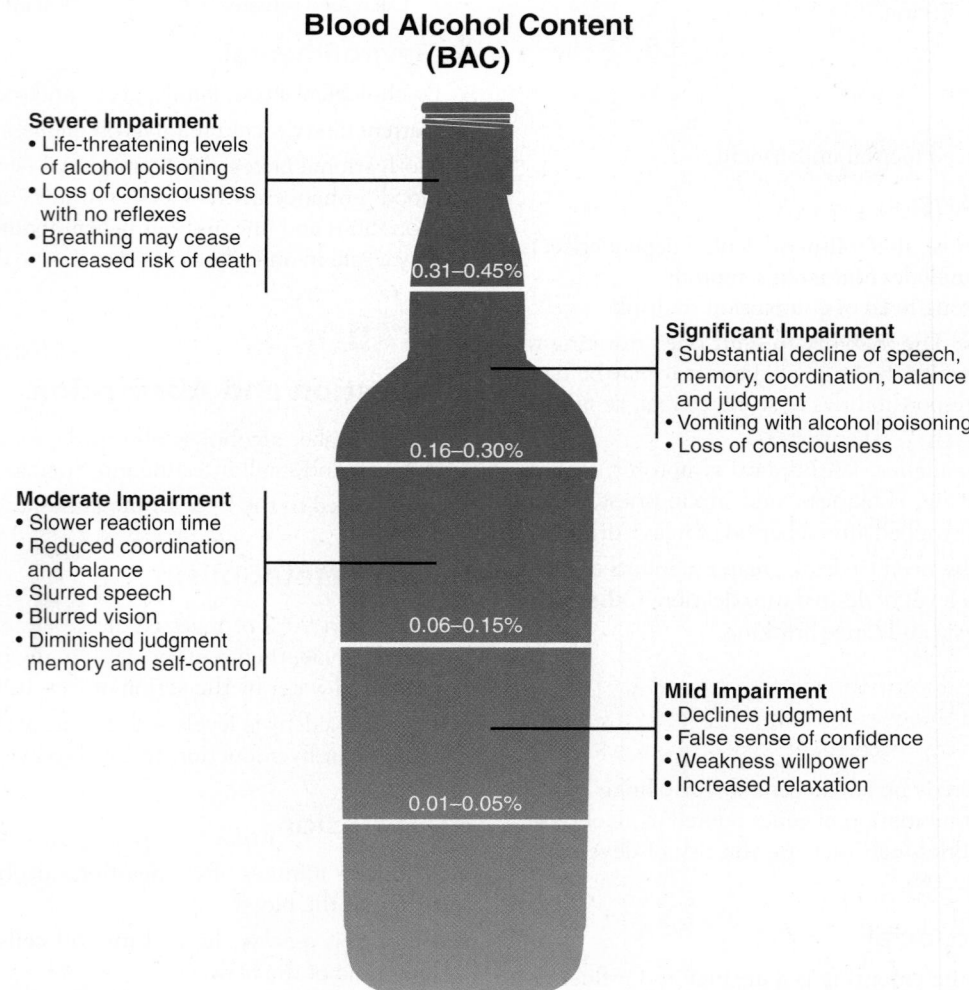

Blood Alcohol Content (BAC)

Severe Impairment
• Life-threatening levels of alcohol poisoning
• Loss of consciousness with no reflexes
• Breathing may cease
• Increased risk of death

0.31–0.45%

Significant Impairment
• Substantial decline of speech, memory, coordination, balance and judgment
• Vomiting with alcohol poisoning
• Loss of consciousness

0.16–0.30%

Moderate Impairment
• Slower reaction time
• Reduced coordination and balance
• Slurred speech
• Blurred vision
• Diminished judgment memory and self-control

0.06–0.15%

Mild Impairment
• Declines judgment
• False sense of confidence
• Weakness willpower
• Increased relaxation

0.01–0.05%

FIGURE 59-2 • Blood Alcohol Concentration (BAC) Levels Represent the Percent of Your Blood That Is Concentrated with Alcohol. A BAC of 0.10 means that 0.1% of your bloodstream is composed of alcohol. Legal intoxication level in most states is 0.080 BAC. (From Graphic designed by Anthony Portillo. Adapted from: Aware Awake Alive. Retrieved from https://awareawakealive.org/educate/blood-alcohol-content.)

II. Heart

Drinking excessively for a long period will lead to damage to the heart such as[11]:

- Cardiomyopathy.
- Arrhythmias.
- Stroke.
- High blood pressure.

III. Liver Disease

Chronic alcohol abuse is the most frequent cause of morbidity and mortality from liver diseases. Alcoholic liver disease (ALD) includes the following conditions[11,12]:

- Fatty liver with degeneration: early stages are reversible with abstinence.
- Alcoholic hepatitis: inflammation of the liver.
- Early fibrosis: healthy cells replaced by scar tissue.
- Cirrhosis: scarring of the liver with irreversible damage.
- Individuals with hepatitis C virus (HCV) are more susceptible to ALD.

IV. Digestive System

- Alcohol ingestion alters the stomach mucosa, stimulates gastric acid secretion, and affects gastric function.
- Desquamation of the stomach lining (acute gastritis) may result in bleeding lesions.
- Alcohol causes the pancreas to produce toxic substances that can eventually lead to pancreatitis.
- Injury to small intestines: diarrhea, weight loss, and vitamin deficiencies.

V. Nutritional Deficiencies

- Alcohol provides an excess of caloric intake. With the intake of large quantities of alcohol, the individual loses interest in nutritious food, which leads to many deficiencies.
- Deficiencies result from malabsorption of vitamins and essential nutrients.
- Secondary malnutrition develops from direct effects of alcohol on the gastrointestinal tract; malabsorption and maldigestion occur after cellular changes in the intestinal wall.

VI. Cancer Risk

Excessive alcohol use can increase the risk of developing certain cancers, including cancers of the[11]:

- Oral cavity.
- Esophagus.
- Pharynx.
- Liver.
- Breast.

VII. Immunity and Infection

- Those who abuse alcohol have a diminished immune response, suppression of immune system defense, and disturbed function of neutrophils.
- Risk for many bacterial infections is increased, particularly pulmonary diseases (pneumonia, TB) and viral infections (hepatitis B and C).[11]

VIII. Nervous System

A. Central and Peripheral

- Early changes affect intellectual actions, judgment, and learning ability.
- Long-term alcohol abuse combined with malnutrition can lead to damage of both central and peripheral nervous systems.
- Prolonged and heavy alcohol consumption leads to chronic brain damage.

B. Wernicke–Korsakoff's Syndrome

Wernicke–Korsakoff's syndrome is a brain disorder of the cerebellum resulting in a vitamin B1 (thiamine) deficiency associated with chronic alcohol consumption. Two syndromes are involved as follows[13]:

- *Wernicke encephalopathy* causes brain damage in lower parts of the brain (thalamus and hypothalamus) leading to symptoms of mental confusion, ocular dysfunction, and gait disturbances.
- *Korsakoff's psychosis*: results in permanent brain damage resulting in persistent knowledge and memory problems characterized by forgetfulness, easy frustration, lack of muscle coordination, and amnesia.

IX. Reproductive System

- Alcohol affects every branch of the endocrine system, directly and indirectly, through the body's organization of the endocrine hormones.
- Female: increased risk for menstrual disturbances, infertility, and miscarriage, stillbirth, or premature delivery.[14]
- Male: diminished testicular function and male hormone production resulting in increased risk for impotence, infertility, and reduction of secondary sex characteristics.[15]

FETAL ALCOHOL SPECTRUM DISORDERS (FASDS)

- FASDs are a group of conditions that can occur in an individual whose mother drank alcohol during pregnancy.
- These conditions include issues with the individual's cognitive, physical, or behavioral abilities.[16]

I. Alcohol Use during Pregnancy

◆ There is no known safe amount of alcohol use during pregnancy. There is no safe form of alcohol during pregnancy; all forms of alcohol are harmful.

◆ Complete abstinence during pregnancy is safest to prevent FASD.

◆ Prenatal alcohol exposure is cited as the leading preventable cause of birth defects and intellectual disability.[17]

◆ Box 59-1 lists terminology and abbreviations for FASD.

A. Why Alcohol Is Dangerous during Pregnancy

◆ Alcohol passes freely across the placenta.

◆ Increased incidence of spontaneous abortions and stillbirths associated with alcohol consumption.

◆ Alcohol consumption anytime during pregnancy can inhibit the fetus to grow properly (low birth weight), and negatively affect proper development of the brain or central nervous system. Consumption during the first 3 months of pregnancy can cause the infant to have facial dysmorphology as shown in Figure 59-3.

◆ An infant born with FAD will have to overcome several impairments such as physical, social, psychological, and intellectual disabilities.[17]

◆ Common characteristics associated with FASD are listed in Box 59-2.

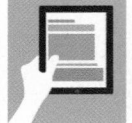

FIGURE 59-3 • Facial Features of Fetal Alcohol Syndrome. Child presenting with the characteristic pattern of abnormal facial features diagnostic for fetal alcohol spectrum disorders, including short palpebral fissure lengths, smooth philtrum, and thin upper lip. (Porth, Carol Mattson. *Essentials of Pathophysiology: Concepts of Altered Health States*, 4e. Lippincott Williams & Wilkins.)

Labels on figure: Microcephaly · Epicanthal folds · Smooth philtrum · Small chin · Flat nasal bridge · Small palpebral fissures · Short nose · Thin vermilion border (upper lip)

B. Other Factors

◆ Other poor health habits often accompany the use of alcohol, including inadequate diet and use of tobacco.

◆ The use of prescription or illicit drugs with alcohol can increase the risk of adverse outcomes.

BOX 59-1
Fetal Alcohol Spectrum Disorders (FASD) Terminology and Abbreviations

• **Fetal Alcohol Syndrome (FAS):** FAS represents the most involved end of the FASD spectrum. Fetal death is the most extreme outcome from drinking alcohol during pregnancy. People with FAS might have abnormal facial features, growth problems, and central nervous system (CNS) problems. People with FAS can have problems with learning, memory, attention span, communication, vision, or hearing. They might have a mix of these problems. People with FAS often have a hard time in school and trouble getting along with others.

• **Alcohol-Related Neurodevelopmental Disorder (ARND):** People with ARND might have intellectual disabilities and problems with behavior and learning. They might do poorly in school and have difficulties with math, memory, attention, judgment, and poor impulse control.

• **Alcohol-Related Birth Defects (ARBD):** People with ARBD might have problems with the heart, kidneys, or bones or with hearing. They might have a mix of these.

Source: Centers for Disease Control and Prevention (CDC). Fetal Alcohol Spectrum Disorders (FASD). Facts About FASDs. https://www.cdc.gov/ncbddd/fasd/facts.html. Accessed April 2, 2018.

BOX 59-2
Characteristics of an Individual with Fetal Alcohol Spectrum Disorder

• Abnormal facial features, such as a smooth philtrum and thin upper lip
• Small head size
• Shorter-than-average height
• Low body weight
• Poor coordination
• Hyperactive behavior
• Difficulty with attention
• Poor memory
• Difficulty in school (especially with math)
• Learning disabilities
• Speech and language delays
• Intellectual disability or low IQ
• Poor reasoning and judgment skills
• Sleep and sucking problems as a baby
• Vision or hearing problems
• Problems with the heart, kidneys, or bones

Source: Centers for Disease Control and Prevention (CDC). Fetal Alcohol Spectrum Disorders (FASD). Facts About FASDs. https://www.cdc.gov/ncbddd/fasd/facts.html. Accessed April 2, 2018.

ALCOHOL WITHDRAWAL SYNDROME

◆ Withdrawal syndrome consists of disturbances that occur after abrupt cessation of alcohol intake in the alcohol-dependent person.
◆ Withdrawal signs appear within a few hours after drinking has stopped.
◆ Even a relatively small decline in blood concentration can precipitate the syndrome.

I. Predisposing Factors

◆ Malnutrition, fatigue, depression, and physical illnesses aggravate withdrawal symptoms.

II. Signs and Symptoms

◆ Tremor of hands, tongue, and eyelids.
◆ Nervousness and irritation; anxiety.
◆ Malaise, weakness, and headache.
◆ Dry mouth.
◆ Autonomic hyperactivity: sweating, rapid pulse rate, and elevated blood pressure.
◆ Transient visual, tactile, or auditory hallucinations.
◆ Insomnia.
◆ Grand mal seizures.
◆ Nausea or vomiting.

III. Complications

A. Alcohol Hallucinosis

◆ Auditory and visual hallucinations can develop within 48 hours after the abrupt stop or reduction of heavy alcohol intake of long-standing dependency.
◆ Symptoms: may last weeks or months.
◆ Impairment is severe with schizophrenic symptoms, although schizophrenia is not a predisposing factor.
◆ Delirium is not present.

B. Alcohol Withdrawal Delirium or Delirium Tremens

Alcohol withdrawal delirium tremens symptoms include:
◆ A more severe reaction to a reduction in blood alcohol levels.
◆ May occur within 1 week of cessation of heavy alcohol intake.
◆ Features: marked autonomic hyperactivity: rapid heartbeat, hypertension, fever, and sweating.
◆ Vivid hallucinations (visual, auditory, tactile).
◆ Delusions and agitated behavior; tremor.
◆ Confusion and disorientation.

TREATMENT FOR AUD

I. Types of Treatment

There are different types of treatment for AUD.
◆ Behavioral treatments
  • Individual therapy to help the patient develop skills to stop drinking as well as coping skills to avoid relapse.
  • Marital and family counseling to help the patient build a strong social support system.
◆ Medications
  • Naltrexone (ReVia®) pill form taken once a day or to reduce craving for alcohol. Naltrexone is an opiate antagonist which interferes with the neurotransmitter system. Therefore, if a patient drinks alcohol while on Naltrexone, euphoria will not result.[18]
  • Acamprosate (Campral®) is a pill taken three times a day to alleviate negative symptoms of prolonged abstinence such as insomnia, anxiety, and restlessness.[19]
  • Disulfiram (Antabuse®) is a pill taken daily that will cause nausea/vomiting, flushing, and heart palpations if taken with alcohol. Disulfiram is used as a deterrent to alcohol consumption.[19]
◆ Mutual-support groups
  • Alcoholics Anonymous and other 12-step programs provide peer support for individuals who are trying to quit drinking or have quit and are trying not to relapse.

II. Treatment Settings

◆ There are different treatment settings:
  • Inpatient.
  • Outpatient.
◆ Patients with AUD should start with their primary physician for overall health assessment and assistance in determining the appropriate treatment option and resources.[20]

ABUSE OF PRESCRIPTION AND STREET DRUGS

◆ With the legalization of medical and recreational marijuana in many states and the opioid crisis occurring in many regions in our nation, every dental hygienist in current practice will encounter a patient with a chemical dependence issue and should be able to provide care in a safe manner for this patient.

RISK MANAGEMENT FOR PRESCRIPTION DRUGS OF ABUSE

◆ A major problem facing health care is the diversion of prescription medications with a high potential for abuse.

◆ Substances are classified in the U.S. Drug Enforcement Administration drug schedule according to use and abuse potential as listed in Box 59-3.

I. Prevention of Opioid Addiction in the Dental Office

◆ All members of the dental team should take responsibility to prevent opioid addiction.[21]

- Dentists should register with and utilize prescription drug monitoring programs to promote the appropriate use of controlled substances. Prescription pads are not recommended for use to avoid alterations and abuse.

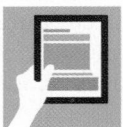

BOX 59-3
U.S. Drug Enforcement Administration Drug Schedule Classifications

Schedule I

No accepted medical use; extremely high potential for abuse; high potential for psychological and physical dependency. Some examples of Schedule I drugs are: heroin, lysergic acid diethylamide, marijuana (cannabis), 3,4-methylenedioxymethamphetamine (ecstasy), methaqualone, and peyote.

Schedule II

Has medical use but high potential for abuse; relative potential for psychological and physical dependency. Some examples of Schedule II drugs are: cocaine, methamphetamine, methadone, oxycodone (OxyContin), fentanyl.

Schedule III

Has medical use; moderate abuse potential but less than Schedule II. Some examples of Schedule III drugs are: Tylenol with codeine, ketamine, anabolic steroids, testosterone.

Schedule IV

Abuse potential exists, but less than Schedule III. Some examples of Schedule IV drugs are: Xanax, Soma, Darvon, Darvocet, Valium, Ativan, Talwin, Ambien, Tramadol.

Schedule V

Abuse potential exists, but less than Schedule IV. Some examples of Schedule V drugs are: cough preparations with less than 200 milligrams of codeine or per 100 milliliters (Robitussin AC), Lomotil, Motofen, Lyrica, Parepectolin.

Source: U.S. Drug Enforcement Administration. Drug Scheduling. https://www.dea.gov /druginfo/ds.shtml. Accessed April 2, 2018.

◆ Dentists should consider nonsteroidal anti-inflammatory analgesics as the first-line therapy for acute pain management.
◆ Patients should be educated regarding their responsibilities for preventing misuse, abuse, storage, and disposal of prescription opioids.
◆ All members of the dental team should seek continuing education in addictive disease and pain management.

MOST COMMON DRUGS OF ABUSE

The most common drugs of abuse are alcohol and those found in the categories in this section. Examples of the substance names in each category and the commercial and street names are listed in Table 59-1.

I. Cannabinoids (Marijuana)

◆ Despite cannabis use being illegal at the federal government level, as of January 2018, 30 states and the District of Columbia have legalized marijuana for either medical or recreational use.[22]
◆ The three basic types of cannabis, used for recreational or medicinal purposes, are called marijuana/weed, hash, or hash oil.[23]
◆ All three types contain more than 85 cannabinoids found within the plant, with tetrahydrocannabinol (THC) and cannabidiol (CBD) being the two best known cannabinoids.[24]
◆ THC is the primary psychoactive compound of the plant which can make a person feel paranoid or anxious. CBD is nonpsychoactive, so patients do not feel "high" using cannabis with this strain, rather gain the medicinal and therapeutic benefits cannabis can offer for medical relief.[24]

A. Medical Marijuana Use

◆ Patients use medical marijuana as an alternative to manage pain, anxiety, depression, migraine headaches, and sleep problems.[25]
◆ Synthetic oral (THC) medications such as nabilone (Cesamet®) and dronabinol (Marinol®) can be prescribed to reduce nausea and vomiting symptoms related to chemotherapy treatment or AIDS-related conditions.[26,27]
◆ Nabiximol oromucosal sprays (Sativex®) containing THC can help reduce pain and muscle spasticity in patients suffering from multiple sclerosis, spinal cord injuries, fibromyalgia, or rheumatoid arthritis.[27]
◆ Children and adolescents with drug-resistant epilepsy have experienced a decrease in seizure occurrences with CBD added into their therapy.[28]

B. Different Forms of Marijuana

◆ Inhaled[29,30]
- Cigarette forms called *joints*.
- Cigars hollowed out and filled with cannabis called *blunts*.

TABLE 59-1 • Most Commonly Abused Prescription Drugs

DRUG CATEGORY AND DEA SCHEDULE	STREET NAME AND COMMERCIAL NAME	HOW UTILIZED	HEALTH RISKS
Cannabinoids (marijuana) DEA Schedule I	Blunt, Bud, Dope, Ganja, Grass, Green, Herb, Joint, Mary Jane, Pot, Reefer, Sinsemilla, Skunk, Smoke, Trees, Weed; Hashish: Boom, Gangster, Hash, Hemp	Inhaled, smoked, vaped, dapping Edibles Pill form Topical Other forms: suppositories, inserted vaginally	Short term: Enhanced sensory perception and euphoria followed by drowsiness/relaxation; slowed reaction time; problems with balance and coordination; increased heart rate and appetite; problems with learning and memory; anxiety. Long term: Mental health problems, chronic cough, frequent respiratory infections.
Depressants: Flunitrazepam DEA Schedule IV	Circles, Date Rape Drug, Forget Pill, Forget-Me Pill, La Rocha, Lunch Money, Mexican Valium, Mind Eraser, Pingus, R2, Reynolds, Rib, Roach, Roach 2, Roaches, Roachies, Roapies, Rochas Dos, Roofies, Rope, Rophies, Row-Shay, Ruffies, Trip-and-Fall, Wolfies Rohypnol®	Swallowed (as a pill or dissolved in a drink), snorted	Drowsiness, sedation, sleep; amnesia, **blackout**; decreased anxiety; muscle relaxation, impaired reaction time and motor coordination; impaired mental functioning and judgment; confusion; aggression; excitability; slurred speech; headache; slowed breathing and heart rate.
Barbiturates: pentobarbital DEA Schedule II, III, IV	Barbs, Phennies, Red Birds, Reds, Tooies, Yellow Jackets, Yellows Nembutal®	Swallowed, injected	Drowsiness, slurred speech, poor concentration, confusion, dizziness, problems with movement and memory, lowered blood pressure, slowed breathing.
Benzodiazepines: alprazolam DEA Schedule IV	Candy, Downers, Sleeping Pills, Tranks Xanax®, Valium®, Ativan®	Swallowed, snorted	Drowsiness, slurred speech, poor concentration, confusion, dizziness, problems with movement and memory, lowered blood pressure, slowed breathing.
Dissociative anesthetics: Ketamine DEA Schedule III	Cat Valium, K, Special K, Vitamin K Ketalar®	Injected, snorted, smoked (powder added to tobacco or marijuana cigarettes), swallowed	Short term: Problems with attention, learning, and memory; dream-like states, hallucinations; sedation; confusion; loss of memory; raised blood pressure; unconsciousness; dangerously slowed breathing. Long term: Ulcers and pain in the bladder; kidney problems; stomach pain; depression; poor memory.
Hallucinogens: *Lysergic acid diethylamide* DEA Schedule I	Acid, Blotter, Blue Heaven, Cubes, Microdot, Yellow Sunshine *No commercial uses	Swallowed, absorbed through mouth tissues (paper squares)	Short term: Rapid emotional swings; distortion of a person's ability to recognize reality, think rationally, or communicate with others; raised blood pressure, heart rate, body temperature; dizziness; loss of appetite; tremors; enlarged pupils. Long term: Frightening flashbacks (called hallucinogen persisting perception disorder); ongoing visual disturbances, disorganized thinking, paranoia, and mood swings.
MDMA (Ecstasy/Molly) DEA Schedule I	Adam, Clarity, Eve, Lover's Speed, Peace, Uppers *No commercial uses	Swallowed, snorted	Short term: Lowered inhibition; enhanced sensory perception; increased heart rate and blood pressure; muscle tension; nausea; faintness; chills or sweating; sharp rise in body temperature leading to kidney failure or death.

(Continues)

TABLE 59-1 • Most Commonly Abused Prescription Drugs (*Continued*)

DRUG CATEGORY AND DEA SCHEDULE	STREET NAME AND COMMERCIAL NAME	HOW UTILIZED	HEALTH RISKS
Opioids: Fentanyl DEA Schedule II	Apache, China Girl, China Town, Dance Fever, Friend, Goodfellas, Great Bear, He-Man, Jackpot, King Ivory, Murder 8, and Tango & Cash.	Injected, snorted/sniffed, smoked, taken orally by pill or tablet, and spiked onto blotter paper	Relaxation, euphoria, pain relief, sedation, confusion, drowsiness, dizziness, nausea, vomiting, urinary retention, pupillary constriction, and respiratory depression.
Heroin DEA Schedule I	Brown sugar, China White, Dope, H, Horse, Junk, Skag, Skunk, Smack, White Horse *No commercial uses	Injected, smoked, snorted	Short term: euphoria; dry mouth; itching; nausea; vomiting; analgesia; slowed breathing and heart rate. Long term: collapsed veins; abscesses (swollen tissue with pus); infection of the lining and valves in the heart; constipation and stomach cramps; liver or kidney disease; pneumonia.
Stimulants: Cocaine DEA Schedule II	Blow, Bump, C, Candy, Charlie, Coke, Crack, Flake, Rock, Snow, Toot Cocaine hydrochloride topical solution	Snorted, smoked, injected	Short term: Narrowed blood vessels; enlarged pupils; increased body temperature, heart rate, and blood pressure; headache; abdominal pain and nausea; euphoria; increased energy, alertness; insomnia, restlessness; anxiety; erratic and violent behavior, panic attacks, paranoia, psychosis; heart rhythm problems, heart attack; stroke, seizure, coma. Long term: Loss of sense of smell, nosebleeds, nasal damage, and trouble swallowing from snorting; infection and death of bowel tissue from decreased blood flow; poor nutrition and weight loss; lung damage from smoking.
Methamphetamine DEA Schedule II	Crank, Chalk, Crystal, Fire, Glass, Go Fast, Ice, Meth, Speed Desoxyn®	Swallowed, snorted, smoked, injected	Short term: Increased wakefulness and physical activity; decreased appetite; increased breathing, heart rate, blood pressure, temperature; irregular heartbeat. Long term: Anxiety, confusion, insomnia, mood problems, violent behavior, paranoia, hallucinations, delusions, weight loss, severe dental problems (meth mouth), intense itching leading to skin sores from scratching.
Other compounds: Steroids DEA Schedule III	Juice, Gym Candy, Pumpers, Roids Oxandrin®, Anadrol®, Depo-testosterone®	Injected, swallowed, applied to skin	Short term: Builds muscles, improved athletic performance, acne, fluid retention (especially in the hands and feet), oily skin, yellowing of the skin, infection. Long term: Kidney damage or failure; liver damage; high blood pressure, enlarged heart, or changes in cholesterol leading to increased risk of stroke or heart attack, even in young people; aggression; extreme mood swings; anger (roid rage); extreme irritability; delusions; impaired judgment.

TABLE 59-1 • Most Commonly Abused Prescription Drugs (*Continued*)

DRUG CATEGORY AND DEA SCHEDULE	STREET NAME AND COMMERCIAL NAME	HOW UTILIZED	HEALTH RISKS
Inhalants Not scheduled	Poppers, snappers, whippets, laughing gas	Inhaled through the nose or mouth	Confusion; nausea; slurred speech; lack of coordination; euphoria; dizziness; drowsiness; lightheadedness, hallucinations/delusions; headaches; sudden sniffing death due to heart failure (from butane, propane, and other chemicals in aerosols); death from asphyxiation, suffocation, convulsions or seizures, coma, or choking.
Emerging Drugs: synthetic cathinones (bath salts) Not scheduled	Bloom, Cloud Nine, Cosmic Blast, Flakka, Ivory Wave, Lunar Wave, Scarface, Vanilla Sky, White Lightning No commercial uses for ingested "bath salts"	Swallowed, snorted, injected	Short term: Increased heart rate and blood pressure; euphoria; increased sociability and sex drive; paranoia, agitation, and hallucinations; violent behavior; sweating; nausea, vomiting; insomnia; irritability; dizziness; depression; panic attacks; reduced motor control; cloudy thinking. Long term: death.
Krokodil DEA Schedule I	Russian Magic, Cheornaya, Himiya, Crocodil Desomorphine	Injected	Blood vessel damage, open ulcers, gangrene, phlebitis, skin and soft tissue infections, limb amputations, blood poisoning, infected gums/tooth loss, blood-borne virus transmission (HIV/HCV due to needle sharing), bone infections (osteomyelitis), speech and motor skills impairment, memory loss and impaired concentration, liver and kidney damage, death.

Source: National Institute on Drug Abuse. *Commonly Abused Drugs.* https://d14rmgtrwzf5a.cloudfront.net/sites/default/files/commonly_abused_drugs.pdf. Accessed April 2, 2018.

- Can use a hookah pipe or bong which filters the smoke through water.
- Vaping—a fine mist is inhaled instead of smoking the cannabis to reduce a person's exposure to carcinogens.
- Dabbing uses hash oil (most potent type) in a wax form.

◆ Oral
- Edibles are when marijuana is added to foods or beverages.
  - Edibles take longer for the person to feel the effect (up to 2 hours) because it must be digested and metabolized.
  - Edibles can present a dosing challenge for some users, and the intensity of edibles is much greater causing full-body, psychoactive effects with much longer lasting duration times of several hours.
  - Many edible users prefer consumption before bedtime to aid with sleeping and wake up not feeling high but pain free.[31]

- Pill or capsule forms of marijuana (discussed in "Medical Marijuana Use" section).
- Oral tinctures (liquid cannabis) or oromucosal sprays (also discussed in the "Medical Marijuana Use" section) are applied sublingually for a rapid response (5–30 minutes).[30,31]

◆ Topical
- There are forms of cannabis delivery that can provide medicinal benefits without cerebral stimulation.
- Examples are topical creams or oils for localized pain relief or reduction of inflammation to an area.[32]

◆ Alternative
- For more general body distribution with nonpsychoactive effects, there are cannabis suppositories that can be inserted vaginally like a tampon.
- This provides an alternative for those who cannot tolerate the edibles or for patients who do not want to be exposed to the carcinogens of smoking, vaping, or dabbing.
- Rectal cannabis suppositories take only 10–15 minutes to take effect, directing the cannabinoids into

the bloodstream, bypassing metabolism in the liver, and allowing the therapeutic effects to last 4–8 hours without impairing the user's cognition.[32]

◆ Individuals who utilize the inhalation forms of marijuana, similar to tobacco use, are associated with increased risk of cancer, lung damage, and oral health disease, such as oral cancers, periodontitis, and dental caries.[33,34]

II. Depressants

◆ A drug that suppresses the central nervous system to calm or sedate the patient.

◆ Depressants are taken to relieve anxiety, promote sleep, and manage seizure activity.

◆ Examples are *downers*, *sleeping pills*, *ludes*, *rophies*, *alcohol*.

III. Dissociative Anesthetics

◆ A form of general anesthesia that promotes dissociation from the environment but not necessarily complete unconsciousness. Sometimes used for short diagnostic or surgical procedures.

◆ Drugs such as synthetic cannabinoids, synthetic cathinones, ketamine, piperazines, and some plant-based drugs such as khat and kratom are examples of new psychoactive substances (NPS).

◆ In the past few decades, ketamine has gained popularity as a *club drug* due to its euphoric qualities.

◆ Street names: *angel dust*, *Special K*.

IV. Hallucinogens

◆ Chemical substances that produce mind-altering or mental perception-altering properties.

◆ These drugs act on the central nervous system leading to the user seeing and hearing phenomena that do not exist.

◆ A disorder associated with the use of these substances can produce hallucinogen persisting perception disorder, commonly known as "flashbacks."

◆ 3,4-methylenedioxymethamphetamine (*MDMA*) or *Ecstasy* or *Molly*, a popular drug among teens and young adults, widely used at nightclubs and bars (also used as a club drug).

◆ Molly, which is slang for *molecular*, refers to the pure crystalline powder form of ecstasy.

◆ *MDMA* is classified as a stimulant, but is known for its hallucinogenic effects.

◆ Examples are *lysergic acid diethylamide (LSD)*, *peyote*, *dimethyltryptamine*, and *magic mushrooms*.

V. Opioids and Morphine Derivatives

◆ Narcotic substances made from the Asian poppy or produced as synthetic drugs with the effects of opium: they result in analgesic and euphoric effects.

◆ Opioids are one of the most commonly prescribed as analgesics, anesthetics, antidiarrheal agents, and cough suppressants.

◆ *Heroin* is one of the most commonly abused drugs of this class: it can be injected, smoked, or snorted. Heroin use changes the functioning of the brain, increasing dependence of the drug.

◆ Other opioid drugs include morphine, OxyContin® (oxycodone), Vicodin® (hydrocodone), Percodan® (oxycodone), and Percocet® (oxycodone). Although these opioids are prescribed legally for medical use to treat pain, the medications can lead to addiction resulting in similar harmful consequences as illegal heroin use.

◆ Vicodin® (hydrocodone) is a schedule III drug and its potency is between codeine and oxycodone. It is an analgesic and pain reliever, and has a high risk for addiction and dependence.

◆ OxyContin® (oxycodone) is a schedule II drug, a narcotic pain reliever to treat moderate to severe pain. Has high risk for addiction and dependence with use.

◆ Percodan® (oxycodone/aspirin) is a schedule II drug and a nonsteroidal anti-inflammatory drug, narcotic, and analgesic used to treat moderate to severe pain. High risk for addiction and dependence exists with use.

◆ Percocet® (oxycodone/acetaminophen) is a schedule II drug and a pain reliever to treat moderate to moderately severe pain. High risk for addiction and dependence exists with use.

◆ Fentanyl is an opioid that is 80 times more potent than morphine and 50 times more potent than heroin.
  • Intravenous Fentanyl can be used as an anesthetic and analgesic for surgical procedures.
  • Duragesic® is a Fentanyl transdermal patch used to manage chronic pain by slowly releasing fentanyl through the skin into the bloodstream over 48–72 hours.
  • Actiq® dissolves quickly and is absorbed through the sublingual mucosa to provide rapid analgesia. This is especially beneficial for patients undergoing cancer treatment to treat pain that has a rapid onset with intensity.[35]

◆ Street-produced Fentanyl, which is produced in China and trafficked through Mexico, has generated the opioid and heroin crisis in many American cities which has led to fatalities.[35]
  • Fentanyl users do not fit the typical illicit drug user characteristic, since many became addicted from a surgical procedure or to treat chronic pain conditions, and became addicted to opioids as a result.[35]

◆ Naloxone (Narcan®) is a nasal spray that blocks the effects of opioids in overdose situations.
  • Many first responders carry Narcan®, especially in cities where opioid overdosing is prevalent.
  • Individuals or families with a family member battling an opioid addiction are encouraged to carry Narcan® to counter an opioid overdose situation and many dental offices and clinics include it in the emergency kit.

VI. Stimulants

- A class of drugs that enhances brain activity.
  - Stimulants cause an increase in mental alertness, attention, and energy; they improve motor skills and elicit a general sense of well-being.
  - They increase cardiac and respiratory function and speed up metabolism.
  - Stimulants include drugs such as cocaine, crack cocaine, amphetamine, and methamphetamine.
- *Cocaine hydrochloride powder* can be "snorted" through the nostrils, or, when mixed with water, can be injected intravenously.
  - *Crack cocaine* is a cocaine alkaloid in the form of a small rock.
  - *Crack* is cocaine that has been processed from cocaine hydrochloride to a free base for smoking. It is easily vaporized and inhaled and exhibits an extremely rapid onset of effects.
- *Amphetamines* are prescription medication used to treat attention-deficit hyperactivity disorder and narcolepsy. They increase alertness, focus, and energy.
  - Common prescription stimulants are dextroamphetamine (Dexedrine®), dextroamphetamine/amphetamine (Adderall®), methylphenidate (Ritalin®, Concerta®).
  - Slang terms for prescription stimulants include *Speed, Uppers,* and *Vitamin R*.
- *Methamphetamine* (*meth, speed*) is taken orally, intranasally (snorting the powder), by intravenous injection, or by smoking. Meth users are resistant to local anesthesia.[26]
  - *Ice,* a very pure form of methamphetamine (seen as crystals under high magnification), produces an immediate and powerful stimulant when smoked.

VII. Other Compounds

A. Anabolic Steroids

- Used to build muscles and for increased performance.
- May produce a feeling of well-being or euphoria, followed by lack of energy and irritability.
- Short-term effects may lead to mental problems such as paranoia, extreme irritability, delusions, impaired judgment, and violent outbursts.
  - Long-term effects include depression, kidney decline or failure, liver damage, enlarged heart, hypertension, and elevated blood cholesterol levels which increase the risk of stroke and heart attack, even if the user is of a young age.
  - Gender-specific effects in males can cause shrinking testicles, decreased sperm count, baldness, development of breasts, and increased risk for prostate cancer. In females, steroids can cause growth of facial hair or excess body hair, male-pattern baldness, changes in or stop in the menstrual cycle, enlarged clitoris, and a deepened voice.

- Age-specific effects in teenagers can result in stunted growth if steroids are used before the teen's growth spurt.

B. Inhalants

- A breathable chemical vapor that produces psychoactive effects.
- Capable of producing intoxication, abuse, and dependence.
- Inhalants can come in different forms: solvents, aerosol sprays, gases, or nitrites.
  - Available in a wide variety of commercial products: paint thinners, gasoline, glue, spray paint, computer cleaning dusters, liquid aroma, leather cleaner, or balloons filled with nitrous oxide are just a few common household examples.
  - Nitrous oxide used in medical and dental settings also presents a risk for abuse.
- A substance-soaked cloth (called huffing) or substance placed in a paper or plastic bag (called bagging) is applied to the nose and mouth and vapors are inhaled.
- Intoxication is characterized by mild euphoria and a change in the perception of time.
- Causes relaxation of the smooth muscle and a decrease in oxygen-carrying capacity of the blood.
- Toxic reactions: vomiting, headache, hypotension, and dizziness.

VIII. Emerging Drugs

A. Synthetic Cathinones (Bath Salts)

- Bath salts contain two man-made stimulants mephedrone and methylone which effect the brain much like MDMA (Ecstasy).
- Bath salts are usually in the form of white or brown crystal-like powder which can be swallowed, snorted, smoked, or injected.
- Synthetic cathinones are part of a group of drugs called "NPS."
- Synthetic cathinone affects the brain similar to cocaine, but is 10 times more powerful.
- Bath salts can produce such effects as paranoia, hallucinations, increased sex drive, panic attacks, or excited delirium.
- Bath salts are marketed as an inexpensive alternative to methamphetamine or cocaine.
- Synthetic cathinones consumers can purchase products online and in drug paraphernalia stores under a variety of brand names, which include Bliss, Cloud Nine, Lunar Wave, Vanilla Sky, or White Lightning.

B. Desomorphine (Krokodil)

- Desomorphine is a synthetic opioid first synthesized in the U.S. in 1932 and used for surgical procedures because it was 8–10 times more potent than morphine with a fast onset. It was later discontinued as other medications were found to be more effective and longer lasting.

- A street form of desomorphine reemerged in the early 2000s in Russia called krokodil, with the name being related to its chemical name α-chlorocodide, and for the damage that occurs to the skin with intravenous use, resembling crocodile leather.[36,37]

- Homemade production of krokodil is inexpensive compared to heroin use, but very toxic. The user will mix 5–10 codeine tablets with paint thinner, gasoline or lighter fluid, hydrochloric acid, iodine, and red phosphorus. The drug is injected and since no filtration process has occurred, skin, blood vessels, muscles, and bones in the injected area are immediately damaged and eventually necrosis of the area occurs. These conditions usually lead to amputation or death. Since desomorphine has a short half-life, krokodil users have to inject often to obtain their high, decreasing their life span to 1–2 years from their initial injection without intervention.[38,39]

  - The first reported case in the U.S. was seen in the emergency department of John Hopkins School of Medicine in Baltimore, MD. The patient was a 23-year-old female who complained of pain and nonhealing ulcers in her forearms where she had injected krokodil 12 months previously. The patient grew more concerned as the area of injection initially had purulent drainage, but had become malodorous as the area became necrotic.[40]

  - Due to the use of red phosphorus in the street form, cases of jaw osteonecrosis in both maxillary and mandibular jaws have been reported in users of krokodil. The necrotic areas leave exposed alveolar bone with empty dental sockets. Surgical removal of the necrotized areas in krokodil users who have gone through withdrawal has had some cases with low rates of reoccurrence.[41,42]

MEDICAL EFFECTS OF DRUG ABUSE

I. Cardiovascular Effects

- Studies show illicit drug abuse has an adverse effect on the cardiovascular system. Intravenous drug use can lead to collapsed veins and bacterial infections of the arterial system and heart valves.[43]

- Cocaine in particular causes vasoconstriction in the coronary arteries increasing blood pressure, atherosclerotic phenomena, thrombus formation, and myocardial infarction.[44]

II. Neurologic Effects

- All addictive drugs target the reward centers in the brain allowing the user to experience euphoria.

- Repeated drug abuse will alter the structure of the brain making it more difficult for the user to reach euphoric

levels, requiring increased levels of the drug which increases the dependency.[45] These alterations in the brain can lead to:

- Memory lapses.
- Decision-making or attention problems.
- Lack of impulse control.
- Increase in mental health issues which include depression, suicidal thoughts and behaviors, anxiety, paranoia, aggression, or hallucinations.[45]
- Users of addictive drugs are twice as likely to suffer from mood and anxiety disorders than the general population.[46]
- Chronic abuse of volatile solvents, such as toluene, damages the protective sheath around certain nerve fibers in the brain and peripheral nervous system. This extensive destruction of nerve fibers is clinically similar to that seen with neurologic diseases such as multiple sclerosis.[47]

III. Gastrointestinal Effects

- Cocaine in particular has been associated with gastrointestinal complications and abdominal pain.[48]

- Cocaine reduces blood flow to the intestines which can lead to ulcerations and even severe bowel gangrene.[44]

- Many drugs of abuse have been known to cause nausea and vomiting leading to appetite loss, malnourishment, and significant weight loss.[48]

IV. Kidney Damage

- Chronic drug use causes toxicity to several organs including the kidney.

- Drugs affect renal function either through the toxic effects of the drug or by a reduction in kidney function.

- Pain medications, alcohol, antibiotics, and illegal drugs can all cause kidney damage if not used properly. In addition, substance abusers tend not to keep hydrated with water which negatively impacts the proper function of the kidneys.

- Chronic use of drugs that increase blood pressure will lead to renal failure.

- Shared needles or nonsterile injecting techniques increase the user's risk for contracting infections such as viral hepatitis.[49]

V. Liver Damage

The liver detoxifies drugs, chemicals, and alcohol that are ingested.

- Changes in liver function due to drug abuse decrease the metabolism of drugs: when not able to break down properly, the drug can remain at a toxic level.

- Chronic abuse of heroin, inhalants, and steroids may cause significant liver damage.[50]

- The consumption of alcohol and cocaine together compound the danger each drug poses.

◆ The liver combines cocaine and alcohol to form a toxic metabolite called cocaethylene.[51]

◆ Cocaethylene intensifies cocaine's euphoric effects, potentially increases the risk of sudden death.

VI. Musculoskeletal Effects

Steroid use during childhood or adolescence increases sex hormone levels, which signal the bones to stop growing. This will result in the steroid user having stunted growth, unable to reach their full height potential.[52]

◆ Other drugs such as MDMA (Molly) or methamphetamine may cause severe muscle cramping and overall weakness.[52]

VII. Respiratory Effects

Drug abuse can lead to a variety of respiratory problems:

◆ Inhaling cannabis can lead to the same respiratory effects as smoking cigarettes or cigars; increased risk for bronchitis, emphysema, and/or cancer.

◆ Smoking crack cocaine can cause lung damage and severe respiratory conditions.

◆ Opioid use may cause breathing to slow and block air from entering the lungs. If the user suffers from asthma, opioids will increase breathing complications.

◆ Inhalants are comprised of toxic chemicals that damage sensitive lung tissue when inhaled.[53]

VIII. Prenatal Effects

◆ Prenatal drug abuse has been associated with:
  • Miscarriage.
  • Premature birth.
  • Low birth weight.
  • Increase of behavioral and cognitive problems in the child.[54]

◆ Drug use such as heroin during pregnancy can cause a condition in the infant called neonatal abstinence syndrome (NAS) in which the infant is born dependent on opioids.
  • An infant born with NAS requires hospitalization to treat symptoms such as seizures, fever, and weight loss or dehydration.
  • The infant is typically treated with opioid replacement, either oral morphine solution or methadone.
  • Emerging studies show sublingual buprenorphine was found to be superior to morphine or methadone. Infants treated with buprenorphine had a significantly shorter course of treatment and decreased hospital stay.[55]

◆ Inhalant abuse by expectant women can result in fetal solvent syndrome with abnormalities similar to those occurring in FASD.[56]

IX. Infections

◆ Infections have been recognized as one of the most serious complications among drug users.

◆ There are many reasons why drug users are at greater risk for infections such as the following:
  • Unsterile injection techniques and/or contaminated drug paraphernalia.
  • Adulterants (or cutting agents) may be deliberately added to street drugs to enhance their effects, resulting in lower purity of the drug. This will also increase cutaneous abscesses in the drug users.
  • Unsafe sex practices and/or multiple sex partners.
  • Living conditions such as overcrowded housing or homeless shelters or in unsanitary environments such as living on the streets.
  • Malnourishment in conjunction with the toll of the drugs on the body leads to a weakened immune system.
  • Poor hygiene.

◆ The type of infections drug users are at risk for are multiple. The following are a few examples[57,58]:
  • Pulmonary TB and respiratory tract infections including community-acquired pneumonia.
  • Endovascular—infective endocarditis.
  • Skin and soft tissue—abscesses and cellulitis located at injection sites.
  • Bone and joint—septic arthritis and osteomyelitis (an extension of soft tissue infection).
  • Sexually transmitted infections—gonorrhea, chancroid, herpes simplex virus-2, bacterial vaginosis, trichomoniasis, candidiasis, human immunodeficiency virus, hepatitis B virus, and HCV.[57,58]

TREATMENT METHODS

Chronic drug addiction causes changes in the brain involved in reward and motivation, learning and memory, and control over behavior.

◆ Drug addiction can be treated but it is complex. Successful treatment should include the following steps[59]:
  • Detoxification.
  • Behavioral therapies.
  • Medication (for opioid, tobacco, or alcohol addiction).
  • Evaluation and treatment for co-occurring mental health issues such as depression and anxiety.
  • Long-term follow-up to prevent relapse.

The principles that characterize the most effective drug abuse treatment can be found in Box 59-4.

I. Behavioral Therapies

◆ Behavioral therapies help patients modify their attitudes and behaviors toward drug use and encourage healthier life choices.

◆ Behavioral therapy sessions can be provided in an outpatient or inpatient setting. Inpatient settings are more structured and supervised. The following are examples of behavioral therapies[59]:

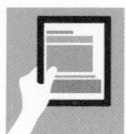

BOX 59-4
Principles of Drug Addiction Treatment

1. Addiction is a complex but treatable disease that affects brain function and behavior.
2. No single treatment is appropriate for everyone.
3. Treatment needs to be readily available.
4. Effective treatment attends to multiple needs of the individual, not just his or her drug abuse.
5. Remaining in treatment for an adequate period of time is critical.
6. Behavioral therapies—including individual, family, or group counseling—are the most commonly used forms of drug abuse treatment.
7. Medications are an important element of treatment for many patients, especially when combined with counseling and other behavioral therapies.
8. An individual's treatment and services plan must be assessed continually and modified as necessary to ensure that it meets his or her changing needs.
9. Many drug-addicted individuals also have other mental disorders.
10. Medically assisted detoxification is only the first stage of addiction treatment and by itself does little to change long-term drug abuse.
11. Treatment does not need to be voluntary to be effective.
12. Drug use during treatment must be monitored continuously, as lapses during treatment do occur.
13. Treatment programs should test patients for the presence of HIV/AIDS, hepatitis B and C, tuberculosis, and other infectious diseases as well as provide targeted risk-reduction counseling, linking patients to treatment if necessary.

Source: National Institute on Drug Abuse. *Principles of Drug Addiction Treatment: A Research-Based Guide.* 3rd ed. Principles of Effective Treatment. https://www.drugabuse.gov/publications/principles-drug-addiction-treatment-research-based-guide-third-edition/principles-effective-treatment. Accessed April 2, 2018.

- Cognitive-behavioral therapy helps patients recognize, avoid, and cope with the situations in which they are most likely to use drugs.
- Multidimensional family therapy—designed to help improve family functioning if patient still lives at home and include the family in the recovery plan.
- Motivational incentives (contingency management), which uses positive reinforcement to encourage abstinence from drugs.

II. Drug Withdrawal Medications

Medications and devices can help suppress withdrawal symptoms during the detoxification process.

- In November 2017, the Food and Drug Administration approved an electronic stimulation device called the NSS-2 Bridge. This device is placed behind the ear and sends electrical pulses to stimulate certain brain nerves to help with opioid withdrawal symptoms.[59]
- Medications such as methadone can be used to manage withdrawal symptoms, prevent relapse, and treat co-occurring conditions.

A. Methadone (Dolophine®, Methadose®)

- A full opioid agonist meaning it is an opioid that can reduce withdrawal symptoms and cravings by activating opioid receptors in the brain without producing the euphoric high.
  - Misuse of this narcotic medication can increase addiction or result in overdose or death.
- It is used in long-term maintenance for patients recovering from heroin or opioid addiction.
- Methadone can be administered 2.5–10 mg intravenously, intramuscularly, or subcutaneously every 8–12 hours. Can also be administered orally initially, 20–30 mg for the initial dose, additional 5–10 mg given every 2–4 hours. The goal is to get the patient to a 40 mg/day maintenance level.[59–61]

B. *Buprenorphine* (Subutex®) Buprenorphine/Naloxone (Suboxone®)

- A partial opioid agonist meaning it is an opioid that can activate and block opioid receptors in the brain to reduce or eliminate withdrawal symptoms without producing the euphoric high.
- Buprenorphine is a schedule III drug versus methadone which is a schedule II drug; therefore, the potential for abuse is lower.
- It is available for sublingual administration both in a stand-alone formulation (Subutex®) or in combination with naloxone (marketed as Suboxone®).
- Buprenorphine is administered in 2 or 8 mg tablets taken once or twice a day sublingually.[59–62]

C. Naltrexone (Vivitrol®/ReVia®)

- This medication is not an opioid, it is an opioid antagonist, blocking the brain's opioid receptors preventing the user from reaching the euphoric phase, and making the potential for misuse less.
- Vivitrol® is injected once a month or ReVia® can be taken orally one 50 mg tablet a day.
- Naltrexone/ReVia® is also prescribed for patients recovering from alcoholism.
- It does require full detoxification to use (usually 3–10 days of no opioid use).[59,61]

D. Other Medications

Additional medications may be prescribed during the detoxification phase including:

- Benzodiazepines—to reduce anxiety and irritability.

◆ Antidepressants—like Prozac or Zoloft to counter depression.

◆ Clonidine—reduces sweating, cramps, muscle aches, and anxiety. It can also stop tremors and seizures.

DENTAL HYGIENE PROCESS OF CARE

Every patient appreciates an atmosphere with open communication, but this is especially important in caring for patients who are chemically dependent. The clinician should assure the patient that any information shared will be kept confidential in accordance to Health Insurance Portability and Accountability Act laws, but in order to treat the patient safely, the clinician has to know what substances are in the patient's system. It is imperative that a thorough assessment be completed and documented. If the patient is cognitively impaired by a substance, legally the patient cannot consent to care and cannot be treated.

I. Assessment

A. Patient History

◆ The medical health history questionnaire should inquire about substances used, how patient administers the substance (i.e., intravenously, smoked), quantity, and time of the last dosage.

◆ Identify all current medications (both prescription and substances of abuse) in order to investigate drug–drug interactions with any medications that may be used in the oral health setting such as local anesthesia (see Chapter 11).

◆ A medical consult with the patient's physician and/or addiction specialist should be conducted prior to any dental care to determine the patient's readiness for treatment and to determine if there are any conditions requiring antibiotic prophylaxis.

◆ Conduct the medical health history examination utilizing a motivational interviewing approach to establish a nonjudgmental environment and encourage the patient to communicate openly and freely with the clinician (see Chapter 24).

B. Screening: National Institute on Drug Abuse (NIDA) Quick Screen

◆ NIDA has developed a screening tool for health professionals to assess if a patient is abusing alcohol, tobacco, prescription medications for nonmedical purposes, or illegal substances.

- The NIDA Quick Screen tool incorporates the Five A's (Ask, Advise, Assess, Assist, Arrange) Steps to Intervention.

◆ The NIDA website provides an online interactive form to complete on a mobile device or chairside. A paper version is also available for the patient to complete, along with Clinicians Resource and Reference Guides.

- The NIDA website can be found at https://www.drugabuse.gov/ and the screening tools can be found by going to the *Medical and Health Professionals* link and finding the *Drug Screening and Assessment Resources* which contains a chart with links to a variety of screening. One tool easily used online for assessment is the NIDA-Modified ASSIST, https://www.drugabuse.gov/nmassist/.

C. Vital Signs

◆ Record information in patient record.

◆ Blood pressure frequently is increased when alcohol and other drugs like stimulants are used; fluctuations can be particularly significant.

◆ Increase in heart rate with cannabis use.

D. Clinical Examination

◆ Information in the patient history may not reveal the extent of a patient's drug use.

◆ Clinical observations along with the medical history may provide a high degree of suspicion.

◆ Observations to note during the interview could include:

- Inability to focus or recall simple concepts like phone number or address.
- May exhibit rapid mood swings or display paranoia or disorientation.
- May start to complain about dental pain requesting a prescription for specific pain medications.

◆ Depression, suicidal/homicidal thoughts, or agitation could indicate a drug overdose and requires immediate emergency care.

E. Extraoral Examination

◆ Alcohol signs

- *Breath and body odor of alcohol and of tobacco*: Many alcohol users are also heavy tobacco users.
- *Tremor of hands, tongue, eyelids*: Signs of withdrawal.
- *Skin*: Redness of forehead, cheeks, dilated blood vessels that produce spider petechiae on the nose; may worsen preexisting acne rosacea.
- *Face color*: Light yellowish brown may indicate jaundice from liver disease.
- *Eyes*: Red, baggy eyes or puffy facial features; bloated appearance.
- *Evidences of trauma*: Facial injuries related to falls when intoxicated. Alcohol abusers are especially prone to traumatic accidents.
- *Lips*: Angular cheilitis related to poor nutrition.
- *Parotid glands*: Swelling.

◆ Personal appearance

- Does the patient look much older than their age stated on their health history form?
- Lack of interest in proper dress and personal hygiene.
- Wears long sleeves to cover needle marks.
- Dramatic weight loss and/or emaciated appearance.

- Head and neck
  - Patients smoking or vaping substances are at greater risk for cancers in the head and neck region.
- Eyes
  - Wears sunglasses to conceal dilated or constricted pupils and eye redness, or to avoid bright light because of eye sensitivity.
  - Pupils dilated (amphetamine, LSD, cocaine, marijuana).
  - Pupils constricted (heroin, morphine, methadone), as shown in Figure 59-4.
  - Red, inflamed, bloodshot (only if cannabis contains THC).
- Nose
  - Inhaled or snorted substances can damage nasal structures causing frequent nosebleeds or patients may constantly be sniffing or wiping their noses.
  - Nasal septum perforation (cocaine snorting).
- Arms
  - Needle marks may be noted when assessing blood pressure.
  - Heroin use can cause subcutaneous abscesses called "popping" that leaves scarring.
- Behavior
  - Sneezing, itching.
  - Tendency to gaze into space; moodiness.
  - Drowsiness, yawning; may sleep long hours.
  - Appearance of intoxication or lethargic with or without the odor of alcohol.
  - Slurred speech.
  - Changes in habits, such as irregular attendance at appointments by one who was previously prompt.

CONSTRICTED PUPILS	DILATED PUPILS
HEROIN MORPHINE OXYCODONE FENTANYL METHADONE CODEINE HYDROCODONE	AMPHETAMINES METHAMPHETAMINE COCAINE OR CRACK HALLUCINOGENS MARIJUANA

FIGURE 59-4 • Examination of the Pupils. Pupil on left: Pinpoint or constricted; occurs in the use of morphine, opioids, and heroin. Pupil on the right: Dilated; occurs in shock, heart failure, other emergencies, and in the use of hallucinogens, cocaine, marijuana, methamphetamines, and amphetamines. (From Graphic designed by Anthony Portillo. Adapted from: National RX Drug Abuse Summit: Orlando, FL. 2012. Retrieved from http://nationalrxdrugabusesummit.org/2012-summit/.)

- Possession of pills or capsules.
- Hallucinations or convulsions indicate need for immediate emergency care.

II. Intraoral Examination

- Mucosa, lips, tongue
  - Dry; drug-induced xerostomia, soft tissue abnormalities.
  - Tongue coated; glossitis related to nutritional deficiencies.
  - Burns and sores on lips from smoking crack or meth.
  - Taste impairment.
- Gingiva
  - Generalized poor oral hygiene; heavy biofilm is typical.
  - Calculus deposits may be generalized, depending on patient neglect.
  - Moderate to severe gingival inflammation.
  - Gingival enlargement.
  - Gingiva that bleeds spontaneously or on probing.
  - Gingival lesions resulting from the direct application of cocaine.
  - Higher incidence of periodontal disease, particularly destructive periodontitis.[63]
  - Necrotizing gingivitis.
- Palate
  - Perforation of palate due to chronic cocaine snorting (Figure 59-5).
- Teeth
  - Chipped and fractured from falls and injuries; stained from tobacco use.
  - Attrition secondary to bruxism especially among cocaine and meth users with increased tooth sensitivity.
  - Erosion secondary to frequent vomiting, exposure to substances with low pH levels (oral application of cocaine, meth).

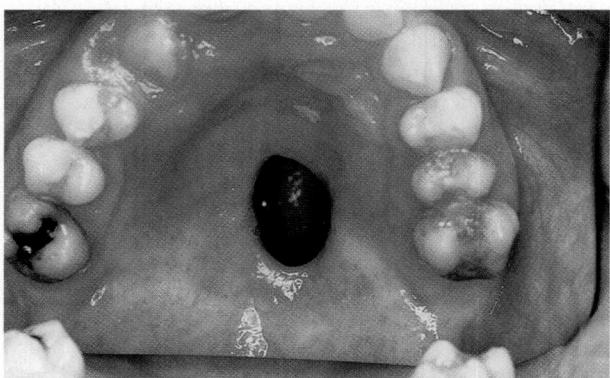

FIGURE 59-5 • Nasopalatal Defect. Problems due to chronic cocaine snorting began to manifest themselves as nosebleeds followed by recurring sinus infections. Within 4 months, the patient discovered a pinhole in his palate. Each time he tried to swallow liquid it came out of his nose. (Photo courtesy of Peter Villa, DDS, FRDC.)

- Removable or fixed partial dentures: chipped or broken, may require frequent repairs.
◆ Dental caries
  - Increased risk factors: poor diet, lack of dental care, accumulation of biofilm, and xerostomia.[63]
  - Diet high in cariogenic substances.
  - Generalized tooth decay especially on smooth and cervical surfaces and fewer restorations suggesting not accessing dental care on a regular basis.[63]
◆ Open rampant carious lesions: abuse of methamphetamine, diet of sweets, alcohol, and sugar-sweetened beverages with decreased salivary secretion as shown in Figure 59-6.
  - Tooth loss.
◆ Oral pathologies
  - Oral candidiasis can be present with substance abuse due to immunosuppression.
  - Due to immunosuppression and inadequate nutrition, tissue healing is poor.
  - Leukoplakia and hyperkeratosis (referred as cannabis stomatitis) that can develop into malignant neoplasias.
  - Erythroplakia.
  - Oral papilloma.
  - Mucosal infections.
  - Complaints of "burning mouth."
  - Xerostomia.[64]
◆ Temporomandibular joint (TMJ)
  - TMJ tenderness due to grinding, clenching, or bruxism (hallucinogen users).
  - Difficulty with opening and chewing.

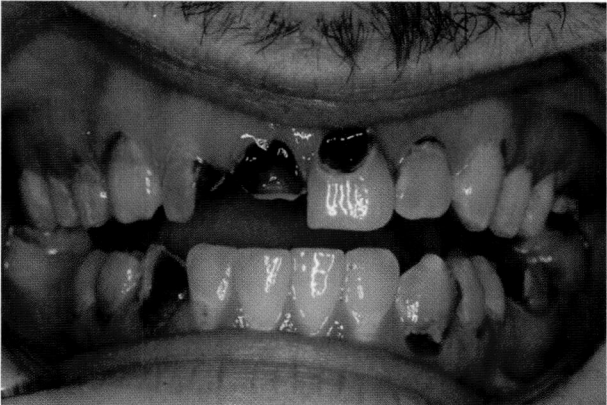

FIGURE 59-6 • **Rampant Dental Caries Due to Methamphetamine Use in a 24-Year-Old Patient Who Presented for Treatment After Serving Time In Prison and Going to Rehab; Patient Started Using Meth at Age 16, Initially Snorting the Powder and Progressed to Smoking the Drug.** Although some teeth could have been saved, the patient chose to have all the remaining teeth extracted in order to receive full dentures. (Photo courtesy of Kessler BH, Dinnen M. Methamphetamine: oral effects and treatment. *Inside Dent.* 2010;6(2):44-46.)

◆ Indirect effects of drugs on oral health[63]
  - Substance abuse patients may delay dental and dental hygiene care due to dental anxiety and/or stigma of drug use.
  - Any available money is used in the purchase of drugs; low priority on oral health.
  - Dental care is on an emergency basis to alleviate any pain or discomfort, and to obtain prescriptions for drugs.
◆ Specific oral manifestations are associated with particular drugs. Examples can be found in Box 59-5.

BOX 59-5
Oral Manifestations of Abused Drugs

A. "Meth mouth": key ingredients used in meth manufacturing are corrosive[64-66]
  - Meth smoker swirls heated, vaporized substances in the mouth.
  - Oral mucosa is irritated and burned, creating sores and leading to infection.
  - Rampant caries "meth mouth" resembles early childhood caries seen in young children; black, decayed teeth often fractured to the gumline.
  - Distinctive pattern of decay is on the buccal and cervical smooth tooth surfaces and proximal surfaces of the anterior teeth.
  - Snorting meth also causes chemical damage to teeth.
  - Symptoms: xerostomia, dryness of the mouth from a lack of normal secretions.
  - Rampant dental caries on proximal surfaces and at the gingival margin.
  - Cracked teeth, excessive wear, tooth sensitivity, and difficulty in mastication from grinding and/or clenching.
  - Enamel erosion: corrosive acids in ingredients.
  - Periodontal infection: reduced blood supply and tissue breakdown.

B. Cocaine abuse[64]
  - Cocaine snorting is associated with perforation of the nasal septum and/or perforation of the palate (Figure 59-5).
  - Saddlenose deformity.
  - Erosive carious lesions from low pH level of cocaine powder.
  - Oral administration may result in gingival lesions, recession, and mucosal ulcerations.
  - Trismus.
  - Dental attrition due to bruxism.
  - Crack-cocaine smoking produces burns and sores on labial mucosa; open lesions expose user to infections.

C. Lysergic acid diethylamide and "ecstasy," hallucinogen drugs[64,67]

- Xerostomia.
- Tooth wear associated with chewing and grinding.
- Temporomandibular joint tenderness (ecstasy users).
- Bruxism leading to trismus.
- Rampant dental caries.
- Topical use of ecstasy may result in tissue necrosis and mucosal fenestration.

D. Cannabis users[34,64,68-70]

- Increased xerostomia.
- Increased smooth-surface caries; higher decayed-missing-filled scores.
- Increased periodontal infections.
- Leukoedema.
- Premalignant lesions of the oral mucosa.
- Leukoplakia.
- Increased oral infections due to immunosuppressive effects.
- Inhaled cannabis users at higher risk for oropharyngeal cancers.

III. Dental Hygiene Diagnosis

◆ The patient who is actively dependent on a substance will probably not seek dental care except for emergency needs.

◆ The dental hygienist cannot provide care until the patient is in recovery.

◆ The patient's oral needs could be extensive. The dental hygienist should assess for the following diseases/conditions[63]:

- Head/neck swelling (lymph nodes).
- TMJ or occlusion issues.
- Oral cancer/pathologies.
- Xerostomia.
- Dental caries.
- Periodontal infections.
- Nutritional deficiencies.

IV. Care Planning

◆ Develop strategies to meet the individual needs of the patient as identified from the risk assessment and dental hygiene diagnosis.

◆ Recovering addicts may have some anxiety about taking medications in their attempt to achieve total body health. This could pose a problem if pain control is needed for extensive dental hygiene care. Therefore, pain control for procedures provided in the office and postoperative pain at home should be coordinated with the patient's primary physician and/or addiction specialist.

◆ The following are care planning considerations:

- Oral self-care instruction beginning with daily toothbrushing. Once the patient can brush effectively, an appropriate interdental technique can be introduced. As the patient moves through their recovery, they may become more motivated and open to additional biofilm removal techniques.
- Use of fluoride toothpaste and fluoride mouthrinse without alcohol. Prescription fluorides may be necessary depending on patient caries risk.
- Office fluoride applications such as fluoride varnish and custom trays for home use if the patient will be compliant.
- A nightguard may be recommended if bruxism is present.
- Increase of water consumption, xylitol gum, or mints to address xerostomia.
- Nutrition counseling may be necessary to address poor nutrition and/or caries risk. A 24-hour diet recall along with MyPlate can be used by the hygienist and the patient to identify goals to improve diet. Proper nutrition will be critical for adequate healing and to decrease the risk for dental caries.
- Short appointments may be needed if patient has anxiety.
- The patient should understand the importance of informing the clinician of any substances in their system that could potentially have a negative interaction with local anesthesia or other therapeutics the clinician may provide to the patient.
- Anesthesia and pain control may be more difficult to achieve because many substance abusers build up tolerance to various pain reducing effects. A consultation with the patient's primary physician should provide the best method to plan for pain control.

V. Implementation

◆ The clinical procedures for dental hygiene care are greatly influenced by the many health problems resulting from drug use.

◆ If short appointments are required, the dental hygienist may only be able to complete limited care at each appointment.

◆ The dental hygienist should implement good stress reduction protocols for patients who are experiencing anxiety.

A. Preparation for Treatment

◆ Caution is needed for potential drug–drug interactions.

◆ Avoid pre-procedural rinse, antibacterial agents, and oral hygiene products containing alcohol for all patients with a past history or current alcohol use problem.

- The smallest amount of alcohol ingested by a patient being treated with disulfiram can cause an emergency.
- Additionally, any patient suffering from xerostomia should avoid any product containing alcohol.

B. Periodontal Debridement

- ◆ Careful periodontal debridement to reduce the bacterial load and support healing is essential.
- ◆ Use of anesthesia: drug interactions, use of epinephrine, should have been approved during the consultation with the patient's physician prior to treatment.
  - • Contraindications for the use of nitrous oxide/oxygen and medical considerations for local anesthesia with or without epinephrine are provided in Chapter 36.

C. Response to Therapy

The usual oral tissue response expected following periodontal instrumentation may be limited by the following:

- ◆ Prolonged bleeding time; impaired clotting mechanism from chronic liver disease.
- ◆ Inability to obtain profound anesthesia.
- ◆ Impaired healing.
- ◆ Interference with collagen formation and deposition.
- ◆ Decreased immune system function.
- ◆ Increased susceptibility to postoperative care infection.

VI. Evaluation

- ◆ The evaluation of dental hygiene care occurs 6–8 weeks after initial debridement.
- ◆ Evaluate treatment plans and goals with the patient.
- ◆ Make changes according to the patient's progress.
- ◆ Evaluate to determine the frequency of continuing care appointment; typically set at 3 months but should depend on many factors such as tissue response, patient's level of motivation.

DOCUMENTATION

- ◆ Patient record medical alert box for possible substance abuse alerts dental personnel to:
  - • Use a nonalcoholic mouthrinse.
  - • Results of drug and alcohol screening.
  - • Any alerts or contraindications for treatment, that is, epinephrine in local anesthetic.
  - • Inappropriate behavior during appointments, such as aggressive or belligerent behavior.
- ◆ Document early oral signs/symptoms of substance abuse such as:
  - • *Oral examination*: ulcerations, infections, and xerostomia.
  - • *Dental examination*: dental caries in unusual sites or more extensive than previously documented.
  - • *Periodontal examination*: rapid changes in periodontal status.
  - • *Patient education*: relapse of previously good oral hygiene.
  - • *Psychological reactions and/or aggressive behavior.*
- ◆ Example documentation for a patient with substance abuse is found in Box 59-6.

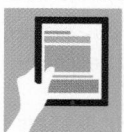

BOX 59-6
Example Documentation: Patient with Substance Abuse

S—A 65-year-old male patient presents for nonsurgical periodontal therapy with local anesthesia appointment. Patient admitted to daily marijuana use to control his arthritic pain, and drinks 4–5 beers most nights to unwind.

O—BP 205/110 mmHg, pulse 89 bpm, and patient stated he has not seen his primary physician in years.

A—Possible hypertension. The quick results of the NIDA Modified screening tool reveals Mr. Keile is an at-risk drinker. The patient is also at risk for illegal drug use with marijuana use that is not prescribed by his physician.

P—Referred patient for medical consult to discuss possible hypertension and substance use addiction. Patient became upset upon finding out that no treatment could be initiated today with the patient's blood pressure significantly elevated. Patient stormed out of the operatory and building before the medical consultation referral could be completed or any follow-up appointments could be scheduled.

Signed: _____, RDH

Date: _____

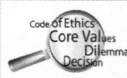

EVERYDAY ETHICS

Mr. Keile is a 65-year-old man and a new patient to the practice. Dr. Jones has diagnosed Mr. Keile with Stage III Grade B periodontitis and recommends four quadrants of nonsurgical periodontal therapy with local anesthesia. At the initial dental hygiene appointment, the dental hygienist Sean assesses Mr. Keile's medical history. Significant findings include the following: (1) BP 205/110 mmHg, pulse 89 bpm; (2) Mr. Keile states he smokes marijuana on a daily basis for pain control to manage his arthritis; (3) Mr. Keile has not seen his primary physician in years and was unaware of his hypertension status; (4) Mr. Keile drinks 4–5 beers most nights to unwind.

Sean uses the NIDA Modified screening tool (https://www.drugabuse.gov/nmassist/) plugging in Mr. Keile's substance use information. The quick results reveal Mr. Keile is an at-risk drinker. One or more days of heavy drinking places a patient at risk. With the patient's daily use of marijuana, the patient is at risk for illegal drug use, especially since his primary physician did not prescribe the marijuana for him.

Sean expresses his concern about Mr. Keile's blood pressure and tells Mr. Keile he is referring him to his primary care provider for a complete physical examination. When Sean tries to dismiss Mr. Keile, Mr. Keile expresses his frustration that no treatment would be provided to him today, "I took time off from work to be here and you are telling me you are not going to clean my teeth?" In addition, Mr. Keile states, "I feel like I am being discriminated against for my marijuana use." Sean tries to explain that he cannot treat him while his blood pressure is elevated without a medical consultation from Mr. Keile's primary physician. Before Sean can walk Mr. Keile to the front reception area, Mr. Keile angrily gets up out of the dental chair and storms out of the building. Sean records the interaction and patient's behavior in the patient's chart.

Questions for Consideration

1. Does the decision to postpone treatment for today violate Mr. Keile's rights? Why or why not?

2. If Dr. Jones and Sean decide to terminate their practitioner–client relationship with Mr. Keile could this be considered "abandonment" or "discrimination" as Mr. Keile accused?

3. What ethical and legal considerations does Dr. Jones and Sean must consider when treating a patient who smokes marijuana and drinks alcohol heavily daily?

Factors to Teach the Patient

▶ Explain how the substance use has affected the patient's oral and general health. Discuss in a positive manner what the patient can do to improve their oral and general health.

▶ Emphasize the importance of regular dental and dental hygiene care. Also, point out their important role in daily biofilm removal at home.

▶ Encourage the patient to maintain a healthy diet. Proper nutrition will be crucial to their healing process. Discuss ways to modify diet to reduce caries risk such as replacing some or all sugar-sweetened beverages with water, use of xylitol-containing mints or gum, rinsing with water after a snack or sugar-sweetened beverage if brushing is not possible.

▶ Recommend daily topical fluoride if the patient is at high risk for caries. Avoid alcohol-containing products if the patient exhibits xerostomia or is recovering from alcohol.

▶ Illicit drug use during pregnancy can pose serious risks for unborn babies.

ENHANCE YOUR UNDERSTANDING

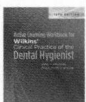

ONLINE RESOURCES
(see the inside front cover for access information)
- Audio glossary
- Appendices

SUPPORT FOR LEARNING
(available separately)
- *Active Learning Workbook for Wilkins' Clinical Practice of the Dental Hygienist, 13th Edition*

INDIVIDUALIZED REVIEW
- Customized practice quizzing with Navigate 2 TestPrep for *Wilkins' Clinical Practice of the Dental Hygienist*

References

1. National Institute on Drug Abuse. *Drugs, Brain, and Behavior: The Science of Addiction.* 2014. https://www.drugabuse.gov/publications/drugs-brains-behavior-science-addiction. Accessed February 25, 2018.

2. National Institute on Alcohol Abuse and Alcoholism. *Drinking Levels Defined.* n.d. https://www.niaaa.nih.gov/alcohol-health/overview-alcohol-consumption/moderate-binge-drinking. Accessed April 14, 2018.

3. National Institute on Alcohol Abuse and Alcoholism. *Alcohol Use Disorder.* n.d. https://www.niaaa.nih.gov/alcohol-health/overview-alcohol-consumption/alcohol-use-disorders. Accessed April 15, 2018.

4. World Health Organization. *Global Status Report on Alcohol and Health 2014.* 2014. http://www.who.int/substance_abuse/publications/global_alcohol_report/en/. Accessed February 25, 2018.

5. National Institute on Alcohol Abuse and Alcoholism. *Underage Drinking.* 2017. https://pubs.niaaa.nih.gov/publications/UnderageDrinking/UnderageFact.htm. Accessed February 25, 2018.

6. U.S. National Library of Medicine. *Alcoholism and Alcohol Abuse.* 2018. https://medlineplus.gov/alcoholismandalcoholabuse.html. Accessed February 25, 2018.

7. National Bureau of Economic Research. *Mental Illness and Substance Abuse.* 2018. https://www.nber.org/digest/apr02/w8699.html. Accessed February 25, 2018.

8. U.S. National Library of Medicine. *Alcohol Use Disorder.* 2018. https://ghr.nlm.nih.gov/condition/alcohol-use-disorder#inheritance. Accessed February 25, 2018.

9. Cederbaum AI. Alcohol metabolism. *Clinics in Liver Disease.* 2012;16(4):667-685.

10. National Center for Statistics and Analysis. Alcohol-impaired driving: 2014 data. In: U.S. Department of Transportation, ed. Washington, DC: National Highway Traffic Safety Administration; 2015.

11. National Institute on Alcohol Abuse and Alcoholism. *Alcohols Affect on the Body.* 2017. https://www.niaaa.nih.gov/alcohol-health/alcohols-effects-body. Accessed February 25, 2018.

12. Rehm J, Shield KD. Alcohol and mortality: global alcohol-attributable deaths from cancer, liver cirrhosis, and injury in 2010. *Alcohol Res.* 2014;35(2):174-183.

13. U.S. National Library of Medicine. *Wernicke-Korsakoff Syndrome.* 2018. https://medlineplus.gov/ency/article/000771.htm. Accessed February 25, 2018.

14. Centers for Disease Control and Prevention. *Alcohol and Public Health: Fact Sheets - Excessive Alcohol Use and Risks to Women's Health.* 2016. https://www.cdc.gov/alcohol/fact-sheets/womens-health.htm. Accessed February 25, 2018.

15. Centers for Disease Control and Prevention. *Alcohol and Public Health: Fact Sheets- Excessive Alcohol Use and Risks to Men's Health.* 2016. https://www.cdc.gov/alcohol/fact-sheets/mens-health.htm. Accessed February 25, 2018.

16. Centers for Disease Control and Prevention. *Facts About FASDs.* 2017. https://www.cdc.gov/ncbddd/fasd/facts.html. Accessed April 2, 2018.

17. Centers for Disease Control and Prevention. *Alcohol Use in Pregnancy.* 2016. https://www.cdc.gov/ncbddd/fasd/alcohol-use.html. Accessed February 27, 2018.

18. Substance Abuse and Mental Health Services Administration. Clinical advances in non-agonist therapies. In: U.S. Department of Health and Human Services, ed. Rockville, MD: National Institutes of Health 2016:50.

19. Substance Abuse and Mental Health Services Administration and National Institute on Alcohol Abuse and Alcoholism. Medication for the Treatment of Alcohol Use Disorder. In: U.S. Department of Health and Human Services, ed. Washington, DC; 2015:14.

20. National Institute on Alcohol Abuse and Alcoholism. Treatment for alcohol problems: finding and getting help. In: U.S. Department of Health and Human Services, ed. Washington, DC: National Institutes of Health; 2014.

21. American Dental Association. *Policies and Recommendations on Substance Use Disorders.* 2016. https://www.ada.org/en/about-the-ada/ada-positions-policies-and-statements/policies-and-recommendations-on-substance-use-disorders. Accessed February 27, 2018.

22. Govering the States and Localities. *State Marijuana Laws in 2018 Map.* 2018. http://www.governing.com/gov-data/state-marijuana-laws-map-medical-recreational.html. Accessed January 29, 2018.

23. Versteeg PA, Slot DE, van der Velden U, van der Weijden GA. Effect of cannabis usage on the oral environment: a review. *Int J Dent Hyg.* 2008;6(4):315-320.

24. Rella JG. Recreational cannabis use: pleasures and pitfalls. *Cleve Clin J Med.* 2015;82(11):765-772.

25. Ogborne AC, Smart RG, Weber T, Birchmore-Timney C. Who is using cannabis as a medicine and why: an exploratory study. *J Psychoactive Drugs.* 2000;32(4):435-443.

26. Bostwick JM. Blurred boundaries: the therapeutics and politics of medical marijuana. *Mayo Clin Proc.* 2012;87(2):172-186.

27. Howard P, Twycross R, Shuster J, Mihalyo M, Wilcock A. Cannabinoids. *J Pain Symptom Manage.* 2013;46(1):142-149.

28. Devinsky O, Marsh E, Friedman D, et al. Cannabidiol in patients with treatment-resistant epilepsy: an open-label interventional trial. *Lancet Neurol.* 2016;15(3):270-278.

29. Drug Enforcement Administration. *Drug Fact Sheet-Marijuana.* n.d.:1-2.

30. National Institute on Drug Abuse. *Marijuana.* December 12, 2017. https://www.drugabuse.gov/publications/research-reports/marijuana. Accessed December 29, 2017.

31. Huestis MA. Human cannabinoid pharmacokinetics. *Chem Biodivers.* 2007;4(8):1770-1804.

32. Hutton H. Beyond THC: exploring the topical uses of cannabis. *J Am Herbalists Guild.* 2014;12(3):40-44.

33. Cho CM, Hirsch R, Johnstone S. General and oral health implications of cannabis use. *Aust Dent J.* 2005;50(2):70-74.

34. Rawal SY, Tatakis DN, Tipton DA. Periodontal and oral manifestations of marijuana use. *J Tenn Dent Assoc.* 2012;92(2):26-31; quiz 31-22.

35. U.S. Drug Enforcement Administration. *Drug Fact Sheets-Fentanyl.* n.d. https://www.dea.gov/druginfo/concern_fentanyl.shtml. Accessed March 28, 2018.

36. Grund JP, Latypov A, Harris M. Breaking worse: the emergence of krokodil and excessive injuries among people who inject drugs in Eurasia. *Int J Drug Policy.* 2013;24(4):265-274.

37. Florez DH, Dos Santos Moreira AM, da Silva PR, et al. Desomorphine (Krokodil): an overview of its chemistry, pharmacology, metabolism, toxicology and analysis. *Drug Alcohol Depend.* 2017;173:59-68.

38. Gahr M, Freudenmann RW, Hiemke C, Gunst IM, Connemann BJ, Schonfeldt-Lecuona C. "Krokodil": revival of an old drug with new problems. *Subst Use Misuse.* 2012;47(7):861-863.

39. U.S. Drug Enforcement Administration. *Desomorphine.* 2013. https://www.deadiversion.usdoj.gov/drug_chem_info/desomorphine.pdf. Accessed March 28, 2018.

40. Haskins A, Kim N, Aguh C. A new drug with a nasty bite: a case of krokodil-induced skin necrosis in an intravenous drug user. *JAAD Case Reports.* 2016;2(2):174-176.

41. Hakobyan K, Poghosyan Y. Spontaneous bone formation after mandible segmental resection in "krokodil" drug-related jaw osteonecrosis patient: case report. *Oral Maxillofac Surg.* 2017;21(2):267-270.

42. Poghosyan YM, Hakobyan KA, Poghosyan AY, Avetisyan EK. Surgical treatment of jaw osteonecrosis in "Krokodil" drug addicted patients. *J Craniomaxillofac Surg.* 2014;42(8):1639-1643.

43. National Institute on Drug Abuse. *Health Consequences of Drug Misuse: Cardiovascular Effects.* 2017. https://www.drugabuse.gov/publications/health-consequences-drug-misuse/cardiovascular-effects. Accessed March 28, 2018.

44. Riezzo I, Fiore C, De Carlo D, et al. Side effects of cocaine abuse: multiorgan toxicity and pathological consequences. *Curr Med Chem.* 2012;19(33):5624-5646.

45. National Institute on Drug Abuse. *Health Consequences of Drug Misuse: Neurological Effects.* 2017. https://www.drugabuse.gov/publications/health-consequences-drug-misuse/neurological-effects. Accessed March 28, 2018.

46. Bose J HS, Lipari RN, Park-Lee E, Parker JD, Pemberton MR. Key substance use and mental health indicators in the United States: results from the 2015 national survey on drug use and health. 2016:1-74. Retrieved from https://www.samhsa.gov/data/sites/default/files/NSDUH-FFR1-2015/NSDUH-FFR1-2015/NSDUH-FFR1-2015.pdf. Accessed November 16, 2017.

47. National Institute on Drug Abuse. *Inhalants.* 2012. https://www.drugabuse.gov/publications/research-reports/inhalants/what-are-other-medical-consequences-inhalant-abuse. Accessed March 28, 2018.

48. National Institute on drug Abuse. *Health Consequences of Drug Misuse: Gastrointestinal Effects.* 2017. https://www .drugabuse.gov/publications/health-consequences-drug -misuse/gastrointestinal-effects. Accessed March 28, 2018.

49. National Institute on Drug Abuse. *Health Consequences of Drug Misuses: Kidney Damage.* 2017. https://www.drugabuse .gov/publications/health-consequences-drug-misuse/kidney -damage. Accessed March 28, 2018.

50. National Institute on Drug Abuse. *Health Consequences of Drug Misuse: Liver Damage.* 2017. https://www.drugabuse .gov/publications/health-consequences-drug-misuse/liver -damage. Accessed March 28, 2018.

51. Dasgupta A. 4—Combined alcohol and drug abuse: a potentially deadly mix. In: *Alcohol, Drugs, Genes and the Clinical Laboratory.* Amsterdam, Netherlands: Academic Press; 2017:75-88.

52. National Institute on Drug Abuse. *Health Consequences of Drug Misuse: Musculoskeletal Effects.* 2017. https://www .drugabuse.gov/publications/health-consequences-drug -misuse/musculoskeletal-effects. Accessed March 28, 2018.

53. National Institute on Drug Abuse. *Health Consequences of Drug Misuse: Respiratory Effects.* 2017. https://www.drugabuse .gov/publications/health-consequences-drug-misuse/respiratory -effects. Accessed March 28, 2018.

54. National Institute on Drug Abuse. *Health Consequences of Drug Misuse: Prenatal Effects.* 2017. https://www.drugabuse .gov/publications/health-consequences-drug-misuse/prenatal -effects. Accessed March 29, 2018.

55. McQueen K, Murphy-Oikonen J. Neonatal abstinence syndrome. *N Engl J Med.* 2016;375(25):2468-2479.

56. White KM, Sabatino JA, He M, Davis N, Tang N, Bearer CF. Toluene disruption of the functions of L1 cell adhesion molecule at concentrations associated with occupational exposures. *Pediatr Res.* 2016;80(1):145-150.

57. National Institute on Drug Abuse. *Health Consequences of Drug Misuse: HIV, Hepatitis, and other Infectious Diseases.* 2017. https://www.drugabuse.gov/publications/health-consequences -drug-misuse/hiv-hepatitis-other-infectious-diseases. Accessed March 30, 2018.

58. Wurcel AG, Merchant EA, Clark RP, Stone DR. Emerging and underrecognized complications of illicit drug use. *Clin Infect Dis.* 2015;61(12):1840-1849.

59. National Institute on Drug Abuse. *Treatment Approaches for Drug Addiction.* 2018. https://www.drugabuse.gov/publications /drugfacts/treatment-approaches-drug-addiction. Accessed March 30, 2018.

60. Srivastava A, Kahan M, Nader M. Primary care management of opioid use disorders: abstinence, methadone, or buprenorphine-naloxone? *Can Fam Physician.* 2017;63(3):200-205.

61. Uebelacker LA, Bailey G, Herman D, Anderson B, Stein M. Patients' beliefs about medications are associated with stated preference for methadone, buprenorphine, naltrexone, or no medication-assisted therapy following inpatient opioid detoxification. *J Subst Abuse Treat.* 2016;66:48-53.

62. Dunlop AJ, Brown AL, Oldmeadow C, et al. Effectiveness and cost-effectiveness of unsupervised buprenorphine-naloxone for the treatment of heroin dependence in a randomized waitlist controlled trial. *Drug Alcohol Depend.* 2017;174:181-191.

63. Baghaie H, Kisely S, Forbes M, Sawyer E, Siskind DJ. A systematic review and meta-analysis of the association between poor oral health and substance abuse. *Addiction.* 2017;112(5):765-779.

64. Shekarchizadeh H, Khami MR, Mohebbi SZ, Ekhtiari H, Virtanen JI. Oral health of drug abusers: a review of health effects and care. *Iran J Public Health.* 2013;42(9): 929-940.

65. Boyer EM, Thompson N, Hill T, Zimmerman MB. The relationship between methamphetamine use and dental caries and missing teeth. *J Dent Hyg.* 2015;89(2):119-131.

66. Hamamoto DT, Rhodus NL. Methamphetamine abuse and dentistry. *Oral Dis.* 2009;15(1):27-37.

67. Taghi KM, Arghavan T, Maryam A, Pourya B, Elham MG, Gelareh T. Drug addiction and oral health; a comparison of hallucinogen and non-hallucinogen drug users. *Int J Dent Oral Health.* 2016;2(6):1-6.

68. Rechthand MM, Bashirelahi N. What every dentist needs to know about cannabis. *Gen Dent.* 2016;64(1):40-43.

69. Grafton SE, Huang PN, Vieira AR. Dental treatment planning considerations for patients using cannabis: a case report. *J Am Dent Assoc.* 2016;147(5):354-361.

70. Schulz-Katterbach M, Imfeld T, Imfeld C. Cannabis and caries—does regular cannabis use increase the risk of caries in cigarette smokers? *Schweiz Monatsschr Zahnmed.* 2009;119(6):576-583.

60

The Patient with a Respiratory Disease

Lisa F. Mallonee, RDH, RD, LD, MPH, Valerie G. Herring RDH, BsM, MEd, and Katherine A. Yee, RDH, BSDH, MPH

CHAPTER OUTLINE

THE RESPIRATORY SYSTEM
I. Anatomy
II. Physiology
III. Function of the Respiratory Mucosa
IV. Respiratory Assessment
V. Classification

UPPER RESPIRATORY TRACT DISEASES
I. Modes of Transmission
II. Dental Hygiene Care

LOWER RESPIRATORY TRACT DISEASES

ACUTE BRONCHITIS

PNEUMONIA
I. Etiology
II. Symptoms
III. Categories and Role of Oral Bacteria
IV. Medical Management
V. Dental Hygiene Care

TUBERCULOSIS
I. Etiology
II. Transmission
III. Disease Development
IV. Diagnosis
V. Medical Management
VI. Oral Manifestations
VII. Dental Hygiene Care

ASTHMA
I. Etiology
II. Atopic (Allergic) Asthma
III. Asthma Attack
IV. Medical Management
V. Oral Manifestations
VI. Dental Hygiene Care

CHRONIC OBSTRUCTIVE PULMONARY DISEASE
I. Chronic Bronchitis
II. Emphysema

III. Medical Management
IV. Oral Manifestations
V. Dental Hygiene Care

CYSTIC FIBROSIS
I. Disease Characteristics
II. Medical Management
III. Dental Hygiene Care

SLEEP-RELATED BREATHING DISORDERS
I. Etiology
II. Signs and Symptoms
III. Medical Management
IV. Dental Hygiene Care

DOCUMENTATION

EVERYDAY ETHICS

FACTORS TO TEACH THE PATIENT

REFERENCES

LEARNING OBJECTIVES

After studying the chapter, the student will be able to:

1. Identify and define key terms and concepts related to respiratory diseases.

2. Differentiate between upper and lower respiratory diseases.

3. Describe the etiology, symptoms, and management of respiratory diseases.

4. Plan and document dental hygiene care and oral hygiene instructions for patients with compromised respiratory function.

Patients with respiratory diseases have increased risks for complications due to decreased breathing function and treatment–drug interactions.

◆ *Tobacco cessation*:

- Many respiratory diseases are caused or aggravated by use of tobacco products.
- Dental hygienists have a unique opportunity to educate their patients about this health hazard.

◆ *Emergency treatment*: Patients with respiratory distress may need emergency care, which dental hygienists are prepared to prevent or provide when necessary.

- Signs and symptoms and medical emergency procedures for local anesthesia reactions, respiratory failure, airway obstruction, asthma attack, hyperventilation, anaphylaxis, and allergic reactions are found in Chapter 9.

◆ *Oral–systemic link*: Scientific evidence shows dental biofilm and microorganisms from periodontal infections can contribute to the initiation and/or progression of certain respiratory infections.[1] Dedication of the dental hygienist to the prevention and control of periodontal infections can have a major influence on the overall health of the patient.

THE RESPIRATORY SYSTEM

I. Anatomy

Structures: sinuses, nasal cavity, larynx, pharynx, trachea, bronchi, lungs, and pleura (Figure 60-1A).[2]

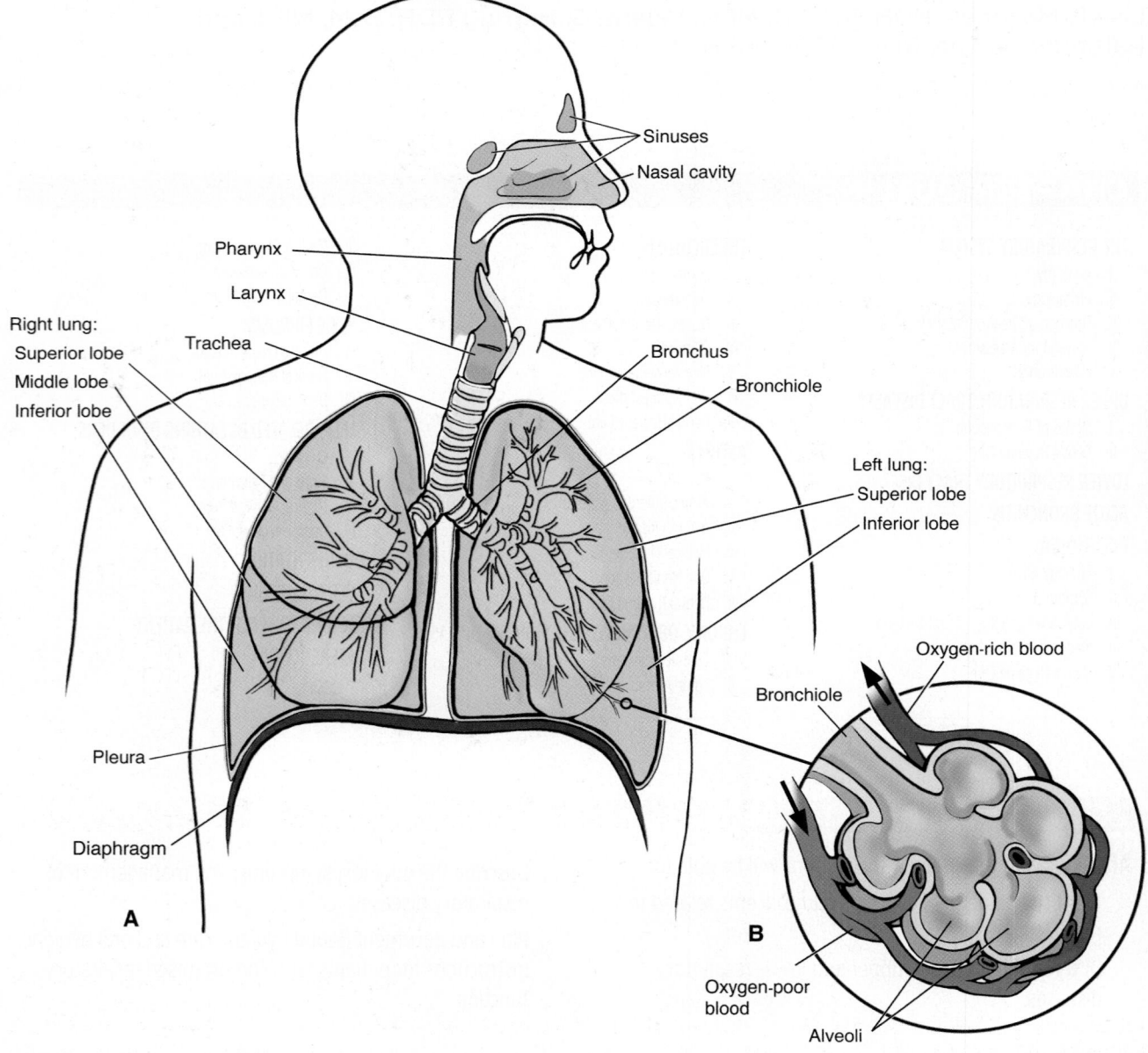

FIGURE 60-1 • Structures of the Respiratory System. A: Structures. The major anatomic structures of the respiratory system are shown. Each bronchus branches out to the bronchioles. **B:** Gas exchange. Exchange of oxygen and carbon dioxide occurs in the alveoli of the bronchioles.

II. Physiology

The respiratory tract from nasal cavity to lungs serves as a passageway for air exchange (Figure 60-1A).

- *Inhaled fresh air*: warmed and filtered in the nasal cavity, enters the lungs.
- *Exhaled air*: with carbon dioxide, leaves the body.
- *Gas exchange*: at the cellular level, occurs in the alveoli at the ends of the bronchioles, as shown in Figure 60-1B.
- *Cardiovascular system*: functions with the respiratory system to pump oxygenated blood from the lungs to every cell in the body and deoxygenated blood back to the lungs for exhalation.

III. Function of the Respiratory Mucosa

Figure 60-2 shows ciliated epithelial cells and mucus-secreting goblet cells that line the respiratory tract to make up the respiratory mucosa.

- Mucus secreted from goblet cells moistens inspired air, prevents delicate alveolar walls from becoming dry, and traps dust and other airborne particles.
- Cilia assist in removing foreign material and contaminated mucus by a constant beating and wavelike motion that propels this material back into the larger bronchi and trachea where it can be coughed up and expectorated or swallowed.
- Lack of function results when the inflammatory process of asthma and chronic bronchitis initiates an overabundance of mucus. Congestion is created, and the cilia are prevented from assisting with normal breathing.

IV. Respiratory Assessment

Respiratory disease assessment includes several objective measures.

A. Vital Signs

- Determination of vital signs (body temperature, pulse, respiratory rate, blood pressure) and also smoking status is considered standard procedure in dental patient care.
- Methods of determining vital signs are described in Chapter 12. Tobacco use is discussed in Chapter 32.

B. Spirometry

- Medical test that measures various aspects of breathing and lung function.
- Used to diagnose and monitor many lower respiratory tract diseases.
- Performed with a spirometer, a device that registers the amount of air a person inhales or exhales and the rate at which air is moved in and out of the lungs.
- Figure 60-3 shows the use of a spirometer to evaluate lung function.

C. Pulse Oximetry

- Medical test that measures blood oxygen saturation levels.[3]

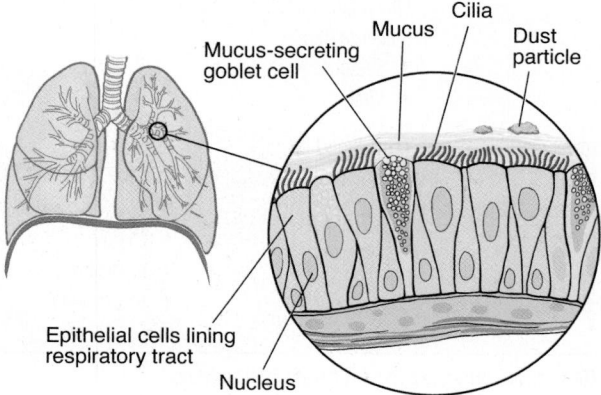

FIGURE 60-2 • Lining of the Respiratory Mucosa. Ciliated epithelial cells and mucus secreted by goblet cells help to remove foreign objects (dust particles). The material is coughed up and either expectorated or swallowed.

Mucus-secreting goblet cell
Mucus
Cilia
Dust particle
Epithelial cells lining respiratory tract
Nucleus

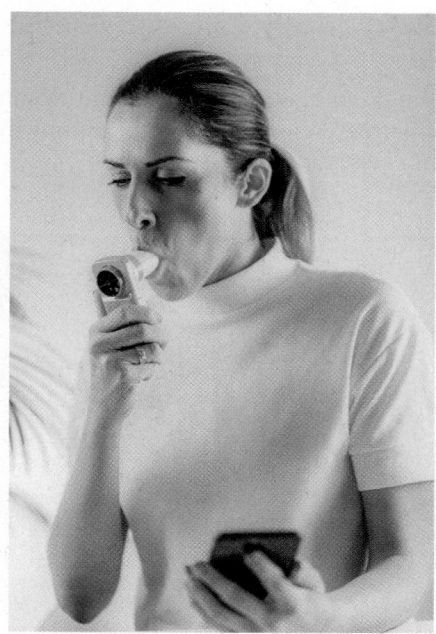

FIGURE 60-3 • Use of a Spirometer to Evaluate Lung Function. Person being tested takes in a full breath, seals their lips over the mouthpiece of the spirometer, and then blows out as hard and as fast as possible for at least 6 seconds. Nose clips may be applied to ensure no air escapes through the nose. (© Microgen/Shutterstock)

◆ Performed with a pulse oximeter.
  • Color of blood varies depending upon the amount of oxygen it contains.
  • Pulse oximeter emits a light through the finger to calculate the percentage of oxygen.
  • Any finger (excluding the thumb) can be used. Nail polish or a skin callous may interfere with reading.
  • Intended only as an adjunct in patient assessment along with other methods of assessing clinical signs and symptoms.
  • Healthy patients have an oxygen saturation of 97%–100%.
  • Saturation of 91% or below signifies poor oxygen exchange.
◆ Figure 60-4 shows the use of a pulse oximeter to measure blood oxygen saturation levels.

D. Chest Radiography (Imaging)

◆ Indicates presence of pathologic density (radiopacity) in the lungs.
◆ *Standard chest radiograph:* shows a two-dimensional view of lung tissues.
◆ *Computed axial tomography radiograph or computed tomography scan:* shows a three-dimensional cross section of lung tissues.

E. Blood Gas Analysis

◆ Blood test to determine acid–base balance, alveolar ventilation, arterial oxygen saturation, and carbon dioxide elimination.

F. Cytology (Body Cells and Fluids) and Hematology Evaluation

◆ Examination of body cells, blood, and other fluids to determine the presence of microorganisms that cause respiratory diseases.

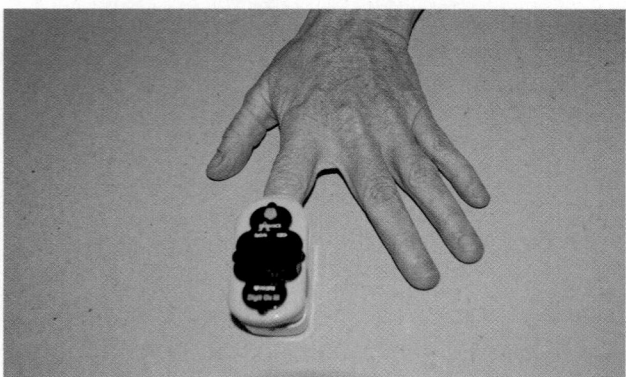

FIGURE 60-4 • Use of a Pulse Oximeter to Measure Blood Oxygen Saturation Level. Color of blood varies depending on the amount of oxygen it contains. The pulse oximeter clips on any finger (except the thumb) and emits a light through the finger to calculate the percentage of oxygen in the blood. Nail polish and a skin callous may interfere with reading.

◆ Samples are taken from sputum, pleural cavity fluid, bronchial biopsy, or blood.

V. Classification

Classification of respiratory diseases is listed in Table 60-1.

UPPER RESPIRATORY TRACT DISEASES

The more common disorders of the upper respiratory tract are caused by infections or allergic reactions that result in inflammation.

◆ Signs and symptoms, etiology, medical treatment, and clinical evaluation assessment are summarized in Table 60-2.

I. Modes of Transmission

◆ Inhalation of airborne droplets.[4]
◆ Indirectly by contaminated hands or articles freshly soiled with discharge of nose or throat of infected person.[4]

II. Dental Hygiene Care

A. Disease Prevention

◆ All healthcare professionals are encouraged to obtain immunizations for seasonal viral influenza.

TABLE 60-1 • Classification of Respiratory Diseases		
LOCATION/ STRUCTURES	ACUTE	CHRONIC
Upper respiratory tract	Diseases of the nose, sinuses, pharynx, larynx Rhinitis (common cold) Sinusitis Pharyngitis/tonsillitis Influenza (flu) • Seasonal • Viral	Allergic rhinitis (hay fever)
Lower respiratory tract Diseases of the trachea, lungs	Acute bronchitis Pneumonia	TB Asthma COPD • Chronic bronchitis • Emphysema CF

COPD, chronic obstructive pulmonary disease; TB, tuberculosis.
Source: Centers for Disease Control and Prevention. National Center for Immunization and Respiratory Diseases (NCIRD). Atlanta, GA: Centers for Disease Control and Prevention. http://www.cdc.gov/ncird/overview/websites.html. Updated July 26, 2017. Accessed February 2, 2019.

TABLE 60-2 • Summary of Upper Respiratory Diseases: Signs/Symptoms, Etiology, Medical Management, and Dental Hygiene Care—Clinical Evaluation Assessment

SIGNS/SYMPTOMS	ETIOLOGY	MEDICAL MANAGEMENT	CLINICAL EVALUATION ASSESSMENT
Upper Respiratory Infections—Infectious Rhinitis (Common Cold)			
• Sneezing • Nasal • Congestion • Nasal discharge (**coryza**) • Headache • Watering of the eyes	• Viral	• **Analgesic** for sore throat, muscle ache • Anticholinergic agent to decrease nasal discharge • Oral decongestant to decrease nasal congestion • Antihistamine for itching, sneezing, "runny nose" • Fluids	• May observe small round erythematous lesions on soft palate, enlarged tonsils, erythema multiforme, acute ulcerative gingivitis • Decongestants and mouth breathing may cause dry mouth
Allergic Rhinitis (Hay Fever)			
• Watering, burning eyes • Sneezing • Nasal congestion	• Seasonal triggers (grass, trees, pollen) or perennial triggers (dust mites, mold spores, animal dander) result in immunoglobulin E–mediated hypersensitivity reactions	• Avoidance of the allergen • Pharmacotherapy medication: antihistamines, decongestants • Immunotherapy: allergy injections increase tolerance to allergens and reduce symptoms	• Dry mouth • Oral candidiasis from long-term use of topical corticosteroids
Sinusitis			
• Nasal obstruction • Fever, chills • Constant midface head pain, more severe when lying down • Palpation over sinus area: tenderness, swelling	• Bacterial infection of the epithelial lining of the sinus • Triggers include upper respiratory infections, dental infections, direct trauma	• Antibiotics • Decongestants • Fluids	• Dry mouth • Sinus congestion creates pressure on nearby maxillary molar roots and may cause symptoms of toothache; *important to determine whether pain originates from tooth or sinus infection*
Pharyngitis/Tonsillitis			
• Sore throat	• Mostly viral • Rarely bacterial: Group A beta-hemolytic streptococcus infection	• Viral: treat symptoms • Bacterial: antibiotics • Patient is no longer infective after 1 day on antibiotics	• Enlarged tonsils • Erythematous tissues
Influenza (Flu)			
• Chills, fever • Headache, coryza • Sore throat • Nonproductive dry cough • **Myalgia, malaise**	• Viral • Mode of transmission: airborne (coughing, sneezing) or direct (contact with contaminated surface) • Diagnostic testing is required to distinguish between types of influenza viruses	• Bed rest, fluids • Analgesics, antivirals (amantadine, rimantadine, zanamivir, oseltamivir) • Monitor for secondary bacterial infection • Prevent with vaccine • For information on infection control, vaccinations, prevention, treatment, and updates, see: www.cdc.gov/flu/professionals	• Dry mouth

Source: Centers for Disease Control and Prevention. *Get Smart: Know When Antibiotics Work (Treatment Guidelines for Upper Respiratory Tract Infections)*. Atlanta, GA: Centers for Disease Control and Prevention. http://www.cdc.gov/getsmart/campaign-materials/treatment-guidelines.html. Updated September 26, 2017. Accessed February 2, 2019.

◆ Observe standard precautions including respiratory hygiene and cough etiquette as listed in Table 60-3 to prevent transmission of pathogens from patient to clinician and to prevent healthcare-associated infections to the patient.[5]

B. Appointment Management

◆ Delay treatment until patient is no longer infectious.
◆ Noninfectious status is determined by temperature returning to normal and regression of oral lesions such as

TABLE 60-3 • Respiratory Hygiene and Cough Etiquette in Healthcare Settings

To prevent transmission of *all* respiratory infections in healthcare settings, incorporate the following infection control practices as one component of standard precautions:

Visual alerts	• Post visual alerts: symptoms of respiratory infection and respiratory hygiene and cough etiquette.
Respiratory hygiene and cough etiquette	• Use tissue to cover coughs and sneezes and discard in no-touch receptacle. • Perform hand hygiene (hand washing with nonantimicrobial soap and water, alcohol-based rub, or antiseptic hand wash) after contact with respiratory secretions or contaminated objects.
Masking and separation of persons with respiratory symptoms	• Offer masks to persons who are coughing and encourage coughing persons to sit at least 3 feet away from others in common waiting areas.
Droplet precautions	• Observe droplet precautions (wearing a surgical or procedure mask for close contact) in addition to standard precautions when examining a patient with symptoms of a respiratory infection, particularly when a fever is present.

Source: Centers for Disease Control and Prevention. *Respiratory Hygiene/Cough Etiquette*. Atlanta, GA: Centers for Disease Control. https://www.cdc.gov/oralhealth/infectioncontrol/faqs/respiratory-hygiene.html. Updated March 25, 2016. Accessed February 2, 2019.

erythematous lesions of the soft palate and erythema multiforme.[6]

C. Bacterial Resistance to Antibiotics

◆ Bacteria may become resistant to antibiotics within 14 days.[7]

◆ For patients currently prescribed an antibiotic for a nondental condition (such as acute bacterial bronchitis or sinus infection): a different category of antibiotic will be necessary to treat an odontogenic (dental origin) infection.

LOWER RESPIRATORY TRACT DISEASES

◆ Considered to be a more serious infection.

◆ Diseases of the lower respiratory tract are listed in Table 60-1.

ACUTE BRONCHITIS

◆ An acute respiratory infection that involves large airways (trachea, bronchi).[8]

◆ Primary symptom: cough with or without phlegm; may last up to 3 weeks.

◆ Lower respiratory tract disease symptoms: wheezing, shortness of breath, or chest tightness.

◆ Differentiated from pneumonia: no significant findings on chest radiography.

◆ A comparison of acute viral and bacterial bronchitis is listed in Table 60-4.

PNEUMONIA

◆ An infection and subsequent inflammation of the lungs that may be caused by viruses, bacteria, fungi, mycoplasma, or parasites.[9]

◆ The respiratory tract of a healthy person is able to defend against organisms aspirated into the lungs.

◆ With diminished salivary flow, decreased cough reflex, swallowing disorders, poor ability to perform good oral hygiene, or other physical disabilities, there is an increased risk of aspiration and respiratory infection.

I. Etiology

A. Viral and Bacterial

◆ Comparison of viral and bacterial pneumonias is listed in Table 60-5.

B. Fungal

◆ Etiologic agent of *pneumocystis* pneumonia is *Pneumocystis jirovecii* (yee-row-vetsee).

TABLE 60-4 • Comparison of Acute Viral and Bacterial Bronchitis

ITEM	VIRAL	BACTERIAL
Occurrence	• Most prevalent	• Least prevalent
Medical treatment	• Supportive: bed rest, fluids • May need inhaled bronchodilators and/or cough suppressant	• Antibiotics: amoxicillin, macrolides, cephalosporin

Source: Centers for Disease Control and Prevention. *Get Smart: Know When Antibiotics Work (Treatment Guidelines for Upper Respiratory Tract Infections)*. Atlanta, GA: Centers for Disease Control and Prevention. http://www.cdc.gov/getsmart/campaign-materials/treatment-guidelines.html. Updated September 26, 2017. Accessed February 2, 2019.

TABLE 60-5 • Comparison of Viral and Bacterial Pneumonias

ITEM	VIRAL	BACTERIAL
Occurrence	• Most prevalent	• Least prevalent

Causative agent	• Virus	Bacteria
		Nosocomial
		Aerobic gram-negative bacilli
		Example: *Pseudomonas aeruginosa*
		  Escherichia coli
		  Klebsiella pneumonia
		  Gram-positive cocci
		Example: *Staphylococcus aureus*
		  Methicillin-resistant
		  S. aureus
		Community acquired
		Gram-negative cocci
		Example: *Haemophilus influenzae*
		  Gram-positive cocci
		Example: *Streptococcus pneumonia*

Signs and symptoms	• Mild symptoms • Cough, sputum • Mild fever • Dyspnea	• Sudden onset • Cough, purulent sputum • High fever • Dyspnea, tachypnea • Pleuritic chest pain
Diagnosis	• Patient history • Physical findings • Chest radiography	• Patient history • Physical findings • Chest radiography • Sputum sample
Medical treatment	• Supportive: bed rest, fluids	• Antibiotics

Source: American Lung Association. *Symptoms, Diagnosis and Treatment*. Chicago, IL: American Lung Association; 2018. http://www.lung.org/lung-disease/pneumonia/symptoms-diagnosis-and.html. Updated October 15, 2018. Accessed February 2, 2019.

◆ Susceptibility is enhanced by chronic debilitating disease in which immune mechanisms are impaired, such as in HIV/AIDS.

II. Symptoms

◆ Fever greater than 100.4° F.
◆ Productive cough.
◆ Chest pain.
◆ Shortness of breath.
◆ Visible on chest x-ray.

III. Categories and Role of Oral Bacteria

Pneumonia is often categorized by location and/or procedure.

A. Community-Acquired Pneumonia

◆ Infection occurring in an individual in the community (not in a healthcare facility).[10]
◆ Person-to-person transmission.

B. Healthcare-Associated (Nosocomial) Pneumonia

◆ Infection occurring 48–72 hours after admission to a healthcare facility.
◆ A major cause of death in hospitalized patients.
◆ Commonly multidrug-resistant pathogens.
◆ More common in the very elderly >80 years and those with comorbidities.
◆ Bacteria in periodontal pockets may serve as a reservoir for lung infection, especially in institutional settings.
◆ Bacteria from oral biofilm are released into saliva and can be aspirated into the lungs.
◆ Contributing factors:
  • Poor oral health, dependence on others to perform daily oral hygiene
  • Oral colonization of periodontal and respiratory pathogens
  • Influenced by periodontitis, are associated with nosocomial pneumonia.
◆ *Nursing home–acquired pneumonia*
  • Owing to dysphagia from decrease in saliva, cough reflex, and/or swallowing disorders.
  • Aspiration of saliva can be the main route of bacteria into the lungs and may lead to aspiration pneumonia.
◆ *Hospital-acquired pneumonia*
  • Ventilator-associated pneumonia: mechanically ventilated patients in the immediate care unit with no ability to clear oral secretions by swallowing or coughing.
  • Nonventilator-associated pneumonia: biofilm forms on endotracheal tubes, catheters.

IV. Medical Management

◆ *Viral*: supportive treatment of bed rest and fluids.
◆ *Bacterial*: antibiotic therapy.
◆ *Fungal*: sulfa drugs.

V. Dental Hygiene Care

Control of oral disease and periodontal disease for patients in nursing homes and hospitals will help prevent aspiration pneumonia.

◆ Use 0.12% chlorhexidine gluconate rinse prior to beginning treatment to reduce the bacterial load.[11]
◆ Avoid use of ultrasonic scalers due to the production of aerosols.

TUBERCULOSIS

◆ Tuberculosis (TB) is a chronic, infectious, and communicable disease with worldwide public health significance as a cause of disability and death, especially in developing countries.[12]

◆ Groups at high risk for exposure to TB include those who have been recently infected with TB bacteria or persons with medical conditions that weaken the immune system. Those at risk include[13]:

  • Close contact with people infected with TB.
  • Residing and working in institutional settings (prisons, nursing homes).
  • From countries with a high TB incidence/prevalence.
  • Injection drug users.
  • People who abuse alcohol.
  • Persons with HIV.
  • Patients with diabetes, severe kidney disease, organ transplants head neck cancer.
  • Patients undergoing specialized treatment for Crohn disease or rheumatoid arthritis.
  • Malnourished or low body weight.
  • Medical/dental care providers for any of the aforementioned high-risk groups.

I. Etiology

Mycobacterium tuberculosis, a rod-shaped bacterium (tubercle bacillus), is the most common causative agent.

II. Transmission

◆ Tubercle bacilli travel in airborne droplet nuclei in infected saliva or mucus from persons with pulmonary or laryngeal TB during forceful expirations (coughing, sneezing, talking, singing).

◆ The airborne droplet nuclei can remain suspended in the air for hours.[14]

◆ Inhalation and other modes of transmission are described in Chapter 5.

III. Disease Development

◆ Inhaled tubercle bacilli travel to the lung alveoli where local infection begins.

◆ While TB can affect any organ or tissue, M. *tuberculosis* is an aerobe and survives best in an environment of high oxygen tension, such as the lungs.

◆ Latent tuberculosis infection (LTBI)

  • Within 2–10 weeks following exposure, immune response will limit further growth of M. *tuberculosis*, although not all bacilli will be eliminated.

  • At this stage, the infected person is categorized as having LTBI.

  • Approximately 5%–10% of people infected with M. *tuberculosis* and not treated for LTBI will develop TB disease during their lifetime.[13,15]

• Comparison of LTBI and active TB disease including signs/symptoms, diagnosis, and medical treatment with TB drugs is listed in Table 60-6.

IV. Diagnosis

A. Latent tuberculosis infection

Two tests are available to determine exposure to M. *tuberculosis*.

◆ Tuberculin skin test (TST).

  • Also known as Mantoux test, purified protein derivative (PPD) test.

  • PPD is injected under the skin on the forearm. After 72 hours, the circumference of induration (hard swelling) is measured to determine exposure.

  • A negative TST does not exclude TB disease in a person with signs and symptoms of TB disease.

◆ Interferon-gamma release assay (IGRA).

  • Blood test to determine exposure to M. *tuberculosis*.

  • IGRA blood test, as with TST, cannot differentiate LTBI from active TB disease. Laboratory sputum smear and culture is required.

B. Active TB Disease

When tests to determine exposure to M. *tuberculosis* are positive, further examination is required to rule out active TB disease.

◆ Chest radiograph.

◆ Physical examination and evaluation of signs and symptoms.

◆ *Preliminary diagnosis*: Perform microscopic examination of sputum smears for acid-fast bacilli (AFB).

  • The waxy cell wall of tubercle bacilli does not absorb the traditional water-soluble Gram stain and cannot be identified.

  • However, when treated with an acid stain, the organisms appear pink and are named AFB.

◆ *Definitive diagnosis*: When AFB are seen on a stained smear of sputum, or other clinical specimen, a diagnosis of TB disease is *suspected*. However, the diagnosis is *not confirmed* until a laboratory culture is grown and identified as M. *tuberculosis*.

V. Medical Management

A. Commonly Prescribed Drugs

Commonly prescribed TB drugs are included in Table 60-6.

B. Directly Observed Therapy

Observing the patient swallow anti-TB drugs is recommended for all LTBI and TB disease patients and will result in:

◆ High medication compliance.

◆ Prevention of multidrug-resistant bacterial development.

◆ Prevention of multidrug-resistant TB (MDR-TB) disease, which is more severe and difficult to treat.

TABLE 60-6 • Comparison of LTBI and Active TB Disease: Signs/Symptoms, Diagnosis, and Medical Management with TB Drugs

ITEM	LTBI	ACTIVE TB DISEASE
Signs and symptoms of pulmonary TB	None	*Early onset:* Low-grade fever Nonproductive cough lasting 3 wk or longer Fatigue Unexplained weight loss Sweating at night *Later onset:* Fever Chills Persistent cough with purulent sputum Hemoptysis Hoarseness (associated with pharyngeal TB) Chest pain Dyspnea
Wellness of patient	Does not feel sick	Usually feels sick
Infectivity	Does not infect others	May infect others
TST, PPD, or Mantoux	Positive	May be positive
IGRA blood test	Positive	Positive
Sputum sample for AFB and culture	Negative	May be positive
Chest radiograph	Normal	Abnormal
Medical management for adults: commonly prescribed TB drugs	300-mg isoniazid (INH) taken daily for 9 mo (twice weekly if Directly Observed Therapy (DOT) is available). Alternate options include a 6 mo course of INH (twice weekly if DOT is available); a 3-mo regimen of INH and rifapentine once weekly OR rifampin (RIF) taken daily for 4 mo.	Various combinations of drugs taken daily for a minimum of 6 mo Drugs commonly prescribed: INH RIF Ethambutol (EMB) Pyrazinamide (PZA) Therapy for multidrug-resistant TB Bedaquiline fumarate

AFB, acid-fast bacilli; IGRA, interferon-gamma release assay; LTBI, latent tuberculosis infection; PPD, purified protein derivative; TB, tuberculosis; TST, tuberculin skin test.
Source: Centers for Disease Control and Prevention. *Treatment for TB Disease.* Atlanta, GA: Centers for Disease Control and Prevention. https://www.cdc.gov/tb/topic/treatment/tbdisease.htm. Updated April 5, 2016. Accessed February 2, 2019; Centers for Disease Control and Prevention, National Center for HIV Viral Hepatitis STD and TB Prevention. *Fact Sheet: Treatment Options for Latent Tuberculosis Infection.* Atlanta, GA: Center for Disease Control and Prevention; 2016. https://www.cdc.gov/tb/publications/factsheets/treatment/ltbitreatmentoptions_revised.pdf. Accessed February 28, 2019.

C. Drug Resistance

TB bacteria can become resistant (drugs are no longer effective in killing the bacteria).[12]

- Types of resistance[16]
  - Primary resistance: individuals who have not been previously exposed to anti-TB drug treatments.
  - Acquired resistance: individuals who have been previously exposed to anti-TB drug treatments. This is occurs frequently when a full course of anti-TB drug treatments is not completed.
- MDR-TB: TB bacterial resistance to at least two of the first-line (most preferred) drugs, isoniazid and rifampin.[17]
- Extensively drug-resistant TB: TB bacterial resistance to isoniazid, rifampin, any fluoroquinolone, and at least one of three injectable second-line drugs.

VI. Oral Manifestations

- TB infrequently appears in the oral cavity from pulmonary organisms in infected sputum brought to the mouth by coughing.[13,14]
- Classic mucosal lesion: painful, deep, irregular ulcer on dorsum of the tongue as seen in Figure 60-5.
- Lesions can also occur on palate, lips, buccal mucosa, and gingiva.
- A biopsy and laboratory culture of an oral lesion that reveals M. *tuberculosis* confirms a diagnosis of TB.
- Glandular swelling: cervical or submandibular lymph nodes infected with TB. Nodes may become enlarged.

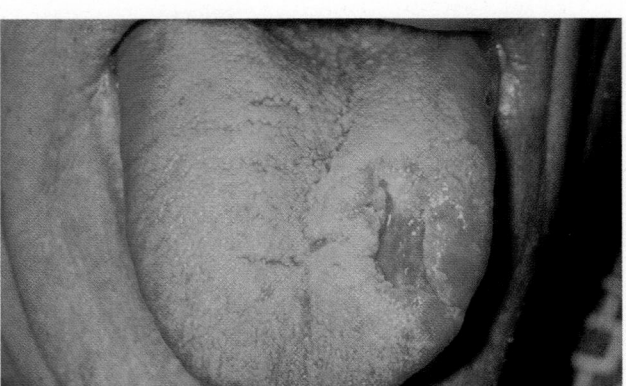

FIGURE 60-5 • Oral Ulcer on Tongue Caused by *Mycobacterium tuberculosis.* The classic oral mucosal lesion is a painful, deep, irregular ulcer on the dorsum of the tongue. (Courtesy of the United States Department of Veteran's Affairs. From DeLong L and Burkhart N. *General and Oral Pathology for Dental Hygienists.* Baltimore, MD: Lippincott Williams & Wilkins; 2008.)

VII. Dental Hygiene Care

A. Implementation of Infection Control Measures

- Update medical history.
- Recognize signs and symptoms of TB as listed in Table 60-6.
- Refer to the web resource for CDC guidelines on infection control and prevention of transmission of TB in healthcare settings.
- Create and routinely update written office/clinic protocols for:
  - Educating and training staff.
  - Instrument reprocessing and operatory cleanup.
  - Identifying, managing, and referring patients with active TB disease.
  - Assessing, managing, and investigating dental staff with positive TST (PPD).

B. Management of Patients with Symptoms or History of TB

Potential infectivity dictates decisions regarding whether to treat a patient or refer to a physician for medical clearance.[13]

- Active TB disease and sputum-positive TB
  - Do not treat in the dental office or any outpatient facility.
  - Treatment needs to be performed in a hospital with appropriate isolation, sterilization, and engineering controls.
- History of TB
  - Use caution, obtain history of disease, treatment duration, and discuss signs and symptoms of disease.
  - Consult with physician before treatment.

- Also consult with physician if adequate treatment time/appropriate medical follow-up is unclear or patient presents with signs or symptoms of relapse.
- Recent conversion to positive TST or blood test. Treatment is permitted after:
  - Patient is free of clinically active disease
  - Evaluation by physician to rule out active TB disease
  - Verification by physician of receiving isoniazid for 6 months to 1 year to prevent active TB disease.
- When the patient has signs and symptoms of TB, postpone nonemergency treatment and refer to physician.

ASTHMA

Asthma is a chronic respiratory disease consisting of recurrent episodes of dyspnea, coughing, and wheezing, leading to bronchial inflammation and muscle contraction.[18]

I. Etiology

The exact cause of asthma is not completely understood. The following types are based on pathophysiology.

A. Extrinsic (Allergic or **Atopic**): Allergic Triggers from Outside the Body

- Most common type of asthma.[19]
- Exaggerated inflammatory response triggered by inhalation of an environmental allergen (dust, pollen, tobacco smoke, mold, dust mites, or animal dander).
- Allergic stimulus leads to activation of airway epithelial mast cells.[19]
- Steps of an immunoglobulin E (IgE)-mediated hypersensitivity reaction are shown in Figure 60-6.

B. Intrinsic (Nonallergic): Nonallergic Triggers from within the Body

- Intrinsic triggers: emotional stress, gastroesophageal reflux disease (GERD).[20]
- Trigger may be unidentified.
- Obesity.
- Usually seen in adults.[20]

C. Drug- or Food-Induced (Nonallergenic, Nonatopic)

- Aspirin.
- Nonsteroidal anti-inflammatory drugs (NSAIDs).
- Beta-blockers.
- Food substances: nuts, shellfish, milk, and strawberries.
- Tartrazine (yellow food dye).
- Metabisulfite preservative in food (wine, beer, shrimp, dried fruit).
- Metabisulfite preservative in drugs (local anesthetic with epinephrine).

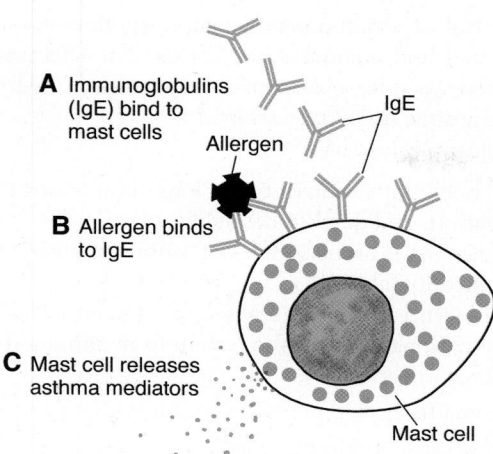

FIGURE 60-6 • Steps of an Immunoglobulin E (IgE)-mediated Hypersensitivity Reaction. A: Initial exposure. On initial exposure to an allergen (dust, pollen), immunoglobulins (IgE) are produced and bind to mast cells. **B:** Subsequent exposure. On subsequent exposures, allergen binds to IgE on the mast cell. **C:** Mast cells respond by releasing asthma mediators (histamines, leukotrienes, prostaglandins). The asthma mediators cause bronchoconstriction, vasodilation, and mucus production, resulting in coughing, wheezing, and dyspnea.

D. Exercise Induced

- Vigorous physical activity: usually affects young people due to their level of activity.
- Thermal changes during inhalation of cold air may provoke mucosal irritation and airway hyperactivity.

E. Infection Induced

- Lung infections caused by viruses, bacteria, or fungi may provoke asthmatic symptoms.
- Treatment of the infection improves breathing.

II. Atopic (Allergic) Asthma

Atopic asthma is one type of IgE-mediated hypersensitivity reaction.

A. Immunoglobulin E

- One of the five types of antibodies produced by the body.
- Provides the primary defense against environmental allergens (pollen, tobacco smoke, and food substances).

B. Normal Inflammatory Reaction

- IgE breaks down the allergens and removes them from the body.
- Normally, such activity does not produce noticeable symptoms.

C. Asthmatic Hypersensitivity Reaction

- People with asthma are believed to "hyper-react" and produce more IgE antibodies than normal.

- The results can be symptoms of asthma: wheezing, coughing, and dyspnea.

D. How Allergens Trigger Asthma

Steps in an IgE-mediated hypersensitivity reaction (Figure 60-6):

- On initial exposure to an allergen (dust, pollen, food), immunoglobulins (IgE) are produced and bind to mast cells (Figure 60-6A).
- On subsequent exposures, the antigen binds to the IgE on the mast cell (Figure 60-6B).
- Mast cells release asthma mediators, such as histamines, leukotrienes, and prostaglandins (Figure 60-6C).
- Asthma mediators cause bronchoconstriction, vasodilation, and mucus production. The result is wheezing, coughing, and dyspnea.

E. Summary of IgE-Mediated Hypersensitivity Reactions

- Local anaphylaxis:
  - Allergen binds to mast cell in nasal cavity: results in allergic rhinitis (hay fever).
  - Allergen binds to mast cell in bronchiole: results in asthma.
- Systemic anaphylaxis: Allergen (penicillin, bee venom, food substance) binds to mast cells throughout the body: results in a reaction sometimes referred to as anaphylactic shock.

III. Asthma Attack

A. Recognize Signs and Symptoms of Severe or Worsening Asthma Attack

- Chest tightness, sense of suffocation.
- Ineffectiveness of bronchodilator to relieve dyspnea.
- Wheezing, cough.
- Flushed appearance, sweating.
- Confusion due to lack of oxygen.
- Dilated pupils.
- Inability to complete a sentence in one breath.
- Tachypnea.
- Tachycardia.

B. Prepare for Possible Emergency Care

- Recognize signs and symptoms.
- Stop dental hygiene treatment.
- Rule out foreign-body obstruction.
- Assist with patient's own bronchodilator inhaler.
- Administer supplemental oxygen by nasal cannula.
- Assist with the administration of subcutaneous injection or inhalation of epinephrine.
- Monitor vital signs.
- Call emergency medical service and initiate emergency procedures described in Chapter 9.

IV. Medical Management

A. Diagnosis

Conduct physical examination and lung function assessment (spirometry).[18]

B. Achieve and Maintain Asthma Control

◆ Assess and monitor asthma severity and asthma control.[18]

◆ The National Asthma Education and Prevention Program classification is based on four levels of severity and frequency of symptoms as well as pulmonary function assessment (spirometry).[19]

- Intermittent.
- Persistent–mild.
- Persistent–moderate.
- Persistent–severe.

◆ Education: Patients are advised to have a written control plan from the physician explaining the process of disease, treatment options, and how to treat exacerbations (worsening of symptoms).

◆ Control of environmental factors (pollutants and allergens) and comorbid conditions that affect asthma (GERD, obesity, obstructive sleep apnea [OSA], rhinitis/sinusitis, stress/depression).

◆ Medications:

- There are two main types: long-term control medications and quick-relief medications.
- Categories and examples of asthma medications are listed in Table 60-7.

◆ People with asthma are advised to get seasonal influenza vaccinations and may also benefit from immunotherapy (allergy injections).

◆ Asthma triggers: potentially harmful drugs to avoid

- Aspirin-containing medications (use acetaminophen).
- Sulfite-containing local anesthetic solution, such as epinephrine.
- NSAIDs.

◆ Avoid drugs that decrease respiratory function such as narcotics and barbiturates.

◆ Avoid harmful drug-to-drug interactions.

TABLE 60-7 • Types, Categories, and Examples of Asthma Medications

Long-Term Control: Used Daily for Persistent Asthma

Corticosteroids • Anti-inflammatory • Decreases airway hyperresponsiveness. *Preferred:* inhaled corticosteroid for all levels of persistent asthma: oral–systemic corticosteroid for severe, persistent asthma	Beclomethasone dipropionate (Vanceril) (Prednisone)
Mast cell stabilizers: for mild persistent asthma	Cromolyn sodium (Intal)
Immunomodulators: for severe persistent asthma with sensitivity to allergens • Prevents binding of immunoglobulin E to basophils and mast cells	Omalizumab
Leukotriene receptor antagonist: also known as leukotriene modifiers • Interferes with leukotriene mediators that are released from mast cells, eosinophils, and basophils. *Alternative:* for mild persistent asthma	Montelukast (Singulair) (Zafirlukast)
Long-acting beta-2 agonists • Inhaled bronchodilator with 12-hr duration • Used in combination with other medications	Salmeterol, Formoterol
Methylxanthines: for mild persistent asthma • Bronchodilator to relax smooth muscle	Sustained-release theophylline (Theolair, Theo-24)
Combination medication • Anti-inflammatory medication used in combination with bronchodilator medication	

Short-Term Control: Quick-Relief Medication

Short-acting beta-2 agonists (SABA): home use for relief of acute symptoms • Bronchodilator to relax smooth muscle	Albuterol (Ventolin, Levalbuterol, Pirbuterol)
Anticholinergics • Used in hospital emergency room and in inhalers	
Systemic corticosteroids • For exacerbations used with SABAs to speed recovery and prevent reoccurrence of exacerbations	

Source: American Lung Association. *Understand Your Medication.* Chicago, IL: American Lung Association; 2018. http://www.lung.org/lung-disease/asthma/taking-control-of-asthma/understand-your-medication.html. Updated June 4, 2018. Accessed February 27, 2019.

- Macrolide antibiotics (such as erythromycin) if patient takes theophylline.
- Erythromycin inhibits metabolism of theophylline, which can result in an increase in serum level and possible overdose.
- Discontinue cimetidine 24 hours before intravenous sedation in patients taking theophylline.

V. Oral Manifestations

- Beta-2 agonist inhalers:
  - Cause a decrease in salivary flow and dental biofilm pH.
  - Are associated with xerostomia and a possible increase in caries and gingivitis in patients with inadequate biofilm control.
- Increase in GERD with use of beta-2 agonists and theophylline, which may contribute to enamel erosion.
- Oral candidiasis may occur with high dosage or frequency of inhaled corticosteroids.
  - Occurrence may decrease with use of a "spacer" or aerosol-holding chamber attached to metered-dose inhaler.
  - Rinse mouth with water after each use.

VI. Dental Hygiene Care

Table 60-8 summarizes dental hygiene care before, during, and after treatment.[19,20]

CHRONIC OBSTRUCTIVE PULMONARY DISEASE

- The term "chronic obstructive pulmonary disease (COPD)" is used to describe pulmonary disorders that obstruct airflow.[21,22]
- Two of the most common diseases are chronic bronchitis and emphysema.
- Progressive disease that is not fully reversible.[22]
- Characterized by chronic inflammation in the lungs and airways and a continual airflow limitation.[22]
- The primary etiology is inhaling tobacco smoke with occupational and environmental pollutants as contributing factors.
- Tobacco use accounts for 8 of 10 COPD-related deaths.[23,24]
- Motivating a patient with COPD to begin a tobacco cessation program can be one of the most rewarding aspects of dental hygiene practice.

I. Chronic Bronchitis

A. Etiology

Chronic bronchitis is defined as excessive respiratory tract mucus production sufficient to cause a cough, with expectoration (coughing up mucus) for at least 3 months of the year for 2 years or more.

TABLE 60-8 • Dental Hygiene Care for the Patient with Asthma	
TIME	DENTAL HYGIENE CARE

Before treatment	• Remind the patient to bring inhaler (rescue drug) and/or other medications.
	• Assess risk level: Review medical history, frequency/severity of acute episodes, and triggering agents.
	• Questions to ask: In the past 2 wk, how many times have you:
	  • Had problems with coughing, wheezing, shortness of breath, or chest tightness during the day?
	  • Awakened at night from sleep because of coughing or other asthma symptoms?
	  • Awakened in the morning with asthma symptoms?
	  • Had asthma symptoms that did not improve within 15 min of using inhaled medication?
	  • Had symptoms while exercising or playing?
	• Evaluate current symptoms: Reappoint if symptoms are not well controlled.
	• Review current medications. See Table 60-7 for commonly prescribed asthma medications.
	• Ask if all prescription medication has been taken.
	• Schedule morning appointments for patients with nocturnal asthma (symptoms worsen at night).
	• Have bronchodilator and oxygen available. May use patient's bronchodilator as a preventive measure before the appointment.
	• Obtain a medical consultation for patients with unstable or severe acute asthma or if on corticosteroid to determine necessity of steroid replacement and/or antibiotics to prevent infection.
	• Provide a stress-free environment.

During treatment	• Prevent triggering a hypersensitive airway by properly placing cotton rolls, fluoride trays, and suction tip. • Use local anesthetic without sulfites. • Fluoride treatment for all patients with asthma, especially those using beta-2 agonists. • If asthma attack occurs, stop treatment, rule out foreign-body obstruction, initiate emergency procedures shown in Chapter 9.
After treatment	• Home care instructions: advise patient to rinse mouth with water after using inhaler to decrease oral candidiasis. • Analgesic drug of choice is acetaminophen (aspirin or nonsteroidal anti-inflammatory drugs may trigger attack).

◆ Obstruction caused by narrowing of small airways, increased sputum (phlegm), and mucus plugging.

◆ Difficulty breathing present on *inspiration* (breathing in) and *expiration* (breathing out).

B. Signs and Symptoms

◆ Chronic cough.

◆ Copious sputum.

◆ Chest radiograph abnormalities.

◆ Sedentary, overweight, cyanotic, edematous, and breathless, leading to the term "blue bloater."

II. Emphysema

A. Etiology

Emphysema is defined as a distension (widening) of the air spaces distal to terminal bronchioles due to destruction of alveolar walls (septa).

◆ Smoke injures alveolar epithelium destroying alveolar walls and creating large air spaces.

◆ Difficulty breathing only on *expiration*.

B. Signs and Symptoms

◆ Difficulty in breathing on exertion.

◆ Minimal, nonproductive cough (dry, no mucus).

◆ Barrel chest (enlarged chest walls) due to increased use of respiratory chest muscles.

◆ Weight loss.

◆ Chest radiograph abnormalities.

◆ Purses lips to forcibly expel air, leading to the term "pink puffer."

III. Medical Management

There is no cure for COPD. To decrease exacerbations, patients are encouraged to stop smoking, eliminate exposure to environmental pollutants, have adequate nutrition, drink water, and exercise regularly.[21] Four medical intervention strategies are described as follows.[21,22]

A. Assess and Monitor Disease

◆ Confirm diagnosis with spirometry and determine severity.

◆ COPD is classified into five stages: at-risk, mild, moderate, severe, and very severe.

• *At-risk* stage is defined by normal spirometry, but patients have chronic symptoms of cough and sputum production.

• *Mild, moderate, and severe* COPD has evidence of increasing airway obstruction on spirometry in each progressive stage.

• *Very severe* COPD is defined by severe airway obstruction with chronic respiratory failure. At this stage, quality of life is significantly impaired, and exacerbations may be life-threatening.

B. Reduce Risk Factors

◆ Tobacco cessation.

◆ Reduction of exposure to environmental indoor/outdoor pollutants.

◆ Examples: Ozone and industrial air pollution, automobile emissions, household cleaning products.

◆ Vaccinations for influenza and pneumococcal.[21]

◆ Education on self-management.

◆ Periodontal infection, inadequate biofilm control, and lack of oral health knowledge are associated with increased risk of COPD.[21,23]

C. Manage Stable COPD

◆ Relief of symptoms: aerosol bronchodilators, inhaled corticosteroids, and other medications similar to those used to treat asthma.

◆ Pneumonia and seasonal influenza vaccinations.

◆ Antibiotics for infectious exacerbations.

◆ Pulmonary rehabilitation including a structured exercise program to relieve symptoms and improve quality of life.

◆ Surgery.

• In severe emphysema, the removal of part of one or both lungs may result in more space for the remaining lungs to function.

• Lung transplant.

• Oxygen therapy: A patient who uses oxygen (as shown in Figure 60-7) to improve breathing function may hold a portable unit during treatment.

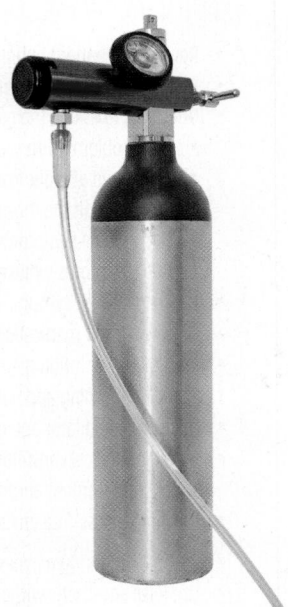

FIGURE 60-7 • Portable Oxygen Tank. A patient who uses oxygen to improve breathing function may hold a portable unit during treatment. (© rCarner/Shutterstock)

- Types: *Continuous flow*: oxygen flows at a determined rate of liters per minute.
- *On demand*: oxygen flows during inhalation only, extending the period of time between oxygen tank refills.
- Precautions: oxygen promotes rapid burning. Keep away from heat, flame, or other ignition source (cigarettes, Bunsen burner).

D. Prevent and Manage Exacerbations

◆ Infections, inhalation of irritants, and nonadherence to management programs lead to exacerbations.

IV. Oral Manifestations

◆ Similar to patients with asthma.

◆ Patients who use any form of tobacco have an increased risk of the following oral conditions[24,25]:
- Oral cancer.
- Nicotine stomatitis.
- Halitosis.
- Periodontal infections.
- Extrinsic tooth stain.

V. Dental Hygiene Care

A. Before Treatment

◆ Precautions are needed when concurrent cardiovascular disease is present. Emergency procedures are outlined in Chapter 9. The following should be considered prior to initiating treatment[25]:
- Assess severity of COPD and breathing difficulty.
- Treatment may be performed on stable patients with adequate breathing.
- Identify patients who may experience exacerbation of symptoms under emotional stress.
- Monitor blood pressure.
- Appointment length may need to be modified.
- Chair positioning: upright or semi-upright to facilitate breathing, as shown in Chapter 8.

B. During Treatment

◆ Use antimicrobial preprocedural rinse.

◆ Avoid the use of power-driven scalers and air polishers.

◆ Administer local anesthesia without epinephrine.

◆ Nitrous oxide–oxygen inhalation sedation: avoid with severe COPD and emphysema.

C. Patient Education

◆ Encourage patients to stop smoking. Tobacco cessation strategies are described in Chapter 32.

◆ Promote oral care and oral health knowledge in prevention and treatment of COPD.

◆ Discuss oral–systemic link between periodontitis and COPD.

◆ Teach and promote oral cancer self-examination.

◆ Schedule frequent periodontal and maintenance visits.

CYSTIC FIBROSIS

Cystic fibrosis (CF) is an autosomal recessive gene disorder. Both parents must carry the genetic mutation for the disease to be transmitted to their children.[26]

◆ CF is progressive and ultimately fatal.

◆ With improved multifaceted health care, many people now live beyond 30–40 years of age.

◆ Clinical signs and symptoms are shown in Box 60-1.

I. Disease Characteristics

The gene disorder affects the movement of salt and water in and out of epithelial cells in the respiratory tract and exocrine glands (respiratory, pancreas, gastrointestinal) and results in thickened secretions. Main systems affected are described as follows.

A. Respiratory Tract

Airways are filled with phlegm, similar to pus, leading to:
◆ Chronic sinusitis.
◆ Opportunistic bacterial lung infection.

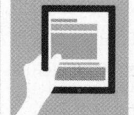

BOX 60-1
Clinical Signs and Symptoms of Cystic Fibrosis (CF)

Early Stage
- In infancy, failure to thrive
- Persistent cough and wheezing
- Recurrent pneumonia
- Excessive appetite but poor weight gain
- Salty skin or sweat
- Bulky, foul-smelling stools (undigested lipids)

Late Stage with Pulmonary Involvement
- Tachypnea (rapid breathing)
- Sustained chronic cough with mucus production and vomiting
- Barrel chest
- Cyanosis and digital (finger) clubbing
- Exertional dyspnea with decreased exercise capacity
- **Pneumothorax**
- Right heart failure secondary to **pulmonary hypertension**

Cystic Fibrosis Foundation. *What Is Cystic Fibrosis.* Bethesda, MD: Cystic Fibrosis Foundation. http://www.cff.org/AboutCF/. Accessed February 27, 2019.

Both are difficult to eradicate, even with antibiotics, due to the ability of *Pseudomonas aeruginosa* to form biofilm.[26]

B. Pancreas and Intestinal Tract

◆ Thick mucus clogs pancreatic ducts.

◆ Clogged ducts prevent the release of pancreatic enzymes into the intestinal tract.

◆ Without enzymes, food is not properly digested or absorbed.

II. Medical Management

Patients are encouraged to have regular physical activity and to adjust their diet to include pancreatic enzyme supplements, fat-soluble vitamins, liquids with high-salt intake, and caloric supplementation. Comprehensive medical care includes[26]:

◆ Antibiotics including inhalation solution: tobramycin sulfate nebulizer.

◆ Bronchodilators and anti-inflammatory agents.

◆ Chest physiotherapy.
  • Postural drainage: patient is placed in various body positions to allow mucus to drain from the airway.
  • Percussion (tapping): to loosen secretions.

III. Dental Hygiene Care

A. Oral Manifestations

◆ No specific oral lesions related to CF.

◆ Gingivitis associated with dry mouth.

B. To Facilitate Breathing

◆ Adapt chair positioning.

◆ Avoid use of rubber dam.

C. Summary Guidelines for Dental Hygiene Care

Summary guidelines for dental hygiene care for a patient with a respiratory disease are listed in Table 60-9.

TABLE 60-9 • Summary Guidelines for Oral Hygiene Care for Patients with a Respiratory Disease	
ITEM	**DENTAL HYGIENE CARE**
Medical consultation required when:	• Signs or symptoms suggest respiratory disease. Examples: Cough/dyspnea at rest, hemoptysis, sputum, **wheeze**, chest pain, oxygen saturation level of 91% or lower as determined by pulse oximetry, or positive TB skin test (TST, PPD, Mantoux). • The clinician is uncertain of the patient's medical status, severity of disease, or level of control. • Patient with systemic conditions has not seen a primary care provider within the past year. • Patient has American Society of Anesthesiologists risk status class III or higher, as shown in Chapter 22. • Patient has taken corticosteroids within the past 12 mo. Patient unsure of medications and dosages.
Stress reduction protocol	• Prevent asthma attack; helpful for patients with COPD. • Short morning appointments. • Avoid precipitating factors.
Chair position	• Semi-reclined or upright position may make breathing easier.
Anxiety and pain control	• Local anesthetic: avoid epinephrine for patients with asthma/COPD. • Nitrous oxide–oxygen may be contraindicated: • For patients with upper respiratory infection or moderate/severe COPD. • With upper respiratory tract obstruction or infection if nose breathing would be difficult or breathing apparatus cannot be sterilized or replaced. • Be prepared to handle an emergency.
Analgesia	• Avoid aspirin, aspirin-containing analgesics, and other NSAIDs as 10% of patients with asthma have aspirin-induced asthma.
Antibiotics	• Patients with extrinsic asthma may have allergy to antibiotics.
Infection control	• Standard precautions including respiratory hygiene and cough etiquette.
Emergency protocol	• Recognize symptoms of respiratory distress. • Terminate treatment. • Emergency protocol is shown in Chapter 9.
Use of equipment that produces aerosols	• Ultrasonic, sonic scalers, and polishing may be contraindicated. Septic material and microorganisms from biofilm and periodontal pockets can be aspirated into the lungs. For additional contraindications, see Chapter 39.

COPD, chronic obstructive pulmonary disease; NSAIDs, nonsteroidal anti-inflammatory drugs; PPD, purified protein derivative; TB, tuberculosis; TST, tuberculin skin test.
Source: Lozano AC, Perez MGS, Esteve CG. Dental Considerations in patients with respiratory problems. *J Clin Exp Dent.* 2011;3(3):e222-e227. Available from: http://www.medicinaoral .com/odo/volumenes/v3i3/jcedv3i3p222.pdf. Accessed February 2, 2019.

SLEEP-RELATED BREATHING DISORDERS

◆ Usually due to chronic airway obstruction.[27]

◆ Primary snoring and OSA syndrome are common SRBDs.[27]

I. Etiology

◆ Repetitive narrowing and closure of the of upper airway during sleep.

◆ Pharyngeal airway obstruction.

◆ In children, the most common cause is tonsillar hypertrophy.[28]

II. Signs and Symptoms

◆ Interruption in sleep patterns.

◆ Snoring may cause tissue inflammation.

◆ Wake up with a dry mouth or sore throat.

◆ Associated with comorbidities, motor vehicle accidents, and occupational accidents.

III. Medical Management

◆ Continuous positive airway pressure (CPAP) machine (shown in Figure 60-8) increases air pressure in the throat so that the airway does not collapse when inhaling.[29]

◆ Oral appliance therapy (OAT) is an effective treatment for mild-to-moderate sleep apnea and for severe sleep apnea when a CPAP is not tolerated by the patient.[29,30]

◆ The mandibular advancement device shown in Figure 60-9 is the most common form of oral appliance used in clinical practice.

◆ The mandibular advancement splint moves the mandible slightly forward and tightens the soft tissue and muscles of the upper airway to prevent obstruction of the airway during sleep.[30–32]

◆ Contraindications to OAT include periodontal disease, temporomandibular disorders, and insufficient number of teeth.[33]

◆ Positional therapy to prevent postural drainage.

◆ Weight loss.

◆ Surgery.

IV. Dental Hygiene Care

◆ Assessment of oral tissues at each maintenance visit.

◆ Assessment of temporomandibular joint.

◆ Recommend non-alcohol–based mouth moisturizer/rinse.

◆ Bring mandibular advancement device to each continuing care appointment for evaluation.

DOCUMENTATION

Include in the patient's permanent record:

◆ Alerts for dental personnel to the possibility of disease transmission or a medical emergency due to medical condition or allergy.

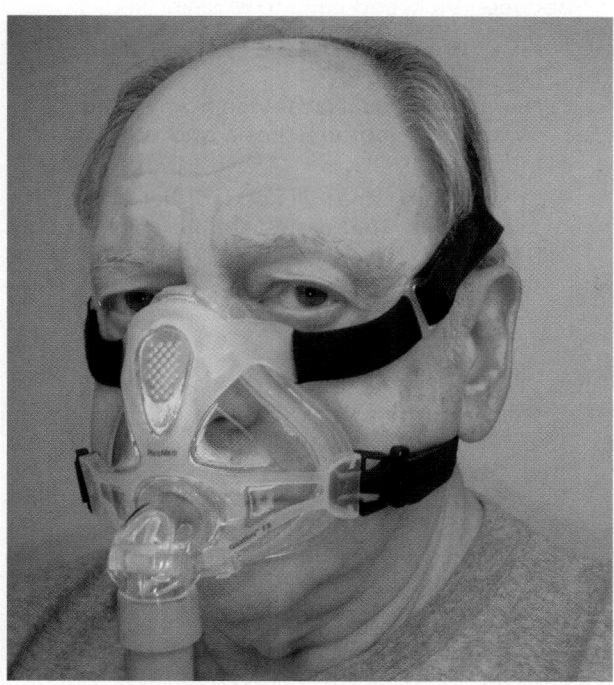

FIGURE 60-8 · Continuous Positive Airway Pressure (CPAP). This machine is attached by a hose to the nose mask that is held in place while sleeping by straps. The CPAP machine increases the air pressure in the throat so the airway does not collapse when inhaling. (Picture courtesy of Dennis Freeman, DDS.)

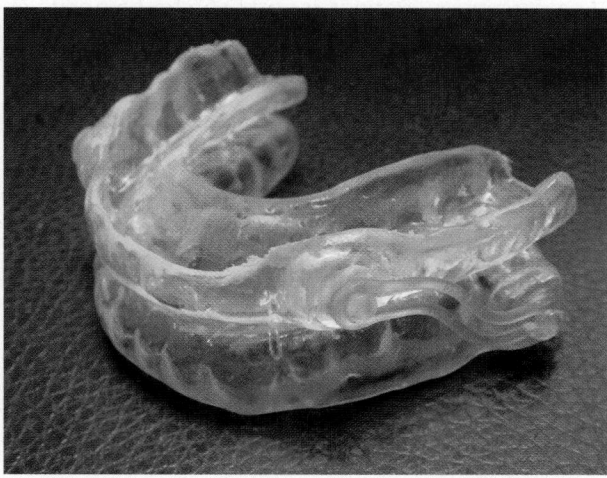

FIGURE 60-9 · Mandibular Advancement Splint (MAS). A splint that moves the mandible slightly forward that tightens the soft tissue and muscles of the upper airway to prevent obstruction of the airway during sleep.

BOX 60-2
Examples of Medical Alert Notifications

Medical alert notifications should not be visible on the outside of the patient record.

Medical Alert: Asthma

Medical Alert: **XDR-TB**

♦ *Paper records*: to protect patient confidentiality, place the medical alert box inside front cover.

♦ *Electronic records*: insert in a prominent area.

♦ Box 60-2 shows an example of medical alert notifications.

♦ *Medical consultation*: file written reports and document telephone conversations.

♦ *Patient's current health status*: especially related to signs and symptoms of respiratory disease, known allergies, current medications.

♦ *Vital signs*: including pulse oximetry.

♦ *Oral examination*: with attention to oral cancer screening and periodontal evaluation.

♦ *Patient education*: especially issues about dry mouth, tobacco cessation, and medication compliance.

♦ *Changes in respiratory signs and symptoms during treatment and interventions performed.*

♦ A sample progress note for a patient with a positive TST is shown in Box 60-3.

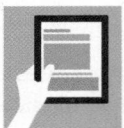

BOX 60-3
Example Documentation:
Patient with a Positive TST

S—A 36-year-old patient presents for new patient examination. Patient reports she had a positive TST test 1 year ago. She states that she was treated and is not contagious.

O—Called patient's physician (Dr. Roberts). Spoke with nurse (Becky) who provided verbal summary and will also send written report to include in the patient's record. Patient successfully completed regime of isoniazid for 9 months. Latest medical examination findings:

• Chest radiograph—negative

• Sputum smear and culture—negative

• Signs and symptoms—none

A—No signs of active TB disease; patient may receive any medical dental treatment without restriction.

P—Proceeded with patient assessment and dental prophylaxis.

Signed: _____, RDH

Date: _____

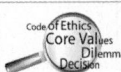

EVERYDAY ETHICS

On a beautiful spring day, Lana Thomas arrived for her 3-month continuing care visit. Vicki, the dental hygienist, noticed a labored breathing pattern as they walked down the hall to the dental hygiene treatment room. She rechecked the patient history before beginning the intraoral assessment but found the information unremarkable.

Lana reported taking an over-the-counter product for seasonal allergies, but it didn't seem to be helping with her nasal and chest congestion. The patient also requested that she should not be placed so far back in the dental chair because it was difficult for her to breathe. Vicki began to reconsider her plan to use the ultrasonic scaler given the patient's current condition.

Questions for Consideration

1. What are the ethical responsibilities of a primary healthcare clinical dental hygienist when a patient presents with symptoms such as those of Lana Thomas?

2. How does each of the dental hygiene core values have an application as Vicki prepares her care plan for the immediate appointment?

3. Pair up with a partners to plan a conversation between Vicki and Lana to explain:

• Procedures they will follow for this appointment,

• Need for medical clearance from Lana's physician for using anesthesia and other treatments, and

• Special care Lana will need for her daily care because of the oral–systemic relationship that exists.

Factors to Teach the Patient

▶ Attention to respiratory hygiene and cough etiquette.

▶ The need for frequent hand washing to help prevent transmission of respiratory disease.

▶ The need for thorough daily cleaning and drying of toothbrushes to help prevent spread of infections.

▶ How using a new toothbrush and cleaning dentures/orthodontic appliances after bacterial infections can decrease possibility of reinfection.

▶ For elderly patients and those with chronic respiratory or cardiovascular disease, diabetes, or immunosuppressed conditions, the need for pneumonia and seasonal influenza immunization.

▶ To improve compliance in taking all prescribed medications, maintain a medication list and use pill containers that open easily and are labeled with large type.

▶ Options to combat medication-induced dry mouth.

▶ Educate the patient help avoid resistant bacteria by not requesting or taking antibiotics for a respiratory infection unless the infection has been determined by their physician to be bacterial rather than viral.[34,35]

 ENHANCE YOUR UNDERSTANDING

ONLINE RESOURCES
(see the inside front cover for access information)
- Audio glossary
- Appendices

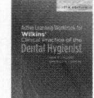

SUPPORT FOR LEARNING
(available separately)
- *Active Learning Workbook for Wilkins' Clinical Practice of the Dental Hygienist, 13th Edition*

INDIVIDUALIZED REVIEW
- Customized practice quizzing with Navigate 2 TestPrep for *Wilkins' Clinical Practice of the Dental Hygienist*

References

1. Sabharwal A, Gomes-Filho IS, Stellrecht E, Scannapieco FA. Role of periodontal therapy in management of common complex systemic diseases and conditions: an update. *Periodontol 2000*. 2018;78(1):212-226.

2. McLafferty E, Johnstone C, Hendry C, et al. Respiratory system part 1: pulmonary ventilation. *Nurs Stand*. 2013;27(22):40-47.

3. Jubran A. Pulse oximetry. *Crit Care*. 2015;19:272. doi:10.1186/s13054-015-0984-8.

4. Seto WH, Conly JM, Pessoa-Silva CL, et al. Infection prevention and control measures for acute respiratory infections in healthcare settings: an update. *East Mediterr Health J*. 2013;19(suppl 1):S39-S47.

5. Centers for Disease Control and Prevention. *Respiratory Hygiene/Cough Etiquette*. Atlanta, GA: Centers for Disease Control. https://www.cdc.gov/oralhealth/infectioncontrol/faqs/respiratory-hygiene.html. Updated March 25, 2016. Accessed February 2, 2019.

6. Agado BE, Crawford B, DeLaRosa J, et al. Effects of periodontal instrumentation on quality of life and illness in patients with chronic obstructive pulmonary disease: a pilot study. *J Dent Hyg*. 2012;86(3):204-214.

7. Davies J, Davies D. Origins and evolution of antibiotic resistance. *Microbiol Mol Biol Rev*. 2010;74(3):417-433.

8. Kinkade S, Long NA. Acute bronchitis. *Am Fam Physician*. 2016;94(7):560-565.

9. Thompson AE. Pneumonia. JAMA. 2016;315(6):626.

10. Franco J. Community-acquired pneumonia. *Radiol Technol*. 2017;88(6):621-636.

11. Gupta G, Mitra D, Ashok KP, et al. Efficacy of preprocedural mouth rinsing in reducing aerosol contamination produced by ultrasonic scaler: a pilot study. *J Periodontol*. 2014;85:562-568.

12. Centers for Disease Control and Prevention (CDC). *Reported Tuberculosis in the United States, 2017*. Atlanta, GA: U.S. Department of Health and Human Services, CDC; 2018. https://www.cdc.gov/tb/statistics/reports/2017/2017_Surveillance_FullReport.pdf. Accessed February 27, 2019.

13. TB Risk Factors. *Centers for Disease Control and Prevention*. https://www.cdc.gov/tb/topic/basics/risk.htm. Updated March 18, 2016. Accessed February 27, 2019.

14. Petti S. Tuberculosis: Occupational risk among dental healthcare workers and risk for infection among dental patients. A meta-narrative review. *J Dent*. 2016;49(suppl C):1-8.

15. Lewinsohn DM, Leonard MK, LoBue PA, et al. Official American Thoracic Society/Infectious Diseases Society of America/Centers for Disease Control and Prevention Clinical Practice Guidelines: diagnosis of tuberculosis in adults and children. *Clin Infect Dis*. 2017;15;64(2):111-115.

16. Kanabus A. Information about tuberculosis. *Global Health Education (GHE)*. 2018. www.tbfacts.org. Accessed February 28, 2019.

17. Seaworth BJ, Griffith DE. Therapy of multidrug resistant and extensively drug-resistant tuberculosis. *Microbiol Spectr*. 2017;5(2). doi:10.1128/microbiolspec.

18. U.S. Department of Health and Human Services; National Institutes of Health; National Heart, Lung, and Blood Institute. *Asthma Care Quick Reference Diagnosing and Managing Asthma*. Bethesda, MD: NHLBI Health Information Center; 2002. Revised 2012. NIH Publication No. 12-5075.

19. Rabe, FK. Update in asthma 2015. *Am J Respir Crit Care Med*. 2016;194(3).

20. U.S. Department of Health and Human Services; National Institutes of Health; National Heart, Lung, and Blood Institute. *Expert Panel Report 3: Guidelines for the Diagnosis and Management of Asthma. Full Report*. Bethesda, MD: NHLBI Health Information Center; 2007:417. NIH Publication No. 07-4051.

21. Devlin J. Patients with chronic obstructive pulmonary disease: management considerations for the dental team. *Br Dent J*. 2014;217(5):235-237.

22. Global Initiative for Chronic Obstructive Lung Disease. *Global Strategy for the Diagnosis, Management and Prevention of Chronic Obstructive Pulmonary Disease*. Revised 2018. https://goldcopd.org/wp-content/uploads/2017/11/GOLD-2018-v6.0-FINAL-revised-20-Nov_WMS.pdf. Accessed March 2, 2019.

23. Shen TC, Chang PY, Lin CL et al. Periodontal treatment reduces risk of adverse respiratory events in patients with chronic obstructive pulmonary disease: a propensity-matched cohort study. *Medicine (Baltimore)*. 2016;95(20):e3735. doi:10.1097/MD.0000000000003735

24. U.S. Department of Health and Human Services. *The Health Consequences of Smoking—50 Years of Progress: A Report of the Surgeon General*. Atlanta: U.S. Department of Health and Human Services, Centers for Disease Control and Prevention, National Center for Chronic Disease Prevention and Health Promotion, Office on Smoking and Health, 2014. Accessed February 27, 2019.

25. Lozano AC, Perez MGS, Esteve CG. Dental considerations in patients with respiratory problems. *J Clin Exp Dent.* 2011;3(3):e222-e227.

26. Cystic Fibrosis Foundation. *Frequently Asked Questions.* Bethesda, MD: Cystic Fibrosis Foundation. https://www.cff .org/What-is-CF/About-Cystic-Fibrosis/. Updated August 10, 2016. Accessed February 2, 2019.

27. Carstensen S. Obstructive sleep apnea's connections with clinical dentistry. *Sleep Med Clin.* 2018;13:521-529.

28. Pinto JA, Kohler R, Wambier H, et al. Laryngeal pathologies as an etiologic factor of obstructive sleep apnea syndrome in children. *Int J Pediatr Ororhinolaryngol.* 2013;77:573-575.

29. Marklund M. Update on oral appliance therapy for OSA. *Curr Sleep Med Rep.* 2017;3(3):143-151.

30. Wojda M, Jurkowski P, Lewandowska A, Mierzwińska-Nastalska E, Kostrzewa-Janicka J. Mandibular advancement devices in patients with symptoms of obstructive sleep Apnea: a review. *Adv Exp Med Biol.* 2019. doi: 10.1007/5584_2019_334.

31. Policy statement on the role of dentistry in the treatment of sleep-related breathing disorders. American Dental Association; 2018. https://www.ada.org/~/media/ADA/Member%20Center /FIles/The-Role-of-Dentistry-in-Sleep-Related-Breathing -Disorders.pdf?la=en. Accessed March 5, 2019.

32. ADA Evidence Brief: Oral Appliances for Sleep-Related Breathing Disorders. https://www.ada.org/~/media/ADA /Member%20Center/FIles/ADA_SCI_OralAppl_SRBD _Brief_Final_15.pdf?la=en. Accessed March 5, 2019

33. Minichbauer BC, Sheats RD, Wilder RS, Phillips CL, Essick GK. Sleep medicine content in dental hygiene education. *J Dent Educ.* 2015;79(5):484-492. http://www.jdentaled.org /content/jde/79/5/484.full.pdf

34. Martínez-González NA, Coenen S, Plate A, et al. The impact of interventions to improve the quality of prescribing and use of antibiotics in primary care patients with respiratory tract infections: a systematic review protocol. *BMJ Open.* 2017;7(6):e016253. doi:10.1136/bmjopen-2017-016253.

35. Centers for Disease Control and Prevention. *Antibiotic Use in the United States, 2017: Progress and Opportunities.* Atlanta, GA: U.S. Department of Health and Human Services, CDC; 2017.

The Patient with Cardiovascular Disease

Dianne Smallidge, RDH, BS, MDH, EdD, and Linda D. Boyd, RDH, RD, EdD

CHAPTER OUTLINE

CLASSIFICATION

INFECTIVE ENDOCARDITIS
  I. Description
  II. Etiology
  III. Disease Process
  IV. Prevention

CONGENITAL HEART DISEASES
  I. The Normal Healthy Heart
  II. Anomalies
  III. Etiology
  IV. Types of Defects
  V. Prevention
  VI. Clinical Considerations

RHEUMATIC HEART DISEASE
  I. Rheumatic Fever
  II. The Course of Rheumatic Heart Disease

MITRAL VALVE PROLAPSE
  I. Description
  II. Symptoms

HYPERTENSION
  I. Etiology
  II. Blood Pressure Levels

  III. Clinical Symptoms of Hypertension
  IV. Treatment
  V. Hypertension in Children

ISCHEMIC HEART DISEASE
  I. Etiology
  II. Manifestations of Ischemic Heart Disease

ANGINA PECTORIS
  I. Precipitating Factors
  II. Treatment

MYOCARDIAL INFARCTION
  I. Etiology
  II. Symptoms
  III. Management during an Attack
  IV. Treatment after Acute Symptoms

HEART FAILURE
  I. Etiology
  II. Clinical Manifestations
  III. Treatment during Chronic Stages
  IV. Emergency Care for Heart Failure and Acute Pulmonary Edema

CARDIAC ARRHYTHMIAS
  I. Etiology
  II. Symptoms
  III. Treatment

LIFESTYLE MANAGEMENT FOR THE PATIENT WITH CARDIOVASCULAR DISEASE

SURGICAL TREATMENT
  I. Revascularization
  II. Cardiac Resynchronization Therapy
  III. Dental Considerations

ANTITHROMBOTIC THERAPY
  I. Anticoagulant Therapy
  II. Direct Oral Anticoagulants
  III. Antiplatelet Therapy

DOCUMENTATION

EVERYDAY ETHICS

FACTORS TO TEACH THE PATIENT

REFERENCES

LEARNING OBJECTIVES

After studying this chapter, the student will be able to:

1. Identify the cardiovascular conditions that may be encountered in patients seeking oral health care.

2. Discuss the etiology, symptoms, and risk factors associated with cardiovascular conditions.

3. Discuss the impact of cardiovascular diseases on the oral cavity and their relationship to oral health.

4. Plan dental hygiene treatment modifications for the patient with cardiovascular disease.

INTRODUCTION

Cardiovascular disease (CVD) includes conditions and diseases affecting the heart and blood vessels.

◆ Patients with cardiovascular conditions are encountered frequently in a dental office or clinic and may be from any age group, although the highest incidence is among older people.

◆ Although a causal relationship between periodontal disease and coronary heart disease (CHD) has not been proven, current data suggest the presence of periodontal disease may be a marker for CHD risk.[1]

◆ Dental hygienists need to take responsibility to inform patients of the significant relationship between oral and systemic health and the related need for maintenance of healthy oral tissues and prevention of periodontal disease.

◆ The major CVDs are included in this chapter, with their principle symptoms and treatments as well as applications for dental hygiene care.

CLASSIFICATION

◆ *Anatomic classification*
  • Diseases of the heart: pericardium, myocardium, endocardium, and heart valves.
  • Diseases of the blood vessels and peripheral circulation.

◆ *Etiologic classification*
  • Congenital anomalies.
  • Atherosclerosis, hypertension.
  • Infectious agents, immunologic mechanisms.

INFECTIVE ENDOCARDITIS

Infective endocarditis (IE) is a microbial infection of the heart valves or endocardium with a high mortality rate.

I. Description

◆ IE is a serious disease, the prognosis of which depends on the degree of cardiac damage, the valves involved, duration of the infection, and treatment.

◆ IE is characterized by the formation of bacterial vegetations on the heart valves or surface of the heart lining (endocardium).

◆ When IE develops, it directly affects the function of the heart.

II. Etiology[2]

◆ *Microorganisms*
  • Streptococci and staphylococci are responsible for IE in most cases, with alpha-hemolytic streptococci being the most prevalent.
  • As yeast, fungi, and viruses have been implicated, the choice of the name "infective" endocarditis is more inclusive than "bacterial" endocarditis.
  • Incidence related to dental procedures: The majority of IE cases related to oral microflora are random bacteremias resulting from routine daily activities. An exceedingly small number of cases are believed to result from dental procedures.

◆ *Risk factors*[2,3]
  • Preexisting cardiac abnormalities: Bacteria lodge on the endocardial (valvular) surface during bacteremia.
  • Prosthetic (artificial) heart valves: There is an increased number of patients who have had valve replacement surgery who are susceptible. Patients who have had prosthetic valve replacements have a risk of developing prosthetic valve endocarditis.
  • History of previous endocarditis.
  • Intravenous drug abuse. Infected material is injected by contaminated needles directly into the bloodstream. Intravenous drug abusers are at high risk for endocarditis, which can initiate on previously normal valves.

◆ *Precipitating factors*
  • Self-induced bacteremia: In the oral cavity, self-induced bacteremias may result from eating, bruxism, chewing gum, or any activity that can force bacteria through the wall of a diseased sulcus or pocket. Interdental aids for oral hygiene can also cause self-induced bacteremia.
  • Infection at portals of entry: Infections at sites where microorganisms may enter the circulating blood provide a constant source of potential infectious microorganisms. In the oral cavity, organisms enter the blood by way of periodontal and gingival pockets, where many species of microorganisms are harbored. An open area of infection, such as an ulcer caused by an ill-fitting denture, may also provide a site of entry. Patients are exposed daily to bacteremias.
  • Trauma to tissues by instrumentation: Bacteremias are created during general or oral surgery, endodontic procedures, periodontal therapy, scaling, and any therapy that results in bleeding.

III. Disease Process

◆ *Transient bacteremia initiated*[4]

- Trauma to a mucosal surface such as the gingival sulcus during instrumentation releases bacteria into the bloodstream.
- Ease of entry of organisms directly relates to the severity of tissue trauma, quantity of bacterial biofilm, and the severity of inflammation or infection such as periodontitis.

◆ *Bacterial adherence*[4]

- Circulating microorganisms attach to a damaged heart valve, prosthetic valve, or other susceptible area on the endocardium.

◆ *Proliferation of bacteria*[4]

- Microorganisms proliferate to form vegetative lesions containing masses of plasma cells, fibrin, and bacteria.
- Heart valve becomes inflamed, and function is diminished.
- Clumps of microorganisms (emboli) may break off and spread by way of the general circulation (embolism); complications result.

◆ *Clinical course*[4]

- A small number of patients are symptomatic within 2 days, but usually symptoms appear within 2 weeks.
- Severe symptoms of fever, loss of appetite and weight loss, weakness, arthralgia, and heart murmurs require hospitalization. Diagnosis is based on symptoms, echocardiography, blood cell count, and positive blood cultures.
- Complications lead to eventual susceptibility to reinfection with IE, congestive heart failure (CHF), and cerebrovascular disease.

IV. Prevention

The basic areas for attention in dental and dental hygiene care that contribute to the prevention of IE are as follows:

◆ *Patient history*

- Special content: Specific questions need to be directed to elicit any history of congenital heart defects, cardiac transplant, the presence of prosthetic valves, acquired valvular defects, or previous episode of IE.
- Consultation with patient's physician: Consultation is necessary for all patients with a history of heart defects and any other condition suggesting the need for prophylactic antibiotic premedication.
- Withhold instrumentation: The use of a probe or explorer during assessment of the patient should be delayed until the medical status is cleared.

◆ *Prophylactic antibiotic premedication*

- There exists no conclusive evidence that confirms the effectiveness or ineffectiveness of antibiotic premedication for the prevention of IE.[4]
- Recommended regimens: Follow the current recommendations of the American Heart Association.[2,3]

- Specific information can be found in Chapter 11.
- When antibiotic prophylaxis is indicated, verify the antibiotic was taken as prescribed. In the patient record, document the name of the antibiotic, time, and dosage taken by the patient.

◆ *Dental hygiene care*

- Oral health: Prevention and management of oral disease is necessary for each patient susceptible to IE.
- Education: Instruction in oral self-care such as brushing and interdental cleaning at initial appointments can be provided while the patient is under antibiotic coverage.
- Sequence of treatment: Biofilm removal instruction precedes instrumentation for scaling to bring the tissues to a healthy state. The more severe the gingival or periodontal inflammation, the higher the incidence of bacteremia during and following instrumentation.
- Instrumentation: Reduce the microbial population about the teeth and on the oral mucosa prior to instrumentation by having the patient brush, floss, and rinse thoroughly with an antimicrobial mouth rinse such as 0.12% chlorhexidine.

CONGENITAL HEART DISEASES

I. The Normal Healthy Heart

◆ A diagram of the normal heart is shown in Figure 61-1 to provide a comparison with the anatomic changes that may appear in a defective heart.

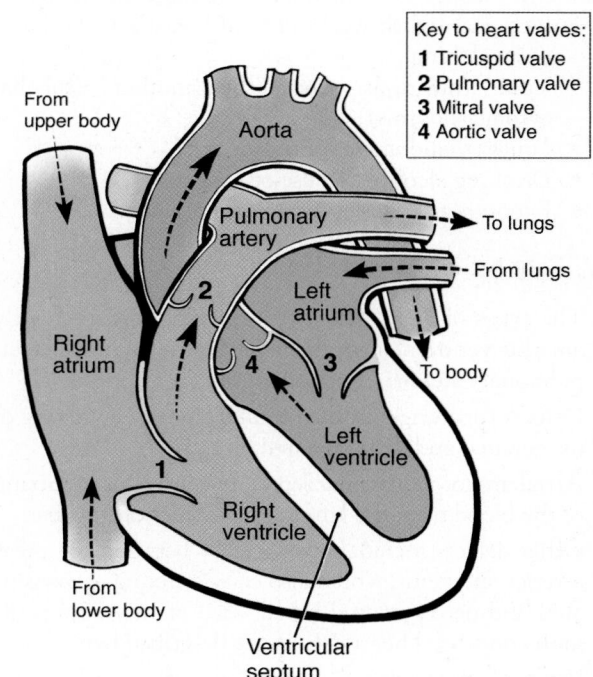

Key to heart valves:
1 Tricuspid valve
2 Pulmonary valve
3 Mitral valve
4 Aortic valve

FIGURE 61-1 • **The Normal Heart.** The major vessels and the location of the tricuspid, pulmonary, aortic, and mitral valves are shown.

◆ In the healthy heart, the blood flows in one direction as each chamber contracts, with the valves acting as trap doors that snap shut after each contraction to prevent backflow of blood.

◆ The right side of the heart contains deoxygenated blood from the body cells on its way to the lungs for reoxygenation. The left side of the heart contains oxygenated blood from the lungs being pumped out to the aorta on its way to the cells of the body. The septal wall divides the left and right sides of the heart.

II. Anomalies

◆ Anomalies of the anatomic structure of the heart or major blood vessels result following irregularities of development during the first 9 weeks in utero.

◆ The fetal heart is completely developed by the ninth week.

◆ Early diagnosis is necessary, but not all defects require treatment.

◆ Treatment usually involves surgical correction.

III. Etiology

Causes may be genetic or environmental or a combination of both. Many are unknown.

◆ *Genetic*[5,6]
  • Heredity is apparent in some types of defects.
  • An example of a chromosomal defect is Down syndrome in which congenital heart anomalies occur frequently.

◆ *Environmental*[5,6]
  • Most congenital anomalies originate between the fifth and eighth weeks of fetal life, when the heart is developing.
  • Viral infections from the mother (rubella, cytomegalovirus).
  • Drugs (thalidomide, isotretinoin).
  • Drinking alcohol and use of cocaine.
  • Exposure to industrial chemical solvents.

IV. Types of Defects

◆ The types of heart defects that occur most frequently are the ventricular septal defect, atrial septal defect, pulmonary **stenosis**, and patent ductus arteriosis.[5]

◆ Defects (openings) in the septal wall cause a mixing of oxygenated and deoxygenated blood.

◆ Atrial and/or ventricular septal defects result in mixing of the blood from the left and right sides of the heart.

◆ Other defects include a passageway between the great arteries and veins, which also causes mixing of oxygenated and deoxygenated blood. Two of the more common congenital heart defects are described here.

◆ *Ventricular septal defect*[5]
  • In this type of defect, the left and right ventricles exchange blood through an opening in their dividing wall (septum).

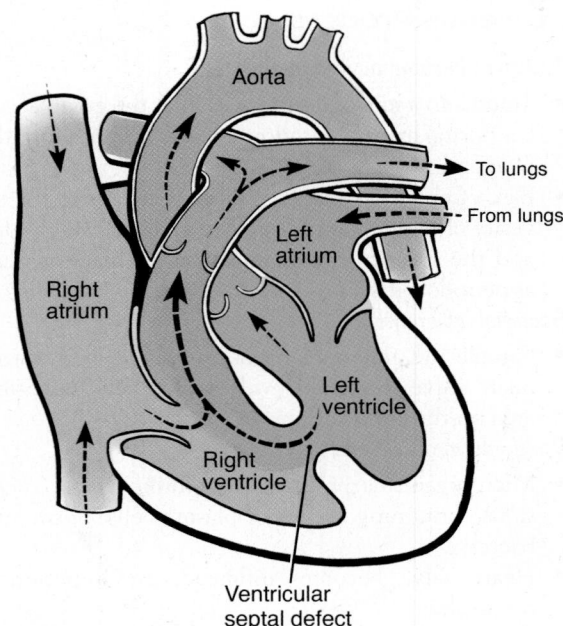

FIGURE 61-2 • Ventricular Septal Defect. The right and left ventricles are connected by an opening that permits oxygenated blood from the left ventricle to shunt across to the right ventricle and then recirculate to the lungs. Compare with Figure 61-1, in which the septum separates the ventricles.

  • The oxygenated blood from the lung, which is normally pumped by the left ventricle to the aorta and then to the entire body, can pass across to the right ventricle through the septal defect, as shown in Figure 61-2.
  • The severity of symptoms is directly related to the specific location and size of the defect. Small defects may close without surgical correction.

◆ *Patent ductus arteriosus*[5]
  • A patent ductus arteriosus means the passageway (**shunt**) is open between the two great arteries that arise from the heart, namely, the aorta and the pulmonary artery.
  • Normally, the opening closes during the first few weeks after birth.
  • When the opening does not close, blood from the aorta can pass back to the lungs, as shown in Figure 61-3.
  • The heart compensates in the attempt to provide the body with oxygenated blood and becomes overburdened.

V. Prevention

Prevention of congenital heart defects includes[6]:

◆ Rubella vaccination for women of childbearing age is highly advised for those not vaccinated in childhood or those without confirmation of immunity by a laboratory test.
  • For women of childbearing age who are health care providers, two measles, mumps, and rubella

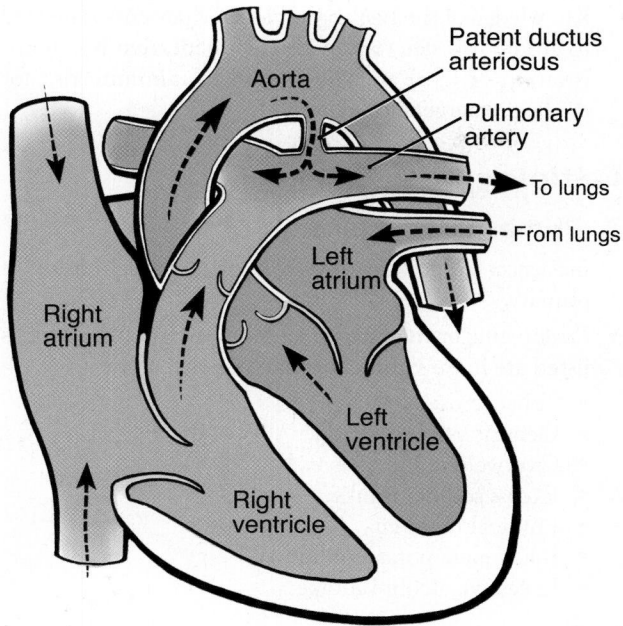

FIGURE 61-3 • Patent Ductus Arteriosus. An open passageway between the aorta and the pulmonary artery permits oxygenated blood from the aorta to pass back into the lungs. Arrows show directions of flow through the patent ductus. Compare with normal anatomy in Figure 61-1.

(MMR) doses at least 28 days apart (or one dose is one dose of MMR was previously administered) is recommended by the Centers for Disease Control and Prevention.

◆ No medications, including over-the-counter and herbal medications, are to be taken during pregnancy without prior consultation with the physician.

◆ Avoid tobacco use at least 1 month before pregnancy and throughout the pregnancy.

◆ Attain and maintain a healthy weight prior to pregnancy.

◆ Genetic counseling.

VI. Clinical Considerations

◆ *Signs and symptoms of congenital heart disease*
  • Easy fatigue.
  • Exertional dyspnea, fainting.
  • Cyanosis of lips and nail beds.
  • Poor growth and development.
  • Heart murmurs.
  • CHF.
◆ *Dental hygiene concerns*
  • Prevention of IE: Certain defective heart valves are at risk for endocarditis from bacteremia produced during oral treatments. The American Heart Association recommendations for antibiotic prophylaxis are consulted for procedure with this group of patients.[4]
  • Elimination of oral disease: Prevention and management of oral disease.

RHEUMATIC FEVER AND HEART DISEASE[7]

Rheumatic heart disease is a complication following rheumatic fever. A rather high percent of patients with a history of rheumatic fever have permanent heart valve damage.[7]

I. Rheumatic Fever

◆ *Incidence*[7]
  • Frequency of this condition in developed countries has declined significantly in the past several decades and is not common in the United States.
  • Primarily effects children between the ages of 5 and 15 years.
◆ *Etiology*[7]
  • The onset of acute rheumatic fever usually appears 2–3 weeks after a beta-hemolytic group A streptococcal pharyngeal infection.
  • Rheumatic fever and rheumatic heart disease are believed to be immunologic disorders caused by sensitization to antigens of beta-hemolytic group A streptococci.
◆ *Prevention*[7]
  • The persistence and severity of the pharyngeal infection are significant factors in determining whether rheumatic fever follows.
  • Early diagnosis and treatment of streptococcal throat and pharyngeal infections are necessary.
◆ *Symptoms of acute rheumatic fever*[7]
  • Low-grade fever.
  • Abdominal pain.
  • Shortness of breath and chest pain related to cardiac issues.
  • Joint pain with arthritis present in the ankles, knees, elbows and wrists as well as joint swelling with redness and warmth.
  • Nosebleeds.
  • Skin rash on trunk and upper parts of the arms and legs or nodules on skin.
  • Emotional instability.
  • Muscle weakness with quick uncontrolled jerky movements affecting the face, feet, and hands.

II. The Course of Rheumatic Heart Disease

Following the acute stage of rheumatic fever, symptoms do not usually persist, except the effects of the valvular deformity.

◆ *Symptoms*
  • Stenosis or incompetence of valves; most commonly, the aortic and mitral valves.
  • Heart murmur influenced by the amount of scarring of the valves and myocardium.
  • Cardiac arrhythmias (CAs).

- Late symptoms include shortness of breath, angina pectoris, endocarditis, pericarditis, elevation of diastolic blood pressure (BP), enlargement of the left ventricle, and increasing signs of CHF.
- *Practice applications*
  - The American Heart Association no longer recommends antibiotic prophylaxis prior to dental treatment for patients with this condition due to minimal risk of developing IE.[4]

MITRAL VALVE PROLAPSE[8,9]

I. Description

- The mitral valve is between the left atrium and the left ventricle (Figure 61-1).
- Oxygenated blood from the lungs passes from the pulmonary vein into the left ventricle, where it is pumped through the aortic valve and into the aorta for distribution to the body cells.
- When the mitral valve leaflets are damaged, the closure is imperfect and oxygenated blood can backflow or regurgitate.
- Mitral valve prolapse is the most common disorder of the valve that causes regurgitation.[8,9]
- The mitral valve is prolapsed (becomes misaligned) backward into the atrium during systole.[8,9]

II. Symptoms

- Most patients with mitral valve prolapse are asymptomatic.[8,9]
  - A small number of cases will have symptoms of palpitations, fatigue, atypical chest pain, and a late systolic murmur.
- When there is more severe involvement, an increase in frequency of palpitations and progressive mitral regurgitation is apparent along with a systolic click and murmur.[8,9]
- Initial suspicion for diagnosis of valvular heart disease is the recognition of a heart murmur.
- The American Heart Association no longer recommends antibiotic prophylaxis during dental treatment for patients with this condition.

HYPERTENSION

Hypertension means an abnormal elevation of Arterial Blood Pressure. It has been called the "silent killer." Hypertension is responsible for more deaths from CVD than any other modifiable risk factor for CVD.[10]

- Detection of BP for dental and dental hygiene patients has become an essential step in patient assessment prior to treatment.
- Early detection, with referral for additional diagnosis and treatment when indicated, can prove to be lifesaving for certain people.

- Knowledge of the health problems of patients is needed to ensure it is safe to provide treatment, that is, administration of local anesthesia, and to minimize risk for medical emergencies.

I. Etiology

A. Primary Hypertension

- *Incidence*: Approximately 90% of all hypertension is primary.[10]
- *Predisposing or risk factors*: Combinations of the factors listed are more significant than any one alone[10]:
  - Tobacco use.
  - Genetic predisposition.
  - Overweight and obesity.
  - Excess sodium intake.
  - Physical inactivity.
  - Inadequate potassium intake.
  - Excessive alcohol intake.

B. Secondary Hypertension

- *Incidence*: About 10% of all hypertension is secondary to other underlying medical conditions.[10]
- *Causes* of secondary hypertension may include[10]:
  - Renal disease.
  - Obstructive sleep apnea.
  - Drug or alcohol induced.
  - Endocrine conditions, such as Cushing syndrome, hypothyroidism and hyperthyroidism hyperparathyroidism.
  - Medications such as amphetamines, antidepressants, caffeine, herbal supplements (e.g., St. John wart), immunosuppressants, oral contraceptives,[8] corticosteroids, recreational drugs.

II. Blood Pressure Levels

A. Normal and High Blood Pressure

Table 61-1 lists the normal readings for BP and the stages of hypertension for adults aged 18 years and older.[10]

B. Low Blood Pressure

- Many healthy people, with no evident clinical problems, have a normal systolic pressure under 90 mm Hg.
- A marked sudden drop in BP is usually associated with an emergency, such as severe blood loss, shock, Myocardial infarction, sepsis, or other medical problem.
- Procedures to follow during specific medical emergencies can be found in Chapter 9.

III. Clinical Symptoms of Hypertension

Hypertension is frequently recognized only by BP readings and may go unrecognized because of the lack of clinical symptoms.

TABLE 61-1 • Classification of Blood Pressure for Adults Aged 18 Years or Older

BLOOD PRESSURE CATEGORY	SYSTOLIC (mm Hg)	DIASTOLIC (mm Hg)
Normal	<120	<80
Elevated	120–129	<80
Stage 1 hypertension	130–139	80–89
Stage 2 hypertension	≥140	≥90
Hypertensive crisis	>180	>120

Source: Whelton PK, Carey RM, Aronow WS, Casey DE Jr, Collins KJ, Dennison Himmelfarb C, et al. 2017 ACC/AHA/AAPA/ABC/ACPM/AGS/APhA/ASH/ASPC/NMA/PCNA guideline for the prevention, detection, evaluation, and management of high blood pressure in adults: a Report of the American College of Cardiology/American Heart Association Task Force on Clinical Practice Guidelines. *Hypertension.* 2018;71(6):e13-e115.

◆ Those who have early symptoms may describe them as[10]:
  • Dizziness.
  • Snoring.
  • Muscle cramps and weakness.
  • Pallor.
  • Edema.
  • Fatigue.
◆ *Major sequela of long-standing elevation of BP*[10]:
  • Cerebral vascular accident or stroke.
  • End-stage renal disease.
  • CHD.
  • Heart failure.
◆ *Hypertension crisis*[10]
  • Malignant hypertension is life-threatening, is sudden, and characterized by extremely high BP.
  • *Activate emergency* procedures as the situation can be fatal if not treated immediately or may result in damage to multiple body systems.

IV. Treatment of Hypertension

Treatment depends on risk factors and stage of hypertension.[11]
◆ Patients diagnosed or at risk for CVD should a target BP below 130/80.
◆ Pharmacotherapy is recommended for patients with a systolic reading greater than or equal to 140, or a diastolic reading of greater than or equal to 90.
  • Medications to treat hypertension may include diuretics, calcium channel blockers, beta-blockers, and/or angiotensin-converting enzyme (ACE) inhibitors.

A. Goals
◆ *Primary hypertension*
  • Achieve and maintain diastolic pressure level below 80 mm Hg.
  • Lower the risk of serious complications and premature death.

B. Lifestyle Changes (Box 61-1)
◆ *Weight and exercise*: Control weight and exercise daily.
◆ *Diet*: Sodium restriction, in those who are salt sensitive, and modest weight loss of 5%–10% of body weight may control mild elevations of BP.
◆ *Tobacco use*: All forms of tobacco must be eliminated.
◆ *Other risk factors*: In addition to factors listed in Box 61-1, life activity contributing to stress and tension need to be minimized.

V. Hypertension in Children[12]
◆ Children aged 3 years and older need to have BP determinations made at least annually.
◆ Prevalence of hypertension is higher in children who suffer from obesity, sleep disorders, kidney disease, and those who were born prematurely.
◆ If the BP of a child or adolescent is greater than or equal to the 90th percentile, the BP measurement should be repeated twice during the visit to determine whether the patient is hypertensive (see Chapter 12 for BP values for children and adolescents).

ISCHEMIC HEART DISEASE

Ischemic heart disease is an acute and chronic cardiac disability, arising from reduction or arrest of blood supply to the myocardium.
◆ The heart muscle (myocardium) is supplied through the coronary arteries, which are branches of the descending aorta.

BOX 61-1

Lifestyle Modifications for Hypertension Control and/or Overall Cardiovascular Risk

• If overweight, lose weight 5%–10% of body weight.
• Heart healthy diet such as DASH (Dietary Approaches to Stop Hypertension) diet.
• Limit alcohol intake to no more than "standard" drink = 1–12 ounce beer or 1.5 ounces distilled spirits or 5 ounces of wine.
• Physical activity daily.
• Reduce sodium intake.
• Possible potassium supplementation, check with primary care provider.
• Stop use of tobacco.

Source: Whelton PK, Carey RM, Aronow WS, et al. 2017 ACC/AHA/AAPA/ABC/ACPM/AGS/APhA/ASH/ASPC/NMA/PCNA guideline for the prevention, detection, evaluation, and management of high blood pressure in adults: a Report of the American College of Cardiology/American Heart Association Task Force on Clinical Practice Guidelines. *Hypertension.* 2018;71(6):e13-e115.

◆ Because of the relationship to the coronary arteries, the disease is often referred to as coronary heart disease (CHD) or coronary artery disease (CAD).

◆ Ischemia is defined as oxygen deprivation in a local area from a reduced passage of fluid into the area.

◆ Ischemic heart disease is the result of an imbalance of the oxygen supply and demand of the myocardium resulting from a narrowing or blocking of the lumen of the coronary arteries.

I. Etiology

Other factors may be involved, but the principal cause of reduction of blood flow to the heart muscle is *atherosclerosis* of the vessel walls, which narrows the lumen, thus obstructing the flow of blood.

◆ *Definition of atherosclerosis*[13]

  • Atherosclerosis is an inflammatory disease of medium and large arteries in which atheromas deposit and thicken the intimal layer of the involved blood vessel.

  • An atheroma is a fibro-fatty deposit or plaque containing several lipids, especially cholesterol.

  • With time, the plaques continue to thicken and, eventually, close the vessel (Figure 61-4).

  • Some plaques calcify, whereas others may develop an overlying thrombus.

◆ Risk factors for atherosclerosis[13,14]

  • Inflammation plays a significant role in the formation of atheromas. Low-grade chronic inflammation in other parts of the body, including chronic periodontitis, has been shown to have a relationship to adverse cardiovascular outcomes.

  • Pathogenic microorganisms from these inflammatory processes have been associated with atheroma formation in the blood and the subsequent progression of atherosclerosis.

  • Many risk factors for periodontal disease are also risk factors for atherosclerosis.[14]

  • Each risk factor can contribute to the condition; however, when factors occur in combination, the risk of atherosclerosis, and ischemic heart disease, is increased.

  • Risk factors include elevated levels of blood lipids, the result of an increased dietary intake of cholesterol, saturated fat, carbohydrate (especially sucrose), alcohol, and calories.

  • Tobacco use, diabetes, unhealthy blood cholesterol levels, obesity, insufficient physical activity, increased tensions, emotional stress, older age, and family history may also be risk factors.

  • Prevention depends on educational programs along with early identification of persons at risk.

II. Manifestations of Ischemic Heart Disease

◆ Angina pectoris.

◆ Myocardial infarction.

◆ CHF.

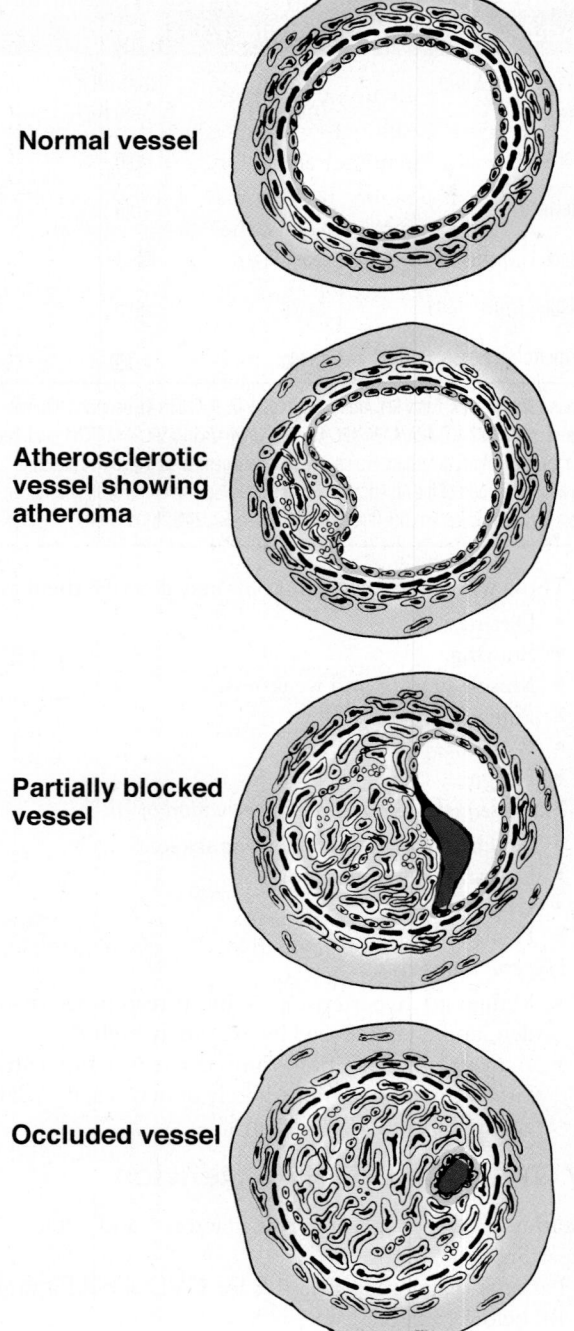

Normal vessel

Atherosclerotic vessel showing atheroma

Partially blocked vessel

Occluded vessel

FIGURE 61-4 • Atherosclerosis. An atheroma develops within the lining of the normal blood vessel. The atheroma is made of a fatty deposit containing cholesterol. At first, the atheroma is small, and no symptoms are apparent, but eventually, it enlarges and completely blocks the vessel, thus depriving the area served by the vessel of oxygen. (Source: National Institute of Health. *Report of the Working Group on Arteriosclerosis of the National Heart, Lung, and Blood Institute, National Institutes of Health, United States Department of Health and Human Services.* Bethesda, MD: National Institute of Health; 1981. NIH Publication No. 81-2034.)

ANGINA PECTORIS

◆ Angina pectoris is chest pain, the most common symptom of coronary atherosclerotic heart disease, and is caused by a reduction of blood flow to the heart.

◆ The pain is described as a heavy, squeezing pressure or tightness in the mid-chest region.

◆ The pain may radiate to the arms, neck, shoulder, or the mandible. On rare occasions, the pain may be limited to one of these areas and not occur in the chest area at all.

◆ The patient may be pale and also experience faintness, sweating, difficulty in breathing, anxiety, or fear. The pain lasts 1–5 minutes if precipitating factors are eliminated.

I. Precipitating Factors

◆ *Stable angina* may be precipitated by exertion or exercise, emotion, or a heavy meal. In the dental office or clinic, a preventive atmosphere of calmness and quiet can do much to alleviate stress. Stable angina is predictable and consistent in frequency, intensity, and duration.[15]

◆ *Unstable angina* occurs without exertion or other precipitating factors. The pain may occur while the patient is at rest, and it may vary in intensity at each attack.[15]

II. Treatment

◆ A vasodilator, usually nitroglycerin, is administered sublingually (see Chapter 9).[15]

◆ Basic life support that includes supplemental oxygen is part of the treatment provided in a dental office or clinic.

◆ If the patient does not report relief from the nitroglycerin, the emergency medical system (911) should be implemented.

◆ Thoroughly document the events that occurred and assessment data collected in the patient's chart for future reference.

MYOCARDIAL INFARCTION

◆ Myocardial infarction is the most extreme manifestation of ischemic heart disease.

◆ Other names: heart attack, coronary occlusion, or coronary thrombosis.

◆ The infarction results from a sudden reduction or arrest of coronary blood flow.

◆ The most common artery associated with a myocardial infarction is the anterior descending branch of the left coronary artery and is also the most common site of advanced atherosclerosis.[16]

I. Etiology

◆ Immediate cause: a thrombosis blocking an artery already narrowed by atherosclerosis.

◆ The blockage creates an infarct, leading to tissue necrosis.

◆ Necrosis of the area can occur within a few hours.

◆ A few patients die immediately or within a few hours. Sudden death may be caused by ventricular fibrillation.[16]

II. Symptoms

◆ *Pain*[16]

• Location: Pain symptoms may start under the sternum, with feelings of indigestion, or in the middle to upper sternum. Pain may last for extended periods, even hours.

• When the pain is severe, it gives a pressing or crushing heavy sensation and is not relieved by rest or nitroglycerin.

• Onset: The pain may have a sudden onset, sometimes during sleep or following exercise. The pain may be radial, similar to angina pectoris, which extends to the left or right arm, neck, and mandible.

◆ *Other symptoms*[16]

• Cold sweat, weakness and faintness, shortness of breath, nausea, and vomiting may occur.

• BP falls below baseline.

• Women do not always present with symptoms similar to men and may not experience chest pain; fainting, pain in the upper back and lower abdomen, and extreme fatigue are chief symptoms.[17]

III. Management during an Attack

◆ Review Chapter 9 for medical management of a heart attack.

◆ *Terminate treatment*

• Sit the patient up for comfortable breathing.

• Give nitroglycerin, and reassure the patient.

◆ *Summon medical assistance*

• Apply basic life support measures, if indicated, while waiting for medical assistance.

IV. Treatment after Acute Symptoms

◆ *Medical supervision*[18]

• Current medical care for heart attack calls for a shortened rest period with increased activity, in keeping with the strength and progress of the patient.

• Most patients experience extreme fatigue during their convalescence.

◆ *Lifestyle changes*[18]

• Cardiac rehabilitation in a medically supervised program is required to learn about the lifestyle changes needed, which include supervised exercise training and education on heart healthy choices, including diet, quitting use of tobacco, and management of stress.

◆ *Subsequent appointments*

• Consultation with the cardiologist is needed to determine when the patient can have elective dental treatment. Elective dental treatment may need to be postponed for at least 6 months following a heart attack.[19] This is in part due to the greatest mortality rate being in the first 6 months after a myocardial infarction.[19]

HEART FAILURE

Heart failure, often referred to as congestive heart failure (CHF), is a syndrome in which an abnormality of cardiac function is responsible for the inability or failure of the heart to pump blood at a rate necessary to meet the oxygen needs of the body tissues.[20]

I. Etiology

- CHF is a chronic, progressive condition resulting from many forms of CVDs and can be related to a number of other systemic conditions including[20,21]:
  - CHD.
  - Myocardial infarction (heart attack).
  - Hypertension.
  - Diabetes.
  - Arrhythmias.
  - Congenital heart disease.
  - Thyroid disorders.
  - Sleep apnea.
  - Alcohol or illegal drug use such as cocaine.
  - HIV/AIDS.

II. Clinical Manifestations

- The clinical manifestations coincide with the parts of the heart involved.
- Signs and symptoms are different, depending, in general, on whether the left or the right side of the heart or both are affected. The most common symptoms include[20,21]:
  - Fatigue or feeling lightheaded.
  - Shortness of breath or trouble breathing.
  - Chronic coughing or wheezing.
  - Swelling or edema of legs, ankles, abdomen, and veins in the neck.
  - Confusion or impaired thinking.
  - Nausea or lack of appetite.
  - High heart rate.

A. Left Heart Failure

- The left side of the heart receives oxygenated blood from the lungs and pumps the blood into the aorta to the rest of the body. The left ventricle is larger because it supplies most of the heart's pumping power.[21]
  - Left-sided heart failure is a pathologic condition of the left ventricle, resulting in failure to properly pump oxygen-rich blood to the body.[21]
- Clinical symptoms are more prominent at night. The patient rests better in a sitting or semi-upright sitting position with more than one pillow.[20]

- Signs and symptoms of left heart failure include the following:
  - Weakness, fatigue.
  - Dyspnea, particularly evident on exertion. Shortness of breath when lying supine, relieved when sitting up.
  - Cough and expectoration.
  - Nocturia.
  - Pallor; sweating, cold skin.
  - Diastolic BP increased.
  - Heart rate rapid.
  - Anxiety, fear.

B. Right Heart Failure

- The right heart receives the venous blood from the vena cava and pumps it to the lungs for oxygenation.[20]
- Right-sided heart failure usually occurs as a result of left-sided heart failure.[21]
  - Loss of pumping power by the left ventricle results in blood (fluid) backing up into the lungs and eventually damages the right ventricle.
- Signs and symptoms of right heart failure include the following[21]:
  - Weakness, fatigue.
  - Swelling of the feet and/or ankles. The edema progresses to the thighs and abdomen (ascites) in advanced stages of heart failure.
  - Cold hands and feet.
  - Clubbing of fingers.
  - Cyanosis of mucous membranes and nail beds.
  - Prominent jugular veins.
  - Congestion with edema in various organs: enlarged spleen and liver. gastrointestinal distress with nausea and vomiting. and central nervous system involvement with headache and irritability.
  - Anxiety, fear.

III. Treatment during Chronic Stages

A patient with an appointment in a dental office or clinic may be receiving a variety of medical treatments. These are revealed by questioning during preparation of histories and consultation with the cardiologist of primary care provider is recommended. Heart failure patients may be using one or more of the following approaches to treatment[20,21]:

- *Drug therapy*
  - ACE inhibitors, such as Lisinopril (Prinivil) or Enalapril (Vasotec).
  - Angiotensin receptor blockers, such as Losartan (Cozaar) or Valsartan (Diovan).
  - Beta-blockers, such as metoprolol (Toprol).
  - Digoxin.
  - Diuretics, such as furosemide (Lasix).
  - Aldosterone antagonists such as, spironolactone (Aldactone).
- *Lifestyle modifications*

- Achieve or maintain a healthy weight.
- Track fluid intake.
- Limit sodium intake.
- Make healthy diet choices.
- Tobacco cessation.
- Manage stress.
- Monitor BP.
- Adequate sleep.
- Physical activity under medical supervision.
- ◆ *Surgery may be indicated and include one of the following:*
  - Pacemaker.
  - Heart transplant.

IV. Emergency Care for Heart Failure and Acute Pulmonary Edema

A patient with heart failure or acute pulmonary edema is usually conscious at the time a cardiac medical emergency occurs. See Chapter 9 for emergency procedures to follow.

CARDIAC ARRHYTHMIAS

The contractions of the heart are controlled by a complex electronic circuitry system. Impulses within this system send messages to the heart muscle, triggering contraction. The interruption of the conduction of the impulse, causing a delay or block, results in an abnormal heart rhythm or arrhythmia.[22]

I. Etiology

- ◆ Arrhythmias such as atrial fibrillation (AF) may result from a number of cause including[22,23]:
  - Heart failure or a heart attack may damage the heart muscle.
  - Age can increase the risk.
  - Congenital heart conditions.
  - Chemical agents, such as alcohol, cigarettes, cocaine, and other addictive substances.
  - Hypertension.
  - Diabetes.
  - Chronic obstructive pulmonary disease, such as emphysema and asthma.
  - Thyroid disorders.
  - Sleep apnea.

II. Symptoms

- ◆ A CA may be symptomatic or asymptomatic; patients with an asymptomatic CA may still be at risk for stroke.
- ◆ Symptoms of a CA may include the following[22,23]:
  - Heart palpitations.
  - Slow or irregular heartbeat.
  - Dizziness or lightheadedness.
  - Feeling faint/syncope.
  - Fatigue.
  - Dyspnea.
  - Sweating.

III. Treatment

- ◆ Most arrhythmias do not require treatment.[22]
- ◆ *Drug therapy for AF may include:*
  - Beta-blockers, such as atenolol and metoprolol.
  - Calcium channel blockers, such as diltiazem.
  - Digoxin.
  - Anticoagulants such as warfarin (Coumadin®) and antiplatelets may be used to reduce risk of blood clots and stroke prevention.
- ◆ *Lifestyle modifications*[24]
  - Consume a heart healthy diet, for example, the Dietary Approaches to Stop Hypertension (DASH) diet[25]:
    - High in vegetables, fruits, whole grains, low-fat dairy, lean poultry and fish, legumes, and nuts.
    - Limit sodium, added sugars, solid fats, and refined grains.
  - Maintain blood cholesterol and BP at normal levels.
  - Tobacco cessation.
  - Be physically active.
  - Achieve and maintain a healthy weight.
- ◆ *Medical procedures*[24]
  - Placement of a pacemaker, which is also called an implantable cardioverter defibrillator (ICD).
  - Catheter ablation (a thin tube is inserted in an arm or groin blood vessel and guided to the heart).
- ◆ *Surgery may be indicated.*

LIFESTYLE MANAGEMENT FOR THE PATIENT WITH CARDIOVASCULAR DISEASE

The recommendation for the following is appropriate for all patients with CVD[26]:

- ◆ *Education:* Education on lifestyle modifications reduces the risk of recurrence of cardiovascular events such as a heart attack.
- ◆ *Lifestyle modifications* from the American College of Cardiology and American Heart Association include (Box 61-1):
  - Consume a heart healthy diet, including fruits, vegetables, whole grains, low-fat dairy products, poultry, fish, legumes, and nuts. DASH diets and Mediterranean diet patterns are recommended.
  - Limit added sugars, saturated fat, trans fat, and red meats.
  - As previously noted in the second on CHF, some cardiac conditions may require monitoring of fluid intake.
  - For those with hypertension, consume no more than 2,400 mg of sodium.

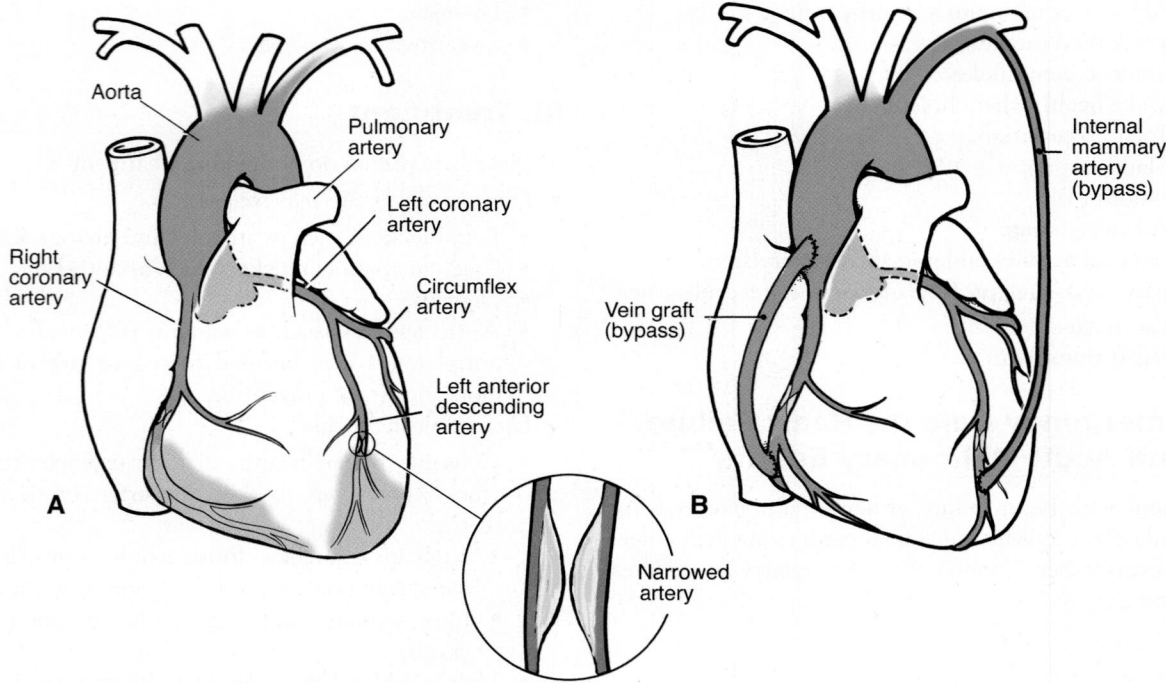

FIGURE 61-5 • Coronary Bypass Surgery. A: Heart showing infarcted (shaded) areas created by coronary arteries narrowed by atherosclerosis. **B:** Vein graft from saphenous vein connected with aorta to bypass narrowed area of right coronary artery, and internal mammary artery used to bypass narrowed left anterior descending artery.

- Engage in physical activity 3–4 times/week for an average of 40 minutes/session. NOTE: For patients with recent cardiac events, cardiac rehabilitation will aid the patient in increasing their stamina to engage in physical activity under supervision.

SURGICAL TREATMENT

I. Revascularization

Revascularization in CAD is done to improve survival and relieve symptoms and only recommended in more severe cases of stenosis.[27]

A. Percutaneous Coronary Intervention[27,28]

- ◆ Also known as coronary angioplasty, it is nonsurgical procedure to open the coronary arteries.
- ◆ A contrast dye is injected, and a catheter is inserted through either a wrist or groin blood vessel and guided to the blocked coronary blood vessel, where an inflatable balloon at the end of the catheter widens the narrowed lumen.
- ◆ A stent may be inserted into the artery to provide a semi-rigid scaffolding within the lumen, which helps prevent restenosis or re-narrowing of the lumen.
  - The stent may be impregnated with a drug to prevent return of the coronary blockage and called a drug-eluting stent.

B. Coronary Artery Bypass Grafting

- ◆ Coronary bypass is recommended in patients with more complex multivessel CAD and those with CAD and diabetes.[27]
- ◆ A healthy artery or vein is grafted to go around or bypass the blocked portion of an artery.
- ◆ The beneficial effects are reduced mortality, relief from angina pain, less workload for the heart, and an increase in oxygen and blood supply to the myocardium.[27]
- ◆ Figure 61-5 shows the use of a saphenous vein graft and the internal mammary artery for bypasses.

II. Cardiac Resynchronization Therapy

For those with heart failure or an arrhythmia (irregular heartbeat), cardiac resynchronization therapy (CRT) may be indicated. CRT helps to improve the heart rhythm and involves surgically implanting a pacemaker or defibrillator.[29]

- ◆ Natural pacemaker function.
  - The natural pacemaker, or center where the normal heartbeat is initiated, is the sinoatrial node located in the right atrium.
  - From that node, impulses are sent along the muscle walls to stimulate and regulate the contractions of the ventricles, which pump the blood throughout the body.

- When the natural pacemaker cells are not able to maintain a reliable rhythm, or when the impulses are interrupted because of heart block, cardiac arrest, various arrhythmias, or other disease conditions, treatment by a cardiologist may include the placement of an artificial pacemaker.

A. Cardiac Pacemaker

- Cardiac pacemaker purpose[29]
  - A cardiac pacemaker is an electronic stimulator used to send a specified electrical current to the myocardium to monitor heart rate irregularities, and tiny electrical pulses are emitted to correct the heart rate.
  - The pulse generator is a half dollar size device implanted under the skin just below the collarbone. The area selected depends on the individual condition as determined by the cardiologist (Figure 61-6).

B. Implantable Cardioverter Defibrillator

- An ICD is indicated to prevent sudden cardiac death.[30,31]
  - Those with pacemaker were at 64% higher risk of all-cause death than those with an ICD in a recent systematic review and meta-analysis.[31] This suggests the benefit of an ICD over a pacemaker in individuals needing CRT.
- An ICD is a battery-powered pulse generator about the size of a pocket watch surgically placed in the chest or abdomen, often just below the collarbone.[29]
- The ICD may be single (defibrillator only) or dual chamber (pacemaker and defibrillator).[29]
  - A dual-chamber ICD can detect when the heartbeat is too slow and deliver an electric signal to the heart as well as deliver defibrillation shocks for abnormal rhythm to normalize it.

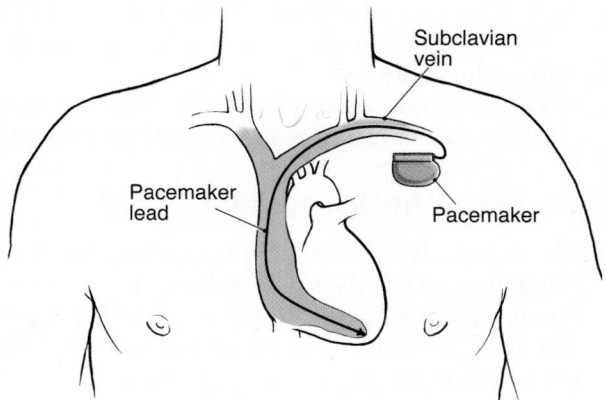

FIGURE 61-6 • Cardiac Pacemaker. The pulse generator is implanted under the skin in the thorax or upper abdomen. The lead electrodes may go to the ventricle or to the atrium or both to provide the necessary stimulus for regulation of the heartbeat.

C. Devices That May Interfere with CRT Devices

- Devices emitting electromagnetic waves may impact the function of pacemaker or ICD devices.
- Use of ultrasonic and piezo power scalers for patients with pacemakers and ICDs has previously been discouraged due to concerns regarding electromagnetic interference and its disruption to pacemakers and ICDs.
- The American Heart Association lists ultrasonic scalers, cleaners, pulp testers, electrosurgery devices, lasers, and drills as posing minimal risk if precautions are taken in relation to the proper use and distance from the CRT device.[32,33] However, the dental literature remains inconsistent.
  - Ultrasonic scalers may cause minor electromagnetic interference, but not impact the defibrillator pacing or sensing functions when used less than 15–18 inches from the IED.[34,35]
  - In vivo research found little or no risk from electric toothbrushes, pulp testers, or pulp testers.[33]
  - Risk for interference also varied by the type and model of CRT device with newer shielded devices finding less interference.[36]
- The American Dental Association (ADA) recommends patients with pacemakers or ICDs inform their health care providers about the presence of their device and a consultation with the cardiologist who placed the device to determine whether ultrasonic devices can be used safely.[33]
  - If it is determined that ultrasonic equipment can be used, the ADA recommends they not be waved over the implant area and that the equipment should be turned off when not in use.

D. Prophylactic Antibiotic Premedication

- The American Heart Association issued a statement that there is no scientific evidence for the use of antibiotic prophylaxis for those with cardiac implantable electronic devices.[37]
- Although evidence suggests the patient with a pacemaker is at low risk for endocarditis, consult with the cardiologist to verify whether they choose to use prophylactic antibiotics for dental and dental hygiene procedures.

III. Dental Considerations

Patients in dental offices and clinics who have had or will have cardiac surgery such as coronary artery bypass grafting or heart transplantation need to have their oral health evaluated and managed prior to surgery.

IV. Presurgical Dental Care

- Before elective cardiac surgery, the patient should have a comprehensive dental and periodontal examination.

- All active disease should be treated to resolve any sources of acute or chronic infection, and any nonrestorable teeth should be removed.
- Elimination of potential sources of infection is essential to minimize the risk for IE postsurgery.

V. Postsurgical Dental Care

- Adherence to a regular preventive maintenance program to manage dental biofilm and maintain optimal oral health is essential to minimize risk for oral infections.

A. Prophylactic Antibiotic

- Use of antibiotic prophylaxis is limited to those at highest risk for IE to minimize the risk for development of antibiotic resistance.
- The American Heart Association guidelines for antibiotic prophylaxis were discussed earlier in this chapter.
- Patients with implanted vascular *autografts* generally do not need antibiotic premedication before dental and dental hygiene appointments. An example of an implanted vascular autograft is the use of a patient's own blood vessel to provide a coronary bypass (Figure 61-5).

ANTITHROMBOTIC THERAPY

Antithrombotic therapy prevents embolus or thrombus formation and may include antiplatelet or anticoagulant drugs.

I. Anticoagulant Therapy

- Anticoagulants are used to prevent occurrence or recurrence of blood clots or thrombus and causing a myocardial infarction or stroke.
- *Common anticoagulant drugs*[38]
  - Heparin (hospital-administered intravenously).
    - Heparin inhibits several clotting factors.
  - Vitamin K antagonists include coumarin derivatives such as warfarin.
    - Warfarin (Coumadin®) blocks the vitamin K–dependent clotting pathway.
    - The most significant adverse event related to warfarin is excessive bleeding or hemorrhage.
- *Indications for use*[39]
  - Traditionally, warfarin has been used for long-term anticoagulation, but with the advent of new medications, current guidelines have changed.[38]
    - Guidelines recommend use of warfarin with aspirin for the first 3 months after a myocardial infarction or for someone at high risk for thrombus.
    - Recommendations are to then transition to dual-antiplatelet therapy for 12 months followed by a single antiplatelet.
- *Monitoring of anticoagulant therapy*
  - The international normalized ratio (INR) is used to monitor therapy with anticoagulants with a target therapeutic range of between 2.0 and 3.0.[39]

- The prothrombin time may also be used.
- The partial thromboplastin time may be used to monitor heparin treatment and results with the therapeutic range of 60–70 seconds.

A. Dental Management of Patients Taking Anticoagulants

- Medical history and medication review.
- Consultation with cardiologist and/or primary care provider regarding bleeding risk during dental/dental hygiene procedures.
  - Obtain the most current INR.
  - For a surgical or invasive procedure, the INR may need to be done 24 hours prior to the appointment.
- Discontinuation of anticoagulant therapy is *not* generally recommended for dental procedures.[40,41]
- Treatment should begin with oral self-care education to ensure adequate biofilm removal to minimize bleeding.
- Local anesthetic with a vasoconstrictor for infiltration is recommended, if there are no contraindications to use of a vasoconstrictor, to minimize bleeding. Use of nerve blocks should be minimized to avoid hemorrhage.[42]
- Following nonsurgical periodontal therapy (NSPT), local hemostasis may include[42]:
  - Minimize tissue trauma.
  - Apply pressure with gauze or sponges against the bleeding area or pack interdentally until bleeding is controlled. If the bleeding is not controlled, the dentist may use a hemostatic dressing like Gelfoam®.
  - Do *not* dismiss the patient until bleeding has stopped.
- Postprocedural instructions may include the following[42]:
  - Contact the patient the evening after the procedures to follow up.
  - Avoid rinsing for 24 hours.
  - Advise to avoid vigorous toothbrushing for several hours or until the next day.
  - Provide the patient with extra gauze or sponges to use to apply pressure should bleeding resume.
  - Avoid hot liquid and hard foods for the rest of the day. A soft diet may be suggested, but typically, this is not necessary for NSPT.
  - Provide contact information for the dentist or emergency contact if there is excessive or prolonged bleeding.

Direct Oral Anticoagulants

- The newest classification of anticoagulants are direct oral anticoagulants (DOACs) and have more targeted action and less risk of life-threatening bleeding events than the older anticoagulant drugs like warfarin.[43] The mechanism of action varies for each drug.
- *Common DOAC drugs*[41,43]
  - Dabigatran (Pradaxa®).
  - Rivaroxaban (Xarelto®).
  - Apixaban (Eliquis®).
  - Edoxaban (Savaysa®, Lixiana®).

◆ *Indications for use*[43]
- Prevention of venous thromboembolism.
- Prevention of stroke in patient with AF.

◆ *Monitoring of DOAC therapy*
- Routine monitoring is not required.
- At this time, an ideal test for measuring DOAC is not widely available, and no established therapeutic ranges have been identified for these drugs.[44]

A. Dental Management of Patients Taking Direct Oral Anticoagulants

◆ Medical history and medication review.

◆ Consultation with cardiologist and/or primary care provider regarding bleeding risk during dental/dental hygiene procedures.

◆ Discontinuation of DOAC therapy is *not* generally recommended for dental procedures.[41]

◆ Treatment should begin with oral self-care education to ensure adequate biofilm removal to minimize bleeding.

◆ Local measures to manage bleeding and maintain homeostasis may include local anesthesia with a vasoconstrictor for infiltration, minimize tissue trauma, apply pressure to control bleeding, and monitor patient prior to dismissing.

Antiplatelet Therapy

◆ Antiplatelet medications impact aggregation of platelets, which affects the ability for the blood to clot.

◆ Antiplatelet drugs may be used in combination such as aspirin and clopidogrel.[39]

◆ *Common antiplatelet drugs*
- Aspirin is used for those at risk to prevent cardiovascular events as well as in dual-antiplatelet therapy.
- Clopidogrel (Plavix®).
- Ticlopidine (Ticlid®).
- Ticagrelor (Brilinta®).

◆ *Indications for use*[39]
- Established CAD.
- Coronary stenosis.
- Evidence of cardiac ischemia.

◆ *Monitoring of antiplatelet therapy*
- Platelet function testing is used to evaluate the effectiveness of antiplatelet therapy, but there are no recommendations to assess this prior to most routine dental treatment.[45,46]

A. Dental Management of Patients Taking Antiplatelet Therapy

◆ Medical history and medication review.

◆ Consultation with cardiologist and/or primary care provider regarding bleeding risk during dental/dental hygiene procedures may be indicated in a patient taking multiple antiplatelet medications and/or with complex medical conditions.

◆ Discontinuation of antiplatelet therapy is *not* generally recommended for dental procedures.[41,42,47,48]

◆ Education to attain optimal oral self-care to ensure adequate biofilm removal to minimize bleeding is an important part of the treatment plan.

◆ Local measures to manage hemostasis should be implemented as previously noted for anticoagulants and DOACs.

DOCUMENTATION

Documentation for a routine dental hygiene continuing care or periodontal maintenance appointment for a patient with a cardiovascular illness would need to include a minimum of the following items:

◆ Note and record the responses to health history review questions about visitations to the cardiologist, the patient's reported state of health, and physician updates that could influence dental procedures.

◆ Record all findings and compare to previous assessment outcomes regarding vital signs, extraoral and intraoral examination, and gingival and periodontal clinical examinations.

◆ An example documentation note may be reviewed in Box 61-2.

BOX 61-2
Example Documentation: Patient with Uncontrolled Hypertension

S—A 46-year-old African American patient arrives in the dental office for a 3-month periodontal continuing care appointment. He reports he has been diagnosed with high blood pressure (BP) and is taking Procardia.

O—Vital signs: blood pressure: 180/100. Patient reports he cannot afford his medication so he takes it every other day. Contact his cardiologist and/or primary care provider to ensure it is safe to proceed with treatment. The providers give permission, but recommend no vasoconstrictor in the local anesthetic until the BP is under control.

A—A comprehensive periodontal and caries examination findings include localized Stage II, Grade B periodontitis with bleeding on probing in molar areas along with recurrent caries MO-#14, MO-#15.

P—Oral self-care is reviewed with a focus on use of an interdental brush in posterior interproximal areas. Periodontal maintenance is completed, except for in the area of #14–15 where localized nonsurgical periodontal therapy (NSPT) with local anesthesia is recommended. Patient to follow up with his primary care provider and return for localized NSPT once BP is controlled. Office will follow up in 2 weeks.

Signed: _____, RDH

Date: _____

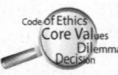

EVERYDAY ETHICS

Leo is a 68-year-old, black male with a history of hypertension obesity, and high cholesterol. He reminds Kerstin, the dental hygienist, that he has an extreme dental anxiety as he grasps very tightly to the armrests of the dental chair.

During the medical history review, Leo admits he usually remembers to take his BP medications, but since he has not been feeling well after taking his cholesterol-lowering medication, he has not been taking it regularly. Kerstin takes his BP using his right arm and obtains a reading of 165/90 mm Hg. Kerstin observes Leo rubbing his left arm, and when she asks him how he is feeling, Leo says he is experiencing heartburn as a result of a spicy food consumed the previous night. He also reports soreness in his left arm, which he believes is the result of yard work performed a couple of days ago.

Questions for Consideration

1. What medical, legal, and ethical questions should be taken into account with a patient like Leo who presents with a complicated medical history, multiple medications, his current symptoms, and dental anxiety?

2. Which of the dental hygiene core values should be considered when dealing with this scenario? How do these core values guide Kerstin's planned treatment for this patient?

3. Using the legal and ethical guidelines, prepare at least three possible responses and actions Kerstin should consider as she makes decisions for her patient regarding his planned care.

Factors to Teach the Patient

► Encourage patients to continue their prescribed medications.

► Assess level of dental anxiety using an assessment tool such as the Modified Dental Anxiety Scale to help the patient identify the things that create anxiety and develop a plan for management. Establishing rapport and building trust is an important part of managing dental anxiety.

► Good communication about treatment options and what the patient can expect can help to minimize anxiety.

► If dental anxiety is moderate to high, the following are suggested as part of a stress reduction protocol:

• Select an optimum appointment time for the patient with respect to the time of the day that might work best for the patient. Note: Most anxious patients prefer a morning appointment.

• Encourage patient to get adequate sleep and rest.

• Eat meals and snacks on usual schedule, and take medications as directed.

• If a sedative is prescribed, the patient should follow the directions carefully and will require someone to drive them to and from the appointment.

• Allow time to get to the dental office or clinic so they do not feel rushed.

• Suggest bringing their own headphones and a portable device to listen to music while waiting for and during the appointment. Some offices have headphones, media such as movies, and so on that the patient can use as an audiovisual distraction.

• Nitrous oxide may also be a part of stress reduction.

• Ensure patient knows how to signal the dental clinician in the case of a problem.

ENHANCE YOUR UNDERSTANDING

ONLINE RESOURCES
(see the inside front cover for access information)

• Audio glossary
• Appendices

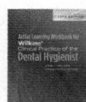

SUPPORT FOR LEARNING
(available separately)

• *Active Learning Workbook for Wilkins' Clinical Practice of the Dental Hygienist, 13th Edition*

INDIVIDUALIZED REVIEW

• Customized practice quizzing with Navigate 2 TestPrep for *Wilkins' Clinical Practice of the Dental Hygienist*

References

1. Humphrey L, Fu R, Buckley D, et al. Periodontal disease and coronary heart disease incidence: a systematic review and meta-analysis. *J Gen Intern Med.* 2008;23(12):2079-2086.

2. Wilson W, Taubert KA, Gewitz M, et al. Prevention of infective endocarditis: guidelines from the American Heart Association Rheumatic Fever, Endocarditis, and Kawasaki Disease Committee, Council on Cardiovascular Disease in the Young, and the Council on Clinical Cardiology, Council on Cardiovascular Surgery and Anesthesia, and the Quality of Care and Outcomes Research Interdisciplinary Working Group. *Circulation.* 2007. http://circ.ahajournals.org/content/116/15/1736.full. Accessed August 2013.

3. Nishimura RA, Otto CM, Bonow RO, et al. 2017 AHA/ACC focused update of the 2014 AHA/ACC guideline for the management of patients with valvular heart disease: a Report of the American College of Cardiology/American Heart Association Task Force on clinical practice guidelines. *J Am Coll Cardiol.* 2017;70(2):252-289.

4. Glenny AM, Oliver R, Roberts GJ, et al. Antibiotics for the prophylaxis of bacterial endocarditis in dentistry. *Cochrane Database Syst Rev.* 2013;10:CD003813.

5. National Institutes of Health; National Heart, Lung and Blood Institute. *Congenital Heart Defects.* https://www.nhlbi.nih.gov/health-topics/congenital-heart-defects. Accessed May 24, 2018.

6. Centers for Disease Control and Prevention. *Facts about Congenital Heart Defects.* http://www.cdc.gov/ncbddd/heartdefects/facts.html. Updated March 12, 2018. Accessed May 24, 2018.

7. National Institutes of Health, National Library of Medicine, Medline Plus. *Rheumatic Fever.* http://www.nlm.nih.gov/medlineplus/ency/article/003940.htm. Updated April 30, 2018. Accessed May 29, 2018.

8. National Institutes of Health, U.S. National Library of Medicine: MedlinePlus. *Mitral Valve Prolapse.* http://www.nhlbi.nih.gov/health/health-topics/topics/mvp/. Updated April 23, 2018. Accessed May 29, 2018.

9. American Heart Association. *Problem: Mitral Valve Prolapse.* http://www.heart.org/HEARTORG/Conditions/More/HeartValveProblemsandDisease/Problem-Mitral-Valve-Prolapse_UCM_450441. Updated May 2016. Accessed May 29, 2018.

10. Whelton PK, Carey RM, Aronow WS, et al. 2017 ACC/AHA/AAPA/ABC/ACPM/AGS/APhA/ASH/ASPC/NMA/PCNA guideline for the prevention, detection, evaluation, and management of high blood pressure in adults: a Report of the American College of Cardiology/American Heart Association Task Force on Clinical Practice Guidelines. *Hypertension.* 2018;71(6):e13-e115.

11. Cifu AS, Davis AM. Prevention, detection, evaluation, and management of high blood pressure in adults. *JAMA.* 2017;318(21):2132-2134.

12. Flynn JT, Kaelber DC, Baker-Smith CM, et al. Clinical practice guideline for screening and management of high blood pressure in children and adolescents. *Pediatrics.* 2017;140(3):pii: e20171904.

13. National Institutes of Health, National Heart, Lung, and Blood Institute. *Atherosclerosis.* https://www.nhlbi.nih.gov/health-topics/atherosclerosis. Accessed May 29, 2018.

14. Lockhart PB, Bolger AF, Papapanou PN, et al. Periodontal disease and atherosclerotic vascular disease: does the evidence support an independent association?: a scientific statement from the American Heart Association. *Circulation.* 2012;125(20):2520-2544.

15. American Heart Association. *Angina Pectoris.* http://www.heart.org/HEARTORG/Conditions/HeartAttack/SymptomsDiagnosisofHeartAttack/Angina-Pectoris-Chest-Pain_UCM_437515_Article.jsp. Updated August 21, 2017. Accessed May 29, 2018.

16. National Institutes of Health, National Library of Medicine, Medline Plus. *Heart Attack.* https://www.nlm.nih.gov/medlineplus/ency/article/000195.htm. Updated April 30, 2018. Accessed May 29, 2018.

17. American Heart Association. *Heart Attack Symptoms in Women.* http://www.heart.org/HEARTORG/Conditions/HeartAttack/WarningSignsofaHeartAttack/Heart-Attack-Symptoms-in-Women_UCM_436448_Article.jsp. Updated July 2015. Accessed May 29, 2018.

18. American Heart Association. *Prevention and Treatment of Heart Attack.* http://www.heart.org/HEARTORG/Conditions/HeartAttack/PreventionTreatmentofHeartAttack/Prevention-and-Treatment-of-Heart-Attack_UCM_002042_Article.jsp. Updated March 2017. Accessed May 29, 2018.

19. Rose LF, Mealey B, Minsk L, Cohen DW. Oral care for patients with cardiovascular disease and stroke. *J Am Dent Assoc.* 2002;133(suppl):37S-44S.

20. National Institutes of Health, National Heart, Lung, and Blood Institute. *Heart Failure.* http://www.nhlbi.nih.gov/health/health-topics/topics/hf/. Accessed May 29, 2018.

21. American Heart Association. *Types of Heart Failure.* http://www.heart.org/HEARTORG/Conditions/HeartFailure/Heart-Failure_UCM_002019_SubHomePage.jsp. Updated May 2017. Accessed July 21, 2018.

22. National Institutes of Health, National Heart, Lung, and Blood Institute. *Arrhythmia.* https://www.nhlbi.nih.gov/health-topics/arrhythmia. Accessed July 22, 2018.

23. American Heart Association. Arrhythmia. http://www.heart.org/HEARTORG/Conditions/Arrhythmia/Arrhythmia_UCM_002013_SubHomePage.jsp. Updated September 2016. Accessed May 29, 2018.

24. NIH, NHLBI. *Arrhythmia.* https://www.nhlbi.nih.gov/health-topics/arrhythmia. Accessed August 3, 2018.

25. National Institutes of Health, National Heart, Lung, and Blood Institute. *What Is the DASH Eating Plan?* http://www.nhlbi.nih.gov/health/health-topics/topics/dash/. Accessed May 29, 2018.

26. Eckel RH, Jakicic JM, Ard JD, et al. 2013 AHA/ACC guideline on lifestyle management to reduce cardiovascular risk: a report of the American College of Cardiology/American Heart Association Task Force on Practice Guidelines. *Circulation.* 2014;129(25, suppl 2):S76-S99.

27. Fihn SD, Blankenship JC, Alexander KP, et al. 2014 ACC/AHA/AATS/PCNA/SCAI/STS focused update of the guideline for the diagnosis and management of patients with stable ischemic heart disease: a report of the American College of Cardiology/American Heart Association Task Force on Practice Guidelines, and the American Association for Thoracic Surgery, Preventive Cardiovascular Nurses Association, Society for Cardiovascular Angiography and Interventions, and Society of Thoracic Surgeons. *J Am Coll Cardiol.* 2014;64(18):1929-1949.

28. National Institute of Health, National Heart, Lung, and Blood Institute. *Percutaneous Coronary Intervention: Overview.* https://www.nhlbi.nih.gov/health-topics/percutaneous-coronary-intervention. Accessed August 18, 2018.

29. National Institutes of Health, National Heart, Lung and Blood Institute. *Cardiac Resynchronization Therapy (CRT).* http://www.heart.org/HEARTORG/Conditions/HeartFailure/Cardiac-Resynchronization-Therapy_UCM_452920_Article.jsp#.W3h_1Gct1jY. Accessed August 18, 2018.

30. Russo AM, Stainback RF, Bailey SR, et al. ACCF/HRS/AHA/ASE/HFSA/SCAI/SCCT/SCMR 2013 appropriate use criteria for implantable cardioverter-defibrillators and cardiac resynchronization therapy: a report of the American College of Cardiology Foundation appropriate use criteria task force, Heart Rhythm Society, American Heart Association, American Society of Echocardiography,

Heart Failure Society of America, Society for Cardiovascular Angiography and Interventions, Society of Cardiovascular Computed Tomography, and Society for Cardiovascular Magnetic Resonance. *J Am Coll Cardiol.* 2013;61(12):1318-1368.

31. Barra S, Providência R, Tang A, Heck P, Virdee M, Agarwal S. Importance of implantable cardioverter-defibrillator back up in cardiac resynchronization therapy recipients: a systematic review and meta-analysis. *J Am Heart Assoc.* 2015;4(11):e002539.

32. American Heart Association. *Devices that May Interfere with ICDs and Pacemakers.* September 30, 2016. https://www.heart.org/en/health-topics/arrhythmia/prevention-treatment-of-arrhythmia/devices-that-may-interfere-with-icds-and-pacemakers. Accessed August 19, 2018.

33. American Dental Association, Center for Scientific Information, ADA Science Institute. *Oral Health Topics: Cardiac Implanted Devices and Electronic Dental Instruments.* October 13, 2017. https://www.ada.org/en/member-center/oral-health-topics/cardiac-implanted-devices-and-electronic-dental-instruments. Accessed August 19, 2018.

34. Elayi CS, Lusher S, Meeks Nyquist JL, et al. Interference between dental electrical devices and pacemakers or defibrillators: results from a prospective clinical study. *J Am Dent Assoc.* 2015;146(2):121-128.

35. Lahor-Soler E, Miranda-Rius J, Brunet-Llobet L, Sabaté de la Cruz X. Capacity of dental equipment to interfere with cardiac implantable electrical devices. *Eur J Oral Sci.* 2015;123(3):194-201.

36. Miranda-Rius J, Lahor-Soler E, Brunet-Llobet L, Sabaté de la Cruz X. Risk of electromagnetic interference induced by dental equipment on cardiac implantable electrical devices. *Eur J Oral Sci.* 2016;124(6):559-565.

37. Baddour LM, Epstein AE, Erickson CC, et al.; American Heart Association Rheumatic Fever, Endocarditis, and Kawasaki Disease Committee of the Council on Cardiovascular Disease in the Young; Council on Cardiovascular Surgery and Anesthesia; Council on Cardiovascular Nursing; Council on Clinical Cardiology; Interdisciplinary Council on Quality of Care and Outcomes Research. A summary of the update on cardiovascular implantable electronic device infections and their management: a scientific statement from the American Heart Association. *J Am Dent Assoc.* 2011;142(2):159-165.

38. Harter K, Levine M, Henderson SO. Anticoagulation drug therapy: a review. *Western J Emer Med.* 2015;16(1):11-17.

39. Vandvik PO, Lincoff AM, Gore JM, et al. Primary and secondary prevention of cardiovascular disease: antithrombotic therapy and prevention of thrombosis, 9th ed: American College of Chest Physicians Evidence-Based Clinical Practice Guidelines. *Chest.* 2012;141(2 suppl):e637S-e668S.

40. Nematullah A, Alabousi A, Blanas N, Douketis JD, Sutherland SE. Dental surgery for patients on anticoagulant therapy with warfarin: a systematic review and meta-analysis. *J Can Dent Assoc.* 2009;75(1):41.

41. American Dental Association, Center for Scientific Information, ADA Science Institute. *Anticoagulant and Antiplatelet Medications and Dental Procedures.* March 15, 2018. https://www.ada.org/en/member-center/oral-health-topics/anticoagulant-antiplatelet-medications-and-dental-. Accessed August 25, 2018.

42. United Kingdom National Health Service. Surgical Management of the Primary Care Dental Patient on Antiplatelet Medication. National Electronic Library of Medicines: 2007. http://www.app.dundee.ac.uk/tuith/Static/info/antiplatelet.pdf. Accessed August 25, 2018.

43. Levy JH, Spyropoulos AC, Samama CM, Douketis J. Direct oral anticoagulants: new drugs and new concepts. *JACC Cardiovasc Interv.* 2014;7(12):1333-1351.

44. Samuelson BT, Cuker A, Siegal DM, Crowther M, Garcia DA. Laboratory assessment of the anticoagulant activity of direct oral anticoagulants: a systematic review. *Chest.* 2017;151(1):127-138.

45. Lordkipanidzé M, So D, Tanguay JF. Platelet function testing as a biomarker for efficacy of antiplatelet drugs. *Biomark Med.* 2016;10(8):903-918.

46. Zhou Y, Wang Y, Wu Y, et al. Individualized dual antiplatelet therapy based on platelet function testing in patients undergoing percutaneous coronary intervention: a meta-analysis of randomized controlled trials. *BMC Cardiovasc Disord.* 2017;17:157.

47. Napeñas JJ, Oost FC, DeGroot A, et al. Review of postoperative bleeding risk in dental patients on antiplatelet therapy. *Oral Surg Oral Med Oral Pathol Oral Radiol.* 2013;115(4):491-499.

48. van Diermen DE, van der Waal I, Hoogstraten J. Management recommendations for invasive dental treatment in patients using oral antithrombotic medication, including novel oral anticoagulants. *Oral Surg Oral Med Oral Pathol Oral Radiol.* 2013;116(6):709-716.

62

The Patient with a Blood Disorder

Lisa Welch, RDH, BS, MSDH

CHAPTER OUTLINE

NORMAL BLOOD
I. Composition
II. Origin of Blood Cells

PLASMA

RED BLOOD CELLS (ERYTHROCYTES)
I. Description
II. Functions
III. Hemoglobin

WHITE BLOOD CELLS (LEUKOCYTES)
I. Types of Leukocytes
II. Functions
III. Agranulocytes
IV. Granulocytes

PLATELETS (THROMBOCYTES)

ANEMIA
I. Classification by Cause
II. Clinical Characteristics of Anemia

IRON DEFICIENCY ANEMIA
I. Characteristics
II. Causes

III. Signs and Symptoms
IV. Therapy

MEGALOBLASTIC ANEMIA
I. Pernicious Anemia
II. Folate-Deficiency Anemia

SICKLE CELL DISEASE
I. Disease Process
II. Clinical Course
III. Treatment and Disease Management
IV. Oral Implications
V. Appointment Management

POLYCYTHEMIAS
I. Polycythemia Vera (Primary Polycythemia)
II. Secondary Polycythemia

DISORDERS OF WHITE BLOOD CELLS
I. Neutropenia
II. Lymphocytopenia
III. Leukocytosis

PLATELET DISORDERS
I. Thrombocytopenia (Decrease in Platelets)
II. Reactive Thrombocytosis (Overproduction of Platelets)
III. Platelet Dysfunction

BLEEDING OR COAGULATION DISORDERS
I. Oral Findings Suggestive of Bleeding Disorders
II. Disorders of Coagulation

DENTAL HYGIENE CARE PLAN
I. Preparation for Clinical Appointment
II. Patient History
III. Consultation with Physician/Hematologist
IV. Examination
V. Treatment Care Plan
VI. Treatment

DOCUMENTATION

EVERYDAY ETHICS

FACTORS TO TEACH THE PATIENT

REFERENCES

LEARNING OBJECTIVES

After studying this chapter, the student will be able to:

1. Describe the major types of blood disorders.

2. Explain the general and oral signs and symptoms of the major types of blood disorders.

3. Identify clinical implications of selected blood values including the INR (international normalized ratio), platelet count, and neutrophil count.

4. Provide examples of dental hygiene treatment modifications necessary for the patient with a blood disorder.

NORMAL BLOOD

Oral soft tissue changes, lowered resistance to infection, and bleeding tendencies are major factors to be considered for a patient with a blood disorder. Oral manifestations of blood disorders are generally exaggerated in the presence of dental biofilm and local predisposing factors.

I. Composition

- Blood is composed of 45% formed elements and 55% fluid termed plasma.[1]
- The 45% formed elements consist of[1]:
  - 44% erythrocytes (red blood cells or corpuscles).
  - 1% leukocytes (white blood cells) and platelets.
- Figure 62-1 shows cell forms and nuclei.
  - Hematocrit, a test commonly used in health examinations, indicates the amount of blood cells present in a sample of blood expressed as a percentage.
  - Reference values for blood cell counts are listed in Table 62-1 with examples of conditions in which increases and decreases in the normal values occur.

II. Origin of Blood Cells

- Adult blood cells originate in bone marrow.
- Hemocytoblasts are the stem cells of origin.
- Erythrocytes and granulocytes leave the bone marrow as mature cells and enter the circulating blood.
- Agranulocytes (lymphocytes and monocytes) leave the bone marrow as immature cells and migrate to the lymphoid tissues to mature.
- Certain blood diseases and cancers are characterized by the predominance of immature cells.

PLASMA

- Blood is a connective tissue: Thus, plasma has similar constituents to that of connective tissue fluid.
- Plasma is composed of 90% water.
- Plasma proteins make up the other 10% and include:
  - Albumin (functions to maintain tissue fluid balance within the vascular system).
  - Gamma globulins (circulating antibodies essential to the immune system).
  - Beta globulins (aid in transport of hormones, metallic ions, and lipids).

- Fibrinogen and prothrombin (essential for blood clotting).
- Inorganic salts include: sodium, potassium, calcium, bicarbonate, and chloride.
- Gases include: dissolved oxygen, carbon dioxide, and nitrogen.
- Substances being transported include: hormones, nutrients, waste products, and enzymes.
- If either plasma or whole blood is allowed to clot, the remaining fluid devoid of clotting factors is termed serum.

RED BLOOD CELLS (ERYTHROCYTES)

I. Description

- Red blood cells are more properly termed "corpuscles" because they have no nuclei (Figure 62-1).
- They are flexible biconcave discs containing hemoglobin, which can change shape as they pass through small capillaries.

II. Functions

- Transport hemoglobin, which facilitates the transport of oxygen to the cells in the form of oxyhemoglobin and waste carbon dioxide from the cells in the form of carbaminohemoglobin.

III. Hemoglobin

- Hemoglobin is the iron-containing protein in red blood cells.
- Measured in grams (g) per 100 milliliters (mL).
- Normal values range from 12 to 17.5 g/mL depending on gender (Table 62-1).[2]
- Values below normal reflect an anemic state; pathologic conditions may result when values increase above normal.

WHITE BLOOD CELLS (LEUKOCYTES)

I. Types of Leukocytes

- White blood cells are divided into two general groups, the granulocytes and the agranulocytes.

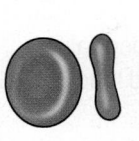 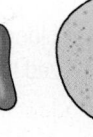 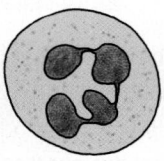 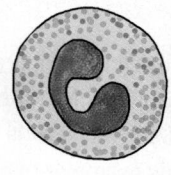 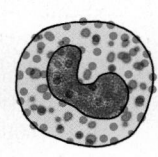 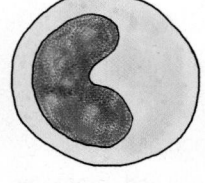 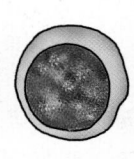 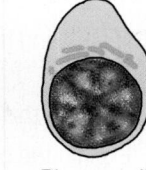

Erythrocytes   Neutrophil   Eosinophil   Basophil   Monocyte   Lymphocyte   Plasma cell

FIGURE 62-1 • Red and White Blood Cells. Diagram shows normal cell forms drawn to scale for comparison of cell size. Note the shape of nuclei in each of the white blood cells. The erythrocyte or red blood cell does not have a nucleus; its biconcave disc shape is shown in the lateral view second from the left.

TABLE 62-1 • Laboratory Values and Clinical Implications

TEST	NORMAL RANGE[a]	CLINICAL IMPLICATIONS	CAUSES OF DEVIATIONS
Prothrombin time (PT)	11–15 sec	Routine care can be performed when PT is <20 sec	Prolonged in: Prothrombin deficiency Anticoagulant therapy Vitamin K deficiency Liver diseases Aspirin use
International normalized ratio (INR)	<2.5	Routine care can be performed when INR 2–3, MD consult when INR >3.0	Prolonged in: Polycythemia vera Prothrombin deficiency Anticoagulant therapy Vitamin K deficiency Liver diseases Aspirin use
Activated partial thromboplastin time (aPTT)	25–35 sec	Routine care when aPTT is <1.5 × normal, MD consult when >57 sec	Prolonged in: Hemophilia and von Willebrand disease Anticoagulant therapy
Platelet count	140,000–400,000/mm³	Routine care can be provided when values are >50,000/mm³ MD consult needed when values <10,000/mm³—potentially life threatening	Thrombocytopenia: <20,000 mm³
Hemoglobin (g/dL)	Males: 13.6–17.2 g/100 mL Females: 12–15 g/100 mL	Delivers O_2 through circulation to body tissues and returns CO_2 from tissues to lungs	Increased in: Polycythemia Dehydration Decreased in: Anemias Hemorrhage Leukemias
Hematocrit (volume of packed red cells) (percentage)	Males: 39%–49% Females: 33%–43%	Indicates relative proportions of plasma and red blood cells	Increased in: Polycythemia Dehydration Decreased in: Anemias Hemorrhage Leukemias
Absolute neutrophil count (ANC)	Normal ANC: 2,500–6,000	Measure of the number of infection fighting white blood cells. Routine care 50,000/mm³; <500/mm³—potentially life threatening	Decreased in: Anemias Chemotherapy

[a]Ranges vary among health facilities and laboratories. The reference ranges of the facility providing the results are used in interpreting the test result.

◆ Granulocytes have granules in their cytoplasm, whereas the agranulocytes do not.

◆ They are further subdivided into the following categories:
  • Granulocytes: neutrophils, eosinophils, and basophils.
  • Agranulocytes: lymphocytes, monocytes.

II. Functions

◆ Phagocytic, immunologic, and other functions related to the inflammatory process in the connective tissue.

◆ Blood functions as a transport medium for the white cells as they pass to areas in the connective tissue where they are needed.

◆ They pass through the walls at the terminal ends of capillaries and into the connective tissue.

◆ Numbers and proportions in the blood maintain a constant level in health, as listed in Table 62-2.

◆ Differential cell count of the white blood cells is used in the detection and monitoring of disease states. Increases and decreases of each cell type can be associated with certain conditions.

TABLE 62-2 • Blood Cell Reference Values

An examination of a blood smear (or film) may be requested by a physician in response to abnormality in blood counts.

CELL TYPE	NORMAL VALUE	CAUSES OF INCREASE	CAUSES OF DECREASE
Red blood cells (erythrocytes)	Males: 4.3–5.9 million/mm^3 Females: 3.5–5.0 million/mm^3	Polycythemia dehydration	Anemias Leukemias Hemorrhage
Platelets (thrombocytes) (cell fragments essential for the process of blood clotting)	150,000–400,000/mm^3 Wintrobe method: 140,000–440,000/mm^3	Polycythemia vera Chronic myelocytic leukemia Sickle cell anemia Rheumatic fever Hemolytic anemias Bone fractures	Acute severe infections Cirrhosis of the liver Thrombocytopenic purpura Acute leukemias Aplastic anemias Pernicious anemia
White blood cells (leukocytes)	5,000–10,000/mm^3	Inflammation Overexertion Polycythemia vera Leukemia	Aplastic anemia Granulocytopenia Drug poisoning Thrombocytopenia Radiation Severe infections HIV/AIDS
Differential white cell count granulocytes • Neutrophils • Eosinophils • Basophils	60%–70% 1%–3% 1%	Acute infections Myelogenous leukemia Poisoning Erythroblastosis Allergic diseases Dermatitis Hodgkin disease Scarlet fever Certain chronic infections	Aplastic anemia Granulocytopenia Typhoid fever
Agranulocytes • Lymphocytes • Monocytes	20%–35% 2%–6%	Lymphocytic leukemia Chronic infections Viral diseases Monocytic leukemias Tuberculosis Infective endocarditis Hodgkin disease	Aplastic anemia Myelogenous leukemia Radiation

◆ A large number of cells will migrate into the area of an injury.

◆ Neutrophils arrive first and are active in the phagocytosis of foreign material and microorganisms.

III. Agranulocytes

◆ Lymphocytes
  • Small round cells with a large round nucleus surrounded with a narrow rim of cytoplasm (Figure 62-1).
  • Can move back and forth between the vessels and the extravascular tissues.
  • Capable of reverting to blast-like cells of origin and then multiplying as the immunologic need arises.

◆ Monocytes
  • Large cells with a bean-shaped or indented nucleus.
  • Actively phagocytic.
  • In connective tissue, monocytes differentiate into macrophages, which are important in immunologic processes.

IV. Granulocytes

◆ Neutrophils
  • Also called polymorphonuclear leukocytes.
  • Most numerous of all the white blood cells.
  • Nucleus has three to five lobes connected by thin chromatin threads.

- Cells are round in circulation.
- Amoeboid (move and change shape) in the tissues and function in phagocytosis.
- Part of the first line of defense of the body.

◆ Eosinophils
  - Two-lobed nucleus and larger, coarser granules than those of a neutrophil.
  - Microscopically, the cells stain a distinct bright pink; are readily recognized.
  - Few in number; increase during allergic conditions.

◆ Basophils
  - Nucleus has a "U" or "S" form.
  - Function is to increase vascular permeability during inflammation so phagocytic cells can pass into the area.

PLATELETS (THROMBOCYTES)

◆ Small round or oval formed element without a nucleus.

◆ Approximately one-fourth the size of a red blood cell.

◆ Active in blood clotting mechanism.

◆ Essential in the maintenance of the integrity of blood capillaries by repairing them at the time of injury.

◆ Participate in clot dissolution after healing.

ANEMIA

Anemia is the reduction in the number and/or the amount of hemoglobin present in red blood cells such that oxygen-carrying capacity of the blood is diminished.[3]

I. Classification by Cause

A. Caused by Blood Loss

◆ Acute: Blood loss from trauma or disease.

◆ Chronic: An internal lesion with constant slow bleeding, usually of gastrointestinal or gynecologic origin, can lead to a chronic loss of blood. Iron deficiency anemia can result.

B. Caused by Increased Hemolysis

Hemolysis means the destruction of red blood cells; also called hemolytic anemia because it is attributed to cell destruction.

◆ Hereditary hemolytic disorders
  - Sickle cell disease (SCD), which belongs to the group of hereditary disorders called hemoglobinopathies.

◆ Acquired hemolytic disorders
  - Drugs, infections, and certain physical and chemical agents may cause red cell destruction.
  - Erythroblastosis fetalis (hemolytic disease of the newborn), a form of antibody-mediated anemia that occurs when an expectant mother is Rh positive and the fetus is Rh negative.

C. Caused by Diminished Production of Red Blood Cells

◆ Nutritional deficiency
  - Inadequate intake of necessary nutrients for erythrocyte production.
  - Defective absorption from the gastrointestinal tract.
  - Examples: iron deficiency anemia, which may occur during pregnancy or during a growth spurt; celiac disease (sprue), which results from sensitivity to dietary gluten; and pernicious anemia, which results from a B_{12} vitamin absorption deficiency.
  - Increased demand for nutrients such as in growth or pregnancy.

◆ Bone marrow failure
  - Aplastic anemia (which can be inherited) can occur without apparent cause or when the bone marrow is injured by medications, radiation, chemotherapy, or infection.
  - In aplastic anemia, a combination of anemia, neutropenia (reduction in white blood cells), and thrombocytopenia (reduction in number of platelets) occurs, which leads to a quantitative decrease in all cells formed in the bone marrow.
  - Consult with physician to determine if antibiotic premedication would be indicated.

D. Anemia of Chronic Diseases[4]

◆ Second most prevalent anemia after iron deficiency anemia.

◆ Anemia is associated with many chronic systemic diseases.

E. Caused by Genetic Blood Disorders

◆ Thalassemia is a diverse group of genetic blood disorders characterized by defects in the synthesis of normal hemoglobin.[5]

◆ It typically affects people of Mediterranean, African, Middle Eastern, and Southeast Asian descent.

◆ The condition can range in severity from mild to life threatening.

◆ The most severe form is beta thalassemia major (Cooley anemia).

◆ Blood counts are evaluated and monitored for delayed wound healing.

◆ Treatment[5]
  - May require periodic and lifelong blood transfusions and chelation therapy.
  - Folic acid supplements.
  - Bone marrow transplant, hematopoietic (blood forming) stem cell transplantation, has the potential to cure thalassemia.
  - Novel treatments including gene therapy are under investigation.[5]

II. Clinical Characteristics of Anemia[3]

When a patient's medical history shows the presence of anemia, certain general signs and symptoms may be identified through additional questions or clinical observation including:

- Pale skin, nails, buccal mucosa.
- Weakness, malaise, easy fatigability.
- Dyspnea on slight exertion, faintness.
- Brittle nails with loss of convexity referred to as spooning of the nails.

IRON DEFICIENCY ANEMIA

I. Characteristics

Iron deficiency anemia is a hypochromic microcytic anemia, which means that:

- Hemoglobin content is deficient (hypochromic).
- Red blood cells are smaller than normal (microcytic).
- Occurs more in younger than older people and more in females than in males.
- Diagnosis is by laboratory test that shows low hemoglobin and a reduced hematocrit value.

II. Causes[6,7]

- Low intake
  - Malnutrition.
  - Vegans.
- Chronic infection.
- Decreased intestinal absorption.
  - Bariatric surgery (gastric bypass).
  - Celiac disease.
  - Inflammatory bowel diseases, for example, Crohn disease.
- Increased body demand for iron over and above the daily intake, for example, during pregnancy.
- Acute or chronic blood loss due to:
  - Excessive menstrual flow.
  - Frequent blood donations.
  - Bleeding disorders.
  - Major surgery.
  - Malignancy.
- Internal bleeding due to:
  - Gastrointestinal diseases, such as ulcer and colon or stomach cancer.
  - Drugs, notably aspirin.
  - Hemorrhoids.
  - Chronic alcoholism.

III. Signs and Symptoms

- General
  - General weakness, pallor.
  - Fatigue on slight exertion.

- Decreased immune function and increased risk for infection.
- Oral findings
  - Pallor of the mucosa and gingiva.
  - Tongue changes: atrophic glossitis with loss of filiform papillae. In moderate and severe anemia, the tongue may be smooth and shiny. The patient may have burning, painful sensations (glossodynia).
  - Secondary irritations to the thinned, atrophic mucosa may result from smoking, mechanical trauma, or hot, spicy foods.
  - Angular cheilitis.
  - Increased risk of candidiasis.

IV. Therapy

- Treatment of underlying cause to prevent further blood loss.
- Treated with oral ferrous iron tablets with vitamin C to aid absorption; to be taken on empty stomach for best absorption rates.
- Intravenous (IV) iron therapy may be indicated for certain patients.[6]
- Folic acid supplements may be indicated if there is an underlying folate deficiency.
- Nutritional counseling: recommend foods high in iron.
- Liquid preparations, which are sometimes used for children, may stain the teeth. Administering the medicine by way of a straw is advised.

MEGALOBLASTIC ANEMIA

Characterized by abnormally large (megalo-) red blood cells, many of which are oval shaped resulting from a deficiency of vitamin B_{12} (cobalamin) and/or folate, both necessary for the production of healthy red blood cells.

I. Pernicious Anemia

- Etiologic factors[8–12]
  - Considered an autoimmune disease causing atrophy of the gastric mucosa and destruction of stomach parietal cells (intrinsic factor [IF]).
  - Stomach parietal cells produce IF necessary for the absorption of vitamin B_{12}.
  - Deficiency of vitamin B_{12} can also be caused by:
    - Malabsorption due to gastrointestinal disorders such as celiac disease and Crohn disease.
    - Inadequate intake due to dietary choices may cause deficiency, for example, strict vegans who do not consume animal sources.
    - Chronic atrophic gastritis (e.g., older adults) or surgical removal of part or all of the stomach (e.g., gastric bypass) decreased hydrochloric acid production, decreasing absorption.
    - Long-term use of histamine (H_2) receptor antagonists, proton pump inhibitors, or metformin.[11,12]

◆ Age characteristics
- Pernicious anemia is primarily a disease of adults and occurs with increasing frequency in those over age 60 years, although about half of patients are less than 60 years.[8]

◆ Signs and symptoms: general
- Fatigue and weakness.
- Loss of appetite and weight loss.
- Poor memory.

◆ Signs and symptoms: neurologic involvement[8]
- Sclerosis of the spinal cord.
- Peripheral neuropathy (numbness and painful tingling of hands and feet).
- Optical neuropathy.
- Psychiatric manifestations.
- Autonomic dysfunction, which may include dizziness or fainting on standing (orthostatic hypotension).

◆ Signs and symptoms: oral findings
- Glossitis (Hunter glossitis), slick or bald tongue, loss of filiform papillae, and burning sensation with certain foods.
- Sensitivity to hot or spicy foods.
- Gingiva and mucosa: pale, atrophic similar to vitamin B deficiency.

◆ Treatment
- For individuals with IF deficiency and/or malabsorption, vitamin B_{12} is administered by injection daily until the condition is controlled.
- Once controlled, administration will continue monthly for life or until the underlying condition causing the deficiency is managed.
- For patients with inadequate IF production, oral supplementation of vitamin B_{12} is the treatment of choice.
- Vitamin B_{12} is only found in foods from animal sources and fortified foods. Good dietary sources of vitamin B_{12} are meat, clams, liver, fortified breakfast cereals, fish, poultry, milk, cheese, and eggs.

II. Folate-Deficiency Anemia[13]

Folate-deficiency anemia has the same characteristics as pernicious anemia, except no clinical neurologic changes are evident.

◆ Etiologic factors
- Decreased intake.
- Inadequate intake: Severely restricted diets or diets influenced by such factors as poverty, food faddism, or alcoholism, when the use of alcohol takes precedence over food.
- Impaired absorption.

◆ Individuals at risk of folate inadequacy:
- Women of childbearing age.
- Pregnant women.
- Patients with alcohol dependence.
- Individuals with malabsorption disorders (e.g., postgastric surgery, celiac disease, and inflammatory bowel disease).

- Certain treatment regimens impair the utilization of folate, for example, cancer chemotherapy, rheumatoid arthritis, and medications such as methotrexate and dilantin.

◆ Dietary factors: sources
- In 1998, the Food and Drug Administration required fortification of cereals, breads, flours, pastas, and other grain products with folate.
- Dietary sources can be found in Chapter 33.

◆ Fetal development
- Women with inadequate folic acid intake are at increased risk of having a baby with neural tube defects.
- Spina bifida (myelomeningocele): a severe condition affecting the formation of the nerves of the spinal cord and resulting in infant paralysis. Spina bifida is described in Chapter 52.

SICKLE CELL DISEASE

◆ SCD is a hereditary form of hemolytic anemia, resulting from a defective hemoglobin molecule.[14–16]

◆ The name is derived from the crescent or "sickle" shape assumed by the erythrocytes when the defective hemoglobin loses oxygen (Figure 62-2).[14–16]

◆ It is an autosomal recessive trait. Those with sickle cell trait demonstrate few symptoms unless placed under severe stress.[14–16]

I. Disease Process

Occurs primarily in the African-American population and to a lesser degree in Hispanic, Middle Eastern, or Asian Indian populations.[14–16]

◆ Diagnosis[14,15]
- Prenatal diagnosis can be made with 100% accuracy and genetic counseling provided for the parents.
- A simple blood test will detect SCD or sickle cell trait (parental carrier). Newborn screening is mandatory in most states in the United States.

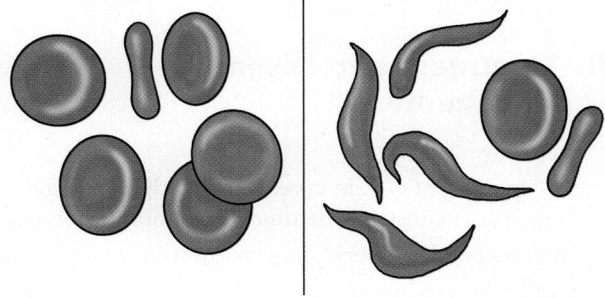

FIGURE 62-2 • **Sickle Cell Disease.** Left, diagrammatic drawing of normal red blood cells. Right, sickle shapes of red blood cells of a patient with sickle cell disease.

II. Clinical Course[14,16]

◆ Anemia
- Life span of red blood cells is significantly reduced from a normal lifespan of approximately 90–120 days to about 10–15 days.
- Anemia appears within the first 6 months.
- Growth and development may be impaired during the early years.
- Increased susceptibility to severe bacterial infection, especially pneumococcal infections in young children.
- Multiple blood transfusions putting patients at risk of blood-borne pathogens (e.g., hepatitis C).

◆ Vaso-occlusion
- Mortality is primarily from repeated vaso-occlusions (blood vessel blockage), resulting in infarctions, organ damage, and/or stroke.
- Progressive changes to blood vessels as a result of damage by the sickle-shaped red blood cells that result in the blood vessel blockage.
- Progressive organ damage resulting in a shortened life expectancy, with most patients only living into their thirties.

◆ Pain crises (sickle cell crisis)
- Repeated episodes of unpredictable acute pain, which results in hospitalization.
- Often preceded by a viral or bacterial infection.

◆ Most people with SCD will experience progressive organ damage.
- Neurologic damage results in impaired cognition and hemorrhagic strokes.
- Cardiopulmonary damage impairs lung function and results in dilation of the left ventricle of the heart and heart murmurs.
- Hepatobiliary damage results in abnormal liver function and increases the likelihood of gallstones.
- Genitourinary damage may result in kidney failure.
- Skeletal damage may result in necrosis of the hips and shoulders, with a need for joint replacement.
- Skin effects may result in chronic ulceration.
- Ocular damage in sickle cell anemia is the leading cause of blindness in patients of African ancestry.

III. Treatment and Disease Management[16]

◆ Supportive
- Management of pain crises remains challenging.

◆ Oxygen is a mainstay of treatment to minimize hypoxia.

◆ Pain relief without depressing breathing.

◆ Avoid substance abuse.

◆ Management of febrile episodes.

◆ Antibiotics for infectious diseases to avoid sepsis.

◆ Prevention of sickling.

- Pharmacologic therapy using a chemotherapy agent (Hydroxyurea) to increase hemoglobin F decreases the permanent formation of sickle cells.
- Stem cell transplant may be an option.
- Use of prophylactic penicillin to prevent pneumonia and meningococcal sepsis.
- Regular blood transfusions.
- Chemotherapy and gene therapy show promise in the future.

IV. Oral Implications[17]

◆ Radiographic findings
- Coarse trabecular pattern appearing as horizontal rows between teeth ("step ladder"), with large marrow spaces.
- Osteoporotic changes.

◆ Oral manifestations[17]
- Necrosis of the dental pulp.
- Osteomyelitis of the mandible.
- Enamel hypomineralization.
- Overgrowth of the facial bones, resulting in protrusion of the maxilla causing malocclusion.
- Pallor of buccal mucosa.
- Numb chin syndrome (mental nerve neuropathy).
- Facial and dental pain.

V. Appointment Management

◆ Thoroughly review the comprehensive medical history. Gather patient information regarding:
- Related complications specific to organ damage and other problems since birth.
- Characteristics of pain control (frequency, duration, average number, date of last crisis).
- Past and current medical treatment (surgeries, transfusions, medications, allergies).
- Presence of venous access catheters and joint replacement.
- Growth and development issues.

◆ Consultation with the patient's primary care provider recommended to:
- Determine disease control including complete blood count.

◆ Determine if the antibiotic prophylaxis is indicated before any form of tissue manipulation, which could create a bacteremia, is performed because the patient is highly susceptible to infection. A stress reduction protocol is necessary to prevent precipitation of a sickle cell crisis.

◆ Implement a comprehensive preventive program to minimize oral infection and control oral disease risk factors.

◆ Avoid long complicated dental appointments by maintaining good oral health with frequent preventive care appointments with the dental hygienist.

◆ Use local anesthesia with low doses of vasoconstrictors to avoid intravascular occlusion of red blood cells.

POLYCYTHEMIAS

Polycythemia implies an increase in the number and concentration of red blood cells above the normal level. There are two categories of polycythemia: primary and secondary.

I. Polycythemia Vera (Primary Polycythemia)[18,19]

◆ Cause
  • Polycythemia vera is a neoplasm caused by a genetic mutation increasing the sensitivity of bone marrow cells to erythropoietin, resulting in an increased production of red blood cells.[18,19]
  • Blood viscosity increases, affecting oxygen transport to tissues.
◆ Clinical signs and symptoms[18,19]
  • Average age at diagnosis is 60 years.
  • Increased bleeding risk with spontaneous bleeding of the gingiva.
  • Bruise easily, resulting in submucosal petechiae and hematoma formation.
  • Risk of fatal and nonfatal blood clot formation, leading to heart attack, stroke, and pulmonary embolism.
  • Migraines.
  • Vertigo.
  • Fatigue.
  • Purplish or red areas on the oral mucosa, gingiva, lips, or tongue.
◆ Treatment[18,19]
  • Chemotherapy.
  • Phlebotomy (blood drawing), to reduce the total volume, particularly the red cell volume, of the blood.
  • Low-dose aspirin (<100 mg/daily) as an antiplatelet.
◆ Dental hygiene treatment considerations
  • Thorough review of the medical history due to the increased risk of bleeding, bruising, cerebral vascular accident, and myocardial infarction.
  • Consult with the hematologist and/or primary care provider about disease management and patient's blood test results, especially hemoglobin and hematocrit.
  • Careful attention to oral self-care and preventive maintenance is required to maintain good oral health.
  • Carefully monitor bleeding and monitor clotting during and following instrumentation.
  • Provide careful postoperative instructions for early identification of bleeding that does not stop after applying pressure.

II. Secondary Polycythemia[19]

◆ Secondary polycythemia is also called erythrocytosis (an increase in the number of red blood cells).

◆ Increased red cell production can result from hypoxia due to chronic obstructive pulmonary disease, cyanotic heart disease, emphysema, tobacco smoking, or residing at high altitudes.

◆ Bleeding tendencies may be partially controlled with control of gingival irritants.

DISORDERS OF WHITE BLOOD CELLS

◆ Disorders may occur because of a decrease (leukopenia) or an increase (leukocytosis) of numbers of white blood cells.

◆ The types of white blood cells are described in Table 62-2 and illustrated in Figure 62-1.

I. Neutropenia[20]

A decrease in the total number of neutrophils results when cell production cannot keep pace with the turnover rate or when there is an accelerated rate of removal of cells, as in certain disease states.

A. Etiology[20]

◆ Defects in myeloid cells possibly due to genetics.

◆ Secondary neutropenia may develop in the following conditions: alcohol abuse, autoimmune disease (e.g., human immunodeficiency virus [HIV]/acquired immunodeficiency syndrome [AIDS]), chemotherapy or radiation therapy, folate or vitamin B_{12} deficiency, infection, or bone marrow transplant.

B. Signs and Symptoms[20]

◆ Oral stomatitis and lymph node enlargement may present in patients with neutropenias, resulting from defects in myeloid cells.

◆ Frequent, severe, or unusual infections such as pneumonia.

C. Diagnosis[20]

◆ Moderate neutropenia (500–1,000/μL of blood)

◆ Severe neutropenia (<500/μL)
  • When values drop below 500/μL, even normal microbial flora in the mouth can cause infection.

D. Dental Treatment Considerations

◆ Thorough review of the medical history is essential.

◆ Consultation with the primary care provider is necessary to determine if neutrophil count is at a safe level.

◆ Antibiotic prophylaxis may be needed.

II. Lymphocytopenia

Abnormally low number of lymphocytes in the blood.

A. Etiology[20]

◆ Acquired lymphocytopenia may be caused by protein–energy malnutrition, AIDS, chemotherapy, radiation therapy, or infectious disease such as hepatitis, influenza, and tuberculosis.

◆ Hereditary lymphocytopenia may be associated with inherited immunodeficiency disorders.

B. Signs and Symptoms[20]

◆ Pallor.

◆ Bruising (petechiae).

◆ Mouth ulcers.

C. Dental Treatment Considerations

◆ The same as for neutropenia.

III. Leukocytosis

Leukocytosis is an increase in the number of circulating white blood cells.

◆ Caused by inflammatory and infectious states, trauma, exertion, and other conditions listed in Table 62-2.

◆ The most extreme cause of leukocytosis is leukemia.[21]

• Leukemias are malignant neoplasms of immature white blood cells that multiply uncontrollably.

• Cancer cells located within the circulating blood and in bone marrow infiltrate into other body tissues and organs such as the spleen and lymph nodes.

• Leukemias can be acute, such as acute lymphocytic leukemia, or chronic, such as chronic lymphocytic leukemia.

• Oral manifestations may include bruising and bleeding of the gingiva.

PLATELET DISORDERS[22]

Platelets function in the clotting system. Disorders include abnormal increases or decreases in numbers of platelets and/or platelet dysfunction.

◆ When the number of platelets decreases, the risk for bleeding increases.

• Risk of bleeding increases when platelet count is below 50,000/μL.

I. Thrombocytopenia (Decrease in Platelets)

◆ A lower number of platelets may be caused by decreased production in the bone marrow.

◆ Bone marrow depression may be due to drugs, such as hydrochlorothiazide (used to treat high blood pressure) and acetaminophen, infections like HIV and hepatitis, or blood transfusions.

◆ If severe, a platelet transfusion may be necessary.

II. Reactive Thrombocytosis (Overproduction of Platelets)

◆ Overproduction is due to another disorder.

◆ Causes include acute infection, chronic inflammatory disorders, iron deficiency, and certain cancers.

◆ Not usually with increased risk of thrombosis.

III. Platelet Dysfunction

◆ Acquired platelet dysfunction

• Causes of acquired platelet dysfunction include cirrhosis, systemic lupus erythematosus, and certain drugs.

◆ Hereditary platelet dysfunction

• Dysfunction may occur because of a disease such as von Willebrand disease (a coagulation disorder).

BLEEDING OR COAGULATION DISORDERS

◆ Blood clotting or hemostasis is the body's mechanism for stopping bleeding from injured blood vessels while preventing intravascular clots, which can cause serious health problems.[23]

◆ The three main processes of blood clotting include constriction of bleeding vessels, activity of platelets, and activity of blood clotting factors.

◆ A history or suspicion of a bleeding problem requires careful evaluation before treatment can be started.

◆ Spontaneous bleeding occurs as small hemorrhages into the skin or mucous membranes and other tissues and appears as petechiae or purpura.

◆ People with bleeding disorders have the tendency to exhibit spontaneous bleeding and moderate to excessive bleeding following trauma, surgical procedure, or dental hygiene therapy, including nonsurgical instrumentation.

I. Oral Findings Suggestive of Bleeding Disorders

◆ Early signs of systemic conditions frequently appear in the oral soft tissues and clinical examination may identify these changes.

◆ Referral for medical examination may lead to diagnosis and treatment of a serious disease.

◆ Laboratory blood tests may provide essential information for safe and effective dental hygiene care.

◆ Oral soft tissue changes observed in patients with blood diseases are not necessarily exclusive to systemic blood disorders.

◆ It is necessary to recognize change in a previously healthy patient or an apparently exaggerated response in a patient being examined at an initial appointment.

◆ Findings suggesting a blood disorder include the following[24–26]:

• Gingival bleeding, spontaneously or excessive bleeding on gentle probing.

- History of difficulty in controlling bleeding by usual procedures.
- History of bruising easily, with large ecchymoses.
- Numerous petechiae.
- Marked pallor of the mucous membranes.
- Atrophy of the papillae of the tongue (atrophic glossitis) or magenta tongue.
- Angular stomatitis.
- Persistent sore or painful tongue (glossodynia).
- Acute or chronic infections, such as candidiasis, that do not respond to usual treatment.
- Severe ulcerations associated with a lack of response to treatment.
- Exaggerated gingival response to local irritants, sometimes with characteristics of necrotizing ulcerative gingivitis (ulceration, necrosis, bleeding, pseudomembrane).
- Vascular fragility is increased; petechial and purpuric hemorrhages appear in the skin or mucous membranes, including the gingiva.

II. Disorders of Coagulation

Abnormal bleeding can be due to acquired, drug-related, or hereditary factors including disorders of the coagulation system, of platelets, and/or of blood vessels.

A. Acquired Bleeding Disorders[24–26]

- Vitamin K deficiency
  - Vitamin K is essential in the synthesis of prothrombin and clotting factors VII, IX, and X.
  - Food sources of vitamin K may be found in Chapter 33. Vitamin K is also produced in the alimentary tract by intestinal bacteria.
  - Excessive exposure to antibiotic therapy or prolonged gastrointestinal disturbances may affect vitamin K production.
- Liver disease: Most clotting factors are produced in the liver. When the liver is not functioning properly, production of clotting factors may be altered.
  - May occur in cirrhosis.
- Renal disease: erythropoietin is produced by the kidneys, which is involved in the stimulation of red blood cell production in bone marrow.
- Bone marrow disorders: impact red and white blood cell production.

B. Drug-Related Acquired Bleeding Disorders[27]

- Anticoagulation drugs: Following are the examples of some common medications
  - Antiplatelet drugs such as aspirin, nonsteroidal anti-inflammatory drugs (NSAIDs) and clopidogrel (Plavix).
  - Anticoagulants such as coumadin (warfarin) and heparin.
  - Corticosteroids.
  - Chemotherapy.

C. Hereditary Bleeding Disorders[28]

At least 30 hereditary coagulation disorders exist, each resulting from a deficiency or abnormality of a plasma protein.

- Hemophilia

Hemophilias are the oldest known hereditary bleeding disorders caused by low levels or complete absence of blood proteins essential for clotting.

- Etiology[25]
  - Results from mutation or deletion affecting the factor VIII or IX gene.
  - Hemophilia is an X-linked recessive genetic disease. The defective gene is located on the X chromosome; thus, the disorder occurs primarily in males.
- Treatment[25]
  - Most patients do well with appropriate medical management involving the administration of drugs to decrease bleeding or the infusion of platelets or plasma containing clotting factors.
- Effects and long-term complications[25]
  - Bleeding and bruising from minor trauma vary depending on the severity of the disease.
  - Bleeding into the soft tissue of joints (hemarthroses) of knees, ankles, and elbows begins in the very young with severe hemophilia.
  - Hemorrhage into the muscles (intramuscular hemorrhage) is accompanied by pain and limitation of motion.
  - Bleeding from the gingiva is common and more extensive when periodontal infection is more severe.
- Management of uncontrolled bleeding
  - The hematologist should be consulted prior to performing dental procedures with a risk of postoperative bleeding, including subgingival debridement and scaling.[27]
  - In someone with mild bleeding disorders, the clinician should implement the following:
    - If clotting does not occur within a few minutes, apply digital pressure to area with sterile gauze.
    - If needed, local hemostatic agents can be applied, such as absorbable gelatin sponge. Absorbs for 3–5 days.
  - Medical attention required if bleeding is not controlled.

DENTAL HYGIENE CARE PLAN

I. Preparation for Clinical Appointment

- Certain blood tests may be needed prior to treatment and should be documented.
  - Prothrombin time.
  - International Normalized Ratio (INR) ideally should be measured within 24–72 hours of any invasive procedure.[26]

- Basic tests are listed in Table 62-1 with their ranges or values.
- Indications for screening and preappointment tests:
  - When the patient reports a history of a bleeding problem.
  - Clinical examination reveals signs of a bleeding disorder.
  - Patient is being treated with anticoagulants, chemotherapy, or corticosteroids.

II. Patient History

A. Medical History Review

The medical history needs to include information regarding the type, severity, medical treatment, medications, and family history of the blood clotting defect.

- Question patient specifically regarding bleeding after previous clinical and surgical procedures, such as tooth extractions.
- Question about blood or plasma transfusions as individuals who received them prior to 1990 are at risk for hepatitis B and C as well as HIV.
- Patients with bleeding disorders have many emotional stresses related to the condition, including ongoing anxiety, so it is important to understand the patient's psychosocial situation.

B. Medication Review

A careful review of a patient's drug, supplements, and herb use is critical to determine potential oral and physiologic effects.

- The primary purpose of the drug and potential side effects needs careful review in a current drug reference guide.
- A variety of drugs and herbs may be factors in increased bleeding.[26]
  - Herbs and supplements associated with increased bleeding are listed in Box 62-1.
  - It is recommended to carefully review any herbs and supplements the patient may be taking, which could be associated with an increased risk of bleeding and to discontinue for at least a week prior to receiving invasive surgical procedures.
- Patients taking coumadin (for prevention of recurrent thrombosis), heparin (for short-term use following a total joint replacement procedure), or medication for long-term anticoagulation (such as aspirin) may need special consultation.
  - The most common side effect of both warfarin and heparin is hemorrhage.
  - Hemorrhages may present as gingival bleeding or submucosal bleeding with hematoma formation.
- Cancer chemotherapeutic agents may secondarily induce profound thrombocytopenia ($<20,000$ mm^3) or neutropenia (<500 mm^3).
- Antithrombotic agents such as aspirin and clopidogrel (Plavix®) alter the ability of platelets to stick or clump together and form a clot.

BOX 62-1
Herbs and Supplements Associated with Increased Bleeding

Alfalfa	Cat's claw	Garlic
Allspice	Chamomile	Ginkgo
Antiplatelet activity		Coumarin-containing herbs
Bilberry	Ginseng	Chamomile
Dong quai	Feverfew	Fenugreek
Feverfew	Meadowsweet	Horse chestnut
Garlic	Turmeric	Motherwort
Ginger	White willow	Red clover
Ginkgo biloba		

Sources: Barbara A. Bleeding and thrombosis. In: Kasper D, Fauci A, Hauser S, Longo D, Jameson J, Loscalzo J, eds. *Harrison's Principles of Internal Medicine.* 19th ed. New York, NY: McGraw-Hill; 2014; Baatsch B, Zimmer S, Rodrigues Recchia D, Büssing A. Complementary and alternative therapies in dentistry and characteristics of dentists who recommend them. *Complement Ther Med.* 2017;35:64-69.

C. Dental History Review

Discuss previous dental care and perceived treatment needs when developing the current care plan with the patient.

D. Risk Assessment

The patient with a bleeding disorder may be at high risk for dental caries and periodontal disease, so modifiable risk factors need to be addressed in the treatment care plan.

- Early prevention of oral disease should be initiated at a young age, including regular professional preventive care, meticulous oral self-care, appropriate use of fluorides, and pit and fissure sealants.

III. Consultation with Physician/Hematologist

- Consultation with the primary care provider/hematologist is necessary to obtain complete and accurate information.
- Anticoagulant therapy is seldom discontinued for most dental treatments because the risk for intravascular clot formation is greater than the risk for hemorrhage.[26]
- A joint policy advising healthcare providers who perform invasive or surgical procedures to contact the cardiologist and discuss patient management before discontinuing antiplatelet drugs has been developed by[29]:
  - American Dental Association.
  - American Heart Association.
  - American College of Cardiology.
  - Society for Cardiovascular Angiography and Interventions.
  - American College of Surgeons.

- Consult primary care provider/hematologist to determine whether antibiotic prophylaxis is required during dental procedures to prevent infection in joint prostheses and/or indwelling catheter.[30,31]
- In inherited bleeding disorder, many procedures require factor replacement therapy immediately preceding the dental appointment.[28]
- Request reports of current blood tests.

IV. Examination

- Use a preprocedural chlorhexidine mouthrinse to reduce the bacterial load prior to beginning examination or treatment.
- Radiographic imaging: Films/sensor (infection control barriers) can cut and press on the mucous membranes. Exercise care in placement to avoid bleeding and/or a hematoma.
- The dental and periodontal examination can be conducted once a consultation with the primary care provider or specialist has assessed the need for antibiotic prophylaxis or pretreatment to prevent bleeding.

V. Treatment Care Plan

- Select age-appropriate preventive measures based on risk assessment including, but not limited to:
  - Oral self-care instruction.
  - Nutrition counseling.
  - Preventive agents including fluoride treatments, remineralizing agents, and/or sealants.
  - Prophylaxis or nonsurgical periodontal therapy (NSPT).
  - Restorative care.
  - Referral as needed.
  - Continuing care recommendations.

VI. Treatment

- Nutritional assessment and counseling are recommended for caries control and periodontal health to stress choosing foods that provide a healthy, well-balanced diet.
- Provide patient education to enhance oral self-care at the initial appointment and reinforce at each session to minimize bleeding during instrumentation.
  - Spontaneous oral bleeding problems can be partially controlled by the elimination of oral inflammation and infection.
  - A soft toothbrush is indicated. If patient indicates using a power brush, proper demonstration of technique is necessary.
  - Choose the appropriate interdental aid(s) and teach the patient correct use to prevent tissue injury.
  - Patients with limited manual dexterity can benefit from adaptive oral hygiene aids.

- Stress reduction protocol: Prevention or reduction of stress begins before the appointment and throughout treatment.
- Local anesthesia.[26]
  - Use local anesthesia with a vasoconstrictor.
  - Infiltration injections are preferred.
  - Block anesthesia, especially the inferior alveolar and posterior superior nerve blocks, increase the risk of bleeding. In inherited bleeding disorders, preoperative infusion to prevent bleeding is necessary for block anesthesia.[28]
- NSPT requires a consult with the medical provider to ensure the patient is managed properly to prevent an emergency.
  - Scheduling of appointments may be dependent on whether preprocedural medication is needed to prevent bleeding. If IV infusion is used, it may be necessary to complete the NSPT and restorative treatment in fewer appointments to minimize the need for IV infusions.[28]
  - Minimize tissue trauma as much as possible.
  - Exercise caution with the use of suction to prevent trauma and hematomas to the buccal, sublingual, or other mucosal tissues.
- Postoperative: Monitor to ensure bleeding has stopped postoperatively.
  - Never recommend aspirin or NSAIDs for a patient with a bleeding disorder.
  - Ideally call the patient the evening after treatment to ensure they are having no bleeding issues.
- Frequency of continuing care: Frequent appointments can aid in keeping the oral tissues in an optimum state of health and help to prevent the need for complex or lengthy dental appointments.

DOCUMENTATION

Documentation in the permanent record for each appointment with a blood disorder includes a minimum of the following factors:

- Review or update medical history thoroughly. Document laboratory findings.
- Document extra- and intraoral examination findings. Use written description and an intraoral picture when possible.
- Note treatment planning considerations such as shorter appointments, stress reduction protocols that need to be implemented, and oral hygiene considerations.
- Note consultations with other health professionals involved in the patient's care.
- Reference any difficulties with bleeding control during appointment.
- A sample progress note is provided in Box 62-2.

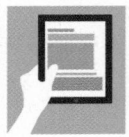

BOX 62-2
Example Documentation:
Patient with a Blood Disorder

S—A 70-year-old white man presents for a new patient examination. He reports having a stroke a year ago and currently taking coumadin (warfarin). Patient states that his INR last week was 2.8.

O—Oral cancer examination: all tissues appear normal. Full-mouth series of radiographs and caries examination reveal no new caries. Periodontal examination: generalized 4–5 mm pocket depths with localized bleeding on probing. Plaque score: 50%.

A—Increased risk for oral bleeding following dental hygiene treatment.

P—Disclosed plaque biofilm and reviewed technique for oral hygiene aids. Stressed need for meticulous oral self-care to prevent infection and associated bleeding. NSPT completed maxillary and mandibular right quadrants with 2 carpules 2% xylocaine with 1:100,000 epinephrine. Areas monitored to verify bleeding had stopped within 5 minutes following completion of instrumentation. Postoperative instruction given to contact the office should he be unable to stop bleeding.

Next appointment: Complete NSPT with local anesthesia and apply fluoride varnish.

Signed: _____, RDH

Date: _____

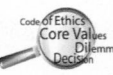

EVERYDAY ETHICS

As Dena, the dental hygienist, begins to periodontally probe Mr. Bennett, a new patient in the practice, the receptionist interrupts to give Dena a medical clearance form that has been faxed from the patient's physician. As Dena reviews the information, she understands that the patient has a blood disorder but is unclear as to its extent from the laboratory values in the report. She briefly questions Mr. Bennett about any medical tests and he indicates that he was in the hospital 4 days the previous month.

As Dena continues periodontal probing, she notices considerable bleeding with oozing around the gingival margins.

Questions for Consideration

1. What action, if any, does Dena need to take to ensure she is performing beneficently on behalf of this patient?

2. It appears that Mr. Bennett has not given sufficient information about his medical condition prior to this continuing care appointment. What obligation does a patient have to update the medical history at each appointment? And what obligation does the professional person have to help the patient understand this obligation?

3. While Dena quietly acknowledges to herself that she used to know the information about bleeding conditions, she is currently uncertain of the meaning of the laboratory values in this patient's report. Ethically, how can this realization be assessed? What is the immediate need? What can be done to prevent such a situation from occurring in the future?

Factors to Teach the Patient

► Meticulous oral hygiene techniques to practice daily: toothbrushing, interdental cleaning, and other appropriate oral hygiene aids.

► How to self-evaluate the oral cavity for deviations from normal. Watching for changes in size, shape, and color and contacting oral health professional when lesions last longer than 2 weeks.

► Selection of noncariogenic foods to prevent caries and knowledge about the diet's relationship to health.

► Avoid use of salicylates (aspirin) and NSAIDs.

► Importance of informing the dental provider of any changes to the medical history, including drugs, herbs, supplements, and hospitalizations and providing recent laboratory values before beginning treatment.

ENHANCE YOUR UNDERSTANDING

ONLINE RESOURCES
(see the inside front cover for access information)
- Audio glossary
- Appendices

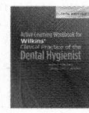

SUPPORT FOR LEARNING
(available separately)
- *Active Learning Workbook for Wilkins' Clinical Practice of the Dental Hygienist, 13th Edition*

INDIVIDUALIZED REVIEW
- Customized practice quizzing with Navigate 2 TestPrep for *Wilkins' Clinical Practice of the Dental Hygienist*

References

1. Mesher AL. Blood. In: Mescher AL, eds. *Junqueira's Basic Histology*. 14th ed. New York, NY: McGraw-Hill. http://accessmedicine.mhmedical.com.p.atsu.edu/content.aspx?bookid=1687&sectionid=108453529. Accessed May 31, 2018.

2. American Association for Clinical Chemistry. Hemoglobin. https://labtestsonline.org/tests/hemoglobin. Accessed June 17, 2018.

3. Buhn FH. Introduction to anemia and red cell disorders. In: Aster JC, Bunn H, eds. *Pathophysiology of Blood Disorders*. 2nd ed. New York, NY: McGraw-Hill; 2017. http://accessmedicine.mhmedical.com.p.atsu.edu/content.aspx?bookid=1900&sectionid=137391675. Accessed May 31, 2018.

4. Damon LE, Andreadis C. Blood disorders. In: Papadakis MA, McPhee SJ, Rabow MW, eds. *Current Medical Diagnosis & Treatment 2018*. New York, NY: McGraw-Hill; 2018:chap 13. http://accessmedicine.mhmedical.com.p.atsu.edu/content.aspx?bookid=2192&sectionid=167993948. Accessed May 31, 2018.

5. Rund D. Thalassemia 2016: modern medicine battles an ancient disease. *Am J Hematol*. 2016;91(1):15-21.

6. Camaschella C. New insights into iron deficiency and iron deficiency anemia. *Blood Rev*. 2017;31(4):225-233.

7. Office of Dietary Supplements. *Iron: Fact Sheet for Health Professionals*. Bethesda, MD: National Institutes of Health. http://ods.od.nih.gov/factsheets/Iron-HealthProfessional/. Accessed May 31, 2018.

8. Rojas Hernandez CM, Oo TH. Advances in mechanisms, diagnosis, and treatment of pernicious anemia. *Discov Med*. 2015;19(104):159-168.

9. Office of Dietary Supplements. *Vitamin B₁₂: Fact Sheet for Health Professionals*. Bethesda, MD: National Institutes of Health. http://ods.od.nih.gov/factsheets/VitaminB12-HealthProfessional/. Accessed May 31, 2018.

10. Hoffbrand A. Megaloblastic anemias. In: Kasper D, Fauci A, Hauser S, Longo D, Jameson J, Loscalzo J, eds. *Harrison's Principles of Internal Medicine*. 19th ed. New York, NY: McGraw-Hill; 2014. http://accessmedicine.mhmedical.com.p.atsu.edu/content.aspx?bookid=1130&sectionid=79731307. Accessed May 31, 2018.

11. Jung SB, Nagaraja V, Kapur A, Eslick GD. Association between vitamin B12 deficiency and long-term use of acid-lowering agents: a systematic review and meta-analysis. *Intern Med J*. 2015;45(4):409-416.

12. Ahmed MA. Metformin and Vitamin B12 deficiency: where so we stand? *J Pharm Pharm Sci*. 2016;19(3):382-398.

13. Office of Dietary Supplements. *Folate: Dietary Supplement Fact Sheet*. Bethesda, MD: National Institutes of Health. http://ods.od.nih.gov/factsheets/Folate-HealthProfessional/. Accessed May 31, 2018.

14. Bunn H. Sickle cell disease. In: Bunn H, Aster JC, eds. *Pathophysiology of Blood Disorders*. New York, NY: McGraw-Hill; 2017:chap 9. http://accessmedicine.mhmedical.com.p.atsu.edu/content.aspx?bookid=1900&sectionid=137391675. Accessed May 30, 2018.

15. Sheth S, Licursi M, Bhatia M. Sickle cell disease: time for a closer look at treatment options? *Br J Haematol*. 2013;162(4):455-464.

16. Yawn BP, Buchanan GR, Afenyi-Annan AN, et al. Management of sickle cell disease: summary of the 2014 evidence-based report by expert panel members. JAMA. 2014;312(10):1033-1048.

17. da Fonseca M, Oueis HS, Casamassimo PS. Sickle cell anemia: a review for the pediatric dentist. *Pediatr Dent*. 2007;29(2):159-169.

18. Squizzato A, Romualdi E, Passamonti F, et al. Antiplatelet drugs for polycythaemia vera and essential thrombocythaemia. *Cochrane Database Syst Rev*. 2013;(4):CD006503.

19. Tefferi A, Barbui T. Polycythemia vera and essential thrombocythemia: 2015 update on diagnosis, risk stratification and management. *Am J Hematology*. 2015;90(2):162-173. https://www.cancer.gov/types/myeloproliferative/hp/chronic-treatment-pdq. Accessed May 31, 2018.

20. Territo M. Overview of white blood cell disorders. *The Merck Manual—Professional Edition*. https://www.merckmanuals.com/professional/SearchResults?query=Overview+of+White+Blood+Cell+Disorders&icd9=MM334. Accessed May 31, 2018.

21. Rytting ME. Chronic myelogenous leukemia. *The Merck Manual—Professional Edition*. http://www.merckmanuals.com/professional/hematology-and-oncology/leukemias/chronic-myelogenous-leukemia-cml. Accessed May 31, 2018.

22. Kuter DJ. Overview of platelet disorders. *The Merck Manual—Professional Edition*. http://www.merckmanuals.com/professional/hematology_and_oncology/thrombocytopenia_and_platelet_dysfunction/overview_of_platelet_disorders. Accessed May 30, 2018.

23. Moake JL. Overview of hemostasis. *The Merck Manual—Professional Edition*. https://www.merckmanuals.com/professional/hematology-and-oncology/hemostasis/overview-of-hemostasis. Accessed May 30, 2018.

24. Moake JL. Overview of coagulation disorders. *The Merck Manual—Professional Edition*. https://www.merckmanuals.com/professional/hematology-and-oncology/hemostasis/overview-of-hemostasis. Accessed May 30, 2018.

25. Moake JL. Hemophilia. *The Merck Manual—Professional Edition*. http://www.merckmanuals.com/professional/hematology_and_oncology/coagulation_disorders/hemophilia. Accessed May 30, 2018.

26. Nizarali N, Rafique S. Special care dentistry: part 2. Dental management of patients with drug-related acquired bleeding disorders. *Dent Update*. 2013;40(9):711-712, 714-716, 718.

27. Nizarali N, Rafique S. Special care dentistry: part 3. Dental management of patients with medical conditions causing acquired bleeding disorders. *Dent Update*. 2013;40(10):805-808, 810-812.

28. Rafique S, Fiske J, Palmer G, Daly B. Special care dentistry: part 1. Dental management of patients with inherited bleeding disorders. *Dent Update*. 2013;40(8):613-616, 619-622, 625-626 passim.

29. American Dental Association. Oral health topics, anticoagulant and antiplatelet medications and dental procedures. https://www.ada.org/en/member-center/oral-health-topics/anticoagulant-antiplatelet-medications-and-dental-. Accessed May 31, 2018.

30. Sollecito TP, Abt E, Lockhart PB, et al. The use of prophylactic antibiotics prior to dental procedures in patients with prosthetic joints: evidence-based clinical practice guideline for dental practitioners—a report of the American Dental Association Council on Scientific Affairs. *J Am Dent Assoc*. 2015;146(1):11-16.

31. Abed H, Ainousa A. Dental management of patients with inherited bleeding disorders: a multidisciplinary approach. *Gen Dent*. 2017;65(6):56-60.

63

The Patient with an Autoimmune Disease

Robin L. Kerkstra, RDH, MSDH, and Linda D. Boyd, RDH, RD, EdD

CHAPTER OUTLINE

OVERVIEW OF AUTOIMMUNE DISEASES
I. Immune System Basics
II. Prevalence of Autoimmune Diseases
III. Etiology
IV. Classification
V. Treatment Modalities

CONNECTIVE TISSUE AUTOIMMUNE DISEASES

ORAL LICHEN PLANUS
I. Prevalence
II. Etiology
III. Clinical Presentation
IV. Treatment
V. Dental Hygiene Care

RHEUMATOID ARTHRITIS
I. Prevalence
II. Etiology
III. Clinical Presentation
IV. Treatment
V. Dental Hygiene Care

SCLERODERMA
I. Prevalence
II. Etiology
III. Clinical Presentation
IV. Treatment
V. Dental Hygiene Care

GASTROINTESTINAL TRACT AUTOIMMUNE DISEASES

CELIAC DISEASE
I. Prevalence
II. Etiology
III. Clinical Presentation
IV. Treatment
V. Dental Hygiene Care

CROHN'S DISEASE
I. Prevalence
II. Etiology
III. Clinical Presentation
IV. Treatment
V. Dental Hygiene Care

ULCERATIVE COLITIS
I. Prevalence
II. Etiology
III. Clinical Presentation
IV. Treatment
V. Dental Hygiene Care

NEUROLOGIC SYSTEM AUTOIMMUNE DISEASES

MULTIPLE SCLEROSIS
I. Prevalence
II. Etiology
III. Clinical Presentation
IV. Treatment
V. Dental Hygiene Care

MYASTHENIA GRAVIS
I. Prevalence
II. Etiology
III. Clinical Presentation
IV. Treatment
V. Dental Hygiene Care

SYSTEMIC AUTOIMMUNE DISEASES

SJÖGREN'S SYNDROME
I. Prevalence
II. Etiology
III. Clinical Presentation
IV. Treatment
V. Dental Hygiene Care

SYSTEMIC LUPUS ERYTHEMATOSUS
I. Prevalence
II. Etiology
III. Clinical Presentation
IV. Treatment
V. Dental Hygiene Care

DOCUMENTATION

EVERYDAY ETHICS

FACTORS TO TEACH THE PATIENT

REFERENCES

LEARNING OBJECTIVES

After studying this chapter, the student should be able to:

1. Describe how autoimmune diseases affect the immune system.

2. Identify various types of autoimmune diseases and the identifying symptoms and treatment.

3. Plan dental hygiene care modifications for the patient with an autoimmune disease.

OVERVIEW OF AUTOIMMUNE DISEASES

Autoimmune diseases occur when the immune system has problems fighting viruses, bacteria, and infection because immune cells attack parts of the body instead of protecting it.

I. Immune System Basics

- ◆ The immune system consists of two parts called the acquired and innate immune systems (Figure 63-1).
  - • As a person grows, so does their acquired immune system and its ability to recognize invaders in the body and remember them for future immune response.
  - • Acquired immune cells activate antibodies that attach themselves to invaders to be destroyed.

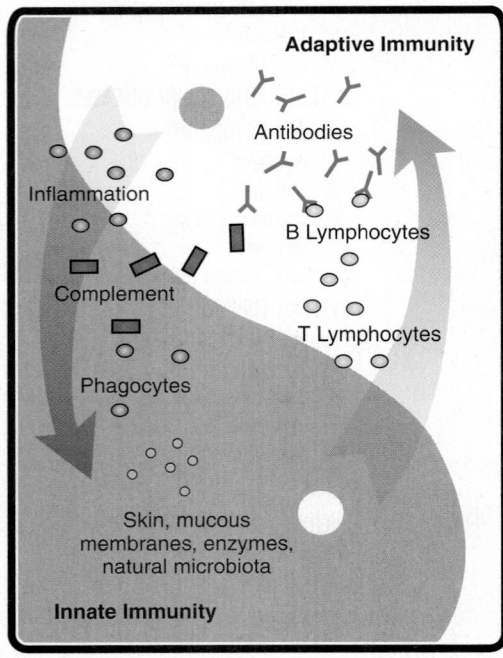

FIGURE 63-1 • Overview of the Immune System. As part of the innate immunity, the human body has natural measures to prevent entry of microbes. When these barriers are overcome, a foreign invader first encounters phagocytes. Inflammation may develop. If the innate immune system cannot destroy the invader, the adaptive immune system is activated with T and B lymphocytes. Although the innate and adaptive immune systems are characterized by contrasting functions and timing, they work closely together and rely on each other to succeed in removing the invading pathogens.

- ◆ Immune cells associated with adaptive immunity, called lymphocytes, develop in the bone marrow and specialize in protecting the body against any foreign invader.
  - • There are two major types of lymphocytes: B lymphocytes which mature in the bone marrow and T lymphocytes that mature in the thymus.

II. Prevalence of Autoimmune Diseases

- ◆ Worldwide prevalence of autoimmune diseases is between 7.6% and 9.4%.[1]
- ◆ Immune diseases affect an estimated 4.5% (14.7 million) of the United States population, with 2.7% men and 6.4% women affected.[2]
  - • Systemic lupus erythematosus (SLE) and Sjögren's syndrome (SS) affect females predominantly versus males (9:1).[3]
  - • Multiple sclerosis (MS) is the most common neurologic autoimmune disease and two-thirds of women account for all cases.[3]
  - • Graves' disease and Hashimoto thyroiditis tends to favor women as well.[3]
- ◆ The most common age of onset of autoimmune diseases is 40–50 years.[2]

III. Etiology

- ◆ Multifactorial etiology includes a genetic predisposition for activation of self-antigen specific T lymphocytes resulting in the formation of autoantibodies.
- ◆ Factors that may modify the autoimmune response include biologic (e.g., gender, pregnancy, and age) and environmental variables (e.g., infectious agents, diet, tobacco, and chemicals).[3,4]
- ◆ Autoantibodies cause damage and dysfunction of tissues that are targeted.
- ◆ Some autoimmune diseases tend to co-occur and may have a genetic predisposition such as type 1 diabetes, rheumatoid arthritis (RA), and thyroiditis.[1]
- ◆ Connective tissue autoimmune diseases have higher comorbidity than other types of autoimmune diseases.[1]

IV. Classification

- ◆ There are 80–100 autoimmune diseases and the most common ones can be found in Table 63-1 along with the organ system affected.[4]

TABLE 63-1 • Types of Autoimmune Diseases

	ORGAN AFFECTED	EXAMPLES OF AUTOIMMUNE DISEASES
Organ-specific autoimmune diseases	Skin	• Psoriasis • Pemphigus
	Pancreas	• Type 1 diabetes mellitus • Autoimmune pancreatitis
	Gastrointestinal system	• Celiac disease • Ulcerative colitis • Crohn's disease
	Neurologic system	• Multiple sclerosis • Myasthenia gravis • Narcolepsy
	Thyroid and para-thyroid gland	• Graves' disease • Hashimoto autoimmune thyroiditis • Autoimmune hypoparathyroidism
	Connective tissue	• Rheumatoid arthritis • Scleroderma • Ankylosing spondylitis
Systemic (organ nonspecific) autoimmune diseases	Lungs, liver, kidneys, central nervous system, salivary, and lacrimal glands	• Sjögren's syndrome
	Heart, joints, skin, lungs, blood vessels, liver, kidneys, and nervous system	• Systemic lupus erythematosus

◆ Various classification systems have been proposed and will likely be refined in future years.

A. Organ-Specific Autoimmune Diseases

◆ In organ-specific diseases, the antibodies and T-cells reach with self-antigens in specific tissue.[4] Examples include:
   • Gastrointestinal (GI) autoimmune diseases: Crohn's disease, celiac disease (CD), and ulcerative colitis (UC).
   • Connective tissue autoimmune diseases: RA and scleroderma. These two autoimmune diseases may also be systemic if they extend beyond their target tissue/organ.
   • Neurologic system autoimmune diseases: MS and myasthenia gravis.

B. Systemic Autoimmune Diseases

◆ Autoimmune disease is considered systemic when immune cells react to self-antigens throughout the body and in various tissues.[4]

◆ Examples of systemic autoimmune diseases include SLE and SS. Both these conditions can affect several organ systems including the lungs, liver, and nervous system.

V. Treatment Modalities

◆ There is a wide range of treatment options classified into the following categories:
   • Nonsteroidal anti-inflammatory drugs (NSAIDs).
   • Glucocorticosteroid medications.
   • Immunosuppressive medications.
   • Therapeutic monoclonals.
   • Immunoglobulin replacement therapy.
   • Medications to replace hormones secreted by the target organ, such as thyroxine in autoimmune thyroid disease.

CONNECTIVE TISSUE AUTOIMMUNE DISEASES

◆ Connective tissue autoimmune diseases are a diverse group of conditions affecting a variety of organs.[5]
◆ Most connective tissue diseases have significant genetic risk factors.
◆ A few connective tissue autoimmune diseases will be reviewed here including oral lichen planus (OLP), RA, and scleroderma.

ORAL LICHEN PLANUS

◆ The cause of OLP is not understood, but some research points toward it being an autoimmune disorder in which the cells lining the mouth are attacked by the body's own white blood cells.[6]
◆ OLP is a chronic inflammatory disease that affects the inside of the oral cavity on any mucosal surface as well as cheeks, tongue, and gingiva.[6]

I. Prevalence

◆ Approximately 0.5%–2% of the population is affected.[7]
◆ OLP tends to mostly commonly affect women between the ages of 30 and 60 years.[7]

II. Etiology

◆ May have a genetic component.
◆ Sometimes associated with other systemic diseases.
◆ Frequently associated with hepatitis C virus (HCV).

III. Clinical Presentation

◆ Six types of OLP[6]:
   • Reticular: characteristic Wickham striae: mossy, lacy white threads that are slightly raised found on the buccal mucosa (Figure 63-2).

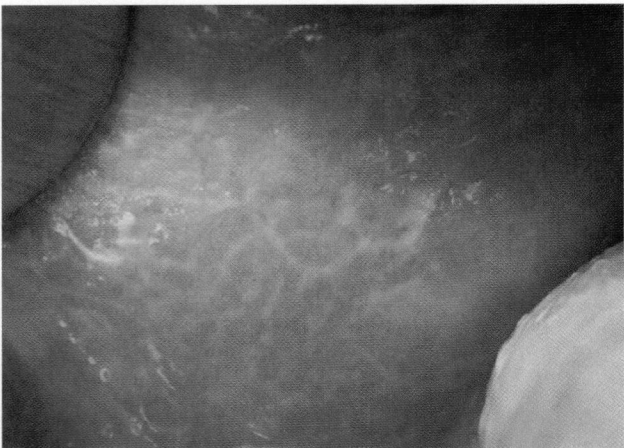

FIGURE 63-2 • Wickham Striae of Oral Lichen Planus. A white, lacy network of lesions and erosions is present on the buccal mucosa.

- Plaque-like: occurs more frequently on the dorsal surface of the tongue and may look like oral leukoplakia.
- Papular: appear as papules on the oral mucosa, especially the buccal mucosa.
- Atrophic/erosive: may resemble oral erythroleukoplakia lesion, but is typically bilateral and symmetric.
- Ulcerative: similar to erosive OLP, but there is central ulceration in the lesion.
- Bullous: bulla or a separation of the oral epithelium from the underlying connective tissue is present.
- The condition tends to have periods of remission and flare-ups.

IV. Treatment

- OLP can be definitively diagnosed with a biopsy which will also rule out the possibility of malignancy.
  - OLP can be confused with leukoplakia and lichenoid reactions which have the potential for progression to oral cancer.[6]
- There is no definitive treatment for OLP and management of symptoms is the usual approach to care.[8]
- When erosive or ulcerative lesions are present, pain is possible when eating or drinking with temperature extremes, acidic, coarse, or spicy foods.
- Symptoms may be managed by topical corticosteroids for mild and moderate symptomatic lesions.[6]
- Systemic corticosteroids, such as prednisolone, may also be needed for those with a severe outbreak of lesions.
- A healthy lifestyle of a well-balanced diet, exercise, and stress reduction may help with flare-ups.
  - Many OLP patients have deficiencies of iron, vitamin B_{12}, and folic acid; so ensuring an adequate intake and possibly supplementation may help in management.[6]
- Avoid oral risk factors for OLP such as betel quid chewing, cigarette smoking, and alcohol.[6]

V. Dental Hygiene Care

- Avoid food and drink that aggravate OLP.
- Painful lesions may limit a patient's ability to adequately remove oral biofilm.
- Palliative care for painful lesions may be required and include viscous lidocaine mouthrinses.
- For erosive or ulcerated lesions, it may be best to avoid toothpastes with pyrophosphates and mouthrinses with alcohol.

RHEUMATOID ARTHRITIS

- RA is an autoimmune disease resulting in joint inflammation and ultimately destruction of the joint and loss of cartilage.[9]
- Systematic reviews of the literature suggest an association between periodontal disease and RA possibly due to commonalities in the inflammatory processes.[10]

I. Prevalence

- The prevalence in the United States is around 55% with 1.28–1.36 million people affected by RA and continues to increase.[11]
- More than twice as many women are affected with RA when compared to men.[9]
- Peak incidence is at age 50 years.[9]

II. Etiology

- Presence of autoantibodies (rheumatoid factor) can be found even in early RA.[9]
- Genetic risk factors:
  - Genetic risk factors determine 50%–60% of the risk for RA.
  - Family history of RA triples the risk for developing RA.[9]
- Environmental risk factors:
  - Cigarette smoking has the strongest association with development of RA.[9]
  - Other environmental risk factors include: obesity, lower educational level, high birth weight, and exposure to pollutants.[9]
  - Periodontal bacteria, such as *Porphyromonas gingivalis* and *Aggregatibacter actinomycetemcomitans*, may contribute to RA autoantibody production.[12]

III. Clinical Presentation

- Swelling and pain in multiple joints for 6 weeks or more with morning stiffness lasting an hour or more.
- As joint destruction progresses, deformity with limited motion and muscle atrophy occurs in severely involved joints (Figure 63-3).
- Arthralgia is a nonspecific symptom that may be suggestive of RA.[9]

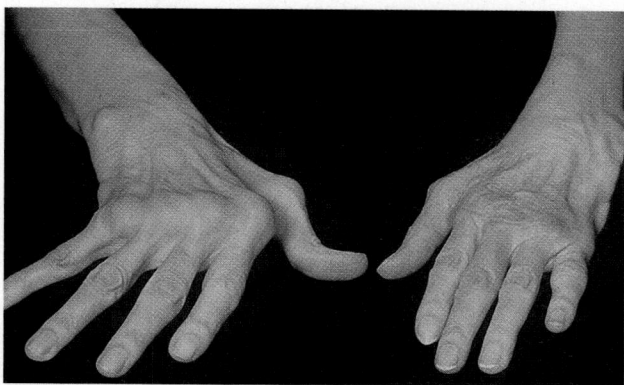

FIGURE 63-3 • Rheumatoid Arthritis. Deformity to the hands caused by rheumatoid arthritis.

- May experience weakness, loss of motor control, or difficulty making a fist.[13]
- As many as 50% of those with RA may have involvement of the temporomandibular joint (TMJ) resulting in pain, stiffness, joint sounds, and limitations in opening.[14]

IV. Treatment

- Early intervention is essential to limit destruction and progression of the disease.[9]
- Pharmacologic management includes[15]:
  - Disease modifying antirheumatic drugs (DMARDs) are the cornerstone of RA treatment and methotrexate is a first-line DMARD.
  - Corticosteroids may be used early in the disease along with DMARDs to reduce progression.
  - NSAIDs may be used over a short term.
- Nonpharmacologic management includes:
  - Consumption of a Mediterranean diet has been shown to reduce pain and improve quality of life in those with RA.[16]
  - Physical activity including cardio, muscle strength, flexibility and neuromotor exercise is recommended and may reduce pain and improve function.[17]
  - Weight loss for those who are overweight or obese.
  - Smoking cessation.

V. Dental Hygiene Care

- Although more research is needed, nonsurgical periodontal therapy to eliminate periodontal inflammation may reduce severity of RA in addition to standard medical care.[12]
- Adaptations for decreased manual dexterity may include:
  - Power toothbrushes.
  - Floss holders or interdental brushes.
  - Modification of the toothbrush handle to make it larger for easier grasp.

- Dental professionals also need to support healthy eating, weight management, and tobacco cessation.

SCLERODERMA

- Systemic scleroderma, also called systemic sclerosis, is an autoimmune disease affecting connective tissue associated with the skin, blood vessels, heart, lungs, kidneys, GI tract, and musculoskeletal system.
  - Fibrosis, or hardening, of the skin, internal organs, and vasculopathy may occur.[18]
- There are three types of systemic scleroderma[19]:
  - Limited cutaneous systemic scleroderma, also known as CREST syndrome (see Box 63-1), is the milder form of scleroderma and usually involves thick skin on the fingers and/or face.
  - Diffuse cutaneous systemic scleroderma involves large areas of the skin on the arms, legs, and trunk that are thick and tight.
  - Diffuse scleroderma affects internal organs and worsens more quickly than the other types.
  - Systemic scleroderma affects one or more internal organs, but not the skin.

I. Prevalence

- Prevalence in the United States is estimated to be 50–300 cases per million.[19]
- Women are four times more likely than men to develop scleroderma.[19]
- Diffuse scleroderma seems to occur more commonly in African American women.[20]

II. Etiology

- Genetic factors leading to the production of autoantibodies increase the risk for development of systemic scleroderma.[19,21]
- Environmental factors include[21]:
  - Infectious agents.
  - Drugs.
  - Chemicals, silica dust, and solvents.

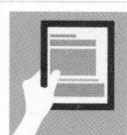

BOX 63-1
CREST Syndrome

C—calcium deposits under the skin and in tissues (calcinosis).

R—Raynaud's phenomenon.

E—esophageal dysmotility that causes heartburn, which is very common in CREST patients.

S—sclerodactyly that is thick skin on the fingers.

T—telangiectasias that appear as red spots on the face and other parts of the body.

III. Clinical Presentation

◆ Raynaud's phenomenon is one of the first clinical signs of scleroderma.[21]

   • Loss of blood supply to the fingers characterized by sensitivity to cold and change of skin color (white or clear) on fingers.

◆ GI manifestations may include[21,22]:

   • Gastroesophageal reflux disease (GERD).

   • Severe weight loss and nutrient deficiencies due to malabsorption.

◆ Skin manifestations include[21]:

   • Thickening and tightening of the skin (sclerodactyly) on the fingers and possible fingertip lesions (Figure 63-4).

   • Puffy and swollen fingers.

◆ Fatigue.[21]

◆ Organ-based manifestations may include[21]:

   • Lung fibrosis.

   • Pulmonary arterial hypertension.

   • Renal failure.

◆ More than 80% of those with systemic sclerosis experience orofacial manifestations which may include[22,23]:

   • Fibrosis of the facial skin results in a mask-like appearance.

   • Hypo- or hyperpigmentation.

   • Microstomia from sclerosis of the lips and skin around the mouth reduces the mouth opening (Figure 63-5).

   • Telangiectases result from dilation of small blood vessels in the skin and appear as small red macular areas. They may appear on the cheeks, nose, lips, and the oral mucosa.

   • Gingiva may appear pale and sclerotic.

   • Burning mouth syndrome.

   • Impaired tongue mobility due to tongue fibrosis.

   • Xerostomia due to salivary gland involvement appears in 25%–71% of cases increasing caries risk.

   • Bone resorption and TMJ involvement.

   • Individuals with systemic sclerosis have a worse measure of periodontal health including probing depths, bleeding on probing, and plaque index.

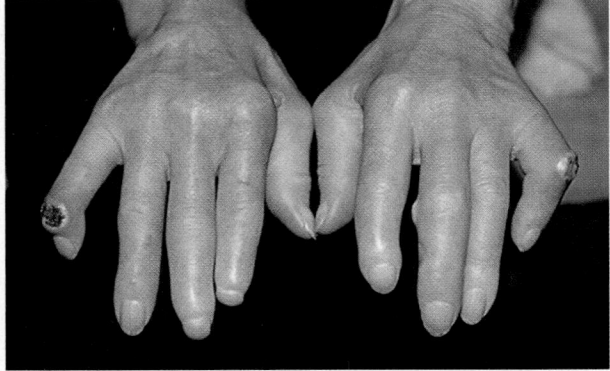

FIGURE 63-4 • Scleroderma. Hard, tight skin with ulcerations.

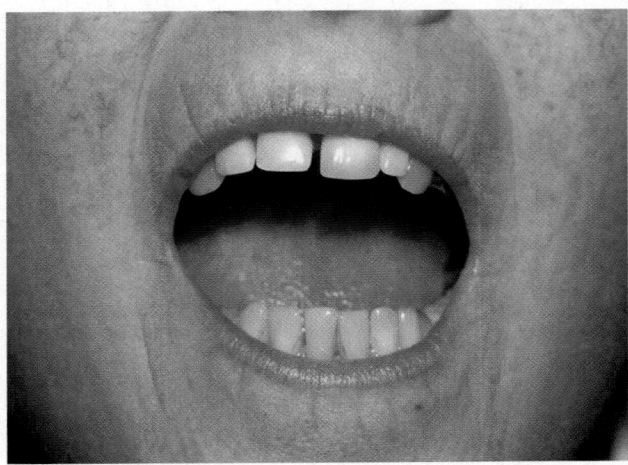

FIGURE 63-5 • Oral Manifestation of Scleroderma. Linear furrows on the lips and decreased oral aperture are common.

   • Widening of the periodontal ligament is a common radiographic finding.

   • Trigeminal neuropathy.

IV. Treatment

◆ Early diagnosis and risk assessment to determine those who may develop new organ complications is ideal to manage progression of systemic sclerosis.[24]

◆ Treatment will depend on the organ involved; so it can be quite variable.

◆ Pharmacologic management includes[24]:

   • *Raynaud's disease:* calcium channel blockers such as nifedipine.

   • *Ulcers on fingers or toes:* intravenous (IV) iloprost, phosphodiesterase type 5 inhibitors, and bosentan.

   • *Renal:* angiotensin converting enzyme inhibitors.

   • *GI:* proton pump inhibitors.

   • *Skin and lung disease:* methotrexate, cyclophosphamide (in progressive disease), hematopoietic stem cell transplantation in severe disease.

◆ Nonpharmacologic recommendations have extremely limited evidence and include[25]:

   • Physical therapy and regular physical activity, including stretching and cardio, may help keep joints flexible, including orofacial exercises to maintain and possibly improve mouth opening.

   • Dietary modifications to minimize GERD may also be helpful.

   • Protect skin from excessive dryness and cold by using multiple layers to cover skin and a humidifier to keep air moist. Creams and soaps designed for dry skin are recommended.

V. Dental Hygiene Care

◆ Tight facial skin, microstomia, and TMJ involvement may make oral self-care as well as professional care difficult due to limited mouth opening and access. Due to the challenges in providing restorative or surgical dental care, prevention of oral disease is crucial.[22,23]

- Xerostomia increases the risk of dental caries and management may include[22,23]:
  - Office and home fluorides (see Chapter 34).
  - Keep the mouth moist with saliva substitute sprays, water, saliva stimulants such as sugar-free candy and gum, and medications such as pilocarpine.
  - Recommend xylitol products sparingly as they may irritate the GI tract.
  - Avoid dental products with alcohol.
- Finger lesions and tight skin resulting in hand weakness and reduced grip strength may make oral self-care challenging; so a power toothbrush or other modifications may be needed along with more frequent continuing care (see Chapter 51).[22,23]
- Tobacco cessation is strongly recommended.[22]

GASTROINTESTINAL TRACT AUTOIMMUNE DISEASES

- Several autoimmune diseases have effects on the GI tract, but several primarily affect the GI tract through an organ-specific autoantibody.[26]
- As in other autoimmune diseases, these also have a significant genetic component moderated by environmental factors.
- A few GI tract autoimmune diseases will be reviewed in this section including celiac disease (CD), and inflammatory bowel diseases (IBD): Crohn's disease and ulcerative colitis (UC).[26]

CELIAC DISEASE

- CD results in damage to the villi of the small intestine with exposure to dietary gluten.
- Inflammation and destruction of the intestinal villi result in chronic malabsorption of nutrients such as iron, folic acid, fat-soluble vitamins, and vitamin B_{12}.[26]

I. Prevalence

- Prevalence in the United States is estimated to be 0.7%.[27]
- Occurs more frequently in women and non-Hispanic whites.[28]
- CD is five times more common in individuals living in northern latitudes of 35°–39° of the United States versus southern latitudes.[27]
  - This could be related to differences in vitamin D levels which is involved in modulating the immune response in CD.

II. Etiology

- Genetic predisposition:
  - A first-degree family member increases the risk of CD as does having more than one family member with CD.[28]

- Environmental factors[28]:
  - Gluten is the primary trigger.
  - CD is more common in individuals with type 1 diabetes mellitus.
  - Higher education level and socioeconomic status are associated with CD; however, the reason for this association is unclear.[27]

III. Clinical Presentation

- Some individuals may have no symptoms.
- GI symptoms include: diarrhea, steatorrhea, weight loss, bloating, flatulence, and abdominal pain.[28]
  - Oral symptoms may include oral aphthous ulcers and discolored teeth or developmental enamel abnormalities.[28]
- Non-GI abnormalities may include: abnormal liver function tests, iron deficiency anemia, bone disease, skin disorders, thyroid disease, and many other atypical manifestations.[28]

IV. Treatment

- The only effective treatment is a gluten free diet.[28]
  - Dietary sources of gluten include wheat, barley, rye, and sometimes oats dependent on processing.
  - Referral to a registered dietitian/nutritionist specializing in CD is recommended.[28]
- Management of nutrient deficiencies is essential to minimize long-term consequences such low bone mass.

V. Dental Hygiene Care

- Children with enamel defects and aphthous ulcers should be referred for evaluation for possible undiagnosed CD.[29]
- Little research has been done on recurrent aphthous ulcers (RAU) in adults with CD, but patients with RAU may want to be evaluated for possible CD.
- Malabsorption of nutrients may result in angular cheilosis and glossitis; so continued support for a healthy diet should be provided by the dental hygienist.[30]
  - In children, malabsorption may result in delayed growth including tooth eruption and malocclusion so they may need referral to an orthodontist for evaluation.
- Typically, dental products do not contain gluten, but care should be taken to ensure gluten free products are used.
- Palliative treatment of oral lesions with mouthrinses containing lidocaine and possibly topical steroids.
- Assist the patient in tobacco cessation (see Chapter 32).

CROHN'S DISEASE

- Crohn's disease is a chronic, progressive, destructive inflammatory condition impacting any part of the GI tract from the mouth to the anus.

I. Prevalence

- ◆ Prevalence estimates in the United States are that 1.3% or about 3 million individuals have a diagnosis of Crohn's disease.[31]
- ◆ Slight higher prevalence in women.[31]
- ◆ More common in those of Ashkenazi Jewish origin.

II. Etiology

- ◆ Genetic predisposition:
  - • 10%–25% of those with Crohn's disease have a first-degree relative diagnosed with the disease.[31]
- ◆ Environmental triggers include[31,32]:
  - • Smoking not only doubles the risk of Crohn's disease, but may also lead to a more aggressive form of the disease.
  - • Antibiotic use increases the odds nearly three-fold of developing Crohn's disease.
  - • Oral contraceptives.
  - • Diet triggers seem to include high animal protein intake and high linoleic acid intake which may impact the gut microbiome.
- ◆ Protective factors include[32]:
  - • Breastfeeding for at least 12 months seems to provide a protective effect.
  - • High dietary zinc, fiber, and fish intake.

III. Clinical Presentation

- ◆ Hallmark symptoms include[31,33]:
  - • Abdominal pain.
  - • Chronic diarrhea.
  - • Nausea and vomiting.
  - • Weight loss.
  - • Growth failure in children/adolescents.
  - • Fever.
  - • Fatigue: may be a result of anemia or other nutrient deficiencies along with the effect from the body of trying to manage the inflammation.
  - • Iron deficiency.
- ◆ Extraintestinal manifestations may include: osteonecrosis, metabolic bone disease, ankylosing spondylitis, etc.[33]
- ◆ Orofacial manifestations (Figure 63-6)[34]:
  - • Diffuse labial and buccal swelling.
  - • Hyperplastic plaques on the buccal mucosa with a cobblestone appearance.
  - • Mucosal tissue tags.
  - • Deep linear ulcerations.
  - • Aphthous ulcers which are shallow round or oval as compared to the linear ulcerations previously mentioned.
  - • Prevalence of periodontitis may be higher.
  - • Angular cheilitis and/or glossitis due to nutritional deficiencies.

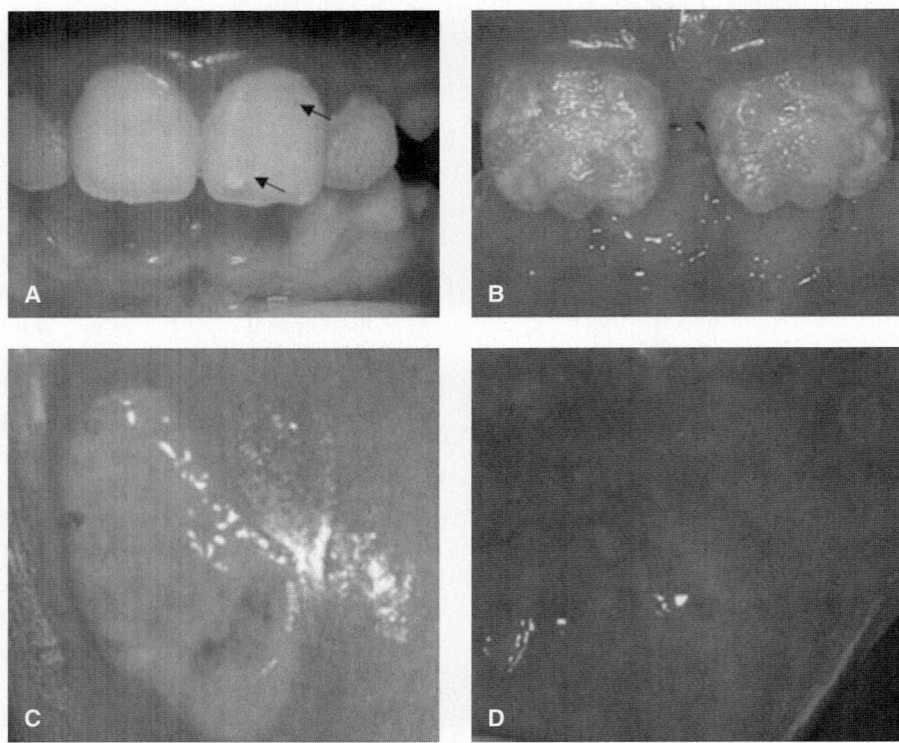

FIGURE 63-6 • Dental Enamel Hypoplasia in Celiac Disease. A: Enamel defects of upper incisors (arrows indicate the color changes). **B:** Enamel defects of upper incisors (structural changes). **C:** Major types of recurrent aphthous stomatitis. **D:** Numerous minor-type lesions of recurrent aphthous stomatitis. (Reproduced from Campisi G. Oral pathology in untreated coeliac disease. *Aliment Pharmacol Ther.* 2007;26:1529-1536.)

- Crohn's disease may be associated with other autoimmune conditions such as CD, RA, and MS.[33]
- Bowel obstructions may also occur and require surgical intervention.

IV. Treatment

- Treatment depends on the severity, location, and subtype of Crohn's disease and can be complex.[31,33]
  - Remission and maintenance of remission is a goal of the treatment.
- Pharmacologic therapies may include:
  - Methotrexate, azathioprine, and 6-mercaptopurine may be used for active Crohn's disease.
  - Biologic therapies like antitumor necrosis factor (anti-TNF) have been most effective in moderate-to-severe Crohn's disease and in maintenance.[31,33]
- Surgical intervention:
  - Eighty percent of those with long-term Crohn's disease will require surgery and many may require multiple surgeries over their lifetime.[31,33]

V. Dental Hygiene Care

- Avoid use of NSAIDs as they may exacerbate disease activity.
- Encourage and assist with tobacco cessation (see Chapter 32).
- Quality of life may be impacted by stress, anxiety, and depression in those with IBD and referral to a mental health specialist may be necessary.[33]
- Working closely with the interprofessional team providing care is important to manage oral health given the complexity of the disease.
- Dietary assessment and counseling may be indicated if frequency of sugar intake impacts caries risk and to support adequate intake of nutrients (see Chapter 33).[34]
- Palliative treatment of oral lesions as needed to relieve pain which may include a topical agent or mouthrinse with lidocaine and/or topical steroids.[34]
- Management of oral biofilm is essential to manage caries and periodontal risk.
- Optimal use of home and office fluorides to manage caries risk (see Chapter 34).

ULCERATIVE COLITIS

- UC is an autoimmune IBD affecting primarily the colon.

I. Prevalence

- More common in industrialized countries, particularly North America and Western Europe.[35]
- Prevalence is about 7.6–245 cases per 100,000 per year.[35]
- Tends to present during ages 20–30 years.[35]
- Slightly more common in men.

II. Etiology

- Genetic disposition[34,35]:
  - Family history increases risk 10- to 15-fold.
  - More common in those of Jewish origin.
- Environmental risk triggers may include[32,35]:
  - Alterations of the gut microbiome.
  - Possible infectious agent.
  - Being a former smoker.
  - Hormone replacement therapy and oral contraceptive use.
  - Higher dose and long-term use of NSAIDs.
- Protective factors include[32]:
  - Breastfeeding for at least 12 months appears to reduce the risk.
  - High intake of omega-3 fatty acids.

III. Clinical Presentation

- Intestinal symptoms include[35]:
  - Bloody diarrhea.
  - Abdominal pain/cramps.
- Extraintestinal manifestations may include[35]:
  - Colitis-associated arthritis is the most common.
  - Skin lesions.
  - Liver conditions including portal hypertension and cirrhosis.
  - Optic neuritis.
  - Osteoporosis.
  - Reduced growth in children.
  - Increased risk for colorectal cancer.
- Orofacial manifestations include[34]:
  - Pyostomatitis vegetans which consists of multiple small yellow and white pustules on an erythematous and edematous mucosal base (Figure 63-7).
  - Aphthous ulcers.

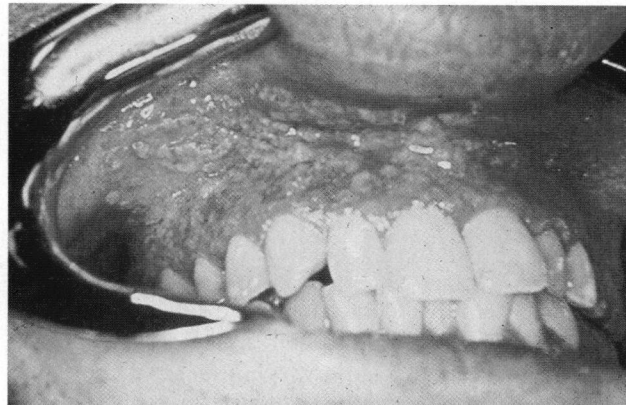

FIGURE 63-7 • Pyostomatitis Vegetans. Multiple small white pustules on mucosa with erythematosus. (From Corman ML, Veidenheimer MC, Nugent FW, et al. *Diseases of the Anus, Rectum and Colon. Part II: Non-Specific Inflammatory Bowel Disease.* New York, NY: Medcom; 1976.)

- Gingivitis and periodontitis.
- Possible taste changes.

IV. Treatment

- Treatment depends on the severity and extent of the disease and continues to evolve.
- Pharmacologic therapy[36]:
  - Mild to moderate UC: medication such as oral aminosalicylates, topical mesalamine, or topical steroids.
  - With more extensive mild to moderate UC the following may be used: corticosteroids, IV monoclonal antibody to TNF.
  - Severe UC: IV steroids and colectomy may be necessary if pharmacologic approaches fail or the patient experiences toxicity.
- Surgical treatment may be required.
- Nonpharmacologic recommendations[37]:
  - Monitor for depression and anxiety.
  - Increased risk for cancers including colon, cervical, melanoma, and nonmelanoma requires regular screening.
  - Monitor bone health for steroid-induced osteoporosis.
  - It is important for an individual with UC to keep their vaccinations current due to immunosuppression.

V. Dental Hygiene Care

- Palliative treatment for oral lesions to help reduce discomfort, that is, 2% viscous lidocaine or a steroid gel.[34]
- Avoid prescribing NSAIDs as they may trigger a flare-up of the UC.[34]
- Education to enhance dental biofilm removal along with regular preventive services and periodontal maintenance are essential due to the increased risk for periodontal disease.

NEUROLOGIC SYSTEM AUTOIMMUNE DISEASES

- Autoimmune conditions affect the central nervous system which may include the brain, spinal cord, and/or peripheral nervous system.

MULTIPLE SCLEROSIS

- MS is a chronic demyelinating disease of the central nervous system characterized by progressive disability with motor, sensory, cognitive, and emotional changes.[38]

I. Prevalence

- Affects an estimated 100 per 100,000 persons in the United States and 2–3 million worldwide.[38]

- Prevalence tends to be higher in North American and northern European countries.
- Usually adult onset occurs between 20 and 50 years of age, may occur in children up to age 18 and older adults as well.[38]
- Prevalence higher among Caucasians.[38]
  - However, in Hispanic and black Americans with MS, the disease tends to progress faster.
- Higher incidence in females than males.[38]

II. Etiology

- Genetic predisposition has a significant role in the development of MS.[38]
- Environmental factors include[38]:
  - Vitamin D deficiency.
  - Obesity in early life results in a two-fold increase in risk.
  - Smoking.
  - Exposure to infectious agents.

III. Clinical Presentation

A. Clinical Forms of MS

There are four clinical forms of MS and relapsing–remitting accounts for 85% of cases.[39]

- *Relapsing–remitting*: acute episodes worsening with some recovery over weeks to months with no changes in neurologic functioning between attacks.
- *Secondary progressive*: gradual neurologic deterioration with or without superimposed acute relapses in a patient.
- *Primary progressive*: gradual, nearly continuous neurologic deterioration from the onset of symptoms.
- *Progressive relapsing*: gradual neurologic deterioration from the onset of symptoms but with subsequent superimposed relapses (uncommon).

B. Symptoms

- MS can affect any area of the brain, optic nerve, or spinal cord and cause a wide variety of neurologic signs and symptoms (Figure 63-8). Symptoms fluctuate, and several years may elapse between bouts of symptoms.
- Symptoms may include[38]:
  - Initial symptoms often fluctuate: transient difficulty in coordination, tremor, or fatigue.
  - May have a sudden onset with paralysis or marked weakness of one or more extremities.
  - Sensory changes.
  - Changes in bowel or bladder function.
  - Involuntary motion of eyes (nystagmus); the individual may later become partially or completely blind.
  - Speech disorders; dysarthria and possible loss of speech in the advanced stages.
  - Changes in muscular coordination and gait; loss of balance; spasms.

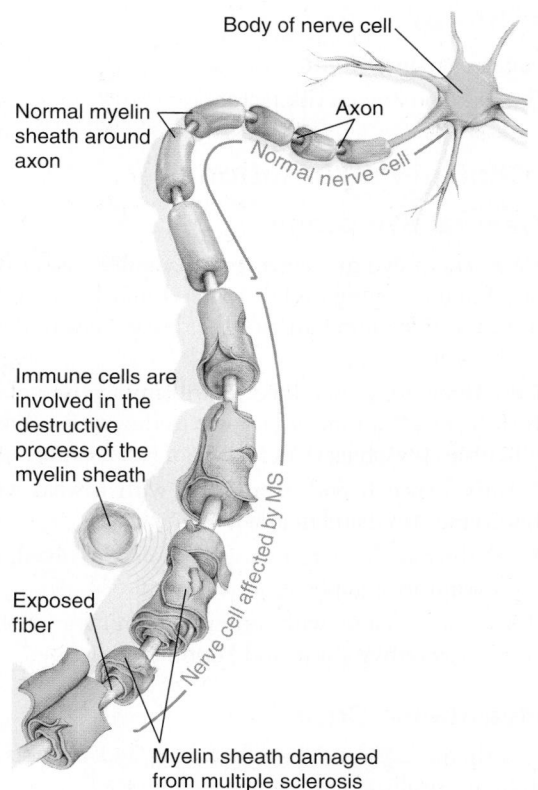

Body of nerve cell

Axon

Normal myelin sheath around axon

Normal nerve cell

Immune cells are involved in the destructive process of the myelin sheath

Nerve cell affected by MS

Exposed fiber

Myelin sheath damaged from multiple sclerosis

FIGURE 63-8 • Multiple Sclerosis. Nerve cell damage.

- Susceptibility to infection, particularly upper respiratory.
- Cognitive impairment.
- Depression.
- Orofacial manifestations[40]:
  - TMJ disorder.
  - Facial palsy.
  - Trigeminal neuralgia usually is bilateral.
  - Dysphagia.
  - In females, there is twice the risk of periodontal disease.[41]
  - Immunosuppressants may result in aphthous ulcers and opportunistic infections such as *Candida*.
- Course of Disease:
  - *Relapses and remissions:* An attack may last several days or weeks and be followed by a symptom-free period. The condition worsens with each relapse.
  - *Longevity:* Close to normal life span; approximately 80% have functional limitations after 15 years.

IV. Treatment

- Diagnosis is based on history, clinical, imaging (magnetic resonance imaging), and laboratory findings.[38]
- Prompt diagnosis and early treatment are crucial to deter neurologic damage.[38]
- Pharmacologic therapy includes a wide range of medications, but only eight have been U.S. Food and Drug Administration approved (Box 63-2).[39]

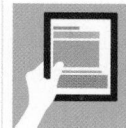

BOX 63-2
Medications Used to Treat Multiple Sclerosis

Generic Name	Brand Names	Drug Action
Interferon beta 1a/1b	Rebif Avonex Betaseron Extavia	Reduces relapse rate, decreases progression and disability, and MRI evidence of disease progression.
Glatiramer acetate	Copaxone Gilenya	Reduces or prevents relapse.
Monoclonal antibodies (natalizumab and rituximab*)	Tysabri Rituxan	Reduces rate of relapse and disability.
Cytotoxic agents (mitoxantrone, cyclophosphamide*, azathioprine*, methotrexate*, and mycophenolate mofetil*)	Novantrone	Immunosuppression, these are not the first-line agents for use in MS.
Methylprednisolone*		Potent anti-inflammatory effects and used in acute relapses.
IV immunoglobulin		Decrease in relapse rate, improved disability scores, and reduces deterioration.
Cladribine*		Lower relapse rate and reduction in MRI evidence of MS activity.

*Used off label or pending FDA approval.
MRI: magnetic resonance imaging; MS: multiple sclerosis; IV: intravenous; FDA: U.S. Food and Drug Administration.
Source: Loma I, Heyman R. Multiple sclerosis: pathogenesis and treatment. *Curr Neuropharmacol.* 2011;9(3):409-416.

- Although some disease modifying medications such as steroids are used, there is no evidence supporting their effectiveness in reducing the progression of MS.[38]
- In addition, medications to treat the various symptoms such as bladder dysfunction may be required.
- Nonpharmacologic recommendations include[42]:
  - Exercise, physiotherapy, and hydrotherapy.
  - Occupational therapy may be necessary to assist in the management of activities of daily living as disability progresses.
  - Cognitive and behavioral therapy.
  - Tobacco cessation.
  - Vitamin D supplementation as needed to bring levels to normal.

- A plant-based, anti-inflammatory diet rich in vegetables, fruit, whole grains, low-fat dairy, high fiber foods, lean proteins, and omega-3 fatty acids is suggested although evidence is limited.
  - Maintenance of a healthy weight.
  - Management of mental health and stress.
- Some individuals with MS will try alternative medicine approaches and special diets that may not have good evidence of benefit and may cause harm such as malnutrition.

V. Dental Hygiene Care

Factors to consider when planning dental hygiene care for a patient with MS include:

- Medical consultation needs to be the first step to determine patient readiness for dental care.[40]
  - Immunosuppressants and other MS medications used may result in neutropenia; so a white blood cell count is essential prior to care.
  - If a patient has been on steroids over a long term, they may need additional steroids to prevent an adrenal crisis.
- Palliative treatment for symptom relief for oral lesions such as mouthrinses with viscous lidocaine or topical steroid agents.
- Orofacial manifestations, such as intermittent headaches, facial pain, numbness, palsy, and spasms.
- Oral self-care education will need to be individualized based on patient needs and oral condition.
  - Visual disturbances and changes in motor function may impact the ability to adequately manage dental biofilm.
- Prevention will be recommended based on the risk for oral disease such as home and office fluorides (see Chapter 34), diet counseling (see Chapter 33).
- Oral and systemic effects of medications used for treatment may require management, such as candidiasis.
- The increased risk for periodontal disease may require more frequent continuing care appointments, particularly if the patient is having issues with motor function.

MYASTHENIA GRAVIS

- Myasthenia gravis is an autoimmune neuromuscular disease characterized by weakness and abnormal fatigability due to defective transmission of nerve impulses to the skeletal muscles.[43]

I. Prevalence

- Prevalence of individuals with the condition is around 200 per million individuals in the United States.[43]
- Early onset before the age of 50 years tends to occur more frequently in women. Between ages 50 and 60 there is no difference between genders, but in those over age 60 the condition is more common in men.[43]

II. Etiology

- Genetic predisposition.
- There are no known risk factors.

III. Clinical Presentation

A. General Symptoms

- Weakness of eye movements with double vision (diplopia) and drooping eyelids (ptosis) may be the initial indicator. In certain patients, the disease may not progress further.[44]
- If the disease is generalized, it will involve muscles of the face, mastication, and tongue leading to swallowing difficulties (dysphagia) and a lack of facial expression.[44]
- Disturbed speech and expression, with a weak voice that sounds tired and muffled, are typical.
- When the muscles of respiration become involved, serious respiratory complications can result.[44]
- May be associated with other autoimmune diseases such as hyperthyroidism and Hashimoto disease.[43]

B. Myasthenic Crisis

- Myasthenic crisis is life-threatening and impacts the ability to swallow and respiratory muscles.[44]
- This is an emergency and **911** must be called immediately and basic life support (see Chapter 9) provided until medical assistance arrives.

IV. Treatment

- Pharmacologic therapy may include[44]:
  - Anticholinesterase agents are used to improve neuromuscular transmission and increase muscle strength.
  - Immunosuppressive medications include corticosteroids, azathioprine (when corticosteroids are contraindicated), and cyclosporine.
- Surgical treatment:
  - Therapy for attempting to induce remission can include surgical removal of the thymus gland, particularly if a tumor of the gland develops, and drug therapy is ineffective.

V. Dental Hygiene Care

Factors to consider when planning dental hygiene care for the patient with myasthenia gravis[45]:

- Schedule short dental or dental hygiene appointments in the morning when the patient may not be as fatigued.
- Consultation with the medical provider may be necessary to determine the safety of providing care for the patient.
- Use anxiety management strategies to keep the patient calm to minimize the risk of myasthenic crisis.

◆ Risk for choking may require adjustment of the dental chair to a semi-upright position and minimal use of water to avoid aspiration.

◆ A mouth prop may help the individual who has difficulty holding the mouth open for treatment.

◆ Allow for rest periods.

◆ Speech difficulties may compromise the patient's ability to communicate.

◆ Because of the lack of facial expression, distress may be difficult for the patient to convey.

◆ Due to fatigue and muscle weakness, the patient may have difficulty performing adequate dental biofilm removal.

  • A power toothbrush and dividing the mouth into multiple sessions when performing oral self-care may be helpful.

  • The patient may need to support the hand with the toothbrush either by leaning on a counter or possibly an assistive device of which a number are available (see Chapter 51).

◆ More frequent preventive care may be needed depending on the patient's motor abilities and oral health status.

SYSTEMIC AUTOIMMUNE DISEASES

◆ In systemic autoimmune diseases, autoantibodies affect various tissues throughout the body causing destruction.

SJÖGREN'S SYNDROME

◆ Sjogren's syndrome (SS) is a chronic, systemic autoimmune disease in which autoantibodies attack healthy cells in the exocrine glands followed by many other organs.

  • Exocrine glands are responsible for producing moisture for the mouth, eyes, nose, throat, and skin.

I. Prevalence

◆ Primary SS prevalence globally is estimated to be 62 per 100,000 individuals.[46]

◆ The ratio of female to male individuals with SS is 10.72:1.[46]

II. Etiology

◆ Genetic predisposition: 20-fold higher risk for SS if a first-degree relative is affected.[47]

◆ Environmental trigger[47]:

  • Viral infection of the glands such as HCV and Epstein–Barr virus.

III. Clinical Presentation

◆ Glandular manifestations include[48,49]:

  • Dry eyes.
  • Parotid enlargement.

• Dry mouth (xerostomia): reduced quantity and quality of saliva.
• Angular cheilitis.

◆ Extraglandular manifestations include:

  • Lungs: recurrent bronchitis or pneumonia, pulmonary fibrosis, and chronic dry cough.
  • Kidney: glomerulonephritis.
  • Liver.
  • Skin: xeroderma (dry skin), urticaria (rashes), etc.
  • Rheumatologic: myalgia (muscle pain), arthralgia (joint pain), and Raynaud's phenomenon.
  • Peripheral neuropathy.
  • GI: esophageal dysmotility, GERD, etc.
  • Fatigue.

◆ Dental manifestations:

  • Increased caries risk.
  • Increased biofilm accumulations with higher numbers of cariogenic bacteria.
  • Oral candidiasis.

IV. Treatment

◆ Pharmacologic therapy may include[49]:

  • Artificial tears/saliva, gels, and ointments.
  • DMARDS may include methotrexate, short-or long-term corticosteroids, hydroxychloroquine, cyclosporine, etc.
  • Biologic therapies such as TNF-α inhibitors.

◆ Nonpharmacologic recommendations may include[49]:

  • Physical activity to reduce fatigue.

V. Dental Hygiene Care

◆ An interprofessional approach to care is needed to manage SS and improve the patient's overall quality of life.

◆ Oral self-care education to aid the patient in developing optimal dental biofilm removal is crucial to manage the risk for oral disease.

◆ Assess dietary intake and counsel on minimizing intake of fermentable carbohydrates, particularly between meals (see Chapter 33).

◆ Recommend sugar-free chewing gum, mints, or hard candy containing xylitol for salivary stimulation.

◆ Saliva substitutes with glycerol may help the mouth feel moist.[48]

◆ Encourage the patient to carry a water bottle to aid in relieving mouth dryness.

◆ Antifungal rinse or lozenges for oral candidiasis.

◆ Recommend at-home fluoride therapy which may include rinses, gels (see Chapter 34). Custom fluoride trays or mouthguard may also be considered.[49]

◆ Avoid use of toothpaste with pyrophosphates or sodium laurel sulfate.[48]

◆ Antimicrobial rinse such as chlorhexidine may aid in managing caries risk.[49]

◆ Non-fluoride remineralizing preparations with calcium phosphate may aid in reducing caries risk.[49]

◆ More frequent continuing care may be required to maintain oral health.

SYSTEMIC LUPUS ERYTHEMATOSUS

SLE is a chronic autoimmune disease causing widespread inflammation which can affect internal organs and glands by causing tissue damage (Figure 63-9).

I. Prevalence

◆ Prevalence globally varies from 9 to 241 per 100,000 individuals.[50]

◆ In the United States prevalence varies from 80 to 103 per 100,000 indivduals.[50]

  • In some populations like American Indian and Alaska Native groups the prevalence is 178 per 100,000.

◆ The female to male ratio varies across the lifespan from 7 to 15:1.[50]

◆ Hispanic and South/East Asian populations tend to experience more severe disease and organ damage.[50]

II. Etiology

◆ Genetic predisposition imparts about 40%–50% of the risk for SLE.[50]

◆ Environmental risks may include[50]:

  • Smoking.
  • Endometriosis.
  • Moderate alcohol consumption (≥ 5g or half a drink per day).
  • Silica exposure.

◆ Possible environmental triggers needing more research include[50]:

  • Low vitamin D status.
  • Air pollution.
  • Diet impact on the gut microbiome.
  • Infectious agents such as Epstein–Barr virus.

III. Clinical Presentation

◆ Skin manifestations include[52]:

  • Butterfly-shaped rash on nose and cheeks (malar rash) (Figure 63-10).
  • Erythema on skin exposed to sun (photosensitivity).
  • Alopecia (hair loss).
  • Raynaud's phenomenon.

◆ Oral lesions may include[50,51]:

  • Oral discoid lesions (Figure 63-11).
  • Petechia-like lesions.
  • Gingival bleeding such as desquamative gingivitis.
  • Erosive mucosal lesions in as many as 40% of individuals.

◆ Arthritis: joint pain, tenderness, swelling, and morning stiffness.[52]

◆ Lung involvement: pleuritis.

◆ Renal disorder: high creatinine/protein in urine.[52]

◆ Neurologic disorders: neuropathy, seizure disorder, etc.[52]

◆ Hematologic disorder: hemolytic anemia, leukopenia, and thrombocytopenia.[52]

◆ Immunologic changes: positive blood test for antinuclear antibodies.[52]

◆ Neuropsychiatric disorders: anxiety, mood disorder, psychosis, cognitive dysfunction.[52]

◆ Fatigue.

IV. Treatment

◆ Management is complex and requires an interprofessional team with the goal to control disease activity and prevent organ damage.

◆ Pharmacologic therapy may include[51]:

  • NSAIDs.

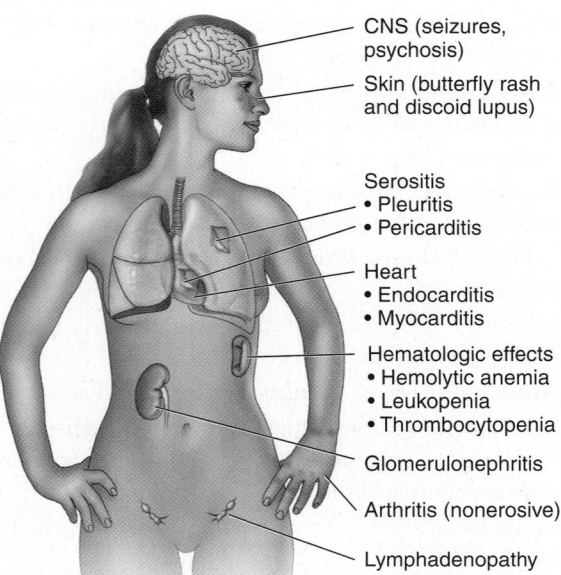

CNS (seizures, psychosis)

Skin (butterfly rash and discoid lupus)

Serositis
• Pleuritis
• Pericarditis

Heart
• Endocarditis
• Myocarditis

Hematologic effects
• Hemolytic anemia
• Leukopenia
• Thrombocytopenia

Glomerulonephritis

Arthritis (nonerosive)

Lymphadenopathy

FIGURE 63-9 • Systemic Lupus Erythematosus: Systemic Effects.

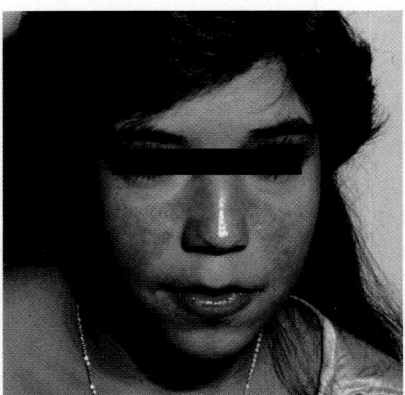

FIGURE 63-10 • Systemic Lupus Erythematosus. This young girl has the classic "butterfly" rash of lupus.

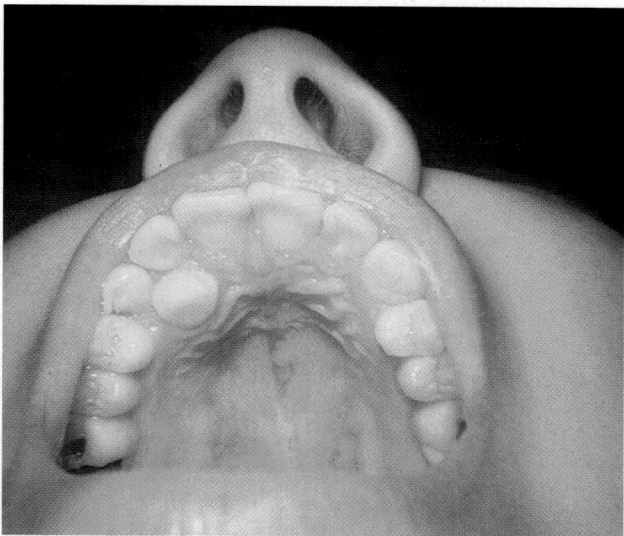

FIGURE 63-11 • Systemic Lupus Erythematosus. The dental professional may be the first to observe the manifestations of some autoimmune disorders because they may present in the oral cavity prior to any cutaneous manifestations. Ulceration is present on the hard palate in this individual with systemic lupus erythematosus. (From Goodheart HP. *Goodheart's Photoguide of Common Skin Disorders.* 2nd ed. Philadelphia, PA: Lippincott Williams & Wilkins, 2003.)

- Antimalarial drugs believed to help reduce lupus related symptoms of joint pain, rashes, fatigue, and mouth sores.
- Corticosteroids.
- Immunosuppressive therapy such as azathioprine and cyclosporine.
- Biologic agents such as belimumab.
♦ Nonpharmacologic recommendations include:
  - Protection from ultraviolet radiation.
  - Stress management such as meditation.
  - Physical activity.
  - Psychological interventions to improve coping abilities and any mental neuropsychiatric conditions.
  - Acupuncture.
  - Healthy diet.
  - Achieve and maintain a healthy weight.

V. Dental Hygiene Care

♦ Consultation with the interprofessional team is crucial to assess the level of immune suppression and any possible risks for dental care.

♦ Periodontal health must be carefully monitored due to the risk for steroid inducing bone loss with long-term use of corticosteroids.

♦ Oral self-care education to aid the patient in optimal daily dental biofilm removal for management of gingivitis.

♦ Preventive services based on oral disease risk and medications which may include office/home fluorides (see Chapter 34), diet counseling (see Chapter 33), saliva substitutes, etc.

♦ For patients with mobility and dexterity issues due to SLE-associated arthritis modifications to oral self-care techniques and oral health aids (see Chapter 51) may be required.

♦ For oral lesions, palliative treatment may be necessary such as viscous lidocaine.

♦ Tobacco cessation (see Chapter 32).

DOCUMENTATION

♦ Record the chief complaint and compare findings with previous recordings which may include intra and extraoral examinations, digital photos, and periodontal assessment.

♦ The patient with an autoimmune disease must provide their thorough health history including any symptoms that may be affecting their oral health.

♦ Review all medications and document any oral side effects.

♦ Carefully document the medical providers' patient care recommendations.

♦ Record recommendations for oral self-care and treatment provided.

♦ An example documentation may be reviewed in Box 63-3.

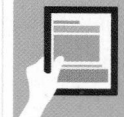

BOX 63-3
Example Documentation: Patient with Autoimmune Disease

S—A 52-year-old female patient arrives in the dental office for an appointment for hygiene care. It has been 3 years since her last prophylaxis and reports her teeth feel "dirty and my gums bleed when I brush."

O—Medical history reveals diagnosis of rheumatoid arthritis 8 years ago. Medications include corticosteroids to help with joint inflammation. Patient states she cannot grasp a toothbrush or floss due to her contralateral joint pain. Biofilm scores greater than 50%.

A—A comprehensive periodontal and caries examination including a complete mouth radiographic series indicates generalized stage II grade B periodontitis with heavy calculus, plaque, and bleeding.

P—The dental hygiene care plan includes quadrant NSPT with local anesthetic. Patient education includes a thorough explanation of periodontal disease and why NSPT is recommended. Oral hygiene instruction is reviewed and tailored to help with toothbrush and flossing dexterity. A power brush is recommended with a modification to the handle to make it larger and easier to grasp. Floss holders are also demonstrated to help with interproximal access. Patient will return to begin NSPT.

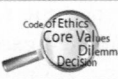

EVERYDAY ETHICS

Mary reluctantly arrives for her appointment with a hygienist. She knows she is overdue and is not looking forward to the embarrassment of admitting her fears and difficulties with her oral care. It has been her dream to have beautiful teeth, but since her autoimmune disease diagnosis, she has had chronic pain in her joints that has prevented her from being able to take care of herself the way she would like. Mary is also fearful because she has had some of her friends tell her she should not have her teeth "scraped under the gums" because it is very painful.

Teri, Mary's dental hygienist, greets Mary with a smile and welcomes her into her operatory. Teri encourages Mary to share her concerns regarding treatment and acknowledges Mary's autoimmune disease noted in the health history. Mary tells Teri she does not want her teeth "scraped under the gums." Upon evaluation of the radiographs, Teri identifies generalized heavy subgingival calculus with moderate bone loss. Upon clinical assessment, Teri confirms Mary will need quadrant nonsurgical periodontal therapy to treat her oral condition due to generalized moderate clinical attachment loss. Teri thinks about how she will address Mary's fears and her oral disease.

Questions for Consideration

1. Which dental hygiene core values will Teri have to consider in this scenario?

2. Mary has told Teri she does not want to have her teeth scaled subgingivally. Which dental hygiene core value does Teri have to consider when presenting the dental hygiene care plan? Why?

3. Discuss how core values veracity and fidelity in this scenario must be addressed by Teri and how applying those to Mary's education may lead to a better treatment outcome for Mary.

Factors to Teach the Patient

▶ Maintain recommended re-care intervals to keep biofilm at a low level.

▶ Stay connected with autoimmune disease specialists to help control symptoms.

▶ What are the autoimmune disease specific oral manifestations?
  • For example: Wickham striae, xerostomia, candidiasis, mouth ulcers.

▶ What can be done at home to reduce symptoms?
  • For example: reduce stress, maintain a healthy weight, stop smoking and alcohol consumption.

▶ How to adapt preventive aids to help with dexterity and access.

▶ The dental office is a safe place to share concerns and ask questions.

ENHANCE YOUR UNDERSTANDING

ONLINE RESOURCES
(see the inside front cover for access information)
• Audio glossary
• Appendices

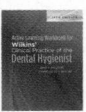

SUPPORT FOR LEARNING
(available separately)
• *Active Learning Workbook for Wilkins' Clinical Practice of the Dental Hygienist, 13th Edition*

INDIVIDUALIZED REVIEW
• Customized practice quizzing with Navigate 2 TestPrep for *Wilkins' Clinical Practice of the Dental Hygienist*

References

1. Cooper GS, Bynum ML, Somers EC. Recent insights in the epidemiology of autoimmune diseases: improved prevalence estimates and understanding of clustering of diseases. *J Autoimmun.* 2009;33(3-4):197-207.

2. Hayter SM, Cook MC. Updated assessment of the prevalence, spectrum and case definition of autoimmune disease. *Autoimmun Rev.* 2012;11(10):754-765.

3. Ngo ST, Steyn FJ, McCombe PA. Gender differences in autoimmune disease. *Front Neuroendocrinol.* 2014;35(3):347-369.

4. Wang L, Wang FS, Gershwin ME. Human autoimmune diseases: a comprehensive update. *J Intern Med.* 2015;278(4):369-395.

5. Jog NR, James JA. Biomarkers in connective tissue diseases. *J Allergy Clin Immunol.* 2017;140(6):1473-1483.

6. Chiang CP, Yu-Fong Chang J, Wang YP, Wu YH, Lu SY, Sun A. Oral lichen planus—differential diagnoses, serum autoantibodies, hematinic deficiencies, and management. *J Formos Med Assoc.* 2018;117(9):756-765.

7. Alrashdan MS, Cirillo N, McCullough M. Oral lichen planus: a literature review and update. *Arch Dermatol Res.* 2016;308(8):539-551.

8. Cheng S, Kirtschig G, Cooper S, Thornhill M, Leonardi-Bee J, Murphy R. Interventions for erosive lichen planus affecting mucosal sites. *Cochrane Database Syst Rev.* 2012;(2):CD008092.

9. Van der Woude D, van der Helm-Van M. Update on the epidemiology, risk factors, and disease outcomes of rheumatoid arthritis. *Best Pract Res Clin Rheumatol.* 2018;32(2):174-187.

10. Kaur S, White S, Bartold PM. Periodontal disease and rheumatoid arthritis: a systematic review. *J Dent Res.* 2013;92(5):399-408.

11. Hunter TM, Boytsov NN, Zhang X, Schroeder K, Michaud K, Araujo AB. Prevalence of rheumatoid arthritis in the United States adult population in healthcare claims databases, 2004-2014. *Rheumatol Int.* 2017;37(9):1551-1557.

12. Cheng Z, Meade J, Mankia K, Emery P, Devine DA. Periodontal disease and periodontal bacteria as triggers for rheumatoid arthritis. *Best Pract Res Clin Rheumatol.* 2017;31(1):19-30.

13. Jutley GS, Latif ZP, Raza K. Symptoms in individuals at risk of rheumatoid arthritis. *Best Pract Res Clin Rheumatol.* 2017;31(1):59-70.

14. Rehan OM, Saleh HAK, Raffat HA, Abu-Taleb NS. Osseous changes in the temporomandibular joint in rheumatoid arthritis: a cone-beam computed tomography study. *Imaging Sci Dent.* 2018;48(1):1-9.

15. Lau CS, Chia F, Harrison A, et al; Asia Pacific League of Associations for Rheumatology. APLAR rheumatoid arthritis treatment recommendations. *Int J Rheum Dis.* 2015;18(7):685-713.

16. Forsyth C, Kouvari M, D'Cunha NM, et al. The effects of the Mediterranean diet on rheumatoid arthritis prevention and treatment: a systematic review of human prospective studies. *Rheumatol Int.* 2018;38(5):737-747.

17. Rausch Osthoff AK, Juhl CB, Knittle K. Effects of exercise and physical activity promotion: meta-analysis informing the 2018 EULAR recommendations for physical activity in people with rheumatoid arthritis, spondyloarthritis and hip/knee osteoarthritis. *RMD Open.* 2018;4(2):e000713.

18. Denton CP, Khanna D. Systemic sclerosis. *Lancet.* 2017;390(10103):1685-1699.

19. U.S. National Library of Medicine, National Institutes of Health. Genetics Home Reference. Systemic scleroderma. January 15, 2019. https://ghr.nlm.nih.gov/condition/systemic-scleroderma. Accessed January 20, 2019.

20. Mayes MD. Scleroderma epidemiology. *Rheum Dis Clin North Am.* 2003;29(2):239-254.

21. Asano Y. Systemic sclerosis. *J Dermatol.* 2018;45(2):128-138.

22. Jung S, Martin T, Schmittbuhl M, Huck O. The spectrum of orofacial manifestations in systemic sclerosis: a challenging management. *Oral Dis.* 2017;23(4):424-439.

23. Veale BJ, Jablonski RY, Frech TM, Pauling JD. Orofacial manifestations of systemic sclerosis. *Br Dent J.* 2016;221(6):305-310.

24. Kowal-Bielecka O, Fransen J, Avouac J, et al; EUSTAR Coauthors. Update of EULAR recommendations for the treatment of systemic sclerosis. *Ann Rheum Dis.* 2017;76(8):1327-1339.

25. Willems LM, Vriezekolk JE, Schouffoer AA, et al. Effectiveness of nonpharmacologic interventions in systemic sclerosis: a systematic review. *Arthritis Care Res.* 2015;67(10):1426-1439.

26. Di Sabatino A, Lenti MV, Giuffrida P, Vanoli A, Corazza GR. New insights into immune mechanisms underlying autoimmune diseases of the gastrointestinal tract. *Autoimmun Rev.* 2015;14(12):1161-1169.

27. Unalp-Arida A, Ruhl CE, Choung RS, Brantner TL, Murray JA. Lower Prevalence of celiac disease and gluten-related disorders in persons living in southern vs northern latitudes of the United States. *Gastroenterology.* 2017;152(8):1922.e2-1932.e2.

28. Rubio-Tapia A, Hill ID, Kelly CP, Calderwood AH, Murray JA; American College of Gastroenterology. ACG clinical guidelines: diagnosis and management of celiac disease. *Am J Gastroenterol.* 2013;108(5):656-676.

29. Nieri M, Tofani E, Defraia E, Giuntini V, Franchi L. Enamel defects and aphthous stomatitis in celiac and healthy subjects: systematic review and meta-analysis of controlled studies. *J Dent.* 2017;65:1-10.

30. Macho VMP, Coelho AS, Veloso E Silva DM, de Andrade DJC. Oral manifestations in pediatric patients with coeliac disease—a review article. *Open Dent J.* 2017;11:539-545.

31. Feuerstein JD, Cheifetz AS. Crohn disease: epidemiology, diagnosis, and management. *Mayo Clin Proc.* 2017;92(7):1088-1103.

32. Bernstein CN. Review article: changes in the epidemiology of inflammatory bowel disease—clues for aetiology. *Aliment Pharmacol Ther.* 2017;46(10):911-919.

33. Lichtenstein GR, Loftus EV, Isaacs KL, Regueiro MD, Gerson LB, Sands BE. ACG clinical guideline: management of Crohn's disease in adults. *Am J Gastroenterol.* 2018;113(4):481-517.

34. Tan CX, Brand HS, de Boer NK, Forouzanfar T. Gastrointestinal diseases and their oro-dental manifestations: Part 1: Crohn's disease. *Br Dent J.* 2016;221(12):794-799.

35. Feuerstein JD, Cheifetz AS. Ulcerative colitis: epidemiology, diagnosis, and management. *Mayo Clin Proc.* 2014;89(11):1553-1563.

36. Kornbluth A, Sachar DB; Practice Parameters Committee of the American College of Gastroenterology. Ulcerative colitis practice guidelines in adults: American College Of Gastroenterology, Practice Parameters Committee. *Am J Gastroenterol.* 2010;105(3):501-524.

37. Farraye FA, Melmed GY, Lichtenstein GR, Kane SV. ACG clinical guideline: preventive care in inflammatory bowel disease. *Am J Gastroenterol.* 2017;112(2):241-258.

38. Thompson AJ, Baranzini SE, Geurts J, Hemmer B, Ciccarelli O. Multiple sclerosis. *Lancet.* 2018;391(10130):1622-1636.

39. Loma I, Heyman R. Multiple sclerosis: pathogenesis and treatment. *Curr Neuropharmacol.* 2011;9(3):409-416.

40. Danesh-Sani SA, Rahimdoost A, Soltani M, Ghiyasi M, Haghdoost N, Sabzali-Zanjankhah S. Clinical assessment of orofacial manifestations in 500 patients with multiple sclerosis. *J Oral Maxillofac Surg.* 2013;71(2):290-294.

41. Sheu JJ, Lin HC. Association between multiple sclerosis and chronic periodontitis: a population-based pilot study. *Eur J Neurol.* 2013;20(7):1053-1059.

42. Moss BP, Rensel MR, Hersh CM. Wellness and the role of comorbidities in multiple sclerosis. *Neurotherapeutics.* 2017;14(4):999-1017.

43. Berrih-Aknin S, Frenkian-Cuvelier M, Eymard B. Diagnostic and clinical classification of autoimmune myasthenia gravis. *J Autoimmun.* 2014;48-49:143-148.

44. Sieb JP. Myasthenia gravis: an update for the clinician. *Clin Exp Immunol.* 2014;175(3):408-418.

45. Tamburrini A, Tacconi F, Barlattani A, Mineo TC. An update on myasthenia gravis, challenging disease for the dental profession. *J Oral Sci.* 2015;57(3):161-168.

46. Qin B, Wang J, Yang Z, et al. Epidemiology of primary Sjögren's syndrome: a systematic review and meta-analysis. *Ann Rheum Dis.* 2015;74(11):1983-1989.

47. García-Carrasco M, Fuentes-Alexandro S, Escárcega RO, Salgado G, Riebeling C, Cervera R. Pathophysiology of Sjögren's syndrome. *Arch Med Res.* 2006;37(8):921-932.

48. Bolstad AI, Skarstein K. Epidemiology of Sjögren's syndrome-from an oral perspective. *Curr Oral Health Rep.* 2016;3(4):328-336.

49. Vivino FB, Carsons SE, Foulks G, et al. New treatment guidelines for Sjögren's disease. *Rheum Dis Clin North Am.* 2016;42(3):531-551.

50. Gergianaki I, Bortoluzzi A, Bertsias G. Update on the epidemiology, risk factors, and disease outcomes of systemic lupus erythematosus. *Best Pract Res Clin Rheumatol.* 2018;32(2):188-205. doi: 10.1016/j.berh.2018.09.004.

51. Saccucci M, Di Carlo G, Bossù M, Giovarruscio F, Salucci A, Polimeni A. Autoimmune diseases and their manifestations on oral cavity: diagnosis and clinical management. *J Immunol Res.* 2018;2018:6061825.

52. Yu C, Gershwin ME, Chang C. Diagnostic criteria for systemic lupus erythematosus: a critical review. *J Autoimmun.* 2014;48-49:10-13.

Glossary

Chapter 1: The Professional Dental Hygienist

ADHA: American Dental Hygienists' Association.

ADHP: Advanced Dental Hygiene Practitioner. The dental hygiene–based, alternative workforce model, proposed by the American Dental Hygienists' Association, would be a registered dental hygienist with additional training who could autonomously provide additional oral health services.

Collaborative practice: the science of the prevention and treatment of oral disease through the provision of educational, assessment, preventive, clinical, and other therapeutic services in a collaborative working relationship with a consulting dentist, with general supervision.

Competency: the skills, understanding, and professional values of an individual ready for beginning professional practice.

Continuing education: Post-licensure short-term educational experiences for refresher, updating, and renewal; continuing education units may be required for relicensure.

Core values: basic values of a profession; guide to choices or actions by implying a preference for what is deemed to be acceptable in the profession.

Co-therapist: term used to describe the relationships between patient, dentist, and dental hygienist when coordinating the efforts to attain and maintain the oral health of the patient.

Dental hygiene care: the science and practice of the prevention of oral diseases; the integrated preventive and treatment services administered for a patient by a dental hygienist.

Dental hygiene care plan: the services within the framework of the total treatment plan to be carried out by the dental hygienist, patient, and caregiver.

Dental hygiene diagnosis: identification of an existing or a potential oral health problem that a dental hygienist is qualified and licensed to treat.

Dental hygiene process of care: an organized, systematic group of activities that provides the framework for delivering quality dental hygiene care.

Dental hygienist: oral health specialist whose primary concern is the maintenance of oral health and the prevention of oral disease (see also opening section of this chapter).

Dental therapist: a midlevel oral healthcare provider with expanded training who provides direct patient care under an expanded scope of practice that includes the ability to diagnose and perform restorative services. Dental therapists provide safe, quality dental care in many countries around the world.

Direct access: allows a dental hygienist to initiate dental hygiene treatment based on assessment of the patient's needs and without the specific authorization or presence of a dentist.

Ethical dilemma: a problem that involves two morally correct choices or courses of action. There may not be a single answer, and, depending on the choice, the outcomes can differ.

Ethical issue: a common problem wherein a solution is readily grounded in the governing practice act, recognized laws, or acceptable standards of care. Decisions involving ethical issues are generally more clearly defined than are dilemmas.

Ethics: a sense of moral obligation; a system of moral principles that governs the conduct of a professional group, planned by them for the common good of people; principles of morality.

Health: state of physical, mental, and social well-being, not only the absence of disease.

Health promotion: the process of enabling people to improve their health through self-care, mutual aid, and the creation of a healthy environment.

Interprofessional collaborative practice: comprehensive healthcare delivered by multiple healthcare providers with different professional backgrounds who work together with each other, the patient, the family, and other caregivers to meet the patient's needs.

Moral: a principle or habit with respect to right or wrong behavior.

Profession: occupation or calling that
- requires specialized knowledge, methods, and skills
- requires preparation, from an institution of higher learning, in the scholarly, scientific, and historic principles underlying such methods and skills
- continuously enlarges its body of knowledge

- functions autonomously in formulation of policy
- maintains high standards of achievement and conduct.

Rights: expectations by the patient that correlate with the duties of a professional person when providing care.

Supervision: term applied to a legal relationship between dentist and dental team members in practice. Each state practice act defines the type of supervision required for dental hygiene practice.

Chapter 2: Evidence-Based Dental Hygiene Practice

Best practices: approaches or interventions that have consistently shown results (outcomes) superior to those achieved with other means; used as a benchmark based on repeatable research over time on large diverse groups of people.

Biomedical database: organized collection of medically related journal articles, systematic reviews, research reports, theses, and/or dissertations typically in digital form.

Biostatistics: a branch of statistics directed toward application in the discipline of health sciences.

Clinical practice guidelines: statements that include recommendations intended to optimize patient care.

Clinical significance: practical or observed difference expected in patient care outcomes following a clinical intervention; in research, a clinically observable difference rather than statistical difference.

Confidence interval: a range of values defining a specific probability that the value of a factor lies within it.

Context: personal and environmental factors that influence patient care.

Descriptive statistics: use of numbers to describe the main features or characteristics of a particular person, event, or group; to determine the frequency with which something occurs; or to categorize information.

Evidence: source of information used to support, determine, or demonstrate the truth of a statement.

Evidence-based decision-making (EBDM): process of making decisions grounded in best available research, professional experience, and contextual factors.

Evidence-based dental hygiene (EBDH) practice: a scientific, research-supported approach to decide dental hygiene interventions for each patient.

Evidence-based practice (EBP): the practical application of evidence-based decision-making in diverse professions, including healthcare contexts.

Human subjects: living individuals whom an investigator conducts research about and obtains.

Inferential statistics: numerical data designed to allow generalization from a sample to a population.

Informed consent: process of adequately explaining research to prospective patients and ensuring that they understand what will happen to them, especially associated risks and benefits.

Institutional review board (IRB): an independent ethics committee formally designated to approve, monitor, and review biomedical and behavioral research involving humans.

Levels of evidence pyramid: visual hierarchy for making clinical judgments related to patient care based on the strength and types of research studies.

Literature review: summary and critical analysis of published sources on a particular topic.

Peer review: review of a journal article by a panel of experts prior to publication.

Post hoc fallacy: understanding that correlation does not mean causation between multiple variables.

Probability value (*p* value): calculated probability of finding the observed results when the null hypothesis is true.

Randomized controlled clinical trial: controlled experiment where researchers aim to predict and/or test causal relationships.

Reliability: the ability of a measurement instrument or test to get the same results repeatedly.

Research question: answerable inquiry into a specific concern or issue.

Scientific evidence: evidence repeatedly tested through research with valid and reliable methods.

Statistical significance: identifies the extent to which the results are not due to chance; indicated in research by the "*p* value" notation.

Validity: ability to measure what was intended.

Variable: factors in a research study that can be manipulated and measured; includes dependent, independent, and extraneous variables.

Chapter 3: Effective Health Communication

Affect: as used by mental health professionals, refers to an expressed or observed emotional response or lack of expression or emotional response (flat or restricted affect).

Aphasia: communication disorder caused by damage to certain parts of brain, making it difficult for an individual to read, write, express, or understand language.

Communication: a process of defining the meaning of a message shared between a sender and one or more intended recipients.

> **Nonverbal communication:** sending and receiving wordless messages; usually refers to body language, gestures, facial expressions, eye contact, and verbal elements such as rhythm and intonation.

Verbal communication: sending and receiving messages using words; usually defined as spoken or written communication.

Culture: a learned set of beliefs, values, attitudes, convictions, and behaviors that are common to a group (especially an ethnic group) of people and usually passed down from generation to generation.

Cultural competence: a set of congruent attitudes, skills, behaviors, and policies that enable effective cross-cultural communication for delivery of oral health services.

Cultural rapport: actions that foster understanding, empathy, and enhanced communication between individuals with different cultural backgrounds.

Cultural sensitivity: making an effort to understand the language, culture, and behaviors of diverse individuals and groups.

Culturally effective health care: refers to a dynamic relationship between provider and patient, resulting in culturally relevant and culturally specific healthcare recommendations; delivery of healthcare services in a way respectful of and responsive to the cultural norms and linguistic needs of individual patients.

Decoding: the reverse process of encoding; the receiver takes the words, gestures, or other signs to recreate the thought.

Dysarthria: a motor/speech disorder that weakens or paralyzes the muscles of the face, mouth, larynx, and vocal cords, causing slurred, slow, and difficult-to-understand speech.

Encoding: the translation of a thought into words, gestures, or other linguistic signs that will allow thoughts to be expressed in some understandable way to another; encoding can be verbal or nonverbal, oral, visual, or tactile.

Feedback: the receiver's direct response to a communicated message.

Health literacy: the ability of a patient to obtain, process, understand, and respond to health messages, and be motivated to make health decisions that promote and maintain good health.

Media communication: the use of tools or technology to convey information.

Motivational interviewing: a patient-centered communication approach to changing health behaviors (see Chapter 24).

Nonvocal: a type of cue, such as body position, movement of body parts, eye movements, and facial expression, that occurs during communication.

Plain language: verbal or written health information provided using simplified terminology, clear and to the point sentence structure, pictures, or any other method that can enhance understanding for patients with limited language proficiency or health literacy.

Social determinants of health: social, environmental, and physical circumstances that have an effect on health status; these conditions are shaped by the distribution of power, money, and resources at a global, national, or local level.

Stereotypes: attitudes or judgments (either positive or negative) made about people that are usually not based on personal experience but rather on what has been learned from other sources; seeing individuals from a population group as having no individuality as though all have the same characteristics.

Vocal: a type of cue, such as accent, loudness, tempo, pitch, cadence, and tone that occurs during communication.

Chapter 4: Dental Hygiene Care in Alternative Settings

ADL/IADL (activities of daily living/instrumental activities of daily living): a measure of ability to carry out the basic tasks needed for self-care.

Chronically ill: a condition or disease that persists for a long period of time, usually more than 3 months. Can be maintained, but not often cured.

Cognitively impaired: difficulty remembering, learning new things, concentrating, or making decisions that affect everyday life. Ranges from mild to severe.

Collaborative practice: an alternative oral care delivery model in which dental hygienists collaborate autonomously with members of interprofessional teams to provide dental hygiene services in a variety of nontraditional settings.

Critically ill patient: survival of the patient is at stake. Intensive care or hospitalization is usually required.

Custodial care: nonmedical care provided by nonlicensed caregivers. Often at home, but can be in a nursing facility.

Depression: temporary mental state or chronic disorder characterized by feelings of sadness and low self-esteem.

Direct access: ability to maintain a direct patient provider relationship; allows dental hygienist to deliver care without the specific or previous authorization of a dentist and provide treatment without the presence of a dentist.

Disability: physical, mental, or functional impairment that restricts a major activity; may be partial or complete.

Frail elderly: medically and/or physically fragile, delicate, or weak older person; usually refers to those older than 80 years.

Functional dependence: inability to perform one or more ADL without help; the level of functional dependence is based on the level of assistance needed to perform ADL or the number of activities for which assistance is needed.

Hospice: an interprofessional practice program providing a continuum of home and inpatient palliative and supportive care to meet the physical, emotional, spiritual, social, and economic needs experienced by terminally ill individuals and their families during the final stages of illness and during dying and bereavement.

Interprofessional healthcare teams: patient care team consists of specialists from many fields; combines expertise and resources to provide insight into all aspects of the patient's needs.

Long-term care: assistance with physical, mental, and emotional needs for an extended period of time due to terminal condition, disability, illness, injury, or frailness of old age. Can be custodial or skilled care.

Nonambulatory: inability to walk or move about freely.

Nurse practitioner (NP): a licensed registered nurse who has had advanced preparation for practice that includes clinical experience in diagnosis and treatment of illness; NPs may work in collaborative practice with physicians or independently in private practice or nursing clinics; in some states, NPs can prescribe medications.

Palliative care: affording relief, but not cure.

Residence-bound (homebound): inability to leave home due to illness or injury; leaving requires considerable and taxing effort. Can be temporary or permanent situation.

Silver diamine fluoride: colorless liquid containing silver particles and fluoride ion. Used for the prevention and nonsurgical arrest of caries.

Skilled nursing: medically necessary care that can only be provided by or under the supervision of licensed medical professional. Often in a nursing facility, but can be delivered at a home.

Sordes: foul matter that collects on the lips, teeth, and oral mucosa in patients with low fevers or dehydration; consists of debris, microorganisms, epithelial elements, and food particles; forms a crust.

Teledentistry: a model of healthcare delivery that uses web-based technology to send electronic information such as patient history and digital radiographs, between on-site and off-site practitioners; this model can be used to support collaborative practice between dentists and dental hygienists who are caring for patients in nontraditional settings.

Terminally ill patient: a person who is experiencing the end stages of a life-threatening disease and for whom there is no longer hope of a cure.

Triage: screening and classification of individuals in order to make optimal use of treatment resources; sorting and allocating relative priority for patient treatment needs.

Chapter 5: Infection Control: Transmissible Diseases

Antibody: a soluble protein molecule produced and secreted by body cells in response to an antigen; it is capable of binding to that specific antigen.

Antigen: a substance capable, under appropriate conditions, of inducing a specific immune response and of reacting with the products of that specific antibody.

Asymptomatic carrier: an individual who harbors pathogenic organisms without clinically recognizable symptoms; a carrier may infect those contacted.

Carrier: a person who harbors a specific infectious agent in the absence of discernible clinical disease and serves as a potential source of infection. The carrier state may be temporary, transient, or chronic.

CDC: US Centers for Disease Control and Prevention, Department of Health and Human Services, Public Health Service, Atlanta, GA 30333. www.cdc.gov.

CFU: colony-forming unit.

Communicable: an infectious agent may be transferred directly or indirectly from an infected person to another person.

DHCP: dental healthcare personnel.

Endemic: the constant presence of a disease or an infectious agent within a geographic area.

Immunity: the resistance that a person has against disease; it may be natural or acquired.

Incubation period: the time interval between the initial contact with an infectious agent and the appearance of the first clinical sign or symptom of the disease.

Infection: a state caused by the invasion, development, or multiplication of an infectious agent into the body.

> **Latent infection:** persistent infection following a primary infection in which the causative agent remains inactive within certain cells.
>
> **Primary infection:** first time; no preexisting antibodies.
>
> **Recurrent infection:** symptomatic reactivation of a latent infection.

Infectious agent: organism capable of producing an infection.

Opportunistic infectious agent: capable of causing disease only when the host's resistance is lowered.

Pandemic: widespread epidemic usually affecting the population of an extensive region, several countries, or sometimes the entire globe.

Parenteral: injection by a route other than the alimentary tract, such as subcutaneous, intramuscular, or intravenous.

Pathogen: a virus, microorganism, or other substance that causes disease.

Percutaneous: by way of, or through, the skin.

Planktonic: microscopic organisms floating or swimming in a liquid environment.

Sequestrum: a piece of dead bone tissue.

Seroconversion: after exposure to the etiologic agent of a disease, the blood changes from negative ("seronegative") to positive ("seropositive") for the serum marker for that disease; the time interval for conversion is specific for each disease.

Standard precautions: an approach to infection control to protect healthcare providers and patients from pathogens that can be spread by blood or any other body fluid, secretion, or excretion.

Susceptible host: host not possessing resistance against an infectious agent.

Viral shedding: presence of virus in body secretions, in excretions, or in body surface lesions with potential for transmission.

Virus: a subcellular genetic entity capable of gaining entrance into a limited range of living cells and capable of replication only within such cells; a virus contains either DNA or RNA, but not both.

Chapter 6: Exposure Control: Barriers for Patient and Clinician

Aeroallergen: Inhalation of the allergen when the powder (or cornstarch) from the gloves becomes airborne.

Allergen: substance, protein or nonprotein, capable of inducing allergy or specific hypersensitivity; can enter the body by being inhaled, swallowed, touched, or injected.

Antimicrobial soap: a soap containing an active ingredient against skin microorganisms.

Antiseptic: a substance that prevents or arrests the growth or action of microorganisms either by inhibiting their activity or by destroying them; term used especially for preparation applied topically to living tissue.

Barrier protection: refers to placing a physical barrier between the patient's body fluids (such as blood and saliva) and the healthcare personnel (HCP) to prevent disease transmission.

Contamination: introduction of microorganisms, blood, or other potentially infectious material or agent onto a surface or into tissue.

Cross-contamination: the transfer of microorganisms, blood, or other potentially infectious material or agent onto a surface or into tissue.

Hand hygiene: a general term that applies to either handwashing, **antiseptic** handwash, **antiseptic** hand rub, or surgical hand antisepsis.

Immunization: the process of rendering a subject immune to a particular disease by stimulation with a specific antigen to promote antibody formation in the body.

Latex allergy: an acquired hypersensitivity reaction to the proteins found in natural rubber latex (NRL).

Occupational exposure: reasonably anticipated skin, eye, mucous membrane, or parenteral contact with blood or other potentially infectious materials that may result from the performance of one's usual duties.

Chapter 7: Infection Control: Clinical Procedures

Antimicrobial agent: any agent that kills or suppresses the growth of microorganisms.

Antiseptic: mouth rinses are rinses containing antimicrobial substances that decrease the number of intraoral bacteria.

Asepsis: free from contamination with microorganisms; includes sterile conditions in tissues and on materials, as obtained by exclusion, removing, or killing organisms.

Biofilm: the surface film that contains microorganisms and other biologic substances.

Biohazard: a substance that poses a biologic risk because it is contaminated with biomaterial that has a potential for transmitting infection.

Biologic monitor: a preparation of nonpathogenic microorganisms, usually bacterial spores, carried by an ampule or a specially impregnated paper enclosed within a package during sterilization and subsequently incubated to verify that the sterilizer is functioning properly.

Chain of asepsis: a procedure that avoids transfer of infection. The "chain" implies that each step, related to the previous one, continues to be carried out without contamination.

Chemical indicator: a color change stripe or other mark, often on autoclave tape or bag, used to monitor the process of sterilization; color change indicates that the package has been brought to a specific temperature, but color change is not an indicator of sterilization.

Contamination: introduction of microorganisms, blood, or other potentially infectious material or agent onto a surface or into tissue.

Disinfectant: an agent, usually a chemical, but may be a physical agent, such as x-rays or ultraviolet light, that destroys microorganisms but may not kill bacterial spores; refers to substances applied to inanimate objects.

EPA: US Environmental Protection Agency.

EPA registered: number on a label indicates that the product has the acceptance of EPA.

FDA: US Food and Drug Administration regulates food, drugs, biologic products, medical devices, and radiologic products.

Infection control: the selection and use of procedures and products to prevent the spread of infectious disease.

PPE: personal protective equipment.

Sanitation: the process by which the number of organisms on inanimate objects is reduced. It does not imply freedom from microorganisms and generally refers to a cleaning process.

Shelf life: stability of an item after it has been prepared; length of time a substance or preparation can be kept without changes occurring in its chemical structure or other properties.

Sterilization: process by which all forms of life, including bacterial spores, are destroyed by physical or chemical means.

Waste

   Contaminated waste: items that have contacted blood or other body secretions.

   Hazardous waste: poses a risk to humans or the environment.

   Infectious waste: capable of causing an infectious disease; contaminated with blood, saliva, or other substances; potentially or actually infected with pathogenic material; officially called "regulated" waste.

   Regulated waste: liquid blood or saliva, sharps contaminated with blood or saliva, and nonsharp solid waste saturated with or caked with liquid or semisolid blood or saliva or tissue including teeth.

Chapter 8: Patient Reception and Ergonomic Practice

Ergonomics: study of designing and arranging the working environment around the worker for the most efficient and safe function.

Fatigue: a state of physical exhaustion triggered by stress, overwork, and other factors.

Kyphosis: naturally occurring curve of the back in the thoracic region of spine that, when viewed from the side, is curved outward.

Lordosis: the normal curvature of the cervical and lumbar regions of the spine that, when viewed from the side, is curved inward.

Musculoskeletal disorder, cumulative trauma disorder, repetitive stress injury: terms used to describe disorders of the musculoskeletal, autonomic, and peripheral nervous system caused by repeated, forceful, and awkward movements of the human body, as well as by exposure to mechanical stress, vibration, and cold temperatures; often work related.

Neutral working position: the position of the body in which the normal curvatures of the spine are maintained and the muscles and joints are naturally aligned to allow for reduction of muscles and joints fatigue during work activities.

Postural hypotension: also called orthostatic hypotension; a sudden drop in blood pressure often associated with dizziness, syncope, and blurred vision that occurs upon moving from lying down to standing up position.

Risk factor: an element that puts the clinician or the patient at risk or increases their susceptibility to exposure to an identified hazard.

Safe work practice: any work practice that improves clinician and patient safety. This includes, but is not limited to, decreased physical demands, improved layout, environmental factors, and work process organization.

Stress: a physical, chemical, or emotional factor that causes physical or mental tension and may be a factor in disease causation or fatigue.

Supine: flat face-up position with head and feet on the same level.

Trendelenburg position: the modified supine position when the head is lower than the heart.

Chapter 9: Emergency Care

Adrenal crisis: also known as Addisonian crisis and acute adrenal insufficiency. A medical emergency and potentially life-threatening situation requiring immediate emergency treatment. It is a constellation of symptoms that indicate severe adrenal insufficiency caused by insufficient levels of the hormone cortisol.

Analgesics: any member of the group of drugs used to achieve relief from pain. Act on the peripheral and central nervous systems.

Anaphylaxis: a severe, potentially life-threatening allergic reaction. It can occur within seconds or minutes of exposure to an allergen. Anaphylaxis causes your immune system to release a flood of chemicals that may lead to shock—your blood pressure drops suddenly and your airways narrow, blocking breathing. Signs and symptoms include a rapid, weak pulse; a skin rash; and nausea and vomiting.

Angina pectoris (stable angina): Chest pain or discomfort due to coronary heart disease. It occurs when the heart muscle is lacking blood, usually because of blocked arteries (ischemia).

Angioedema: swelling of the lower layer of skin and tissue just under the skin or mucous membranes. It may occur in the face, tongue, larynx, abdomen, or arms and legs. Often associated with hives and onset is over minutes to hours.

Baseline: an initial known value that is used for comparison with later data.

Cannula: tube for insertion into a duct or cavity.

Crepitation: dry crackling sound, such as that produced by the grating of the ends of a fractured bone.

Cricothyrotomy: incision through the skin and the cricothyroid membrane to secure a patent airway for emergency relief of upper airway obstruction.

Cyanosis: bluish or purplish discoloration of the skin or mucous membranes due to low oxygen saturation of the tissues near the skin surface.

Dyspnea: labored or difficult breathing; indication of inadequate ventilation or of insufficient oxygen in the circulating blood.

Ecchymoses: discoloration of the skin resulting from bleeding underneath.

Emphysema: a lung condition that causes shortness of breath, reducing the amount of oxygen that reaches the bloodstream.

Erythema: redness of the skin or mucous membranes caused by increased blood flow in superficial capillaries. Occurs with injury, infection, or inflammation.

Hypoglycemia: when blood sugar decreases to below normal levels.

Kussmaul breathing: loud, slow, labored breathing common to patients in diabetic coma.

Myocardial infarction: irreversible necrosis of heart muscle secondary to prolonged lack of oxygen supply (ischemia). Commonly known as heart attack.

Nasal cannula: a semicircle of plastic tubing with two plastic tips that fit into the patient's nostrils.

Orthostatic hypotension: a drop in systolic and diastolic blood pressure due to change in body position, usually from lying back or sitting to a standing position. The resulting reduction in blood flow can cause temporary shortage of oxygen to the brain and a feeling of light-headedness or syncope.

Paresthesia: abnormal sensation such as tingling, tickling, prickling, numbness, or burning of a person's skin with no apparent physical cause. May be transient or chronic. Multiple possible causes.

Paroxysmal: a sudden, violent recurrence or intensification of symptoms, such as a spasm or seizure.

Premedication: antibiotics prescribed in advance of dental procedures in patients known to be at high risk for an adverse medical outcome.

Premonitory: when symptoms give warning of a more serious attack, such as headache or "funny feeling" shortly before the onset of a seizure.

Pruritis: itching.

Syncopal episodes (syncope): temporary loss of consciousness caused by a sudden fall in blood pressure; can have serious consequences, particularly in patients with a cardiovascular disease; commonly referred to as *fainting*.

Tonic–clonic seizure: also known as convulsion or "grand mal." Usually begins on both sides of the brain, but can start in one side and spread to the whole brain. Last 1 to 3 minutes and have a longer recovery period.

Trendelenburg position: the patient is supine with the heart higher than the head on a surface inclined downward about 45°.

Urticaria: vascular reaction of the skin with transient appearance of slightly elevated patches (wheals) that are redder or paler than the surrounding skin; may be accompanied by severe itching; also called hives.

Vaporoles: a brand of smelling salts or aromatic ammonia in a small capsule-type container that is crushed and put under the syncope victim's nose to stimulate respiration.

Chapter 10: Documentation for Dental Hygiene Care

Chart: a form/graphic representation used as a component of a patient's permanent health record.

Charting: the process of tabulating clinical information on a graphic form.

Electronic patient record: in a computerized database management system, a record is a complete set of information. Records are composed of electronic fields, each of which contains space for one item of information.

Encryption: translation of computerized data into a secret code; the most effective way to achieve data security; in order to read an encrypted file, the reader needs access to a secret key or password that enables changing the "cipher text" into plain text.

Forensic: pertaining to or used in legal proceedings.

Malpractice: professional negligence; an act or omission by a healthcare provider that causes injury to a patient; a deviation from acceptable standards of care.

Multidisciplinary team: professional individuals from different backgrounds/specialties working together for the benefit of the patient.

Odontogram: a graphic representation of the patient's hard and soft tissues.

Patient record: a written document that contains information identifying an individual patient, such as a patient's name, address, and phone number, as well as information related to that particular patient's care, such as health history information, dental charting items, treatment dates, and treatment codes.

Sign: objective, observable evidence of an illness or disorder; a physical manifestation of a disorder that is apparent to a trained healthcare provider and sometimes to the patient.

Symptom: any change in the body or its function that is perceived by the patient; the subjective experience of a disease or disorder.

Chapter 11: Medical, Dental, and Psychosocial Histories

Antibiotic premedication: provision of an effective antibiotic before invasive clinical procedures that can create a transient bacteremia, which, in turn, can cause IE or other serious infection.

Bacteremia: presence of microorganisms in the bloodstream.

Immunocompromised: when the immune response is attenuated by administration of immunosuppressive drugs, by irradiation, by malnutrition, or by certain disease processes.

Infective endocarditis (IE): infection of the heart lining; previously termed subacute bacterial endocarditis (SBE).

Informed consent: a medicolegal document that holds providers responsible for ensuring that patients understand the risks and benefits of a procedure or medication before it is administered.

Premedication: preliminary medication; may be for the purpose of allaying apprehension, preventing bacteremia, or otherwise facilitating the clinical procedure.

Sequelae: a condition that may happen as a result of a previous disease or injury.

Chapter 12: Vital Signs

Anoxia: oxygen deficiency; a reduction of oxygen in the tissues can lead to deep respirations, cyanosis, increased pulse rate, and impairment of coordination.

Apnea: temporary cessation of breathing; absence of spontaneous respirations.

Auscultation: listening for sounds produced within the body; may be performed directly or with a stethoscope.

Bradycardia: unusually slow heartbeat evidenced by slowing of the pulse rate.

Diastole: the phase of the cardiac cycle in which the heart relaxes between contractions and the two ventricles are dilated by the blood flowing into them; diastolic pressure is the lowest blood pressure.

Hypertension: systolic blood pressure of 140 mm Hg or greater and diastolic blood pressure of 90 mm Hg or greater.

Hyperthermia: higher-than-normal body temperature.

Hypotension: systolic blood pressure of 90 mm Hg or lower and diastolic blood pressure of 60 mm Hg or lower.

Hypothermia: lower-than-normal body temperature.

Korotkoff sounds: the sounds heard during the determination of blood pressure; sounds originating within the blood passing through the vessel or produced by vibratory motion of the arterial wall.

Normotensive: normal tension or tone; of or pertaining to having normal blood pressure.

Postural hypotension: a decrease in standing systolic blood pressure greater than 10 mm Hg; associated with dizziness or fainting: more frequently seen in older patients with systolic hypertension and those taking certain prescription medications.

Pulse pressure: the difference between systolic and diastolic blood pressure; normally 40 mm Hg.

Pyrexia: an abnormal elevation of the body temperature above 37.0°C (98.6°F).

Stethoscope: instrument used to hear and amplify the sounds produced by the heart, lungs, and other internal organs.

Systole: the contraction, or phase of contraction, of the heart, especially the ventricles, during which blood is forced into the aorta and the pulmonary artery; systolic pressure is the highest, or greatest, pressure.

Tachycardia: unusually fast heartbeat; at a rate greater than 100 bpm.

White-coat hypertension: elevated blood pressure as a result of feeling anxious in a medical environment.

Chapter 13: Extraoral and Intraoral Examination

Aphtha: a little white or reddish ulcer.

Corium: the dermis or true skin just beneath the epidermis; well supplied with nerves and blood vessels.

Crust: outer scablike layer of solid matter formed by drying of a body exudate or secretion.

Cyst: a closed, epithelial-lined sac, normal or pathologic, that contains fluid or other material.

Dorsal: back surface; opposite of ventral.

Epidermis: outermost and nonvascular layers of the skin composed of basal layer, spinous layer, granular layer, and horny layer.

Erosion: soft-tissue slightly depressed lesion in which the epithelium above the basal layer is denuded.

Erythema: red area of variable size and shape; reaction to irritation, radiation, or injury.

Exophytic: growing outward.

Exostosis: a benign bony growth projecting from the surface of bone.

Fissure: a narrow slit or cleft in the epidermis where infected ulceration, inflammation, and pain can result.

Forensic: pertaining to or used in legal proceedings.

Idiopathic: of unknown etiology.

Indurated: hardened; abnormally hard.

Lymphadenopathy: disease of the lymph nodes; regional lymph node enlargement.

Morphology: science that deals with form and structure.

Palpation: perceiving by sense of touch.

Papillary: small, nipple-shaped projection or elevation (papillary: adjective).

Patch: circumscribed flat lesion larger than a macule; differentiated from surrounding epidermis by color and/or texture.

Pedunculated: elevated lesion attached by a thin stalk.

Petechia: hemorrhagic nonraised spot of pinpoint to pinhead size.

Polyp: any growth or mass protruding from a mucous membrane.

Pseudomembrane: a loose membranous layer of exudate that contains microorganisms, precipitated fibrin, necrotic cells, and inflammatory cells produced during an inflammatory reaction on the surface of a tissue.

Punctate: marked with points or punctures differentiated from the surrounding surface by color, elevation, or texture.

Purulent: containing, forming, or discharging pus.

Rubefacient: reddening of the skin.

Scar: cicatrix; mark remaining after healing of a wound or healing following a surgical intervention.

Sclerosis: induration or hardening.

Sessile: elevated lesion with a broad base.

Temporomandibular disorder (TMD): a collective term that includes a wide range of disorders of the masticatory system characterized by one or more of the following: pain in the preauricular area, temporomandibular joint (TMJ), and muscles of mastication, with limitation or deviation in mandibular motion and TMJ sounds during mandibular function.

Torus/tori (pl): bony elevation or prominence usually located on the midline of the hard palate (torus palatinus) and the lingual surface of the mandible in the premolar area (torus mandibularis).

Trismus: motor disturbance of the trigeminal nerve, especially spasm of the masticatory muscles with difficulty in opening the mouth.

Ventral: inferior surface; opposite of dorsal.

Verruca: verrucous (verrucose), a wartlike growth.

Chapter 14: Family Violence

Abuse: the nonaccidental physical, emotional (psychological), or sexual acts against a child.

Cachexia: ill health, malnutrition, wasting (emaciating).

Condyloma acuminatum: multiple papillary or focal sessile-based lesions caused by the human papilloma virus (HPV6 or HPV11).

Dental neglect: the willful failure of a parent or guardian to seek and follow through with treatment necessary to ensure a level of oral health essential for adequate function and freedom from pain and infection.

Differential diagnosis: determining the probability of one disease or condition versus another by comparing and contrasting the symptoms.

Domestic violence: violent or aggressive behavior within the home, typically involving the violent abuse of a spouse or partner.

Ecchymosis: discoloration on the skin that is blue-black with irregularly formed hemorrhagic areas. Color changes with time to yellow or greenish brown.

Edema: swelling.

Financial exploitation: improper, illegal, or unethical exploitation of resources or assets.

Forensic dentistry: aspect of dental science that relates and applies dental facts to legal problems; encompasses dental identification, malpractice litigation, legislation, peer review, and dental licensure.

Human trafficking: human trafficking is the trade of humans for the purpose of forced labor, sexual slavery, or commercial sexual exploitation for the trafficker or others.

Idiopathic thrombocytopenia purpura: hemorrhages on the skin caused by abnormal decrease in the number of blood platelets with unknown etiology.

Intimate partners: marriage partners, partners living together, dating relationships, and former spouses, partners, and boyfriends/girlfriends.

Lichenification: area of skin that has thickened and hardened from continuous irritation.

Munchausen syndrome by proxy (MSBP): a form of child abuse and mental health problem in which a caregiver makes up or causes an illness or injury in a person under his or her care, such as a child, an elderly adult, or a person who has a disability.

Neglect: the intentional or unintentional failure to provide basic physical, emotional, educational, and medical/dental needs.

Pathognomonic: (of a sign or symptom) specifically characteristic or indicative of a particular disease.

Raccoon sign: bilateral periorbital ecchymosis, which can occur as a result of a basilar skull fracture.

Scale photography: a method of photography to record bite marks; the use of a metric scale placed directly above or below the injury to indicate scale; use of grid photographic film.

Sexual abuse: sexual contact with an individual who is unable to consent or otherwise nonconsensual sexual contact or exploitation.

Traumatic alopecia: an area of baldness on the head caused by pulling out the hair at the roots.

Chapter 15: Dental Radiographic Imaging

Absorbed dose: the amount of energy imparted by ionizing radiation to a unit mass of irradiated material at a specific exposure point; the unit of absorbed dose is the Gray (Gy).

Analog: continuous and variable representation of an image as opposed to digital, which is a binary representation (0's and 1's) of an image. An analog image will include all levels of clarity and will not be enhanced as the digital representation.

Backscatter: radiation deflected by scattering processes at angles greater than 90° to the original direction of the beam of radiation.

Cassette: a light-tight plastic, cardboard, or metal container in which x-ray image receptors are placed for exposure to x-radiation; usually backed with lead to reduce the effect of backscatter radiation and contain intensifying screen(s).

Digital sensors: include CCD, CMOS, and PSP plates.

Digitize: to convert an image into a digital form that can be used by the computer using a grid of pixels.

Dose equivalent: the product of absorbed dose and modifying factors, such as the quality factor, distribution factor, and any other necessary factors; different types of radiation cause differing biologic effects; the unit of dose equivalence is the Sievert (Sv).

Electromagnetic ionizing radiation: forms of energy propagated by wave motion as photons; the radiations differ widely in wavelength, frequency, and photo energy; examples are infrared waves, visible light, ultraviolet radiation, x-rays, gamma rays, and cosmic radiation.

Gamma radiation: short-wavelength electromagnetic radiation of nuclear origin similar to x-rays but usually of higher energy.

Image receptors: traditional film and digital sensors used to capture and record a radiographic image.

Impulse: the burst of radiation generated during a half cycle of alternating current (AC); film exposure time is measured in impulses.

Irradiation: exposure to radiation; one speaks of radiation therapy and irradiation of a body part.

Latent image: the invisible change produced in an x-ray film emulsion by the action of x-radiation or light from which the visible image is subsequently developed and fixed chemically.

Leakage radiation: the radiation that escapes through the protective shielding of the x-ray unit tube head; it may be detected at the sides, top, bottom, or back of the tube head.

Penumbra: the secondary shadow that surrounds the periphery of the primary shadow; in radiography, it is the blurred margin of an image detail (geometric unsharpness).

Photon: a finite bundle of energy of visible light or electromagnetic radiation.

Pixel: the smallest discrete component of an image or a picture on a screen that makes up the overall picture; usually dots arranged in rows and columns.

Primary radiation: all radiation coming directly from the target of the anode of an x-ray tube.

Radiation: the emission and propagation of energy through space or a material medium in the form of waves or particles.

Radiograph: a visible image on a radiation-sensitive film emulsion or a digitized image on a computer monitor after exposure of the image receptor to ionizing radiation that has passed through an area, region, or substance of interest.

Radiography: the art and science of making radiographs.

Radiology: a branch of science that deals with the use of radiant energy in the diagnosis and treatment of disease.

Rare earth intensifying screen: commonly used to refer to intensifying screens containing rare earth elements in the form of a plastic sheet coated with fluorescent material positioned singly or in pairs in a cassette. When the cassette is exposed to x-radiation, the visible light from the fluorescent image on the screen adds to the latent image produced directly by x-radiation.

Secondary radiation: particles or photons produced by the interaction of primary radiation with matter. Scatter radiation is a form of secondary radiation.

Sensor: a small detector that is placed intraorally to capture a radiographic image.

Verruca vulgaris: common warts; a benign lesion of skin and mucous membranes caused by human papillomovirus (HPV).

Chapter 16: Hard-Tissue Examination of the Dentition

Amelogenesis imperfecta: disorder of production and development of enamel.

Avulsion: the tearing away or forcible separation of a structure or part. Tooth avulsion is the traumatic separation of a tooth from the alveolus.

Bruxism: an oral habit of grinding, clenching, or clamping the teeth; involuntary, rhythmic, or spasmodic movements outside the chewing range; may damage teeth and attachment apparatus.

Cariogenic: *adj.* conducive to dental caries.

Carious: *adj.* used to define a carious lesion.

Cavitation: when an incipient lesion breaks through the surface of the tooth surface.

Centric occlusion (or habitual occlusion): the maximum intercuspation or contact of the teeth of the opposing arches; also called habitual occlusion.

Dental caries: disease of the mineralized structures of the teeth characterized by demineralization of the hard components and dissolution of the organic matrix.

> **Arrested caries:** carious lesion that has become stationary and does not show a tendency to progress further; frequently has a hard surface and takes on a dark brown or reddish brown color.
>
> **Incipient caries:** early signs of a carious lesion.
>
> **Rampant caries:** widespread formation of chalky white areas and incipient lesions that may increase in size over a comparatively short time.
>
> **Recurrent caries:** occurs on a surface adjacent to a restoration; may be a continuation of the original lesion; also called secondary caries.
>
> **Root caries:** occurs on root surfaces.

Dentinogenesis imperfecta: is a genetic defect in dentin formation during tooth development.

Dentition: the natural teeth in the dental arch.

Primary (deciduous) dentition: the first teeth; normally will be shed and replaced by permanent teeth.

Permanent dentition: the natural 32 teeth that serve throughout life.

Mixed dentition: combination of primary and permanent teeth between the ages of 6 and 12 when primary teeth are being replaced; starts with the eruption of the first permanent tooth.

Diastema: a space between two adjacent teeth in the same arch.

Edentulous: without teeth; referred to as partially edentulous when some, but not all, teeth are missing.

Endogenous: having an internal cause or origin.

Exfoliation: loss of primary teeth following physiologic resorption of root structure.

Exogenosis: related to external factors.

Exogenosis: related to external factors.

Exfoliation: loss of primary teeth following physiologic resorption of root structure.

Facet: a small flattened surface on a hard body, such as a tooth; a wear facet can result from attrition or repeated parafunctional contact.

Fremitus: tooth vibration that can be felt due to occlusal trauma typically occurring on the upper front teeth when the patient taps teeth together.

Hypomaturation: a defect in the enamel crystal structure as it forms.

Hypomineralization: deficiency in mineralization of the tooth enamel.

Hypoplasia: incomplete development or underdevelopment of a tissue or an organ.

Enamel hypoplasia: incomplete or defective formation of the enamel of either primary or permanent teeth. The result may be an irregularity of tooth form, color, or surface.

Interocclusal record: a registration of the positional relationship of the opposing teeth or dental arches made in a plastic material, such as a soft baseplate wax; also called the maxillomandibular relationship record or wax-bite.

Luxation: loosening or dislocation of the tooth.

Occlusal plane: the average plane established by the incisal and occlusal surfaces of the teeth; generally not actually a plane, but the planar mean of the curvature of those surfaces

Occlusal trauma: injury to the periodontium that results from occlusal forces in excess of the reparative capacity of the attachment apparatus; also called occlusal traumatism.

Oral microbiome: the complex community of microbes composed of bacteria, fungi, and so on, inhabiting the oral cavity.

Parafunctional: abnormal or deviated function, as in bruxism.

Pathologic migration: the movement of a tooth out of its natural position as a result of periodontal infection; contrasts with mesial migration, which is the physiologic process maintained by tooth proximal contacts in the normal dental arches.

Primate space: space or gap in the tooth row occasionally observed in the human primary dentition. It is characteristic of nearly all species of primates except man. The maxillary primate spaces accommodate the mandibular canines, and the mandibular primate spaces accommodate the maxillary canines when the teeth are in occlusion. As a reduction in the length of canines accompanied man's evolution, the canines no longer protruded beyond the occlusal level. The diastema (primate space) was no longer functional.

Pulp vitality testing: a test to determine whether the nerves in the pulp are healthy.

Resorption: gradual dissolution of the mineralized tissue, that is the root of the tooth; may be internal or external; occurs during exfoliation of a primary tooth and from the pressure of orthodontic treatment.

Study model: a positive life-size reproduction of the teeth and adjacent tissues usually formed pouring dental plaster or stone into a matrix or impression. Used in the study of a patient's oral condition in preparation for treatment planning and patient education.

Succedaneous: the permanent teeth that erupt into the positions of exfoliated primary teeth.

Supernumerary tooth: a condition where extra teeth are present.

Tongue thrust: the infantile pattern of suckle-swallow movement in which the tongue is placed between the incisor teeth or alveolar ridges; may result in an anterior open bite, deformation of the jaws, and abnormal function.

Chapter 17: Dental Soft Deposits, Biofilm, Calculus, and Stains

Acellular: not made up of or containing cells.

Adsorption: attachment of one substance to the surface of another; the action of a substance in attracting and holding other materials or particles on its surface.

Aerobe: heterotrophic microorganism that can live and grow in the presence of free oxygen; some are obligate, others facultative; *adj.* aerobic.

Amelogenesis imperfecta: imperfect formation of enamel; hereditary condition in which the ameloblasts fail to lay down the enamel matrix properly or at all.

Amorphous: without definite shape or visible differentiation in structure.

Anaerobe: heterotrophic microorganism that lives and grows in complete (or almost complete) absence of oxygen; some are obligate, others facultative; *adj.* anaerobic.

Apatite: crystalline mineral component of bones and teeth that contains calcium and phosphate.

Biofilm: dynamic, complex, multispecies communities of microorganisms that colonize the oral cavity. Unique characteristics allow biofilms to adapt to a variety of every changing environments; characteristics include tenacious adherence to surfaces, protective EPS, three-dimensional structures with complex nutrient, and communication pathways.

Cariogenic: adjective to indicate a conduciveness to the initiation of dental caries, such as a cariogenic biofilm or a cariogenic food.

Chlorophyll: green plant pigment essential to photosynthesis.

Chromogenic: producing color or pigment.

Chronologic: the order a series of events occurs. Often refers to timing as related to age.

Dental calculus: also referred to as "tartar," calculus is dental biofilm that has been mineralized primarily with calcium and phosphorus and occurs on the teeth and prosthetic appliances worn in the mouth.

Dentinogenesis imperfecta: hereditary disorder of dentin formation in which the odontoblasts lay down an abnormal matrix; can occur in both primary and permanent dentitions.

Endogenous: produced within or caused by factors within.

Exogenous: originating outside or caused by factors outside.

Extracellular polymeric substance (EPS): extracellular polymeric substances are compounds secreted by microorganisms and form a matrix for biofilm.

Extrinsic: derived from or situated on the outside; external.

Extrinsic stain: tooth discoloration or staining on the surface of the tooth surface.

Flora: the collective organisms of a given locale.

Oral flora: the various bacteria and other microorganisms that inhabit the oral cavity. The mouth has an indigenous flora, meaning those organisms that are native to that area of the body. Certain organisms specifically reside in certain parts, for example, on the tongue, on the mucosa, or in the gingival sulcus.

Food impaction: the forceful wedging of food into the periodontium by occlusal forces.

Hypoplasia: incomplete development or underdevelopment of an organ or a tissue.

Infection: invasion and multiplication of a microorganism in body tissues.

Insoluble: incapable of being dissolved.

Intrinsic: situated entirely within.

Leukocyte: white blood corpuscle capable of amoeboid movement; functions to protect the body against infection and disease.

Materia alba: white or cream-colored "cheesy" mass that can collect over dental biofilm on unclean, neglected teeth; it is composed of food debris, mucin, and bacteria sloughed epithelial cells.

Matrix: a surrounding framework, enabling development in a structured manner.

Maturation: stage or process of attaining maximal development; become mature.

Microorganism: minute living organisms, usually microscopic; includes bacteria, rickettsiae, viruses, fungi, and protozoa.

Mineralization: addition of mineral elements, such as calcium and phosphorus, to the body or a part thereof with resulting hardening of the tissue.

Nidus: nucleus, focus, point of origin.

Oral microbiome: microorganisms, their genetic makeup, and the environments they inhabit in the oral cavity.

Pathogen: disease-producing agent or microorganism; *adj.* pathogenic.

Planktonic: free floating single bacteria such as in saliva gingival crevicular fluid.

Polymeric: repeating molecular structures; in biofilms, the polymers are glycoprotein polysaccharides.

Pyrophosphate: inhibitor of calcification that occurs in parotid saliva of humans in variable amounts; anticalculus component of "tartar-control" dentifrices.

Quid: a portion of a substance, like tobacco, to be chewed, but not swallowed.

Quorum sensing: bacteria produce chemical signal molecules, resulting in development of the plaque biofilm.

Sharpey's fibers: connective tissue with bundles of fibers that connect bone to the periosteum covering the bone.

Supersaturated: a solution containing more of an ingredient that can be held in solution permanently.

Chapter 18: The Periodontium

Anoxemia: deficiency of oxygen in arterial blood.

Attachment apparatus: the cementum, periodontal ligament (PDL), and the alveolar bone.

Attached gingiva: gingiva attached to the underlying alveolar bone.

Biologic width: the distance from the base of the sulcus to the alveolar bone.

Bulbous: bulging or rounded.

Col: a depression between the buccal and lingual inter-proximal papilla.

Diastema: a space between two natural adjacent teeth.

Edematous: enlargement caused by fluids in inflamed tissues.

Embrasure: a triangular shaped space below the contact area of two adjacent teeth.

Epithelium: specialized single layer (simple) or multiple (stratified) layers of cells that form on the surface of skin, mucosa, or serous membranes.

> **Oral epithelium:** the tissue serving as a liner for the intraoral mucosal surfaces.

> **Squamous epithelium:** composed of a layer of flat, scale-like cells; or may be stratified.

Exudate: fluid and dead cells produced during inflammation, which can vary in color, thickness, and odor.

Fibrotic: fibroblasts (fiber-producing cells) of the connective tissue produce a change in the texture of the tissue, especially the gingiva, because of chronic inflammation; fibrotic gingiva may appear outwardly healthy and not bleed on probing, thus masking underlying disease.

Free gingiva: the part of the gingiva exposed to the oral cavity that surrounds the tooth and is not attached to the tooth.

Free gingival groove: a shallow line or groove that may be visible between the free and attached gingiva.

Frenum: a membrane that supports or restricts movement, that is labial frenum.

Friable: gingival tissue may become fragile and easily traumatized during examination and instrumentation.

GCF (gingival crevicular fluid): fluid secreted from the gingival crevice or sulcus around the tooth.

Gingival sulcus: crevice or space between the free gingiva and the tooth extending from the free gingival margin to the JE.

Hemidesmosome: half of a desmosome that forms a site of attachment between junctional epithelial cells and the tooth surface.

Hyperkeratosis: abnormal thickening of the keratin layer (stratum corneum) of the epithelium.

Interdental gingiva (interdental papilla): the unattached gingiva found in the space between teeth.

Junctional epithelium (JE): epithelium that is at the base or bottom of the sulcus.

Keratinized: a horny layer of flattened epithelial cells containing keratin.

Masticatory force: created by the action of the masticatory muscles during chewing.

MGJ (mucogingival junction): the line where mucosa from the cheeks or floor of the mouth and attached gingiva come together.

Non-keratinized mucosa: lining mucosa in which the stratified squamous epithelial cells retain their nuclei and cytoplasm.

Periodontium: tissues surrounding and supporting the teeth are divided into two sections the gingival unit, composed of the free and attached gingiva and the alveolar mucosa, and the attachment apparatus, which includes the cementum, PDL, and alveolar process.

Periodontal ligament (PDL): connective tissue connecting the cementum covering the root to the alveolar bone.

Probing depth: the distance from the gingival margin to the location of the periodontal probe tip inserted for gentle probing to the attachment.

Sharpey's fibers: penetrating connective-tissue fibers by which the tooth is attached to the adjacent alveolar bone; the fiber bundles penetrate cementum on one side, and alveolar bone on the other.

Stippled: the pitted, orange-peel appearance frequently seen on the surface of the attached gingiva.

Suppuration (or pus): formation of a fluid product or process of discharging pus as a result of inflammation. The fluid contains leukocytes, degenerated tissue elements, tissue fluids, and microorganisms. Color may range vary from blood tinged to white, yellow, or green.

Chapter 19: Periodontal Disease Development

Collagen: white fibers of the connective tissue.

Desquamation: shedding of the outer epithelial layer of the stratified squamous epithelium of skin or mucosa.

Edema: an accumulation of excessive fluid in cells, tissues, or a serous cavity.

Gingivitis: inflammation of the gingival tissues.

Iatrogenic: resulting from treatment by a professional person.

Impaction: forceful wedging of food, floss, and so on into the periodontium by occlusal forces.

Infiltration: the diffusion or accumulation in a tissue or cells of substances not normal to it or in amounts in excess of normal.

Lesion: any pathologic or traumatic discontinuity of tissue or loss of function of a part; broad term including wounds, sores, ulcers, tumors, and any other tissue damage.

Nonsurgical periodontal therapy (NSPT): includes dental biofilm removal and biofilm control (by patient); supragingival and subgingival scaling; root planing; and the adjunctive use of chemotherapeutic agents for control of bacterial infection, desensitizing hypersensitive exposed root surfaces, and dental caries prevention as related to the health of the periodontium.

Periodontitis: inflammation in the periodontium, affecting gingival tissues, periodontal ligament, cementum, and supporting bone.

Permeable: permitting passage of a fluid.

Periodontal risk assessment (PRA): periodontal risk assessment web-based tool based on tooth loss, and genetic and systemic conditions to predict risk for disease.

Periodontal risk calculator (PRC): periodontal risk calculator is a web-based periodontal risk assessment tool based on factors such as smoking, diabetes, and periodontal history to predict risk for disease.

Xerostomia: dryness of the mouth from a lack of normal secretions.

Chapter 20: Periodontal Examination

Calibration: determination of the accuracy of an instrument by measurement of its variation from a standard.

Clinical attachment level (CAL): probing depth (PD) as measured from the cementoenamel junction (CEJ) (or other fixed point) to the location of the probe tip at the coronal level of attached periodontal tissues.

Explorer: an instrument with a fine flexible, sharp point used for examination of the surfaces of the teeth to detect irregularities.

Fremitus: a vibration perceptible by palpation.

Periodontal probe: instrument with a rounded tip calibrated in millimeter increments to facilitate measurement of the pocket depth.

Probing depth (PD): the distance from the gingival margin (GM) to the location of the periodontal probe tip at the base of the sulcus.

Tactile: pertaining to the touch.

Tension test: application of tension at the mucogingival junction (MGJ) by retracting cheek, lip, and tongue to tighten the alveolar mucosa and test for the presence of attached gingiva; area of missing attached gingiva is revealed when the alveolar mucosa and frena are connected directly to the free gingiva.

Chapter 21: Indices and Scoring Methods

Calibrate: determine accuracy and consistency between examiners in order to standardize procedures and gain reliability of recorded findings.

Data: pieces of information collected using measurements and/or counts.

Data collection: the process of gathering information (through the use of tools such as dental indices).

Determinant: a factor that can influence the outcome of some process. Health determinants include physical and social factors that influence the health outcomes of an individual or in a community.

Epidemiology: the study of the relationships of various factors that determine the frequency and distribution of diseases in the human community; study of health and disease in populations.

Incidence: the rate at which a certain event occurs, as the number of new cases of a specific disease occurring during a certain period of time.

Index: a graduated, numeric scale with upper and lower limits; scores on the scale correspond to a specific criterion for individuals or populations; *pl.* indices or indexes.

> **Dental index:** describes oral status by expressing clinical observations as numeric values.

Indicator: a factor that typically characterizes a disease or health condition; a factor measured and analyzed to describe health status. Dental indices described in this chapter measure oral health indicators.

Prevalence: the total number of cases of a specific disease or condition in existence in a given population at a certain time.

Ramfjord index teeth: teeth used for epidemiologic studies of periodontal diseases: the maxillary right and mandibular left first molars, maxillary left and mandibular right first premolars, and maxillary left and mandibular right central incisors.

Reliability: ability of an index or a test procedure to measure consistently at different times and under a variety of conditions, reproducibility, and consistency.

Sample: a portion or subset of an entire population.

Screening: assessment of characteristics in individuals that indicate need for additional examination or, if performed on many individuals, can disclose the incidence or prevalence of specific diseases in a population.

Status: refers to the state or condition of an individual or population.

Surveillance: the ongoing systematic collection, analysis, and interpretation of outcome-specific data for use in planning, implementing, and evaluating the effect of public health programs and practices.

Validity: ability of an index or a test procedure to measure what it is intended to measure.

Chapter 22: Dental Hygiene Diagnosis

ADLs (activities of daily living): a measure of the ability to carry out the basic tasks needed for self-care.

Anticipatory guidance: patient education and oral hygiene instructions that anticipate potential oral and systemic health problems associated with risk factors identified during patient assessment.

ASA: American Society of Anesthesiologists; originally developed the ASA classifications to determine modifications necessary to provide general anesthetic to patients during surgical procedures.

Assessment: the critical analysis and evaluation or judgment of a particular condition, situation, or other subject of appraisal.

Best practice: a procedure or treatment intervention that has been shown by research and experience to produce optimal results and is established as a standard suitable for widespread adoption.

Chief complaint: the patient's concern as stated during the initial health history preparation; may be the reason for seeking professional care; a complaint such as pain or discomfort may require emergency dental diagnosis.

Diagnosis: a statement of the problem; a concise technical description of the cause, nature, or manifestations of a condition, situation, or problem; identification of a disease or deviation from normal condition by recognition of characteristic signs and symptoms.

> **Dental hygiene diagnosis:** identification of an existing or a potential oral health problem that a dental hygienist is qualified and licensed to treat.

> **Dental hygiene prognosis:** a judgment regarding the results (outcomes) expected to be achieved from oral treatment provided by a dental hygienist.

Evidence-based approach: providing oral care based on relevant, scientifically sound research.

Genetic susceptibility: an increased likelihood of developing a particular disease based on a person's genetic makeup.

Health literacy: determining an individual's capacity to obtain, process, and understand basic oral health information and services needed to make appropriate health decisions and follow through with them.

IADLs (instrumental activities of daily living): a measure of the ability to perform more of the complex tasks necessary to function in our society; tasks that require a combination of physical and cognitive ability.

Prognosis: prediction of outcome; a forecast of the probable course and outcome of a disease and the prospects of recovery as expected by the nature of the specific condition and the symptoms of the case.

Risk factor: an attribute or exposure that increases the probability of disease, such as an aspect of personal behavior, environmental exposure, or an inherited characteristic associated with health-related conditions.

> **Modifiable risk factor:** a determinant that can be modified by intervention, thereby reducing the probability of disease.

Chapter 23: The Dental Hygiene Care Plan

Consent: voluntary agreement to an action proposed by another.

Dental hygiene care plan: the services within the framework of the total treatment plan to be carried out by the dental hygienist.

Implied consent: the granting of permission of healthcare without a formal agreement between the patient and the healthcare provider.

Informed consent: a patient's voluntary agreement to a treatment plan after details of the proposed treatment have been presented and comprehended by the patient.

Informed refusal of care: a patient's decision to refuse recommended treatment after all options, potential risks, and potential benefits have been thoroughly explained.

Lifestyle factors: the habits, attitudes, moral standards, economic status that together constitute a mode of living that are often associated with disease. Examples would be physical inactivity, obesity, unhealthy diet, tobacco smoking, risky alcohol consumption.

Intervention: to happen or take place between other events; to intervene, as with a specific treatment.

Prioritize: to arrange in order of importance.

Sequence: a continuous or related series of things (such as dental hygiene interventions) following in a certain order or succession.

Chapter 24: Preventive Counseling and Behavior Change

Affirmation: to validate or confirm; commending a patient's efforts toward change.

Ambivalence: simultaneous conflict or uncertainty toward making a change.

Autonomy: individual's right to make their own decisions.

Behavior: manner in which an individual acts or manages himself or herself.

Behavior change: transition in the way a patient acts or manages himself or herself.

Change talk: any self-expressed language that is an argument for change.

Communication: verbal or nonverbal interaction or interchange.

Communication style: attitude and approach to assisting patients, a way of talking with them that describes the clinician's relationship with the patient.

Compliance: extent to which a person's health behaviors coincide with dental/medical counseling.

Elicit: to draw forth or bring out.

Evaluation: assessment of changes in patient's behavior or oral health status.

Evocation: eliciting or drawing out from patient through open-ended questions.

Learning: acquiring knowledge or skills though study, instruction, or experience.

Listening: to make an attempt to hear what someone is saying.

Active listening: a listening style of maintaining focus and remaining engaged with what the patient is saying and reacting by demonstrating you are listening and have understood the patient either through reflection of the main points or summarizing what has been said.

Reflective listening: response to what the patient is conveying with a statement or summary that is more than repeating verbatim what the patient has said.

Motivation: internal driving force that prompts an individual to act to satisfy a need or desire or to accomplish a particular goal.

Motivational interviewing (MI): is a person-centered, goal-directed method of communication for eliciting and strengthening intrinsic motivation for positive change.

Preventive counseling: professional guidance and support to assist a patient with acting ahead regarding oral health through the utilization of MI methods.

Spirit of MI: the underlying perspective with which one practices MI.

Sustain talk: the individuals own arguments for not changing.

Chapter 25: Protocols for Prevention and Control of Dental Caries

Acidogenic bacteria: bacteria in dental biofilm capable of metabolizing fermentable carbohydrates into acids.

Aciduric bacteria: bacteria in dental biofilm capable of thriving in an acidic oral environment.

Buffer: a substance that by its presence in solution is capable of neutralizing alkali or acid.

CAMBRA® (Caries Assessment and Management by Risk Assessment): procedure to assess risk for future dental caries development and identify approaches to managing caries risk.

Cavitated carious lesion: advanced lesion with break through the tooth surface; contrast with noncavitated carious lesion, when a dull probe passed over a white demineralized area detects no roughness or breakthrough.

Cavitation: breakthrough of the enamel surface; final stage in the caries process.

Cavitated lesion: a loss of the integrity of the surface enamel with exposure of dentin.

CRA (caries risk assessment): procedure to predict future dental caries development before the clinical onset of the disease.

Demineralization: major stage in the dental caries process in which minerals, primarily calcium and phosphorous, are removed from tooth structure by acids formed by acidogenic bacteria, primarily *mutans streptococci* and lactobacilli.

Dental caries: infectious disease of teeth caused by acidogenic bacteria with dissolution of enamel and dentin (coronal caries) and cementum and dentin (root caries).

Hyposalivation: reduced salivary flow rates due to medication or medical-related effect on the salivary gland function.

ICCMS™ (International Caries Classification and Management System): a caries management system based on evidence and a consensus of international experts.

ICDAS™ (International Caries Detection and Assessment System): a caries classification system created by a consensus of international experts.

Remineralization: healing process in which minerals are redeposited in the demineralized tooth structure; accomplished by the protective factors of the saliva and the action of fluoride to inhibit demineralization and interfere with the enzymatic requirements of bacteria.

White spot lesion: early stage of the caries process when demineralization causes a change in the enamel to appear chalky white.

Xerostomia: dry mouth from reduced or absent salivary flow. May be related to medical conditions, head and neck radiation, or medications.

Chapter 26: Oral Infection Control: Toothbrushes and Toothbrushing

Abrasion (gingiva): lesion of the gingiva resulting from mechanical removal of the surface epithelium.

Abrasion (tooth): loss of tooth structure produced by a mechanical cause (such as a hard-bristled toothbrush used with excessive pressure and an abrasive dentifrice); abrasion contrasts with erosion, which involves a chemical process.

Bristle: individual short stiff, natural hair of an animal; historically, toothbrush bristles were taken from hog or wild boar, but current toothbrush bristles are made of nylon and are called filaments.

Bristle stiffness: the reaction force exerted per unit area of the brush during deflection; the term stiffness is used interchangeably with firmness of toothbrush bristles or filaments; the stiffness depends primarily on the length and diameter of the filaments.

Dysgeusia: impairment or unpleasant change in taste of food.

End-rounded: characteristic shape of each toothbrush filament; a special manufacturing process removes all sharp edges and provides smooth, rounded ends to prevent injury to gingiva or tooth structure during use.

Filament: individual synthetic fiber; a single element of a tuft fixed into a toothbrush head.

Halitosis: bad breath or unpleasant odor or smell from the mouth.

Mechanical dental biofilm control: oral hygiene methods for removal of dental biofilm from tooth surfaces using a toothbrush and selected devices for interdental cleaning; contrasts with chemotherapeutic biofilm control in which an antimicrobial agent is used.

Mucositis: painful inflammation with ulcerations of mucous membranes found in the gastrointestinal tract including the mouth. Oral mucositis is a debilitating complication of cancer therapies including chemotherapy and radiotherapy and can lead to increased morbidity and mortality.

Neutropenia: abnormally low neutrophils; a type of white blood cell that prevents infection. Neutrophil counts of less than 1,500 neutrophils/microliter (μL) of blood are considered neutropenia, but when risk of serious infection increases as the absolute neutrophil count (ANC) falls to less than 500/μL.

Power toothbrush: a brush driven by electricity or battery; also called power-assisted, automatic, or electric.

Sulcular brushing: a method in which the end-round filament tips are directed into the gingival sulcus at approximately 45° for the purpose of loosening and removing dental biofilm from both the gingival sulcus and the tooth surface just below the gingival margin.

Toothbrush head: the part of the toothbrush composed of the tufts and the stock (extension of the handle where the tufts are attached).

Trismus: inability to open the mouth fully.

Tuft: a cluster of bristles or filaments secured together in one hole in the head of a toothbrush.

Chapter 27: Oral Infection Control: Interdental Care

Col: the depression in the gingival tissue under a contact area between the lingual (palatal) papilla and the facial papilla.

Embrasure: V-shaped spillway space next to the contact area of adjacent teeth, narrowest at the contact and widening toward the facial, lingual (palatal), and occlusal contacts.

Floss cleft: a cleft in the gingival margin usually at a mesial or distal line angle of a tooth where dental floss was repeatedly applied incorrectly. The lining of the cleft can be completely lined with epithelium.

Floss cut: unintentional incision at the gingival margin due to incorrect positioning and placement of dental floss.

Interproximal space: the triangular region bounded by the proximal surfaces of contacting teeth and the alveolar bone between the teeth, which forms the base of the triangle; the space is normally filled with the interdental papilla; also called the interdental area.

Irrigant: substance used for irrigation.

Irrigation: flushing of a specific area or site with a stream of fluid; application of a continuous or pulsated stream of fluid to a part of the body for a cleansing or therapeutic purpose.

Supragingival irrigation: the point of delivery of the irrigation is at, or coronal to, the free gingival margin.

Subgingival irrigation: the point of the delivery of the irrigation is placed in the sulcus or pocket and may reach the base of the pocket depending on its probing depth.

Keratinized epithelium: outer, protective surface of stratified squamous epithelium; covers the masticatory mucosa; interdental col area is not normally keratinized.

Chapter 28: Dentifrices and Mouthrinses

Antimicrobial agent: chemical that is bacteriostatic or bactericidal.

Astringent: a substance that causes contraction or shrinkage and arrests discharges.

Chemotherapeutic agent: a chemical that is used for therapeutic reasons.

CHX: chlorhexidine.

Copolymer: a substance with a high molecular weight that results from chemically combining two or more monomers.

Efficacy: the benefits of a product or procedure that lead to intended results, such as reduction in gingivitis.

Humectant: substance contained in a product (such as in a dentifrice) to retain moisture and prevent hardening upon exposure to air.

Substantivity: the ability of an agent to bind to the pellicle, tooth surface, and soft tissue and be released over an extended period of time with the retention of its potency.

Therapeutic: a chemical with therapeutic properties that is delivered by rinsing or irrigation device.

Chapter 29: The Patient with Orthodontic Appliances

Aligner system: a series of customized transparent and removable aligners utilized in orthodontic therapy to align or straighten teeth.

Appliance: any device designed to influence the shape and/or function of the mouth/jaw system.

Arch wire: curved wire positioned in the brackets around the dental arch and held in place by elastomers or ligatures.

Band: preformed stainless-steel ring fitted around a tooth and cemented in place; available in shapes for each tooth form; each band has a bracket attached on the facial side, which is the mode of attachment for the arch wire.

Bonding: process by which orthodontic brackets are affixed to the tooth surface; a fluoride-releasing, light-activated resin is frequently used.

Bracket: attachment that is bonded to the enamel for the purpose of holding the arch wire.

Ceramic: alumina (Al_2O_3) used as a single-crystal material or as a polycrystalline material.

Debonding: removal of brackets and residual adhesive, after which the tooth surface is returned to its normal contour.

Elastomer: elastoplastic ring or latex elastic used to hold an arch wire in a bracket wing.

Fixed appliance: a bonded or banded appliance affixed to individual teeth or groups of teeth.

Hawley retainer: a removable plastic and wire appliance used to stabilize teeth; may be modified for special applications during or after orthodontic therapy.

Orthodontic appliance: device used to influence growth and/or position of teeth and jaws.

Retainer: an orthodontic appliance, fixed or removable, used to maintain the position of the teeth following corrective treatment.

Shear bond strength (SBS): the amount of force needed for a restoration or bonded material to be broken or fractured from a tooth surface.

Chapter 30: Care of Dental Prosthesis

Abutment: a tooth or an implant used for the support or retention of a fixed or removable prosthesis.

Angular cheilitis: inflammation on the corners of the mouth typically affecting the vermillion border and perioral skin. The cause may be nutrient deficiency, fungal or yeast infection, and overclosure or loss of vertical dimension.

Anodontia: a rare condition characterized by congenital absence of all teeth, primary and permanent.

Complete denture: dental prosthesis that replaces the entire dentition and associated structures; may be a complete maxillary denture or a complete mandibular or both.

Denture: artificial substitute for missing natural teeth and adjacent tissues.

Denture adhesive: a soft material used to adhere a denture to the underlying mucosa; also referred to as an adherent.

Denture foundation area: the surfaces of the oral structures available to support a denture.

Denture insertion: the process of directing a prosthesis to a desired oral location; introduction of a prosthesis into a patient's mouth; other terms used are denture delivery or denture placement.

Denture stomatitis: an inflammation of the oral mucosa that bears a complete or partial removable dental prosthesis, typically a denture.

Edentulous: lacking or missing teeth.

Fixed partial denture: a replacement for one or more missing teeth that is securely cemented to natural teeth and/or dental implant abutments that furnish the primary support for the prosthesis; also called a fixed prosthesis or bridge.

Immediate denture: any removable dental prosthesis fabricated for placement immediately following the removal of a natural tooth/teeth.

Interim denture: a fixed or removable dental prosthesis designed to enhance esthetics, stabilization, and/or function for a limited period, after which it is to be replaced by a definitive dental or maxillofacial prosthesis. Also referred to as provisional prosthesis, provisional restoration.

Obturator: a prosthesis used to close a congenital or acquired opening, such as for a cleft palate, an area lost due to trauma, or after surgery for removal of a diseased area.

Occlusal vertical dimension: the distance measured between two points when the occluding members are in contact.

Overclosure: the vertical relationship between the jaws is impaired due to missing teeth.

Overdenture: a removable denture that covers and is partially supported by one or more remaining natural teeth, roots, and/or dental implants and the soft tissue of the residual alveolar ridge; also called overlay denture.

Pontic: an artificial tooth on a partial denture that replaces a missing natural tooth, restores its function, and usually occupies the space previously filled by the natural crown.

Precision attachment: a type of connector that consists of a metal receptacle and a close-fitting part; the metal receptacle is usually included within the restoration of an abutment tooth, and the close-fitting part is attached to a pontic or RPD framework.

Prosthesis: artificial replacement of an absent part of the body; may be a therapeutic device to improve or alter function; may be a device employed to aid in accomplishing a desired surgical result.

Removable partial denture (RPD): a dental prosthesis that supplies teeth and/or associated structures in a partially edentulous jaw and can be removed and replaced at will.

Residual ridges: the portion of the alveolar bone and its soft-tissue covering that remains after the removal of teeth.

Supererupt: a tooth will continue to migrate occlusally if there is no opposing tooth for it to occlude with.

Ultrasonic cleaner: a device, in which a denture is placed in water or some type of solvent cleaner, that uses ultrasonic waves to dislodge debris on a denture.

Chapter 31: The Patient with Dental Implants

Abutment: segment connecting the submerged implant body to the prosthetic component. The abutment enters the oral cavity, providing a platform for attaching crowns or bridges.

Alloplast: an inert foreign body used for implantation within tissue.

Augmentation: to increase the size beyond the existing size; in alveolar ridge or maxillary sinus augmentation, to increase the bone to accommodate a dental implant.

Biologic or permucosal seal: functional soft-tissue barrier at the base of the peri-implant sulcus; characterized by adhesion of junctional epithelium in the absence of Sharpey fibers, making it more susceptible to bacterial invasion by periodontal pathogens.

Endosseous or root form dental implant: tooth root replacement with a cylindrical or conical shape similar to a natural tooth root.

Fibrous encapsulation: layer of fibrous connective tissue between the implant and surrounding bone. Also called fibrous integration; indicative of failed osseointegration.

Osseointegration: the direct attachment or connection of osseous tissue to an inert alloplastic material without intervening connective tissue.

Peri-implant mucositis: reversible inflammation of the periodontal tissues around an implant with no subsequent bone loss; similar to gingivitis in a natural tooth.

Peri-implantitis: destructive inflammatory process of the periodontal tissues around an implant characterized by progressive bone loss in addition to soft-tissue inflammation with hemorrhage and/or exudate; similar to periodontitis in a natural tooth.

Root form: endosseous implant shaped in the approximate form of a tooth root.

Sinus augmentation (sinus lift): site preparation procedure that elevates the floor of the maxillary sinus to accommodate a dental implant by increasing the vertical height of bone via grafting/augmentation.

Subperiosteal: the periosteum that is tacked in place on the bone with a few small implant screws to support an overdenture.

Titanium: a uniquely biocompatible metal used for implants either in the commercially pure form or as an alloy.

Titanium alloy: a common titanium alloy (Ti-6A1-4V) used for dental implants that contains 6% aluminum to increase strength and decrease weight and 4% vanadium to prevent corrosion.

Transosseous: dental devices implanted through the bone.

Tomography: a three-dimensional image of the internal structures of a solid object like the mandible.

Chapter 32: The Patient with Nicotine Use Disorders

Addiction: a chronic disorder leading to negative physical, psychological, or social consequences from compulsive use of substance; characterized by continued use despite negative effects encountered by use.

Alternative tobacco products (ATPs): tobacco products besides cigarettes, including e-cigarettes, vape pens, water pipe/hookah, and smokeless tobacco.

Carcinogen: substance or chemical that has been known to cause cancer.

Cotinine: a by-product of nicotine found in body fluids; cotinine levels are used in behavioral research to determine recent use of nicotine-containing products or recent contact with passive smoke and in clinical research to determine correlations between cotinine levels and oral disease.

Electronic cigarette: see electronic nicotine delivery system (ENDS).

Electronic nicotine delivery system (ENDS): also called an ENDS, electronic cigarette or e-cigarette, the nicotine liquid is heated to deliver vaporized nicotine through a device that is made to look similar to a regular cigarette but comes in a variety of shapes, including one that looks like a USB jump drive. E-cigarettes come as disposable or rechargeable models with a variety of flavors. May also be called vaping.

Environmental tobacco smoke (ETS) or passive smoke: tobacco smoke present in room air resulting from ignited tobacco products burning in an ashtray or exhaled by a smoker (people who are currently smoking are also exposed to other smokers' sidestream smoke).

Mainstream smoke: smoke inhaled directly into the user's lungs.

Nicotine: a poisonous, addictive stimulant that is the chief psychoactive ingredient in tobacco.

Nitrosamines: cancer-causing chemicals found in tobacco.

Psychoactive drug: possessing the ability to alter mood, behavior, cognitive processes, or mental tension.

Sidestream smoke: the aerosol emitted directly into the surrounding air from the lit end of a smoldering tobacco product; may be inhaled by the user; is a major component of environmental smoke.

Smokeless (spit) tobacco: term used to define all forms of tobacco that are not ignited or inhaled.

Third-hand smoke: tobacco smoke residue absorbed by furnishings.

Transdermal: method of drug delivery by patch on skin; a mode for slow release over extended time.

Transmucosal: type of drug delivery by infiltration of mucosal lining.

Water pipe (or hookah): a water pipe used to smoke specially made flavored tobacco.

Chapter 33: Diet and Dietary Analysis

AIs (adequate intakes): the recommended nutrient intake utilized when there is not enough information to establish an EAR.

Anticariogenic: substance in foods that inhibits or arrests dental caries formation.

Antioxidant: a compound that stops the damaging effects of reactive substances seeking an electron (oxidizing agent).

Ariboflavinosis: a condition resulting from a lack of riboflavin.

Body mass index (BMI): a measure of body fat based on height in centimeters (cm) and weight in kilograms (kg).

Cariogenic: foods and beverages that lower oral pH and are conducive to dental caries; the degree of cariogenicity depends on many factors, including physical form, texture, and consistency of the carbohydrate-containing food; its retention and clearance time from the oral cavity and the frequency of use.

Diet: customary amount and kind of food and drink taken by an individual from day to day.

Dietary assessment: assessment of quality of food intake, whether an individual is consuming an adequate diet, and where modifications are needed to promote optimum health.

DRIs (Dietary Reference Intakes): a comprehensive term for categories of reference values that concentrate on maintaining a healthy state for the healthy general population to avoid overeating and prevent chronic disease.

EARs (Estimated Average Requirements): estimates the nutrient requirements of the average individual.

Malnutrition: poor nourishment resulting from improper diet or some defect of metabolism that prevents the body from utilizing the intake of food properly.

Meal plan: a selectively planned or prescribed regimen of food to meet certain needs of the individual.

Noncariogenic: does not support or promote bacterial growth responsible for caries formation.

Nutrient: a chemical substance in foods needed by the body for growth and repair; the six classes of nutrients are proteins, fats, carbohydrates, minerals, vitamins, and water.

> **Macronutrients:** energy-yielding nutrients needed in larger amounts in the diet: carbohydrate, protein, and fat.
>
> **Micronutrients:** nutrients needed in small amounts in the diet and are not energy yielding: vitamins and minerals.

Nutrient or Nutritional Deficiency: inadequacy of nutrients in the tissues; the result of inadequate dietary intake or impairment of digestion, absorption, transport, or metabolism.

Nutrient-dense: food with high content of vitamins and minerals, but comparatively low in calories.

Nutrition: sum of processes involved in taking nutrients into the body, assimilating and utilizing them; includes ingestion, digestion, absorption, transport, utilization of nutrients, and excretion of waste products.

RDAs (Recommended Dietary Allowances): recommendations for the average amounts of nutrients recommended to be consumed daily by healthy people to achieve adequate nutrient intake to prevent deficiency.

Registered dietitian or Registered dietitian nutritionist (RD or RDN): a healthcare professional with a minimum of a bachelor's degree in nutrition or dietetics who has attended an internship program or equivalent and passed the registration examination, all under the approval of the American Dietetic Association. Continuing education is required to keep credentials current.

ULs (Tolerable Upper Intake Levels, or Upper Levels): maximum intake by an individual that is unlikely to create risks of adverse health effects in almost all healthy individuals.

USDA: U.S. Department of Agriculture.

Vegan diet: a diet consisting of only plant foods. Other varieties of the vegan diet are the fruitarian: fruits, nuts, honey, and vegetable oils; lacto-vegetarian: vegan based with the inclusion of dairy products; lacto-ovo-vegetarian: vegan based with the inclusion of dairy products and eggs.

Chapter 34: Fluorides

AAPD: American Association of Pediatric Dentistry.

Abrasive system: cleaning or polishing substances used in dentifrice; best when compatible with fluoride compounds and other ingredients, and does not alter the tooth structure unfavorably.

ADA: American Dental Association.

Apatite: a group of minerals of the general formula $Ca_{10}(PO_4)X_2$, wherein the X might include hydroxyl (OH), carbonate (CO), fluoride (F), or oxygen (O); crystalline mineral component of hard tissues (bones and teeth).

APF: acidulated phosphate fluoride.

Cariostatic: exerting an inhibitory action on the progress of dental caries.

CDC: Centers for Disease Control and Prevention.

Defluoridation: lowering the amount of fluoride in fluoridated water to an optimum level for the prevention of dental caries and dental fluorosis.

Demineralization: breakdown of the tooth structure with a loss of mineral content, primarily calcium and phosphorus.

DMFT/dmft: decayed, missing, and filled teeth (permanent and primary dentition, respectively).

Efficacy: with reference to a product, an efficacious product produces a statistically and clinically significant benefit under ideal testing conditions in carefully controlled clinical trials.

FDA: Food and Drug Administration.

Fluorapatite: the form of hydroxyapatite in which fluoride ions have replaced some of the hydroxyl ions; with fluoride, the apatite is less soluble and, therefore, more resistant to the acids formed from carbohydrate intake.

Fluoride: a salt of hydrofluoric acid; the ionized form of fluorine that occurs in many tissues and is stored primarily in bones and teeth.

Fluorosis: form of enamel hypomineralization due to excessive ingestion of fluoride during the development and mineralization of the teeth; depending on the length of exposure and the concentration of the fluoride, the fluorosed area may appear as a small white spot or as severe brown staining with pitting.

Gel: semisolid or solid phase of a colloidal solution.

Halo or diffusion effect: occurs when foods and beverages processed in a fluoridated community are imported and consumed in a nonfluoridated community.

Hydroxyapatite: $Ca_{10}(PO_4)_6(OH)_2$; the form of apatite that is the principal mineral component of teeth, bones, and calculus.

Maturation: stage or process of becoming mature or attaining maximal development; with respect to tooth development, maturation results from the continuous dynamic exchange of ions into the surface of the enamel from pellicle, dental biofilm, and oral fluids.

NaF: neutral sodium fluoride.

OTC: over-the-counter.

ppm (parts per million): measure used to designate the amount of fluoride used for optimum level in fluoridated water, dentifrice, and other fluoride-containing preparations (1 ppm is equivalent to 1 mg/L).

Prevented fraction: the proportion of disease occurrence in a population that is averted due to an intervention.

Remineralization: restoration of mineral elements in a tooth surface; enhanced by the presence of fluoride; remineralized lesions are more resistant to initiation of dental caries than is normal tooth structure.

Rx: prescription.

SnF$_2$: stannous fluoride.

Thixotropic: type of gel that sets in a gel-like state but becomes fluid under stress; the fluid form permits the solution to flow into interdental areas.

USPHS: US Public Health Services.

White spot: term used to describe a small area on the surface of enamel that contrasts in appearance with the rest of the surface and may be visible only when the tooth is dried; two types of white spots can be differentiated: an area of demineralization and an area of fluorosis (also referred to as an "enamel opacity").

Chapter 35: Sealants

Acid etch: in sealant placement, the enamel surface is prepared by the application of phosphoric acid, which etches the surface to provide mechanical retention for the sealant.

Articulating paper: paper treated with dye or wax used to mark points of contact (occlusion) between the maxillary and mandibular teeth.

Bibulous pad: absorbent; a flat bibulous pad, placed in the cheek over the opening of Stensen duct, is used to aid in maintaining a dry field while placing sealants.

Bis-GMA (bisphenol A glycidyl methylacrylate): plastic material used for dental sealants.

Bond strength: expression of the degree of adherence between the tooth surface and the sealant.

Bonding (mechanical): physical adherence of one substance to another; the adherence of a sealant to the enamel surface is accomplished by an acid-etching technique that leaves microspaces between the enamel rods; the sealant becomes mechanically locked (bonded) in these microspaces.

Curing: the process is used for **polymerization** of resin-based sealant and composites so that the material hardens by which plastic becomes rigid.

Filled sealant: contains, in addition to bis-GMA, microparticles of glass, quartz, silica, and other fillers used in composite restorations; fillers make the sealant more resistant to abrasion.

Incipient caries: early or beginning caries, caries not limited to the enamel.

Micropores: tiny openings.

Polymer: a compound of high molecular weight formed by a combination of a chain of simpler molecules (monomers).

Polymerization: a reaction in which a high-molecular-weight product is produced by successive additions of a simpler compound.

>**Autopolymerized:** self-curing; a reaction in which a high-molecular-weight product is produced by successive additions of a simpler compound; hardening process of pit-and-fissure sealants.

>**Photopolymerized:** polymerization with the use of an external light source.

Sealant: organic polymer that bonds to an enamel surface by mechanical retention accommodated by projections of the sealant into micropores created in the enamel by etching; the two types of sealants, filled and unfilled, both are composed of bis-GMA.

Viscosity: in general, the resistance to flow or alteration of shape by any substance as a result of molecular cohesion.

Chapter 36: Anxiety and Pain Control

Absolute contraindication: under no circumstances should the local anesthetic or vasoconstrictor be administered.

Ambient air: atmospheric air in its natural state.

Analgesia: reduction or elimination of pain in the conscious patient.

Anesthesia: loss of feeling or sensation, especially loss of tactile sensitivity, with or without loss of consciousness.

Anxiety: a negative, emotional response to an anticipated event, the outcome of which is unknown. This is a learned response from personal experience or the stories of others.

ASA classification: developed by the American Society of Anesthesiologists, is a grading system to assess the patient's medical and physical state prior to receiving anesthesia or undergoing surgery.

Aspiration: recommended technique for preventing injection of local anesthetic directly into circulatory system. Negative pressure is created in anesthetic cartridge. If needle tip is in artery or vein, blood will be visible in cartridge.

Block anesthesia: induced by injecting the anesthetic close to a nerve trunk; may be at some distance from the area to be treated; involves multiple teeth and surrounding hard and soft tissues.

Conscious sedation: the combination of medications to help a patient relax (sedation) and block pain (anesthesia) during a medical or dental procedure.

Diffusion hypoxia: lack of adequate amounts of oxygen that can result from the rapid diffusion of nitrous oxide molecules from the bloodstream into the lungs.

Epinephrine: a hormone secreted by the adrenal medulla that, among many functions, causes vasodilation of blood vessels of skeletal muscles, vasoconstriction of arterioles of skin and mucous membranes, and stimulation of heart action; used in local anesthetics for its vasoconstrictive action.

Extravascular: not occurring or contained in body vessels.

General anesthesia: the elimination of all sensations, accompanied by the loss of consciousness.

Half-life: the time it takes for the plasma concentration of a drug to reach half of its original concentration; the time it takes for half of the dose to be eliminated from the bloodstream.

Iatrosedation: reduction of anxiety as a result of the clinician's behavior or actions. A psychosomatic method of pain control.

Idiosyncratic: unusual feature of a person; unusual or exaggerated response.

Infiltration anesthesia: induced by injecting the anesthetic directly into or around the area to be anesthetized; anesthetizes the smaller terminal nerve endings of the tooth.

Local anesthesia: loss of sensation, especially pain, in a circumscribed area without loss of consciousness; also called regional anesthesia.

Maximum recommended dose (MRD): the highest amount of an anesthetic agent that can be given safely and without complication to a patient.

Occupational exposure: subject to an action or influence, usually negative, as a result of one's occupation or work environment.

Pain threshold: point at which a sensation starts to be painful and a response results. Varies between individuals based on interpretation of sensation. May be altered by some drugs.

Potency: strength of a drug. Amount of a medication or drug necessary to achieve a desired effect.

Prostaglandin synthesis: the process of making lipid compounds that takes place in the cells; chemical messengers that mediate biologic processes, such as inflammation, and are important in the normal function of many different tissues.

Psychogenic reaction: having an emotional or psychological origin.

Relative contraindication: the offending drug (either local anesthetic or vasoconstrictor) can be administered after careful review of the medical history and assessment of risk factors. Use minimal effective amount; stay below the MRD.

Titration: a technique for individualization of drug dose. Administration of small, incremental dose of a drug until the desired clinical action is observed.

Vasoconstrictor: a drug that constricts blood vessels. An additive to most local anesthetic solutions to offset the vasodilating actions of the local anesthetic.

Chapter 37: Instruments and Principles for Instrumentation

Acoustic turbulence: agitation in the fluids surrounding a rapidly vibrating ultrasonic tip; has potential to disrupt the bacterial matrix.

Activation: the action of an instrument in the performance of the task for which it was designed; consists of a series of strokes.

Adaptation: relationship between the working end of an instrument and the tooth surface being treated.

Amplitude: the distance of power scaler tip movement measured in micrometers.

Angulation: the angle formed by the working end of an instrument with the surface to which the instrument is applied for treatment.

Blade: working end of an instrument with special design for a particular clinical treatment.

Cavitation: action created by the formation and collapse of bubbles in the water by high-frequency sound waves surrounding an ultrasonic tip.

Curet: a curved, rounded dental instrument utilized primarily for subgingival scaling and root planing.

    Area-specific curet: a specialized instrument designed with specific angles in the shank for adaptation to a certain group of tooth surfaces.

Universal curet: a curet designed for use on any tooth surface where the adaptation, angulation, and other principles of instrumentation can be correctly and effectively accomplished.

Dominant hand: the hand generally used for performing tasks, such as writing and holding instruments for scaling.

Ferromagnetic: type of rod with unusually high magnetic permeability used in magnetostrictive ultrasonic unit inserts.

Finger rest: for an intraoral rest, the place on a tooth or teeth where the third or ring finger of the hand holding the instrument is placed to provide stabilization and control during activation of the instrument.

Frequency: the speed of tip movement, measured in cycles per second (CPS).

Fulcrum: the support upon which a lever rests while force intended to produce motion is exerted.

Kilohertz (kHz): a unit of energy equal to 1,000 cps.

Lateral pressure: the minimal pressure that is required of an instrument against the tooth to accomplish the objective of the assessment or treatment.

Lavage: the therapeutic washing of the pocket and root surface to remove endotoxins and loose debris.

Magnetostrictive: ultrasonic scaling device that generates a magnetic field and produces tip vibrations by the expansion and contraction of a metal stack or rod.

Nondominant hand: the hand that is often times used for essential supplementary functions to assist the dominant hand.

Offset blade: the blade of an area-specific Gracey curet in which the lower shank is at a 70° angle to the face of the blade; contrasts with a universal curet blade, which is at a 90° angle with the lower shank.

Piezoelectric: ultrasonic scaling device activated by dimensional changes in crystals housed in the handpiece.

Scaler: instrument designed for initial removal of supragingival calculus, prior to finishing with a curet.

Scaling: instrumentation of a tooth surface to remove calculus and biofilm.

Shank: the part of the instrument between the handle and the working end.

Sonic scaler: type of mechanical power-driven scaler that functions from energy delivered by a vibrating working tip in the frequency of 2,500–7,000 cps; driven by compressed air, the handpiece connects directly to a conventional rotary handpiece tubing.

Stack: magnetostrictive inserts made of flat metal strips stacked, or sandwiched, together; metal in stack acts like an antenna to pick up magnetic field and cause vibration.

Stroke: a single unbroken movement made by an instrument against a tooth surface during an examination or treatment procedure to accomplish a particular objective; the motion made for activation of an instrument.

Terminal (lower) shank: the part of the shank next to the blade.

Transducer: a device that converts energy or power from one form to another.

Ultrasonic scaler: power-driven scaling instrument that operates in a frequency range between 25,000 and 50,000 cps to convert a high-frequency electrical current into mechanical vibrations.

Working end: the part of an instrument used to carry out the purpose and function of the instrument.

Chapter 38: Instrument Care and Sharpening

Arkansas stone: fine-grained sharpening stone quarried from natural mineral deposits.

Bevel: a sloping surface; for an instrument, it refers to reducing the share angle of the cutting edge to a sloping surface.

Burnish: to smooth and polish; an effect that can result when a dull scaler or curet is passed over tenacious calculus in an attempt to remove the deposit.

Cutting edge: the fine line formed where the face and lateral surfaces of a scaler or curet meet when the instrument is sharp; when the instrument is dull, the line has thickness and may even reflect light.

Sharpness: when a scaler or curet is sharp, the cutting edge is a fine line that does not reflect light.

Testing stick: plastic 1/4-inch rod, 3 inches long, used to test the sharpness of a scaler or a curet.

Chapter 39: Nonsurgical Periodontal Therapy and Adjunctive Therapy

Antibiotic: a form of antimicrobial agent produced by or obtained from microorganisms that can kill other microorganisms or inhibit their growth; may be specific for certain organisms or may cover a broad spectrum.

Antimicrobial therapy: use of specific chemical or pharmaceutical agents for the control or destruction of microorganisms, either systemically or at specific sites.

Bacteremia: presence of bacteria in the blood.

Bioabsorbable: available for absorption by the body.

Biodegradable: susceptible of degradation by biologic processes, either by bacterial or other enzymatic action.

Cannula: tubular instrument placed in a cavity to introduce or withdraw fluid.

Chemotherapeutic: treatment by means of chemical or pharmaceutical agents to treat disease.

Controlled release: local delivery of a chemotherapeutic agent to a site-specific area; may be a patch worn on the skin or a polymeric fiber, such as that used to deliver an agent to a periodontal pocket.

Endoscope: a minimally invasive diagnostic procedure used in medicine to examine inaccessible tissues by inserting a fiberoptic tube into the body.

Endotoxin: LPS complex found in the cell wall of many gram-negative microorganisms; contained superficially within periodontally involved cementum.

Instrumentation zone: area on tooth where instrumentation is confined; area where calculus and altered cementum are located and treatment is required.

New attachment: the union of connective tissue or epithelium with a root surface that has been deprived of its original attachment apparatus; the new attachment may be epithelial adhesion and/or connective-tissue adaptation or attachment, and it may include new cementum.

Nonsurgical periodontal therapy (NSPT): dental biofilm removal and control, supragingival and subgingival scaling, root debridement, and adjunctive treatments such as the use of chemotherapy; the basic objectives are to restore periodontal health; arrest or slow the progression of early periodontal disease; or, for more advanced disease, to prepare the tissues for surgical periodontal therapy.

Periodontal debridement: disruption and removal of dental biofilm and associated endotoxins along with calculus from the root.

Refractory: not responding to usual treatment.

Scaling: instrumentation of the crown or root surfaces to remove dental biofilm and calculus.

Superinfection: a second infection superimposed over a first infection and often resistant to the treatment used for the first infection.

Chapter 40: Sutures and Dressings

Alveolectomy: surgical removal of a portion of the alveolar bone to allow for fitting of a prosthesis.

Border mold: the shaping of the edges of a dressing by manual manipulation of the tissue adjacent to the borders (e.g., lips, cheeks) to duplicate the contour and size of the vestibule.

Chemical cure: mode of self-cure or setting of a dressing in which the ingredients unite in a chemical process that starts as soon as the blending is complete; the setting time is influenced by warm temperature and the addition of an accelerator.

Coapt: to approximate, as the edges of a wound; bring edge to edge with no overlap.

Eugenol: constituent of clove oil; used in early periodontal dressings with zinc oxide for its alleged antiseptic and anodyne properties; more recently found to be toxic, to elicit allergic reactions, and to hinder, more than promote, healing.

Hemostasis: the termination of bleeding by mechanical or chemical means or by the complex coagulation process of the body that consists of vasoconstriction, platelet aggregation, and thrombin and fibrin synthesis.

Hydrolysis: a process in which water slowly penetrates the suture filaments, causing breakdown of the suture's polymer chain. Hydrolyzation yields a lesser degree of tissue reaction.

Ligation: application of a wire or thread (suture) to hold or constrict tissue.

Suture: a stitch or series of stitches made to secure apposition of the edges of a surgical or traumatic wound.

Swaged: the fusion of a suture material to the needle, allowing for a smooth eyeless attachment. The suture will then pass through the tissue as smoothly as possible.

Tensile strength: amount of strength the suture material will retain throughout the healing period. As the wound gains strength, the suture loses strength.

Visible light–cure: light activation using a photocure system; shorter curing time than self-cure (chemical cure); does not start setting until the light is activated, thereby allowing longer working time for adapting the dressing material.

Chapter 41: Dentinal Hypersensitivity

Abfraction: wedge- or V-shaped cervical lesion created by the stresses of lateral or eccentric tooth movements during occlusal function, bruxing, or parafunctional activity, resulting in enamel microfractures.

Dentinal hypersensitivity: transient pain arising from exposed dentin, typically in response to a stimulus, which cannot be explained as arising from any other form of dental defect or pathology and subsides quickly when stimulus is removed.

Hydrodynamic theory: currently accepted mechanism for pain impulse transmission to the pulp as a result of fluid movement within the dentinal tubule, which stimulates the nerve endings at the dentinopulpal interface.

Intratubular or peritubular dentin: increased deposition of minerals into tubules that become more mineralized with increasing age, resulting in thicker, sclerotic dentin.

Neural depolarization mechanism (sodium/potassium pump): reduction of the resting potential of the nerve membrane so that a nerve impulse is fired. At rest, the inner surface of the nerve fiber is negatively charged and impermeable to sodium ions. A stimulus temporarily alters the membrane, making it permeable so that potassium leaks out and sodium rushes into the nerve fiber. This mechanism is known as the sodium–potassium pump. The reversal of electrical charge, or depolarization, creates the nerve impulse. The process then reverses, and the membrane potential is restored, or repolarized.

Osmotic: alteration of pressure in dentinal tubules through a selective membrane.

Patent: open, unobstructed; a patent dentinal tubule allows fluid flow to signal pain; many desensitizing agents work by decreasing the patency of the tubule.

Randomized clinical trials (RCT): a specific type of scientific experiment that is the gold standard for a clinical trial. RCTs are often used to test the efficacy and/or effectiveness of various types of interventions within a patient population.

Secondary dentin: dentin that is secreted slowly over time after root formation to "wall off" the pulp from fluid flow within dentinal tubules following a stimulus; results in narrower pulp chamber and root canals.

Smear layer: has been referred to as "grinding debris" from instrumentation or other devices applied to the tooth; consists of microcrystalline particles of cementum, dentin, tissue, and cellular debris; serves to plug tubule orifices.

Tertiary/reparative dentin: a type of dentin formed along the pulpal wall or root canal as a protective mechanism in response to trauma or irritation, such as caries or a traumatic cavity preparation.

Chapter 42: Extrinsic Stain Removal

Abrasion: wearing away of surface material by friction.

Abrasive: a material composed of particles of sufficient hardness and sharpness to cut or scratch a softer material when drawn across its surface; available in various particle sizes.

Air-powder polisher: air-powered device using air and water pressure to deliver a controlled stream of specially processed sodium bicarbonate slurry through the handpiece nozzle; also called air abrasive, airpolishing, airpowered abrasive, or airbrasive.

Cleaning agent: round, flat nonabrasive particles that do not scratch surface materials.

Coronal polishing: polishing of the anatomic crowns of the teeth to remove dental biofilm and extrinsic stains; does not involve calculus removal.

Glycerin: clear, colorless, syrupy fluid used as a vehicle and sweetening agent for drugs and as a solvent and vehicle for abrasive agents.

Glycine: an amino acid–based water-soluble powder used for airpolishing.

Grit: with reference to abrasive agents, grit is the particle size.

Polishing: the production, especially by friction, of a smooth, glossy, mirror-like surface that reflects light.

Polishing agent: an abrasive used to achieve a smooth, lustrous finish to a tooth surface.

rpm: revolutions per minute.

Three-body abrasive polishing: involves loose abrasive particles that move in the interface space between the surface being polished and the polishing application device.

Tribiology: tribiology incorporates the study and application of the principles of friction, lubrication, and wear as they apply to polishing.

Two-body abrasive polishing: involves abrasive particles attached to a medium (polishing application device) that move directly against the surface being polished.

Chapter 43: Tooth Bleaching

Amorphous calcium phosphate: a compound used on the teeth as an artificial hydroxyapatite.

Bleaching: a cosmetic dental procedure that uses free radicals and breakdown of pigments to whiten teeth.

Bleaching trays: synonym for night guard vital bleaching, which requires development of a custom tray that allows for administration and containment of tooth bleaching material such as carbamide peroxide or hydrogen peroxide.

Block-out resin: light-cured resin materials that can be used as a rubber dam substitute during bleaching procedure or on study models to create space to hold bleaching material on custom trays.

Color: a phenomenon of light or visual perception that enables the differentiation of otherwise identical objects. Usually determined visually by measurement of hue, saturation, and luminous reflectance of light.

Esthetic: pertaining to the study of beauty and the sense of beautiful; objectifies beauty and attractiveness, elicits pleasure.

Extrinsic: external, extraneous, as originating from or on the outside.

Intrinsic: from within, incorporation of a colorant within a material.

Microabrasion: a proven method for treating tooth discolorations by microreduction of superficial enamel through various methods of mechanical and/or chemical actions.

Potassium nitrate: active ingredient in many antisensitivity dentifrices.

Surfactant: a wetting agent.

Translucency: having the appearance between complete opacity and complete transparency; partially opaque.

Whitening: use of abrasive agents in the dentifrice that results in whitening of teeth. Often used interchangeably with the term bleaching, but not actually the same procedure.

Chapter 44: Principles of Evaluation

Evaluation design: a description of the purpose, plans, and strategies that will be needed to gather, process, and interpret the data used to determine treatment outcomes.

Expert witness: a person licensed to perform treatment in a specific health profession or with specialized knowledge, beyond that of the average person, in an area of treatment; a source for determining legal professional standard of care in a court case.

Feedback: communication that occurs among all individuals participating in the patient's care, including the dentist, the dental hygienist, the patient, and the patient's physician or caregiver, if necessary. Giving and receiving feedback creates trust and ensures that those involved in all aspects of patient care stay informed at every step.

Formative evaluation: ongoing evaluation to monitor each step in the dental hygiene process of care; ongoing feedback that determines any needed changes in the dental hygiene care plan prior to the completion of a treatment sequence.

Indicators: measurable information used to assess whether a treatment or program is achieving the expected outcomes.

Impact evaluation: assesses long-term effectiveness of dental hygiene care in achieving health goals.

Indicators: benchmarks used to measure or test changes. In evaluating dental hygiene interventions, indicators can be quantitative (measurement of probing depth or plaque scores) or qualitative (patient expressions of satisfaction or ability to perform self-care routines).

Outcome evaluation: a measure of the effectiveness of dental hygiene clinical and educational interventions in meeting oral health goals identified in the patient care plan.

Process evaluation: Ongoing evaluation to determine whether dental hygiene services are being implemented as intended.

Standard of care: criteria or protocols that define the minimal quality of care required to defend against a legal dispute against the practice of one's profession; usually established by federal laws, state, and local statutes and codes and/or testimony from an "expert witness" and is supported by guidelines or recommendations documents published by professional associations.

Chapter 45: Continuing Care

Compliance: action in accordance with request; extent to which a person's health behaviors coincide with dental/medical health advice. Also called *adherence*.

Continuing care: system of appointments for the long-term maintenance phase of patient care; the system is carried out by computer, telephone, and/or mail. Also called recare or maintenance.

Disease activity: ongoing dynamic process that results in loss of clinical attachment and alveolar supporting bone; an area is quiescent when a diseased site becomes inactive or stable without treatment.

PM (periodontal maintenance): also called preventive maintenance, supportive periodontal therapy (SPT); procedures performed at selected intervals as an extension of periodontal therapy to assist the patient in maintaining oral health; includes complete assessment, review of and/or additional instruction in dental biofilm control, and such clinical procedures as scaling and root planing.

Refractory: resistant, not responding to routine therapy.

Risk factor: a characteristic, habit, or predisposing condition that makes an individual susceptible to, or in danger of acquiring, a certain disease or disability.

Chapter 46: The Pregnant Patient and Infant

Anticipatory guidance: anticipatory guidance is the process of providing practical, developmentally appropriate information about children's health to prepare parents for the significant physical, emotional, and psychological milestones.

Dental home: an ongoing relationship between the dentist and the patient, including all aspects of oral healthcare delivered in a comprehensive, continuously accessible, coordinated, and family-centered way.

Early childhood caries (ECC): the presence of one or more decayed (noncavitated or cavitated lesions), missing (due to caries), or filled tooth surfaces in any primary tooth in a child younger than 6 years.

Fetus: an unborn offspring, from the embryo stage until birth.

Gestation: gestation is the period of time between conception and birth.

Gestational diabetes: diabetes with initial onset or recognition during pregnancy.

Low birth weight: as weight at birth less than 2,500 g (5.5 lb).

Severe early childhood caries (S-ECC): the presence of any area of smooth surface decay in a child younger than 3 years.

Xylitol: a natural sugar-alcohol that is approved for use in food by the US Food and Drug Administration.

Chapter 47: The Pediatric Patient

Adolescent: child from 12 years of age to 18 years of age; considered teen or young adult.

Anticipatory guidance: provide information to parents and caregivers on what to expect in a child's current and next developmental stage so that the child's needs can be anticipated and properly managed.

CAMBRA: acronym that refers to the phrase "caries management by risk assessment."

Dental home: a dentist of record in the community established early in childhood for continuous and comprehensive preventive interventions, dental hygiene, and dental care.

Infant: child younger than 1 year.

Interim therapeutic restoration (ITR): a provisional placement of a fluoride-releasing glass ionomer restoration without using local anesthesia and utilizing a spoon excavator to remove most—all caries; purpose is to prevent the progression of dental caries in young patients, uncooperative patients, patients with special healthcare needs, and situations in which traditional cavity preparation and/or placement of traditional dental restorations are not feasible. It is necessary to "recharge" the glass ionomer material using fluoridated toothpaste daily and regular 3–6-month professional fluoride applications.

Main caregiver: the person who has primary daily care of the child.

Nonnutritive sucking: sucking fingers, thumb, pacifiers, or other objects for comfort.

Obstructive sleep apnea (OSA): occurs when the muscles in the back of the throat relax, causing the airway to narrow on inspiration that lowers the oxygen levels in the blood and triggers the brain to wake the person. This causes disruptive sleep patterns and possible intermittent periods of suspended breathing.

Pediatric obstructive sleep apnea (POSA): a disorder of breathing characterized by prolonged, partial upper airway obstruction and/or intermittent/complete obstruction (obstructive apnea) that disrupts normal ventilation during sleep and normal sleep patterns.

Preschooler: child 3–5 years of age; may or may not be attending a preschool program.

PSR (periodontal screening and recording): used as a screening procedure to determine the need for comprehensive periodontal evaluation; described in Chapter 21.

School-age: child from 6 to 12 years of age, considered middle childhood.

Sippy cup: a special cup with a lid that may have a straw or a drinking projection to teach a young child to drink.

Toddler: child from age 1 year to 3 years of age.

Chapter 48: The Older Adult Patient

Aging: the continuous process (biologic, psychological, social) beginning with conception and ending with death, in which the organ systems age.

Alzheimer disease: a form of irreversible dementia, usually occurring in older adulthood, characterized by gradual deterioration of memory, disorientation, and other features of dementia.

Biologic age: the anatomic or physiologic age of a person as determined by changes in organismic structure and function; takes into account features such as posture, skin texture, strength, speed, and sensory acuity.

Chronologic age: the actual measure of time elapsed since a person's birth.

Dementia: severe mental deterioration involving impairment of mental ability; organic loss of intellectual function.

Functional age: how well an older adult performs.

Gerontology: study of the aging process; includes the biologic, psychological, and sociologic sciences.

Lifestyle: relatively permanent organization of activities, including work, leisure, and associated social activities, characterizing an individual.

Osteoporosis: low bone mass resulting from an excess of bone resorption over bone formation, with resultant bone fragility and increased risk of fracture.

Polypharmacy: concurrent use of a large number of drugs.

Presbycusis: progressive loss of hearing due to the normal aging process.

Presbyopia: a condition of farsightedness (hyperopia) resulting from a loss of elasticity of the lens of the eye due to the normal aging process.

Sjögren syndrome: an immunologic disorder characterized by insufficient production of the lacrimal gland to produce tears and the salivary glands to produce saliva, resulting in abnormally dry eyes and mouth.

Tinnitus: ringing, buzzing, tinkling, or hissing sounds in the ear.

Chapter 49: The Patient with a Cleft Lip and/or Palate

Bifid uvula: cleft of the uvula of the soft palate that divides the uvula into two parts (Figure 49-1, Class 2).

Cleft lip: a unilateral or bilateral congenital fissure of the upper lip, usually lateral to the midline; can extend into one nostril or both and may involve the alveolar process; caused by defect in the fusion of the maxillary and globular processes.

Cleft palate: a congenital fissure of the palate caused by failure of the palatal shelves to fuse; may extend to connect with unilateral or bilateral cleft lip.

Congenital: present at and existing since birth.

Craniofacial: pertaining to the cranium, the part of the skull that encloses the brain, and the face.

Dentally dysfunctional: abnormal functioning of dental structures.

Grafting: tissue that is transplanted and expected to become a part of the host tissue.

Interdisciplinary: relating to more than one branch of knowledge.

Multifactorial: pertaining to, or arising through the action of, many factors.

Nasoalveolar molding technique (NAM): treatment used for unilateral and bilateral cleft palate to reduce the severity of the cleft in the maxillary gingiva or alveolar ridges and to reduce the deformity of the nose.

Obturator: a prosthesis designed to close a congenital or an acquired opening, such as a cleft of the hard palate.

Orthopedics: branch of surgery dealing with the preservation and restoration of function of the skeletal system, its articulations, and associated structures.

Premaxillary: anterior part of maxilla that contains the incisor teeth; bilateral cleft lips separate the premaxilla from its normal fusion with the entire maxilla.

Prosthesis: an artificial replacement of an absent part of the human body; a therapeutic device to improve or alter function.

Rehabilitation: the process of restoring a person's ability to live and work as normally as possible after a disabling injury or illness; aims to help the individual to achieve maximum possible physical and psychological fitness and to regain ability to carry out personal care.

Rhinoplasty: plastic surgery of nose.

Speech aid prosthesis: a prosthetic device with a posterior section to assist with palatopharyngeal closure; also called bulb, speech bulb, or prosthetic speech appliance.

Syndrome: a combination of symptoms either resulting from a single cause or occurring so commonly together as to constitute a distinct clinical picture.

Chapter 50: The Patient with a Neurodevelopment Disorder

Adaptive behavior: conceptual, social, and practical skills learned by individuals to support the ability to function in everyday life.

Autism spectrum disorder: a developmental disorder, generally evident before age 3, affecting verbal and non-verbal communications and social interaction.

Comorbid: existing simultaneously with and usually independently of another medical condition; coexisting or additional disease processes. Comorbidity may affect the ability to function or survive.

Dysmorphic: abnormality in morphologic development.

Epicanthic fold: a vertical fold of skin on either side of the nose, sometimes covering the inner canthus; a normal characteristic in persons of certain races.

Hyperactivity: abnormally increased activity.

Intellectual functioning: a broad term that takes adaptive behavior, mental health, opportunities to participate in life activities, and the context in which a life is lived into consideration.

Intelligence quotient (IQ): a score derived from one of several standardized tests used to assess intellectual ability.

Macroglossia: very large tongue.

Microcephalus: abnormally small head size in relation to the rest of the body.

Neurodevelopmental disability: physical, behavioral, and/or ID, that first manifests symptoms during developmental period (before age 21) and leads to intellectual, social, and/or physical impairment in everyday life activities.

Pathognomonic: characteristic or indicative of a particular disease or syndrome; especially one or more typical symptoms.

Pervasive: throughout entire individual, entire development is severely and markedly impaired, as in ASD.

Stereotypic movement disorder: repetitive, nonfunctional motor behavior that interferes with normal activities and may result in bodily injury.

Tic: an involuntary, sudden, rapid, recurrent, nonrhythmic, stereotyped motor movement or vocal sound.

Chapter 51: The Patient with a Disability

American sign language: is a visual/gestural language with a unique grammar and syntax.

Americans with Disabilities Act (ADA) or (AwDA): prohibits discrimination on the basis of a disability and requires public and commercial facilities to meet standards of accessibility by removing architectural, transportation, and communication barriers.

Applied behavioral analysis: is a scientific discipline concerned with applying techniques based on the principles of learning to change behavior of social significance. The name "applied behavior analysis" has replaced behavior modification because the latter approach suggested attempting to change behavior without clarifying the relevant behavior–environment interactions. In contrast, ABA tries to change behavior by first assessing the functional relationship between a targeted behavior and the environment.

Barrier free: area freely accessible to all without discrimination on the basis of a disability; obstacles to passage or communication have been removed.

Blind: no perception of visual stimuli; lack or loss of ability to see.

Braille: a system of writing and printing by means of raised points representing letters; enables people with a visual disability to read by touch.

Cataract: clouding or opacity of the lens of an eye.

Cochlear implants: is a surgically **implanted** electronic device that provides a sense of sound to a person who is profoundly deaf or severely hard of hearing in both ears.

Colostomy bag: a removable, disposable bag that attaches to the exterior opening of a colostomy(stoma) to permit sanitary collection and disposal of bodily wastes.

Communicative Disability: any disorder that affects an individual's ability to comprehend, detect, or apply language and speech to engage in discourse effectively with others. The delays and disorders can range from simple sound substitution to the inability to understand or use one's native language.

Comorbidities: the simultaneous presence of two chronic diseases or conditions in a patient.

Computer screen reader: software programs that allow visually impaired individuals to read data displayed on a computer screen with a speech synthesizer.

Desensitization techniques: a **technique** used in behavior therapy to treat phobias and other behavior problems involving anxiety: desensitization to accept dental treatment might consist, for example, of short exposures to the dental chair, instruments, air syringe, and sound of a handpiece along with building trust in the dental team members.

Developmental disability: a substantial handicap of indefinite duration with onset before the age of 18 years. Examples include autism and cerebral palsy.

Disability: (individual dimension) restriction or lack of ability (resulting from an impairment) to perform an activity in the manner or within the range considered normal for a human being of the same age, sex, and background.

Food pouching: trapping of food in the mouth between cheek and teeth, commonly seen in individuals with poor control of facial muscles.

Glaucoma: group of diseases of the eye characterized by intraocular pressure from pathologic.

Hearing: the sense by which sounds are perceived; conversion of sound waves into nerve impulses, which are then interpreted by the brain.

Hearing aids: an electronic device worn in or behind the ear. It amplifies and shapes sound waves that enter the external auditory canal

Hearing impairment: a full or partial reduction in the ability to understand or detect any sounds.

Impairment: in health, any loss or abnormality of physiologic, psychological, or anatomic structure or function, whether permanent or temporary.

Legal blindness is less than 20/200 vision with corrective eyeglasses.

Musculoskeletal disability: are conditions that can affect your muscles, bones, and joints. They include conditions such as tendinitis and carpal tunnel syndrome.

Neurologic disabilities: are caused by damage to the nervous system (including the brain and spinal cord) that results in the loss of some bodily or mental functions. Heart attacks, infections, genetic **disorders**, and lack of oxygen to the brain may also result in a **neurologic disability**.

Retinopathy of prematurity: a condition peculiar to premature infants; characterized by opaque tissue behind the lens resulting from a high concentration of oxygen, which causes spasm of the retinal vessels, leads to retinal detachment, and arrests eye growth and development; prevented

by keeping oxygen administration as low as possible and discontinuing the oxygen as soon as possible.

Sensory disability: is a disability of the senses (e.g., sight, hearing, smell, touch, taste).

Speech reading: recognizing spoken words by watching the speaker's lips, face, and gestures.

Survival rate: is the percentage of people in a study or treatment group still alive for a given period of time after diagnosis.

Vision: the faculty or state of being able to see.

Visual impairment: a visual condition that impacts a person's abilities to succeed normal everyday activities during life.

Chapter 52: Neurologic Disorders and Stroke

Akinesia: absence or loss of power of voluntary motion.

ALS: atropic lateral sclerosis.

Ankylosis: immobility due to direct union between parts.

Aphasia: defect in, or loss of power of, expression by speech, writing, or signs, or of comprehension of spoken or written language.

Apoptosis: cell death activated by a biochemical reaction; sometimes referred to as "programmed cell death."

Atrophy: wasting; decrease in size; occurs when muscle fibers are not used or are deprived of their blood supply, or when the nerve connection is interrupted.

Bradykinesia: abnormal slowness of movements.

Cerebrovascular accident (CVA): a focal neurologic disorder caused by destruction of brain substance because of intracerebral hemorrhage, thrombosis, embolism, or vascular insufficiency; also called stroke.

Decubitus ulcer: ulcer that usually occurs over a bony prominence as a result of prolonged, excessive pressure from body weight; also called pressure sore or bed sore.

Dysarthria: impairment of oral, lingual, or pharyngeal muscles that causes verbal clumsiness or impairment.

Hemiparesis: slight or incomplete paralysis of one side of the body.

Hemiplegia: paralysis of one side of the body; usually caused by CVA or a brain lesion.

Hypercholesterolemia: excess of cholesterol in the blood.

Hypertriglyceridema: raised triglyceride blood level.

Ischemia: deficiency of blood caused by functional constriction or actual obstruction of a blood vessel.

Kyphosis: abnormally increased convexity in the curvature of the thoracic spine (viewed from the side).

Orthosis: orthopedic appliance or apparatus used to support, align, prevent, or correct deformities or to improve the function of a movable part of the body.

Pallidotomy: surgical excision or destruction of part of the globus pallidus in the basal ganglia to prevent symptoms of Parkinsonism, including tremor, muscular rigidity, and bradykinesia.

Paralysis: a symptom of the loss or impairment of motor function in a body part caused by a lesion of the neural or muscular mechanism.

Shunt: passage between two natural channels; to bypass or drain an area.

Sialorrhea: excessive secretion of saliva.

Spinal shock: immediately after the injury, spinal shock causes a complete loss of reflex activity. The result is a flaccid paralysis below the level of injury that may last from several hours to several months.

TIA (transient ischemic attack): brief episode of cerebral ischemia that results in no permanent neurologic damage; symptoms are warning signals of impending CVA (stroke).

Ventriculoatrial shunt: surgical creation of a communication between a cerebral ventricle and a cardiac atrium by means of a plastic tube; for relief of hydrocephalus.

Ventriculoperitoneal shunt: communication between a cerebral ventricle and the peritoneum by means of a plastic tube; for relief of hydrocephalus.

Chapter 53: The Patient with an Endocrine Condition

Adolescence: the period extending from the time the secondary sex characteristics appear to the end of somatic growth, when the individual is mature.

Congenital hypothyroidism: partial or complete lack of production of thyroid hormone in infants from birth.

Endocrine: pertaining to secretion of a substance directly into blood or lymph rather than into a duct; the opposite of exocrine.

Endometrium: the lining of the uterus.

Epinephrine: a catecholamine hormone that causes the "fight-or-flight" response to physical or emotional stress; increased secretion produces marked dilation of bronchioles and increased blood pressure, blood glucose level, and heart rate.

Gland: organ or structure that secretes or excretes substances.

Gonad: sex gland in which reproductive cells form.

Homeostasis: the tendency of biologic systems to maintain constant internal stability while continually adjusting to external changes.

Hormone: a chemical product of an organ or of certain cells within the organ that has a specific regulatory effect upon cells elsewhere in the body.

Hyperkalemia: a higher-than-normal level of potassium in the bloodstream.

Hypernatremia: elevated sodium level in the bloodstream.

Hypokalemia: a lower-than-normal level of potassium in the bloodstream.

Insulin resistance: when the insulin does not adequately absorb blood glucose and thus produces higher quantities of insulin to maintain balance.

Libido: sexual urge or desire.

Macrocephaly: head circumference that is greater than 2 standard deviations larger than the average for a given age and sex.

Macrognathia: enlargement or elongation of the jaw.

Mastalgia: fullness, soreness, or pain in the breast.

Menarche: onset of menstruation; may occur from ages 9 to 17 years.

Menopause: the time of life when a woman ceases menstruation; defined as a period of 12 months of amenorrhea in a woman over 45 years of age.

Menses: menstruation.

Myxedema: a disease caused by decreased activity of the thyroid gland characterized by dry skin, swellings around the lips and nose.

Myxedema coma: blunting of the senses and intellect, labored speech, swelling all over the body associated with hypothyroidism. Condition is life-threatening.

Norepinephrine: a catecholamine that functions as a neurotransmitter, sending signals from one neuron to another neuron or to a muscle cell.

Premenstrual syndrome: a cluster of behavioral, somatic, affective, and cognitive disorders that appear in the premenstrual (luteal) phase of the menstrual cycle and that resolve rapidly with the onset of menses.

Puberty: period during in which adolescents reach sexual maturity and become capable of reproduction.

Thyroiditis: inflammation of the thyroid.

Thyrotoxic crisis (thyroid storm): potentially life-threatening condition for people with hyperthyroidism. The thyroid suddenly releases large amounts of thyroid hormone.

Xerostomia: dry mouth.

Chapter 54: The Patient with Diabetes Mellitus

A1c (A One C): common abbreviation for glycosylated hemoglobin (HbA1c)

Beta cells: insulin-producing cells of the islets of Langerhans in the pancreas.

Charcot joints: a joint that is deprived of any pain or position sense due to severe osteoarthritis or as a result of disease such as diabetic neuropathy.

Diabetic ketoacidosis (DKA): diabetic coma; too little insulin; accumulation of ketone bodies in the blood. Occurs primarily in type 1 diabetes mellitus.

Exogenous insulin: insulin delivered from a source outside the body, such as by injection.

Fasting plasma glucose (FPG): measurement of blood glucose taken at least 8 hours after a meal.

Gastroparesis: delayed gastric emptying. Occurs when the vagus nerve is damaged or stops functioning normally and movement of food is slowed or stopped.

Gestational diabetes mellitus (GDM): diabetes that occurs during pregnancy.

Glycated or glycosylated hemoglobin (HbA1c): the primary assay for assessing long-term glycemic control. Indicates blood glucose levels for the previous 2–3 months.

Glycemia: presence of glucose in blood.

HbA$_{1c}$: see glycated or glycosylated hemoglobin.

Hyperglycemia: high blood glucose: opposite of hypoglycemia.

Hyperpnea: abnormal increase in depth and rate of respiration.

Hypogeusia: abnormally diminished acuteness of the sense of taste.

Hypoglycemia: an abnormally low level of glucose in the blood.

Hyperinsulinemia: excess insulin relative to the level of glucose in the blood.

Hypoinsulinemia: abnormally low levels of insulin he blood.

Impaired fasting glucose (IFG): A prediabetes state when the fasting blood glucose level is consistently above normal, but not in the range for a diagnosis of diabetes.

Impaired glucose tolerance (IGT): A prediabetes state of hyperglycemia associated with insulin resistance.

Insulin: a powerful hormone secreted by the beta cells in the islets of Langerhans of the pancreas; the major fuel-regulating hormone; enters the blood in response to a rise in concentration of blood glucose and is transported immediately to bind with cell surface receptors throughout the body.

Insulin-dependent diabetes mellitus (IDDM): former name for type 1 diabetes mellitus that is no longer used because some people with type 2 diabetes mellitus also use insulin.

Insulin resistance: lower or diminished response to insulin, impairing the ability to "unlock" the cell to allow glucose from the blood into the cell.

Ketones: normal metabolic products of lipid (fat) within the liver; excess production leads to urinary excretion of these acidic chemicals.

LDL (low-density lipoprotein): is a carrier of cholesterol in the body, which leads to buildup of cholesterol in the arteries causing an increased risk for cardiovascular disease. Sometimes called the "bad" cholesterol.

NIDDM (noninsulin-dependent diabetes mellitus): former name for type 2 diabetes mellitus, but it is no longer used since people with type 2 diabetes may use insulin.

Oral glucose tolerance test (OGTT): a test of the body's ability to utilize carbohydrates; aid to the diagnosis of diabetes mellitus. After ingestion of a specific amount of glucose solution, the fasting blood glucose rises promptly in a nondiabetic person, then falls to normal within an hour. In diabetes mellitus, the blood glucose rise is greater, and the return to normal is prolonged.

Polycystic ovarian syndrome (PCOS): Hormonal disorder where the ovaries or adrenal glands produce more male hormones than normal. Women with PCOS are at risk for diabetes, metabolic syndrome, cardiovascular disease, and hypertension.

Polydipsia: excessive thirst.

Polyphagia: excessive ingestion of food.

Polyuria: excessive excretion of urine.

Postprandial: after a meal.

Prediabetes: IFG (impaired fasting glucose) and IGT (impaired glucose tolerance) are risk factors for future diabetes and cardiovascular disease.

Retinopathy: noninflammatory degenerative disease of the retina; called diabetic retinopathy when it occurs with diabetes of long standing.

Self-monitoring of blood glucose (SMBG): regular home blood glucose testing for diabetic people to understand diabetes control and possible changes needed to improve blood glucose.

Chapter 55: The Patient with Cancer

Alimentation: providing nutrition.

Alopecia: a loss of hair.

Anaplasia: an irreversible alteration in adult cells toward more primitive (embryonic) cell types; characteristic of tumor cells.

Benign: not malignant.

Biotherapy: use of biologic agents to treat cancer.

Carcinoma: a malignant tumor of epithelial origin.

Chemotherapy: treatment of illness by chemical means, that is, by medication or drugs.

Dysgeusia: distortion of the sense of taste.

Hematopoiesis: formation and development of blood cells.

Leukemia: an acute or chronic progressive malignant neoplasm of the blood-forming organs, marked by diffuse proliferation of immature white blood cells (leukocytes); subsequent reduction in erythrocytes and platelets results.

Malignant: tending to become progressively worse and to result in death; having the properties of anaplasia, invasiveness, and metastasis; said of tumors

Metastasis: transfer of disease from one organ or part to another not directly connected with it; for example, regional or distant spread of cancer cells from the site primarily involved.

Neoplasm: any new and abnormal growth, specifically one in which cell multiplication is controlled and progressive; may be benign or malignant.

Oncology: the study of tumors; the sum of knowledge regarding tumors.

Oral mucositis/stomatitis: inflammation and ulceration of the oral mucous membranes; can increase the risk for pain, oral and systemic infection, and nutritional compromise.

Osteonecrosis of the jaw (ONJ): occurs when the jaw bone is exposed and begins to starve from a lack of blood.

> **Antiresorptive drug-related osteonecrosis of the jaw (ARONJ):** is exposed bone in maxilla or mandible that can occur when a patient is treated with a bisphosphonate or other antiresorptive drug with no history of radiation to the head/neck tissues.

> **Medication-related osteonecrosis of the jaw (MRONJ):** equivalent term for exposed bone in maxilla or mandible that can occur when a patient is taking other antiresorptive or antiangenic medications that are not bisphosphonates.

Osteoradionecrosis: blood vessel compromise and necrosis of bone exposed to high-dose radiation therapy, resulting in decreased ability to heal if traumatized and in extreme susceptibility to infection.

Palliative/palliation: affording relief, but does not cure.

Pancytopenia: abnormal depression of all cellular elements of the blood.

Radiation therapy: the treatment of disease by ionizing radiation; may be external megavoltage or internal by use of interstitial implantation of an isotope (radium).

Radium: a highly radioactive chemical element found in uranium minerals; used in the treatment of malignant tumors in the form of needles or pellets for interstitial implantation.

Relapse: the return of a disease weeks or months after its apparent cessation.

Remission: diminution or abatement of the symptoms of a disease; the period during which such diminution occurs.

Salivary gland hypofunction: objective reduction in the production of saliva, often a long-term complication of head/neck radiation.

Sarcoma: a tumor, often highly malignant, composed of cells derived from connective tissue such as bone and cartilage, muscle, blood vessel, or lymphoid tissue.

Staging: the succinct, standardized description of a tumor with regard to origin and spread. This clinical classification is based on physical assessments, biopsy, imaging, and endoscopy. Each stage (I–IV) consists of three components: T (size of tumor); N (lymph node involvement); and M (presence or absence of distant metastasis).

Trismus: limitations of opening because of spasm and/or fibrosis of the muscles of mastication and/or temporomandibular joint located in the field of radiation.

Xerostomia: subjective report of oral dryness—saliva may appear thick or reduced, or increases the risk for infection and compromises chewing, and swallowing. Chronic dry mouth increases the risk for dental caries.

Chapter 56: The Oral and Maxillofacial Surgery Patient

Alveolitis: infection and inflammation after extraction of a tooth due to the loss of the blood clot.

Biopsy: sample of tissue taken from the body to determine extent, cause, or presence of disease.

> **Incisional biopsy:** surgeon removes a part of the lesion along with some normal tissue.

> **Excisional biopsy:** surgeon removes the entire lesion along with some normal tissue.

> **Exfoliative biopsy:** removes surface epithelial cells; commonly known as oral brush biopsy.

Cone-beam computed tomography (CBCT): radiographic technology that produces three-dimensional (3-D) images of teeth, soft tissues, nerve pathways, and bone in a single scan.

Ecchymosis: a hemorrhagic spot, larger than a petechia, in the skin or mucous membrane caused by extravasation of blood; forms a nonelevated, rounded, or irregular purplish patch.

Exodontics: branch of dentistry dealing with the surgical removal of teeth.

Intermaxillary fixation (IMF): fixation of the maxilla in occlusion with the mandible held in place by means of wires and elastic bands; the healing parts are stabilized following fracture or surgery.

Maxillofacial: pertaining to the jaws and the face.

Maxillofacial prosthetics: the branch of prosthodontics concerned with the restoration of the mouth and jaws and associated facial structures that have been affected by disease, injury, surgery, or a congenital defect.

Miniplate osteosynthesis: a method of internal fixation of mandibular fractures utilizing miniaturized metal plates and screws formerly made of titanium or stainless steel and currently made primarily of biodegradable or resorbable synthetic materials.

Orthognathic surgery: surgery to alter relationships of the dental arches and/or supporting bone; usually coordinated with orthodontic therapy.

Osteosynthesis: internal fixation of a fracture by mechanical means, such as metal plates, pins, or screws.

Trismus: motor disturbance of the trigeminal nerve with spasm of masticatory muscles and difficulty in opening the mouth (lockjaw).

Chapter 57: The Patient with a Seizure Disorder

Absence seizure: a type of generalized onset seizure, most often affecting children, producing lapses in awareness, sometimes mistaken for day dreaming.

Antiepileptic/antiseizure: a remedy for epilepsy and/or seizures.

Ataxia: problems with coordination and balance due to defects in the cerebellum of the brain.

Atonic seizure: muscles suddenly become limp, eyelids drop, head may nod forward, and person may drop things. Also called drop-attacks or drop seizures, lasting less than 15 seconds.

Atypical: different, unusual, and not typical.

Automatism: repetitive tapping, lip smacking, picking at clothes, chewing, mumbling, or spitting.

Autonomic symptoms: pale appearance, sweating, pupil dilation, heart arrhythmia, and bladder incontinence.

Aura: is a sensory warning that precedes a seizure; may involve flashing lights, dizziness, peculiar taste or tingling and numbness.

Behavior arrest: lack of movement.

Clonic: sustained rhythmical jerking of parts or the whole body.

Convulsion: violent spasm.

Electroencephalography: EEG is an electrophysiologic monitoring method to record electrical activity of the brain.

Epilepsy: a disease of the brain characterized by recurrent unprovoked (or reflex) seizures.

Epileptic spasm: a sudden flexion and extension of proximal and truncal muscles.

Focal onset: level of awareness a person has when experience a seizure. This seizure originates in one hemisphere of the brain, previously known as partial seizure.

Focal onset aware: the patient is awake and aware during the seizure, formally called simple partial seizure.

Generalized onset: refers to seizures that are generalized from the onset or beginning, can also be described as motor or nonmotor, formerly known as grand mal.

Grand mal: former name for a generalized or major seizure as contrasted with petit mal, a minor or relatively mild seizure.

Hirsutism: abnormal hair growth on the face or body in women.

Ictal (or Ictus): a psychological state or event such as a seizure, stroke, or headache.

Myoclonic: seizures with brief shocklike jerks of an individual or multiple muscles.

Myoclonus: isolated or repetitive shocklike contractions of a muscle or groups of muscles, myoclonic.

Neurologist: a doctor who has special training in disorders of the brain, including epilepsy.

Paroxysm or paroxysmal: sharp spasm or convulsion; sudden recurrence or intensification of symptoms.

Petit mal: attack or brief impairment of consciousness often associated with flickering of the eyelids and mild twitching of the mouth.

Postictal: a period of decreased activity of the brain following a seizure, usually lasting less than 48 hours.

Prodrome: a premonitory symptom; a symptom indicating the onset of a disease or condition; *adj.*, prodromal.

Seizure: is an event, a transient occurrence due to abnormal excessive synchronous neuronal activity in the brain.

Spasm: sudden involuntary contraction of a muscles; may be tonic or clonic; may vary from small twitches to severe convulsions.

Status epilepticus: rapid succession of epileptic seizures without intervals of consciousness; life-threatening; emergency care is urgent.

Tonic: state of continuous, unremitting action of muscular contraction; patient appears stiff.

Tonic–clonic: a seizure involving the whole body with rapid rhythmic, violent shaking movements, person loses consciousness, generally last for 1 to 3 minutes. Formally known as grand mal seizures.

Trigger/signs: factor that precipitate a seizure, usually something that may occur prior to a seizure.

Unclassified: seizures of unknown onset.

Unknown onset: onset was unobserved, or determination of origin is unknown.

Chapter 58: The Patient with a Mental Health Disorder

Affect: emotion or feeling; tone of reaction to persons and events.

Akinesia: loss or impairment in the ability to move muscles voluntarily.

Anxiolytics: medication used to relieve anxiety or emotional tension, also called antianxiety agent.

Bradykinesia: abnormal slowness of movement; sluggish physical and mental responses.

Cognitive: mental process of comprehension, judgment, and memory.

Compensatory behavior: behavior meant to relieve guilt or anxiety over eating.

Decompensate: appearance or exacerbation of a mental disorder, which may include hallucinations, delusion, violent, or bizarre behavior.

Delusion: false belief firmly held, although contradicted by social reality.

Dysarthria: impairment in uttering words due to diseases that affect oral and pharyngeal muscles.

Dysgeusia: changes in sense of taste.

Dystonia: muscles contract uncontrollably.

Electroconvulsive therapy (ECT): electroshock therapy; a form of somatic therapy in which an electric current is used to produce convulsions; primarily used to treat severe depression.

Hallucination: false sensory perception in the absence of an actual external stimulus.

Hyperarousal: an abnormal state of increased sensitivity or responsiveness to stimuli.

Insomnia: wakefulness; inability to sleep in the absence of noise or other disturbance.

Perimolysis: erosion of enamel and dentin as a result of chemical and mechanical effects.

Psychotherapy: treatment of emotional, behavioral, personality, and psychiatric disorders by means of individual or group verbal or nonverbal communication with the patient.

Tardive dyskinesia: involuntary movements of the mouth, lips, tongue, and jaws, usually associated with long-term use of antipsychotic medication.

Chapter 59: The Patient with a Substance-Related Disorder

Abstinence: refraining from an activity that is known to be harmful and addictive. Abstinence involves not taking a particular substance, avoiding areas where this is likely to be offered or adopting a healthier lifestyle.

Acne rosacea: facial skin condition usually characterized by a flushed appearance; often accompanied by puffiness and a "spider-web" effect of broken capillaries seen in individuals with AUD.

Addiction: habitual psychological and physiologic dependence on a substance or practice that is beyond voluntary control.

Alcohol intoxication: results from recent ingestion of excessive amounts of alcohol; characterized by behavioral changes that alter the usual behavior of the individual.

Alcohol use disorder (AUD): also known as alcoholism, is a pattern of alcohol use in which one has difficulty controlling his or her drinking, being preoccupied with alcohol, continuing to use alcohol even when it causes problems, having to drink more to get the same effect, or having withdrawal symptoms when blood alcohol levels decrease or if one ceases to drink.

Amnesia: impairment of long-term and/or short-term memory.

Analgesia: loss of sensibility to pain without loss of consciousness.

Antabuse: brand name of the generic drug disulfiram; used to deter consumption of alcohol by persons being treated for alcohol dependency by inducing vomiting.

Binge drinking: occurs when an individual excessively drinks in a short period, typically 4 drinks for women and 5 drinks for men in about a 2-hour period, increasing blood alcohol concentration (BAC) levels to 0.08 g/dL.

Blackout: temporary amnesia occurring during periods of intensive drinking; person is not unconscious.

Blood alcohol concentration (BAC): refers to the percent of alcohol in a person's blood stream. A BAC of 0.10% means that an individual's blood supply contains one-part alcohol for every 1,000 parts blood. In most states, an individual is legally intoxicated if he or she has a BAC of 0.08% or higher.

Delirium: extreme mental and usually motor excitement marked by a rapid succession of confused and unconnected ideas; often with illusions and hallucinations; may be accompanied by tremors.

Delirium tremens: (DTs): a serious acute condition associated with the last stages of alcohol withdrawal. Usually lasting 2 or 3 days, the individual can experience hallucinations, shaking, shivering, irregular heart rates, sweating, hyperthermia, or seizures that could result in death.

Dependence: dependence develops when the neurons in the brain adapt to the repeated substance exposure and only function normally in the presence of the substance. When the substance is withdrawn, several physiologic reactions can occur from mild to life-threatening (withdrawal syndrome).

> **Chemical dependence:** the use of substances, alters an individual's brain making the brain more dependent on the chemical substance to operate.
>
> **Physical dependence:** occurs when a person requires the substance to function, if the substance is not present in their system, the person could experience physical symptoms ranging from anxiety to seizures.

Detoxification: treatment designed to assist in recovery from the toxic effects of a substance; involves withdrawal and may include pharmacologic and/or nonpharmacologic treatment with psychotherapy and counseling.

Drug Enforcement Administration (DEA) drug schedules: drugs, substances, and certain chemicals used to make drugs are classified by the US Drug Enforcement Administration (DEA) into five distinct categories or schedules depending on the drug's acceptable medical use and the drug's abuse or dependency potential.

Euphoria: feeling of well-being, elation; without fear or worry.

Hallucination: a sensory impression (sight, sound, touch, smell, or taste) that has no basis in external stimulation; may have psychological causes, or may result from the use of drugs, (including alcohol), a brain tumor, senility, or exhaustion.

Illicit: and illegal substance; not authorized, not sanctioned by law.

NIDA Quick Screen: a tool developed by the National Institute on Drug Abuse (NIDA), for providers in healthcare settings to screen for substance use. The NIDA Quick Screen incorporates the Five A's of Intervention (Ask, Advise, Assess, Assist, Arrange), providing an opportunity for the clinician to explain how the patient's substance use is impacting their health and resources available if they would like to assistance in quitting.

Nystagmus: involuntary, rapid, rhythmic movements of the eyeball.

Opiate antagonist: examples include naltrexone and naloxone. These drugs have a high affinity for opiate receptors but do not activate them and block the effect of exogenously administered opioids (e.g., morphine, heroin, and methadone) or of endogenously released endorphins.

Opioid: synthetic narcotic that has opiate-like activities but is not derived from opium.

Prescription drug monitoring programs (PDMP): is statewide electronic database for healthcare providers to see patients' prescribing histories especially for controlled substances, in attempt to reduce the over prescribing of substances such as opioids.

Saddlenose deformity: a collapse of the nasal bridge seen in substance users who snort cocaine.

Substance abuse: refers to the harmful or hazardous use of psychoactive substances, including alcohol and illicit drugs.

Tolerance: is an individual's diminished response to a substance, which occurs when the substance is used repeatedly and the body adapts to the continued presence of the substance, requiring increased amounts to achieve the same effect.

Withdrawal syndrome: a group of signs and symptoms, both physiologic and psychological, that occurs on abrupt discontinuation of a substance use.

Chapter 60: The Patient with a Respiratory Disease

Acute: (of a disease or disease symptom) beginning abruptly with marked intensity or sharpness, then subsiding after a relatively short time; opposite of **chronic.**

AFB: acid-fast bacilli.

Allergen: see antigen.

Analgesic: relieving pain.

Anaphylaxis: an exaggerated life-threatening hypersensitivity reaction to a previously encountered allergen.

Antigen: any substance that is capable of inducing a specific immune response and of reacting with the products of that response, that is, with specific antibody or specifically sensitized T-lymphocytes or both. When used to describe an allergic response, these antigens are called **allergens**.

Atopic: form of allergy in which a hypersensitivity reaction may occur in a part of the body not in contact with the allergen.

Bronchodilator: a drug that relaxes contractions of the smooth muscle of the bronchioles to improve ventilation of the lungs.

Chronic: (of a disease or disorder) developing slowly and persisting for a long period, often for the remainder of a person s lifetime; opposite of **acute.**

Communicable disease: (contagious) any disease transmitted from one person or animal to another. *Direct:* from excreta or other bodily discharges. *Indirect:* from substances or inanimate objects (contaminated drinking glasses, water, insects, or toys).

Comorbid: medical condition(s) existing simultaneously but independently with another condition.

Coryza: profuse discharge from mucous membrane of the nose.

DOT: directly observed therapy.

Dysphagia: difficulty in swallowing. Do not confuse with **dysphasia:** loss of ability to understand language as a result of injury or disease to the brain.

Dyspnea: labored or difficult breathing.

Edematous: abnormal accumulation of fluids in the intercellular spaces of tissues causing swelling.

EMB: ethambutol.

Exacerbation: increase in severity of a disease or any of its symptoms.

Expiration: release of air from the lungs through the nose or mouth. See **inspiration.**

Gastroesophageal reflux disease (GERD): backflow of stomach contents into the esophagus where gastric juices produce a burning sensation.

Goblet cell: specialized epithelial cell that secretes mucus.

Hemoptysis: spitting of blood because of a lesion in the larynx, trachea, or lower respiratory tract.

HIV: human immunodeficiency virus.

Hyperventilation: greater rate and volume of breathing than metabolically necessary for pulmonary gas exchange; may lead to dizziness and possible syncope.

IGRA: interferon-gamma release assay.

INH: isoniazid.

Inspiration: inhaling air into the lungs. See **expiration.**

LTBI: latent tuberculosis infection.

Malaise: a vague uneasy feeling of body weakness, often marking the onset of, and persisting throughout, a disease.

Mast cell: constituent of connective tissue; releases substances in response to injury or infection.

MDR-TB: multidrug-resistant tuberculosis.

Mediator: a substance that effects a change in a disease state.

Mucus: *n.* viscous, slippery secretion of mucous membranes and glands. Contains mucin, white blood cells, inorganic salts, and exfoliated cells.

Myalgia: muscle pain accompanied by malaise.

Mycoplasma: bacteria without a cell wall, more resistant to antibiotics.

Nosocomial: pertaining to, or originating in, a healthcare facility.

Nosocomial pneumonia: pneumonia contracted during confinement in a healthcare facility.

Pathophysiology: disruption of bodily functions due to disease.

Pleura: delicate membrane enclosing the lungs.

Pneumothorax: collection of air or gas causing the lungs to collapse.

PPD: purified protein derivative.

Pulmonary hypertension: condition of abnormally high pressure within the pulmonary circulation.

PZA: pyrazinamide.

RIF: rifampin.

Spirometer: instrument for measuring volume of air entering and leaving the lungs to determine lung function and breathing capacity.

Sputum: matter expectorated (coughed up) from the respiratory system, especially the lungs in a diseased state, composed chiefly of mucus and may contain pus, blood, or microorganisms.

Tachycardia: abnormally high heart rate (>100 beats/minute) for an adult.

Tachypnea: abnormally high respiration rate (>20 breaths/minute) for an adult.

TB: Tuberculosis.

TST: tuberculin skin test.

Wheeze: breathe with difficulty, usually with a whistling sound.

XDR-TB: extensively drug-resistant tuberculosis.

Chapter 61: The Patient with Cardiovascular Disease

Angina pectoris: acute pain in the chest from decreased blood supply to the heart muscle.

Anticoagulant: a substance that suppresses, delays, or nullifies coagulation of the blood.

Apnea: temporary cessation of breathing.

Arrhythmia: variation from the normal rhythm, especially with reference to the heart.

Arterial blood: oxygenated blood carried by an artery away from the heart to nourish the body tissues.

Arthralgia: joint pain.

Atheroma: lipid (cholesterol) deposit on the intima (lining) of an artery; also called atheromatous plaque.

Atherosclerosis: disease process caused by the deposit of atheromas on the inner lining of arteries that results in the obstruction of blood flow.

Coronary heart disease: narrowing of the arteries that supply blood and oxygen to the heart caused by the buildup of plaque in the arteries.

Cyanosis: bluish discoloration of the skin and mucous membranes caused by excess concentration of reduced hemoglobin in the blood.

Dyspnea: labored or difficult breathing.

Echocardiography: recording of the position and motion of the heart walls and internal structures of the heart and neighboring tissue by the echo obtained from beams of ultrasonic waves directed through the chest wall; used to show valvular and other structural deformities; the record produced is called an echocardiogram.

Edema: abnormal accumulation of fluid in the intercellular spaces of the body.

Embolism: the sudden blocking of an artery by a clot of foreign material, an embolus, that has been brought to its site of lodgment by the bloodstream; the embolus may be a blood clot (most frequently) or an air bubble, a clump of bacteria, or a fat globule.

Heparin: anticoagulant; prevents platelet agglutination and thrombus formation.

Infarct: localized area of ischemic necrosis produced by occlusion of the arterial supply or venous drainage of the part.

Ischemia: deficiency of blood to supply oxygen in part resulting from functional constriction or actual obstruction of a blood vessel.

Lumen: the cavity or channel within a tube or tubular organ, such as a blood vessel or the intestine.

Murmur: irregularity of heartbeat caused by a turbulent flow of blood through a valve that has failed to close.

Myocardial infarction: heart attack; a sudden and sometimes fatal occurrence of coronary thrombosis, typically resulting in the death of part of a heart muscle.

Myocardium: the middle and thickest layer of the heart wall, composed of cardiac muscle.

Nocturia: waking at night one or more times to urinate.

Occlusion: blockage; state of being closed.

Prolapse: when an organ falls out of its normal position due to lack of support from ligaments and muscles.

Restenosis: recurrent stenosis.

Shunt: abnormal communication between chambers or blood vessels; *verb*, to bypass, divert.

Stenosis: narrowing or contraction of a body passage or opening.

Thrombus: blood clot attached to the intima of a blood vessel; may occlude the lumen; contrast with embolus, which is detached and carried by the bloodstream.

Venous blood: nonoxygenated blood from the tissues; blood pumped from the heart to the lungs for oxygenation.

Chapter 62: The Patient with a Blood Disorder

Differential cell count: record of the number of white blood cells, including determination of the percentage of each type of cell present; the "differential" is used in the diagnosis of various blood disorders, infections, and other abnormal conditions of the body.

Glossitis: inflammation of the tongue.

Glossodynia: pain in the tongue.

Hemarthrosis: blood in a joint cavity.

Hematocrit: volume percentage of erythrocytes (red blood cells) in whole blood.

Hemoglobin: protein in the erythrocyte that transports molecular oxygen to body cells.

Hemolysis: rupture of erythrocytes with the release of hemoglobin into the plasma.

Hemolytic: destruction of blood cells, resulting in liberation of hemoglobin.

Hypoxia: diminished availability of oxygen to body tissues.

IF (intrinsic factor): produced by the parietal cells in the stomach; aids in vitamin B_{12} absorption.

INR (international normalized ratio): ratio between actual blood coagulation time and the normal coagulation time.

Leukocytosis: increase in the total number of leukocytes.

Leukopenia: reduction in total number of leukocytes in the blood; count under 500/mL.

Neutropenia: diminished number of neutrophils (polymorphonuclear leukocytes or PMNs).

Petechia: minute, pinpoint, round, nonraised, purplish red spot in the skin or mucous membrane, caused by hemorrhage.

Phagocytosis: engulfing of microorganisms and foreign particles by phagocytes, such as macrophages.

Purpura: hemorrhage into the tissues, under the skin, and through the mucous membranes; produces petechiae and ecchymoses.

Vaso-occlusion: blood vessel blockage resulting in organ damage.

Vertigo: dizziness.

Chapter 63: The Patient with an Autoimmune Disease

Arthralgia: joint pain.

Autoantibodies: an antibody produced by the immune system against the individual's own body proteins/tissues.

Diplopia: double vision.

Dysarthria: difficult or unclear speech cause by muscle weakness.

Fibrosis: thickening and scarring of connective tissue.

First-line: refers to a drug or therapy that is the first choice for treatment.

Glucocorticosteroid (or corticosteroid): steroids produced by the adrenal gland (or medication) involved in anti-inflammatory activity through metabolism (catabolism) of proteins, carbohydrates, and fat.

Microstomia: small mouth opening.

Neuritis: inflammation of a peripheral nerve, causing pain and loss of function.

Palliative: minimize or relieve pain without dealing with the cause of the pain.

Ptosis: drooping of the upper eyelid due to paralysis or disease.

Sclerodactyly: localized thickening and tightening on the skin of the fingers or toes.

Steatorrhea: excretion of abnormal quantities of fat with the feces as a result of malabsorption.

Telangiectases: dilation of capillaries making them appear as small red or purple cluster, which may have a "spidery" appearance.

Vasculopathy: this term is applied to any disease affecting blood vessels.

Wickham striae: whitish lines visible on oral mucosa giving a lace-like appearance in oral lichen planus.

Index

Note: Page numbers followed by "*f*", "*t*", and "*b*" refer to figures, tables, and boxes, respectively.

A

A1c, 925, 930
  average blood glucose and, 939*t*
AAPD. *See* American Academy of
  Pediatric Dentistry (AAPD)
ABA (applied behavioral analysis), 876
Abfraction, 262–263, 718, 718*f*
Abrasion, 262, 262*f*, 717, 733
Abrasive agents, 734
Abrasive grits, 730
Abrasive system, 590
Absence seizure, 971
Absolute insulin deficiency, 926
Absolute neutrophil count (ANC), 1063*t*
Absorbed dose, 235
Absorption, alcohol, 1001
Abstinence, 1000
Abuse and neglect, 212
  child. *See* Child abuse and neglect
  elder. *See* Elder abuse and neglect
  reporting, 219
    reportable required information, 220
    reporting laws, 220
    training, 220
Abutment, 518
Acamprosate (Campral), 1005
Acanthosis nigricans, 939*f*
Acceptance, motivational interviewing
  and, 408–409
Accommodative speech, 39
Accurate empathy, 409
Acellular, 281
Acid etch, purposes of, 600, 600*f*
Acid-etchant, 600
Acid-fast bacilli (AFB), 1030
Acid production, 422
Acidogenic bacteria, 422
Acidulated phosphate fluoride (APF), 582
Aciduric bacteria, 422
Acne rosacea, 1015
Acoustic turbulence, 655
ACP (amorphous calcium phosphate),
  724, 749
Acquired hemolytic disorders, 1065
Acquired pellicle, 281, 291
Acquired platelet dysfunction, 1070
Actinomyces, 296
Actiq, 1010
Activated partial thromboplastin time
  (aPTT), 1063*t*
Activation (stroke), 644, 650–651, 650*f*,
  660

Active listening, 409
Active TB disease, 1030, 1031*t*
Activities of daily living (ADL), 386,
  386*t*
Acute bronchitis, 1028
  viral and bacterial, 1028*t*
Acute graft-versus-host disease, 948
Acute neurologic disorders, 892
Acute oral inflammatory, toothbrushing,
  448–449
Acute periodontal lesions
  endo-periodontal lesions, 333
  necrotizing periodontal diseases,
    332–333
  periodontal abscess, 332
Acute pulmonary edema, 1053
Acute respiratory infection, 1028
Acute toxic dose, 592
ADA. *See* American Dental Association
  (ADA)
ADA (Americans with Disability Act),
  866
Adaptation, 644, 649, 659–660
Adaptive behavior, 851
Addiction, 1000
Addison disease. *See* Hypoadrenalism
Additional transmission-based
  precautions, 62
Adequate intakes (AIs), 554
ADHA. *See* American Dental Hygienists'
  Association (ADHA)
Adjunctive therapy
  antimicrobial treatment
    local delivery antimicrobial agents,
      695
    systemic delivery of antibiotics,
      694–695
    systemic subantimicrobial dose
      antibiotics, 695
  indications for use of local delivery
    agents, 695–696
ADL (activities of daily living), 386, 386*t*
Adolescence, stages of, 916
Adolescents, 800, 805
  accident and injury prevention, 817
  communication skills of, 38
  Community Periodontal Index, 368
  dietary and feeding pattern
    recommendations, 816
  oral health considerations for, 818
  psychosocial development of, 805*t*
Adrenal crisis, 140*t*
  symptoms of, 915, 916*b*

Adrenal glands
  adrenal crisis, symptoms of, 916*b*
  hyperadrenalism, 915
  hypoadrenalism, 915–916
Adrenal insufficiency. *See*
  Hypoadrenalism
Adsorption, 281
ADT. *See* Advanced dental therapist (ADT)
Advanced Dental Hygiene Practitioner,
  9–10
Advanced dental therapist (ADT), 9–10
  clinical role of, 10
  impact of, 10
Aeroallergen, 93
Aerobic bacteria, 284
Aerosol, 64, 85
AFB (acid-fast bacilli), 1030
Affect, 34
Affirmation, 409, 412
Agency for Healthcare Research and
  Quality, 25*b*
Agenda setting, motivational
  interviewing and, 411
Aging, 824. *See also* Older adults
Agranulocytes, 1064, 1064*t*
AHA (American Heart Association),
  178–179
Air-powder polishing, 732, 739*f*
  principles of application, 739
  recommendations and precautions, 741
  on restorative materials, 742*t*
  risk patients, 741
  specially formulated powders for use
    in, 739–740
  technique, 740–741, 740*b*, 741*b*
  uses and advantages of, 740
Air-water syringe, 338–339
Airborne infection, 64
Airborne precautions, 62
Akathisia, 992*t*
Akinesia, 899, 992*t*
Alcohol
  consumption, 319
    clinical pattern, 1000–1001
    etiology, 1001
  dependence, 1000
  fetal alcohol spectrum disorders, 1003
    alcohol use during pregnancy, 1004
    characteristics of an individual with,
      1004b
    fetal alcohol syndrome, facial features
      of, 1004f
    terminology and abbreviations, 1004b

Alcohol (*continued*)
 hallucinosis, 1005
 health hazards of
  brain, 1002
  cancer risk, 1003
  digestive system, 1003
  heart, 1003
  immunity and infection, 1003
  liver disease, 1003
  nervous system, 1003
  nutritional deficiencies, 1003
  reproductive system, 1003
 intoxication, 1000–1001
 metabolism of
  blood alcohol level, 1002, 1002f
  diffusion, 1001
  ingestion and absorption, 1001
  liver metabolism, 1001
 mouthrinses, 478
Alcohol-related birth defect (ARBD),
 1004b
Alcohol-related neurodevelopmental
 disorder (ARND), 1004b
Alcohol use disorder (AUD), 1000
 signs of, 1001
 treatment for, 1005
Alcohol withdrawal syndrome, 1005
Alcoholic liver disease (ALD), 1003
Alcoholism. *See also* Alcohol use disorder
 (AUD)
 older adult
  *dental hygiene management
   considerations, 829*
  effects of alcohol use, 828–829
ALD (alcoholic liver disease), 1003
Aligner system, removable, 487
Alimentation, 949t
Allergens, 93, 1032
Allergic rhinitis (hay fever), 1027t
Allergy, local anesthesia and, 626
Allograft, 518
Alloplast, 518
Alopecia, 946
Als (adequate intakes), 554
ALS (Amyotrophic lateral sclerosis), 898
Altered taste sensations, 560t
Aluminum filters, 233
Aluminum trihydroxide, 740
Alveolar bone
 biomechanical force, 518
 classification of, 518
 grafting and regeneration, 518
Alveolar bone, 309
Alveolar mucosa, 307
Alveolar process fracture, 964
Alveolectomy, 706
Alveolitis, 959
Alzheimer disease, 826
 dental hygiene care considerations for,
  828b
 dental hygiene management
  considerations, 827–828
 etiology, 827
 guidelines for caregivers, 828b
 stages of, 827b
 symptoms and stages, 827
 treatment, 827
Ambient air, 616

Ambivalence, exploring
 decisional balance, 413, 413f, 414b
 readiness ruler, 414, 414f, 415b
 sustain talk *vs.* change talk, 413
Amelogenesis imperfecta, 260, 298
American Academy of Pediatric Dentistry
 (AAPD), 580, 800
 caries-risk assessment tool, 424
 caries risk management protocol, 427
American Dental Association (ADA),
 580
 Caries Classification System, 266
 caries risk assessment, 424
 evidence-based dentistry website, 25b
 Seal of Acceptance Program, 479–480,
  481f
 tooth numbering systems, 152, 152f
American Dental Hygienists' Association
 (ADHA), 4, 9f
 Code of Ethics for dental hygienists,
  1095–1098
American Heart Association (AHA),
 178–179
American manual alphabet, 877
American Sign Language (ASL), 877
American Society of Anesthesiologists
 (ASA) physical status classification
 system, 179, 384, 385t, 618
Americans with Disability Act (ADA),
 866
Amide anesthetics, 621
Amnesia, 1001
Amorphous, 292t
Amorphous calcium phosphate (ACP),
 724, 749
Ampere, 227
Amphetamines, 1011
Amplitude, 655
Amputation, 935
Amyotrophic lateral sclerosis (ALS), 898
Anabolic steroids, 1008t, 1011
Anaerobic bacteria, 284
Analgesia, 615, 1010
Analgesics, 130, 1027t
Anaphylaxis, 138t, 1024
Anaplastic features, 945t
ANC (absolute neutrophil count), 1063t
Anemia, 1065–1066
 caused by
  blood loss, 1065
  *diminished production of red blood
   cells, 1065*
  genetic blood disorders, 1065
  increased hemolysis, 1065
 of chronic diseases, 1065
 clinical characteristics of, 1066
 iron deficiency, 1066
 megaloblastic anemia
  folate-deficiency anemia, 1067
  pernicious anemia, 1066–1067
Aneroid sphygmomanometer, 187
Anesthesia, 621. *See also specific entries*
 reversal agent, 638
Anesthetics
 buffered local, 638
 intranasal dental, 638–639
Angina, local anesthesia and, 627
Angina pectoris, 130, 1048, 1051

Angioedema, 141t
Angular cheilitis, 512–513, 560t, 990,
 991f
Angulation, 649–650, 650f
Ankylosis, 904
Anorexia nervosa, 987–988, 987f
 characteristics of, 987b
 dental hygiene care, 989–990
Anoxia, 187
Antabuse. *See* Disulfiram
Antibacterial therapeutic mouthrinses,
 808
Antibiotic prophylaxis, 1056
 AHA guidelines, 178–179
 medical conditions, 179, 179b
 recommendations based on principles,
  179
 recommended antibiotic protocol,
  179, 180t
Antibiotics, 680
 bacterial resistance to, 1028
 systemic delivery of, 694–695
 systemic subantimicrobial dose, 695
Antibody, 70
Anticalculus dentifrice, 293
Anticariogenic food, 567
Anticholinergics, 992t, 1034t
Anticipatory guidance, 384, 790, 791t,
 800, 814
 accident and injury prevention, 817
 dietary and feeding pattern
  recommendations, 815–816
 digit habits, 817, 817f
 oral health considerations for
  adolescents, 818
 oral health considerations for toddlers/
  pre-schoolers, 816
 oral malodor (halitosis), 817
 referral, 818
 6 years of age to adolescent, 815t
 speech and language development,
  816f, 817
 tobacco/obstructive sleep apnea/
  piercings/substance abuse, 818
 12 months to 6 years of age,
  812–813t
Anticoagulants
 for cardiac arrhythmias, 1053
 for cardiovascular disease, 1056
 for stroke, 897b
Antidepressants, 1015
 for bipolar disorder, 986
 for feeding and eating disorders, 989
 for posttraumatic stress disorder, 983
Antiepileptic drugs, 972
 for stroke, 897b
Antigen, 1033
Antigen/antibody tests, 76
Antihyperglycemic therapy, for type 2
 diabetes, 934, 934t
Antihypertensives, for stroke, 897b
Antimicrobial agent, 106, 296–297, 476
Antimicrobial soap, 91
Antimicrobial therapy, 694
Antimicrobials
 adjunctive therapy, 694–695
 local delivery agents, 695, 696t
Antiplatelet therapy, 1057

Antipsychotics
for bipolar disorder, 986
effects of, 992t
for schizophrenia, 992
Antiresorptive drug-related osteonecrosis
of the jaw, 946
Antiretroviral therapy (ART), 784
Antiseizure medications, 972, 973t
Antiseptic hand rub, 91
Antiseptic handwash, 90–91
Antiseptic mouthrinse, 110
Antithrombotic therapy
anticoagulant therapy, 1056
antiplatelet therapy, 1057
direct oral anticoagulants, 1056–1057
Anxiety disorders, 617
dental hygiene care, 983–984
and pain control. See Pain
treatment, 983
types and symptoms of, 982–983
Anxiolytics, for posttraumatic stress
disorder, 983
Apatite, 289, 575
APF (acidulated phosphate fluoride),
582
Aphasia, 39, 896b
Aphtha, 206
Apnea, 187, 1048
Apoptosis, 892
Appliances, orthodontic. See Orthodontic
appliances
Applied behavioral analysis (ABA), 876
Apron, 238, 238f
aPTT (activated partial thromboplastin
time), 1063t
ARBD (alcohol-related birth defect),
1004b
Arch wire, 486, 487
Area-specific curets, 653
Aripiprazole, 857
Arkansas stone, 668
ARND (alcohol-related
neurodevelopmental disorder), 1004b
Arrested caries, 258t
Arrhythmia, 1053
ART (antiretroviral therapy), 784
Arterial BP, 1048
Arteries of arm, 186f
Arthralgia, 1045, 1080
Arthritis. See also specific arthritis
degenerative joint disease
adult hand compromised by, 905f
medical treatment, 905
occurrence, 904
symptoms of, 904–905
dental hygiene care, 905
Articaine HCl, 623
Articulating paper, 607
Articulation, 896b
Artificial nails, 89
Ascorbic acid, 559t
ASD. See Autism spectrum disorder (ASD)
Ask, Validate, Document, Refer (AVDR)
Tutorial for Dentists, 220
ASL (American Sign Language), 877
Asperger disorder, 856b
Aspiration, 632
Assessment, 384

Asthma
atopic (allergic), 1033
attack, 1033
dental hygiene care, 1035, 1035t
etiology of, 1032–1033, 1033f
medical management, 1034–1035
medications, types, categories, and
examples of, 1034t
oral manifestations, 1035
Asthmatic hypersensitivity reaction, 1033
Astringent, 475
Asymmetric tonic neck reflex, 900
Asymptomatic carrier, 62
At-home bleaching trays, 759f
At-home products, bleaching, 755
Ataxia, 973
Ataxic palsy, 900
Atheromas, 1050
Atherosclerosis, 1044, 1050, 1050f
Atonic seizures, 971
Atopic (allergic) asthma, 1032, 1033
Atrophy, 899
Attached gingiva, 306–307
significance of, 326
Attachment apparatus, 303
Attention-deficit/hyperactivity disorder,
850b
Attrition, 261, 261f, 717
Atypical plasma cholinesterase, 627
Atypical seizure, 970t
AUD. See Alcohol use disorder (AUD)
Augmentation, 518
Aura, 971, 972
Auscultation, 188
Autism Speaks dental tool kit, 858
Autism spectrum disorder (ASD), 850,
850b, 856b
approaches to dental care, 858
characteristics, 856–857
etiology of, 856
factors significant for dental hygiene
care, 858
levels of severity, 857b
prevalence of, 855–856
treatment interventions, 857–858
Autistic disorder, 856b
Autoantibodies, 1078
Autograft, 518
Autoimmune disease
classification of, 1078–1079
connective tissue, 1079
oral lichen planus, 1079–1080, 1080f
rheumatoid arthritis, 1080–1081,
1081f
documentation, 1091, 1091b
etiology, 1078
everyday ethics, 1092
factors to teach patient, 1092
gastrointestinal tract, 1083
celiac disease, 1083
Crohn's disease, 1083–1085, 1084f
ulcerative colitis, 1085–1086, 1085f
immune system, 1078, 1078f
neurologic system, 1086
multiple sclerosis, 1086–1088,
1087b, 1087f
myasthenia gravis, 1088–1089
organ-specific, 1079

prevalence of, 1078
scleroderma
clinical presentation, 1082, 1082f
CREST syndrome, 1081b
dental hygiene care, 1082–1083
etiology of, 1081
prevalence of, 1081
treatment for, 1082
systemic, 1079
systemic autoimmune diseases, 1089
Sjogren's syndrome, 1089–1090
systemic lupus erythematosus,
1090–1091, 1091–1092f
treatment modalities, 1079
types of, 1079t
Automatisms, 970t
Autonomic dysreflexia, 893, 895
Autonomic neuropathy, 935
Autonomic seizure, 970t
Autonomy, 407
support, 409
Autopolymerized, 600
Autotransformer, 227
Avulsion, 263

B

B complex, 560
BAC (blood alcohol concentration),
1000, 1002, 1002f
Backscatter, 235
Bacteremia, 178, 450, 684
Bacterial bronchitis, 1028t
Bacterial invasion, 284f
Bacterial pneumonias, 1028, 1029t
Bag mask, 136t
Bands, 486
Barrier-free environment
external features, 870
internal features, 870
treatment room, 871
Barrier protection, 85
Barriers and surface covers, 107, 107f,
108f
Baseline, 128
Basic life support (BLS), 136
Basophils, 1065
Bass methods, 440–441, 440f
BD. See Bipolar disorder (BD)
Becker muscular dystrophy, 902
Behavior arrest, 970t
Behavior change, 407
patient motivation and
health behavior change model, 407,
407t
health behavior change, motivation
for, 408
transtheoretical model, 408
Behavioral therapies, 1013–1014
Bell's palsy, 892, 897
Benign neoplasms, 944, 945t
Benzocaine, 636
Benzodiazepines, 1014
Best practice, 20, 384
Beta-blockers, for posttraumatic stress
disorder, 983
Beta cells, 925
Betel/areca, 297

Beveled edge, 668
Bibulous pad, 606
Bidigital palpation, 196, 196f
Bilateral palpation, 197, 197f
Bimanual palpation, 196–197, 197f
Binders (thickeners), 473
Binge drinking, 1000
Binge-eating disorder, 988–989
   dental hygiene care, 990
Bioabsorbable polymeric formulation, 698
Biodegradable medication, 695
Bioethics, 29
Biofilm, 109. See also Dental biofilm control
   fluoride in, 576–577
   index, 886
   -induced gingivitis, 809
Biofilm control record, 360f
   procedure, 360
   purpose, 360
   scoring, 360
      calculation, example, 360
      interpretation, 361
   selection of teeth and surfaces, 360
Biofilm-free score, 361, 361f
   papillary bleeding on probing, 362
   procedure, 361–362
   purpose, 361
   scoring, 362
      calculation, 362
      interpretation, 362
   selection of teeth and surfaces, 361
Biohazard, 100
Biologic monitor, 103
Biologic or permucosal seal, 519
Biologic width, 306
Biological age, 824
Biomedical databases, 25, 25b
Biopsy, 207–208, 956b
Biostatistics, 21
Biotherapy, 945
Bipolar disorder (BD)
   dental hygiene care, 986
   signs and symptoms of, 986
   treatment, 986
Bisphenol A–glycidyl methylacrylate (bis-GMA), 600
Bitewing (interproximal) surveys
   image receptor placement, 245, 245f
   image receptor selection for, 242
   positioning, 244–245, 244f
Black-line stain, 295–296
Bladder and bowel paralysis, 903
Blade, 646, 646f
   form dental implant, 520
Bleaching of tooth, 747
   at-home bleaching trays, 759f
   dental hygiene process of care
      dental hygiene care plan, 758
      dental hygiene diagnosis, 758
      digital photographic record of tooth shade, 758f
      evaluation and planning for maintenance, 758
      implementation, 758
      manual selection of tooth shade, 757f, 758b
      patient assessment, 757–758
   documentation, 759, 759b

everyday ethics, 759–760
factors to teach patient, 760
nonvital
      factors associated with efficacy, 757
      history of, 748
      procedure for, 756–757, 756–757b
      vital vs., 747–748
vital
      decision making for, 751t
      desensitization procedures for, 753t
      factors associated with efficacy, 750–752
      history of, 748
      irreversible tooth damage, 753
      materials used for, 748–749, 748f, 749f
      mechanism of, 748
      medications associated with potential photosensitivity and hyperpigmentation, 750b
      modes of, 753–756, 754t
      nonvital vs., 747–748
      over-the-counter bleaching preparations, 756b
      reversible side effects of, 753
      safety, 749–750
      scalloped and unscalloped bleaching tray designs, 755f
      sensitivity, 753
      tooth color change with, 748
   whitening vs., 747
Bleaching trays, 754
Bleeding disorder, 1070–1071
Blind, 868
Block (regional) anesthesia, 625
Block-out resin, 754
Blood alcohol concentration (BAC), 1000, 1002, 1002f
Blood disorder
   anemia, 1065–1066
      iron deficiency, 1066
      megaloblastic, 1066–1067
   bleeding or coagulation disorders, 1070–1071
   blood cell reference values, 6064t
   dental hygiene care plan
      consultation with physician/hematologist, 1072–1073
      examination, 1073
      patient history, 1072, 1072b
      preparation for clinical appointment, 1071–1072
      treatment, 1073
      treatment care plan, 1073
   documentation, 1073, 1074b
   everyday ethics, 1074
   factors to teach patient, 1074
   laboratory values and clinical implications, 1063t
   normal blood, 1062
   plasma, 1062
   platelets, 1065
      disorders, 1070
   polycythemias, 1069
   red blood cells, 1062, 1062f
   sickle cell disease, 1067–1068, 1067f
   white blood cells, 1062–1065, 1062f
      disorders of, 1069–1070

Blood, effects of antipsychotics, 992t
Blood pressure
   classifications, 190t
   components of, 187
   cuff in position, 189f
   equipment for determining, 187–188, 188f
   factors influencing, 187
   follow-up criteria, 191
   hypertension, 190–191, 191t
   procedure for determining, 188–190
   sizes of cuff, 188f
BLS (basic life support), 136
Body temperature
   care of patient with temperature elevation, 185
   indications for taking, 184
   maintenance of, 184
   methods of determining, 184–185
   thermometers, 185, 185f
Bond strength, 601
Bonded brackets
   advantages of, 486
   disadvantages of, 486
   fixed appliance system, 486–487, 486f
   removable aligner system, 487
Bonding, 600
   agent, 486
   clinical procedures for, 487–488
Bone grafting, 845
Border mold, 710
Bordetella pertussis, 66t
Bottle feeding, 792
Bottled water, 580
Brackets, 486, 487. See also Bonded brackets
Bradycardia, 185
Bradykinesia, 898
Braille, 868
Brain, alcohol and, 1002
Brainstorming, 416
Breastfeeding, 792
Bristles. See Filaments
Bronchitis, due to tobacco use, 534
Bronchodilator, 1033
Brown pellicle, 296
Brown stain, 296–297, 297f. See also Dental fluorosis
Brush-on gel, 589–590, 589t
Bruxism, 261, 990
Buffered local anesthetic, 638
Buffering, 423
Bulimia nervosa, 988, 988f
   characteristics of, 988b
   dental hygiene care, 990
Bupivacaine HCl, 623
Buprenorphine (Subutex), 1014
Buprenorphine/naloxone (Suboxone), 1014
Bupropion SR, 540t, 541
Burning mouth syndrome, 918
Burnishing, 668

C

C-CLAD (computer-controlled local anesthesia delivery) system, 629
CA (cardiac arrhythmias), 1053

Cachexia, 218
Calcium, 284
Calcium carbonate (whiting, calcite, chalk), 734, 740
Calcium phosphate, 735
Calcium sodium phosphosilicate (Novamin), 724, 740
Calculus, 286, 287, 287f, 524, 719. See also Subgingival calculus; Supragingival calculus
  attachment of, 291
  clinical characteristics of, 291–292, 292t
  composition, 289–290
  detection tool, 662
  formation, 290–291
  mineralization, 290
  prevention of, 293
  removal, 682
    using manual instruments, 687b
  significance of, 291
  structure of, 290–291
  teeth and bone vs., 290
CAMBRA (Caries Management by Risk Assessment), 239, 425–426, 425–426t, 427, 809
Campral. See Acamprosate
Canadian Dental Hygienists Association, 1101–1103
Cancer
  benign and malignant neoplasms, characteristics of, 945t
  chemotherapy
    agents used for, 946b
    indications, 946
    objectives, 945
    oral complications of, 946
    systemic side effects of, 946
    types of, 946
  dental hygiene care plan
    objectives, 949
    oral care protocol, 949–951, 949t, 950t
    personal factors, 949
  description of, 944
  documentation, 951, 952b
  everyday ethics, 952
  factors to teach patient, 953
  hematopoietic stem cell transplantation
    acute complications, 948
    chronic complications, 948
    stages of transplantation process, 947–948
    types, 947
  incidence and survival, 944
  mucositis management
    prevention/oral health maintenance, 948
    treatment of established mucositis, 948–949
  multidisciplinary team for care, 944b
  radiation therapy
    doses, 947
    indications, 946
    oral complications, 947, 947f
    systemic effects, 947
    types, 946–947, 947f

risk, alcohol and, 1003
risk factors, 944
signs and symptoms of, 945t
surgery, 945
and tobacco use, 534
treatment of, 945
types of, 945
Candida albicans, 67t
Candidiasis, 56, 560t
Cannabinoids (marijuana) abuse, 1006, 1007t, 1009–1010
Cannula, 136t, 697
Carbamazepine (Tegretol, Carbatrol), 973t
Carbamide peroxide, 748f, 749, 749f
Carbatrol. See Carbamazepine
Carbohydrates, 285
Carbopol, 749
Carcinogen, 530
Carcinomas, 944
Cardiac arrhythmias (CA), 1053
Cardiac pacemaker, 1055, 1055f
Cardiac resynchronization therapy (CRT), 1054–1055
Cardiovascular disease (CVD), 776, 935
  angina pectoris, 1051
  antithrombotic therapy
    anticoagulant therapy, 1056
    antiplatelet therapy, 1057
    direct oral anticoagulants, 1056–1057
  cardiac arrhythmias, 1053
  classification, 1044
  congenital heart diseases
    anomalies, 1046
    clinical considerations, 1047
    etiology of, 1046
    normal heart, 1045–1046
    patent ductus arteriosus, 1047f
    prevention of, 1046–1047
    types of defects, 1046
    ventricular septal defect, 1046f
  documentation, 1057, 1057b
  due to tobacco use, 534
  everyday ethics, 1058
  factors to teach patient, 1058
  heart failure
    clinical manifestations of, 1052
    emergency care for, 1053
    etiology of, 1052
    treatment during chronic stages, 1052–1053
  hypertension
    blood pressure levels, 1048, 1049t
    in children, 1049
    clinical symptoms of, 1048–1049
    etiology of, 1048
    treatment of, 1049, 1049b
  infective endocarditis
    description of, 1044
    disease process, 1045
    etiology of, 1044
    prevention of, 1045
  ischemic heart disease, 1049–1050
    etiology of, 1050, 1050f
    manifestations of, 1050
  lifestyle management for, 1053–1054
  mitral valve prolapse, 1048
  myocardial infarction, 1051–1052

older adult, 830–831
rheumatic fever, 1047
rheumatic heart disease, 1047–1048
surgical treatment
  cardiac pacemaker, 1055, 1055f
  cardiac resynchronization therapy, 1054–1055
  coronary artery bypass grafting, 1054
  dental considerations, 1055
  implantable cardioverter defibrillator, 1055
  percutaneous coronary intervention, 1054
  postsurgical dental care, 1056
  presurgical dental care, 1055–1056
  revascularization, 1054
Cardiovascular effects
  of antipsychotics, 992t
  of drug abuse, 1012
Cardiovascular system, changes due to aging, 825
Care of sharpening equipment
  care of tanged file, 676
  flat sharpening stone, 675–676
  manufacturer's directions, 676
Care plan records, 157
Caregivers
  communication with, 42–43
  instruction for, 55, 885, 886f
  main, 809
  motivational interview, 417, 417b
  teaching, disabilities, 889
Caries Classification System (CCS), 266
Caries Management by Risk Assessment (CAMBRA), 239, 425–426, 425–426t, 427, 809
Caries risk assessment (CRA)
  American Academy of Pediatric Dentistry Caries-Risk Assessment Tool, 424
  American Dental Association, 424
  Caries Management by Risk Assessment, 425–426, 425–426t
  Cariogram, 424–425
  International Caries Classification and Management System, 426
  pediatrics
    classification of, 810–811
    early childhood caries, 811, 814, 814f
    levels, 811b
    principles, 809–810
    and protective factors to assess at each dental visit, 810t
    purpose, 809, 811f
    steps, 810, 812–813t
    white-spot lesions, 814f
  in process of care, 427
Caries-risk assessment tool (CAT), 424
Caries risk management systems
  AAPD caries risk management protocol, 427
  Caries Management by Risk Assessment, 427
  International Caries Classification and Management System, 427, 428f
Cariogenic dental biofilm, 266
Cariogenic exposure, 568f
Cariogenic food, 561

Cariogram, 424–425
Cariostatic agent, 586
Carious lesion, 264
　　assessment, 257, 259
　　classification of, 264–266
　　formation, stages in, 266, 266f
Carriers, 62
Case reports, 28
Case studies, 28
Case–control studies, 28
Casein phosphopeptide (CPP), 724
Cassette, 243, 246
CAT (caries-risk assessment tool), 424
Cataracts, 868
Cavitated carious lesion, 423
Cavitation, 266, 424, 655
CBCT (cone beam computed
　　tomography), 957
CBT. See Cognitive behavioral therapy
　　(CBT)
CCS (Caries Classification System), 266
CD. See Celiac disease (CD)
CDC. See Centers for Disease Control
　　and Prevention (CDC)
Celiac disease (CD), 1083
　　dental enamel hypoplasia in, 1084f
Cemented bands, 486–487
Cementum, 308–309
　　enamel and, 309f
　　fluoride in, 576
　　loss, 717
Centers for Disease Control and
　　Prevention (CDC), 68, 546, 577
Centric occlusion, 269
Ceramic brackets, 486
Cerebral palsy, 899–900
　　accompanying conditions, 900
　　classifications of, 900. See also specific
　　　　types
　　dental hygiene care, 901
　　medical treatment, 900
　　oral characteristics, 901
Cerebrovascular accident (CVA). See
　　Stroke
CF. See Cystic fibrosis (CF)
CFU (colony-forming units), 65
CGM (continuous glucose monitoring),
　　932
Chain of asepsis, 102
Change talk
　　eliciting and recognizing, 414
　　　　mobilizing, 415b, 416
　　　　preparatory, 415–416, 415b
　　sustain talk vs., 413
Charcot joints, 935
Charters method, 442–443, 443f
Charting of hard and soft tissues, 154
　　forms used for, 154
　　periodontal and dental, 155f
　　purpose of, 154
　　sequence for, 154–155
CHD. See Coronary heart disease (CHD)
Chemical-cure dressing, 709
Chemical dependence, 1005
Chemical disinfectants
　　categories of, 106
　　criteria for selection of chemical agent,
　　　　106–107

manufacturer's information, 106
　　principles of action, 106
　　properties of, 107b
　　uses of, 106
Chemical indicator, 102, 102f
Chemical liquid sterilization, 105
Chemical vapor sterilizer, 105
Chemotherapeutic agent, 472, 475
　　characteristics of, 478b
　　functions of, 475b
Chemotherapeutics, 681
Chemotherapy, 944
　　agents used for, 946b
　　indications, 946
　　objectives, 945
　　oral care protocol, 951
　　oral complications of, 946
　　systemic side effects of, 946
　　types of, 946
Chest radiography, for respiratory disease,
　　1026
Chewing tobacco, 531
Child abuse and neglect
　　consequences of, 212
　　definitions of, 212
　　extraoral wounds and signs of trauma,
　　　　215, 215t
　　intraoral signs of, 216
　　parental attitude, 216
　　risk factors, 212
　　signs of
　　　　behavioral features, 213
　　　　cognitive features, 215
　　　　emotional well-being, 215
　　　　indicators and features of, 213–214t
　　　　physical indicators, 213
　　　　social behavior, 215
Child dental visits, 800–801
Child-sized sunglasses, 87
Childhood disintegrative disorder, 856b
Childhood-onset fluency disorder
　　(stuttering), 850b
Children
　　chemotherapy and/or radiation
　　　　therapy, 951
　　environmental tobacco smoke, impact
　　　　in, 535
　　hypertension in, 1049
Chlorhexidine (CHX), 475–476, 476f,
　　523, 698–699, 699f
Chlorophyll, 295
Chromogenic bacteria, 295
Chronic bronchitis, 1025
Chronic graft-versus-host disease,
　　948
Chronic obstructive pulmonary disease
　　(COPD), 534
　　chronic bronchitis, 1035–1036
　　dental hygiene care, 1037
　　due to tobacco use, 534
　　emphysema, 1036
　　medical management, 1036–1037,
　　　　1036f
　　oral manifestations, 1037
Chronic toxicity, 592–593
Chronologic hypoplasia, 298. See also
　　Enamel hypoplasia
Chronological age, 824

CHX (chlorhexidine), 475–476, 476f,
　　523, 698–699, 699f
Cigar, 530
Cigarette, 530
CINAHL (Cumulative Index to Nursing
　　and Allied Health Literature), 25b
Circuit voltmeter, 227
Circuits, 227, 228f
Clasp brush, 508f
Cleaning
　　agents, 730, 733
　　effects of, 730–731, 731f
　　ingredients, 735
　　and polishing agents (abrasives), 473
Cleft lip and/or palate, 842
　　classification of, 842, 842f
　　dental hygiene care, 846–847
　　documentation, 847, 847b
　　etiology
　　　　embryology, 842–843, 842f
　　　　risk factors, 843
　　everyday ethics, 848
　　factors to teach patient, 848
　　general physical characteristics
　　　　airway and breathing, 843
　　　　congenital anomalies, 843
　　　　facial deformities, 843, 843f
　　　　hearing loss, 843
　　　　infections, 843
　　　　speech, 843
　　oral characteristics, 844, 844f
　　treatment, 844–846, 845b
Clinical assessment findings, dental
　　hygiene diagnosis
　　chief complaint, 384
　　oral healthcare literacy level, 386
　　patient's self-care ability, 386, 386t
　　physical status, 384, 385t
　　risk factors, 384
　　tobacco use, 386
Clinical attire, 84
　　hair and head covering, 85
　　protective clothing, 85, 85f
Clinical periodontal health, 328
Clinical practice guidelines, 27
Clinical significance, 26
Clinical trial
　　purpose, 358
　　uses, 358
Clinician–patient positioning, 119,
　　119f
Clonapam (Klonopin), 973t
Clonic seizure, 970
Clonidine, 1015
Clorazepate (Tranxene), 973t
Closed neural tube defect, 903
Closed reduction, 962
Clostridium tetani, 64
CMV (cytomegalovirus), 66t, 72, 74
Coagulation disorder, 1071
Coapting, 707
Cobalamin, 559t
Cocaine hydrochloride powder, 1011
Cochlear implants, 869
Cochrane Library, 25b
Code of Ethics, 13
　　American Dental Hygienists'
　　　　Association, 1095–1098

Canadian Dental Hygienists Association, 1101–1103

International Federation of Dental Hygienists, 1105–1106

National Dental Hygienists' Association, 1099

Cognitive behavioral therapy (CBT), 857
  for bipolar disorder, 986
  for posttraumatic stress disorder, 983

Cognitive change, 826, 826t

Cognitive disability, 776

Cognitive impairment, cerebral palsy and, 900

Cognitive processing therapy (CPT), 983

Cohort studies, 28

Col, 305, 305f, 456

Cold sterile. See Chemical liquid sterilization

Collaborative practice, 6, 7b, 47

Collagen, 323
  dressing, 710

Collimation, 232, 233f
  of beam, 237

Collimator, 232

Colony-forming units (CFU), 65

Color change, tooth, 748

Colostomy bag, 883

Combined fluoride program, 591

Communicable disease, 62, 1030

Communication, 408. See also Health communication
  definition of, 34
  media, 34
  modes of, 876–877
  nonverbal, 34
  oral, 877
  suggestions for effective, 130
  telephone numbers for medical aid, 130–131
  verbal, 34

Communicative impairment, 866

Community-acquired pneumonia, 1029

Community-based delivery of services, 869

Community-based settings for alternative dental hygiene practice, 49

Community periodontal index (CPI), 366–368, 366f
  adolescents, 368
  for adults, 367–368
  for children, 368
  LOA codes, 368, 369f
  procedure, 368
  purpose, 366–367
  selection of teeth, 367

Community surveillance of oral health, 358

Comorbid, 853

Comorbid conditions, 1034

Comorbidities, 866

Compassion, motivational interviewing and, 409

Compensatory behaviors, 988

Competency, 10

Complete denture prosthesis, 501–502, 501f
  components of, 501–502

patient self-care procedures for, 510–511

professional care procedures for, 509–510

types of, 501

Complete history, 164

Completed radiographs, analysis of
  anatomic landmarks, 250
  identification of errors, 250, 251t
  interpretation, 250
  mounting, 249

Compliance, 407, 773

Comprehensive Patient Assessment and Diagnosis Worksheet, 389, 390f

Computer-controlled local anesthesia delivery (C-CLAD) system, 629

Computer screen readers, 868

Condyloma acuminatum, 216

Cone beam computed tomography (CBCT), 957

"Cone-cut" of image receptor, 232

Confidence intervals, 26

Congenital anomalies, 843

Congenital heart diseases
  anomalies, 1046
  clinical considerations, 1047
  etiology of, 1046
  patent ductus arteriosus, 1047f
  prevention of, 1046–1047
  types of defects, 1046
  ventricular septal defect, 1046f

Congenital syphilis, hypoplasia of, 260

Congestive heart failure (CHF). See Heart failure

Connective tissue
  autoimmune disease, 1079
    oral lichen planus, 1079–1080, 1080f
    rheumatoid arthritis, 1080–1081, 1081f

Conscious sedation, 615

Consent, 400. See also Informed consent

Consultations, 786

Contact lenses, 87

Contact precautions, 62

Contaminated waste, 100

Contamination, 84, 102

Context, 20

Continuing care, 773
  appointment intervals, 776
  appointment procedures
    assessment, 774
    care plan, 775
    criteria for referral during periodontal maintenance, 776
    criteria for referral to periodontist, 775–776
    dental caries control, 775
    oral hygiene instruction/motivation, 775
    periodontal disease, recurrence of, 775
    periodontal instrumentation and debridement, 775
    referral from general practice, 775
    supplemental care procedures, 775
  dental caries, 429
  documentation, 777, 777b

everyday ethics, 777
  factors to teach patient, 777
  goals of, 773–774
  monthly reminder method, 776
  periodontal maintenance, 774, 774b
  prebook or preschedule method, 776
  short- and long-term, 406

Continuous glucose monitoring (CGM), 932

Continuous Numbers 1–32, 152, 152f

Continuous positive airway pressure (CPAP), 1039, 1039f

Controlled release, 698

Convulsion, 970

COPD. See Chronic obstructive pulmonary disease (COPD)

Copolymer, 472

Copper, 560t

Cords, managing, 121

Core skills, motivational interviewing and, 411–413, 412b

Core values, 13
  ethical duty, 14
  patient first, 14
  personal values, 14
  in professional practice, 13, 13b

Coronal polishing, 735–736

Coronary artery bypass grafting, 1054, 1054f

Coronary heart disease (CHD), 1044
  local anesthesia and, 626

Correlational research, 27

Corticosteroids, 1080
  for asthma, 1034t
  for Bell's palsy, 897

Corynebacterium diphtheria, 66t

Coryza, 1027t

Cotherapist, 16

Cotinine, 531

Cotton pliers, 662

CPAP (continuous positive airway pressure), 1039, 1039f

CPI. See Community periodontal index (CPI)

CPP (casein phosphopeptide), 724

CPT (Cognitive processing therapy), 983

CRA. See Caries risk assessment (CRA)

Crack cocaine, 1011

Craniofacial anomalies, 842

Craniopharyngiomas, 913

Crepitation, 143t

CREST syndrome, 1081b

Cricothyrotomy, 131t

"Critical incident" approach, 769

Critically ill/unconscious patient, 54
  caregivers, instructions for, 55
  strategies for prevention and management, 50t
  toothbrush with suction attachment, 55, 55b, 55f

Crohn's disease, 1083–1085, 1084f

Cross-contamination, 84

Cross-cultural communication, 40
  nonverbal communication and, 41t

Crossbites, 271, 271f

CRT (cardiac resynchronization therapy), 1054–1055

Crust, 206

Cultural competence, 41
    attaining, 41
    and dental hygiene process of care,
        41–42
Cultural considerations
    health communication, 40b
        cross-cultural communication, 40,
            41t
        cultural competence, 41–42
        culture and health, 39–40
Cultural rapport, 36
Cultural sensitivity, 36
Culturally effective health care, 40
Culture, 33
Cumulative Index to Nursing and Allied
    Health Literature (CINAHL), 25b
Cumulative index, types of, 359
Cumulative trauma
    disorders, 116
    preventing, 662, 662–663f
    risk factors for, 662
Curets, 644
    advanced area-specific, 653–654, 653f
    area-specific, 653
    design, 652
    internal angles of, 652f
    selection of cutting edges to sharpen,
        671
    -specific instrumentation, 654
    technique objectives, 671
    universal, 653, 653f
    uses of, 652
Curing, 600
Cushing syndrome. See Hyperadrenalism
Custodial care, 48
Cutting edge, 667
    selection of, 668
CVD. See Cardiovascular disease (CVD)
Cyanosis, 138t, 1047
Cyst, 206
Cystic fibrosis (CF)
    clinical signs and symptoms of, 1037b
    dental hygiene care, 1038, 1038t
    disease characteristics
        pancreas and intestinal tract, 1038
        respiratory tract, 1037–1038
    medical management, 1038
    –related diabetes, 929
Cytomegalovirus (CMV), 66t, 72, 74

D

D-termined program (DTP), 858
Daily functional movement exercises,
    123–124
Database of Promoting Health
    Effectiveness Reviews (DoPHER), 25b
DD (diabetes distress), 935
Dean's fluorosis index, 375
    procedure, 375
    purpose, 375
    scoring, 375, 376t
    selection of teeth, 375
Debonding, 486
    clinical procedures for, 490, 490–492f,
        491b
Decayed, indicated for extraction, and
    filled (df and def), 373

Decayed, missing, and filled (dmf),
    373–374
Decayed, missing, and filled teeth
    (DMFT)/surfaces (DMFS), 371–372
    calculation and interpretation, 372
    procedures, 372
    purpose, 371
    scoring, 372
    selection of teeth and surfaces,
        371–372
Decisional balance
    balancing act, 413
    pro–con matrix, 413, 413f, 414b
Decoding, 34
Decompensates, 993
Decubitus ulcers, 893
Defluoridation, 579
Degenerative joint disease
    adult hand compromised by, 905f
    medical treatment, 905
    occurrence, 904
    symptoms of, 904–905
Degenerative neural disorders, 892
Delirium, 1005
Delirium tremens, 1005
Delta hepatitis. See Hepatitis D virus
    (HDV)
Delusions, 991
Demand valve resuscitation, 136t
Dementia, 826
Demineralization, 422, 423, 492, 575,
    576–577, 576f
Dental abrasion, 450
Dental biofilm, 280, 281–282, 282f
    accumulation in protected areas,
        285f
    –associated gingivitis, 328
    bacterial invasion, 284f
    bacterial multiplication and
        colonization, 282
    cariogenic microorganisms in, 286
    changes in microorganisms, 282–284,
        283f
    clinical aspects of, 285
    composition of
        inorganic elements, 284
        organic elements, 285
    control program, 835–837, 836t
        dentinal hypersensitivity, 723
        effect of tobacco, 536, 543
        implant systems, 522
        pregnancy, 788
    dental caries, 286, 286f
    detection of, 285
    distribution of, 285
    effect of diet on, 286
    growth, 282
    matrix formation, 282
    maturation, 282
    pH of, 286
    removal
        disabilities, 872–875
        positions for child or disabled patient
            during, 886f
        teaching techniques for, 885
    stages in formation, 282
    subgingival, 284
    supragingival, 284

Dental caries, 262, 286, 422, 990, 991
    caries classification system, 266
    caries risk assessment systems
        ADA caries risk assessment, 424
        American Academy of Pediatric
            Dentistry Caries-Risk Assessment
            Tool, 424
        Caries Management by Risk
            Assessment, 425–426, 425–426t
        Cariogram, 424–425
        International Caries Classification
            and Management System, 426
    caries risk management systems
        AAPD caries risk management
            protocol, 427
        Caries Management by Risk
            Assessment, 427
        International Caries Classification
            and Management System, 427,
            428f
    carious lesions, classification of,
        264–266
    classifications, 423–424
    and consistency of food, 562
    continuing care, 429
    control, 837
    counseling for, 562
    defined, 263–264
    development of, 264
    development of, 286f
    diabetes mellitus, 925
    dietary assessment and counseling for,
        562
    documentation, 429, 429b
    everyday ethics, 430
    G.V. Black's classification, 264–265,
        264f
    indices for measuring experience
        decayed, indicated for extraction, and
            filled, 373
        decayed, missing, and filled, 373–374
        decayed, missing, and filled teeth/
            surfaces, 371–372
        early childhood caries, 374, 374t
        root caries index, 374–375
    international caries classification and
        management system, 265–266, 265f
    management, 422
    meal pattern and, 568
    patient teaching, 430
    planning care for patient's caries risk
        level, 427–428
        patient with high and extreme caries
            risk, 429
        patient with low caries risk, 428
        patient with moderate caries risk, 429
    pregnancy, 789
    process
        acid production, 422
        acidogenic and aciduric bacteria, 422
        demineralization, 423
        fermentable carbohydrates, role of,
            422
        remineralization, 423, 423f
    risk factors for, 384
    risk level, 388
    role of cariogenic foods, 561
Dental carious lesion, stages of, 424, 424f

Dental chair, 98, 117
    escort patient to, 116
    use of, 118
Dental chart, 154, 257, 276f
Dental deposits
    acquired pellicle, 281
    calculus, 287f
        attachment of, 291
        clinical characteristics of, 291–292,
            292t
        composition, 289–290
        formation, 290–291
        mineralization, 290
        prevention of, 293
        significance of, 291
        structure of, 290–291
        subgingival, 287–288t, 288–289,
            289f
        supragingival, 287–288, 287–288t,
            288f
        teeth and bone vs., 290
    dental biofilm. *See* Dental biofilm
    dental stains and discolorations. *See*
        Dental stains and discolorations
    documentation, 300, 300b
    everyday ethics, 300–301
    factors to teach patient, 301
    food debris, 287
    materia alba
        clinical appearance and content, 286
        prevention, 287
Dental extraction, toothbrushing after,
    449
Dental floss and tape
    floss, types of, 459
    prevention of injuries, 461
    procedure, 460–461, 460–461f
Dental fluorosis, 298, 577
    indices for measuring
        Dean's fluorosis index, 375
        tooth surface index of fluorosis, 375,
            376t
Dental home, 800
    for infants, 790
Dental hygiene care, 8
    additional considerations, 54
    in alternative practice settings
        barriers to access, 48
        community-based settings, 49
        eliminating barriers, 48
        portable delivery of care, 48
        private homes, 48
        residence-bound patients, 48–49, 48b
        residential facilities, 48–49, 49b
    approach to patient, 53
    assessment and care planning, 54
    assistance for ambulatory patient, 906
    charting symbols and standardized
        abbreviations, 1123–1124
    cleft lip and/or palate, 846–847
    considerations during clinical care, 906
    critically ill/unconscious patient, 54
        caregivers, instructions for, 55
        toothbrush with suction attachment,
            55, 55b, 55f
    documentation, 56–57, 57b
    everyday ethics, 56
    factors to teach patient, 57

four-handed dental hygiene, 906
instruments and equipment, 52b
neurodevelopmental disorder, 858–859
    appointment considerations, 859–860
    dental hygiene care plan, 859
    dental staff preparation, 859
    oral health problems, 859
objectives of care, 49
for older adults, 834
    assessment, 835
    barriers to care, 835
    dental biofilm control, 835–837, 836t
    dental caries control, 837
    diet and nutrition, 837–838
    periodontal care, 837
    preventive care plan, 835
    xerostomia, relief for, 837
oral and maxillofacial surgery
    diet, 964–966, 965f
    diet selection, 958
    before general surgery, 966–967
    instrumentation, 964
    personal oral care procedures, 966
    postsurgical care, 959, 959b
    presurgery treatment planning,
        957–958
    presurgical instructions, 958–959
    problems, 964
oral health to overall health,
    significance of, 49
oral problems and conditions, 49
orthodontic appliances
    disease control, 488–490, 489f
    risk factors, 488
patient in bed, 53–54
patient in wheelchair, 54, 54f
patient positioning and body
    stabilization, 906
personal factors affecting self-care,
    906–907
portable equipment, sources for, 51b
preparation for appointments,
    905–906
residence-based delivery of care, 907
residential visit, preparation for, 51–53
strategies for prevention and
    management, 50t, 54
terminally ill patient, 56
treatment location, 53–54, 53f
wheelchair transfer, 906
Dental hygiene care plan, 12, 394
cancer
    objectives, 949
    oral care protocol, 949–951, 949t,
        950t
    personal factors, 949
consultation with physician/
    hematologist, 1072–1073
description of, 394, 394t
documentation, 401, 401b
everyday ethics, 402
examination, 1073
factors to teach patient, 402
informed consent, 401b
    additional considerations, 401
    criteria for adequate content in, 400b
    informed refusal, 401
    procedures, 400

objectives, 394–395
pain and anxiety control, 398
parts of, 395
patient history, 1072, 1072b
patient, role of, 398
preparation of, 394–395, 1071–1072
presenting plan
    to collaborating dentist, 399–400
    to patient, 400
rationale, 394
sequencing and prioritizing patient
    care
    factors affecting sequence of care, 399
    objectives, 398–399
treatment, 1073
treatment care plan, 1073
vital signs, 183–184
written care plan, components of,
    396–397f
    appointment plan, 398
    assessment findings and risk factors,
        395
    caries risk status, 395
    demographic data, 395
    diagnostic statements, 397
    evaluation methods, 398
    expected outcomes, 398
    patient-centered oral health goals, 397
    periodontal diagnosis and status, 395
    planned interventions, 397
    re-evaluation, 398
Dental hygiene diagnosis, 11, 12, 12b, 384
basis for, 388
clinical assessment findings
    chief complaint, 384
    oral healthcare literacy level, 386
    patient's self-care ability, 386, 386t
    physical status, 384, 385t
    risk factors, 384
    tobacco use, 386
Comprehensive Patient Assessment
    and Diagnosis Worksheet, 389,
    390f
dental caries risk level, 388
dental hygiene care plan, 391
dental hygiene interventions, selection
    of, 389, 391
diagnostic statements, 388, 388t
documentation, 391, 391b
evaluation of assessment data, 389
everyday ethics, 390
factors to teach patient, 391
periodontal disease
    classification of, 386, 386t, 388
    description of past and current
        conditions, 386
    parameters of care, 387t, 388
prognosis, 388–389, 389b
Dental hygiene ethics, 13
Dental hygiene interventions, 397–398
expected outcomes following, 766b
selection of, 389, 391
Dental hygiene practice, 4–5. *See also*
    Evidence-based dental hygiene
    (EBDH)
advanced practice dental hygiene,
    9–10
alternative practice settings, 8, 9f

Dental hygiene practice (*continued*)
  clinical services
    educational services, 6
    preventive services, 6, 8b
    therapeutic services, 8
  dental hygiene specialties, 8
  dental hygienist, role of, 5–6, 7t
  interprofessional collaborative patient
    care, 10–11, 10b
  oral health, advocacy for, 11
  patient education, 8
  supervision and scope of, 6, 7b
Dental hygiene process of care, 11
  assessment, 12
  components of, 12f
  cultural competence and, 41–42
  dental hygiene care plan, 12, 12b, 758
  dental hygiene diagnosis, 12, 758
  digital photographic record of tooth
    shade, 758f
  evaluation and planning for
    maintenance, 12, 758
  implementation, 12, 758
  manual selection of tooth shade, 757f,
    758b
  patient assessment, 757–758
  purposes of, 12
  substance-related disorder
    assessment, 1015–1016, 1016f
    care planning, 1018
    dental hygiene diagnosis, 1018
    evaluation, 1019
    implementation, 1018–1019
    intraoral examination, 1016–1017,
      1017b, 1017f
    nasopalatal defect, 1016f
Dental hygiene specialties, 8
Dental hygiene visit
  components of, pediatrics, 805
    *child and family medical/dental
      history*, 806
    dental hygiene treatment, 808
    *dentition, occlusion, and
      temporomandibular*, 806–807
    dietary assessment, 808
    initial interview/new patient visit, 806
    intraoral and extraoral examination,
      806
    prevention, 808–809
    *primary teeth, developmental
      disturbance of*, 807f
    radiographic assessment, 807–808
    *second primary molar, premature loss
      of*, 807f
    tooth development and eruption, 806
Dental hygienist, 4. *See also* Professional
  dental hygienist
  with disability, 887
  in intimate partner violence, 219
  role of, 5–6, 7t
Dental hypersensitivity, 991
Dental implants, 925
  appointments following placement,
    523–524
  documentation, 525–526, 526b
  effect of tobacco, 536
  everyday ethics, 525
  factors to teach patient, 526

implant-supported restorations, 522
  interfaces, 518–519
    implant/bone, 518
    implant/soft tissue, 519, 519f
  long-term success of an implant, 523
  need for, 518
  patient selection
    local factors, 521
    systemic health, 521
  peri-implant care, 522–523
    antimicrobial use, 523
    care of natural teeth, 522
    disease control program, 522
    implant biofilm, 522
    *maintenance of implant-supported
      restoration*, 522
    using fluoride preparations, 523
  professional maintenance and
    monitoring, 523–524
    continuing care appointment,
      523–524
    frequency of appointments, 523
    probing of dental implants, 523, 523f
  types of, 519–520, 521f
    endosseous (endosteal) implant, 520,
      520f
    subperiosteal, 519–520, 519f
    transosseous (transosteal), 520, 520f
Dental light, 120, 120f
Dental loupes, 87, 88f
Dental neglect, 212
Dental radiographic imaging
  acceptable radiographic image,
    characteristics of, 231t
    radiolucency, 231
    radiopacity, 231
  bitewing (interproximal) surveys
    image receptor placement, 245, 245f
    image receptor selection for, 242
    positioning, 244–245, 244f
  completed radiographs, analysis of
    anatomic landmarks, 250
    identification of errors, 250, 251t
    interpretation, 250
    mounting, 249
  digital radiography
    advantages of, 230
    digital imaging and sensors, 229
    digital imaging principles, 229
    direct digital imaging, 229, 229f
    disadvantages of, 230
    evaluation, 230–231
    indirect digital imaging, 229, 229f
    steps in production of, 229–230, 230f
  documentation, 252, 252b
  everyday ethics, 252
  factors influencing finished radiograph,
    231, 231–232b
    collimation, 232, 233f
    distance, 234
    filtration, 232–233
    image receptors, 234–235
    kilovoltage, 233
    milliampere seconds, 233–234
  factors to teach patient, 253
  handheld X-ray devices, 249, 249f
  image receptor placement and angulation
    of central ray, 241–242, 242f

image receptor selection for intraoral
    surveys, 242–243
  infection control
    basic procedures, 247, 247b
    *no-touch method for films and
      photostimulable phosphor plates*,
      248, 248f
    practice policy, 247
  occlusal surveys
    image receptor selection for, 242–243
    *mandibular topographic and cross-
      sectional projection*, 246
    *maxillary midline topographic
      projection*, 246
    uses and purposes, 245
  ownership, 250
  panoramic radiographic images
    limitations of, 246–247
    procedures, 247
    technique, 246
    uses of, 246, 247b
  periapical surveys
    bisecting-angle technique, 245
    image receptor selection for, 242
    paralleling technique, 243–244
  radiation
    exposure, 235–236, 236t
    factors influencing biologic effects of,
      235b
    ionizing radiation, 235
    risk of injury from, 237–241
    sensitivity of cells, 236–237, 236b
    units, 236t
  shadow casting, 242b
  traditional film processing
    automated processing, 248
    darkroom lighting, 248
    image production, 248
    manual processing, 248–249
  X-ray production, 226
    circuits, 227, 228f
    machine control devices, 227–228
    properties of, 226b
    steps in, 228–229
    transformers, 227
    X-ray tube, 227, 227f
Dental records, 157
Dental stains and discolorations, 293
  classification of, 293–294
  extrinsic stains
    black-line stain, 295–296
    brown stains, 296–297, 297f
    green stain, 295
    metallic stains, 297
    orange and red stains, 297
    tobacco stain, 296, 296f
    yellow stain, 294, 294f
  intrinsic stains
    endogenous, 297–299, 298f
    exogenous, 299, 299f, 300f
  recognition and identification, 294
  removal, 294
  significance of, 293–294
Dental therapist, 9
Dentally dysfunctional, 842
Dentifrices, 724
  active components of, 474
  for child, 817f

components of
  binders, 473
  cleaning and polishing agents, 473
  detergents, 473
  flavoring agents, 474
  humectants, 474
  preservatives, 474
cosmetic effects of
  extrinsic stain, removal of, 472
  oral malodor, reduction of, 473
fluoride, 590–591
ingredients and function of
  commercially available, 473t
preventive and therapeutic benefits
  of, 472
selection of, 474
therapeutic active ingredients in, 473t
Dentin, 716, 716f
  -bonding agents, 725
  developmental defects of, 261
  fluoride in, 576
  open tubules, 718f
  partially occluded tubules, 719f
  sclerosis of, 718–719
  secondary, 717, 719
  stain in, 299
  tertiary/reparative, 717
Dentin hypersensitivity, 735
  behavioral changes for, 723
  characteristics of pain from, 716
  defined, 716
  dental biofilm control, 723
  dentin exposure
    abfraction, 718, 718f
    attrition, abrasion, and erosion, 717
    enamel and cementum loss, 717
    gingival recession and subsequent root
      exposure, 717, 717f
    other factors, 718
  desensitization, mechanisms of, 722
  desensitizing agents for
    calcium phosphate technology, 724
    fluorides, 724
    glutaraldehyde, 724
    oxalates, 724
    potassium salts, 723
  dietary modifications, 723
  differential diagnosis, 720
    data collection by interview, 721, 721b
    diagnostic techniques and tests, 721
    differentiation of pain, 721
  documentation, 726, 726b
  etiology of, 716–718
  everyday ethics, 726–727
  factors to teach patient, 727
  hydrodynamic theory, 718, 718f, 719f
  management of
    assessment components, 721–722
    educational considerations, 722
    ideal desensitizing agent, 722b
    reassessment, 722
    subjective pain assessment form, 722b
    treatment hierarchy, 722
  natural desensitization
    calculus, 719
    sclerosis of dentin, 718–719
    secondary dentin, 719
    smear layer, 719

oral hygiene care and treatment
  interventions, 722–726
pain of
  pain experience, 719–720
  patient profile, 719
parafunctional habits, eliminating, 723
periodontal debridement
  considerations, 725
prevalence of, 719
professionally applied measures, 725
reduction of, 472
research developments, 726
self-applied measures, 724–725
stimuli eliciting pain reaction, 716
tooth structures, anatomy of
  dentin, 716, 716f
  nerves, 717
  pulp, 716–717, 716f
tooth whitening–induced sensitivity,
  725–726
toothbrush type and technique, 723
Dentinogenesis imperfecta, 261, 298
Dentofacial orthopedics, 844
Denture brush, 508f
Denture-induced oral mucosal lesions
  (OMLs), 511–513
  contributing factors, 511–512
  types of, 512–513
Denture stomatitis, 512
Depakote. See Valproic acid/valproate
Depressants, 1007t, 1010
Depressed lesions, 204, 205f, 206
Depression, 53
  during pregnancy, 789–790
Depressive disorders
  dental hygiene care, 985
  signs and symptoms of, 984
  treatment, 984–985
  types of, 984
Descriptive research, 27
Descriptive statistics, 26
Desensitization, 879
  mechanisms of, 722
  natural
    calculus, 719
    sclerosis of dentin, 718–719
    secondary dentin, 719
    smear layer, 719
  procedures for bleaching, 753t
Desensitizers, 749
Desomorphine (krokodil), 1009t,
  1011–1012
Desquamated epithelial cells, 324
Detergents (foaming agents or
  surfactants), 473
Detoxification, 1013
Developmental coordination disorder,
  850b
Developmental enamel lesions
  enamel hypoplasia, 260, 260f, 261f
  hypomaturation, 260
  hypomineralization, 260
Developmental impairment, 866, 892
Dexterity development
  mouth mirror and cotton pliers,
    661–662
  pen/pencil exercises, 661
  squeezing, 660

stretching exercises, 660–661, 661f
tactile sensitivity, increasing, 662, 662f
Diabetes distress (DD), 935
Diabetes mellitus, 319, 776
  classification of, 928–930
  complications of
    amputation, 935
    cardiovascular disease, 935
    infection, 934
    mental health, 935
    nephropathy, 935
    neuropathy, 935
    pregnancy complications, 935
    retinopathy, 935
  cystic fibrosis–related, 929
  definition of, 924
  dental caries, 925
  dental hygiene care plan, 935
    appointment planning, 936, 936f
    consultation with primary care
      provider, 937
    continuing care, 938
    dental hygiene assessment and
      treatment, 937
    patient history, 937
  dental implants, 925
  diagnosis of, 930, 931f
  documentation, 939, 939b
  endodontic infections, 925
  everyday ethics, 940
  extraoral/intraoral findings associated
    with, 924t
  factors to teach patient, 940
  gestational, 786, 929
  insulin
    absolute insulin deficiency, 926
    definition of, 925
    description of, 925, 925f
    functions of, 926, 926b
    hyperglycemia, 927, 927t
    hypoglycemia, 926, 926b, 927t
    impaired secretion/action of insulin, 926
    types and action of, 933t
  local anesthesia and, 627
  medical history questions to screen
    for, 937b
  monogenic diabetes syndromes, 929
  oral health implications of, 924–925
  and periodontal disease, 925
  pharmacologic therapy
    antihyperglycemic therapy, 934, 934t
    insulin therapy, 933–934
  posttransplantation, 930
  prediabetes, 928
  prevalence, of, 924
  questions to ask patient with, 938b
  risk factors, 927–928
  standards of medical care for
    early diagnosis, 930
    habits, 933
    medical nutrition therapy, 932–933
    physical activity, 933
    prediabetes, management of, 930
    psychosocial issues, 933
    self-management education, 930,
      932, 932f
  type 1, 928t, 929
  type 2, 928t, 929

Diabetes Prevention Program (DPP), 928
Diabetes Risk Test, 924, 930, 931f
Diabetic coma. See Hyperglycemia
Diabetic ketoacidosis (DKA), 926
Diabulimia, 989
Diagnosis, 384
Diamond-coated finishing file, 655f
Diamond particles, 734
Diastema, 258t, 314
Diastolic pressure, 187
Diet and dietary analysis, 319–320
    ChooseMyPlate guidelines, 555f
    counseling for, 566–569
    dietary assessment
        forms used, 562, 563t, 564t
        preliminary preparation, 562
        purpose, 562
        using food diary, 563–565, 563b
    dietary standards, 554
    for disabilities, 876
    documentation, 569, 570b
    evaluation of progress, 569
    everyday ethics, 570
    factors to teach patient, 570
    food intake pattern recommendations,
      555
    "Food Pyramid" by United States
      Department of Agriculture, 555
    frequency and time of exposure, 568
    government standards, 554
    guidelines for Americans, 554, 555b
    nutrient standards for diet adequacy
      in, 553–572
    and nutrition, 837–838
    oral and maxillofacial surgery, 964–965
        liquid diet, 965, 965f
        methods of feeding, 965
        nutritional needs, 965
        selection, 958
        soft diet, 965, 965f
        suggestions for nonhospitalized
          patient, 965–966
    and oral health relationships, 555,
      560–561
        dental caries, 561
        dietary assessment for periodontal
          conditions, 562–566
        periodontal tissues, 560–561
        skin and mucous membrane, 555
        tooth structure and integrity, 561
    pregnancy, 788–789
    recommendations, 569
    retention, 568
Dietary assessment, 561
Dietary calcium, 560
Dietary fluoride supplements, 580–581,
  580t
Dietary modifications, dentinal
  hypersensitivity, 723
Dietary reference intakes (DRIs), 554
Dietary standards, 554
Differential cell count, 1063
Differential diagnosis, 213
Difficult-to-reach areas, brushing, 445,
  445f
Diffusion, alcohol, 1001
Diffusion hypoxia, 616

Digestive system, alcohol and, 1003
Digital palpation, 196
Digital radiography
    advantages of, 230
    digital imaging
        direct, 229, 229f
        principles, 229
        and sensors, 229
    disadvantages of, 230
    evaluation, 230–231
    indirect digital imaging, 229, 229f
    steps in production of, 229–230, 230f
Digital sensors, 234–235
Digitized image, 230
Dilantin. See Phenytoin
Diplopia, 1088
Direct access, 53
    care, 8, 9f
    supervision, 7b
Direct digital imaging, 229, 229f, 230f
Direct oral anticoagulants (DOACs),
  1056–1057
Direct supervision, 7b
Directly observed therapy (DOT), 1030,
  1031t
Disabilities, 49, 866
    Americans with Disability Act, 866
    barrier-free environment
        external features, 870
        internal features, 870
        treatment room, 871
    basic planning questions for, 888b
    caregivers, instruction for, 885, 886f
    community-based delivery of services,
      trends in, 869
    definitions and classifications, 866,
      867–868t
    dental hygienist with, 887
    documentation, 887–888, 888b
    everyday ethics, 888
    factors to teach patient and caregiver,
      889
    group in-service education, 885–886
    oral disease prevention and control
        dental biofilm removal, 872–875,
          873–875f
        diet instruction, 876
        fluoride program, 875–876
        objectives, 872
        pit and fissure sealants, 876
        preventive care introduction, 872
    oral health services, access to, 869,
      870t
    patient management
        ambulatory patient, assistance for,
          880
        appointment scheduling, 878–879
        clinical settings, 879–880, 880f
        continuing care appointments, 880
        four-handed dental hygiene, 882
        instrumentation, 882
        modes of communication, 876–877
        objectives, 876
        pain and anxiety control, 882
        patient positioning, 880–881
        pretreatment planning, 877–878,
          877–878b

        supportive and protective stabilization,
          881, 882f
    physical and intellectual disabilities,
      868
    risk assessment
        functional ability, 871, 872b
        medical status, 872
        oral manifestations, 871
    sensory disabilities, 868–869
    types of conditions, 866
    wheelchair transfer
        patient who can assist, 883, 883f
        patient who is immobile, 883–884
        preparation for, 882–883
        sliding board transfer, 884, 884f
        wheelchair used during treatment,
          884, 884f
Discontinued fluoridation, 579
Disease activity, 776
Disease transmission, 63–64, 63f
Disinfectant, 98
Dislocated mandible, treatment for, 144f
Disposal of waste, 111, 111f
Dissociative anesthetics, 1007t, 1010
Distance, 234
Disulfiram (Antabuse), 1005
DKA (diabetic ketoacidosis), 926
DMD (Duchenne muscular dystrophy),
  901–902
DMFT (decayed, missing, and filled teeth)
  index, 358, 579
DOACs (direct oral anticoagulants),
  1056–1057
Documentation
    anxiety and pain control, 639
    autoimmune disease, 1091, 1091b
    blood disorder, 1073, 1074b
    cancer, 951, 952b
    cardiovascular disease, 1057, 1057b
    care plan records, 157
    charting of hard and soft tissues
        forms used for, 154
        periodontal and dental, 155f
        purpose of, 154
        sequence for, 154–155
    cleft lip and/or palate, 847, 847b
    continuing care, 777, 777b
    dental caries, 429, 429b
    dental deposits, 300, 300b
    dental hygiene care, 56–57, 57b
    dental hygiene care plan, 401, 401b
    dental hygiene diagnosis, 391, 391b
    dental records, 157
    dentinal hypersensitivity, 726, 726b
    diabetes mellitus, 939, 939b
    diet and dietary analysis, 569, 570b
    disabilities, 887–888, 888b
    emergency care, 145b
        comprehensive record keeping, 137
        consults, 144
        new entries, 144
    endocrine gland disorders, 919, 919b
    everyday ethics, 159
    evidence-based dental hygiene, 30, 30b
    exposure control, 94, 94b
    extra- and intraoral examination, 152,
      208, 208b

extrinsic stain removal, 743, 743b
evaluation
    patient care outcomes, 769, 770b
    self-assessment and reflection, 769
factors to teach patient, 159
family violence, 221b
    content of record, 221
    thorough and accurate, 221
fluorides, 593, 594b
hard tissue examination, 275, 276b
health communication, 43, 43b
Health Insurance Portability and
    Accountability Act
    privacy rule, 151
    security rule, 151–152
implant systems, 525–526, 526b
indices, 377, 378b
infection control, 79, 79b
clinical procedures, 112, 113b
informed consent, 157
instrument care and sharpening, 676,
    676b
instruments and principles for
    instrumentation, 663, 663b
interdental care, 467, 467b
mental health disorders, 994, 994b
motivational interview, 418, 418b
mouthrinse, 480–481, 481b
neurodevelopmental disorder, 860,
    860b
nonsurgical periodontal therapy, 699,
    699b
older adults, 838, 838b
oral and maxillofacial surgery, 967,
    967b
orthodontic appliances, 493, 494b
patient care progress notes, 252, 252b
patient history, 180, 180–181b
patient records
    components of, 150
    electronic records, 150–151
    handwritten records, 150
    purposes and characteristics of, 150
patient reception and ergonomic
    practice, 124, 125b
patient visits
    progress notes, 157, 158b
    purpose of, 157
    risk reduction and legal considerations,
        158–159
    SOAP approach, 157–158, 158b, 158t
pediatrics, 819, 819b
periodontal disease, 333, 334b
periodontal examination, 355, 355b
periodontal records, 155–156
charting, 156
    deposits, 156
    factors related to occlusion, 156
    gingiva, clinical observations of,
        155–156
    periodontal disease, severity of, 156
    radiographic findings, 156
periodontium, 315, 315b
physical impairment, 907, 907b
pregnancy, 794, 794b
prosthesis, 513, 513–514b
radiation exposure history, 252

respiratory disease, 1039–1040, 1040b
sealants, 608, 608b
seizure disorder, 978, 978b
substance-related disorder, 1019,
    1019b
sutures and dressings, 713, 713b
tobacco use, 547, 547b
toothbrush selection and
    toothbrushing method, 451, 451b
tooth numbering systems
    Continuous Numbers 1–32, 152, 152f
    Fédération Dentaire Internationale
        system, 152–153, 153f
    Palmer Notation System, 153–154, 153f
vital signs, 191, 191b
vital tooth bleaching, 759, 759b
Dolophine. See Methadone
Domestic violence (DV). See also
    Intimate partner violence (IPV)
    during pregnancy, 790
Dominant hand, 646
Dopamine, 1000
Dopamine norepinephrine reuptake
    inhibitor, 985
DoPHER (Database of Promoting Health
    Effectiveness Reviews), 25b
Dose equivalent, 235
DOT (directly observed therapy), 1030,
    1031t
Down syndrome (DS), 850
    child with, 854f
    cognitive and behavioral
        characteristics, 853
    comorbidity and health considerations,
        853
    eye characteristics, 853f
    factors significant for dental hygiene
        care, 854
    hand, 853f
    oral findings, 853–854
    physical characteristics, 852
Doxycycline hyclate, 697–698, 698f
DPP (Diabetes Prevention Program), 928
Dressings. See Periodontal dressings
DRIs (dietary reference intakes), 554
Droplet precautions, 62
Drug enforcement administration drug
    schedule, 1006, 1006b
Drug-induced gingival enlargement, 328
Drug-induced stains and discolorations,
    298–299
Drug-related acquired bleeding disorders,
    1071
Drug-resistant tuberculosis, 67
Drug/food-induced asthma, 1032
Dry heat, 104–105
DS. See Down syndrome (DS)
DTP (D-termined program), 858
Duchenne muscular dystrophy (DMD),
    901–902
Duragesic, 1010
Dust-borne infectious agents, 64
Dyclonine HCl, 637
Dysarthria, 39, 898, 992t, 1086
Dysgeusia, 449, 947
Dyskinetic/athetoid palsy, 900
Dysmorphic features, 852

Dysphagia, 1029
Dyspnea, 141t, 1032, 1047, 1052
Dystonia, 992t

E

Early childhood caries (ECC), 267, 267f,
    374, 374t, 790, 811, 814
    progression of, 814f
EARs (estimated average requirements),
    554
Eastman interdental bleeding index
    (EIBI), 370, 370f
    areas examined, 370
    calculation, 370
    number of bleeding sites, 370
    percentage scores, 370
    procedure, 370
    purpose, 370
    scoring, 370
Eating habits, disabilities, 876
EBDH. See Evidence-based dental
    hygiene (EBDH)
EBDM (evidence-based decision making),
    20
EBP (evidence-based practice), 20
EBV (Epstein–Barr virus), 66t, 71, 73–74
ECC. See Early childhood caries (ECC)
Ecchymosis, 143t, 215, 960
Echocardiography, 1045
Edema, 215, 328, 1052
Edematous, 1036
Edentulous, 275
Edentulous mouth, 498–499
    bone, 498
    mucous membrane, 498–499
Edge-to-edge bite, 271, 271f
Editorials, 28–29
EEG (electroencephalography), 971
Efficacy, 472, 579
EIBI. See Eastman interdental bleeding
    index (EIBI)
Elastomers, 486, 487
Elder abuse and neglect, 212
    definitions, 217–218
    general considerations, 217
    general signs of, 218
    orofacial signs of, 218
    physical signs of, 218, 218f
Electrical pulp tester, 268f, 269
Electroconvulsive therapy, 985
Electroencephalography (EEG), 971
Electromagnetic ionizing radiation, 226
Electronic records, 150–151
Electronic sphygmomanometer, 187
Electronic thermometer, 185, 185f
Electronic timer, 228
Elevated lesions, 204, 205f, 206f
Elicit, 408
Elicit-provide-elicit (EPE) approach, 411
Embolic stroke, 895
Embolism, 1045
Embrasure, 304
Emergencies, prevention of, 128, 128b
Emergency care
    abbreviations, 128b
    basic life support certification, 136

Emergency care (*continued*)
documentation, 145*b*
  comprehensive record keeping, 137
  consults, 144
  new entries, 144
emergencies, prevention of, 128, 128*b*
emergency materials and preparation
  care of drugs, 132
  equipment, 131, 131f, 131t
  medical emergency report form, 132,
    133f
  practice and drill, 132–135, 134f, 135f
  telephone numbers for medical aid,
    130–131
emergency preparedness, 128
emergency reference chart, 138–143*t*
everyday ethics, 144
factors to teach patient, 144
oxygen administration
  equipment, 136–137
  oxygen delivery systems, 136f, 136t
  oxygen tank, 137b
  positive pressure, 137
  supplemental oxygen, 137
patient assessment
  extraoral and intraoral examinations,
    129
  increased risk factors, recognition of,
    129–130
  medical history, 129
  for routine treatment, 128–129
  vital signs, 129
seizure disorder
  differential diagnosis of seizure, 977
  emergency procedure, 977–978
  objectives, 977
  postictal phase, 978
  preparation for appointment, 977
  status epilepticus, 978
specific emergencies, 137
stress minimization, 130
Emergency preparedness, 128
Emerging drugs, 1009*t*, 1011–1012
Emery (corundum), 734
Emery–Dreifuss muscular dystrophy, 902
Emotional maltreatment, 214*t*
Emphysema, 136
due to tobacco use, 534
Enamel caries
formation of carious lesion, stages in,
  266, 266*f*
nomenclature by surfaces, 266
types of dental caries, 266–267
Enamel erosion, 300*f*
in pregnancy, 785
Enamel hypomineralization, 298
Enamel hypoplasia, 260, 260*f*, 298
crown forms of, 261*f*
Encoding, 34
Encryption, 152
End-rounded filaments, 435, 437*f*
End-to-end bite, 271, 271*f*
End-tuft brush. *See* Single-tuft brush
Endemic, hepatitis B virus, 68
Endo-periodontal lesions, 333
Endocarditis prophylaxis, 179*b*
Endocrine gland disorders
adrenal glands
  adrenal crisis, symptoms of, 916b

hyperadrenalism, 915
hypoadrenalism, 915–916
documentation, 919, 919*b*
everyday ethics, 920
factors to teach patient, 920
pancreas, 916
parathyroid glands, 914
  hyperparathyroidism, 915
  hypoparathyroidism, 915
pituitary gland, 913
puberty
  patient management considerations,
    917
  pubertal changes, 916–917
  stages of adolescence, 916
thyroid gland
  hyperthyroidism, 914, 914t
  hypothyroidism, 913–914, 914t
women's health
  hormonal contraceptives, 918
  menopause, 918–919
  menstrual cycle, 917, 917f
  patient management considerations,
    919
Endocrine system, 916
changes due to aging, 825
glands of, 912, 912*f*, 912*t*
hormones, 912*t*
  and functions, 912
  regulation of, 912–913
Endodontic infections, 925
Endodontic therapy, 299
Endogenous erosion, 262
Endogenous stains, 294, 297–299, 298*f*
Endometrium, 917
Endoscope, 689
-assisted periodontal debridement,
  690–691, 690*f*
Endosseous or root form dental implant,
  519
bone physiology, 520–521
definition, 520, 520*f*
description, 520
parts of, 520*f*
Endotoxins, 680
Environmental Protection Agency
  (EPA)-registered hospital disinfectant,
  98
Environmental tobacco smoke (ETS),
  530, 534
cardiovascular effects, 534
impact in children, 535
infants and, 535
lung and respiratory effects, 535
toxicity, 535
in utero, 535
Eosinophils, 1065
EPE (elicit-provide-elicit) approach,
  411
Epicanthic fold, 852
Epidemiologic surveys
purpose, 358
use, 358
Epilepsy, 970
Epileptic cry, 971
Epileptic spasms, 970*t*
Epinephrine (Adrenalin), 622, 623–624
Epithelial desquamation, 635
Epithelium, 306

EPS (extracellular polymeric substance),
  281
Epstein–Barr virus (EBV), 66*t*, 71, 73–74
Ergonomics, 116. *See also under* Patient
  reception
Erosion, 206, 262, 262*f*, 717
Erythema, 141*t*, 206
Erythrocytes. *See* Red blood cells
Erythroplakia, 207
Ester anesthetics, 621
Esthetic, 747
Estimated average requirements (EARs),
  554
Estrogen, 918
Ethambutol (EMB), 1031*t*
Ethical dilemma, 14, 14*b*
Ethical issue, 14, 14*b*
Ethics, 11. *See also* Code of Ethics
dental hygiene, 13
in research
  ethical research involving human
    subjects, 29
  ethical standards, 29
  informed consent for, 29–30
  Institutional Review Board, 30
Ethosuximide (Zarontin), 973*t*
ETS. *See* Environmental tobacco smoke
  (ETS)
Eugenol, 709
Euphoria, 1005
Evaluation, 406
based on goals and outcomes, 766,
  766*b*
of clinical (treatment) outcomes, 767
comparison of assessment findings,
  767, 768*b*
design, 766
documentation
  patient care outcomes, 769, 770b
  self-assessment and reflection, 769
everyday ethics, 770
factors to teach patient, 770
of health behavior outcomes, 767
interview evaluation, 767
periodontal examination, 767
principles of, 765–766
process, 766
purposes of, 765
self-assessment and reflective practice
  "critical incident" approach, 769
  purpose, 768
  skills and methods, 768–769
standard of care, 767–768, 768*b*
tactile evaluation, 767
types of, 766*t*
visual examination, 767
Evidence, 20
Evidence-based approach, 384
Evidence-based decision making
  (EBDM), 20
Evidence-based dental hygiene (EBDH),
  2
definition of, 20
documentation, 30, 30*b*
everyday ethics, 30–31
factors to teach patient, 31
model, 20–21, 20*f*
need for, 20
purposes of, 20

research
    designs, 27
    ethics in, 29–30
    evidence sources, 27
    levels of evidence, 27–29, 28f
    time intervals, 29
    types, 27
skills needed for, 21, 21b
systematic approach, 22f
    clinical issue assessment, 21
    clinically evaluation of evidence,
        25–26
    evaluating outcomes, 26
    integration and application of
        evidence, 26
    research question development, 21,
        22t, 23
    scientific evidence. See Scientific
        evidence, search for
Evidence-based, individualized patient
    care, 398
Evidence-based practice (EBP), 20
Evocation, 408
    motivational interviewing and, 409
Exacerbations, 1034
Excisional biopsy, 956b
Exercise induced asthma, 1033
Exfoliation, 273
Exfoliative biopsy, 956b
Exodontics, 956b
Exogenous erosion, 262
Exogenous insulin, 929
Exogenous stains, 294, 299, 299f, 300f
Exophytic, defined, 206
Experimental research, 27
Expert witnesses, 768b
Expiration, 1036
Explorers, 339–340, 339f
    procedures for, 339–340
        tooth surface irregularities,
            339–340
        types of stimuli, 340
        usage of sensory stimuli, 339
    purpose and use, 339
    subgingival procedures, 340
    supragingival procedures, 340
        facial and lingual surfaces, 340
        proximal surfaces, 340
        usage of vision, 340
    usage of special, 339
Exposure control
    clinical attire, 84
        hair and head covering, 85
        protective clothing, 85, 85f
    documentation, 94, 94b
    everyday ethics, 94
    face mask
        aerosols, 85
        characteristics of, 85b
        efficiency, 85–86
        removal of, 86f
        respiratory hygiene, 86
        use of, 86
    factors to teach patient, 94
    gloves and gloving
        factors affecting integrity, 92–93
        procedures of, 92
        selection of treatment/examination
            gloves, 91–92

steps for removal of, 92f
types of, 92
hand care, 87–88
    artificial nails, 89
    bacteriology of skin, 88
    fingernails, 89
    gloves, 89
    wristwatch and jewelry, 89
hand hygiene
    methods of, 89–91, 90b
    principles, 89
infection control, 84
latex hypersensitivity, 93–94
personal protection for dental team, 84
protective eyewear, 86
    face shield, 87
    general features of, 87
    indications for use of, 87
    suggestions for clinical application, 87
    types of, 87, 88f
Extensively drug-resistant tuberculosis, 67
External skeletal fixation, 963, 963f
External validity, 26
Extracellular polymeric substance (EPS),
    281
Extraoral and intraoral examination
    child abuse and neglect, 215–216,
        215t
    components of, 196–198
    documentation, 152, 208, 208b
    emergency care, 129
    everyday ethics, 208
    factors to teach patient, 208–209
    methods for
        auscultation, 197
        electrical test, 197
        instrumentation, 197
        palpation. See Palpation
        percussion, 197
        visual examination, 196
    morphologic categories
        depressed lesions, 204, 205f, 206
        elevated lesions, 204, 205f, 206f
        flat lesions, 206, 206f
    oral cancer, 206–207
    oral cavity, anatomic landmarks of,
        198, 199f, 200b, 200f
    oral lesions, clinical recommendations
        for evaluation of, 207–208
    preparation for, 198
    rationale for, 196
    sequence of, 198–199, 201–202t
        cervical node palpation, 202f
        documentation of findings, 203–204
        extraoral examination, 199, 202–203
        intraoral examination, 203
        lymph nodes, 202f
        probe, use of, 204f
        record form for clinical findings, 203f
        tongue, examination of, 203f
    signs and symptoms, 197–198
    tobacco use, 542
    types of, 196
Extrinsic asthma, 1032
Extrinsic stain, 281, 293, 747
    black-line stain, 295–296
    brown stains, 296–297, 297f
    green stain, 295
    metallic stains, 297

orange and red stains, 297
removal, 472
    air-powder polishing, 739–741, 739f,
        740–741b, 742t
    cleaning and polishing agents,
        733–735, 734t
    clinical application of, 732–733
    coronal polishing, 735–736
    documentation, 743, 743b
    effects of cleaning and polishing,
        730–731, 731f
    everyday ethics, 744
    factors to teach patient, 744
    indications for, 731–732
    polishing proximal surfaces,
        741–743
    porte polisher, 743
    power-driven instruments, 736–738,
        736t, 737f
    procedures for, 735–736
    prophylaxis angle, use of, 738–739
    purposes for, 730
    science of polishing, 730
    tobacco stain, 296, 296f
    yellow stain, 294, 294f
Exudate, 309
Eyewear. See also Protective eyewear
    with curved frames, 87, 88f
    with side shields, 87, 88f

F

Face mask, 136t
    aerosols, 85
    characteristics of, 85b
        removal of, 86f
        respiratory hygiene, 86
        use of, 86
    efficiency, 85–86
Face shield, 87
Facet, 261
Facial paralysis, 635
Facial profiles, types of, 270
Facioscapulohumeral muscular dystrophy,
    902
Family decision making, 40
Family violence (FV)
    abuse and neglect
        child. See Child abuse and neglect
        elder. See Elder abuse and neglect
        reporting, 219–220
    categories of, 212
    documentation, 221b
        content of record, 221
        thorough and accurate, 221
    everyday ethics, 222
    factors to teach patient, 222
    forensic dentistry
        in abuse cases, 220–221
        other uses of, 221
    human trafficking, 217
    intimate partner violence
        dental hygienist, role of, 219
        general health consequences of, 219
        orofacial impact of, 219
        physical injury from, 219
        prevalence of, 218–219
    Munchausen syndrome by proxy,
        216–217
    types of, 212, 212f

FAS. *See* Fetal alcohol syndrome (FAS)
FASDs. *See* Fetal alcohol spectrum
    disorders (FASDs)
Fasting plasma glucose (FPG), 930
Fatigue, 116
FDA. *See* Food and Drug Administration
    (FDA)
Fear, effects of, 130
Federal Drug Authority (FDA), 102
Fédération Dentaire Internationale
    system, 152–153, 153*f*
Feedback, 34, 765
Feeding and eating disorders
    dental hygiene care, 989–991
    medical complications, 989
    treatment, 989
    types and symptoms of, 987–989
Felbamate (Felbatol), 973*t*
Fentanyl, 1010
Fermentable carbohydrates, role of, 422
Ferromagnetic units, 657
Fetal alcohol spectrum disorders (FASDs),
    1003
    alcohol use during pregnancy, 1004
    characteristics of an individual with,
        1004*b*
    fetal alcohol syndrome, facial features
        of, 1004*f*
    terminology and abbreviations, 1004*b*
Fetal alcohol syndrome (FAS), 1004*b*
    facial features of, 1004*f*
Fetal development
    factors harming fetus, 782–784
        drugs of abuse and dependence, 784
        herbal dietary supplements, 784
        infections and, 782
        pharmacological considerations for,
            782–784, 783t
    first trimester, 782
    second and third trimesters, 782
Fetus, 782
Fibrosis, 1081
Fibrotic tissue, 313
Fibrous encapsulation, 518
Filament step-down transformer, 227
Filaments (bristles), 434, 435–436
    natural and synthetic, 437*t*
    stiffness of, 439
File scaler sharpening, 675, 675*f*
Filled sealants, 607
Filtration, 232–233
Financial exploitation, 212, 218
FINER criteria, 21, 23
Fingernails, 89
Finishing files, 654–655, 655*f*
First-line agents, 1086*b*
First trimester, 782
5% glutaraldehyde, 725
Fixed appliance system, 486–487, 486*f*,
    488
Flash sterilization. *See* Intermediate-use
    steam sterilization
Flat affect, 991
Flat lesions, 206, 206*f*
Flavoring agents (sweeteners), 474
Flora, 284
Floss cleft, 312, 461
Floss cuts, 461

Floss holder, 462, 463*f*
Floss threader, 461–462, 461*f*, 506*f*
Fluorapatite, 575
Fluoridation
    discontinued, 579
    effects and benefits of, 578–579
    historical aspects, 577–578
    research cities, 578*b*
    school, 579
    water supply adjustment, 578
Fluorides, 284, 475, 559*t*
    absorption, 574
    acquisition after eruption, 576*f*
    action, 577
    in biofilm and saliva, 576–577
    bottled water, 580
    brush-on gel, 589–590, 589*t*
    calculation, 593, 593*f*
    in cementum, 576
    combined fluoride program, 591
    demineralization–remineralization,
        576–577, 576*f*
    dentifrices, 590–591
    in dentin, 576
    dentinal hypersensitivity, 724
        gels, 724
        tray-delivered agents, 725
        varnish, 725
    dietary supplements, 580–581, 580*t*
    distribution and retention, 574
    documentation, 593, 594*b*
    in enamel, 576
    everyday ethics, 594
    excretion, 574
    factors to teach patient, 594
    fluoridation
        discontinued, 579
        effects and benefits of, 578–579
        historical aspects, 577–578
        research cities, 578b
        school, 579
        water supply adjustment, 578
    in foods, 579–580
    halo/diffusion effect, 580
    home tray application, 587–588, 588*b*
    for implant systems, 523
    infant formula, 580
    intake, 574
    mechanisms of action, 423
    metabolism, 574
    mouthrinses, 588–589, 589*t*
    orthodontic appliances, 493
    partial defluoridation, 579
    pediatrics, 808
    professional topical fluoride
        applications, 581–583, 582t
        clinical procedures, 583–586, 583b,
            584–585t, 585–586f, 587t
    program, 875–876
        pregnancy, 789
    prophylaxis pastes, 735
    -releasing bonding system, 488
    safety
        acute toxic dose, 592
        chronic toxicity, 592–593
        emergency treatment, 592
        risk management, 591
        toxicity, 591–592

    salt, 580
    self-applied, 587
    and tooth development, 574
        maturation stage, 575
        mineralization stage, 575, 575f
        posteruptive, 575–576
    tooth surface, 576
    water filters, 580
Fluorosis, 575, 592–593, 751–752
Focal onset aware, 971
Focal onset seizure, 970*t*, 971
Folate, 559*t*
    -deficiency anemia, 1067
Fones (or circular) method, 443,
    444*f*
Food and Drug Administration (FDA),
    479, 480*t*, 583
    pregnancy categories, 622*b*
Food debris, 287
Food diary
    analysis of diet consistency, 566
    benefits of, 566
    instructions, 563*b*
    nutritional analysis, 565
Food impaction, 287, 321
Food pouching, 871
Foods, fluorides in, 579–580
Forensic dentistry, 150, 220
    in abuse cases, 220–221
    other uses of, 221
Formative evaluation, 766, 766*t*
Four-handed dental hygiene, 882,
    906
FPG (fasting plasma glucose), 930
Fractured jaw
    causes of, 960
    emergency care, 960
    recognition, 960
    treatment, 961–962
    types, 960–961, 961*f*
Fractures, of teeth, 263, 263*f*
Fragile X syndrome (FXS), 855*f*
    cognitive and behavioral
        characteristics, 855
    comorbidity and health considerations,
        855
    factors significant for dental hygiene
        care, 855
    oral findings, 855
    physical characteristics, 854
Free gingiva (marginal gingiva), 303–304
Free gingival groove, 303
Fremitus, 274, 351–352
Frenum, 307
Frequency, 655
Friable, 312
Fulcrum, 647, 659
    alternative, 649
    extraoral, 648–649
    intraoral, 648
    purpose of, 648
Functional ability, 871, 872*b*
Functional age, 824
Functional contacts, occlusion, 274
Functionally dependent, 48
Furcations
    anatomic variations of, 685*f*
    examination, 342*f*, 352–353

involvement, periodontal disease, 325, 325f, 326f
FV. See Family violence (FV)
FXS. See Fragile X syndrome (FXS)

G

Gabapentin (Neurontin), 973t
Gabitril. See Tiagabine
Gagging, causes of, 241
Gamma, 235
Gamma-knife radiosurgery, 973
Gastroesophageal reflux disease (GERD), 1032
Gastrointestinal effects of drug abuse, 1012
Gastrointestinal tract
    autoimmune diseases, 1083
        celiac disease, 1083
        Crohn's disease, 1083–1085, 1084f
        ulcerative colitis, 1085–1086, 1085f
    changes due to aging, 825
Gastroparesis, 935
Gauze strip, 462, 463f
GBI. See Gingival bleeding index (GBI)
GCF (gingival crevicular fluid), 304
GDM (gestational diabetes mellitus), 786, 929
Gel, 582
General anesthesia, 615
General supervision, 7b
Generalized anxiety disorder, 982
Generalized onset seizure, 970t, 971
Genetic susceptibility, 384
Genital herpes, 73
GERD (gastroesophageal reflux disease), 1032
Gerontology, 824
Gestation, 782
Gestational diabetes mellitus (GDM), 786, 929
GI. See Gingival index (GI)
Gingiva
    alveolar mucosa, 307
    attached gingiva, 306–307
    clinical observations of, 155–156
    free gingiva, 303–304
    gingival sulcus, 304
    gingival tissues, 304f, 305f
    interdental gingiva, 304–305, 306f
    junctional epithelium, 305–306
    mucogingival junction, 307
    parts of, 304f, 307f
    after periodontal surgery, 314–315
    of young children, 314
Gingival abrasion, 439, 449–450
Gingival and periodontal health, indices for
    community periodontal index, 366
    Eastman interdental bleeding index, 370
    gingival bleeding index, 368–370
    periodontal screening and recording, 365–366
    sulcus bleeding index, 368
Gingival and periodontal infections, 77
Gingival bleeding index (GBI), 368–370
    areas examined, 369

criteria, 369
instruments, 369
procedure, 369
purpose, 368
scoring, 370
steps, 369
Gingival conditions, in pregnancy, 784
Gingival crevicular fluid (GCF), 304
Gingival description, 309
    bleeding, 314
    color, 311, 311f
    consistency, 312–313, 313f
    exudate, 314
    gingival clinical markers, 309–310t
    position, 313
    shape, 311–312, 312f
    size, 311
    surface texture, 313
Gingival embrasure (Class II), 456f
Gingival enlargement, pregnancy, 785
Gingival fiber groups, 308, 308f
Gingival grafting surgery, 315
Gingival hyperplasia, phenytoin and, 320f
Gingival index (GI), 359, 370–371, 371f, 886
    for area, 371
    calculation and interpretation, 371
    for group, 371
    for individual, 371
    procedure, 370
    purpose, 370
    scoring, 371
    selection of teeth and gingival areas, 370
    for tooth, 371
Gingival overgrowth/gingival hyperplasia
    complicating factor, 975
    differential diagnosis of medications causing, 975
    effects, 974
    mechanism, 974
    occurrence, 974
    phenytoin-induced gingival enlargement, 974f
    phenytoin-induced gingival overgrowth, 975f
    tissue characteristics, 974–975
    treatment, 975
Gingival pocket, 324, 325f
Gingival recession, 717, 717f
Gingival sulcus, 303, 304
Gingivectomy, 975
Gingivitis, 319, 386, 536
    classification of, 328–329, 332f
    plaque (or biofilm)-induced, 681
    pregnancy, 784–785
    reduction of, 472
Glands, 912
Glass ionomer sealants, dentinal hypersensitivity, 725
Glaucoma, 868
    local anesthesia and, 627
Global developmental delay, 850b
Glossitis, 560t, 1066
Glossodynia, 560t, 1066
Gloves and gloving, 89
    factors affecting integrity, 92–93
    procedures of, 92

selection of treatment/examination, 91–92
steps for removal of, 92f
types of, 92
Glucocorticosteroids, 1079
Glucose meter (glucometer), 932
Glutaraldehyde, 724
Glycated/glycosylated hemoglobin, 930
Glycemia, 930
Glycerin, 732, 749
Glycine, 740
Goggles, 87, 88f
Gonads, 912
Grafting, 845
Grand mal seizures, 971
Granulocytes, 1064–1065, 1064t
Grasp, 659. See also specific types
Green stain, 295
Grit, 730
Group A streptococci (beta-hemolytic), 67t
Group in-service education, 885–886

H

HAART (highly active antiretroviral therapy), 78
Hair and head covering, 85
Half-life, 623
Halitosis (bad breath), 445. See also Oral malodor
    due to tobacco use, 542
Hallucinations, 991, 1005
Hallucinogens, 1007t, 1010
Halo/diffusion effect, 580
Hand care, 87–88
    artificial nails, 89
    bacteriology of skin, 88
    fingernails, 89
    gloves, 89
    wristwatch and jewelry, 89
Hand hygiene, 85
    methods of, 90b
        antimicrobial soap, 91
        antiseptic hand rub, 91
        antiseptic handwash, 90–91
        indications, 89, 90b
        routine handwash, 90
        surgical antisepsis, 91
    principles, 89
Handheld X-ray devices, 249, 249f
Handle, instrument, 645, 645f
Handpieces, 121
Handwritten records, 150
Hard tissue examination
    dental caries, 263–264
        caries classification system, 266
        carious lesions, classification of, 264–266
        development of, 264
        G.V. Black's classification, 264–265, 264f
        international caries classification and management system, 265–266, 265f
    dental charting of existing restorations, 257
    dentin, developmental defects of, 261

Hard tissue examination (*continued*)
developmental enamel lesions
enamel hypoplasia, 260, 260f, 261f
hypomaturation, 260
hypomineralization, 260
documentation, 275, 276b
early childhood caries, 267, 267f
enamel caries
formation of carious lesion, stages in, 266, 266f
nomenclature by surfaces, 266
types of dental caries, 266–267
everyday ethics, 277
factors to teaching patient, 277
interocclusal record, 275, 275f
mixed or transitional dentition, 256, 256f
noncarious and carious lesions
assessment, 257, 259
noncarious cervical lesions, 261
abfraction, 262–263
abrasion, 262, 262f
erosion, 262, 262f
noncarious dental lesions, 261
attrition, 261, 261f
occlusion, 259–260
dynamic or functional, 274
facial profiles, types of, 270
malocclusion, 269–270, 269f
malrelations of groups of teeth, 271–273, 271–273f
normal, 269, 269f
of primary teeth, 273–274, 273f
trauma from, 274–275
permanent dentition, 256, 257t
primary (deciduous) dentition, 256
primary teeth occlusion
malocclusion of, 274
normal, 273, 273f
pulp vitality testing
causes of loss of vitality, 268
electrical pulp tester, 268f, 269
indications for, 268
response to pulp testing, 268
thermal pulp testing, 268
root caries, 267f
risk factors for, 267–268
stages in formation of, 267
study models, 275, 275f
teeth, 257, 257f
examination of, 258–259t
fractures of, 263, 263f
terminology for malposition of, 273
Hawley retainer, 493, 493f
Hazardous material, universal label for, 111, 111f
Hazardous waste, 111
HbA1c, 930
HBV (hepatitis B virus), 65t, 68–70, 69t
HCV (hepatitis C virus), 65t, 70
HDV (hepatitis D virus), 65t, 70
Health, 4
Health behavior, 406
change model, 407, 408t. *See also* Behavior change
motivation for, 408
Health communication
barriers to effective, 35, 35t

with caregivers, 42–43
cultural considerations, 40b
cross-cultural communication, 40, 41t
cultural competence, 41–42
culture and health, 39–40
documentation, 43, 43b
effective health communicators, skills and attributes of, 34
effective health information, attributes of, 34–35
everyday ethics, 43
factors influencing, 35–36
factors to teach patient, 43
health literacy and
assessing and addressing, 36, 37f, 38f
health learning capacity, 36, 36t
interprofessional communication, 42
across lifespan
adolescents, 38
infants, 37
older adults, 39, 39b
preschoolers, 37–38
school-age children, 38
tips, 38b
toddlers, 37–38
social and economic aspects of, 39
web-based health messages, 35
Health hazards of alcohol
brain, 1002
cancer risk, 1003
digestive system, 1003
heart, 1003
immunity and infection, 1003
liver disease, 1003
nervous system, 1003
nutritional deficiencies, 1003
reproductive system, 1003
Health Insurance Portability and Accountability Act (HIPAA), 886
privacy rule, 151
security rule, 151–152
Health learning capacity, 36, 36t
Health literacy, 34, 386
assessing and addressing, 36, 37f, 38f
health learning capacity, 36, 36t
Health promotion, 11
nutrient standards for diet adequacy in, 553–571
Healthcare-associated (nosocomial) pneumonia, 1029, 1029t
Healthy People 2020, 358
Hearing aids, 869
Hearing impairment, 868, 869
clinical settings, introduction of, 879–880
Heart
alcohol and, 1003
normal, 1045–1046, 1045f
surgery, local anesthesia and, 626
Heart failure
clinical manifestations of, 1052
emergency care for, 1053
etiology of, 1052
local anesthesia and, 626
treatment during chronic stages, 1052–1053
Hemarthroses, 1071

Hematocrit, 1062, 1063t
Hematoma (bruise), 634
Hematopoietic stem cell transplantation
acute complications, 948
chronic complications, 948
oral care protocol, 951
stages of, 947–948
types, 947
Hemidesmosomes, 306
Hemiparesis, 895
Hemiplegia, 896
Hemoglobin, 1062, 1063t
Hemolysis, 1065
Hemolytic anemia, 1065
Hemophilia, 1071
local anesthesia and, 627
Hemoptysis, 1031t
Hemorrhagic stroke, 895
Hemostasis, 704
Heparin, 1056
Hepatitis B virus (HBV), 65t, 68–70, 69t
Hepatitis C virus (HCV), 65t, 70
Hepatitis D virus (HDV), 65t, 70
Hepatitis E virus (HEV), 65t, 70
Hereditary bleeding disorders, 1071
Hereditary hemolytic disorders, 1065
Hereditary platelet dysfunction, 1070
Heroin, 1010
Herpes labialis, 72–73
Herpes lymphotropic virus
HLV-6A, 74
HLV-6B, 74
Herpes simplex virus
type 1 (HSV-1), 65t, 71, 72
type 2 (HSV-2), 65t, 71
Herpetic whitlow, 73
HEV (hepatitis E virus), 65t, 70
HHVs. *See* Human herpes virus diseases (HHVs)
High blood pressure (HBP). *See* Hypertension (HTN)
High-voltage step-up transformer, 227
Highly active antiretroviral therapy (HAART), 78
HIPAA. *See* Health Insurance Portability and Accountability Act (HIPAA)
Hirsutism, 973
HIV/AIDS infection, 65t, 1029
dental hygiene management, 78–79
etiology of oral lesions associated with, 77t
oral manifestations of, 76–78
pregnancy, 784
prescribed medications, 78t
prevention and treatment, 78
testing for diagnosis and staging of infection, 76
transmission, 75–76
Home tray bleaching treatment, 755, 755f
Homeostasis, 912
Horizontal (or scrub) method, 443
Hormonal contraceptives, 918
Hormones, 912, 912t
and functions, 912
regulation of, 912–913
Hospices, 47
Hospital-acquired pneumonia, 1029

HPV (human papillomavirus), 66t, 75
HTN. *See* Hypertension (HTN)
Human herpes virus diseases (HHVs), 70–71, 71t
  clinical management for, 72–75
  general characteristics, 71–72
  HHV-1 (HSV-1), 72–73, 73f
  HHV-2 (HSV-2), 73
  HHV-3 (VZV), 73
  HHV-4 (EBV), 73–74
  HHV-5 (CMV), 74
  HHV-6A, 74
  HHV-6B, 74
  HHV-7, 74
  HHV-8 (Kaposi's sarcoma–associated herpesvirus), 74–75
  periodontal infections, relation to, 72
Human papillomavirus (HPV), 66t, 75
Human subjects, 29
Human trafficking, 217
Humectants (moisture stabilizers), 473t, 474
Hydrocephalus, 903, 903f
  shunt for treatment, 904f
Hydrodynamic theory, 718, 718f, 719f
Hydrogen peroxide, 748f, 749, 749f
Hydrolysis, 704
Hydroxyapatite, 575
Hyperactivity, 855
Hyperadrenalism, 915
Hyperarousal symptoms, 983
Hypercholesterolemia, 896
Hyperglycemia, 927, 927t
Hyperinsulinemia, 926
Hyperkalemia, 916
Hyperkeratosis, 313
Hypernatremia, 916
Hyperparathyroidism, 915
Hyperpnea, 927t
Hypersensitive teeth, 990
Hypertension (HTN), 190–191
  blood pressure levels, 1048, 1049t
  in children, 1049
  clinical symptoms of, 1048–1049
  etiology of, 1048
  lifestyle modifications for management, 191t
  local anesthesia and, 627
  primary, 1048
  pulmonary, 1037b
  secondary, 1048
  treatment of, 1049, 1049b
  white-coat, 190
Hyperthermia, 184
Hyperthyroidism, 914, 914t
  local anesthesia and, 626
Hypertriglyceridemia, 896
Hyperventilation, 1024
Hypoadrenalism, 915–916
Hypogeusia, 924t
Hypoglycemia, 130, 926, 926b, 927t, 936f
Hypoinsulinemia, 927
Hypokalemia, 915
Hypomaturation, 260
Hypomineralization, 260
Hypoparathyroidism, 915
Hypoplasia, 258t, 298
Hyposalivation, 423

Hypotension, 190t
Hypothermia, 184
Hypothyroidism, 913–914, 914t
Hypoxia, 1068

I

IADL (instrumental activities of daily living), 386, 386t
Iatrogenic factor, 320
Iatrosedation, 615
ICCMS (International Caries Classification and Management System), 265, 265f, 266, 423, 426, 427, 428f
ICD (implantable cardioverter defibrillator), 1055
ICDAS (International Caries Detection and Assessment System), 427
Ictus, 971
Idiopathic temporary facial paralysis. *See* Bell's palsy
Idiosyncratic reactions, 619
IDs. *See* Intellectual disabilities (IDs)
IE. *See* Infective endocarditis (IE)
IF (intrinsic factor), 1066
IGRA (interferon-gamma release assay), 1030
Illicit drugs, 1004
Image receptor, 226, 234–235
IMF (intermaxillary fixation), 959–960, 962, 962f
Immune system, 1078, 1078f
  changes due to aging, 825
Immunity, 64
  and infection, alcohol and, 1003
Immunizations, 84
Immunocompromised patient, 179
Immunoglobulin E, 1033
Impact evaluation, 766, 766t
Impaction, 320
Impaired fasting glucose, 928
Impaired glucose tolerance, 928
Impairment, 866. *See also* Disabilities
Implant surgery, 315
Implantable cardioverter defibrillator (ICD), 1055
Implantitis, 536
Implied consent, 400
Impulses, 228
IMRT (intensity-modulated radiation therapy), 946–947
Incipient caries, 267, 601
Incisional biopsy, 956b
Incubation periods, 65, 79
Independent practice, 7b
Indicators (evaluation measures), 766
Indices, 358–359
  for community-based oral health surveillance
    Association of State and Territorial Dental Directors Basic Screening Survey, 377t, 378t
    World Health Organization Basic Screening Survey, 376
  cumulative, 359
  descriptive categories of, 358–359

DMFT index, 358
documentation, 377, 378b
everyday ethics, 377
factors to teach patient/members of community, 378
general categories, 358–359
for gingival and periodontal health
  community periodontal index, 366–368
  Eastman interdental bleeding index, 370
  gingival bleeding index, 368–370
  gingival index, 359, 370–371
  periodontal screening and recording, 365–366
  sulcus bleeding index, 368
gingival and periodontal indices, 365–371
irreversible, 359
for measuring dental caries experience
  decayed, indicated for extraction, and filled, 373
  decayed, missing, and filled, 373–374
  decayed, missing, and filled teeth/surfaces, 371–372
  early childhood caries, 374, 374t
  root caries index, 374–375
for measuring dental fluorosis
  Dean's fluorosis index, 375
  tooth surface index of fluorosis, 375, 376t
measuring oral hygiene
  biofilm control record, 360–361
  biofilm-free score, 361–362
  patient hygiene performance, 362–363
  plaque index, 359
  simplified oral hygiene index, 363–365
presence of dental biofilm, 360
reversible, 359
selection criteria, 359
simple, 358
Indirect digital imaging, 229, 229f
Indirect supervision, 7b
Individual assessment score
  purpose, 358
  uses, 358
Indurated, defined, 206
Infants, 800
  communication skills of, 37
  and environmental tobacco smoke, 535
  formula, 580
  knee-to-knee examination, 793f
  oral health
    anticipatory guidance, 790, 791t
    birth to age 12 months, 791t
    daily oral hygiene care, 790–791
    examination, 793f
    feeding patterns (birth to 1 year), 791–792
    first dental visit, components of, 792–794, 793f
    nonnutritive sucking, 792, 792f
    oral soft and hard tissue conditions/pathology in, 793t

Infarct, 1051
Infection, 62, 298
  diabetes mellitus, 934
  drug abuse, 1013
  induced asthma, 1033
Infection control, 98
  basic procedures, 247, 247b
  clinical procedures
    barriers and surface covers, 107,
      107f, 108f
    basic considerations for safe practice,
      98
    care of sterile instruments, 105–106
    chemical disinfectants, 106–107,
      107b
    chemical liquid sterilization, 105
    chemical vapor sterilizer, 105
    disposal of waste, 111, 111f
    documentation, 112, 113b
    dry heat, 104–105
    everyday ethics, 112
    factors to teach patient, 113
    instrument packing and management
      system, 102, 102f
    instrument processing center, 100,
      100f
    intermediate-use steam sterilization,
      105
    moist heat, 104
    objectives, 98
    occupational postexposure
      management, 112
    patient preparation, 110
    precleaning procedures, 100–102,
      101f
    standard procedures, 110–111
    sterilization, 102–104, 103t
    supplemental recommendations,
      111–112
    treatment room features, 98–100, 99f
    treatment room preparation,
      107–110, 109t
  documentation, 79, 79b
  everyday ethics, 80
  factors to teach patient, 80
  guidelines in dental healthcare settings
    blood-borne pathogens, preventing
      transmission of, 1108
    contact dermatitis and latex
      hypersensitivity, 1110
    dental unit waterlines, biofilm, and
      water quality, 1112–1113
    environmental infection control,
      1111–1112
    hand hygiene, 1108–1109
    infection-control program, personnel
      health elements of, 1107–1108
    personal protective equipment,
      1109–1110
    special considerations, 1113–1115
    sterilization and disinfection of
      patient-care items, 1110–1111
  HIV/AIDS infection
    dental hygiene management, 78–79
    oral manifestations of, 76–78, 77t
    prevention and treatment, 78, 78t
    testing for diagnosis and staging of
      infection, 76

    transmission, 75–76
  human herpesvirus diseases, 70–71, 71t
    clinical management for, 72–75
    general characteristics, 71–72
    periodontal infections, relation to, 72
  human papillomavirus, 75
  infectious process
    airborne infection, 64
    disease transmission, 63–64, 63f
    transmission, prevention of, 64–65
  methicillin-resistant Staphylococcus
    aureus, 79
  no-touch method for films and
    photostimulable phosphor plates,
    248, 248f
  oral cavity
    microorganisms of, 62
    pathogens transmissible from, 65,
      65–67t
  practice policy, 247
  standard precautions, 62
  tuberculosis
    clinical management, 68
    transmission, 67–68, 68f
  viral hepatitis
    hepatitis B virus, 68–70, 69t
    hepatitis C virus, 70
    hepatitis D virus, 70
Infectious agents, 62
Infectious process
  airborne infection, 64
  disease transmission, 63–64, 63f
  transmission, prevention of, 64–65
Infectious rhinitis (common cold), 1027t
Infectious waste, 111
Infective endocarditis (IE), 175
  description of, 1044
  disease process, 1045
  etiology of, 1044
  prevention of, 1045
Inferential statistics, 26
Infiltration, 323, 625
Influenza (flu), 1027t
Influenza viruses (A, B, C), 67t
Informed consent, 29–30, 157, 180, 400,
  401b
  additional considerations, 401
  criteria for adequate content in, 400b
  informed refusal, 401
  procedures, 400
Informed refusal of care, 401
Ingestion, alcohol, 1001
Inhalants, 1009t, 1011
Inorganic content, in calculus, 289–290
INR (international normalized ratio),
  1063t, 1071
Insoluble coating, 281
Insomnia, 984
Inspiration, 1036
Institutional Review Board (IRB), 30
Instrument care and sharpening,
  667–668
  angulation, 670
  care of sharpening equipment
    care of tanged file, 676
    flat sharpening stone, 675–676
    manufacturer's directions, 676
  care of sharpening stone, 670

  curets and scalers
    selection of cutting edges to sharpen,
      671
    technique objectives, 671
  documentation, 676, 676b
  dynamics of, 668, 668f
  evaluation of technique, 670–671
  everyday ethics, 676
  factors to teach patient, 676
  file scaler, 675, 675f
  instrument handling, 669
  instrument wear, 671
  maintain control, 670
  moving flat stone, stationary
    instrument, 671–674, 672f, 673f
  plastic testing stick, 670f
  preparation of stone for sharpening,
    669
  stationary flat stone, moving
    instrument, 674–675, 674f
  sterilization of sharpening stone, 669
  tests for instrument sharpness, 670
  types of devices
    power-driven or mechanical
      sharpening devices, 669
    stones, 668–669, 669f
  visual or glare test, 670
  wire edge after sharpening, 671
Instrument packing and management
  system, 102, 102f
Instrument processing center, 100, 100f
Instrument washer, 100–101, 101f
Instrument wear, 671
Instrumental activities of daily living
  (IADL), 386, 386t
Instrumentation. See also Periodontal
  instruments
  activation (stroke), 650–651, 650f
  adaptation, 649
  advanced instrumentation
    channel scaling, 688f, 689
    definitions, 686
    instrument adaptation, 688f
    location of, 686f
    subgingival anatomical considerations,
      686
    technique, 687–689, 687b
  angulation, 649–650, 650f
  dominant hand, 646
  effect on pocket microflora, 681t
  formulate strategy for, 686
  fulcrum, 647
    alternative, 649
    extraoral, 648–649
    intraoral, 648
    purpose of, 648
  modified pen grasp, 647, 647f
  neutral wrist, 647, 648f
  nondominant hand, 647
  palm grasp, 647, 647f
  specialized debridement instruments
    advanced ultrasonic tips, 689
    endoscope-assisted periodontal
      debridement, 690–691, 690f
    furcation debridement, 689
    laser therapy, 692
    microultrasonics, 689–690, 689f
    subgingival air polishing, 691–692, 691f

Insulin, 924
 absolute insulin deficiency, 926
 complications
  hyperglycemia, 927, 927t
  hypoglycemia, 926, 926b, 927t
 definition of, 925
 -dependent diabetes mellitus, 929
 description of, 925, 925f
 dosage, 933
 functions of, 926, 926b
 impaired secretion/action of insulin, 926
 methods for administration, 933–934
 pump, 932f
 resistance, 916, 929
 shock. *See* Hypoglycemia
 therapy, 933–934
 types and action of, 933, 933t
Intact periodontium, 328
Intellectual disabilities (IDs), 868. *See also* Intellectual disorders
 classification of, 851
 definition of, 850
 etiology of, 851
 factors significant for dental hygiene care, 852
 general characteristics, 852
 models of human functioning and disability, 850
 supportive interventions, 851
 treatment, 852
Intellectual functioning, 851
Intelligence quotient (IQ), 851
Intensity-modulated radiation therapy (IMRT), 946–947
Interdental area, 456, 456f
Interdental biofilm removal, 457
Interdental care
 biofilm removal, 457
 brushes
  care of brushes, 459
  indications for use, 458
  procedure, 458–459, 459f
  types, 457–458, 458f
 dental floss and tape, 459–461, 460–461f
 documentation, 467, 467b
 everyday ethics, 468
 factors to teach patient, 468
 flossing, aids for
  floss holder, 462, 463f
  floss threader, 461–462, 461f
  gauze strip, 462, 463f
  tufted dental floss, 462, 462f
 interdental tip, 464, 464f
 oral irrigation, 466–467, 466–467f
 planning
  dental hygiene care plan, 457
  patient assessment, 456–457
 power flossers, 463–464, 463f
 single-tuft brush, 464, 464f
 toothpick in holder, 465, 465f
 wooden interdental cleaner, 465–466, 465f
Interdental gingiva, 304–305, 306f
Interdental papilla. *See* Interdental gingiva
Interdental tip, 464, 464f

Interdisciplinary team, 842, 845b
Interferon-gamma release assay (IGRA), 1030
Interim therapeutic restoration, 812t
Intermaxillary fixation (IMF), 959–960, 962, 962f
Intermediate-use steam sterilization, 105
Internal bleaching. *See* Nonvital tooth bleaching
Internal validity, 26
International Caries Classification and Management System (ICCMS), 265, 265f, 266, 423, 426, 427, 428f
International Caries Detection and Assessment System (ICDAS), 427
International Federation of Dental Hygienists Code of Ethics, 1105–1106
International normalized ratio (INR), 1063t, 1071
International system. *See* Fédération Dentaire Internationale system
Internet, 24–25, 24b
Interocclusal record, 275, 275f
Interpersonal and social rhythm therapy (IPSRT), 986
Interpreter, 40
Interprofessional collaborative practice, 10, 10b
Interprofessional communication, 42
Interprofessional healthcare teams, 54
Interproximal space, 456
Interventions, 394
Interview, 167
 advantages of, 168
 disadvantages of, 168
 form, 168
 participants, 168
 pointers for, 168
 setting, 168
Intestinal tract, cystic fibrosis and, 1038
Intimate partner violence (IPV), 212
 dental hygienist, role of, 219
 general health consequences of, 219
 orofacial impact of, 219
 physical injury from, 219
 prevalence of, 218–219
Intimate partners, 219
Intranasal dental anesthetic, 638–639
Intraoral surveys. *See specific surveys*
Intratubular dentin, 719
Intrinsic (nonallergic) asthma, 1032
Intrinsic factor (IF), 1066
Intrinsic stains, 293, 747
 endogenous, 297–299, 298f
 exogenous, 299, 299f, 300f
Ionizing radiation, 235
IPSRT (interpersonal and social rhythm therapy), 986
IPV. *See* Intimate partner violence (IPV)
IQ (intelligence quotient), 851
IRB (Institutional Review Board), 30
Iron, 559t
Iron deficiency anemia, 1066
Irradiation, 235
Irreversible tooth damage, 753
Irrigant, 466
Irrigation, oral, 466

Ischemia, 892
 defined, 1050
Ischemic heart disease, 1049–1050
 etiology of, 1050, 1050f
 manifestations of, 1050
Ischemic stroke, 895
Isoniazid (INH), 1031t

J

Jacquettes, 651, 652f
JE (junctional epithelium), 303, 305–306
Journals/magazines, commercial-based, 24
Junctional epithelium (JE), 303, 305–306

K

Kaposi's sarcoma (KS), 77
 –associated herpesvirus, 74–75
Keppra. *See* Levetiracetam
Keratinized epithelium, 307, 456
Ketoacidosis, 927
Ketogenic diet, 973
Ketones, 926
Kidney damage
 drug abuse, 1012
 local anesthesia and, 626
Kilohertz (kHz), 658
Kilovoltage, 233
Klonopin. *See* Clonapam
Knee-to-knee infant examination, 793, 793f
Knots
 characteristics, 706
 management, 706
Korotkoff sounds, 189
Korsakoff's psychosis, 1003
KS. *See* Kaposi's sarcoma (KS)
Kussmaul breathing, 138t
kVp (selector), 227
 advantages of, 233
 affecting radiographic image, 233
 disadvantages of, 233
Kyphosis, 118, 903

L

Lactation, local anesthesia and, 627
Lamotrigine (Lamictal), 973t
Language disorder, 850b
Language proficiency, 40
Laser therapy, 692
Laser treatment, dentinal hypersensitivity, 725
Latent image, 248
Latent tuberculosis infection (LTBI), 1030, 1031t
Lateral pressure, 650
Latex allergy, 93
Latex hypersensitivity, 93–94
Lavage, 655
LDL (low-density lipoprotein), 935
Le Fort classification of facial fractures, 961, 962f
Learning, 406
Legal blindness, 868
Leonard's (or vertical) method, 443–444
Lesions, 319
Leucocytosis, 1069
Leukemia, 946
Leukocytes. *See* White blood cells

Leukocytosis, 1070
Leukopenia, 1069
Leukoplakia, 207
Leukotriene receptor antagonist, for
    asthma, 1034t
Levels of evidence pyramid, 27
Levetiracetam (Keppra), 973t
Levonordefrin (Neo-Cobefrin), 624
Levothyroxine (Synthroid), 913
Libido, 918
Lichenification, 215
Lidocaine HCl, 621, 636–637
Lifestyle, 824
    factors, 398
Ligation, 707
Light-activated bleaching, 752b
Limb-girdle muscular dystrophy, 902
Lips, scars of, 973–974
Listening, 407
Literature review, 23
Liver
    damage, drug abuse, 1012–1013
    disease, alcohol and, 1003
    metabolism, alcohol, 1001
Local anesthesia, 620–621
    advantages, 635
    adverse drug reactions, 634
    amide drugs, 621–623
    armamentarium for
        additional, 629
        C-CLAD System, 629
        cartridge or carpule, 628–629
        needle, 628, 628f
        sequence of syringe assembly, 629,
            629f
        syringe, 627–628, 628f
    clinical procedures for administration
        areas anesthetized, 630, 631f
        aspiration, 632
        injection(s) selection, 630, 630–631t
        sharps management, 632, 632–634f
        steps in administration, 631–632b
    color code for, 629b
    contents of, 621
    criteria for selection, 624
    disadvantages, 635
    documentation, 630b, 639
    duration of, 625t
    ester and amide anesthetic drugs, 621
    factors to teach patient, 639
    indications for, 624
    local complications, 634–635
    patient assessment, 625–626
        allergy, 626
        angina, 627
        atypical plasma cholinesterase, 627
        coronary heart disease, 626
        diabetes, 627
        glaucoma, 627
        heart failure, 626
        heart surgery, 626
        hemophilia, 627
        hypertension, 627
        hyperthyroidism, 626
        impaired liver/kidney function, 626
        malignant hyperthermia, 626
        methemoglobinemia, 626
        myocardial infarction, 626

    potential drug interactions, 627
    pregnancy and lactation, 627
    stroke, 626
prepare for, 684–685
psychogenic reactions, 634
vasoconstrictors, 623–624, 624t
Local delivery agents
    advantages of, 695
    antimicrobials, 695
    chlorhexidine gluconate, 698–699,
        699f
    doxycycline hyclate, 697–698, 698f
    limitations to, 695
    minocycline hydrochloride, 696–697,
        697f
Local enamel hypoplasia, 260
Long-acting beta-2 agonists, for asthma,
    1034t
Long-term care, 47
Lordosis, 118
Lou Gehrig's disease. See Amyotrophic
    lateral sclerosis
Low birth weight, 785
Low-density lipoprotein (LDL), 935
Lower respiratory tract diseases, 1028
LTBI (latent tuberculosis infection),
    1030, 1031t
Lumen, 1050
Luminal. See Phenobarbital
Lung cancer and tobacco use, 534
Luxation, 263
Lymphocytes, 1064
Lymphocytopenia, 1069–1070

M

Machine control devices, 227–228
Macrocephaly, 913
Macroglossia, 852
Macrognathia, 913
Macronutrients, 554
Magnesium, 559t
Magnetostrictive scalers, 656, 657–658,
    658f
Magnification, 120–121
Mainstream smoke, 530
Maintenance appointments
    professional, for implant systems,
        523–524
        continuing care appointment,
            523–524
        frequency of appointments, 523–524
        probing of dental implants, 523, 523f
Major depressive disorder, 984
Malaise, 1027t
Malignant hyperthermia (MH), 626
Malignant neoplasms, 944, 945t
Malnutrition, 560
    effect on immune system, 560
Malocclusion, 269–270, 269f
Malpractice, 158
Mandibular advancement splint (MAS),
    1039, 1039f
Mandibular fractures
    closed reduction, 962
    external skeletal fixation, 963, 963f
    intermaxillary fixation, 962, 962f
    open reduction, 963, 963f

Manual scrubbing, 100
Manufacturer's Safety Data Sheet
    (MSDS), 106
Marijuana abuse, 1006, 1007t, 1009–1010
MAS (mandibular advancement splint),
    1039, 1039f
Masses, 207
Mast cells, 1032
    stabilizers, for asthma, 1034t
Mastalgia, 917
Masticatory forces, 308
Masticatory mucosa, 198
Materia alba, 280
    clinical appearance and content, 286
    prevention, 287
Matrix, 281
Maturation, 281, 575
Maxillofacial prosthetics, 956b
Maxillofacial surgery, 956
    oral and. See Oral and maxillofacial
        surgery
Maximum recommended dose (MRD),
    621
Meal plan, 569
Measles virus (Morbillivirus), 67t
Mechanical dental biofilm control, 436
Media communication, 34
Mediators, 1033
Medical Alert Box, use of, 129
Medical consultation, 176–177
Medical emergency
    emergency reference chart, 138–142t
    report form, 132, 133f
Medical impairment, 866
Medical nutrition therapy, 932–933
Medication-related osteonecrosis of the
    jaw, 946
MEDLINE (PubMed), 25, 25b, 26b
Megaloblastic anemia
    folate-deficiency anemia, 1067
    pernicious anemia, 1066–1067
Meningocele, 903
Menopause, 918–919
Menses, 917
Menstrual cycle, 917, 917f
Mental function, 896b
Mental health disorders
    anxiety disorders
        dental hygiene care, 983–984
        treatment, 983
        types and symptoms of, 982–983
    bipolar disorder, 986
    depressive disorders
        dental hygiene care, 985
        signs and symptoms of, 984
        treatment, 984–985
        types of, 984
    documentation, 994, 994b
    everyday ethics, 995
    factors to teach patient, 995
    feeding and eating disorders
        dental hygiene care, 989–991
        medical complications, 989
        treatment, 989
        types and symptoms of, 987–989
    mental health emergency
        intervention, 993–994
        patients at risk for, 993

preparation for, 993
prevention of, 993
psychiatric, 993
panic attack, symptoms of, 983*b*
prevalence of, 982
schizophrenia
dental hygiene care, 991–993
signs and symptoms of, 991
treatment, 991
Mepivacaine HCl, 622
Mercury sphygmomanometer, 187
Meta-analysis, 27–28
Metabolic syndrome, 319
Metallic stain, 297
Metastasis, 944
Methadone (Dolophine, Methadose), 1014
Methadose. *See* Methadone
Methamphetamine, 1011, 1017*f*
Methemoglobinemia, 626
Methicillin-resistant *Staphylococcus aureus* (MRSA), 79
Methylxanthines, for asthma, 1034*t*
MGJ (mucogingival junction), 306, 307
MH (malignant hyperthermia), 626
MI. *See* Motivational interviewing (MI)
Microabrasion, 752
Microcephalus, 852
Micronutrients, 554
Microorganisms, 281
Micropores, 600
Microstomia, 1082
Microultrasonics, 689–690, 689*f*
Midfacial fractures, 964
Milliammeter, 227
Milliampere seconds, 233–234
Mineralization, 290
Mineralized, biofilm, 287
Miniplate osteosynthesis, 963
Minocycline, 299
    staining, 751
Minocycline hydrochloride, 696–697, 697*f*
Missing teeth, 498
Mitral valve prolapse, 1048
Mixed/transitional dentition, 256, 256*f*
Mobility examination, tooth, 351, 351*f*
Modifiable risks factors, 384
Modified Bass methods, 440–441, 440*f*
Modified pen grasp, 647, 647*f*
Modified Stillman method, 441–442, 441*f*
Moist heat, 104
Monoamine oxidase inhibitors, for depressive disorders, 985
Monocytes, 1064
Monogenic diabetes syndromes, 929
Mononucleosis, 73
Monthly reminder method, 776
Mood stabilizers, for bipolar disorder, 986
Moral, 14
Morphology, 203
Motivation, 406
Motivational interviewing (MI), 34
    basic components of, 408*t*
    clinician checklist of four processes of, 410*b*, 410*f*
    documentation, 418, 418*b*

eliciting and recognizing change talk, 414, 415*b*
    mobilizing change talk, 416, 416t
    preparatory change talk, 415–416
everyday ethics, 418–419
exploring ambivalence
    decisional balance, 413, 413f, 414b
    readiness ruler, 414, 414f, 415b
    sustain talk versus change talk, 413
guiding principles, 409
implementation
    agenda setting, 411
    core skills, 411–413, 412b
    information exchange, 410, 411b
patient teaching, 419
with pediatric patients and caregivers, 417, 417*b*
processes of, 410
spirit, elements of
    acceptance, 408–409
    compassion, 409
    evocation, 409
    partnership, 408
strengthening commitment (the plan), 416, 417*b*
training and coaching, 418
Mouth mirror, 338, 661
    procedure, 338
    purpose and use, 338
Mouthrinses, 293, 724
    American Dental Association Seal of Acceptance Program, 479–480, 481*f*
    commercial ingredients
        active ingredients, 477–478
        contraindications, 478
        inactive ingredients, 478
        patient-specific mouthrinse recommendations, 478
    documentation, 480–481, 481*b*
    emerging alternative practices, 479
    everyday ethics, 481
    factors to teach patient, 482
    fluoride
        benefits, 589
        indications, 588
        limitations, 588
        patient-applied, 589t
        preparations, 588–589
    formulation, 478*t*
    oil pulling, 479
    preventive and therapeutic agents of
        chlorhexidine, 475–476, 476f
        fluoride, 475
        oxidizing agents, 477
        oxygenating agents, 477
        phenolic-related essential oils, 477
        quaternary ammonium compounds, 477
        triclosan, 476
    procedure for rinsing, 478, 479*b*
    purposes and uses of, 475
    United States Food and Drug Administration, 479, 480*t*
MRD (maximum recommended dose), 621
MRSA (methicillin-resistant *Staphylococcus aureus*), 79

MS. *See* Multiple sclerosis (MS)
MSBP (Munchausen syndrome by proxy), 216–217
MSDS (Manufacturer's Safety Data Sheet), 106
Mucogingival deformities, 326–327, 327*f*
Mucogingival examination, 342*f*, 349–351, 350*f*
Mucogingival involvement, periodontal disease, 326–327, 326*f*, 327*f*
Mucogingival junction (MGJ), 306, 307
Mucositis, 56, 449, 560*t*
    prevention/oral health maintenance, 948
    treatment, 948–949
Mucus-secreting goblet cells, 1025
Multidisciplinary team, 151
Multidrug-resistant tuberculosis, 67, 1031
Multifactorial genetic and environmental factors, 843
Multiple sclerosis (MS), 1087*f*
    clinical forms of, 1086
    dental hygiene care, 1088
    etiology of, 1086
    medications used to treat, 1087*b*
    prevalence of, 1086
    symptoms, 1086–1087
    treatment, 1087–1088
Mumps virus (paramyxovirus), 66*t*
Munchausen syndrome by proxy (MSBP), 216–217
Murmurs, 1045
Muscular dystrophies
    Becker, 902
    dental hygiene care, 902
    Duchenne, 901–902
    Emery–Dreifuss, 902
    facioscapulohumeral, 902
    limb-girdle, 902
    medical treatment, 902
    myotonic, 902
    oculopharyngeal and myotonic dystrophies, 902
Musculoskeletal disorders, 116
    affecting dental hygienists, 122*t*
Musculoskeletal effects of drug abuse, 1013
Musculoskeletal impairment, 866
Musculoskeletal system, changes due to aging, 825
Myalgia, 1027*t*
Myasthenia gravis, 1088–1089
Myasthenic crisis, 1088
Mycobacterium tuberculosis, 66*t*, 67, 1032*f*
Mycoplasma, 1028
Myelomeningocele, 902–903
    deformities, types of, 903
    dental hygiene care, 904
    medical treatment
        neurosurgery, 903–904
        orthopedic surgery, 904
    physical characteristics, 903
Myocardial infarction (MI), 140*t*, 626, 1048, 1051–1052
Myocardium, 1044
Myoclonic seizure, 970*t*
Myoclonus, 971
Myotonic dystrophies, 902

Myotonic muscular dystrophy, 902
Mysoline. *See* Primidone
Myxedema coma, 914, 914*b*

N

NAF (neutral sodium fluoride), 582
Naloxone (Narcan), 1010
Naltrexone (Vivitrol/ReVia), 1005, 1014
Narcan. *See* Naloxone
Narrative reviews, 28
Nasal cannula, 131*t*
Nasoalveolar molding technique, 844
Nasopalatal defect, 1016*f*
National Dental Hygienists' Association
    Code of Ethics, 1099
National Institute on Drug Abuse
    (NIDA), 1015
National Institutes of Health, 25*b*
National Standards for Diabetes
    Education and Support guidelines, 930
NCCLs. *See* Noncarious cervical lesions
    (NCCLs)
Necrotizing gingivitis (NG), 77
Necrotizing periodontal diseases (NPDs),
    77, 329, 332–333
Necrotizing stomatitis (NS), 77
Needles
    characteristics, 705–706, 706*f*
    components, 705, 705*f*
Neglect, 212
Neisseria gonorrhoeae, 66*t*
Neonatal herpes, 73
Nephropathy, 935
Nerves, 717
Nervous system, alcohol and, 1003
Neural depolarization mechanism
    (sodium–potassium pump), 717
Neuritis, 1085
Neurodevelopmental disabilities, 850
Neurodevelopmental disorder, 850*b*
    autism spectrum disorder, 856*b*
        approaches to dental care, 858
        characteristics, 856–857
        etiology of, 856
        *factors significant for dental hygiene
            care, 858*
        levels of severity, 857b
        prevalence of, 855–856
        treatment interventions, 857–858
    dental hygiene care, 858–859
        *appointment considerations,
            859–860*
        dental hygiene care plan, 859
        dental staff preparation, 859
        oral health problems, 859
    documentation, 860, 860*b*
    everyday ethics, 860
    factors to teach patient, 860
    fragile X syndrome, 855*f*
        *cognitive and behavioral
            characteristics, 855*
        *comorbidity and health considerations,
            855*
        *factors significant for dental hygiene
            care, 855*
        oral findings, 855
        physical characteristics, 854

intellectual disorders
    classification of, 851
    definition of, 850
    etiology of, 851
    *factors significant for dental hygiene
        care, 852*
    general characteristics, 852
    *models of human functioning and
        disability, 850*
    supportive interventions, 851
    treatment, 852
Down syndrome
    child with, 854f
    *cognitive and behavioral
        characteristics, 853*
    *comorbidity and health considerations,
        853*
    eye characteristics, 853f
    *factors significant for dental hygiene
        care, 854*
    hand, 853f
    oral findings, 853–854
    physical characteristics, 852
Neurologic disorders, 892
Neurologic effects of drug abuse, 1012
Neurologic impairment, 866
Neurologic system
    autoimmune diseases, 1086
        *multiple sclerosis, 1086–1088,
            1087b, 1087f*
        myasthenia gravis, 1088–1089
Neurontin. *See* Gabapentin
Neuropathy, 935
Neutral seated position, 118, 119*f*
Neutral sodium fluoride (NAF), 582
Neutral working position (NWP)
    clinician–patient positioning, 119, 119*f*
    effects of, 118
    neutral seated position, 118, 119*f*
    objectives, 118
Neutral wrist, 647, 648*f*
Neutropenia, 449, 1065, 1069
Neutrophils, 1064–1065
New attachment, 682
NG (necrotizing gingivitis), 77
Niacin, 559*t*
Nicotine, 530
    absorption
        distribution, 531
        intestinal, 533
        in lungs, 531
        oral cavity, 531
    addiction, 536–538
    combination medications therapy, 541
    dependency, 537, 537*b*
    electronic delivery devices of, 533
    free therapy, 541
    gum, 540*t*, 541
    inhaler, 533*f*, 540*t*, 541
    levels of various tobacco products, 531*t*
    lozenge, 533*f*, 540*t*, 541
    metabolism, 530–531
    nasal spray, 540*t*, 541
    patch, 540*t*, 541
    peak blood plasma concentrations for,
        531, 533*f*
    pharmacotherapies used for addiction,
        539–541

second-line medications, 541
    stains, 752
    withdrawal symptoms, 538, 538*t*
Nicotine replacement therapies (NRTs),
    539–541
NIDA (National Institute on Drug
    Abuse), 1015
NIDA Quick Screen, 1015
Nidus, 281
Nitrosamines, 531
Nitrous oxide
    anesthetic, analgesic, and anxiolytic
        properties, 615–616
    blood solubility, 616
    chemical and physical properties, 616
    equipment for, 616
    pharmacology of, 616
Nitrous oxide–oxygen conscious sedation
    anesthesia, 62
    clinical procedures for administration
        completion of sedation, 619–620
        equipment preparation, 618
        patient preparation, 618
        steps in, 618b
        technique for gas delivery, 618–619
    documentation, 619*b*, 639
    equipment for
        compressed gas cylinders, 616
        gas delivery system, 616
        maintenance, 617, 617f
        nasal hood, nose piece, and mask, 616
        safety feature, 617
        scavenger system, 616
    factors to teach patient, 639
    signs and symptoms of, 619*t*
Nocturia, 1052
Non-Hodgkin lymphoma, 77
Non-plaque (biofilm)-induced gingivitis,
    328–329
Nonblisterform lesions, 204, 206*f*
Noncariogenic food, 567
Noncarious and carious lesions
    assessment, 257, 259
Noncarious cervical lesions (NCCLs),
    261
    abfraction, 262–263
    abrasion, 262, 262*f*
    erosion, 262, 262*f*
Noncarious dental lesions, 261
Nondominant hand, 647
Noninjectable anesthesia, 635–636, 637*t*
Noninsulin-dependent diabetes mellitus,
    929
Nonkeratinized mucosa, 305
Nonnutritive sucking, 792, 792*f*, 813*t*
Nonopioid analgesics, 615
Nonrebreather mask, 136*t*
Nonsurgical periodontal therapy (NSPT),
    333, 680, 937
    advanced instrumentation, 686–689
    appointment planning, 682
    calculus removal, 682
        using manual instruments, 687b
    components of, 680, 682
    definitive, 683–684
    dental biofilm removal, 682
    dental hygiene treatment care plan for
        periodontal debridement, 682

documentation, 699, 699b
effects and benefits of, 680–681, 681t
everyday ethics, 700
factors to teach patient, 700
formulate strategy for instrumentation, 686
full-mouth disinfection, 683
indications for use of local delivery agents, 695–696
multiple appointments, 683
outcomes, 680
post-op instruction for periodontal debridement appointments, 692–693
preparation for, 684–686
preventive services, 682
re-evaluation of, 693–694
restorative biofilm-retentive factors, 682
single appointment, 683
specialized debridement instruments
    advanced ultrasonic tips, 689
    endoscope-assisted periodontal debridement, 690–691, 690f
    furcation debridement, 689
    laser therapy, 692
    microultrasonics, 689–690, 689f
    subgingival air polishing, 691–692, 691f
subgingival examination, 685–686, 685f
supragingival examination, 685
treatment goals
    mild-to-moderate periodontitis, 681
    moderate-to-severe periodontitis, 681
    plaque (or biofilm)-induced gingivitis, 681
    poor response to initial or maintenance therapy, 681
    surgical or other advanced periodontal therapy, 682
Nonverbal communication, 34
    and cross-cultural communication, 40, 41t
Nonvital tooth bleaching
    factors associated with efficacy, 757
    history of, 748
    procedure for, 756–757, 756–757b
    vital tooth bleaching vs., 747–748
Nonvocal communication, 34
Normotensive, 190t
Nosocomial pneumonia, 1029, 1029t
Novamin. See Calcium sodium phosphosilicate
NPDs (necrotizing periodontal diseases), 77, 329, 332–333
NRTs (nicotine replacement therapies), 539–541
NS (necrotizing stomatitis), 77
NSPT. See Nonsurgical periodontal therapy (NSPT)
Nurse practitioners, 48
Nursing home–acquired pneumonia, 1029
Nutrients, 554
    relevant to oral health, 558–560t
Nutrition, 554
Nutritional deficiencies, 555
    alcohol and, 1003

and oral manifestations, 560t
    periodontal infections, 560–561
NWP. See Neutral working position (NWP)
Nystagmus, 1001

O
OAT (oral appliance therapy), 1039
Obesity, 319
Object–image receptor distance, 234
Obsessive-compulsive disorder, 982
Obstructive sleep apnea (OSA), 818
Obturator, 503, 844, 844f
    clinical applications, 503
    description, 503
    professional continuing care, 503
    purpose and use, 503
Occlusal brushing, 444–445, 444f
Occlusal plane, 261
Occlusal surveys
    image receptor selection for, 242–243
    mandibular topographic and cross-sectional projection, 246
    maxillary midline topographic projection, 246
    uses and purposes, 245
Occlusal trauma, 274–275
Occlusion, 259–260, 1051
    dynamic or functional, 274
    facial profiles, types of, 270
    factors related to, 156
    malocclusion, 269–270, 269f
    malrelations of groups of teeth
        crossbites, 271, 271f
        edge-to-edge bite, 271, 271f
        end-to-end bite, 271, 271f
        open bite, 271, 271f
        overbite, 272–273, 272f
        overjet, 271–272, 272f
        underjet, 272, 272f
    normal, 269, 269f
    of primary teeth, 273–274, 273f
    trauma from, 274–275
Occupational exposure, 93
    potential hazards of, 620
Occupational postexposure management, 112
Ocular/ophthalmic herpes, 73
Oculopharyngeal dystrophies, 902
Odontogram, 154
Offset blade, 653
OHI-S. See Simplified oral hygiene index (OHI-S)
Older adults
    aging, 824
    biological and chronological age, 824
    chronic conditions associated with aging
        alcoholism, 828–829
        Alzheimer disease, 826–828, 827b, 828b
        cardiovascular disease, 830–831
        osteoarthritis, 828
        osteoporosis, 829–830, 829f
        respiratory disease, 830
        sexually transmitted diseases, 830
    classification by function, 824
    communication skills of, 39, 39b

dental hygiene care for, 834
    assessment, 835
    barriers to care, 835
    dental biofilm control, 835–837, 836t
    dental caries control, 837
    diet and nutrition, 837–838
    periodontal care, 837
    preventive care plan, 835
    xerostomia, relief for, 837
documentation, 838, 838b
everyday ethics, 838
factors to teach patient, 839
normal physiologic aging, 824–825
    cardiovascular system, 825
    central nervous system, 825
    cognitive change, 826, 826t
    endocrine system, 825
    gastrointestinal system, 825
    immune system, 825
    musculoskeletal system, 825
    peripheral nervous system, 825
    respiratory system, 825
    sensory systems, 825
oral changes associated with aging
    periodontium, 832, 834
    soft tissues, 831–832, 832b
    teeth, 832, 833–834f
pathology and disease, 826, 826b
primary, secondary, and optimal aging, 824
OLP (oral lichen planus), 1079–1080, 1080f
Oncology, 944b
Open bite, 271, 271f
Open-ended versus closed questions, 411–412
Open reduction, 963, 963f
Opiate antagonist, 1005
Opioids, 1005
    and morphine derivatives, 1008t, 1010
Opportunistic infectious agents, 72
Optimal aging, 824
Oral and maxillofacial surgery
    alveolar process fracture, 964
    categories of, 956b
    dental hygiene care
        diet, 964–966, 965f, 958
        before general surgery, 966–967
        instrumentation, 964
        personal oral care procedures, 966
        postsurgical care, 959, 959b
        presurgery treatment planning, 957–958
        presurgical instructions, 958–959
        problems, 964
    documentation, 967, 967b
    everyday ethics, 967
    factors to teach patient, 967
    fractured jaw
        causes of, 960
        emergency care, 960
        recognition, 960
        treatment of fractures, 961–962
        types of fractures, 960–961, 961f
    intermaxillary fixation, 959–960
    mandibular fractures
        closed reduction, 962
        external skeletal fixation, 963, 963f

Oral and maxillofacial surgery (continued)
  intermaxillary fixation, 962, 962f
  open reduction, 963, 963f
  midfacial fractures, 964
  patient preparation
    objectives, 956–957
    personal factors, 957
  tray setup for extraction of teeth, 956f
Oral appliance therapy (OAT), 1039
Oral cancer, 206–207
  risk factors for, 384
Oral candidiasis, HIV-associated, 77
Oral cavity
  anatomic landmarks of, 198, 199f, 200b, 200f
  microorganisms of, 62
  Parkinson's disease, 899
  pathogens transmissible from, 65, 65–67t
Oral epithelium, 306
Oral flora, 283
Oral glucose tolerance test, 930
Oral hairy leukoplakia, 73–74
  HIV-associated, 77
Oral health
  advocacy for, 11
  implications of, 924–925
  infants
    anticipatory guidance, 790, 791t
    birth to age 12 months, 791t
    daily oral hygiene care, 790–791
    examination, 793f
    feeding patterns (birth to 1 year), 791–792
    first dental visit, components of, 792–794, 793f
    nonnutritive sucking, 792, 792f
    oral soft and hard tissue conditions/pathology in, 793t
  to overall health, significance of, 49
Oral Health in America, 358
Oral health services, access to, 869, 870t
Oral hygiene status, 359–365
  biofilm control record, 360–361, 360f
  biofilm-free score, 361–362, 361f
  biofilm index, 359–360
  patient hygiene performance, 362–363, 363f
  simplified oral hygiene index, 363–365, 364f
Oral irrigation, 466–467, 466–467f
Oral lichen planus (OLP), 1079–1080, 1080f
Oral malodor (halitosis), 473, 817
Oral microbiome, 264, 281
Oral mucosa, 198
Oral mucositis/stomatitis, 946
Oral self-care, 872b
Oral, Systemic, Capability, Autonomy, and Reality (OSCAR) Planning Guide, 384, 385t
Oral ulcer on tongue, 1032f
Orange stain, 297
Organic content, in calculus, 290
Orthodontic appliances, 844, 846
  band removal, clinical procedures for, 490

bonded brackets
    advantages of, 486
    disadvantages of, 486
    fixed appliance system, 486–487, 486f
    removable aligner system, 487
  cemented bands, 486–487
  clinical procedures for bonding, 487–488
  debonding, clinical procedures for, 490, 490–492f, 491b
  dental hygiene care, 488–490, 489f
  documentation, 493, 494b
  everyday ethics, 494
  factors to teach patient, 494
  orthodontic retention, 493
  postdebonding evaluation
    demineralization, 492
    enamel loss, 492
    etched enamel not covered by adhesive, 493
  postdebonding preventive care, 493
  as predisposing factor for periodontal disease, 322f
Orthodontic retention, 493
Orthodontic therapy, 776
Orthognathic surgeries, 960
Orthorexia nervosa, 989
Orthosis, 895
Orthostatic hypotension, 130
OSA (obstructive sleep apnea), 818
Osseointegrated implant, use of, 845
Osseointegration, 518
Osteoarthritis, older adult, 828
Osteoporosis
  of jaw, 946
  older adult, 829f
    causes of, 829
    medications, 830
    prevention, 829, 830
    relationship to periodontal disease, 829
    risk factors, 829
    symptoms, 829
Osteoradionecrosis, 947
Osteosynthesis, 963
Outcome evaluation, 766, 766t
Over-the-counter (OTC) products, bleaching, 755–756, 756b
Overbite, 272–273, 272f
Overdenture prosthesis, 502, 502f
  implant-supported overdenture, 502
  root-supported overdenture, 502
Overjet, 271–272, 272f
Overlay prosthesis, 501
Ownership, radiographs, 250
Oxalates, 724
Oxcarbazepine (Trileptal), 973t
Oxidizing agents, 477
Oxycodone (OxyContin), 1010
Oxycodone/acetaminophen (Percocet), 1010
Oxycodone/aspirin (Percodan), 1010
OxyContin. See Oxycodone
Oxygen administration
  equipment, 136–137
  oxygen delivery systems, 136f, 136t

oxygen tank, 137b
  positive pressure, 137
  supplemental oxygen, 137
Oxygenating agents, 477

P

Pacifiers, 792, 792f
Pain
  anesthesia reversal agent, 638
  and anxiety control, 398
  buffered local anesthetic, 638
  components of, 614
  control mechanisms
    depressing central nervous system, 615
    new developments, 638
    painful stimulus removal, 615
    pathway of pain message, 615
    prevent pain reaction by raising pain reaction threshold, 615
    psychosedation methods, 615
  documentation, 639
  everyday ethics, 639
  factors to teach patient, 639
  intranasal dental anesthetic, 638–639
  local anesthesia. See Local anesthesia
  nitrous oxide
    anesthetic, analgesic, and anxiolytic properties, 615–616
    blood solubility, 616
    chemical and physical properties, 616
    equipment for, 616
    pharmacology of, 616
  nitrous oxide–oxygen conscious sedation. See Nitrous oxide–oxygen conscious sedation
  noninjectable anesthesia, 635–636, 637t
  nonopioid analgesics, 615
  oxygen, equipment for, 616
  patient selection
    contraindications, 617–618
    indications, 617
  perception, 614
  potential hazards of occupational exposure, 620
  reaction, 614
  threshold, 614
  topical anesthesia. See Topical anesthesia
Palliative care, 49, 1080
Palliative/palliation, 945
Pallidotomy, 899
Palm grasp, 647, 647f
Palmer Notation System, 153–154, 153f
Palpation, 196
  bidigital, 196, 196f
  bilateral, 197
  bimanual, 196–197, 197f
  digital, 196
Pancreas, 916
  cystic fibrosis and, 1038
Pancytopenia, 948
PANDA (Prevent Abuse and Neglect through Dental Awareness), 220
Pandemic, 75
Panic disorder, 982, 983b

Panoramic radiographic images
  limitations of, 246–247
  procedures, 247
  technique, 246
  uses of, 246, 247b
Papillae, 198, 198f
Papillary, defined, 206
Parafunctional contacts, occlusion, 274
Paralysis, 892, 896b
Parathyroid glands, 914
  hyperparathyroidism, 915
  hypoparathyroidism, 915
Parathyroid hormone (PTH), 914
Parental attitude, 216
Parenteral, HIV transmission, 75
Parents teaching, 820
Paresthesia, 139t, 634–635
Parkinson-like syndrome, 992t
Parkinson's disease
  characteristics, 899
  dental hygiene care, 899
  occurrence, 898–899
  treatment, 899
Parotid gland, 990
Paroxysmal, 970
Paroxysmal pain, 140t, 970
Partial defluoridation, 579
Partnership, motivational interviewing
    and, 408
Parts per million (ppm), 577
Passive smoke, 535
Patch, 207
Patent, 723
Patent ductus arteriosus, 1046, 1047f
Pathogen, 77
Pathogenic microorganisms, 283, 286
Pathognomonic, intellectual disorders,
    852
Pathognomonic of abuse, 215
Pathologic migration, 274
Pathophysiology, 1032
Patient-centered oral health goals, 397
Patient counseling, 406–407
Patient history
  American Society of Anesthesiologists
      Determination, 179
  application of
    medical consultation, 176–177
    prophylactic premedication, 178, 178b
    radiation, 178
  documentation, 180, 180–181b
  everyday ethics, 181
  factors to teach patient, 181
  interview, 167
    advantages of, 168
    disadvantages of, 168
    form, 168
    participants, 168
    pointers for, 168
    setting, 168
  introduction to patient, 165
  items included in, 168
    dental history, 169, 169–170t
    medical history, 170–175, 170–174t,
        176f
    psychosocial history, 175–176, 175t,
        177f
  limitations of, 165

methods for preparation, 164
pretreatment antibiotic prophylaxis
    AHA guidelines, 178–179
    medical conditions, 179, 179b
    recommendations based on principles,
        179
    recommended antibiotic protocol,
        179, 180t
  purpose of, 164
  questionnaire
    advantages of, 166
    disadvantages of, 167
    questions, types of, 165–166, 166f,
        167f
  record forms, 164–165
  review and update of, 180
  significance of, 164
Patient hygiene performance (PHP), 362
  of mandibular molars, 362
  of maxillary molars, 362
  procedure, 362
  purpose, 362
  scoring, 363
    calculation and interpretation, 363
    debris score for individual tooth, 363
    PHP for group, 363
    PHP for individual, 363
  selection of teeth and surfaces,
      363–364
Patient motivation
  behavior change and
    health behavior change model, 407,
        407t
    health behavior change, motivation
        for, 408
    transtheoretical model, 408
Patient reception
  documentation, 124, 125b
  and ergonomic practice
    ergonomic dental hygiene, scope of,
        121
    ergonomic risk factors, 122, 123t
    factors to consider for, 121b
    related occupational problems, 122,
        122t
    self-care for dental hygienist,
        123–124
  escort patient to dental chair, 116
  everyday ethics, 124
  factors to teach patient, 124
  neutral working position
    clinician–patient positioning, 119,
        119f
    effects of, 118
    neutral seated position, 118, 119f
    objectives, 118
  position of clinician, 118
  position of patient
    dental chair, 117–118
    semi-upright, 116, 117f
    supine, 117, 117f
    trendelenburg, 117, 117f
    upright, 116, 117f
  preparation for patient, 116
  treatment area
    clinician's chair, 120
    cords, 121
    handpieces, 121

    lighting, 120, 120f
    magnification, 120–121
Patient records, 150
  components of, 150
  electronic records, 150–151
  handwritten records, 150
  purposes and characteristics of, 150
Patient-specific dental hygiene care plan,
    395, 396–397f
Patient teaching, 760
  anxiety and pain control, 639
  autoimmune disease, 1092
  bleaching of tooth, 759, 759b
  blood disorder, 1074
  cancer, 953
  cardiovascular disease, 1058
  cleft lip and/or palate, 848
  continuing care, 777
  dental caries, 430
  dental deposits, 301
  dental hygiene care, 57
  dental hygiene care plan, 402
  dental hygiene diagnosis, 391
  dental implants, 526
  dental radiographic imaging, 253
  dentinal hypersensitivity, 727
  diabetes mellitus, 940
  diet and dietary analysis, 570
  disabilities, 889
  documentation, 159
  emergency care, 144
  endocrine gland disorders, 920
  evaluation, 770
  evidence-based dental hygiene, 31
  exposure control, 94
  extraoral and intraoral examination,
      208–209
  extrinsic stain removal, 744
  family violence, 222
  fluorides, 594
  hard tissue examination, 277
  health communication, 43
  indices, 378
  infection control, 80
    clinical procedures, 113
  instrument care and sharpening, 676
  instruments and principles for
      instrumentation, 664
  interdental care, 468
  mental health disorders, 995
  motivational interview, 419
  mouthrinse, 482
  neurodevelopmental disorder, 860
  nonsurgical periodontal therapy, 700
  older adults, 839
  oral and maxillofacial surgery, 967
  orthodontic appliances, 494
  patient history, 181
  patient reception and ergonomic
      practice, 124
  periodontal disease, 333
  periodontal examination, 356
  periodontium, 315
  physical impairment, 908
  pregnancy, 794–795
  professional dental hygienist, 16
  prosthesis, 514
  respiratory disease, 1040–1041

Patient teaching (continued)
  sealants, 609
  seizure disorder, 979
  substance-related disorder, 1020
  sutures and dressings, 713
  tobacco use, 547
  toothbrush selection and
    toothbrushing method, 452
  vital signs, 192
Patient visits
  progress notes, 157, 158b
  purpose of, 157
  risk reduction and legal considerations,
    158–159
  SOAP approach, 157–158, 158b, 158t
Patient's rights, 14
PDD-NOS (pervasive developmental
  disorder, not otherwise specified), 856b
PDL. See Periodontal ligament (PDL)
Pediatric dentistry, specialty of, 800
Pediatric OSA, 818
Pediatrics
  adolescents, 805
    psychosocial development of, 805t
  American Academy of Pediatric
    Dentistry, 800
  anticipatory guidance, 814
    accident and injury prevention, 817
    dietary and feeding pattern
      recommendations, 815–816
    digit habits, 817, 817f
    oral health considerations for
      adolescents, 818
    oral health considerations for toddlers/
      pre-schoolers, 816
    oral malodor (halitosis), 817
    referral, 818
    6 years of age to adolescent, 815t
    speech and language development,
      816f, 817
    tobacco/obstructive sleep apnea/
      piercings/substance abuse, 818
    12 months to 6 years of age,
      812–813t
  barriers to dental care, 800
  caries risk assessment
    classification of, 810–811
    early childhood caries, 811, 814
    levels, 811b
    principles, 809–810
    and protective factors to assess at each
      dental visit, 810t
    purpose, 809, 811f
    steps, 810, 812–813t
    white-spot lesions, 814f
  child dental visits, 800–801
  child development, 12 months to 5
    years, 803–805t
  child-friendly substitution words for
    dental terminology, 801b
  dental home, 800
  dental hygiene visit, components of,
    805
    child and family medical/dental
      history, 806
    dental hygiene treatment, 808
    dentition, occlusion, and
      temporomandibular, 806–807

  dietary assessment, 808
  initial interview/new patient visit, 806
  intraoral and extraoral examination,
    806
  prevention, 808–809
  primary teeth, developmental
    disturbance of, 807f
  radiographic assessment, 807–808
  second primary molar, premature loss
    of, 807f
  tooth development and eruption, 806
dentifrices, 474
documentation, 819, 819b
everyday ethics, 819–820
factors to teach parents, 820
motivational interview, 417, 417b
oral soft and hard tissue conditions/
  pathology in children 6 months to
  5 years, 802t
periodontal risk assessment, 809
preschoolers, 801
school-age children, 801–805
specialty of pediatric dentistry, 800
toddlers, 801
treatment planning and consent, 819
Pedunculated lesion, 204
Peer-reviewed (refereed) publications, 24
Percocet. See Oxycodone/acetaminophen
Percodan. See Oxycodone/aspirin
Percutaneous coronary intervention, 1054
Peri-implant care, 522–523
Peri-implant mucositis, 524–525
Peri-implantitis, 525, 696
Periapical surveys
  bisecting-angle technique, 245
  image receptor selection for, 242
  paralleling technique
    features of, 244
    image receptor placement and central
      ray angulation, 243–244, 243f,
      244b
    patient position, 243
Perimolysis, 990, 991
Periodontal abscess, 332
Periodontal care, 837
Periodontal chart form, 348f
Periodontal debridement, 680
Periodontal disease
  acute periodontal lesions
    endo-periodontal lesions, 333
    necrotizing periodontal diseases,
      332–333
    periodontal abscess, 332
  association with systemic conditions,
    384
  classification of, 386, 386t, 388
  complications resulting from
    progression
    furcation involvement, 325, 325f,
      326f
    mucogingival involvement, 326–327,
      326f, 327f
  description of past and current
    conditions, 386
  development, recurrence of, 775
  diabetes mellitus and, 925
  documentation, 333, 334b
  etiology of, 318–319

  everyday ethics, 333
  factors to teach patient, 333
  gingival pocket or pseudopocket, 324,
    325f
  gingivitis, classification of, 328–329,
    332f
  individual risk factors for, 384
  parameters of care, 387t, 388
  pathogenesis of
    acute inflammatory response, 323
    gingival and periodontal infection,
      323–324
  periodontal health, classification of,
    328, 332f
  periodontal pocket, 324, 325f
  periodontal-systemic disease
    connection, 318
  periodontitis, 329–330, 332f
    clinical changes in, 318f
    as manifestation of systemic disease,
      329
    necrotizing periodontitis, 329
    terminology for grading, 331–332,
      331f
    terminology for staging, 330–331,
      330f
  recognition of gingival and
    periodontal infections
    clinical examination, 327
    signs and symptoms, 327
    tissue changes, causes of, 327–328
  remission, 328
  risk assessment, 318
  risk factors
    local factors, 320–323, 321f, 322f
    modifiable risk factors, 319–320,
      319f, 320f
    nonmodifiable risk factors, 320
  severity of, 156
  stability, 328
  tooth surface irregularities, 324–325
Periodontal dressings
  characteristics of, 709, 710, 711f
  chemical-cured dressing, 709
  collagen dressing, 710
  documentation, 713, 713b
  everyday ethics, 713
  factors to teach patient, 713
  follow-up, 711
  material, characteristics of, 709
  patient dismissal and instructions, 710,
    712t
  patient examination, 710
  patient oral self-care instruction,
    710–711
  placement, 710
  procedure for removal, 710
  purposes and uses, 709
  replacement procedure, 710
  visible light–cure dressing, 709
  zinc oxide with eugenol dressing, 709
Periodontal examination
  air-water syringe, 338–339
  care for, 345–353
    clinical attachment level, 349
    fremitus, 351–352
    furcation examination, 352–353
    mobility examination, 351

mucogingival examination, 349–351,
    350f
  probing procedure, 345–349
documentation, 355, 355b
everyday ethics, 356
explorers, 339–340
  procedures for, 339–340
  purpose and use, 339
  subgingival procedures, 340
  supragingival procedures, 340
  usage of special, 339
factors to teach patient, 356
instruments required for, 338
mouth mirror, 338
  procedure, 338
  purpose and use, 338
preliminary assessment prior to,
  344–345
  dental and psychosocial history, 345
  dental examination, 345
  extraoral/intraoral examination, 345
  hard and soft deposits, 345
  medical history, 345
  radiographic examination, 345
  risk assessment, 345
  vital signs, 345
probe, 340–344
  guide to, 343–344
  manual, description of, 343
  purpose and use, 342
  types of, 341–342f, 342–343, 343t
radiographic changes, 353–355
  bone level, 353, 353f
  crestal lamina dura, 354, 354f
  furcation involvement, 354, 354f
  periodontal ligament space, 354–355
  shape of remaining bone, 353, 354f
radiographic findings, 355
  calculus, 355
  overhanging restorations, 355
Periodontal files, 654–655
Periodontal flap procedure, 975
Periodontal health, classification of, 328,
  332f
Periodontal infections, 785
  and diet, 560–561
  nutritional deficiencies and, 560–561,
    560t
  obesity and, 561
Periodontal instruments
  adaptation, 648f
  assessment, 644
  classification of, 644
  cumulative trauma
    preventing, 662, 662–663f
    risk factors for, 662
  curets
    advanced area-specific, 653–654,
      653f
    area-specific, 653
    blade, parts of, 646f
    design, 652
    internal angles of, 652f
    -specific instrumentation, 654
    universal, 653, 653f
    uses of, 652
  design, 644, 645–646, 645f
    name, 644

number, 644
dexterity development
  exercises for, 661f
  mouth mirror and cotton pliers,
    661–662
  pen/pencil exercises, 661
  squeezing, 660
  stretching, 660–661
  tactile sensitivity, increasing, 662,
    662f
documentation, 663, 663b
everyday ethics, 663–664
factors to teach patient, 664
finishing files, 654–655, 655f
handle, 645, 645f
identification of, 644
parts of, 645f
periodontal files, 654–655
powered instrumentation technique,
  659–660, 659f, 660f
powered instruments, 655–657, 655f,
  657f
removal, 644
scalers
  design of, 651
  internal angles of, 651f
  magnetostrictive, 657–658, 658f
  piezoelectric, 658, 658f
  sonic, 657
  -specific instrumentation, 652
  types of, 651, 652f
  uses of, 651
shank, 645–646
working end, 646
working files, 654, 654f
Periodontal ligament (PDL), 307–308,
  307f
  gingival fiber groups, 308, 308f
  principal fiber groups, 308, 308f
Periodontal maintenance (PM), 774
  criteria for referral during, 776
  purposes and outcomes of, 774b
Periodontal pocket, 324, 325f
Periodontal probe, 340–344, 341f
  circumferential, 347
  guide to, 343–344
  insertion, 345–346
  manual, description of, 343
  measurment, 346–347
  purpose and use, 342
  sources of error in, 349
  types of, 341–342f, 342–343, 343t
Periodontal records, 155–156
  charting, 156
  deposits, 156
  gingiva, clinical observations of,
    155–156
  occlusion, factors related to, 156
  periodontal disease, severity of, 156
  radiographic findings, 156
Periodontal risk assessment (PRA), 318,
  809
Periodontal risk calculator (PRC), 318
Periodontal screening and recording
  (PSR), 365–366, 366f, 809
  calculation and interpretation, 366
  procedure
    criteria, 366

  probe application, 365–366
  recording, 365–366
  WHO Periodontal Probe, 365, 366f
  purpose, 365
  scoring, 366
  selection of teeth, 365
Periodontal surgery, 314–315, 956
  toothbrushing after, 449
Periodontal-systemic disease connection,
  318
Periodontitis, 329–330, 332f, 388, 925
  clinical changes in, 318f
  as manifestation of systemic disease,
    329
  necrotizing periodontitis, 329
  nonsurgical periodontal therapy, 681
  risk factors for, 809
  terminology for grading, 331–332, 331f
  terminology for staging, 330–331, 330f
  in tobacco users, 536
Periodontium, 303
  alveolar bone, 309
  cementum, 308–309, 309f
  changes associated with aging, 832,
    834
  documentation, 315, 315b
  everyday ethics, 315
  factors to teach patient, 315
  gingiva
    alveolar mucosa, 307
    attached gingiva, 306–307
    free gingiva, 303–304
    gingival sulcus, 304
    gingival tissues, 304f, 305f
    interdental gingiva, 304–305, 306f
    junctional epithelium, 305–306
    mucogingival junction, 307
    parts of, 304f, 307f
    after periodontal surgery, 314–315
    of young children, 314
  gingival description, 309
    bleeding, 314
    color, 311, 311f
    consistency, 312–313, 313f
    exudate, 314
    gingival clinical markers, 309–310t
    position, 313
    shape, 311–312, 312f
    size, 311
    surface texture, 313
  periodontal ligament, 307–308, 307f
    gingival fiber groups, 308, 308f
    principal fiber groups, 308, 308f
Peripheral nervous system, changes due to
  aging, 825
Peripheral neuropathy, 935
Peritubular dentin, 719
Permanent dentition, 256, 257t
Permanent teeth
  average measurements of, 1117
  dental caries, 578–579
  development and eruption, 257t
Permeable, 323
Pernicious anemia, 1066–1067
Personal factors, 896b
Personal protection for dental team, 84
Personal protective equipment (PPE), 107
Personal supervision, 7b

Pervasive developmental disorder, not otherwise specified (PDD-NOS), 856b
Pervasive impairment, 856b
Petechiae, 206, 1069
Petit mal, 971
Phagocytosis, 1064
Pharyngitis/tonsillitis, 1027t
Phenobarbital (Luminal), 973t
Phenolic-related essential oils, 477
Phenytoin (Dilantin), 973t
    -induced gingival enlargement, 974f
    -induced gingival overgrowth, 975f
    therapy, 977
Phosphorus, 284, 559t
Photons, 227
Photopolymerized, 601
PHP. See Patient hygiene performance (PHP)
Physical abuse, 213t, 217
Physical activity, 933
Physical dependence, 1001
Physical disability, 776, 868
Physical impairment
    amyotrophic lateral sclerosis, 898
    arthritis
        degenerative joint disease, 904–905, 905f
        dental hygiene care, 905
    Bell's palsy, 897
    cerebral palsy, 899–900
        accompanying conditions, 900
        classifications of, 900
        dental hygiene care, 901
        medical treatment, 900
        oral characteristics, 901
    cerebrovascular accident, 896f
        categories and purposes of medications used to treat, 897b
        dental hygiene care, 897
        etiologic factors, 895–896
        medical treatment, 896–897
        signs and symptoms, 896, 896b
    dental hygiene care
        assistance for the ambulatory patient, 906
        considerations during clinical care, 906
        four-handed dental hygiene, 906
        patient positioning and body stabilization, 906
        personal factors affecting self-care, 906–907
        preparation for appointments, 905–906
        residence-based delivery of care, 907
        wheelchair transfer, 906
    documentation, 907, 907b
    everyday ethics, 907
    factors to teach patient, 908
    muscular dystrophies
        Becker, 902
        dental hygiene care, 902
        Duchenne, 901–902
        Emery–Dreifuss, 902
        facioscapulohumeral, 902
        limb-girdle, 902
        medical treatment, 902
        myotonic, 902

    oculopharyngeal and myotonic dystrophies, 902
    myelomeningocele, 902–903
        deformities, types of, 903
        dental hygiene care, 904
        medical treatment, 903–904
        physical characteristics, 903
    neurologic disorders, 892
    Parkinson's disease
        characteristics, 899
        dental hygiene care, 899
        occurrence, 898–899
        treatment, 899
    postpolio syndrome, 899
    spinal cord injury, 892–893
        characteristics/effects of, 893
        dental hygiene care, 895
        levels of, 894f
        mouth-held implements, 895
        occurrence, 893
        potential secondary complications, 893–895
Physical neglect, 214t, 217
Pica, 987
PICO criteria, 21, 22t
PID. See Position-indicating device (PID)
Piercings, 818
Piezoelectric scalers, 656, 658, 658f
Pigmentation, 207
Pigtail or Cowhorn explorer, 339, 339f
Pipe tobacco, 533
Pit and fissure sealant, 876
    placement of, 732
Pituitary gland, 913
Pituitary tumors, 913
Pixels, 229
Placenta previa, 535
Plain language, 34
Planktonic bacteria, 281, 282
Planktonic microorganisms, 65
Plaque (biofilm)-induced gingivitis, 328
Plaque control record. See Biofilm control record
Plaque-free score. See Biofilm-free score
Plaque index (PL I), 359
Plasma, 1062
Plastic testing stick, 670, 670f
Platelets
    count, 1063t
    decrease in, 1070
    disorders
        platelet dysfunction, 1070
        reactive thrombocytosis, 1070
        thrombocytopenia, 1070
    dysfunction, 1070
    overproduction of, 1070
    reference values, 1064t
Pleura, 1024
PM. See Periodontal maintenance (PM)
Pneumonia
    categories and role of oral bacteria, 1029
    community-acquired, 1029
    dental hygiene care, 1029
    etiology of, 1028–1029
    fungal, 1028–1029
    healthcare-associated (nosocomial), 1029

    hospital-acquired, 1029
    medical management of, 1029
    nursing home–acquired, 1029
    symptoms of, 1029
    viral vs. bacterial, 1028, 1029t
Pneumothorax, 1037b
Pocket depth (PD), 343f
Pocket epithelium, 323
Pocket reduction surgery, 314, 314f
Poliovirus types 1, 2, 3, 66t
Polishing, 730
    agents, 730, 733–734
    air-powder, 739–741, 739f, 740–741b, 742t
    coronal, 735–736
    effect on gingiva, 731
    effect on teeth, 730–731
    porte polisher, 743
    proximal surfaces, 741–742
        dental tape and floss, 742
        finishing strips, 742–743
    proximal surfaces, 741–743
    science of, 730
Polyarthritis, 904
Polycystic ovarian syndrome, 928
Polycythemia vera (primary polycythemia), 1069
Polydipsia, 930
Polymer, 600
Polymerization, 601
Polyp, 206
Polyphagia, 930
Polypharmacy, 826
Polyuria, 930
Portable oxygen tank, use of, 1036f
Porte polisher, 743
Position-indicating device (PID), 234
    type of, 237
Post hoc fallacy, 27
Postdebonding evaluation
    demineralization, 492
    enamel loss, 492
    etched enamel not covered by adhesive, 493
Postdebonding preventive care, 493
Postictal phase, 971, 978
Postmydriatic spectacles, 87, 88f
Postpartum depression (PPD), 984
Postpolio syndrome, 899
Postprandial, 938b
Postsurgical dental care, 1056
Posttransplantation diabetes mellitus (PTDM), 930
Posttraumatic stress disorder (PTSD), 982–983
Postural hypotension, 118, 190t
Potassium nitrate, 749
Potassium salts, 723
Potency, 620
Power-driven instruments
    handpiece, 736
    prophylaxis angles
        attachments, 737, 737f
        types of, 736–737, 736t, 737f
        uses for attachments, 737–738
Power-driven/mechanical sharpening devices, 669
Power flossers, 463–464, 463f

Power toothbrush, 434
Powered instrumentation technique, 659–660, 659f, 660f
Powered instruments, 655–657, 655f, 657f. *See also specific types*
PPE (personal protective equipment), 107
PRA (periodontal risk assessment), 318, 809
PRC (periodontal risk calculator), 318
Prebook/preschedule method, 776
Preclinical trials (in vitro and in vivo), 29
Prediabetes, 928
  management of, 930
Pregnancy
  alcohol use during, 1004
  complications, diabetes mellitus, 935
  dental biofilm control, 788
  dental caries control, 789
  depression during, 789–790
  diet, 788–789
  documentation, 794, 794b
  domestic violence, 790
  everyday ethics, 794
  factors to teach patient, 794–795
  fetal development
    drugs of abuse and dependence, 784
    factors harming fetus, 782–784
    first trimester, 782
    herbal dietary supplements, 784
    infections and, 782
    pharmacological considerations for, 782–784, 783t
    second and third trimesters, 782
  fluoride program, 789
  local anesthesia and, 627
  oral findings during
    enamel erosion, 785
    gingival conditions, 784
    gingival enlargement, 785, 785f
    gingivitis, 784–785
    periodontal infections, 785
  patient care, aspects of
    assessment, 785–786
    dental hygiene care, 787–788
    overall treatment considerations, 786–787
    prenatal patient, appointment adaptations for, 787t
    radiography, 786
  positions during, 788f
  "pyogenic" granuloma, 785, 785f
  transitioning to infancy, 790
Premaxillary region, 842
Premedication, 130, 180
Premenstrual syndrome, 917
Premonitory dizziness, 139t
Prenatal care, 782
Prenatal effects of drug abuse, 1013
Preschoolers, 800, 801
  communication skills of, 37–38
  dietary and feeding pattern recommendations, 815
  oral health considerations for, 816, 817f
Prescription (Rx), 587
  drug abuse, 1005
    risk management for, 1005–1006
  drug monitoring programs, 1006

Preservatives, 474
Presurgical dental care, 1055–1056
Prevent Abuse and Neglect through Dental Awareness (PANDA), 220
Prevented fraction, 582
Preventive counseling, 406
Preventive program, 406
Prilocaine HCl, 622–623
Primary (deciduous) dentition, 256
Primary aging, 824
Primary herpetic gingivostomatitis, 72
Primary teeth
  average measuraements of, 1118
  dental caries, 579
  occlusion
    malocclusion of, 274
    normal, 273, 273f
Primate space, 273
Primidone (Mysoline), 973t
Principal fiber groups, 308, 308f
Prioritize, 394
Pristine periodontal health, 328
Probability value (p-value), 26
Probing depth (PD), 304, 342
Probing procedure, 345–349
Process evaluation, 766, 766t
Prodrome, 976b
Profession of dental hygiene, 4, 4–5b, 6f
Professional dental hygienist
  code of ethics, 13
  core values, 13
    ethical duty, 14
    patient first, 14
    personal values, 14
    in professional practice, 13, 13b
  dental hygiene ethics, 13
  dental hygiene practice, 4–5
    advanced practice dental hygiene, 9–10
    alternative practice settings, 8, 9f
    clinical services, types of, 6, 8, 8b
    dental hygiene specialties, 8
    dental hygienist, role of, 5–6, 7t
    interprofessional collaborative patient care, 10–11, 10b
    oral health, advocacy for, 11
    patient education, 8
    supervision and scope of, 6, 7b
  dental hygiene process of care, 11
    assessment, 12
    components of, 12f
    dental hygiene care plan, 12
    dental hygiene diagnosis, 12, 12b
    evaluation, 12
    implementation, 12
    purposes of, 12
  dental hygiene profession, 4, 4–5b, 6f
  ethical applications, 14–15, 14b
  everyday ethics, 15
  factors to teach patient, 16
  legal factors in practice, 15
  objectives for, 11
  professionalism, 15–16
  standards for, 11
Professional journals, 24
Professional topical fluoride
  applications, 582t
    compounds, 582–583

    historical perspectives, 581
    indications, 582
  clinical procedures
    objectives, 583, 583b
    patient and/or parent counseling, 584
    preparation of teeth for topical application, 583–584
    silver diamine fluoride, 586, 587t
    tray technique, 584, 584t, 585–586f
    varnish technique, 584, 585t
Professionalism, 15–16
Progestin, 918
Prognosis, dental hygiene, 388–389
  criteria for various prognoses, 389, 389b
  factors in assigning, 389
Progress notes, 157, 158b
Prolapse, 1048
Prolonged exposure (PE) therapy, 983
Prophylactic antibiotic premedication, 164, 179, 1055
Prophylactic premedication, 178, 178b
Prophylaxis angle
  attachments, 737, 737f
  effects on tissues, 738
  procedure, 738–739
  types of, 736–737, 736t, 737f
  use of, 738–739
Prostaglandin synthesis, 615
Prosthesis, 845
  complete denture, 501–502
    components of, 501–502
    patient self-care procedures for, 510–511
    professional care procedures for, 509–510
    types of, 501
  complete overdenture, 502
    implant-supported overdenture, 502
    root-supported overdenture, 502
  denture-induced oral mucosal lesions (OMLs), 511–513
    contributing factors, 511–512
    types of, 512–513
  denture marking for identification, 503–504
    criteria for, 504
    inclusion methods, 504
    information to include, 504
    surface markers, 504
  documentation, 513, 513–514b
  edentulous mouth, 498–499
    bone, 498
    mucous membrane, 498–499
  everyday ethics, 514
  factors to teach patient, 514
  fixed
    patient self-care procedures for, 505–506
    professional care procedures for, 505
  fixed partial denture, 499–500
    criteria for, 500
    description, 499–500
    types, 500
  missing teeth, 498
  obturator, 503
    clinical applications, 503
    description, 503

Prosthesis (*continued*)
  professional continuing care, 503
  purpose and use, 503
  purpose of wearing, 499
  removable partial denture, 500, 501*f*
    description, 500
    types of, 500
  removal partial
    patient self-care procedures for, 507–509
    professional care procedures for, 506–507
Prosthodontics, 845–846
Protective clothing, 85, 85*f*
Protective eyewear, 86
  face shield, 87
  general features of, 87
  indications for use of, 87
  suggestions for clinical application, 87
  types of, 87, 88*f*
Proteins, 285
Prothrombin time (PT), 1063*t*
Provisional prosthesis, 501
Proximal contacts, occlusion, 274
Proximal surface probing, 344*f*
Pseudohypertrophic muscular dystrophy. *See* Duchenne muscular dystrophy (DMD)
Pseudomembrane, 206
Pseudopocket, 324, 325*f*
PSR. *See* Periodontal screening and recording (PSR)
Psychiatric emergency, 993
Psychoactive drug, 542
Psychogenic reaction, 634
Psychological abuse, 218
Psychological neglect, 218
Psychosedation methods, 615
Psychosocial factors, 320
Psychotherapy, for depressive disorders, 985
PT (prothrombin time), 1063*t*
PTDM (posttransplantation diabetes mellitus), 930
PTH (parathyroid hormone), 914
Ptosis, 1088
PTSD (posttraumatic stress disorder), 982–983
Puberty
  patient management considerations, 917
  pubertal changes, 916–917
  stages of adolescence, 916
Pulmonary diseases, due to tobacco use, 534
Pulmonary hypertension, 1037*b*
Pulp vitality testing
  causes of loss of vitality, 268
  electrical pulp tester, 268*f*, 269
  indications for, 268
  response to pulp testing, 268
  thermal pulp testing, 268
Pulpless/traumatized teeth, 297–298
Pulse
  normal, maintenance of, 185
  pressure, 187
  procedure for determining rate, 185–186, 186*f*

Pulse oximetry, for respiratory disease, 1025–1026, 1026*f*
Pumice, 734
Punctate, 206
Pupils, Examination of, 1016*f*
Purging-type eating disorders, oral manifestations of, 990*f*
Purified protein derivative (PPD) test, 1030
Purpura, 1070
Purulent, defined, 206
"Pyogenic" granuloma, 785, 785*f*
Pyostomatitis vegetans, 1085, 1085*f*
Pyrazinamide (PZA), 1031*t*
Pyrexia, 184
Pyridoxine, 559*t*
Pyrophosphate salts, 290

Q

Quasi-experimental research, 27
Quaternary ammonium compounds, 477
Questionnaire
  advantages of, 166
  culture oriented, 165–166
  disadvantages of, 167
  disease oriented, 165
  questions, types of, 165–166, 166*f*, 167*f*
  symptom oriented, 165
  system oriented, 165
Quid, 297, 531
Quorum sensing, 282

R

RA (rheumatoid arthritis), 1080–1081, 1081*f*
Raccoon sign, 215
Radiation, 178, 226
  assessment, 239, 240–241*t*
  clinician protection
    from leakage radiation, 237
    from primary radiation, 237
    from secondary radiation, 237–238, 237f
  exposure, 235–236, 236*t*
  factors influencing biologic effects of, 235*b*
  ionizing radiation, 235
  patient protection
    body shields, 238
    collimation, 238
    filtration, 238
    image receptors, 238
    processing, 238
    protective apron, 238, 238f
    thyroid cervical collar, 238, 239f
    total exposure, 238
  protection, rules for, 237
  quantity of, 233–234
  risk of injury from, 237–241
  risk reduction, 239, 241
  sensitivity of cells, 236–237, 236*b*
  units, 236*t*
Radiation therapy, 944
  doses, 947
  indications, 946
  oral care protocol, 949, 951
  oral complications, 947, 947*f*

  systemic effects, 947
  types, 946–947, 947*f*
Radiographic changes
  periodontal examination, 353–355
    bone level, 353, 353f
    crestal lamina dura, 354, 354f
    furcation involvement, 354, 354f
    periodontal ligament space, 354–355
Radiographic charting, 154–155
Radiographic image, 226, 231
Radiographic survey, 231
Radiography, 229
Radiology, 226
Radiolucency, 231
Radiopacity, 231
Radium, 947
Rampant caries, 267
Randomized controlled trial (RCT), 28, 722
Rare earth intensifying screens, 246
Rathke cleft cysts, 913
RCI. *See* Root caries index (RCI)
RCT (randomized controlled trial), 28, 722
RDAs (recommended dietary allowances), 554
Reactive thrombocytosis, 1070
Readiness ruler, 414, 414*f*, 415*b*
Recommended dietary allowances (RDAs), 554
Record keeping, comprehensive, 137
Red areas of cancer, 207
Red blood cells, 1062, 1062*f*
  anemia caused by diminished production of, 1065
  reference values, 1064*t*
Red stain, 297
Reduced periodontium, 328
Reflective listening, 411, 412, 413–414*b*
Refractory, 695, 775
Registered dietitian, 562
Regulated waste, 111
Rehabilitation, 842
Relapse, 947
Reliability, 20
Remineralization, 422, 423, 423*f*, 575, 576–577, 576*f*
Remissions, 947
Remote supervision, 7*b*
Removable partial denture prosthesis, 500, 501*f*
  description, 500
  patient self-care procedures for, 507–509
  professional care procedures for, 506–507
  types of, 500
Repetitive stress injuries, 116
Reproductive system, alcohol and, 1003
Research
  approaches to
    designs, 27
    ethics in. See Ethics
    evidence sources, 27
    levels of evidence, 27–29, 28f
    time intervals, 29
    types. See specific types
  question, 21, 22*t*, 23

Residence-based delivery of care, 907
Residence-bound patients, 48–49, 48b
  strategies for prevention and
    management, 50t
Residential visit, preparation for, 51–53
  instruments and equipment, 51, 52b
  sources for portable equipment, 51b
Resist Righting Reflex, 409
Resorption, 259
Respiration
  normal, maintenance of, 186–187
  procedures for observing, 187
Respiratory disease
  acute bronchitis, 1028, 1028t
  assessment
    blood gas analysis, 1026
    chest radiography, 1026
    cytology and hematology evaluation,
      1026
    pulse oximetry, 1025–1026, 1026f
    spirometry, 1025, 1025f
    vital signs, 1025
  asthma
    atopic (allergic), 1033
    attack, 1033
    dental hygiene care, 1035
    etiology of, 1032–1033
    medical management, 1034–1035
    oral manifestations, 1035
  chronic obstructive pulmonary disease
    chronic bronchitis, 1035–1036
    dental hygiene care, 1037
    emphysema, 1036
    medical management, 1036–1037
    oral manifestations, 1037
  classification of, 1026, 1026t
  cystic fibrosis
    clinical signs and symptoms of, 1037b
    dental hygiene care, 1038
    disease characteristics, 1037–1038
    medical management, 1038
  documentation, 1039–1040, 1040b
  everyday ethics, 1040
  factors to teach patient, 1040–1041
  lower tract, 1026t, 1028
  medical alert notifications, 1040b
  older adult, 830
  pneumonia, 1029t
    categories and role of oral bacteria,
      1029
    dental hygiene care, 1029
    etiology of, 1028–1029
    medical management of, 1029
    symptoms of, 1029
  sleep-related breathing disorders, 1039
  tuberculosis
    dental hygiene care, 1032
    diagnosis of, 1030
    disease development, 1030
    etiology of, 1030
    medical management, 1030–1031
    oral manifestations, 1031, 1032f
    transmission of, 1030
  upper tract, 1026t, 1027t, 1028t
    dental hygiene care, 1026–1028
    modes of transmission, 1026
Respiratory effects of drug abuse, 1013
Respiratory function, impaired, 893

Respiratory mucosa, function of, 1025, 1025f
Respiratory protection, 85–86
Respiratory system
  anatomy of, 1024, 1024f
  changes due to aging, 825
  physiology of, 1025
  respiratory mucosa, function of, 1025,
    1025f
Restenosis, 1054
Restorative dentistry, 846
Retainers, 487
Retinopathy, 924, 935
  of prematurity, 868
Rett disorder, 856b
Revascularization, 1054
ReVia. See Naltrexone
Review, 27
Revolutions per minute (rpm), 736
Rheumatic fever, 1047
Rheumatic heart disease, 1047–1048
Rheumatoid arthritis (RA), 1080–1081,
  1081f
Riboflavin, 558t
Rifampin (RIF), 1031t
Rinsing, 110
Risk factors, 384, 386, 775
  ergonomic, 122, 123t
Risperidone, 857
Roll/rolling stroke method, 442
Root caries, 267f, 579
  older adults, 832
  risk factors for, 267–268
  stages in formation of, 267
Root caries index (RCI), 374–375
  calculation and interpretation, 375
  procedure, 374
  purpose, 374
  scoring, 375
  selection of teeth, 374
Root form dental implant, 519
Rouge (Jeweler's rouge), 734
Rubber bite blocks, 881, 882f
Rubber interdental cleaners, 458
Rubefacient, 206
Rubella virus (Togavirus), 67t
Rx. See Prescription (Rx)

S
Saddlenose deformity, 1017b
Safe work practices, 123
Saliva, 423, 423f
  fluoride in, 576–577
Salivary gland hypofunction, 946
Salivation, 896b
Salts, fluoridated, 580
Sanitation, 111
Sarcomas, 944
SBI. See Sulcus bleeding index (SBI)
Scale photography, 221
Scalers, 644. See also specific scalers
  design of, 651
  internal angles of, 651f
  selection of cutting edges to sharpen,
    671
  -specific instrumentation, 652
  technique objectives, 671
  types of, 651, 652f
  uses of, 651

Scaling, 644, 681
Scavenger system, 616
SCD. See Sickle cell disease (SCD)
Schizophrenia
  dental hygiene care, 991–993
  signs and symptoms of, 991
  treatment, 991
School-age children, 800, 801–805
  accident and injury prevention, 817
  communication skills of, 38
  dietary and feeding pattern
    recommendations, 815–816
School-based dental sealant programs,
  608, 608f
School fluoridation, 579
SCI. See Spinal cord injury (SCI)
Scientific evidence, 20
  search for
    biomedical databases, 25, 25b
    Cochrane collaboration database,
      25
    evidence resources, strength of, 23f
    information sources, 23
    online information, 24–25, 24b
    publications, 23–24, 24b
Sclerodactyly, 1082
Scleroderma, 1081–1083, 1082f
  clinical presentation, 1082, 1082f
  crest syndrome, 1081b
  dental hygiene care, 1082–1083
  etiology of, 1081
  prevalence of, 1081
  treatment for, 1082
Sclerosis, 207
Scoring methods, 357–358
  clinical trial, 358
  community surveillance, 358
  epidemiologic survey, 358
  individual assessment score, 358
  types, 357–358
SDF (silver diamine fluoride), 583, 586,
  587t
Sealants, 600, 776, 808. See also specific
  entries
  acid etch, purposes of, 600, 600f
  clinical procedures, 603–607,
    604–605t, 606–607f
    acid etch, 606–607
    additional isolation options, 606
    complete etching, evaluate for, 607
    cotton-roll isolation, 606
    cure sealant, 607
    follow-up, 607
    occlusion, 607
    patient preparation, 603
    place sealant material, 607, 607f
    rinse and air dry tooth, 607
    rubber dam isolation, 606
    steps for placement of a dental
      sealant, 604–605t
    tooth isolation, 603
    tooth preparation, 603
  development of, 600
  documentation, 608, 608b
  everyday ethics, 609
  factors to teach patient, 609
  indications for placement, 601,
    601–602f

Sealants (*continued*)
 maintenance, 607–608
 materials
  classification of, 600–601
  criteria for ideal sealant, 600
 penetration of
  amount of, 603
  contents of pit or fissure, 603
  effect of cleaning, 603
  pit and fissure anatomy, 601, 602f,
   603
 purposes of, 600
 school-based dental sealant programs,
  608, 608f
Second trimester, 782
Secondary aging, 824
Secondary polycythemia, 1069
Secondary radiation, 232
Sedation, effects of antipsychotics, 992t
Seizure disorder, 970
 aura, 972
 cerebral palsy and, 900
 classification of, 970, 970t
 clinical manifestations, 972
 definition of, 970
 dental hygiene care plan, 975–976
  care plan, 976–977
  information to obtain, 976, 976b
  patient approach, 976
  patient history, 976
 diagnosis of, 971
 documentation, 978, 978b
 emergency care
  differential diagnosis of seizure, 977
  emergency procedure, 977–978
  objectives, 977
  postictal phase, 978
  preparation for appointment, 977
  status epilepticus, 978
 etiology, 971–972
 everyday ethics, 979
 factors to teach patient, 979
 implications, 972
 oral findings
  effects of accidents with seizures,
   973–974
  gingival overgrowth/gingival
   hyperplasia, 974–975, 974–975f
 precipitating factors and trigger signs,
  972
 prevention of injuries, 972
 prognosis, 972
 treatment
  ketogenic diet, 973
  medications, 972–973, 973t
  surgery, 973
 types of, 971
Selective serotonin reuptake inhibitors,
 985
Self-applied fluoride, 587
Self-care
 ability, 386
 caregivers, 885
 for dental hygienist, 123–124
 mouthrinses, 475
 of neutropenic patient, 449
 oral, 872b
 orthodontic appliances, 488–489

personal factors affecting, 906–907
Self-directed products, bleaching, 755
Self-history, 164
Self-inflicted soft-tissue injury, 635
Self-monitoring of blood glucose
 (SMBG), 932
Self-neglect, 218
Semi-upright position, 116, 117f
Sensation, loss of, 903
Sensitivity, vital bleaching, 753
Sensor, 229
Sensory disorders, 868–869. *See also*
 specific disorders
 cerebral palsy and, 900
Sensory impairment, 866
Sensory loss, 896b
Sensory stimuli, usage of, 339
Sensory systems, changes due to aging,
 825
Sequelae, 165
Sequence, 394
 and prioritizing patient care
  factors affecting sequence of care,
   399
  objectives, 398–399
Sequestrum, 77
Seroconversion, 78
Serotonin and noradrenergic reuptake
 inhibitors, 985
Sessile lesion, 204
Severe ECC, 792
Sexual abuse, 212, 214t
 definition of, 218
 signs of, 216
Sexually transmitted diseases, older adult,
 830
Shadow casting, 241, 242b
Shank, 645
Sharpey's fibers, 291, 308
Sharpness, 668
Sharps management, 632, 632–634f
Sharps precautions, 62
Shear bond strength, 486
Shelf life, 106
Shepherd hook explorer, 339, 339f
Short-acting beta-2 agonists (SABA), for
 asthma, 1034t
Shunt, 904, 1046
Sialorrhea, 898
Sickle cell disease (SCD), 1067f
 appointment management, 1068
 clinical course, 1068
 disease process, 1067
 oral implications, 1068
 treatment and disease management,
  1068
Sickles, 651, 652f
Sidestream smoke, 534
SIDS (sudden infant death syndrome),
 535
Signs, 150
Silex (silicon dioxide), 734
Silver amalgam, 299
Silver diamine fluoride (SDF), 583, 586,
 587t
Simple index, types of, 358
Simplified calculus index (CI-S), 363
Simplified debris index (DI-S), 363

Simplified oral hygiene index (OHI-S),
 363–365, 363f, 364f
 calculation and interpretation, 363
 calculus score, 364
 components, 363
 debris score, 364
 location and tooth surface areas
  scored, 364–365
 procedure, 364
 purpose, 363
 scoring
  group, 366
  individual, 364
 selection of teeth and surfaces,
  363–364
Single-tuft brush, 464, 464f
Sinus augmentation (sinus lift), 518
Sinusitis, 1027t
Sippy cup, 814
Sjogren's syndrome (SS), 1089–1090
Skilled nursing, 47
Skin, bacteriology of, 88
SLE (systemic lupus erythematosus),
 1090–1091, 1091–1092f
Sleep-related breathing disorders
 dental hygiene care, 1039
 etiology of, 1039
 medical management, 1039, 1039f
 signs and symptoms of, 1039
Sliding board transfer, 884, 884f
Smear layer, 717, 719
SMEs. *See* Subject matter experts (SMEs)
Smokeless tobacco, 531–533
Snuff, 531
Snus, 531
SOAP approach, 157–158, 158b, 158t
Social (pragmatic) communication
 disorder, 850b
Social and economic factors, 39
Social determinants of health, 39
Sodium bicarbonate, 739–740
Sodium bisulfite, 623
Sodium fluoride (NaF), 578
Sodium hydroxide, 749
Soft tissues. *See also* Charting of hard and
 soft tissues
 changes associated with aging,
  831–832, 832b
  lips, 831
  oral candidiasis, 831–832
  oral mucosa, 831
  tongue, 831
  xerostomia, 831
 grafts, dentinal hypersensitivity, 725
 lesions, adverse effects of
  toothbrushing, 449–450
Sonic scalers, 655, 657
Sordes, 55
Sore or burning tongue, 560t
Spasms, 970
Spastic palsy, 900
Spatter, 64
Specific learning disorder, 850b
Speech and language disorders, 900
Speech sound disorder, 850b
Speech therapy, 846
Speechreading, 877
Spina bifida occulta, 903

Spinal cord injury (SCI), 892–893
  characteristics/effects of, 893
  dental hygiene care, 895
  levels of, 894f
  mouth-held implements, 895
  occurrence, 893
  potential secondary complications
    autonomic dysreflexia, 893, 895
    body temperature, 893
    cardiovascular instability, 893
    decubitus ulcers, 893
    impaired respiratory function, 893
    neurogenic bladder and bowel, 893
    spasticity, 893
    vulnerability to infection, 893
Spinal shock, 893
Spirometer, 1025
Spirometry, for respiratory disease, 1025,
  1025f
Spore testing, 103–104, 103t
Sputum, 1026
Squamous epithelium, 306
Squeezing, 660
SS (Sjogren's syndrome), 1089–1090
St. John's Wart, 985
Stack, 657
Staging, 944
Standard drink, 1001f
Standard of care, 767–768, 768b
Standard precautions, 62, 84
Standard procedures, 110–111
Stannous fluoride, 296
Staphylococcus aureus, 67t
Staphylococcus epidermidis, 67t
Startle reflex, 900
Statistical significance, 26
Status epilepticus, 971, 978
Steatorrhea, 1083
Steinert disease. *See* Myotonic muscular
  dystrophy
Stenosis, 1046
Stereotypes, 41
Stereotypic movement disorder, 850b
Sterilization, 98, 102–104. *See also specific
  methods*
  care of sterile instruments, 105–106
  comparison of methods for, 103t
Steroids, for stroke, 897b
Stethoscope, 187, 188, 189f, 190f
Stillman method, 441–442, 441f
Stillman's cleft, 312, 312f
Stimulants, 1008t, 1011
Stimuli, types of, 340
Stippled, 313
Stones, sharpening
  dry, 669
  lubricated, 669
  moving flat stone, stationary
    instrument, 671–674, 672f, 673f
  preparation for sharpening, 669
  as sharpening devices, 668–669, 670f
  stationary flat stone, moving
    instrument, 674–675, 674f
  sterilization of, 669
  water on, 669
Street drug abuse, 1005
Strengthening commitment (the plan),
  416, 417b

Streptococcus pneumonia, 67t
Streptococcus pyogenes, 67t
Stress, 116
  minimization, 130
Stretching exercises, 660–661, 661f
Stroke, 650, 660, 896f
  categories and purposes of medications
    used to treat, 897b
  dental hygiene care, 897
  direction, 650, 650f
  etiologic factors, 895–896
  exploratory/assessment, 651
  lateral pressure, 650
  local anesthesia and, 626
  medical treatment, 896–897
  root debridement, 651
  scaling/calculus removal, 651
  signs and symptoms, 896, 896b
  walking, 650
Study models, 275, 275f
Styrofoam disposable film/photostimulable
  phosphor (PSP) holder, 243f
Subgingival air polishing, 691–692, 691f
Subgingival bacterial flora, 681
Subgingival biofilm, 284, 287–288f
Subgingival calculus, 288–289, 289f, 345,
  364f
Subgingival irrigation, 466
Subgingival pellicle, 281
Subgingival procedures, 340, 341f
Subject matter experts (SMEs), 24
  opinions, 28–29
Suboxone. *See* Buprenorphine/naloxone
Subperiosteal frame dental implant, 519
Substance abuse, 818, 1000
Substance-related disorder. *See also*
  Alcohol use disorder (AUD)
  alcohol use. *See* Alcohol
  alcohol withdrawal syndrome, 1005
  dental hygiene process of care
    assessment, 1015–1016, 1016f
    care planning, 1018
    dental hygiene diagnosis, 1018
    evaluation, 1019
    implementation, 1018–1019
    *intraoral examination, 1016–1017,
      1017–1018b, 1017f*
    nasopalatal defect, 1016f
  documentation, 1019, 1019b
  drug abuse
    anabolic steroids, 1011
    *cannabinoids (marijuana) abuse,
      1006, 1009–1010*
    cardiovascular effects of, 1012
    depressants, 1010
    desomorphine, 1011–1012
    dissociative anesthetics, 1010
    emerging drugs, 1011–1012
    gastrointestinal effects of, 1012
    hallucinogens, 1010
    infections, 1013
    inhalants, 1011
    kidney damage, 1012
    liver damage, 1012–1013
    musculoskeletal effects of, 1013
    neurologic effects of, 1012
    *opioids and morphine derivatives,
      1010*

    prenatal effects of, 1013
    respiratory effects of, 1013
    stimulants, 1011
    synthetic cathinones, 1011
  drug enforcement administration drug
    schedule, 1006, 1006b
  everyday ethics, 1019–1020
  factors to teach patient, 1020
  prescription drug abuse, 1005
    risk management for, 1005–1006
  street drug abuse, 1005
  treatment methods, 1014b
    behavioral therapies, 1013–1014
    *drug withdrawal medications,
      1014–1015*
Substance-use disorder (SUD), 991
Substantivity, 472
Subutex. *See* Buprenorphine
Succedaneous teeth, 256
Suction toothbrush, 55, 55b
SUD (substance-use disorder), 991
Sudden infant death syndrome (SIDS),
  535
Sulcular brushing, 440, 489
Sulcus bleeding index (SBI), 368
  for area, 368
  for individual, 368
  procedure, 368
  purpose, 368
  scoring, 368
  for tooth, 368
Superinfection, 697
Supernumerary teeth, 257
Supersaturation, 290
Supervision, in dental hygiene practice, 6,
  7b. *See also specific types*
Supine hypotensive syndrome, 786
Supine position, 117, 117f
  contraindications for, 118
Suppuration (or pus), 314
Supragingival biofilm, 284, 287–288f
Supragingival calculus, 287–288, 288f,
  345
  formation, reduction of, 472
Supragingival irrigation, 466
Supragingival pellicle, 281
Supragingival procedures, 340
Surfactants, 749
Surgical antisepsis, 91
Surgical scrub. *See* Surgical antisepsis
Survival rate, 866
Susceptible host, 64
Sustain talk *vs.* change talk, 413
Sutures, 704
  characteristics of, 704
  classification of, 704
  documentation, 713, 713b
  everyday ethics, 713
  factors to teach patient, 713
  functions of, 704
  ideal material, 704
  procedures
    blanket (continuous lock), 706
    circumferential, 707
    continuous uninterrupted, 707
    interdental, 707
    interrupted, 707
    sling or suspension, 707

Sutures (*continued*)
  removal of
    preparation of patient, 707
    review previous documentation, 707
    steps for, 707–708, 708f
    sterile clinic tray setup, 707
  selection of, 705, 705*b*
  types of, 706–707*f*
Swaged, needles, 705
Swimmer stain, 297
Symptoms of disease, 152
Syncopal episodes, 130
Syndrome, 842
Synthetic cathinones (bath salts), 1009*t*, 1011
Synthroid. *See* Levothyroxine
Systematic reviews, 27–28
Systemic autoimmune diseases, 1089
  Sjogren's syndrome, 1089–1090
  systemic lupus erythematosus, 1090–1091, 1091–1092*f*
Systemic lupus erythematosus (SLE), 1090–1091, 1091–1092*f*
Systole phase, 187

T

Tachycardia, 185, 1033
Tachypnea, 1033
Tactile sensitivity, increasing, 662, 662*f*
Tanged file, care of, 676
Tardive dyskinesia, 992, 992*t*
Target–image receptor distance, 234
Taste perception, 990
TB. *See* Tuberculosis (TB)
TCP (tricalcium phosphate), 274
Teeth, 257, 257*f*. *See also* Permanent teeth; Primary teeth
  examination of, 258–259*t*
  fractures of, 263, 263*f*, 974
  hypersensitive, 990
  malrelations of groups of, 271–273, 271–273*f*
  missing, 498
  pulpless/traumatized, 297–298
  succedaneous, 256
  terminology for malposition of, 273
Tegretol. *See* Carbamazepine
Telangiectases, 1082
Teledentistry, 48
Temporal artery thermometer, 185, 185*f*
Temporomandibular joint
  assessment of, 198*f*
  disorders, 990
Tensile strength, 704
Tension test procedure, 349
Terminal (lower) shank, 653
Terminal shank, 645
Terminally ill patients, 56
  strategies for prevention and management, 50*t*
Testing stick, 669
Tetracaine HCl, 636
Tetracycline, 298–299, 783–784
  staining, 751, 752*f*
Textbooks, 24
Therapeutic rinses, 475
Thermal disinfector, 100–101
Thermal pulp testing, 268

Thermometers, 185, 185*f*. *See also specific types*
Third trimester, 782
Thixotropic gel, 584
Three-body abrasive polishing, 730
Three-person emergency team, duties for, 132, 135*f*
Thrombocytes. *See* Platelets
Thrombocytopenia, 1070
Thrombolytics, for stroke, 897*b*
Thrombotic stroke, 895
Thrombus, 1050
Thyroid cervical collar, 238, 239*f*
Thyroid gland
  hyperthyroidism, 914, 914*t*
  hypothyroidism, 913–914, 914*t*
Tiagabine (Gabitril), 973*t*
Tic disorders, 850*b*
Time-delay switch, 228
Tin oxide (putty powder, stannic oxide), 734
Tissue hyperplasia, 513, 513*f*
Titanium, 519
Titanium alloy, 520
Titration, 618
Tobacco cessation methods, 544*f*. *See also* Tobacco use
  assisted strategies, 539
  community oral health program, 547
  "5 A's," 543–546
  motivational interviewing, 543
  pharmacotherapies, 540*t*
  program for, 543
  public health policy, 546
  reasons for quitting, 538–539
  self-help interventions, 539
  sources for educational materials, 545*t*
  team approach, 546
Tobacco-free environment, 546
Tobacco-specific nitrosamines, 531
Tobacco stain, 296, 296*f*
Tobacco use, 818
  among children and adolescents, 543
  components of tobacco product, 530
  dental clinical treatment
    biofilm control, 543
    diet and nutrition planning, 543
    nonsurgical periodontal therapy, 543
  dental hygiene care for, 541–542
  disease consequences of, 534*t*
  documentation, 547, 547*b*
  factors to teach patient, 547
  and halitosis, 542
  health hazards, 530
    life expectancy, 530
  implant system and, 521
  nicotine metabolism, 530–531
  oral effects of, 535–536, 536*t*
  patient assessment
    extraoral examination, 542
    form, 542f
    intraoral examination, 542f
  periodontal diseases, 319, 319*f*
  as risk factor for periodontal diseases, 536
  systemic effects of, 534
  use of alcohol with, 534
  and use of other drugs, 534
Tobacco user tracking system, 546

Toddlers, 800, 801
  accident and injury prevention, 817
  communication skills of, 37–38
  dietary and feeding pattern recommendations, 815
  oral health considerations for, 816, 817*f*
Tolerance, 537, 1001
Tongue
  cleaning, 445–446, 446*f*
  examination of, 203*f*
  papillae of, 198*f*
  scars of, 973–974
  thrust, 259*t*
Tonic-clonic seizure, 971
Tonic labyrinthine reflex, 900
Tonic seizure, 970
Tooth abrasion, 439
Tooth development
  disturbances in, 298
  fluorides, 574
    maturation stage, 575
    mineralization stage, 575, 575f
    posteruptive, 575–576
Tooth numbering systems
  Continuous Numbers 1–32, 152*f*
    permanent teeth, 152
    primary/deciduous teeth, 152
  Fédération Dentaire Internationale system
    permanent teeth, 152–153, 153f
    primary/deciduous teeth, 153
    two digit, 152
  Palmer Notation System
    permanent teeth, 153, 153f
    primary/deciduous teeth, 154
Tooth shade
  digital photographic record of, 758*f*
  manual selection of, 757*f*, 758*b*
Tooth structures, anatomy of
  dentin, 716, 716*f*
  nerves, 717
  pulp, 716–717, 716*f*
Tooth surface fluoride, 576
Tooth surface index of fluorosis (TSIF), 375, 376*t*
Tooth surface irregularities, 324–325
Tooth whitening, 735
  –induced sensitivity, 725–726
Toothbrushes
  care of, 450–451
  characteristics of, 439
  cleaning, 450–451
  composition, 435
  contamination, 450
  dimensions, 435
  disinfection, 450–451
  documentation, 451, 451*b*
  early, 434
  everyday ethics, 451
  factors to teach patient, 452
  grasp, 446
  head, 435
  historical perspective on toothbrushing instruction, 434*b*
  for implant systems, 522
  influencing factors, 439
  interdental
    care of brushes, 459

indications for use, 458
procedure, 458–459, 459*f*
types, 457–458, 458*f*
manual
brush head, 435
characteristics of effective, 434–435
filaments (bristles), 435–436, 437*t*
general description, 435
handle, 435
trim profiles, 436*f*
origins of, 434
orthodontic Bi-level, 489, 489*f*
parts, 435, 435*f*
power
child, 438*f*
description, 437–439
effectiveness, 436
motions, 437*t*
purposes and indications, 436–437
trim profiles, 438*f*
replacement, 450
selection of, 439
shape, 435
stiffness of filaments or bristles, 439
storage, 451
supply of, 450
type and technique, 723
Toothbrushing, 110
acute oral inflammatory or traumatic lesions, 448–449
adverse effects of
bacteremia, 450
hard tissue lesions, 450
soft tissue lesions, 449–450
following dental extraction, 449
documentation, 451, 451*b*
duration of, 447
everyday ethics, 451
factors to teach patient, 452
force, 447–448
frequency of, 447
guidelines for instructions, 446–448
manual, 439
Bass and modified Bass methods, 440–441, 440*f*
Charters method, 442–443, 443*f*
fones (or circular) method, 443, 444*f*
horizontal (or scrub) method, 443
Leonard's (or vertical) method, 443–444
roll/rolling stroke method, 442
Stillman and Modified Stillman methods, 441–442, 441*f*
oral self-care of neutropenic patient, 449
for orthodontic appliances, 489, 489*f*
patient education, 448
following periodontal surgery, 449
power, 444
procedure, 448
sequence, 447
supplemental brushing methods
brushing difficult-to-reach areas, 445, 445*f*
occlusal brushing, 444–445, 444*f*
tongue cleaning, 445–446, 446*f*
Toothpick in holder, 465, 465*f*
Topamax. *See* Topiramate

Topical anesthesia, 637*t*
action of, 636
adverse reactions of, 637
agents used, 636–637
application of
completion of, 638
patient preparation, 637
techniques, 637
factors to teach patient, 639
indications for use, 636
topical drug mixtures, 637
Topiramate (Topamax), 973*t*
Torus, 196, 206
Toxicity, 591–592
Traditional film processing
automated processing, 248
darkroom lighting, 248
image production, 248
manual processing, 248–249
Trafficking in persons. *See* Human trafficking
Transducers, 658
Transformers, 227
Transient ischemic attack, 896
Translucency, 748
Transtheoretical model, 408, 408*t*
Tranxene. *See* Clorazepate
Trauma from occlusion, 274–275
Traumatic alopecia, 215, 218
Traumatic injuries, emergency reference chart, 142–143*t*
Traumatic lesions, toothbrushing, 448–449
Tray technique, 584, 584*t*, 585–586*f*
home tray application, 587–588, 588*b*
Treatment room
features, 99*f*
contact surfaces, 98–99
housekeeping surfaces, 99–100
preparation of, 107
clean and disinfect environmental surfaces[1], 109
objective, 108
preliminary planning, 108, 109*t*
surface disinfection procedure, 108–109
unit water lines, 109–110
Trendelenburg position, 117, 117*f*, 139*t*
Treponema pallidum, 66*t*
Triage, 48, 49
Tribiology, 730
Tricalcium phosphate (TCP), 724
Triclosan, 476
Triggers, 970
Trileptal. *See* Oxcarbazepine
Trismus, 449, 634, 947, 959
TSIF (tooth surface index of fluorosis), 375, 376*t*
TST (tuberculin skin test), 1030
Tuberculin skin test (TST), 1030
Tuberculosis (TB)
active TB disease, 1030, 1031*t*
clinical management, 68
dental hygiene care, 1032
diagnosis of, 1030
disease development, 1030
etiology of, 1030
latent tuberculosis infection, 1030, 1031*t*
medical management, 1030–1031

oral manifestations, 1031, 1032*f*
transmission, 67–68, 68*f*
transmission of, 1030
Tufted dental floss, 462, 462*f*
Tufts, 435
Two-body abrasive polishing, 730
2-hour plasma glucose, 930
Tympanic thermometer, 185, 185*f*
Type 1 diabetes, 926, 928*t*, 929
Type 2 diabetes, 926, 928*t*, 929

U

Ulcerative colitis (UC), 1085–1086, 1085*f*
Ulcers, 207
ULs (upper intake levels), 554
Ultrasonic denture cleaner, 507*f*
Ultrasonic processing, 101–102
Ultrasonic scalers, 655, 656
magnetostrictive, 657–658, 658*f*
piezoelectric, 658, 658*f*
Unclassified seizures, 971
Underjet, 272, 272*f*
United States Department of Agriculture (USDA), 554
United States Department of Health and Human Services (USDHHS), 554
Universal curets, 653, 653*f*
Unknown onset seizure, 970, 970*t*, 971
Unspecified intellectual disability, 850*b*
Upper intake levels (ULs), 554
Upper respiratory tract disease
dental hygiene care
appointment management, 1027–1028
bacterial resistance to antibiotics, 1028
disease prevention, 1026–1027
modes of transmission, 1026
respiratory hygiene and cough etiquette, 1028*t*
signs and symptoms, etiology, medical treatment, and clinical evaluation assessment, 1027*t*
Upright position, 116, 117*f*
Urinary bag, 883
Urticaria, 141*t*
U.S. Public Health Service (USPHS), 577
USDA (United States Department of Agriculture), 554
USDHHS (United States Department of Health and Human Services), 554
USPHS (U.S. Public Health Service), 577

V

Validity, 20
evidence for, 26
Valproic acid/valproate (Depakote), 973*t*
Vaporole, 131*t*
Varenicline tartrate, 541
Variables, 26
Varicella–zoster virus (VZV), 66*t*, 71–72, 73
Varnish technique, 584, 585*t*
Vasculopathy, 1081
Vaso-occlusion, 1068

Vasoconstrictors, 623–624, 624*t*
Vasodilators, for stroke, 897*b*
Venous blood, 1052
Ventricular septal defect, 1046, 1046*f*
Ventriculoatrial shunt, 904, 904*f*
Ventriculoperitoneal shunt, 904, 904*f*
Verbal communication, 34
Verruca, 206
Verruca vulgaris, 216
Vertigo, 1069
Viral bronchitis, 1028*t*
Viral hepatitis
    hepatitis B virus, 68–70, 69*t*
    hepatitis C virus, 70
    hepatitis D virus, 70
Viral pneumonias, 1028, 1029*t*
Virus, 62
Viscosity, 600
Visible light–cure (VIC) dressing
    (Barricaid), 709
Visual impairment, 868–869
    clinical settings, introduction of, 879
    escorting, 880*f*
Visual impairment, 896*b*
Vital signs
    blood pressure
        classifications, 190*t*
        components of, 187
        equipment for determining, 187–188,
            188*f*
        factors influencing, 187
        follow-up criteria, 191
        hypertension, 190–191, 191*t*
        procedure for determining, 188–190,
            188*f*, 189*f*, 190*f*
    body temperature
        care of patient with temperature
            elevation, 185
        indications for taking, 184
        maintenance of, 184
        methods of determining, 184–185
        thermometers, 185*f*
    dental hygiene care planning, 183–184
    documentation, 191, 191*b*
    everyday ethics, 192
    factors to teach patient, 192
    patient preparation and instruction,
        183
    pulse
        normal, maintenance of, 185
        procedure for determining rate,
            185–186, 186*f*
    respiration
        normal, maintenance of, 186–187
        procedures for observing, 187
    resting ranges infant through older
        adult, 184*t*
Vital tooth bleaching
    decision making for, 751*t*
    desensitization procedures for, 753*t*
    factors associated with efficacy, 750
        extrinsic, 752
        intrinsic, 751–752
        longevity of results, 752
    history of, 748
    irreversible tooth damage, 753
    materials used for, 748–749
        carbamide peroxide, 748*f*, 749, 749*f*
        desensitizers, 749

hydrogen peroxide, 748*f*, 749, 749*f*
        others, 749
    mechanism of, 748
    modes of, 754*t*
        over-the-counter products, 755–756,
            756*b*
        professionally applied bleaching,
            753–754
        professionally dispensed/professionally
            monitored bleaching, 754–755,
            755*f*
    nonvital tooth bleaching vs.,
        747–748
    over-the-counter bleaching
        preparations, 756*b*
    reversible side effects of, 753
    safety
        cautions and contraindications, 750
        potential photosensitivity and
            hyperpigmentation, medications
            associated with, 750*b*
        restorative materials, 749–750
        soft tissue, 749
        systemic factors, 750
        tooth structure, 749
    scalloped and unscalloped bleaching
        tray designs, 755*f*
    sensitivity, 753
    tooth color change with, 748
Vitamin A, 558*t*
Vitamin C, 559*t*, 560*t*
Vitamin D, 558*t*
Vitamin E, 558*t*
Vitamin K, 558*t*, 1056, 1071
Vivitrol. See Naltrexone
Vocal communication, 34
VZV (varicella–zoster virus), 66*t*, 71–72,
    73

W

Walking bleach method, 748. See also
    Nonvital tooth bleaching
Water filters, 580
Water flosser, 466, 466*f*
Water, mouthrinses, 478
Web-based health messages, 35
Wernicke encephalopathy, 1003
Wernicke–Korsakoff's syndrome, 1003
Wheelchair transfer, 54, 54*f*
    dental hygiene care, 906
    patient who can assist, 883, 883*f*
    patient who is immobile, 883–884
    preparation for, 882–883
    sliding board transfer, 884
    wheelchair used during treatment, 884
Wheeze, 1038*t*
White areas of cancer, 207
White blood cells, 284, 286
    agranulocytes, 1064
    disorders of, 1069–1070
    disorders of
        leukocytosis, 1070
        lymphocytopenia, 1069–1070
        neutropenia, 1069
    functions, 1063–1064
    granulocytes, 1064–1065
    reference values, 1064*t*
    types of, 1062–1063
White-coat hypertension, 190

White spots, 593
    lesion, 422, 492
Whitening, bleaching vs., 747
WHO. See World Health Organization
    (WHO)
Wickham striae, 1079, 1080*f*
Wire edge, after sharpening, 671, 671*f*
Withdrawal syndrome, 1005
Women's health
    hormonal contraceptives, 918
    menopause, 918–919
    menstrual cycle, 917, 917*f*
    patient management considerations,
        919
Wooden interdental cleaner, 465–466,
    465*f*
Working end, 645, 646
Working files, 654, 654*f*
World Health Organization (WHO)
    Basic Screening Survey, 376
    child abuse and neglect, 212
    oral mucositis scale, 949*t*
Wound healing, 560*t*
Wrinkle or fold test, 350*f*
Wrist, anatomy of, 124*f*
Wrist/finger devices, 187
Wristwatch and jewelry, 89
Writing, 877
Written care plan, components of,
    396–397*f*
    appointment plan, 398
    assessment findings and risk factors, 395
    caries risk status, 395
    demographic data, 395
    diagnostic statements, 397
    evaluation methods, 398
    expected outcomes, 398
    patient-centered oral health goals, 397
    periodontal diagnosis and status, 395
    planned interventions, 397
    re-evaluation, 398

X

X-ray production, 226
    circuits, 227, 228*f*
    machine control devices, 227–228
    properties of, 226*b*
    steps in, 228–229
    transformers, 227
    X-ray tube, 227, 227*f*
X-ray timer, 228
X-ray tube, 227, 227*f*
Xerostomia, 56, 328, 423, 919, 946, 991
    relief for, 837
Xylitol, 472, 785

Y

Yellow stain, 294, 294*f*
Young children
    gingiva, 314

Z

Zarontin. See Ethosuximide
Zinc, 560*t*
Zinc oxide with eugenol dressing, 709
Zonegran. See Zonisamide
Zonisamide (Zonegran), 973*t*
Zoster (shingles) infection, 73